a LANGE medical book

Morgan & Mikhail's Clinical Anesthesiology

SEVENTH EDITION

John F. Butterworth IV, MD
Former Professor and Chairman
Department of Anesthesiology
Virginia Commonwealth University School of Medicine
VCU Health System
Richmond, Virginia

David C. Mackey, MD
Professor
Department of Anesthesiology and Perioperative Medicine
University of Texas MD Anderson Cancer Center
Houston, Texas

John D. Wasnick, MD, MPH
Steven L. Berk Endowed Chair for Excellence in Medicine
Professor and Chair
Department of Anesthesia
Texas Tech University Health Sciences Center
School of Medicine
Lubbock, Texas

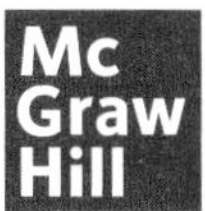

New York Chicago San Francisco Athens London Madrid Mexico City
Milan New Delhi Singapore Sydney Toronto

Morgan & Mikhail's Clinical Anesthesiology, Seventh Edition

4 5 6 7 8 LBC 28 27 26 25 24

ISBN 978-1-260-47379-7
MHID 1-260-47379-1
ISSN 1058-4277

This book was set in Minion pro by KnowledgeWorks Global Ltd.
The editors were Jason Malley and Christie Naglieri.
The production supervisor was Richard Ruzycka.
Project management was provided by Warishree Pant, KnowledgeWorks Global Ltd.
The cover designer was W2 Design.
This book is printed on acid-free paper.

Contents

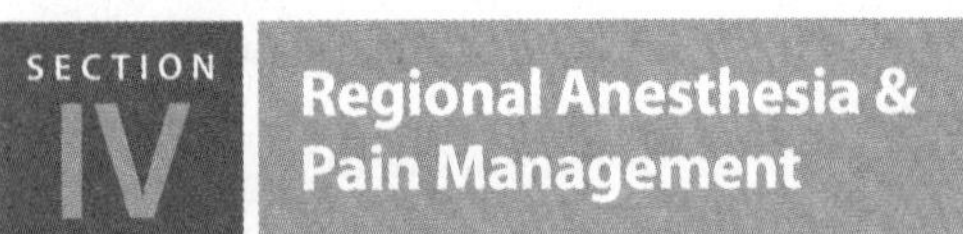
SECTION IV
Regional Anesthesia & Pain Management

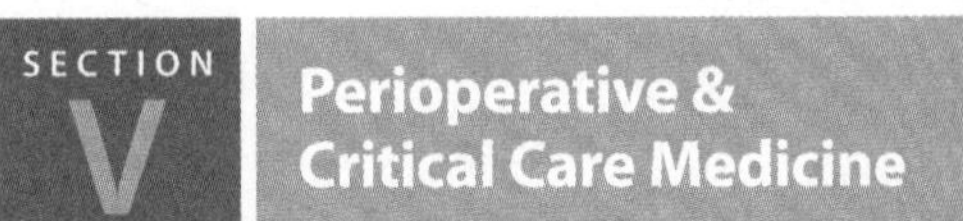
SECTION V
Perioperative & Critical Care Medicine

Chapter Authors

Gabriele Baldini, MD, MSc
Associate Professor
Medical Director, Montreal General Hospital Preoperative Centre
Department of Anesthesia
McGill University Health Centre
Montreal General Hospital
Montreal, Quebec, Canada

John F. Butterworth IV, MD
Former Professor and Chairman
Department of Anesthesiology
Virginia Commonwealth University School of Medicine
VCU Health System
Richmond, Virginia

Seamas Dore, MD
Assistant Professor
Department of Anesthesiology
Virginia Commonwealth University
School of Medicine, Richmond, Virginia

John J. Finneran IV, MD
Associate Professor of Anesthesiology
University of California, San Diego

Michael A. Frölich, MD, MS
Tenured professor
Department of Anesthesiology and Perioperative Medicine
University of Alabama at Birmingham
Birmingham, Alabama

Brian M. Ilfeld, MD, MS (Clinical Investigation)
Professor of Anesthesiology, In Residence
Division of Regional Anesthesia and Pain Medicine
Department of Anesthesiology
University of California at San Diego
San Diego, California

Jody C. Leng, MD, MS
Department of Anesthesiology and Perioperative Care Service, Virginia
Palo Alto Health Care System, Palo Alto, California
Department of Anesthesiology, Perioperative and Pain Medicine, Stanford University School of Medicine, Stanford, California

David C. Mackey, MD
Professor
Department of Anesthesiology and Perioperative Medicine
University of Texas MD Anderson Cancer Center
Houston, Texas

Edward R. Mariano, MD, MAS
Professor
Department of Anesthesiology, Perioperative & Pain Medicine
Stanford University School of Medicine
Chief, Anesthesiology & Perioperative Care Service
Associate Chief of Staff, Inpatient Surgical Services
Veterans Affairs Palo Alto Health Care System
Palo Alto, California

Nirvik Pal, MD
Associate Professor
Department of Anesthesiology
Virginia Commonwealth University
School of Medicine, Richmond, Virginia

Michael Ramsay, MD, FRCA
Chairman, Department of Anesthesiology
Baylor University Medical Center
Baylor Scott and White Health Care System
Professor
Texas A&M University Health Care Faculty
Dallas, Texas

Pranav Shah, MD
Assistant Professor
Department of Anesthesiology
VCU School of Medicine
Richmond, Virginia

Bruce M. Vrooman, MD, MS, FIPP
Associate Professor of Anesthesiology
Geisel School of Medicine at Dartmouth
Dartmouth-Hitchcock Medical Center
Lebanon, New Hampshire

John D. Wasnick, MD, MPH
Steven L. Berk Endowed Chair for Excellence in Medicine
Professor and Chair
Department of Anesthesia
Texas Tech University Health Sciences Center
School of Medicine
Lubbock, Texas

George W. Williams, MD, FASA, FCCP
Associate Professor of Anesthesiology and Surgery & Vice Chair for Critical Care Medicine, Department of Anesthesiology
Medical Co-Director, Surgical Intensive Care Unit- Lyndon B. Johnson General Hospital
Medical Director, Donor Specialty Care Unit- Memorial Hermann Hospital TMC
Chair, American Society of Anesthesiologists Committee on Critical Care Medicine

Kimberly Youngren, MD
Clinical Assistant Professor of Anesthesiology
Geisel School of Medicine
Program Director, Pain Medicine Fellowship
Dartmouth Hitchcock. Lebanon

Past Contributors

Kallol Chaudhuri, MD, PhD
Professor
Department of Anesthesia
West Virginia University School of Medicine
Morgantown, West Virginia

Swapna Chaudhuri, MD, PhD
Professor
Department of Anesthesia
Texas Tech University Health Sciences Center
Lubbock, Texas

Lydia Conlay, MD
Professor
Department of Anesthesia
Texas Tech University Health Sciences Center
Lubbock, Texas

Johannes De Riese, MD
Assistant Professor
Department of Anesthesiology
Texas Tech University Health Sciences Center
Lubbock, Texas

Seamas Dore, MD
Assistant Professor
Department of Anesthesiology
Virginia Commonwealth University
School of Medicine, Richmond, Virginia

Suzanne N. Northcutt, MD
Associate Professor
Department of Anesthesia
Texas Tech University Health Sciences Center
Lubbock, Texas

Aschraf N. Farag, MD
Assistant Professor
Department of Anesthesia
Texas Tech University Health Sciences Center
Lubbock, Texas

Pranav Shah, MD
Assistant Professor
Department of Anesthesiology
VCU School of Medicine
Richmond, Virginia

Robert Johnston, MD
Associate Professor
Department of Anesthesia
Texas Tech University Health Sciences Center
Lubbock, Texas

Sabry Khalil, MD
Assistant Professor
Department of Anesthesiology
Texas Tech University Health Sciences Center
Lubbock, Texas

Sanford Littwin, MD
Assistant Professor
Department of Anesthesiology
St. Luke's Roosevelt Hospital Center and Columbia University College of Physicians and Surgeons
New York, New York

Alina Nicoara, MD
Associate Professor
Department of Anesthesiology
Duke University Medical Center
Durham, North Carolina

Nirvik Pal, MD
Associate Professor
Department of Anesthesiology
Virginia Commonwealth University
School of Medicine, Richmond, Virginia

Nitin Parikh, MD
Associate Professor
Department of Anesthesia
Texas Tech University Health Sciences Center
Lubbock, Texas

Cooper W. Phillips, MD
Assistant Professor
Department of Anesthesiology
UT Southwestern Medical Center
Dallas, Texas

Elizabeth R. Rivas, MD
Assistant Professor
Department of Anesthesiology
Texas Tech University Health Sciences Center
Lubbock, Texas

Bettina Schmitz, MD, PhD
Associate Professor
Department of Anesthesia
Texas Tech University Health Sciences Center
Lubbock, Texas

Christiane Vogt-Harenkamp, MD, PhD
Assistant Professor
Department of Anesthesia
Texas Tech University Health Sciences Center
Lubbock, Texas

Denise J. Wedel, MD
Professor of Anesthesiology
Mayo Clinic
Rochester, Minnesota

Foreword

It hardly seems any time since we had the 6th edition of this popular textbook of anesthesia. Yet the world has greatly changed and so has the field of anesthesia. The authors, John Butterworth, David Mackey and John Wasnick, have maintained the same layout with Key Concepts beginning each chapter in order to focus the reader's attention on the important points. They have updated chapters and references notably those on enhanced recovery after anesthesia (ERAS), and cardiovascular anesthesia, with increasing emphasis on percutaneous valvular replacement.

Clinical Anesthesiology is one of the best-selling textbooks of anesthesia around the world. The last edition was translated into 10 languages. It is popular with anesthesia residents, nurse anesthetists and trainees everywhere. It is not meant to be all encompassing but to provide a solid basic knowledge of the specialty on which one can effectively build. The authors have succeeded in their objectives.

Congratulations to the authors and editors on a very fine textbook.

Angela Enright OC, MB, FRCPC
Former President World Federation of Societies of Anesthesiologists

Preface

The past few years have been busy times for health care providers in general and anesthesia personnel in particular, thanks to waves of corona virus variants and the continuing evolution of our field. The former necessitated new approaches to respiratory failure. The latter has led to the need for this 7th edition of this textbook.

The textbook reflect the continuing importance of enhanced recovery after surgery (ERAS), critical care of the surgical patient, pain management and imaging in our field.

We have done our best to eliminate unnecessary references. We assume the intelligence of our readers who we know are fluent with internet search engines and PubMed.

Once again we provide a listing of Key Concepts at the beginning of each chapter and include images and artwork when needed.

We thank the sharp-eyed readers who notified us about typographical errors in the 6th edition. We hope that you will be equally vigilant as you read the 7th edition. Please email us at mm7edition@gmail.com if you suspect an error so that we can correct them in subsequent printings.

John F. Butterworth, IV, MD
David C. Mackey, MD
John D. Wasnick, MD, MPH

CHAPTER 1

The Practice of Anesthesiology

KEY CONCEPTS

1. In 1846, Oliver Wendell Holmes was the first to propose the use of the term *anesthesia* to denote the state that incorporates amnesia, analgesia, and narcosis to make painless surgery possible.
2. Ether was used for frivolous purposes ("ether frolics"), but it was not used as an anesthetic agent in humans until 1842 when Crawford W. Long and William E. Clark independently used it on patients. On October 16, 1846, William T.G. Morton conducted the first publicized demonstration of general anesthesia for surgical operation using ether.
3. The original application of modern local anesthesia is credited to Carl Koller, at the time a house officer in ophthalmology, who demonstrated topical anesthesia of the eye with cocaine in 1884.
4. Curare greatly facilitated tracheal intubation and muscle relaxation during surgery. For the first time, operations could be performed on patients without the requirement that relatively deep levels of inhaled general anesthetic be used to produce muscle relaxation.
5. John Snow, often considered the father of the anesthesia specialty, was the first to scientifically investigate ether and the physiology of general anesthesia.
6. The "captain of the ship" doctrine, which held the surgeon responsible for every aspect of the patient's perioperative care (including anesthesia), is no longer a valid notion when an anesthesiologist is present.

The Greek philosopher Dioscorides first used the term *anesthesia* in the first century AD to describe the narcotic-like effects of the plant *mandragora*. The term was defined in 18th century references as "a defect of sensation" or as "privation of the senses."

1 In 1846, Oliver Wendell Holmes was the first to propose the use of the term to denote the state that incorporates amnesia, analgesia, and narcosis to make painless surgery possible. In the United States, the use of the term *anesthesiology* to denote the practice or study of anesthesia was first proposed in the second decade of the 20th century to emphasize the growing scientific basis of the medical specialty.

Although anesthesia now rests on scientific foundations comparable with those of other medical specialties, the practice of anesthesia remains very much a mixture of science and art. Moreover, the practice has expanded well beyond rendering patients insensible to pain during surgery or obstetric delivery (Table 1–1). Anesthesiologists require a working familiarity with a long list of other specialties, including surgery and its subspecialties, internal medicine, pediatrics, palliative care, and obstetrics, as well as imaging techniques (particularly ultrasound), clinical pharmacology, applied physiology, safety science, process improvement,

TABLE 1–1 Aspects of the practice of medicine that are included within the scope of anesthesiology.

Assessment of, consultation for, and preparation of patients for anesthesia.
Relief and prevention of pain during and following surgical, obstetric, therapeutic, and diagnostic procedures.
Monitoring and maintenance of normal physiology during the perioperative or periprocedural period.
Management of critically ill patients.
Diagnosis and treatment of acute, chronic, and cancer-related pain.
Management of hospice and palliative care.
Clinical management and teaching of cardiac, pulmonary, and neurological resuscitation.
Evaluation of respiratory function and application of respiratory therapy.
Conduct of clinical, translational, and basic science research.
Supervision, teaching, and evaluation of performance of both medical and allied health personnel involved in perioperative or periprocedural care, hospice and palliative care, critical care, and pain management.
Administrative involvement in health care facilities, health care organizations, and medical schools, as appropriate to the American Board of Anesthesiology's mission.

Data from the American Board of Anesthesiology Primary Certification Policy Book (Booklet of Information), 2017.

and biomedical technology. Advances in the scientific underpinnings of anesthesia make it an intellectually stimulating and rapidly evolving profession. Many physicians entering residency positions in anesthesiology will already have multiple years of graduate medical education and perhaps certification in other medical specialties.

This chapter reviews the history of anesthesia, emphasizing its British and American roots, and considers the current scope of the specialty.

The History of Anesthesia

The medical specialty of anesthesia began in the mid-19th century and became firmly established in the following century. Ancient civilizations had used opium poppy, coca leaves, mandrake root, alcohol, and even phlebotomy (to the point of unconsciousness) to allow surgeons to operate. Ancient Egyptians used the combination of opium poppy (containing morphine) and hyoscyamus (containing scopolamine) for this purpose. A similar combination, morphine and scopolamine, was widely used for premedication until recent times. What passed for regional anesthesia in ancient times consisted of compression of nerve trunks (nerve ischemia) or the application of cold (cryoanalgesia). The Incas may have practiced local anesthesia as their surgeons chewed coca leaves and applied them to operative wounds, particularly prior to trephining for headache.

The evolution of modern surgery was hampered not only by a poor understanding of disease processes, anatomy, and asepsis but also by the lack of reliable and safe anesthetic techniques. These techniques evolved first with inhalation anesthesia, followed by local and regional anesthesia, intravenous anesthesia, and neuromuscular blockers. The development of surgical anesthesia is considered one of the most important discoveries in human history, and it was introduced to practice without a supporting randomized clinical trial.

INHALATION ANESTHESIA

Because the hypodermic needle was not invented until 1855, the first general anesthetics were destined to be inhalation agents. Diethyl ether (known at the time as "sulfuric ether" because it was produced by a simple chemical reaction between ethyl alcohol and sulfuric acid) was originally prepared in
2 1540 by Valerius Cordus. Ether was used for frivolous purposes ("ether frolics"), but it was not used as an anesthetic agent in humans until 1842, when Crawford W. Long and William E. Clark independently used it on patients for surgery and dental extraction, respectively. However, neither Long nor Clark publicized his discovery. Four years later, in Boston, on October 16, 1846, William T.G. Morton conducted the first publicized demonstration of general anesthesia for surgical operation using ether. The dramatic success of that exhibition led the operating surgeon to exclaim to a skeptical audience: "Gentlemen, this is no humbug!"

Chloroform was independently prepared by Moldenhawer, von Liebig, Guthrie, and Soubeiran around 1831. Although first used by Holmes Coote in 1847, chloroform was introduced into clinical practice by the Scot Sir James Simpson, who administered it to his patients to relieve the pain of labor. Ironically, Simpson had almost abandoned his medical practice after witnessing the terrible despair and agony of patients undergoing operations without anesthesia.

Joseph Priestley produced nitrous oxide in 1772, and Humphry Davy first noted its analgesic properties in 1800. Gardner Colton and Horace Wells are credited with having first used nitrous oxide as an anesthetic for dental extractions in humans in 1844. Nitrous oxide's lack of potency (an 80% nitrous oxide concentration results in analgesia but not surgical anesthesia) led to clinical demonstrations that were less convincing than those with ether.

Nitrous oxide was the least popular of the three early inhalation anesthetics because of its low potency and its tendency to cause asphyxia when used alone (see Chapter 8). Interest in nitrous oxide was revived in 1868 when Edmund Andrews administered it in 20% oxygen; its use was, however, overshadowed by the popularity of ether and chloroform. Ironically, nitrous oxide is the only one of these three agents still in use today. Chloroform superseded ether in popularity in many areas (particularly in the United Kingdom), but reports of chloroform-related cardiac arrhythmias, respiratory depression, and hepatotoxicity eventually caused practitioners to abandon it in favor of ether, particularly in North America.

Even after the introduction of other inhalation anesthetics (ethyl chloride, ethylene, divinyl ether, cyclopropane, trichloroethylene, and fluroxene), ether remained the standard inhaled anesthetic until the early 1960s. The only inhalation agent that rivaled ether's safety and popularity was cyclopropane (introduced in 1934). However, both are highly combustible and have since been replaced by a succession of nonflammable potent fluorinated hydrocarbons: halothane (developed in 1951; released in 1956), methoxyflurane (developed in 1958; released in 1960), enflurane (developed in 1963; released in 1973), and isoflurane (developed in 1965; released in 1981).

Currently, sevoflurane is by far the most popular inhaled agent in developed countries. It is far less pungent than isoflurane and has low blood solubility. Ill-founded concerns about the potential toxicity of its degradation products delayed its release in the United States until 1994 (see Chapter 8). These concerns have proved to be theoretical. Sevoflurane is very suitable for inhaled inductions and has largely replaced halothane in pediatric practice. Desflurane (released in 1992) has many of the desirable properties of isoflurane as well as more rapid uptake and elimination (nearly as fast as nitrous oxide). Sevoflurane, desflurane, and isoflurane are the most commonly used inhaled agents in developed countries worldwide.

LOCAL & REGIONAL ANESTHESIA

The medicinal qualities of coca had been recognized by the Incas for centuries before its actions were first observed by Europeans. Cocaine was isolated from coca leaves in 1855 by Gaedicke and was purified in 1860 by Albert Niemann. Sigmund Freud performed
3 seminal work with cocaine. Nevertheless, the original application of cocaine for anesthesia is credited to Carl Koller, at the time a house officer in ophthalmology, who demonstrated topical anesthesia of the eye in 1884. Later in 1884 William Halsted used cocaine for intradermal infiltration and nerve blocks (including blocks of the facial nerve, brachial plexus, pudendal nerve, and posterior tibial nerve). August Bier is credited with administering the first spinal anesthetic in 1898. He was also the first to describe intravenous regional anesthesia (Bier block) in 1908. Procaine was synthesized in 1904 by Alfred Einhorn, and within a year it was used clinically as a local anesthetic by Heinrich Braun. Braun was also the first to add epinephrine to prolong the duration of local anesthetics. Ferdinand Cathelin and Jean Sicard introduced caudal epidural anesthesia in 1901. Lumbar epidural anesthesia was described first in 1921 by Fidel Pages and again (independently) in 1931 by Achille Dogliotti. Additional local anesthetics subsequently introduced include dibucaine (1930), tetracaine (1932), lidocaine (1947), chloroprocaine (1955), mepivacaine (1957), prilocaine (1960), bupivacaine (1963), and etidocaine (1972). The most recent additions, ropivacaine (1996) and levobupivacaine (1999), have durations of action similar to bupivacaine but less cardiac toxicity

(see Chapter 16). Another, chemically dissimilar local anesthetic, articaine, has been widely applied for dental anesthesia.

INTRAVENOUS ANESTHESIA

Induction Agents

Intravenous anesthesia required the invention of the hypodermic syringe and needle by Alexander Wood in 1855. Early attempts at intravenous anesthesia included the use of chloral hydrate (by Oré in 1872), chloroform and ether (Burkhardt in 1909), and the combination of morphine and scopolamine (Bredenfeld in 1916). Barbiturates were first synthesized in 1903 by Fischer and von Mering. The first barbiturate used for induction of anesthesia was diethylbarbituric acid (barbital), but it was not until the introduction of hexobarbital in 1927 that barbiturate induction became popular. Thiopental, synthesized in 1932 by Volwiler and Tabern, was first used clinically by John Lundy and Ralph Waters in 1934, and for many years it remained the most common agent for the intravenous induction of anesthesia. Methohexital was first used clinically in 1957 by V.K. Stoelting. Methohexital continues to be very popular for brief general anesthetics for electroconvulsive therapy. After chlordiazepoxide was discovered in 1955 and released for clinical use in 1960, other benzodiazepines—diazepam, lorazepam, and midazolam—came to be used extensively for premedication, conscious sedation, and induction of general anesthesia. Ketamine was synthesized in 1962 by Stevens and first used clinically in 1965 by Corssen and Domino; it was released in 1970 and continues to be popular today, particularly when administered in combination with other agents for general anesthesia or when infused in low doses to awake patients with painful conditions. Etomidate was synthesized in 1964 and released in 1972. Initial enthusiasm over its relative lack of circulatory and respiratory effects was tempered by evidence of adrenal suppression, reported after even a single dose. The release of propofol in 1986 (1989 in the United States) was a major advance in outpatient anesthesia because of its short duration of action (see Chapter 9). Propofol is currently the most popular agent for intravenous induction worldwide.

Neuromuscular Blocking Agents

The introduction of curare by Harold Griffith and Enid Johnson in 1942 was a milestone in anesthesia. 4 Curare greatly facilitated tracheal intubation and muscle relaxation during surgery. For the first time, operations could be performed on patients without the requirement for relatively deep planes of inhaled general anesthetic to produce muscle relaxation. Such deep planes of general anesthesia often resulted in excessive cardiovascular and respiratory depression as well as prolonged emergence. Moreover, deep planes of inhalation anesthesia often were not tolerated by frail patients.

Succinylcholine was synthesized by Bovet in 1949 and released in 1951; it remains a standard agent for facilitating tracheal intubation during rapid sequence induction. Until recently, succinylcholine remained unchallenged in its rapid onset of profound muscle relaxation, but its side effects prompted the search for a comparable substitute. Other neuromuscular blockers (NMBs; discussed in Chapter 11)—gallamine, decamethonium, metocurine, alcuronium, and pancuronium—were subsequently introduced. Unfortunately, these agents were often associated with side effects (see Chapter 11), and the search for the ideal NMB continued. Recently introduced agents that more closely resemble an ideal NMB include vecuronium, atracurium, rocuronium, mivacurium, and *cis*-atracurium.

Opioids

Morphine, first isolated from opium in between 1803 and 1805 by Sertürner, was also tried as an intravenous anesthetic. The adverse events associated with opioids in early reports caused many anesthetists to favor pure inhalation anesthesia. Interest in opioids in anesthesia returned following the synthesis and introduction of meperidine in 1939. The concept of *balanced anesthesia* was introduced in 1926 by Lundy and others and evolved to include thiopental for induction, nitrous oxide for amnesia, an opioid for analgesia, and curare for muscle relaxation. In 1969, Lowenstein rekindled interest in "pure" opioid anesthesia by reintroducing the concept of large doses of opioids as complete anesthetics. Morphine was the first agent so employed, but fentanyl and sufentanil have been preferred by a large margin as sole agents. As experience grew with this technique, its multiple limitations—unreliably preventing patient awareness, incompletely suppressing autonomic responses during surgery, and prolonged respiratory depression—were realized. Remifentanil, an opioid subject to rapid degradation by nonspecific plasma and tissue esterases, permits profound levels of opioid analgesia to be employed without concerns regarding the need for postoperative ventilation, albeit with an increased risk of acute opioid tolerance.

EVOLUTION OF THE SPECIALTY

British Origins

Following its first public demonstration in the United States, ether anesthesia quickly was adopted
5 in England. John Snow, often considered the father of the anesthesia specialty, was the first physician to take a full-time interest in this new anesthetic. He was the first to scientifically investigate ether and the physiology of general anesthesia. Of course, Snow was also a pioneer in epidemiology who helped stop a cholera epidemic in London by proving that the causative agent was transmitted by ingestion of contaminated well water rather than by inhalation. In 1847, Snow published the first book on general anesthesia, *On the Inhalation of Ether*. When the anesthetic properties of chloroform were made known, he quickly investigated and developed an inhaler for that agent as well. He believed that an inhaler should be used in administering ether or chloroform to control the dose of the anesthetic. His second book, *On Chloroform and Other Anaesthetics*, was published posthumously in 1858.

After Snow's death, Dr. Joseph T. Clover took his place as England's leading anesthetist. Clover emphasized continuously monitoring the patient's pulse during anesthesia, a practice that was not yet standard at the time. He was the first to use the jaw-thrust maneuver for relieving airway obstruction, the first to insist that resuscitation equipment always be available during anesthesia, and the first to use a cricothyroid cannula (to save a patient with an oral tumor who developed complete airway obstruction). After Clover, Sir Frederic Hewitt became England's foremost anesthetist in the 1890s. He was responsible for many inventions, including the oral airway. Hewitt also wrote what many consider to be the first true textbook of anesthesia, which went through five editions. Snow, Clover, and Hewitt established the tradition of physician anesthetists in England, but it was Hewitt who made the most sustained and strongest arguments for educating specialists in anesthesia. In 1893, the first organization of physician specialists in anesthesia, the London Society of Anaesthetists, was formed in England by J.F. Silk.

The first elective tracheal intubations during anesthesia were performed in the late 19th century by surgeons Sir William MacEwen in Scotland, Joseph O'Dwyer in the United States, and Franz Kuhn in Germany. Tracheal intubation during anesthesia was popularized in England by Sir Ivan Magill and Stanley Rowbotham in the 1920s.

North American Origins

In the United States, only a few physicians had specialized in anesthesia by 1900. The task of providing general anesthesia was often delegated to junior surgical house officers, medical students, or general practitioners.

The first organization of physician anesthetists in the United States was the Long Island Society of Anesthetists, formed in 1905, which, as it grew, was renamed the New York Society of Anesthetists in 1911. The group now known as the International Anesthesia Research Society (IARS) was founded in 1922, and in that same year the IARS-sponsored scientific journal *Current Researches in Anesthesia and Analgesia* (now called *Anesthesia and Analgesia*) began publication. In 1936, the New York Society of Anesthetists became the American Society of Anesthetists, and later, in 1945, the American Society of Anesthesiologists (ASA). The scientific journal *Anesthesiology* was first published in 1940.

Harold Griffith and others founded the Canadian Anesthetists Society in 1943, and Griffith (now better known for introducing curare) served as its first president. Twelve years later the journal now known as the *Canadian Journal of Anesthesia* was first published. Five physicians stand out in the early development of anesthesia in the United States after 1900: James Tayloe Gwathmey, F.H. McMechan,

Arthur E. Guedel, Ralph M. Waters, and John S. Lundy. Gwathmey was the author (with Charles Baskerville) of the first major American textbook of anesthesia in 1914 and was the highly influential first president of the New York State Society of Anesthetists. McMechan, assisted by his wife, was the driving force behind both the IARS and *Current Researches in Anesthesia and Analgesia* and until his death in 1939 tirelessly organized physicians specializing in anesthesia into national and international organizations. Guedel was the first to describe the signs and four stages of general anesthesia. He advocated cuffed tracheal tubes and introduced artificial ventilation during ether anesthesia (later termed *controlled respiration* by Waters). Ralph Waters made a long list of contributions to the specialty, probably the most important of which was his insistence on the proper education of specialists in anesthesia. Waters developed the first academic department of anesthesiology at the University of Wisconsin in Madison. Lundy, working at the Mayo Clinic in Minnesota, was instrumental in the formation of the American Board of Anesthesiology (1937) and chaired the American Medical Association's Section on Anesthesiology for 17 years.

Because of the scarcity of physicians specializing in anesthesia in the United States, surgeons at both the Mayo Clinic and Cleveland Clinic began training and employing nurses as anesthetists in the early 1900s. As the number of nurse anesthetists increased, a national organization was formed in 1932. It was formerly called the American Association of Nurse Anesthetists but was recently (and controversially) renamed the American Association of Nurse Anesthesiology (AANA) . The AANA first offered a certification examination in 1945. In 1969 two Anesthesiology Assistant programs began accepting students, and in 1989 the first certification examinations for anesthesiologist assistants were administered. Certified registered nurse anesthetists and anesthesiologist assistants represent important members of the anesthesia workforce in the United States and in other countries.

Official Recognition

In 1889 Henry Isaiah Dorr, a dentist, was appointed Professor of the Practice of Dentistry, Anaesthetics and Anaesthesia at the Philadelphia College of Dentistry. Thus, he was the first known professor of anesthesia worldwide. Thomas D. Buchanan, of the New York Medical College, was the first physician to be appointed Professor of Anesthesia (in 1905). When the American Board of Anesthesiology was established in 1938, Dr. Buchanan served as its first president. Certification of specialists in anesthesia was first available in Canada in 1946. In England, the first examination for the Diploma in Anaesthetics took place in 1935, and the first Chair in Anaesthetics was awarded to Sir Robert Macintosh in 1937 at Oxford University. Anesthesia became an officially recognized specialty in England only in 1947, when the Royal College of Surgeons established its Faculty of Anaesthetists. In 1992 an independent Royal College of Anaesthetists was granted its charter. Momentous changes occurred in Germany during the 1950s, progress likely having been delayed by the isolation of German medical specialists from their colleagues in other countries that began with World War I and continued until the resolution of World War II. First, the journal *Der Anaesthetist* began publication in 1952. The following year, requirements for specialist training in anesthesia were approved, and the German Society of Anesthetists was founded.

The Scope of Anesthesiology

The practice of anesthesia has changed dramatically since the days of John Snow. The modern anesthesiologist must be both a perioperative consultant and a deliverer of care to patients. In general, anesthesiologists are responsible for nearly all "noncutting" aspects of the patient's medical care in the immediate
6 perioperative period. The "captain of the ship" doctrine, which held the surgeon responsible for every aspect of the patient's perioperative care (including anesthesia), is no longer a valid notion when an anesthesiologist is present. The surgeon and anesthesiologist must function together as an effective team, and both are ultimately answerable to the patient rather than to each other.

The modern practice of anesthesia is not confined to rendering patients insensible to pain

(**Table 1–1**). Anesthesiologists monitor, sedate, and provide general or regional anesthesia outside the operating room for various imaging procedures, endoscopy, electroconvulsive therapy, and cardiac catheterization. Anesthesiologists such as Peter Safar have been pioneers in cardiopulmonary resuscitation, and anesthesiologists continue to be integral members of resuscitation teams.

An increasing number of practitioners pursue subspecialty fellowships in anesthesia for cardiac surgery in adults (see Chapter 22); critical care (see Chapter 57); neuroanesthesia (see Chapter 27); obstetric anesthesia (see Chapter 41); pediatric anesthesia (see Chapter 42); palliative care, regional anesthesia, and acute pain management (see Chapters 45, 46, 48); and chronic pain medicine (see Chapter 47). Certification requirements for special competence in critical care, pediatric anesthesia, and chronic pain medicine already exist in the United States. Fellowship programs in Adult Cardiac Anesthesia, Critical Care Medicine, Pediatric Anesthesiology, Obstetric Anesthesiology, Regional Anesthesia and Acute Pain Management, Sleep Medicine, Palliative Care, and Chronic Pain have specific accreditation requirements. Education and certification in anesthesiology can also be used as the basis for certification in Sleep Medicine or in Palliative Medicine.

Anesthesiologists are actively involved in the administration and medical direction of many ambulatory surgery facilities, operating room suites, intensive care units, and respiratory therapy departments. They lead Enhanced Recovery programs at their hospitals. They have also assumed administrative and leadership positions on the medical staff of many hospitals and ambulatory care facilities. They serve as deans of medical schools and chief executives of health systems. In the United States, they have served in state legislatures, in the U.S. Congress, and as the Surgeon General. The future of the specialty has never looked brighter.

SUGGESTED READINGS

American Board of Anesthesiology Policies , 2021. Available at: http://www.theaba.org Accessed September 29, 2021.

Bacon DR. The promise of one great anesthesia society. The 1939–1940 proposed merger of the American Society of Anesthetists and the International Anesthesia Research Society. *Anesthesiology*. 1994;80:929.

Bergman N. *The Genesis of Surgical Anesthesia*. Wood Library-Museum of Anesthesiology; 1998.

Eger E III, Saidman L, Westhorpe R, eds. *The Wondrous Story of Anesthesia*. Springer; 2014.

Keys TE. *The History of Surgical Anesthesia*. Schuman Publishing; 1945.

Reves JG, Greene NM. Anesthesiology and the academic medical center: place and promise at the start of the new millennium. *Int Anesthesiol Clin*. 2000;38:iii.

Shepherd D. *From Craft to Specialty: A Medical and Social History of Anesthesia and Its Changing Role in Health Care*. Xlibris Corporation; 2009.

Sykes K, Bunker J. *Anaesthesia and the Practice of Medicine: Historical Perspectives*. Royal Society of Medicine Press; 2007.

CHAPTER 2

The Operating Room Environment

KEY CONCEPTS

1. A pressure of 1000 pounds per square inch (psig) indicates an E-cylinder that is approximately half full and represents 330 L of oxygen.
2. The only reliable way to determine the residual volume of nitrous oxide is to weigh the cylinder.
3. To discourage incorrect cylinder attachments, cylinder manufacturers have adopted a pin index safety system.
4. A basic principle of radiation safety is to keep exposure "as low as reasonably practical" (ALARP). The principles of ALARP optimize protection from radiation exposure by the use of *time*, *distance*, and *shielding*.
5. The magnitude of a leakage current is normally imperceptible to touch (<1 milliampere [mA] and well below the fibrillation threshold of 100 mA). If the current bypasses the high resistance offered by skin, however, and is applied directly to the heart (*microshock*), current as low as 100 microamperes (μA) may be fatal. The maximum leakage allowed in operating room equipment is 10 μA.
6. To reduce the chance of two coexisting electrical faults, a line isolation monitor measures the potential for current flow from the isolated power supply to the ground. Basically, the line isolation monitor determines the degree of isolation between the two power wires and the ground and predicts the amount of current that *could* flow if a second short circuit were to develop.
7. Almost all surgical fires can be prevented. Unlike medical complications, fires are a product of simple physical and chemical properties. Occurrence is guaranteed given the proper combination of factors but can be almost entirely eliminated by understanding the basic principles of fire risk.
8. The most common risk factor for surgical fire relates to the open delivery of oxygen.
9. Administration of oxygen in concentrations of greater than 30% should be guided by the clinical presentation of the patient and not by protocols or habits.
10. The sequence of stopping gas flow and removal of the endotracheal tube when a fire occurs in the airway is not as important as ensuring that both actions are performed immediately.
11. Before laser surgery is begun, the laser device should be in the operating room, warning signs should be posted on the doors, and protective eyewear should be issued. The anesthesia provider should ensure that the warning signs and eyewear match the labeling on the device because laser protection is specific to the type of laser.

Anesthesiologists, who spend more time in operating rooms than any other physician specialty, are responsible for protecting patients and operating room personnel from a multitude of dangers. Some of these threats are unique to the operating room. As a result, the anesthesiologist may be responsible for ensuring the proper functioning of the operating room's medical gases, fire prevention and management, environmental factors (eg, temperature, humidity, ventilation, noise), and electrical safety. Anesthesiologists often coordinate or assist with the layout, design, and workflow of surgical and procedural suites. This chapter describes the major operating room features that are of special interest to anesthesiologists and the potential hazards associated with these systems.

Culture of Safety

Patients often think of the operating room as a safe place where the care given is centered around protecting the patient. Anesthesia providers, surgeons, nurses, and other medical personnel are responsible for carrying out critical tasks safely and efficiently. Unless members of the operating room team remain vigilant, errors can occur that may result in harm to the patient or to members of the operating room team. The best way to prevent serious harm to the patient or the operating room team is by creating a *culture of safety*, which identifies and stops unsafe acts before harm occurs.

One tool that fosters the culture of safety is the use of a surgical safety checklist. Such checklists must be used prior to incision on every case and include components agreed upon by the facility as crucial. Many surgical checklists are derived from the surgical safety checklist published by the World Health Organization (WHO). For checklists to be effective, they must first be used, and all members of the surgical team must be focused on the checklist when it is being used. Checklists are most effective when performed in an interactive fashion. An example of a suboptimally executed checklist is one that is read in entirety, after which the surgeon asks whether everyone agrees. This format makes it difficult to identify possible problems. A better method is to elicit a response after each checkpoint. For example, the surgeon may begin by asking, "Does everyone agree this patient is John Doe?" and then ask, "Does everyone agree we are performing a removal of the left kidney?" Optimal checklists do not attempt to cover every possibility, but they address key components, which allows them to be completed in less than 90 seconds.

Some practitioners argue that checklists waste too much time, failing to realize that cutting corners to save time often leads to problems, loss of time, and harm to the patient. If safety checklists were followed in every case, there would be reductions in the incidence of preventable surgical complications such as wrong-site surgery, procedures on the wrong patient, retained foreign objects, or administration of a medication to a patient with a known allergy to that medication. Anesthesia providers have been leaders in patient safety initiatives and should take a proactive role to use checklists and other activities that foster the culture of safety.

Medical Gas Systems

The medical gases commonly used in operating rooms are oxygen, nitrous oxide, air, and nitrogen. Although technically not a gas, vacuum exhaust for disposal or scavenging of waste anesthetic gas and surgical suction must also be provided because these are considered integral parts of the medical gas system. Patients are endangered if medical gas systems, particularly oxygen, are misconfigured or malfunction. The anesthesia provider must understand the sources of the gases and the means of their delivery to the operating room to prevent or detect medical gas depletion or supply line misconnection. Estimates of a particular hospital's peak demand determine the type of medical gas supply system required. Design and standards follow National Fire Protection Association (NFPA) 99 in the United States and HTM 2022 in the United Kingdom.

SOURCES OF MEDICAL GASES

Oxygen

A reliable supply of oxygen is a critical requirement in any surgical area. Medical grade oxygen (99% or

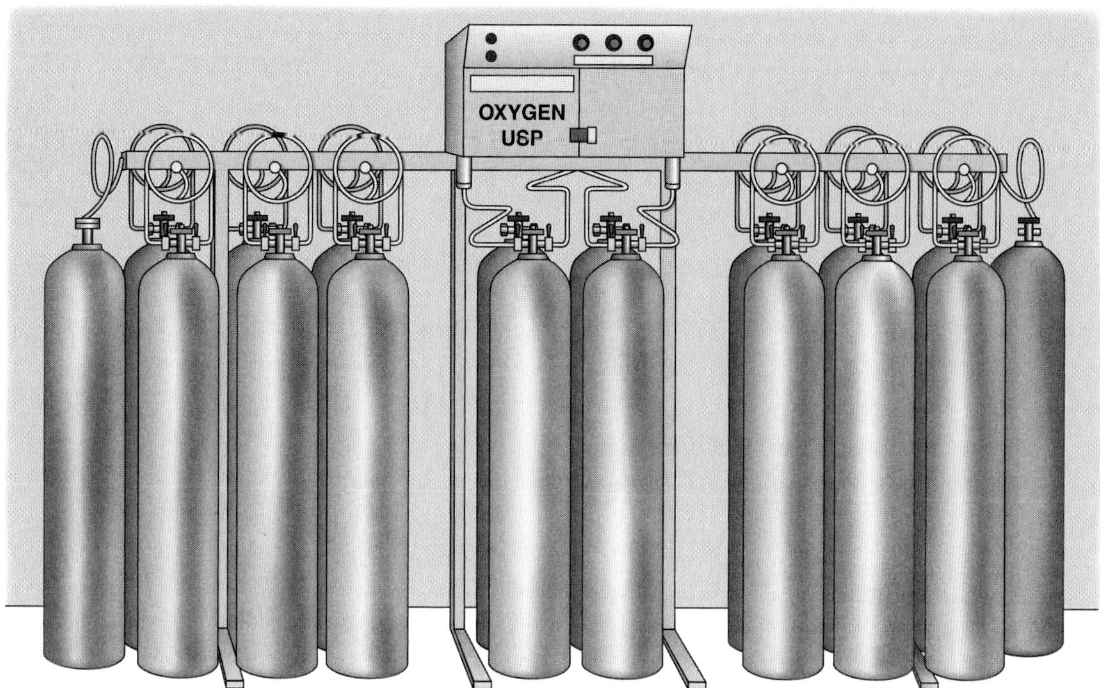

FIGURE 2–1 A bank of oxygen H-cylinders connected by a manifold.

99.5% pure) is manufactured by fractional distillation of liquefied air. Oxygen is stored as a compressed gas at room temperature or refrigerated as a liquid. Most small hospitals store oxygen in two separate banks of high-pressure cylinders (H-cylinders) connected by a manifold (Figure 2–1). Only one bank is used at a time. The number of cylinders in each bank depends on the anticipated daily demand. The manifold contains valves that reduce the *cylinder pressure* (approximately 2000 pounds per square inch [psig]) to *line pressure* (55 ± 5 psig) and automatically switch banks when one group of cylinders is exhausted.

A liquid oxygen storage system (Figure 2–2) is more economical for large hospitals. Liquid oxygen must be stored well below its critical temperature of −119°C because gases can be liquefied by pressure *only* if they are stored below their critical temperature. A large hospital may have a smaller liquid oxygen supply or a bank of compressed gas cylinders that can provide one day's oxygen requirements as a reserve. To guard against a hospital gas-system failure, the anesthesiologist must always have an emergency (E-cylinder) supply of oxygen available during anesthesia.

Most anesthesia machines accommodate E-cylinders of oxygen (Table 2–1). As oxygen is expended, the cylinder's pressure falls in proportion

1 to its content. A pressure of 1000 psig indicates an E-cylinder that is approximately half full and represents 330 L of oxygen at atmospheric pressure and a temperature of 20°C. If the oxygen is exhausted at a rate of 3 L per minute, a cylinder that is half full will be empty in 110 minutes. Oxygen cylinder pressure should be assessed prior to use and periodically during use. Anesthesia machines usually also accommodate E-cylinders for medical air and nitrous oxide, and they may accept cylinders of helium. Compressed medical gases use a pin index safety system for these cylinders to prevent inadvertent crossover and connections for different gas types. As a safety feature, oxygen E-cylinders have a "plug" made from *Wood's metal*. This alloy has a low melting point, allowing dissipation of pressure in a fire that might otherwise heat the cylinder to the

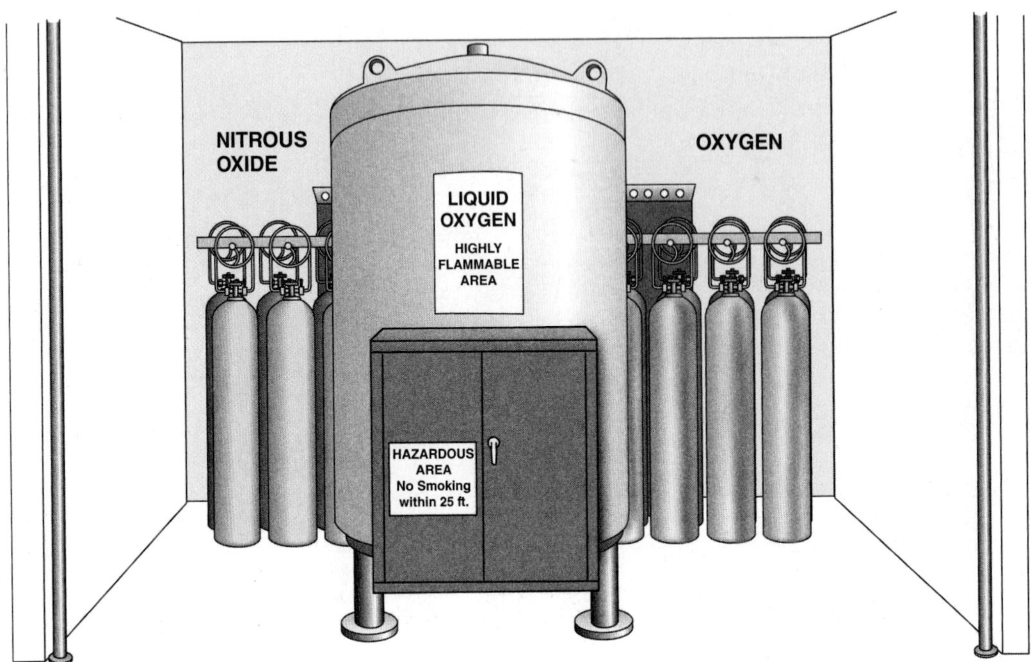

FIGURE 2–2 A liquid storage tank with reserve oxygen tanks in the background.

point of explosion. This pressure-relief "valve" is designed to rupture at 3300 psig, well below the pressure E-cylinder walls should be able to withstand (more than 5000 psig), preventing "overfilling" of the cylinder.

Nitrous Oxide

Nitrous oxide is almost always stored by hospitals in large H-cylinders connected by a manifold with an automatic crossover feature. Bulk liquid storage of nitrous oxide is economical only in very large institutions.

Because the critical temperature of nitrous oxide (36.5°C) is above room temperature, it can be kept liquefied without an elaborate refrigeration system. If the liquefied nitrous oxide rises above its critical temperature, it will revert to its gaseous phase. Because nitrous oxide is not an ideal gas and is easily compressible, the transformation into a gaseous phase is not accompanied by a great rise

TABLE 2–1 Characteristics of medical gas cylinders.

Gas	E-Cylinder Capacity[1] (L)	H-Cylinder Capacity[1] (L)	Pressure[1] (psig at 20°C)	Color (USA)	Color (International)	Form
O_2	625–700	6000–8000	1800–2200	Green	White	Gas
Air	625–700	6000–8000	1800–2200	Yellow	White and black	Gas
N_2O	1590	15,900	745	Blue	Blue	Liquid
N_2	625–700	6000–8000	1800–2200	Black	Black	Gas

[1]Depending on the manufacturer.

N_2O, nitrous oxide; O_2, oxygen.

in tank pressure. Nonetheless, as with oxygen cylinders, all nitrous oxide E-cylinders are equipped with a Wood's metal plug to prevent explosion under conditions of unexpectedly high gas pressure (eg, unintentional overfilling or during a fire).

Although a disruption in nitrous oxide supply is not catastrophic, most anesthesia machines have reserve nitrous oxide E-cylinders. Because these smaller cylinders also contain nitrous oxide in its liquid state, the volume remaining in a cylinder is *not* proportional to cylinder pressure. By the time the liquid nitrous oxide is expended and the tank pressure begins to fall, only about 400 L of nitrous oxide remains. **If liquid nitrous oxide is kept at a constant temperature (20°C), it will vaporize at the same rate at which it is consumed and will maintain a constant pressure (745 psig) until the liquid is exhausted.**

2 The only reliable way to determine the residual volume of nitrous oxide is to weigh the cylinder. For this reason, the tare weight (TW), or empty weight, of cylinders containing a liquefied compressed gas (eg, nitrous oxide) is often stamped on the shoulder of the cylinder. The pressure gauge of a nitrous oxide cylinder should not exceed 745 psig at 20°C. A higher reading implies gauge malfunction, tank overfill (liquid fill), or a cylinder containing a gas other than nitrous oxide.

Because energy is consumed in the conversion of a liquid to a gas (the latent heat of vaporization), liquid nitrous oxide cools during vaporization. The drop in temperature results in lower vapor pressure and lower cylinder pressure. The cooling is so pronounced at high flow rates that there is often frost on the tank, and the pressure regulator may freeze in such circumstances.

Medical Air

The use of air is becoming more frequent in anesthesiology as the popularity of nitrous oxide and the use of unnecessarily high concentrations of oxygen have declined. Cylinder air is medical grade and is obtained by blending oxygen and nitrogen. Dehumidified (but unsterile) air is provided to the hospital pipeline system by compression pumps. The inlets of these pumps must be distant from vacuum exhaust vents and machinery to minimize contamination. Because the critical temperature of air is −140.6°C, it exists as a gas in cylinders whose pressures fall in proportion to their content.

Nitrogen

Although compressed nitrogen is not administered to patients, it may be used to drive operating room equipment, such as saws, drills, and surgical handpieces. Nitrogen supply systems incorporate either the use of H-cylinders connected by a manifold or a wall system supplied by a compressor-driven central supply.

Vacuum

A central hospital vacuum system usually consists of independent suction pumps, each capable of handling peak requirements. Traps at every user location prevent contamination of the system with foreign matter. The medical-surgical vacuum system may be used for waste anesthetic gas disposal (WAGD) as long as it does not affect the performance of the system. Medical vacuum receptacles are usually black in color with white lettering. A dedicated WAGD vacuum system is required with modern anesthesia machines. The WAGD outlet may incorporate the use of a suction regulator with a float indicator that should be maintained between the designated markings. Excess suction may result in inadequate patient ventilation, and insufficient suction levels may result in failure to evacuate waste anesthetic gases. WAGD receptacles and tubing are usually lavender in color.

Carbon Dioxide

Many surgical procedures are performed using laparoscopic or robotic-assisted techniques requiring insufflation of body cavities with carbon dioxide, an odorless, colorless, nonflammable, and slightly acidic gas. Large cylinders containing carbon dioxide, such as M-cylinders or LK-cylinders, are frequently found in the operating room; *these cylinders share a common-size orifice and thread with oxygen cylinders and can be inadvertently interchanged.*

DELIVERY OF MEDICAL GASES

Medical gases are delivered from their central supply source to the operating room through a network of pipes that are sized such that the pressure drop

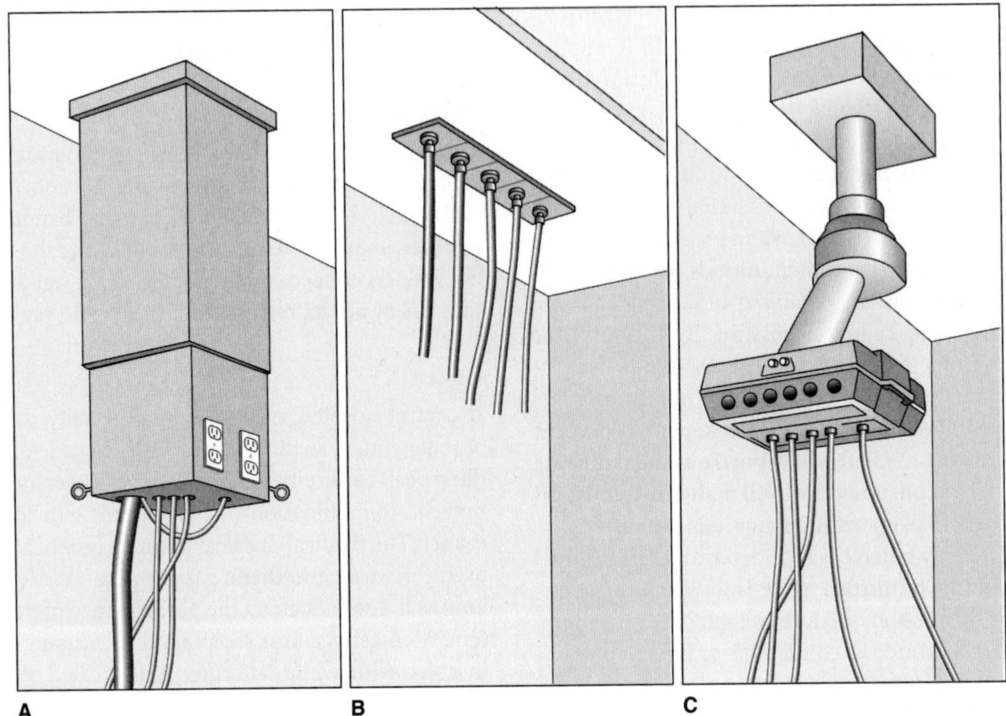

FIGURE 2–3 Typical examples of **A:** gas columns, **B:** ceiling hose drops, and **C:** articulating arms. One end of a color-coded hose connects to the hospital medical gas supply system by way of a quick-coupler mechanism. The other end connects to the anesthesia machine through the diameter index safety system.

across the whole system never exceeds 5 psig. Gas pipes are usually constructed of seamless copper tubing using a special welding technique. Internal contamination of the pipelines with dust, grease, or water must be avoided. The hospital's gas delivery system appears in the operating room as hose drops, gas columns, or elaborate articulating arms (Figure 2–3). Operating room equipment, including the anesthesia machine, connects to pipeline system outlets by color-coded hoses. Quick-coupler mechanisms, which vary in design with different manufacturers, connect one end of the hose to the appropriate gas outlet. The other end connects to the anesthesia machine through a noninterchangeable diameter index safety system fitting that prevents incorrect hose attachment.

3 E-cylinders of oxygen, nitrous oxide, and air attach directly to the anesthesia machine. To discourage incorrect cylinder attachments, cylinder manufacturers have adopted a *pin index safety system*. Each gas cylinder (sizes A–E) has two holes in its cylinder valve that mate with corresponding pins in the yoke of the anesthesia machine (Figure 2–4).

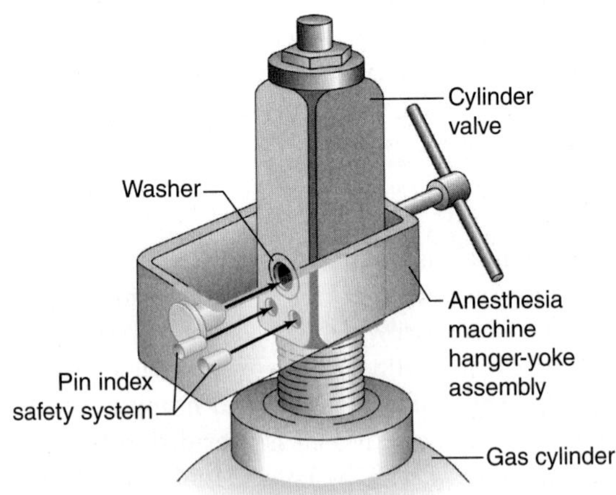

FIGURE 2–4 Pin index safety system interlink between the anesthesia machine and gas cylinder.

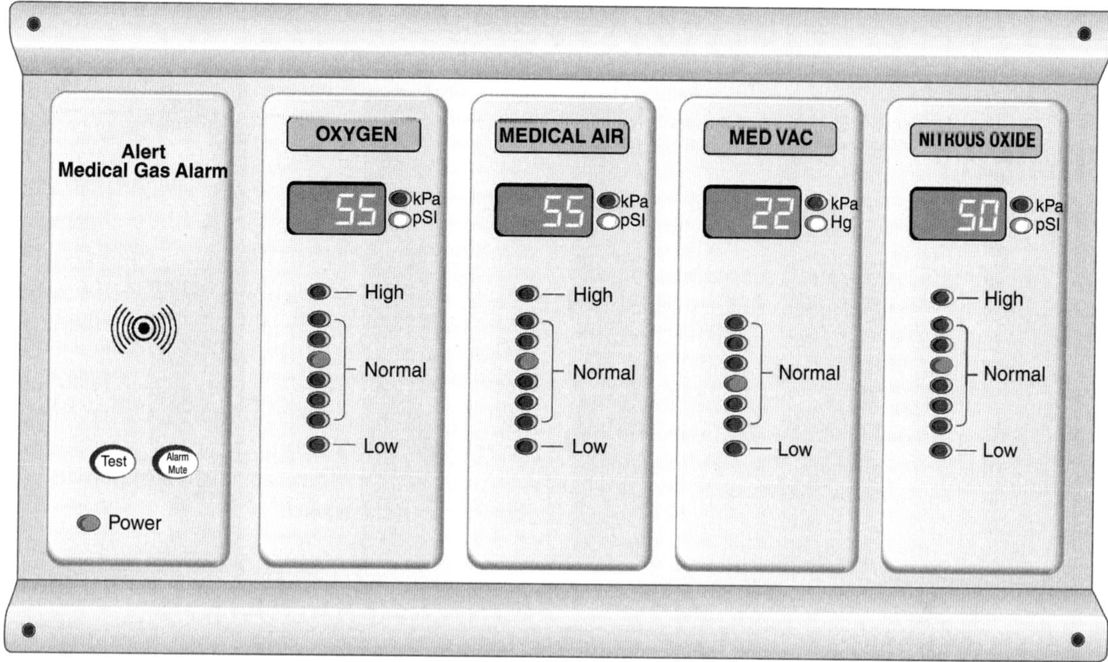

FIGURE 2–5 An example of a master alarm panel that monitors gas line pressure.

The relative positioning of the pins and holes is unique for each gas. Multiple washers placed between the cylinder and yoke prevent proper engagement of the pins and holes, defeating the pin index system, and thus must not be used. The pin index safety system is also ineffective if yoke pins are damaged or if the cylinder is filled with the incorrect gas.

The functioning of medical gas supply sources and pipeline systems is constantly monitored by central and area alarm systems. Indicator lights and audible signals warn of the changeover to secondary gas sources and abnormally high (eg, pressure regulator malfunction) or low (eg, supply depletion) pipeline pressures (Figure 2–5).

Modern anesthesia machines and anesthetic gas analyzers continuously measure the fraction of inspired oxygen (Fio_2). Analyzers have a variable threshold setting for the minimal Fio_2 but must be configured to prevent disabling this alarm. The monitoring of Fio_2 does not reflect the oxygen concentration distal to the monitoring port and thus should not be used to reference the oxygen concentration within distal devices such as endotracheal tubes. Due to gas exchange, flow rates, and shunting, a marked difference may exist between the indicated supply Fio_2 and the actual oxygen concentration at the tissue level.

Environmental Factors in the Operating Room

TEMPERATURE

The temperature in most operating rooms seems uncomfortably cold to many conscious patients and, at times, to anesthesia providers. However, scrub nurses and surgeons stand in surgical garb for hours under hot operating room lights. As a general principle, the comfort of operating room personnel must be reconciled with patient care, and for adult patients, ambient room temperature should be maintained between 68°F (20°C) and 75°F (24°C). The impact of environmental temperature on patient core temperature must be monitored, as hypothermia is associated with wound infection, impaired coagulation, greater intraoperative blood loss, and prolonged hospitalization (see Chapter 52).

HUMIDITY

In previous decades, the maintenance of adequate operating room humidity was important because static discharges were a feared source of ignition when flammable anesthetic gases such as ether and cyclopropane were used. Now, humidity control is more relevant to infection control practices, and ambient operating room humidity should be maintained between 20% and 60%. Below this range, the dry air facilitates airborne mobility of particulate matter, which can be a vector for infection. At high humidity, dampness can affect the integrity of barrier devices such as sterile cloth drapes and pan liners.

VENTILATION

A high rate of operating room airflow decreases contamination of the surgical site. These flow rates, usually achieved by blending up to 80% recirculated air with fresh air, are engineered in a manner to decrease turbulent flow and to be unidirectional. Although recirculation conserves energy costs associated with heating and air conditioning, it is unsuitable for WAGD. Therefore, a separate waste anesthetic gas scavenging system must always supplement operating room ventilation. The operating room should maintain a slightly positive pressure to drive away gases that escape scavenging and should be designed so fresh air is introduced through, or near, the ceiling and air return is handled at, or near, floor level. Ventilation considerations must address both air quality and volume changes. The National Fire Protection Agency (NFPA) recommends 20 air volume exchanges per hour to decrease the risk of stagnation and bacterial growth. Air quality should be maintained by adequate air filtration using a 90% filter, defined simply as one that filters out 90% of particles presented. Although high-efficiency particulate filters (HEPA) are frequently used, these are not required by engineering or infection control standards.

NOISE

Multiple studies have demonstrated that exposure to noise can have a detrimental effect on human cognitive function, and prolonged exposure may result in hearing impairment. Operating room noise has been measured at 70 to 80 decibels (dB) with frequent sound peaks exceeding 80 dB. As a reference, if the speaking voice has to be raised above conversational level, ambient noise is approximated at 80 dB. Noise levels in the operating room approach the time-weighted average (TWA) for which the Occupational Safety and Health Administration (OSHA) requires hearing protection. Orthopedic air chisels and neurosurgical drills can approach noise levels of 125 dB, the level at which most human subjects begin to experience pain.

IONIZING RADIATION

Anesthesia providers are exposed to radiation as a component of either diagnostic imaging or radiation therapy; examples include fluoroscopy, linear accelerators, computed tomography, directed beam therapy, proton therapy, and diagnostic radiographs. The effects of radiation on humans are measured by units of absorbed doses such as the gray (Gy) and rads, or by equivalent dose units such as the Sievert (Sv) and Roentgen equivalent in man (REM). Radiation-sensitive organs such as eyes, thyroid, and gonads must be protected, as well as blood, bone marrow, and the fetus. Radiation levels must be monitored if individuals are exposed to greater than 40 REM, and the most common method of measurement is by film badge. Radiation badges should be worn routinely by anesthesia providers who work even intermittently in areas where fluoroscopy or other ionizing radiation devices are used. Lifetime exposure can be tabulated by a required database of film badge wearers.

4 A basic principle of radiation safety is to keep exposure "as low as reasonably practical" (ALARP). The principles of ALARP optimize protection from radiation exposure by the use of *time*, *distance*, and *shielding*. The length of time of exposure is usually not an issue for simple radiographs such as chest films but can be prolonged in

fluoroscopic procedures, such as those commonly performed in interventional radiology or pulmonary procedural areas, during c-arm use, and in a diagnostic gastroenterology center. Exposure can be reduced to the provider by increasing the distance between the beam and the provider. Radiation exposure over distance follows the inverse square law. To illustrate, intensity is represented as $1/d^2$ (where d = distance) so that 100 millirads (mrads) at 1 cm will be 0.01 mrads at 100 cm. Shielding is the most reliable form of radiation protection; typical personal shielding is in the form of leaded aprons, thyroid collars, and glasses. Physical shields are usually incorporated into radiology suites and can be as simple as a wall to stand behind or a rolling leaded shield to place between the beam and the provider. Although most modern facilities are designed in a very safe manner, providers can still be exposed to scattered radiation as atomic particles are bounced off shielding. For this reason, radiation protection should be donned whenever ionizing radiation is used.

As the use of reliable shielding has increased, the incidence of radiation-associated diseases of sensitive organs has decreased, with the exception of radiation-induced cataracts. Because protective eyewear has not been consistently used to the same degree as other types of personal protection, the incidence of radiation-induced cataracts is increasing among employees working in interventional radiology suites. Anesthesia providers who work in these environments should consider the use of leaded goggles or glasses to decrease the risk of such problems.

Electrical Safety

THE RISK OF ELECTROCUTION

The use of electronic medical equipment subjects patients and health care personnel to the risk of shock and electrocution. Anesthesia providers must have an understanding of electrical hazards and their prevention.

Body contact with two conductive materials at different voltage potentials may complete a circuit and result in an electrical shock. Usually, one point of exposure is a live 120-V or 240-V conductor, with the circuit completed through a ground contact. For example, a grounded person need contact only one live conductor to complete a circuit and receive a shock. The live conductor could be the frame of a patient monitor that has developed a fault to the hot side of the power line. A circuit is now complete between the power line (which is earth grounded at the utility company's pole-top transformer) through the victim and back to the ground (Figure 2–6). The physiological effect of electrical current depends on the location, duration, frequency, and magnitude (more accurately, current density) of the shock.

Leakage current is present in all electrical equipment as a result of capacitive coupling, induction between internal electrical components, or defective insulation. Current can flow as a result of capacitive coupling between two conductive bodies (eg, a circuit board and its casing) even though they are not physically connected. Some monitors are doubly insulated to decrease the effect of capacitive coupling. Other monitors are designed to be connected to a low-impedance ground (the safety ground wire) that should divert the current away from a person touching the instrument's case. The magnitude of
5 such leaks is normally imperceptible to touch (<1 milliampere [mA] and well below the fibrillation threshold of 100 mA). If the current bypasses the high resistance offered by skin, however, and is applied directly to the heart, current as low as 100 microamperes (μA) (*microshock*) may be fatal. The maximum leakage allowed in operating room equipment is 10 μA.

Cardiac pacing wires and invasive monitoring catheters provide a direct conductive pathway to the myocardium, and blood and normal saline can also serve as electrical conductors. The exact amount of current required to produce fibrillation depends on the timing of the shock relative to the vulnerable period of heart repolarization (the T wave on the electrocardiogram). Even small differences in potential between the ground connections of two electrical outlets in the same operating room can place a patient at risk for microelectrocution.

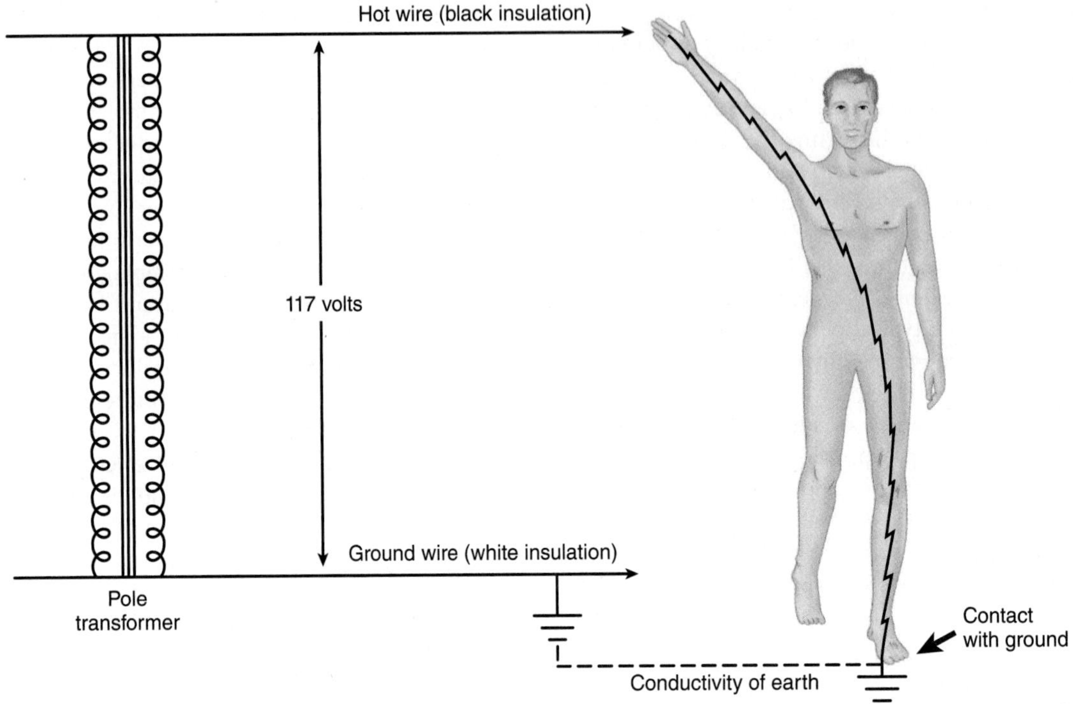

FIGURE 2–6 The setting for most electric shocks. An accidentally grounded person simultaneously contacts the hot wire of the electric service, usually via defective equipment that provides a pathway linking the hot wire to an exposed conductive surface. The complete electrical loop originates with the secondary of the pole transformer (the voltage source) and extends through the hot wire, the victim and the victim's contact with a ground, the earth itself, the neutral ground rod at the service entrance, and back to the transformer via the neutral (or ground) wire. (Modified with permission from Bruner J, Leonard PF. *Electricity, Safety, and the Patient*. St Louis, MO: Mosby Year Book; 1989.)

PROTECTION FROM ELECTRICAL SHOCK

Most patient electrocutions are caused by current flow from the live conductor of a grounded circuit through the body and back to a ground (**Figure 2–6**). This would be prevented if everything in the operating room were grounded except the patient. Although direct patient grounds should be avoided, complete patient isolation is not feasible during surgery. Instead, the operating room power supply can be isolated from grounds by an **isolation transformer** (Figure 2–7).

Unlike the utility company's pole-top transformer, the secondary wiring of an isolation transformer is not grounded and provides two live ungrounded voltage lines for operating room equipment. Equipment casings—but not the electrical circuits—are grounded through the longest blade of a three-pronged plug (the *safety ground*). If a live wire is then unintentionally contacted by a grounded patient, the current will not flow through the patient because no circuit back to the secondary coil has been completed (Figure 2–8).

Of course, if both power lines are contacted, a circuit is completed, and a shock is possible. In addition, if either power line comes into contact with a ground through a fault, contact with the other power line will complete a circuit through a grounded patient. 6 To reduce the chance of two coexisting faults, a *line isolation monitor* measures the potential for current flow from the isolated power supply to the ground (Figure 2–9). Basically, the line isolation monitor determines the degree of isolation between the two power wires and the ground and predicts the amount of current that *could* flow if a second short

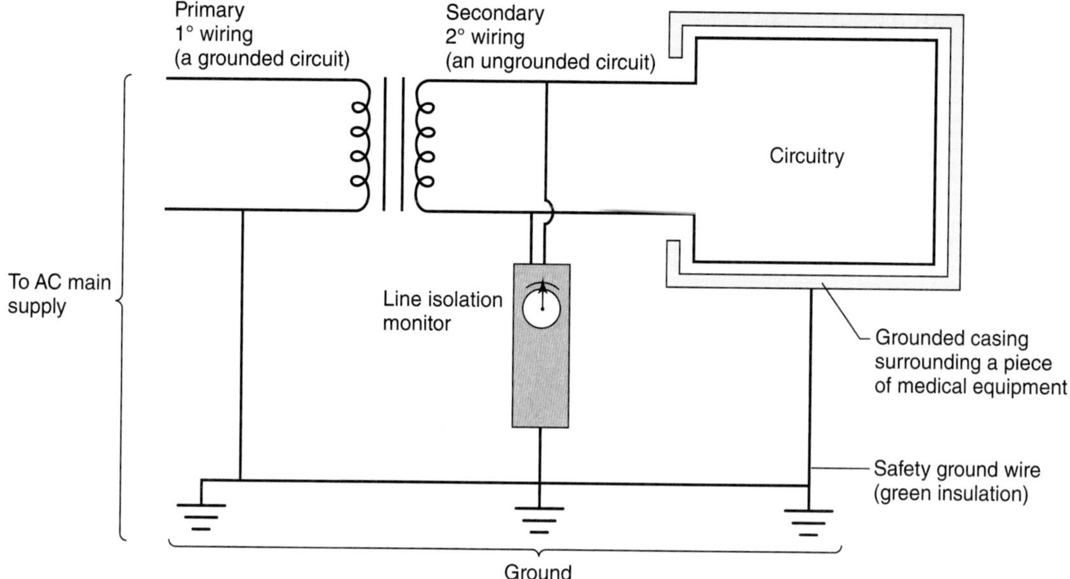

FIGURE 2–7 A circuit diagram of an isolation transformer and monitor.

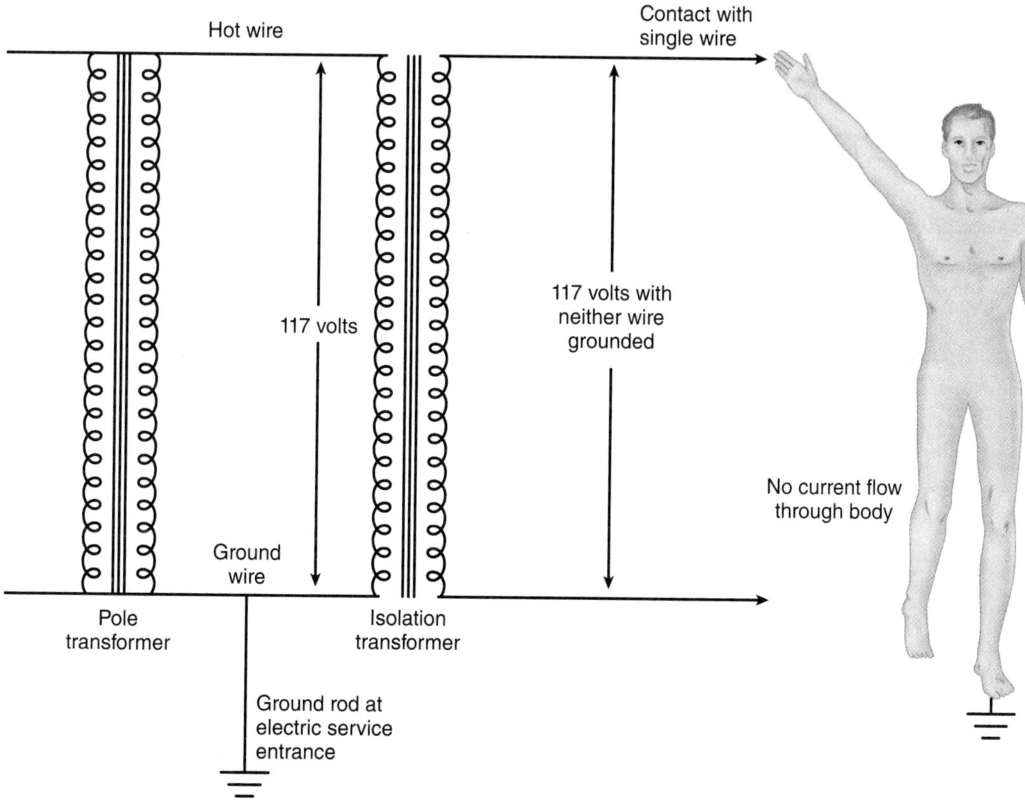

Hot wire
Contact with
single wire
117 volts
117 volts with
neither wire
grounded
No current flow
through body
Ground
wire
Pole
transformer
Isolation
transformer
Ground rod at
electric service
entrance

FIGURE 2–8 Even though a person is grounded, no shock results from contact with one wire of an isolated circuit. The individual is in simultaneous contact with two separate voltage sources but does not close a loop including either source. (Modified with permission from Bruner J, Leonard PF. *Electricity, Safety, and the Patient*. Mosby Year Book; 1989.)

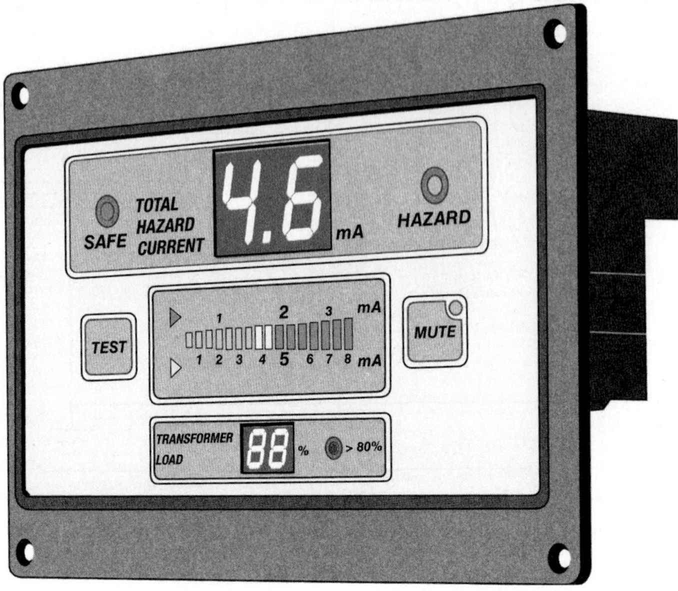

FIGURE 2–9 A line isolation monitor.

circuit were to develop. An alarm is activated if an unacceptably high current flow to the ground becomes possible (usually 2 mA or 5 mA), but power is not interrupted unless a ground-fault circuit interrupter is also activated. The latter, a common feature in household bathrooms and kitchens, is usually not installed in locations such as operating rooms, where discontinuation of life support systems (eg, cardiopulmonary bypass machine) is more hazardous than the risk of electrical shock. The alarm of the line isolation monitor merely indicates that the power supply has partially reverted to a grounded system. In other words, although the line isolation monitor warns of the existence of a single fault (between a power line and a ground), two faults are required for a shock to occur. Since the line isolation monitor alarms when the sum of leakage current exceeds the set threshold, the last piece of equipment added is usually the defective one; however, if this item is life-sustaining, other equipment can be removed from the circuit to evaluate whether the life safety item is truly at fault.

Even isolated power circuits do not provide complete protection from the small currents capable of causing microshock fibrillation. Furthermore, the line isolation monitor cannot detect all faults, such as a broken safety ground wire within a piece of equipment. There are, however, modern equipment designs that decrease the possibility of microelectrocution. These include double insulation of the chassis and casing, ungrounded battery power supplies, and patient isolation from equipment-connected grounds by using optical coupling or transformers.

In the latest edition of the U.S. NPFA 99 Health Care Facilities Code, building system requirements for facilities—including electrical systems—are based upon a risk assessment carried out by facilities personnel with the input of health care providers. The risk levels are categorized in levels as follows:

Category 1—Facility systems in which failure of such equipment or system is likely to cause major injury or death of patients or caregivers

Category 2—Facility systems in which failure of such equipment is likely to cause minor injury to patients or caregivers

Category 3—Facility systems in which failure of such equipment is not likely to cause injury to patients or caregivers but can cause patient discomfort

Category 4—Facility systems in which failure of such equipment would have no impact on patient care

Category 1 locations and systems will have the greatest amount of reliability and redundancy; lesser categories will have less stringent requirements. Under the electrical code, operating rooms are defined as a wet location requiring electrical systems that reduce the risk of electrical shock hazards. If an operating room is used for procedures without liquid exposure, such as rooms used for central line placement or eye procedures, facilities can perform a risk assessment and reclassify the operating room as a nonwet area.

SURGICAL DIATHERMY (ELECTROCAUTERY, ELECTROSURGERY)

Electrosurgical units (ESUs) generate an ultrahigh-frequency electrical current that passes from a small active electrode (the cautery tip) through the patient and exits by way of a large plate electrode (the dispersal pad, or return electrode). The high current density at the cautery tip is capable of tissue coagulation or cutting, depending on the electrical waveform. Ventricular fibrillation is prevented by the use of ultrahigh electrical frequencies (0.1–3 MHz) compared with that of line power (50–60 Hz). The large surface area of the low-impedance return electrode avoids burns at the current's point of exit by providing a low current density (the concept of current *exit* is technically incorrect because the current is alternating rather than direct). The high power levels of ESUs (up to 400 W) can cause inductive coupling with monitor cables, leading to electrical interference.

Malfunction of the dispersal pad may result from disconnection from the ESU, inadequate patient contact, or insufficient conductive gel. In these situations, the current will find another place to exit (eg, electrocardiogram pads or metal parts of the operating table), which may result in a burn (Figure 2–10). Precautions to prevent diathermy

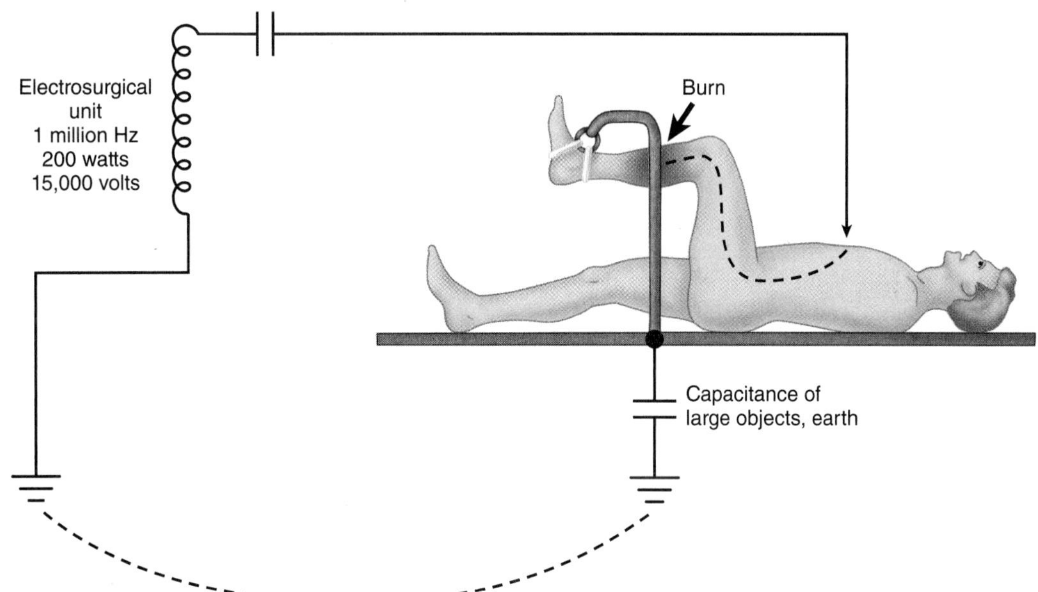

FIGURE 2–10 Electrosurgical burn. If the intended path is compromised, the circuit may be completed through other routes. Because the current is of high frequency, recognized conductors are not essential; capacitances can complete gaps in the circuit. Current passing through the patient to a contact of small area may produce a burn. (A leg drape would not offer protection in the situation depicted.) The isolated output electrosurgical unit (ESU) is much less likely than the ground-referenced ESU to provoke burns at ectopic sites. *Ground-referenced* in this context applies to the ESU output and has nothing to do with isolated versus grounded power systems. (Modified with permission from Bruner J, Leonard PF. *Electricity, Safety, and the Patient.* St Louis, MO: Mosby Year Book; 1989.)

burns include proper return electrode placement, avoiding prostheses and bony protuberances, and elimination of patient-to-ground contacts. Current flow through the heart may lead to the malfunction of an implanted cardiac pacemaker or cardioverter defibrillator. This risk can be minimized by placing the return electrode as close to the surgical field and as far from the implanted cardiac device as practical.

Newer ESUs are isolated from grounds using the same principles as the isolated power supply (*isolated output* versus *ground-referenced* units). Because this second layer of protection provides ESUs with their own isolated power supply, the operating room's line isolation monitor may not detect an electrical fault. Although some ESUs are capable of detecting poor contact between the return electrode and the patient by monitoring impedance, many older units trigger the alarm only if the return electrode is unplugged from the machine. Bipolar electrodes confine current propagation to a few millimeters, eliminating the need for a return electrode. Because pacemaker and electrocardiogram interference is possible, pulse or heart sounds should be closely monitored when any ESU is used. Automatic implanted cardioverter defibrillator devices may need to be suspended if monopolar ESU is used, and any implanted cardiac device should be interrogated after use of a monopolar ESU to verify that its settings have not been altered by electrical interference.

Surgical Fires & Thermal Injury

FIRE PREVENTION & PREPARATION

Surgical fires are relatively rare, with an incidence of about 1 in 87,000 cases, which is close to the incidence rate of other events such as retained foreign objects
7 after surgery and wrong-site surgery. Almost all surgical fires can be prevented (Figure 2–11). Unlike medical complications, fires are a product of simple physical and chemical properties. Occurrence is guaranteed given the association of fundamental combustion factors, but it can be almost entirely eliminated by understanding and heeding
8 the basic principles of fire risk. The most common risk factor for surgical fire relates to the open delivery of oxygen.

Situations classified as carrying a high risk for a surgical fire are those that involve an ignition source in close proximity to an oxidizer. The simple chemical combination required for any fire is commonly referred to as the *fire triad* or *fire triangle.* The triad is composed of fuel, oxidizer, and ignition source (heat). Table 2–2 lists potential contributors to fires and explosions in the operating room. *Surgical fires can be managed and possibly avoided completely by incorporating education, fire drills, preparation, prevention, and response into educational programs regularly provided to operating room personnel.*

For anesthesia providers, fire prevention education should place a heavy emphasis on the risks of open delivery of oxygen. The Anesthesia Patient Safety Foundation has developed an educational video and online teaching module that provides fire safety education from the perspective of the anesthesia provider.

Operating room fire drills increase awareness of the fire hazards associated with surgical procedures. In contrast to the typical institutional fire drill, these drills should be specific to the operating room and should place a greater emphasis on the particular risks associated with that setting. For example, consideration should be given to both vertical and horizontal evacuation of surgical patients, movement of patients requiring ventilatory assistance, and unique situations such as prone or lateral positioning and movement of patients who may be fixed in neurosurgical pins.

Surgical fire preparedness can be incorporated into the time-out process of the universal protocol. Team members should be introduced by name and specific roles agreed upon should a fire erupt. Items needed to properly manage a fire can be assembled or identified beforehand (eg, ensuring the proper endotracheal tube for patients undergoing laser surgery; having water or saline ready on the surgical field; identifying the location of fire extinguishers, gas cutoff valves, and escape routes). A poster or flowsheet to standardize this preparation is beneficial.

Preventing catastrophic fires in the operating room begins with a strong level of communication

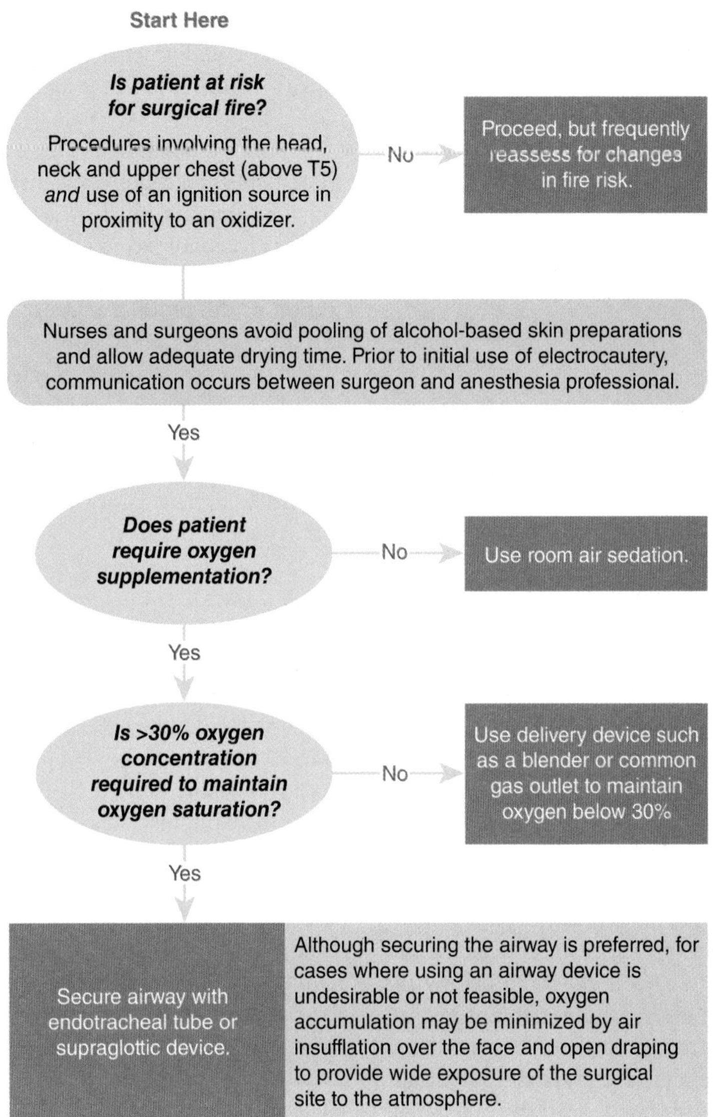
Start Here
Is patient at risk for surgical fire?
Procedures involving the head, neck and upper chest (above T5) and use of an ignition source in proximity to an oxidizer.
No
Proceed, but frequently reassess for changes in fire risk.
Nurses and surgeons avoid pooling of alcohol-based skin preparations and allow adequate drying time. Prior to initial use of electrocautery, communication occurs between surgeon and anesthesia professional.
Yes
Does patient require oxygen supplementation?
No
Use room air sedation.
Yes
Is >30% oxygen concentration required to maintain oxygen saturation?
No
Use delivery device such as a blender or common gas outlet to maintain oxygen below 30%
Yes
Secure airway with endotracheal tube or supraglottic device.
Although securing the airway is preferred, for cases where using an airway device is undesirable or not feasible, oxygen accumulation may be minimized by air insufflation over the face and open draping to provide wide exposure of the surgical site to the atmosphere.

FIGURE 2–11 Operating Room Fire Prevention Algorithm. (©Anesthesia Patient Safety Foundation. Used with permission.)

among all members of the surgical team. Different aspects of the fire triad are typically under the domain of particular surgical team members. Fuels such as alcohol-based solutions, adhesive removers, and surgical drapes and towels are typically controlled by the circulating nurse. Ignition sources such as electrocautery, lasers, drills, burrs, and light sources for headlamps and laparoscopes are usually controlled by the surgical team. The anesthesia provider(s) maintains control of the oxidizer concentration of oxygen and nitrous oxide. Communication between operating room personnel is exemplified by a surgeon verifying the oxygen concentration before using electrocautery in or near an airway or by an anesthesia provider asking the operating room circulator to configure drapes to prevent

TABLE 2–2 Potential contributors to operating room fires and explosions.

Flammable agents (fuels)		
	Solutions, aerosols, and ointments	
		Alcohol
		Chlorhexidine
		Benzoin
		Mastisol
		Acetone
		Petroleum products
	Surgical drapes (paper and cloth)	
	Surgical gowns	
	Surgical sponges and packs	
	Surgical sutures and mesh	
	Plastic/polyvinyl chloride/latex products	
		Endotracheal tubes
		Masks
		Cannulas
		Tubing
	Intestinal gases	
	Hair	
Gases supporting combustion (oxidizers)		
	Oxygen	
	Nitrous oxide	
Ignition sources (heat)		
	Lasers	
	Electrosurgical units	
	Fiberoptic light sources (distal tip)	
	Drills and burrs	
	External defibrillators	

the accumulation of oxygen in a case that involves the use of nasal cannula oxygen delivery.

9 Administration of oxygen in concentrations of greater than 30% should be guided by the clinical presentation of the patient and not by protocols or habits. Increased flows of oxygen delivered via nasal cannula or face mask are potentially dangerous. When enriched oxygen levels are needed, especially when the surgical site is above the level of the xiphoid, the airway should be secured by either an endotracheal tube or a supraglottic airway device.

When the surgical site is in or near the airway and a flammable endotracheal tube is present, the oxygen concentration should be reduced for a sufficient period of time before the use of an ignition device (eg, laser or cautery) to allow adequate reduction of oxygen concentration at the site. Laser airway surgery should incorporate either jet ventilation without an endotracheal tube or the appropriate protective endotracheal tube specific for the wavelength of the laser. Precautions for laser cases are outlined below.

Alcohol-based skin preparations are extremely flammable and require adequate drying time. Pooling of solutions must be avoided. Large prefilled swabs of alcohol-based solution should be used with caution on the head or neck to avoid both oversaturation of the product and excess flammable waste. Product inserts are a good source of information about these preparations. Surgical gauze and sponges should be moistened with sterile water or saline if used in close proximity to an ignition source.

Should a fire occur in the operating room, it is important to determine whether the fire is located *on the patient, in the airway,* or *elsewhere in the operating room.* For fires occurring in the airway, the delivery of fresh gases to the patient must be stopped immediately. Stopping fresh gas flow to the patient can be accomplished by turning off flowmeters, disconnecting the circuit from the machine, or disconnecting the circuit from the endotracheal tube. The endotracheal tube should be removed, and either sterile water or saline should be poured into the airway
10 to extinguish any burning tissue or foreign material. The sequence of stopping gas flow and removal of the endotracheal tube when a fire occurs in the airway is not as important as ensuring that both actions are performed immediately. The two tasks can be accomplished at the same time and by the same individual. If carried out by different team members, the personnel should act without waiting for a predetermined sequence of events. After these actions are carried out, ventilation may be resumed, preferably using room air and avoiding oxygen or nitrous oxide–enriched gases. The endotracheal tube should be examined for missing pieces. The airway should be reestablished and, if indicated, carefully examined with a fiberoptic bronchoscope. Treatment for smoke inhalation and transfer to a burn center should be considered.

For fires on the patient, the flow of oxidizing gases should be stopped, the surgical drapes removed, and the fire extinguished by water or smothering. The patient should be assessed for injury. If the fire is not immediately extinguished by first attempts, then a carbon dioxide (CO_2) fire extinguisher may be used. Further actions may include evacuation of the patient and activation of the nearest alarm pull station. As noted previously, prior to an actual emergency, the location of fire extinguishers, emergency exits, and fresh gas cutoff valves should be verified by the operating room team.

Fires that result in injuries requiring medical treatment or death must be reported to the fire marshal who retains jurisdiction over the facility. Providers should gain basic familiarity with local reporting standards, which can vary according to location.

Cases in which supplemental oxygen delivery is used and the surgical site is above the xiphoid constitute the most commonly reported scenario for surgical fires. Frequently, the face or airway is involved, resulting in life-threatening or severely disfiguring injuries. These fires can almost always be avoided by the elimination of the open delivery of oxygen.

FIRE EXTINGUISHERS

For fires not suppressed by initial attempts, or those in which evacuation may be hindered by the location or intensity of the fire, the use of a portable fire extinguisher is warranted. A CO_2 extinguisher is safe for fires on the patient in the operating room. CO_2 readily dissipates, is not toxic, and is not likely to result in thermal injury. FE-36, a more expensive DuPont product, also can be used.

"A"-rated extinguishers contain water, which makes their use in the operating room problematic because of the presence of electrical equipment. A water mist "AC"-rated extinguisher is excellent but requires time and an adequate volume of mist over multiple attempts to extinguish the fire. Furthermore, these devices are large and difficult to maneuver. Both A and AC fire extinguishers can be constructed relatively inexpensively as nonferromagnetic devices, making them the best choice for fires involving magnetic resonance imaging equipment. Halon extinguishers, though very effective, are being phased out because of concerns about depletion of the ozone layer and because of the hypoxic atmosphere that results for rescuers. *Halotrons* are halon-type extinguishers that have a lower environmental impact and do not leave a residue.

LASER SAFETY

Lasers are commonly used in operating rooms and procedure areas. When lasers are used in the airway or for procedures involving the neck and face, the case should be considered high risk for surgical fire and managed as previously discussed. The type of laser (CO_2, neodymium–yttrium aluminum garnet [Nd:YAG], or potassium titanyl phosphate [KTP]), wavelength, and focal length are all important considerations for the safe operation of medical lasers. Without this vital information, operating room personnel cannot adequately protect themselves or the
11 patient from harm. Before laser surgery is begun, the laser device should be in the operating room, warning signs should be posted on the doors, and protective eyewear should be issued. The American National Standards Institute (ANSI) standards specify that eyewear and laser devices must be labeled for the wavelength emitted or the protection offered. The anesthesia provider should ensure that the warning signs and eyewear match the labeling on the device because protection is specific to the type of laser. Some ophthalmologic lasers and vascular mapping lasers have such a short focal length that protective eyewear is not needed. For other devices, protective goggles should be worn by personnel at all times during laser use, and eye protection in the form of either goggles or protective eye patches should be used on the patient.

Laser endotracheal tube selection should be based on laser type and wavelength. The product insert and labeling for each type of tube should be compared with the type of laser used. Endotracheal tubes less than 4 mm in diameter are not compatible with the Nd:YAG or argon laser, and Nd:YAG-compatible tubes are not available in half sizes. Attempts to wrap conventional endotracheal tubes with foil should be avoided. This obsolete method is not approved by either manufacturers or the U.S. Food and Drug Administration; it often leads to breaking or unraveling, and it does not confer complete protection against laser penetration. Alternatively, jet ventilation without an endotracheal tube can offer a reduced risk of airway fire.

CREW RESOURCE MANAGEMENT: CREATING A CULTURE OF SAFETY IN THE OPERATING ROOM

Crew resource management (CRM) was developed in the aviation industry to promote teamwork and allow personnel to intervene or call for investigation of any situation thought to be unsafe. CRM is comprised of seven principles, and its goal is to avoid errors caused by human actions. In the airline model, CRM gives any crew member the authority to question situations that fall outside the range of normal practice. Before the implementation of CRM, crew members other than the captain had little input on aircraft operations. After CRM was instituted, anyone identifying a safety issue could take steps to ensure adequate resolution of the situation. The benefit of this method in the operating room is clear given the potential for a deadly mistake to be made.

The seven principles of CRM are (1) adaptability/flexibility, (2) assertiveness, (3) communication, (4) decision making, (5) leadership, (6) analysis, and (7) situational awareness. *Adaptability/flexibility* refers to the ability to alter a course of action when new information becomes available. For example, if a major blood vessel is unintentionally cut in a routine procedure, the anesthesiologist must recognize that the anesthetic plan has changed and volume resuscitation must be made even in the presence of medical conditions that typically contraindicate large-volume fluid administration.

Assertiveness is the willingness and readiness to actively participate, state, and maintain a position until convinced by the facts that other options are better; this requires the initiative and the courage to act. For instance, if a senior and well-respected surgeon tells the anesthesiologist that the patient's aortic stenosis is not a problem because it is a chronic condition and the procedure will be relatively quick, the anesthesiologist should respond by voicing concerns about the management of the patient and should not proceed until a safe anesthetic and surgical plan have been agreed upon.

Communication is defined simply as the clear and accurate sending and receiving of information, instructions, or commands and providing useful feedback. Communication is a two-way process and should continue in a loop fashion.

Decision making is the ability to use logic and sound judgment to make decisions based on available information. Decision-making processes are involved when a less experienced clinician seeks out the advice of a more experienced clinician or when a person defers important clinical decisions because of fatigue. Good decision making is based on the realization of personal limitations.

Leadership is the ability to direct and coordinate the activities of other crew members and encourage the crew to work together as a team.

Analysis refers to the ability to develop short-term, long-term, and contingency plans, as well as to coordinate, allocate, and monitor crew and operating room resources.

The last, and most important, principle is *situational awareness*, that is, the accuracy with which a person's perception of the current environment reflects reality. In the operating room, lack of situational awareness can cost precious minutes, as when readings from a monitor (eg, capnograph or arterial line) suddenly change and the operator focuses on the monitor rather than on the patient. One must decide whether the monitor is correct and the patient is critically ill or the monitor is incorrect and the patient is fine. The problem-solving method used should consider both possibilities but quickly eliminate one. In this scenario, tunnel vision can result in catastrophic mistakes. Furthermore, if the sampling line has become dislodged and the capnograph indicates low end-tidal CO_2, this finding does not exclude the possibility that at the same time a pulmonary embolus may occur, resulting in decreased end-tidal CO_2.

If all members of the operating room team apply these seven principles, problems arising from human factors can almost entirely be eliminated. These seven principles serve no purpose when applied in a suppressive operating room environment. Anyone with a concern must be able to speak up without fear of repercussion. Chapter 59 provides further discussion of these and other issues relating to patient safety.

ROLES OF ACCREDITATION AGENCIES & REGULATORY BODIES

In the United States, the Centers for Medicare and Medicaid Services (CMS) drive many of the mandated policies and procedures carried out by facilities. Efforts to reduce fraudulent claims and disparities in levels of care include the requirement of certification of an accrediting agency such as The Joint Commission (TJC), Det Norske Veritas/ Germanischer Lloyd (DNV GL), and others. These accreditation agencies examine processes and procedures and determine whether facilities have appropriate policies and whether those policies are actually followed. The process may involve a self-study submitted by a facility and a site visit carried out by a team of various medical professionals who inspect a facility, observe operations, and compare observations with the policies and self-studies.

Accreditors use laws, codes, and standards to determine if a facility is carrying out care in alignment with current best practices. Many accreditation agencies maintain policies prohibiting the use of anything other than standards or codes to determine accreditation. Anesthesia providers should be apprised that guidelines, recommendations, and advisories typically should not be used by accreditors to determine a best practice. Recommendations, advisories, and guidelines are often educated opinions and, as such, carry a lesser degree of evidence than a standard. Facilities should be cautioned that sometimes the site visitors may issue a citation incorrectly based upon these opinions. All accrediting agencies maintain an appeal process for citations, and if seemingly unwarranted citations are issued, facility administrators may wish to consider this option.

Site visitors frequently cite anesthesiologists for unlocked anesthesia carts and wearing certain attire deemed to be an infection risk. With regard to the locked cart, a more appropriate assessment is whether an anesthesia cart is secure. Since most operating rooms are within an access-controlled suite, this is considered a secure area, and as long as the operating rooms are not left unattended, this scenario should be in compliance with security concerns regarding medications.

Regarding operating room attire, site visitors may reference the Association of Perioperative Registered Nurses (AORN) recommendation for operating room attire, which limits the wearing of personal scrubs and jackets and requires that surgical attire be laundered at the health care facility. However, such a recommendation is merely a professional opinion. Organizations such as the American Society of Anesthesiologists (ASA) and the American College of Surgeons (ACS) have position statements and focused committees to assist with clarification when accrediting citations conflict with clinical evidence (or lack thereof).

Codes and regulations are not subject to such opinions, and accreditation citations based upon conflict with a code or regulation are usually valid. However, codes and regulations regularly undergo review and revision, and site accreditation inspectors may not be using the latest version as a reference.

Safety is best driven by culture, and attempts to regulate safe behavior by merely creating policy should be avoided. Our experience suggests that most errors or safety breaches are due to factors such as poor engineering, production pressure, inconsistent processes, or a combination of these. Design improvements and examination and remedy of system faults are far more effective in promoting patient and team safety than creating a policy.

FUTURE DESIGN OF OPERATING ROOMS

Safety Interlock Technology

Despite heightened awareness of safety and increased educational efforts among operating room personnel, harm to patients still remains unacceptably frequent. Similarly, despite threats of payment withholding, public scoring of physicians and hospitals, provider-rating websites, and punitive legal consequences, medical errors and the human factors that lead to errors have not been eliminated. In the future, safety-engineered designs may assist in the reduction of medical errors. One developing area is the use of interlock devices that cannot be operated until a defined sequence of events occurs. Anesthesia personnel use interlock technology with anesthesia vaporizers that prevent the use of more than one vaporizer at a time. Expansion of this technology might prevent the release of a drug from an automated dispensing device until a barcode is scanned from a patient's hospital armband or, at a minimum, the patient's drug allergies have been entered into the machine's database. Other applications might include a laser that could not be used when the FiO_2 is greater than 30%, thus minimizing the risk of fire. Similarly, computers, monitors, and other devices could be designed to be inoperable until patient identification is confirmed.

Workflow Design

Coordinating the activities of surgeons, anesthesia providers, operating room nurses, technicians, and environmental services personnel is essential to the running of a surgical suite. Clinical directors in facilities must accommodate procedures of varying durations, requiring varying degrees of surgical skill and efficiency, while allowing for unplanned or emergency operations. The need to optimize scheduling and staffing prompted the development of software systems that anticipate and record the timing of surgical events.

Some surgical suites improve workflow by incorporating separate induction areas to decrease nonsurgical time spent in operating rooms. Although uncommon in the United States, induction rooms have long been employed in the United Kingdom. One induction room model uses rotating anesthesia teams. One team is assigned to the first patient of the day; a second team induces anesthesia for the next patient in an adjacent area while the operating room is being turned over. The second team continues caring for that patient after transfer to the operating room, leaving the first team available to induce anesthesia in the third patient as the operating room is being turned over. The advantage of this model is continuity of care; the disadvantage is the need for two anesthesia teams for every operating room.

Another model uses separate induction and anesthesia teams. The induction team induces anesthesia for all patients on a given day and then transfers care to the anesthesia team, which is assigned to an individual operating room. The advantage of this model is the reduction in anesthesia personnel to staff induction rooms; disadvantages include failure to maintain continuity of care and staffing log jams when several patients must undergo induction concurrently. This model can use either a separate induction room adjacent to each operating room or one common induction room that services multiple operating rooms.

The final model uses several staffed operating rooms, one of which is kept open. After the first patient of the day is transferred to the initial room, subsequent patients always proceed to the open room, thus eliminating the wait for room turnover and readiness of personnel. All of these models assume that the increased cost of additional anesthesia personnel can be justified by the increased surgical productivity.

Lean Methodology

Many hospitals are exploring methods of applying *lean methodology* to the surgical environment. Lean examination systems seek to find and eliminate waste and duplicate activity. The most notable company to apply lean methodology is Toyota, which has branded a lean system, the *Toyota Production System* (TPS), that many health care systems incorporate into their perioperative settings. TPS centers on three concepts: muda, muri, and mura. *Muda* (from the Japanese term for "waste") is created by *muri* and *mura*. *Muri* is waste created by overburden and production pressure, and *mura* is the waste created by uneven work patterns or lack of load leveling.

TPS also incorporates a set of five processes, referred to as *5S*, into improvement efforts. These key processes, which begin with the sound of the letter "S" in the original Japanese, have since been translated into synonymous S-words in English.

- *Sort*—Eliminate excess, remove items that are not in use, and remove the unneeded or unwanted items.
- *Set in Order*—Arrange items in use for easy selection and in an organized manner. Make the workflow easier and natural.

- *Shine*—The workplace should be clean.
- *Standardize*—Workstations should be alike, and variability should be reduced or eliminated. Every process should have a standard.
- *Sustain*—Work should be goal driven; no one should be told to work, but rather all should do the work without asking.

With the elimination of waste and application of the 5S methodology, daily operations should become safer, standardized, and more efficient.

Radio Frequency Identification

Radio frequency identification (RFID) technology utilizes a chip with a small transmitter whose signal is read by a reader; each chip yields a unique signal. The technology has many potential applications in the perioperative environment. Using RFID in employee identification (ID) badges may enable surgical control rooms to keep track of nursing, surgeons, and anesthesia personnel, obviating the need for paging and telephony to establish the location of key personnel. Incorporating the technology in patient ID bands and hospital gurneys allows a patient's flow to be tracked through an entire facility. The ability to project an identifying signal to hospital systems would offer an additional degree of safety for patients unable to communicate with hospital personnel. Finally, RFID can be incorporated into surgical instruments and sponges, allowing surgical counts to be performed by identification of the objects as they are passed on and off the surgical field. In the event that counts are mismatched, a wand could then be placed over the patient to screen for retained objects.

CASE DISCUSSION

Monitored Anesthesia Care with Oxygen Supplementation

You are asked to provide monitored anesthesia care for a patient undergoing simple removal of a lesion on the cheek. The patient is morbidly obese and has a history of sleep apnea. He states, "It bothers me when people are working on my face," and indicates that he does not want to remember anything about the surgery. The surgeon assures you the procedure will not last more than 5 minutes. The patient's partner mentions that they are from out of town and have made flight arrangements to return home soon after the procedure.

What features of this case indicate a high risk for surgical fire?

Patients with a clinical history of obstructive sleep apnea usually have a sensitivity to sedating medications, especially opioids. Administration of even small doses of opioids may lead to upper airway obstruction and hypoventilation, resulting in hypercapnia and hypoxemia. In obese patients, upper airway obstruction, hypoventilation, and decreased functional reserve capacity may result in rapid oxygen desaturation. Most anesthesia providers respond by increasing the amount of oxygen supplementation delivered via face mask or nasal cannula. Open delivery of oxygen in concentrations greater than 30% is one of the elements of the fire triad. Another consideration is the anatomic location of the procedure. A location above the xiphoid process in this patient would place an ignition source (if used) in close proximity to the open delivery of an oxidizer.

What is the safest manner in which to proceed?

There are three strategies that can be implemented to improve safety in this scenario: avoid oxygen supplementation, secure the airway with an endotracheal tube or supraglottic device, or avoid the use of an ignition source.

Are there any concerns relating to airway management or selection of the delivery device?

As previously noted, the patient is likely to manifest airway changes associated with obstructive sleep apnea and obesity. Selection of a delivery device should take into consideration the need to prevent the open delivery of oxygen.

How would the length of the procedure affect the management of anesthesia?

Practically speaking, if the patient requires a lengthy procedure, local anesthetics may wear off; the cumulative dose of narcotics provided may exacerbate the patient's obstructive sleep apnea and increase recovery time. Additionally, more complex surgical excision may result in bleeding requiring the use of cautery.

Does the patient's expectation of discharge soon after the procedure affect your anesthesia plans?

The expectation of an accelerated recovery period may not be feasible if the patient requires general anesthesia or significant amounts of opioids. The American Society of Anesthesiologists (ASA) has published a practice advisory providing direction for the safe postoperative assessment and discharge of patients with obstructive sleep apnea. See www.asahq.org.

What if the surgeon thinks your plans are "overkill"?

The first and most effective means for conflict resolution is to communicate your specific concerns to the surgeon. If this fails, the procedure must not be allowed to proceed as long as any team member has a legitimate safety concern. Many ASA safety-related guidelines and advisories are also endorsed by professional societies such as the American College of Surgeons (ACS). Anesthesia providers should also develop familiarity with their facility's methods of dispute resolution before an event occurs.

SUGGESTED READINGS

Dorsch JA, Dorsch SE. *Understanding Anesthesia Equipment*. 5th ed. Lippincott Williams & Wilkins; 2008. A detailed discussion of compressed gases and medical gas delivery systems, but many other chapters are approaching obsolescence.

Ehrenwerth J, Eisenkraft JB, Berry JM. *Anesthesia Equipment: Principles and Applications*. 3rd ed. Elsevier; 2021.

National Fire Protection Association (NFPA). *Standard for Health Care Facilities*. NFPA; 2021. An updated version of NFPA 99 standards.

WEBSITES

The American National Standards Institute is the reference source for laser standards and many other protective engineering standards. http://www.ansi.org

The Anesthesia Patient Safety Foundation provides resources and a newsletter that discusses important safety issues in anesthesia. The website also contains a link to view or request the video *Prevention and Management of Operating Room Fires*, which is an excellent resource to gain information concerning the risks and prevention of surgical fires. http://www.apsf.org

The American Society of Anesthesiologists (ASA) website contains the ASA practice parameters and advisories. Many are oriented around patient safety issues, and all can be printed for review. http://www.asahq.org

The Compressed Gas Association and its website are dedicated to the development and promotion of safety standards and safe practices in the industrial gas industry. http://www.cganet.com

The ECRI (formerly the Emergency Care Research Institute) is an independent nonprofit health services research agency that focuses on health care technology, health care risk and quality management, and health care environmental management. http://www.ecri.org

The U.S. Food and Drug Administration (FDA) has an extensive website covering many broad categories. Two major divisions address patient safety: the Center for Devices and Radiological Health (CDRH), which regulates and evaluates medical devices, and the Center for Drug Evaluation and Research (CDER), which regulates and evaluates drugs. http://www.fda.org

The National Fire Protection Association (NPFA) has a website with a catalog of publications on fire, electrical, and building safety issues. Some areas require a subscription to access. http://www.nfpa.org

The Patient Safety Authority maintains data collected from the mandatory reporting of incidents of harm or near harm in the Commonwealth of Pennsylvania. Some data such as surgical fires data can be extrapolated to determine the likely incidence for the entire United States. http://patientsafetyauthority.org

The Virtual Anesthesia Machine website has extensive interactive modules to facilitate understanding of many processes and equipment. The site, which contains high-quality graphic illustrations and animation, requires free registration. http://vam.anest.ufl.edu/

The Society of American Gastrointestinal and Endoscopic Surgeons (SAGES) has created an educational program, the Fundamental Use of Surgical Energy (FUSE), which is an educational and certification program for all surgical personnel. The educational content is (as of October, 2021) available without charge, and the certification and continuing education process is available for a reasonable fee. The course covers all types of electrical surgical units in the operating room and makes recommendations for their correct use and safety precautions. http://www.fuseprogram.org/

REFERENCES

Bree K, Barnhill S, Rundell W. The dangers of electrosurgical smoke to operating room personnel. A review. *Workplace Health Saf.* 2017;65:517.

Burgess RC. Electrical safety. *Handb Clin Neurol.* 2019;160:67.

Dexter F, Parra MC, Brown JR, Loftus RW. Perioperative COVID-19 defense: an evidence-based approach for optimization of infection control and operating room management. *Anesth Analg.* 2020;131:37.

Gui JL, Nemergut EC, Forkin KT. Distraction in the operating room: a narrative review of environmental and self-initiated distractions and their effect on anesthesia providers. *J Clin Anesth.* 2021;68:110110.

Haugen AS, Sevdalis N, Søfteland E. Impact of the World Health Organization surgical safety checklist on patient safety. *Anesthesiology.* 2019;131:420.

Jung JJ, Elfassy J, Jüni P, Grantcharov T. Adverse events in the operating room: definitions, prevalence, and characteristics. A systematic review. *World J Surg.* 2019;43:2379.

Katz JD. Control of the environment in the operating room. *Anesth Analg.* 2017;125:1214.

Koch A, Burns J, Catchpole K, Weigl M. Associations of workflow disruptions in the operating room with surgical outcomes: a systematic review and narrative synthesis. *BMJ Qual Saf.* 2020;29:1033.

Kyriazanos I, Kalles V, Stefanopoulos A, et al. Operating personnel safety during administration of hyperthermic intraperitoneal chemotherapy (HIPEC). *Surg Oncol.* 2016;25:30.

Mowbray NG, Ansell J, Horwood J, et al. Safe management of surgical smoke in the age of COVID-19. *Br J Surg.* 2020;107:1406.

Papadakis M, Meiwandi A, Grzybowski A. The WHO safer surgery checklist time out procedure revisited: strategies to optimize compliance and safety. *Int J Surg.* 2019;69:19.

Pattni N, Arzola C, Malavade A, et al. Challenging authority and speaking up in the operating room environment: a narrative synthesis. *Br J Anaesth.* 2019;122:233.

Prakash L, Dhar SA, Mushtaq M. COVID-19 in the operating room: a review of evolving safety protocols. *Patient Saf Surg.* 2020;14:30.

Rhea EB, Rogers TH, Riehl JT. Radiation safety for anaesthesia providers in the orthopaedic operating room. *Anaesthesia.* 2016;71:455.

Roy S, Smith LP. Preventing and managing operating room fires in otolaryngology-head and neck surgery. *Otolaryngol Clin N Am.* 2019;52:163.

Wahr JA, Abernathy JH III, Lazarra EH, et al. Medication safety in the operating room: literature and expert-based recommendations. *Br J Anaesth.* 2017;118:32.

Wakeman D, Langham MR Jr. Creating a safer operating room: groups, team dynamics and crew resource management principles. *Semin Pediatr Surg.* 2018;27:107.

Wheeler DS, Sheets AM, Ryckman FC. Improving transitions of care between the operating room and intensive care unit. *Transl Pediatr.* 2018;7:299.

CHAPTER 3

Breathing Systems

KEY CONCEPTS

1. Because insufflation avoids any direct patient contact, there is no rebreathing of exhaled gases if the flow is high enough. Ventilation cannot be controlled with this technique, however, and the inspired gas contains unpredictable amounts of entrained atmospheric air.

2. Long breathing tubes with high compliance increase the difference between the volume of gas delivered to a circuit by a reservoir bag or ventilator and the volume actually delivered to the patient.

3. The adjustable pressure-limiting (APL) valve should be fully open during spontaneous ventilation so that circuit pressure remains negligible throughout inspiration and expiration.

4. Because a fresh gas flow equal to minute ventilation is sufficient to prevent rebreathing, the Mapleson A design is the most efficient Mapleson circuit for spontaneous ventilation.

5. The Mapleson D circuit is efficient during controlled ventilation because fresh gas flow forces alveolar air away from the patient and toward the APL valve.

6. Increasing the hardness of soda lime by adding silica minimizes the risk of inhalation of sodium hydroxide dust and also decreases the resistance of gas flow.

7. Malfunction of either unidirectional valve in a circle system may allow rebreathing of carbon dioxide, resulting in hypercapnia.

8. With an absorber, the circle system prevents rebreathing of carbon dioxide at fresh gas flows that are considered low (fresh gas flow ≤1 L) or even fresh gas flows equal to the uptake of anesthetic gases and oxygen by the patient and the circuit itself (closed-system anesthesia).

9. Because of the unidirectional valves, apparatus dead space in a circle system is limited to the area distal to the point of inspiratory and expiratory gas mixing at the Y-piece. Unlike Mapleson circuits, the circle system tube length does not directly affect dead space.

10. The fraction of inspired oxygen (FIO_2) delivered by a resuscitator breathing system to the patient is directly proportional to the oxygen concentration and flow rate of the gas mixture supplied to the resuscitator (usually 100% oxygen) and inversely proportional to the minute ventilation delivered to the patient.

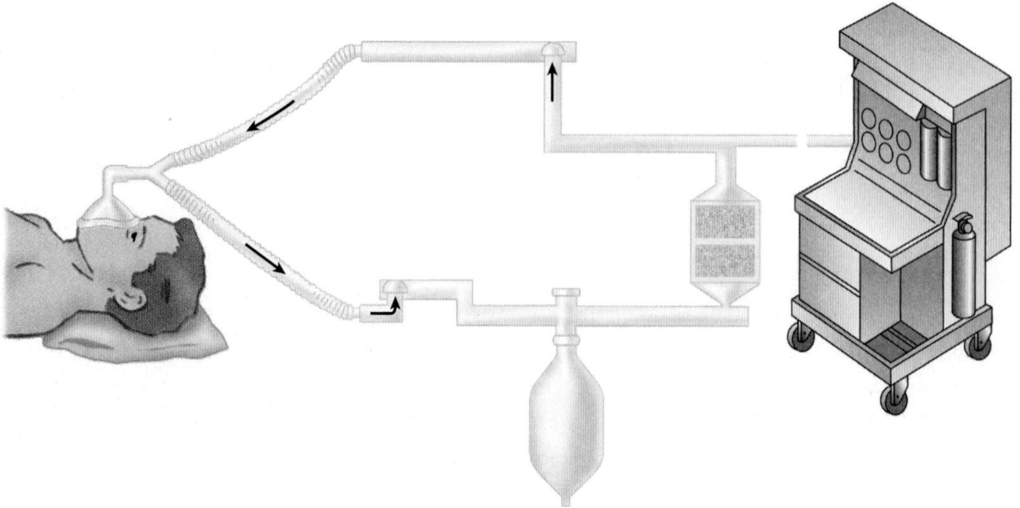

FIGURE 3–1 The relationship between the patient, the breathing system, and the anesthesia machine.

Breathing *systems* provide the final conduit for the delivery of anesthetic gases to the patient. Breathing *circuits* link a patient to an anesthesia machine (Figure 3–1). Many different circuit designs have been developed, each with varying degrees of efficiency, convenience, and complexity. This chapter reviews the most important breathing systems: insufflation, draw-over, Mapleson circuits, the circle system, and resuscitation systems.

Most classifications of breathing systems artificially consolidate functional characteristics (eg, the extent of rebreathing) with physical characteristics (eg, the presence of unidirectional valves). Because these seemingly contradictory classifications (eg, open, closed, semi-open, semi-closed) often tend to confuse rather than aid understanding, they are avoided in this discussion.

INSUFFLATION

The term *insufflation* usually denotes the blowing of anesthetic gases across a patient's face. Although insufflation is categorized as a breathing system, it is perhaps better considered a technique that avoids direct connection between a breathing circuit and a patient's airway. Because children often resist the placement of a face mask (or an intravenous line), insufflation is particularly valuable during inductions with inhalation anesthetics in children (Figure 3–2). It is useful in other situations as well. Carbon dioxide (CO_2) accumulation under head and neck draping is a hazard of ophthalmic surgery performed with local anesthesia. Insufflation of air across the patient's face at a high flow rate (>10 L/min)

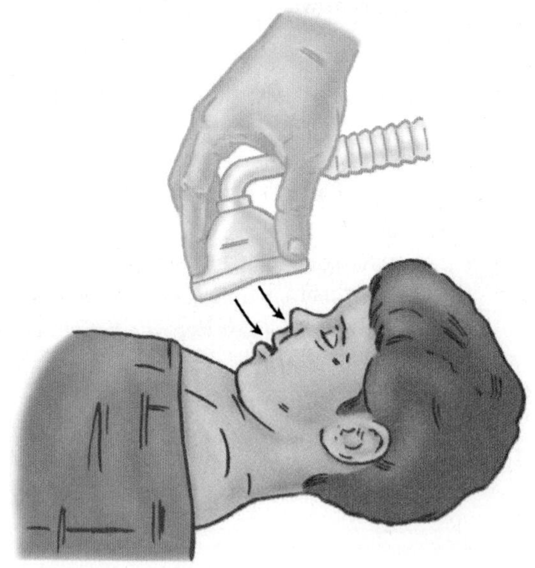

FIGURE 3–2 Insufflation of an anesthetic agent across a child's face during induction.

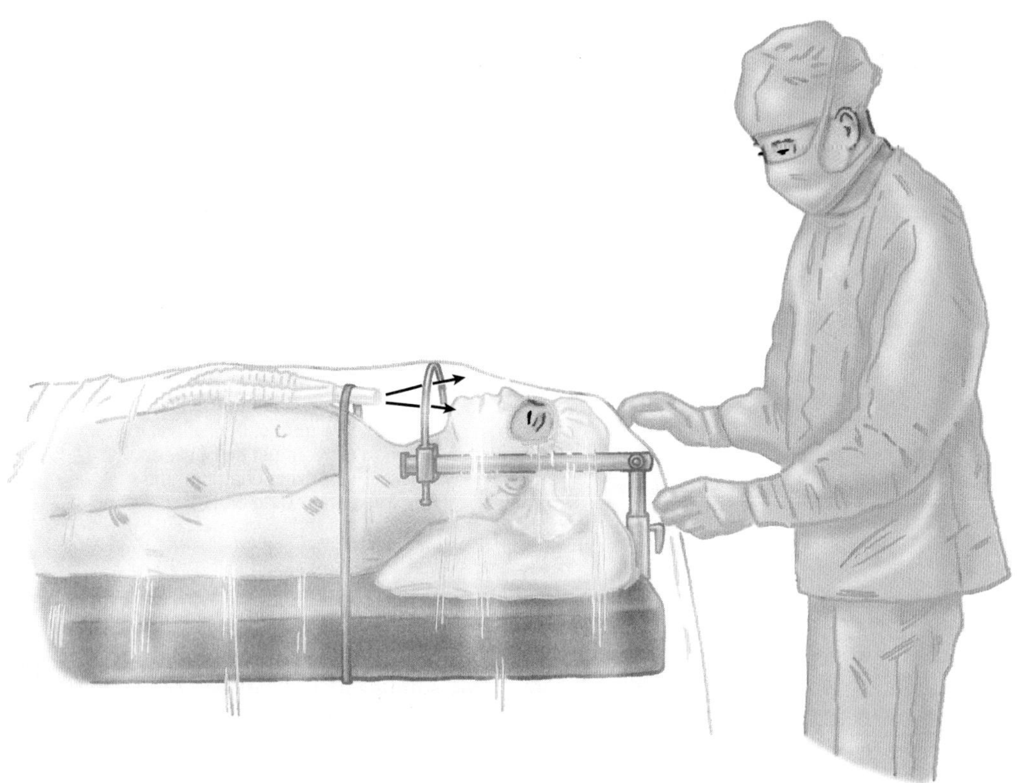

FIGURE 3–3 Insufflation of oxygen and air under a head drape.

avoids this problem while not increasing the risk of fire from the accumulation of oxygen (Figure 3–3). 1 Because insufflation avoids any direct patient contact, there is no rebreathing of exhaled gases if the flow is high enough. Ventilation cannot be controlled with this technique, however, and the inspired gas contains unpredictable amounts of entrained atmospheric air.

Insufflation can also be used to maintain arterial oxygenation during brief periods of apnea (eg, during bronchoscopy). Instead of blowing gases across the face, oxygen is directed into the lungs through a device placed in the trachea.

OPEN-DROP ANESTHESIA

Although open-drop anesthesia is not used in modern medicine, its historic significance warrants a brief description here. A highly volatile anesthetic—historically, ether or chloroform—was dripped onto a gauze-covered mask (Schimmelbusch mask) applied to the patient's face. As the patient inhales, air passes through the gauze, vaporizing the liquid agent and carrying high concentrations of anesthetic to the patient. The vaporization lowers mask temperature, resulting in moisture condensation and a drop in anesthetic vapor pressure (vapor pressure is proportional to temperature).

A modern derivative of open-drop anesthesia uses draw-over vaporizers that depend on the patient's inspiratory efforts to draw ambient air through a vaporization chamber. This technique may be used in locations or situations in which compressed medical gases are unavailable (eg, battlefields).

DRAW-OVER ANESTHESIA

Draw-over devices have non-rebreathing circuits that use ambient air as the carrier gas, though supplemental oxygen can be used if available. The devices

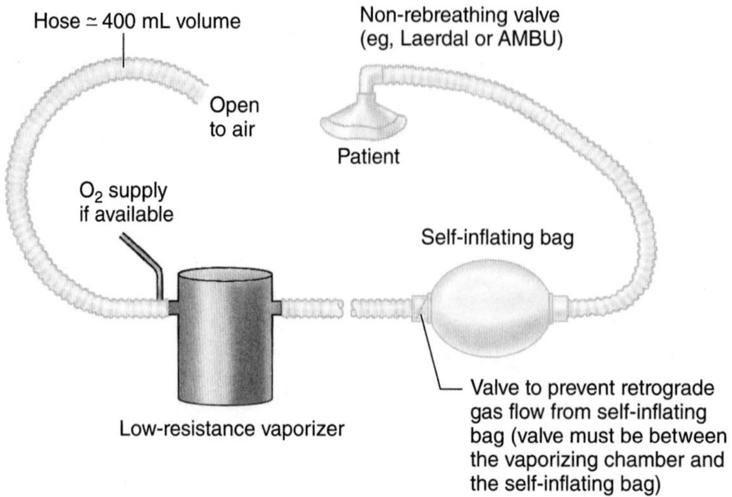

FIGURE 3–4 Schematic diagram of a draw-over anesthesia device/circuit. O_2, oxygen.

can be fitted with connections and equipment that allow intermittent positive-pressure ventilation (IPPV) and passive scavenging, as well as continuous positive airway pressure (CPAP) and positive end-expiratory pressure (PEEP).

In its most basic application (Figure 3–4), air is drawn through a low-resistance vaporizer as the patient inspires. Patients spontaneously breathing room air and a potent halogenated agent often manifest an oxygen saturation (Spo_2) less than 90%, a situation treated with IPPV, supplemental oxygen, or both. The fraction of inspired oxygen (Fio_2) can be supplemented using an open-ended reservoir tube of about 400 mL, attached to a T-piece at the upstream side of the vaporizer. Across the clinical range of tidal volume and respiratory rate, an oxygen flow rate of 1 L/min gives an Fio_2 of 30% to 40%, or with 4 L/min, an Fio_2 of 60% to 80%. There are several commercial draw-over systems available that share common properties (Table 3–1).

TABLE 3–1 Properties of draw-over devices.

Portable
Low resistance to gas flow
Usable with any agent[1]
Controllable vapor output

[1]Halothane cannot be used with the Epstein Mackintosh Oxford device.

The greatest advantage of draw-over systems is their simplicity and portability, making them useful in locations where compressed gases or ventilators are not available.

MAPLESON CIRCUITS

The insufflation and draw-over systems have several disadvantages: poor control of inspired gas concentration (and, therefore, poor control of depth of anesthesia), mechanical drawbacks during head and neck surgery, and pollution of the operating room with large volumes of waste gas. The **Mapleson systems** solve some of these problems by incorporating additional components (breathing tubes, fresh gas inlets, adjustable pressure-limiting [APL] valves, reservoir bags) into the breathing circuit. The relative location of these components determines circuit performance and is the basis of the Mapleson classification (Table 3–2).

Components of Mapleson Circuits

A. Breathing Tubes

Corrugated tubes connect the components of the Mapleson circuit to the patient (Figure 3–5). The large diameter of the tubes (22 mm) creates a low-resistance pathway and a potential reservoir for

TABLE 3–2 Classification and characteristics of Mapleson circuits.

Mapleson Class	Other Names	Configuration[1]	Required Fresh Gas Flows: Spontaneous	Required Fresh Gas Flows: Controlled	Comments
A	Magill attachment	FGI, Breathing tube, APL valve, Breathing bag, Mask	Equal to minute ventilation (≈80 mL/kg/min)	Very high and difficult to predict	Poor choice during controlled ventilation. Enclosed Magill system is a modification that improves efficiency. Coaxial Mapleson A (Lack breathing system) provides waste gas scavenging.
B		FGI, APL valve	2 × minute ventilation	2–2½ × minute ventilation	
C	Waters' to-and-fro	FGI, APL valve	2 × minute ventilation	2–2½ × minute ventilation	
D	Bain circuit	APL valve, FGI	2–3 × minute ventilation	1–2 × minute ventilation	Bain coaxial modification: fresh gas tube inside breathing tube (see Figure 3–7).
E	Ayre's T-piece	FGI	2–3 × minute ventilation	3 × minute ventilation (I:E-1:2)	Exhalation tubing should provide a larger volume than tidal volume to prevent rebreathing. Scavenging is difficult.
F	Jackson-Rees' modification	FGI, APL valve	2–3 × minute ventilation	2 × minute ventilation	A Mapleson E with a breathing bag connected to the end of the breathing tube to allow controlled ventilation and scavenging.

[1]APL, adjustable pressure-limiting (valve); FGI, fresh gas inlet.

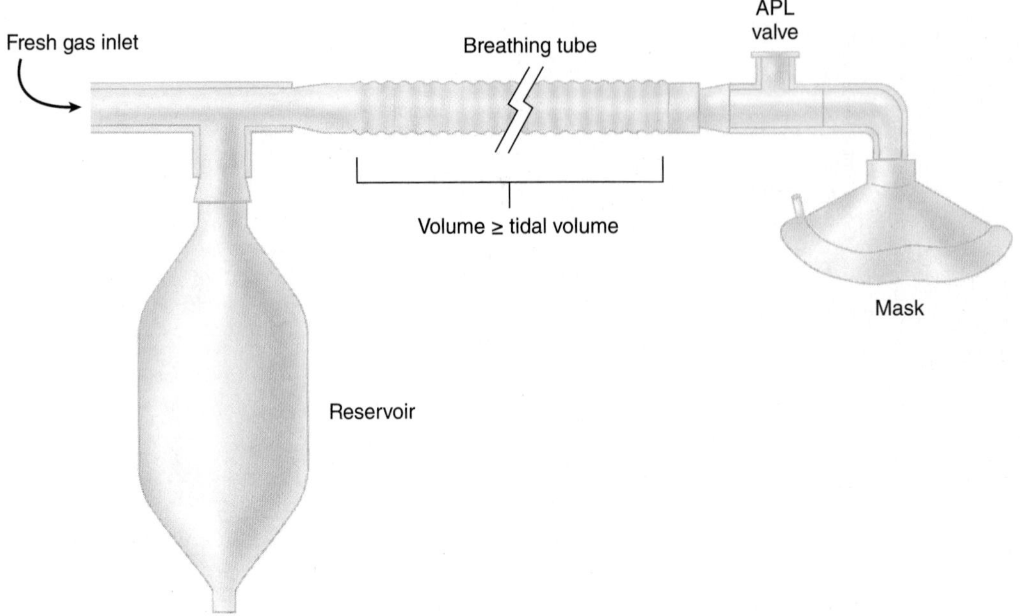

FIGURE 3–5 Components of a Mapleson circuit. APL, adjustable pressure-limiting (valve).

anesthetic gases. To minimize fresh gas flow requirements, the volume of gas within the breathing tubes in most Mapleson circuits should be at least as great as the patient's tidal volume.

The compliance of the breathing tubes largely determines the compliance of the circuit. (Compliance is defined as the change of volume produced by a change in pressure.) 2 Long breathing tubes with high compliance increase the difference between the volume of gas delivered to a circuit by a reservoir bag or ventilator and the volume actually delivered to the patient. For example, if a breathing circuit with a compliance of 8 mL gas/cm H_2O is pressurized during delivery of a tidal volume to 20 cm H_2O, 160 mL of the tidal volume will be lost to the circuit. The 160 mL represents a combination of gas compression and breathing-tube expansion. This is an important consideration in any circuit delivering positive-pressure ventilation through expandible breathing tubes (eg, circle systems).

B. Fresh Gas Inlet

Gases (anesthetics mixed with oxygen or air) from the anesthesia machine continuously enter the circuit through the fresh gas inlet. As discussed below, the relative position of the fresh gas inlet is a key differentiating factor among Mapleson circuits.

C. Adjustable Pressure-Limiting Valve (Pressure-Relief Valve, Pop-Off Valve)

As anesthetic gases enter the breathing circuit, pressure will rise if the gas inflow is greater than the combined uptake of the patient and the circuit. Gases may exit the circuit through an APL valve, controlling this pressure buildup. Exiting gases enter the operating room atmosphere or, preferably, a waste-gas scavenging system. All APL valves allow a 3 variable pressure threshold for venting. The APL valve should be fully open during spontaneous ventilation so that circuit pressure remains negligible throughout inspiration and expiration. Assisted and controlled ventilation requires positive pressure during inspiration to expand the lungs. Partial closure of the APL valve limits gas exit, permitting positive circuit pressures during reservoir bag compressions.

D. Reservoir Bag (Breathing Bag)

Reservoir bags function as a reservoir of anesthetic gas and a method of generating positive-pressure

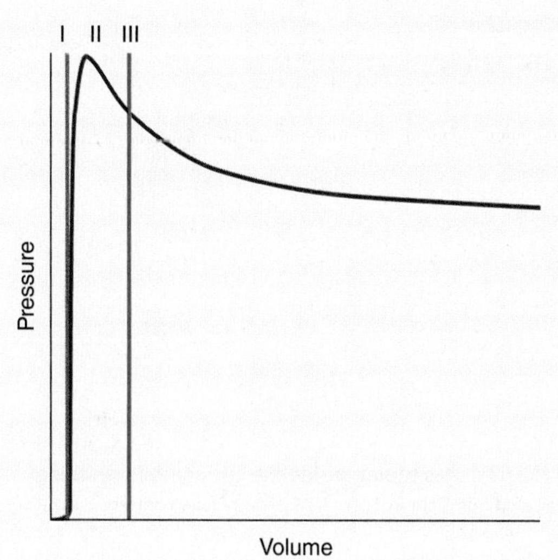

FIGURE 3–6 The increasing compliance and elasticity of breathing bags as demonstrated by three phases of filling (see text). (Reproduced with permission from Johnstone RE, Smith TC. Rebreathing bags as pressure limiting devices. *Anesthesiology.* 1973 Feb;38(2):192-194.)

ventilation. They are designed to increase in compliance as their volume increases. Three distinct phases of reservoir bag filling are recognizable (Figure 3–6). After the nominal 3-L capacity of an adult reservoir bag is achieved (phase I), pressure rises rapidly to a peak (phase II). Further increases in volume result in a plateau or even a slight decrease in pressure (phase III). This ceiling effect provides some minimal protection of the patient's lungs against high airway pressures if the APL valve is unintentionally left in the closed position while fresh gas continues to flow into the circuit.

Performance Characteristics of Mapleson Circuits

Mapleson circuits are lightweight, inexpensive, and simple. Breathing-circuit efficiency is measured by the fresh gas flow required to reduce CO_2 rebreathing to a negligible value. Because there are no unidirectional valves or CO_2 absorption in Mapleson circuits, rebreathing is prevented by adequate fresh gas flow into the circuit and venting exhaled gas through the APL valve before inspiration. There is usually some rebreathing in any Mapleson circuit. The total fresh gas flow into the circuit controls the amount. High fresh gas flows are required to attenuate rebreathing. The APL valve in Mapleson A, B, and C circuits is located near the face mask, and the reservoir bag is located at the opposite end of the circuit.

Reexamine the drawing of a Mapleson A circuit in **Figure 3–5**. During spontaneous ventilation, alveolar gas containing CO_2 will be exhaled into the breathing tube or directly vented through an open APL valve. Before inhalation occurs, if the fresh gas flow exceeds alveolar minute ventilation, the inflow of fresh gas will force the alveolar gas remaining in the breathing tube to exit from the APL valve. If the breathing tube volume is equal to or greater than the patient's tidal volume, the next inspiration will

4 contain only fresh gas. Because a fresh gas flow equal to minute ventilation is sufficient to prevent rebreathing, the Mapleson A design is the most efficient Mapleson circuit for *spontaneous* ventilation.

Positive pressure during *controlled* ventilation, however, requires a partially closed APL valve. Although some alveolar and fresh gas exits through the valve during inspiration, no gas is vented during expiration because the exhaled gas stagnates during the expiratory phase of positive-pressure ventilation. As a result, very high fresh gas flows (greater than three times minute ventilation) are required to prevent rebreathing with a Mapleson A circuit during controlled ventilation. The fresh gas inlet is in close proximity to the APL valve in a Mapleson B circuit.

Interchanging the position of the APL valve and the fresh gas inlet transforms a Mapleson A into a

5 **Mapleson D circuit** (Table 3–2). The Mapleson D circuit is efficient during controlled ventilation because fresh gas flow forces alveolar air *away* from the patient and *toward* the APL valve. Thus, simply moving components completely alters the fresh gas requirements of the Mapleson circuits.

The **Bain circuit** is a coaxial version of the Mapleson D system that incorporates the fresh gas inlet tubing inside the breathing tube (Figure 3–7). This modification decreases the circuit's bulk and retains heat and humidity better than a conventional

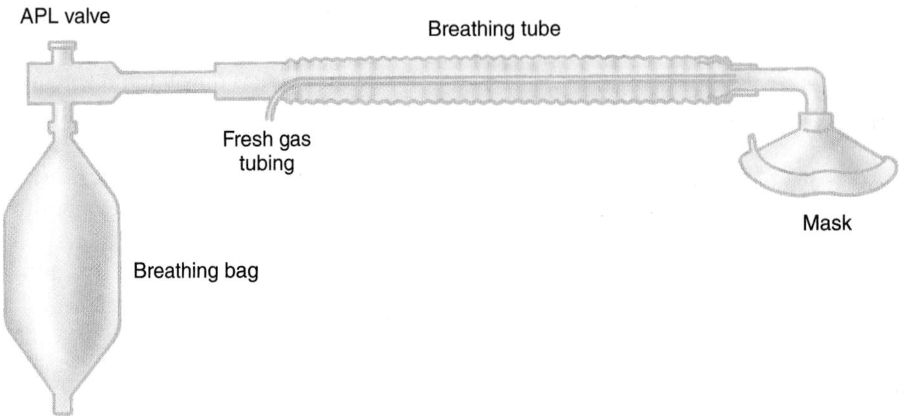

FIGURE 3–7 A Bain circuit is a Mapleson D circuit design with the fresh gas tubing inside the corrugated breathing tube. APL, adjustable pressure-limiting (valve). (Reproduced with permission from Bain JA, Spoerel WE. Flow requirements for a modified Mapleson D system during controlled ventilation. *Can Anaesth Soc J.* 1973 Sep;20(5):629-636.)

Mapleson D circuit as a result of partial warming of the inspiratory gas by countercurrent exchange with the warmer expired gases. A disadvantage of this coaxial circuit is the possibility of kinking or disconnection of the fresh gas inlet tubing. Periodic inspection of the inner tubing is mandatory to identify this complication; if unrecognized, either of these mishaps could result in significant rebreathing of exhaled gas.

THE CIRCLE SYSTEM

Although Mapleson circuits overcome some of the disadvantages of the insufflation and draw-over systems, the high fresh gas flows required to prevent rebreathing of CO_2 result in waste of anesthetic agent, pollution of the operating room environment, and loss of patient heat and humidity (Table 3–3). In an attempt to avoid these problems, the **circle system** adds more components to the breathing system.

The components of a circle system include: (1) a CO_2 absorber containing CO_2 absorbent; (2) a fresh gas inlet; (3) an inspiratory unidirectional valve and inspiratory breathing tube; (4) a Y-connector; (5) an expiratory unidirectional valve and expiratory breathing tube; (6) an APL valve; and (7) a reservoir (Figure 3–8).

Components of the Circle System

A. Carbon Dioxide Absorber and the Absorbent

Rebreathing alveolar gas conserves heat and humidity. However, the CO_2 in exhaled gas must be eliminated to prevent hypercapnia. CO_2 chemically combines with water to form carbonic acid. CO_2 absorbents (eg, soda lime or calcium hydroxide lime)

TABLE 3–3 Characteristics of breathing circuits.

	Insufflation and Open Drop	Mapleson	Circle
Complexity	Very simple	Simple	Complex
Control of anesthetic depth	Poor	Variable	Good
Ability to scavenge	Very poor	Variable	Good
Conservation of heat and humidity	No	No	Yes[1]
Rebreathing of exhaled gases	No	No[1]	Yes[1]

[1]These properties depend on the rate of fresh gas flow.

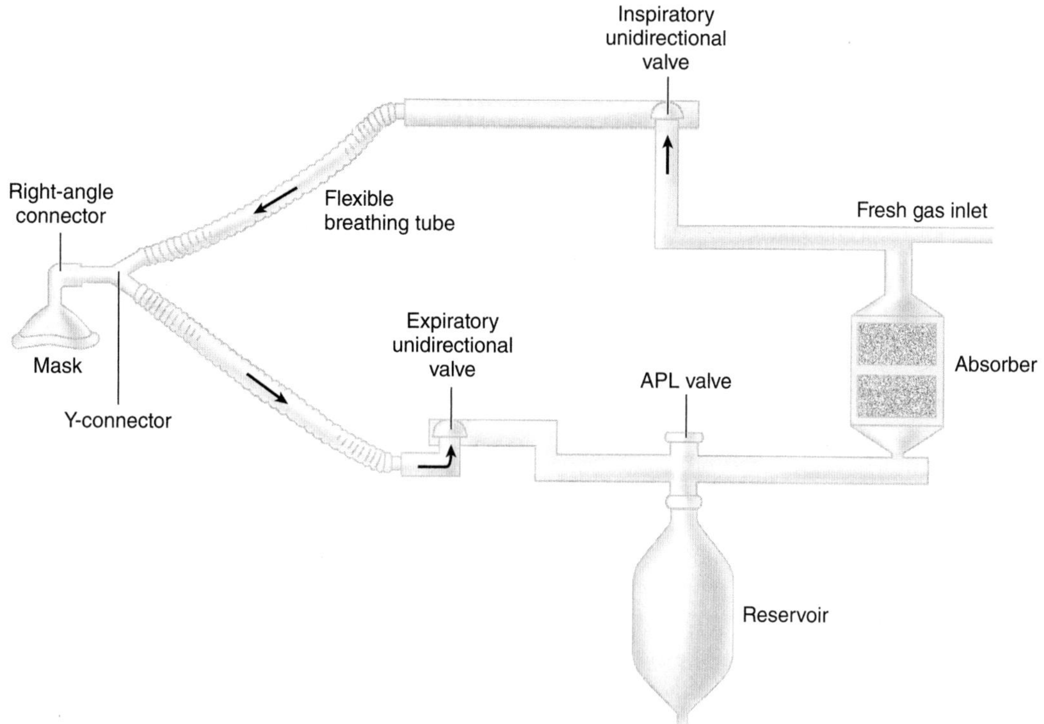

FIGURE 3–8 A circle system. APL, adjustable pressure-limiting (valve).

contain hydroxide salts that are capable of neutralizing carbonic acid. Reaction end products include heat (the heat of neutralization), water, and calcium carbonate. **Soda lime** is an absorbent and is capable of absorbing up to 23 L of CO_2 per 100 g of absorbent. It consists primarily of calcium hydroxide (80%), along with sodium hydroxide, water, and a small amount of potassium hydroxide. Its reactions are as follows:

$$CO_2 + H_2O \rightarrow H_2CO_3$$

$$H_2CO_3 + 2NaOH \rightarrow Na_2CO_3 + 2H_2O + \text{Heat}$$

(a fast reaction)

$$Na_2CO_3 + Ca(OH)_2 \rightarrow CaCO_3 + 2NaOH$$

(a slow reaction)

Note that the water and sodium hydroxide initially required are regenerated. Another absorbent, barium hydroxide lime, is no longer used because of the possible increased hazard of fire in the breathing system.

A pH indicator dye (eg, ethyl violet) changes color from white to purple as a consequence of increasing hydrogen ion concentration and absorbent exhaustion. Absorbent should be replaced when 50% to 70% has changed color. Although exhausted granules may revert to their original color if rested, no significant recovery of absorptive capacity occurs. The granule size is a compromise between the higher absorptive surface area of small granules and the lower resistance to the gas flow of larger granules. The granules commonly used as a CO_2 absorbent are between 4 and 8 mesh; the mesh number corresponds to the number of holes per square inch of a screen. The hydroxide salts are irritating to the skin and mucous membranes. Increasing the hardness of soda lime by adding silica minimizes the risk of inhalation of sodium hydroxide dust and also decreases the resistance of gas flow. Additional water is added to the absorbent during packaging to provide optimal conditions for carbonic acid formation. Commercial soda lime has a water content of 14% to 19%.

Absorbent granules can absorb and later release
6 medically active amounts of volatile anesthetic. The drier the soda lime, the more likely it will absorb and degrade volatile anesthetics. Volatile anesthetics can be broken down to carbon monoxide by dry absorbent (eg, sodium or potassium hydroxide) sufficiently to cause clinically measurable carboxyhemoglobin concentrations. The formation of carbon monoxide is greatest with desflurane; with sevoflurane, it occurs at a higher temperature.

Amsorb is a CO_2 absorbent consisting of calcium hydroxide and calcium chloride (with calcium sulfate and polyvinylpyrrolidone added to increase hardness). It possesses greater inertness than soda lime, resulting in less degradation of volatile anesthetics (eg, sevoflurane into compound A or desflurane into carbon monoxide).

Compound A is one of the byproducts of degradation of sevoflurane by absorbent. Higher concentrations of sevoflurane, prolonged exposure, and low-flow anesthetic technique seem to increase the formation of compound A. Compound A has been shown to produce nephrotoxicity in certain animals but has never been associated with ill effects in humans.

The granules of absorbent are contained within one or two canisters that fit snugly between a head and base plate. Together, this unit is called an absorber (Figure 3–9). Although bulky, double canisters permit complete CO_2 absorption, require less frequent absorbent changes, and lower gas flow resistance. To ensure complete absorption, the anesthesia provider should ensure that a patient's tidal volume does not exceed the air space between absorbent granules, which is roughly equal to 50% of the absorber's capacity. The indicator dye color is monitored through the absorber's transparent walls. Absorbent exhaustion typically occurs first where exhaled gas enters the absorber and along the canister's smooth inner walls. Channeling through areas of loosely packed granules is minimized by a baffle system, which directs gas flow through the center, thereby allowing greater use of the absorbent. A trap at the base of the absorber collects dust and moisture.

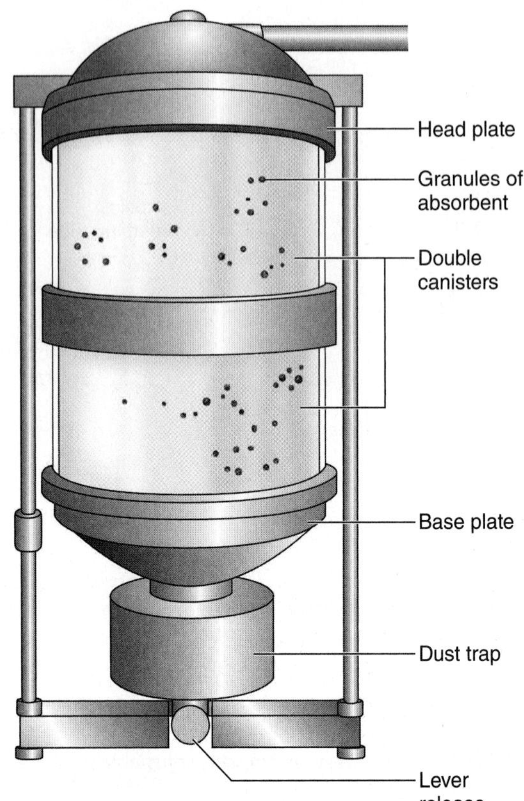

FIGURE 3–9 A carbon dioxide absorber.

B. Unidirectional Valves

Unidirectional valves, which function as check valves, contain a ceramic or mica disk resting horizontally on an annular valve seat (Figure 3–10). Forward flow displaces the disk upward, permitting the gas to proceed through the circuit. Reverse flow pushes the disk against its seat, preventing reflux. Valve incompetence is usually due to a warped disk or seat irregularities. The expiratory valve is exposed to the humidity of alveolar gas. Condensation and resultant moisture formation may prevent upward displacement of the disks, resulting in the incomplete escape of expired gases and rebreathing.

Inhalation opens the inspiratory valve, allowing the patient to breathe a mixture of fresh and exhaled gas that has passed through the CO_2 absorber. Simultaneously, the expiratory valve closes to prevent rebreathing of exhaled gas that still contains CO_2. The subsequent flow of gas away from the patient during exhalation opens the expiratory valve. This gas is vented through the APL valve or rebreathed by the patient after passing through

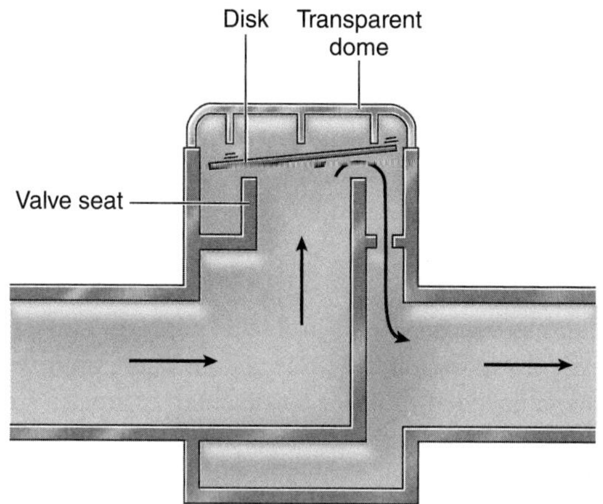

FIGURE 3–10 A unidirectional valve. CO_2, carbon dioxide.

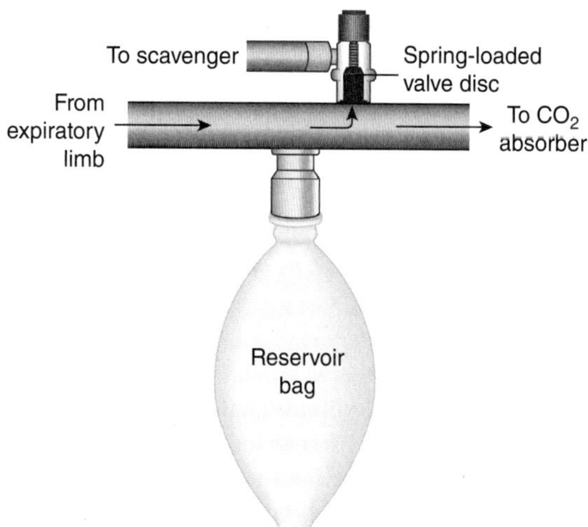

FIGURE 3–11 Adjustable pressure-limiting (APL) valve. CO_2, carbon dioxide. (Reproduced with permission from Rose G, McLarney JT: *Anesthesia Equipment Simplified.* New York, NY: McGraw Hill; 2014.)

the absorber. Closure of the inspiratory valve during exhalation prevents expiratory gas from mixing with fresh gas in the inspiratory limb. 7 Malfunction of either unidirectional valve may allow rebreathing of CO_2, resulting in hypercapnia.

Optimization of Circle System Design

Although the major components of the circle system (unidirectional valves, fresh gas inlet, APL valve, CO_2 absorber, and a reservoir bag) can be placed in several configurations, the following arrangement is preferred (Figure 3–8):

- Unidirectional valves are relatively close to the patient to prevent backflow into the inspiratory limb if a circuit leak develops. However, unidirectional valves are not placed in the Y-piece, as that makes it difficult to confirm or maintain proper orientation and intraoperative function.
- The fresh gas inlet is placed between the absorber and the inspiratory valve. Positioning it downstream from the inspiratory valve would allow fresh gas to bypass the patient during exhalation and be wasted. Fresh gas introduced between the expiratory valve and the absorber would be diluted by recirculating gas. Furthermore, inhalation anesthetics may be absorbed or released by soda lime granules, thus slowing induction and emergence.
- The APL valve is usually placed between the absorber and the expiratory valve and close to the reservoir bag (Figure 3–11). Positioning the APL valve in this location (ie, before the absorber) helps conserve absorption capacity and minimizes the venting of fresh gas. The APL valve regulates the flow of gas from the expiratory limb of the circuit into the gas scavenger system.
- Resistance to exhalation is decreased by locating the reservoir bag in the expiratory limb.

Performance Characteristics of the Circle System

A. Fresh Gas Requirement

8 With an absorber, the circle system prevents rebreathing of CO_2 at reduced fresh gas flows (≤1 L) or even fresh gas flows equal to the uptake of anesthetic gases and oxygen by the patient and the circuit itself (closed-system anesthesia). At fresh gas flows greater than 5 L/min, rebreathing is so minimal that a CO_2 absorber is usually unnecessary.

With low fresh gas flows, concentrations of oxygen and inhalation anesthetics can vary markedly between fresh gas (ie, gas in the fresh gas inlet) and inspired gas (ie, gas in the inspiratory limb of the breathing tubes). The latter is a mixture of fresh gas and exhaled gas that has passed through the absorber. The greater the fresh gas flow rate, the less time it will take for a change in fresh gas anesthetic concentration to be reflected in a change in inspired gas anesthetic concentration. Higher flows speed induction and recovery and can compensate for leaks in the circuit.

B. Dead Space

That part of a tidal volume that does not undergo alveolar ventilation is referred to as *dead space.* Thus, any increase in dead space must be accompanied by a corresponding increase in tidal volume if alveolar ventilation is to remain unchanged. 9 Because of the unidirectional valves, apparatus dead space in a circle system is limited to the area distal to the point of inspiratory and expiratory gas mixing at the Y-piece. Unlike Mapleson circuits, the circle system corrugated breathing tube length does not affect dead space. Like Mapleson circuits, length does affect circuit compliance and thus the amount of tidal volume lost to the circuit during positive-pressure ventilation. Pediatric circle systems may have both a septum dividing the inspiratory and expiratory gas in the Y-piece and low-compliance breathing tubes to further reduce dead space, and they are lighter in weight.

C. Resistance

The unidirectional valves and absorber increase circle system resistance, especially at high respiratory rates and large tidal volumes. Nonetheless, even premature neonates can be successfully ventilated using a circle system.

D. Humidity and Heat Conservation

Medical gas delivery systems supply dehumidified gases to the anesthesia circuit at room temperature. Exhaled gas, on the other hand, is saturated with water at body temperature. Therefore, the heat and humidity of inspired gas depend on the relative proportion of rebreathed gas to fresh gas. High flows are accompanied by low relative humidity, whereas reduced flows allow greater water saturation. CO_2-absorbent granules provide a significant source of heat and moisture in the circle system.

E. Bacterial Contamination

The minimal risk of microorganism retention in circle system components could theoretically lead to respiratory infections in subsequent patients. For this reason, bacterial filters are incorporated into the inspiratory or expiratory breathing tubes or at the Y-piece.

Disadvantages of the Circle System

Although most of the problems of Mapleson circuits are solved by the circle system, these improvements have led to other disadvantages: greater size and less portability; increased complexity, resulting in a greater risk of disconnection or malfunction; complications related to use of absorbent; and the difficulty of predicting inspired gas concentrations during low fresh gas flows.

RESUSCITATION BREATHING SYSTEMS

Resuscitation bags (AMBU bags or bag-mask units) are commonly used for emergency ventilation because of their simplicity, portability, and ability to deliver almost 100% oxygen (Figure 3–12). Bag-mask ventilation maintains higher oxygen saturations during tracheal intubation in critically ill adult patients. A resuscitator is unlike a Mapleson circuit or a circle system because it contains a **nonrebreathing valve**. (Remember that a Mapleson system is considered valveless even though it contains an APL valve, whereas a circle system contains unidirectional valves that direct flow through an absorber but allow rebreathing of exhaled gases.)

High concentrations of oxygen can be delivered to a mask or tracheal tube during spontaneous or controlled ventilation if a source of high fresh gas flow is connected to the inlet nipple. The patient valve opens during controlled or spontaneous inspiration to allow gas flow from the ventilation bag to the patient. Rebreathing is prevented by venting exhaled gas to the atmosphere through exhalation ports in this valve. The compressible, self-refilling ventilation bag also contains an intake valve. This valve closes during bag compression, permitting positive-pressure ventilation. The bag is refilled by flow through the fresh gas inlet and across the intake valve. Connecting a

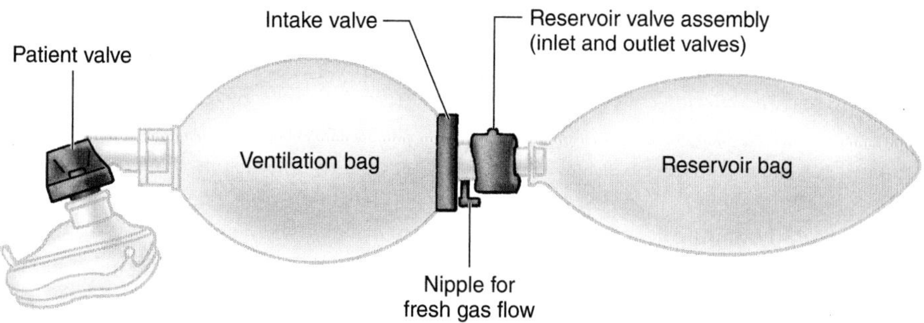

FIGURE 3–12 The Laerdal resuscitator. (Reproduced with permission from Laerdal Medical Corp.)

reservoir to the intake valve helps prevent the entrainment of room air. The reservoir valve assembly is really two unidirectional valves: the inlet valve and the outlet valve. The inlet valve allows ambient air to enter the ventilation bag if fresh gas flow is inadequate to maintain reservoir filling. Positive pressure in the reservoir bag opens the outlet valve, which vents oxygen if fresh gas flow is excessive.

There are several disadvantages to resuscitator breathing systems. First, they require high fresh gas
10 flows to achieve a high Fio_2. Fio_2 is directly proportional to the oxygen concentration and flow rate of the gas mixture supplied to the resuscitator (usually 100% oxygen) and inversely proportional to the minute ventilation delivered to the patient. Although a normally functioning patient valve has low resistance to inspiration and expiration, exhaled moisture can cause valve sticking. Finally, venting exhaled gas into the atmosphere can lead to local contamination if the expiratory gases are contaminated with infectious agents.

CASE DISCUSSION

Unexplained Light Anesthesia

An extremely obese but otherwise healthy 5-year-old child presents for inguinal hernia repair. After uneventful induction of general anesthesia and tracheal intubation, the patient is placed on a ventilator set to deliver a tidal volume of 6 mL/kg at a rate of 16 breaths/min. Despite the delivery of high concentrations of sevoflurane in 50% oxygen in air, tachycardia (145 beats/min) and mild hypertension (144/94 mm Hg) are noted. Fentanyl (3 mcg/kg) is administered to increase anesthetic depth. Heart rate and blood pressure continue to rise and are accompanied by frequent premature ventricular beats.

What should be considered in the differential diagnosis of this patient's cardiovascular changes?

The combination of tachycardia and hypertension during general anesthesia should always alert the anesthesiologist to the possibility of hypercapnia or hypoxia, both of which produce signs of increased sympathetic activity. These life-threatening conditions should be quickly and immediately ruled out by end-tidal CO_2 monitoring, pulse oximetry, or arterial blood gas analysis.

A common cause of intraoperative tachycardia and hypertension is an inadequate level of anesthesia. Normally, this is confirmed by movement. If the patient is paralyzed, however, there are few reliable indicators of light anesthesia. The lack of a response to a dose of an opioid should alert the anesthesiologist to the possibility of other, perhaps more serious, causes.

Malignant hyperthermia is rare but must be considered in cases of unexplained tachycardia, especially if accompanied by premature atrial or ventricular contractions. Certain drugs used in anesthesia (eg, ketamine, ephedrine) stimulate the sympathetic nervous system and can produce or exacerbate tachycardia and hypertension. Patients with diabetes who become hypoglycemic from the administration of insulin or long-acting oral hypoglycemic agents can have similar cardiovascular changes. Other endocrine abnormalities (eg, pheochromocytoma, thyroid storm, carcinoid) should also be considered.

Could any of these problems be related to an equipment malfunction?

Gas analysis can confirm the delivery of anesthetic gases to the patient. An empty vaporizer would certainly lead to inadequate anesthesia, tachycardia, and hypertension but would not cause hypercapnia.

A misconnection of the ventilator could result in hypoxia or hypercapnia. In addition, a malfunctioning unidirectional valve will increase circuit dead space and allow rebreathing of expired CO_2. Soda lime exhaustion could also lead to rebreathing in the presence of a low fresh gas flow. Rebreathing of CO_2 can be detected during the inspiratory phase on a capnograph. If rebreathing appears to be due to an equipment malfunction, the patient should be disconnected from the anesthesia machine and ventilated with a resuscitation bag until repairs are possible.

What are some other consequences of hypercapnia?

Hypercapnia has a multitude of effects, most of them masked by general anesthesia. Cerebral blood flow increases proportionately with arterial CO_2. This effect is dangerous in patients with increased intracranial pressure (eg, from brain trauma or tumor). Extremely high levels of CO_2 (>80 mm Hg) can cause unconsciousness related to a decrease in cerebrospinal fluid pH. CO_2 depresses the myocardium, but this direct effect is usually overshadowed by activation of the sympathetic nervous system. During general anesthesia, hypercapnia usually results in increased cardiac output, an elevation of arterial blood pressure, and a propensity for arrhythmias.

Elevated serum CO_2 concentrations can overwhelm the blood's buffering capacity, leading to respiratory acidosis. This causes other cations such as Ca^{2+} and K^+ to shift extracellularly. Acidosis also shifts the oxyhemoglobin dissociation curve to the right.

CO_2 is a powerful respiratory stimulant. In fact, for each mm Hg rise of $Paco_2$ above baseline, normal awake subjects increase their minute ventilation by about 2 to 3 L/min. General anesthesia markedly decreases this response, and paralysis eliminates it. Finally, severe hypercapnia can produce hypoxia by displacement of oxygen from alveoli.

SUGGESTED READINGS

Casey JD, Janz DR, Russell DW, et al. Bag-mask ventilation during tracheal intubation of critically ill adults. *New Engl J Med.* 2019;380:811.

Dobson MB. Anaesthesia for difficult locations—developing countries and military conflicts. In: Prys-Roberts C, Brown BR, eds. *International Practice of Anaesthesia*. Butterworth Heinemann; 1996.

Gegel B. A field expedient Ohmeda Universal Portable Anesthesia Complete draw-over vaporizer setup. *AANA J.* 2008;76:185.

Levy RJ. Anesthesia-related carbon monoxide exposure: toxicity and potential therapy. *Anesth Analg.* 2016;123:670.

Rose, G, McLarney JT. *Anesthesia Equipment Simplified.* McGraw-Hill; 2014.

CHAPTER 4

The Anesthesia Workstation

KEY CONCEPTS

1. Equipment-related adverse outcomes are rarely due to device malfunction or failure; rather, misuse of anesthesia gas delivery systems is three times more prevalent among closed claims. An operator's lack of familiarity with the equipment, an operator's failure to verify machine function prior to use, or both are the most frequent causes. Such mishaps accounted for about 1% of cases in the ASA Closed Claims Project database from 1990 to 2011.

2. The anesthesia machine receives medical gases from a gas supply, controls the flow and reduces the pressure of desired gases to a safe level, vaporizes volatile anesthetics into the final gas mixture, and delivers the gases to a breathing circuit that is connected to the patient's airway. A mechanical ventilator attaches to the breathing circuit but can be excluded with a switch during spontaneous or manual (bag) ventilation.

3. Whereas the oxygen supply can pass directly to its flow control valve, nitrous oxide, air, and other gases must first pass through safety devices before reaching their respective flow control valves. These devices permit the flow of other gases only if there is sufficient oxygen pressure in the safety device and help prevent accidental delivery of a hypoxic mixture in the event of oxygen supply failure.

4. Another safety feature of anesthesia machines is a linkage of the nitrous oxide gas flow to the oxygen gas flow; this arrangement helps ensure a minimum oxygen concentration of 25%.

5. All modern vaporizers are agent specific and temperature corrected, capable of delivering a constant concentration of agent regardless of temperature changes or flow through the vaporizer.

6. A rise in airway pressure may signal worsening pulmonary compliance, an increase in tidal volume, or an obstruction in the breathing circuit, endotracheal tube, or the patient's airway. A drop in pressure may indicate an improvement in compliance, a decrease in tidal volume, or a leak in the circuit.

7. Traditionally ventilators on anesthesia machines have a double-circuit system design and are pneumatically powered and electronically controlled. Newer machines also incorporate microprocessor controls and sophisticated pressure and flow sensors. Some anesthesia machines have ventilators that use a single-circuit piston design.

8. The major advantage of a piston ventilator is its ability to deliver accurate tidal volumes to patients with very poor lung compliance and to very small patients.

9. Whenever a ventilator is used, "disconnect alarms" must be passively activated. Anesthesia workstations should have at least three disconnect alarms: low peak inspiratory pressure, low exhaled tidal volume, and low exhaled carbon dioxide.

—*Continued next page*

Continued—

10 Because the ventilator's spill valve is closed during inspiration, fresh gas flow from the machine's common gas outlet normally contributes to the tidal volume delivered to the patient.

11 Use of the oxygen flush valve during the inspiratory cycle of a ventilator must be avoided because the ventilator spill valve will be closed and the adjustable pressure-limiting (APL) valve is excluded; the surge of oxygen (600–1200 mL/s) and circuit pressure will be transferred to the patient's lungs.

12 Large discrepancies between the set and actual tidal volume are often observed in the operating room during volume-controlled ventilation. Causes include breathing circuit compliance, gas compression, ventilator–fresh gas flow coupling, a preset ventilator peak airway pressure limit, and leaks in the anesthesia machine, the breathing circuit, or the patient's airway.

13 Waste-gas scavengers dispose of gases that have been vented from the breathing circuit by the APL valve and ventilator spill valve. Pollution of the operating room environment with anesthetic gases may pose a health hazard to surgical personnel.

14 A routine inspection of anesthesia equipment before each use increases operator familiarity and confirms proper functioning. The U.S. Food and Drug Administration has made available a generic checkout procedure for anesthesia gas machines and breathing systems.

No piece of equipment is more intimately associated with the practice of anesthesiology than the anesthesia machine (Figure 4–1). The anesthesiologist uses the anesthesia machine to control the patient's ventilation and the oxygen concentration delivered to the patient and to administer inhalation anesthetics. Proper functioning of the machine is crucial for patient safety. Modern anesthesia machines incorporate many built-in safety features and devices, monitors, and multiple microprocessors. Moreover, modular machine designs allow a variety of configurations and features within the same product line. The term *anesthesia workstation* is therefore often used for modern anesthesia machines. Anesthesia providers should be familiar with the operation manuals of all the machines in their clinical practice. Figure 4-1A displays the typical external layout of an anesthesia workstation. Figure 4-1B provides schematics of various modern anesthesia machines.

Much progress has been made in reducing the number of adverse outcomes arising from anesthetic
1 gas delivery. Equipment-related adverse outcomes are rarely due to device malfunction or failure; rather, misuse of anesthesia gas delivery systems is three times more prevalent among closed claims. Equipment misuse includes errors in the preparation, maintenance, or deployment of a device. Preventable anesthetic mishaps are frequently traced to an operator's lack of familiarity with the equipment, an operator's failure to verify machine function prior to use, or both. Such mishaps accounted for about 1% of cases in the American Society of Anesthesiologists' (ASA) Closed Claims Project database from 1990 to 2011. Severe injury was found to be related to provider errors involving, in particular, improvised oxygen delivery systems and breathing circuit failures, supplemental oxygen supply problems outside of the operating room, and problems with an anesthesia ventilator. In 35% of such claims, an appropriate preanesthetic machine check (see the ASA's 2008 Recommendations for Pre-Anesthesia Checkout) would likely have prevented the adverse event. Although patient injuries secondary to anesthesia equipment have decreased both in number and in average severity over the past decades, claims for awareness during general anesthesia have increased.

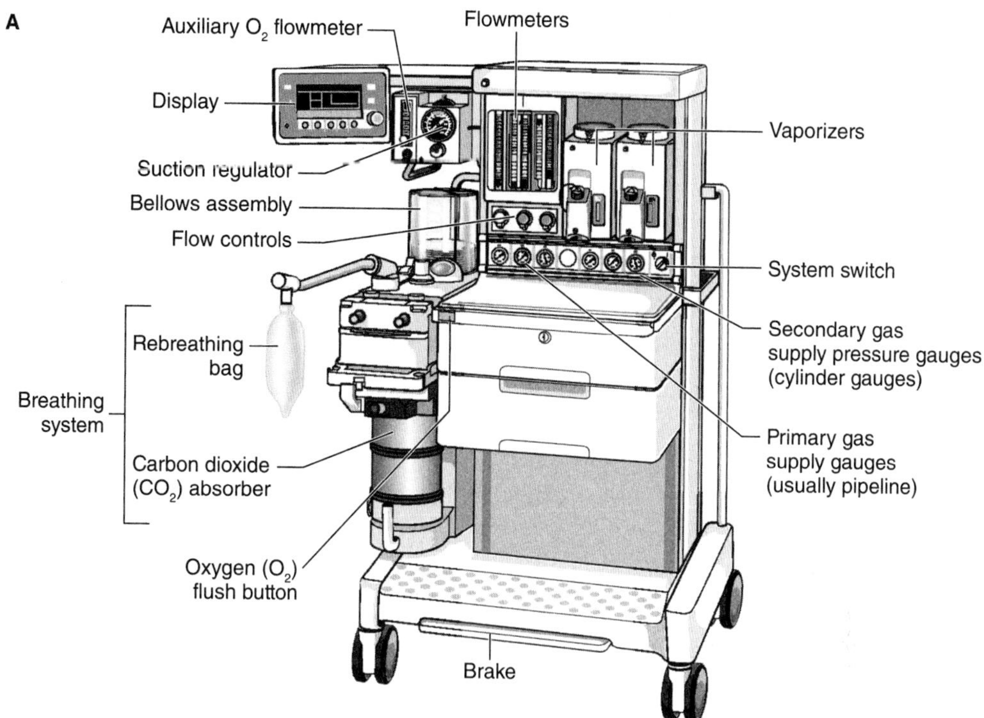

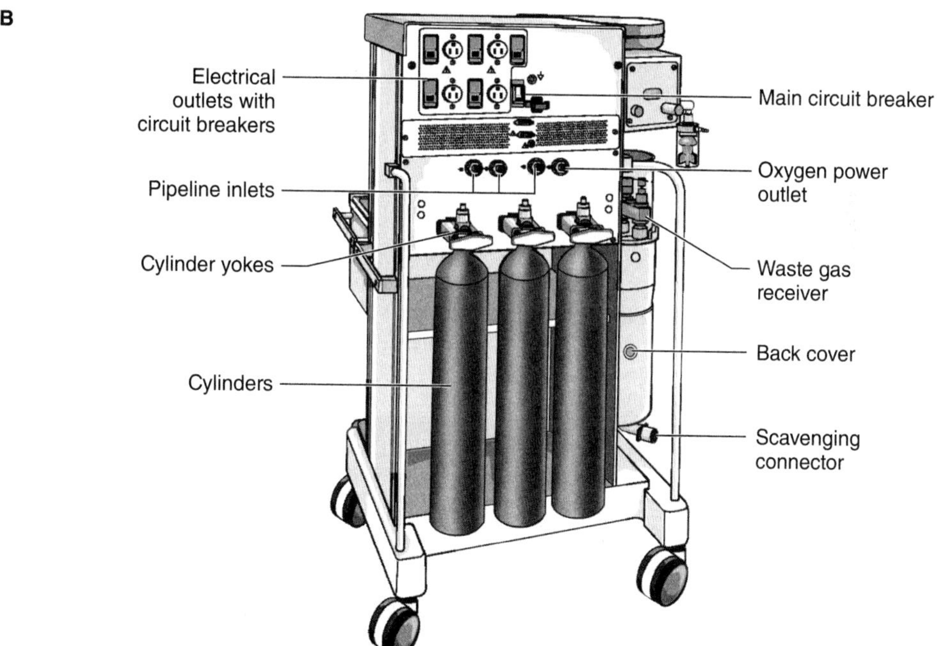

FIGURE 4–1A Modern anesthesia machine (Datex-Ohmeda Aestiva). **A**: Front. **B**: Back.

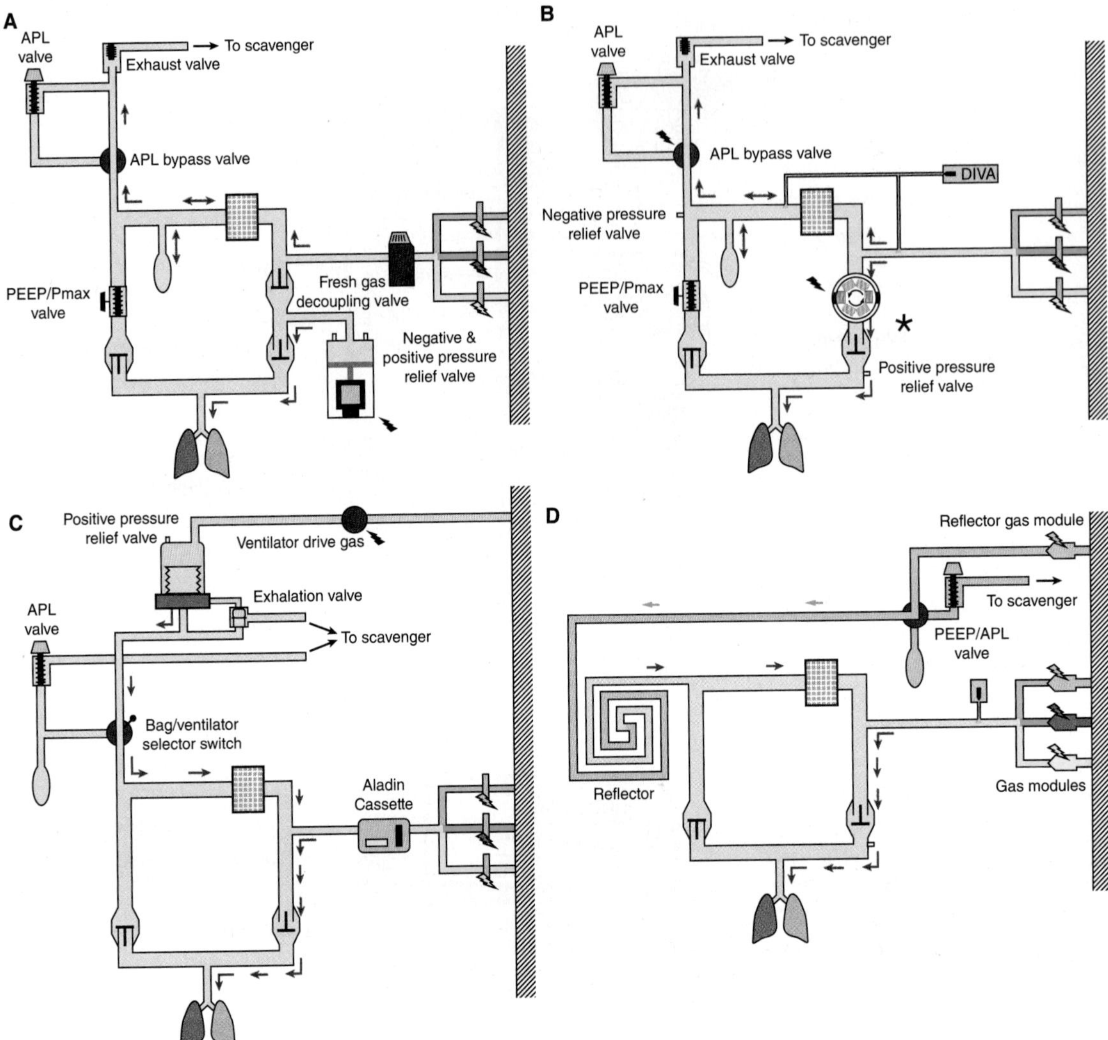

FIGURE 4-1B Circuit configuration of modern anesthesia machines. From the wall outlets, carrier gases (O_2 = green; air = yellow; N_2O = blue) pass through pressure regulators at the entrance of the anesthesia machine. Their flow into the breathing circuit is controlled by electronic flowmeters (colored lightning rods), except in the FLOW-i, where gas modules are used. During spontaneous or assisted ventilation, excess gas is vented via the adjustable pressure-limiting (APL) valve. Because all machines are depicted during the inspiratory phase of a mechanical breath (*blue arrows*, the direction of fresh gas flow [FGF]; *red arrows*, gas flow generated by the ventilator), the APL valve is excluded from the circle system. In addition, the inspiratory valve is open, and the expiratory valve is closed. **A**: Dräger Fabius (Apollo and Primus have similar circuit configurations). Fresh gas flows through a conventional vaporizer. A fresh gas decoupling valve directs the FGF during the inspiratory phase to the reservoir bag and, once that is filled, to the exhaust valve to make tidal volume delivery by the electronically driven piston ventilator independent from the FGF. At no point along their trajectory do the red and blue arrows overlap during inspiration. The negative- and positive-pressure relief valves (in the ventilator) and the Pmax valves are safety valves that will open only with negative and very high positive pressure in the ventilator or circuit. **B**: Dräger Zeus (Perseus has a similar circuit, except that the FG inlet is located between the turbine and the inspiratory valve [see asterisk] and it has a conventional vaporizer). The fresh gas enters the circle system via an inlet separated from the liquid agent injector (DIVA). An electronically driven turbine mixes the gases in the system (shortening response times), ventilates the patient (considering and adjusting for the continuous inflow of fresh gas), and helps apply

The American National Standards Institute and subsequently ASTM International (formerly known as the American Society for Testing and Materials, F1850–00) have published standard specifications for anesthesia machines and their components. Table 4–1 lists essential features of a modern anesthesia workstation.

OVERVIEW

2 In its most basic form, the anesthesia machine receives medical gases from a gas supply, controls the flow and reduces the pressure of desired gases to a safe level, vaporizes volatile anesthetics into the final gas mixture, and delivers the gases at the common gas outlet to the breathing circuit connected to the patient's airway (Figures 4–2 and 4–3). A mechanical ventilator attaches to the breathing circuit but can be excluded with a switch during spontaneous or manual (bag) ventilation. An auxiliary oxygen supply and suction regulator are also usually built into the workstation. In addition to standard safety features (**Table 4–1**), top-of-the-line anesthesia machines have additional safety features and built-in computer processors that integrate and monitor all components, perform automated machine checkouts, and provide options such as automated record-keeping and networking interfaces to external monitors and hospital information systems. Work is ongoing in the development of anesthesia delivery systems capable of increasingly autonomous or "closed-loop" anesthetic management. Some machines are designed specifically for mobility, magnetic resonance imaging (MRI) compatibility, or compactness.

GAS SUPPLY

Most machines have gas inlets for oxygen, nitrous oxide, and air. Compact models often lack air inlets, whereas other machines may have a fourth inlet for helium, heliox, carbon dioxide (CO_2), or nitric oxide. Separate inlets are provided for the primary pipeline gas supply that passes through the walls of health care facilities and the secondary cylinder gas supply. Machines, therefore, have two gas inlet pressure gauges for each gas: one for pipeline pressure and another for cylinder pressure.

Pipeline Inlets

Oxygen and nitrous oxide (and often air) are delivered from their central supply source to the operating room through a piping network. The tubing is color coded and connects to the anesthesia machine through a noninterchangeable **diameter-index safety system (DISS)** fitting that prevents incorrect hose attachment. Interchangeability is prevented by making the bore diameter of the body and that of the connection nipple specific for each supplied gas. A filter helps trap debris from the wall supply, and a one-way check valve

positive end-expiratory pressure (PEEP). The turbine rotations are induced by alternating the current through pairwise positioned coils, successively magnetizing them and thus attracting them to the magnets (black) enclosed in the turbine housing. **C**: GE Aisys. The electronic controls of the draw over variable bypass vaporizer determine the proportion of the FGF that passes through the vaporizing chamber (Aladin cassette). The resulting anesthetic gas mixture enters the circle system proximally from the inspiratory valve. Compressed gas from the wall outlet is used to drive the bellows of the ventilator and generate the tidal volume. The pressure in the bellows housing surrounding the bellows is controlled by an electronically controlled valve, and excessive pressure around the bellows is vented via the ventilator positive-pressure relief valve. The Aisys uses FGF compensation: the tidal volume delivered by the bellows is adjusted (decreased) by the amount of fresh gas that enters the inspiratory limb during the inspiratory cycle. **D**: Getinge FLOW-i. Fresh gas is delivered via three gas modules, one for each gas (O_2, air, N_2O), and vapor is added from a vaporizer by injecting a liquid agent into the heated vaporizing chamber. Exhaled gas is temporarily stored in a long piece of tubing called the *volume reflector* (it redirects or "reflects" a volume of exhaled gas back to the circle system). The inspired tidal volume consists of gas from the volume reflector pushed out by the reflector gas module and fresh gas from the three fresh gas modules with an agent added by the injector. The lower the FGF, the more exhaled gas will be pushed back into the circle system. Gas mixing within the volume reflector is minimal. The APL/PEEP valve is physical the same valve and has no opening pressure. (Reproduced with permission from Hendrickx JFA, De Wolf AM. The Anesthesia Workstation: Quo Vadis? *Anesth Analg*. 2018 Sep;127(3):671-675.)

TABLE 4–1 Essential safety features on a modern anesthesia workstation.

Essential Features	Purpose
Noninterchangeable gas-specific connections to pipeline inlets (DISS)[1] with pressure gauges, filter, and check valve	Prevent incorrect pipeline attachments; detect failure, depletion, or fluctuation
Pin index safety system for cylinders with pressure gauges and at least one oxygen cylinder	Prevent incorrect cylinder attachments; provide backup gas supply; detect depletion
Low oxygen pressure alarm	Detect oxygen supply failure at the common gas inlet
Minimum oxygen/nitrous oxide ratio controller device (hypoxic guard)	Prevent delivery of less than 21% oxygen
Oxygen failure safety device (shut-off or proportioning device)	Prevent administration of nitrous oxide or other gases when the oxygen supply fails
Oxygen must enter the common manifold downstream to other gases	Prevent hypoxia in event of proximal gas leak
Oxygen concentration monitor and alarm	Prevent administration of hypoxic gas mixtures in event of a low-pressure system leak; precisely regulate oxygen concentration
Automatically enabled essential alarms and monitors (eg, oxygen concentration)	Prevent use of the machine without essential monitors
Vaporizer interlock device	Prevent simultaneous administration of more than one volatile agent
Capnography and anesthetic gas measurement	Guide ventilation; prevent anesthetic overdose; help reduce awareness
Oxygen flush mechanism that does not pass through vaporizers	Rapidly refill or flush the breathing circuit
Breathing circuit pressure monitor and alarm	Prevent pulmonary barotrauma and detect sustained positive, high peak, and negative airway pressures
Exhaled volume monitor	Assess ventilation and prevent hypo- or hyperventilation
Pulse oximetry, blood pressure, and electrocardiogram monitoring	Provide minimal standard monitoring
Mechanical ventilator	Control alveolar ventilation more accurately and during muscle paralysis for prolonged periods
Backup battery	Provide temporary electrical power (>30 min) to monitors and alarms in event of power failure
Scavenger system	Prevent contamination of the operating room with waste anesthetic gases

[1]DISS, diameter-index safety system.

prevents the retrograde flow of gases into the pipeline supplies. It should be noted that most modern machines have an oxygen (pneumatic) power outlet that may be used to drive the ventilator or provide an auxiliary oxygen flowmeter. The DISS fittings for the oxygen inlet and the oxygen power outlet are identical and should not be mistakenly interchanged. The approximate pipeline pressure

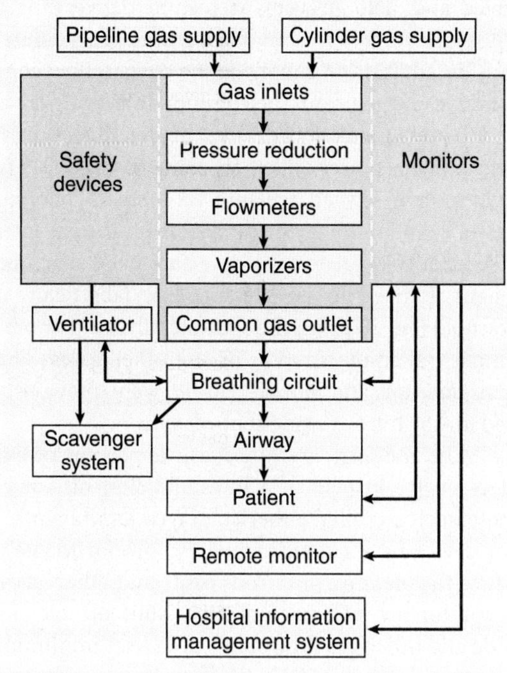

FIGURE 4–2 Functional schematic of an anesthesia machine/workstation.

of gases delivered to the anesthesia machine is 50 psig (pounds per square inch gauge).

Cylinder Inlets

Cylinders attach to the machine via hanger-yoke assemblies that use a **pin index safety system** to prevent accidental connection of a wrong gas cylinder. The yoke assembly includes index pins, a washer, a gas filter, and a check valve that prevents retrograde gas flow. The gas cylinders are also color coded for specific gases to allow for easy identification. In North America, the following color-coding scheme is used: oxygen = green; nitrous oxide = blue; CO_2 = gray; air = yellow; helium = brown; nitrogen = black. Color codes differ around the world; therefore, practitioners must be aware of the coding scheme in use where they practice. The E-cylinders attached to the anesthesia machine are a high-pressure source of medical gases and are generally used only as a backup supply in case of pipeline failure. The pressure of gas supplied from the cylinder to the anesthesia machine is 45 psig. Some machines have two oxygen cylinders so one cylinder can be used while

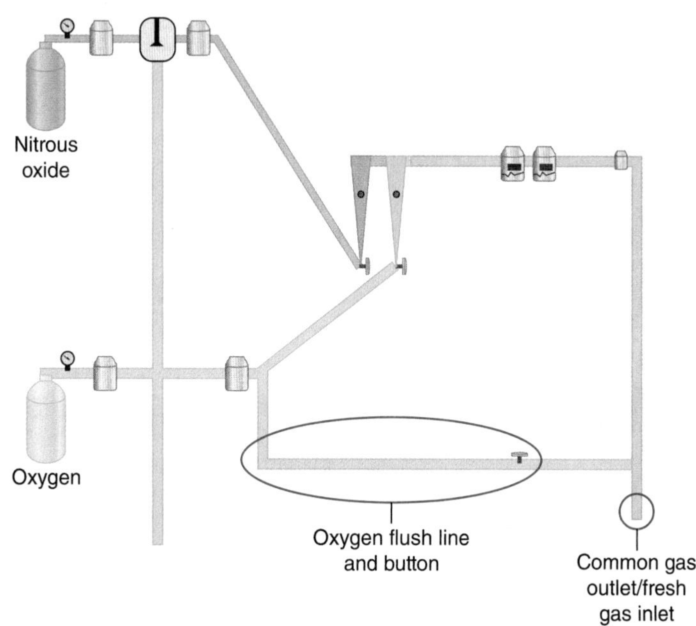

FIGURE 4–3 The anesthesia machine reduces the pressure from the gas supply, vaporizes anesthetic agents, and delivers the gas mixture to the common gas outlet. The oxygen flush line bypasses the vaporizers and directs oxygen directly to the common gas outlet. (Reproduced with permission from Rose G, McLarney JT: *Anesthesia Equipment Simplified.* New York, NY: McGraw Hill; 2014.)

the other is changed. At 20°C, a full E-cylinder contains 600 L of oxygen at a pressure of 1900 psig or 1590 L of nitrous oxide at 745 psig.

FLOW CONTROL CIRCUITS

Pressure Regulators

Unlike the relatively constant pressure of the pipeline gas supply, the high and variable gas pressure in cylinders makes flow control difficult and potentially dangerous. To enhance safety and ensure optimal use of cylinder gases, machines use a pressure regulator to reduce the cylinder gas pressure to 45 to 47 psig.[1] This pressure, which is slightly lower than the pipeline supply, allows preferential use of the pipeline supply if a cylinder is left open (unless pipeline pressure drops below 45 psig). After passing through pressure gauges and check valves, the pipeline gases share a common pathway with the cylinder gases. A high-pressure relief valve provided for each gas is set to open when the supply pressure exceeds the machine's maximum safety limit (95–110 psig), as might happen with a regulator failure on a cylinder. Some machines also use a second regulator to drop both pipeline and cylinder pressure further (two-stage pressure regulation). A second-stage pressure reduction may also be needed for an auxiliary oxygen flowmeter, the oxygen flush mechanism, or the drive gas to power a pneumatic ventilator.

Oxygen Supply Failure Protection Devices

3 Whereas the oxygen supply can pass directly to its flow control valve, nitrous oxide, air (in some machines), and other gases must first pass through safety devices before reaching their respective flow control valves. In other machines, air passes directly to its flow control valve; this allows the administration of air even in the absence of oxygen. These devices permit the flow of other gases only if there is sufficient oxygen pressure in the safety device and help prevent accidental delivery of a hypoxic mixture in the event of oxygen supply failure. Thus, in addition to supplying the oxygen flow control valve, oxygen from the common inlet pathway is used to pressurize safety devices, oxygen flush valves, and ventilator power outlets (in some models). Safety devices sense oxygen pressure via a small "piloting pressure" line that may be derived from the gas inlet or secondary regulator. In some anesthesia machine designs, if the piloting pressure line falls below a threshold (eg, 20 psig), the shut-off valves close, preventing the administration of any other gases. The terms *fail-safe* and *nitrous cut-off* were previously used for the nitrous oxide shut-off valve.

Most modern machines use a proportioning safety device instead of a threshold shut-off valve. These devices, called either an *oxygen failure protection device* or a *balance regulator*, proportionately reduce the pressure of nitrous oxide and other gases except for air. (They completely shut off nitrous oxide and other gas flow only below a set minimum oxygen pressure [eg, 0.5 psig for nitrous oxide and 10 psig for other gases]).

All machines also have an oxygen supply low-pressure sensor that activates alarm sounds when inlet gas pressure drops below a threshold value (usually 20–30 psig). It must be emphasized that these safety devices do *not* protect against other possible causes of hypoxic accidents (eg, gas line misconnections) in which threshold pressure may be maintained by gases containing inadequate or no oxygen.

Flow Valves & Meters

Once the pressure has been reduced to a safe level, each gas must pass through flow control valves and is measured by flowmeters before mixing with other gases, entering the active vaporizer, and exiting the machine's common gas outlet. **Gas lines proximal to flow valves are considered to be in the high-pressure circuit, whereas those between the flow valves and the common gas outlet are considered part of the low-pressure circuit of the machine.** Touch- and color-coded control knobs make it more difficult to turn the wrong gas off or on. As a safety feature, the oxygen knob is usually fluted and larger, and it usually protrudes farther than other knobs.

[1]Pressure unit conversions: 1 kiloPascal (kP) = kg/m · s2 = 1000 N/m2 = 0.01 bar = 0.1013 atmospheres = 0.145 psig = 10.2 cm H2O = 7.5 mm Hg.

By convention, in modern machines, the oxygen flowmeter is positioned furthest to the right, downstream to the other gases; this arrangement helps prevent hypoxia if there is leakage from a flowmeter positioned upstream.

Flow control knobs adjust gas entry into the flowmeters via a needle valve. Flowmeters on anesthesia machines are classified as either constant-pressure variable-orifice (rotameter) or electronic. In constant-pressure variable-orifice flowmeters, an indicator ball, bobbin, or float is supported by the flow of gas through a tube (Thorpe tube) whose bore (orifice) is tapered. Near the bottom of the tube, where the diameter is small, a low flow of gas will create sufficient pressure under the float to raise it in the tube. As the float rises, the (variable) orifice of the tube widens, allowing more gas to pass around the float. The float will stop rising when its weight is just supported by the difference in pressure above and below it. If the flow is increased, the pressure under the float increases, raising it higher in the tube until the pressure drop again just supports the float's weight. This pressure drop is constant regardless of the flow rate or the position in the tube and depends on the float weight and the cross-sectional tube area.

Flowmeters are calibrated for specific gases, as the flow rate across a constriction depends on the gas's viscosity at low laminar flows (Poiseuille's law) and its density at high turbulent flows. Floats are designed to rotate constantly so that they remain centered in the tube, thus minimizing the effect of friction with the tube's wall. Coating the tube's interior with a conductive substance grounds the system and reduces the effect of static electricity. Some flowmeters have two glass tubes, one for low flows and another for high flows (Figure 4–4A); the two tubes are in a series and are still controlled by one valve. A dual taper design can allow a single flowmeter to

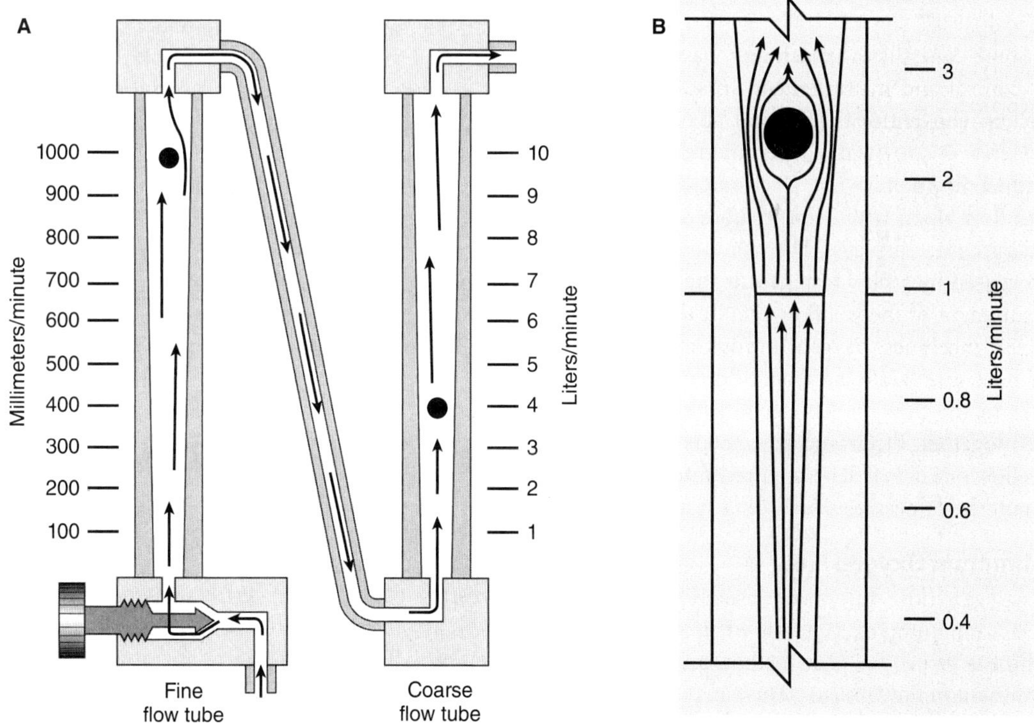

FIGURE 4–4 Constant-pressure variable-orifice flowmeters (Thorpe type). **A:** Two tube design. **B:** Dual taper design.

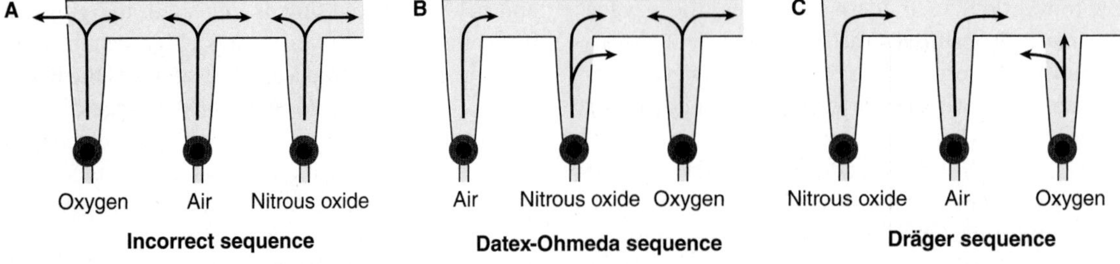

FIGURE 4–5 Sequence of flowmeters in a three-gas machine. **A**: An unsafe sequence. **B**: Typical Datex-Ohmeda sequence. **C**: Typical Dräger sequence. Note that regardless of sequence, a leak in the oxygen tube or further downstream can result in the delivery of a hypoxic mixture.

read both high and low flows (Figure 4–4B). **Causes of flowmeter malfunction include debris in the flow tube, vertical tube misalignment, and sticking or concealment of a float at the top of a tube.**

Should a leak develop within or downstream from an oxygen flowmeter, a hypoxic gas mixture can be delivered to the patient (Figure 4–5). Oxygen flowmeters are *always* positioned downstream to all other flowmeters (nearest to the vaporizer) to reduce this risk.

Some anesthesia machines have electronic flow control and measurement. In such instances, a backup conventional (Thorpe) auxiliary oxygen flowmeter is provided. Other models have conventional flowmeters but electronic measurement of gas flow along with Thorpe tubes and digital or digital/graphic displays. The amount of pressure drop caused by a flow restrictor is the basis for the measurement of the gas flow rate in these systems. In these machines, oxygen, nitrous oxide, and air each have a separate electronic flow measurement device in the flow control section before they are mixed together. Electronic flowmeters are required if gas flow rate data will be acquired automatically by computerized anesthesia recording systems.

A. Minimum Oxygen Flow

The oxygen flow valves are usually designed to deliver a minimum oxygen flow when the anesthesia machine is turned on. One method involves the use of a minimum flow resistor. This safety feature helps ensure that some oxygen enters the breathing circuit even if the operator forgets to turn on the oxygen flow.

B. Oxygen/Nitrous Oxide Ratio Controller

4 Another safety feature of anesthesia machines is a linkage of the nitrous oxide gas flow to the oxygen gas flow; this arrangement helps ensure a minimum oxygen concentration of 25%. The oxygen/nitrous oxide ratio controller links the two flow valves either pneumatically or mechanically.

Vaporizers

Volatile anesthetics (eg, halothane, isoflurane, desflurane, sevoflurane) must be vaporized before being delivered to the patient. Vaporizers have concentration-calibrated dials that precisely add volatile anesthetic agents to the combined gas flow from all flowmeters. They must be located between the flowmeters and the common gas outlet. Moreover, unless the machine accepts only one vaporizer at a time, all anesthesia machines should have an interlocking or exclusion device that prevents the concurrent use of more than one vaporizer.

A. Physics of Vaporization

At temperatures encountered in the operating room, the molecules of a volatile anesthetic in a closed container are distributed between the liquid and gaseous phases. The gas molecules bombard the walls of the container, creating the saturated vapor pressure of that agent. Vapor pressure depends on the characteristics of the volatile agent and the temperature. The greater the temperature, the greater the tendency for the liquid molecules to escape into the gaseous phase and the greater the vapor pressure (Figure 4–6). Vaporization requires energy

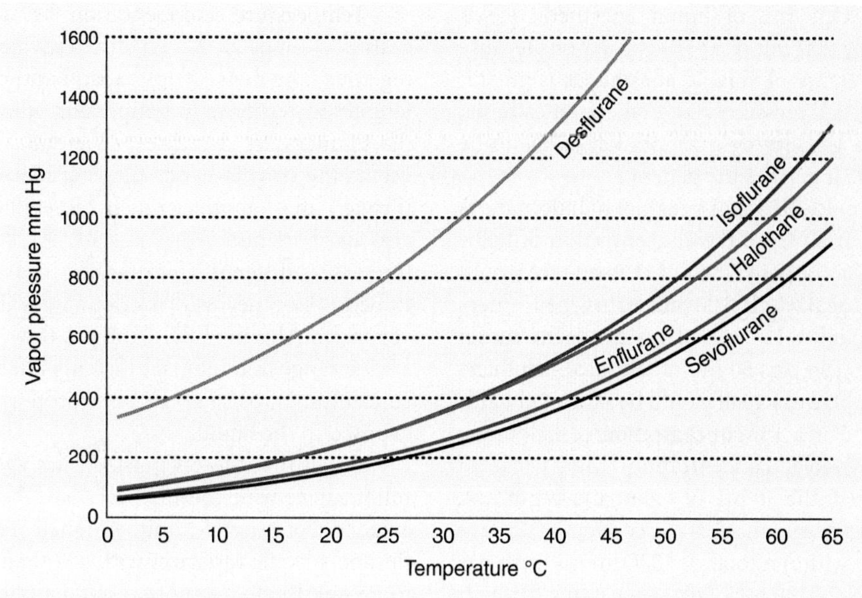

FIGURE 4–6 The vapor pressure of anesthetic gases.

(the latent heat of vaporization), which results in a loss of heat from the liquid. As vaporization proceeds, the temperature of the remaining liquid anesthetic drops and the vapor pressure decreases unless heat is readily available to enter the system. Vaporizers contain a chamber in which a carrier gas becomes saturated with the volatile agent.

A liquid's boiling point is the temperature at which its vapor pressure is equal to the atmospheric pressure. As the atmospheric pressure decreases (as in higher altitudes), the boiling point also decreases. Anesthetic agents with low boiling points are more susceptible to variations in barometric pressure than agents with higher boiling points. Among the commonly used agents, desflurane has the lowest boiling point (22.8°C at 760 mm Hg).

B. Copper Kettle

The copper kettle vaporizer is no longer used in clinical anesthesia; however, understanding how it works provides invaluable insight into the delivery of volatile anesthetics (Figure 4–7). It is classified as a measured-flow vaporizer (or flowmeter-controlled vaporizer). In a copper kettle, the amount of carrier gas bubbled through the volatile anesthetic is controlled by a dedicated flowmeter. This valve is turned off when the vaporizer circuit is not in use. Copper is used as the construction metal because its relatively high specific heat (the quantity of heat required to raise the temperature of 1 g of substance by 1°C) and high thermal conductivity (the speed of heat conductance through a substance) enhance the vaporizer's ability to maintain a constant temperature. All the gas entering the vaporizer passes through the anesthetic liquid and becomes saturated

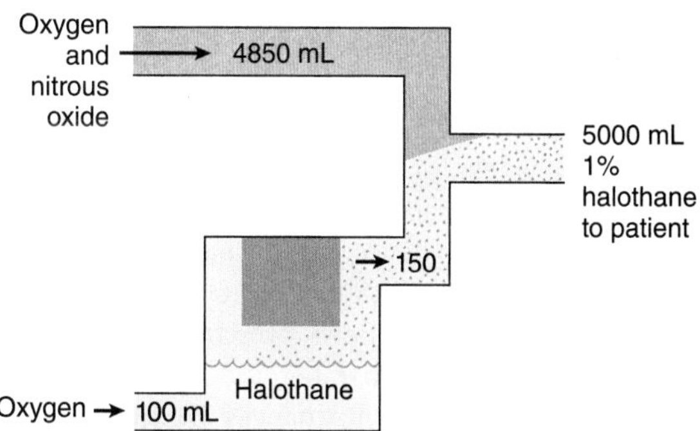

FIGURE 4–7 Schematic of a copper kettle vaporizer. Note that 50 mL/min of halothane vapor is added for each 100 mL/min oxygen flow that passes through the vaporizer.

with vapor. One mL of liquid anesthetic yields approximately 200 mL of anesthetic vapor. Because the vapor pressure of volatile anesthetics is greater than the partial pressure required for anesthesia, the saturated gas leaving a copper kettle has to be diluted before it reaches the patient.

For example, the vapor pressure of halothane is 243 mm Hg at 20°C, so the concentration of halothane exiting a copper kettle at 1 atmosphere would be 243/760, or 32%. If 100 mL of oxygen enters the kettle, roughly 150 mL of gas exits (the initial 100 mL of oxygen plus 50 mL of saturated halothane vapor), one-third of which would be saturated halothane vapor. For a 1% concentration of halothane (minimum alveolar concentration [MAC] 0.75%) to be delivered, the 50 mL of halothane vapor and 100 mL of carrier gas that left the copper kettle have to be diluted within a total of 5000 mL of fresh gas flow. Thus, every 100 mL of oxygen passing through a halothane vaporizer translates into a 1% increase in concentration if the total gas flow into the breathing circuit is 5 L/min. Therefore, when the total flow is fixed, the flow through the vaporizer determines the ultimate concentration of the anesthetic. Isoflurane has an almost identical vapor pressure, so the same relationship between copper kettle flow, total gas flow, and anesthetic concentration exists. However, if total gas flow decreases without an adjustment in copper kettle flow (eg, exhaustion of a nitrous oxide cylinder), the delivered volatile anesthetic concentration rises rapidly to potentially dangerous levels.

C. Modern Conventional Vaporizers

5 All modern vaporizers are agent specific and temperature corrected, capable of delivering a constant concentration of agent regardless of temperature changes or flow through the vaporizer. Turning a single calibrated control knob counterclockwise to the desired percentage diverts an appropriately small fraction of the total gas flow into the carrier gas, which flows over the liquid anesthetic in a vaporizing chamber, leaving the balance to exit the vaporizer unchanged (Figure 4–8). Because some of the entering gas is never exposed to anesthetic liquid, this type of agent-specific vaporizer is also known as a *variable-bypass vaporizer*.

Temperature compensation is achieved by a strip composed of two different metals welded together. The metal strips expand and contract differently in response to temperature changes. When the temperature decreases, differential contraction causes the strip to bend, allowing more gas to pass through the vaporizer. Such bimetallic strips are also used in home thermostats. As the temperature rises, differential expansion causes the strip to bend the other way, restricting gas flow into the vaporizer. Altering total fresh gas flow rates within a wide range does not significantly affect anesthetic concentration because the same proportion of gas is exposed to the liquid.

Given that these vaporizers are agent specific, filling them with the incorrect anesthetic must be avoided. For example, unintentionally filling a sevoflurane-specific vaporizer with halothane could lead to an anesthetic overdose. First, halothane's higher vapor pressure (243 mm Hg versus 157 mm Hg) will cause a 40% greater amount of anesthetic vapor to be released. Second, halothane is more than twice as potent as sevoflurane (MAC 0.75 versus 2.0). Conversely, filling a halothane vaporizer with sevoflurane will cause an anesthetic underdosage. Modern vaporizers offer agent-specific, keyed filling ports to prevent filling with an incorrect agent.

Variable-bypass vaporizers compensate for changes in ambient pressures (ie, altitude changes maintaining relative anesthetic gas partial pressure). It is the partial pressure of the anesthetic agent that determines its concentration-dependent physiological effects. Thus, there is no need to increase the selected anesthetic concentration when using a variable-bypass vaporizer at altitude because the partial pressure of the anesthetic agent will be largely unchanged. Although at lower ambient pressures gas passing through the vaporizer is exposed to increased vaporizer output, because of Dalton's law of partial pressure, the partial pressure of the anesthetic vapor will remain largely unaffected compared with partial pressures obtained at sea level.

D. Electronic Vaporizers

Electronically controlled vaporizers must be utilized for desflurane and may be used for all volatile anesthetics in some anesthesia machines.

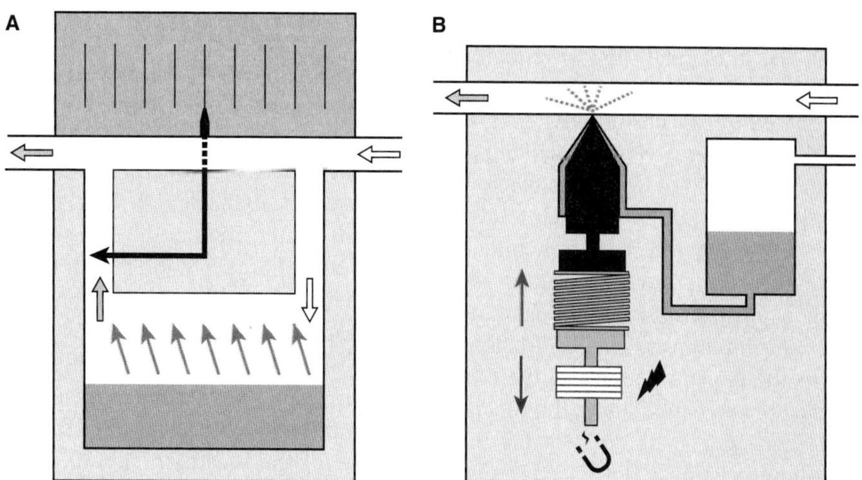

FIGURE 4–8 Vaporizer technology. **A**: General principle of variable bypass vaporizer. When the wheel (dial) is turned, more or less fresh gas is directed through the vaporizing chamber containing the liquid agent (orange). Gas exiting the vaporizing chamber is saturated with an agent (at the prevailing temperature) and mixes with gas bypassing the vaporizing chamber. Desflurane cannot be administered with this type of vaporizer because it boils at room temperature. **B**: Injector principle. The DIVA vaporizer of the Zeus and the FLOW-i vaporizer both use fuel injector technology in their systems. The liquid agent (orange) is pressurized, which makes the system also suitable for desflurane. The liquid agent is injected into a heated chamber (where it evaporates and mixes with fresh gas) or directly into the breathing system (in the Zeus in target control mode) via a nozzle. In the resting position, a spring (green) pushes the ferromagnetic plunger (yellow) into the nozzle. When the microprocessor directs current through the coiled wire surrounding the ferromagnetic plunger (yellow), the plunger is moved backward (red arrow), and a liquid agent is injected. (Reproduced with permission from Hendrickx JFA, De Wolf AM. The Anesthesia Workstation: Quo Vadis? *Anesth Analg.* 2018 Sep;127(3):671-675.)

1. **Desflurane vaporizer**—Desflurane's vapor pressure is so high that at sea level it almost boils at room temperature (Figure 4–6). **This high volatility, coupled with a potency of only one-fifth that of other volatile agents, presents unique delivery problems.** First, the vaporization required for general anesthesia produces a cooling effect that would overwhelm the ability of conventional vaporizers to maintain a constant temperature. Second, because it vaporizes so extensively, a tremendously high fresh gas flow would be necessary to dilute the carrier gas to clinically relevant concentrations. These problems have been addressed by the development of specific desflurane vaporizers. A reservoir containing desflurane (desflurane sump) is electrically heated to 39°C (significantly higher than its boiling point), creating a vapor pressure of 2 atmospheres. Unlike a variable-bypass vaporizer, no fresh gas flows through the desflurane sump. Rather, pure desflurane vapor joins the fresh gas mixture before exiting the vaporizer. The amount of desflurane vapor released from the sump depends on the concentration selected by turning the control dial and the fresh gas flow rate. Although the Tec 6 Plus maintains a constant desflurane concentration over a wide range of fresh gas flow rates, it cannot automatically compensate for changes in elevation like the variable-bypass vaporizers can. Decreased ambient pressure (eg, high elevation) does not affect the concentration of the agent delivered, but it decreases the partial pressure of the agent. Thus at high elevations, one must manually increase the desflurane concentration control.

2. **Aladin (GE) cassette vaporizer**—Gas flow from the flow control is divided into bypass flow and liquid chamber flow. The latter is conducted into an agent-specific, color-coded cassette (Aladin cassette) in which the volatile anesthetic is vaporized. The machine accepts only one cassette at a time and recognizes the cassette through magnetic labeling.

The cassette does not contain any bypass flow channels; therefore, unlike traditional vaporizers, liquid anesthetic cannot escape during handling, and the cassette can be carried in any position. After leaving the cassette, the now anesthetic-saturated liquid chamber flow reunites with the bypass flow before exiting the fresh gas outlet. A flow restrictor valve near the bypass flow helps adjust the amount of fresh gas that flows to the cassette. Adjusting the ratio between the bypass flow and liquid chamber flow changes the concentration of volatile anesthetic agent delivered to the patient. Sensors in the cassette measure pressure and temperature, thus determining agent concentration in the gas leaving the cassette. Correct liquid chamber flow is calculated based on desired fresh gas concentration and determined cassette gas concentration.

Common (Fresh) Gas Outlet

In contrast to the multiple gas inlets, the anesthesia machine has only one common gas outlet that supplies gas to the breathing circuit. The term *fresh gas outlet* is also often used because of its critical role in adding new gas of fixed and known composition to the circle system. Unlike older models, some newer anesthesia machines measure and report common outlet gas flows. An antidisconnect retaining device is used to prevent accidental detachment of the gas outlet hose that connects the machine to the breathing circuit.

The oxygen flush valve provides a high flow (35–75 L/min) of oxygen directly to the common gas outlet, bypassing the flowmeters and vaporizers. It is used to rapidly refill or flush the breathing circuit, but because the oxygen may be supplied at a line pressure of 45 to 55 psig, there is a real potential for lung barotrauma to occur. For this reason, the flush valve must be used cautiously whenever a patient is connected to the breathing circuit. Moreover, inappropriate use of the flush valve (or a situation of a stuck valve) may result in the backflow of gases into the low-pressure circuit, causing dilution of inhaled anesthetic concentration. Some machines use a second-stage regulator to drop the oxygen flush pressure to a lower level. A protective rim around the flush button limits the possibility of unintentional activation

THE BREATHING CIRCUIT

In adults, the breathing system most commonly used with anesthesia machines is the circle system, though a Bain circuit is occasionally used. The components and use of the circle system were previously discussed (see Chapter 3). It is important to note that gas composition at the common gas outlet can be controlled precisely and rapidly by adjustments in flowmeters and vaporizers. In contrast, gas composition, especially volatile anesthetic concentration, in the breathing circuit is significantly affected by other factors, including anesthetic uptake in the patient's lungs, minute ventilation, total fresh gas flow, the volume of the breathing circuit, and the presence of gas leaks. The use of high gas flow rates during induction and emergence decreases the effects of such variables and can diminish the magnitude of discrepancies between the fresh gas outlet and circle system anesthetic concentrations. Measurement of inspired and expired anesthetic gas concentration also greatly facilitates anesthetic management.

Oxygen Analyzers

General anesthesia must not be administered without an oxygen analyzer in the breathing circuit. **Three types of oxygen analyzers are available: polarographic (Clark electrode), galvanic (fuel cell), and paramagnetic.** The first two techniques use electrochemical sensors that contain cathode and anode electrodes embedded in an electrolyte gel separated from the sample gas by an oxygen-permeable membrane (usually Teflon). As oxygen reacts with the electrodes, a current is generated that is proportional to the oxygen partial pressure in the sample gas. The galvanic and polarographic sensors differ in the composition of their electrodes and electrolyte gels. The components of the galvanic cell are capable of providing enough chemical energy so that the reaction does not require an external power source.

Although the initial cost of paramagnetic sensors is greater than that of electrochemical sensors, paramagnetic devices are self-calibrating and have no consumable parts. In addition, their response time is fast enough to differentiate between inspired and expired oxygen concentrations.

All oxygen analyzers should have a low-level alarm that is automatically activated by turning on the anesthesia machine. The sensor should be placed into the inspiratory or expiratory limb of the circle system's breathing circuit—but *not* into the fresh gas line. As a result of the patient's oxygen consumption, the expiratory limb has a slightly lower oxygen partial pressure than the inspiratory limb, particularly at low fresh gas flows. The increased humidity of expired gas does not significantly affect most modern sensors.

Spirometers

Spirometers, also called *respirometers*, are used to measure exhaled tidal volume in the breathing circuit on all anesthesia machines, typically near the exhalation valve. Some anesthesia machines also measure the inspiratory tidal volume just past the inspiratory valve or the actual delivered and exhaled tidal volumes at the Y-connector that attaches to the patient's airway.

A common method employs a rotating vane of low mass in the expiratory limb in front of the expiratory valve of the circle system (vane anemometer or Wright respirometer).

The flow of gas across vanes within the respirometer causes their rotation, which is measured electronically, photoelectrically, or mechanically.

During positive-pressure ventilation, changes in exhaled tidal volumes usually represent changes in ventilator settings, but they can also be due to circuit leaks, disconnections, or ventilator malfunction. These spirometers are prone to errors caused by inertia, friction, and water condensation. For example, Wright respirometers under-read at low flow rates and over-read at high flow rates. Moreover, measurements of "exhaled" tidal volumes at this location in the expiratory limb include gas that expanded the corrugated tubing in the circuit (and was not delivered to the patient). The difference between the volume of gas delivered to the circuit and the volume of gas actually reaching the patient becomes very significant with long, compliant breathing tubes; rapid respiratory rates; and increased airway pressures.

Circuit Pressure

Breathing-circuit pressure is always measured somewhere between the expiratory and inspiratory unidirectional valves; the exact location depends on the model of anesthesia machine. Breathing-circuit pressure usually reflects airway pressure if it is measured as close to the patient's airway as possible. The most accurate measurements of both inspiratory and expiratory pressures can be obtained from the
6 Y-connection. A rise in airway pressure may signal worsening pulmonary compliance, an increase in tidal volume, or an obstruction in the breathing circuit, endotracheal tube, or the patient's airway. A drop in pressure may indicate an improvement in pulmonary compliance, a decrease in tidal volume, or a leak in the circuit. If circuit pressure is being measured at the CO_2 absorber, however, it will not always mirror the pressure in the patient's airway. For example, clamping the expiratory limb of the breathing tubes during exhalation will prevent the patient's breath from exiting the lungs. Despite this buildup in airway pressure, a pressure gauge at the absorber will read zero because of the intervening one-way valve. Some machines have incorporated auditory feedback for pressure changes during ventilator use.

Adjustable Pressure-Limiting Valve

The adjustable pressure-limiting (APL) valve, sometimes referred to as the *pressure relief* or *pop-off valve*, is usually fully open during spontaneous ventilation but must be partially closed during manual or assisted bag ventilation. The APL valve often requires fine adjustments. If it is not closed sufficiently, excessive loss of circuit volume due to leaks prevents manual ventilation. At the same time, if it is closed too much or is fully closed, a progressive rise in pressure could result in pulmonary barotrauma (eg, pneumothorax) or hemodynamic compromise, or both. As an added safety feature, the APL valves on modern machines act as true pressure-limiting devices that can never be completely closed; the upper limit is usually 70 to 80 cm H_2O.

Humidifiers

Absolute humidity is defined as the weight of water vapor in 1 L of gas (ie, mg/L). Relative humidity is the ratio of the actual mass of water present in a volume of gas to the maximum amount of water possible at a particular temperature. At 37°C and 100% relative humidity, absolute humidity is 44 mg/L, whereas at room temperature (21°C and 100% humidity), it is 18 mg/L. Inhaled gases in the operating room are normally administered at room temperature with little or no humidification. Gases must therefore be warmed to body temperature and saturated with water by the upper respiratory tract. Tracheal intubation and high fresh gas flow bypass this normal humidification system and expose the lower airways to dry (<10 mg H_2O/L), room temperature gases.

Prolonged humidification of gases by the lower respiratory tract leads to dehydration of mucosa, altered ciliary function, and, if excessively prolonged, could potentially lead to inspissation of secretions, atelectasis, and even ventilation/perfusion mismatching. Body heat is also lost as gases are warmed and, even more importantly, as water is vaporized to humidify the dry gases. The heat of vaporization for water is 560 cal/g of water vaporized. Fortunately, this heat loss accounts for about only 5% to 10% of total intraoperative heat loss, is not significant for a short procedure (<1 h), and usually can easily be compensated for with a forced-air warming blanket. Humidification and heating of inspiratory gases may be most important for small pediatric patients and older patients with severe underlying lung pathology (eg, cystic fibrosis).

A. Passive Humidifiers

Humidifiers added to the breathing circuit minimize water and heat loss. The simplest designs are condenser humidifiers or heat and moisture exchanger (HME) units (Figure 4–9). These passive devices do not add heat or vapor but rather contain a hygroscopic material that traps exhaled humidification and heat, which is released upon subsequent inhalation. Depending on the design, they may substantially increase apparatus dead space (more than 60 mL^3), which can cause significant rebreathing in pediatric patients. They can also increase breathing-circuit resistance and the work of breathing during spontaneous respirations. Excessive saturation of an HME with water or secretions can obstruct the breathing circuit. Some condenser humidifiers also act as effective filters that may protect the breathing circuit and anesthesia machine from bacterial or viral cross-contamination. This may be particularly important when ventilating patients with respiratory infections or compromised immune systems.

B. Active Humidifiers

Active humidifiers are more effective than passive ones in preserving moisture and heat. Active humidifiers add water to gas by passing the gas over a water chamber (passover humidifier) or through a saturated wick (wick humidifier), bubbling it through water (bubble-through humidifier), or mixing it with vaporized water (vapor-phase humidifier). Because increasing temperature increases the capacity of a gas to hold water vapor, heated humidifiers with thermostatically controlled elements are most effective.

The hazards of heated humidifiers include thermal lung injury (inhaled gas temperature should be monitored and should not exceed 41°C), nosocomial infection, increased airway resistance from excess water condensation in the breathing circuit, interference with flowmeter function, and an increased likelihood of circuit disconnection. The use of these humidifiers is particularly valuable in children as they help prevent both hypothermia and the plugging of small tracheal tubes by dried secretions. Of course, any design that increases airway dead space should be avoided in pediatric patients. Unlike passive humidifiers, active humidifiers do not filter respiratory gases.

VENTILATORS

All modern anesthesia machines are equipped with a ventilator. Historically, ventilators used in the operating room were simpler and more compact than their intensive care unit (ICU) counterparts. This distinction has become blurred due to advances in technology and an increasing need for "ICU-type" ventilators as more critically ill patients come to the operating room. The ventilators on some modern machines have the same capabilities as those in the ICU. Indeed, during the COVID-19 pandemic, anesthesia workstations were employed to provide mechanical ventilation when traditional ICU ventilators were unavailable. A complete discussion of mechanical ventilation and ventilator design is contained in Chapter 57.

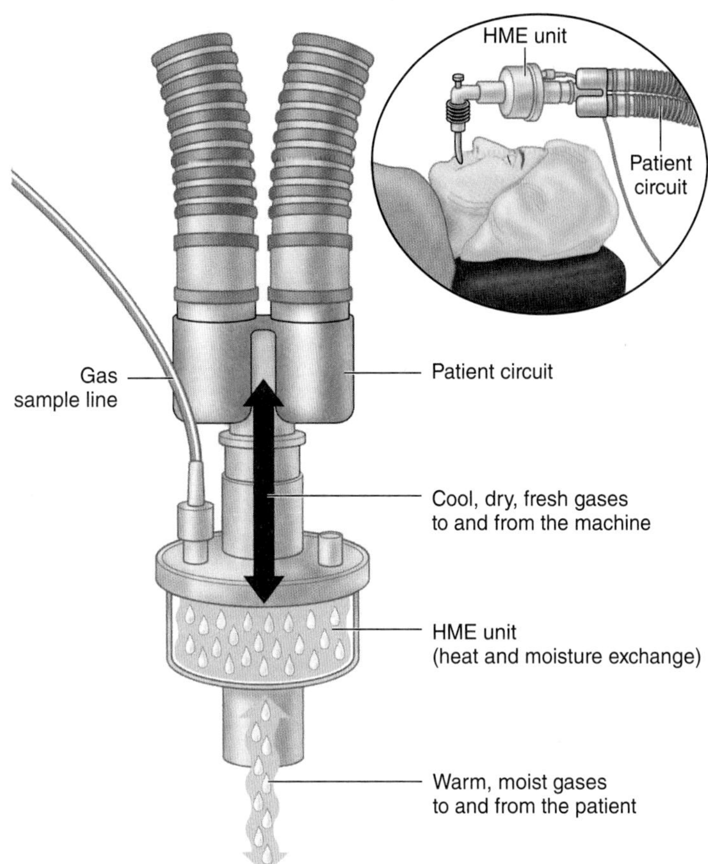

FIGURE 4–9 The heat and moisture exchanger (HME) functions as an "artificial nose" that attaches between the tracheal tube and the right-angle connector of the breathing circuit.

Overview

Ventilators generate gas flow by creating a pressure gradient between the proximal airway and the alveoli. Ventilator function is best described in relation to the four phases of the ventilatory cycle: inspiration, the transition from inspiration to expiration, expiration, and the transition from expiration to inspiration. Although several classification schemes exist, the most common is based on inspiratory phase characteristics and the method of cycling from inspiration to expiration.

A. Inspiratory Phase

During inspiration, ventilators generate tidal volumes by producing gas flow along a pressure gradient. The machine generates either a constant pressure (constant-pressure generators) or a constant gas flow rate (constant-flow generators) during inspiration, regardless of changes in lung mechanics (Figure 4–10). Nonconstant generators produce pressures or gas flow rates that vary during the cycle but remain consistent from breath to breath. For instance, a ventilator that generates a flow pattern resembling a half cycle of a sine wave (eg, rotary piston ventilator) would be classified as a nonconstant-flow generator. An increase in airway resistance or a decrease in lung compliance would increase peak inspiratory pressure but would not alter the flow rate generated by this type of ventilator (Figure 4–11).

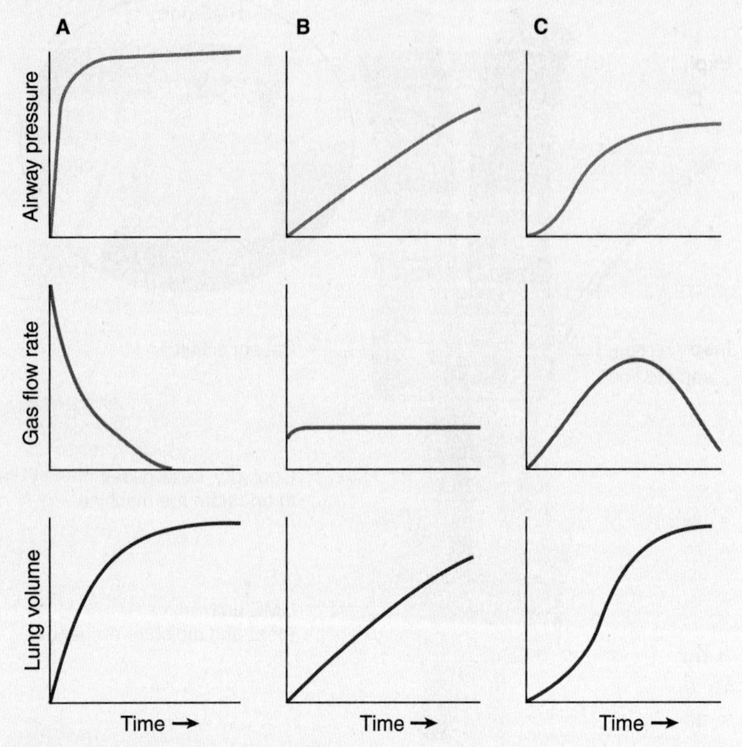

FIGURE 4–10 Pressure, volume, and flow profiles of different types of ventilators. **A**: Constant pressure. **B**: Constant flow. **C**: Nonconstant generator.

B. Transition Phase from Inspiration to Expiration

Termination of the inspiratory phase can be triggered by a preset limit of time (fixed duration), a set inspiratory pressure that must be reached, or a predetermined tidal volume that must be delivered. Time-cycled ventilators allow tidal volume and peak inspiratory pressure to vary depending on lung compliance. Tidal volume is adjusted by setting inspiratory duration and inspiratory flow rate. Pressure-cycled ventilators will not cycle from the inspiratory phase to the expiratory phase until a preset pressure is reached. If a large circuit leak decreases peak pressures significantly, a pressure-cycled ventilator may remain in the inspiratory phase indefinitely. On the other hand, a small leak may not markedly decrease tidal volume because cycling will be delayed until the pressure limit is met. Volume-cycled ventilators vary the inspiratory duration and pressure to deliver a preset volume. In reality, modern ventilators overcome the many shortcomings of classic ventilator designs by incorporating secondary cycling parameters or other limiting mechanisms.

C. Expiratory Phase

The expiratory phase of ventilators normally reduces airway pressure to atmospheric levels or some preset value of positive end-expiratory pressure (PEEP). Exhalation is therefore passive. Flow out of the lungs is determined primarily by airway resistance and lung compliance. Expired gases fill up the bellows; excess is relieved to the scavenging system.

D. Transition Phase from Expiration to Inspiration

Transition into the next inspiratory phase may be based on a preset time interval or a change in pressure. The behavior of the ventilator during this

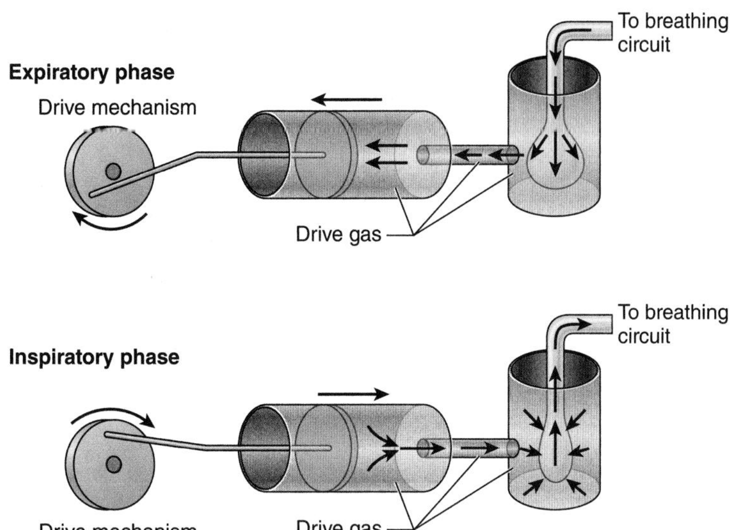

FIGURE 4–11 Rotary piston ventilator.

phase, together with the type of cycling from inspiration to expiration, determines ventilator mode. During controlled ventilation, the most basic mode of all ventilators, the next breath always occurs after a preset time interval. Thus, tidal volume and rate are fixed in volume-controlled ventilation, whereas peak inspiratory pressure and rate are fixed in pressure-controlled ventilation (Figure 4–12).

Ventilator Circuit Design

7 Traditionally, ventilators on anesthesia machines have a double-circuit system design and are pneumatically powered and electronically controlled (Figure 4–13). Newer machines also incorporate microprocessor controls and sophisticated and precise pressure and flow sensors to achieve multiple ventilatory modes, PEEP, accurate tidal volumes, and enhanced safety features.

A. Double-Circuit System Ventilators

In a double-circuit system design, tidal volume is delivered from a bellows assembly that consists of a bellows in a clear rigid plastic enclosure (Figure 4–13). A standing (ascending) bellows is preferred as it readily draws attention to a circuit disconnection by collapsing. Hanging (descending) bellows are rarely used and must not be weighted; older ventilators with weighted hanging bellows continue to fill by gravity despite a disconnection in the breathing circuit.

The bellows in a double-circuit design ventilator takes the place of the breathing bag in the anesthesia circuit. Pressurized oxygen or air from the ventilator power outlet (45–50 psig) is routed to the space between the inside wall of the plastic enclosure and the outside wall of the bellows. Pressurization of the plastic enclosure compresses the pleated bellows inside, forcing the gas inside into the breathing circuit and patient. In contrast, during exhalation, the bellows ascend as the pressure inside the plastic enclosure drops and the bellows fills up with the exhaled gas. A ventilator flow control valve regulates drive gas flow into the pressurizing chamber. This valve is controlled by ventilator settings in the control box (Figure 4–13). Ventilators with microprocessors also utilize feedback from flow and pressure sensors. If oxygen is used for pneumatic power, it will be consumed at a rate at least equal to minute ventilation. Thus, if oxygen fresh gas flow is 2 L/min and a ventilator is delivering 6 L/min to the circuit, a total of at least 8 L/min of oxygen is being consumed. This should be kept in mind if the hospital's medical gas system fails and cylinder oxygen is required. Some anesthesia machines reduce oxygen consumption by

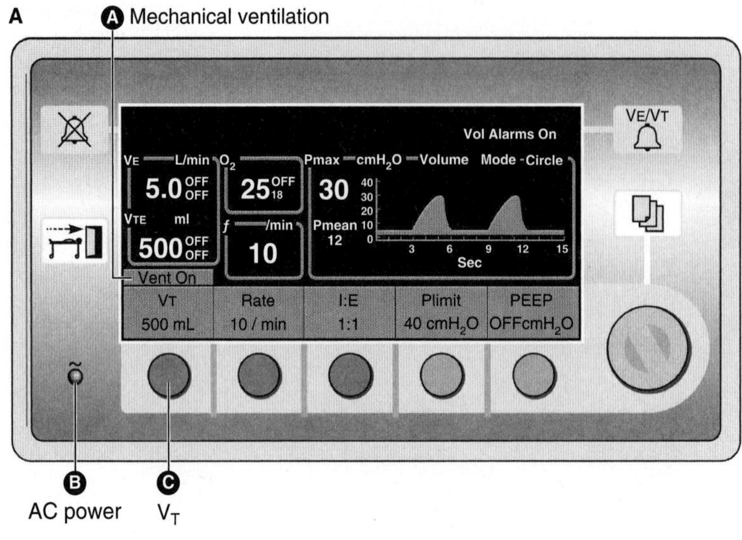

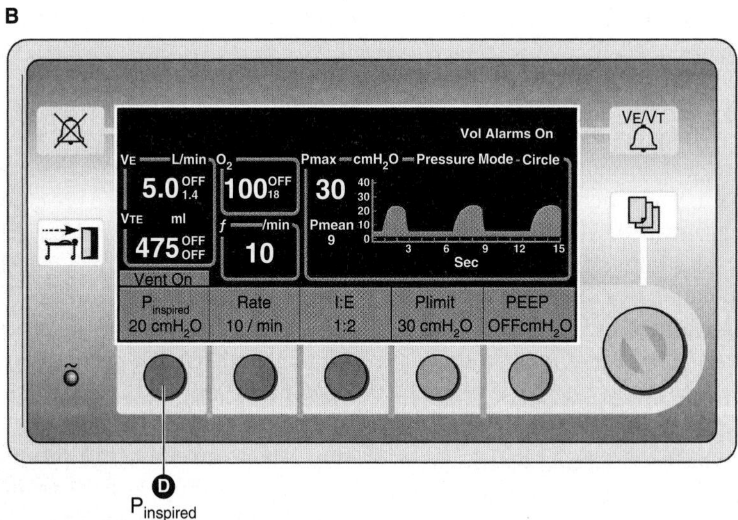

FIGURE 4–12 Ventilator controls (Datex-Ohmeda). **A**: Volume control mode. **B**: Pressure control mode.

incorporating a Venturi device that draws in room air to provide air/oxygen pneumatic power. Newer machines may offer the option of using compressed air for pneumatic power. A leak in the ventilator bellows can transmit high gas pressure to the patient's airway, potentially resulting in pulmonary barotrauma. **This may be indicated by a higher than expected rise in inspired oxygen concentration (if oxygen is the sole pressurizing gas).** Some machine ventilators have a built-in drive gas regulator that reduces the drive pressure (eg, to 25 psig) for added safety.

Double-circuit design ventilators also incorporate a free breathing valve that allows outside air to enter the rigid drive chamber and the bellows to collapse if the patient generates negative pressure by taking spontaneous breaths during mechanical ventilation.

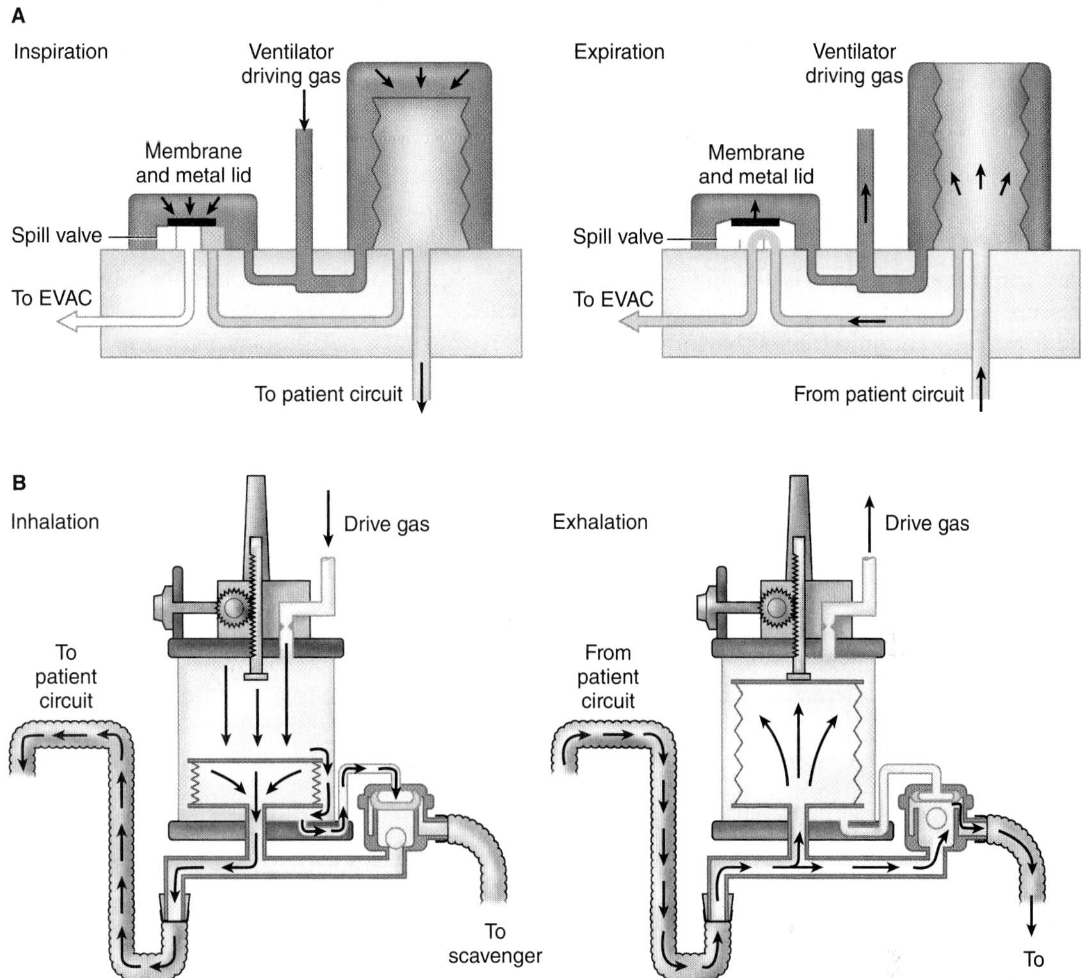

FIGURE 4–13 Double-circuit pneumatic ventilator design. **A**: Datex-Ohmeda. **B**: Dräger.

B. Piston Ventilators

In a piston design, the ventilator substitutes an electrically driven piston for the bellows, and the ventilator requires either minimal or no pneumatic (oxygen) power. The major advantage of a piston ventilator is its ability to deliver accurate tidal volumes to patients with very poor lung compliance and to very small patients.

8

C. Spill Valve

Whenever a ventilator is used on an anesthesia machine, the circle system's APL valve must be functionally removed or isolated from the circuit. A bag/ventilator switch typically accomplishes this. When the switch is turned to "bag," the ventilator is excluded, and spontaneous/manual (bag) ventilation is possible. When it is turned to "ventilator," the breathing bag and the APL are excluded from the breathing circuit. The APL valve may be automatically excluded in some newer anesthesia machines when the ventilator is turned on. The ventilator contains its own pressure-relief (pop-off) valve, called the *spill valve*, which is pneumatically closed during inspiration so that positive pressure can be generated (Figure 4–13). During exhalation, the pressurizing gas is vented out, and the ventilator spill valve is no longer closed.

The ventilator bellows or piston refills during expiration; when the bellows is completely filled, the increase in circle system pressure causes the excess gas to be directed to the scavenging system through the spill valve. Sticking of this valve can result in abnormally elevated airway pressure during exhalation.

Pressure & Volume Monitoring

Peak inspiratory pressure is the highest circuit pressure generated during an inspiratory cycle, and it provides an indication of dynamic compliance. Plateau pressure is the pressure measured during an inspiratory pause (a time of no gas flow), and it mirrors static compliance. During normal ventilation of a patient without lung disease, peak inspiratory pressure is equal to or only slightly greater than plateau pressure. An increase in both peak inspiratory pressure and plateau pressure implies an increase in tidal volume or a decrease in pulmonary compliance. An increase in peak inspiratory pressure without any change in plateau pressure signals an increase in airway resistance or inspiratory gas flow rate (Table 4–2). Thus, the shape of the breathing-circuit pressure waveform can provide important airway information. Many anesthesia machines graphically display breathing-circuit pressure (Figure 4–14). Airway secretions or kinking of the tracheal tube can be easily ruled out with the use of a suction catheter. Flexible fiberoptic bronchoscopy usually provides a definitive diagnosis.

TABLE 4–2 Causes of increased peak inspiratory pressure (PIP), with or without an increased plateau pressure (PP).

Increased PIP and PP
Increased tidal volume
Decreased pulmonary compliance
Pulmonary edema
Trendelenburg position
Pleural effusion
Ascites
Abdominal packing
Peritoneal gas insufflation
Tension pneumothorax
Endobronchial intubation
Increased PIP and Unchanged PP
Increased inspiratory gas flow rate
Increased airway resistance
Kinked endotracheal tube
Bronchospasm
Secretions
Foreign body aspiration
Airway compression
Endotracheal tube cuff herniation

Ventilator Alarms

Alarms are an integral part of all modern anesthesia
9 ventilators. Whenever a ventilator is used, "disconnect alarms" must be passively activated. Anesthesia workstations should have at least three disconnect alarms: low peak inspiratory pressure, low exhaled tidal volume, and low exhaled CO_2. The first is always built into the ventilator, whereas the latter two may be in separate modules. A small leak or partial breathing-circuit disconnection may be detected by subtle decreases in peak inspiratory pressure, exhaled volume, or end-tidal CO_2 before alarm thresholds are reached. Other built-in ventilator alarms include high peak inspiratory pressure, high PEEP, sustained high airway pressure, negative pressure, and low oxygen supply pressure. Most modern anesthesia ventilators also have integrated spirometers and oxygen analyzers that provide additional alarms.

Problems Associated with Anesthesia Ventilators

A. Ventilator–Fresh Gas Flow Coupling

10 From the previous discussion, it is important to appreciate that because the ventilator's spill valve is closed during inspiration, fresh gas flow from the machine's common gas outlet normally contributes to the tidal volume delivered to the patient. For example, if the fresh gas flow is 6 L/min, the inspiratory-expiratory (I:E) ratio is 1:2, and the respiratory rate is 10 breaths/min, each tidal volume will include an extra 200 mL in addition to the ventilator's output:

$$\frac{(6000 \text{ mL/min})(33\%)}{10 \text{ breaths/min}} \approx 200 \text{ mL/breath}$$

Thus, increasing fresh gas flow increases tidal volume, minute ventilation, and peak inspiratory pressure. To avoid problems with ventilator–fresh gas flow coupling, airway pressure and exhaled tidal volume must be monitored closely, and excessive fresh gas

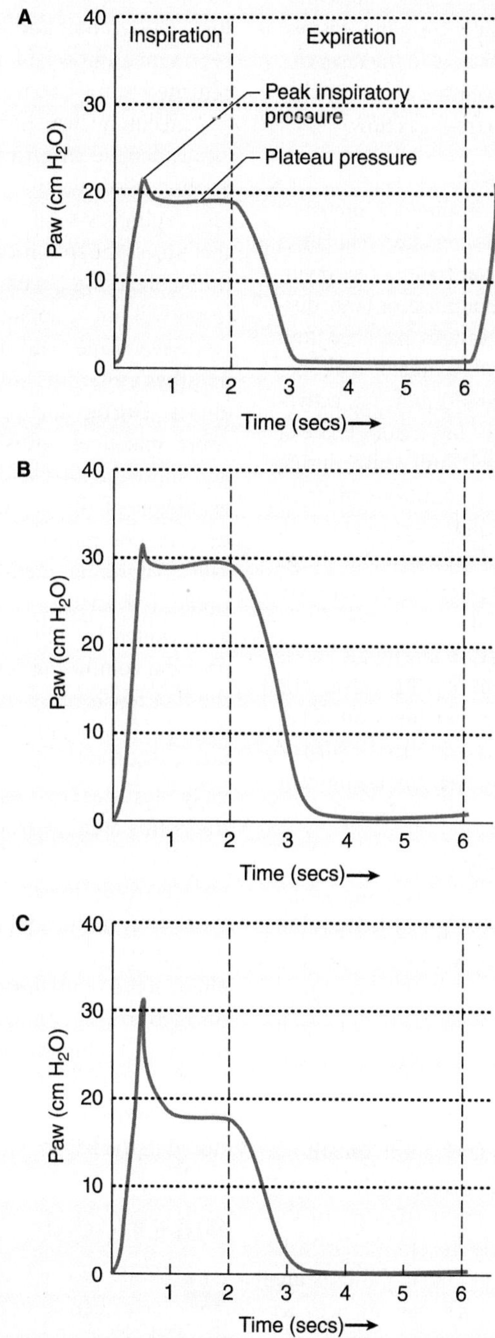

FIGURE 4–14 Airway pressures (Paw) can be diagrammatically presented as a function of time. **A**: In normal persons, the peak inspiratory pressure is equal to or slightly greater than the plateau pressure. **B**: An increase in peak inspiratory pressure and plateau pressure (the difference between the two remains almost constant) can be due to an increase in tidal volume or a decrease in pulmonary compliance. **C**: An increase in peak inspiratory pressure with little change in plateau pressure signals an increase in inspiratory flow rate or an increase in airway resistance.

flows must be avoided. Current ventilators automatically compensate for fresh gas flow coupling. Piston-style ventilators redirect fresh gas flow to the reservoir bag during inspiration, thus preventing augmentation of the tidal volume secondary to fresh gas flow.

B. Excessive Positive Pressure

Intermittent or sustained high inspiratory pressures (>30 mm Hg) during positive-pressure ventilation increase the risk of pulmonary barotrauma (eg, pneumothorax) or hemodynamic compromise, or both, during anesthesia. Excessively high pressures may arise from incorrect settings on the ventilator, ventilator malfunction, fresh gas flow coupling (discussed above), or activation of the oxygen flush during the inspiratory phase of the ventilator. Use of the oxygen flush valve during
11 the inspiratory cycle of a ventilator *must be avoided* because the ventilator spill valve will be closed and the APL valve is excluded; the surge of oxygen (600–1200 mL/s) and circuit pressure will be transferred to the patient's lungs.

In addition to a high-pressure alarm, all ventilators have a built-in automatic or APL valve. The mechanism of pressure limiting may be as simple as a threshold valve that opens at a certain pressure or electronic sensing that abruptly terminates the ventilator inspiratory phase.

C. Tidal Volume Discrepancies

12 Large discrepancies between the set and actual tidal volume that the patient receives are often observed in the operating room during volume-controlled ventilation. Causes include breathing-circuit compliance, gas compression, ventilator–fresh gas flow coupling (described above), and leaks in the anesthesia machine, the breathing circuit, or the patient's airway.

The compliance for standard adult breathing circuits is about 5 mL/cm H_2O. Thus, if peak inspiratory pressure is 20 cm H_2O, about 100 mL of set tidal volume is lost to expanding the circuit. For this reason, breathing circuits for pediatric patients are designed to be much stiffer, with compliances as small as 1.5 to 2.5 mL/cm H_2O.

Compression losses, normally about 3%, are due to gas compression within the ventilator bellows and may be dependent on breathing-circuit volume. Thus, if tidal volume is 500 mL, another 15 mL of the set tidal gas may be lost. Gas sampling for capnography and anesthetic gas measurements represent additional losses unless the sampled gas is returned to the breathing circuit.

Accurate detection of tidal volume discrepancies is dependent on where the spirometer is placed. Sophisticated ventilators measure both inspiratory and expiratory tidal volumes. It is important to note that unless the spirometer is placed at the Y-connector in the breathing circuit, compliance and compression losses will not be apparent.

Several mechanisms have been built into newer anesthesia machines to reduce tidal volume discrepancies. During the initial electronic self-checkout, some machines measure total system compliance and subsequently use this measurement to adjust the excursion of the ventilator bellows or piston; leaks may also be measured but are usually not compensated. The actual method of tidal volume compensation or modulation varies according to manufacturer and model. In one design, a flow sensor measures the tidal volume delivered at the inspiratory valve for the first few breaths and adjusts subsequent metered drive gas flow volumes to compensate for tidal volume losses (feedback adjustment). Another design continually measures fresh gas and vaporizer flow and subtracts this amount from the metered drive gas flow (preemptive adjustment). Alternately, machines that use electronic control of gas flow can decouple fresh gas flow from the tidal volume by delivery of fresh gas flow only during exhalation. Lastly, the inspiratory phase of the ventilator–fresh gas flow may be diverted through a decoupling valve into the breathing bag, which is excluded from the circle system during ventilation. During exhalation, the decoupling valve opens, allowing the fresh gas that was temporarily stored in the bag to enter the breathing circuit.

WASTE-GAS SCAVENGERS

13 Waste-gas scavengers dispose of gases that have been vented from the breathing circuit by the APL valve and ventilator spill valve. Pollution of the operating room environment with anesthetic gases may pose a health hazard to surgical personnel. Although it is difficult to define safe levels of exposure, the National Institute for Occupational

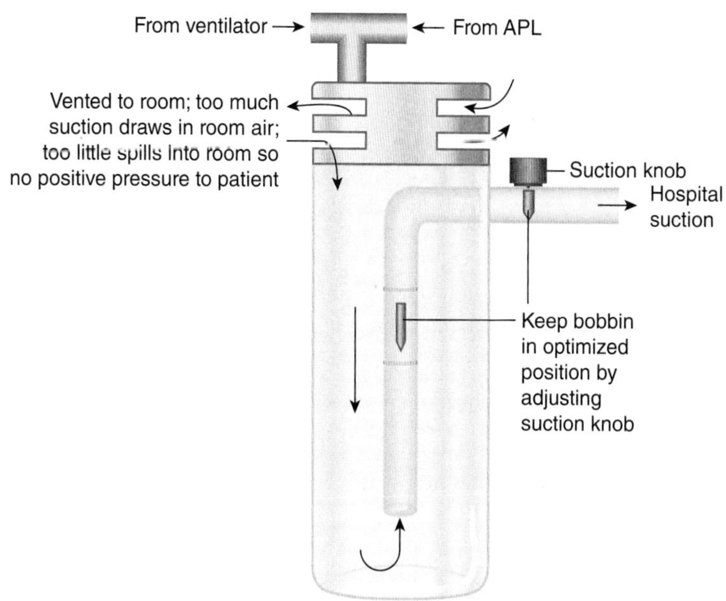

FIGURE 4–15 Open interface scavenger system. (Reproduced with permission from Rose G, McLarney JT: *Anesthesia Equipment Simplified.* New York, NY: McGraw Hill; 2014.)

Safety and Health (NIOSH) recommends limiting the room concentration of nitrous oxide to 25 ppm and halogenated agents to 2 ppm (0.5 ppm if nitrous oxide is also being used) in time-integrated samples. Reduction to these trace levels is possible only with properly functioning waste-gas scavenging systems.

To avoid the buildup of pressure, the excess gas volume is vented through the APL valve in the breathing circuit and the ventilator spill valve. Both valves should be connected to hoses (transfer tubing) leading to the scavenging interface, which may be inside the machine or an external attachment. The pressure immediately downstream to the interface should be kept between 0.5 and +3.5 cm H_2O during normal operating conditions. The scavenging interface may be described as either open or closed.

An open interface is open to the outside atmosphere and usually requires no pressure relief valves (Figure 4–15). In contrast, a closed interface is closed to the outside atmosphere and requires negative- and positive-pressure relief valves that protect the patient from the negative pressure of the vacuum system and positive pressure from an obstruction in the disposal tubing, respectively. The outlet of the scavenging system may be a direct line to the outside via a ventilation duct beyond any point of recirculation (passive scavenging) or a connection to the hospital's vacuum system (active scavenging). A chamber or reservoir bag accepts waste-gas overflow when the capacity of the vacuum is exceeded. The vacuum control valve on an active system should be adjusted to allow the evacuation of 10 to 15 L of waste gas per minute. This rate is adequate for periods of high fresh gas flow (ie, induction and emergence) yet minimizes the risk of transmitting negative pressure to the breathing circuit during lower flow conditions (maintenance). Unless an open interface is used correctly, the risk of occupational exposure for health care providers is greater with an open interface. Some machines may come with both active and passive scavenger systems.

ANESTHESIA MACHINE CHECKOUT LIST

Misuse or malfunction of anesthesia gas delivery equipment can cause major morbidity or mortality. 14 A routine inspection of anesthesia equipment before each use increases operator familiarity

TABLE 4–3 Anesthesia apparatus checkout recommendations.[1]

This checkout, or a reasonable equivalent, should be conducted before the administration of anesthesia. These recommendations are valid only for an anesthesia system that conforms to current and relevant standards and includes an ascending bellows ventilator and at least the following monitors: capnograph, pulse oximeter, oxygen analyzer, respiratory volume monitor (spirometer), and breathing-system pressure monitor with high- and low-pressure alarms. Users are encouraged to modify this guideline to accommodate differences in equipment design and variations in local clinical practice. Such local modifications should have appropriate peer review. Users should refer to the appropriate operator manuals for specific procedures and precautions.

Emergency Ventilation Equipment

*1. Verify that backup ventilation equipment is available and functioning.

High-Pressure System

*2. Check the O_2 cylinder supply.
   a. Open the O_2 cylinder, and verify it is at least half full (about 1000 psig).
   b. Close the cylinder.

*3. Check central pipeline supplies; check that hoses are connected and pipeline gauges read about 50 psig.

Low-Pressure System

*4. Check the initial status of the low-pressure system.
   a. Close flow control valves and turn vaporizers off.
   b. Check the fill level and tighten vaporizers' filler caps.

*5. Perform a leak check of the machine's low-pressure system.
   a. Verify that the machine master switch and flow control valves are off.
   b. Attach the suction bulb to the common (fresh) gas outlet.
   c. Squeeze the bulb repeatedly until fully collapsed.
   d. Verify the bulb stays *fully* collapsed for at least 10 seconds.
   e. Open one vaporizer at a time, and repeat steps c and d.
   f. Remove the suction bulb, and reconnect the fresh gas hose.

*6. Turn on the machine master switch and all other necessary electrical equipment.

*7. Test flowmeters.
   a. Adjust the flow of all gases through their full range, checking for smooth operation of floats and undamaged flow tubes.
   b. Attempt to create a hypoxic O_2/N_2O mixture, and verify the correct changes in the flow or alarm.

Scavenging System

*8. Adjust and check the scavenging system.
   a. Ensure proper connections between the scavenging system and both the APL (pop-off) valve and the ventilator relief valve.
   b. Adjust the waste-gas vacuum (if possible).
   c. Fully open the APL valve and occlude the Y-piece.
   d. With minimum O_2 flow, allow the scavenger reservoir bag to collapse completely, and verify that the absorber pressure gauge reads about zero.
   e. With the O_2 flush activated, allow the scavenger reservoir bag to distend fully, and then verify that the absorber pressure gauge reads <10 cm H_2O.

Breathing System

*9. Calibrate the O_2 monitor.
   a. Ensure the monitor reads 21% in room air.
   b. Verify that the low-O_2 alarm is enabled and functioning.
   c. Reinstall the sensor in the circuit and flush the breathing system with O_2.
   d. Verify that the monitor now reads greater than 90%.

10. Check the initial status breathing system.
   a. Set the selector switch to Bag mode.
   b. Check that the breathing circuit is complete, undamaged, and unobstructed.
   c. Verify that CO_2 absorbent is adequate.
   d. Install the breathing-circuit accessory equipment (eg, humidifier, PEEP valve) to be used during the case.

11. Perform a leak check of the breathing system.
   a. Set all gas flows to zero (or minimum).
   b. Close the APL (pop-off) valve, and occlude the Y-piece.
   c. Pressurize the breathing system to about 30 cm H_2O with O_2 flush.
   d. Ensure that the pressure remains fixed for at least 10 seconds.
   e. Open the APL (pop-off) valve and ensure that pressure decreases.

Manual and Automatic Ventilation Systems

12. Test ventilation systems and unidirectional valves.
   a. Place a second breathing bag on the Y-piece.
   b. Set appropriate ventilator parameters for the next patient.
   c. Switch to automatic-ventilation (ventilator) mode.
   d. Turn the ventilator on, and fill the bellows and breathing bag with O_2 flush.
   e. Set O_2 flow to minimum and other gas flows to zero.
   f. Verify that during inspiration the bellows delivers the appropriate tidal volume and that during expiration the bellows fills completely.
   g. Set the fresh gas flow to about 5 L min^{-1}.
   h. Verify that the ventilator bellows and simulated lungs fill and empty appropriately without sustained pressure at end expiration.
   i. Check for proper action of unidirectional valves.
   j. Exercise breathing circuit accessories to ensure proper function.
   k. Turn the ventilator off, and switch to manual ventilation (Bag/APL) mode.
   l. Ventilate manually, and ensure inflation and deflation of artificial lungs and appropriate feel of system resistance and compliance.
   m. Remove the second breathing bag from the Y-piece.

(*continued*)

TABLE 4–3 Anesthesia apparatus checkout recommendations.[1] (Continued)

Monitors 13. Check, calibrate, or set alarm limits of all monitors: capnograph, pulse oximeter, O_2 analyzer, respiratory-volume monitor (spirometer), and pressure monitor with high and low airway-pressure alarms.	*Final Position* 14. Check the final status of the machine. a. Vaporizers off b. APL valve open c. Selector switch to Bag mode d. All flowmeters to zero (or minimum) e. Patient suction level adequate f. Breathing system ready to use

[1]Data from the U.S. Food and Drug Administration and the U.S. Department of Health and Human Services.

[2]APL, adjustable pressure-limiting; CO_2, carbon dioxide; H_2O, water; O_2, oxygen; PEEP, positive end-expiratory pressure.

*If an anesthesia provider uses the same machine in successive cases, these steps need not be repeated, or they can be abbreviated after the initial checkout.

and confirms proper functioning. The U.S. Food and Drug Administration (FDA) has made available a generic checkout procedure for anesthesia gas machines and breathing systems (Table 4–3). This procedure should be modified as necessary, depending on the specific equipment being used and the manufacturer's recommendations. Note that although the entire checkout does not need to be repeated between cases on the same day, the conscientious use of an abbreviated checkout list is mandatory before each anesthetic procedure. A mandatory check-off procedure increases the likelihood of detecting anesthesia machine faults. Some anesthesia machines provide an automated system check that requires a variable amount of human intervention. These system checks may include nitrous oxide delivery (hypoxic mixture prevention), agent delivery, mechanical and manual ventilation, pipeline pressures, scavenging, breathing circuit compliance, and gas leakage.

CASE DISCUSSION

Detection of a Leak

After induction of general anesthesia and intubation of a 70-kg patient for elective surgery, a standing bellows ventilator is set to deliver a tidal volume of 500 mL at a rate of 10 breaths/min. Within a few minutes, the anesthesiologist notices that the bellows fails to rise to the top of its clear plastic enclosure during expiration. Shortly thereafter, the disconnect alarm is triggered.

Why has the ventilator bellows fallen and the disconnect alarm sounded?

Fresh gas flow into the breathing circuit is inadequate to maintain the circuit volume required for positive-pressure ventilation. In a situation in which there is no fresh gas flow, the volume in the breathing circuit will slowly fall because of the constant uptake of oxygen by the patient (metabolic oxygen consumption) and absorption of expired CO_2. An absence of fresh gas flow could be due to exhaustion of the hospital's oxygen supply (remember the function of the fail-safe valve) or failure to turn on the anesthesia machine's flow control valves. These possibilities can be ruled out by examining the oxygen pressure gauge and the flowmeters. A more likely explanation is a gas leak that exceeds the rate of fresh gas flow. Leaks are particularly important in closed-circuit anesthesia.

How can the size of the leak be estimated?

When the rate of fresh gas inflow equals the rate of gas outflow, the circuit's volume will be maintained. Therefore, the size of the leak can be estimated by increasing fresh gas flows until there is no change in the height of the bellows from one expiration to the next. If the bellows collapse despite a high rate of fresh gas inflow, a complete circuit disconnection should be considered. The site of the disconnection must be determined immediately and repaired to prevent hypoxia and hypercapnia. A resuscitation bag must be immediately available and can be used to ventilate the patient if there is a delay in correcting the situation.

Where are the most likely locations of a breathing-circuit disconnection or leak?

Frank disconnections occur most frequently between the right-angle connector and the tracheal tube, whereas leaks are most commonly traced to the base plate of the CO_2 absorber. In the intubated patient, leaks often occur in the trachea around an uncuffed tracheal tube or an inadequately filled cuff. There are numerous potential sites of disconnection or leak within the anesthesia machine and the breathing circuit, however. Every addition to the breathing circuit, such as a humidifier, provides another potential location for a leak.

How can these leaks be detected?

Leaks may occur before the fresh gas outlet (ie, within the anesthesia machine) or after the fresh gas inlet (ie, within the breathing circuit). Large leaks within the anesthesia machine are less common and can be ruled out by a simple test. Pinching the tubing that connects the machine's fresh gas outlet to the circuit's fresh gas inlet creates a back pressure that obstructs the forward flow of fresh gas from the anesthesia machine. This is indicated by a drop in the height of the flowmeter floats. When the fresh gas tubing is released, the floats should briskly rebound and settle at their original height. If there is a substantial leak within the machine, obstructing the fresh gas tubing will not result in any back pressure, and the floats will not drop. A more sensitive test for detecting small leaks that occur before the fresh gas outlet involves attaching a suction bulb at the outlet, as described in step 5 of Table 4–3. Correcting a leak within the machine will usually require removing it from service.

Leaks within a breathing circuit not connected to a patient are readily detected by closing the APL valve, occluding the Y-piece, and activating the oxygen flush until the circuit reaches a pressure of 20 to 30 cm H_2O. A gradual decline in circuit pressure indicates a leak within the breathing circuit (Table 4–3, step 11).

How are leaks in the breathing circuit located?

Any connection within the breathing circuit is a potential site of a gas leak. A quick survey of the circuit may reveal a loosely attached breathing tube or a cracked oxygen analyzer adaptor. Less obvious causes include detachment of the tubing used by the disconnect alarm to monitor circuit pressures, an open APL valve, or an improperly adjusted scavenging unit. Leaks can usually be identified audibly or by applying a soap solution to suspect connections and looking for bubble formation.

Leaks within the anesthesia machine and breathing circuit are usually detectable if the machine and circuit have undergone an established checkout procedure. For example, steps 5 and 11 of the FDA recommendations (Table 4–3) will reveal most leaks.

SUGGESTED READINGS

Haina KMK Jr. Use of anesthesia machines in a critical care setting during the coronavirus disease 2019 pandemic. *A Pract.* 2020;14:e01243.

Hendrickx JFA, De Wolf AM. The anesthesia workstation: quo vadis? *Anesth Analg.* 2018;127:671.

Kuck K, Johnson KB. The three laws of autonomous and closed-loop systems in anesthesia. *Anesth Analg.* 2017;124:377.

Mehta S, Eisenkraft J, Posner K, Domino K. Patient injuries from anesthesia gas delivery equipment. *Anesthesiology.* 2013;119:788.

Rose G, McLarnery J, eds. *Anesthesia Equipment Simplified.* McGraw-Hill Education; 2014.

Sherwin MA, Eisenkraft JB. Anesthesia hazards: what is the role of the anesthesia machine? *Int Anesthesiol Clin.* 2020;58:27.

WEBSITES

The Anesthesia Patient Safety Foundation website provides resources and a newsletter that discusses important safety issues in anesthesia. http://www.apsf.org/

The website of the American Society of Anesthesiologists includes a link to the 2008 ASA Recommendations for Pre-Anesthesia Checkout (https://www.asahq.org/resources/clinical-information/2008-asa-recommendations-for-pre-anesthesia-checkout). https://www.asahq.org/clinical/fda.aspx

CHAPTER 5

Cardiovascular Monitoring

KEY CONCEPTS

1. The tip of the central venous pressure catheter should not be allowed to migrate into the heart chambers.
2. Although the pulmonary artery (PA) catheter can be used to guide goal-directed hemodynamic therapy to ensure organ perfusion in shock states, other less invasive methods to determine hemodynamic performance are available, including transpulmonary thermodilution cardiac output (CO) measurements, pulse contour analyses of the arterial pressure waveform, and methods based on bioimpedance measurements across the chest.
3. Relative contraindications to PA catheterization include left bundle-branch block (because of the concern about complete heart block) and conditions associated with a greatly increased risk of arrhythmias.
4. Pulmonary artery pressure should be continuously monitored to detect an overwedged position indicative of catheter migration.
5. Accurate measurements of CO depend on rapid and smooth injection, precisely known injectant temperature and volume, correct entry of the calibration factors for the specific type of PA catheter into the CO computer, and avoidance of measurements during electrocautery.

Vigilant perioperative monitoring of the cardiovascular system is one of the primary duties of anesthesia providers. The American Society of Anesthesiologists has established standards for basic anesthesia monitoring, which includes continuous monitoring of oxygenation, ventilation, circulation, and temperature throughout the anesthetic. This chapter focuses on the specific monitoring devices and techniques used to monitor cardiac function and circulation in healthy and nonhealthy patients alike.

ARTERIAL BLOOD PRESSURE

The rhythmic contraction of the left ventricle, ejecting blood into the arterial tree, results in pulsatile arterial pressures. The peak left ventricular end-systolic pressure (in the absence of aortic valve stenosis) approximates the systolic arterial blood pressure (SBP); the lowest arterial pressure during diastolic relaxation is the diastolic blood pressure (DBP). Pulse pressure is the difference between the systolic and diastolic pressures. The time-weighted average of arterial pressures during a pulse cycle is the **mean arterial pressure (MAP).** MAP can be estimated by application of the following formula:

$$\text{MAP} = \frac{(\text{SBP}) + 2(\text{DBP})}{3}$$

Arterial blood pressure varies depending upon where within the vasculature the pressure is measured. **As a pulse moves peripherally through the arterial tree, wave reflection distorts the pressure**

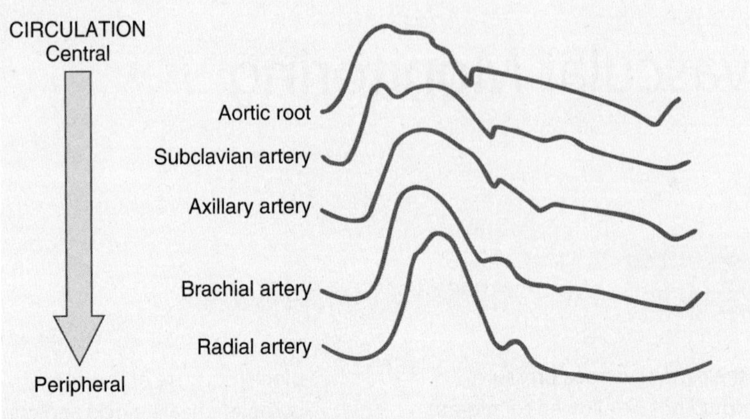

FIGURE 5–1 Changes in configuration as a waveform moves peripherally. (Reproduced with permission from Lake CL, Hines RL, Blitt CD. *Clinical Monitoring: Practical Applications in Anesthesia and Critical Care Medicine.* Philadelphia, PA: WB Saunders; 2001.)

waveform, leading to an exaggeration of systolic and pulse pressures (Figure 5–1). For example, radial artery systolic pressure is usually greater than aortic systolic pressure because of its more distal location. In contrast, radial artery systolic pressures often underestimate more "central" pressures immediately following hypothermic cardiopulmonary bypass because of changes in hand vascular resistance. Vasodilating drugs may accentuate this discrepancy. The level of the sampling site relative to the heart affects the measurement of blood pressure because of the effect of gravity (Figure 5–2). In patients with severe peripheral vascular disease, there may be significant differences in blood pressure measurements among the extremities. The greater value should be used in these patients.

Because noninvasive (palpation, Doppler, auscultation, oscillometry, plethysmography, volume clamp) and invasive (arterial cannulation) methods of blood pressure determination differ greatly, they are discussed separately.

1. Noninvasive Arterial Blood Pressure Monitoring

Indications

The use of any anesthetic is an indication for arterial blood pressure measurement. The techniques and frequency of pressure determination will depend on the patient's condition and the type of surgical procedure. A noninvasive blood pressure measurement every 3 to 5 minutes is adequate in most cases.

Contraindications

Although some method of blood pressure measurement is mandatory, techniques that rely on a blood pressure cuff are best avoided in extremities with vascular abnormalities (eg, dialysis shunts) or with intravenous lines. It rarely may prove impossible to monitor blood pressure in patients (eg, those who have burns) who have no accessible site from which the blood pressure can be safely recorded.

Techniques & Complications

A. Palpation

SBP can be determined by (1) locating a palpable peripheral pulse, (2) inflating a blood pressure cuff proximal to the pulse until flow is occluded, (3) releasing cuff pressure by 2 or 3 mm Hg per heartbeat, and (4) measuring the cuff pressure at which pulsations are again palpable. This method tends to underestimate systolic pressure, however, because of the insensitivity of touch and the delay between flow under the cuff and distal pulsations. Palpation does not provide a diastolic pressure or MAP. The equipment required is simple and inexpensive.

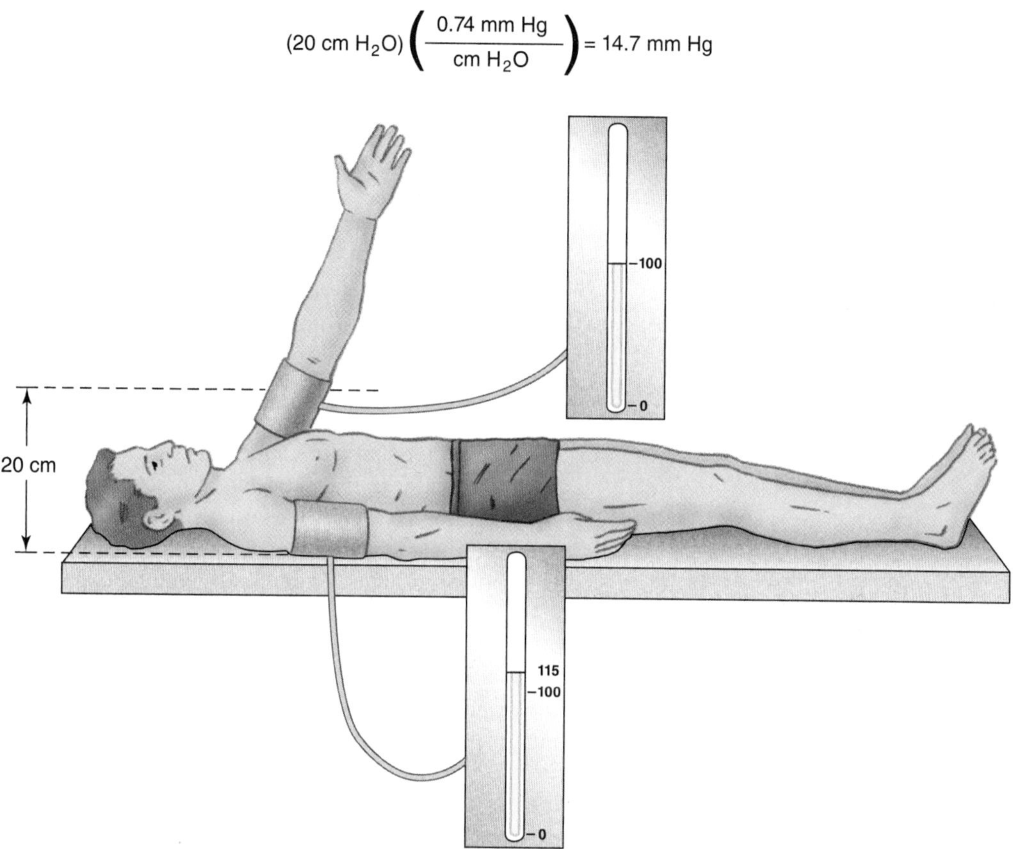

FIGURE 5–2 The difference in blood pressure (mm Hg) at two different sites of measurement equals the height of an interposed column of water (cm H_2O) multiplied by a conversion factor (1 cm H_2O = 0.74 mm Hg).

B. Doppler Probe

When a Doppler probe is substituted for the anesthesiologist's finger, arterial blood pressure measurement becomes sensitive enough to be useful in obese patients, pediatric patients, and patients in shock (Figure 5–3). The **Doppler effect** is the shift in the frequency of sound waves when their source moves relative to the observer. For example, the pitch of a train's whistle increases as a train approaches and decreases as it departs. Similarly, the reflection of sound waves off of a moving object causes a frequency shift. A Doppler probe transmits an ultrasonic signal that is reflected by underlying tissue. As red blood cells move through an artery, a Doppler frequency shift will be detected by the probe. The difference between transmitted and received frequency causes the characteristic swishing sound, which indicates blood flow. Because air reflects ultrasound, a coupling gel (but not corrosive electrode jelly) is applied between the probe and the skin. Note that only systolic pressures can be reliably determined with the Doppler technique.

C. Auscultation

Inflation of a blood pressure cuff to a pressure between systolic and diastolic pressures will partially collapse an underlying artery, producing turbulent flow and the characteristic Korotkoff sounds. These sounds are audible through a stethoscope placed under—or just distal to—the distal third of the blood pressure cuff. The clinician measures pressure with an aneroid or mercury manometer.

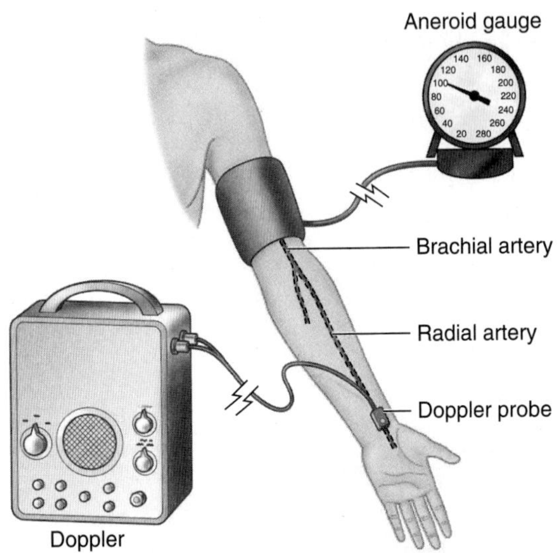

FIGURE 5–3 A Doppler probe secured over the radial artery will sense red blood cell movement as long as the blood pressure cuff is below systolic pressure. (Reproduced with permission from Parks Medical Electronics.)

Occasionally, Korotkoff sounds cannot be heard through part of the range from systolic to diastolic pressure. This auscultatory gap is most common in hypertensive patients and can lead to an inaccurate diastolic pressure measurement. Korotkoff sounds are often difficult to auscultate in noisy patient care environments and during episodes of hypotension or marked peripheral vasoconstriction.

D. Oscillometry

Arterial pulsations cause oscillations in cuff pressure. These oscillations are small if the cuff is inflated above systolic pressure. When the cuff pressure decreases to systolic pressure, the pulsations are transmitted to the entire cuff, and the oscillations markedly increase. Maximal oscillation occurs at the MAP, after which oscillations decrease. Because some oscillations are present above and below arterial blood pressure, a mercury or aneroid manometer provides an inaccurate and unreliable measurement. Automated blood pressure monitors electronically measure the pressures at which the oscillation amplitudes change (Figure 5–4). A microprocessor derives systolic, mean, and diastolic pressures using an algorithm. Machines that require identical consecutive pulse waves for measurement confirmation may be unreliable during arrhythmias (eg, atrial fibrillation). Oscillometric monitors should not be used on patients on cardiopulmonary bypass. Nonetheless, the speed, accuracy, and versatility of oscillometric

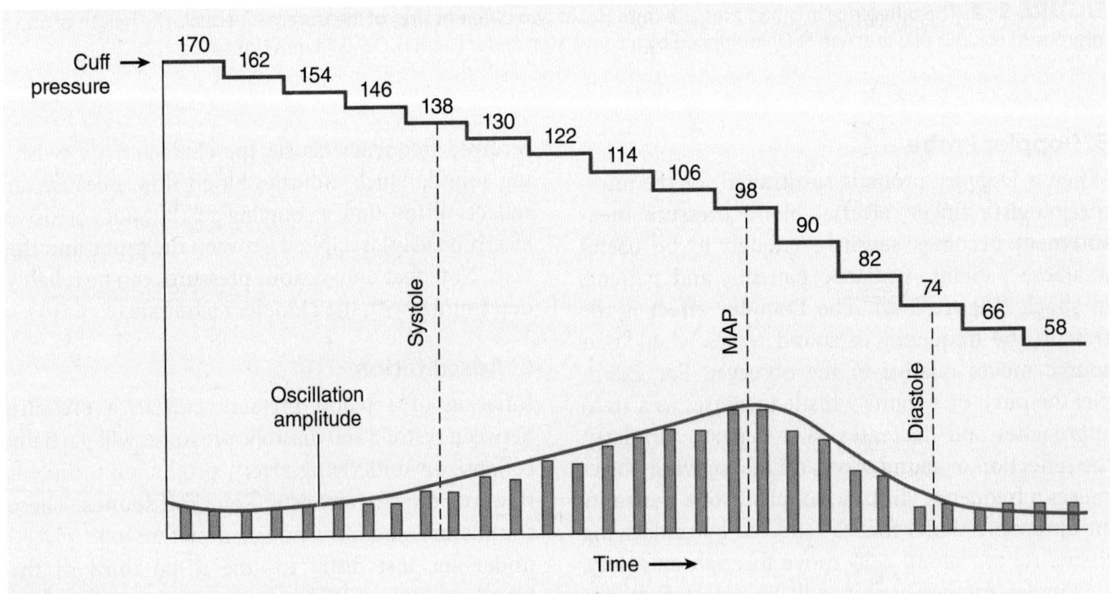

FIGURE 5–4 Oscillometric determination of blood pressure. MAP, mean arterial pressure.

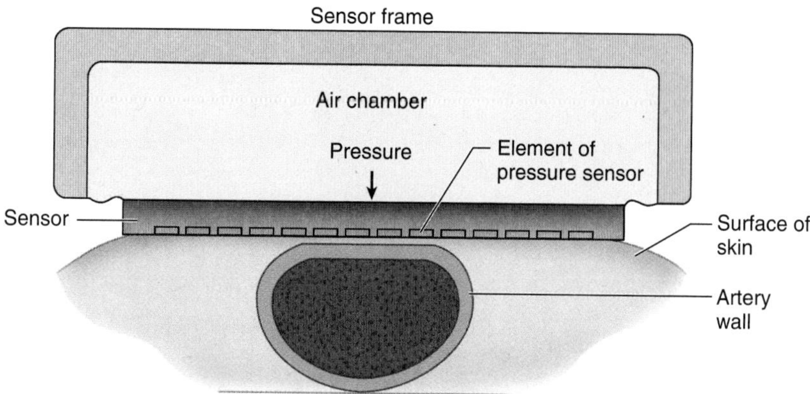

FIGURE 5–5A Tonometry is a method of continuous (beat-to-beat) arterial blood pressure determination. The sensors must be positioned directly over the artery.

devices have greatly improved, and they have become the preferred noninvasive blood pressure monitors in the United States and worldwide.

E. Arterial Tonometry and the Finger Cuff Method

Arterial tonometry measures beat-to-beat arterial blood pressure by sensing the pressure required to partially flatten a superficial artery that is supported by a bony structure (eg, radial artery). A tonometer consisting of several independent pressure transducers is applied to the skin overlying the artery (Figure 5–5A). The contact stress between the transducer directly over the artery and the skin reflects intraluminal pressure. Continuous pulse recordings produce a tracing very similar to an invasive arterial blood pressure waveform. Limitations to this technology include sensitivity to movement artifact and the need for frequent calibration.

The finger cuff method uses an inflatable finger cuff and an infrared light detector measure the changing finger diameter to generate a pressure waveform (Figure 5–5B). These devices apply pressure to the finger to determine MAP and generate a

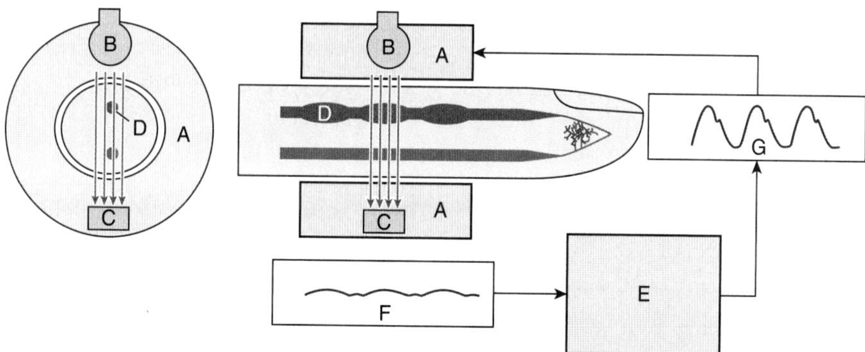

FIGURE 5–5B Finger cuff method (vascular unloading technique, volume clamp method). Schematic illustration showing the measurement principle of the finger cuff method. An inflatable finger cuff **(A)** with an integrated infrared photodiode **(B)** and light detector **(C)** applies pressure to the finger and measures the diameter (ie, blood volume) of the finger artery **(D)**. The cuff pressure is adjusted automatically using a control system **(E)** to keep the diameter of the finger artery constant (and the arterial wall "unloaded"). From the pressure needed to keep the volume in the finger artery constant **(F)** throughout the cardiac cycle, the arterial blood pressure waveform can be derived indirectly **(G)**. With this blood pressure waveform, cardiac output can be estimated using pulse wave analysis. (Reproduced with permission from Saugel B, Dueck R, Wagner JY. Measurement of blood pressure, *Best Pract Res Clin Anaesthesiol.* 2014 Dec;28(4):309-322.)

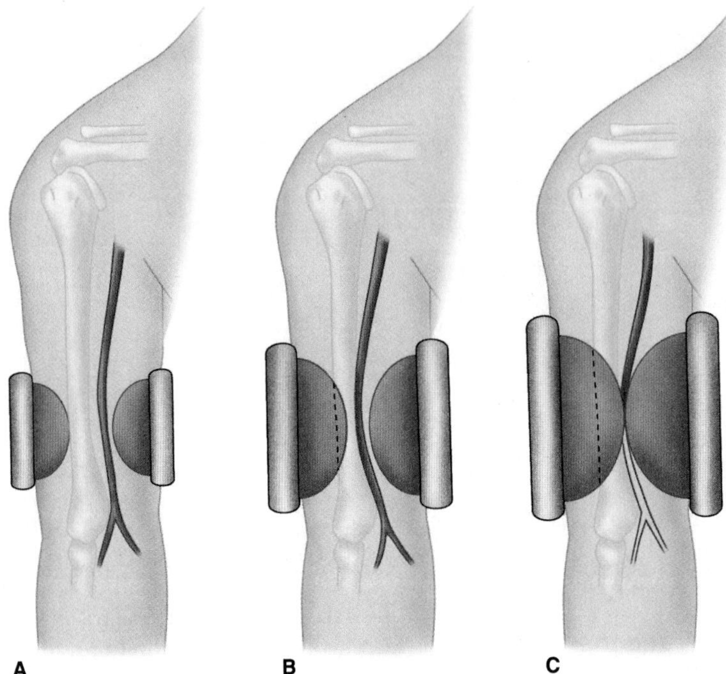

FIGURE 5–6 Blood pressure cuff width influences the pressure readings. The narrowest cuff **(A)** will require more pressure and the widest cuff **(B)** normal cuff size **(C)** will require less pressure to occlude the brachial artery for the determination of systolic pressure. Too narrow a cuff may produce a large overestimation of systolic pressure. Whereas the wider cuff may underestimate the systolic pressure, the error with a cuff 20% too wide is not as significant as the error with a cuff 20% too narrow. (Reproduced with permission from Gravenstein JS, Paulus DA. *Clinical Monitoring Practice.* 2nd ed. Philadelphia, PA: Lippincott Williams & Wilkins; 1987.)

waveform from which a cardiac output (CO) measurement is calculated. A 2018 study demonstrated that patients who had continuous noninvasive blood pressure monitoring experienced reduced duration and severity of intraoperative hypotension compared with patients who had intermittently monitored blood pressure.

Clinical Considerations

Adequate oxygen delivery to vital organs must be maintained during anesthesia. Unfortunately, instruments to monitor specific organ perfusion and oxygenation are complex, expensive, and often unreliable, and for that reason, an adequate arterial blood pressure is assumed to predict adequate organ blood flow. However, flow also depends on vascular resistance:

$$\text{Flow} = \frac{\text{Pressure}}{\text{Resistance}}$$

Even if the pressure is high, when the resistance is also high, flow can be low. Thus, arterial blood pressure should be viewed as an indicator—but not a measure—of organ perfusion.

The accuracy of any method of blood pressure measurement that involves a blood pressure cuff depends on proper cuff size (Figure 5–6). The cuff's bladder should extend at least halfway around the extremity, and the width of the cuff should be 20% to 50% greater than the diameter of the extremity.

Automated blood pressure monitors, using one or a combination of the methods described previously, are frequently used in anesthesiology. A self-contained air pump inflates the cuff at set intervals. Incorrect placement or too-frequent cycling of these automated devices has resulted in nerve palsies, and when they are placed on the same extremity as an intravenous catheter, there can be extravasation of intravenously administered fluids or blood products.

2. Invasive Arterial Blood Pressure Monitoring

Indications

Indications for invasive arterial blood pressure monitoring by catheterization of an artery include current or anticipated hypotension or wide blood pressure deviations, end-organ disease necessitating beat-to-beat blood pressure regulation, and the need for multiple arterial blood gas or other blood analyses.

Contraindications

If possible, catheterization should be avoided in smaller end arteries lacking collateral blood flow or in extremities where there is a suspicion of preexisting vascular insufficiency.

A. Selection of Artery for Cannulation

Several arteries are available for percutaneous catheterization.

1. The **radial artery** is commonly cannulated because of its superficial location and substantial collateral flow (in most patients, the ulnar artery is larger than the radial, and there are connections between the two via the palmar arches). Five percent of patients have incomplete palmar arches and lack adequate collateral blood flow. The Allen test is a simple but not reliable method for assessing the safety of radial artery cannulation. In this test, the patient exsanguinates their hand by making a fist. While the operator occludes the radial and ulnar arteries with fingertip pressure, the patient relaxes the blanched hand. Collateral flow through the palmar arterial arch is confirmed by flushing of the thumb within 5 seconds after pressure on the ulnar artery is released. Delayed return of normal color (5–10 s) indicates an equivocal test or insufficient collateral circulation (>10 s). The Allen test is of such questionable utility that many practitioners routinely avoid it. Alternatively, blood flow distal to the radial artery occlusion can be detected by palpation, Doppler probe, plethysmography, or pulse oximetry. Unlike the Allen test, these methods of determining the adequacy of collateral circulation do not require patient cooperation.
2. **Ulnar artery** catheterization is usually more difficult than radial catheterization because of the ulnar artery's deeper and more tortuous course. Because of the risk of compromising blood flow to the hand, ulnar catheterization would not normally be considered if the ipsilateral radial artery has been punctured but unsuccessfully cannulated.
3. The **brachial artery** is large and easily identifiable in the antecubital fossa. Its proximity to the aorta provides less waveform distortion. However, being near the elbow predisposes brachial artery catheters to kinking.
4. The **femoral artery** is prone to atheroma formation and pseudoaneurysm but often provides excellent access. The femoral site has been associated with an increased incidence of infectious complications and arterial thrombosis. Aseptic necrosis of the head of the femur is a rare but tragic complication of femoral artery cannulation in children.
5. The **dorsalis pedis and posterior tibial arteries** are some distance from the aorta and therefore have the most distorted waveforms.
6. The **axillary artery** is surrounded by the axillary plexus, and nerve damage can result from a hematoma or traumatic cannulation. Air or thrombi can quickly gain access to the cerebral circulation during vigorous retrograde flushing of axillary artery catheters. Nevertheless, in extensively burned patients, the axillary artery may be the best option.

B. Technique of Radial Artery Cannulation

One technique of radial artery cannulation is illustrated in Figure 5–7. Supination and extension of the wrist optimally position the radial artery. The pressure–tubing–transducer system should be nearby and already flushed with saline to ensure an easy and quick connection after cannulation. The radial pulse is palpated, and the artery's course is determined by lightly pressing the *tips* of the index and middle fingers of the nondominant hand over the

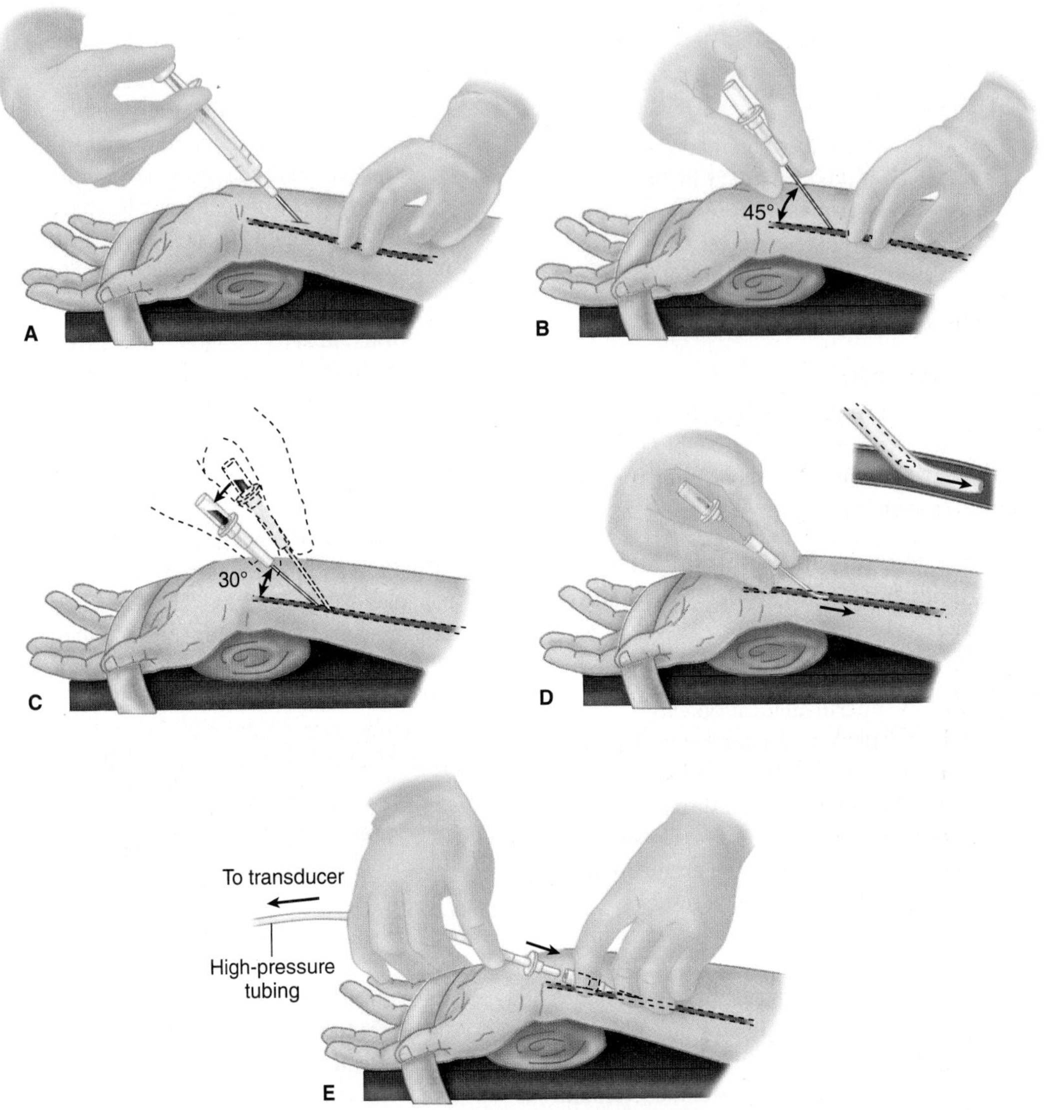

FIGURE 5–7 Cannulation of the radial artery. **A**: Proper positioning and palpation of the artery are crucial. After skin preparation, a local anesthetic is infiltrated with a 25-gauge needle. **B**: A 20- or 22-gauge catheter is advanced through the skin at a 45° angle. **C**: Flashback of blood signals entry into the artery, and the catheter–needle assembly is lowered to a 30° angle and advanced 1–2 mm to ensure an intraluminal catheter position. **D**: The catheter is advanced over the needle, which is withdrawn. **E**: Proximal pressure with the middle and ring fingers prevents blood loss, while the arterial tubing Luer-lock connector is secured to the intraarterial catheter.

area of maximal impulse or by use of ultrasound (the authors' preferred technique when any difficulty is encountered). After the skin is cleansed with chlorhexidine or other prep solution using aseptic technique, 1% lidocaine is infiltrated in the skin of awake patients, directly above the artery, with a small gauge needle. A larger 18-gauge needle can then be used as a skin punch, facilitating the entry of a 20- or 22-gauge catheter over a needle through the skin at a 45° angle, directing it toward the point of palpation. Upon blood flashback, a guidewire may be advanced through the catheter into the artery, and the catheter can be advanced over the guidewire. Alternatively, the needle is lowered to a 30° angle and advanced another 1 to 2 mm to make certain that the tip of the catheter is well into the vessel lumen. The catheter is advanced off the needle into the arterial lumen, after which the needle is withdrawn. Applying firm pressure over the artery proximal to the catheter insertion site prevents blood from spurting from the catheter while the tubing is connected. Waterproof tape or sutures can be used to hold the catheter in place, and a sterile dressing should be applied over the insertion site.

C. Complications

Complications of intraarterial monitoring include hematoma, bleeding (particularly with catheter tubing disconnections), vasospasm, arterial thrombosis, embolization of air bubbles or thrombi, pseudoaneurysm formation, necrosis of skin overlying the catheter, nerve damage, infection, necrosis of extremities or digits, and unintentional intraarterial drug injection. Factors associated with an increased rate of complications include prolonged cannulation, repeated insertion attempts, extracorporeal circulation, the use of larger catheters in smaller vessels, the use of vasopressors, and hyperlipidemia.

Clinical Considerations

Because intraarterial cannulation allows continuous beat-to-beat blood pressure measurement, it is considered the optimal blood pressure monitoring technique. The quality of the transduced waveform, however, depends on the dynamic characteristics of the catheter–tubing–transducer system. False readings can lead to inappropriate therapeutic interventions.

A complex waveform, such as an arterial pulse wave, can be expressed as a summation of simple harmonic waves (according to the Fourier theorem). For accurate measurement of pressure, the catheter–tubing–transducer system must be capable of responding adequately to the highest frequency of the arterial waveform (Figure 5–8A **and** 5–8B). Stated another way, the natural frequency of the measuring system must exceed the natural frequency of the arterial pulse (approximately 16–24 Hz).

Most transducers have frequencies of several hundred Hz (>200 Hz for disposable transducers). The addition of tubing, stopcocks, and air in the line all decrease the frequency of the system. If the frequency response is too low, the system will be overdamped and will not faithfully reproduce the arterial waveform, underestimating the systolic pressure. Underdamping is also a serious problem, leading to overshoot and a falsely high SBP.

Catheter–tubing–transducer systems must also prevent **hyperresonance,** an artifact caused by reverberation of pressure waves within the system. A **damping coefficient** (β) of 0.6 to 0.7 is optimal. Arterial blood pressure measurements are improved by minimizing

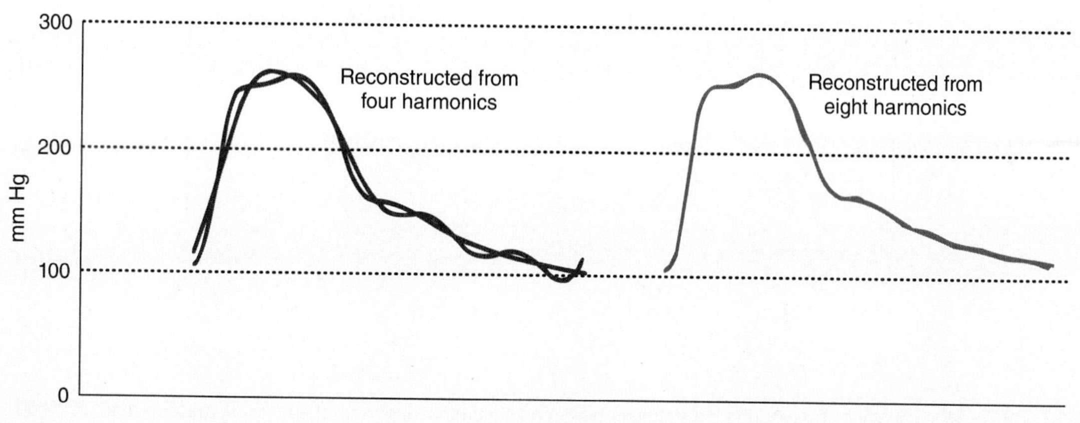

FIGURE 5–8A An original waveform overlays a four-harmonic reconstruction (*left*) and an eight-harmonic reconstruction (*right*). Note that the higher harmonic plot more closely resembles the original waveform. (Reproduced with permission from Saidman LS, Smith WT. *Monitoring in Anesthesia.* Philadelphia, PA: Butterworth-Heinemann; 1985.)

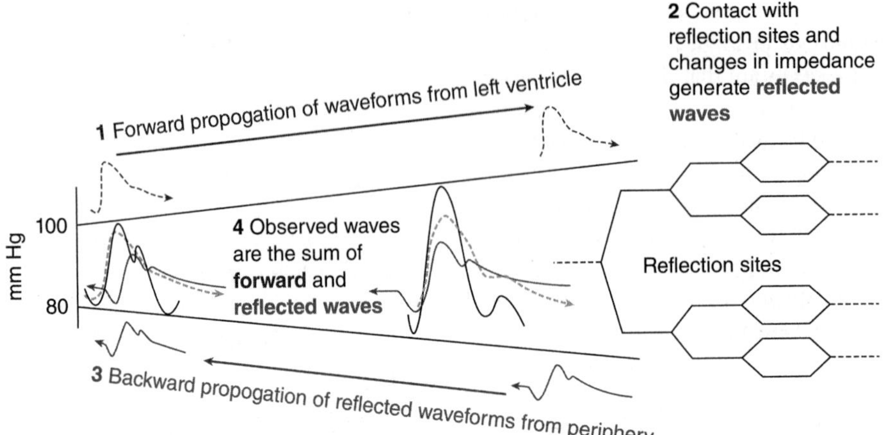

FIGURE 5–8B The arterial waveform is the summation of both forward- and backward-traveling pressure waveforms. The phase difference between these two waveforms, as well as diminution over time, can lead to complex shapes. Note that, in this example, as in many humans, the pulse pressure increases as one moves toward the periphery (the mean arterial pressure, however, must decrease). (Reproduced with permission from Roach JK, Thiele RH. Perioperative blood pressure monitoring. *Best Pract Res Clin Anaesthesiol.* 2019 Jun;33(2):127-138.)

tubing length, eliminating unnecessary stopcocks, removing air bubbles, and using low-compliance tubing. Although smaller-diameter catheters lower natural frequency, they improve under-dampened systems and are less apt to result in vascular complications.

Transducers contain a diaphragm that is distorted by an arterial pressure wave. The mechanical energy of a pressure wave is converted into an electric signal. Most transducers are resistance types that are based on the **strain gauge** principle: stretching a wire or silicone crystal changes its electrical resistance. The sensing elements are arranged as a "Wheatstone bridge" circuit so that the voltage output is proportionate to the pressure applied to the diaphragm (Figure 5–8C).

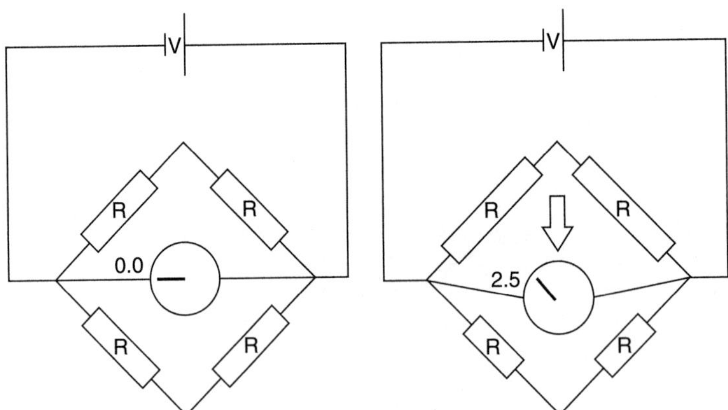

FIGURE 5–8C The Wheatstone bridge is a simple engineering circuit that allows for the accurate measurement of blood pressure. Mechanical forces bend the Wheatstone bridge, changing the resistance of its elements, which, when unmatched, lead to a small voltage differential that can be detected (and converted to units of pressure). (Reproduced with permission from Roach JK, Thiele RH. Perioperative blood pressure monitoring. *Best Pract Res Clin Anaesthesiol.* 2019 Jun;33(2):127-138.)

Transducer accuracy depends on correct calibration and zeroing procedures. A stopcock at the level of the desired point of measurement—usually the midaxillary line—is opened, and the zero trigger on the monitor is activated. If the patient's position is altered by raising or lowering the operating table, the transducer must either be moved in tandem or zeroed to the new level of the midaxillary line. In a seated patient, the arterial pressure in the brain differs significantly from left ventricular pressure. In this circumstance, cerebral pressure is determined by setting the transducer to zero at the level of the ear, which approximates the circle of Willis. The transducer's zero should be verified regularly as some transducer measurements can "drift" over time.

Digital readouts of systolic and diastolic pressures are a running average of the highest and lowest measurements within a certain time interval. Because motion or cautery artifacts can result in some very misleading numbers, the arterial waveform should always be monitored. The shape of the arterial wave provides clues to several hemodynamic variables. The rate of upstroke indicates contractility, the rate of downstroke indicates peripheral vascular resistance, and exaggerated variations in size during the respiratory cycle suggest hypovolemia or excessive tidal volumes. Intraarterial catheters also provide access for intermittent arterial blood gas sampling and analysis. Analysis of the arterial pressure waveform allows for the estimation of CO and other hemodynamic parameters. These devices are discussed in the section on CO monitoring.

ELECTROCARDIOGRAPHY

Indications & Contraindications

All patients must have continuous intraoperative monitoring of their electrocardiogram (ECG), as mandated by the American Society of Anesthesiologists standards for basic anesthetic monitoring. There are no contraindications.

Techniques & Complications

Lead selection determines the diagnostic sensitivity of the ECG. ECG leads are positioned on the chest and extremities to provide different perspectives of the electrical potentials generated by the heart. At the end of diastole, the atria contract, which provides the atrial contribution to CO, generating the "P" wave. Following atrial contraction, the ventricle is loaded, awaiting systole. The QRS complex begins the electrical activity of systole following the 120 to 200 msec atrioventricular (AV) nodal delay. Depolarization of the ventricle proceeds from the AV node through the interventricular system via the His–Purkinje fibers. The normal QRS lasts approximately 120 msec, which can be prolonged in patients with cardiomyopathies and heart failure. The T wave represents repolarization as the heart prepares to contract again. Prolongation of the QT interval secondary to electrolyte imbalances or drug effects can potentially lead to life-threatening arrhythmias (torsades de pointes).

The electrical axis of lead II is approximately 60° from the right arm to the left leg, which is parallel to the electrical axis of the atria, resulting in the largest P-wave voltages of any surface lead. This orientation enhances the diagnosis of arrhythmias and the detection of inferior wall ischemia. Lead V_5 lies over the fifth intercostal space at the anterior axillary line; this position is a good compromise for detecting anterior and lateral wall ischemia. A true V_5 lead is possible only on operating room ECGs with at least five lead wires, but a modified V_5 can be monitored by rearranging the standard three-limb lead placement (Figure 5–9). Ideally, because each lead provides unique information, leads II and V_5 should be monitored simultaneously. If only a single-channel machine is available, the preferred lead for monitoring depends on the location of any prior infarction or ischemia and whether arrhythmia or ischemia appears to be the greater concern.

Electrodes are placed on the patient's body to monitor the ECG. Conductive gel lowers the skin's electrical resistance, which can be further decreased by cleansing the site with alcohol. Needle electrodes are used only if the disks are unsuitable (eg, with an extensively burned patient).

Clinical Considerations

The ECG is a recording of the electrical potentials generated by myocardial cells. Its routine use allows arrhythmias, myocardial ischemia, conduction abnormalities, pacemaker malfunction, and electrolyte

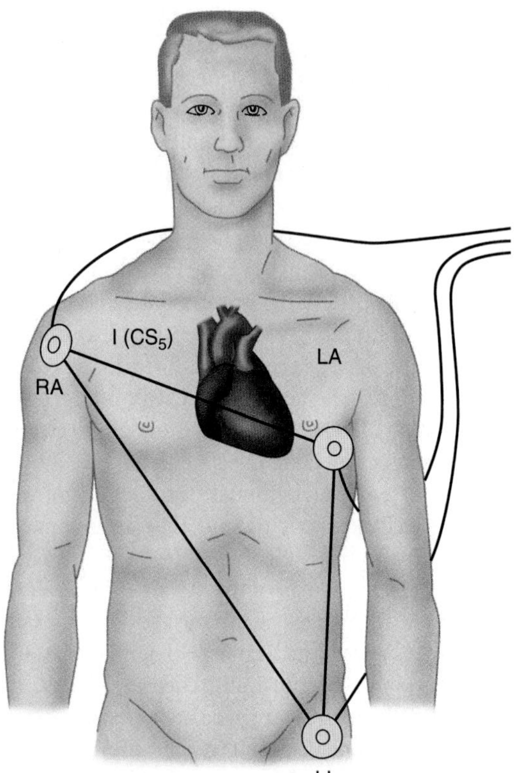

FIGURE 5–9 Rearranged three-limb lead placement. Anterior and lateral ischemia can be detected by placing the left arm lead (LA) at the V_5 position. When lead I is selected on the monitor, a modified V_5 lead (CS_5) is displayed. Lead II allows detection of arrhythmias and inferior wall ischemia. LL, left leg; RA, right arm.

disturbances to be detected (Figure 5–10). Because of the small voltage potentials being measured, artifacts remain a major problem. Patient or lead-wire movement, use of electrocautery, 60-Hz interference from nearby alternating current devices, and faulty electrodes can simulate arrhythmias. Monitoring filters incorporated into the amplifier to reduce "motion" artifacts will lead to distortion of the ST segment and may impede the diagnosis of ischemia. Digital readouts of the heart rate (HR) may be misleading because of monitor misinterpretation of artifacts or large T waves—often seen in pediatric patients—as QRS complexes.

Commonly accepted criteria for diagnosing myocardial ischemia require that the ECG be recorded in "diagnostic mode" and include a flat or downsloping ST-segment depression exceeding 1 mm, 80 msec after the J point (the end of the QRS complex), particularly in conjunction with T-wave inversion. ST-segment elevation with peaked T waves can also represent ischemia. Wolff–Parkinson–White syndrome, bundle-branch blocks, extrinsic pacemaker capture, and digoxin therapy may preclude the use of ST-segment information. The audible beep associated with each QRS complex should be loud enough to detect rate and rhythm changes when the anesthesiologist's visual attention is directed elsewhere. Some ECGs are capable of storing aberrant QRS complexes for further analysis, and some can even interpret and diagnose arrhythmias. The interference caused by electrocautery units limits the usefulness of automated arrhythmia analysis in the operating room.

CENTRAL VENOUS CATHETERIZATION

Indications

Central venous catheterization is indicated for monitoring central venous pressure (CVP), the administration of fluid to treat hypovolemia and shock, the infusion of caustic drugs and total parenteral nutrition, aspiration of air emboli, the insertion of transcutaneous pacing leads, and gaining venous access in patients with poor peripheral veins. With specialized catheters, central venous catheterization can be used for continuous monitoring of central venous oxygen saturation ($Scvo_2$). $Scvo_2$ is used as a measure to assess the adequacy of oxygen delivery. Decreased $Scvo_2$ (normal >65%) alerts to the possibility of inadequate delivery of oxygen to the tissues (eg, low CO, low hemoglobin, low arterial oxygen saturation, increased oxygen consumption). An elevated $Scvo_2$ (>80%) may indicate arterial/venous shunting or impaired cellular oxygen utilization (eg, cyanide poisoning).

Contraindications

Relative contraindications include tumors, clots, or tricuspid valve vegetations that could be dislodged

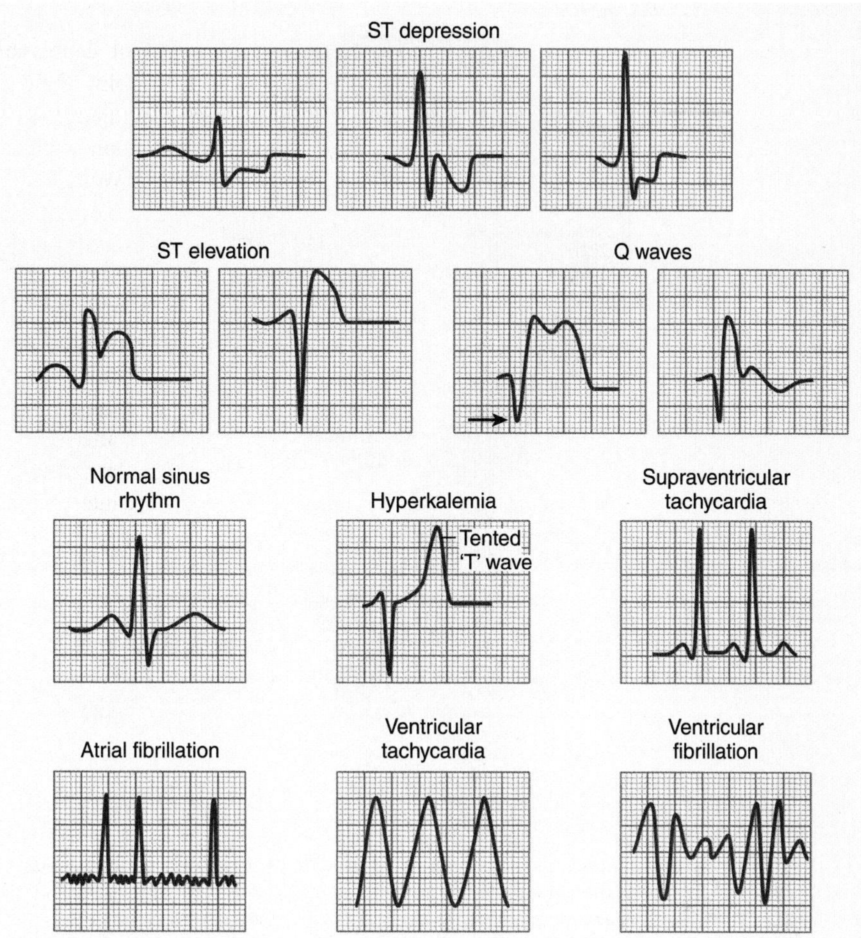

FIGURE 5–10 Common ECG findings during cardiac surgery. (Reproduced with permission from Wasnick J, Hillel Z, Kramer D, et al. *Cardiac Anesthesia & Transesophageal Echocardiography.* New York, NY: McGraw Hill; 2011.)

or embolized during cannulation. Other contraindications relate to the potential cannulation site (eg, infection).

Techniques & Complications

Central venous cannulation involves introducing a catheter into a vein so that the catheter's tip lies with the venous system within the thorax. Generally, the optimal location of the catheter tip when the catheter is inserted via the jugular, subclavian, or brachial veins is just superior to or at the junction of the superior vena cava and the right atrium. When the catheter tip is located within the thorax, inspiration will increase or decrease CVP, depending on whether ventilation is controlled or spontaneous. CVP pressure should be measured during end expiration.

Various sites can be used for cannulation (Figure 5–11). All cannulation sites have an increased risk of infection the longer the catheter remains in place. Compared with other sites, the subclavian vein is associated with a greater risk of pneumothorax during insertion but a reduced risk of other complications during prolonged cannulations (eg, in critically ill patients). The right

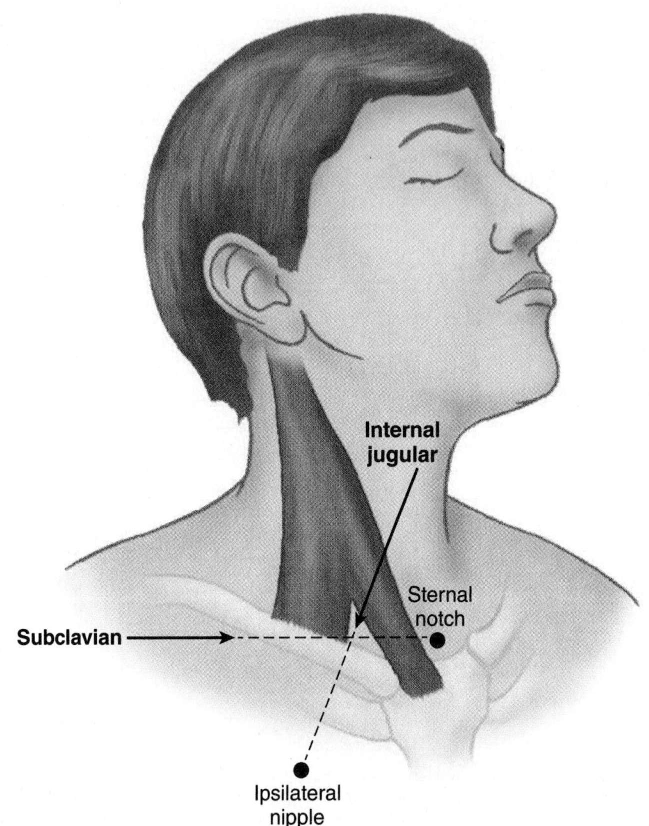

FIGURE 5–11 The subclavian and internal jugular veins are both used for central access perioperatively with the sternal notch and ipsilateral nipple in the direction of needle passage for each, respectively. (Reproduced with permission from Wasnick J, Hillel Z, Kramer D, et al. *Cardiac Anesthesia & Transesophageal Echocardiography.* New York, NY: McGraw Hill; 2011.)

internal jugular vein provides a combination of accessibility and safety. Left-sided internal jugular vein catheterization has an increased risk of pleural effusion and chylothorax. The external jugular veins can also be used as entry sites, but because of the acute angle at which they join the great veins of the chest, using them is associated with a greater likelihood of failure to gain access to the central circulation compared with using the internal jugular veins. Femoral veins can also be cannulated, but using them is associated with an increased risk of line-related sepsis. There are at least three cannulation techniques: a catheter over a needle (similar to peripheral catheterization), a catheter through a needle (requiring a large-bore needle stick), and a catheter over a guidewire (Seldinger technique; Figure 5–12). The overwhelming majority of central lines are placed using the Seldinger technique.

The following scenario describes the placement of an internal jugular venous line. The patient is placed in the Trendelenburg position to decrease the risk of air embolism and to distend the internal jugular (or subclavian) vein. Central venous catheterization requires full aseptic technique, including hand scrub, sterile gloves, gown, mask, hat, bactericidal skin preparation (alcohol-based solutions are preferred), and sterile drapes. The two heads of the sternocleidomastoid muscle and the clavicle form the three sides of a triangle (Figure 5–12A). A 25-gauge needle is used

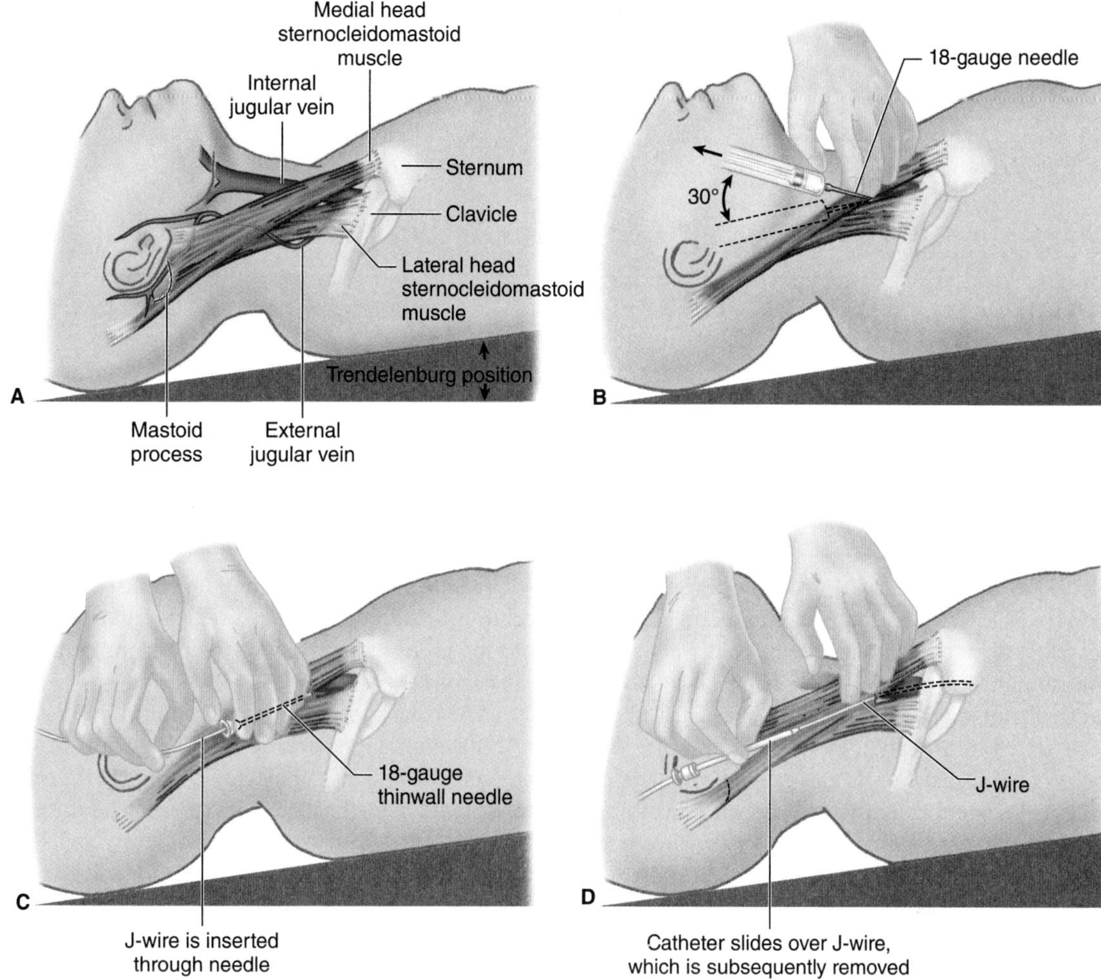

FIGURE 5–12 Right internal jugular cannulation with the Seldinger technique (see text).

to infiltrate the apex of the triangle with a local anesthetic. The internal jugular vein can be located using ultrasound, and we strongly recommend that it be used whenever possible (Figure 5–13A). Many institutions mandate the use of ultrasound whenever internal jugular vein cannulation is performed (Figure 5–13B). Alternatively, the vein may be located by advancing the 25-gauge needle—or a 23-gauge needle in heavier patients—along the medial border of the lateral head of the sternocleidomastoid, toward the ipsilateral nipple, at an angle of 30° to the skin, aiming just lateral to the carotid artery pulse. Aspiration of venous blood confirms the vein's location. It is essential that the vein (and not the artery) be cannulated. Cannulation of the carotid artery can lead to hematoma, stroke, airway compromise, and possibly death. An 18-gauge thin-wall needle or an 18-gauge catheter over needle is advanced along the same path as the locator needle (Figure 5–12B), and with the latter apparatus, the needle is removed from the catheter once the catheter has been advanced into the vein. After obtaining free blood flow, we usually confirm central venous versus arterial pressure (using intravenous

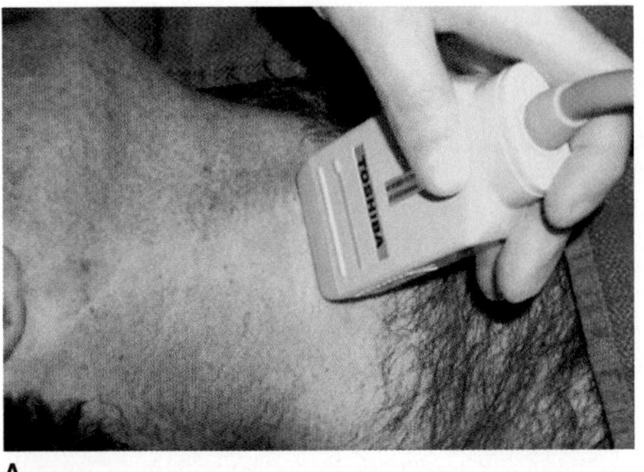

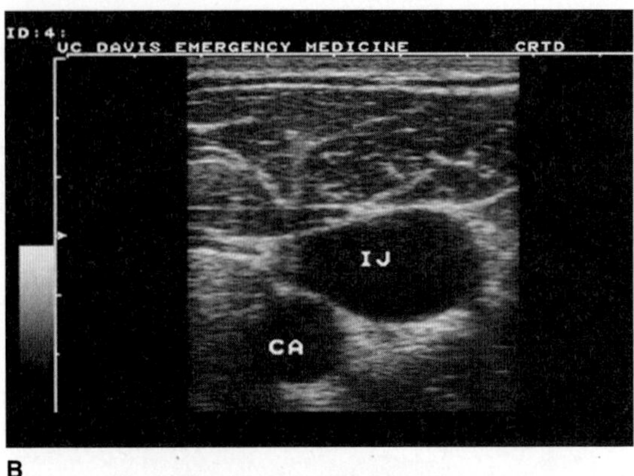

FIGURE 5–13 **A**: Probe position for ultrasound of the large internal jugular vein with deeper carotid artery and **B**: corresponding ultrasound image. CA, carotid artery; IJ, internal jugular vein. (Reproduced with permission from Tintinalli JE, Stapczynski J, Ma OJ, et al. *Tintinalli's Emergency Medicine: A Comprehensive Study Guide,* 7th ed. New York, NY: McGraw Hill; 2011.)

extension tubing) before introducing a guidewire (Figure 5–12C). We strongly recommend that correct placement of the guidewire be confirmed using ultrasound. The needle (or catheter) is removed, and a dilator is advanced over the wire. The catheter is prepared for insertion by flushing all ports with saline, and all distal ports are "capped" or clamped, except the one through which the wire must pass. Next, the dilator is removed, and the final catheter is advanced over the wire (Figure 5–12D). Do not lose control of the external tip of the guidewire. The guidewire is removed, with a thumb placed over the catheter hub to prevent aspiration of air until the intravenous catheter tubing is connected to it. The catheter is then secured, and a sterile dressing is applied. Correct location is confirmed with a chest
1 radiograph. The tip of the catheter should not be allowed to migrate into the heart chambers.

As mentioned, the likelihood of accidental placement of the vein dilator or catheter into the carotid artery can be decreased by measuring the vessel's pressure from the introducer needle (or catheter, if a catheter over needle has been used) before passing the wire (most simply accomplished by using a sterile intravenous extension tubing as a manometer). Blood color and pulsatility can be misleading or inconclusive and should not be used as a guide to determine venous cannulation. More than one confirmation method should be used. In cases where either surface ultrasound or transesophageal echocardiography (TEE) are used, the guidewire can be seen in the jugular vein or right atrium, confirming venous entry (Figure 5–14).

The risks of central venous cannulation include line infection, bloodstream infection, air or thrombus embolism, arrhythmias (indicating that the catheter tip is in the right atrium or ventricle), hematoma, pneumothorax, hemothorax, hydrothorax, chylothorax, cardiac perforation, cardiac tamponade, trauma to nearby nerves and arteries, and thrombosis.

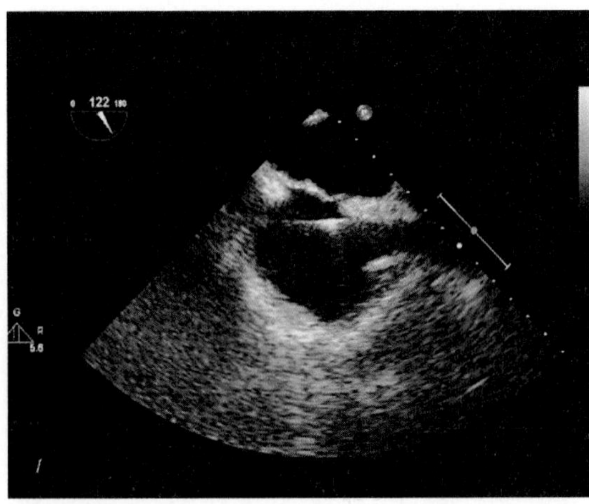

FIGURE 5–14 A wire is seen on this transesophageal echocardiography image of the right atrium.

Clinical Considerations

Normal cardiac function requires adequate ventricular filling. CVP approximates right atrial pressure. Ventricular volumes are related to pressures through compliance. Highly compliant ventricles accommodate volume with minimal changes in pressure. Noncompliant systems have larger swings in pressure with fewer volume changes. Consequently, any CVP measurement will reveal only limited information about ventricular volumes and filling. Although a very low CVP may indicate a volume-depleted patient, a moderate to high pressure reading may reflect volume overload, poor ventricular compliance, or both. Changes in CVP associated with volume administration coupled with other measures of hemodynamic performance (eg, stroke volume, CO, blood pressure, HR, urine output) may be a better indicator of the patient's volume responsiveness.

The shape of the central venous waveform corresponds to the events of cardiac contraction (Figure 5–15): *a* waves from *a*trial contraction are absent in atrial fibrillation and are exaggerated in junctional rhythms ("cannon" *a* waves); *c* waves are due to tricuspid valve elevation during early ventricular contraction; *v* waves reflect *v*enous return against a closed tricuspid valve; and the *x* and *y* descents are probably caused by the downward displacement of the tricuspid valve during systole and tricuspid valve opening during diastole.

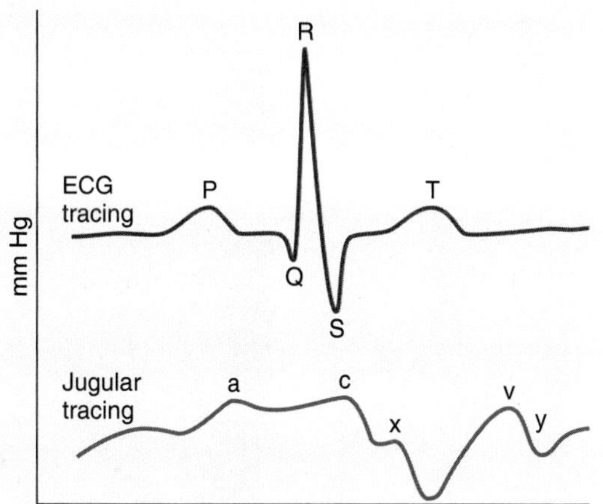

FIGURE 5–15 The upward waves (*a, c, v*) and the downward descents (*x, y*) of a central venous tracing in relation to the electrocardiogram (ECG).

PULMONARY ARTERY CATHETERIZATION

Indications

The pulmonary artery (PA) catheter (or Swan-Ganz catheter) was introduced into routine practice in operating rooms and in coronary and critical care units in the 1970s. It quickly became common for sicker patients undergoing major surgery to be managed with PA catheterization. The catheter provided measurements of both CO and PA occlusion pressures and was used to guide hemodynamic therapy, especially when patients became unstable. Determination of the PA occlusion or wedge pressure permitted (in the absence of mitral stenosis) an estimation of the left ventricular end-diastolic pressure (LVEDP) and, depending upon ventricular compliance, ventricular volume. Through the ability of the PA catheter to perform measurements of CO, the patient's stroke volume (SV) was also determined.

$$\text{CO} = \text{SV} \times \text{HR}$$
$$\text{SV} = \text{CO/HR}$$
$$\text{Blood pressure} = \text{CO} \times \text{systemic vascular resistance (SVR)}$$

Consequently, hemodynamic monitoring with the PA catheter attempted to discern why a patient was unstable so that therapy could be directed at the underlying problem.

If the SVR is diminished, such as in states of vasodilatory shock (sepsis), the SV may increase. Conversely, a reduction in SV may be secondary to poor cardiac performance or hypovolemia. Determination of the "wedge" or pulmonary capillary occlusion pressure (PCOP) by inflating the catheter balloon estimates the LVEDP. A decreased SV in the setting of a low PCOP/LVEDP indicates hypovolemia and the need for volume administration. A "full" heart, reflected by a high PCOP/LVEDP and low SV, indicates the need for a positive inotropic drug. Conversely, a normal or increased SV in the setting of hypotension could be treated with the administration of vasoconstrictor drugs to restore SVR in a vasodilated patient.

Although patients can and do present concurrently with hypovolemia, sepsis, and heart failure, the aforementioned shock treatment approach using the PA catheter to guide therapy became more or less synonymous with perioperative intensive care and cardiac anesthesia. However, several large observational studies have shown that patients managed with PA catheters had worse outcomes than similar patients who were managed without PA catheters. Other studies seem to indicate that although PA catheter-guided patient management may do no harm, it offers no specific benefits. Although the PA catheter can be used to guide goal-directed hemodynamic therapy to ensure organ perfusion in shock states, other less invasive methods to determine hemodynamic performance are available, including transpulmonary thermodilution CO measurements, pulse contour analyses of the arterial pressure waveform, and methods based on bioimpedance measurements across the chest. All these methods permit calculation of the SV as a guide for hemodynamic management. Moreover, right atrial blood oxygen saturation, as opposed to mixed venous saturation (normal is 75%), can be used as an alternative measure to discern tissue oxygen extraction and the adequacy of tissue oxygen delivery.

2

Despite numerous reports of its questionable utility and the increasing number of alternative methods to determine hemodynamic parameters, the PA catheter is still employed perioperatively more often in the United States than elsewhere. Although echocardiography can readily determine if the heart is full, compressed, contracting, or empty, a trained individual is required to obtain and interpret the images. Alternative hemodynamic monitors have gained wide acceptance in Europe and are increasingly used in the United States, further decreasing the use of PA catheters.

PA catheterization can be considered whenever cardiac index, preload, volume status, or the degree of mixed venous blood oxygenation need to be known. These measurements might prove particularly important in surgical patients at greatest risk for hemodynamic instability or during surgical procedures associated with a greatly increased incidence of hemodynamic complications. However, the authors prefer transesophageal echocardiography in these situations.

Contraindications

3

Relative contraindications to PA catheterization include left bundle-branch block (because of the concern about complete heart block) and conditions associated with a greatly increased risk of arrhythmias. A catheter with pacing capability is better suited to these situations. A PA catheter may serve as a nidus of infection in bacteremic patients or of thrombus formation in patients prone to hypercoagulation.

Techniques & Complications

Although various PA catheters are available, the most popular design integrates five lumens into a 7.5F catheter, 110-cm long, with a polyvinylchloride body (Figure 5–16). The lumens house the following: wiring to connect the thermistor near the catheter tip to a thermodilution CO computer; an air channel for inflation of the balloon; a proximal port

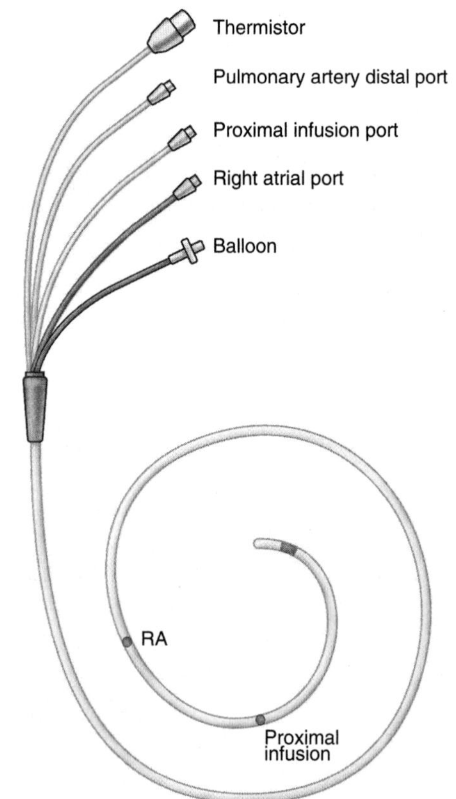

FIGURE 5–16 Balloon-tipped pulmonary artery flotation catheter (Swan–Ganz catheter). RA, right atrium.

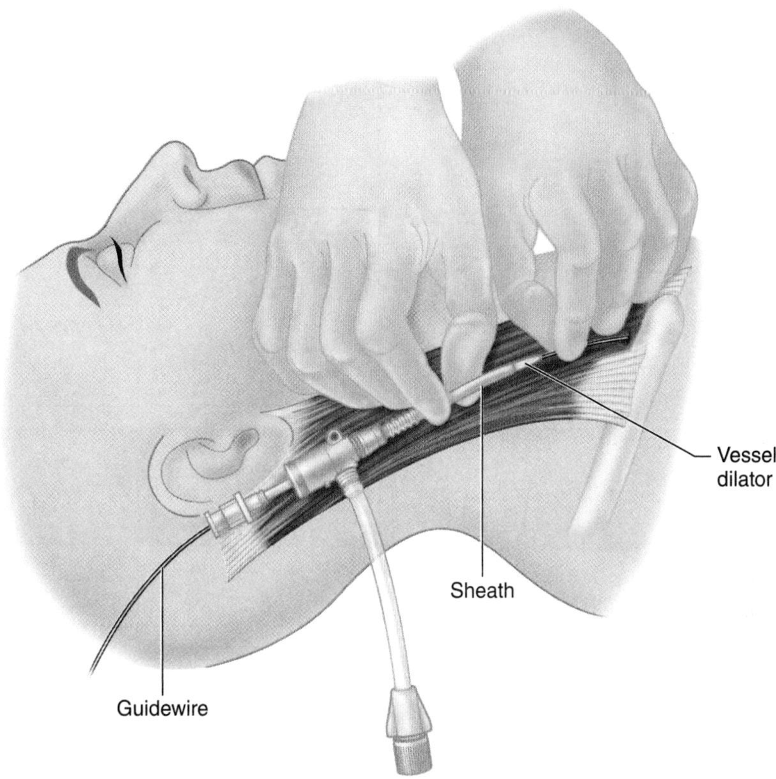

FIGURE 5–17 A percutaneous introducer consisting of a vessel dilator and a sheath passed over the guidewire.

30 cm from the tip for infusions, CO injections, and measurements of right atrial pressures; a ventricular port at 20 cm for infusion of drugs; and a distal port for aspiration of mixed venous blood samples and measurements of PA pressure.

Insertion of a PA catheter requires central venous access, which can be accomplished using the previously described Seldinger technique. Instead of a central venous catheter, a dilator and sheath are threaded over the guidewire. The sheath lumen accommodates the PA catheter after removal of the dilator and guidewire (Figure 5–17).

Prior to insertion, the PA catheter is checked by inflating and deflating its balloon and filling all three lumens with intravenous fluid. The distal port is connected to a transducer that is zeroed to the patient's midaxillary line.

The PA catheter is advanced through the introducer and into the internal jugular vein. At approximately 15 cm, the distal tip should enter the right atrium, and a central venous tracing that varies with respiration confirms an intrathoracic position. The balloon is then inflated with air according to the manufacturer's recommendations (usually 1.5 mL) to protect the endocardium from the catheter tip and to allow flow through the right ventricle to direct the catheter forward. The balloon is always deflated during withdrawal. During catheter advancement, the ECG should be monitored for arrhythmias. Transient ectopy from irritation of the right ventricle by the balloon and catheter tip is common and rarely requires treatment. A sudden increase in the *systolic* pressure on the distal tracing indicates a right ventricular location of the catheter tip (Figure 5–18). Entry into the pulmonary artery normally occurs by 35 to 45 cm and is heralded by a sudden increase in *diastolic* pressure.

The balloon should be deflated and the catheter withdrawn if pressure changes do not occur at

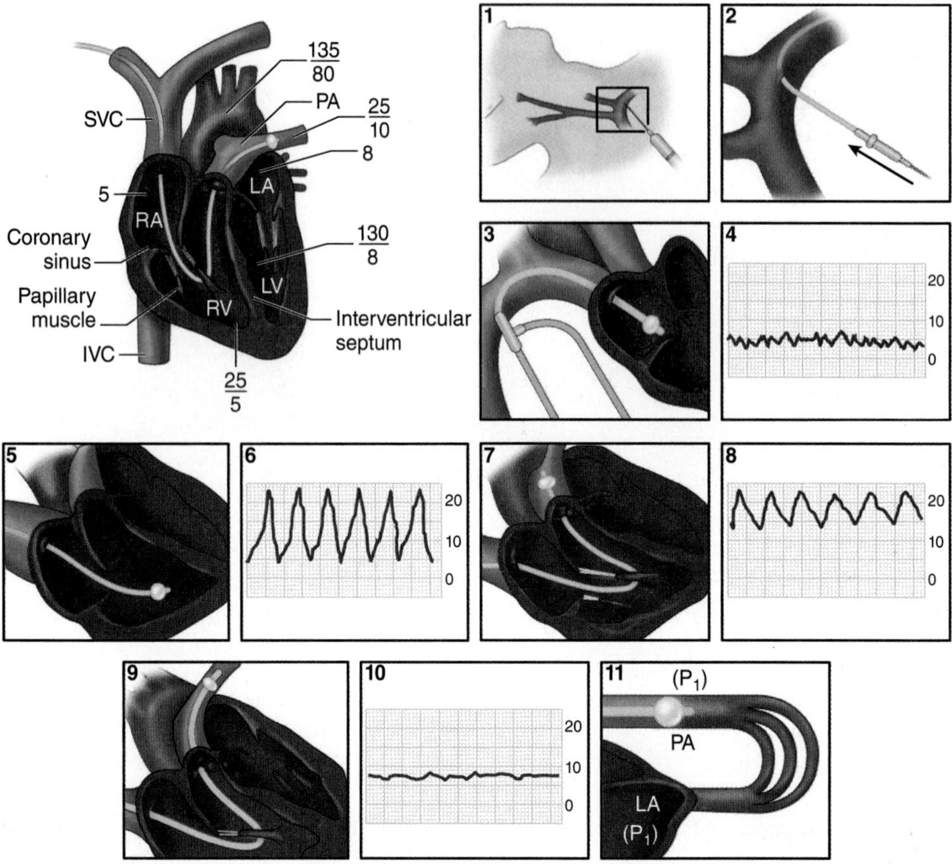

FIGURE 5–18 Although their utility is increasingly questioned, pulmonary artery (PA) catheters continue to be a part of perioperative management of the cardiac surgery patient. Following placement of a sheath introducer in the central circulation (**panels 1 and 2**), the PA catheter is floated. Central line placement should always be completed using rigorous sterile technique, full body draping, and only after multiple, redundant confirmations of the correct localization of the venous circulation. Pressure guidance is used to ascertain the localization of the PA catheter in the venous circulation and the heart. Upon entry into the right atrium (RA; **panels 3 and 4**), the central venous pressure tracing is noted. Passing through the tricuspid valve (**panels 5 and 6**), right ventricular pressures are detected. At 35 to 50 cm, depending upon patient size, the catheter will pass from the right ventricle (RV) through the pulmonic valve into the pulmonary artery (**panels 7 and 8**). This is noted by the measurement of diastolic pressure once the pulmonic valve is passed. Lastly, when indicated, the balloon-tipped catheter will wedge or occlude a pulmonary artery branch (**panels 9, 10, and 11**). When this occurs, the pulmonary artery pressure equilibrates with that of the left atrium (LA), which, barring any mitral valve pathology, should reflect left ventricular end-diastolic pressure. IVC, inferior vena cava; SVC, superior vena cava. (Reproduced with permission from Soni N. *Practical Procedures in Anaesthesia and Intensive Care.* Philadelphia, PA: Butterworth Heinemann; 1994.)

the expected distances to prevent catheter knotting. Occasionally, the insertion may require fluoroscopy or TEE for guidance.

After the catheter tip enters the PA, minimal additional advancement results in a pulmonary artery occlusion pressure (PAOP) waveform. The PA tracing should reappear when the balloon is deflated. Wedging before maximal balloon inflation signals an overwedged position, and the catheter should be slightly withdrawn (with the balloon deflated). Because **PA rupture** from balloon overinflation may cause hemorrhage and mortality, wedge readings should be obtained infrequently. 4 PA pressure should be continuously monitored to detect an overwedged position indicative of catheter migration. Correct PA catheter position is confirmed by a chest radiograph.

The numerous complications of PA catheterization include all those associated with central venous cannulation plus endocarditis, thrombogenesis, pulmonary infarction, PA rupture, and hemorrhage (particularly in patients taking anticoagulants, older adult or female patients, or patients with pulmonary hypertension), catheter knotting, arrhythmias, conduction abnormalities, and pulmonary valvular damage. Even trace hemoptysis should not be ignored because it may herald PA rupture. If the latter is suspected, prompt placement of a double-lumen tracheal tube may maintain adequate oxygenation by the unaffected lung. The risk of complications increases with the duration of catheterization, which usually should not exceed 72 hours.

Clinical Considerations

PA catheters allow more precise estimation of left ventricular preload than either CVP or physical examination (but not as precise as TEE), as well as the sampling of mixed venous blood. Catheters with self-contained thermistors (discussed later in this chapter) can be used to measure CO, from which a multitude of hemodynamic values can be derived (Table 5–1). Some catheter designs incorporate electrodes that allow intracavitary ECG recording and pacing. Optional fiberoptic bundles allow continuous measurement of the oxygen saturation of mixed venous blood.

Starling demonstrated the relationship between left ventricular function and left ventricular end-diastolic muscle fiber length, which is usually proportionate to end-diastolic volume (see Chapter 20). If compliance is not abnormally decreased (eg, by myocardial ischemia, overload, ventricular hypertrophy, or pericardial tamponade), LVEDP should reflect fiber length. In the presence of a normal mitral valve, left atrial pressure approaches left ventricular pressure during diastolic filling. The left atrium connects with the right side of the heart through the pulmonary vasculature. The distal lumen of a correctly wedged PA catheter is isolated from right-sided pressures by balloon inflation. Its distal opening is exposed only to capillary pressure, which—in the absence of high airway pressures or pulmonary vascular disease—equals left atrial pressure. In fact,

TABLE 5–1 Hemodynamic variables derived from pulmonary artery catheterization data.[1]

Variable	Formula	Normal	Units
Cardiac index	$\frac{\text{Cardiac output (L/min)}}{\text{Body surface area (m}^2\text{)}}$	2.2–4.2	L/min/m^2
Total peripheral resistance	$\frac{(\text{MAP} - \text{CVP}) \times 80}{\text{Cardiac output (L/min)}}$	1200–1500	dynes • s cm^{-5}
Pulmonary vascular resistance	$\frac{(\overline{\text{PA}} - \text{PAOP}) \times 80}{\text{Cardiac output (L/min)}}$	100–300	dynes • s cm^{-5}
Stroke volume	$\frac{\text{Cardiac output (L/min)} \times 1000}{\text{Heart rate (beats/min)}}$	60–90	mL/beat
Stroke index (SI)	$\frac{\text{Stroke volume (mL/beat)}}{\text{Body surface area (m}^2\text{)}}$	20–65	mL/beat/m^2
Right ventricular stroke-work index	$0.0136\ (\overline{\text{PA}} - \text{CVP}) \times \text{SI}$	30–65	g-m/beat/m^2
Left ventricular stroke-work index	$0.0136\ (\text{MAP} - \text{PAOP}) \times \text{SI}$	46–60	g-m/beat/m^2

[1]g-m, gram meter; CVP, central venous pressure; MAP, mean arterial pressure; $\overline{\text{PA}}$, mean pulmonary artery pressure; PAOP, pulmonary artery occlusion pressure.

aspiration through the distal port during balloon inflation samples arterialized blood. PAOP is an indirect measure of LVEDP, which, depending upon ventricular compliance, approximates left ventricular end-diastolic volume.

Whereas CVP may reflect right ventricular function, a PA catheter may be indicated if either ventricle is markedly depressed, causing disassociation of right- and left-sided hemodynamics. CVP is poorly predictive of pulmonary capillary pressures, especially in patients with abnormal left ventricular function. Even the PAOP does not always predict LVEDP. The relationship between left ventricular end-diastolic volume (actual preload) and PAOP (estimated preload) can become unreliable during conditions associated with changing left atrial or ventricular compliance, mitral valve function, or pulmonary vein resistance. These conditions are common immediately following major cardiac or vascular surgery and in critically ill patients who are receiving inotropic agents or experiencing septic shock.

Ultimately, the value of the information provided by the PA catheter is dependent upon its correct interpretation by the patient's caregivers. Thus, the PA catheter is only a tool to assist in goal-directed perioperative therapy. Given the increasing number of less invasive methods now available to obtain similar information, we anticipate that PA catheterization will become mostly of historical interest.

CARDIAC OUTPUT

Indications

CO measurement to permit calculation of the SV is one of the primary reasons for PA catheterization. Currently, there are a number of alternative, less invasive methods to estimate ventricular function to assist in goal-directed therapy.

Techniques & Complications

A. Thermodilution

The injection of a quantity (2.5, 5, or 10 mL) of fluid that is below body temperature (usually room temperature or iced) into the right atrium changes the temperature of blood in contact with the thermistor at the tip of the PA catheter. The degree of change is inversely proportional to CO: Temperature change is minimal if there is a high blood flow, whereas temperature change is greater when flow is reduced. After injection, one can plot the temperature as a function of time to produce a **thermodilution curve** (Figure 5–19). CO is determined by a computer program that integrates the area under the curve.

5 Accurate measurements of CO depend on rapid and smooth injection, precisely known injectant temperature and volume, correct entry of the calibration factors for the specific type of PA catheter into the CO computer, and avoidance of measurements during electrocautery. Tricuspid regurgitation and cardiac shunts invalidate results because only right ventricular output into the PA is actually being measured. Rapid infusion of the iced injectant has rarely resulted in cardiac arrhythmias.

A modification of the thermodilution technique allows continuous CO measurement with a special catheter and monitor system. The catheter contains a thermal filament that introduces small pulses of heat into the blood proximal to the pulmonic valve and a thermistor that measures changes in PA blood temperature. A computer in the monitor determines CO by cross-correlating the amount of heat input with the changes in blood temperature.

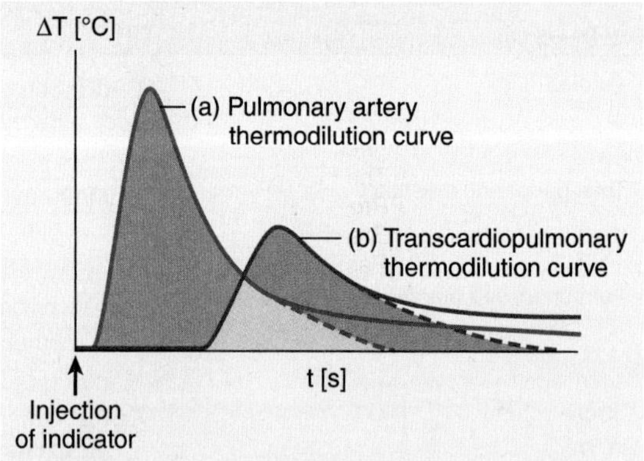

FIGURE 5–19 Comparison of thermodilution curves after injection of cold saline into the superior vena cava. The peak temperature change arrives earlier when measured in the pulmonary artery (a) than if measured in the femoral artery (b). Thereafter, both curves soon reapproximate baseline. (Reproduced with permission from Reuter D, Huang C, Edrich T, et al. Cardiac output monitoring using indicator dilution techniques: Basics, limits and perspectives. *Anesth Analg*. 2010 Mar 1;110(3):799-811.)

Transpulmonary thermodilution (PiCCO® system, VolumeView™ system) relies upon the same principles of thermodilution, but it does not require PA catheterization. A central line and a thermistor equipped arterial catheter (usually placed in the femoral artery) are necessary to perform transpulmonary thermodilution. Thermal measurements from radial artery catheters have been found to be invalid. Transpulmonary thermodilution measurements involve the injection of a cold indicator into the superior vena cava via a central line (Figure 5–20). A thermistor notes the change in temperature in the arterial

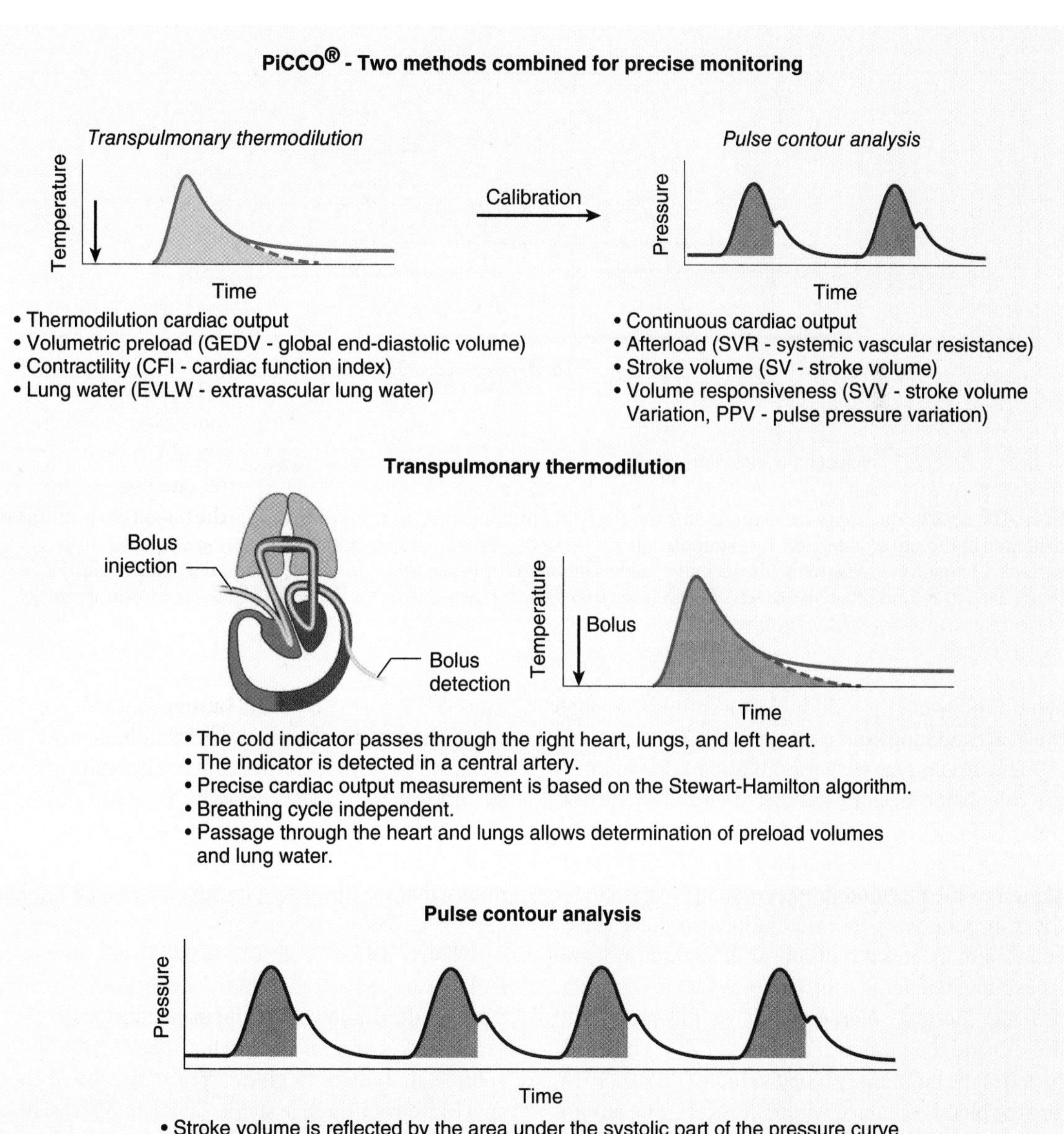

FIGURE 5–20 Two methods combined for precise monitoring. (Reproduced with permission from Royal Philips Electronics.)

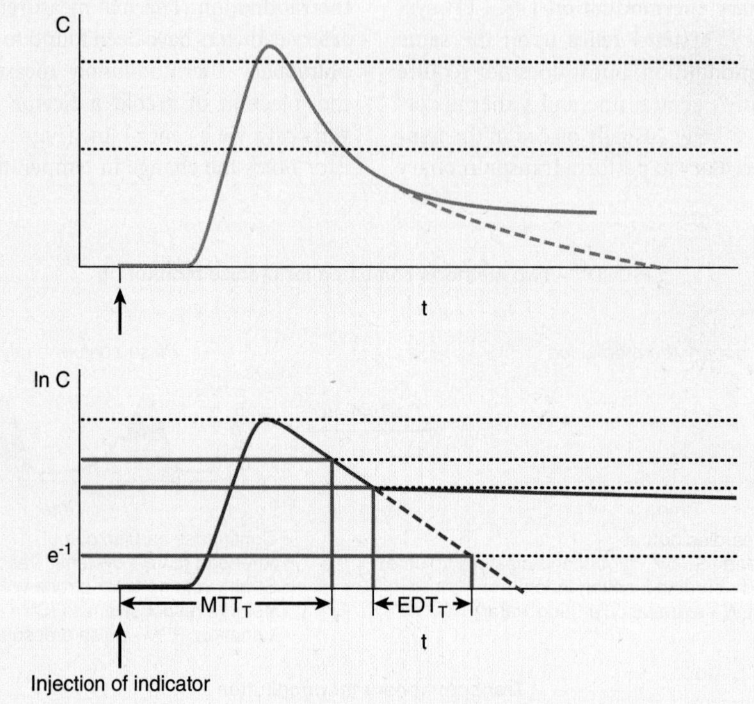

FIGURE 5–21 The upper curve represents the classic thermodilution curve, showing the concentration of an indicator over time at the site of detection. By extrapolation of the curve (dashed line), potential recirculation phenomena are excluded. Logarithmic illustration (lower curve) allows defining the mean transit time (MTT_T) and the exponential decay time (EDT_T) of the indicator. (Reproduced with permission from Reuter D, Huang C, Edrich T, et al. Cardiac output monitoring using indicator dilution techniques: Basics, limits and perspectives. *Anesth Analg.* 2010 Mar 1;110(3):799-811.)

system following the cold indicator's transit through the heart and lungs and estimates the CO.

Transpulmonary thermodilution also permits the calculation of both the global end-diastolic volume (GEDV) and the extravascular lung water (EVLW). Through mathematical analysis and extrapolation of the thermodilution curve, it is possible for the transpulmonary thermodilution computer to calculate both the mean transit time of the indicator and its exponential decay time (Figure 5–21). The intrathoracic thermal volume (ITTV) is the product of the CO and the mean transit time (MTT). The ITTV includes the pulmonary blood volume (PBV), EVLW, and the blood contained within the heart. The pulmonary thermal volume (PTV) includes both the EVLW and the PBV and is obtained by multiplying the CO by the exponential decay time (EDT). Subtracting the PTV from the ITTV gives the GEDV (Figure 5–22). The GEDV is a hypothetical volume that assumes that all of the heart's chambers are simultaneously full in diastole. With a normal index between 640 and 800 mL/m^2, the GEDV can assist in determining volume status. An extravascular lung water index of less than 10 mL/kg is normative. The EVLW is the ITTV minus the intrathoracic blood volume (ITBV). The ITBV = GEDV × 1.25.

Thus, EVLW = ITTV – ITBV. An increased EVLW can be indicative of fluid overload. Through mathematical analysis of the transpulmonary thermodilution curve, it is therefore possible to obtain volumetric indices to guide fluid replacement therapy. Moreover, these systems calculate SV variation and pulse pressure variation through pulse contour analysis, both of which can be used to determine fluid responsiveness. Both SV and pulse pressure are decreased during positive-pressure ventilation.

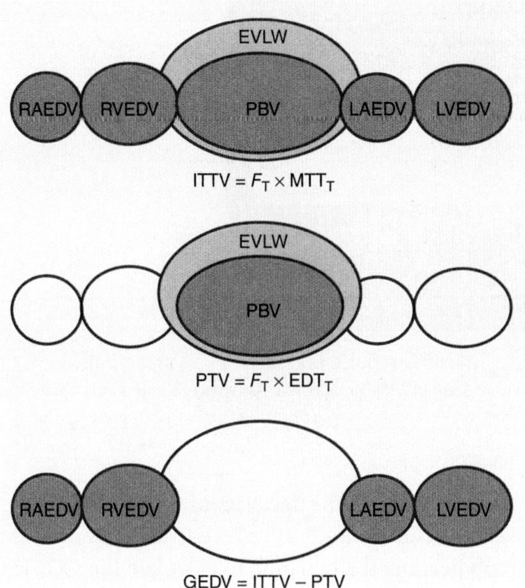

FIGURE 5–22 Assessment of global end-diastolic volume (GEDV) by transcardiopulmonary thermodilution. **Upper row**: The intrathoracic thermal volume (ITTV) is the complete volume of distribution of the thermal indicator, including the right atrium end-diastolic volume (RAEDV), the right ventricle (RVEDV), the left atrium (LAEDV), the left ventricle (LVEDV), the pulmonary blood volume (PBV), and the extravascular lung water (EVLW). It is calculated by multiplying cardiac output (F_T) with the mean transit time (MTT_T) of the indicator. **Middle row**: The pulmonary thermal volume (PTV) represents the largest mixing chamber in this system and includes the PBV and the EVLW and is assessed by multiplying F_T with the exponential decay time (EDT_T) of the thermal indicator. **Bottom row:** The GEDV, including the volumes of the right and the left heart, is now calculated by subtracting PTV from ITTV. (Reproduced with permission from Reuter D, Huang C, Edrich T, et al. Cardiac output monitoring using indicator dilution techniques: Basics, limits and perspectives. *Anesth Analg.* 2010 Mar 1;110(3):799-811.)

The greater the variations over the course of positive-pressure inspiration and expiration, the more likely the patient is to improve hemodynamic measures following volume administration. Figure 5–23 demonstrates that patients located on the steeper portion of the curve will be more responsive to volume administration compared with those whose volume status is already adequate. Dynamic measures such as SV and pulse pressure variation assist in the identification of individuals likely to respond to volume administration (Figures 5-24 and 5-25).

Pulse pressure variation is the change in pulse pressure that occurs throughout the respiratory cycle in patients supported by positive-pressure ventilation. As volume is administered, pulse pressure variation decreases. Variation greater than 12% to 13% is suggestive of fluid responsiveness. Dynamic measures such as pulse pressure variation and stroke volume variation become less reliable when arrhythmias are present. Unfortunately, many of the validation studies using these dynamic measures were performed prior to the routine use of low tidal

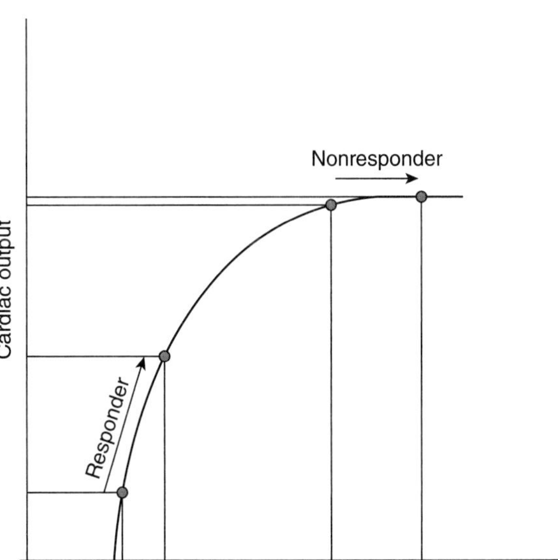

FIGURE 5–23 The fluid responder located on the steep portion of the right atrial pressure (RAP)/cardiac output (CO) curve will augment CO with minimal change in RAP when administered a fluid challenge. Conversely, the nonresponder will see little change in CO; however, RAP will likely increase. (Reproduced with permission from Cherpanath T, Aarts L, Groeneveld J, Geerts B. Defining fluid responsiveness: A guide to patient tailored volume titration. *J Cardiothorac Vasc Anesth.* 2014 Jun;28(3):745-754.)

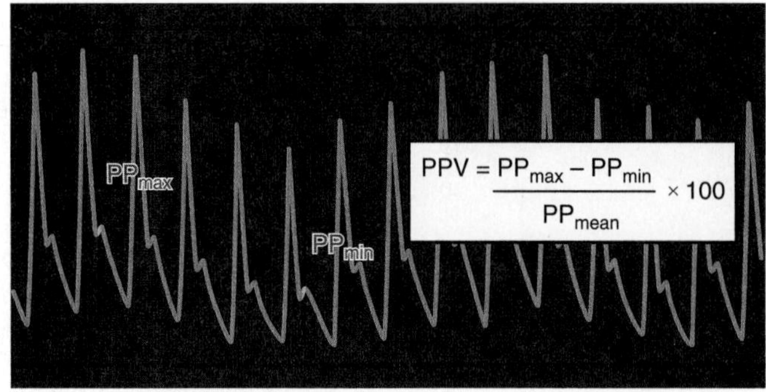

FIGURE 5–24 Calculation of pulse pressure variation (PPV). PP_{max}, maximum pulse pressure; PP_{mean}, mean pulse pressure; PP_{min}, minimum pulse pressure. (Reproduced with permission from Scott MC, Mallemat H, eds. Assessing volume status. *Emerg Med Clin N Am.* 2014 Nov;32(4):811-822.)

volume (6 mL/kg) lung-protective ventilation strategies during positive-pressure ventilation.

B. Dye Dilution

If indocyanine green dye (or another indicator such as lithium) is injected through a central venous catheter, its appearance in the systemic arterial circulation can be measured by analyzing arterial samples with an appropriate detector (eg, a densitometer for indocyanine green). The area under the resulting **dye indicator curve** is related to CO. By analyzing arterial blood pressure and integrating it with CO, systems that use lithium (LiDCO™) also calculate beat-to-beat SV. In the LiDCO™ system, a small bolus of lithium chloride is injected into the circulation. A lithium-sensitive electrode in an arterial catheter measures the decay in lithium concentration over time. Integrating the concentration over a time graph permits the machine to calculate the CO. The LiDCO™ device, like the PiCCO® thermodilution device, employs pulse contour analysis of the arterial waveform to provide ongoing beat-to-beat determinations of CO and other calculated parameters. Lithium dilution determinations can be made in patients who have only peripheral venous access. Lithium should not be administered to patients in the first trimester of pregnancy. The dye dilution technique, however, introduces the problems of indicator recirculation, arterial blood sampling, and background tracer buildup, potentially limiting the use of such approaches perioperatively. Nondepolarizing neuromuscular blockers may affect the lithium sensor.

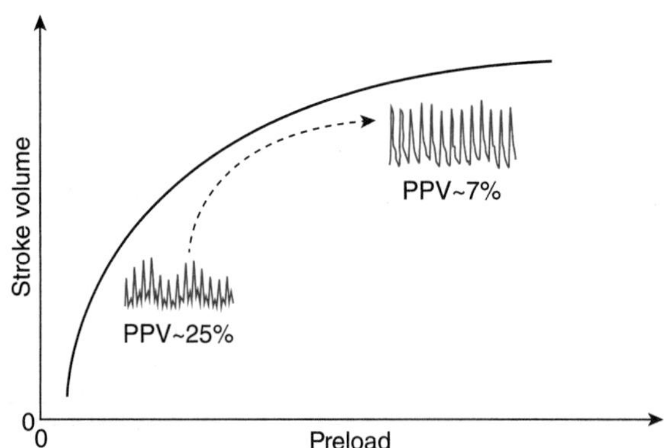

FIGURE 5–25 Pulse pressure variation (PPV) decreases as volume is administered. (Reproduced with permission from Ramsingh D, Alexander B, Cannesson M. Clinical review: Does it matter which hemodynamic monitoring system is used? *Crit Care.* 2013 Mar 5;17(2):208.)

C. Pulse Contour Devices

Pulse contour devices use arterial pressure tracing to estimate the CO and other dynamic parameters, such as pulse pressure and SV variation with mechanical ventilation. These indices are used to help determine if hypotension is likely to respond to fluid therapy.

Pulse contour devices rely upon algorithms that measure the area of the systolic portion of the arterial pressure trace from end diastole to the end of ventricular ejection. The devices then incorporate a calibration factor for the patient's vascular compliance, which is dynamic and not static. Some pulse contour devices rely first on transpulmonary thermodilution or lithium thermodilution to calibrate the machine for subsequent pulse contour measurements. The FloTrac sensor (Edwards Lifesciences) does not require calibration with another measure and relies upon a statistical analysis of its algorithm to account for changes in vascular compliance occurring as a consequence of changed vascular tone.

D. Esophageal Doppler

Esophageal Doppler relies upon the Doppler principle to measure the velocity of blood flow in the descending thoracic aorta. The Doppler principle is integral in perioperative echocardiography. The Doppler effect has been described previously in this chapter. Blood in the aorta is in relative motion compared with the Doppler probe in the esophagus. As red blood cells travel, they reflect a frequency shift, depending upon both the direction and velocity of their movement. When blood flows toward the transducer, its reflected frequency is higher than that which was transmitted by the probe. When blood cells move away from the transducer, the frequency is lower than that which was initially sent by the probe. By using the Doppler equation, it is possible to determine the velocity of blood flow in the aorta. The equation is:

Velocity of blood flow = {frequency change/ cosine of angle of incidence between Doppler beam and blood flow} × {speed of sound in tissue/ 2 (source frequency)}

For Doppler to provide a reliable estimate of velocity, the angle of incidence should be as close to zero as possible since the cosine of 0 is 1. As the angle approaches 90°, the Doppler measure is unreliable, as the cosine of 90° is 0.

The esophageal Doppler device calculates the velocity of flow in the aorta. As the velocities of the cells in the aorta travel at different speeds over the cardiac cycle, the machine obtains a measure of all of the velocities of the cells moving over time. Mathematically integrating the velocities represents the distance that the blood travels. Next, using nomograms, the monitor approximates the area of the descending aorta. The monitor thus calculates both the distance the blood travels, as well as the area: area × length = volume.

Consequently, the SV of blood in the descending aorta is calculated. Knowing the HR allows calculation of that portion of the CO flowing through the descending thoracic aorta, which is approximately 70% of total CO. Correcting for this 30% allows the monitor to estimate the patient's total CO. Esophageal Doppler is dependent upon many assumptions and nomograms, which may hinder its ability to accurately reflect CO in a variety of clinical situations.

E. Thoracic Bioimpedance

Changes in thoracic volume cause changes in thoracic resistance (bioimpedance) to low-amplitude, high-frequency currents. If thoracic changes in bioimpedance are measured following ventricular depolarization, SV can be continuously determined. This noninvasive technique requires six electrodes to inject microcurrents and to sense bioimpedance on both sides of the chest. Increasing fluid in the chest results in less electrical bioimpedance. Mathematical assumptions and correlations are then used to calculate CO from changes in bioimpedance. Disadvantages of thoracic bioimpedance include susceptibility to electrical interference and motion artifacts.

F. Fick Principle

The amount of oxygen consumed by an individual (Vo_2) equals the difference between arterial and venous (a–v) oxygen content (C) (Cao_2 and Cvo_2) multiplied by CO. Therefore,

$$CO = \frac{\text{Oxygen consumption}}{a - vO_2 \text{ content difference}} = \frac{\dot{V}o_2}{Cao_2 - Cvo_2}$$

Mixed venous and arterial oxygen content is easily determined if a PA catheter and an arterial line are in place. Oxygen consumption can also be calculated from the difference between the oxygen content in inspired and expired gas. Variations of the Fick principle are the basis of all indicator–dilution methods of determining CO.

G. Echocardiography

There are no more powerful tools to diagnose and assess cardiac function perioperatively than transthoracic (TTE) and transesophageal echocardiography (TEE). Both TTE and TEE can be employed preoperatively and postoperatively. TTE has the advantage of being completely noninvasive; however, acquiring the "windows" to view the heart can be difficult. In the operating room, limited access to the chest makes TEE an ideal option to visualize the heart. Disposable TEE probes are now available that can remain in position in critically ill patients for days, during which intermittent TEE examinations can be performed.

Echocardiography can be employed by anesthesia staff in two ways, depending upon degrees of training and certification. Basic (or hemodynamic) TEE permits the anesthesiologist to discern the primary source of a patient's hemodynamic instability. Whereas in past decades the PA flotation catheter would be used to determine why the patient might be hypotensive, the anesthetist performing TEE is attempting to determine if the heart is adequately filled, contracting appropriately, not externally compressed, and devoid of any grossly obvious structural defects. At all times, information obtained from TEE must be correlated with other information as to the patient's general condition.

Anesthesiologists performing advanced (diagnostic) TEE make therapeutic and surgical recommendations based upon their TEE interpretations. Various organizations and boards have been established worldwide to certify individuals in all levels of perioperative echocardiography. More importantly, individuals who perform echocardiography should be aware of the credentialing requirements of their respective institutions.

Echocardiography has many uses, including:

- Diagnosis of the source of hemodynamic instability, including myocardial ischemia, systolic and diastolic heart failure, valvular abnormalities, hypovolemia, and pericardial tamponade
- Estimation of hemodynamic parameters, such as SV, CO, and intracavitary pressures
- Diagnosis of structural diseases of the heart, such as valvular heart disease, shunts, aortic diseases
- Guiding surgical interventions, such as mitral valve repair

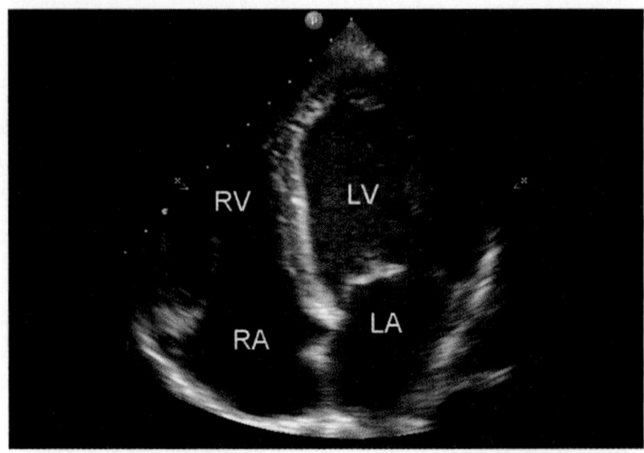

FIGURE 5–26 Normal apical four-chamber view. LA, left atrium; LV, left ventricle; RA, right atrium; RV, right ventricle. (Reproduced with permission from Carmody KA, Moore CL, Feller-Kopman D: *Handbook of Critical Care and Emergency Ultrasound.* New York, NY: McGraw Hill; 2011.)

Various echocardiographic modalities are employed perioperatively by anesthesiologists, including TTE, TEE, epiaortic and epicardial ultrasound, and three-dimensional echocardiography. Some advantages and disadvantages of the modalities are as follows:

- TTE has the advantage of being noninvasive and essentially risk free. Limited scope TTE examinations are now increasingly common in the intensive care unit (Figure 5–26). Bedside TTE exams such as the FATE (focus-assessed transthoracic echocardiography) or FAST (focused assessment with sonography in trauma) protocols can readily assist in hemodynamic diagnosis. It is possible to identify various common cardiac pathologies perioperatively using pattern recognition (Figures 5–27 and 5–28).

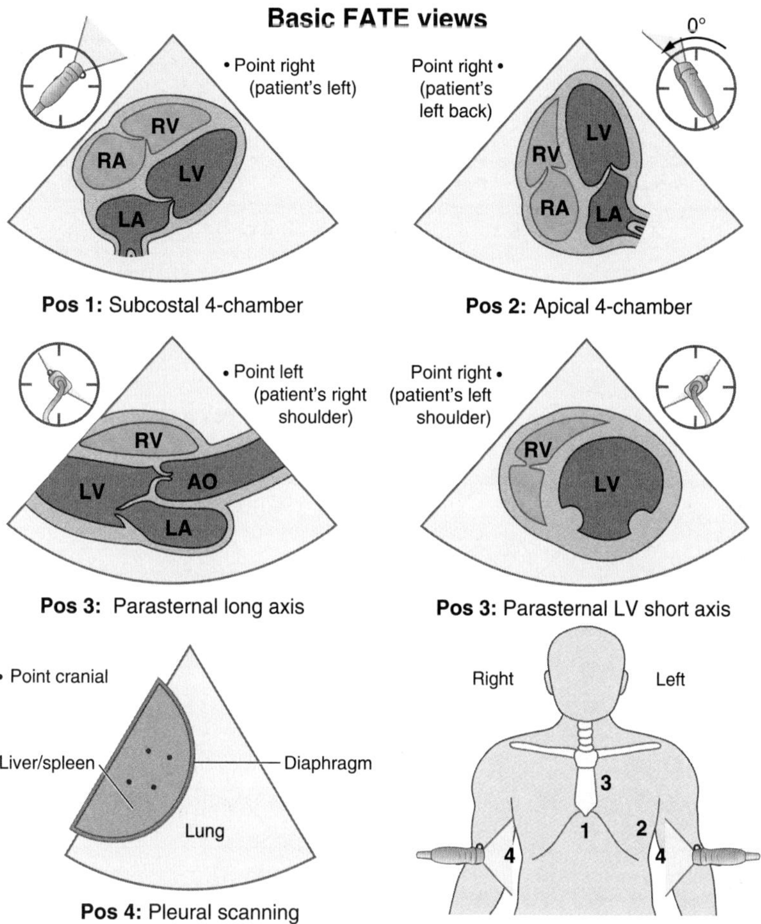

FIGURE 5–27 The FATE examination. AO, aorta; LA, left atrium; LV, left ventricle; RA, right atrium; RV, right ventricle. (Reproduced with permission from UltraSound Airway Breathing Circulation Dolor (USABCD) and Prof. Erik Sloth. http://usabcd.org/node/35.)

- Unlike TTE, TEE is an invasive procedure with the potential for life-threatening complications (esophageal rupture and mediastinitis) (Figure 5–29). The close proximity of the esophagus to the left atrium eliminates the problem of obtaining "windows" to view the heart and permits great detail. TEE has been used frequently in the cardiac surgical operating room over the past decades. Its use to guide therapy in general cases has been limited by both the cost of the equipment and the learning necessary to correctly interpret the images. Both TTE and TEE generate two-dimensional images of the three-dimensional heart. Consequently, it is necessary to view the heart through many two-dimensional image planes and windows to mentally recreate the three-dimensional anatomy. The ability to interpret these images at the advanced certification level requires much training.

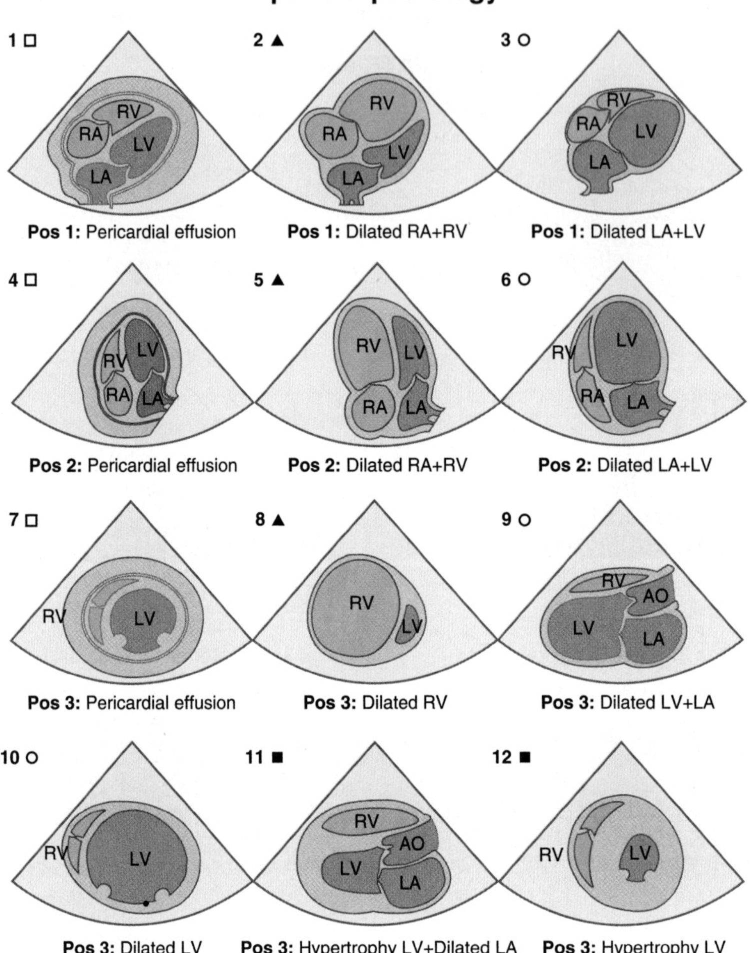

FIGURE 5–28 Important pathological conditions identified with the FATE examination. AO, aorta; LA, left atrium; LV, left ventricle; RA, right atrium; RV, right ventricle. (Reproduced with permission from UltraSound Airway Breathing Circulation Dolor (USABCD) and Prof. Erik Sloth. http://usabcd.org/node/35.)

- Epiaortic and epicardiac ultrasound imaging techniques employ an echo probe wrapped in a sterile sheath and manipulated by thoracic surgeons intraoperatively to obtain views of the aorta and the heart. The air-filled trachea prevents TEE imaging of the ascending aorta. Because the aorta is manipulated during cardiac surgery, detection of atherosclerotic plaques permits the surgeon to potentially minimize the incidence of embolic stroke. Imaging of the heart with epicardial ultrasound permits intraoperative echocardiography when TEE is contraindicated because of esophageal or gastric pathology.

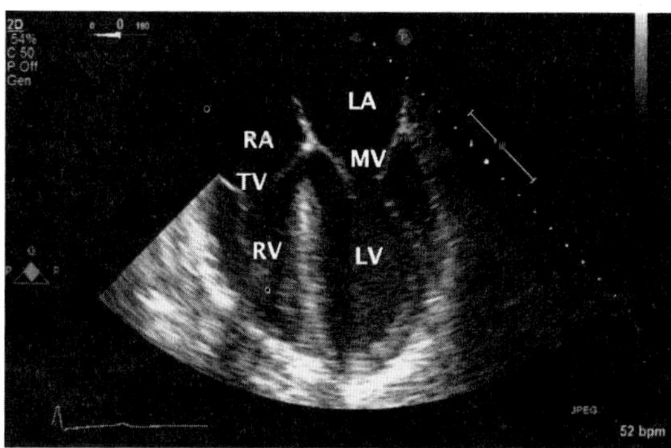

FIGURE 5–29 The structures of the heart as seen on a midesophageal four-chamber view, including the right atrium (RA), tricuspid valve (TV), right ventricle (RV), left atrium (LA), mitral valve (MV), and left ventricle (LV). (Reproduced with permission from Wasnick J, Hillel Z, Kramer D, et al. *Cardiac Anesthesia & Transesophageal Echocardiography.* New York, NY: McGraw Hill; 2011.)

- Three-dimensional echocardiography (TTE and TEE) has become available in recent years (Figure 5–30). These techniques provide a three-dimensional view of the heart's structure. In particular, three-dimensional images can better quantify the heart's volumes and can generate a surgeon's view of the mitral valve to aid in guiding valve repair.

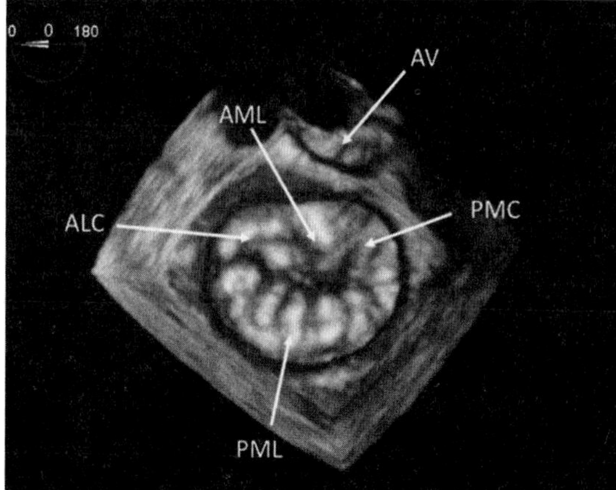

FIGURE 5–30 Three-dimensional echocardiography of the mitral valve demonstrates the anterior leaflet (AML), the posterior leaflet (PML), the anterolateral commissure (ALC), and the posteromedial commissure (PMC). The aortic valve (AV) is also seen. (Reproduced with permission from Wasnick J, Hillel Z, Kramer D, et al. *Cardiac Anesthesia & Transesophageal Echocardiography.* New York, NY: McGraw Hill; 2011.)

Echocardiography employs ultrasound (sound at frequencies greater than normal hearing) from 2 to 10 MHz. A Piezoelectric sensor in the probe transducer converts electrical energy delivered to the probe into ultrasound waves. These waves then travel through the tissues, encountering the blood, the heart, and other structures. Sound waves pass readily through tissues of similar acoustic impedance; however, when they encounter different tissues, they are scattered, refracted, or reflected back toward the ultrasound probe. The echo wave then interacts with the ultrasound probe, generating an electrical signal that can be reconstructed as an image. The machine knows the time delay between the transmitted and the reflected sound wave. By knowing the time delay, the location of the source of the reflected wave can be determined and the image generated. The TEE probe contains myriad crystals generating and processing waves, which then create the echo image. The TEE probe can generate images through multiple planes and can be physically manipulated in the stomach and esophagus, permitting visualization of heart structures (Figure 5–31). These views can be used to determine if the walls of the heart are receiving an adequate blood supply (Figure 5–32). In the healthy heart, the walls thicken and move inwardly with each beat. Wall motion abnormalities, in which the heart walls fail to thicken during systole or move in a dyskinetic fashion, can be associated with myocardial ischemia.

The Doppler effect is routinely used in echocardiographic examinations to determine both the direction and the velocity of blood flow and tissue movement. Blood flow in the heart follows the law of the conservation of mass. Therefore, the volume of blood that flows through one point (eg, the left ventricular outflow tract) must be the same volume that passes through the aortic valve. When the pathway through which the blood flows becomes narrowed (eg, aortic stenosis), the blood velocity must increase to permit the volume to pass. The increase in velocity as blood moves toward an esophageal echo probe is detected. The Bernoulli equation (pressure change = $4V^2$) allows echocardiographers to determine the pressure gradient between areas of different velocities, where v represents the area of maximal velocity (Figure 5–33). Using continuous-wave

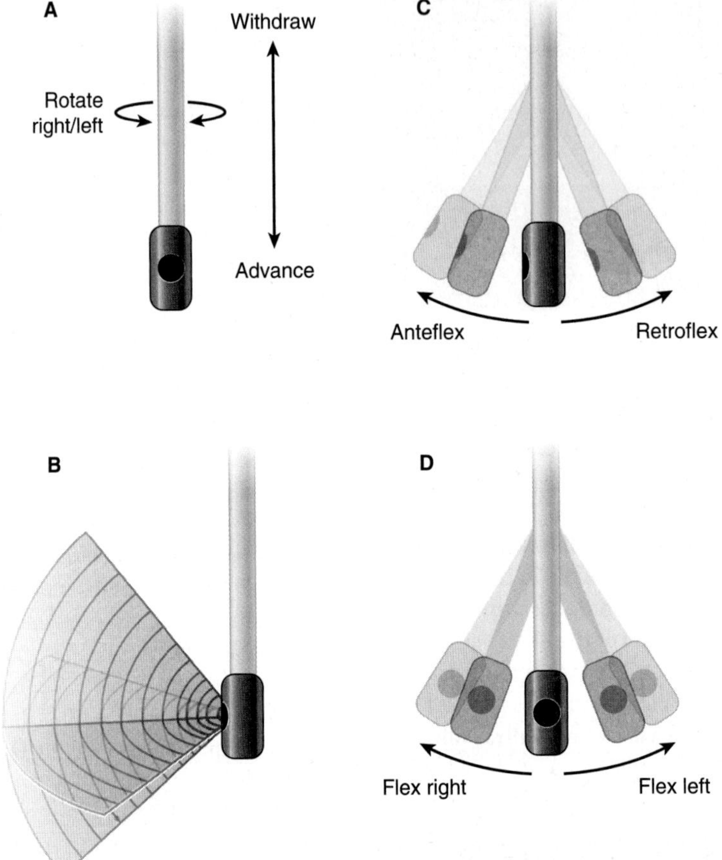

FIGURE 5–31 The echo probe is manipulated by the examiner in multiple ways to create the standard images that constitute the comprehensive perioperative transesophageal echocardiography (TEE) examination. Never force the probe; if resistance is encountered, abandon the examination. Echocardiographic information can be provided by an intraoperative epicardial and epiaortic examination. Advancing the probe in the esophagus permits the upper, mid, and transgastric examinations (**A**). The probe can be turned in the esophagus from left to right to examine both left- and right-sided structures (**A**). Using the button located on the probe permits the echocardiographer to rotate the scan beam through 180°, thereby creating various two-dimensional imaging slices of the three-dimensional heart (**B**). Lastly, panels **C** and **D** demonstrate manipulation of the tip of the probe to permit the beam to be directed to best visualize the image. (Modified with permission from Shanewise JS, Cheung AT, Aronson S, et al. ASE/SCA guidelines for performing a comprehensive intraoperative multiplane transesophageal echocardiography examination; recommendations of the American Society of Echocardiography Council for Intraoperative Echocardiography and the Society for Cardiovascular Anesthesiologists Task Force for Certification in Perioperative Transesophageal Echocardiography. *Anesth Analg.* 1999 Oct;89(4):870-884.)

Doppler, it is possible to determine the maximal velocity as blood accelerates through a pathological heart structure. For example, a blood flow of 4 m/s reflects a pressure gradient of 64 mm Hg between an area of slow flow (the left ventricular outflow tract) and a region of high flow (a stenotic aortic valve).

The Bernoulli equation permits echocardiographers to estimate PA and other intracavitary pressures.

$$\text{Assume } P_1 >> P_2$$

Blood flow proceeds from an area of high pressure (P_1) to an area of low pressure (P_2).

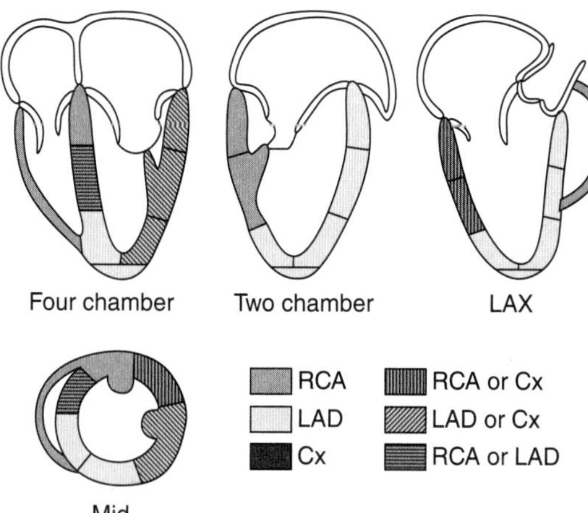

FIGURE 5–32 Typical distributions of the right coronary artery (RCA), the left anterior descending (LAD) coronary artery, and the circumflex (Cx) coronary artery from transesophageal views of the left ventricle. The arterial distribution varies among patients. Some segments have variable coronary perfusion. (Adapted with permission from Lang RM, Bierig M, Devereux RB, et al. Recommendations for chamber quantification: a report from the American Society of Echocardiography's Guidelines and Standards Committee and the Chamber Quantification Writing Group, developed in conjunction with the European Association of Echocardiography, a branch of the European Society of Cardiology, *J Am Soc Echocardiogr.* 2005 Dec;18(12):1440-1463.)

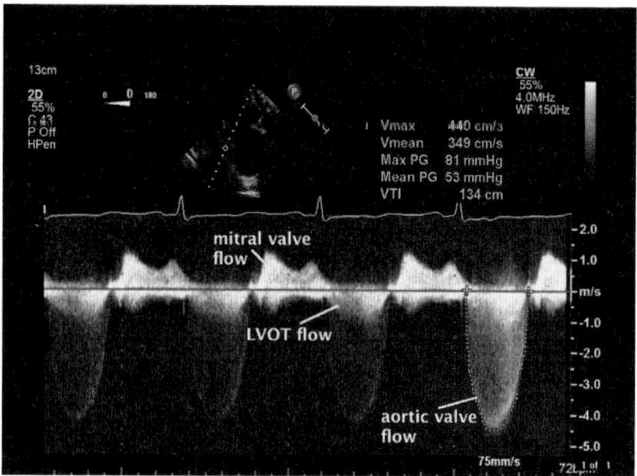

FIGURE 5–33 The time-velocity interval (TVI) of the aortic valve is calculated using continuous-wave Doppler, while pulsed-wave Doppler is useful for measurements at lower blood velocities. This continuous-wave Doppler has been aligned parallel to that aortic valve flow as imaged using the deep transgastric view. Of note, the blood velocity across the aortic valve is greater than 4 m/s. (Reproduced with permission from Wasnick J, Hillel Z, Kramer D, et al. *Cardiac Anesthesia & Transesophageal Echocardiography.* New York, NY: McGraw Hill; 2011.)

The pressure gradient = $4V^2$, where V is the maximal velocity measured in meters per second.

Thus,

$$4V^2 = P_1 - P_2$$

Thus, assuming that there is a jet of regurgitant blood flow from the left ventricle into the left atrium and that left ventricular systolic pressure (P_1) is the same as systemic blood pressure (eg, no aortic stenosis), it is possible to calculate left atrial pressure (P_2). In this manner, echocardiographers can estimate intracavitary pressures when there are pressure gradients, measurable flow velocities between areas of high and low pressure, and knowledge of either P_1 or P_2 (Figure 5–34).

Color flow Doppler is used by echocardiographers to identify areas of abnormal flow. Color flow Doppler creates a visual picture by assigning a color code to the blood velocities in the heart. Blood flow directed away from the echocardiographic transducer is blue, whereas that which is moving toward the probe is red. The higher the velocity of flow, the lighter the color hue (Figure 5–35). When the velocity of blood flow becomes greater than that which the machine can measure, flow toward the probe is misinterpreted as flow away from the probe, creating images of turbulent flow and "aliasing" of the image. Such changes in flow pattern are used by echocardiographers to identify areas of pathology.

Doppler can also be used to provide an estimate of SV and CO. Similar to the esophageal Doppler probes previously described, TTE and TEE can be used to estimate CO. Assuming that the left ventricular outflow tract is a cylinder, it is possible to measure its diameter (Figure 5–36). Knowing this, it is possible to calculate the area through which blood flows using the following equation:

$$\text{Area} = \pi r^2 = 0.785 \times \text{diameter}^2$$

Next, the time velocity integral is determined. A Doppler beam is aligned in parallel with the left

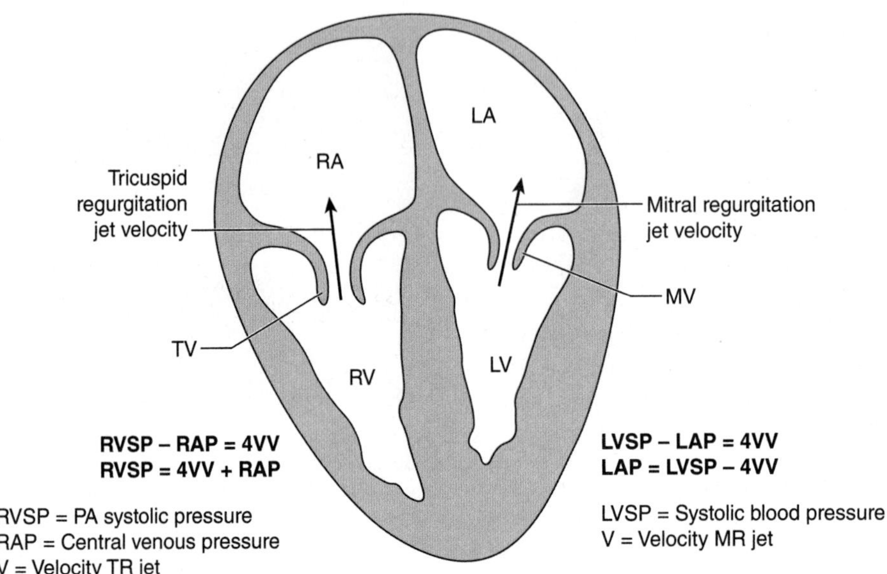

FIGURE 5–34 Intracavity pressures can be calculated using known pressures and the Bernoulli equation when regurgitant jets are present. The pulmonary artery (PA) systolic pressure is obtained when tricuspid regurgitation is present and the right atrial pressure is known. Assuming no pulmonic valve disease, the right ventricular systolic pressure (RVSP) and the pulmonary systolic pressure are the same. The left atrial pressure can be similarly calculated if mitral regurgitation is present. Again, assuming no valvular disease, left ventricular systolic pressure (LVSP) should equal systemic systolic blood pressure. Subtracting $4V^2$ from the LVSP estimates the left atrial pressure (LAP). (Reproduced with permission from Wasnick J, Hillel Z, Kramer D, et al. *Cardiac Anesthesia & Transesophageal Echocardiography.* New York, NY: McGraw Hill; 2011.)

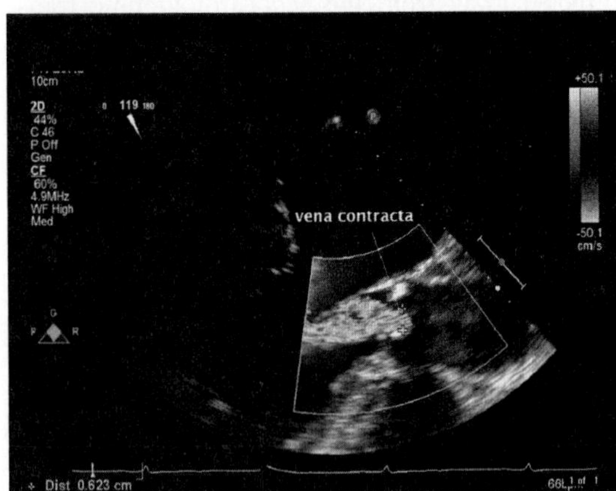

FIGURE 5–35 The color flow Doppler image of the midesophageal aortic valve long-axis view demonstrates measurement of the vena contracta of aortic regurgitation. The vena contracta represents the smallest diameter of the regurgitant jet at the level of the aortic valve. A vena contracta of 6.2 mm grades the aortic regurgitation in this case as severe. (Reproduced with permission from Wasnick J, Hillel Z, Kramer D, et al. *Cardiac Anesthesia & Transesophageal Echocardiography.* New York, NY: McGraw Hill; 2011.)

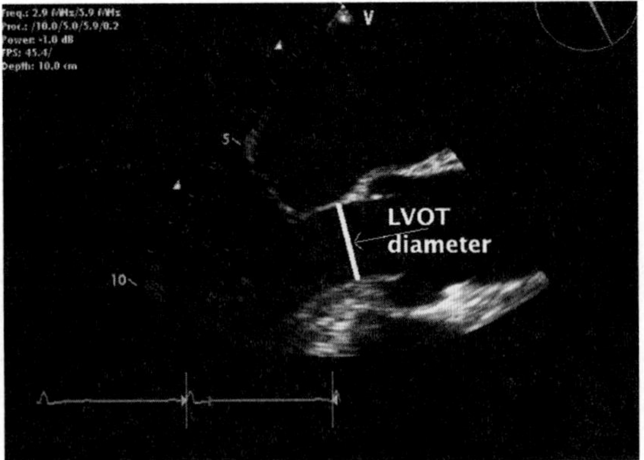

FIGURE 5–36 The midesophageal long-axis view is employed in this image to measure the diameter of the left ventricular outflow tract (LVOT). Knowing the diameter of the LVOT permits the calculation of the LVOT area. (Reproduced with permission from Wasnick J, Hillel Z, Kramer D, et al. *Cardiac Anesthesia & Transesophageal Echocardiography.* New York, NY: McGraw Hill; 2011.)

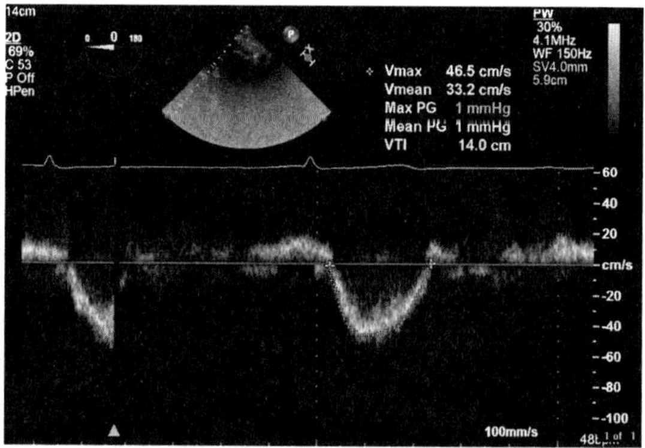

FIGURE 5–37 Pulsed-wave Doppler is employed in this deep transgastric view interrogation of the left ventricular outflow tract (LVOT). Blood is flowing in the LVOT away from the esophagus. Therefore, the flow velocities appear below the baseline. Flow velocity through the LVOT is 46.5 cm/s. This is as expected when there is no pathology noted as blood is ejected along the LVOT. Tracing the flow envelope (*dotted lines*) identifies the time-velocity interval (TVI). In this example, the TVI is 14 cm. (Reproduced with permission from Wasnick J, Hillel Z, Kramer D, et al. *Cardiac Anesthesia & Transesophageal Echocardiography.* New York, NY: McGraw Hill; 2011.)

ventricular outflow tract (Figure 5–37). The velocities passing through the left ventricular outflow tract are recorded, and the machine integrates the velocity/time curve to determine the distance the blood traveled.

$$\text{Area} \times \text{length} = \text{volume}$$
In this instance, the SV is calculated:
$$\text{SV} \times \text{HR} = \text{CO}$$

Lastly, Doppler can be used to examine the movement of the myocardial tissue. Tissue velocity is normally 8 to 15 cm/s (much less than that of blood, which is 100 cm/s). It is possible to discern both the directionality and velocity of the heart's movement using the tissue Doppler function of the echo machine. During diastolic filling, the lateral annulus myocardium will move toward a TEE probe. Reduced myocardial velocities (<8 cm/s) are associated with impaired diastolic function and higher left ventricular end-diastolic pressures.

Ultimately, echocardiography can provide comprehensive cardiovascular monitoring. Its routine use outside of the cardiac operating room has been hindered by both the costs of the equipment and the training required to correctly interpret the images. It is likely that anesthesia staff will perform an increasing number of echocardiographic examinations perioperatively. All anesthesiology trainees should acquire basic echocardiography skills. When questions arise beyond those related to hemodynamic guidance, interpretation by an individual credentialed in diagnostic echocardiography is warranted.

CASE DISCUSSION

Hemodynamic Monitoring and Management of a Complicated Patient

A 68-year-old patient presents with a perforated colon secondary to diverticulitis. Vital signs are as follows: heart rate, 120 beats/min; blood pressure, 80 mm Hg/55 mm Hg; respiratory rate, 28 breaths/min; and body temperature, 38C°. The patient is scheduled for an emergency exploratory laparotomy. The patient's history includes placement of a drug-eluting stent in the left anterior descending artery 2 weeks earlier. The patient's medications include metoprolol and clopidogrel.

What hemodynamic monitors should be employed?

This patient presents with multiple medical issues that could lead to perioperative hemodynamic instability. The patient has a history of coronary artery disease treated with stents. Any previous and current ECGs should be reviewed for signs of new ST- and T-wave changes, heralding ischemia. The patient is both tachycardic and febrile and thus may be concurrently ischemic, vasodilated, and hypovolemic. All of these conditions could complicate perioperative management.

Arterial cannulation and monitoring will provide beat-to-beat blood pressure determinations intraoperatively and will also provide for blood gas measurements in a patient likely to be acidotic and hemodynamically unstable. Central venous access is obtained to permit volume resuscitation and to provide a port for the delivery of fluid for transpulmonary measurements of CO and SV variation. Alternatively, pulse contour analysis can be employed from an arterial trace to determine volume responsiveness should the patient become hemodynamically unstable. Echocardiography can be used to determine ventricular function, filling pressures, and CO and provide surveillance for the development of ischemia-induced wall motion abnormalities.

A PA catheter could also be placed to measure CO and pulmonary capillary occlusion pressure; however, we would use TEE if we were unable to manage the patient well with an arterial line, a CVP catheter, and a monitor for CO (eg, pulse contour analysis, transpulmonary thermodilution).

The choice of hemodynamic monitors remains with the individual physician and the availability of various monitoring techniques. It is important to also consider which monitors can be used post-operatively to ensure the continuation of goal-directed therapy.

SUGGESTED READINGS

Alhashemi JA, Cecconi M, della Rocca G, Cannesson M, Hofer CK. Minimally invasive monitoring of cardiac output in the cardiac surgery intensive care unit. *Curr Heart Fail Rep.* 2010;7(3):116.

Beaulieu Y, Marik P. Bedside ultrasonography in the ICU: part 1. *Chest.* 2005;128:881.

Beaulieu Y, Marik P. Bedside ultrasonography in the ICU: part 2. *Chest.* 2005;128:1766.

Bein B, Renner J. Best practice & research clinical anaesthesiology: advances in haemodynamic monitoring for the perioperative patient: perioperative cardiac output monitoring. *Best Pract Res Clin Anaesthesiol.* 2019;33:139.

Breukers RM, Groeneveld AB, de Wilde RB, Jansen JR. Transpulmonary versus continuous thermodilution cardiac output after valvular and coronary artery surgery. *Interact Cardiovasc Thorac Surg.* 2009;9:4.

Chatterjee K. The Swan Ganz catheters: past, present, and future. A viewpoint. *Circulation.* 2009;119:147.

Cherpanath TG, Aarts LP, Groeneveld JA, Geerts BF. Defining fluid responsiveness: a guide to patient-tailored volume titration. *J Cardiothorac Vasc Anesth.* 2014;28:745.

De Backer D, Vincent JL. The pulmonary artery catheter: is it still alive? *Curr Opin Crit Care.* 2018;24:204.

Fayad A, Shillcutt SK. Perioperative transesophageal echocardiography for non-cardiac surgery. *Can J Anaesth.* 2018;65:381.

Funk D, Moretti E, Gan T. Minimally invasive cardiac monitoring in the perioperative setting. *Anesth Analg.* 2009;108:887.

Geisen M, Spray D, Fletcher S. Echocardiography-based hemodynamic management in the cardiac surgical intensive care unit. *J Cardiothorac Vasc Anesth.* 2014;28:733.

Goepfert MS, Reuter DA, Akyol D, Lamm P, Kilger E, Goetz AE. Goal-directed fluid management reduces vasopressor and catecholamine use in cardiac surgery patients. *Intensive Care Med.* 2007;33:96.

Hadian M, Kim H, Severyn D, Pinsky M. Cross comparison of cardiac output trending accuracy of LiDCO, PiCCO, FloTrac and pulmonary artery catheters. *Crit Care.* 2010;14:R212.

Hett D, Jonas M. Non-invasive cardiac output monitoring. *Curr Anaesth Crit Care.* 2003;14:187.

Joshi R, de Witt B, Mosier J. Optimizing oxygen delivery in the critically ill: the utility of lactate and central venous oxygen saturation ($SCVO_2$) as a roadmap of resuscitation in shock. *J Emerg Med.* 2014;47:493.

Kobe J, Mishra N, Arya VK, Al-Moustadi W, Nates W, Kumar B. Cardiac output monitoring: technology and choice. *Ann Card Anaesth.* 2019;22:6.

Maheshwari K, Khanna S, Bajracharya GR, et al. A randomized trial of continuous noninvasive blood pressure monitoring during noncardiac surgery. *Anesth Analg.* 2018;127:424.

Marik P. Noninvasive cardiac output monitors: a state of the art review. *J Cardiovasc Thorac Anesth.* 2013;27:121.

McGuinness S, Parke R. Using cardiac output monitoring to guide perioperative haemodynamic therapy. *Curr Opin Crit Care.* 2015;21:364.

Michard F, Alaya S, Zarka V, Bahloul M, Richard C, Teboul JL. Global end-diastolic volume as an indicator of cardiac preload in patients with septic shock. *Chest.* 2003;124:1900.

Monnet X, Teboul JL. Transpulmonary thermodilution: advantages and limits. *Crit Care.* 2017;21:147.

Ramsingh D, Alexander B, Cannesson M. Clinical review: does it matter which hemodynamic monitoring system is used? *Crit Care.* 2013;17:208.

Renner J, Grünewald M, Bein B. Monitoring high-risk patients: minimally invasive and non-invasive possibilities. *Best Pract Res Clin Anaesthesiol.* 2016;30:201.

Reuter DA, Huang C, Edrich T, Shernan SK, Eltzschig HK. Cardiac output monitoring using indicator-dilution techniques: basics, limits, and perspectives. *Anesth Analg.* 2010;110:799.

Rex S. Brose S, Metzelder S, et al. Prediction of fluid responsiveness in patients during cardiac surgery. *Br J Anaesth.* 2004;93:782.

Roach JK, Thiele RH. Perioperative blood pressure monitoring. *Best Pract Res Clin Anaesthesiol.* 2019;33:127.

Saugel B, Cecconi M, Hajjar LA. Noninvasive cardiac output monitoring in cardiothoracic surgery patients: available methods and future directions. *J Cardiothorac Vasc Anesth.* 2019;33:1742.

Schmidt C, Berggreen AE, Heringlake M. Perioperative hemodynamic monitoring: still a place for cardiac filling pressures? *Best Pract Res Clin Anaesthesiol.* 2019;33:155.

Shanewise J, Cheung A, Aronson S, et al. ASE/SCA guidelines for performing a comprehensive intraoperative multiplane transesophageal echocardiography examination: recommendations of the American Society of Echocardiography Council for Intraoperative Echocardiography and the Society of Cardiovascular Anesthesiologists Task Force for Certification in Perioperative Transesophageal Echocardiography. *Anesth Analg.* 1999;89:870.

Singer M. Oesophageal Doppler monitoring: should it be routine for high-risk surgical patients? *Curr Opin Anesthesiol.* 2011;24:171.

Singh K, Mayo P. Critical care echocardiography and outcomes in the critically ill *Curr Opin Crit Care.* 2018;24:316.

Skubas N. Intraoperative Doppler tissue imaging is a valuable addition to cardiac anesthesiologists' armamentarium: a core review. *Anesth Analg.* 2009;108:48.

Strumwasser A, Frankel H, Murthi S, Clark D, Kirton O; American Association for the Surgery of Trauma Committee on Critical Care. Hemodynamic monitoring of the injured patient: from central venous pressure to focused echocardiography. *J Trauma Acute Care Surg.* 2016;80:499.

Vincent JL. Fluid management in the critically ill. *Kidney Int.* 2019;96:52.

WEBSITE

The American Society of Anesthesiologists standards for basic anesthesia monitoring can be found on the organization's website. http://www.asahq.org

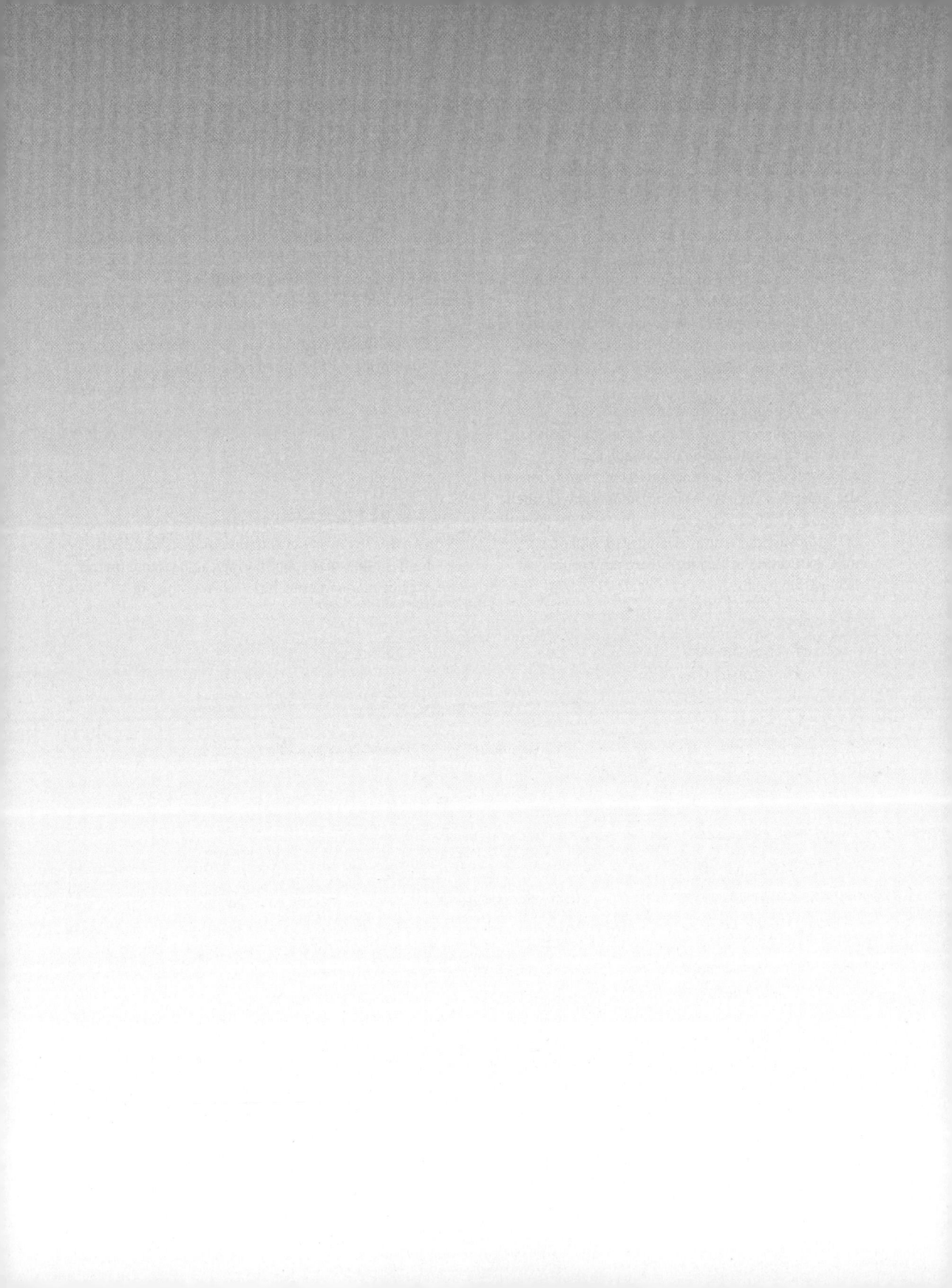

CHAPTER 6

Noncardiovascular Monitoring

KEY CONCEPTS

1 Capnographs rapidly and reliably detect esophageal intubation—a cause of anesthetic catastrophe—but do not reliably detect mainstem bronchial intubation.

2 Postoperative residual paralysis remains a problem in postanesthesia care, producing potentially injurious airway and respiratory function compromise and increasing length of stay and cost in the postanesthesia care unit (PACU).

The previous chapter reviewed the routine hemodynamic monitoring used in anesthesia practice. This chapter examines the vast array of techniques and devices used perioperatively to monitor neuromuscular transmission, neurological condition, respiratory gas exchange, and body temperature.

Respiratory Gas Exchange Monitors

PRECORDIAL & ESOPHAGEAL STETHOSCOPES

Indications

Prior to the routine availability of gas exchange monitors, anesthesiologists used a precordial or esophageal stethoscope to ensure that the lungs were being ventilated, to monitor for circuit disconnections, and to auscultate heart tones to confirm a beating heart. Although largely supplanted by other modalities, the finger on the pulse and auscultation remain frontline monitors, especially when technology fails. Chest auscultation remains the primary method to confirm bilateral lung ventilation in the operating room, even though detection of an end-tidal carbon dioxide (CO_2) waveform is definitive to exclude esophageal intubation.

Contraindications

Esophageal stethoscopes and esophageal temperature probes should be avoided in patients with esophageal varices or strictures.

Techniques & Complications

A precordial stethoscope (Wenger chest piece) is a heavy, bell-shaped piece of metal placed over the chest or suprasternal notch. Although its weight tends to maintain its position, double-sided adhesive disks maintain an acoustic seal to the patient's skin. Various chest pieces are available, but the child size works well for most patients. The bell is connected to the anesthesia provider's earpiece by extension tubing.

The esophageal stethoscope is a soft plastic catheter (8–24F) with balloon-covered distal openings (Figure 6–1). Although the quality of breath and heart sounds is much better than with a precordial stethoscope, its use is limited to intubated patients. Temperature probes, electrocardiogram (ECG) leads, ultrasound probes, and even atrial

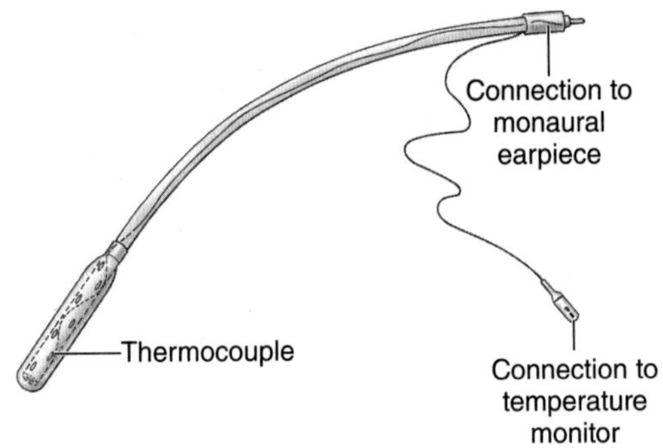

FIGURE 6–1 Esophageal stethoscope.

pacemaker electrodes have been incorporated into esophageal stethoscopes. Placement through the mouth or nose can occasionally cause mucosal irritation and bleeding. Rarely, the stethoscope slides into the trachea instead of the esophagus, resulting in a gas leak around the tracheal tube cuff.

Clinical Considerations

The information provided by a precordial or esophageal stethoscope includes confirmation of ventilation, quality of breath sounds (eg, stridor, wheezing), regularity of heart rate, and quality of heart tones (muffled tones are associated with decreased cardiac output). The confirmation of bilateral breath sounds after tracheal intubation, however, is best made with a binaural stethoscope.

PULSE OXIMETRY

Indications & Contraindications

Pulse oximeters are mandatory monitors for any anesthetic, including cases of moderate sedation. There are no contraindications.

Techniques & Complications

Pulse oximeters combine the principles of oximetry and plethysmography to noninvasively measure oxygen saturation in arterial blood. A sensor containing light sources (two or three light-emitting diodes) and a light detector (a photodiode) is placed across a finger, toe, earlobe, or any other perfused tissue that can be transilluminated. When the light source and detector are opposite one another across the perfused tissue, transmittance oximetry is used. When the light source and detector are placed on the same side of the patient (eg, the forehead), the backscatter (reflectance) of light is recorded by the detector.

Oximetry depends on the observation that oxygenated and reduced hemoglobin differ in their absorption of red and infrared light (Lambert–Beer law). Specifically, oxyhemoglobin (Hbo_2) absorbs more infrared light (940 nm), whereas deoxyhemoglobin absorbs more red light (660 nm) and thus appears blue, or cyanotic, to the naked eye. The change in light absorption during arterial pulsations is the basis of oximetric determinations (Figure 6–2). The ratio of the absorptions at the red and infrared wavelengths is analyzed by a microprocessor to provide the oxygen saturation (Spo_2) of arterial blood based on established norms. The greater the ratio of red to infrared absorption, the lower the arterial hemoglobin oxygen saturation. Arterial pulsations are identified by plethysmography, allowing corrections for light absorption by nonpulsating venous blood and tissue. The heat from the light source or

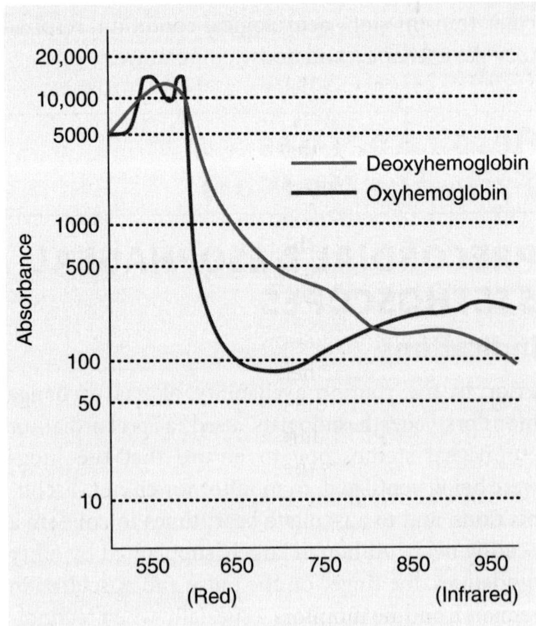

FIGURE 6–2 Oxyhemoglobin and deoxyhemoglobin differ in their absorption of red and infrared light.

sensor pressure may, in extraordinarily rare circumstances, cause tissue damage. No user calibration is required.

Clinical Considerations

In addition to Spo_2, pulse oximeters provide an indication of tissue perfusion (pulse amplitude) and measure heart rate. Depending on a particular patient's oxygen–hemoglobin dissociation curve, a 90% saturation may indicate a Pao_2 of less than 65 mm Hg. Clinically detectable cyanosis usually corresponds to Spo_2 of less than 80%. Mainstem bronchial intubation will usually go undetected by pulse oximetry in the absence of lung disease or low fraction of inspired oxygen (Fio_2) concentrations.

Because carboxyhemoglobin (COHb) and Hbo_2 absorb light at 660 nm, pulse oximeters that compare only two wavelengths of light will register a falsely high reading in patients with carbon monoxide poisoning. Methemoglobin has the same absorption coefficient at both red and infrared wavelengths. The resulting 1:1 absorption ratio corresponds to a saturation reading of 85%. **Thus, methemoglobinemia causes a falsely low saturation reading when Sao_2 is actually greater than 85% and a falsely high reading if Sao_2 is actually less than 85%.**

Most pulse oximeters are inaccurate at low Spo_2, and all demonstrate a delay between changes in Sao_2 and Spo_2. **Other causes of pulse oximetry artifact include excessive ambient light, motion, methylene blue dye, venous pulsations in a dependent limb, low perfusion (eg, low cardiac output, profound anemia, hypothermia, increased systemic vascular resistance), a malpositioned sensor, and leakage of light from the light-emitting diode to the photodiode, bypassing the arterial bed (optical shunting).** Nevertheless, pulse oximetry can be an invaluable aid to the rapid diagnosis of hypoxia, which may occur in unrecognized esophageal intubation, and it furthers the goal of monitoring oxygen delivery to vital organs. In the recovery room, pulse oximetry helps identify postoperative pulmonary problems, such as hypoventilation, bronchospasm, and atelectasis. Advanced examination of the photoplethysmographic waveform can aid in the assessment of volume responsiveness in mechanically ventilated patients.

Two extensions of pulse oximetry technology are mixed venous blood oxygen saturation (Svo_2) and noninvasive brain oximetry. The former requires the placement of a pulmonary artery catheter containing fiberoptic sensors that continuously determine Svo_2 in a manner analogous to pulse oximetry. Because $Svo_2/Scvo_2$ varies with changes in hemoglobin concentration, cardiac output, arterial oxygen saturation, and whole-body oxygen consumption, its interpretation is somewhat complex. Impaired oxygen delivery to the tissues (reduced arterial oxygen saturation, reduced cardiac output, increased tissue oxygen demand) results in lower venous oxygen saturation. Higher venous oxygen concentrations occur when tissue oxygen delivery exceeds tissue demand or arteriovenous shunting occurs. Measurement of central venous oxygen saturation ($Scvo_2$) is frequently used as a surrogate for Svo_2. Svo_2 measures the saturation of venous blood returning from the upper body, the cardiac circulation, and the lower body. Normally, Svo_2 is approximately 70%. $Scvo_2$ is usually a few percentage points higher as it does not reflect venous return from the cardiac circulation.

Noninvasive brain oximetry monitors regional oxygen saturation (rSo_2) of hemoglobin in the brain. A sensor placed on the forehead emits light of specific wavelengths and measures the light reflected back to the sensor (near-infrared optical spectroscopy). Unlike pulse oximetry, brain oximetry measures venous and capillary blood oxygen saturation in addition to arterial blood saturation. Thus, its oxygen saturation readings represent the average oxygen saturation of all regional microvascular hemoglobin (approximately 70%). Cardiac arrest, cerebral embolization, and severe hypoxia cause a dramatic decrease in rSo_2. Cerebral oximetry is routinely employed in the perioperative management of patients undergoing cardiopulmonary bypass. (See the section "Neurological System Monitors.")

CAPNOGRAPHY

Indications & Contraindications

Determination of end-tidal CO_2 ($ETco_2$) concentration to confirm adequate ventilation is mandatory during all anesthetic procedures. Increases in alveolar dead space ventilation (eg, pulmonary thromboembolism, venous air embolism, decreased pulmonary perfusion) produce a decrease in ETCO_2 compared with arterial CO_2 concentration (PaCO_2). Generally, ETCO_2 and PaCO_2 increase or decrease depending upon the balance of CO_2 production and CO_2 elimination (ventilation). A rapid fall of ETCO_2 is a sensitive indicator of air embolism, in which both an increase in dead space ventilation and a decrease in cardiac output may occur. Capnography is also used to gauge the success of ongoing resuscitation, where improvements in perfusion will be heralded by increases in end-tidal CO_2. There are no contraindications.

Techniques & Complications

Capnography is a valuable monitor of the pulmonary, cardiovascular, and anesthetic breathing systems. Capnographs in common use rely on the absorption of infrared light by CO_2. As with oximetry, absorption of infrared light by CO_2 is governed by the Beer–Lambert law.

Diverting (sidestream) capnographs continuously suction gas from the breathing circuit into a sample cell within the bedside monitor. CO_2 concentration is determined by comparing infrared light absorption in the sample cell with a chamber free of CO_2. Continuous aspiration of anesthetic gas essentially represents a leak in the breathing circuit that will contaminate the operating room unless it is scavenged or returned to the breathing system. High aspiration rates (up to 250 mL/min) and low-dead-space sampling tubing usually increase sensitivity and decrease lag time. However, if tidal volumes (VT) are small (eg, pediatric patients), a high rate of aspiration may entrain fresh gas from the circuit and dilute ETCO_2 measurement. Low aspiration rates (<50 mL/min) can retard ETCO_2 measurement and underestimate it during rapid ventilation. Diverting units are prone to water precipitation in the aspiration tube and sampling cell that can cause obstruction of the sampling line and erroneous readings. Expiratory valve malfunction and depleted CO_2-absorbent media are detected by the presence of CO_2 in inspired gas. Although inspiratory valve failure also results in rebreathing CO_2, this is not as readily apparent because part of the inspiratory volume will still be free of CO_2, causing the monitor to read zero during part of the inspiratory phase.

Clinical Considerations

1 Capnographs rapidly and reliably detect esophageal intubation—a cause of anesthetic catastrophe—but do not reliably detect mainstem bronchial intubation. Although there may be some CO_2 in the stomach from swallowed expired air, this should be washed out within a few breaths. Sudden cessation of CO_2 during the expiratory phase may indicate a circuit disconnection. The increased metabolic rate caused by malignant hyperthermia causes a marked rise in ETCO_2.

The gradient between PaCO_2 and ETCO_2 (normally 2–5 mm Hg) reflects alveolar dead space (alveoli that are ventilated but not perfused). Any significant reduction in lung perfusion (eg, air embolism, decreased cardiac output, or decreased blood pressure) increases alveolar dead space, dilutes expired CO_2, and lessens ETCO_2. Capnographs display a waveform of CO_2 concentration that allows recognition of a variety of conditions (Figure 6–3).

ANESTHETIC GAS ANALYSIS

Indications

Analysis of anesthetic gases is essential during any procedure requiring inhalation anesthesia. There are no contraindications to analyzing these gases.

Techniques

Techniques for analyzing multiple anesthetic gases include mass spectrometry, Raman spectroscopy, infrared spectrophotometry, or piezoelectric crystal (quartz) oscillation. Most of these methods are primarily of historical interest, as most anesthetic gases are now measured by infrared absorption analysis.

Infrared units use a variety of techniques similar to that described for capnography. These devices are all based on the Beer–Lambert law, which provides a formula for measuring an unknown gas within inspired gas because the absorption of infrared light passing through a solvent (inspired or expired gas) is proportional to the amount of the unknown gas. Oxygen and nitrogen do not absorb infrared light. There are a number of commercially available devices that use a single- or dual-beam infrared light source and positive or negative filtering.

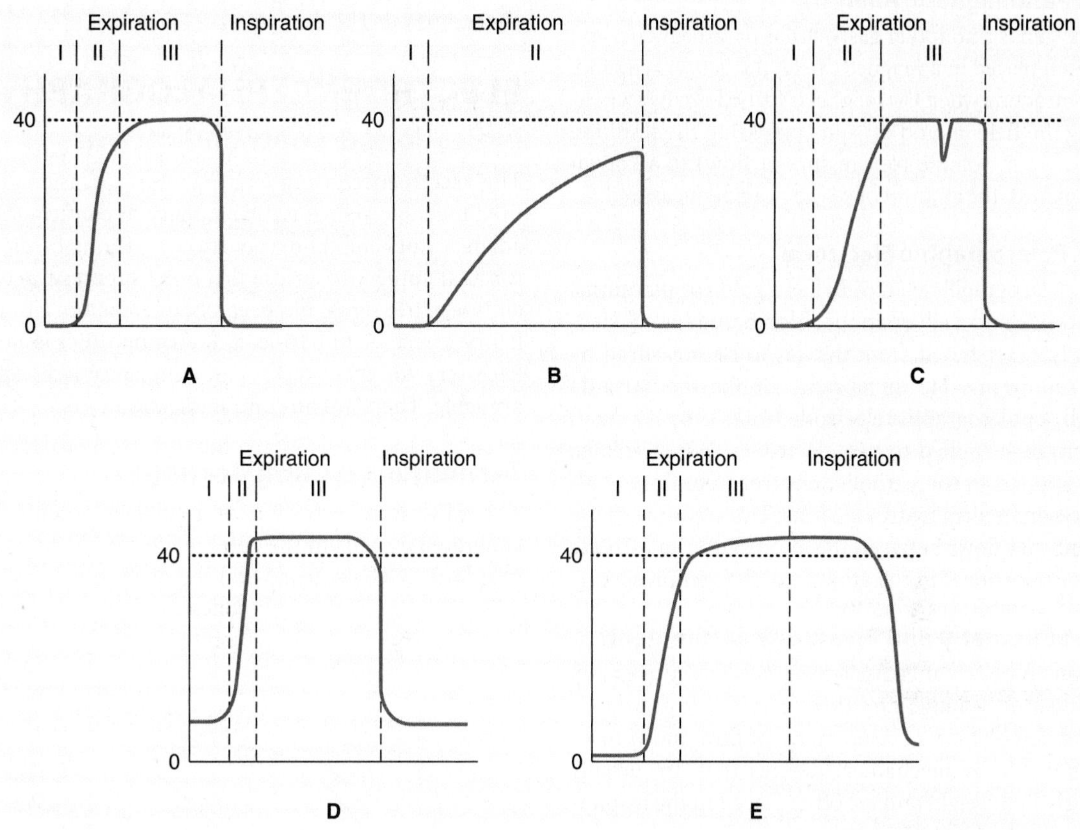

FIGURE 6–3 **A**: A normal capnograph demonstrating the three phases of expiration: phase I—dead space; phase II—a mixture of dead space and alveolar gas; phase III—alveolar gas plateau. **B**: Capnograph of a patient with severe chronic obstructive pulmonary disease. No plateau is reached before the next inspiration. The gradient between end-tidal carbon dioxide (CO_2) and arterial CO_2 is increased. **C**: Depression during phase III indicates spontaneous respiratory effort. **D**: Failure of the inspired CO_2 to return to zero may represent an incompetent expiratory valve or exhausted CO_2 absorbent. **E**: The persistence of exhaled gas during part of the inspiratory cycle signals the presence of an incompetent inspiratory valve.

Because oxygen molecules do not absorb infrared light, their concentration cannot be measured with monitors that rely on infrared technology, and hence oxygen concentration must be measured by other means (see below).

Clinical Considerations

A. Oxygen Analysis

To measure the Fio_2 of inhaled gas, manufacturers of anesthesia machines have relied on various technologies.

B. Galvanic Cell

Galvanic cell (fuel cell) contains a lead anode and gold cathode bathed in potassium chloride. At the gold terminal, hydroxyl ions are formed that react with the lead electrode (thereby gradually consuming it) to produce lead oxide, causing current, which is proportional to the amount of oxygen being measured, to flow. Because the lead electrode is consumed, monitor life can be prolonged by exposing it to room air when not in use. These are the oxygen monitors used on many anesthesia machines in the inspiratory limb.

C. Paramagnetic Analysis

Oxygen is a nonpolar gas, but it is paramagnetic, and when placed in a magnetic field, the gas will expand, contracting when the magnet is turned off. By switching the field on and off and comparing the resulting change in volume (or pressure or flow) to a known standard, the amount of oxygen can be measured.

D. Polarographic Electrode

A polarographic electrode has a gold (or platinum) cathode and a silver anode, both bathed in an electrolyte, separated from the gas to be measured by a semipermeable membrane. Unlike the galvanic cell, a polarographic electrode works only if a small voltage is applied to two electrodes. When voltage is applied to the cathode, electrons combine with oxygen to form hydroxide ions. The amount of current that flows between the anode and the cathode is proportional to the amount of oxygen present.

E. Spirometry and Pressure Measurements

Contemporary anesthesia machines measure airway pressures, volume, and flow to calculate resistance and compliance. Measurements of flow and volume are made by mechanical devices that are usually fairly lightweight and are often placed in the inspiratory limb of the anesthesia circuit.

The most fundamental detected abnormalities include low peak inspiratory pressure and high peak inspiratory pressure, which indicate either a ventilator or circuit disconnect or an airway obstruction, respectively. By measuring V_T and breathing frequency (*f*), exhaled minute ventilation (V_E) can be calculated, providing some sense of security that ventilation requirements are being met.

Spirometric loops are usually displayed as flow versus volume and volume versus pressure (Figure 6–4). There are characteristic changes with obstruction, bronchial intubation, reactive airways disease, and so forth. If a normal loop is observed shortly after induction of anesthesia and a subsequent loop is different, the observant anesthesia provider is alerted to the fact that pulmonary or airway compliance, or both, may have changed. Mechanical ventilation and ventilators are discussed more completely in Chapter 57. (Chapter 23 reviews respiratory physiology).

Neurological System Monitors

ELECTROENCEPHALOGRAPHY

Indications & Contraindications

The electroencephalogram (EEG) is occasionally used during cerebrovascular surgery to confirm the adequacy of cerebral oxygenation or during cardiovascular surgery to ensure that burst suppression or an isoelectric signal has been obtained before circulatory arrest. A full 16-lead, 8-channel EEG is not necessary for these tasks, and simpler systems are available. There are no contraindications.

Techniques & Complications

The EEG is a recording of electrical potentials generated by cells in the cerebral cortex. Although standard ECG electrodes can be used, silver disks

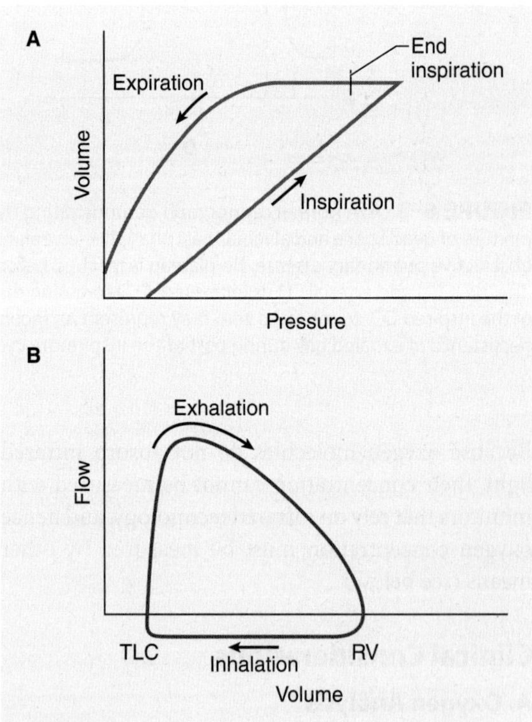

FIGURE 6–4 **A**: Normal volume–pressure loop. **B**: Normal flow–volume loop.

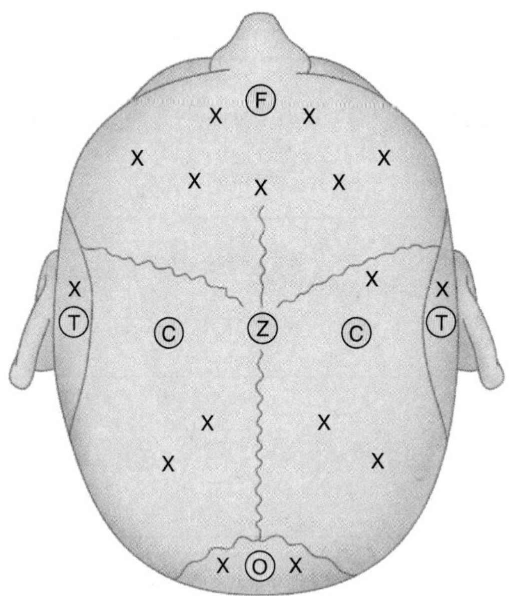

FIGURE 6–5 International 10–20 system. Montage letters refer to cranial location. C, coronal; F, frontal; O, occipital; T, temporal; Z, middle.

containing a conductive gel are preferred. Platinum or stainless steel needle electrodes traumatize the scalp and have high impedance (resistance); however, they can be sterilized and placed in a surgical field. Electrode position (montage) is governed by the international 10–20 system (Figure 6–5). Electric potential differences between combinations of electrodes are filtered, amplified, and displayed by an oscilloscope or pen recorder. EEG activity occurs mostly at frequencies between 1 and 30 cycles/sec (Hz). Alpha waves have a frequency of 8 to 13 Hz and are often found in a resting adult with the eyes closed. Beta waves at 8 to 13 Hz are found in concentrating individuals and, at times, in individuals under anesthesia. Delta waves have a frequency of 0.5 to 4 Hz and are found in brain injury, seizure disorders, deep sleep, and anesthesia. Theta waves (4–7 Hz) are also found in sleeping individuals and during anesthesia. EEG waves are also characterized by their amplitude, which is related to their potential (high amplitude, >50 microV; medium amplitude, 20–50 microV; and low amplitude, <20 microV). Lastly, the EEG is examined for symmetry between the left and right hemispheres.

Examination of a multichannel EEG is at times performed intraoperatively to detect areas of cerebral ischemia, such as during carotid endarterectomy. Likewise, it can be used to detect EEG isoelectricity and maximal cerebral protection during hypothermic arrest. The strip chart EEG is cumbersome in the operating room, and often the EEG is processed using power spectral analysis. Frequency analysis divides the EEG into a series of sine waves at different frequencies and then plots the power of the signal at each frequency, allowing for a presentation of EEG activity in a more easily interpreted form than the raw EEG (Figure 6–6).

As inhalational anesthesia progressively deepens, initial beta activation is followed by slowing, burst suppression, and isoelectricity. Intravenous agents, depending on dose and drug used, can produce a variety of EEG patterns.

Awareness during general anesthesia remains a vexing concern for anesthesia practitioners. Devices have been developed that process two-channel EEG signals and display a dimensionless variable to indicate the level of wakefulness. The bispectral index (BIS) is most commonly used in this regard. BIS monitors examine four components within the EEG that are associated with the anesthetic state: (1) low frequency, as found during deep anesthesia; (2) high-frequency beta activation found during "light" anesthesia; (3) suppressed EEG waves; and (4) burst suppression. Other devices attempt to include measures of spontaneous muscle activity, as influenced by the activity of subcortical structures not contributing to the EEG to further provide an assessment of anesthetic depth. Various devices, each with its own algorithm to process the EEG or incorporate other variables to ascertain patient wakefulness, may become available in the future (Table 6–1).

So far, the medical literature provides very limited support for the efficacy of these devices in preventing awareness. Some studies have demonstrated a reduced incidence of awareness when these devices were used, whereas other studies have failed to reveal any advantage over the use of end-tidal inhalational gas measurements to ensure

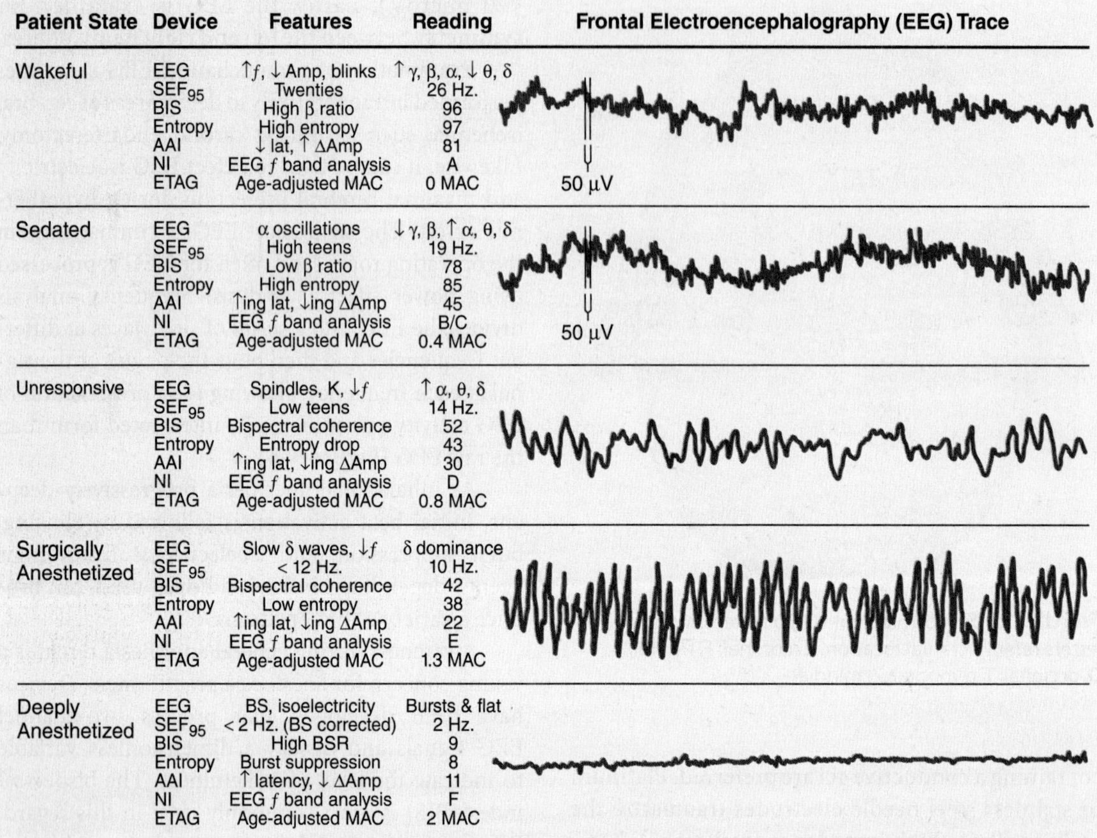

Patient State	Device	Features	Reading	Frontal Electroencephalography (EEG) Trace
Wakeful	EEG	↑f, ↓Amp, blinks	↑γ, β, α, ↓θ, δ	
	SEF_{95}	Twenties	26 Hz.	
	BIS	High β ratio	96	
	Entropy	High entropy	97	
	AAI	↓lat, ↑ΔAmp	81	
	NI	EEG f band analysis	A	
	ETAG	Age-adjusted MAC	0 MAC	50 μV
Sedated	EEG	α oscillations	↓γ, β, ↑α, θ, δ	
	SEF_{95}	High teens	19 Hz.	
	BIS	Low β ratio	78	
	Entropy	High entropy	85	
	AAI	↑ing lat, ↓ing ΔAmp	45	
	NI	EEG f band analysis	B/C	
	ETAG	Age-adjusted MAC	0.4 MAC	50 μV
Unresponsive	EEG	Spindles, K, ↓f	↑α, θ, δ	
	SEF_{95}	Low teens	14 Hz.	
	BIS	Bispectral coherence	52	
	Entropy	Entropy drop	43	
	AAI	↑ing lat, ↓ing ΔAmp	30	
	NI	EEG f band analysis	D	
	ETAG	Age-adjusted MAC	0.8 MAC	
Surgically Anesthetized	EEG	Slow δ waves, ↓f	δ dominance	
	SEF_{95}	< 12 Hz.	10 Hz.	
	BIS	Bispectral coherence	42	
	Entropy	Low entropy	38	
	AAI	↑ing lat, ↓ing ΔAmp	22	
	NI	EEG f band analysis	E	
	ETAG	Age-adjusted MAC	1.3 MAC	
Deeply Anesthetized	EEG	BS, isoelectricity	Bursts & flat	
	SEF_{95}	< 2 Hz. (BS corrected)	2 Hz.	
	BIS	High BSR	9	
	Entropy	Burst suppression	8	
	AAI	↑latency, ↓ΔAmp	11	
	NI	EEG f band analysis	F	
	ETAG	Age-adjusted MAC	2 MAC	

FIGURE 6–6 Patient states, candidate depth of anesthesia devices or approaches, key features of different monitoring approaches, and possible readings at different depths of anesthesia. The readings shown represent examples of possible readings that may be seen in conjunction with each frontal electroencephalography trace. The electroencephalography traces show 3-second epochs (x-axis), and the scale (y-axis) is 50 μV. AAI, A-Line Autoregressive Index (a proprietary method of extracting the midlatency auditory evoked potential from the electroencephalogram); Amp, amplitude of an EEG wave; BIS, bispectral index scale; blinks, eye blink artifacts; BS, burst suppression; BSR, burst suppression ratio; EEG, electroencephalography; ETAG, end-tidal anesthetic gas concentration; *f*, frequency; *γ, β, α, θ, δ*, EEG waves in decreasing frequencies (*γ*, >30 hertz [Hz]; *β*, 12–30 Hz; *α*, 8–12 Hz; *θ*, 4–8 Hz; *δ*, 0–4 Hz); K, K complexes; lat, latency between an auditory stimulus and an evoked EEG waveform response; MAC, minimum alveolar concentration; NI, Narcotrend index; SEF_{95}, spectral edge frequency below which 95% of the EEG frequencies reside; Spindles, sleep spindles. (Reproduced with permission from Mashour GA, Orser BA, Avidan MS. Intraoperative awareness: From neurobiology to clinical practice. *Anesthesiology.* 2011 May;114(5):1218-1233.)

an adequate concentration of volatile anesthetic. Because individual EEG responsiveness to anesthetic agents and level of surgical stimulus are variable, EEG monitoring to assess anesthesia depth or titrate anesthetic delivery may not always ensure the absence of wakefulness. Moreover, many monitors have a delay, which might only indicate a risk for the patient being aware after he or she had already become conscious (Table 6–2).

Clinical Considerations

To perform a bispectral analysis, data measured by EEG are taken through a number of steps (Figure 6–7) to calculate a single number that correlates with the depth of anesthesia/hypnosis.

BIS values of 65 to 85 have been advocated as a measure of sedation, whereas values of 40 to 65 have been recommended for general anesthesia (Figure 6–8).

TABLE 6–1 Characteristics of the commercially available monitors of anesthetic depth.

Parameters	Machine/ Manufacturer	Consumable	Physiologic Signals	Recommended Range of Values for Anesthesia	Principles of Measurement
Bispectral index (BIS)	A-2000/Aspect Medical Systems, Newton, MA	BIS sensor	Single-channel EEG[2]	40–60	BIS is derived from the weighted sum of three EEG parameters: relative α/β ratio; bio-coherence of the EEG waves; and burst suppression. The relative contribution of these parameters has been tuned to correlate with the degree of sedation produced by various sedative agents. BIS ranges from 0 (asleep) to 100 (awake).
Patient state index (PSI)	Patient state analyzer (PSA 400)/ Physiometrix, Inc., N. Billerica, MA	PSArray	4-channel EEG	25–50	PSI is derived from progressive discriminant analysis of several quantitative EEG variables that are sensitive to changes in the level of anesthesia but insensitive to the specific agents producing such changes. It includes changes in power spectrum in various EEG frequency bands; hemispheric symmetry; and synchronization between brain regions and the inhibition of regions of the frontal cortex. PSI ranges from 0 (asleep) to 100 (awake).
Narcotrend stage Narcotrend index	Nacrotrend monitor/ Monitor-Technik, Bad Bramstedt, Germany	Ordinary ECG electrode	1–2-channel EEG	Narcotrend stage D_{0-2} to C_1, which corresponds to an index of 40–60	The Narcotrend monitor classifies EEG signals into different stages of anesthesia (A = awake; B_{0-2} = sedated; C_{0-2} = light anesthesia; D_{0-2} = general anesthesia; $E_{0,1}$ = general anesthesia with deep hypnosis; $F_{0,1}$ = burst suppression). The classification algorithm is based on a discriminant analysis of entropy measures and EEG spectral variables. More recently the monitor converts the Narcotrend stages into a dimensionless number from 0 (asleep) to 100 (awake) by nonlinear regression.
Entropy	S/5 Entropy Module, M-ENTROPY/ Datex-Ohmeda, Instrumentarium Corp., Helsinki, Finland	Special entropy sensor	Single-channel EEG	40–60	Entropy described the "irregularity" of the EEG signal. As the dose of anesthetic is increased, EEG becomes more regular and the entropy value approaches zero. M-ENTROPY calculates the entropy of the EEG spectrum (spectral entropy). To shorten the response time, it uses different time windows according to the corresponding EEG frequencies. Two spectral parameters are calculated: state entropy (frequency band 0–32 Hz) and response entropy (0–47 Hz), which also includes muscle activity. Both entropy variables have been rescaled so that 0 is asleep and 100 is awake.
Aline autoregressive index (AAI)	AEP/2 monitor/ Danmeter A/S, Odense, Demark	Ordinary ECG electrode	AEP	10–25	AAI is derived from the middle latency AEP (20–80 ms). AAI is extracted from an autoregressive model with exogenous input (ARX model) so that only 18 sweeps are required to reproduce the AEP waveform in 2–6 seconds. The resultant waveform is then transformed into a numeric index (0–100) that describes the shape of the AEP. AAI >60 is awake, AAI of 0 indicates deep anesthesia.
Cerebral state index (CSI)	Cerebral state monitor (CSM), Danmeter A/S, Odense, Demark	Ordinary ECG electrode	Single-channel EEG	40–60	CSI is a weighted sum of (1) α ratio, (2) β ratio, (3) difference between the two and (4) burst suppression. It correlates with the degree of sedation by an "adaptive neuro-fuzzy inference system." CSI ranges from 0 (asleep) to 100 (awake).

[1]AEP, auditory evoked potential; ECG, electrocardiogram; EEG, electroencephalogram.

Reproduced with permission from Chan MTV, Gin T, Goh KYC. Interventional neurophysiologic monitoring. *Curr Opin Anaesthesiol.* 2004 Oct;17(5):389-396.

TABLE 6–2 Checklist for preventing awareness.

- ✓ Check all equipment, drugs, and dosages; ensure that drugs are clearly labeled and that infusions are running into veins.
- ✓ Consider administering an amnesic premedication.
- ✓ Avoid or minimize the administration of muscle relaxants. Use a peripheral nerve stimulator to guide minimal required dose.
- ✓ Consider using the isolated forearm technique if intense paralysis is indicated.
- ✓ Choose potent inhalation agents rather than total intravenous anesthesia, if possible.
- ✓ Administer at least 0.5–0.7 minimum alveolar concentration (MAC) of the inhalation agent.
- ✓ Set an alarm for a low anesthetic gas concentration.
- ✓ Monitor anesthetic gas concentration during cardiopulmonary bypass from the bypass machine.
- ✓ Consider alternative treatments for hypotension other than decreasing anesthetic concentration.
- ✓ If it is thought that sufficient anesthesia cannot be administered because of concern about hemodynamic compromise, consider the administration of benzodiazepines or scopolamine for amnesia.
- ✓ Supplement hypnotic agents with analgesic agents such as opioids or local anesthetics, which may help decrease the experience of pain in the event of awareness.
- ✓ Consider using a brain monitor, such as a raw or processed electroencephalogram, but do not try to minimize the anesthetic dose based on the brain monitor because there currently is insufficient evidence to support this practice.
- ✓ Monitor the brain routinely if using total intravenous anesthesia.
- ✓ Evaluate known risk factors for awareness, and if specific risk factors are identified, consider increasing the administered anesthetic concentration.
- ✓ Re-dose intravenous anesthesia when delivery of inhalation anesthesia is difficult, such as during a long intubation attempt or during rigid bronchoscopy.

Reproduced with permission from Mashour GA, Orser BA, Avidan MS. Intraoperative awareness: from neurobiology to clinical practice. *Anesthesiology.* 2011 May;114(5):1218-1233.

Many of the initial studies of BIS were not prospective, randomized, controlled trials but were observational, underpowered, and not masked. The monitor costs several thousand dollars, and the single-use electrodes cost approximately $10 to $15 per anesthetic. Unfortunately, some patients with awareness have had a BIS of less than 65, calling into question the value of this measurement. Detection of awareness can often minimize its consequences. Questions during postoperative visits can identify a potential awareness event. Ask patients to recall the following:

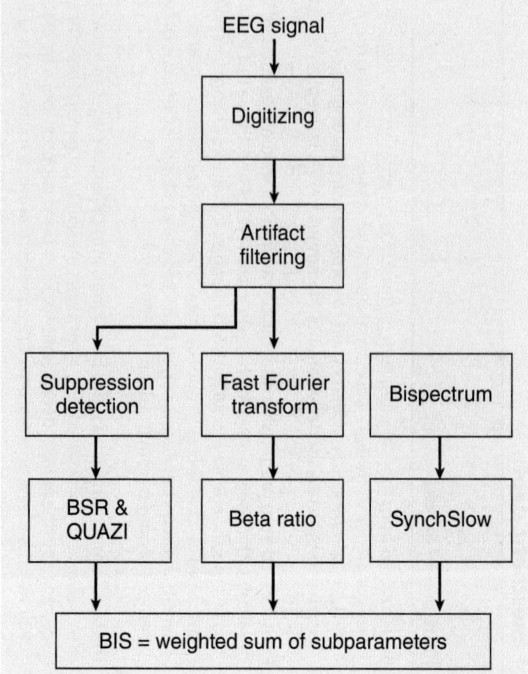

FIGURE 6–7 Calculation of the bispectral index. BIS, bispectral index scale; BSR, burst suppression ratio; EEG, electroencephalogram. (Reproduced with permission from Rampil IJ: A primer for EEG signal processing in anesthesia. *Anesthesiology.* 1998 Oct;89(4):980-1002.)

- What do you remember before going to sleep?
- What do you remember right when awakening?
- Do you remember anything in between going to sleep and awakening?
- Did you have any dreams while asleep?

Close follow-up and involvement of mental health experts may avoid the traumatic stress that can be associated with intraoperative awareness events. Increasingly, patients are managed with regional anesthesia and propofol sedation. Patients undergoing such anesthetics should be made aware that they might recall perioperative events. Clarification of the techniques used may prevent patients

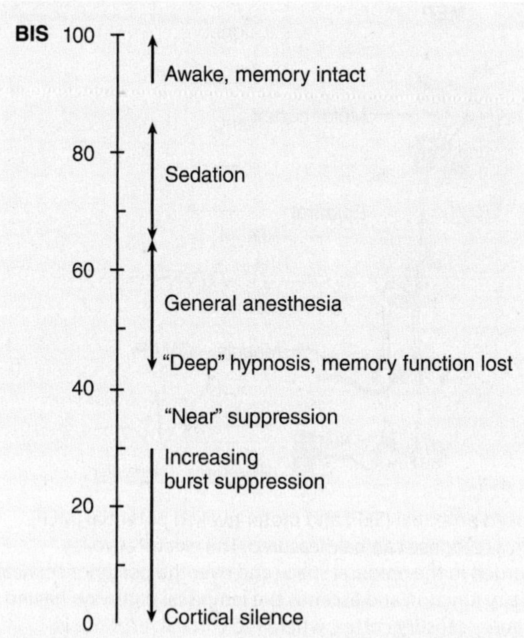

FIGURE 6–8 The bispectral index (BIS versions 3.0 and higher) is a dimensionless scale from 0 (complete cortical electroencephalographic suppression) to 100 (awake). BIS values of 65 to 85 have been recommended for sedation, whereas values of 40 to 65 have been recommended for general anesthesia. At BIS values lower than 40, cortical suppression becomes discernible in a raw electroencephalogram as a burst suppression pattern. (Reproduced with permission from Johansen JW et al: Development and clinical application of electroencephalographic bispectrum monitoring. *Anesthesiology.* 2000 Nov;93(5):1337-1344.)

so managed from the belief that they "were awake" during anesthesia.

Does BIS associate with outcomes? Some investigators have suggested that hospital stay and mortality are increased in patients experiencing the so-called "triple low" of low mean arterial blood pressure, low BIS score, and low minimum alveolar concentration of volatile anesthetics. Other investigations have failed to identify such an association.

EVOKED POTENTIALS

Indications

Indications for intraoperative monitoring of **evoked potentials** (EPs) include surgical procedures associated with possible neurological injury: spinal fusion with instrumentation, spine and spinal cord tumor resection, brachial plexus repair, thoracoabdominal aortic aneurysm repair, epilepsy surgery, and (in some cases) cerebral tumor resection. Ischemia in the spinal cord or cerebral cortex can be detected by EPs. Auditory EPs have also been used to assess the effects of general anesthesia on the brain. The middle latency auditory EP may be a more sensitive indicator than BIS in regard to anesthetic depth. The amplitude and latency of this signal following an auditory stimulus are influenced by anesthetics.

Contraindications

Although there are no specific contraindications for somatosensory evoked potentials (SEPs), this modality is severely limited by the availability of monitoring sites, equipment, and trained personnel. Sensitivity to anesthetic agents can also be a limiting factor, particularly in children. Motor evoked potentials (MEPs) are contraindicated in patients with retained intracranial metal, skull defects, or implantable devices, as well as after seizures and any major cerebral insult. Brain injury secondary to repetitive stimulation of the cortex and inducement of seizures is a concern with MEPs.

Techniques & Complications

EP monitoring noninvasively assesses neural function by measuring electrophysiological responses to sensory or motor pathway stimulation. Commonly monitored EPs are brainstem auditory evoked responses (BAERs), SEPs, and increasingly, MEPs (Figure 6–9).

For SEPs, a brief electrical current is delivered to a sensory or mixed peripheral nerve by a pair of electrodes. If the intervening pathway is intact, a nerve action potential will be transmitted to the contralateral sensory cortex to produce an EP. This potential can be measured by cortical surface electrodes but is usually measured by scalp electrodes. Multiple responses are averaged and background noise is eliminated to distinguish the cortical response to a specific stimulus. EPs are represented by a plot of voltage versus time. The resulting waveforms are

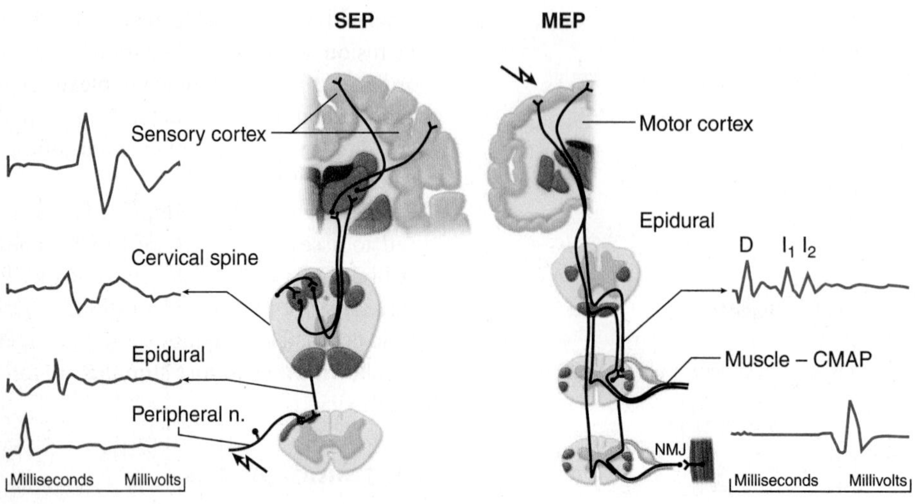

FIGURE 6–9 Neuroanatomic pathways of somatosensory evoked potential (SEP) and motor evoked potential (MEP). The SEP is produced by stimulation of a peripheral nerve, wherein a response can be measured. The electrical volley ascends the spinal cord by the posterior columns and can be recorded in the epidural space and over the posterior cervical spine. It crosses the mid-line after synapsing at the cervicomedullary junction and ascends the lemniscal pathways having a second synapse in the thalamus. From there, it travels to the primary sensory cortex, where the cortical response is measured. The MEP is produced by stimulation of the motor cortex leading to an electrical volley that descends to the anterior horn cells of the spinal cord via the corticospinal tract. After synapsing there, it travels via a peripheral nerve and crosses the neuromuscular junction (NMJ) to produce a muscle response. The MEP can be measured in the epidural space as D and I waves produced by direct and indirect (via internuncial neurons) stimulation of the motor cortex, respectively. It can also be measured as a compound muscle action potential (CMAP) in the muscle. n, nerve. (Reproduced with permission from Sloan TB, Janik D, Jameson L. Multimodality monitoring of the central nervous system using motor-evoked potentials. *Curr Opin Anaesthesiol.* 2008 Oct;21(5):560-564.)

analyzed for their poststimulus latency (the time between stimulation and potential detection) and peak amplitude. These are compared with baseline tracings. Technical and physiological causes of a change in an EP must be distinguished from changes due to neural damage. Complications of EP monitoring are rare but include skin irritation and pressure ischemia at the sites of electrode application.

Clinical Considerations

EPs are altered by many variables other than neural damage. The effect of anesthetics is complex and not easily summarized. **In general, intravenous anesthetic techniques (with or without nitrous oxide) cause minimal changes, whereas volatile agents (sevoflurane, desflurane, and isoflurane) are best avoided or used at a constant low concentration**. Early-occurring (specific) EPs are less affected by anesthetics than are late-occurring (nonspecific) responses. Changes in BAERs may provide a measure of the depth of anesthesia. Physiological (eg, blood pressure, temperature, and oxygen saturation) and pharmacologic factors should be kept as constant as possible.

Persistent obliteration of EPs is predictive of postoperative neurological deficit. Although SEPs usually identify spinal cord damage, because of their different anatomic pathways, *sensory* (dorsal spinal cord) EP preservation does not guarantee normal *motor* (ventral spinal cord) function (false negative). Furthermore, SEPs elicited from posterior tibial nerve stimulation cannot distinguish between peripheral and central ischemia (false positive). Techniques that elicit MEPs by using transcranial magnetic or electrical stimulation of the cortex allow the detection of action potentials in the muscles if the neural pathway is intact. The advantage of using MEPs as opposed to SEPs for spinal cord monitoring

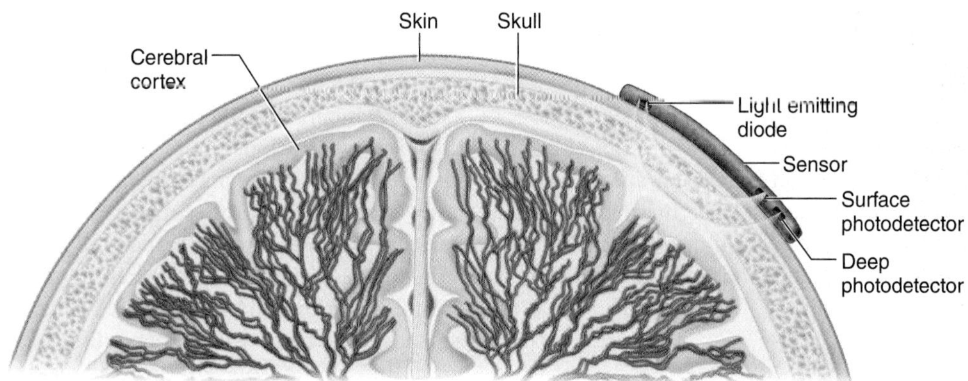

FIGURE 6–10 Principle of the INVOS® near-infrared spectroscopy technique. (Reproduced with permission from Rubio A, Hakami L, Münch F, et al. Noninvasive control of adequate cerebral oxygenation during low-flow antegrade selective cerebral perfusion on adults and infants in the aortic arch surgery. *J Card Surg.* 2008 Sep-Oct;23(5):474-479.)

is that MEPs monitor the ventral spinal cord, and if sensitive and specific enough, they can be used to indicate which patients might develop a postoperative motor deficit. MEPs are more sensitive to spinal cord ischemia than SEPs. The same considerations for SEPs are applicable to MEPs in that they are reduced in amplitude by volatile inhalational agents, high-dose benzodiazepines, and moderate hypothermia (temperatures <32°C). MEPs require monitoring of the level of neuromuscular blockade. Close communication with a neurophysiologist or monitoring technician is essential before the start of any case where these monitors are used. These are cases in which inhaled anesthetics (if used at all) must be maintained at a constant end-tidal concentration to ensure monitoring reliability.

CEREBRAL OXIMETRY AND OTHER MONITORS OF THE BRAIN

Cerebral oximetry uses near-infrared spectroscopy (NIRS). Near-infrared light is emitted by a probe on the scalp (Figure 6–10). Receptors are positioned to detect the reflected light from both deep and superficial structures. As with pulse oximetry, oxygenated hemoglobin and deoxygenated hemoglobin absorb light at different frequencies. Likewise, cytochrome absorbs infrared light in the mitochondria. The NIRS saturation largely reflects the absorption of venous hemoglobin, as it does not have the ability to identify the pulsatile arterial component. Regional saturations of less than 40% on NIRS measures, or changes of greater than 25% of baseline measures, may herald neurological events secondary to decreased cerebral oxygenation.

Reduced jugular venous bulb saturation can also provide an indication of increased cerebral tissue oxygen extraction or decreased cerebral oxygen delivery. Direct tissue oxygen monitoring of the brain can be accomplished by the placement of a probe in or on brain tissue. Interventions to preserve brain tissue oxygenation are called for when oxygen tissue tension is less than 20 mm Hg. Such interventions improve oxygen delivery by increasing Fio_2, increasing hemoglobin, improving cardiac output, decreasing oxygen demand (for example, with sedative/hypnotic drugs), or a combination of these methods.

Other Monitors

TEMPERATURE

Indications

The temperature of patients undergoing anesthesia should be monitored during all but the shortest anesthetics. Postoperative temperature is increasingly used as a measurement of anesthesia quality. Hypothermia is associated with delayed drug metabolism, hyperglycemia, vasoconstriction, impaired coagulation, postoperative shivering accompanied by tachycardia and hypertension, and increased risk of surgical site infections. Hyperthermia can lead to tachycardia, vasodilation, and neurological injury. Consequently, temperature must be measured and recorded perioperatively.

Contraindications

There are no contraindications, though a particular monitoring site may be unsuitable in certain patients.

Techniques & Complications

Intraoperatively, temperature is usually measured using a thermistor or thermocouple. Thermistors are semiconductors whose resistance decreases predictably with warming. A thermocouple is a circuit of two dissimilar metals joined so that a potential difference is generated when the metals are at different temperatures. Disposable thermocouple and thermistor probes are available for monitoring the temperature of the tympanic membrane, nasopharynx, esophagus, bladder, rectum, and skin. Infrared sensors estimate temperature from the infrared energy that is produced. Tympanic membrane temperatures reflect core body temperature; however, the devices used may not reliably measure the temperature at the tympanic membrane. Complications of temperature monitoring are usually related to trauma caused by the probe (eg, rectal or tympanic membrane perforation).

Clinical Considerations

Each monitoring site has advantages and disadvantages. The tympanic membrane theoretically reflects brain temperature because the auditory canal's blood supply is the external carotid artery. Trauma during insertion and cerumen insulation detract from the routine use of tympanic probes. Rectal temperature probes have a slow response to changes in core temperature. Nasopharyngeal probes are prone to cause epistaxis, but they accurately measure core temperature if placed adjacent to the nasopharyngeal mucosa. The thermistor in a pulmonary artery catheter also measures core temperature. There is a variable correlation between axillary temperature and core temperature, depending on skin perfusion. Liquid crystal adhesive strips placed on the skin are inadequate indicators of core body temperature during surgery. Esophageal temperature sensors, often incorporated into esophageal stethoscopes, provide the best combination of economy, performance, and safety. The temperature sensor should be positioned behind the heart in the lower third of the esophagus to avoid measuring the temperature of tracheal gases. Conveniently, heart sounds are most prominent at this location. For more on the clinical considerations of temperature control, see Chapter 52.

URINARY OUTPUT

Indications

Urinary bladder catheterization is the most reliable method of monitoring urinary output. Catheterization is routine in some complex and prolonged surgical procedures such as cardiac surgery, aortic or renal vascular surgery, craniotomy, major abdominal surgery, or procedures in which large fluid shifts are expected. Lengthy surgeries and intraoperative diuretic administration are other possible indications. Occasionally, postoperative bladder catheterization is indicated in patients who have difficulty voiding in the recovery room after general or regional anesthesia.

Contraindications

Foley catheters should be removed as soon as feasible to minimize the risk of catheter-associated urinary tract infections.

Techniques & Complications

Bladder catheterization is usually performed by surgical or nursing personnel. The urologist may be needed to catheterize patients with strictures and other abnormal urethral anatomy. A soft rubber Foley catheter is inserted into the bladder transurethrally and connected to a disposable calibrated collection chamber. To avoid urine reflux and minimize the risk of infection, the collection chamber should remain at a level below the bladder. Complications of catheterization include urethral trauma and urinary tract infections. Rapid decompression of a distended bladder can cause hypotension. Suprapubic drainage of the bladder with tubing inserted through a large-bore needle is an uncommon alternative.

Clinical Considerations

An additional advantage of placing a Foley catheter is the ability to include a thermistor in the catheter tip so that bladder temperature can be monitored. As long as urinary output is high, bladder temperature accurately reflects core temperature. An added value of the more widespread use of urometers is the ability to electronically monitor and record urinary output and temperature.

Urinary output is an imperfect reflection of kidney perfusion and function and of renal, cardiovascular, and fluid volume status. Noninvasive monitors of cardiac function and output (including echocardiography) provide more reliable assessments of the adequacy of intravascular volume. Inadequate urinary output (oliguria) is often arbitrarily defined as a urinary output of less than 0.5 mL/kg/h but actually is a function of the patient's concentrating ability and osmotic load. Urine electrolyte composition, osmolality, and specific gravity aid in the differential diagnosis of oliguria.

PERIPHERAL NERVE STIMULATION

Indications

Because of the variation in patient sensitivity to neuromuscular blocking agents, the neuromuscular function of all patients receiving intermediate- or long-acting neuromuscular blocking agents must be monitored. In addition, peripheral nerve stimulation is helpful in detecting the onset of paralysis during anesthesia inductions or the adequacy of the block during continuous infusions with short-acting agents.

Contraindications

There are no contraindications to neuromuscular monitoring, though certain sites may be precluded by the surgical procedure. Additionally, atrophied muscles in areas of hemiplegia or nerve damage may appear refractory to neuromuscular blockade secondary to the proliferation of receptors. Determining the degree of neuromuscular blockade using such an extremity could lead to the potential overdosing of competitive neuromuscular blocking agents.

Techniques & Complications

A peripheral nerve stimulator delivers current (60–80 mA) to a pair of either ECG silver chloride pads or subcutaneous needles placed over a peripheral motor nerve. The evoked mechanical or electrical response of the innervated muscle is observed. Although electromyography provides a fast, accurate, and quantitative measure of neuromuscular transmission, visual or tactile observation of muscle contraction is usually relied upon in clinical practice. Ulnar nerve stimulation of the adductor pollicis muscle and facial nerve stimulation of the orbicularis oculi are most commonly monitored (Figure 6–11). Because it is the inhibition of the neuromuscular receptor that needs to be monitored, direct stimulation of muscle should be avoided by placing electrodes over the course of the nerve and not over the muscle itself. Peripheral nerve stimulators must be capable of generating at least a 50-mA current across a 1000-Ω load to deliver a supramaximal stimulation to the underlying nerve. This current is uncomfortable for a conscious patient. Complications of nerve stimulation are limited to skin irritation and abrasion at the site of electrode attachment.

Because of concerns for residual neuromuscular blockade, increased attention has been focused on providing quantitative measures of the degree of neuromuscular blockade perioperatively. Acceleromyography uses a piezoelectric transducer on the muscle to be stimulated. The movement of the muscle generates an electrical current that can be quantified and displayed. Indeed, acceleromyography can better predict residual paralysis, compared with routine tactile train-of-four monitoring used in most operating rooms, if it is calibrated from the beginning of the operative period to establish baselines before administration of neuromuscular blocking agents.

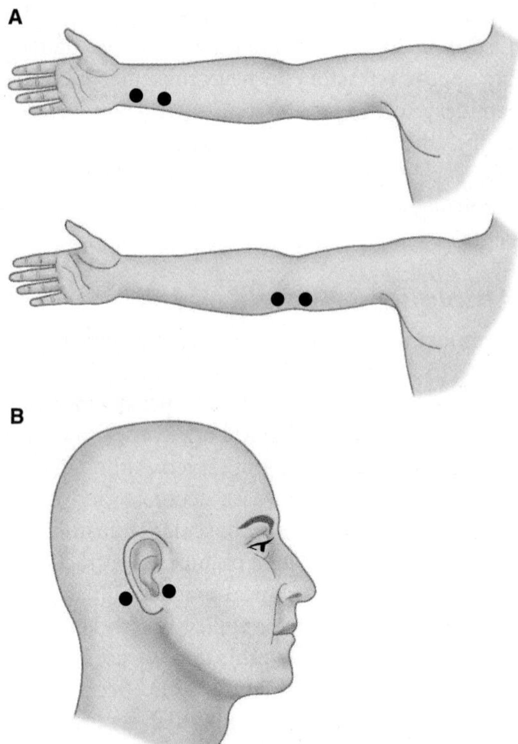

FIGURE 6–11 **A**: Stimulation of the ulnar nerve causes contraction of the adductor pollicis muscle. **B**: Stimulation of the facial nerve leads to orbicularis oculi muscle contraction. The orbicularis oculi muscle recovers from neuromuscular blockade before the adductor pollicis. (Reproduced with permission from Dorsch JA, Dorsch SE. Understanding Anesthesia Equipment. 4th ed. Philadelphia, PA: Lippincott Williams & Wilkins; 1999.)

Clinical Considerations

The degree of neuromuscular blockade is monitored by applying various patterns of electrical stimulation (Figure 6–12). All stimuli are 200 μs in duration and of square-wave pattern and equal current intensity. A twitch is a single pulse that is delivered from every 1 to every 10 seconds (1–0.1 Hz). Increasing block results in decreased evoked response to stimulation.

Train-of-four stimulation denotes four successive 200-μs stimuli in 2 seconds (2 Hz). The twitches in a train-of-four pattern progressively fade as nondepolarizing muscle relaxant block increases. The ratio of the responses to the first and fourth twitches is a sensitive indicator of nondepolarizing muscle paralysis. Because it is difficult to estimate the train-of-four ratio, it is more convenient to visually observe the sequential disappearance of the twitches, as this also correlates with the extent of blockade. The disappearance of the fourth twitch represents a 75% block, the third twitch an 80% block, and the second twitch a 90% block. Clinical relaxation usually requires 75% to 95% neuromuscular blockade.

Tetany at 50 or 100 Hz is a sensitive test of neuromuscular function. Sustained contraction for 5 seconds indicates adequate, but not necessarily complete, reversal from neuromuscular blockade. Double-burst stimulation (DBS) represents two variations of tetany that are less painful to the patient. The $DBS_{3,3}$ pattern of nerve stimulation consists of three short (200-μs) high-frequency bursts separated by 20 ms intervals (50 Hz) followed 750 ms later by another three bursts. $DBS_{3,2}$ consists of three 200-μs impulses at 50 Hz followed 750 ms later by two such impulses. DBS is more sensitive than train-of-four stimulation for the clinical (ie, visual) evaluation of fade.

Because muscle groups differ in their sensitivity to neuromuscular blocking agents, use of the peripheral nerve stimulator cannot replace direct observation of the muscles (eg, the diaphragm) that need to be relaxed for a specific surgical procedure. Furthermore, recovery of adductor pollicis function does not exactly parallel recovery of muscles required to maintain an airway. **The diaphragm, rectus abdominis, laryngeal adductors, and orbicularis oculi muscles recover from neuromuscular blockade sooner than the adductor pollicis**. Other indicators of adequate recovery include sustained (≥5 s) head lift, the ability to generate an inspiratory pressure of at least −25 cm H_2O, and a forceful hand grip. Twitch tension is reduced by hypothermia of the monitored muscle group (6%/°C). Decisions regarding the adequacy of reversal of neuromuscular blockade, as well as the timing of extubation, should be made only by considering the patient's clinical presentation and assessments determined by peripheral nerve stimulation.

2 Postoperative residual paralysis remains a problem in postanesthesia care, producing potentially injurious airway and respiratory function compromise and increasing length of stay and cost in the postanesthesia care unit (PACU). Reversal of neuromuscular blocking agents is warranted, as is

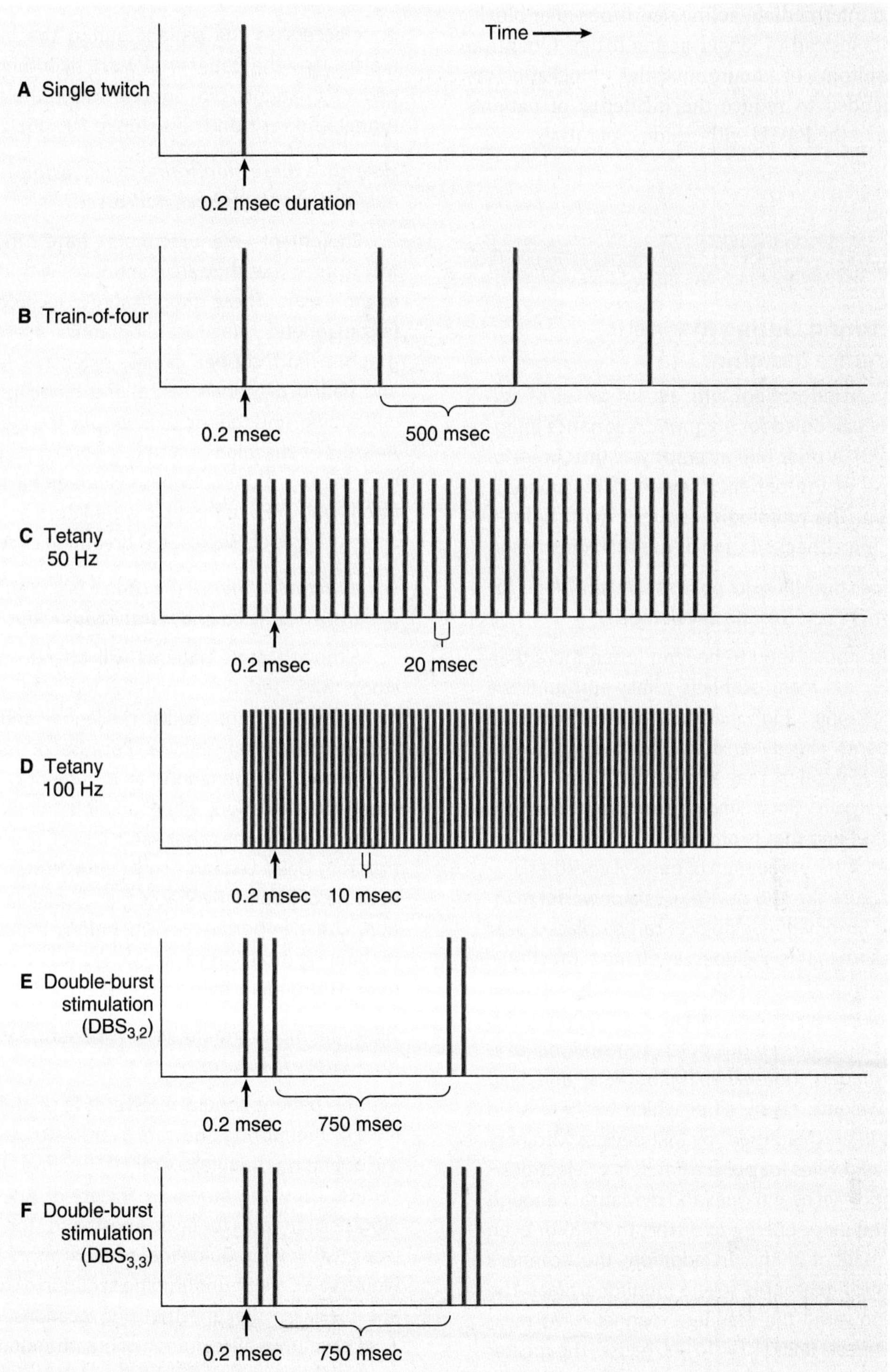

FIGURE 6–12 Peripheral nerve stimulators can generate various patterns of electrical impulses.

the use of intermediate-acting neuromuscular blocking agents instead of longer-acting drugs. Quantitative monitors of neuromuscular blockade are recommended to reduce the incidence of patients admitted to the PACU with residual paralysis.

CASE DISCUSSION

Monitoring During Magnetic Resonance Imaging

A 50-year-old patient with recent onset of seizures is scheduled for magnetic resonance imaging (MRI). A prior MRI attempt was unsuccessful because of the patient's severe claustrophobic reaction. The radiologist requests your help in providing either sedation or general anesthesia.

Why does the MRI suite pose special problems for the patient and the anesthesiologist?

MRI studies tend to be long (often more than 1 hour), and many scanners totally surround the body, causing a high incidence of claustrophobia in patients already anxious about their health. Patient discomfort may also be amplified by preexisting pain. Good imaging requires immobility, something that is difficult to achieve in many patients without sedation or general anesthesia.

Because the MRI device uses a powerful magnet, no ferromagnetic objects can be placed near the scanner. This includes implanted prosthetic joints, artificial pacemakers, surgical clips, batteries, ordinary anesthesia machines, watches, pens, credit cards, intravenous poles, conventional oxygen cylinders, housekeeping buckets, and lead ankle weights, nearly all of which we have seen drawn in and "captured" by MRI devices. Ordinary metal lead wires for pulse oximeters or electrocardiography act as antennas and may attract enough radiofrequency energy to distort the MRI or even cause patient burns. In addition, the scanner's magnetic field causes severe monitor artifact. The more powerful the scanner's magnet is, as measured in Tesla units (1 T = 10,000 gauss), the greater the potential problem. Other problems include poor access to the patient during the imaging (particularly the patient's airway), hypothermia in pediatric patients, dim lighting within the patient tunnel, and very loud noise (up to 100 dB).

How have these monitoring and anesthesia machine problems been addressed?

Equipment manufacturers have modified monitors so that they are compatible with the MRI environment. These modifications include nonferromagnetic electrocardiographic electrodes, graphite and copper cables, extensive filtering and gating of signals, extra-long blood pressure cuff tubing, and the use of fiberoptic technologies. Anesthesia machines with no ferromagnetic components (eg, aluminum gas cylinders) have been fitted with MRI-compatible ventilators and long circle systems or Mapleson D breathing circuits.

What factors influence the choice between general anesthesia and intravenous sedation?

Although most patients will tolerate an MRI study with sedation, head-injured and pediatric patients present special challenges and often require general anesthesia. Because of machine and monitoring limitations, an argument could be made that sedation, when possible, would be a safer choice. On the other hand, loss of airway control from deep sedation could prove catastrophic because of poor patient access and delayed detection. Other important considerations include the monitoring modalities available at a particular facility and the general medical condition of the patient.

Which monitors should be considered mandatory in this case?

The patient should receive at least the same level of monitoring and care in the MR suite as in the operating room for a similarly noninvasive procedure. Thus, the American Society of Anesthesiologists Standards for Basic Anesthetic Monitoring (see the following Guidelines section) apply as they would to a patient undergoing sedation or general anesthesia in other anesthetizing locations.

Continuous auscultation of breath sounds with a plastic (not metal) precordial stethoscope can help identify airway obstruction caused by excessive sedation. Palpation of a peripheral pulse or listening for Korotkoff sounds is impractical in this setting. Ensuring adequacy of circulation depends on electrocardiographic and oscillometric blood pressure monitoring. End-tidal CO_2 analyzers can be adapted to sedation cases by connecting the sampling line to a site near the patient's mouth or nose if a nasal cannula with a CO_2 sampling channel is not available. Because room air entrainment precludes exact measurements, this technique provides a qualitative indicator of ventilation. Whenever sedation is planned, equipment for emergency conversion to general anesthesia (eg, tracheal tubes, resuscitation bag) must be immediately available. Although MRI suites are often located in remote areas far from the operating room suite, appropriate equipment and medication must still be immediately available for anesthesia-related emergencies such as a difficult airway or malignant hyperthermia.

Is the continuous presence of qualified anesthesia personnel required during these cases?

Absolutely yes. Sedated patients must have continuously monitored anesthesia care to prevent a multitude of unforeseen complications, such as apnea or emesis.

GUIDELINES

American Society of Anesthesiologists Standards for Basic Anesthetic Monitoring.

SUGGESTED READINGS

Avidan M, Zhang L, Burnside B, et al. Anesthesia awareness and bispectral index. *New Eng J Med.* 2008;358:1097.

Bergeron EJ, Mosca MS, Aftab M, Justison G, Reece TB. Neuroprotection strategies in aortic surgery. *Cardiol Clin.* 2017;35:453.

Brull SJ, Kopman AF. Current status of neuromuscular reversal and monitoring: challenges and opportunities. *Anesthesiology.* 2017;126:173.

Chan ED, Chan MM, Chan MM. Pulse oximetry: understanding its basic principles facilitates appreciation of its limitations. *Respir Med.* 2013;107:789.

Fahy BG, Chau DF. The technology of processed electroencephalogram monitoring devices for assessment of depth of anesthesia. *Anesth Analg.* 2018;126:111.

Hajat Z, Ahmad N, Andrzejowski J. The role and limitations of EEG-based depth of anaesthesia monitoring in theatres and intensive care. *Anaesthesia.* 2017;72(suppl 1):38.

Kasman N, Brady K. Cerebral oximetry for pediatric anesthesia: why do intelligent clinicians disagree? *Pediatr Anaesth.* 2011;21:473.

Kertai M, White W, Gan T. Cumulative duration of "triple low" state of low blood pressure, low bispectral index, and low minimum alveolar concentration of volatile anesthesia is not associated with increased mortality. *Anesthesiology.* 2014;121:18.

Kirkman MA, Smith M. Brain oxygenation monitoring. *Anesthesiol Clin.* 2016;34:537.

Lam T, Nagappa M, Wong J, Singh M, Wong D, Chung F. Continuous pulse oximetry and capnography monitoring for postoperative respiratory depression and adverse events: a systematic review and meta-analysis. *Anesth Analg.* 2017;125:2019.

Lien CA, Kopman AF. Current recommendations for monitoring depth of neuromuscular blockade. *Curr Opin Anesthesiol.* 2014;27:616.

Mashour G, Orser B, Avidan M. Intraoperative awareness. *Anesthesiology.* 2011;114:1218.

Messina AG, Wang M, Ward MJ, et al. Anaesthetic interventions for prevention of awareness during surgery. *Cochrane Database Syst Rev.* 2016;10:CD007272.

Moritz S, Kasprzak P, Arit M, et al. Accuracy of cerebral monitoring in detecting cerebral ischemia during carotid endarterectomy. *Anesthesiology.* 2007;107:563.

Myles P, Leslie K, McNeil J. Bispectral function monitoring to prevent awareness during anaesthesia. The B-Aware randomized controlled trial. *Lancet.* 2004;363:1757.

Naguib M, Koman A, Ensor J. Neuromuscular monitoring and postoperative residual curarization: a meta-analysis. *Br J Anaesth.* 2007;98:302.

Nwachuku EL, Balzer JR, Yabes JG, et al. Diagnostic value of somatosensory evoked potential changes during carotid endarterectomy: a systematic review and meta-analysis. *JAMA Neurol.* 2015;72:73.

Punjasawadwong Y, Chau-In W, Laopaiboon M, Punjasawadwong S, Pin-On P. Processed electroencephalogram and evoked potential techniques for amelioration of postoperative delirium and cognitive dysfunction following non-cardiac and non-neurosurgical procedures in adults. *Cochrane Database Syst Rev.* 2018;5:CD011283.

Rabai F, Sessions R, Seubert CN. Neurophysiological monitoring and spinal cord integrity. *Best Pract Res Clin Anaesthesiol.* 2016;30:53.

Sessler D. Temperature monitoring and perioperative thermoregulation. *Anesthesiology*. 2008;109:318.

Sessler D, Sigl J, Keley S, et al. Hospital stay and mortality are increased in patients having a "triple low" of low blood pressure, low bispectral index, and low minimum alveolar concentration of volatile anesthesia. *Anesthesiology*. 2012;116:1195.

Stein EJ, Glick DB. Advances in awareness monitoring technologies. *Curr Opin Anaesthesiol.* 2016;29:711.

Thirumala PD, Thiagarajan K, Gedela S, Crammond DJ, Balzer JR. Diagnostic accuracy of EEG changes during carotid endarterectomy in predicting perioperative strokes. *J Clin Neurosci.* 2016;25:1.

Tusman G, Bohm S, Suarez-Sipmann F. Advanced uses of pulse oximetry for monitoring mechanically ventilated patients. *Anesth Analg.* 2017;124:62.

CHAPTER 7

Pharmacological Principles

KEY CONCEPTS

1. Drug molecules obey the law of mass action. When the plasma concentration exceeds the tissue concentration, the drug moves from the plasma into tissue. When the plasma concentration is less than the tissue concentration, the drug moves from the tissue back to plasma.
2. Most drugs that readily cross the blood–brain barrier (eg, lipophilic drugs like hypnotics and opioids) are avidly taken up in body fat.
3. Biotransformation is the chemical process by which the drug molecule is altered in the body. The liver is the primary organ of metabolism for drugs.
4. Small, unbound molecules freely pass from plasma into the glomerular filtrate. The nonionized (uncharged) fraction of drug is reabsorbed in the renal tubules, whereas the ionized (charged) portion is excreted in urine.
5. Elimination half-life is the time required for the drug concentration to fall by 50%. For drugs described by multicompartment pharmacokinetics (eg, all drugs used in anesthesia), there are multiple elimination half-lives.
6. The offset of a drug's effect cannot be predicted from half-lives. The context-sensitive half-time is a clinically useful concept to describe the rate of decrease in drug concentration and should be used instead of half-lives to compare the pharmacokinetic properties of intravenous drugs used in anesthesia.

The clinical practice of anesthesiology is directly connected to the science of clinical pharmacology. One would think, therefore, that the study of pharmacokinetics and pharmacodynamics would receive attention comparable to with that given to airway assessment, choice of inhalation anesthetic, neuromuscular blockade, or treatment of sepsis in anesthesiology curricula and examinations. Sadly, the frequent misidentification or misuse of pharmacokinetic principles and measurements suggests that this is not yet the case.

PHARMACOKINETICS

Pharmacokinetics defines the relationships among drug dosing, drug concentration in body fluids and tissues, and time. It consists of four linked processes:

absorption, distribution, biotransformation, and excretion.

Absorption

Absorption defines the processes by which a drug moves from the site of administration to the bloodstream. There are many possible routes of drug administration: inhalational, oral, sublingual, transtracheal, rectal, transdermal, transmucosal, subcutaneous, intramuscular, intravenous, perineural, peridural, and intrathecal. Absorption is influenced by the physical characteristics of the drug (solubility, pK_a, diluents, binders, formulation), dose, the site of absorption (eg, gut, lung, skin, muscle), and in some cases (eg, perineural or subcutaneous administration of local anesthetics) by additives such as epinephrine. Bioavailability defines the fraction of the administered dose that reaches the systemic circulation. For example, nitroglycerin is well absorbed by the gastrointestinal tract but has low bioavailability when administered orally. The reason is that nitroglycerin undergoes extensive first-pass hepatic metabolism before reaching the systemic circulation.

Oral drug administration is convenient, inexpensive, and relatively tolerant of dosing errors. However, it requires the cooperation of the patient, exposes the drug to first-pass hepatic metabolism, and permits gastric pH, digestive enzymes, motility, food, and other drugs to potentially reduce the predictability of systemic drug delivery.

Nonionized (uncharged) drugs are more readily absorbed than ionized (charged) forms. Therefore, an acidic environment (stomach) favors the absorption of acidic drugs ($A^- + H^+ \rightarrow AH$), whereas a more alkaline environment (intestine) favors basic drugs ($BH^+ \rightarrow H^+ + B$). Nevertheless, in most cases, the greater aggregate amount of drugs is absorbed from the intestine rather than the stomach because of the greater surface area of the small intestine and longer transit duration.

All venous drainage from the stomach and small intestine flows to the liver. As a result, the bioavailability of highly metabolized drugs may be significantly reduced by first-pass hepatic metabolism. Because the venous drainage from the mouth and esophagus flows into the superior vena cava rather than into the portal system, sublingual or buccal drug absorption bypasses the liver and first-pass metabolism. Rectal administration partly bypasses the portal system and represents an alternative route in small children or patients who are unable to tolerate oral ingestion. However, rectal absorption can be erratic, and many drugs irritate the rectal mucosa.

Transdermal drug administration can provide prolonged continuous administration for some drugs. However, the stratum corneum is an effective barrier to all but small, lipid-soluble drugs (eg, clonidine, nitroglycerin, scopolamine, fentanyl, free-base local anesthetics [EMLA]).

Parenteral routes of drug administration include subcutaneous, intramuscular, and intravenous injection. Subcutaneous and intramuscular absorption depend on drug diffusion from the site of injection to the bloodstream. The rate at which a drug enters the bloodstream depends on both blood flow to the injected tissue and the injectate formulation. Drugs dissolved in solution are absorbed faster than those present in suspensions. Irritating preparations can cause pain and tissue necrosis (eg, intramuscular diazepam). Intravenous injections bypass the process of absorption.

Distribution

Once absorbed, a drug is distributed by the bloodstream throughout the body. Highly perfused organs (the so-called vessel-rich group) receive a disproportionate fraction of the cardiac output (Table 7–1). Therefore, these tissues receive a disproportionate

TABLE 7–1 Tissue group composition, relative body mass, and percentage of cardiac output.

Tissue Group	Composition	Body Mass (%)	Cardiac Output (%)
Vessel-rich	Brain, heart, liver, kidney, endocrine glands	10	75
Muscle	Muscle, skin	50	19
Fat	Fat	20	6
Vessel-poor	Bone, ligament, cartilage	20	0

amount of drug in the first minutes following drug administration. These tissues approach equilibration with the plasma concentration more rapidly than less well-perfused tissues because of the differences in blood flow. However, less well-perfused tissues such as fat and skin may have an enormous capacity to absorb lipophilic drugs, resulting in a large reservoir of drug following long infusions or larger doses.

1 Drug molecules obey the law of mass action. When the plasma concentration exceeds the concentration in tissue, the drug moves from the plasma into tissue. When the plasma concentration is less than the tissue concentration, the drug moves from the tissue back to plasma.

The rate of rise in drug concentration in an organ is determined by that organ's perfusion and the relative drug solubility in the organ compared with blood. The equilibrium concentration in an organ relative to blood depends only on the relative solubility of the drug in the organ relative to blood unless the organ is capable of metabolizing the drug.

Molecules in blood are either free or bound to blood constituents such as plasma proteins and lipids. The free concentration equilibrates between organs and tissues. The equilibration between bound and unbound molecules is instantaneous. As unbound molecules of drug diffuse into tissue, they are instantly replaced by previously bound molecules. Plasma protein binding does not affect the rate of transfer directly, but it does affect the relative solubility of the drug in blood and tissue. When a drug is highly bound in blood, a much larger dose will be required to achieve the same systemic effect. If the drug is highly bound in tissues and unbound in plasma, the relative solubility favors drug transfer into tissue. Put another way, a drug that is highly bound in tissue but not in blood will have a very large free drug concentration gradient driving drug into the tissue. Conversely, if the drug is highly protein bound in plasma and has few binding sites in the tissue, transfer of a small amount of drug may be enough to bring the free drug concentration into equilibrium between blood and tissue. Thus, high levels of binding in blood relative to tissues will increase the rate of onset of drug effect because fewer molecules will need to transfer into the tissue to produce an effective free drug concentration.

Albumin has two main binding sites with an affinity for many acidic and neutral drugs (including diazepam). Highly bound drugs (eg, warfarin) can be displaced by other drugs competing for the same binding site (eg, indocyanine green or ethacrynic acid) with dangerous consequences. α_1-Acid glycoprotein (AAG) binds basic drugs (local anesthetics, tricyclic antidepressants). If the concentrations of these proteins are diminished, the relative solubility of the drugs in blood is decreased, increasing tissue uptake. Kidney disease, liver disease, chronic heart failure, and some malignancies decrease albumin production. Major burns of more than 20% of body surface area lead to albumin loss. Trauma (including surgery), infection, myocardial infarction, and chronic pain increase AAG levels. Pregnancy is associated with reduced AAG concentrations. None of these factors has much relevance to propofol, which is administered with its own binding molecules (the lipid in the emulsion).

Lipophilic molecules can readily transfer between the blood and organs. Charged molecules are able to pass in small quantities into most organs. However, the blood–brain barrier is a special case. Permeation of the central nervous system by ionized drugs is limited by pericapillary glial cells and endothelial
2 cell tight junctions. Most drugs that readily cross the blood–brain barrier (eg, lipophilic drugs like hypnotics and opioids) are avidly taken up in body fat.

The time course of the distribution of drugs into peripheral tissues is complex and is best described using computer models and simulation. Following intravenous bolus administration, rapid distribution of drug from the plasma into tissues accounts for the profound decrease in plasma concentration observed in the first few minutes. For each tissue, there is a point in time at which the apparent concentration in the tissue is the same as the concentration in the plasma. The redistribution phase (from each tissue) follows this moment of equilibration. During *re*distribution, drug returns from tissues back into the plasma. This return of drug back to the plasma slows the rate of decline in plasma drug concentration.

Following administration of a bolus of an induction agent, distribution generally contributes to rapid emergence by removing drug from the plasma for many minutes. Following prolonged infusions of lipophilic anesthetic drugs, *re*distribution generally delays emergence as drug returns from tissue reservoirs to the plasma for many hours.

The complex process of drug distribution into and out of tissues is one reason that half-lives provide almost no guidance for predicting emergence times. The offset of a drug's clinical actions is best predicted by computer models using the *context-sensitive half-time* or *decrement time*. The *context-sensitive half-time* is the time required for a 50% decrease in plasma drug concentration to occur following a pseudo-steady-state infusion (in other words, an infusion that has continued long enough to yield nearly steady-state concentrations). Here, the "context" is the duration of the infusion, which defines the total mass of drug remaining within the subject. The *context-sensitive decrement time* is a more generalized concept referring to any clinically relevant decreased concentration in any tissue, particularly the brain or effect site.

The volume of distribution, V_d, is the *apparent* volume into which a drug has "distributed" (ie, mixed). This volume is calculated by dividing a bolus dose of drug by the plasma concentration at time 0. In practice, the concentration used to define the V_d is often obtained by extrapolating subsequent concentrations back to "0 time" when the drug was injected (this assumes immediate and complete mixing), as follows:

$$V_d = \frac{\text{Bolus dose}}{\text{Concentration}_{\text{time0}}}$$

The concept of a single V_d does not apply to any intravenous drugs used in anesthesia. All intravenous anesthetic drugs are better modeled with at least two compartments: a central compartment and a peripheral compartment. The behavior of many of these drugs is more precisely described using three compartments: a central compartment, a rapidly equilibrating peripheral compartment, and a slowly equilibrating peripheral compartment. The central compartment may be thought of as including the blood and any ultra-rapidly equilibrating tissues such as the lungs. The peripheral compartment is composed of the other body tissues. For drugs with two peripheral compartments, the rapidly equilibrating compartment comprises the organs and muscles, while the slowly equilibrating compartment roughly represents the distribution of the drug into fat and skin. These compartments are designated V_1 (central), V_2 (rapid distribution), and V_3 (slow distribution). The volume of distribution at steady state, V_{dss} is the algebraic sum of these compartment volumes. V_1 is calculated by the above equation showing the relationship between volume, dose, and concentration. The other volumes are calculated through pharmacokinetic modeling.

A small V_{dss} implies that the drug has high aqueous solubility and will remain largely within the intravascular space. For example, the V_{dss} of vecuronium is about 200 mL/kg in adult men and about 160 mL/kg in adult women, indicating that vecuronium is mostly present in body water, with little distribution into fat. However, the typical general anesthetics is lipophilic, resulting in a V_{dss} that exceeds total body water (approximately 600 mL/kg in adult males). For example, the V_{dss} for fentanyl is about 350 L in adults, and the V_{dss} for propofol may exceed 5000 L. V_{dss} does not represent a real volume but rather reflects the volume into which the administered drug dose would need to distribute to account for the observed plasma concentration.

Biotransformation

3 Biotransformation includes the chemical processes by which the drug molecule is altered in the body. The liver is the primary organ of metabolism for most drugs. An exception is the esters, which undergo hydrolysis in the plasma or tissues. The end products of biotransformation are often (but not always) inactive and water soluble. Water solubility allows excretion by the kidneys.

Metabolic biotransformation is frequently divided into phase I and phase II reactions. Phase I reactions convert a parent compound into more polar metabolites through oxidation, reduction, or hydrolysis. Phase II reactions couple (conjugate) a parent drug or a phase I metabolite with an endogenous substrate (eg, glucuronic acid) to form water-soluble metabolites that can be eliminated in the urine or stool. Although this is usually a sequential process, phase I metabolites may be excreted without undergoing phase II biotransformation, and a phase II reaction can precede or occur without a phase I reaction.

Hepatic clearance is the volume of blood or plasma (whichever was measured in the assay) cleared of drug per unit of time. The units of clearance are units of flow: volume per unit time. Clearance may be expressed in milliliters per minute, liters per hour, or any other convenient unit of flow. If every molecule of drug that enters the liver is metabolized, hepatic clearance will equal liver blood flow. This is true for very few drugs, though it is very nearly the case for propofol. For most drugs, only a fraction of the drug that enters the liver is removed. The fraction removed is called the *extraction ratio*. The hepatic clearance can therefore be expressed as the liver blood flow times the extraction ratio. If the extraction ratio is 50%, hepatic clearance is 50% of liver blood flow. The clearance of drugs efficiently removed by the liver (ie, having a high hepatic extraction ratio) is proportional to hepatic blood flow. For example, because the liver removes almost all of the propofol that passes through it, when the hepatic blood flow doubles, the clearance of propofol doubles. Induction of liver enzymes has no effect on propofol clearance because the liver so efficiently removes all of the propofol that passes through it. Even severe loss of liver tissue, as occurs in cirrhosis, has little effect on propofol clearance. Drugs such as propofol, propranolol, lidocaine, morphine, and nitroglycerin have flow-dependent clearance.

Many drugs have low hepatic extraction ratios and are slowly cleared by the liver. For these drugs, the rate-limiting step is not the flow of blood to the liver but rather the metabolic capacity of the liver itself. Changes in liver blood flow have little effect on the clearance of such drugs. However, if liver enzymes are induced, clearance will increase because the liver has more capacity to metabolize the drug. Conversely, if the liver is damaged, less capacity is available for metabolism, and clearance is reduced. Drugs with low hepatic extraction ratios thus have capacity-dependent clearance. The extraction ratios of methadone and alfentanil are 10% and 15%, respectively, making these capacity-dependent drugs.

Excretion

Some drugs and many drug metabolites are excreted by the kidneys. Renal clearance is the rate of elimination of a drug from the body by kidney excretion. This concept is analogous to hepatic clearance, and similarly, renal clearance can be expressed as the renal blood flow times the renal extraction ratio. 4 Small, unbound drugs freely pass from plasma into the glomerular filtrate. The nonionized (uncharged) fraction of drug is reabsorbed in the renal tubules, whereas the ionized (charged) portion remains and is excreted in urine. The fraction of drug ionized depends on the pH; thus, renal elimination of drugs that exist in ionized and nonionized forms depends in part on urinary pH. The kidney actively secretes some drugs into the renal tubules.

Many drugs and drug metabolites pass from the liver into the intestine via the biliary system. Some drugs excreted into the bile are then reabsorbed in the intestine, a process called *enterohepatic recirculation*. Occasionally metabolites excreted in bile are subsequently converted back to the parent drug. For example, lorazepam is converted by the liver to lorazepam glucuronide. In the intestine, β-glucuronidase breaks the ester linkage, converting lorazepam glucuronide back to lorazepam.

Compartment Models

Multicompartment models provide a mathematical framework that can be used to relate drug dose to changes in drug concentrations over time. Conceptually, the compartments in these models are tissues with a similar distribution time course. For example, the plasma and lungs are components of the central compartment. The organs and muscles, sometimes called the *vessel-rich group*, could be the second, or rapidly equilibrating, compartment. Fat and skin have the capacity to bind large quantities of lipophilic drug but are poorly perfused. These could represent the third, or slowly equilibrating, compartment. This is an intuitive definition of compartments, but it is important to recognize that the compartments of a

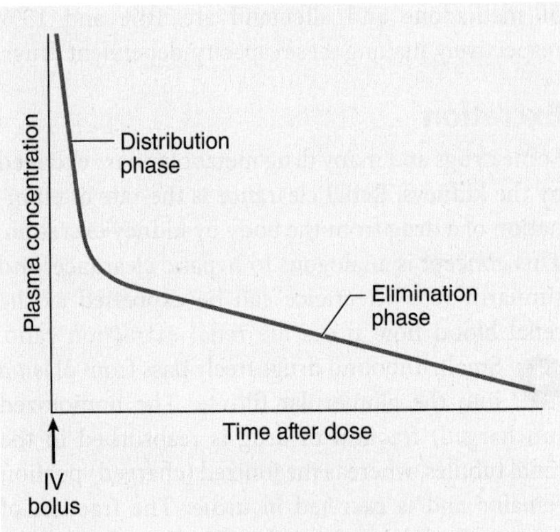

FIGURE 7–1 Two-compartment model demonstrates the changes in drug concentrations in the distribution phase and the elimination phase. During the distribution phase, the drug moves from the central compartment to the peripheral compartment. In the elimination phase, the drug returns from the peripheral compartment to the central compartment and is metabolized and excreted.

pharmacokinetic model are mathematical abstractions that relate dose to observed concentration. A one-to-one relationship does not exist between any "mathematically identified" compartment and any organ or tissue in the body.

Many drugs used in anesthesia are well described by two-compartment models. This is generally the case if the studies used to characterize the pharmacokinetics do not include rapid arterial sampling over the first few minutes (Figure 7–1). Without rapid arterial sampling, the ultrarapid initial drop in plasma concentration immediately after a bolus injection is missed, and the central compartment volume is blended into the rapidly equilibrating compartment. When rapid arterial sampling is used in pharmacokinetic experiments, the results generally support the use of a three-compartment model. Thus, the number of identifiable compartments reported in a pharmacokinetic study may be more a function of the experimental design than a characteristic of the drug.

As previously noted, in compartmental models the instantaneous concentration at the time of a bolus injection is assumed to be the amount of the bolus divided by the central compartment volume. This is not correct. If the bolus is given over a few seconds, the instantaneous concentration is 0 because the drug is all in the vein, still flowing to the heart. It takes a minute or two for the drug to mix in the central compartment volume. This misspecification is common to conventional pharmacokinetic models. More physiologically based models, sometimes called *front-end kinetic models*, can characterize the initial delay in concentration. The additional complexity that these models introduce is useful only if the concentrations over the first few minutes are clinically important. After the first few minutes, front-end models resemble conventional compartmental models.

In the first few minutes following initial bolus administration of a drug, the concentration drops very rapidly as the drug quickly diffuses into peripheral compartments. Concentrations often decline by an order of magnitude over 10 minutes! For drugs with very rapid hepatic clearance (eg, propofol) or those that are metabolized in the blood (eg, remifentanil), metabolism contributes significantly to the rapid initial drop in concentration. Following this very rapid drop, a period of slower decrease in plasma concentration occurs. During this period, the rapidly equilibrating compartment is no longer removing drug from the plasma. Instead, drug returns to the plasma from the rapidly equilibrating compartment. The reversed role of the rapidly equilibrating tissues from extracting drug to returning drug accounts for the slower rate of decline in plasma concentration in this intermediate phase. Eventually, there is an even slower rate of decrease in plasma concentration, which is log-linear until the drug is no longer detectable. This terminal log-linear phase occurs after the slowly equilibrating compartment shifts from net removal of drug from the plasma to net return of drug to the plasma. During this terminal phase, the organ of elimination (typically the liver) is exposed to the body's entire body drug load, which accounts for the very slow rate of decrease in plasma drug concentration during this final phase.

The mathematical models used to describe a drug with two or three compartments are, respectively:

$$Cp(t) = Ae^{-\alpha}t + Be^{-\beta}t$$

and

$$Cp(t) = Ae^{-\alpha t} + Be^{-\beta t} + Ce^{-\gamma t}$$

where $Cp(t)$ equals plasma concentration at time t, and α, β, and γ are the exponents that characterize the very rapid (ie, very steep), intermediate, and slow (ie, log-linear) portions of the plasma concentration over time, respectively. Drugs described by two-compartment and three-compartment models will have two or three half-lives. Each half-life is calculated as the natural log of 2 (0.693), divided by the exponent. The coefficients A, B, and C represent the contribution of each of the exponents to the overall decrease in concentration over time.

The two-compartment model is described by a curve with two exponents and two coefficients, whereas the three-compartment model is described by a curve with three exponents and three coefficients. The mathematical relationships among compartments, clearances, coefficients, and exponents are complex. Every coefficient and every exponent is a function of every volume and every clearance.

5 Elimination half-time is the time required for the drug concentration to fall by 50%. For drugs described by multicompartment pharmacokinetics (eg, fentanyl, sufentanil), there are multiple elimination half-times, in other words, the elimination
6 half-time is context dependent. The offset of a drug's effect cannot be predicted from half-lives alone. Moreover, one cannot easily determine how rapidly a drug effect will disappear simply by looking at coefficients, exponents, and half-lives. For example, the terminal half-life of sufentanil is about 10 h, whereas that of alfentanil is 2 h. This does not mean that recovery from alfentanil will be faster because clinical recovery from clinical dosing will be influenced by all half-lives, not just the terminal one. Computer models readily demonstrate that recovery from an infusion lasting several hours will be faster when the drug administered is sufentanil than it will be when the infused drug is alfentanil. The time required for a 50% decrease in concentration depends on the duration or "context" of the infusion. The context-sensitive half-time, mentioned earlier, captures this concept and should be used instead of half-lives to compare the pharmacokinetic properties of intravenous drugs used in anesthesia.

PHARMACODYNAMICS

Pharmacodynamics, the study of how drugs affect the body, involves the concepts of potency, efficacy, and therapeutic window. The fundamental pharmacodynamic concepts are captured in the relationship between exposure to a drug and physiological response to the drug, often called the *dose–response* or *concentration–response relationship*.

Exposure–Response Relationships

As the body is exposed to an increasing amount of a drug, the response to the drug similarly increases, typically up to a maximal value. This fundamental concept in the exposure versus response relationship is captured graphically by plotting exposure (usually dose or concentration) on the x axis as the independent variable and the body's response on the y axis as the dependent variable. Depending on the circumstances, the dose or concentration may be plotted on a linear scale (Figure 7–2A) or a logarithmic scale (Figure 7–2B), while the response is typically plotted either as the actual measured response (**Figure 7–2A**) or as a fraction of the baseline or maximum physiological measurement (**Figure 7–2B**). For our purposes here, basic pharmacodynamic properties are described in terms of concentration, but any metric of drug exposure (eg, dose, area under the curve) could be used.

The shape of the relationship is typically sigmoidal, as shown in **Figure 7–2**. The sigmoidal shape reflects the observation that often a certain minimal amount of drug must be present before there is any measurable physiological response. Thus, the left side of the curve is flat until the drug concentration reaches a threshold. The right side is also flat, reflecting the maximum physiological response of the body, beyond which the body simply cannot respond to additional drug. Thus, the curve is flat on both the left and right sides. A sigmoidal curve is required to connect the baseline to the asymptote, which is why sigmoidal curves are ubiquitous when modeling pharmacodynamics.

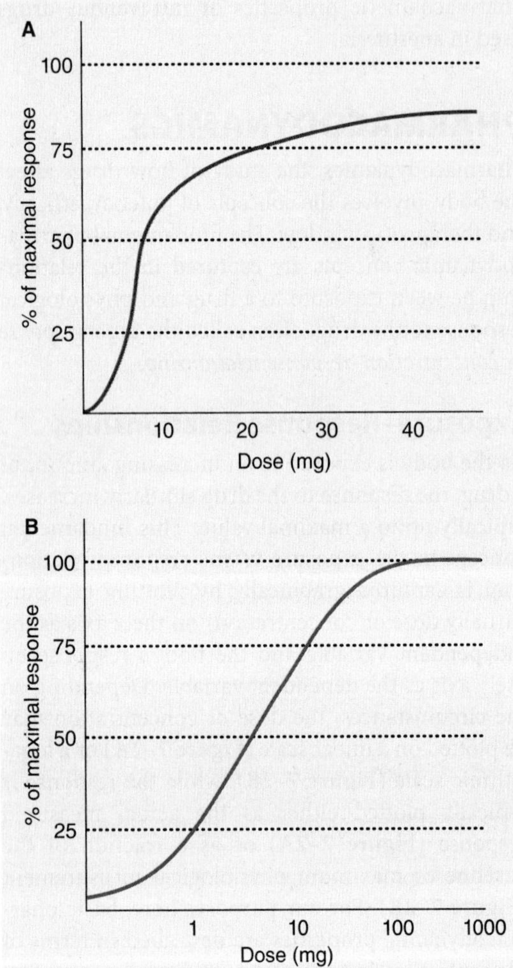

FIGURE 7–2 The shape of the dose (or concentration)–response curve depends on whether the dose or plasma concentration is plotted on a linear (**A**) or logarithmic (**B**) scale.

The sigmoidal relationship between exposure and response is defined by one of two interchangeable relationships:

$$\text{Effect} = E_{max}\frac{C^{\gamma}}{C_{50}^{\gamma} + C^{\gamma}}$$

or

$$\text{Effect} = E_0 + (E_{max} - E_0)\frac{C^{\gamma}}{C_{50}^{\gamma} + C^{\gamma}}$$

In both cases, C is drug concentration, C_{50} is the concentration associated with half-maximal effect, and γ describes the steepness of the concentration versus response relationship (and is also known as the *Hill coefficient*). In the first equation, E_{max} is the maximum physiological measurement, not the maximum change from baseline. For the second equation, E_{max} is the maximum change from the baseline effect (E_0). Once defined in this fashion, each parameter of the pharmacodynamic model speaks to the specific concepts mentioned earlier. E_{max} is related to the intrinsic efficacy of a drug. Highly efficacious drugs have a large maximum physiological effect, characterized by a large E_{max}. For drugs that lack efficacy, E_{max} will equal E_0. C_{50} is a measure of drug potency. Highly potent drugs have a low C_{50}; thus, small amounts produce the drug effect. Drugs lacking potency have a high C_{50}, indicating that a large amount of drug is required to achieve the drug effect. The parameter γ indicates the steepness of the relationship between concentration and effect. A γ value less than 1 indicates a very gradual increase in drug effect with increasing concentration. A γ value greater than 4 suggests that once drug effect is observed, small increases in drug concentration produce large increases in drug effect until the maximum effect is reached.

The curve described above represents the relationship of drug concentration to a continuous physiological response. The same relationship can be used to characterize the probability of a binary (yes/no) response to a drug dose:

$$\text{Probability} = P_0 + (P_{max} - P_0)\frac{C^{\gamma}}{C_{50}^{\gamma} + C^{\gamma}}$$

In this case, the probability (P) ranges from 0 (no chance) to 1 (certainty). P_0 is the probability of a "yes" response in the absence of drug. P_{max} is the maximum probability, necessarily less than or equal to 1. As before, C is the concentration, C_{50} is the concentration associated with half-maximal effect, and γ describes the steepness of the concentration versus response relationship. Half-maximal effect is the same as 50% probability of a response when P_0 is 0 and P_{max} is 1.

The *therapeutic window* for a drug is the range between the concentration associated with a desired therapeutic effect and the concentration associated with a toxic drug response. This range can be measured as either the difference between two points on the same concentration versus response curve (when the toxicity represents an exaggerated form of the desired drug response) or the distance between two distinct curves (when the toxicity represents a different response or process from the desired drug response). For a drug such as sodium nitroprusside, a single concentration versus response curve defines the relationship between concentration and decrease in blood pressure. The therapeutic window might be the difference in the concentration producing a desired 20% decrease in blood pressure and a toxic concentration that produces a catastrophic 60% decrease in blood pressure. However, for a drug such as lidocaine, the therapeutic window might be the difference between the C_{50} for suppression of ventricular arrhythmias and the C_{50} for lidocaine-induced seizures, the two drug effects being described by separate concentration versus response relationships. The therapeutic index is the C_{50} for toxicity divided by the C_{50} for the desired therapeutic effect. Because of the risk of ventilatory and cardiovascular depression (even at concentrations only slightly greater than those producing anesthesia), most inhaled and intravenous hypnotics are considered to have very low therapeutic indices relative to other drugs.

Drug Receptors

Drug receptors are macromolecules (typically proteins) that bind a drug (agonist) and mediate the drug response. Pharmacological antagonists reverse the effects of the agonist but do not otherwise exert an effect of their own. Competitive antagonism occurs when the antagonist competes with the agonist for the same binding site, each potentially displacing the other. Noncompetitive antagonism occurs when the antagonist, through covalent binding or another process, permanently impairs the drug's access to the receptor.

The drug effect is governed by the fraction of receptors that are occupied by an agonist. That fraction is based on the concentration of the drug, the concentration of the receptor, and the strength of binding between the drug and the receptor. This binding is described by the law of mass action, which states that the reaction rate is proportional to the concentrations of the reactants:

$$[D][RU] \underset{k_{\text{off}}}{\overset{k_{\text{on}}}{\rightleftharpoons}} [DR]$$

where $[D]$ is the concentration of the drug, $[RU]$ is the concentration of unbound receptor, and $[DR]$ is the concentration of bound receptor. The rate constant k_{on} defines the rate of ligand binding to the receptor. The rate constant k_{off} defines the rate of ligand unbinding from the receptor. Steady state occurs almost instantly. Because the rate of formation at steady state is 0, it follows that:

$$[D][RU]k_{\text{on}} - [DR]k_{\text{off}}$$

In this equation, k_{d} is the dissociation rate constant, defined as $k_{\text{on}}/k_{\text{off}}$. If we define f, fractional receptor occupancy, as:

$$\frac{[DR]}{[DR]+[RU]}$$

we can solve for receptor occupancy as:

$$f = \frac{[D]}{k_{\text{d}}+[D]}$$

The receptors are half occupied when $[D] = k_{\text{d}}$. Thus, k_{d} is the concentration of drug associated with 50% receptor occupancy.

Receptor occupancy is only the first step in mediating drug effect. Binding of the drug to the receptor can trigger myriad subsequent steps, including opening, closing, or inhibition of an ion channel; activation of a G protein; activation of an intracellular kinase; direct interaction with a cellular structure; or direct binding to DNA.

Like the concentration versus response curve, the shape of the curve relating fractional receptor occupancy to drug concentration is intrinsically sigmoidal. However, the concentration associated with 50% receptor occupancy and the concentration associated with 50% of maximal drug effect are not necessarily the same. Maximal drug effect could occur at very low receptor occupancy or (for partial agonists) at greater than 100% receptor occupancy.

Prolonged binding and activation of a receptor by an agonist may lead to "desensitization" or tolerance. If the binding of an endogenous ligand is chronically blocked or chronically reduced, receptors may proliferate, resulting in hyperreactivity and increased sensitivity. For example, after spinal cord injury, nicotinic acetylcholine receptors are not stimulated by impulses in motor nerves and proliferate in denervated muscle. This can lead to exaggerated responses (including hyperkalemia) to succinylcholine.

SUGGESTED READINGS

Ansari J, Carvalho B, Shafer SL, Flood P. Pharmacokinetics and pharmacodynamics of drugs commonly used in pregnancy and parturition. *Anesth Analg.* 2016;122:786.

Bailey JM. Context-sensitive half-times: what are they and how valuable are they in anaesthesiology? *Clin Pharmacokinet.* 2002;41:793.

Brunton LL, Hilal-Dandan R. Knollman BC, eds. *Goodman & Gilman's The Pharmacological Basis of Therapeutics.* 13th ed. McGraw-Hill; 2017: chap 2.

Shargel L, Yu ABC, eds. *Applied Biopharmaceutics & Pharmacokinetics.* 7th ed. McGraw-Hill; 2016.

CHAPTER 8

Inhalation Anesthetics

KEY CONCEPTS

1. The greater the uptake of anesthetic agent, the greater the difference between inspired and alveolar concentrations and the slower the rate of induction.
2. Three factors affect anesthetic uptake: solubility in the blood, alveolar blood flow, and the difference in partial pressure between alveolar gas and venous blood.
3. Low-output states predispose patients to overdosage with soluble agents as the rate of rise in alveolar concentrations will be markedly increased.
4. Many of the factors that speed induction also speed recovery: elimination of rebreathing, high fresh gas flows, low anesthetic-circuit volume, low absorption by the anesthetic circuit, decreased solubility, high cerebral blood flow, and increased ventilation.
5. The unitary hypothesis proposes that all inhalation agents share a common mechanism of action at the molecular level. This was previously supported by the observation that the anesthetic potency of inhalation agents correlates directly with their lipid solubility (Meyer–Overton rule). The implication is that anesthesia results from molecules dissolving at specific lipophilic sites; however, the correlation is only approximate.
6. The minimum alveolar concentration (MAC) of an inhaled anesthetic is the alveolar concentration that prevents movement in 50% of patients in response to a standardized stimulus (eg, surgical incision).
7. Prolonged exposure to anesthetic concentrations of nitrous oxide can result in bone marrow depression (megaloblastic anemia) and even neurologic deficiencies (peripheral neuropathies).
8. "Halothane hepatitis" is extremely rare. Patients exposed to multiple halothane anesthetics at short intervals, middle-aged obese women, and persons with a familial predisposition to halothane toxicity or a personal history of toxicity are considered to be at increased risk.
9. Isoflurane dilates coronary arteries but not nearly as potently as nitroglycerin or adenosine. Dilation of normal coronary arteries could theoretically divert blood away from fixed stenotic lesions.
10. The low solubility of desflurane in blood and body tissues causes very rapid induction of and emergence from anesthesia.
11. Rapid increases in desflurane concentration lead to transient but sometimes worrisome elevations in heart rate, blood pressure, and catecholamine levels that are more pronounced than occur with isoflurane, particularly in patients with cardiovascular disease.
12. Nonpungency and rapid increases in alveolar anesthetic concentration make sevoflurane an excellent choice for smooth and rapid inhalation inductions in pediatric and adult patients.

Nitrous oxide, chloroform, and ether were the first universally accepted general anesthetics. Currently used inhalation agents include nitrous oxide, halothane, isoflurane, desflurane, and sevoflurane.

The course of a general anesthetic can be divided into three phases: (1) induction, (2) maintenance, and (3) emergence. Inhalation anesthetics, notably halothane and sevoflurane, are particularly useful for the inhalation induction of pediatric patients in whom it may be difficult to start an intravenous line. Although adults are usually induced with intravenous agents, the nonpungency and rapid onset of sevoflurane make inhalation induction practical for them as well. Regardless of the patient's age, anesthesia is often maintained with inhalation agents. Emergence depends primarily upon redistribution of the agent from the brain, followed by pulmonary elimination. Because of their unique route of administration, inhalation anesthetics have useful pharmacological properties not shared by other anesthetic agents.

Pharmacokinetics of Inhalation Anesthetics

Although the mechanism of action of inhalation anesthetics is not yet fully understood, their ultimate effects clearly depend on attaining a therapeutic tissue concentration in the central nervous system (CNS). There are many steps between the anesthetic vaporizer and the anesthetic's deposition in the brain (Figure 8–1).

FACTORS AFFECTING INSPIRATORY CONCENTRATION (F_I)

The fresh gas leaving the anesthesia machine mixes with gases in the breathing circuit before being inspired by the patient. Therefore, the patient is not

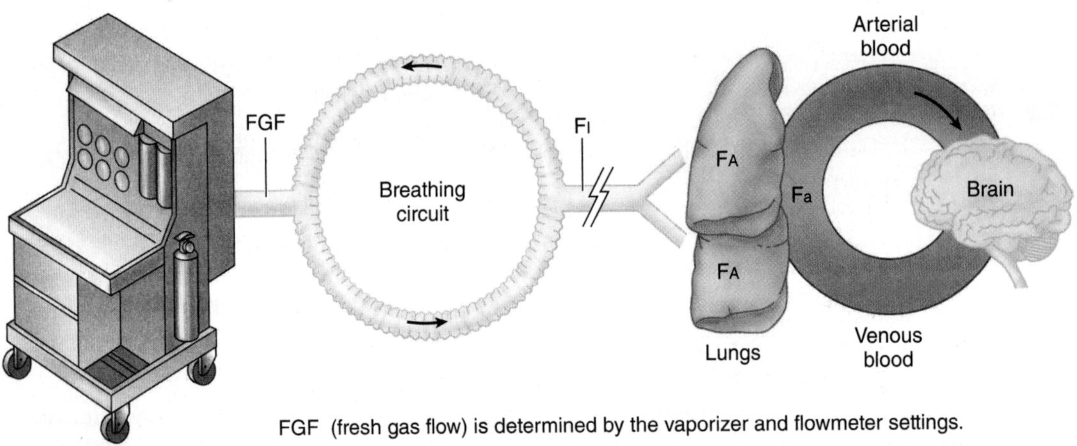

FGF (fresh gas flow) is determined by the vaporizer and flowmeter settings.

FI (inspired gas concentration) is determined by (1) FGF rate; (2) breathing-circuit volume; and (3) circuit absorption.

FA (aveolar gas concentration) is determined by (1) uptake (uptake = λb/g x C(A-V) x Q); (2) ventilation; and (3) the concentration effect and second gas effect:
a) concentrating effect
b) augmented inflow effect

Fa (arterial gas concentration) is affected by ventilation/perfusion mismatching.

FIGURE 8–1 Inhalation anesthetic agents must pass through many barriers between the anesthesia machine and the brain.

necessarily receiving the concentration set on the vaporizer. The actual composition of the inspired gas mixture depends mainly on the fresh gas flow rate, the volume of the breathing system, and any absorption by the machine or breathing circuit. The greater the fresh gas flow rate, the smaller the breathing system volume, and the lower the circuit absorption, the closer the inspired gas concentration will be to the fresh gas concentration.

TABLE 8–1 Partition coefficients of volatile anesthetics at 37°C.[1]

Agent	Blood/ Gas	Brain/ Blood	Muscle/ Blood	Fat/ Blood
Nitrous oxide	0.47	1.1	1.2	2.3
Halothane	2.4	2.9	3.5	60
Isoflurane	1.4	2.6	4.0	45
Desflurane	0.42	1.3	2.0	27
Sevoflurane	0.65	1.7	3.1	48

[1]These values are averages derived from multiple studies and should be used for comparison purposes, not as exact numbers.

FACTORS AFFECTING ALVEOLAR CONCENTRATION (F_A)

Uptake

If there were no uptake of anesthetic agent by the body, the alveolar gas concentration (FA) would rapidly approach the inspired gas concentration (FI). Because anesthetic agents are taken up by the pulmonary circulation during induction, alveolar concentrations lag behind inspired concentrations (FA/FI <1.0). The greater the uptake, the slower the rate of rise of the alveolar concentration and the lower the FA:FI ratio.

Because the concentration of a gas is directly proportional to its partial pressure, the alveolar partial pressure will also be slow to rise. The alveolar partial pressure is important because it determines the partial pressure of anesthetic in the blood and, ultimately, in the brain. Similarly, the partial pressure of the anesthetic in the brain is directly proportional to its brain tissue concentration, which
1 determines the clinical effect. The faster the uptake of anesthetic agent, the greater the difference between inspired and alveolar concentrations and the slower the rate of induction.

2 Three factors affect anesthetic uptake: solubility in the blood, alveolar blood flow, and the difference in partial pressure between alveolar gas and venous blood.

Relatively insoluble agents, such as nitrous oxide, are taken up by the blood less avidly than more soluble agents, such as sevoflurane. As a consequence, the alveolar concentration of nitrous oxide rises and achieves a steady state faster than that of sevoflurane. The relative solubilities of an anesthetic in air, blood, and tissues are expressed as partition coefficients (Table 8–1). Each coefficient is the ratio of the concentrations of the anesthetic gas in each of two phases at steady state. *Steady state* is defined as equal partial pressures in the two phases. For instance, the blood/gas partition coefficient ($\lambda_{b/g}$) of nitrous oxide at 37°C is 0.47. In other words, at steady state, 1 mL of blood contains 0.47 as much nitrous oxide as does 1 mL of alveolar gas, even though the partial pressures are the same. Stated another way, blood has 47% of the capacity for nitrous oxide as alveolar gas. Nitrous oxide is much less soluble in blood than is halothane, which has a blood/gas partition coefficient at 37°C of 2.4. Thus, almost five times more halothane than nitrous oxide must be dissolved to raise the partial pressure of blood by the same amount. The higher the blood/gas coefficient, the greater the anesthetic's solubility and the greater its uptake by the pulmonary circulation. As a consequence of this increased solubility, alveolar partial pressure rises to a steady state more slowly. Because fat/blood partition coefficients are greater than 1, blood/gas solubility is increased by postprandial lipidemia and is decreased by anemia.

The second factor that affects uptake is alveolar blood flow, which—in the absence of pulmonary shunting—is equal to cardiac output. If the cardiac output drops to zero, so will anesthetic uptake. As cardiac output increases, anesthetic uptake increases, the rise in alveolar partial pressure slows, and induction is delayed. The effect of changing cardiac output is less pronounced for insoluble anesthetics, as so little is taken up regardless of alveolar blood flow. 3 Low-output states predispose patients to overdosage with soluble agents as the rate of rise in alveolar concentrations will be markedly increased.

The final factor affecting the uptake of anesthetic by the pulmonary circulation is the partial pressure difference between alveolar gas and venous blood. This gradient depends on tissue uptake. If anesthetics did not pass into organs such as the brain, venous and alveolar partial pressures would become identical, and there would be no pulmonary uptake. The transfer of anesthetic from blood to tissues is determined by three factors analogous to systemic uptake: tissue solubility of the agent (tissue/blood partition coefficient), tissue blood flow, and the difference in partial pressure between arterial blood and the tissue.

To better understand inhaled anesthetic uptake and distribution, tissues have been classified into four groups based on their solubility and blood flow (Table 8–2). The highly perfused vessel-rich group (brain, heart, liver, kidney, endocrine organs) is the first to encounter appreciable amounts of anesthetic. Moderate solubility and small volume limit the capacity of this group, so it is also the first to approach steady state (ie, arterial and tissue partial pressures are equal). The muscle group (skin and muscle) is not as well perfused, so uptake is slower. In addition, it has a greater capacity due to a larger volume, and uptake will be sustained for hours. Perfusion of the fat group nearly equals that of the muscle group, but the tremendous solubility of anesthetic in fat leads to a total capacity (tissue/blood solubility × tissue volume) that would take days to approach steady state. The minimal perfusion of the vessel-poor group (bones, ligaments, teeth, hair, cartilage) results in insignificant uptake.

TABLE 8–2 Tissue groups based on perfusion and solubilities.

Characteristic	Vessel Rich	Muscle	Fat	Vessel Poor
Percentage of body weight	10	50	20	20
Percentage of cardiac output	75	19	6	0
Perfusion (mL/min/100 g)	75	3	3	0
Relative solubility	1	1	20	0

Anesthetic uptake produces a characteristic curve that relates the rise in alveolar concentration to time (Figure 8–2). The shape of this graph is determined by the uptakes of individual tissue groups (Figure 8–3). The initial steep rise of FA/FI is due to unopposed filling of the alveoli by ventilation. The rate of rise slows as the vessel-rich group—and eventually the muscle group—approaches steady-state levels of saturation.

Ventilation

The lowering of alveolar partial pressure by uptake can be countered by increasing alveolar ventilation. In other words, constantly replacing anesthetic taken up by the pulmonary bloodstream results in better maintenance of alveolar concentration. The effect of increasing ventilation will be most obvious in raising the FA/FI for soluble anesthetics because they are more subject to uptake. Because the FA/FI very rapidly approaches 1.0 for insoluble agents, increasing ventilation has minimal effect. In contrast to the effect of anesthetics on cardiac output, anesthetics and other drugs (eg, opioids) that depress spontaneous ventilation will decrease the rate of rise in alveolar concentration and create a negative feedback loop.

Concentration

The slowing of induction due to uptake from alveolar gas can be counteracted by increasing the inspired concentration. Interestingly, increasing the inspired concentration not only increases the alveolar concentration but also increases its rate of rise (ie, increases FA/FI) because of two phenomena (see Figure 8–1) that produce a so-called concentrating effect. First, if 50% of an anesthetic is taken up by the pulmonary circulation, an inspired concentration of 20% (20 parts of anesthetic per 100 parts of gas) will result in an alveolar concentration of 11% (10 parts of anesthetic remaining in a total volume of 90 parts of gas). On the other hand, if the inspired concentration is raised to 80% (80 parts of anesthetic per 100 parts of gas), the alveolar concentration will be 67%

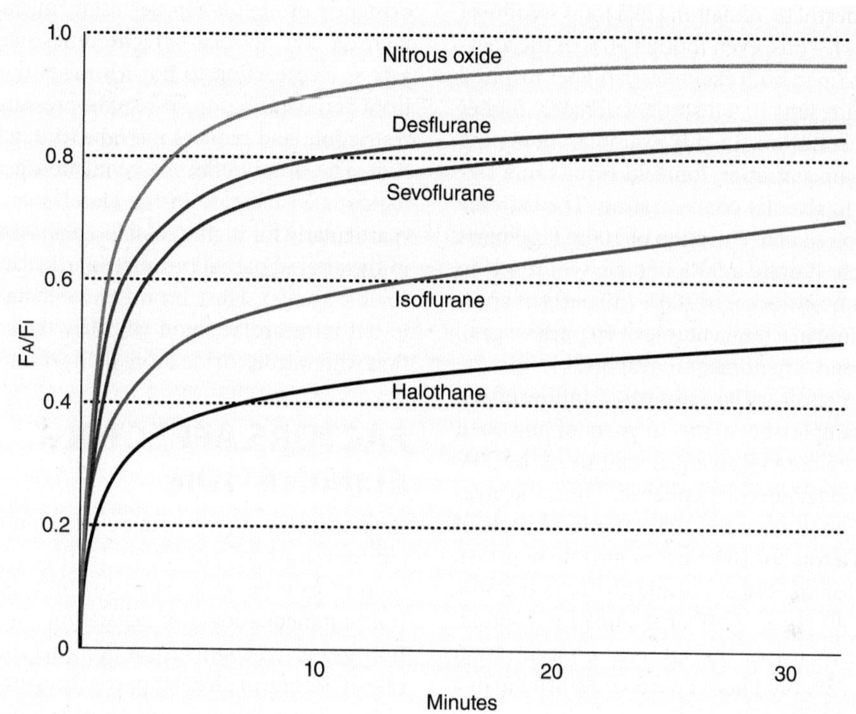

FIGURE 8–2 FA rises toward FI faster with nitrous oxide (an insoluble agent) than with halothane (a soluble agent). See Figure 8–1 for an explanation of FA and FI.

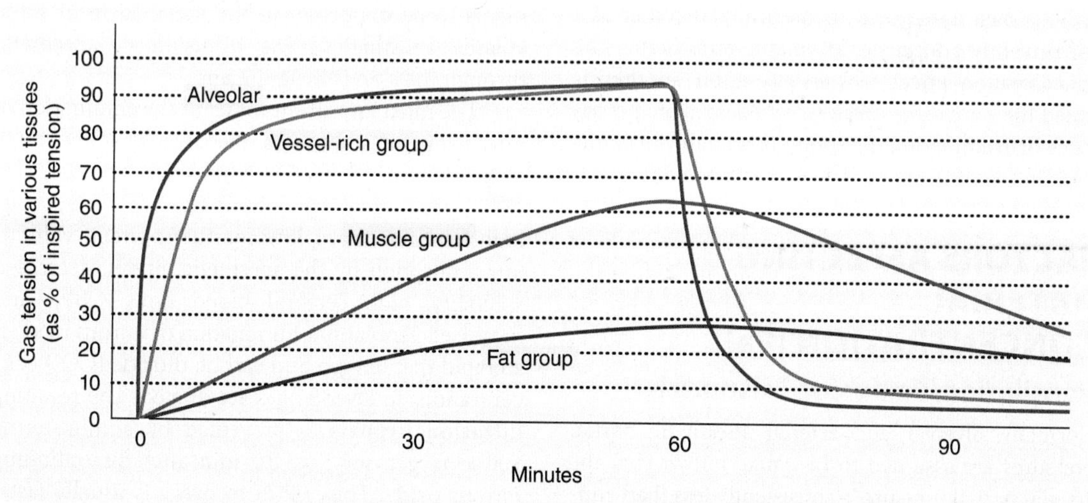

FIGURE 8–3 The rise and fall in alveolar partial pressure precedes that of other tissues. (Modified with permission from Cowles AL, Borgstedt HH, Gillies AJ, et al. Uptake and distribution of inhalation anesthetic agents in clinical practice. *Anesth Analg.* 1968 July-Aug;47(4):404-414.)

(40 parts of anesthetic remaining in a total volume of 60 parts of gas). Thus, even though 50% of the anesthetic is taken up in both examples, a higher inspired concentration results in a disproportionately higher alveolar concentration. In this example, increasing the inspired concentration fourfold results in a sixfold increase in alveolar concentration. The extreme case is an inspired concentration of 100% (100 parts of 100), which, despite a 50% uptake, will result in an alveolar concentration of 100% (50 parts of anesthetic remaining in a total volume of 50 parts of gas).

The second phenomenon responsible for the concentration effect is the augmented inflow effect. Using the example above, the 10 parts of absorbed gas must be replaced by an equal volume of the 20% mixture to prevent alveolar collapse. Thus, the alveolar concentration becomes 12% (10 plus 2 parts of anesthetic in a total of 100 parts of gas). In contrast, after absorption of 50% of the anesthetic in the 80% gas mixture, 40 parts of 80% gas must be inspired. This further increases the alveolar concentration from 67% to 72% (40 plus 32 parts of anesthetic in a volume of 100 parts of gas).

The concentration effect is more significant with nitrous oxide than with volatile anesthetics, as the former can be used in much higher concentrations. Nonetheless, a high concentration of nitrous oxide will augment (by the same mechanism) not only its own uptake but theoretically also that of a concurrently administered volatile anesthetic. The concentration effect of one gas upon another is called the *second gas effect*, which, despite its persistence in examination questions, is probably insignificant in the clinical practice of anesthesiology.

FACTORS AFFECTING ARTERIAL CONCENTRATION (Fa)

Ventilation/Perfusion Mismatch

Normally, alveolar and arterial anesthetic partial pressures are assumed to be equal, but in fact, the arterial partial pressure is consistently less than end-expiratory gas would predict. Reasons for this may include venous admixture, alveolar dead space, and nonuniform alveolar gas distribution. Furthermore, the existence of ventilation/perfusion mismatching will increase the alveolar–arterial difference. Mismatch acts as a restriction to flow: It raises the pressure in front of the restriction, lowers the pressure beyond the restriction, and reduces the flow through the restriction. The overall effect of ventilation/perfusion mismatch is an increase in the alveolar partial pressure (particularly for highly soluble agents) and a decrease in the arterial partial pressure (particularly for poorly soluble agents). Thus, bronchial intubation or a right-to-left intracardiac shunt will slow the rate of induction with nitrous oxide more than with sevoflurane.

FACTORS AFFECTING ELIMINATION

Recovery from anesthesia depends on lowering the concentration of anesthetic in brain tissue. Anesthetics can be eliminated by biotransformation, transcutaneous loss, or exhalation. Biotransformation usually accounts for a minimal increase in the rate of decline of alveolar partial pressure. Its greatest impact is on the elimination of soluble anesthetics that undergo extensive metabolism (eg, methoxyflurane). The greater biotransformation of halothane compared with isoflurane accounts for halothane's faster elimination, even though it is more soluble. The CYP group of isozymes (specifically CYP 2EI) seems to be important in the metabolism of some volatile anesthetics. The diffusion of anesthetic through the skin is insignificant.

The most important route for the elimination of inhalation anesthetics is the alveolar membrane. 4 Many of the factors that speed induction also speed recovery: elimination of rebreathing, high fresh gas flows, low anesthetic-circuit volume, low absorption by the anesthetic circuit, decreased solubility, high cerebral blood flow (CBF), and increased ventilation. Elimination of nitrous oxide is so rapid that oxygen and carbon dioxide (CO_2) concentrations in alveolar gas are diluted. The resulting **diffusion hypoxia** is prevented by administering 100% oxygen for 5 to 10 min after discontinuing nitrous oxide. The rate of recovery is usually faster than induction because tissues that have not reached steady state will continue to take up anesthetic until the alveolar partial pressure falls below the tissue partial pressure. For instance, fat will continue to take up anesthetic and hasten recovery until the partial pressure exceeds the alveolar partial pressure. This redistribution is not as useful after prolonged anesthesia (fat partial pressures of anesthetic will have come "closer" to arterial partial pressures at the time the anesthetic was removed from fresh gas)—thus, the speed of recovery also depends on the length of time the anesthetic has been administered.

Pharmacodynamics of Inhalation Anesthetics

THEORIES OF ANESTHETIC ACTION

General anesthesia is an altered physiological state characterized by reversible loss of consciousness, analgesia, amnesia, and some degree of muscle relaxation. The multitude of substances capable of producing general anesthesia is remarkable: inert elements (xenon), simple inorganic compounds (nitrous oxide), halogenated hydrocarbons (halothane), ethers (isoflurane, sevoflurane, desflurane), and complex organic structures (propofol, etomidate, ketamine). A unifying theory explaining anesthetic action would have to accommodate this diversity of structure. In fact, the various agents probably produce anesthesia by differing sets of molecular mechanisms. Inhalational agents interact with numerous ion channels present in the CNS and peripheral nervous system. Nitrous oxide and xenon are believed to inhibit *N*-methyl-D-aspartate (NMDA) receptors. NMDA receptors are excitatory receptors in the brain. Other inhalational agents (as well as etomidate and midazolam) may interact at other receptors (eg, γ-aminobutyric acid [GABA]-activated chloride channel conductance), leading to anesthetic effects. It is possible that inhalational anesthetics act on multiple protein receptors that block excitatory channels and promote the activity of inhibitory channels affecting neuronal activity. Specific brain areas affected by inhaled anesthetics include the reticular activating system, the cerebral cortex, the cuneate nucleus, the olfactory cortex, and the hippocampus; however, general anesthetics bind throughout the CNS. Anesthetics have also been shown to depress excitatory transmission in the spinal cord, particularly at the level of the dorsal horn interneurons that are involved in pain transmission. Differing aspects of anesthesia may be related to different sites of anesthetic action. For example, unconsciousness and amnesia are probably mediated by cortical anesthetic action, whereas the suppression of purposeful withdrawal from pain likely relates to subcortical structures, such as the spinal cord or brainstem. One study in rats revealed that removal of the cerebral cortex did not alter the potency of the anesthetic! Indeed, measures of minimum alveolar concentration (MAC), the anesthetic concentration that prevents movement in 50% of subjects or animals, are dependent upon anesthetic effects at the spinal cord and not at the cortex.

5 Past understanding of anesthetic action attempted to identify a unitary hypothesis of anesthetic effects. This hypothesis proposes that all inhalation agents share a common mechanism of action at the molecular level. This was previously supported by the observation that the anesthetic potency of inhalation agents correlates directly with their lipid solubility (Meyer–Overton rule). The implication is that anesthesia results from molecules dissolving at specific lipophilic sites. Of course, not all lipid-soluble molecules are anesthetics (some are actually convulsants), and the correlation between anesthetic potency and lipid solubility is only approximate (Figure 8–4).

General anesthetic action could be due to alterations in any one (or a combination) of several cellular systems, including voltage-gated ion channels, ligand-gated ion channels, second messenger functions, or neurotransmitter receptors. There seems to be a strong correlation between anesthetic potency and actions on GABA receptors. Thus, anesthetic action may relate to binding in relatively hydrophobic domains in channel proteins (GABA receptors). Modulation of GABA function may prove to be a principal mechanism of action for many anesthetic drugs. The glycine receptor α_1-subunit, whose function is enhanced by inhalation anesthetics, is another potential anesthetic site of action.

Other ligand-gated ion channels whose modulation may play a role in anesthetic action include nicotinic acetylcholine receptors and NMDA receptors.

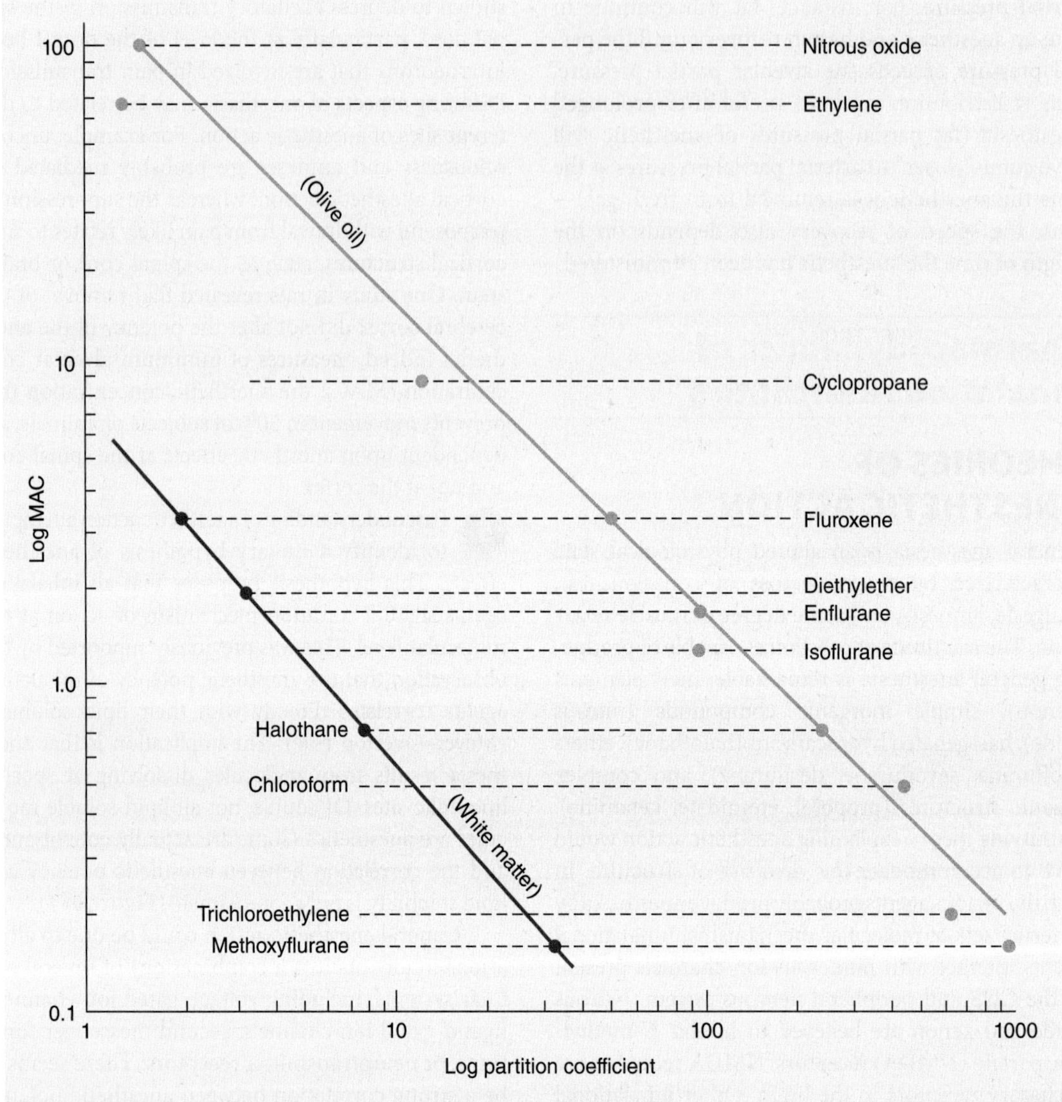

FIGURE 8–4 There is a good but not perfect correlation between anesthetic potency and lipid solubility. MAC, minimum alveolar concentration. (Modified with permission from Lowe HJ, Hagler K. *Gas Chromatography in Biology and Medicine.* Philadelphia, PA: Churchill Livingstone; 1969.)

Investigations into mechanisms of anesthetic action are likely to remain ongoing for many years because many protein channels may be affected by individual anesthetic agents and no obligatory site has yet been identified. Selecting among so many molecular targets for the one(s) that provide optimum effects with minimal adverse actions will be the challenge in designing better inhalational agents.

ANESTHETIC NEUROTOXICITY

In recent years, there has been ongoing concern that general anesthetics damage the developing brain. Concern has been raised that anesthetic exposure affects the development and the elimination of synapses in the infant brain and can promote cognitive impairment in later life. For example, animal studies have demonstrated that isoflurane exposure promotes neuronal apoptosis, altering cellular calcium homeostatic mechanisms with subsequent learning disability.

Human studies exploring whether anesthesia is harmful in children are difficult because conducting a randomized controlled trial for that purpose only would be unethical. Studies that compare populations of children who have had anesthetics with those who have not are also complicated by the reality that the former population is likewise having surgery and receiving the attention of the medical community. Consequently, children receiving anesthetics may be more likely to be diagnosed with learning difficulties in the first place.

Human, animal, and laboratory trials demonstrating or refuting that anesthetic neurotoxicity leads to developmental disability in children are underway. SmartTots, a partnership between the International Anesthesia Research Society and the U.S. Food and Drug Administration (FDA), coordinates and funds research related to anesthesia in infants and young children. As their consensus statement notes: "It is not yet possible to know whether anesthetic drugs are safe for children in a single short-duration procedure. Similarly, it is not yet possible to know whether the use of these drugs poses a risk, and if so, whether the risk is large enough to outweigh the benefit of needed surgery, tests, or other procedures.... Concerns regarding the unknown risk of anesthetic exposure to the child's brain development must be weighed against potential harm associated with cancelling or delaying a needed procedure" (see www.smarttots.org). Of note, the FDA has issued a warning that repeated or prolonged use of general anesthetics or sedatives in children younger than 3 years may affect brain development.

Nevertheless, various clinical studies have failed to demonstrate adverse outcomes from single, brief anesthetic exposures in children, and there is a developing consensus that single anesthetic exposures in infants and young children are very unlikely to result in harm. Some have advocated mitigation strategies to limit anesthetic exposure in children and incorporate dexmedetomidine into anesthetic management. It has been suggested that dexmedetomidine may have neuroprotective properties against anesthetic-induced neurotoxicity. Other investigators are examining the role of xenon in combination with other inhalational anesthetics to promote anti-apoptosis.

Anesthetic agents have also been suggested to contribute to tau protein hyperphosphorylation. Tau hyperphosphorylation is associated with Alzheimer disease (AD), and it has been hypothesized that anesthetic exposures may contribute to AD progression. However, the proposed association between anesthetic delivery, surgery, and AD development has not been sufficiently investigated to draw definitive conclusions.

ANESTHETIC NEUROPROTECTION AND CARDIAC PRECONDITIONING

Although inhalational agents have been suggested as contributing to neurotoxicity, they have also been shown to provide both neurologic and cardiac protective effects against ischemia-reperfusion injury. Ischemic preconditioning implies that a brief ischemic episode protects a cell from future, more pronounced ischemic events. Various molecular mechanisms have been suggested to protect cells preconditioned either through ischemic events or secondary to pharmacologic mechanisms, such as through the use of inhalational anesthetics. In the heart, preconditioning in part arises from actions at adenosine triphosphate (ATP)-sensitive potassium (K_{ATP}) channels.

The exact mechanism of anesthetic preconditioning is likely to be multifocal and includes the opening of K_{ATP} channels, resulting in less mitochondrial calcium ion concentration and reduction of reactive oxygen species (ROS) production. ROS contributes to cellular injury. Anesthetic preconditioning may be the result of increased production of antioxidants following initial anesthesia exposure. Additionally, excitatory NMDA receptors are linked to the development of neuronal injury. NMDA antagonists, such as the noble anesthetic gas xenon, have been shown to be neuroprotective. Xenon has an anti-apoptotic effect that may be secondary to its inhibition of calcium ion influx following cell injury. As with neurotoxicity, the role of inhalational anesthetics in tissue protection is the subject of ongoing investigation. Studies have demonstrated beneficial effects of inhalational anesthetics in coronary artery bypass surgery. Additionally, inhalational anesthetics may offer protection against inflammatory lung injury.

ANESTHETIC IMMUNOMODULATION

Inhaled anesthetics have been shown to have immunosuppressive effects. Although immunosuppression may be desirable in inflammatory conditions (eg, lung inflammation), it may prove deleterious in patients undergoing cancer therapy. As a consequence, avoidance of inhalational anesthetics has been suggested by some in favor of intravenous agents (other than opioids) in the perioperative management of patients with cancer.

MINIMUM ALVEOLAR CONCENTRATION

6 The MAC of an inhaled anesthetic is the alveolar concentration that prevents movement in 50% of patients in response to a standardized stimulus (eg, surgical incision). MAC is a useful measure because it mirrors brain partial pressure, allows comparisons of potency between agents, and provides a standard for experimental evaluations (Table 8–3). Nonetheless, it should be remembered that this is a median value with limited usefulness

TABLE 8–3 Properties of modern inhalation anesthetics.

Agent	Structure	MAC%[1]	Vapor Pressure (mm Hg at 20°C)
Nitrous oxide	N=N \ / O	105[2]	—
Halothane (Fluothane)	F Cl | | F−C−C−H | | F Br	0.75	243
Isoflurane (Forane)	F H F | | | H−C−O−C−C−F | | | F Cl F	1.2	240
Desflurane (Suprane)	F H F | | | H−C−O−C−C−F | | | F F F	6.0	681
Sevoflurane (Ultane)	F | F F−C−F | | H−C−O−C | | H F−C−F | F	2.0	160

[1]These minimum alveolar concentration (MAC) values are for 30- to 55-year-old human subjects and are expressed as a percentage of 1 atmosphere. High altitude requires a higher inspired concentration of anesthetic to achieve the same partial pressure.

[2]A concentration greater than 100% means that hyperbaric conditions are required to achieve 1.0 MAC.

in managing individual patients, particularly during times of rapidly changing alveolar concentrations (cg, induction and emergence).

The MAC values for anesthetic combinations are roughly additive. For example, a mixture of 0.5 MAC of nitrous oxide (53%) and 0.5 MAC of isoflurane (0.6%) produces the same likelihood that movement in response to surgical incision will be suppressed as 1.0 MAC of isoflurane (1.2%) or 1.0 MAC of any other single agent. In contrast to CNS depression, the degree of myocardial depression may not be equivalent at the same MAC: 0.5 MAC of halothane causes more myocardial depression than 0.5 MAC of nitrous oxide. MAC represents only one point on the concentration–response curve—it is the equivalent of a median effective concentration (EC_{50}). MAC multiples are clinically useful if the concentration–response curves of the anesthetics being compared are parallel, nearly linear, and continuous for the effect being predicted. Roughly 1.3 MAC of any of the volatile anesthetics (eg, for halothane: $1.3 \times 0.75\% = 0.97\%$) has been found to prevent movement in about 95% of patients (an approximation of the EC_{95}); 0.3 to 0.4 MAC is associated with awakening from anesthesia (MAC awake) when the inhaled drug is the only agent maintaining anesthetic (a rare circumstance).

MAC can be altered by several physiological and pharmacologic variables (Table 8–4). **One of the most striking is the 6% decrease in MAC per decade of age, regardless of volatile anesthetic.** MAC is relatively unaffected by species, sex, or duration of anesthesia. Further, as noted earlier, MAC is not altered after spinal cord transection in rats, leading to the hypothesis that the site of anesthetic inhibition of motor responses lies in the spinal cord.

Clinical Pharmacology of Inhalation Anesthetics

NITROUS OXIDE

Physical Properties

Nitrous oxide (N_2O; laughing gas) is colorless and essentially odorless. Although nonexplosive and nonflammable, nitrous oxide is as capable as oxygen of supporting combustion. Unlike the potent volatile agents, nitrous oxide is a gas at room temperature and ambient pressure. It can be kept as a liquid under pressure because its critical temperature (the temperature at which a substance cannot be kept as a liquid irrespective of the pressure applied) lies above room temperature. Nitrous oxide is a relatively inexpensive anesthetic; however, concerns regarding its safety have led to continued interest in alternatives such as **xenon** (Table 8–5). As noted earlier, nitrous oxide, like xenon, is an NMDA receptor antagonist.

Effects on Organ Systems

A. Cardiovascular

Nitrous oxide tends to stimulate the sympathetic nervous system. Thus, even though nitrous oxide directly depresses myocardial contractility in vitro, arterial blood pressure, cardiac output, and heart rate are essentially unchanged or slightly elevated *in vivo* because of its stimulation of catecholamines (Table 8–6). Myocardial depression may be unmasked in patients with coronary artery disease or severe hypovolemia. Constriction of pulmonary vascular smooth muscle increases pulmonary vascular resistance, which results in a generally modest elevation of right ventricular end-diastolic pressure. Despite vasoconstriction of cutaneous vessels, peripheral vascular resistance is not significantly altered.

B. Respiratory

Nitrous oxide increases respiratory rate (tachypnea) and decreases tidal volume as a result of CNS stimulation. The net effect is a minimal change in minute ventilation and resting arterial pCO_2. Hypoxic drive, the ventilatory response to arterial hypoxia that is mediated by peripheral chemoreceptors in the carotid bodies, is markedly depressed by even small amounts of nitrous oxide.

C. Cerebral

By increasing CBF and cerebral blood volume, nitrous oxide produces a mild elevation of intracranial pressure. Nitrous oxide also increases cerebral oxygen consumption ($CMRO_2$). Concentrations of nitrous oxide below MAC may provide analgesia in dental surgery, labor, traumatic injury, and minor surgical procedures.

TABLE 8–4 Factors affecting MAC.[1]

Variable	Effect on MAC	Comments
Temperature		
Hypothermia	↓	
Hyperthermia	↓	↑ if >42°C
Age		
Young	↑	
Older adult	↓	
Alcohol		
Acute intoxication	↓	
Chronic abuse	↑	
Anemia		
Hematocrit <10%	↓	
PaO_2		
<40 mm Hg	↓	
$PaCO_2$		
>95 mm Hg	↓	Caused by <pH in CSF
Thyroid		
Hyperthyroid	No change	
Hypothyroid	No change	
Blood pressure		
Mean arterial pressure <40 mm Hg	↓	
Electrolytes		
Hypercalcemia	↓	
Hypernatremia	↑	Caused by altered CSF[2]
Hyponatremia	↓	Caused by altered CSF
Pregnancy	↓	MAC decreased by one-third at 8 weeks' gestation; normal by 72 h postpartum
Drugs		
Local anesthetics	↓	Except cocaine
Opioids	↓	
Ketamine	↓	
Barbiturates	↓	
Benzodiazepines	↓	
Verapamil	↓	
Lithium	↓	
Sympatholytics		
Methyldopa	↓	
Clonidine	↓	
Dexmedetomidine	↓	
Sympathomimetics		
Amphetamine		
Chronic	↓	
Acute	↑	
Cocaine	↑	
Ephedrine	↑	

[1]These conclusions are based on human and animal studies.

[2]CSF, cerebrospinal fluid; MAC, minimum alveolar concentration.

TABLE 8–5 Advantages and disadvantages of xenon (Xe) anesthesia.

Advantages
Inert (probably nontoxic with no metabolism)
Minimal cardiovascular effects
Low blood solubility
Rapid induction and recovery
Does not trigger malignant hyperthermia
Environmentally friendly
Nonexplosive
Disadvantages
High cost
Low potency (MAC = 70%)[1]

[1]MAC, minimum alveolar concentration.

D. Neuromuscular

In contrast to other inhalation agents, nitrous oxide provides no significant muscle relaxation. In fact, at high concentrations in hyperbaric chambers, nitrous oxide causes skeletal muscle rigidity. Nitrous oxide does not trigger malignant hyperthermia.

E. Renal

Nitrous oxide seems to decrease kidney blood flow by increasing renal vascular resistance. This leads to decreased glomerular filtration rate and urinary output.

TABLE 8–6 Clinical pharmacology of inhalational anesthetics.

	Nitrous Oxide	Halothane	Isoflurane	Desflurane	Sevoflurane
Cardiovascular					
Blood pressure	N/C[1]	↓↓	↓↓	↓↓	↓
Heart rate	N/C	↓	↑	N/C or ↑	N/C
Systemic vascular resistance	N/C	N/C	↓↓	↓↓	↓
Cardiac output[2]	N/C	↓	N/C	N/C or ↓	↓
Respiratory					
Tidal volume	↓	↓↓	↓↓	↓	↓
Respiratory rate	↑	↑↑	↑	↑	↑
$PaCO_2$					
Resting	N/C	↑	↑	↑↑	↑
Challenge	↑	↑	↑	↑↑	↑
Cerebral					
Blood flow	↑	↑↑	↑	↑	↑
Intracranial pressure	↑	↑↑	↑	↑	↑
Cerebral metabolic rate	↑	↓	↓↓	↓↓	↓↓
Seizures	↓	↓	↓	↓	↓
Neuromuscular					
Nondepolarizing blockade[3]	↑	↑↑	↑↑↑	↑↑↑	↑↑
Renal					
Renal blood flow	↓↓	↓↓	↓↓	↓	↓
Glomerular filtration rate	↓↓	↓↓	↓↓	↓	↓
Urinary output	↓↓	↓↓	↓↓	↓	↓
Hepatic					
Blood flow	↓	↓↓	↓	↓	↓
Metabolism[4]	0.004%	15–20%	0.2%	<0.1%	5%

[1]N/C, no change.

[2]Controlled ventilation.

[3]Depolarizing blockage is probably also prolonged by these agents, but this is usually not clinically significant.

[4]Percentage of absorbed anesthetic undergoing metabolism.

F. Hepatic

Hepatic blood flow probably falls during nitrous oxide anesthesia, but to a lesser extent than with the volatile agents.

G. Gastrointestinal

The use of nitrous oxide in adults increases the risk of postoperative nausea and vomiting, presumably as a result of activation of the chemoreceptor trigger zone and the vomiting center in the medulla.

Biotransformation & Toxicity

During emergence, almost all nitrous oxide is eliminated by exhalation. A small amount diffuses out through the skin. Biotransformation is limited to the less than 0.01% that undergoes reductive metabolism in the gastrointestinal tract by anaerobic bacteria.

By irreversibly oxidizing the cobalt atom in vitamin B_{12}, nitrous oxide inhibits enzymes that are vitamin B_{12} dependent. These enzymes include methionine synthetase, which is necessary for myelin formation, and thymidylate synthetase, which is necessary for DNA synthesis. 7 Prolonged exposure to anesthetic concentrations of nitrous oxide can result in bone marrow depression (megaloblastic anemia) and even neurologic deficiencies (peripheral neuropathies). However, administration of nitrous oxide for bone marrow harvest does not seem to affect the viability of bone marrow mononuclear cells. Because of possible teratogenic effects, nitrous oxide is often avoided in pregnant patients who are not yet in the third trimester. Nitrous oxide may also alter the immunologic response to infection by affecting chemotaxis and motility of polymorphonuclear leukocytes.

Contraindications

Although nitrous oxide is relatively insoluble in comparison with other inhalation agents, it is 35 times more soluble than nitrogen in blood. Thus, it tends to diffuse into air-containing cavities more rapidly than nitrogen is absorbed by the bloodstream. For instance, if a patient with a 100-mL pneumothorax inhales 50% nitrous oxide, the gas content of the pneumothorax will tend to approach that of the bloodstream. Because nitrous oxide will diffuse into the cavity more rapidly than the air (principally nitrogen) diffuses out, the pneumothorax expands until it contains roughly 100 mL of air and 100 mL of nitrous oxide. If the walls surrounding the cavity are rigid, pressure rises instead of volume. **Examples of conditions in which nitrous oxide might be hazardous include venous or arterial air embolism, pneumothorax, acute intestinal obstruction with bowel distention, intracranial air (pneumocephalus following dural closure or pneumoencephalography), pulmonary air cysts, intraocular air bubbles, and tympanic membrane grafting.** Nitrous oxide will even diffuse into tracheal tube cuffs, increasing the pressure against the tracheal mucosa. Obviously, nitrous oxide is of limited value in patients requiring increased inspired oxygen concentrations.

Drug Interactions

Because the high MAC of nitrous oxide prevents its use as a complete general anesthetic, it is frequently used in combination with the more potent volatile agents. The addition of nitrous oxide decreases the requirements of these other agents (65% nitrous oxide decreases the MAC of the volatile anesthetics by approximately 50%). Although nitrous oxide should not be considered a benign carrier gas, it does attenuate the circulatory and respiratory effects of volatile anesthetics in adults. The concentration of nitrous oxide flowing through a vaporizer can influence the concentration of volatile anesthetic delivered. For example, decreasing nitrous oxide concentration (ie, increasing oxygen concentration) increases the concentration of volatile agents despite a constant vaporizer setting. This disparity is due to the relative solubilities of nitrous oxide and oxygen in liquid volatile anesthetics. The second gas effect was discussed earlier. Nitrous oxide is an ozone-depleting gas with greenhouse effects.

HALOTHANE

Physical Properties

Halothane is a halogenated alkane (see Table 8–3). Carbon–fluoride bonds are responsible for its nonflammable and nonexplosive nature.

Effects on Organ Systems

A. Cardiovascular

A dose-dependent reduction of arterial blood pressure is due to direct myocardial depression; 2.0 MAC of halothane in patients not undergoing surgery results in a 50% decrease in blood pressure and cardiac output. Cardiac depression—from interference with sodium–calcium exchange and intracellular calcium utilization—causes an increase in right atrial pressure. Although halothane is a coronary artery vasodilator, coronary blood flow decreases because of the drop in systemic arterial pressure. Adequate myocardial perfusion is usually maintained as myocardial oxygen demand also drops. Normally, hypotension inhibits baroreceptors in the aortic arch and carotid bifurcation, causing a decrease in vagal stimulation and a compensatory rise in heart rate. Halothane blunts this reflex. Slowing of sinoatrial node conduction may result in a junctional rhythm or bradycardia. In infants, halothane decreases cardiac output by a combination of decreased heart rate and depressed myocardial contractility. Halothane sensitizes the heart to the arrhythmogenic effects of epinephrine, so doses of epinephrine above 1.5 mcg/kg should be avoided. Although organ blood flow is redistributed, systemic vascular resistance is unchanged.

B. Respiratory

Halothane typically causes rapid, shallow breathing. The increased respiratory rate is not enough to counter the decreased tidal volume, so alveolar ventilation drops, and resting $PaCO_2$ is elevated. The **apneic threshold**, the highest $PaCO_2$ at which a patient remains apneic, also rises because the difference between it and resting $PaCO_2$ is not altered by general anesthesia. Similarly, halothane limits the increase in minute ventilation that normally accompanies a rise in $PaCO_2$. Halothane's ventilatory effects are probably due to central (medullary depression) and peripheral (intercostal muscle dysfunction) mechanisms. These changes are exaggerated by preexisting lung disease and attenuated by surgical stimulation. The increase in $PaCO_2$ and the decrease in intrathoracic pressure that accompany spontaneous ventilation with halothane partially reverse the depression in cardiac output, arterial blood pressure, and heart rate described above. The hypoxic drive is severely depressed by even low concentrations of halothane (0.1 MAC).

Halothane is a potent bronchodilator, as it may reverse asthma-induced bronchospasm. This action is not inhibited by β-adrenergic blocking agents. Halothane attenuates airway reflexes and relaxes bronchial smooth muscle by inhibiting intracellular calcium mobilization. Halothane also depresses the clearance of mucus from the respiratory tract (mucociliary function), promoting postoperative hypoxia and atelectasis.

C. Cerebral

By dilating cerebral vessels, halothane lowers cerebral vascular resistance and increases cerebral blood volume and CBF. **Autoregulation**, the maintenance of constant CBF during changes in arterial blood pressure, is blunted. Concomitant rises in intracranial pressure can be prevented by establishing hyperventilation *before* administration of halothane. Cerebral activity is decreased, leading to electroencephalographic slowing and modest reductions in metabolic oxygen requirements.

D. Neuromuscular

Halothane relaxes skeletal muscle and potentiates nondepolarizing neuromuscular-blocking agents (NMBAs). Like the other potent volatile anesthetics, it is a trigger for malignant hyperthermia.

E. Renal

Halothane reduces renal blood flow, glomerular filtration rate, and urinary output. Part of this decrease can be explained by a fall in arterial blood pressure and cardiac output. Because the reduction in renal blood flow is greater than the reduction in glomerular filtration rate, the filtration fraction is increased. Preoperative hydration limits these changes.

F. Hepatic

Halothane decreases hepatic blood flow in proportion to the depression of cardiac output. Hepatic artery vasospasm has been reported during halothane anesthesia. The metabolism and clearance of some drugs (eg, fentanyl, phenytoin, verapamil) seem to be impaired by halothane. Other evidence of hepatic cellular dysfunction includes sulfobromophthalein (BSP) dye retention and minor liver transaminase elevations.

Biotransformation & Toxicity

Halothane is oxidized in the liver by a particular isozyme of CYP (2EI) to its principal metabolite, trifluoroacetic acid. In the absence of oxygen, reductive metabolism may result in a small number of hepatotoxic end products that covalently bind to tissue macromolecules. This is more apt to occur following enzyme induction by chronic exposure to barbiturates.

Postoperative hepatic dysfunction has several causes: viral hepatitis, impaired hepatic perfusion, preexisting liver disease, hepatocyte hypoxia, sepsis, hemolysis, benign postoperative intrahepatic cholestasis, and drug-induced hepatitis. 8 **"Halothane hepatitis"** is extremely rare. Patients exposed to multiple halothane anesthetics at short intervals, middle-aged obese women, and persons with a familial predisposition to halothane toxicity or a personal history of toxicity are considered to be at increased risk. Signs are mostly related to hepatic injury, such as increased serum alanine and aspartate transferase, elevated bilirubin (leading to jaundice), and encephalopathy.

The hepatic lesion seen in humans—centrilobular necrosis—also occurs in rats pretreated with an enzyme inducer (phenobarbital) and exposed to halothane under hypoxic conditions (FiO_2 <14%). This *halothane hypoxic model* implies hepatic damage from reductive metabolites or hypoxia.

Other evidence points to an immune mechanism. For instance, some signs of the disease indicate an allergic reaction (eg, eosinophilia, rash, fever) and do not appear until a few days after exposure. Furthermore, an antibody that binds to hepatocytes previously exposed to halothane has been isolated from patients with halothane-induced hepatic dysfunction. This antibody response may involve liver microsomal proteins that have been modified by trifluoroacetic acid as the triggering antigens (trifluoroacetylated liver proteins such as microsomal carboxylesterase). Other inhalational agents that undergo oxidative metabolism can likewise lead to hepatitis. However, newer agents undergo little to no metabolism and therefore do not form trifluroacetic acid protein adducts or produce the immune response leading to hepatitis.

Contraindications

It is prudent to withhold halothane from patients with unexplained liver dysfunction following previous anesthetic exposure.

Halothane, like all inhalational anesthetics, should be used with care (and only in combination with modest hyperventilation) in patients with intracranial mass lesions because of the possibility of intracranial hypertension secondary to increased cerebral blood volume and blood flow.

Hypovolemic patients and some patients with severe reductions in left ventricular function may not tolerate halothane's negative inotropic effects. Sensitization of the heart to catecholamines limits the usefulness of halothane when exogenous epinephrine is administered (eg, in local anesthetic solutions) or in patients with pheochromocytoma.

Drug Interactions

The myocardial depression seen with halothane is exacerbated by β-adrenergic blocking agents and calcium channel blocking agents. Tricyclic antidepressants and monoamine oxidase inhibitors have been associated with fluctuations in blood pressure and arrhythmias, though neither represents an absolute contraindication. The combination of halothane and aminophylline has resulted in ventricular arrhythmias.

ISOFLURANE

Physical Properties

Isoflurane is a nonflammable volatile anesthetic with a pungent ethereal odor.

Effects on Organ Systems

A. Cardiovascular

Isoflurane causes minimal left ventricular depression *in vivo*. Cardiac output is maintained by an increase in heart rate due to partial preservation of carotid baroreflexes. Mild β-adrenergic stimulation increases skeletal muscle blood flow, decreases

systemic vascular resistance, and lowers arterial blood pressure. Rapid increases in isoflurane concentration lead to transient increases in heart rate, arterial blood pressure, and plasma levels of norepi-
9 nephrine. Isoflurane dilates coronary arteries but not nearly as potently as nitroglycerin or adenosine. Dilation of normal coronary arteries could theoretically divert blood away from fixed stenotic lesions, which was the basis for concern about coronary "steal" with this agent, a concern that has largely been forgotten.

B. Respiratory

Respiratory depression during isoflurane anesthesia resembles that of other volatile anesthetics, except that tachypnea is less pronounced. The net effect is a more pronounced fall in minute ventilation. Even low concentrations of isoflurane (0.1 MAC) blunt the normal ventilatory response to hypoxia and hypercapnia. Despite a tendency to irritate upper airway reflexes, isoflurane is a good bronchodilator, though perhaps not as potent a bronchodilator as halothane.

C. Cerebral

At concentrations greater than 1 MAC, isoflurane increases CBF and intracranial pressure. These effects are thought to be less pronounced than with halothane and are reversed by hyperventilation. In contrast to halothane, hyperventilation does not have to be instituted prior to the use of isoflurane to prevent intracranial hypertension. Isoflurane reduces cerebral metabolic oxygen requirements, and at 2 MAC, it produces an electrically silent electroencephalogram (EEG).

D. Neuromuscular

Isoflurane relaxes skeletal muscle.

E. Renal

Isoflurane decreases renal blood flow, glomerular filtration rate, and urinary output.

F. Hepatic

Total hepatic blood flow (hepatic artery and portal vein flow) may be reduced during isoflurane anesthesia. Hepatic oxygen supply is better maintained with isoflurane than with halothane, however, because hepatic artery perfusion is preserved. Liver function tests are usually not affected.

Biotransformation & Toxicity

Isoflurane is metabolized to trifluoroacetic acid. Although serum fluoride fluid levels may rise, nephrotoxicity is extremely unlikely, even in the presence of enzyme inducers. Prolonged sedation (>24 h at 0.1–0.6% isoflurane) of critically ill patients has resulted in elevated plasma fluoride levels (15–50 μmol/L) without evidence of kidney impairment. Similarly, up to 20 MAC-hours of isoflurane may lead to fluoride levels exceeding 50 μmol/L without detectable postoperative kidney dysfunction. Its limited oxidative metabolism also minimizes any possible risk of significant hepatic dysfunction.

Contraindications

Isoflurane presents no unique contraindications. Patients with severe hypovolemia may not tolerate its vasodilating effects. It can trigger malignant hyperthermia.

Drug Interactions

Epinephrine can be safely administered in doses up to 4.5 mcg/kg. Nondepolarizing NMBAs are potentiated by isoflurane.

DESFLURANE

Physical Properties

The structure of desflurane is very similar to that of isoflurane. In fact, the only difference is the substitution of a fluorine atom for isoflurane's chlorine atom. That "minor" change has profound effects on the physical properties of the drug, however. For instance, because the vapor pressure of desflurane at 20°C is 681 mm Hg, at high altitudes (eg, Denver, Colorado) it boils at room temperature. This problem necessitated the development of a special desflurane vaporizer.
10 Furthermore, the low solubility of desflurane in blood and body tissues causes very rapid induction of and emergence from anesthesia. Therefore, the alveolar concentration of desflurane approaches the inspired concentration more rapidly than with the other volatile agents, providing tighter

control over anesthetic concentrations. **Wakeup times are approximately 50% less than those observed following isoflurane.** This is principally attributable to a blood/gas partition coefficient (0.42) that is even lower than that of nitrous oxide (0.47). Although desflurane is roughly one-fourth as potent as the other volatile agents, it is 17 times more potent than nitrous oxide. A high vapor pressure, an ultrashort duration of action, and moderate potency are the most characteristic features of desflurane.

Effects on Organ Systems

A. Cardiovascular

The cardiovascular effects of desflurane seem to be similar to those of isoflurane. An increase in the concentration is associated with a decline in systemic vascular resistance that leads to a fall in arterial blood pressure. Cardiac output remains relatively unchanged or slightly depressed at 1 to 2 MAC. There is a moderate rise in heart rate, central venous pressure, and pulmonary artery pressure that often does not become apparent at low doses. 11 Rapid increases in desflurane concentration lead to transient elevations in heart rate, blood pressure, and catecholamine levels that are more pronounced than with isoflurane, particularly in patients with cardiovascular disease. These cardiovascular responses to rapidly increasing desflurane concentration can be attenuated by fentanyl, esmolol, or clonidine.

B. Respiratory

Desflurane causes a decrease in tidal volume and an increase in respiratory rate. There is an overall decrease in alveolar ventilation that causes a rise in resting $PaCO_2$. Like other modern volatile anesthetic agents, desflurane depresses the ventilatory response to increasing $PaCO_2$. Pungency and airway irritation during desflurane induction can be manifested by salivation, breath-holding, coughing, and laryngospasm. Airway resistance may increase in children with reactive airway susceptibility. These problems make desflurane a poor choice for inhalation induction.

C. Cerebral

Like the other volatile anesthetics, desflurane directly vasodilates the cerebral vasculature, increasing CBF, cerebral blood volume, and intracranial pressure at normotension and normocapnia. Countering the decrease in cerebral vascular resistance is a marked decline in the cerebral metabolic rate of oxygen ($CMRO_2$) that tends to cause cerebral vasoconstriction and moderate any increase in CBF. The cerebral vasculature remains responsive to changes in $PaCO_2$, however, so that intracranial pressure can be lowered by hyperventilation. Cerebral oxygen consumption is decreased during desflurane anesthesia. Thus, during periods of desflurane-induced hypotension (mean arterial pressure = 60 mm Hg), CBF is adequate to maintain aerobic metabolism despite a low cerebral perfusion pressure. The effect on the EEG is similar to that of isoflurane. Initially, EEG frequency is increased, but as anesthetic depth is increased, EEG slowing becomes manifest, leading to burst suppression at higher inhaled concentrations.

D. Neuromuscular

Desflurane is associated with a dose-dependent decrease in response to train-of-four and tetanic peripheral nerve stimulation.

E. Renal

There is no evidence of any significant nephrotoxic effects caused by exposure to desflurane. However, as cardiac output declines, decreases in urine output and glomerular filtration should be expected with desflurane and all other anesthetics.

F. Hepatic

Hepatic function tests are generally unaffected by desflurane, assuming that organ perfusion is maintained perioperatively. Desflurane undergoes minimal metabolism; therefore, the risk of anesthetic-induced hepatitis is likewise minimal. As with isoflurane and sevoflurane, hepatic oxygen delivery is generally maintained.

Biotransformation & Toxicity

Desflurane undergoes minimal metabolism in humans. Serum and urine inorganic fluoride levels following desflurane anesthesia are essentially unchanged from preanesthetic levels. There is insignificant percutaneous loss. Desflurane, more than other volatile anesthetics, is degraded by desiccated

CO_2 absorbent (particularly barium hydroxide lime, but also sodium and potassium hydroxide) into potentially clinically important levels of carbon monoxide. Carbon monoxide poisoning is difficult to diagnose under general anesthesia, but the presence of carboxyhemoglobin may be detectable by arterial blood gas analysis or lower than expected pulse oximetry readings (though still falsely high). Disposing of dried-out absorbent or use of calcium hydroxide can minimize the risk of carbon monoxide poisoning. Desflurane is the most ozone-depleting of the inhalation anesthetics.

Contraindications

Desflurane shares many of the contraindications of other modern volatile anesthetics: severe hypovolemia, malignant hyperthermia, and intracranial hypertension.

Drug Interactions

Desflurane potentiates nondepolarizing neuromuscular blocking agents to the same extent as isoflurane. Epinephrine can be safely administered in doses up to 4.5 mcg/kg as desflurane does not sensitize the myocardium to the arrhythmogenic effects of epinephrine. Although emergence is more rapid following desflurane anesthesia than after isoflurane anesthesia, switching from isoflurane to desflurane toward the end of anesthesia does not significantly accelerate recovery, nor does faster emergence translate into faster discharge times from the postanesthesia care unit. Desflurane emergence has been associated with delirium in some pediatric patients.

SEVOFLURANE

Physical Properties

Like desflurane, sevoflurane is a fluorinated ether. Sevoflurane's solubility in blood is slightly greater than desflurane ($\lambda_{b/g}$ 0.65 versus 0.42) (see Table 8–1).
12 Nonpungency and rapid increases in alveolar anesthetic concentration make sevoflurane an excellent choice for smooth and rapid inhalation inductions in pediatric and adult patients. In fact, inhalation induction with 4% to 8% sevoflurane in a 50% mixture of nitrous oxide and oxygen can be achieved within 1 min. Likewise, its low blood solubility results in a rapid fall in alveolar anesthetic concentration upon discontinuation and a more rapid emergence compared with isoflurane (though not an earlier discharge from the postanesthesia care unit). Sevoflurane's modest vapor pressure permits the use of a conventional variable bypass vaporizer.

Effects on Organ Systems

A. Cardiovascular

Sevoflurane mildly depresses myocardial contractility. Systemic vascular resistance and arterial blood pressure decline slightly less than with isoflurane or desflurane. Because sevoflurane causes little, if any, rise in heart rate, cardiac output is not maintained as well as with isoflurane or desflurane. Sevoflurane may prolong the QT interval, the clinical significance of which is unknown. QT prolongation may be manifest 60 min following anesthetic emergence in infants.

B. Respiratory

Sevoflurane depresses respiration and reverses bronchospasm to an extent similar to that of isoflurane.

C. Cerebral

Similar to isoflurane and desflurane, sevoflurane causes slight increases in CBF and intracranial pressure at normocarbia, though some studies show a decrease in CBF. High concentrations of sevoflurane (>1.5 MAC) may impair autoregulation of CBF, thus allowing a drop in CBF during hemorrhagic hypotension. This effect on CBF autoregulation seems to be less pronounced than with isoflurane. Cerebral metabolic oxygen requirements decrease, and seizure activity has not been reported.

D. Neuromuscular

Sevoflurane produces adequate muscle relaxation for intubation following an inhalation induction, though most practitioners will deepen anesthesia with various combinations of propofol, lidocaine, or opioids; administer a neuromuscular blocker prior to intubation; or use a combination of these two approaches.

E. Renal

Sevoflurane slightly decreases renal blood flow. Its metabolism to substances associated with impaired renal tubule function (eg, decreased concentrating ability) is discussed below.

F. Hepatic

Sevoflurane decreases portal vein blood flow but increases hepatic artery blood flow, thereby maintaining total hepatic blood flow and oxygen delivery. It is generally not associated with immune-mediated anesthetic hepatotoxicity.

Biotransformation & Toxicity

The liver microsomal enzyme P-450 (specifically the 2E1 isoform) metabolizes sevoflurane at a rate one-fourth that of halothane (5% versus 20%), but 10 to 25 times that of isoflurane or desflurane and may be induced with ethanol or phenobarbital pretreatment. The potential nephrotoxicity of the resulting rise in inorganic fluoride (F^-) was discussed earlier. Serum fluoride concentrations exceed 50 μmol/L in approximately 7% of patients who receive sevoflurane, yet clinically significant kidney dysfunction has not been associated with sevoflurane anesthesia. The overall rate of sevoflurane metabolism is 5%, or 10 times that of isoflurane. Nonetheless, there has been no association with peak fluoride levels following sevoflurane and any renal concentrating abnormality.

Alkali such as barium hydroxide lime or soda lime (but not calcium hydroxide) can degrade sevoflurane, producing a nephrotoxic end product (*compound A*, fluoromethyl-2,2-difluoro-1-[trifluoromethyl]vinyl ether). Accumulation of compound A increases with increased respiratory gas temperature, low-flow anesthesia, dry barium hydroxide absorbent (Baralyme), high sevoflurane concentrations, and anesthetics of long duration. However, compound A should not be a concern for anesthesia providers unless their practice includes laboratory rats. Compound A has no known adverse effects on humans.

No study has associated sevoflurane with any detectable postoperative renal toxicity or injury. Nonetheless, some clinicians recommend that fresh gas flows be at least 2 L/min for anesthetics lasting more than a few hours. Sevoflurane can also be degraded into hydrogen fluoride by metal and environmental impurities present in manufacturing equipment, glass bottle packaging, and anesthesia equipment. Hydrogen fluoride can produce an acid burn on contact with respiratory mucosa. The risk of patient injury has been substantially reduced by inhibition of the degradation process by adding water to sevoflurane during the manufacturing process and packaging it in a special plastic container. Isolated incidents of fire in the respiratory circuits of anesthesia machines with desiccated CO_2 absorbent have been reported when sevoflurane was used.

Contraindications

Contraindications include severe hypovolemia, susceptibility to malignant hyperthermia, and intracranial hypertension.

Drug Interactions

Like other volatile anesthetics, sevoflurane potentiates NMBAs. It does not sensitize the heart to catecholamine-induced arrhythmias.

XENON

Xenon is a noble gas that has long been known to have anesthetic properties. It is an inert element that does not form chemical bonds. Xenon is scavenged from the atmosphere through a costly distillation process. It is an odorless, nonexplosive, naturally occurring gas with a MAC of 71% and a blood/gas coefficient of 0.115, giving it very fast onset and emergence parameters. As previously mentioned, xenon's anesthetic effects seem to be mediated by NMDA inhibition by competing with glycine at the glycine binding site. Xenon seems to have little effect on cardiovascular, hepatic, or renal systems and has been found to be protective against neuronal ischemia. Xenon inhalation combined with hypothermia has been suggested as a protective method to prevent cerebral damage following ischemic brain injury. Additionally, xenon anesthesia has been shown to produce less postoperative delirium compared with sevoflurane anesthesia in patients undergoing off-pump coronary artery bypass graft surgery. As a natural element, it has no effect upon the ozone layer compared with another NMDA antagonist, nitrous oxide. Cost and limited availability have prevented its widespread use.

SUGGESTED READINGS

Al Tmimi L, Van Hemelrijck J, Van de Velde M, et al. Xenon anaesthesia for patients undergoing off-pump coronary artery bypass graft surgery: a prospective randomized controlled pilot trial. *Br J Anaesth.* 2015;115:550.

Alvarado MC, Murphy KL, Baxter MG. Visual recognition memory is impaired in rhesus monkeys repeatedly exposed to sevoflurane in infancy. *Br J Anaesth.* 2017;119:517.

Banks P, Franks N, Dickinson R. Competitive inhibition at the glycine site of the *N*-methyl-D-aspartate receptor mediates xenon neuroprotection against hypoxia ischemia. *Anesthesiology.* 2010;112:614.

Bilotta F, Evered LA, Gruenbaum SE. Neurotoxicity of anesthetic drugs: an update. *Curr Opin Anaesthesiol.* 2017;30:452.

Brown E, Pavone K, Narano M. Multimodal general anesthesia: theory and practice. *Anesth Analg.* 2018;127:1246.

Devroe S, Lemiere J, Van Hese L, et al. The effect of xenon-augmented sevoflurane anesthesia on intraoperative hemodynamics and early postoperative neurocognitive function in children undergoing cardiac catheterization: a randomized controlled pilot trial. *Paediatr Anaesth.* 2018;28:726.

Diaz L, Gaynor J, Koh S, et al. Increasing cumulative exposure to volatile anesthetic agents is associated with poorer neurodevelopmental outcomes in children with hypoplastic left heart syndrome. *J Thorac Cardiovasc Surg.* 2016;52:482.

DiMaggio C, Sun L, Li G. Early childhood exposure to anesthesia and risk of developmental and behavioral disorders in a sibling birth cohort. *Anesth Analg.* 2011;113:1143.

Ebert TJ. Myocardial ischemia and adverse cardiac outcomes in cardiac patients undergoing noncardiac surgery with sevoflurane and isoflurane. *Anesth Analg.* 1997;85:993.

Eden C, Esses G, Katz D, DeMaria S Jr. Effects of anesthetic interventions on breast cancer behavior, cancer-related patient outcomes, and postoperative recovery. *Surg Oncol.* 2018;27:266.

Eger EI 2nd, Bowland T, Ionescu P, et al. Recovery and kinetic characteristics of desflurane and sevoflurane in volunteers after 8-h exposure, including kinetics of degradation products. *Anesthesiology.* 1997;87:517.

Eger EI 2nd, Raines DE, Shafer SL, Hemmings HC Jr, Sonner JM. Is a new paradigm needed to explain how inhaled anesthetics produce immobility? *Anesth Analg.* 2008;107:832.

Herold KF, Sanford RL, Lee W, Andersen OS, Hemmings HC Jr. Clinical concentrations of chemically diverse general anesthetics minimally affect lipid bilayer properties. *Proc Natl Acad Sci U S A.* 2017;114:3109.

Hussain M, Berger M, Eckenhoff R, Seitz D. General anesthetic and risk of dementia in elderly patients: current insights. *Clin Interv Aging.* 2014;9:1619.

Ishizawa Y. General anesthetic gases and the global environment. *Anesth Analg.* 2011;112:213.

Jevtovic-Todorovic V, Absalom A, Blomgren K. Anaesthetic neurotoxicity and neuroplasticity: an expert group report and statement based on the BJA Salzburg Seminar. *Br J Anaesth.* 2013;111:143.

Laitio R, Hynninen M, Arola O, et al. Effect of inhaled xenon on cerebral white matter damage in comatose survivors of out-of-hospital cardiac arrest: a randomized clinical trial. *JAMA.* 2016;315:1120.

Lew V, McKay E, Maze M. Past, present, and future of nitrous oxide. *Br Med Bull.* 2018;125:103.

McCann ME, Soriano SG. Does general anesthesia affect neurodevelopment in infants and children? *BMJ.* 2019;367:l6459.

Njoku D, Laster MJ, Gong DH. Biotransformation of halothane, enflurane, isoflurane, and desflurane to trifluoroacetylated liver proteins: association between protein acylation and hepatic injury. *Anesth Analg.* 1997;84:173.

O'Gara B, Talmor D. Lung protective properties of the volatile anesthetics. *Intensive Care Med.* 2016;42:1487.

Orser BA, Suresh S, Evers AS. SmartTots update regarding anesthetic neurotoxicity in the developing brain. *Anesth Analg.* 2018;126:1393.

Seitz D, Reimer C, Siddiqui N. A review of the epidemiological evidence for general anesthesia as a risk factor for Alzheimer's disease. *Prog Neuropsychopharmacol Biol Psychiatry.* 2013:47:122.

Stollings LM, Jia LJ, Tang P, Dou H, Lu B, Xu Y. Immune modulation by volatile anesthetics. *Anesthesiology.* 2016;125:399.

Stratmann G. Neurotoxicity of anesthetic drugs in the developing brain. *Anesth Analg.* 2011;113:1170.

Sun L, Guohua L, Miller T, et al. Association between a single general anesthesia exposure before age 36 months and neurocognitive outcomes in later childhood. *JAMA.* 2016;315:2312.

Sun X, Su F, Shi Y, Lee C. The "second gas effect" is not a valid concept. *Anesth Analg.* 1999;88:188.

Thomas J, Crosby G, Drummond J, et al. Anesthetic neurotoxicity: a difficult dragon to slay. *Anesth Analg.* 2011;113;969.

Torri G. Inhalational anesthetics: a review. *Minerva Anesthesiol.* 2010;76:215.

Warner DO, Zaccariello MJ, Katusic SK, et al. Neuropsychological and behavioral outcomes after exposure of young children to procedures requiring general anesthesia: the Mayo Anesthesia Safety in Kids (MASK) study. *Anesthesiology.* 2018;129:89.

Wei H. The role of calcium dysregulation in anesthetic-mediated neurotoxicity. *Anesth Analg.* 2011;113:972.

Whittington R, Bretteville A, Dickler M, Planel E. Anesthesia and tau pathology. *Prog Neuropsychopharmacol Biol Psychiatry.* 2013;47:147.

WEBSITE

The SmartTots collaborative research initiative focuses on funding research in pediatric anesthesiology. http://smarttots.org/

CHAPTER

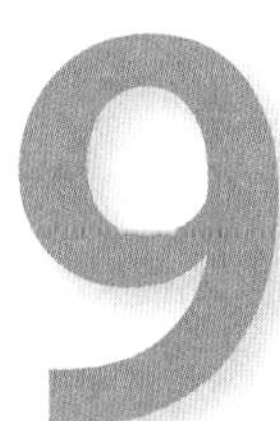

Intravenous Anesthetics

KEY CONCEPTS

1. Repetitive administration of highly lipid-soluble barbiturates (eg, infusion of thiopental for "barbiturate coma" and brain protection) saturates the peripheral compartments, minimizing any effect of redistribution and rendering the duration of action more dependent on elimination. This is an example of context sensitivity.
2. Barbiturates constrict the cerebral vasculature, causing a decrease in cerebral blood flow, cerebral blood volume, and intracranial pressure.
3. Although apnea may be relatively uncommon after benzodiazepine induction, even small intravenous doses of these agents have resulted in respiratory arrest.
4. In contrast to other anesthetic agents, ketamine increases arterial blood pressure, heart rate, and cardiac output, particularly after rapid bolus injections.
5. Induction doses of etomidate transiently inhibit enzymes involved in cortisol and aldosterone synthesis. When used for sedation in the intensive care unit, etomidate produced adrenocortical suppression.
6. Propofol formulations can support the growth of bacteria, so sterile technique must be observed in preparation and handling. Propofol should be administered within 6 h of opening the ampule.

General anesthesia began with inhalation of ether, nitrous oxide, or chloroform, but in current practice, anesthesia and sedation can be induced and maintained with drugs that enter the patient through a wide range of routes. Preoperative or procedural sedation is usually accomplished by way of oral or intravenous routes. Induction of general anesthesia is typically accomplished by inhalation or intravenous drug administration. Alternatively, general anesthesia can be induced and maintained with intramuscular injection of ketamine. General anesthesia is typically maintained with a total intravenous anesthesia (TIVA) technique, an inhalation technique, or a combination of the two. This chapter focuses on the injectable agents used to produce narcosis (sleep), including barbiturates, benzodiazepines, ketamine, etomidate, propofol, and dexmedetomidine.

BARBITURATES

At one time, nearly every general anesthetic in adults was induced with a barbiturate. These agents were also widely used for control of seizures, anxiolysis, and procedural sedation and as sleep-inducing agents. They are now much less widely used in anesthesia.

Mechanisms of Action

Barbiturates depress the reticular activating system in the brainstem, which controls consciousness.

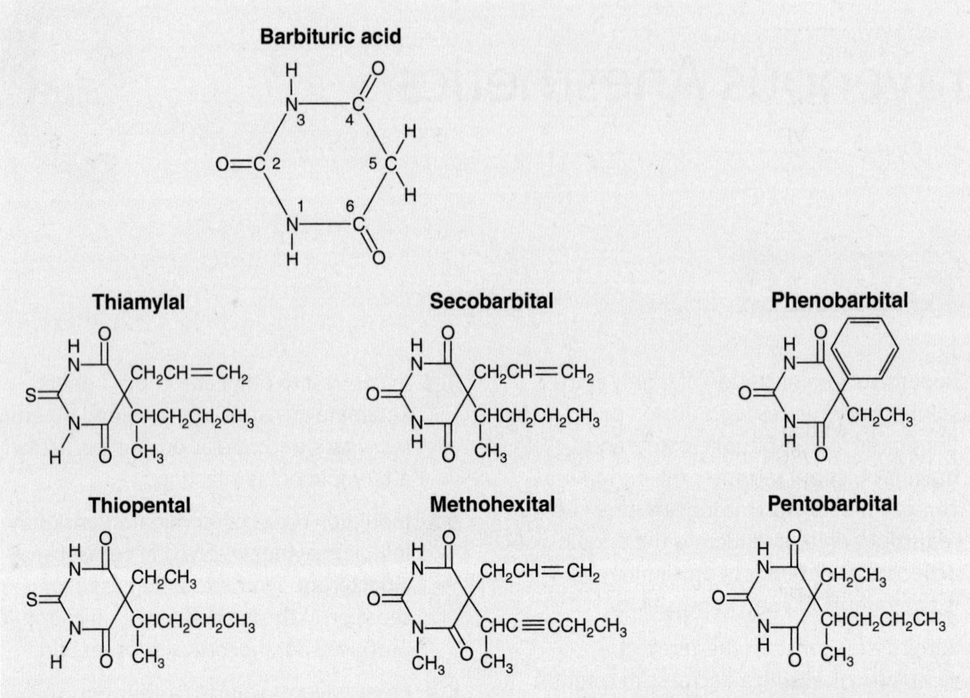

FIGURE 9–1 Barbiturates share the structure of barbituric acid and differ in the C_2, C_5, and N_1 substitutions.

Their primary mechanism of action is through binding to the γ-aminobutyric acid type A ($GABA_A$) receptor. This site is separate from the $GABA_A$ site to which benzodiazepines bind. Barbiturates potentiate the action of GABA in increasing the duration of openings of a chloride-specific ion channel. Barbiturates also inhibit kainate and AMPA receptors.

Structure–Activity Relationships

Barbiturates are derived from barbituric acid (Figure 9–1). Substitution at carbon C_5 determines hypnotic potency and anticonvulsant activity. The phenyl group in *pheno*barbital is anticonvulsive, whereas the methyl group in *metho*hexital is not. Thus methohexital remains useful for providing anesthesia for electroconvulsive therapy wherein a seizure is the objective. Replacing the oxygen at C_2 (*oxy*barbiturates) with a sulfur atom (*thio*barbiturates) increases lipid solubility. As a result, thiopental and thiamylal have a greater potency, more rapid onset of action, and shorter duration of action (after a single "sleep dose") than pentobarbital. The sodium salts of the barbiturates are water soluble but markedly alkaline (pH of 2.5% thiopental ≥10) and relatively unstable (2-week shelf-life for 2.5% thiopental solution).

Pharmacokinetics

A. Absorption

Prior to the introduction of propofol, thiopental, thiamylal, and methohexital were frequently administered intravenously for induction of general anesthesia in adults and children. Rectal methohexital has been used for induction in children.

B. Distribution

The duration of induction doses of thiopental, thiamylal, and methohexital is determined by redistribution, not by metabolism or elimination. Thiopental's great lipid solubility and high nonionized fraction (60%) account for rapid brain uptake (within 30 s). If the central compartment is contracted (eg, hypovolemic

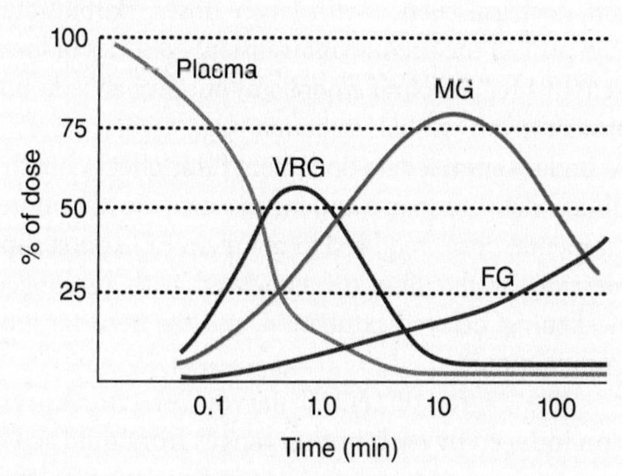

FIGURE 9–2 Distribution of thiopental from plasma to the vessel-rich group (VRG; brain, heart, liver, kidney, endocrine glands), to the muscle group (MG), and finally to the fat group (FG). Propofol follows the same pattern but on a different time scale. (Modified with permission from Price HL, Kovnat PJ, Safer JN, et al. The uptake of thiopental by body tissues and its relation to the duration of narcosis. *Clin Pharmacol Ther.* 1960 Jan;1(1):16-22.)

shock), if the serum albumin is low (eg, severe liver disease or malnutrition), or if the nonionized fraction is increased (eg, acidosis), larger brain and heart concentrations will be achieved for a given dose with greater reduction of blood pressure. Redistribution lowers plasma and brain concentration to 10% of peak levels within 20 to 30 min (Figure 9–2). This pharmacokinetic profile correlates with clinical experience—patients typically lose consciousness within 30 s and awaken within 20 min.

The minimal induction dose of thiopental will depend on body weight and age. Reduced induction doses are required for older adult patients. In contrast to the rapid initial distribution half-life of a few minutes, elimination of thiopental is prolonged (elimination half-life ranges of 10–12 h). Thiamylal and methohexital have similar distribution patterns, whereas less lipid-soluble barbiturates have much longer distribution half-lives and durations of action after a sleep dose. 1 Repetitive administration of highly lipid-soluble barbiturates (eg, infusion of thiopental for "barbiturate coma" and brain protection) saturates the peripheral compartments, minimizing any effect of redistribution and rendering the duration of action more dependent on elimination. This is an example of context sensitivity, which is also seen with other lipid-soluble agents (eg, potent inhaled anesthetics, fentanyl, sufentanil; see Chapter 7).

C. Biotransformation

Barbiturates are principally biotransformed via hepatic oxidation to inactive, water-soluble metabolites. Because of greater hepatic extraction, methohexital is cleared by the liver more rapidly than thiopental. Therefore, full recovery of psychomotor function is also more rapid following methohexital.

D. Excretion

Except for the less protein-bound and less lipid-soluble agents such as phenobarbital, renal excretion is limited to water-soluble end products of hepatic biotransformation. Methohexital is excreted in the feces.

Effects on Organ Systems

A. Cardiovascular

The cardiovascular effects of barbiturates vary markedly, depending on the rate of administration, dose, volume status, baseline autonomic tone, and preexisting cardiovascular disease. A slow rate of injection with adequate preoperative hydration will attenuate or eliminate these changes in most patients. Intravenous bolus induction doses of barbiturates cause a decrease in blood pressure and an increase in heart rate. Depression of the medullary vasomotor center produces vasodilation and peripheral pooling of blood, mimicking reduced blood volume. Tachycardia following administration is probably due to a central vagolytic effect and reflex responses to decreases in blood pressure. Cardiac output is often maintained by an increased heart rate and increased myocardial contractility from compensatory baroreceptor reflexes. Sympathetically induced vasoconstriction of resistance vessels (particularly with intubation under light planes of general anesthesia) may actually increase peripheral vascular resistance. However, in situations where the baroreceptor response will be blunted or absent (eg, hypovolemia, congestive heart failure, β-adrenergic blockade), **cardiac output and arterial blood pressure may fall dramatically due to uncompensated**

peripheral pooling of blood and direct myocardial depression. Patients with poorly controlled hypertension are particularly prone to wide swings in blood pressure during anesthesia induction.

B. Respiratory

Barbiturates depress the medullary ventilatory center, decreasing the ventilatory response to hypercapnia and hypoxia. Apnea often follows an induction dose. During awakening, tidal volume and respiratory rate are decreased. Barbiturates incompletely depress airway reflex responses to laryngoscopy and intubation (much less than propofol), and airway instrumentation may lead to bronchospasm (in asthmatic patients) or laryngospasm in lightly anesthetized patients.

C. Cerebral

2 Barbiturates constrict the cerebral vasculature, causing a decrease in cerebral blood flow, cerebral blood volume, and intracranial pressure. Intracranial pressure often decreases to a greater extent than arterial blood pressure, so cerebral perfusion pressure (CPP) usually increases. (CPP equals cerebral artery pressure minus the greater of jugular venous pressure or intracranial pressure.) Barbiturates induce a greater decline in cerebral oxygen consumption (up to 50% of normal) than in cerebral blood flow; therefore, the decline in cerebral blood flow is not detrimental. Barbiturate-induced reductions in oxygen requirements and cerebral metabolic activity are mirrored by changes in the electroencephalogram (EEG), which progress from low-voltage fast activity with small doses to high-voltage slow activity, burst suppression, and electrical silence with larger doses. Barbiturates may protect the brain from transient episodes of focal ischemia (eg, cerebral embolism) but probably do not protect from global ischemia (eg, cardiac arrest). Abundant animal data document these effects, but the clinical data are sparse and inconsistent. Furthermore, thiopental doses required to maintain EEG burst suppression or flat line are associated with prolonged awakening, delayed extubation, and the need for inotropic support.

The degree of central nervous system depression induced by barbiturates ranges from mild sedation to unconsciousness, depending on the dose administered (Table 9–1). Some patients relate a taste sensation of garlic, onions, or pizza during induction with thiopental. Barbiturates do not impair the perception of pain. Small doses occasionally cause a state of excitement and disorientation. Barbiturates do not produce muscle relaxation, and some induce involuntary skeletal muscle contractions (eg, methohexital). Small doses of thiopental (50–100 mg intravenously) rapidly (but briefly) control most grand mal seizures.

D. Renal

Barbiturates reduce renal blood flow and glomerular filtration rate in proportion to the fall in blood pressure.

E. Hepatic

Hepatic blood flow is decreased. Chronic exposure to barbiturates leads to the induction of hepatic enzymes and an increased rate of metabolism.

TABLE 9–1 Uses and dosages of common barbiturates.

Agent	Use	Route[1]	Concentration (%)	Dose (mg/kg)
Thiopental	Induction	IV	2.5	3–6
Methohexital	Induction	IV	1	1–2
	Sedation	IV	1	0.2–0.4
	Induction	Rectal (children)	10	25
Pentobarbital	Premedication	Oral	5	2–4
		IM		2–4
		Rectal suppository		3

[1]IM, intramuscular; IV, intravenous.

On the other hand, the binding of barbiturates to the cytochrome P-450 enzyme system interferes with the biotransformation of other drugs (eg, tricyclic antidepressants). Barbiturates may precipitate acute intermittent porphyria or variegate porphyria in susceptible individuals.

F. Immunological

Anaphylactic or anaphylactoid allergic reactions are rare. Sulfur-containing thiobarbiturates evoke mast cell histamine release in vitro, whereas oxybarbiturates do not.

Drug Interactions

Contrast media, sulfonamides, and other drugs that occupy the same protein-binding sites may displace thiopental, increasing the amount of free drug available and potentiating the effects of a given dose. Ethanol, opioids, antihistamines, and other central nervous system depressants potentiate the sedative effects of barbiturates.

BENZODIAZEPINES

Mechanisms of Action

Benzodiazepines bind the same set of receptors in the central nervous system as barbiturates but at a different site. Benzodiazepine binding to the $GABA_A$ receptor increases the frequency of openings of the associated chloride ion channel. Benzodiazepine-receptor binding by an agonist facilitates binding of GABA to its receptor. **Flumazenil** (an imidazobenzodiazepine) is a specific benzodiazepine–receptor antagonist that effectively reverses most of the central nervous system effects of benzodiazepines (see Chapter 17).

Structure–Activity Relationships

The chemical structure of benzodiazepines includes a benzene ring and a seven-member diazepine ring (Figure 9–3). Substitutions at various positions on these rings affect potency and biotransformation. The imidazole ring of midazolam contributes to its water solubility at low pH. Diazepam and lorazepam

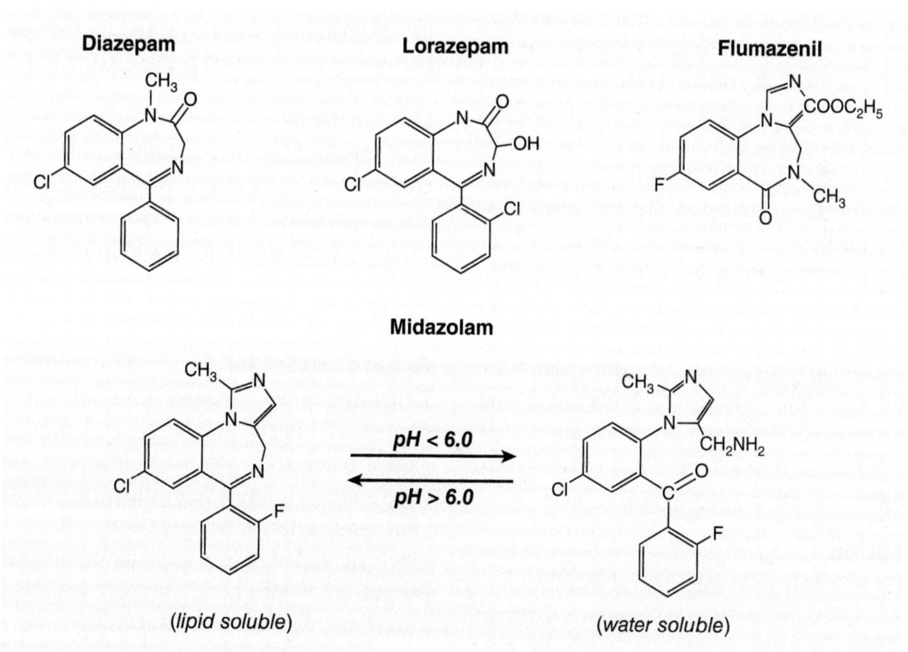

FIGURE 9–3 The structures of commonly used benzodiazepines and their antagonist, flumazenil, share a seven-member diazepine ring. (Modified with permission from White PF. Pharmacologic and clinical aspects of preoperative medication. *Anesth Analg.* 1986 Sep;65(9):963-974.)

TABLE 9–2 Uses and doses of commonly used benzodiazepines.

Agent	Use	Route[1]	Dose (mg/kg)
Diazepam	Premedication	Oral	0.2–0.5
	Sedation	IV	0.04–0.2
Midazolam	Premedication	IM	0.07–0.15
	Sedation	IV	0.01–0.1
	Induction	IV	0.1–0.4
Lorazepam	Premedication	Oral	0.05

[1]IM, intramuscular; IV, intravenous.

are insoluble in water, so parenteral preparations contain propylene glycol, which can produce pain with intravenous or intramuscular injection.

Pharmacokinetics

A. Absorption

Benzodiazepines are commonly administered orally and intravenously (or, less commonly, intramuscularly) to provide sedation (or, less commonly, to induce general anesthesia) (Table 9–2). Diazepam and lorazepam are well absorbed from the gastrointestinal tract, with peak plasma levels usually achieved in 1 and 2 h, respectively. Intravenous midazolam (0.05–0.1 mg/kg) given for anxiolysis before general or regional anesthesia is nearly ubiquitous. Oral midazolam (0.25–1 mg/kg), though not approved by the U.S. Food and Drug Administration for this purpose, is popular for pediatric premedication. Likewise, intranasal (0.2–0.3 mg/kg), buccal (0.07 mg/kg), and sublingual (0.1 mg/kg) midazolam provide effective preoperative sedation.

Intramuscular injections of diazepam are painful and unreliably absorbed. Midazolam and lorazepam are well absorbed after intramuscular injection, with peak levels achieved in 30 and 90 min, respectively.

B. Distribution

Diazepam is relatively lipid soluble and readily penetrates the blood–brain barrier. Although midazolam is water soluble at reduced pH, its imidazole ring closes at physiological pH, increasing its lipid solubility (see Figure 9–3). The moderate lipid solubility of lorazepam accounts for its slower brain uptake and onset of action. Redistribution is fairly rapid for benzodiazepines and, like barbiturates, is responsible for awakening. Although we have used midazolam as an induction agent, none of the benzodiazepines can match the rapid onset and short duration of action of propofol or etomidate. All three benzodiazepines are highly protein bound (90–98%).

C. Biotransformation

The benzodiazepines rely on the liver for biotransformation into water-soluble glucuronidated end products. The phase I metabolites of diazepam are pharmacologically active.

Slow hepatic extraction and a large volume of distribution (V_d) result in a long elimination half-life for diazepam (30 h). Although lorazepam also has a low hepatic extraction ratio, its lower lipid solubility limits its V_d, resulting in a shorter elimination half-life (15 h). Nonetheless, the clinical duration of lorazepam is often quite prolonged due to increased receptor affinity. These differences between lorazepam and diazepam underscore the limited usefulness of pharmacokinetic half-lives in guiding clinical practice (see Chapter 7). Midazolam shares diazepam's V_d, but its elimination half-life (2 h) is the shortest of the group because of its increased hepatic extraction ratio.

D. Excretion

The metabolites of benzodiazepines are excreted chiefly in the urine. Enterohepatic circulation produces a secondary peak in diazepam plasma concentration 6 to 12 h following administration.

Effects on Organ Systems

A. Cardiovascular

Benzodiazepines display minimal left-ventricular depressant effects, even at general anesthetic doses, except when they are coadministered with opioids (these agents interact to produce myocardial depression and arterial hypotension). Benzodiazepines given alone decrease arterial blood pressure, cardiac output, and peripheral vascular resistance slightly and sometimes increase heart rate.

B. Respiratory

Benzodiazepines depress the ventilatory response to carbon dioxide (CO_2). This depression is usually

insignificant unless the drugs are administered
3 intravenously or given with other respiratory depressants. Although apnea may be relatively uncommon after benzodiazepine induction, even small intravenous doses of these agents have resulted in respiratory arrest. The steep dose–response curve and delayed onset (compared with propofol or etomidate) necessitate titration to avoid overdosage and apnea, particularly when these agents are used for procedural sedation. Ventilation must be monitored in all patients receiving intravenous benzodiazepines (we and national advisory panels recommend end-tidal CO_2 monitoring), and resuscitation equipment and a practitioner with airway skills must be present.

C. Cerebral

Benzodiazepines reduce cerebral oxygen consumption, cerebral blood flow, and intracranial pressure but not to the extent the barbiturates do. They are effective in controlling grand mal seizures. Sedative doses often produce anterograde amnesia. The mild muscle-relaxing property of these drugs is mediated at the spinal cord level. The antianxiety, amnestic, and sedative effects seen at lower doses progress to stupor and unconsciousness at anesthetic doses. Compared with propofol or etomidate, induction with benzodiazepines is associated with a slower rate of loss of consciousness and a longer recovery. Benzodiazepines have no direct analgesic properties.

Drug Interactions

Cimetidine binds to cytochrome P-450 and reduces the metabolism of diazepam. Erythromycin inhibits the metabolism of midazolam and causes a two- to threefold prolongation and intensification of its effects.

As previously mentioned, the combination of opioids and benzodiazepines markedly reduces arterial blood pressure and peripheral vascular resistance. This synergistic interaction has often been observed in patients undergoing cardiac surgery who received benzodiazepines before or during induction with larger doses of opioids.

Benzodiazepines reduce the minimum alveolar concentration of volatile anesthetics by as much as 30%. Ethanol, barbiturates, and other central nervous system depressants potentiate the sedative effects of benzodiazepines.

KETAMINE

Mechanisms of Action

Ketamine has multiple effects throughout the central nervous system, and it is well recognized to inhibit *N*-methyl-D-aspartate (NMDA) channels. Investigators have studied ketamine actions on a long list of other ion channels and receptors; however, actions on none other than NMDA receptors appear medically important. Ketamine functionally "dissociates" sensory impulses from the limbic cortex (which is involved with the awareness of sensation). Clinically, this state of dissociative anesthesia may cause the patient to appear conscious (eg, eye opening, swallowing, muscle contracture) but unable to process or respond to sensory input. Ketamine may have additional actions on endogenous analgesic pathways.

Ketamine has effects on mood, and preparations of this agent and its single enantiomer esketamine are now widely used to treat severe, treatment-resistant depression, particularly when patients have suicidal ideation. Small infusion doses of ketamine are also being used to supplement general anesthesia and to reduce the need for opioids both during and after the surgical procedure. Low-dose infusions of ketamine have been used for analgesia ("sub-anesthetic" doses) in postoperative patients and others who are refractory to conventional analgesic approaches. Ketamine has been identified by the World Health Organization as an "essential medicine."

Structure–Activity Relationships

Ketamine (Figure 9–4) is a structural analog of phencyclidine (a veterinary anesthetic and a drug of abuse). It is one-tenth as potent, yet it retains many of phencyclidine's psychotomimetic effects. Ketamine is used for intravenous induction of anesthesia, particularly in settings where its tendency to produce sympathetic stimulation is useful (hypovolemia, trauma). When intravenous access is lacking, ketamine is useful for intramuscular induction of general anesthesia in children and uncooperative adults. Ketamine can be combined with other agents (eg, propofol or midazolam) in small bolus doses or infusions for conscious sedation during procedures such as nerve blocks and endoscopy. Even subanesthetic doses of ketamine may cause hallucinations

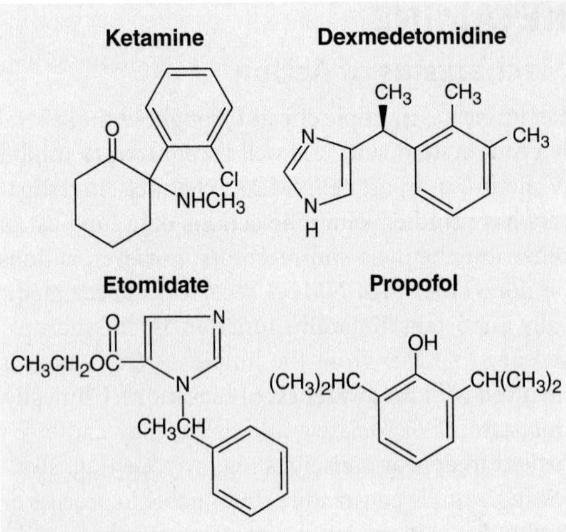

FIGURE 9–4 The structures of ketamine, etomidate, propofol, and dexmedetomidine.

but usually do not do so in clinical practice, where many patients will have received at least a small dose of midazolam (or a related agent) for amnesia and sedation. Ketamine is supplied as the racemic mixture of two optical isomers (enantiomers). The increased anesthetic potency and decreased psychotomimetic side effects of one isomer (S[+] versus R[−]) are the result of stereospecific receptors. The single S(+) stereoisomer preparation is not available in the United States (but widely available elsewhere throughout the world), and it has a considerably greater affinity than the racemic mixture for the NMDA receptor as well as several-fold greater potency as a general anesthetic.

Pharmacokinetics

A. Absorption

Ketamine has been administered orally, nasally, rectally, subcutaneously, and epidurally, but in usual clinical practice, it is given intravenously or intramuscularly (Table 9–3). Peak plasma levels are usually achieved within 10 to 15 min after intramuscular injection.

B. Distribution

Ketamine is highly lipid soluble and, along with a ketamine-induced increase in cerebral blood flow and cardiac output, results in rapid brain uptake and subsequent redistribution (the distribution half-life is 10–15 min). Awakening is due to redistribution from the brain to peripheral compartments.

C. Biotransformation

Ketamine is biotransformed in the liver to several metabolites, one of which (norketamine) retains anesthetic activity. Patients receiving repeated doses of ketamine (eg, for daily changing of dressings on burns) develop tolerance, and this can only be partially explained by induction of hepatic enzymes. Extensive hepatic uptake (hepatic extraction ratio of 0.9) explains ketamine's relatively short elimination half-life (2 h).

TABLE 9–3 Uses and doses of ketamine, etomidate, and propofol.

Agent	Use	Route[1]	Dose
Ketamine	Induction	IV	1–2 mg/kg
		IM	3–5 mg/kg
	Maintenance	IV	10–20 mcg/kg/min
	Analgesia or sedation	IV	2.5–15 mcg/kg/min
Etomidate	Induction	IV	0.2–0.5 mg/kg
Propofol	Induction	IV	1–2.5 mg/kg
	Maintenance infusion	IV	50–200 mcg/kg/min
	Sedation infusion	IV	25–100 mcg/kg/min
Dexmedetomidine	Induction	IV	1 mcg/kg over 10 min
		Nasal	1–2 mcg/kg
	Maintenance	IV	0.2–1.4 mcg/kg/h

[1]IM, intramuscular; IV, intravenous.

D. Excretion

End products of ketamine biotransformation are excreted renally.

Effects on Organ Systems

A. Cardiovascular

4 In contrast to other anesthetic agents, ketamine increases arterial blood pressure, heart rate, and cardiac output (Table 9–4), particularly after rapid bolus injections. These indirect cardiovascular effects are due to central stimulation of the sympathetic nervous system and inhibition of the reuptake of norepinephrine after release at nerve terminals. Accompanying these changes are increases in pulmonary artery pressure and myocardial work. For these reasons, ketamine should be administered carefully to patients with coronary artery disease, uncontrolled hypertension, congestive heart failure, or arterial aneurysms. The **direct myocardial depressant** effects of large doses of ketamine may be unmasked by sympathetic blockade (eg, spinal cord transection) or exhaustion of catecholamine stores (eg, severe end-stage shock).

B. Respiratory

Ventilatory drive is minimally affected by induction doses of ketamine, though combinations of ketamine with opioids may produce apnea. Racemic ketamine is a potent bronchodilator, making it a good induction agent for asthmatic patients; however, S(+) ketamine produces minimal bronchodilation. Upper airway reflexes remain largely intact, but partial airway obstruction may occur, and patients at significant risk for aspiration pneumonia ("full stomachs") should be intubated during ketamine general anesthesia (see Case Discussion, Chapter 17). The increased salivation associated with ketamine can be attenuated by premedication with an anticholinergic agent such as glycopyrrolate.

C. Cerebral

The received dogma about ketamine is that it increases cerebral oxygen consumption, cerebral blood flow, and intracranial pressure. These effects would seem to preclude its use in patients with space-occupying intracranial lesions such as occur with head trauma; however, recent publications offer convincing evidence that when combined with a

TABLE 9–4 Summary of nonvolatile anesthetic effects on organ systems.[1]

	Cardiovascular		Respiratory		Cerebral		
Agent	**HR**	**MAP**	**Vent**	**B'dil**	**CBF**	**$CMRO_2$**	**ICP**
Barbiturates							
Thiopental	↑↑	↓↓	↓↓↓	↓	↓↓↓	↓↓↓	↓↓↓
Methohexital	↑↑	↓↓	↓↓↓	0	↓↓↓	↓↓↓	↓↓↓
Benzodiazepines							
Diazepam	0/↑	↓	↓↓	0	↓↓	↓↓	↓↓
Lorazepam	0/↑	↓	↓↓	0	↓↓	↓↓	↓↓
Midazolam	↑	↓↓	↓↓	0	↓↓	↓↓	↓↓
Ketamine	↑↑	↑↑	↓	↑↑↑	↑↑[2]	↑	↑↑[2]
Etomidate	0	↓	↓	0	↓↓↓	↓↓↓	↓↓↓
Propofol	0	↓↓	↓↓↓	0	↓↓↓	↓↓↓	↓↓↓
Dexmedetomidine	↓	↓	0	?	↓↓	↓↓	↓↓

[1]B'dil, bronchodilation; CBF, cerebral blood flow; $CMRO_2$, cerebral oxygen consumption; HR, heart rate; ICP, intracranial pressure; MAP, mean arterial pressure; Vent, ventilatory drive; 0, no effect; 0/↑, no change or mild increase; ↓, decrease (mild, moderate, marked); ↑, increase (mild, moderate, marked); ?, unknown effect.

[2]Minimal change in CBF and ICP when co-administered with other agents (see text).

benzodiazepine (or another agent acting on the same GABA receptor system) and controlled ventilation (in techniques that exclude nitrous oxide), ketamine is *not* associated with increased intracranial pressure. Myoclonic activity is associated with increased subcortical electrical activity, which is not apparent on surface EEG. Undesirable psychotomimetic side effects (eg, disturbing dreams and delirium) during emergence and recovery are less common in children, in patients premedicated with benzodiazepines, or in those receiving ketamine combined with propofol in a total intravenous anesthesia (TIVA) technique. Of the nonvolatile agents, ketamine comes closest to being a "complete" anesthetic as it induces analgesia, amnesia, and unconsciousness.

Drug Interactions

Ketamine interacts synergistically (more than additive) with volatile anesthetics but in an additive way with propofol, benzodiazepines, and other GABA-receptor–mediated agents. Nondepolarizing neuromuscular blocking agents are dose-dependently, but minimally, potentiated by ketamine (see Chapter 11). Diazepam or midazolam attenuate ketamine's cardiac stimulating effects, and diazepam prolongs ketamine's elimination half-life.

α-Adrenergic and β-adrenergic antagonists (and other agents and techniques that diminish sympathetic stimulation) may unmask the direct myocardial depressant effects of ketamine, which are normally overwhelmed by sympathetic stimulation. Concurrent infusion of ketamine and propofol, often in a fixed infusion (mg:mg) ratio of 1:10, has achieved great popularity for procedural sedation with local and regional anesthesia or intravenous general anesthesia in office-based settings.

ETOMIDATE

Mechanisms of Action

Etomidate depresses the reticular activating system and mimics the inhibitory effects of GABA. Specifically, etomidate—particularly the R(+) isomer—appears to bind to a subunit of the $GABA_A$ receptor, increasing the receptor's affinity for GABA. Etomidate may have disinhibitory effects on the parts of the nervous system that control extrapyramidal motor activity. This disinhibition offers a potential explanation for the 30% to 60% incidence of myoclonus with induction of etomidate anesthesia.

Structure–Activity Relationships

Etomidate contains a carboxylated imidazole and is structurally unrelated to other anesthetic agents (see Figure 9–4). The imidazole ring provides water solubility in acidic solutions and lipid solubility at physiological pH. Therefore, etomidate is dissolved in propylene glycol for injection. This solution often causes pain on injection that can be lessened by a prior intravenous injection of lidocaine.

Pharmacokinetics

A. Absorption

Etomidate is available only for intravenous administration and is used primarily for induction of general anesthesia (see Table 9–3). It is sometimes used for brief production of deep (unconscious) sedation, such as prior to placement of retrobulbar blocks.

B. Distribution

Although it is highly protein bound, etomidate is characterized by a very rapid onset of action due to its great lipid solubility and large nonionized fraction at physiological pH. Redistribution is responsible for decreasing the plasma concentration to awakening levels. Etomidate plasma kinetics are well explained by a two-compartment model.

C. Biotransformation

Hepatic microsomal enzymes and plasma esterases rapidly hydrolyze etomidate to an inactive metabolite.

D. Excretion

The end products of etomidate hydrolysis are primarily excreted in the urine.

Effects on Organ Systems

A. Cardiovascular

Etomidate has no effects on sympathetic tone or myocardial function when given by itself. A mild reduction in peripheral vascular resistance is responsible for a decline in arterial blood pressure. Myocardial contractility and cardiac output are usually unchanged. Etomidate does not release histamine. However, etomidate by itself, even in large doses, produces relatively light anesthesia for laryngoscopy, and marked increases in heart rate and blood pressure may be recorded when etomidate provides the only anesthetic depth for intubation.

B. Respiratory

Ventilation is affected less with etomidate than with barbiturates or benzodiazepines. Even induction doses usually do not result in apnea unless opioids have also been administered.

C. Cerebral

Etomidate decreases cerebral metabolic rate, cerebral blood flow, and intracranial pressure. Because of minimal cardiovascular effects, cerebral perfusion pressure is well maintained. Although changes on EEG resemble those associated with barbiturates, etomidate (like ketamine) increases the amplitude of somatosensory evoked potentials but increases latency and reduces the amplitude of auditory evoked potentials. Postoperative nausea and vomiting are more common following etomidate than following propofol or barbiturate induction. Etomidate lacks analgesic properties.

D. Endocrine

Etomidate pharmacokinetics describes an agent that should be highly efficient for continuous infusion for TIVA or sedation. However, when infused for sedation in the intensive care unit (ICU), etomidate was reported to produce consistent adrenocortical suppression with an increased mortality rate in critically ill (particularly septic) patients.
5 Etomidate is far more potent at inhibiting steroid production than at producing anesthesia. Induction doses of etomidate transiently inhibit CYP11B1 (in the cortisol and corticosterone pathway) and CYP11B2 (in the aldosterone synthesis pathway).

Drug Interactions

Fentanyl increases the plasma level and prolongs the elimination half-life of etomidate. Opioids decrease the myoclonus characteristic of an etomidate induction.

PROPOFOL

Mechanisms of Action

Propofol induction of general anesthesia likely involves the facilitation of inhibitory neurotransmission mediated by $GABA_A$ receptor binding. Propofol allosterically increases the binding affinity of GABA for the $GABA_A$ receptor. This receptor, as previously noted, is coupled to a chloride channel, and activation of the receptor leads to hyperpolarization of the nerve membrane. Propofol (like most general anesthetics) binds multiple ion channels and receptors. Propofol actions are not reversed by the specific benzodiazepine antagonist flumazenil.

Structure–Activity Relationships

Propofol consists of a phenol ring substituted with two isopropyl groups (see Figure 9–4). Propofol is not water soluble, but a 1% aqueous preparation (10 mg/mL) is available for intravenous administration as an oil-in-water emulsion containing soybean oil, glycerol, and egg lecithin. A history of egg allergy does not necessarily contraindicate the use of propofol because most egg allergies involve a reaction to egg white (egg albumin), whereas egg lecithin is extracted from egg yolk. This formulation will often cause pain during injection that can be decreased by prior injection of lidocaine or less effectively by mixing lidocaine with propofol prior to injection (2 mL
6 of 1% lidocaine in 18 mL propofol). Propofol formulations can support the growth of bacteria, so sterile technique must be observed in preparation and handling. Propofol should be administered within 6 h of opening the ampule. Sepsis and death have been linked to contaminated propofol preparations. Current formulations of propofol contain 0.005% disodium edetate or 0.025% sodium metabisulfite to help retard the rate of growth of microorganisms; however, these additives do not render the product "antimicrobially preserved" under United States Pharmacopeia standards.

Pharmacokinetics

A. Absorption

Propofol is available only for intravenous administration for the induction of general anesthesia and for moderate to deep sedation (see Table 9–3).

B. Distribution

Propofol has a rapid onset of action. Awakening from a single bolus dose is also rapid due to a very short initial distribution half-life (2–8 min). Recovery from propofol is more rapid and is accompanied by less "hangover" than recovery from methohexital, thiopental, ketamine, or etomidate. This makes it a good anesthetic for ambulatory surgery. A smaller induction dose is recommended in older adult patients because of their smaller V_d. Age is also a key factor determining required propofol infusion rates for TIVA. In countries other than the United States, a device called the Diprifusor™ is used to provide target (concentration) controlled infusion of propofol. The user must enter the patient's age and weight and the desired target concentration. The device uses these data, a microcomputer, and standard pharmacokinetic parameters to continuously adjust the infusion rate. Unfortunately, this very useful device is not available in the United States.

C. Biotransformation

The clearance of propofol exceeds hepatic blood flow, implying the existence of extrahepatic metabolism. This exceptionally high clearance rate probably contributes to rapid recovery after continuous infusions. Conjugation in the liver results in inactive metabolites that are eliminated by renal clearance. The pharmacokinetics of propofol does not appear to be affected by obesity, cirrhosis, or kidney failure. Use of propofol infusion for long-term sedation of children who are critically ill or young adult neurosurgical patients has been associated with sporadic cases of lipemia, metabolic acidosis, and death, the so-termed *propofol infusion syndrome*.

D. Excretion

Although metabolites of propofol are primarily excreted in the urine, end-stage kidney disease does not affect the clearance of the parent drug.

Effects on Organ Systems

A. Cardiovascular

The major cardiovascular effect of propofol is a decrease in arterial blood pressure due to a drop in systemic vascular resistance (inhibition of sympathetic vasoconstrictor activity), preload, and cardiac contractility. Hypotension following induction is usually reversed by the stimulation accompanying laryngoscopy and intubation. Factors associated with propofol-induced hypotension include large doses, rapid injection, and old age. Propofol markedly impairs the normal arterial baroreflex response to hypotension. Rarely, a marked drop in cardiac filling may lead to a vagally mediated reflex bradycardia (the Bezold–Jarisch reflex). Changes in heart rate and cardiac output are usually transient and insignificant in healthy patients but may be life-threatening in patients at the extremes of age, those receiving β-adrenergic blockers, or those with impaired left ventricular function. Although myocardial oxygen consumption and coronary blood flow usually decrease comparably, coronary sinus lactate production increases in some patients, indicating a mismatch between myocardial oxygen supply and demand.

B. Respiratory

Propofol is a profound respiratory depressant that usually causes apnea following an induction dose. Even when used for conscious sedation in subanesthetic doses, propofol inhibits hypoxic ventilatory drive and depresses the normal response to hypercarbia. As a result, only properly educated and qualified personnel should administer propofol for sedation. Propofol-induced depression of upper airway reflexes exceeds that of thiopental, allowing intubation, endoscopy, or laryngeal mask placement in the absence of neuromuscular blockade. Although propofol can cause histamine release, induction with propofol is accompanied by a lesser incidence of wheezing in both asthmatic and nonasthmatic patients compared with barbiturates or etomidate.

C. Cerebral

Propofol decreases cerebral blood flow, cerebral blood volume, and intracranial pressure. In patients with elevated intracranial pressure, propofol can cause a critical reduction in CPP (<50 mm Hg) unless steps are taken to support mean arterial blood pressure. Propofol and thiopental provide a comparable degree of cerebral protection during experimental focal ischemia. Unique to propofol are its antipruritic properties. Its antiemetic effects provide yet another reason for it to be a preferred drug for outpatient anesthesia. Induction is occasionally accompanied by excitatory phenomena such as muscle twitching, spontaneous movement, opisthotonus, or hiccupping. Propofol has anticonvulsant properties, has been used successfully to terminate status epilepticus, and may safely be administered to epileptic patients. Propofol decreases intraocular pressure. Tolerance does not develop after long-term propofol infusions. Propofol is an uncommon agent of physical dependence or addiction; however, anesthesia personnel, celebrities, and other medically untrained individuals have died while using propofol inappropriately to induce sleep in nonsurgical settings.

Drug Interactions

Many clinicians administer a small amount of midazolam (eg, 30 mcg/kg) prior to induction with propofol; midazolam can reduce the required propofol dose by more than 10%. Propofol is often combined with remifentanil, dexmedetomidine, or ketamine for TIVA.

FOSPROPOFOL

Fospropofol is a water-soluble prodrug that is metabolized in vivo to propofol, phosphate, and formaldehyde. It was released in the United States (2008) and other countries based on studies showing that it produces more complete amnesia and better conscious sedation for endoscopy than midazolam plus fentanyl. It has a slower onset and slower recovery than propofol, offering little reason for anesthesiologists to favor it over propofol. The place (if any) of fospropofol relative to other competing agents has not yet been established in clinical practice.

DEXMEDETOMIDINE

Dexmedetomidine is an α_2-adrenergic agonist similar to clonidine that can be used for anxiolysis, sedation, and analgesia. Strictly speaking, it is not an anesthetic in humans; however, anesthesiologists have used it in combination with other agents to produce anesthesia. It has also been used in combination with local anesthetics to prolong regional blocks.

Most commonly, dexmedetomidine is used for procedural sedation (eg, during awake craniotomy procedures or fiberoptic intubation), ICU sedation (eg, ventilated patients recovering from cardiac surgery), or as a supplement to general anesthesia to reduce the need for intraoperative opioids or to reduce the likelihood of emergence delirium (most often in children) after an inhalation anesthetic. It has also been used to treat alcohol withdrawal and the side effects of cocaine intoxication.

Absorption

This drug is approved only for intravenous injection. Typically, intravenous dexmedetomidine sedation in awake adults is initiated with a 1-mcg/kg loading dose given over 5 to 10 min followed by a maintenance infusion of 0.2 to 1.4 mcg/kg/h. This agent can be used for premedication by nasal (1–2 mcg/kg) or oral (2.5–4 mcg/kg) administration in children, where it compares very favorably with oral midazolam.

Distribution

Dexmedetomidine has very rapid redistribution (minutes) and a relatively short elimination half-life (less than 3 h).

Biotransformation

It is metabolized in the liver by the CYP450 system and through glucuronidation. It should be used with caution in patients with severe liver disease.

Excretion

Nearly all dexmedetomidine metabolites are excreted in the urine.

Effects on Organ Systems

A. Cardiovascular

In research subjects, a loading dose of dexmedetomidine produces a small, transient increase in blood pressure accompanied by reflex bradycardia. Intraoperative infusions of dexmedetomidine typically produce dose-dependent sympatholysis with reduced mean arterial pressure and heart rate. Thus, depending on dose and rate of administration, dexmedetomidine may produce hypertension, hypotension, or bradycardia in any patient. These side effects can be minimized by avoiding rapid bolus dosing.

B. Respiratory

Dexmedetomidine produces no respiratory depression, making it nearly ideal for sedation of patients being weaned from mechanical ventilation. This agent has also been used for sedation during awake tracheal intubations.

C. Cerebral

Dexmedetomidine produces dose-dependent sedation. It is an opioid-sparing agent that can greatly reduce the requirements for general anesthetic drugs. Dexmedetomidine is the agent of choice for sedation of patients undergoing awake craniotomies.

Drug Interactions

Dexmedetomidine may cause exaggerated bradycardia in patients receiving beta-blockers, so it should be dosed carefully in such patients. It will have an additive effect on sedative–hypnotic agents.

CASE DISCUSSION

Premedication of the Surgical Patient

An extremely anxious patient presents for outpatient surgery. The patient demands to be asleep before going to the operating room and does not want to remember anything.

What are the goals of administering preoperative medication?

Anxiety is a normal response to impending surgery. Diminishing anxiety is usually the main purpose for administering premedication. For many patients, the preoperative interview with the anesthesiologist allays fears more effectively than sedative drugs. Preoperative medications may also provide relief of preoperative pain or perioperative amnesia.

There may also be specific medical indications for certain preoperative medications: prophylaxis against postoperative nausea and vomiting ($5\text{-}HT_3$s) and against aspiration pneumonia (eg, nonparticulate antacids) or decreasing upper airway secretions (eg, anticholinergics). The goals of preoperative medication depend on many factors, including the health and emotional status of the patient, the proposed surgical procedure, and the anesthetic plan. For this reason, the choice of anesthetic premedication must be individualized and must follow a thorough preoperative evaluation.

Do all patients require preoperative medication?

Customary levels of preoperative anxiety do not harm most patients; therefore, preoperative sedation is not a requirement for all patients. Some patients dread intramuscular injections, and others find altered states of consciousness more unpleasant than anxiety. If the surgical procedure is brief, the effects of some sedatives may extend into the postoperative period and prolong recovery time. This is particularly troublesome for patients undergoing ambulatory surgery. Specific contraindications for sedative premedication include severe lung disease, hypovolemia, impending airway obstruction, increased intracranial pressure, and depressed baseline mental status. Premedication with sedative drugs should never be given before informed consent has been obtained.

Which patients are most likely to benefit from preoperative medication?

Some patients are quite anxious despite the preoperative interview. Separation of young children from their parents is often a traumatic ordeal for all concerned, particularly if children have undergone multiple prior surgeries. Medical conditions such as coronary artery disease or hypertension may be aggravated by psychological stress.

How does preoperative medication influence the induction of general anesthesia?

Some medications often given preoperatively (eg, opioids) decrease anesthetic requirements and can contribute to a smooth induction. However, intravenous administration of these medications just prior to induction is a more reliable method of achieving the same benefits.

What governs the choice among the preoperative medications commonly administered?

After the goals of premedication have been determined, the clinical effects of the agents dictate the choice. For instance, in a patient experiencing preoperative pain from a femoral fracture, the analgesic effects of an opioid (eg, fentanyl, morphine, hydromorphone) or ketamine will decrease the discomfort associated with transportation to the operating room and positioning on the operating room table. On the other hand, respiratory depression, orthostatic hypotension, and nausea and vomiting may result from opioid premedication.

Benzodiazepines relieve anxiety, often provide amnesia, and are relatively free of side effects; however, they are not analgesics. Diazepam and lorazepam are often administered orally. Intramuscular midazolam has a rapid onset and short duration, but intravenous midazolam has an even better pharmacokinetic profile.

Which factors must be considered in selecting the anesthetic premedication for this patient?

First, it must be made clear to the patient that in most centers, lack of necessary equipment and concern for patient safety preclude anesthesia from being induced in the preoperative holding room. Long-acting agents such as morphine or lorazepam are poor choices for an outpatient procedure. Diazepam can also affect mental function for several hours. In adults, one typically inserts an intravenous line in the preoperative holding area and titrates small doses of midazolam using slurred speech as an endpoint. At that time, the patient can be taken to the operating room. Vital signs—particularly respiratory rate—must be monitored.

SUGGESTED READINGS

Absalom AR, Glen JI, Zwart GJ, Schnider TW, Struys MM. Target-controlled infusion: a mature technology. *Anesth Analg*. 2016;122:70.

Mahmoud M, Mason KP. Dexmedetomidine: review, update, and future considerations of paediatric perioperative and periprocedural applications and limitations. *Br J Anaesth*. 2015;115:171.

Mirrakhimov AE, Voore P, Halytskyy O, Khan M, Ali AM. Propofol infusion syndrome in adults: a clinical update. *Crit Care Res Pract*. 2015;2015:260385.

Newport DJ, Carpenter LL, McDonald WM, et al; APA Council of Research Task Force on Novel Biomarkers and Treatments. Ketamine and other NMDA antagonists: early clinical trials and possible mechanisms in depression. *Am J Psychiatry*. 2015;172:950.

Peltoniemi MA, Hagelberg NM, Olkkola KT, Saari TI. Ketamine: a review of clinical pharmacokinetics and pharmacodynamics in anesthesia and pain therapy. *Clin Pharmacokinet*. 2016;55:1059.

Radvansky BM, Shah K, Parikh A, et al. Role of ketamine in acute postoperative pain management: a narrative review. *Biomed Res Int*. 2015;2015:749837.

Vanlersberghe C, Camu F. Etomidate and other non-barbiturates. *Handb Exp Pharmacol*. 2008;(182):267.

Vanlersberghe C, Camu F: Propofol. *Handb Exp Pharmacol*. 2008;(182):227.

Zhan Z, Wang X, Chen Q, Xiao Z, Zhang B. Comparative efficacy and side-effect profile of ketamine and esketamine in the treatment of unipolar and bipolar depression: protocol for a systematic review and network meta-analysis *BMJ Open*. 2021;11(2): e043457.

CHAPTER 10

Analgesic Agents

KEY CONCEPTS

1. The accumulation of morphine metabolites (morphine 3-glucuronide and morphine 6-glucuronide) in patients with kidney failure has been associated with narcosis and ventilatory depression.
2. Rapid administration of larger doses of opioids (particularly fentanyl, sufentanil, remifentanil, and alfentanil) can induce chest wall rigidity severe enough to make ventilation with bag and mask nearly impossible.
3. Prolonged dosing of opioids can produce "opioid-induced hyperalgesia," in which patients become more sensitive to painful stimuli. Infusion of large doses of (in particular) remifentanil during general anesthesia can produce acute tolerance, in which much larger than usual doses of opioids are required for postoperative analgesia.
4. The neuroendocrine stress response to surgery is measured in terms of the secretion of specific hormones, including catecholamines, antidiuretic hormone, and cortisol. Large doses of opioids inhibit the release of these hormones in response to surgery more completely than volatile anesthetics.
5. Aspirin is unique in that it irreversibly inhibits COX-1 by acetylating a serine residue in the enzyme. The irreversible nature of its inhibition underlies the nearly 1-week persistence of its clinical effects (eg, inhibition of platelet aggregation to normal) after drug discontinuation.

Regardless of how expertly surgical and anesthetic procedures are performed, appropriate use of analgesic drugs such as local anesthetics, opioids, ketamine, gabapentinoids, acetaminophen, and cyclooxygenase (COX) inhibitors can make the difference between a satisfied and an unsatisfied postoperative patient. Moreover, studies have shown that outcomes can be improved when analgesia is provided in a "multimodal" format (typically minimizing opioid use) as one part of a well-organized plan for enhanced recovery after surgery (ERAS; see Chapter 48).

OPIOIDS

Mechanisms of Action

Opioids bind to specific receptors located throughout the central nervous system, gastrointestinal tract, and other tissues. Three major opioid receptor types were first identified (Table 10–1): mu (μ, with subtypes μ_1 and μ_2), kappa (κ), and delta (δ). Additional opioid receptors include nociceptin and the opioid growth factor receptor (also known as *OGFR* or *zeta*). Sigma receptors are no longer

TABLE 10–1 Classification of opioid receptors.[1]

Receptor	Clinical Effect	Agonists
μ	Supraspinal analgesia (μ_1) Respiratory depression (μ_2) Physical dependence Muscle rigidity	Morphine Met-enkephalin[2] β-Endorphin[2] Fentanyl
κ	Sedation Spinal analgesia	Morphine Nalbuphine Butorphanol Dynorphin[2] Oxycodone
δ	Analgesia Behavioral Epileptogenic	Leu-enkephalin[2] β-Endorphin[2]
σ	Dysphoria Hallucinations Respiratory stimulation	Pentazocine Nalorphine Ketamine

[1]Note: The relationships among receptor, clinical effect, and agonist are more complex than indicated in this table. For example, pentazocine is an antagonist at μ receptors, a partial agonist at κ receptors, and an agonist at σ receptors.

[2]Endogenous opioid.

classified as opioid receptors because endogenous opioid peptides do not bind them. All opioid receptors couple to G proteins; the binding of an agonist to an opioid receptor typically causes membrane hyperpolarization. Acute opioid effects are mediated by inhibition of adenylate cyclase (reductions in intracellular cyclic adenosine monophosphate concentrations) and activation of phospholipase C. Opioids inhibit voltage-gated calcium channels and activate inwardly rectifying potassium channels. Opioid effects vary based on the duration of exposure, and opioid tolerance leads to changes in opioid responses.

Although opioids provide some degree of sedation and in some species can produce general anesthesia when given in large doses, they are principally used to provide analgesia. The clinical actions of opioids depend on which receptor is bound (and in the case of spinal and epidural administration of opioids, where the receptor is located in the spinal cord) and the binding affinity of the drug. Agonist–antagonists (eg, nalbuphine, nalorphine, butorphanol, buprenorphine) have less efficacy than full agonists (eg, fentanyl, morphine), and under some circumstances agonist–antagonists will antagonize the actions of full agonists. Pure opioid antagonists (eg, naloxone or naltrexone) are discussed in Chapter 17. Opioid compounds mimic endorphins, enkephalins, dynorphins, nociceptin, and endomorphins, endogenous peptides that bind to opioid receptors.

Opioid receptor activation inhibits the presynaptic release and postsynaptic response to excitatory neurotransmitters (eg, acetylcholine, substance P) released by nociceptive neurons. Transmission of pain impulses can be selectively modified at the level of the dorsal horn of the spinal cord with intrathecal or epidural administration of opioids. Opioid receptors also respond to systemically administered opioids. Modulation through a descending inhibitory pathway from the periaqueductal gray matter to the dorsal horn of the spinal cord may also play a role in opioid analgesia. Although opioids exert their greatest effect within the central nervous system, opioid receptors have also been identified on somatic and sympathetic peripheral nerves. Certain opioid side effects (eg, constipation) are the result of opioid binding to receptors in peripheral tissues (eg, the gastrointestinal tract), and there are now selective antagonists for opioid actions outside the central nervous system (alvimopan and methylnaltrexone). The clinical importance of opioid receptors on primary sensory nerves (if present) remains speculative, despite the persisting practice of compounding opioids in local anesthetic solutions applied to peripheral nerves.

Structure–Activity Relationships

A chemically diverse group of compounds binds opioid receptors. These agents have common structural characteristics, which are shown in Figure 10–1. Small molecular changes convert an agonist into an antagonist. The levorotatory opioid isomers are generally more potent than the dextrorotatory isomers.

Pharmacokinetics

A. Absorption

Rapid and complete absorption follows the intramuscular or subcutaneous injection of hydromorphone,

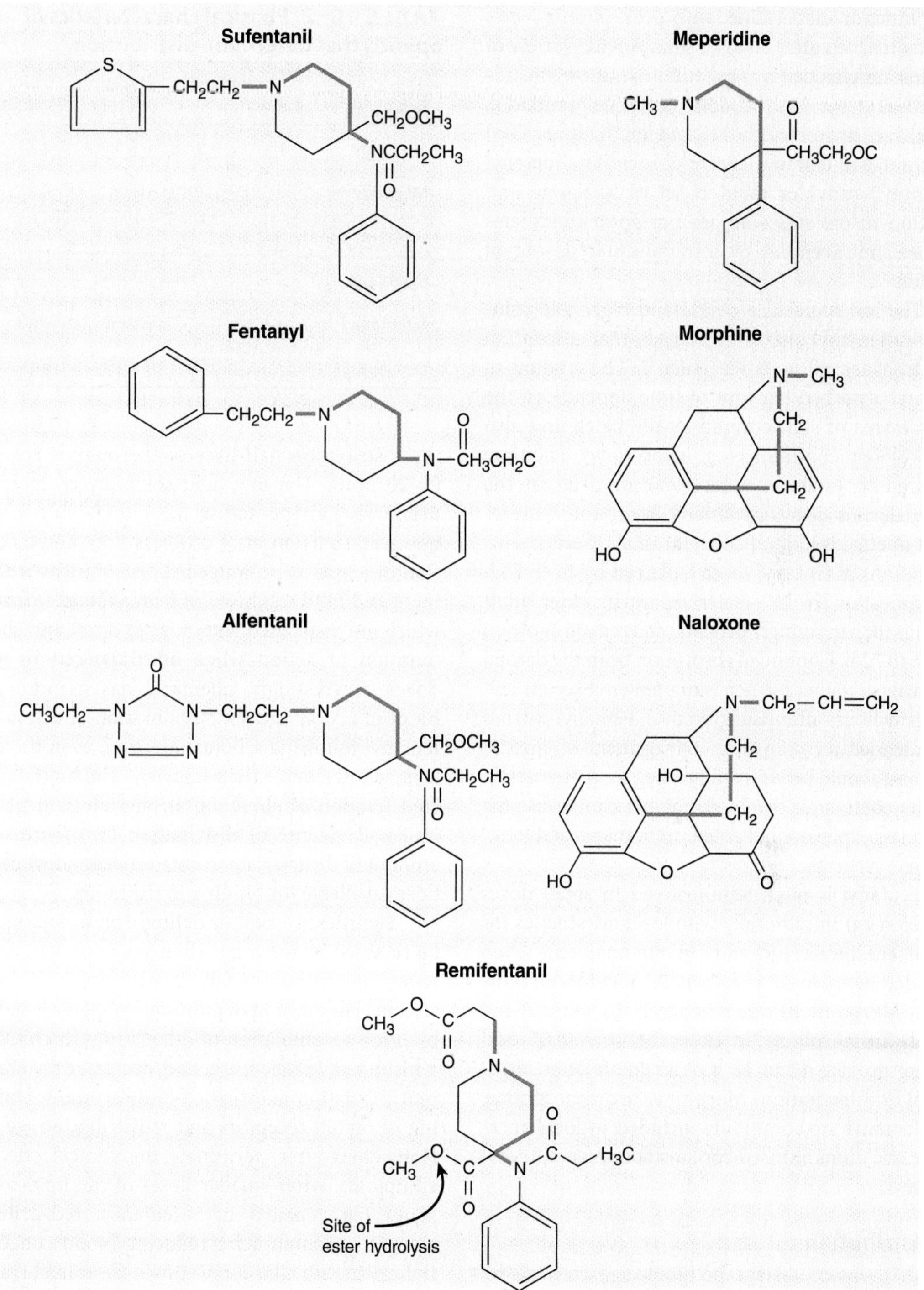

FIGURE 10–1 Opioid agonists and antagonists share part of their chemical structure, which is outlined in cyan.

morphine, or meperidine, with peak plasma levels usually reached after 20 to 60 min. A wide variety of opioids are effective by oral administration, including oxycodone, hydrocodone, codeine, tramadol, morphine, hydromorphone, and methadone. Oral transmucosal fentanyl citrate absorption (fentanyl "lollipop") provides rapid onset of analgesia and sedation in patients who are not good candidates for oral, intravenous, or intramuscular dosing of opioids.

The low molecular weight and high lipid solubility of fentanyl also favor transdermal absorption (the transdermal fentanyl "patch"). The amount of fentanyl absorbed per unit of time depends on the surface area of skin covered by the patch and also on local skin conditions (eg, blood flow). The time required to establish a reservoir of drug in the upper dermis delays by several hours the achievement of effective blood concentrations. Serum concentrations of fentanyl reach a plateau by 14 to 24 h of application (with greater delays in older adult patients than in younger patients) and remain constant for up to 72 h. Continued absorption from the dermal reservoir accounts for persisting fentanyl serum levels many hours after patch removal. Fentanyl patches are intended for outpatient management of chronic pain and should be reserved for the rare patients who require continuous opioid dosing but cannot use the much less expensive but equally efficacious and long-acting oral agents.

Fentanyl is often administered in small doses (10–25 mcg) intrathecally with local anesthetics for spinal anesthesia and adds to the analgesia when included with local anesthetics in epidural infusions. Morphine in doses between 0.1 and 0.5 mg and hydromorphone in doses between 0.05 and 0.2 mg provide 12 to 18 h of analgesia after intrathecal administration. Morphine, hydromorphone, and fentanyl are commonly included in local anesthetic solutions infused for postoperative epidural analgesia.

B. Distribution

Table 10–2 summarizes the physical characteristics that determine the distribution and tissue binding of opioid analgesics. After intravenous administration, the distribution half-lives of the opioids are short (5–20 min). The low lipid solubility of morphine delays its passage across the blood–brain barrier, however, so its onset of action is slow, and its duration of action is prolonged. This contrasts with the increased lipid solubility of fentanyl and sufentanil, which are associated with a faster onset and shorter duration of action **when administered in small doses**. Interestingly, alfentanil has a more rapid onset of action and shorter duration of action than fentanyl following a bolus injection, even though it is less lipid soluble than fentanyl. The high nonionized fraction of alfentanil at physiological pH and its small volume of distribution (V_d) increase the amount of drug (as a percentage of the administered dose) available for binding in the brain.

Significant amounts of lipid-soluble opioids can be retained by the lungs (first-pass uptake). As systemic concentrations fall, they return to the bloodstream. The amount of pulmonary uptake is reduced by prior accumulation of other drugs, increased by a history of tobacco use, and decreased by concurrent inhalation anesthetic administration. Unbinding of opioid receptors and redistribution (of drug from effect sites) terminate the clinical effects of all opioids. After smaller doses of the lipid-soluble drugs (eg, fentanyl or sufentanil), redistribution alone is paramount for reducing blood concentrations, whereas after larger doses, biotransformation becomes an important driver in reducing plasma levels below those that have clinical effects. The time

TABLE 10–2 Physical characteristics of opioids that determine distribution.[1]

Agent	Nonionized Fraction	Protein Binding	Lipid Solubility
Morphine	++	++	+
Meperidine	+	+++	++
Fentanyl	+	+++	++++
Sufentanil	++	++++	++++
Alfentanil	++++	++++	+++
Remifentanil	+++	+++	++

[1]+, very low; ++, low; +++, high; ++++, very high.

required for fentanyl or sufentanil concentrations to decrease by half (the "half-time") is *context sensitive;* the context-sensitive half-time increases as the total dose of drug or duration of exposure, or both, increase (see Chapter 7).

C. Biotransformation

With the exception of remifentanil, all opioids depend primarily on the liver for biotransformation. They are metabolized by the cytochrome P (CYP) system, conjugated in the liver, or both. Because of the high hepatic extraction ratio of opioids, their clearance depends on liver blood flow. Morphine and hydromorphone undergo conjugation with glucuronic acid to form, in the former case, morphine 3-glucuronide and morphine 6-glucuronide, and in the latter case, hydromorphone 3-glucuronide. Meperidine is *N*-demethylated to normeperidine, an active metabolite associated with seizure activity after very large meperidine doses. The end products of fentanyl, sufentanil, and alfentanil are inactive. Norfentanyl, the metabolite of fentanyl, can be measured in urine long after the native compound is no longer detectable in blood to determine chronic fentanyl ingestion. This has its greatest importance in diagnosing fentanyl abuse.

Codeine is a prodrug that becomes active after it is metabolized by CYP2D6 to morphine. Ultrarapid metabolizers of this drug (with genetic variants of CYP2D6) are subject to greater drug effects and side effects; slow metabolizers (including genetic variants and those exposed to inhibitors of CYP2D6 such as fluoxetine and bupropion) experience reduced efficacy of codeine. Similarly, tramadol must be metabolized by CYP to *O*-desmethyltramadol to be active. Hydrocodone is metabolized by CYP2D6 to hydromorphone (a more potent compound) and by CYP3A4 to norhydrocodone (a less potent compound). Oxycodone is metabolized by CYP2D6 and other enzymes to a series of active compounds that are less potent than the parent one.

The ester structure of remifentanil makes it susceptible to hydrolysis (in a manner similar to esmolol) by nonspecific esterases in red blood cells and tissue (see Figure 10–1), yielding a terminal elimination half-life of less than 10 min. Remifentanil

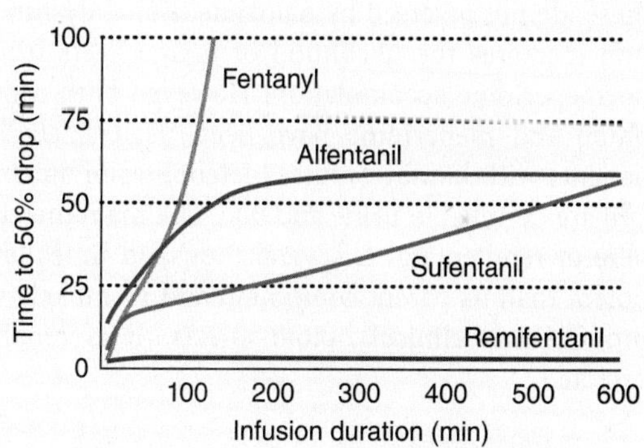

FIGURE 10–2 In contrast to other opioids, the time necessary to achieve a 50% decrease in the plasma concentration of remifentanil (its **half-time**) is very short and is not influenced by the duration of the infusion (it is not **context sensitive**). (Reproduced with permission from Egan TD. The pharmacokinetics of the new short-acting opioid remifentanil [GI87084B] in healthy adult male volunteers. *Anesthesiology.* 1993 Nov;79(5):881-892.)

biotransformation is rapid, and the duration of a remifentanil infusion has little effect on wake-up time (Figure 10–2). The half-time of remifentanil remains approximately 3 min regardless of the dose or duration of infusion. In its lack of accumulation (and lack of context sensitivity), remifentanil differs from other currently available opioids. Hepatic dysfunction requires no adjustment in remifentanil dosing. Finally, patients with pseudocholinesterase deficiency have a normal response to remifentanil (as also appears true for esmolol which is also metabolized by nonspecific esterases).

D. Excretion

The end products of morphine and meperidine biotransformation are eliminated by the kidneys, with less than 10% undergoing biliary excretion. Because 5% to 10% of morphine is excreted unchanged in the urine, kidney failure prolongs morphine duration of action. 1 The accumulation of morphine metabolites (morphine 3-glucuronide and morphine 6-glucuronide) in patients with kidney failure has been associated with prolonged narcosis and ventilatory depression. In fact, morphine 6-glucuronide is a more potent and longer-lasting opioid agonist than morphine. As previously noted, normeperidine at increased concentrations may produce seizures;

these are not reversed by naloxone. Renal dysfunction increases the likelihood of toxic effects from normeperidine accumulation. However, both morphine and meperidine have been used safely in patients with kidney failure. Metabolites of sufentanil are excreted in urine and bile. The main metabolite of remifentanil is several thousand times less potent than its parent compound and is unlikely to produce any clinical opioid effects. It is renally excreted.

Effects on Organ Systems

A. Cardiovascular

In general, opioids have minimal direct effects on the heart. Meperidine tends to increase heart rate (it is structurally similar to atropine and was originally synthesized as an atropine replacement), whereas larger doses of morphine, fentanyl, sufentanil, remifentanil, and alfentanil are associated with a vagus nerve–mediated bradycardia. Opioids do not depress cardiac contractility, provided they are administered alone (which is almost never the case in surgical anesthetic settings). Nonetheless, arterial blood pressure often falls as a result of opioid-induced bradycardia, venodilation, and decreased sympathetic reflexes. The inherent cardiac stability provided by opioids is greatly diminished in practice when other anesthetic drugs, including benzodiazepines, propofol, or volatile agents, are added. For example, sufentanil and fentanyl can be associated with reduced cardiac output when administered in combination with benzodiazepines. Bolus doses of meperidine, hydromorphone, and morphine evoke varying amounts of histamine release that can lead to profound drops in systemic vascular resistance and arterial blood pressure. The potential hazards of histamine release can be minimized by infusing opioids slowly or by pretreatment with H_1 and H_2 antagonists. Histamine side effects can be treated by infusion of intravenous fluid and vasopressors.

Intraoperative hypertension during opioid-based total intravenous or nitrous oxide–opioid anesthesia is common. Such hypertension is often attributed to inadequate anesthetic depth; thus, it is often treated by the addition of other anesthetic agents (benzodiazepines, propofol, or potent inhaled agents). When the depth of anesthesia is adequate, we recommend treating hypertension with antihypertensives rather than additional anesthetics.

B. Respiratory

Opioids depress ventilation, particularly respiratory rate. Thus, respiratory rate and end-tidal CO_2 tension (in contrast to arterial oxygen saturation) provide simple metrics for the early detection of respiratory depression in patients receiving opioid analgesia. Opioids increase the partial pressure of carbon dioxide ($PaCO_2$) and blunt the response to a CO_2 challenge, resulting in a shift of the CO_2 response curve downward and to the right (Figure 10–3). These effects result from opioid binding to neurons in the respiratory centers of the brainstem. **The apneic threshold—the greatest $PaCO_2$ at which a patient remains apneic—rises, and hypoxic drive is decreased**. Respiratory arrest from unintended opioid overdosage is an unfortunate cause of many deaths. Naloxone is increasingly being made available to the public for reversal of opioid-induced apnea outside of medical settings.

2 Morphine and meperidine can cause histamine-induced bronchospasm in susceptible patients. **Rapid administration of larger doses of opioids (particularly fentanyl, sufentanil, remifentanil, and alfentanil) can induce chest wall rigidity**

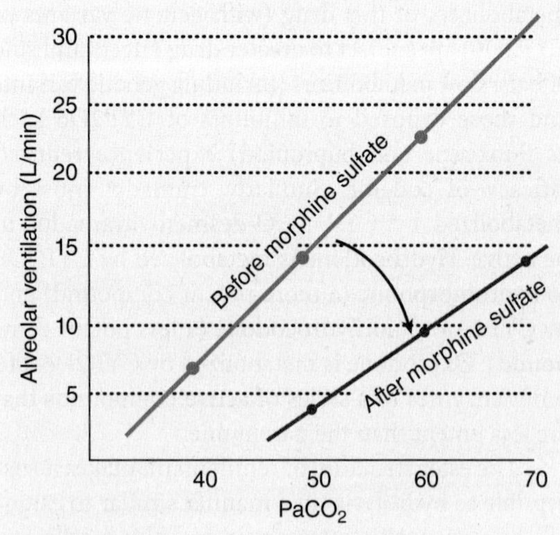

FIGURE 10–3 Opioids depress ventilation. This is graphically displayed by a shift of the carbon dioxide (CO_2) curve downward and to the right.

severe enough to make ventilation with bag and mask nearly impossible. This centrally mediated muscle contraction is effectively treated with neuromuscular blocking agents. This problem is much less frequent now that large-dose opioid anesthesia is no longer prevalent in cardiovascular anesthesia. Opioids can blunt the bronchoconstrictive response to airway stimulation, such as occurs during tracheal intubation.

C. Cerebral

The effects of opioids on cerebral perfusion and intracranial pressure must be separated from any effects of opioids on $PaCO_2$. In general, opioids reduce cerebral oxygen consumption, cerebral blood flow, cerebral blood volume, and intracranial pressure but to a much lesser extent than propofol, benzodiazepines, or barbiturates, provided normocarbia is maintained by artificial ventilation. There are some reports of mild—but transient and almost certainly unimportant—increases in cerebral artery blood flow velocity and intracranial pressure following opioid boluses in patients with brain tumors or head trauma. If combined with hypotension, the resulting fall in cerebral perfusion pressure *could* be deleterious to patients with abnormal intracranial pressure–volume relationships. Nevertheless, the important clinical message is that any trivial opioid-induced increase in intracranial pressure would be much less important than the predictably large increases in intracranial pressure associated with intubation of an inadequately anesthetized patient (from whom opioids were withheld). Opioids usually have almost no effects on the electroencephalogram (EEG), though large doses are associated with slow δ-wave activity. EEG activation and seizures have been associated with the meperidine metabolite normeperidine, as previously noted. Tramadol lowers the seizure threshold in susceptible patients.

Stimulation of the medullary chemoreceptor trigger zone is responsible for opioid-induced nausea and vomiting. Curiously, nausea and vomiting are more common following smaller (analgesic) than very large (anesthetic) doses of opioids. Repeated dosing of opioids (eg, prolonged oral dosing) will reliably produce tolerance, a phenomenon in which progressively larger doses are required to produce the same response. This is not the same as physical dependence or addiction, which may also be associated with repeated opioid administration.

3 Prolonged dosing of opioids can also produce "opioid-induced hyperalgesia," in which patients become more sensitive to painful stimuli. Infusion of large doses of (in particular) remifentanil during general anesthesia can produce acute tolerance, in which much larger than usual doses of opioids will be required for immediate, postoperative analgesia. Relatively large doses of opioids are required to render patients unconscious (Table 10–3). However, even at very large doses opioids will not reliably produce amnesia. The use of opioids in epidural and intrathecal spaces has revolutionized acute and chronic pain management (see Chapters 47 and 48).

Unique among the commonly used opioids, meperidine has minor local anesthetic qualities, particularly when administered into the subarachnoid space. Meperidine's clinical use as a local anesthetic has been limited by its relatively low potency and propensity to cause typical opioid side effects (nausea, sedation, pruritus) at the doses required to induce local anesthesia. **Intravenous meperidine (10–25 mg) is more effective than morphine or fentanyl for decreasing shivering in the postanesthetic care unit, and meperidine appears to be the best agent for this indication.**

D. Gastrointestinal

Opioids slow gastrointestinal motility by binding to opioid receptors in the gut and reducing peristalsis. Biliary colic may result from opioid-induced contraction of the sphincter of Oddi. Biliary spasm, which can mimic a common bile duct stone on cholangiography, is reversed with the opioid antagonist naloxone or by glucagon. Patients receiving long-term opioid therapy (eg, for cancer pain) usually become tolerant to many of the side effects but rarely to constipation. This is the basis for the development of the peripheral opioid antagonists methylnaltrexone, alvimopan, naloxegol, and naldemedine, which promote gastrointestinal motility in patients with varying indications, such as treatment of opioid bowel syndrome, side effects from opioid treatment of noncancer pain, or reduction of ileus in patients receiving intravenous opioids after abdominal surgery.

TABLE 10–3 Uses and doses of common opioids.

Agent	Use	Route[1]	Dose[2]
Morphine	Postoperative analgesia	IM IV	0.05–0.2 mg/kg 0.03–0.15 mg/kg
Hydromorphone	Postoperative analgesia	IM IV	0.02–0.04 mg/kg 0.01–0.02 mg/kg
Fentanyl	Intraoperative anesthesia Postoperative analgesia	IV IV	2–50 mcg/kg 0.5–1.5 mcg/kg
Sufentanil	Intraoperative anesthesia	IV	0.25–20 mcg/kg
Alfentanil	Intraoperative anesthesia Loading dose Maintenance infusion	IV IV	8–100 mcg/kg 0.5–3 mcg/kg/min
Remifentanil	Intraoperative anesthesia Loading dose Maintenance infusion Postoperative analgesia/sedation	IV IV IV	1 mcg/kg 0.05–2 mcg/kg/min 0.05–0.3 mcg/kg/min

[1]IM, intramuscular; IV, intravenous.

[2]Note: The wide range of opioid doses reflects a large therapeutic index and depends upon which other anesthetics are simultaneously administered. For obese patients, dose should be based on ideal body weight or lean body mass, not total body weight. Tolerance can develop rapidly (ie, within 2 h) during IV infusion of opioids, necessitating higher infusion rates. Dose correlates with other variables besides body weight that need to be considered (eg, age). The relative potencies of fentanyl, sufentanil, and alfentanil are estimated to be 1:9:1/7.

E. Endocrine

4 The neuroendocrine stress response to surgery is measured in terms of the secretion of specific hormones, including catecholamines, antidiuretic hormone, and cortisol. Large doses of fentanyl or sufentanil inhibit the release of these hormones in response to surgery more completely than volatile anesthetics. The actual clinical outcome benefit produced by attenuating the stress response with opioids, even in high-risk cardiac patients, remains speculative (and we suspect nonexistent), whereas the many drawbacks of excessive doses of opioids are readily apparent.

Other Effects

A. Cancer Reoccurrence

Retrospective studies have associated general anesthesia (including opioids) with an increased risk of cancer reoccurrence after surgery as compared to techniques that emphasize opioid-sparing regional anesthetic techniques for analgesia. Ongoing clinical trials will likely clarify whether general anesthesia, opioids, both, or neither influence outcomes after cancer surgery.

B. Substance Abuse

There is a well-publicized epidemic of opioid abuse in western democracies, particularly in the United States. Although it comprises less than 5% of the world's population, the United States consumes 80% of the world's prescription opioids (and nearly all of the world's supply of hydrocodone)! Large numbers of patients admit to using prescribed opioids in a recreational fashion, and drug overdosage (most often from prescribed drugs) is the leading cause of accidental death in the United States. Many opioid addicts trace their addiction to opioids prescribed by a physician. There are many causes of this terrible problem, including excessive and misleading marketing of opioids to physicians, unwise prescribing practices by physicians, inappropriate and misleading assertions by "thought leaders" (many with ties to the pharmaceutical industry) regarding opioids, and well-intended but poorly thought out recommendations for assessment and treatment of pain by certifying agencies. In response, the U.S. Centers for Disease Control and Prevention and many other agencies have released guidelines for responsible prescribing of opioids.

Drug Interactions

The combination of meperidine and monoamine oxidase inhibitors may result in hemodynamic instability, hyperpyrexia, coma, respiratory arrest, or death. The cause of this catastrophic interaction is incompletely understood. (The failure to appreciate this drug interaction by a resident physician in the controversial Libby Zion case led to changes in work hour rules for house officers in the United States.)

Propofol, barbiturates, benzodiazepines, inhaled anesthetics, and other central nervous system depressants can have synergistic cardiovascular, respiratory, and sedative effects with opioids.

The clearance of alfentanil may be impaired and the elimination half-life prolonged following treatment with erythromycin.

CYCLOOXYGENASE INHIBITORS

Mechanisms of Action

Many over-the-counter nonsteroidal anti-inflammatory agents (NSAIDs) work through inhibition of cyclooxygenase (COX), the key step in prostaglandin synthesis. COX catalyzes the production of prostaglandin H_1 from arachidonic acid. The two forms of the enzyme, COX-1 and COX-2, have differing distributions in tissue. COX-1 receptors are widely distributed throughout the body, including the gut and platelets. COX-2 is produced in response to inflammation.

COX-1 and COX-2 enzymes differ further in the size of their binding sites: the COX-2 site can accommodate larger molecules that are restricted from binding at the COX-1 site. This distinction is in part responsible for selective COX-2 inhibition. Agents that inhibit COX nonselectively (eg, ibuprofen) will control fever, inflammation, pain, and thrombosis. COX-2 selective agents (eg, celecoxib, etoricoxib) can be used perioperatively without concerns about platelet inhibition or gastrointestinal upset. Curiously, while COX-1 inhibition decreases thrombosis, selective COX-2 inhibition increases the risk of myocardial infarction, thrombosis, and stroke. All NSAIDs except low-dose aspirin increase the risk of stroke or myocardial infarction. Acetaminophen inhibits COX in the brain without binding to the active site of the enzyme (unlike NSAIDs) to produce its antipyretic activities. Acetaminophen analgesia may result from modulation of the endogenous cannabinoid vanilloid receptor systems in the brain, but the actual mechanism of action remains speculative. Acetaminophen has no major effects on COX outside the brain.

Aspirin, the first of the NSAIDs, was formerly used as an antipyretic and analgesic. Now it is used almost exclusively for the prevention of stroke or acute
5 myocardial infarction. Aspirin is unique in that it irreversibly inhibits COX-1 by acetylating a serine residue in the enzyme, resulting in a nearly 1-week persistence of its clinical effects (eg, inhibition of platelet aggregation) after drug discontinuation.

COX inhibitors are most often administered orally. Acetaminophen, ibuprofen, diclofenac, and ketorolac are available for intravenous administration. Unfortunately, intravenous acetaminophen has an acquisition cost that is several orders of magnitude greater than that of oral acetaminophen; therefore, its use is tightly restricted in many medical centers.

"Multimodal" analgesia typically includes the use of acetaminophen, COX inhibitors, possibly a gabapentinoid, regional or local anesthesia techniques, and other approaches aimed at improving the analgesia while reducing the requirement for opioids in postoperative patients. Multimodal analgesia protocols are best used as part of an enhanced recovery after surgery (ERAS) protocol, a topic that is extensively considered in Chapter 48.

Structure–Activity Relationships

The COX enzyme is inhibited by an unusually diverse group of compounds that can be grouped into salicylic acids (eg, aspirin), acetic acid derivatives (eg, ketorolac), propionic acid derivatives (eg, ibuprofen), heterocyclics (eg, celecoxib), and others. Thus, a conventional discussion of structure to potency (and other factors) is not useful for these chemicals, other than to note that the heterocyclics tend to be the compounds with the greatest selectivity for the COX-2 rather than COX-1 form of the enzyme.

Pharmacokinetics

A. Absorption

When taken orally, COX inhibitors will typically achieve their peak blood concentrations in less than 3 h. Some COX inhibitors are formulated for topical application (eg, as a gel to be applied over joints or liquid drops to be instilled on the eye). Ketorolac has been widely used as part of a local anesthetic "cocktail" to be injected around the surgical site and joint after arthroplasty.

B. Distribution

In blood, COX inhibitors are highly bound by plasma proteins, chiefly albumin. Their lipid solubility allows them to readily permeate the blood–brain barrier to produce central analgesia and antipyresis and penetrate joint spaces to produce (with the exception of acetaminophen) an anti-inflammatory effect.

C. Biotransformation

Most COX inhibitors undergo hepatic biotransformation. Acetaminophen at increased doses yields sufficiently large concentrations of *N*-acetyl-*p*-benzoquinone imine to produce hepatic failure.

D. Excretion

Nearly all COX inhibitors are excreted in urine after biotransformation.

Effects on Organ Systems

A. Cardiovascular

COX inhibitors do not act directly on the cardiovascular system. Any cardiovascular effects result from the actions of these agents on coagulation. Prostaglandins maintain the patency of the ductus arteriosus; thus, COX inhibitors have been administered to neonates to promote closure of a persistently patent ductus arteriosus, and prostaglandins have been infused to maintain patency of the ductus in neonates awaiting surgery for ductal-dependent congenital cardiac lesions.

B. Respiratory

At appropriate clinical doses, none of the COX inhibitors have effects on respiration or lung function. Aspirin overdosage has very complex effects on acid–base balance and respiration.

C. Gastrointestinal

The classic complication of COX-1 inhibition is gastrointestinal upset. In its most extreme form, this can cause upper gastrointestinal bleeding. Both complications result from direct actions of the drug, in the former case, on protective effects of prostaglandins in the mucosa, and in the latter case, on the combination of mucosal effects and inhibition of platelet aggregation.

Acetaminophen toxicity is a common cause of fulminant hepatic failure and the need for hepatic transplantation in western societies; it has replaced viral hepatitis as the most common cause of acute hepatic failure.

D. Renal

There is good evidence that NSAIDs, especially selective COX-2 inhibitors, adversely affect renal function in certain patients. Therefore, NSAIDs are generally avoided in patients with reduced creatinine clearance and in others who are dependent upon renal prostaglandin release for vasodilation to avoid hemodynamically mediated acute kidney injury (eg, patients with hypovolemia, heart failure, cirrhosis, diabetic nephropathy, or hypercalcemia).

GABAPENTIN & PREGABALIN

Gabapentin was introduced as an antiepileptic agent but was serendipitously discovered to have analgesic properties. It found its earliest applications in the treatment of chronic neuropathic pain and is now licensed for postherpetic neuralgia. It and the closely related compound pregabalin are also widely prescribed for diabetic neuropathy. These agents are widely used in the treatment of chronic neuropathic pain, and they are included in many multimodal postoperative pain protocols, particularly after total joint arthroplasty. There is no evidence that one agent is predictably more efficacious than the other. Although these agents have been shown to bind to voltage-gated calcium channels and *N*-methyl-D-aspartate (NMDA) receptors, their exact mechanism of action remains speculative. Despite the structural similarities these agents have to γ-aminobutyric acid (GABA), their clinical effects do not appear to arise from binding to GABA receptors or relate in any way to GABA.

When used for the treatment of chronic pain, these agents are generally started at relatively small doses and increased incrementally until side effects of dizziness or sedation appear. An adequate trial of gabapentin can require as much a month to achieve the optimal dosage. Determining the optimal dosage of the more potent pregabalin generally requires less time. When used as part of a multimodal postoperative pain protocol, these agents are generally prescribed in a standard dose that is maintained for the several days during which the protocol runs its course.

SUGGESTED READINGS

Azzam AAH, McDonald J, Lambert DG. Hot topics in opioid pharmacology: mixed and biased opioids. *Br J Anaesth.* 2019;122:e136.

Brunton LL, Knollmann BC, eds. *Goodman & Gilman's The Pharmacological Basis of Therapeutics.* 13th ed. McGraw-Hill; 2018: chaps 18, 34.

Hyland SJ, Brockhaus KK, Vincent et al. Perioperative pain management and opioid stewardship: a practical guide. *Healthcare* (Basel). 2021;9:333.

Jantarada C, Silva C, Guimarães-Pereira L. Prevalence of problematic use of opioids in patients with chronic noncancer pain: a systematic review with meta-analysis. *Pain Pract.* 2021;21:715.

Lee WM. Acetaminophen toxicity: a history of serendipity and unintended consequences. *Clin Liver Dis* (Hoboken). 2020;16(Suppl 1):34.

Rajput K, Vadivelu N. Acute pain management of chronic pain patients in ambulatory surgery centers. *Curr Pain Headache Rep.* 2021;25:1.

WEBSITES

CDC Guideline for Prescribing Opioids for Chronic Pain. http://www.cdc.gov/drugoverdose/prescribing/guideline.html

WHO Treatment Guidelines on Pain. http://www.who.int/medicines/areas/quality_safety/guide_on_pain/en/

American Pain Society Clinical Practice Guidelines. http://americanpainsociety.org/education/guidelines/overview

Practice Guidelines for Chronic Pain Management. https://www.asahq.org/quality-and-practice-management/standards-and-guidelines

Practice Guidelines for Acute Pain Management in the Perioperative Setting. https://www.asahq.org/quality-and-practice-management/standards-and-guidelines

CHAPTER

11

Neuromuscular Blocking Agents

KEY CONCEPTS

1. It is important to realize that muscle relaxation does not ensure unconsciousness, amnesia, or analgesia.
2. Depolarizing muscle relaxants act as acetylcholine (ACh) receptor agonists, whereas nondepolarizing muscle relaxants function as competitive antagonists.
3. Because depolarizing muscle relaxants are not metabolized by acetylcholinesterase, they diffuse away from the neuromuscular junction and are hydrolyzed in the plasma and liver by another enzyme, pseudocholinesterase (nonspecific cholinesterase, plasma cholinesterase, or butyrylcholinesterase).
4. Muscle relaxants owe their paralytic properties to mimicry of ACh. For example, succinylcholine consists of two joined ACh molecules.
5. In contrast to patients with low enzyme levels or heterozygous atypical enzyme in whom blockade duration is doubled or tripled, patients with homozygous atypical enzyme will have a very long blockade (eg, 4–8 h) following succinylcholine administration.
6. Succinylcholine is considered relatively contraindicated in the routine management of children and adolescents because of the risk of hyperkalemia, rhabdomyolysis, and cardiac arrest in children with undiagnosed myopathies.
7. Normal muscle releases enough potassium during succinylcholine-induced depolarization to raise serum potassium by 0.5 mEq/L. Although this is usually insignificant in patients with normal baseline potassium levels, a life-threatening potassium elevation is possible in patients with burn injury, massive trauma, neurological disorders, and several other conditions.
8. Pancuronium and vecuronium are partially excreted by the kidneys, and their action is prolonged in patients with kidney failure.
9. Cirrhotic liver disease and chronic kidney failure often result in an increased volume of distribution and a lower plasma concentration for a given dose of water-soluble drugs, such as muscle relaxants. On the other hand, drugs dependent on hepatic or renal excretion may demonstrate prolonged clearance. Thus, depending on the drug, a greater initial dose—but smaller maintenance doses—might be required in these diseases.
10. Atracurium and cisatracurium undergo degradation in plasma at physiological pH and temperature by organ-independent Hofmann elimination. The resulting metabolites (a monoquaternary acrylate and laudanosine) have no intrinsic neuromuscular blocking effects.

—Continued next page

Continued—

11 Hypertension and tachycardia may occur in patients given pancuronium. These cardiovascular effects are caused by the combination of vagal blockade and catecholamine release from adrenergic nerve endings.

12 After long-term administration of vecuronium to patients in intensive care units, prolonged neuromuscular blockade (up to several days) may be present after drug discontinuation, possibly from accumulation of its active 3-hydroxy metabolite, changing drug clearance, or the development of polyneuropathy.

13 Rocuronium (0.9–1.2 mg/kg) has an onset of action that approaches succinylcholine (60–90 s), making it a suitable alternative for rapid-sequence inductions, but at the cost of a much longer duration of action. The new reversal agent, sugammadex, permits rapid reversal of rocuronium-induced neuromuscular blockade.

Skeletal muscle relaxation can be produced by deep inhalational anesthesia, regional nerve block, or neuromuscular blocking agents (commonly called *muscle relaxants*). In 1942, Harold Griffith published the results of a study using an extract of curare (a South American arrow poison) during anesthesia. Following the introduction of succinylcholine as a "new approach to muscular relaxation," these agents rapidly became a routine part of the anesthesiologist's drug arsenal. However, as noted by Beecher and Todd in 1954: "[m]uscle relaxants given inappropriately may provide the surgeon with optimal [operating] conditions in … a patient [who] is paralyzed but not anesthetized—a state [that] is wholly unacceptable for the patient." In other words,
1 muscle relaxation does not ensure unconsciousness, amnesia, or analgesia. This chapter reviews the principles of neuromuscular transmission and presents the mechanisms of action, physical structures, routes of elimination, recommended dosages, and side effects of several muscle relaxants.

Neuromuscular Transmission

The association between a motor neuron and a muscle cell occurs at the neuromuscular junction (Figure 11–1). The cell membranes of the neuron and muscle fiber are separated by a narrow (20-nm) gap, the synaptic cleft. As a nerve's action potential depolarizes its terminal, an influx of calcium ions through voltage-gated calcium channels into the nerve cytoplasm allows storage vesicles to fuse with the terminal plasma membrane and release their contents (acetylcholine [ACh]). The ACh molecules diffuse across the synaptic cleft to bind with nicotinic cholinergic receptors on a specialized portion of the muscle membrane, the motor end-plate.

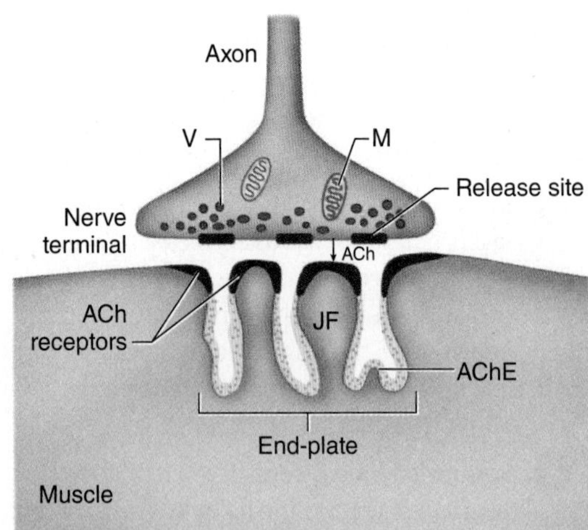

FIGURE 11–1 The neuromuscular junction. ACh, acetylcholine; AChE, acetylcholinesterase; JF, junctional folds; M, mitochondrion; V, transmitter vesicle. (Reproduced with permission from Drachman DB. Myasthenia gravis (1st of 2 parts), *N Engl J Med.* 1978 Jan 19;298(3):136-142.)

Each neuromuscular junction contains approximately 5 million of these receptors, but activation of only about 500,000 receptors is required for normal muscle contraction.

The structure of ACh receptors varies in different tissues and at different times in development. Each ACh receptor in the neuromuscular junction normally consists of five protein subunits: two α subunits, and single β, δ, and ε subunits. Only the two identical α subunits are capable of binding ACh molecules. If both binding sites are occupied by ACh, a conformational change in the subunits briefly (1 ms) opens an ion channel in the core of the receptor (Figure 11–2). The channel will not open if ACh binds to only one site. In contrast to the normal (or mature) junctional ACh receptor, another isoform contains a γ subunit instead of the ε subunit. This isoform is referred to as the fetal or immature receptor because it is in the form initially expressed in fetal muscle. It is also often referred to as *extrajunctional* because, unlike the mature isoform, it may be located anywhere in the muscle membrane, inside or outside the neuromuscular junction, when expressed in adults.

Cations flow through the open ACh receptor channel (sodium and calcium in; potassium out), generating an **end-plate potential**. The contents of a single vesicle, a quantum of ACh (10^4 molecules per quantum), produce a miniature end-plate potential. The number of quanta released by each depolarized

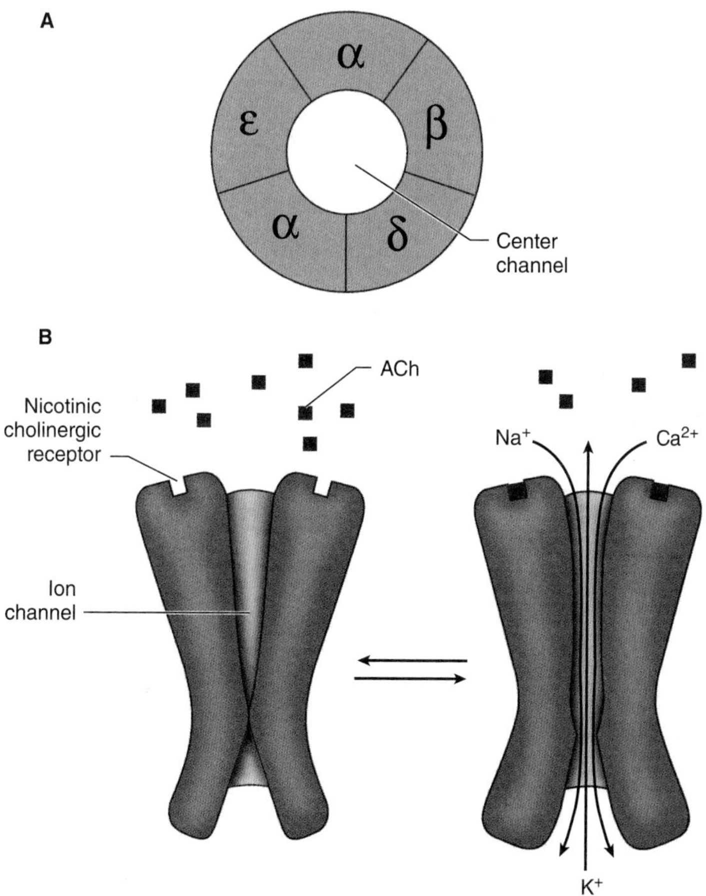

FIGURE 11–2 **A**: Structure of the ACh receptor. Note the two α subunits that actually bind ACh and the center channel. **B**: Binding of ACh to receptors on muscle end-plate causes channel opening and ion flux.

nerve fiber, normally at least 200, is very sensitive to extracellular ionized calcium concentration; increasing calcium concentration increases the number of quanta released. When sufficient receptors are occupied by ACh, the end-plate potential will be strong enough to depolarize the perijunctional membrane. Voltage-gated sodium channels within this portion of the muscle membrane open when a threshold voltage is developed across them, as is true for voltage-gated sodium channels in nerve or heart (Figure 11–3). Perijunctional areas of muscle membrane have a higher density of these sodium channels than other parts of the membrane. The resulting action potential propagates along the muscle membrane and T-tubule system, opening sodium channels and releasing calcium from the sarcoplasmic reticulum. This intracellular calcium allows the contractile proteins actin and myosin to interact, bringing about muscle contraction. The amount of ACh released and the number of receptors subsequently activated with efferent nerve depolarization will normally far exceed the minimum required for the initiation of an action potential in the muscle. The nearly tenfold margin of safety is reduced in Eaton–Lambert myasthenic syndrome (decreased release of ACh) and myasthenia gravis (decreased number of receptors).

ACh is rapidly hydrolyzed into acetate and choline by the substrate-specific enzyme **acetylcholinesterase**. This enzyme is embedded into the motor end-plate membrane immediately adjacent to the ACh receptors. After unbinding ACh, the receptors' ion channels close, permitting the end-plate to repolarize. Calcium is resequestered in the sarcoplasmic reticulum, and the muscle cell relaxes.

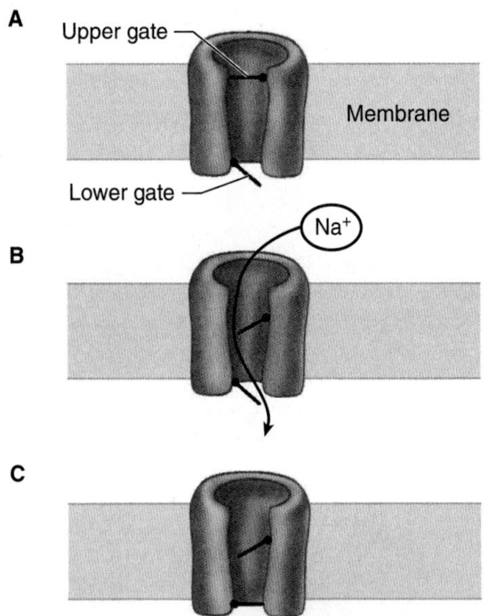

FIGURE 11–3 Schematic of the sodium channel. The sodium channel is a transmembrane protein that can be conceptualized as having two gates. Sodium ions pass only when both gates are open. Opening of the gates is time dependent and voltage dependent; therefore, the channel possesses three functional states. At rest, the lower gate is open, but the upper gate is closed (**A**). When the muscle membrane reaches threshold voltage depolarization, the upper gate opens, and sodium can pass (**B**). Shortly after the upper gate opens, the time-dependent lower gate closes (**C**). When the membrane repolarizes to its resting voltage, the upper gate closes, and the lower gate opens (**A**).

Distinctions Between Depolarizing & Nondepolarizing Blockade

Neuromuscular blocking agents are divided into two classes: depolarizing and nondepolarizing (Table 11–1). This division reflects distinct differences in the mechanism of action, response to peripheral nerve stimulation, and reversal of block.

TABLE 11–1 Depolarizing and nondepolarizing muscle relaxants.

Depolarizing	Nondepolarizing
Short-acting	Short-acting
Succinylcholine	Mivacurium
	Gantacurium[1]
	Intermediate-acting
	Atracurium
	Cisatracurium
	Vecuronium
	Rocuronium
	Long-acting
	Pancuronium

[1]Not yet commercially available in the United States.

MECHANISM OF ACTION

Similar to ACh, all neuromuscular blocking agents are quaternary ammonium compounds whose positively charged nitrogen imparts an affinity for nicotinic ACh receptors. Whereas most agents have two quaternary ammonium atoms, a few have one quaternary ammonium cation and one tertiary amine that is protonated at physiological pH.

Depolarizing muscle relaxants very closely resemble ACh and readily bind to ACh receptors, generating a muscle action potential. Unlike ACh, however, these drugs are *not* metabolized by acetylcholinesterase, and their concentration in the synaptic cleft does not fall as rapidly, resulting in a prolonged depolarization of the muscle end-plate.

Continuous end-plate depolarization causes muscle relaxation because the opening of perijunctional sodium channels is time limited (sodium channels rapidly "inactivate" with continuing depolarization; Figure 11–3). After the initial excitation and opening (Figure 11–3B), these sodium channels inactivate (Figure 11–3C) and cannot reopen until the end-plate repolarizes. The end-plate cannot repolarize as long as the depolarizing muscle relaxant continues to bind to ACh receptors; this is called a *phase I block*. More prolonged end-plate depolarization can cause poorly understood changes in the ACh receptor that result in a *phase II block*, which clinically resembles that of nondepolarizing muscle relaxants.

Nondepolarizing muscle relaxants bind ACh receptors but are incapable of inducing the conformational change necessary for ion channel opening. Because ACh is prevented from binding to its receptors, no end-plate potential develops. Neuromuscular blockade occurs even if only one α subunit is blocked.

Thus, depolarizing muscle relaxants act as ACh
2 receptor agonists, whereas nondepolarizing muscle relaxants function as competitive antagonists. This basic difference in mechanism of action explains their varying effects in certain disease states. For example, conditions associated with a chronic decrease in ACh release (eg, muscle denervation injuries) stimulate a compensatory increase in the number of ACh receptors within muscle membranes. These states also promote the expression of the immature (extrajunctional) isoform of the ACh receptor, which displays low channel conductance properties and prolonged open-channel time. This upregulation causes an exaggerated response to depolarizing muscle relaxants (with more receptors being depolarized) but a resistance to nondepolarizing relaxants (more receptors that must be blocked). In contrast, conditions associated with fewer ACh receptors (eg, downregulation in myasthenia gravis) demonstrate resistance to depolarizing relaxants and increased sensitivity to nondepolarizing relaxants.

OTHER MECHANISMS OF NEUROMUSCULAR BLOCKADE

Some drugs may interfere with the function of the ACh receptor without acting as an agonist or antagonist. They interfere with the normal functioning of the ACh receptor binding site or with the opening and closing of the receptor channel. These may include inhaled anesthetic agents, local anesthetics, and ketamine. The ACh receptor–lipid membrane interface may be an important site of action.

Drugs may also cause either closed or open channel blockade. During closed channel blockade, the drug physically plugs up the channel, preventing passage of cations whether or not ACh has activated the receptor. Open channel blockade is "use dependent" because the drug enters and obstructs the ACh receptor channel only after it is opened by ACh binding. The clinical relevance of open channel blockade is unknown. Based on laboratory experiments, one would expect that increasing the concentration of ACh with a cholinesterase inhibitor would not overcome this form of neuromuscular blockade. Drugs that may cause channel block under laboratory conditions include neostigmine, some antibiotics, cocaine and other local anesthetics, and quinidine. Other drugs may impair the presynaptic release of ACh. Prejunctional receptors play a role in mobilizing ACh to maintain muscle contraction.

Blocking these receptors can lead to a fading of the train-of-four response.

REVERSAL OF NEUROMUSCULAR BLOCKADE

3 Because succinylcholine is not metabolized by acetylcholinesterase, it unbinds the receptor and diffuses away from the neuromuscular junction to be hydrolyzed in the plasma and liver by another enzyme, pseudocholinesterase (nonspecific cholinesterase, plasma cholinesterase, or butyrylcholinesterase). Fortunately, this normally is a fairly rapid process because no specific agent to reverse a depolarizing blockade is available.

With the exception of mivacurium, nondepolarizing agents are not metabolized by either acetylcholinesterase or pseudocholinesterase. Reversal of their blockade depends on unbinding the receptor, redistribution, metabolism, and excretion of the relaxant by the body or administration of specific reversal agents (eg, cholinesterase inhibitors) that inhibit acetylcholinesterase enzyme activity. Because this inhibition increases the amount of ACh that is available at the neuromuscular junction and can compete with the nondepolarizing agent, the reversal agents clearly are of no benefit in reversing a phase I depolarizing block. In fact, by increasing neuromuscular junction ACh concentration and inhibiting pseudocholinesterase-induced metabolism of succinylcholine, *cholinesterase inhibitors can prolong neuromuscular blockade produced by succinylcholine.* The *only* time neostigmine reverses neuromuscular block after succinylcholine is when there is a phase II block (fade of the train-of-four) *and* sufficient time has passed for the circulating concentration of succinylcholine to be negligible.

Sugammadex, a cyclodextrin, is the first selective relaxant-binding agent; it exerts its reversal effect by forming tight complexes in a 1:1 ratio with steroidal nondepolarizing agents (vecuronium, rocuronium, and to a lesser extent, pancuronium). Investigational neuromuscular blocking agents such as gantacurium show promise as ultrashort-acting nondepolarizing agents.

RESPONSE TO PERIPHERAL NERVE STIMULATION

The use of peripheral nerve stimulators to monitor neuromuscular function is discussed in Chapter 6. Four patterns of electrical stimulation with supramaximal square-wave pulses are considered:

Tetany—a sustained stimulus of 50 to 100 Hz, usually lasting 5 s

Single twitch—a single pulse 0.2 ms in duration

Train-of-four—a series of four twitches in 2 s (2-Hz frequency), each 0.2 ms long

Double-burst stimulation (DBS)—three short (0.2 ms) high-frequency stimulations separated by a 20-ms interval (50 Hz) and followed 750 ms later by two ($DBS_{3,2}$) or three ($DBS_{3,3}$) additional impulses

The occurrence of fade, a gradual diminution of evoked response during prolonged or repeated nerve stimulation, is indicative of a nondepolarizing block (Figure 11–4) or a phase II block if only succinylcholine has been administered. Fade may be due to a prejunctional effect of nondepolarizing relaxants that reduces the amount of ACh in the nerve terminal available for release during stimulation (blockade of ACh mobilization). Adequate clinical recovery correlates well with the absence of fade. Because fade is more obvious during sustained tetanic stimulation or double-burst stimulation than following a train-of-four pattern or repeated twitches, the first two patterns are the preferred methods for determining the adequacy of recovery from a nondepolarizing block.

The ability of tetanic stimulation during a partial nondepolarizing block to increase the evoked response to a subsequent twitch is termed *posttetanic potentiation.* This phenomenon may relate to a transient increase in ACh mobilization following tetanic stimulation.

In contrast, a phase I depolarization block from succinylcholine does not exhibit fade during tetanus or train-of-four; neither does it demonstrate posttetanic potentiation. With prolonged exposure to succinylcholine, however, the quality of the block will sometimes change to resemble a nondepolarizing block (phase II block).

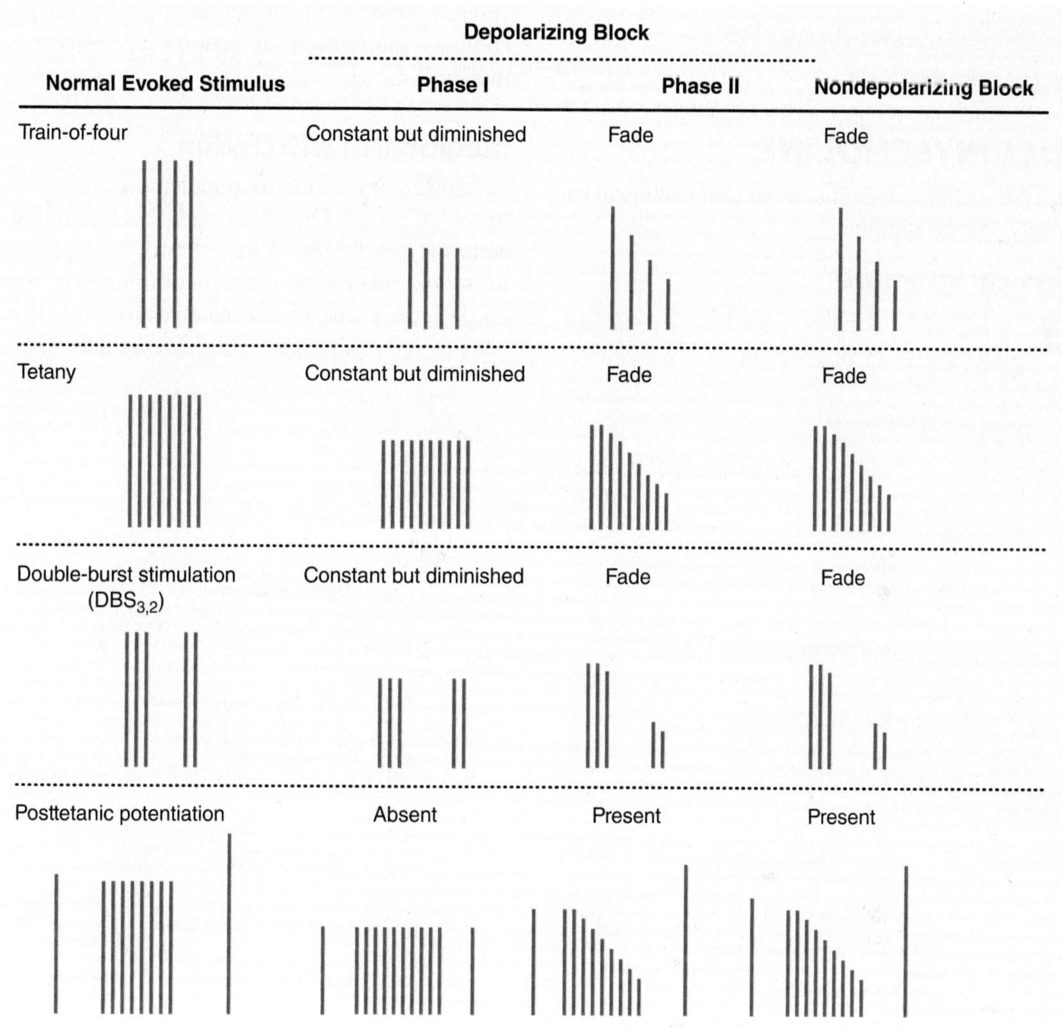

FIGURE 11–4 Evoked responses during depolarizing (phase I and phase II) and nondepolarizing block.

Newer quantitative methods of assessment of neuromuscular blockade, such as acceleromyography, permit the determination of exact train-of-four ratios as opposed to subjective interpretations. Acceleromyography and other objective measures of neuromuscular blockade may reduce the incidence of unexpected postoperative residual neuromuscular blockade. Other technologies have been developed to assess the degree of neuromuscular blockade objectively. A 2018 consensus statement on perioperative use of neuromuscular monitoring recommends objective monitoring and documentation of a train-of-four ratio of greater than or equal to 0.90 as the only monitor that indicates safe recovery from neuromuscular blockade. Residual neuromuscular blockade increases the rate of postoperative intensive care unit admission. Consequently, objective monitoring of the degree of neuromuscular blockade is recommended. Nonetheless, clinicians still employ subjective measures such as head lift and grip strength to assess the return of muscle strength, even though these measures are insensitive assessments.

Depolarizing Muscle Relaxants

SUCCINYLCHOLINE

The only depolarizing muscle relaxant in clinical use today is succinylcholine.

Physical Structure

Succinylcholine—also called suxamethonium—consists of two joined ACh molecules (Figure 11–5). This structure underlies succinylcholine's mechanism of action, side effects, and metabolism.

Metabolism & Excretion

Succinylcholine remains popular due to its rapid onset of action (30–60 s) and short duration of action (typically less than 10 min). Its rapid onset of action relative to other neuromuscular blockers is largely due to the relative overdose that is usually administered. Succinylcholine, like all

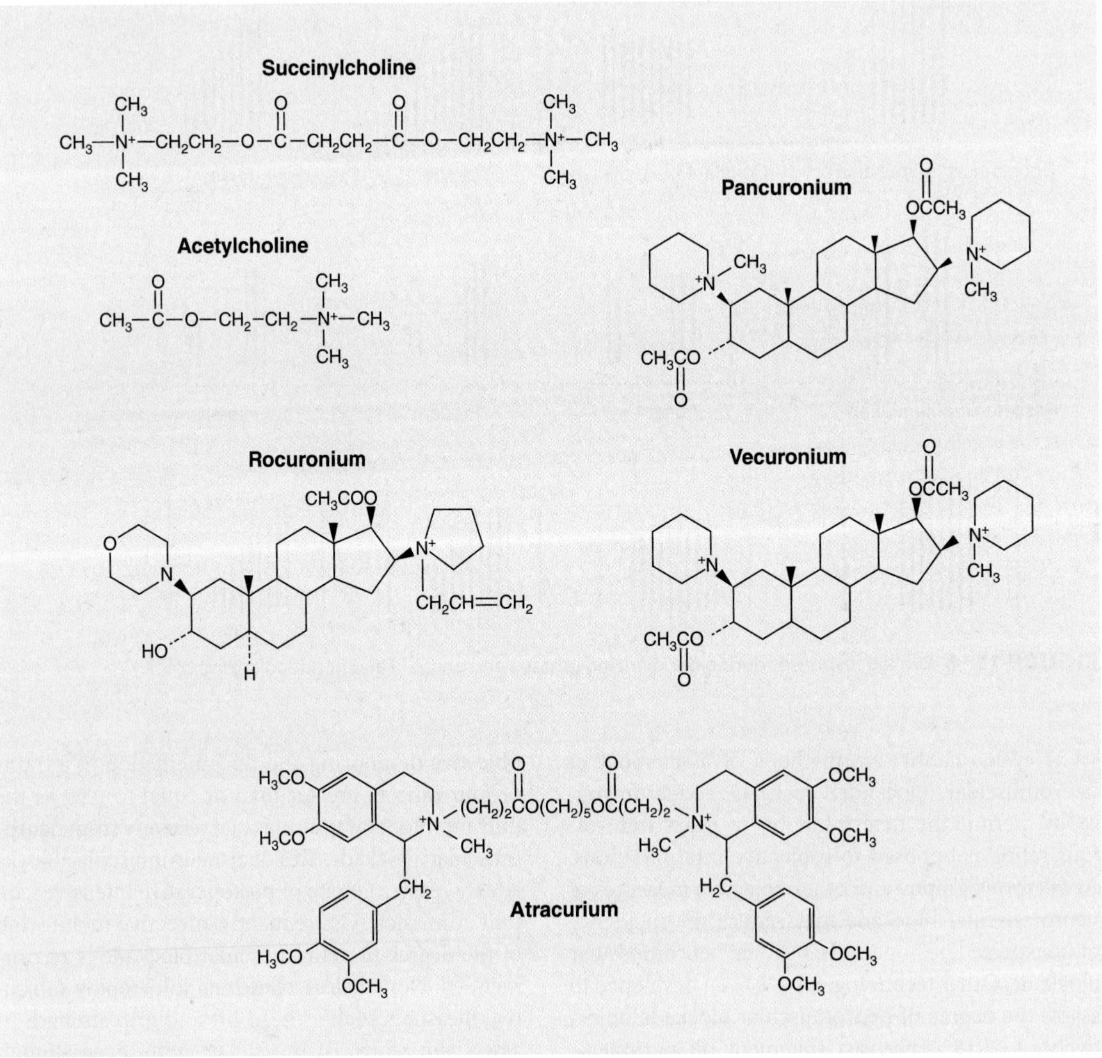

FIGURE 11–5 Chemical structures of neuromuscular blocking agents.

neuromuscular blockers, has a small volume of distribution due to its very low lipid solubility, and this also underlies a rapid onset of action. As succinyl choline enters the circulation, most of it is rapidly metabolized by pseudocholinesterase into succinylmonocholine. This process is so efficient that only a small fraction of the injected dose ever reaches the neuromuscular junction. As drug levels fall in blood, succinylcholine molecules diffuse away from the neuromuscular junction, limiting the duration of action. However, this duration of action can be prolonged by high doses, infusion of succinylcholine, or abnormal metabolism. The latter may result from hypothermia, reduced pseudocholinesterase levels, or a genetically aberrant enzyme. Hypothermia decreases the rate of hydrolysis. Reduced levels of pseudocholinesterase accompany pregnancy, liver disease, kidney failure, and certain drug therapies (Table 11–2). Reduced pseudocholinesterase levels generally produce only modest prolongation of succinylcholine's actions (2–20 min).

Heterozygote patients with one normal and one abnormal (atypical) pseudocholinesterase gene may have slightly prolonged block (20–30 min) following succinylcholine administration. Far fewer (1 in 3000) patients have two copies of the most prevalent abnormal gene (homozygous atypical) that produce an enzyme with little or no affinity for succinylcholine. 5 In contrast to the doubling or tripling of blockade duration seen in patients with low enzyme levels or heterozygous atypical enzyme, patients with homozygous atypical enzyme will have a *very* long blockade (eg, 4–8 h) following administration of succinylcholine. Of the recognized abnormal pseudocholinesterase genes, the dibucaine-resistant (variant) allele, which produces an enzyme that has one-hundredth the normal affinity for succinylcholine, is the most common. Other variants include fluoride-resistant and silent (no activity) alleles.

TABLE 11–2 Drugs known to decrease pseudocholinesterase activity.

Drug	Description
Echothiophate	Organophosphate use for glaucoma
Neostigmine Pyridostigmine	Cholinesterase inhibitors
Phenelzine	Monoamine oxidase inhibitor
Cyclophosphamide	Antineoplastic agent
Metoclopramide	Antiemetic/prokinetic agent
Esmolol	β-Blocker
Pancuronium	Nondepolarizing muscle relaxant
Oral contraceptives	Various agents

Dibucaine, a local anesthetic, inhibits normal pseudocholinesterase activity by 80% but inhibits atypical enzyme activity by only 20%. Serum from an individual who is heterozygous for the atypical enzyme is characterized by an intermediate 40% to 60% inhibition. The percentage of inhibition of pseudocholinesterase activity is termed the dibucaine number. A patient with normal pseudocholinesterase has a dibucaine number of 80; a homozygote for the most common abnormal allele will have a dibucaine number of 20. The dibucaine number measures pseudocholinesterase function, not the amount of enzyme. Therefore, the adequacy of pseudocholinesterase can be determined in the laboratory quantitatively in units per liter (a minor factor) and qualitatively by dibucaine number (the major factor). **Prolonged paralysis from succinylcholine caused by abnormal pseudocholinesterase (atypical cholinesterase) should be treated with continued mechanical ventilation and sedation until muscle function returns to normal by clinical signs.**

Drug Interactions

The effects of muscle relaxants can be modified by concurrent drug therapy (Table 11–3). Succinylcholine is involved in two interactions deserving special comment.

A. Cholinesterase Inhibitors

Although cholinesterase inhibitors reverse nondepolarizing paralysis, they markedly prolong a depolarizing phase I block by two mechanisms. By inhibiting acetylcholinesterase, they lead to a

TABLE 11–3 Potentiation (+) and resistance (–) of neuromuscular blocking agents by other drugs.

Drug	Effect on Depolarizing Blockade[1]	Effect on Nondepolarizing Blockade	Comments
Antibiotics	+	+	Streptomycin, aminoglycosides, kanamycin, neomycin, colistin, polymyxin, tetracycline, lincomycin, clindamycin
Anticonvulsants	?	–	Phenytoin, carbamazepine, primidone, sodium valproate
Antiarrhythmics	+	+	Quinidine, calcium channel blockers
Cholinesterase inhibitors	+	–	Neostigmine, pyridostigmine
Dantrolene	?	+	Used in treatment of malignant hyperthermia (has quaternary ammonium group)
Inhalational anesthetics	+	+	Volatile anesthetics
Ketamine	?	+	
Local anesthetics	+	+	High doses only
Lithium carbonate	+	?	Prolongs onset and duration of succinylcholine
Magnesium sulfate	+	+	Doses used to treat preeclampsia and eclampsia of pregnancy

[1]?, unknown effect.

higher ACh concentration at the nerve terminal, which intensifies depolarization. They also reduce the hydrolysis of succinylcholine by inhibiting pseudocholinesterase. Organophosphate pesticides, for example, cause an irreversible inhibition of acetylcholinesterase and can prolong the action of succinylcholine by 20 to 30 min. Echothiophate eye drops, used in the past for glaucoma, can markedly prolong succinylcholine by this mechanism.

B. Nondepolarizing Relaxants

In general, small doses of nondepolarizing relaxants antagonize a depolarizing phase I block. Because the drugs occupy some ACh receptors, depolarization by succinylcholine is partially prevented. In the presence of a phase II block, a nondepolarizer will potentiate succinylcholine paralysis.

Dosage

Because of the rapid onset, short duration, and low cost of succinylcholine, some clinicians believe that it remains a good choice for routine intubation in adults. The usual adult dose of succinylcholine for intubation is 1 to 1.5 mg/kg intravenously. Doses as small as 0.5 mg/kg usually provide acceptable intubating conditions if a defasciculating dose of a nondepolarizing agent is not used. Repeated small boluses (5–10 mg) or a succinylcholine drip (1 g in 500 or 1000 mL, titrated to effect) can be used during surgical procedures that require brief but intense paralysis (eg, otolaryngological endoscopies). Neuromuscular function should be frequently monitored with a nerve stimulator to prevent overdosing and to watch for phase II block. The availability of intermediate-acting nondepolarizing muscle relaxants has reduced the popularity of succinylcholine infusions. In the past, succinylcholine infusions were a mainstay of ambulatory practice in the United States.

Because succinylcholine is not lipid soluble, it has a small volume of distribution. Per kilogram, infants and neonates have a larger extracellular space than adults. Therefore, on a per-kilogram basis, dosage requirements for pediatric patients are often greater than for adults. If succinylcholine is administered *intramuscularly* to children, a dose as high as 4 to 5 mg/kg does not always produce complete paralysis.

Succinylcholine should be stored under refrigeration (2–8°C) and should generally be used within 14 days after removal from refrigeration and exposure to room temperature.

Side Effects & Clinical Considerations

Succinylcholine is a relatively safe drug—assuming that its many potential complications are under-
6 stood and avoided. Because of the risk of hyperkalemia, rhabdomyolysis, and cardiac arrest in children with undiagnosed myopathies, succinylcholine is considered relatively contraindicated in the routine management of children. Some clinicians have also abandoned the routine use of succinylcholine for adults. Succinylcholine is still useful for rapid sequence induction and for short periods of intense paralysis because none of the presently available nondepolarizing muscle relaxants can match its very rapid onset and short duration. Recent studies have compared succinylcholine and rocuronium for rapid sequence intubation and concluded that succinylcholine may offer slightly improved conditions for intubation. Nonetheless, rocuronium is increasingly employed to facilitate intubation in place of succinylcholine.

A. Cardiovascular

Because of the resemblance of muscle relaxants to ACh, it is not surprising that they affect cholinergic receptors in addition to those at the neuromuscular junction. The entire parasympathetic nervous system and parts of the sympathetic nervous system (sympathetic ganglions, adrenal medulla, and sweat glands) depend on ACh as a neurotransmitter.

Succinylcholine not only stimulates nicotinic cholinergic receptors at the neuromuscular junction, it also stimulates all ACh receptors. The cardiovascular actions of succinylcholine are therefore very complex. Stimulation of nicotinic receptors in parasympathetic and sympathetic ganglia and muscarinic receptors in the sinoatrial node of the heart can increase or decrease blood pressure and heart rate. Low doses of succinylcholine can produce negative chronotropic and inotropic effects, but higher doses usually increase heart rate and contractility and elevate circulating catecholamine levels. In most patients, the hemodynamic consequences are inconsequential in comparison to the effects of the induction agent and laryngoscopy.

Children are particularly susceptible to profound bradycardia following administration of succinylcholine. Bradycardia will sometimes occur in adults when a second bolus of succinylcholine is administered approximately 3 to 8 min after the first dose. The dogma (based on no real evidence) is that the succinylcholine metabolite, succinylmonocholine, sensitizes muscarinic cholinergic receptors in the sinoatrial node to the second dose of succinylcholine, resulting in bradycardia. Intravenous atropine (0.02 mg/kg in children, 0.4 mg in adults) is normally given prophylactically to children prior to the first and subsequent doses and *usually* before a second dose of succinylcholine is given to adults. Other arrhythmias, such as nodal bradycardia and ventricular ectopy, have been reported.

B. Fasciculations

The onset of paralysis by succinylcholine is usually signaled by visible motor unit contractions called *fasciculations*. These can be prevented by pretreatment with a small dose of nondepolarizing relaxant. Because this pretreatment usually antagonizes a depolarizing block, a larger dose of succinylcholine is required (1.5 mg/kg). Fasciculations are typically not observed in young children and older adult patients.

C. Hyperkalemia

7 Normal muscle releases enough potassium during succinylcholine-induced depolarization to increase serum potassium by 0.5 mEq/L. Although this is usually insignificant in patients with normal baseline potassium levels, it can be life-threatening in patients with preexisting hyperkalemia. The increase in potassium in patients with burn injury, massive trauma, neurological disorders, and several other conditions (Table 11–4) can be large and catastrophic. Hyperkalemic cardiac arrest can prove to be quite refractory to routine cardiopulmonary resuscitation, requiring calcium, insulin, glucose, bicarbonate, and even cardiopulmonary bypass to support the circulation while reducing serum potassium levels.

TABLE 11–4 Conditions causing susceptibility to succinylcholine-induced hyperkalemia.

Burn injury
Massive trauma
Severe intraabdominal infection
Spinal cord injury
Encephalitis
Stroke
Guillain–Barré syndrome
Severe Parkinson disease
Tetanus
Prolonged total body immobilization
Ruptured cerebral aneurysm
Polyneuropathy
Closed head injury
Hemorrhagic shock with metabolic acidosis
Myopathies (eg, Duchenne dystrophy)

Following denervation injuries (spinal cord injuries, larger burns), the immature isoform of the ACh receptor may be expressed inside and outside the neuromuscular junction (upregulation). These extrajunctional receptors allow succinylcholine to effect widespread depolarization and extensive potassium release. Life-threatening potassium release is *not* reliably prevented by pretreatment with a nondepolarizer. The risk of hyperkalemia usually seems to peak in 7 to 10 days following the injury, but the exact time of onset and the duration of the risk period vary. The risk of hyperkalemia from succinylcholine is minimal in the first 2 days after spinal cord or burn injury.

D. Muscle Pains

Patients who have received succinylcholine have an increased incidence of postoperative myalgia. The efficacy of nondepolarizing pretreatment is controversial. Administration of rocuronium (0.06–0.1 mg/kg) prior to succinylcholine has been reported to be effective in preventing fasciculations and reducing postoperative myalgias. The relationship between fasciculations and postoperative myalgia is also inconsistent. Myalgia is theorized to be due to the initial unsynchronized contraction of muscle groups; myoglobinemia and increases in serum creatine kinase can be detected following administration of succinylcholine. Perioperative use of nonsteroidal anti-inflammatory drugs and benzodiazepines may reduce the incidence and severity of myalgia.

E. Intragastric Pressure Elevation

Abdominal wall muscle fasciculations increase intragastric pressure, which is offset by an increase in lower esophageal sphincter tone. Therefore, despite being much discussed, there is no evidence that the risk of gastric reflux or pulmonary aspiration is increased by succinylcholine.

F. Intraocular Pressure Elevation

Extraocular muscle differs from other striated muscle in that it has multiple motor end-plates on each cell. Prolonged membrane depolarization and contraction of extraocular muscles following administration of succinylcholine transiently raises intraocular pressure and theoretically could compromise an injured eye. However, there is no evidence that succinylcholine leads to a worsened outcome in patients with "open" eye injuries. The elevation in intraocular pressure is not always prevented by pretreatment with a nondepolarizing agent.

G. Masseter Muscle Rigidity

Succinylcholine transiently increases muscle tone in the masseter muscles. Some difficulty may initially be encountered in opening the mouth because of incomplete relaxation of the jaw. A marked increase in tone preventing laryngoscopy is abnormal and can be a premonitory sign of malignant hyperthermia.

H. Malignant Hyperthermia

Succinylcholine is a potent triggering agent in patients susceptible to malignant hyperthermia, a hypermetabolic disorder of skeletal muscle (see Chapter 52). Although some of the signs and symptoms of neuroleptic malignant syndrome (NMS) resemble those of malignant hyperthermia, the pathogenesis is completely different, and there is no need to avoid the use of succinylcholine in patients with NMS.

I. Generalized Contractions

Patients afflicted with myotonia may develop myoclonus after administration of succinylcholine.

J. Prolonged Paralysis

As previously discussed, patients with reduced levels of normal pseudocholinesterase may have a longer than normal duration of action, whereas patients with atypical pseudocholinesterase will experience markedly prolonged paralysis.

K. Intracranial Pressure

Succinylcholine may lead to an activation of the electroencephalogram and slight increases in cerebral blood flow and intracranial pressure in some patients. Muscle fasciculations stimulate muscle stretch receptors, which subsequently increase cerebral activity. The increase in intracranial pressure can be attenuated by maintaining good airway control and instituting hyperventilation. It can also be prevented by pretreating with a nondepolarizing muscle relaxant and administering intravenous lidocaine (1.5–2.0 mg/kg) 2 to 3 min prior to intubation. The effects of intubation on intracranial pressure far outweigh any increase caused by succinylcholine, and succinylcholine is *not* contraindicated for rapid sequence induction of patients with intracranial mass lesions or other causes of increased intracranial pressure.

L. Histamine Release

Slight histamine release may be observed following succinylcholine in some patients.

Nondepolarizing Muscle Relaxants

Unique Pharmacological Characteristics

In contrast to there being only a single depolarizing muscle relaxant, there is a wide selection of nondepolarizing muscle relaxants (Tables 11–5 and 11–6). Based on their chemical structure, they can be classified as benzylisoquinolinium, steroidal, or other compounds. It is often said that the choice of a particular drug depends on its unique characteristics, which are often related to its structure; however, for most patients, the differences among the intermediate-acting neuromuscular blockers are inconsequential. Steroidal compounds can be vagolytic, most notably pancuronium but inconsequentially with vecuronium or rocuronium. Benzylisoquinolines tend to release histamine. Because of structural similarities, an allergic history to one muscle relaxant strongly suggests the possibility of allergic reactions to other muscle relaxants, particularly those in the same chemical class.

A. Suitability for Intubation

None of the currently available nondepolarizing muscle relaxants equals succinylcholine's rapid onset of action or short duration. However, the onset of

TABLE 11–5 A summary of the pharmacology of nondepolarizing muscle relaxants.

Relaxant	Chemical Structure[1]	Metabolism	Primary Excretion	Onset[2]	Duration[3]	Histamine Release[4]	Vagal Blockade[5]
Atracurium	B	+++	Insignificant	++	++	+	0
Cisatracurium	B	+++	Insignificant	++	++	0	0
Pancuronium	S	+	Renal	++	+++	0	++
Vecuronium	S	+	Biliary	++	++	0	0
Rocuronium	S	Insignificant	Biliary	+++	++	0	+
Gantacurium	C	+++	Insignificant	+++	+	+	0

[1]B, benzylisoquinolone; S, steroidal; C, chlorofumarate.

[2]Onset: +, slow; ++, moderately rapid; +++, rapid.

[3]Duration: +, short; ++, intermediate; +++, long.

[4]Histamine release: 0, no effect; +, slight effect; ++, moderate effect; +++, marked effect.

[5]Vagal blockade: 0, no effect; +, slight effect; ++, moderate effect.

TABLE 11–6 Clinical characteristics of nondepolarizing muscle relaxants.

Drug	ED_{95} for Adductor Pollicis During Nitrous Oxide/Oxygen/Intravenous Anesthesia (mg/kg)	Intubation Dose (mg/kg)	Onset of Action for Intubating Dose (min)	Duration of Intubating Dose (min)	Maintenance Dosing by Boluses (mg/kg)	Maintenance Dosing by Infusion (mcg/kg/min)
Succinylcholine	0.5	1.0	0.5	5–10	0.15	2–15 mg/min
Gantacurium[1]	0.19	0.2	1–2	4–10	N/A	—
Rocuronium	0.3	0.8	1.5	35–75	0.15	9–12
Mivacurium	0.08	0.2	2.5–3.0	15–20	0.05	4–15
Atracurium	0.2	0.5	2.5–3.0	30–45	0.1	5–12
Cisatracurium	0.05	0.2	2.0–3.0	40–75	0.02	1–2
Vecuronium	0.05	0.12	2.0–3.0	45–90	0.01	1–2
Pancuronium	0.07	0.12	2.0–3.0	60–120	0.01	—

[1]Not commercially available in the United States.

nondepolarizing relaxants can be quickened by using either a larger dose or a priming dose. The ED_{95} of any drug is the effective dose of a drug in 95% of individuals. For neuromuscular blockers, one often specifies the dose that produces 95% twitch depression in 50% of individuals. One to two times the ED_{95} or twice the dose that produces 95% twitch depression is usually used for intubation. Although a larger intubating dose speeds onset, it prolongs the duration of blockade. The availability of sugammadex has largely eliminated this concern in regard to the steroidal nondepolarizing muscle relaxants rocuronium and vecuronium (see Chapter 12).

Muscle groups vary in their sensitivity to muscle relaxants. For example, the laryngeal muscles—whose relaxation is important during intubation—recover from blockade more quickly than the adductor pollicis, which is commonly monitored by the peripheral nerve stimulator.

B. Suitability for Preventing Fasciculations

To prevent fasciculations and myalgia, 10% to 15% of a nondepolarizer intubating dose can be administered 5 min before succinylcholine.

C. Maintenance Relaxation

Following intubation, muscle paralysis may need to be maintained to facilitate surgery (eg, abdominal operations), permit a reduced depth of anesthesia, or control ventilation. There is great variability among patients in response to muscle relaxants. Monitoring neuromuscular function with a nerve stimulator helps prevent over- and underdosing and reduces the likelihood of serious residual muscle paralysis in the recovery room. Maintenance doses, whether by intermittent boluses or continuous infusion (Table 11–6), should be guided by the nerve stimulator *and* clinical signs (eg, spontaneous respiratory efforts or movement). In some instances, clinical signs may precede twitch recovery because of differing sensitivities to muscle relaxants between muscle groups or technical problems with the nerve stimulator. Some return of neuromuscular transmission should be evident prior to administering each maintenance dose if the patient needs to resume spontaneous ventilation at the end of the anesthetic. When an infusion is used for maintenance, the rate should be adjusted at or just above the rate that allows some return of neuromuscular transmission so drug effects can be monitored.

D. Potentiation by Inhalational Anesthetics

Volatile agents decrease nondepolarizer dosage requirements by at least 15%. The actual degree of this postsynaptic augmentation depends on the inhalational anesthetic (desflurane > sevoflurane >

isoflurane > halothane > N_2O/O_2/narcotic > total intravenous anesthesia).

E. Potentiation by Other Nondepolarizers

Some combinations of different classes of nondepolarizers (eg, steroidal and benzylisoquinolinium) produce a greater than additive (synergistic) neuromuscular blockade.

F. Autonomic Side Effects

In clinical doses, the nondepolarizers differ in their relative effects on nicotinic and muscarinic cholinergic receptors. Previously used agents (eg, tubocurarine) blocked autonomic ganglia, reducing the ability of the sympathetic nervous system to increase heart contractility and rate in response to hypotension and other intraoperative stresses. In contrast, pancuronium blocks vagal muscarinic receptors in the sinoatrial node, often resulting in tachycardia. All newer nondepolarizing relaxants, including atracurium, cisatracurium, mivacurium, vecuronium, and rocuronium, are devoid of significant autonomic effects in their recommended dosage ranges.

G. Histamine Release

Histamine release from mast cells can result in bronchospasm, skin flushing, and hypotension from peripheral vasodilation. Atracurium and mivacurium are capable of triggering histamine release, particularly at higher doses. Slow injection rates and H_1 and H_2 antihistamine pretreatment ameliorate these side effects.

H. Hepatic Clearance

Only pancuronium, vecuronium, and rocuronium are metabolized to varying degrees by the liver. Active metabolites likely contribute to their clinical effect. Vecuronium and rocuronium depend heavily on biliary excretion. Clinically, liver failure prolongs blockade. Atracurium, cisatracurium, and mivacurium, though extensively metabolized, depend on extrahepatic mechanisms. Severe liver disease does not significantly affect the clearance of atracurium or cisatracurium, but the associated decrease in pseudocholinesterase levels may slow the metabolism of mivacurium.

I. Renal Excretion

8 Pancuronium, vecuronium, and rocuronium are partially excreted by the kidneys. The duration of action of pancuronium and vecuronium is prolonged in patients with kidney failure. The elimination of atracurium and cisatracurium is independent of kidney function. The duration of action of rocuronium and mivacurium is not significantly affected by renal dysfunction.

General Pharmacological Characteristics

Some variables affect all nondepolarizing muscle relaxants.

A. Temperature

Hypothermia prolongs blockade by decreasing metabolism (eg, mivacurium, atracurium, and cisatracurium) and delaying excretion (eg, pancuronium and vecuronium).

B. Acid–Base Balance

Respiratory acidosis potentiates the blockade of most nondepolarizing relaxants and antagonizes its reversal. This could prevent complete neuromuscular recovery in a hypoventilating postoperative patient. Conflicting findings regarding the neuromuscular effects of other acid–base changes may be due to coexisting alterations in extracellular pH, intracellular pH, electrolyte concentrations, or structural differences between drugs (eg, monoquaternary versus bisquaternary; steroidal versus isoquinolinium).

C. Electrolyte Abnormalities

Hypokalemia and hypocalcemia augment a nondepolarizing block. The responses of patients with hypercalcemia are unpredictable. Hypermagnesemia, as may be seen in preeclamptic patients being managed with magnesium sulfate (or after intravenous magnesium administered in the operating room), potentiates a nondepolarizing blockade by competing with calcium at the motor end-plate.

D. Age

Neonates have an increased sensitivity to nondepolarizing relaxants because of their immature neuromuscular junctions (Table 11–7). This sensitivity does not necessarily decrease dosage requirements, as the neonate's greater extracellular space provides a larger volume of distribution.

TABLE 11–7 Additional considerations of muscle relaxants in special populations.

Pediatric	Succinylcholine: should not be used routinely Nondepolarizing agents: faster onset Vecuronium: long-acting in neonates
Older adult	Decreased clearance: prolonged duration, except with cisatracurium
Obese	Dosage 20% more than lean body weight; onset unchanged Prolonged duration, except with cisatracurium
Liver disease	Increased volume of distribution Pancuronium and vecuronium: prolonged elimination due to hepatic metabolism and biliary excretion Cisatracurium: unchanged Pseudocholinesterase decreased; prolonged action may be seen with succinylcholine in severe disease
Kidney failure	Vecuronium: prolonged Rocuronium: relatively unchanged Cisatracurium: safest alternative
Critically ill	Myopathy, polyneuropathy, nicotinic acetylcholine receptor upregulation

E. Drug Interactions

As noted earlier, many drugs augment nondepolarizing blockade (see Table 11–3). They have multiple sites of interaction: prejunctional structures, postjunctional cholinergic receptors, and muscle membranes.

F. Concurrent Disease

The presence of neurological or muscular disease can have profound effects on an individual's response
9 to muscle relaxants (Table 11–8). Cirrhotic liver disease and chronic kidney failure often result in an increased volume of distribution and a lower plasma concentration for a given dose of water-soluble drugs, such as muscle relaxants. On the other hand, drugs dependent on hepatic or renal excretion may demonstrate prolonged clearance (see Table 11–7). Thus, depending on the drug chosen, a greater initial (loading) dose—but smaller maintenance doses—might be required in these diseases.

G. Muscle Groups

The onset and intensity of blockade vary among muscle groups. This may be due to differences in blood flow, distance from the central circulation, or different fiber types. Furthermore, the relative sensitivity of a muscle group may depend on the choice of muscle relaxant. In general, the diaphragm, jaw, larynx, and facial muscles (orbicularis oculi) respond to and recover from muscle relaxation sooner than the thumb. Although they are a fortuitous safety feature, persistent diaphragmatic contractions can be disconcerting in the face of complete adductor pollicis paralysis. Glottic musculature is also quite resistant to blockade, as is often confirmed during laryngoscopy. The dose that produces 95% twitch depression in laryngeal muscles is nearly two times that for the adductor pollicis muscle. Good intubating conditions are usually associated with visual loss of the orbicularis oculi twitch response.

Considering the multitude of factors influencing the duration and magnitude of muscle relaxation, it becomes clear that an individual's response to neuromuscular blocking agents should be monitored. Dosage recommendations, including those in this chapter, should be considered guidelines that require modification for individual patients. Wide variability in sensitivity to nondepolarizing muscle relaxants is often encountered in clinical practice.

ATRACURIUM

Physical Structure

Like all muscle relaxants, atracurium has a quaternary group; however, a benzylisoquinoline structure is responsible for its unique method of degradation. The drug is a mixture of ten stereoisomers.

Metabolism & Excretion

Atracurium is so extensively metabolized that its pharmacokinetics are independent of renal and hepatic function, and less than 10% is excreted unchanged by renal and biliary routes. Two separate processes are responsible for metabolism.

A. Ester Hydrolysis

This action is catalyzed by nonspecific esterases, not by acetylcholinesterase or pseudocholinesterase.

TABLE 11–8 Diseases with altered responses to muscle relaxants.

Disease	Response to Depolarizers	Response to Nondepolarizers
Amyotrophic lateral sclerosis	Contracture/hyperkalemia	Hypersensitivity
Autoimmune disorders Systemic lupus erythematosus Polymyositis Dermatomyositis	Hypersensitivity	Hypersensitivity
Burn injury	Hyperkalemia	Resistance
Cerebral palsy	Slight hypersensitivity	Resistance
Familial periodic paralysis (hyperkalemic)	Myotonia and hyperkalemia	Hypersensitivity?
Guillain–Barré syndrome	Hyperkalemia	Hypersensitivity
Hemiplegia	Hyperkalemia	Resistance on affected side
Muscular denervation (peripheral nerve injury)	Hyperkalemia and contracture	Normal response or resistance
Muscular dystrophy (Duchenne type)	Hyperkalemia and malignant hyperthermia	Hypersensitivity
Myasthenia gravis	Resistance	Hypersensitivity
Myasthenic syndrome	Hypersensitivity	Hypersensitivity
Myotonia	Generalized muscular contractions	Normal or hypersensitivity
Severe chronic infection Tetanus Botulism	Hyperkalemia	Resistance

B. Hofmann Elimination

A spontaneous nonenzymatic chemical breakdown occurs at physiological pH and temperature.

Dosage

A dose of 0.5 mg/kg is administered intravenously for intubation. If succinylcholine is administered for intubation, subsequent intraoperative relaxation using atracurium is achieved with 0.25 mg/kg initially, then in incremental doses of 0.1 mg/kg every 10 to 20 min. An infusion of 5 to 10 mcg/kg/min can effectively replace intermittent boluses.

Although dosage requirements do not significantly vary with age, atracurium may be shorter acting in children and infants than in adults.

Atracurium is available as a solution of 10 mg/mL. It must be stored at 2°C to 8°C because it loses 5% to 10% of its potency for each month it is exposed to room temperature. At room temperature, it should be used within 14 days to preserve potency.

Side Effects & Clinical Considerations

Atracurium triggers a dose-dependent histamine release that becomes significant at doses above 0.5 mg/kg.

A. Hypotension and Tachycardia

Cardiovascular side effects are unusual unless doses in excess of 0.5 mg/kg are administered. Atracurium may also cause a transient drop in systemic vascular resistance and an increase in cardiac index independent of any histamine release. A slow rate of injection minimizes these effects.

B. Bronchospasm

Atracurium should be avoided in patients with asthma. Severe bronchospasm is occasionally seen in patients without a history of asthma.

C. Laudanosine Toxicity

Laudanosine, a tertiary amine, is a breakdown product of atracurium's Hofmann elimination and has been associated with central nervous system excitation, resulting in elevation of the minimum alveolar concentration and even precipitation of seizures. Concerns about laudanosine are probably irrelevant unless a patient has received an extremely large total dose or has hepatic failure. Laudanosine is metabolized by the liver and excreted in urine and bile.

D. Temperature and pH Sensitivity

Because of its unique metabolism, atracurium's duration of action can be markedly prolonged by hypothermia and to a lesser extent by acidosis.

E. Chemical Incompatibility

Atracurium will precipitate as a free acid if it is introduced into an intravenous line containing an alkaline solution such as thiopental.

F. Allergic Reactions

Rare anaphylactoid reactions to atracurium have been described. Proposed mechanisms include direct immunogenicity and acrylate-mediated immune activation. Immunoglobulin E-mediated antibody reactions directed against substituted ammonium compounds, including muscle relaxants, have been described. Reactions to acrylate, a metabolite of atracurium and a structural component of some dialysis membranes, have also been reported in patients undergoing hemodialysis.

CISATRACURIUM

Physical Structure

Cisatracurium is a stereoisomer of atracurium that is four times more potent. Atracurium contains approximately 15% cisatracurium.

Metabolism & Excretion

Like atracurium, cisatracurium undergoes degradation in plasma at physiological pH and temperature by organ-independent Hofmann elimination. The resulting metabolites (a monoquaternary acrylate and laudanosine) have no neuromuscular blocking effects. Because of cisatracurium's greater potency, the amount of laudanosine produced for the same extent and duration of neuromuscular blockade is much less than with atracurium. Metabolism and elimination are independent of kidney or liver failure. Minor variations in pharmacokinetic patterns due to age result in no clinically important changes in the duration of action.

Dosage

Cisatracurium produces good intubating conditions following a dose of 0.1 to 0.15 mg/kg within 2 min and results in muscle blockade of intermediate duration. The typical maintenance infusion rate ranges from 1.0 to 2.0 mcg/kg/min. Thus, it is more potent than atracurium.

Cisatracurium should be stored under refrigeration (2–8°C) and should be used within 21 days after removal from refrigeration and exposure to room temperature.

Side Effects & Clinical Considerations

Unlike atracurium, cisatracurium does not produce a consistent, dose-dependent increase in plasma histamine levels following administration. Cisatracurium does not alter heart rate or blood pressure, nor does it produce autonomic effects, even at doses as high as eight times ED_{95}.

Cisatracurium shares with atracurium the production of laudanosine, pH and temperature sensitivity, and chemical incompatibility.

MIVACURIUM

Mivacurium is a short-acting, benzylisoquinoline, nondepolarizing neuromuscular blocker. It has recently returned to the North American anesthesia market after having been unavailable for a number of years.

Metabolism & Excretion

Mivacurium, like succinylcholine, is metabolized by pseudocholinesterase. Consequently, patients with low pseudocholinesterase concentration or activity may experience prolonged neuromuscular blockade following mivacurium administration. However, like other nondepolarizing agents, cholinesterase inhibitors will antagonize mivacurium-induced neuromuscular blockade. Edrophonium more effectively reverses mivacurium blockade than neostigmine because neostigmine inhibits plasma cholinesterase activity.

Dosage

The usual intubating dose of mivacurium is 0.15 to 0.2 mg/kg.

Side Effects & Clinical Considerations

Mivacurium releases histamine to about the same degree as atracurium. The onset time of mivacurium is approximately 2 to 3 min. The main advantage of mivacurium compared with atracurium is its relatively brief duration of action (20–30 min).

PANCURONIUM

Physical Structure

Pancuronium consists of a steroid structure on which two modified ACh molecules are positioned (a bisquaternary relaxant). In all of the steroid-based relaxants, the steroid "backbone" serves as a "spacer" between the two quaternary amines. Pancuronium resembles ACh enough to bind (but not activate) the nicotinic ACh receptor.

Metabolism & Excretion

Pancuronium is metabolized (deacetylated) by the liver to a limited degree. Its metabolic products have some neuromuscular blocking activity. Excretion is primarily renal (40%), though some of the drug is cleared by the bile (10%). Not surprisingly, elimination of pancuronium is slowed and neuromuscular blockade is prolonged by kidney failure. Patients with cirrhosis may require a larger initial dose due to an increased volume of distribution but have reduced maintenance requirements because of a decreased rate of plasma clearance.

Dosage

A dose of 0.08 to 0.12 mg/kg of pancuronium provides adequate relaxation for intubation in 2 to 3 min. Intraoperative relaxation is achieved by administering 0.04 mg/kg initially, followed every 20 to 40 min by 0.01 mg/kg.

Children may require moderately larger doses of pancuronium. Pancuronium is available as a solution of 1 or 2 mg/mL and is stored at 2°C to 8°C but may be stable for up to 6 months at normal room temperature.

Side Effects & Clinical Considerations

A. Hypertension and Tachycardia

11 These cardiovascular effects are caused by the combination of vagal blockade and sympathetic stimulation. The latter is due to a combination of ganglionic stimulation, catecholamine release from adrenergic nerve endings, and decreased catecholamine reuptake. Large bolus doses of pancuronium should be given with caution to patients in whom an increased heart rate would be particularly detrimental (eg, coronary artery disease, hypertrophic cardiomyopathy, aortic stenosis).

B. Arrhythmias

Increased atrioventricular conduction and catecholamine release increase the likelihood of ventricular arrhythmias in predisposed individuals. The combination of pancuronium, tricyclic antidepressants, and halothane has been reported to be particularly arrhythmogenic.

C. Allergic Reactions

Patients who are hypersensitive to bromides may exhibit allergic reactions to pancuronium (pancuronium bromide).

VECURONIUM

Physical Structure

Vecuronium is pancuronium minus a quaternary methyl group (a monoquaternary relaxant). This minor structural change beneficially alters side effects without affecting potency.

Metabolism & Excretion

Vecuronium is metabolized to a small extent by the liver. It depends primarily on biliary excretion and secondarily (25%) on renal excretion. Although it is a satisfactory drug for patients with kidney failure,

its duration of action will be moderately prolonged. Vecuronium's brief duration of action is explained by its shorter elimination half-life and more rapid
12 clearance compared with pancuronium. After long-term administration of vecuronium to patients in intensive care units, prolonged neuromuscular blockade (up to several days) may be present after drug discontinuation, possibly from accumulation of its active 3-hydroxy metabolite, changing drug clearance. In some patients, this can lead to the development of polyneuropathy. Risk factors seem to include female gender, kidney failure, long-term or high-dose corticosteroid therapy, and sepsis. Thus, these patients must be closely monitored, and the dose of vecuronium must be carefully titrated. Long-term relaxant administration and the subsequent prolonged lack of ACh binding at the postsynaptic nicotinic ACh receptors may mimic a chronic denervation state and cause lasting receptor dysfunction and paralysis. Tolerance to nondepolarizing muscle relaxants can also develop after long-term use. The best approach is to avoid unnecessary paralysis of patients in critical care units.

Dosage

Vecuronium is equipotent with pancuronium, and the intubating dose is 0.08 to 0.12 mg/kg. A dose of 0.04 mg/kg initially followed by increments of 0.01 mg/kg every 15 to 20 min provides intraoperative relaxation. Alternatively, an infusion of 1 to 2 mcg/kg/min produces good maintenance of relaxation.

Age does not affect initial dose requirements, though subsequent doses are required less frequently in neonates and infants. Women seem to be approximately 30% more sensitive than men to vecuronium, as evidenced by a greater degree of blockade and longer duration of action (this has also been seen with pancuronium and rocuronium). The cause for this sensitivity is likely related to gender-related differences in fat and muscle mass and volume of distribution. The duration of action of vecuronium may be further prolonged in postpartum patients due to alterations in hepatic blood flow or liver uptake. As with rocuronium (below), sugammadex permits the rapid reversal of dense vecuronium-induced neuromuscular blockade.

Side Effects & Clinical Considerations

A. Cardiovascular

Even at doses of 0.28 mg/kg, vecuronium is devoid of significant cardiovascular effects. Potentiation of opioid-induced bradycardia may be observed in some patients.

B. Liver Failure

Although it is dependent on biliary excretion, the duration of action of vecuronium is usually not significantly prolonged in patients with cirrhosis unless doses greater than 0.15 mg/kg are given. Vecuronium requirements are reduced during the anhepatic phase of liver transplantation.

ROCURONIUM

Physical Structure

This monoquaternary steroid analogue of vecuronium was designed to provide a rapid onset of action.

Metabolism & Excretion

Rocuronium undergoes no metabolism and is eliminated primarily by the liver and slightly by the kidneys. Its duration of action is not significantly affected by renal disease, but it is modestly prolonged by severe liver failure and pregnancy. Because rocuronium does not have active metabolites, it may be a better choice than vecuronium in the rare patient requiring prolonged infusions in the intensive care unit setting. Older adult patients may experience a prolonged duration of action due to decreased liver mass.

Dosage

Rocuronium is less potent than most other steroidal muscle relaxants (potency seems to be inversely related to the speed of onset). It requires 0.45 to 0.9 mg/kg intravenously for intubation and 0.15 mg/kg boluses for maintenance. Intramuscular rocuronium (1 mg/kg for infants; 2 mg/kg for children) provides adequate vocal cord and diaphragmatic paralysis for intubation, but not until after 3 to 6 min (deltoid injection has a faster onset than quadriceps). The infusion requirements for rocuronium range from 5 to 12 mcg/kg/min. Rocuronium can produce an unexpectedly prolonged duration of action in older adult patients. Initial dosage requirements are modestly increased in patients with advanced liver disease, presumably due to a larger volume of distribution.

Side Effects & Clinical Considerations

13 Rocuronium (at a dose of 0.9–1.2 mg/kg) has an onset of action that *approaches* succinylcholine (60–90 s), making it a suitable alternative for rapid-sequence inductions but at the cost of a much longer duration of action. This intermediate duration of action is comparable to vecuronium or atracurium. Sugammadex permits rapid reversal of dense rocuronium-induced neuromuscular blockade.

Rocuronium (0.1 mg/kg) has been shown to be a rapid (90 s) and effective agent (decreased fasciculations and postoperative myalgias) for precurarization prior to administration of succinylcholine. It has slight vagolytic tendencies.

NEWER MUSCLE RELAXANTS

Gantacurium belongs to a new class of nondepolarizing neuromuscular blockers called *chlorofumarates*. In preclinical trials, gantacurium demonstrated an ultrashort duration of action, similar to that of succinylcholine. Its pharmacokinetic profile is explained by the fact that it undergoes nonenzymatic degradation by two chemical mechanisms: rapid formation of inactive cysteine adduction product and ester hydrolysis. At a dose of 0.2 mg/kg (ED_{95}), the onset of action has been estimated to be 1 to 2 min, with a duration of blockade similar to that of succinylcholine. Its clinical duration of action ranges from 5 to 10 min. Recovery can be accelerated by edrophonium, as well as by the administration of exogenous cysteine. Cardiovascular effects suggestive of histamine release were observed following the use of three times the ED_{95} dosage.

CW002 is another investigational nondepolarizing agent. It is a benzylisoquinolinium fumarate ester-based compound with an intermediate duration of action that undergoes metabolism and elimination similar to that of gantacurium. CW 1759-50 is another short-acting agent reversible by L cysteine. At present, these agents are investigational.

CASE DISCUSSION

Delayed Recovery from General Anesthesia

A 72-year-old patient has undergone general anesthesia for robot-assisted laparoscopic prostatectomy. Twenty min after the conclusion of the procedure, the patient is still intubated and shows no evidence of spontaneous respiration or consciousness.

What is your general approach to this diagnostic dilemma?

Clues to the solution of complex clinical problems are usually found in a pertinent review of the medical and surgical history, the history of drug ingestions, the physical examination, and laboratory results. In this case, the perioperative anesthetic management should also be considered.

What medical illnesses predispose a patient to delayed awakening or prolonged paralysis?

Chronic hypertension alters cerebral blood flow autoregulation and decreases the brain's tolerance to episodes of hypotension. Liver disease reduces hepatic drug metabolism and biliary excretion, resulting in prolonged drug action. Reduced serum albumin concentrations increase free drug (active drug) availability. Hepatic encephalopathy can alter consciousness. Kidney disease decreases the renal excretion of many drugs. Uremia can also affect consciousness. Patients with diabetes are prone to hypoglycemia and hyperosmotic, hyperglycemic, and nonketotic coma. A prior stroke or symptomatic carotid bruit increases the risk of intraoperative cerebral vascular accident. Right-to-left heart shunts, particularly in children with congenital heart disease, allow air emboli to pass directly from the venous circulation to the systemic (possibly cerebral) arterial circulation. A paradoxical air embolism can result in permanent brain damage. Severe hypothyroidism is associated with impaired drug metabolism and, rarely, myxedema coma.

Does an uneventful history of general anesthesia narrow the differential?

Hereditary atypical pseudocholinesterase is ruled out by uneventful prior general anesthesia, assuming succinylcholine was administered. Decreased levels of normal enzyme would not result in postoperative apnea unless the surgery was of very short duration. Malignant hyperthermia does not typically present as delayed awakening, though prolonged somnolence is not unusual. Uneventful prior anesthetics do not, however, rule out malignant hyperthermia. Persons unusually sensitive to anesthetic agents (eg, older adult patients) may have a history of delayed emergence.

How do drugs that a patient takes at home affect awakening from general anesthesia?

Drugs that decrease minimum alveolar concentration, such as methyldopa, predispose patients to anesthetic overdose. Acute ethanol intoxication decreases barbiturate metabolism and acts independently as a sedative. Drugs that decrease liver blood flow, such as cimetidine, will limit hepatic drug metabolism. Antiparkinsonian drugs and tricyclic antidepressants have anticholinergic side effects that augment the sedation produced by scopolamine. Long-acting sedatives, such as benzodiazepines, can delay awakening.

Does anesthetic technique alter awakening?

Preoperative medications can affect awakening. In particular, opioids and benzodiazepines can interfere with postoperative recovery.

Intraoperative hyperventilation is a common cause of postoperative apnea. Because volatile agents and opioids raise the apneic threshold, the $PaCO_2$ level at which spontaneous ventilation ceases, moderate postoperative hypoventilation may be required to stimulate the respiratory centers. Severe intraoperative hypotension or hypertension may lead to cerebral hypoxia and edema.

Hypothermia decreases minimum alveolar concentration, antagonizes muscle relaxation reversal, and limits drug metabolism. Arterial hypoxia or severe hypercapnia ($PaCO_2$ >70 mm Hg) can alter consciousness.

Certain surgical procedures, such as carotid endarterectomy, cardiopulmonary bypass, and intracranial procedures, are associated with an increased incidence of postoperative neurological deficits. Subdural hematomas can occur in severely coagulopathic patients. Transurethral resection of the prostate can be associated with hyponatremia from the dilutional effects of absorbed irrigating solution.

What clues does a physical examination provide?

Pupil size is not always a reliable indicator of central nervous system integrity. Fixed and dilated pupils in the absence of anticholinergic medication or ganglionic blockade, however, may be an ominous sign. Response to physical stimulation, such as a forceful jaw thrust, may differentiate somnolence from paralysis. Peripheral nerve stimulation also differentiates paralysis from coma.

What specific laboratory findings would you order?

Arterial blood gases, plasma glucose, and serum electrolytes may be helpful. Computed tomographic scanning may be necessary if unresponsiveness is prolonged. Increased concentrations of an inhalational agent provided by respiratory gas analysis, as well as processed electroencephalogram (EEG) measurements, may assist in determining if the patient is still under the effects of anesthesia. Slow EEG signals can be indicative of both anesthesia and cerebral pathology. Processed EEG awareness monitors can also be employed with the realization that low numbers on the bispectral index can be caused both by anesthetic suppression of the EEG and ischemic brain injury.

What therapeutic interventions should be considered?

Supportive mechanical ventilation should be continued in the unresponsive patient. Naloxone, flumazenil, and physostigmine may be indicated depending on the probable cause of the delayed emergence and if drug effects are suspected and reversal is considered both safe and desirable.

SUGGESTED READINGS

Brull SJ, Kopman AF. Current status of neuromuscular reversal and monitoring: challenges and opportunities. *Anesthesiology*. 2017;126:173.

deBacker J, Hart N, Fan E. Neuromuscular blockade in the 21st century management of the critically ill patient. *Chest*. 2017;151:697.

Grabitz SD, Rajaratnam N, Chhagani K, et al. The effects of postoperative residual neuromuscular blockade on hospital costs and intensive care unit admission: a population-based cohort study. *Anesth Analg*. 2019;128:1129.

Guihard B, Chollet-Xémard C, Lakhnati P, et al. Effect of rocuronium vs succinylcholine on endotracheal intubation success rate among patients undergoing out-of-hospital rapid sequence intubation: a randomized clinical trial. *JAMA*. 2019;322:2303.

Heerdt PM, Sunaga H, Savarese JJ. Novel neuromuscular blocking drugs and antagonists. *Curr Opin Anaesthesiol*. 2015;28:403.

Madsen MV, Staehr-Rye AK, Gätke MR, Claudius C. Neuromuscular blockade for optimising surgical conditions during abdominal and gynaecological surgery: a systematic review. *Acta Anaesthesiol Scand*. 2015;59:1.

Murphy G. Neuromuscular monitoring in the perioperative period. *Anesth Analg*. 2018;126:464.

Savarese JJ, Sunaga H, McGilvra JD, et al. Preclinical pharmacology in the rhesus monkey of CW 1759-50, a new ultra-short acting nondepolarizing neuromuscular blocking agent, degraded and antagonized by l-cysteine. *Anesthesiology*. 2018;129:970.

Schreiber JU. Management of neuromuscular blockade in ambulatory patients. *Curr Opin Anaesthesiol*. 2014;27:583.

Tran DT, Newton EK, Mount VA, et al. Rocuronium versus succinylcholine for rapid sequence induction intubation. *Cochrane Database Syst Rev*. 2015;(10):CD002788.

CHAPTER 12

Cholinesterase Inhibitors & Other Pharmacological Antagonists to Neuromuscular Blocking Agents

KEY CONCEPTS

1. The primary clinical use of cholinesterase inhibitors is to reverse nondepolarizing neuromuscular blockers.
2. Acetylcholine is the neurotransmitter for the entire parasympathetic nervous system (parasympathetic ganglions and effector cells), parts of the sympathetic nervous system (sympathetic ganglions, adrenal medulla, and sweat glands), some neurons in the central nervous system, and somatic nerves innervating skeletal muscle.
3. Neuromuscular transmission is blocked when nondepolarizing muscle relaxants compete with acetylcholine to bind to nicotinic cholinergic receptors. The cholinesterase inhibitors indirectly increase the amount of acetylcholine available to compete with the nondepolarizing agent, thereby reestablishing neuromuscular transmission.
4. Acetylcholinesterase inhibitors prolong the depolarization blockade of succinylcholine.
5. Any prolongation of action of a nondepolarizing muscle relaxant from renal or hepatic insufficiency will probably be accompanied by a corresponding increase in the duration of action of a cholinesterase inhibitor.
6. The time required to fully reverse a nondepolarizing block depends on several factors, including the choice and dose of cholinesterase inhibitor administered, the muscle relaxant being antagonized, and the extent of the blockade before reversal.
7. A reversal agent should be routinely given to patients who have received nondepolarizing muscle relaxants unless full reversal can be demonstrated or the postoperative plan includes continued intubation and ventilation.
8. Newer quantitative methods for assessing recovery from neuromuscular blockade, such as acceleromyography, may further reduce the incidence of undetected residual postoperative neuromuscular paralysis.
9. Sugammadex exerts its effects by forming tight complexes in a 1:1 ratio with steroidal neuromuscular blocking agents.
10. Cysteine causes the inactivation of gantacurium via metabolic degradation and adduct formation.

Incomplete reversal of neuromuscular blocking agents and residual postprocedure paralysis are associated with morbidity and increased perioperative cost; therefore, careful assessment of neuromuscular blockade and appropriate pharmacological antagonism are strongly recommended whenever muscle relaxants are administered. The
1 primary clinical use of cholinesterase inhibitors is to reverse nondepolarizing neuromuscular blockers. Some of these agents are also used to diagnose and treat myasthenia gravis. More recently, agents such as cyclodextrins and cysteine that have superior ability to reverse neuromuscular blockade from specific agents are being employed or investigated. This chapter reviews cholinergic pharmacology and the mechanisms of acetylcholinesterase inhibition and presents the clinical pharmacology of commonly used cholinesterase inhibitors (neostigmine, edrophonium, pyridostigmine, and physostigmine). It also includes a review of newer reversal agents.

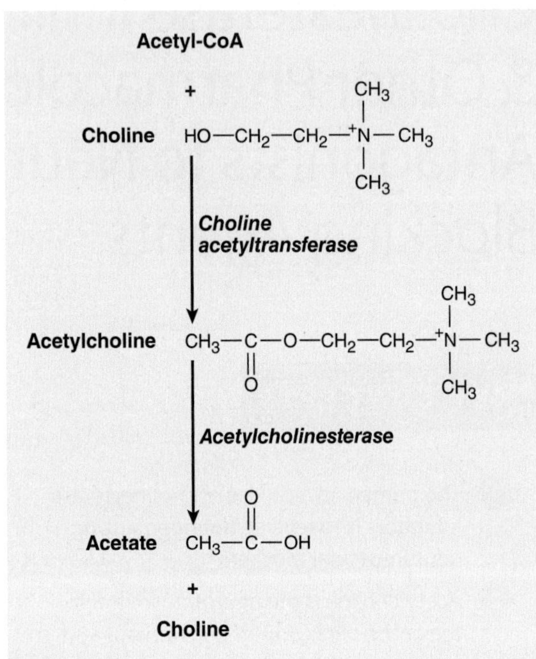

FIGURE 12–1 The synthesis and hydrolysis of acetylcholine.

Cholinergic Pharmacology

The term *cholinergic* refers to the effects of the neurotransmitter acetyl*choline*. Acetylcholine is synthesized in the nerve terminal by the enzyme choline acetyltransferase, which catalyzes the reaction between acetyl coenzyme A and choline (Figure 12–1). After release, acetylcholine is rapidly hydrolyzed by acetylcholinesterase (true cholinesterase) into acetate and choline.

2 Acetylcholine is the neurotransmitter for the entire parasympathetic nervous system (parasympathetic ganglia and effector cells), parts of the sympathetic nervous system (sympathetic ganglia, adrenal medulla, and sweat glands), some neurons in the central nervous system, and somatic nerves innervating skeletal muscle (Figure 12–2).

Cholinergic receptors have been subdivided into two major groups based on their reaction to the alkaloids muscarine and nicotine (Figure 12–3). Nicotine stimulates the autonomic ganglia and skeletal muscle receptors (nicotinic receptors), whereas muscarine activates end-organ effector cells in bronchial smooth muscle, salivary glands, and the sinoatrial node (muscarinic receptors). The central nervous system has both nicotinic and muscarinic receptors. Nicotinic receptors are blocked by muscle relaxants (also called *neuromuscular blockers*), and muscarinic receptors are blocked by anticholinergic drugs such as atropine. Although nicotinic and muscarinic receptors differ in their response to some agonists (eg, nicotine, muscarine) and some antagonists (eg, vecuronium versus atropine), they both respond to acetylcholine (Table 12–1). Clinically available cholinergic agonists antagonize hydrolysis by cholinesterase. Methacholine and bethanechol are primarily muscarinic agonists, whereas carbachol has both muscarinic and nicotinic agonist activities. Methacholine by inhalation has been used as a provocative test in asthma, bethanechol is used for bladder atony, and carbachol may be used topically for wide-angle glaucoma.

When reversing neuromuscular blockade, the goal is to maximize nicotinic transmission with a minimum of muscarinic side effects.

MECHANISM OF ACTION

3 Normal neuromuscular transmission depends on acetylcholine binding to nicotinic cholinergic receptors on the motor end-plate. Nondepolarizing

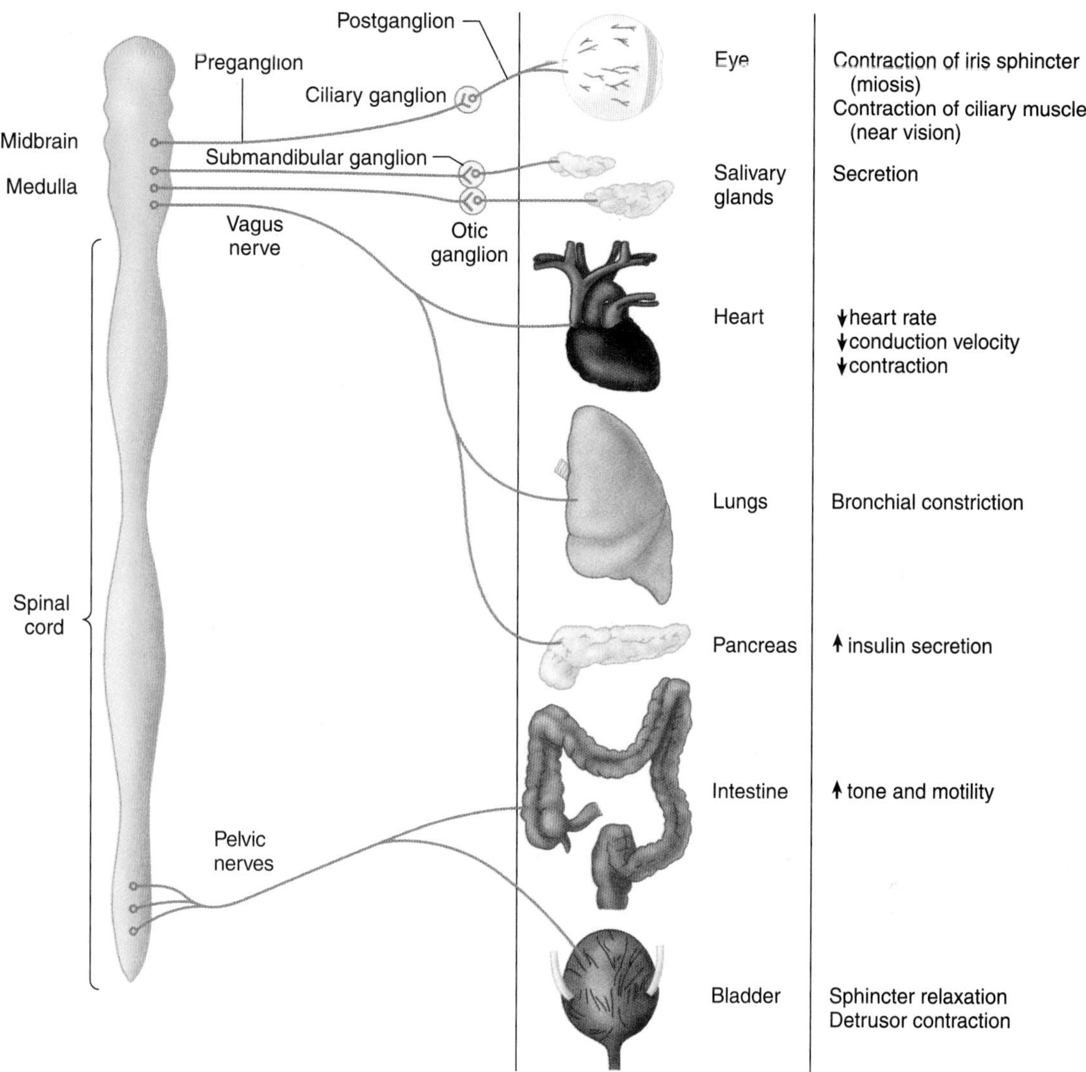

FIGURE 12–2 The parasympathetic nervous system uses acetylcholine as a preganglionic and postganglionic neurotransmitter.

muscle relaxants compete with acetylcholine for these binding sites, thereby blocking neuromuscular transmission. Reversal of blockade depends on diffusion, redistribution, metabolism, and excretion from the body of the nondepolarizing relaxant (*spontaneous reversal*), often assisted by the administration of specific reversal agents (*pharmacological reversal*). Cholinesterase inhibitors *indirectly* increase the amount of acetylcholine available to compete with the nondepolarizing agent, thereby reestablishing normal neuromuscular transmission.

These inhibitors antagonize acetylcholinesterase by reversibly binding to the enzyme. The nature of the binding between the antagonist and enzyme

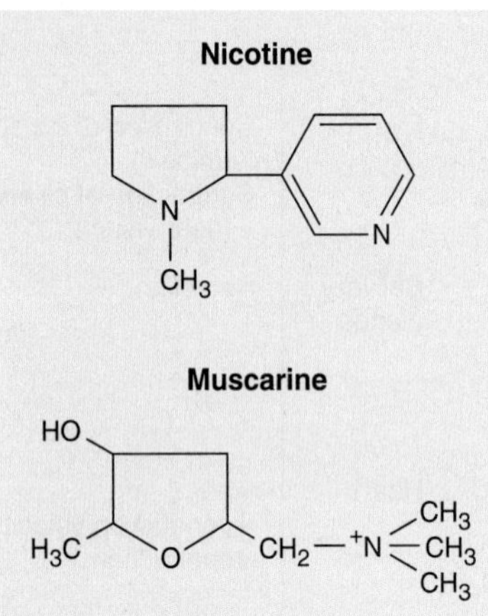

FIGURE 12–3 The molecular structures of nicotine and muscarine. Compare these alkaloids with acetylcholine (Figure 12–1).

influences the antagonist's duration of action. The electrostatic attraction and hydrogen bonding of edrophonium are short-lived; the covalent bonds of neostigmine and pyridostigmine are longer lasting.

Organophosphates, a special class of cholinesterase inhibitors that have been used in ophthalmology

TABLE 12–1 Characteristics of cholinergic receptors.

	Nicotinic	Muscarinic
Location	Autonomic ganglia Sympathetic ganglia Parasympathetic ganglia Skeletal muscle	Glands Lacrimal Salivary Gastric Smooth muscle Bronchial Gastrointestinal Bladder Blood vessels Heart Sinoatrial node Atrioventricular node
Agonists	Acetylcholine Nicotine	Acetylcholine Muscarine
Antagonists	Nondepolarizing relaxants	Antimuscarinics Atropine Scopolamine Glycopyrrolate

and as pesticides, form stable, irreversible bonds to the enzyme for a long-lasting effect that persists long after the drug disappears from the circulation. Chemical warfare nerve agents (eg, VX, sarin) are also organophosphates that produce cholinesterase inhibition. Death occurs secondary to overstimulation of both nicotinic and muscarinic receptors. Cholinesterase inhibitors are also used in the diagnosis and treatment of myasthenia gravis. Other cholinesterase inhibitors (eg, rivastigmine) have been employed to treat cognitive impairment in patients with dementia.

The clinical duration of the cholinesterase inhibitors used in anesthesia is probably most influenced by the rate of drug disappearance from the plasma. Differences in the duration of action can be overcome by dosage adjustments. Thus, the normally short duration of action of edrophonium can be partially overcome by increasing the dosage.

4 Acetylcholinesterase inhibitors prolong the depolarization blockade by succinylcholine. Two mechanisms may explain this latter effect: an increase in acetylcholine (which increases motor end-plate depolarization and receptor desensitization) and inhibition of pseudocholinesterase activity. Neostigmine and, to some extent, pyridostigmine display some limited pseudocholinesterase-inhibiting activity, but their effect on acetylcholinesterase is much greater. Edrophonium has little or no effect on pseudocholinesterase. In astronomical doses, neostigmine is reported to cause a weak neuromuscular blockade.

CLINICAL PHARMACOLOGY

General Pharmacological Characteristics

The increase in acetylcholine caused by cholinesterase inhibitors affects more than the nicotinic receptors of skeletal muscle (Table 12–2). Cholinesterase inhibitors can act at cholinergic receptors of several other organ systems, including the cardiovascular and gastrointestinal systems.

Cardiovascular receptors—The predominant muscarinic effect on the heart is bradycardia that can progress to sinus arrest.

TABLE 12–2 Muscarinic side effects of cholinesterase inhibitors.

Organ System	Muscarinic Side Effects
Cardiovascular	Decreased heart rate, bradyarrhythmia
Pulmonary	Bronchospasm, bronchial secretions
Cerebral	Diffuse excitation[1]
Gastrointestinal	Intestinal spasm, increased salivation
Genitourinary	Increased bladder tone
Ophthalmological	Pupillary constriction

[1]Applies only to physostigmine.

Pulmonary receptors—Muscarinic stimulation can result in bronchospasm (smooth muscle contraction) and increased respiratory tract secretions.

Cerebral receptors—Physostigmine is a cholinesterase inhibitor that crosses the blood–brain barrier and stimulates muscarinic and nicotinic receptors within the central nervous system, reversing the effects of scopolamine or high-dose atropine on the brain. Unlike physostigmine, cholinesterase inhibitors used to reverse neuromuscular blockers do not cross the blood–brain barrier.

Gastrointestinal receptors—Muscarinic stimulation increases peristaltic activity (esophageal, gastric, and intestinal) and glandular secretions (eg, salivary). Postoperative nausea, vomiting, and fecal incontinence have been attributed to the use of cholinesterase inhibitors.

Unwanted muscarinic side effects are minimized by prior or concomitant administration of anticholinergic medications, such as atropine or glycopyrrolate. The duration of action is similar among the cholinesterase inhibitors. Clearance is due to both hepatic metabolism (25–50%) and renal excre-
5 tion (50–75%). Thus, any prolongation of action of a nondepolarizing muscle relaxant from renal or hepatic insufficiency will probably be accompanied by a corresponding increase in the duration of action of a cholinesterase inhibitor.

6 The time required to fully reverse a nondepolarizing block depends on several factors, including the choice and dose of cholinesterase inhibitor administered, the muscle relaxant being antagonized, and the extent of neuromuscular blockade before reversal. Reversal with edrophonium is usually faster than with neostigmine; large doses of neostigmine lead to faster reversal than small doses; intermediate-acting relaxants reverse sooner than long-acting relaxants; and a shallow block is easier to reverse than a deep block. Intermediate-acting muscle relaxants therefore require a lower dose of reversal agent (for the same degree of blockade) than long-acting agents, and concurrent excretion or metabolism provides a proportionally faster reversal of the short- and intermediate-acting agents. These advantages can be lost in conditions associated with severe end-organ disease (eg, the use of vecuronium in a patient with liver failure) or enzyme deficiencies (eg, mivacurium in a patient with homozygous atypical pseudocholinesterase). Depending on the dose of muscle relaxant that has been given, spontaneous recovery to a level adequate for pharmacological reversal may take more than 1 h with long-acting muscle relaxants. Factors associated with faster reversal are also associated with a lower incidence of residual paralysis in the recovery room and a lower risk of postoperative respiratory complications. The absence of any palpable single twitches following 5 s of tetanic stimulation at 50 Hz implies a very intensive blockade that cannot (and should not) be reversed by cholinesterase inhibitors.

A reversal agent should be routinely given to patients who have received nondepolarizing muscle relaxants unless full recovery can be demonstrated or the postoperative plan includes continued intubation and ventilation. In the latter situation, adequate sedation must also be provided.

7 A peripheral nerve stimulator should also be used to monitor the progress and confirm the adequacy of reversal. Clinical signs of adequate reversal vary in sensitivity (sustained head lift > inspiratory force > vital capacity > tidal volume) and are often unreliable. Newer quantitative
8 methods for assessing recovery from neuromuscular blockade, such as acceleromyography, further reduce the incidence of undetected

residual postoperative neuromuscular paralysis and are recommended.

Specific Cholinesterase Inhibitors

NEOSTIGMINE

Physical Structure

Neostigmine consists of a carbamate moiety and a quaternary ammonium group (Figure 12–4). The former provides covalent bonding to acetylcholinesterase. The latter renders the molecule lipid insoluble, so it cannot pass through the blood–brain barrier.

Dosage & Packaging

The maximum recommended dose of neostigmine is 0.08 mg/kg (up to 5 mg in adults), but smaller amounts often suffice, and larger doses have also been given safely (Table 12–3). Neostigmine is most commonly packaged as 10 mL of a 1 mg/mL solution, though 0.5 mg/mL and 0.25 mg/mL concentrations are also available.

Clinical Considerations

The effects of neostigmine (0.04 mg/kg) are usually apparent in 5 min, peak at 10 min, and last more than 1 h. In practice, some clinicians use a dose of 0.04 mg/kg (or 2.5 mg) if the preexisting blockade is mild to moderate and a dose of 0.08 mg/kg (or 5 mg) if intense paralysis is being reversed; other clinicians use the "full dose" for all patients. The duration of action is prolonged in geriatric patients. Muscarinic side effects are minimized by prior or concomitant administration of an anticholinergic agent. The onset of action of glycopyrrolate (0.2 mg glycopyrrolate per 1 mg of neostigmine) is similar to that of neostigmine and is associated with less tachycardia than is experienced with atropine (0.4 mg of atropine per 1 mg of neostigmine). It has been reported that neostigmine crosses the placenta, resulting in fetal bradycardia, but there is no evidence that the choice of atropine versus glycopyrrolate makes any difference in newborn outcomes. Neostigmine is also used to treat myasthenia gravis, urinary bladder atony, and paralytic ileus.

PYRIDOSTIGMINE

Physical Structure

Pyridostigmine is structurally similar to neostigmine except that the quaternary ammonium is incorporated into the phenol ring. Pyridostigmine shares neostigmine's covalent binding to acetylcholinesterase and its lipid insolubility.

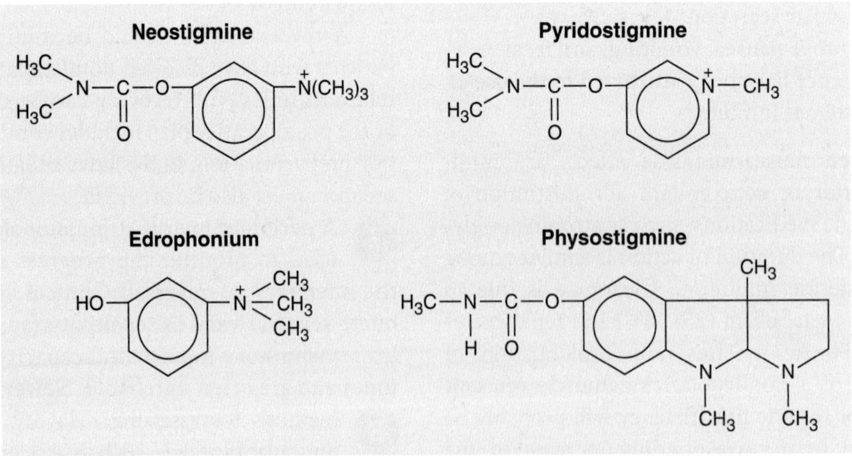

FIGURE 12–4 The molecular structures of neostigmine, pyridostigmine, edrophonium, and physostigmine.

TABLE 12–3 The choice and dose of cholinesterase inhibitor determine the choice and dose of anticholinergic.

Cholinesterase Inhibitor	Usual Dose of Cholinesterase Inhibitor	Recommended Anticholinergic	Usual Dose of Anticholinergic per mg of Cholinesterase Inhibitor
Neostigmine	0.04–0.08 mg/kg	Glycopyrrolate	0.2 mg
Pyridostigmine	0.1–0.25 mg/kg	Glycopyrrolate	0.05 mg
Edrophonium	0.5–1 mg/kg	Atropine	0.014 mg
Physostigmine[1]	0.01–0.03 mg/kg	Usually not necessary	NA[2]

[1]Not used to reverse muscle relaxants.

[2]NA, not applicable

Dosage & Packaging

Pyridostigmine is 20% as potent as neostigmine and may be administered in doses up to 0.25 mg/kg (a total of 20 mg in adults). It is available as a solution of 5 mg/mL.

Clinical Considerations

The onset of action of pyridostigmine is slower (10–15 min) than that of neostigmine, and its duration is slightly longer (>2 h). Glycopyrrolate (0.05 mg per 1 mg of pyridostigmine) or atropine (0.1 mg per 1 mg of pyridostigmine) must also be administered to prevent bradycardia. Glycopyrrolate is preferred because its slower onset of action better matches that of pyridostigmine, again resulting in less tachycardia.

EDROPHONIUM

Physical Structure

Because it lacks a carbamate group, edrophonium must rely on noncovalent bonding to the acetylcholinesterase enzyme. The quaternary ammonium group limits lipid solubility.

Dosage & Packaging

Edrophonium is less than 10% as potent as neostigmine. The recommended dosage is 0.5 to 1 mg/kg.

Clinical Considerations

Edrophonium has the most rapid onset of action (1–2 min) and the shortest duration of effect of any of the cholinesterase inhibitors. Reduced doses should not be used because longer-acting muscle relaxants may outlast the effects of edrophonium. Higher doses prolong the duration of action to more than 1 h. Edrophonium may not be as effective as neostigmine at reversing intense neuromuscular blockade. In equipotent doses, muscarinic effects of edrophonium are less pronounced than those of neostigmine or pyridostigmine, requiring only half the amount of anticholinergic agent. Edrophonium's rapid onset is well matched to that of atropine (0.014 mg of atropine per 1 mg of edrophonium). Although glycopyrrolate (0.007 mg per 1 mg of edrophonium) can also be used, it should be given several minutes prior to edrophonium to avoid the possibility of bradycardia.

PHYSOSTIGMINE

Physical Structure

Physostigmine, a tertiary amine, has a carbamate group but no quaternary ammonium. Therefore, it is lipid soluble and freely passes the blood–brain barrier.

Dosage & Packaging

The dose of physostigmine is 0.01 to 0.03 mg/kg. It is packaged as a solution containing 1 mg/mL.

Clinical Considerations

The lipid solubility and central nervous system penetration of physostigmine limit its usefulness as a reversal agent for nondepolarizing blockade but make it effective in the treatment of central anticholinergic actions of scopolamine or overdoses of atropine. In addition, it reverses some of the central nervous system depression and delirium associated with use of benzodiazepines and volatile anesthetics. Physostigmine (0.04 mg/kg) has been shown to be effective in preventing postoperative shivering. It reportedly partially antagonizes morphine-induced respiratory depression, presumably because morphine reduces acetylcholine release in the brain. These effects are transient, and repeated doses may be required. Bradycardia is infrequent in the recommended dosage range, but atropine should be immediately available. Because glycopyrrolate does not cross the blood–brain barrier, it will not reverse the central nervous system effects of physostigmine. Other possible muscarinic side effects include excessive salivation, vomiting, and convulsions. In contrast to other cholinesterase inhibitors, physostigmine is almost completely metabolized by plasma esterases, so renal excretion is not important.

OTHER CONSIDERATIONS

Recovery from neuromuscular blockade is influenced by the depth of block at the time of antagonism, the clearance and half-life of the relaxant used, and other factors that affect neuromuscular blockade (Table 12–4), such as medications and electrolyte disturbances.

NONCLASSIC REVERSAL AGENTS

Besides cholinesterase inhibitors, additional drugs (calabadion and L-cysteine) are currently under investigation, and sugammadex is increasingly used in the United States. These agents act as selective antagonists of nondepolarizing neuromuscular blockade. Sugammadex is able to reverse aminosteroid-induced neuromuscular blockade, whereas cysteine has been shown to reverse the neuromuscular blocking effects of gantacurium and other fumarates. Calabadion prevents binding to the nicotinic receptor of both benzylisoquinolinium and steroidal nondepolarizing muscle relaxants.

TABLE 12–4 Factors potentiating neuromuscular blockade.

Drugs
Volatile anesthetics
Antibiotics: aminoglycosides, polymyxin B, neomycin, tetracycline, clindamycin
Dantrolene
Verapamil
Furosemide
Lidocaine
Electrolytes and acid–base disorders
Hypermagnesemia
Hypocalcemia
Hypokalemia
Respiratory acidosis
Temperature
Hypothermia

SUGAMMADEX

Sugammadex is a novel selective relaxant-binding agent that is rapidly supplanting neostigmine as the preferred agent for reversal of nondepolarizing neuromuscular blockade. It is a modified γ-cyclodextrin (*su* refers to sugar, and *gammadex* refers to the structural molecule γ-cyclodextrin).

Physical Structure

Its three-dimensional structure resembles a dough-
9 nut with a hydrophobic cavity and a hydrophilic exterior. Hydrophobic interactions trap the drug (eg, rocuronium) in the cyclodextrin cavity (doughnut hole), resulting in the tight formation of a water-soluble guest–host complex in a 1:1 ratio. This restrains the drug in extracellular fluid where it cannot interact with nicotinic acetylcholine receptors to produce a neuromuscular block. Sugammadex is largely eliminated unchanged via the kidneys and does not require coadministration of an antimuscarinic agent.

Clinical Considerations

Sugammadex has been administered in doses of 4 to 8 mg/kg. With an injection of 8 mg/kg, given 3 min after administration of 0.6 mg/kg of rocuronium, recovery of train-of-four ratio to 0.9 was observed within 2 min. It produces a rapid and effective reversal of both shallow and profound rocuronium-induced neuromuscular blockade in a consistent manner.

Sugammadex may impair the contraceptive effect of patients using hormonal contraceptives because of its affinity for compounds with steroidal structure. An alternative, nonhormonal contraceptive should be used for 7 days following sugammadex administration. Toremifene, an estrogen antagonist, has a high affinity for sugammadex and might delay its reversal of neuromuscular block. Because of its renal excretion, sugammadex is not recommended in patients with severe kidney dysfunction (creatine clearance <30 mL/min). Sugammadex may artifactually prolong the activated partial thromboplastin time.

Sugammadex is most effective in the reversal of rocuronium; however, it will bind other steroidal neuromuscular blockers, including vecuronium and pancuronium. Sugammadex is not effective in reversing nondepolarizing neuromuscular blockade secondary to benzylisoquinoline relaxants such as cisatracurium. Moreover, following reversal with sugammadex, subsequent neuromuscular blockade with steroidal neuromuscular blockers may be impaired. Benzylisoquinoline relaxants can be employed as an alternative.

CALABADION

Calabadion 1 and 2 are members of the cucurbituril class of "molecular containers" and are capable of reversing both steroidal and benzylisoquinoline neuromuscular blockers. Calabadions prevent muscle relaxant binding to the nicotinic receptor. Calabadions are currently under investigation.

L-CYSTEINE

L-cysteine is an endogenous amino acid that is often added to total parenteral nutrition regimens to enhance
10 calcium and phosphate solubility. The ultrashort-acting neuromuscular blocker, gantacurium, and other fumarates rapidly combine with L-cysteine in vitro to form less active degradation products (adducts). Exogenous administration of L-cysteine (10–50 mg/kg intravenously) given to anesthetized monkeys 1 min after these neuromuscular blocking agents abolished the block within 2 to 3 min; this antagonism was found to be superior to that produced by anticholinesterases. This unique method of antagonism by adduct formation and inactivation is still in the investigative stage, especially in terms of its safety and efficacy in humans.

CASE DISCUSSION

Respiratory Failure in the Postanesthesia Care Unit

A 66-year-old woman weighing 85 kg is brought to the recovery room following laparoscopic cholecystectomy. The anesthetic technique included the use of isoflurane and vecuronium for muscle relaxation. At the conclusion of the procedure, the anesthesiologist administered 6 mg of morphine sulfate for postoperative pain control and 3 mg of neostigmine with 0.6 mg of glycopyrrolate to reverse any residual neuromuscular blockade. The dose of cholinesterase inhibitor was empirically based on clinical judgment. Although the patient was apparently breathing normally on arrival in the recovery room, her tidal volume progressively diminished. Arterial blood gas measurements revealed a $PaCO_2$ of 62 mm Hg, a PaO_2 of 110 mm Hg, and a pH of 7.26 on a fraction of inspired oxygen (FiO_2) of 40%.

Which drugs administered to this patient could explain her hypoventilation?

Isoflurane, morphine sulfate, and vecuronium all interfere with a patient's ability to maintain a normal ventilatory response to an elevated $PaCO_2$.

Why would the patient's breathing worsen in the recovery room?

Possibilities include the delayed onset of action of morphine sulfate, a lack of sensory stimulation in the recovery area, fatigue of respiratory muscles, the adverse effects of hypoventilation and hypercarbia on neuromuscular function, and splinting as a result of upper abdominal pain.

Could the patient still have residual neuromuscular blockade?

If the dose of neostigmine was not determined by the response to an objective peripheral nerve stimulator, or if the recovery of muscle function was inadequately tested after the reversal drugs were given, persistent neuromuscular blockade is possible. Assume, for example, that the patient had minimal or no response to initial tetanic stimulation at 100 Hz. Even the maximal dose of neostigmine (5 mg) might not yet have adequately reversed the paralysis. Because of enormous patient variability, the response to peripheral nerve stimulation must always be monitored when muscle relaxants are administered. Even if partial reversal is achieved, paralysis may worsen if the patient hypoventilates. **Other factors (in addition to respiratory acidosis) that impair the recovery of neuromuscular function include excessive doses of neuromuscular blockers, electrolyte disturbances (hypermagnesemia, hypokalemia, and hypocalcemia), hypothermia (temperature <32°C), drug interactions (see Table 11–3), metabolic alkalosis (from accompanying hypokalemia and hypocalcemia), and coexisting diseases (see Table 11–7).**

How could the extent of reversal be tested?

Tetanic stimulation is a sensitive but uncomfortable test of neuromuscular transmission in an awake patient. Because of its shorter duration, double-burst stimulation is tolerated better than tetany by conscious patients. Quantitative measures such as acceleromyography are preferred to assess the adequacy of reversal (train of four >0.9) compared with subjective interpretations of twitch. Many other tests of neuromuscular transmission, such as vital capacity and tidal volume, are insensitive as they may still seem normal when 70% to 80% of receptors are blocked. In fact, 70% of receptors may remain blocked despite an apparently ***normal response to train-of-four stimulation.***

What treatment would you suggest?

Ventilation should be assisted to reduce respiratory acidosis. Even if diaphragmatic function seems to be adequate, residual blockade can lead to airway obstruction and poor airway protection. If there is persisting neuromuscular block, additional neostigmine (with an anticholinergic) could be administered up to a maximum recommended dose of 5 mg. Since vecuronium was used, sugammadex is an attractive alternative. If this does not adequately reverse paralysis, mechanical ventilation and airway protection should be instituted and continued until neuromuscular function is fully restored.

SUGGESTED READINGS

Baysal A, Dogukan M, Toman H, et al. The use of sugammadex for reversal of residual blockade after administration of neostigmine and atropine: 9AP1-9 *Eur J Anaesth*. 2013;30:142.

Brull SJ, Kopman AF. Current status of neuromuscular reversal and monitoring: challenges and opportunities. *Anesthesiology*. 2017;126:173.

de Boer HD, Carlos RV. New drug developments for neuromuscular blockade and reversal: gantacurium, CW002, CW011, and calabadion. *Curr Anesthesiol Rep*. 2018;8:119.

Dirkman D, Britten M, Henning P, et al. Anticoagulant effect of sugammadex. *Anesthesiology*. 2016;124:1277.

Haeter F, Simons J, Foerster U, et al. Comparative effectiveness of calabadion and sugammadex to reverse nondepolarizing neuromuscular blocking agents. *Anesthesiology*. 2015;123:1337.

Heerdt P, Sunaga H, Savarese J. Novel neuromuscular blocking drugs and antagonists. *Curr Opin Anesthesiol*. 2015;28:403.

Hoffmann U, Grosse-Sundrup M, Eikermann-Haeter K, et al. Calabadion: a new agent to reverse the effects of benzylisoquinoline and steroidal neuromuscular blocking agents. *Anesthesiology*. 2013;119:317.

Hristovska AM, Duch P, Allingstrup M, Afshari A. Efficacy and safety of sugammadex versus neostigmine in reversing neuromuscular blockade in adults. *Cochrane Database Syst Rev*. 2017;8:CD012763.

Kusha N, Singh D, Shetti A, et al. Sugammadex; a revolutionary drug in neuromuscular pharmacology. *Anesth Essays Res*. 2013:7:302.

Lien CA. Development and potential clinical impact of ultra-short acting neuromuscular blocking agents. *Br J Anaesth*. 2011;107(S1):160.

Meistelman C, Donati F. Do we really need sugammadex as an antagonist of muscle relaxants in anesthesia? *Curr Opin Anesthesiol.* 2016;29:462.

Naguib M. Sugammadex: another milestone in clinical neuromuscular pharmacology. *Anesth Analg.* 2007;104:575.

Taylor P. Anticholinesterase agents. In: Brunton LL, Knollmann BC, Hilal-Dandan R, eds. *Goodman and Gilman's Pharmacological Basis of Therapeutics.* 13th ed. McGraw-Hill, 2018.

CHAPTER

13

Anticholinergic Drugs

KEY CONCEPTS

1. The ester linkage is essential for effective binding of anticholinergics to acetylcholine receptors. This binding competitively blocks binding by acetylcholine and prevents receptor activation. The cellular effects of acetylcholine, which are mediated through second messengers, are inhibited.
2. Anticholinergics relax the bronchial smooth musculature, which reduces airway resistance and increases anatomic dead space.
3. Atropine has particularly potent effects on the heart and bronchial smooth muscle and is the most efficacious anticholinergic for treating bradyarrhythmia.
4. Ipratropium solution (0.5 mg in 2.5 mL) seems to be particularly effective in the treatment of acute chronic obstructive pulmonary disease when combined with a β-agonist drug (eg, albuterol).
5. Scopolamine is a more potent antisialagogue than atropine and causes greater central nervous system effects.
6. Because of its quaternary structure, glycopyrrolate cannot cross the blood–brain barrier and is almost devoid of central nervous system and ophthalmic activity.

One group of cholinergic antagonists has already been discussed: the nondepolarizing neuromuscular blocking agents. These drugs act primarily at the nicotinic receptors in skeletal muscle. This chapter presents the pharmacology of drugs that block muscarinic receptors. Although the classification *anticholinergic* usually refers to this latter group, a more precise term would be *antimuscarinic*.

In this chapter, the mechanism of action and clinical pharmacology are introduced for three common anticholinergics: atropine, scopolamine, and glycopyrrolate. The clinical uses of these drugs in anesthesia relate to their effect on the cardiovascular, respiratory, cerebral, gastrointestinal, and other organ systems (Table 13–1).

MECHANISMS OF ACTION

Anticholinergics are esters of an aromatic acid combined with an organic base (Figure 13–1). **1** The ester linkage is essential for effective binding of the anticholinergics to the acetylcholine receptors. **This competitively blocks binding by acetylcholine and prevents receptor activation.** The cellular effects of acetylcholine, mediated through second messengers, are inhibited. Muscarinic receptors are not homogeneous, and receptor subgroups have been identified, including central nervous system ($M_{1,4,5}$), autonomic ganglia and gastric parietal cells (M_1), cardiac (M_2), and smooth muscle (M_3) receptors. These receptors vary in their affinity for receptor antagonists.

TABLE 13–1 Pharmacological characteristics of anticholinergic drugs.[1]

	Atropine	Scopolamine	Glycopyrrolate
Tachycardia	+++	+	++
Bronchodilatation	++	+	++
Sedation	+	+++	0
Antisialagogue effect	++	+++	+++

[1]0, no effect; +, minimal effect; ++, moderate effect; +++, marked effect.

CLINICAL PHARMACOLOGY

General Pharmacological Characteristics

In normal clinical doses, only muscarinic receptors are blocked by the anticholinergic drugs discussed in this chapter. The clinical response to an anticholinergic drug depends on the degree of baseline vagal tone.

A. Cardiovascular

Blockade of muscarinic receptors in the sinoatrial node produces tachycardia. This effect is especially useful in reversing bradycardia due to vagal reflexes (eg, baroreceptor reflex, peritoneal traction, oculocardiac reflex). A transient slowing of heart rate in response to smaller intravenous doses of atropine (<0.4 mg) has been reported. The mechanism of this paradoxical response is unclear. These agents promote conduction through the atrioventricular node, shortening the P–R interval on the electrocardiogram and antagonizing heart block caused by vagal activity. Atrial arrhythmias and nodal (junctional) rhythms occasionally occur. Anticholinergics generally have little effect on ventricular function or

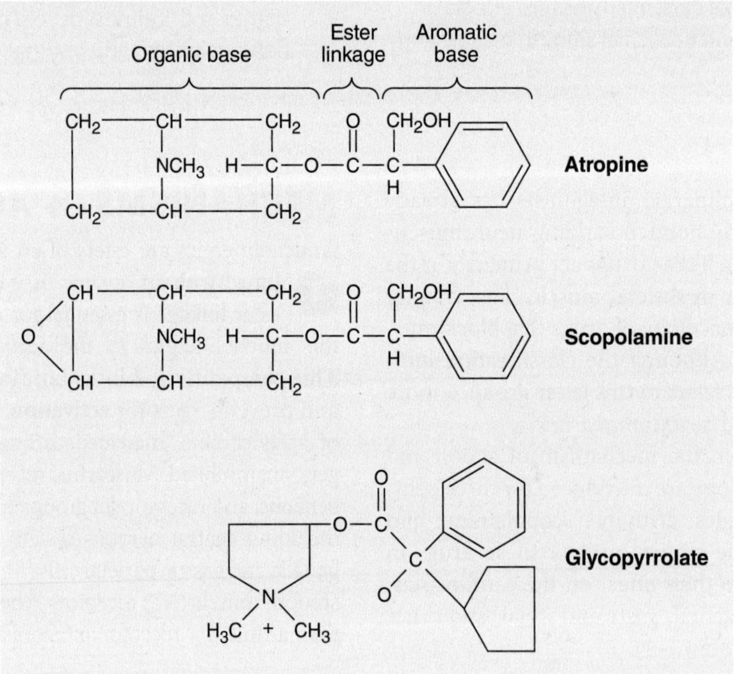

FIGURE 13–1 Physical structures of anticholinergic drugs.

peripheral vasculature because of the paucity of direct cholinergic innervation of these areas despite the presence of cholinergic receptors. Presynaptic muscarinic receptors on adrenergic nerve terminals are known to inhibit norepinephrine release, so muscarinic antagonists may modestly enhance sympathetic activity. Large doses of anticholinergic agents can produce dilation of cutaneous blood vessels (atropine flush).

B. Respiratory

Anticholinergics inhibit respiratory tract secretions, from the nose to the bronchi, a valuable property during endoscopic or surgical procedures on the airway.

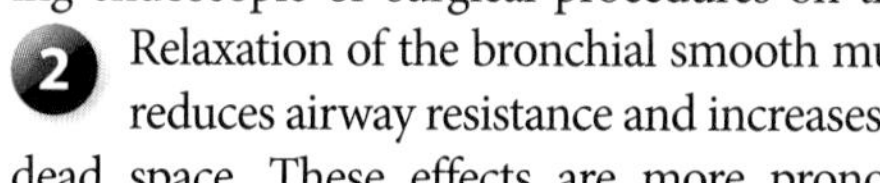

Relaxation of the bronchial smooth musculature reduces airway resistance and increases anatomic dead space. These effects are more pronounced in patients with chronic obstructive pulmonary disease or asthma.

C. Cerebral

Anticholinergic medications can cause a spectrum of central nervous system effects ranging from stimulation to depression, depending on drug choice and dosage. Cerebral stimulation may present as excitation, restlessness, or hallucinations. Cerebral depression, including sedation and amnesia, reliably occurs with scopolamine. Physostigmine, a cholinesterase inhibitor that crosses the blood–brain barrier, promptly reverses anticholinergic actions on the brain.

D. Gastrointestinal

Salivation is markedly reduced by anticholinergic drugs. Gastric secretions are also decreased with larger doses. Decreased intestinal motility and peristalsis prolong gastric emptying time. Lower esophageal sphincter pressure is reduced. Anticholinergic drugs do not prevent aspiration pneumonia.

E. Ophthalmic

Anticholinergics (particularly when dosed topically) cause mydriasis (pupillary dilation) and cycloplegia (an inability to accommodate to near vision). Acute angle-closure glaucoma is unlikely but possible following systemic administration of anticholinergic drugs.

F. Genitourinary

Anticholinergics may decrease ureter and bladder tone as a result of smooth muscle relaxation and lead to urinary retention, particularly in men with prostatic hypertrophy.

G. Thermoregulation

Inhibition of sweat glands may lead to a rise in body temperature (atropine fever).

Specific Anticholinergic Drugs

ATROPINE

Physical Structure

Atropine is a tertiary amine. The levorotatory form is active, but the commercial product is a racemic mixture (see **Figure 13–1**).

Dosage & Packaging

As a premedication, atropine is administered intravenously or intramuscularly in a range of 0.01 to 0.02 mg/kg, up to the usual adult dose of 0.4 to 0.6 mg. Larger intravenous doses of up to 2 mg may be required to completely block the cardiac vagal nerves in treating severe bradycardia. Atropine sulfate is available in a multitude of concentrations.

Clinical Considerations

3 Atropine has particularly potent effects on the heart and bronchial smooth muscle and is the most efficacious anticholinergic for treating bradyarrhythmia. Patients with coronary artery disease may not tolerate the increased myocardial oxygen demand and decreased oxygen supply associated with the tachycardia caused by atropine. A derivative of atropine, ipratropium bromide, is available in a metered-dose inhaler for the treatment of bronchospasm. Its quaternary ammonium structure significantly 4 limits systemic absorption. Ipratropium solution (0.5 mg in 2.5 mL) is effective in the treatment of acute bronchospasm in patients with chronic obstructive pulmonary disease, particularly when combined with a β-agonist drug (eg, albuterol).

The central nervous system effects of atropine are minimal after the usual doses, even though this tertiary amine can rapidly cross the blood–brain barrier. Atropine has been associated with mild postoperative memory deficits, and toxic doses are usually associated with excitatory reactions. An intramuscular dose of 0.01 to 0.02 mg/kg reliably provides an antisialagogue effect. Atropine should be used cautiously in patients with narrow-angle glaucoma, prostatic hypertrophy, or bladder-neck obstruction.

Intravenous atropine is used in the treatment of organophosphate pesticide and nerve gas poisoning. Organophosphates inhibit acetylcholinesterase, resulting in overwhelming stimulation of nicotinic and muscarinic receptors that leads to bronchorrhea, respiratory collapse, and bradycardia. Atropine can reverse the effects of muscarinic stimulation but not the muscle weakness resulting from nicotinic receptor activation. Pralidoxime (2-PAM; 1–2 g intravenously) may reactivate acetylcholinesterase.

SCOPOLAMINE

Physical Structure

Scopolamine, a tertiary amine, differs from atropine by the addition of an epoxide to the heterocyclic ring.

Clinical Considerations

5 Scopolamine is a more potent antisialagogue than atropine and causes greater central nervous system effects. Clinical dosages usually result in drowsiness and amnesia, though restlessness, dizziness, and delirium are possible. The sedative effects may be desirable for premedication but can interfere with awakening following short procedures. Scopolamine has the added virtue of preventing motion sickness. The lipid solubility allows transdermal absorption, and transdermal scopolamine (1 mg patch) has been used to prevent postoperative nausea and vomiting. Because of its pronounced mydriatic effects, scopolamine is best avoided in patients with closed-angle glaucoma.

GLYCOPYRROLATE

Physical Structure

Glycopyrrolate is a synthetic product that differs from atropine in being a quaternary amine and having both cyclopentane and pyridine moieties in the compound.

Dosage & Packaging

The usual dose of glycopyrrolate is one-half that of atropine. For instance, the premedication dose is 0.005 to 0.01 mg/kg up to 0.2 to 0.3 mg in adults. Glycopyrrolate for injection is packaged as a solution of 0.2 mg/mL.

Clinical Considerations

6 Because of its quaternary structure, glycopyrrolate cannot cross the blood–brain barrier and is almost devoid of central nervous system and ophthalmic activity. Potent inhibition of salivary gland and respiratory tract secretions is the primary rationale for using glycopyrrolate as a premedication. Heart rate usually increases after intravenous—but not intramuscular—administration. Glycopyrrolate has a longer duration of action than atropine (2–4 h versus 30 min after intravenous administration).

CASE DISCUSSION

Central Anticholinergic Syndrome

An older adult patient is diagnosed with central anticholinergic syndrome attributed to overuse of eye drops. How many milligrams of atropine is in one drop of a 1% solution?

A 1% solution contains 1 g dissolved in 100 mL, or 10 mg/mL. Eyedroppers vary in the number of drops formed per milliliter of solution but average 20 drops/mL. Therefore, one drop usually contains 0.5 mg of atropine.

How are ophthalmic drops systemically absorbed?

Absorption by vessels in the conjunctival sac is similar to subcutaneous injection. More rapid absorption is possible by the nasolacrimal duct mucosa.

What are the signs and symptoms of anticholinergic poisoning?

Reactions from an overdose of anticholinergic medication involve several organ systems. Central anticholinergic syndrome refers to central nervous system changes that range from unconsciousness to hallucinations. Agitation and delirium are not unusual in older adult patients. Other systemic manifestations include dry mouth, tachycardia, atropine flush, atropine fever, and impaired vision.

What other drugs possess anticholinergic activity that could predispose patients to central anticholinergic syndrome?

Tricyclic antidepressants, antihistamines, and antipsychotics have antimuscarinic properties that could potentiate the side effects of anticholinergic drugs.

What drug is an effective antidote to anticholinergic overdosage?

Cholinesterase inhibitors indirectly increase the amount of acetylcholine available to compete with anticholinergic drugs at the muscarinic receptor. Neostigmine, pyridostigmine, and edrophonium possess a quaternary ammonium group that prevents penetration of the blood–brain barrier. Physostigmine, a tertiary amine, is lipid soluble and effectively reverses central anticholinergic toxicity. An initial dose of 0.01 to 0.03 mg/kg may require redosing after 15 to 30 min.

SUGGESTED READINGS

Brown JH. Muscarinic receptor agonists and antagonists. In: Brunton LL, Knollmann BC, Hilal-Dandan R, eds. *Goodman and Gilman's The Pharmacological Basis of Therapeutics*, 13th ed. McGraw-Hill; 2018.

Eddleston M, Chowdhury F. Pharmacological treatment of organophosphorous insecticide poisoning: the old and the (possible) new. *Br J Clin Pharmacol.* 2015;81:462.

Howard J, Wigley J, Rosen G, D'mello J. Glycopyrrolate: it's time to review. *J Clin Anesth.* 2017;36:51.

Nishtala PS, Salahudeen MS, Hilmer SN. Anticholinergics: theoretical and clinical overview. *Expert Opin Drug Saf.* 2016;15:753.

CHAPTER

14

Adrenergic Agonists & Antagonists

KEY CONCEPTS

1. Adrenergic agonists can be categorized as direct or indirect. Direct agonists bind to the receptor, whereas indirect agonists increase endogenous neurotransmitter activity.
2. The primary effect of phenylephrine is peripheral vasoconstriction with a concomitant rise in systemic vascular resistance and arterial blood pressure.
3. Clonidine decreases anesthetic and analgesic requirements and provides sedation and anxiolysis.
4. Dexmedetomidine has a greater affinity for α_2-receptors than clonidine. It has sedative, analgesic, and sympatholytic effects that blunt many of the cardiovascular responses seen during the perioperative period.
5. Long-term use of these agents, particularly clonidine and dexmedetomidine, leads to super-sensitization and upregulation of receptors; with abrupt discontinuation of either drug, an acute withdrawal syndrome including hypertensive crisis can occur.
6. Ephedrine is commonly used as a vasopressor during anesthesia. As such, its administration should be viewed as a temporizing measure while the cause of hypotension is determined and remedied.
7. At low doses (0.5–3 mcg/kg/min), dopamine (DA) primarily activates dopaminergic receptors. Stimulation of these receptors (specifically, DA_1 receptors) vasodilates the renal vasculature and promotes diuresis.
8. Labetalol lowers blood pressure without reflex tachycardia because of its combination of α and β effects.
9. Esmolol is an ultrashort-acting selective β_1-antagonist that reduces heart rate and, to a lesser extent, blood pressure.
10. Abrupt discontinuation of β-blocker therapy for 24 to 48 h may trigger a withdrawal syndrome characterized by hypertension, tachycardia, and angina pectoris.

Adrenergic agonists and antagonists produce their clinical effects by interacting with the adrenergic receptors (ie, adrenoceptors). The clinical effects of these drugs can be deduced from an understanding of the adrenoceptor physiology and a knowledge of which receptors each drug activates or blocks.

ADRENOCEPTOR PHYSIOLOGY

The term *adrenergic* originally referred to the effects of epinephrine (*adren*aline), though norepinephrine (noradrenaline) is the primary neurotransmitter responsible for most of the adrenergic activity of the sympathetic nervous system. With the exception of

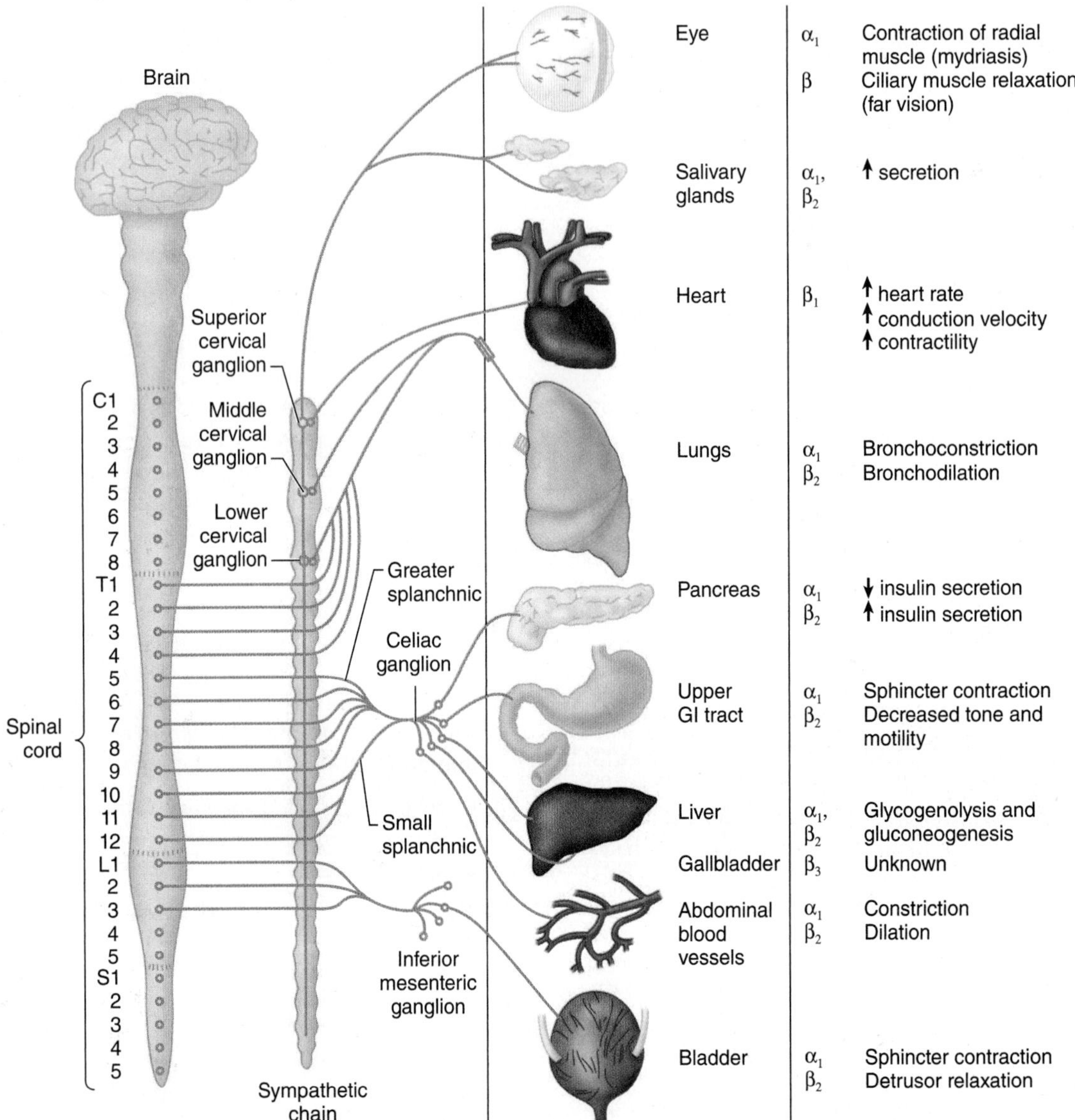

FIGURE 14–1 The sympathetic nervous system. Organ innervation, receptor type, and response to stimulation. The origin of the sympathetic chain is the thoracoabdominal (T1–L3) spinal cord, in contrast to the craniosacral distribution of the parasympathetic nervous system. Another anatomic difference is the greater distance from the sympathetic ganglion to the visceral structures. GI, gastrointestinal.

eccrine sweat glands and some blood vessels, norepinephrine is released by postganglionic sympathetic fibers at end-organ tissues (Figure 14–1). In contrast, acetylcholine is released by preganglionic sympathetic fibers and all parasympathetic fibers.

Norepinephrine is synthesized in the cytoplasm of sympathetic postganglionic nerve endings and stored in the vesicles (Figure 14–2). After release by the process of exocytosis, norepinephrine's actions are primarily terminated by reuptake into the

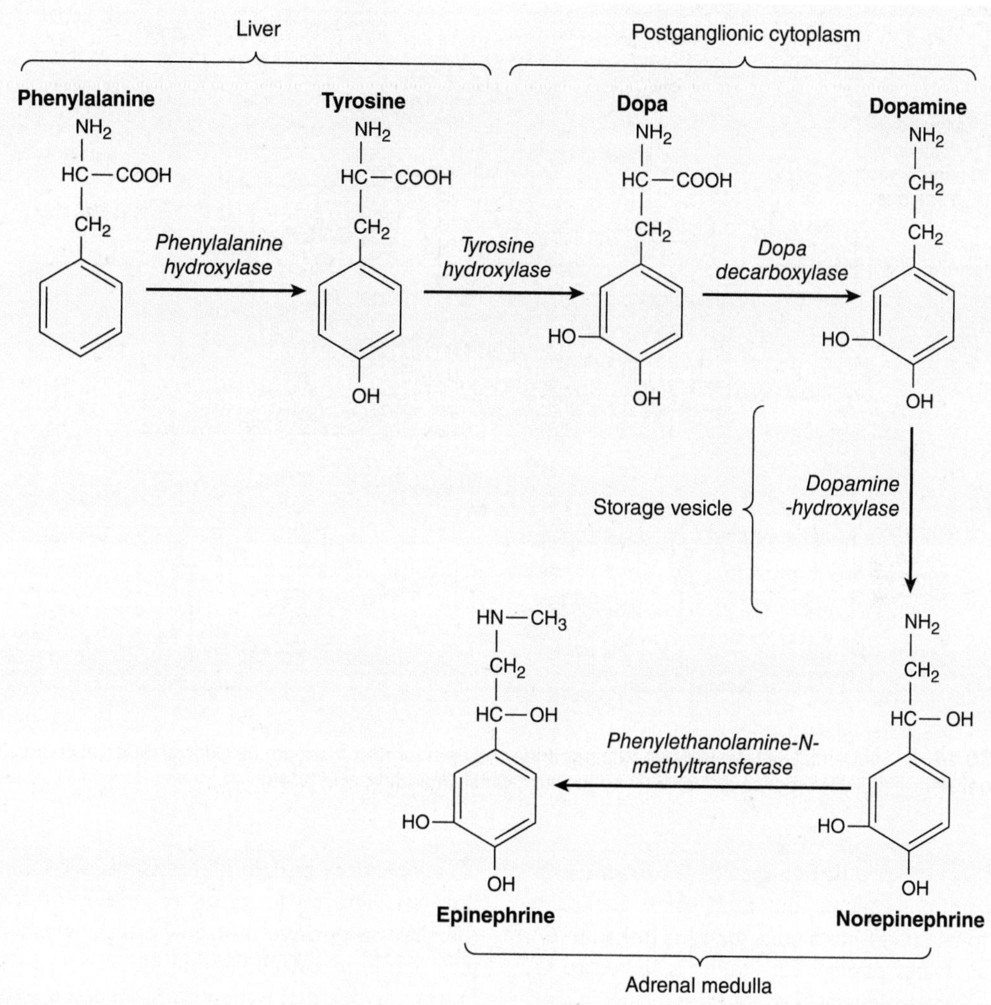

FIGURE 14–2 The synthesis of norepinephrine. Hydroxylation of tyrosine to dopa is the rate-limiting step. Dopamine is actively transported into storage vesicles. Norepinephrine can be converted to epinephrine in the adrenal medulla.

postganglionic nerve ending. The norepinephrine transporter on neuronal cell membranes facilitates the removal of norepinephrine from the synapse. Other transporters facilitate the uptake of dopamine and serotonin. Tricyclic antidepressants, cocaine, and amphetamines inhibit these transporters, leading to their clinical effects. Norepinephrine may diffuse from receptor sites where it is taken up by nonneuronal cells and is metabolized by catechol-*O*-methyltransferase (Figure 14–3). In neurons, norepinephrine may be metabolized by monoamine oxidase or repackaged into vesicles. Prolonged adrenergic activation leads to desensitization and reduced responses and to subsequent stimulation.

Adrenergic receptors are divided into two general categories: α and β. Each of these has been further subdivided into at least two subtypes: α_1 and α_2, and β_1, β_2, and β_3. The α-receptors have been further divided using molecular cloning techniques into α_{1A}, α_{1B}, α_{1D}, α_{2A}, α_{2B}, and α_{2C}. These receptors are linked to G proteins (Figure 14–4)—heterotrimeric receptors with α, β, and γ subunits. The different

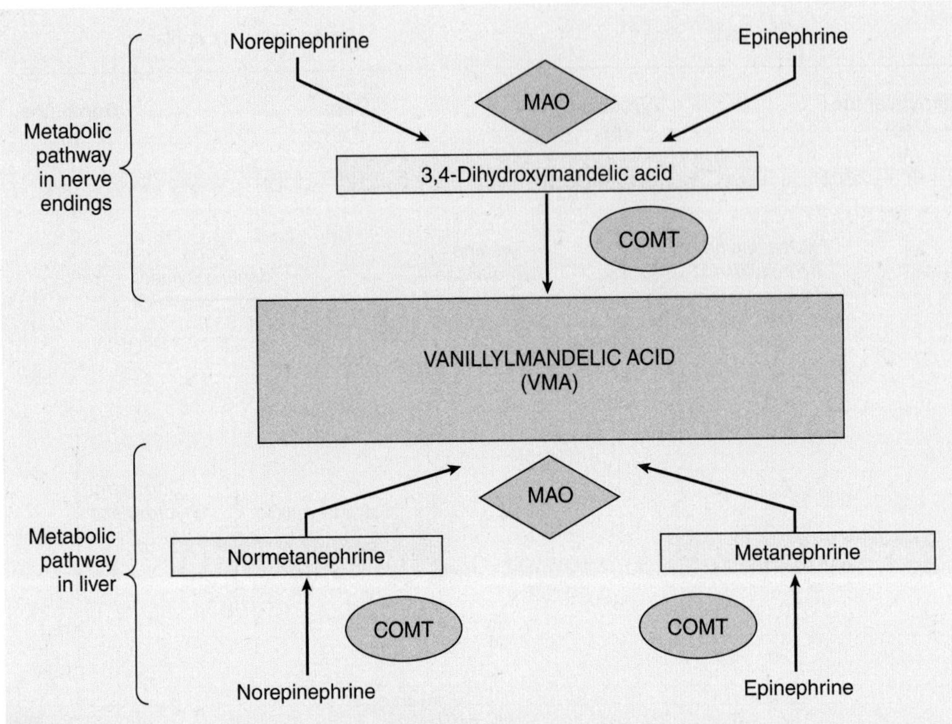

FIGURE 14–3 Sequential metabolism of norepinephrine and epinephrine. Monoamine oxidase (MAO) and catechol-*O*-methyltransferase (COMT) produce a common end product, vanillylmandelic acid (VMA).

adrenoceptors are linked to specific G proteins, each with a unique effector, but each using guanosine triphosphate (GTP) as a cofactor. α_1 is linked to G_q, which activates phospholipases; α_2 is linked to G_i, which inhibits adenylate cyclase (also termed *adenyl* or *adenylyl cyclase*); and β is linked to G_s, which activates adenylate cyclase.

α_1-Receptors

α_1-Receptors are postsynaptic adrenoceptors located in smooth muscle throughout the body (in the eye, lung, blood vessels, uterus, gut, and genitourinary system). Activation of these receptors increases intracellular calcium ion concentration, which leads to the contraction of smooth muscles. Thus, α_1-agonists are associated with mydriasis (pupillary dilation due to contraction of the radial eye muscles), bronchoconstriction, vasoconstriction, uterine contraction, and constriction of sphincters in the gastrointestinal and genitourinary tracts. Stimulation of α_1-receptors also inhibits insulin secretion and lipolysis. The myocardium possesses α_1-receptors that have a positive inotropic effect, which might play a role in catecholamine-induced arrhythmia. During myocardial ischemia, enhanced α_1-receptor coupling with agonists is observed. Nonetheless, the most important cardiovascular effect of α_1 stimulation is vasoconstriction, which increases peripheral vascular resistance, left ventricular afterload, and arterial blood pressure.

α_2-Receptors

In contrast to α_1-receptors, α_2-receptors are located primarily on the presynaptic nerve terminals. Activation of these adrenoceptors inhibits adenylyl cyclase activity. This decreases the entry of calcium ions into the neuronal terminal, which limits subsequent exocytosis of storage vesicles containing norepinephrine. Thus, α_2-receptors create a negative feedback loop that inhibits further norepinephrine

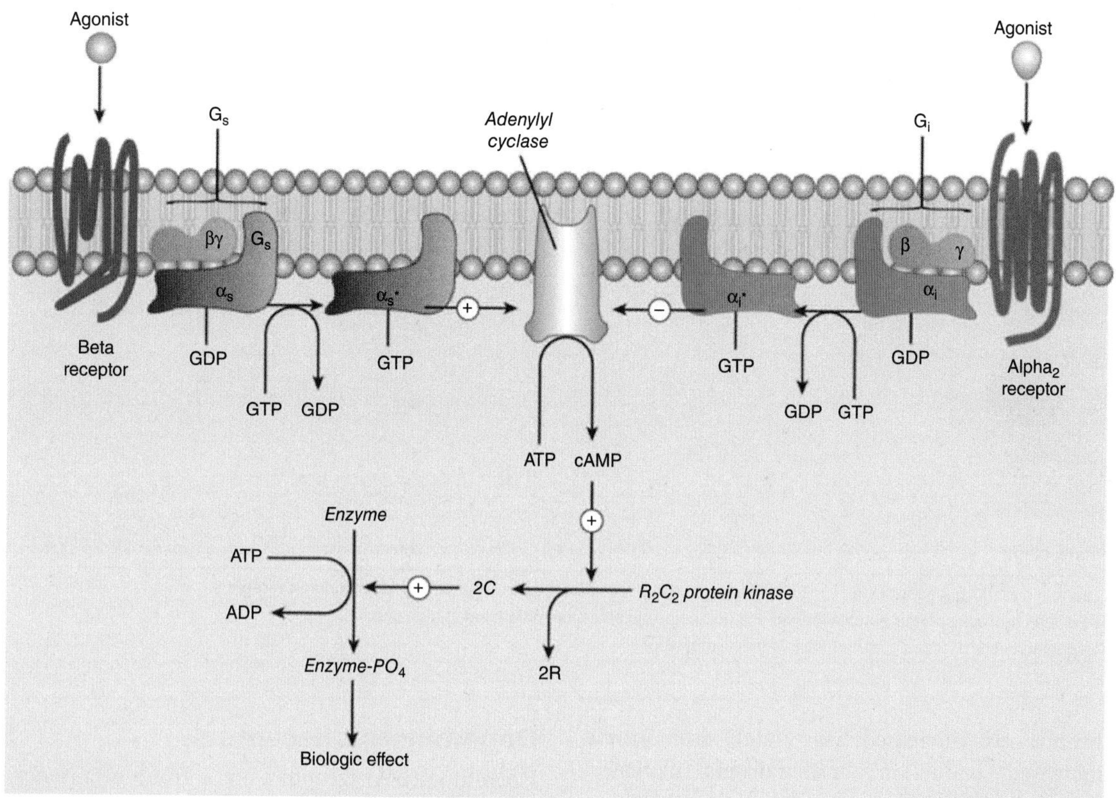

FIGURE 14–4 Activation and inhibition of adenylyl cyclase by agonists that bind to catecholamine receptors. Binding to β-adrenoceptors stimulates adenylyl cyclase by activating the stimulatory G protein, G_s, which leads to the dissociation of its a subunit charged with guanosine triphosphate (GTP). This activated α_s subunit directly activates adenylyl cyclase, resulting in an increased rate of synthesis of cAMP. α_2-Adrenoceptor ligands inhibit adenylyl cyclase by causing dissociation of the inhibitory G protein, G_i, into its subunits (ie, an activated α_i subunit charged with GTP and a β-γ unit). The mechanism by which these subunits inhibit adenylyl cyclase is uncertain. cAMP binds to the regulatory subunit (R) of cAMP-dependent protein kinase, leading to the liberation of active catalytic subunits (C) that phosphorylate specific protein substrates and modify their activity. These catalytic units also phosphorylate the cAMP response element binding protein (CREB), which modifies gene expression. See text for other actions of β- and α_2-adrenoceptors. (Reproduced with permission from Katzung BG, Trevor AJ: *Basic & Clinical Pharmacology,* 13th ed. New York, NY: McGraw Hill; 2015.)

release from the neuron. In addition, vascular smooth muscle contains postsynaptic α_2-receptors that produce vasoconstriction. More importantly, stimulation of postsynaptic α_2-receptors in the central nervous system causes sedation and reduces sympathetic outflow, which leads to peripheral vasodilation and lower blood pressure.

β_1-Receptors

β-Adrenergic receptors are classified into β_1, β_2, and β_3 receptors. Norepinephrine and epinephrine are equipotent on β_1 receptors, but epinephrine is significantly more potent than norepinephrine on β_2 receptors, and in any case, the much more potent actions of norepinephrine on alpha receptors tends to obscure any differences between epinephrine and norepinephrine on β receptors when these drugs are infused in patients.

β_1-receptors are located on the postsynaptic membranes in the heart. Stimulation of these receptors activates adenylyl cyclase, which converts adenosine triphosphate to cyclic adenosine monophosphate and initiates a kinase phosphorylation cascade. Initiation of the cascade has positive

TABLE 14–1 Receptor selectivity of adrenergic agonists.[1]

Drug	α_1	α_2	β_1	β_2	DA_1	DA_2
Phenylephrine	+++	+	0	0	0	0
Clonidine	+	++	0	0	0	0
Dexmedetomidine	+	+++	0	0	0	0
Epinephrine[2]	++	++	+++	++	0	0
Ephedrine[3]	++	?	++	+	0	0
Fenoldopam	0	0	0	0	+++	0
Norepinephrine[2]	++	++	++	0	0	0
Dopamine[2]	++	++	++	+	+++	+++
Dobutamine	0	0	+++	+	0	0
Terbutaline	0	0	+	+++	0	0

[1]0, no/minimal effect; +, agonist effect (mild, moderate, marked); ?, unknown effect; DA_1 and DA_2, dopaminergic receptors.

[2]The α_1 effects of epinephrine, norepinephrine, and dopamine become more prominent at high doses.

[3]The primary mode of action of ephedrine is indirect stimulation.

chronotropic (increased heart rate), dromotropic (increased conduction), and inotropic (increased contractility) effects.

β_2-Receptors

β_2-Receptors are postsynaptic adrenoceptors primarily located in smooth muscle and gland cells, but they are also located in ventricular myocytes. Their relative contribution to the response to intravenous catecholamines increases in patients with chronic heart failure. They share a common mechanism of action with β_1-receptors: adenylyl cyclase activation. Despite this commonality, β_2 stimulation relaxes smooth muscle, resulting in bronchodilation, vasodilation, and relaxation of the uterus (tocolysis), bladder, and gut. Glycogenolysis, lipolysis, gluconeogenesis, and insulin release are stimulated by β_2-receptor activation.

β_3-Receptors

β_3-Receptors are found in the gallbladder and brain adipose tissue. Their role in gallbladder physiology is unknown, but they are thought to play a role in lipolysis, thermogenesis in brown fat, and bladder relaxation.

Dopaminergic Receptors

Dopamine (DA) receptors are a group of adrenergic receptors that are activated by dopamine; these receptors are classified as D_1 and D_2 receptors. Activation of D_1 receptors mediates vasodilation in the kidney, intestine, and heart. D_2 receptors are believed to play a role in the antiemetic action of droperidol, haloperidol, and related agents.

Adrenergic Agonists

Adrenergic agonists interact with varying specificity (selectivity) at α- and β-adrenoceptors (Tables 14–1 and 14–2).

"Overlapping" receptor activity complicates the prediction of clinical effects. For example, epinephrine stimulates α_1-, α_2-, β_1-, and β_2-adrenoceptors. Its net effect on arterial blood pressure depends on the dose-dependent balance between α_1-vasoconstriction, α_2- and β_2-vasodilation, and β_1-inotropic influences (and, to a minor degree, β_2-inotropic influences).

1 Adrenergic agonists can be categorized as direct or indirect. Direct agonists bind to the receptor, whereas indirect agonists increase endogenous

TABLE 14–2 Effects of adrenergic agonists on organ systems.[1]

Drug	Heart Rate	Mean Arterial Pressure	Cardiac Output	Peripheral Vascular Resistance	Bronchodilation	Renal Blood Flow
Phenylephrine	↓	↑↑↑	↓	↑↑↑	0	↓↓↓
Epinephrine	↑↑	↑	↑↑	↑/↓	↑↑	↓↓
Ephedrine	↑↑	↑↑	↑↑	↑	↑↑	↓↓
Fenoldopam	↑↑	↓↓↓	↓/↑	↓↓	0	↑↑↑
Norepinephrine	↓	↑↑↑	↓/↑	↑↑↑	0	↓↓↓
Dopamine	↑/↑↑	↑	↑↑↑	↑	0	↑↑↑
Isoproterenol	↑↑↑	↓	↑↑↑	↓↓	↑↑↑	↓/↑
Dobutamine	↑	↑	↑↑↑	↓	0	↑

[1]0, no/minimal effect; ↑, increase (mild, moderate, marked); ↓, decrease (mild, moderate, marked); ↓/↑, variable effect; ↑/↑↑, mild-to-moderate increase.

neurotransmitter activity. Mechanisms of indirect action include increased release or decreased reuptake of norepinephrine. The differentiation between direct and indirect mechanisms of action is particularly important in patients who have abnormal endogenous norepinephrine stores, as may occur with the use of some antihypertensive medications or monoamine oxidase inhibitors. Intraoperative hypotension in these patients should be treated with direct agonists because their response to indirect agonists will be unpredictable.

Another feature distinguishing adrenergic agonists from each other is their chemical structure. Adrenergic agonists that have a 3,4-dihydroxybenzene structure (Figure 14–5) are known as *catecholamines*. These drugs are typically short-acting because of their metabolism by monoamine oxidase and catechol-*O*-methyltransferase. Patients taking monoamine oxidase inhibitors or tricyclic antidepressants may therefore demonstrate an exaggerated response to catecholamines. The naturally occurring catecholamines are epinephrine, norepinephrine, and DA. Changing the side-chain structure (R_1, R_2, R_3) of naturally occurring catecholamines has led to the development of synthetic catecholamines (eg, isoproterenol and dobutamine) that tend to be more receptor specific.

Adrenergic agonists commonly used in anesthesiology are discussed individually below. Note that the recommended doses for continuous infusion are expressed as mcg/kg/min for some agents and mcg/min (for adult dosing) for others. In either case, these recommendations should be regarded only as guidelines, as individual responses are quite variable.

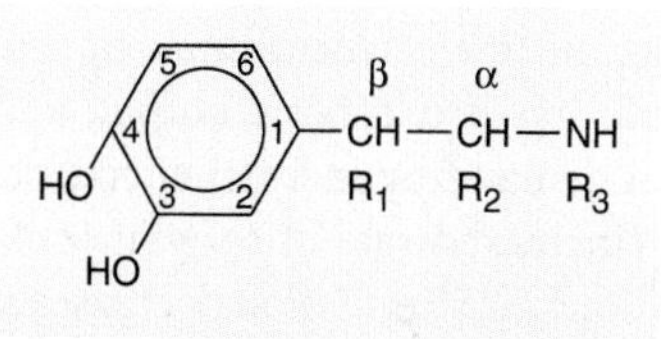

FIGURE 14–5 Adrenergic agonists that have a 3,4-dihydroxybenzene structure are known as *catecholamines*. Substitutions at the R_1, R_2, and R_3 sites affect activity and selectivity.

PHENYLEPHRINE

Phenylephrine is a noncatecholamine with selective **2** α_1-agonist activity. The primary effect of phenylephrine is peripheral vasoconstriction with a concomitant rise in systemic vascular resistance and arterial blood pressure. Reflex bradycardia mediated by the vagus nerve can reduce cardiac output. Phenylephrine is also used topically as a decongestant and a mydriatic agent.

Small intravenous boluses of 50 to 100 mcg (0.5 to 1 mcg/kg) of phenylephrine rapidly reverse reductions in blood pressure caused by peripheral vasodilation (eg, spinal anesthesia) in adults. The duration of action is short, lasting approximately 15 min after administration of a single dose. Tachyphylaxis may occur with phenylephrine infusions and require upward titration of the infusion. Phenylephrine must be diluted from a 1% solution (10 mg/1-mL ampule), usually to a 100 mcg/mL solution and titrated to effect.

α_2-AGONISTS

Clonidine is an α_2-agonist that is commonly used for its antihypertensive and negative chronotropic effects. More recently, it and other α_2-agonists are increasingly being used for their sedative properties. Various studies have examined the anesthetic effects of oral (3–5 mcg/kg), intramuscular (2 mcg/kg), intravenous (1–3 mcg/kg), transdermal (0.1–0.3 mg released per day), intrathecal (15–30 mcg), and perineural or epidural (1–2 mcg/kg) clonidine administration.

3 Clonidine decreases anesthetic and analgesic requirements (decreases minimum alveolar concentration) and provides sedation and anxiolysis. During general anesthesia, clonidine reportedly enhances intraoperative circulatory stability by reducing catecholamine levels. During regional anesthesia, including peripheral nerve block, clonidine prolongs the duration of the block. Direct effects on the spinal cord may be mediated by α_2-postsynaptic receptors within the dorsal horn. Other possible benefits include decreased postoperative shivering, inhibition of opioid-induced muscle rigidity, attenuation of opioid withdrawal symptoms, and the treatment of acute postoperative pain and some chronic pain syndromes. Side effects include bradycardia, hypotension, sedation, respiratory depression, and dry mouth.

Dexmedetomidine has a greater affinity for
4 α_2-receptors than clonidine: the α_2:α_1 receptor specificity ratio is 200:1 for clonidine and 1600:1 for dexmedetomidine. Dexmedetomidine has a shorter half-life (2–3 h) than clonidine (12–24 h). It has sedative, analgesic, and sympatholytic effects that blunt many of the cardiovascular responses seen during the perioperative period. The sedative and analgesic effects are mediated by α_2-adrenergic receptors in the brain (locus ceruleus) and spinal cord. When used intraoperatively, dexmedetomidine reduces intravenous and volatile anesthetic requirements; when used postoperatively, it reduces concurrent analgesic and sedative requirements. Dexmedetomidine is useful in sedating patients in preparation for awake fiberoptic intubation. It is also a useful agent for sedating patients postoperatively in postanesthesia and intensive care units because it does so without significant ventilatory depression. Rapid administration may elevate blood pressure, but hypotension and bradycardia can occur during ongoing therapy. The recommended dosing of dexmedetomidine consists of a loading dose at 1 mcg/kg over 10 min followed by an infusion at 0.2 to 0.7 mcg/kg/h, though we recognize that clinicians administer this agent in a great many ways (including intranasally for sedation in children).

Although these agents are adrenergic agonists, they are also considered to be sympatholytic because
5 sympathetic outflow is reduced. Long-term use of these agents, particularly clonidine and dexmedetomidine, leads to super-sensitization and upregulation of receptors; with abrupt discontinuation of either drug, an acute withdrawal syndrome including hypertensive crisis can occur. This syndrome may manifest after only 48 h of dexmedetomidine infusion when the drug is discontinued. Recent reports have suggested that dexmedetomidine may offer renal protection in the setting of ischemic kidney injury and be of benefit in the treatment of septic shock.

EPINEPHRINE

Epinephrine is an endogenous catecholamine synthesized in the adrenal medulla. Stimulation of β_1-receptors of the myocardium by epinephrine raises blood pressure, cardiac output, and myocardial oxygen demand by increasing contractility and heart rate (increased rate of spontaneous phase IV depolarization). α_1 Stimulation decreases splanchnic and renal blood flow but increases coronary perfusion pressure by increasing aortic diastolic pressure. Systolic blood pressure usually rises, though β_2-mediated vasodilation in skeletal muscle may lower diastolic pressure with lower-dose epinephrine infusions. β_2 Stimulation also relaxes bronchial smooth muscle.

Epinephrine is the principal drug treatment for anaphylaxis and for increasing coronary perfusion pressure during ventricular fibrillation. Complications include cerebral hemorrhage, myocardial ischemia, and ventricular arrhythmias. Volatile anesthetics, particularly halothane, potentiate the arrhythmic effects of epinephrine.

In emergency situations (eg, cardiac arrest and shock), epinephrine is administered as an intravenous bolus of 0.5 to 1 mg, depending on the severity of cardiovascular compromise. In major anaphylactic reactions, epinephrine should be used at a dose of 100 to 500 mcg (repeated, if necessary) followed by infusion. A continuous infusion is prepared (1 mg in 250 mL [4 mcg/mL]) and run at a rate of 2 to 20 mcg/min (30–300 ng/kg/min) to improve myocardial contractility or heart rate. Epinephrine local infiltration is also used to reduce bleeding from the operative sites. Epinephrine is available in vials at a concentration of 1:1000 (1 mg/mL) and prefilled syringes at a concentration of 1:10,000 (0.1 mg/mL [100 mcg/mL]). A 1:100,000 (10 mcg/mL) concentration is available for pediatric use.

EPHEDRINE

The cardiovascular effects of ephedrine, a noncatecholamine sympathomimetic, are similar to those of epinephrine: increase in blood pressure, heart rate, contractility, and cardiac output. Likewise, ephedrine is also a bronchodilator. There are important differences, however: Ephedrine has a longer duration of action, is much less potent, has both indirect and direct actions, and stimulates the central nervous system (it raises minimum alveolar concentration). The indirect agonist properties of ephedrine may be due to peripheral postsynaptic norepinephrine release or inhibition of norepinephrine reuptake.

6 Ephedrine is commonly used as a vasopressor during anesthesia. As such, its administration should be viewed as a temporizing measure while the cause of hypotension is determined and remedied. Unlike direct-acting α_1-agonists, ephedrine did not decrease uterine blood flow in sheep experiments; thus, for many years ephedrine was the preferred vasopressor in obstetric anesthesia. Currently, phenylephrine is widely used in obstetric patients undergoing neuraxial anesthesia because of its faster onset, shorter duration of action, easier titration, and lack of adverse effects on fetal pH relative to ephedrine.

In adults, ephedrine is administered as a bolus of 2.5 to 10 mg; in children, it is given as a bolus of 0.1 mg/kg. Subsequent doses are increased to offset the development of tachyphylaxis, which is probably due to the depletion of norepinephrine stores. Ephedrine is available in 1-mL ampules containing 25 or 50 mg of the agent.

NOREPINEPHRINE

Direct α_1 stimulation with limited β_2 activity (at the doses used clinically) induces intense vasoconstriction of arterial and venous vessels. Increased myocardial contractility from β_1 effects, along with peripheral vasoconstriction, contributes to a rise in arterial blood pressure. Both systolic and diastolic pressures usually rise, but increased afterload and reflex bradycardia may prevent any elevation in cardiac output. Decreased renal and splanchnic blood flow and increased myocardial oxygen requirements are concerns, yet norepinephrine is the agent of choice in the management of refractory (particularly septic) shock. Extravasation of norepinephrine at the site of intravenous administration can cause tissue necrosis.

Norepinephrine is usually administered as a continuous infusion because of its short half-life at a rate of 2 to 20 mcg/min (30–300 ng/kg/min). Ampules contain 4 mg of norepinephrine in 4 mL of solution. In many centers, norepinephrine has replaced phenylephrine as the primary intraoperative vasoconstrictor.

DOPAMINE

The clinical effects of DA, an endogenous nonselective direct and indirect adrenergic and dopaminergic agonist, vary markedly with the dose. At low doses (0.5–3 mcg/kg/min), DA primarily

7

activates dopaminergic receptors (specifically, DA_1 receptors); stimulation of these receptors dilates the renal vasculature and promotes diuresis and natriuresis. Although this action increases renal blood flow, the use of this "renal dose" does not impart any beneficial effect on kidney function. When used in moderate doses (3–10 mcg/kg/min), β_1 stimulation increases myocardial contractility, heart rate, systolic blood pressure, and cardiac output. Myocardial oxygen demand typically increases more than supply. The α_1 effects become prominent at higher doses (10–20 mcg/kg/min), causing an increase in peripheral vascular resistance and a fall in renal blood flow. The exact dose–response curve for dopamine and these several actions is far more unpredictable than the preceding paragraph would suggest! The indirect effects of DA are due to the release of norepinephrine from presynaptic sympathetic nerve ganglion.

DA was formerly a first-line treatment for shock to improve cardiac output, support blood pressure, and maintain renal function. The chronotropic and proarrhythmic effects of DA limit its usefulness in some patients, and it has been replaced by norepinephrine or fenoldopam for many situations in critical illness. DA is administered as a continuous infusion at a rate of 1 to 20 mcg/kg/min. It is most commonly supplied in 5 to 10 mL vials containing 200 or 400 mg of DA.

ISOPROTERENOL

Isoproterenol is of interest because it is a pure β-agonist. β_1 effects increase heart rate, contractility, and cardiac output. Systolic blood pressure may increase or remain unchanged, but β_2 stimulation decreases peripheral vascular resistance and diastolic blood pressure. Myocardial oxygen demand increases while oxygen supply falls, making isoproterenol a poor inotropic choice in most situations.

DOBUTAMINE

Dobutamine is a racemic mixture of two isomers with an affinity for both β_1- and β_2-receptors, with relatively greater selectivity for β_1-receptors. Its primary cardiovascular effect is a rise in cardiac output as a result of increased myocardial contractility. A decline in peripheral vascular resistance caused by β_2 activation usually prevents much of a rise in arterial blood pressure. Left ventricular filling pressure decreases, whereas coronary blood flow increases.

Dobutamine increases myocardial oxygen consumption and should not be routinely used without specific indications to facilitate separation from cardiopulmonary bypass. It is often employed in pharmacological stress testing. Dobutamine is administered as an infusion at a rate of 2 to 20 mcg/kg/min. It is supplied in 20-mL vials containing 250 mg.

FENOLDOPAM

Fenoldopam is a selective D_1-receptor agonist that has many of the benefits of DA but with little or no α- or β-adrenoceptor or D_2-receptor agonist activity. Fenoldopam exerts hypotensive effects characterized by a decrease in peripheral vascular resistance, along with an increase in renal blood flow, diuresis, and natriuresis. It is commonly used in patients undergoing cardiac surgery or aortic aneurysm repair with a potential risk of perioperative kidney impairment. Fenoldopam reduces blood pressure but helps maintain renal blood flow. It is also indicated for patients who have severe hypertension, particularly those with renal impairment. Along with its recommended use in hypertensive emergencies, fenoldopam is also indicated in the prevention of contrast media-induced nephropathy. Fenoldopam has a rapid onset of action and is easily titratable because of its short elimination half-life. The ability of fenoldopam to "protect" the kidney perioperatively remains the subject of ongoing debate, but (as is literature for "renal dose" dopamine) there is no good evidence for efficacy.

Fenoldopam is supplied in 1-, 2-, and 5-mL ampules, 10 mg/mL. It is started as a continuous infusion of 0.1 mcg/kg/min, increased by increments of 0.1 mcg/kg/min at 15- to 20-min intervals until target blood pressure is achieved. Lower doses have been associated with less reflex tachycardia.

Adrenergic Antagonists

Adrenergic antagonists bind but do not activate adrenoceptors. They prevent adrenergic agonist activity. Like the agonists, the antagonists differ in their spectrum of receptor interaction.

α-BLOCKERS: PHENTOLAMINE

Phentolamine produces a competitive (reversible) blockade of both α_1- and α_2-receptors. α_1 Antagonism and direct smooth muscle relaxation are responsible for peripheral vasodilation and a decline in arterial blood pressure. The drop in blood pressure provokes reflex tachycardia. This tachycardia is augmented by antagonism of presynaptic α_2-receptors in the heart because α_2 blockade promotes norepinephrine release by eliminating negative feedback. These cardiovascular effects are usually apparent within 2 min and last up to 15 min. As with all of the adrenergic antagonists, the extent of the response to receptor blockade depends on the degree of existing sympathetic tone. Reflex tachycardia and postural hypotension limit the usefulness of phentolamine to the treatment of hypertension caused by excessive α stimulation (eg, pheochromocytoma, clonidine withdrawal). Prazosin and phenoxybenzamine are examples of other α-antagonists.

Phentolamine is administered intravenously as intermittent boluses (1–5 mg in adults) or as a continuous infusion to prevent or minimize tissue necrosis following extravasation of intravenous fluids containing an α-agonist (eg, norepinephrine), 5 to 10 mg of phentolamine in 10 mL of normal saline can be locally infiltrated.

MIXED ANTAGONISTS: LABETALOL

Labetalol blocks α_1-, β_1-, and β_2-receptors. The ratio of α blockade to β blockade has been estimated to be approximately 1:7 following intravenous administration. This mixed blockade reduces peripheral vascular resistance and arterial blood pressure. Heart rate and cardiac output are usually slightly depressed
8 or unchanged. Thus, labetalol lowers blood pressure without reflex tachycardia because of its combination of α and β effects, which is beneficial to patients with coronary artery disease. Peak effect usually occurs within 5 min after an intravenous dose. Left ventricular failure, paradoxical hypertension, and bronchospasm have been reported.

The initial recommended dose of labetalol is 2.5 to 10 mg administered intravenously over 2 min. After the initial dose, and depending on the response, 5 to 20 mg may be given at 10-min intervals until the desired blood pressure response is obtained.

β-BLOCKERS

β-Receptor blockers have variable degrees of selectivity for the β_1-receptors. Those that are more β_1 selective have less influence on bronchopulmonary and vascular β_2-receptors (Table 14–3). Theoretically,

TABLE 14–3 Pharmacology of β-blockers.[1]

	Selectivity for β_1-Receptors	ISA	α-Blockade	Hepatic Metabolism
Atenolol	+	0	0	0
Esmolol	+	0	0	0
Labetalol		0	+	+
Metoprolol	+	0	0	+
Propranolol		0	0	+

[1]ISA, intrinsic sympathomimetic activity; +, mild effect; 0, no effect.

a selective β_1-blocker would have less of an inhibitory effect on β_2-receptors and, therefore, might be preferred in patients with chronic obstructive lung disease or peripheral vascular disease. Patients with peripheral vascular disease could potentially have a decrease in blood flow if β_2-receptors, which dilate the arterioles, are blocked. β-Receptor blocking agents also reduce intraocular pressure in patients with glaucoma.

β-Blockers are also classified by the amount of intrinsic sympathomimetic activity (ISA) they have. Many of the β-blockers have some agonist activity, though they would not produce effects similar to full agonists (such as epinephrine).

β-Blockers can be further classified as those that are eliminated by hepatic metabolism (such as metoprolol), those that are excreted by the kidneys unchanged (such as atenolol), and those that are hydrolyzed in the blood (such as esmolol).

ESMOLOL

9 Esmolol is an ultrashort-acting selective β_1-antagonist that reduces heart rate and, to a lesser extent, blood pressure. It is used to prevent or minimize tachycardia and hypertension in response to perioperative stimuli, such as intubation, surgical stimulation, and emergence. For example, esmolol (0.5–1 mg/kg) attenuates the rise in blood pressure and heart rate that usually accompanies electroconvulsive therapy without significantly affecting seizure duration. Esmolol is useful in controlling the ventricular rate of patients with atrial fibrillation or flutter. Although esmolol is considered to be cardioselective, at higher doses, it inhibits β_2-receptors in bronchial and vascular smooth muscle. Esmolol administration may contribute to antinociception and opioid-sparing when incorporated into anesthesia delivery, substituting for larger opioid doses.

The short duration of action of esmolol is due to rapid redistribution (distribution half-life is 2 min) and hydrolysis by red blood cell esterase (elimination half-life is 9 min). Side effects can be reversed within minutes by discontinuing its infusion. As with all β_1-antagonists, esmolol should be avoided in patients with sinus bradycardia, heart block greater than first degree, cardiogenic shock, or uncompensated, low ejection fraction heart failure. Esmolol can be used to slow the ventricular rate in patients with supraventricular tachycardia who are not hypotensive.

Esmolol is administered as a bolus (0.2–0.5 mg/kg) for short-term therapy, such as attenuating the cardiovascular response to laryngoscopy and intubation. Long-term treatment is typically initiated with a loading dose of 0.5 mg/kg administered over 1 min, followed by a continuous infusion of 50 mcg/kg/min to maintain therapeutic effect. If this fails to produce a sufficient response within 5 min, the loading dose may be repeated and the infusion increased by increments of 50 mcg/kg/min every 5 min to a maximum of 200 mcg/kg/min.

Esmolol is supplied as multidose vials for bolus administration containing 10 mL of drug (10 mg/mL). Ampules for continuous infusion (2.5 g in 10 mL) are also available but must be diluted prior to administration to a concentration of 10 mg/mL.

METOPROLOL

Metoprolol is a selective β_1-antagonist with no intrinsic sympathomimetic activity. It is available for both oral and intravenous use. It can be administered intravenously in 1 to 5 mg increments every 2 to 5 min, titrated to blood pressure and heart rate. Extended-release metoprolol given orally can be used to treat patients with chronic heart failure.

PROPRANOLOL

Propranolol nonselectively blocks β_1- and β_2-receptors. Arterial blood pressure is lowered by several mechanisms, including decreased myocardial contractility, lowered heart rate, and diminished renin release.

Side effects of propranolol include bronchospasm (β_2 antagonism), acute congestive heart failure, bradycardia, and atrioventricular heart block (β_1 antagonism). Concomitant administration of propranolol and verapamil (a calcium channel blocker) can synergistically depress heart rate, contractility, and atrioventricular node conduction.

Propranolol's elimination half-life of 100 min is quite long compared with that of esmolol. Generally, propranolol is titrated to effect in 0.5 mg increments every 3 to 5 min. Total doses rarely exceed 0.15 mg/kg. Propranolol is supplied in 1-mL ampules containing 1 mg.

NEBIVOLOL

Nebivolol is a newer generation β-blocker with a high affinity for β_1-receptors. The drug is unique in its ability to cause direct vasodilation via its stimulatory effect on endothelial nitric oxide synthase.

CARVEDILOL

Carvedilol is a mixed β- and α-blocker used in the management of chronic heart failure secondary to cardiomyopathy, left ventricular dysfunction following acute myocardial infarction, and hypertension. Carvedilol dosage is individualized and gradually increased up to 25 mg twice daily, as required and tolerated. Bisoprolol and extended-release metoprolol are also used in long-term therapy to reduce mortality in patients with heart failure.

PERIOPERATIVE β-BLOCKER THERAPY

Management of β-blockers perioperatively has been a key anesthesia performance indicator and is closely monitored by various "quality management" agencies. Although studies regarding the perioperative administration of β-blockers have yielded conflicting results as to benefit versus harm, maintenance of β-blockers in patients already being treated with them is essential, unless contraindicated by other clinical concerns. Initial small trials did not demonstrate adverse outcomes from the initiation of perioperative β-blocker therapy. Subsequent studies either demonstrated no benefit or actual harm (eg, stroke) when β blockade was begun perioperatively.

The 2014 American College of Cardiology/American Heart Association (ACC/AHA) guidelines recommend continuation of β-blocker therapy during the perioperative period in patients who are receiving them chronically (class I benefit >>> risk). β-Blocker therapy postoperatively should be guided by clinical circumstances (class IIa benefit >> risk). Irrespective of when β-blocker therapy was started, therapy may need to be temporarily discontinued (eg, bleeding, hypotension, bradycardia). The ACC/AHA guidelines suggest that it may be is reasonable to begin perioperative β-blockers in patients at intermediate or high risk for myocardial ischemia (class IIb benefit ≥ risk). Other conditions such as risk of stroke or uncompensated heart failure should be considered in discerning if β-blockade should be initiated perioperatively. Additionally, in patients with three or more Revised Cardiac Risk Index risk factors (see Chapter 21), it may be reasonable to begin β-blocker therapy before surgery (class IIb). Lacking these risk factors, it is unclear whether preoperative β-blocker therapy is effective or safe. Should it be decided to begin β-blocker therapy, the ACC/AHA guidelines suggest that it is reasonable to start therapy sufficiently in advance of the surgical procedure to assess the safety and tolerability of treatment (class IIb). Lastly, β-blockers should not be initiated in β-blocker naïve patients on the day of surgery (class III: harm).

Abrupt discontinuation of β-blocker therapy for
10 24 to 48 h may trigger a withdrawal syndrome characterized by rebound hypertension, tachycardia, and angina pectoris. This effect seems to be caused by an increase in the number of β-adrenergic receptors (upregulation).

CASE DISCUSSION

Pheochromocytoma

A 45-year-old patient with a history of paroxysmal attacks of headache, hypertension, sweating, and palpitations is scheduled for resection of an abdominal pheochromocytoma.

What is a pheochromocytoma?

A pheochromocytoma is a vascular tumor of chromaffin tissue (most commonly the adrenal medulla) that produces and secretes norepinephrine and epinephrine. The diagnosis and management of pheochromocytoma are based on the effects of abnormally high circulating levels of these endogenous adrenergic agonists.

How is the diagnosis of pheochromocytoma made in the laboratory?

Urinary excretion of vanillylmandelic acid (an end product of catecholamine metabolism), norepinephrine, and epinephrine is often markedly increased. Elevated levels of urinary catecholamines and metanephrines (see Figure 14–3) provide a highly accurate diagnosis. Fractionated plasma-free metanephrine levels may be superior to urinary studies in making the diagnosis. The location of the tumor can be determined by magnetic resonance imaging, computed tomographic scanning, positron emission tomography, or M-iodobenzylguanidine (MIBG) imaging.

What pathophysiology is associated with chronic elevations of norepinephrine and epinephrine?

α_1 Stimulation increases peripheral vascular resistance and arterial blood pressure. Hypertension can lead to intravascular volume depletion (increasing hematocrit), kidney failure, and cerebral hemorrhage. Elevated peripheral vascular resistance also increases myocardial work, predisposing patients to myocardial ischemia, ventricular hypertrophy, and congestive heart failure. Prolonged exposure to epinephrine and norepinephrine may lead to catecholamine-induced cardiomyopathy. Hyperglycemia results from decreased insulin secretion in the face of increased glycogenolysis and gluconeogenesis. β_1 Stimulation increases automaticity and ventricular ectopy.

Which adrenergic antagonists might be helpful in controlling the effects of norepinephrine and epinephrine hypersecretion?

Phenoxybenzamine, an α_1-antagonist, effectively reverses the vasoconstriction, resulting in a drop in arterial blood pressure and an increase in intravascular volume (hematocrit drops). Glucose intolerance is often corrected. Phenoxybenzamine can be administered orally and is longer acting than phentolamine, another α_1-antagonist that is usually administered intravenously. For these reasons, phenoxybenzamine is often administered preoperatively to control symptoms.

Intravenous phentolamine has been used intraoperatively to control hypertensive episodes. Compared with some other hypotensive agents, however, phentolamine has a slow onset and long duration of action; furthermore, the agent is no longer widely available. Other vasodilators can be used in this circumstance.

β_1 Blockade is recommended after the initiation of α blockade for patients with tachycardia or ventricular arrhythmias.

Why should α_1-receptors be blocked with phenoxybenzamine before administration of a β-antagonist?

If β-receptors are blocked first, norepinephrine and epinephrine will produce unopposed α stimulation. β_2-Mediated vasodilation will not be able to offset α_1 vasoconstriction, and peripheral vascular resistance would increase. This may explain the paradoxical hypertension that has been reported in a few patients with pheochromocytoma treated only with labetalol. Finally, the myocardium might not be able to handle its already elevated workload without the inotropic effects of β_1 stimulation.

Which anesthetic agents should be specifically avoided?

Ketamine is a sympathomimetic and might, in theory, exacerbate the effects of adrenergic agonists. Halothane sensitizes the myocardium to the arrhythmogenic effects of epinephrine. Vagolytic drugs (eg, anticholinergics and pancuronium) may contribute to tachycardia. Because histamine provokes catecholamine secretion by the tumor, drugs associated with histamine release (eg, atracurium) are best avoided. Vecuronium and rocuronium are probably the neuromuscular blocking agents of choice.

Would an epidural or spinal technique effectively block sympathetic hyperactivity?

A major regional block—such as an epidural or spinal anesthetic—could block sensory (afferent) nerves and sympathetic (efferent) discharge in the area of the surgical field. However, the catecholamines released from a pheochromocytoma during surgical manipulation would still be able to bind and activate adrenergic receptors throughout the body.

GUIDELINES

Fleisher LA, Fleischmann KE, Auerbach AD, et al. 2014 ACC/AHA guideline on perioperative cardiovascular evaluation and management of patients undergoing noncardiac surgery: executive summary: a report of the American College of Cardiology/American Heart Association Task Force on Practice Guidelines. *Circulation*. 2014;130:2215.

SUGGESTED READINGS

Avni T, Lador A, Lev S, Leibovici L, Paul M, Grossman A. Vasopressors for the treatment of septic shock: systematic review and meta-analysis. *PLoS One*. 2015;10:e0129305.

Bahr MP, Williams BA. Esmolol, antinociception, and its potential opioid-sparing role in routine anesthesia care. *Reg Anesth Pain Med*. 2018;43:815.

Brunton L, Knollman B, Hilal-Dandan R, eds. *Goodman and Gilman's The Pharmacological Basis of Therapeutics*. 13th ed. McGraw-Hill Education; 2018.

Fongemie J, Felix-Getzik E. A review of nebivolol pharmacology and clinical evidence. *Drugs*. 2015;75:1349.

Gu YW, Poste J, Kunal M, Schwarcz M, Weiss I. Cardiovascular manifestations of pheochromocytoma. *Cardiol Rev*. 2017;25:215.

Jørgensen ME, Andersson C, Venkatesan S, Sanders RD. Beta-blockers in noncardiac surgery: did observational studies put us back on safe ground? *Br J Anaesth*. 2018;121:16.

Levy B, Buzon J, Kimmoun A. Inotropes and vasopressors use in cardiogenic shock: when, which and how much? *Curr Opin Crit Care*. 2019;25:384.

Lother A, Hein L. Pharmacology of heart failure: from basic science to novel therapies. *Pharmacol Ther*. 2016;166:136.

Naranjo J, Dodd S, Martin YN. Perioperative management of pheochromocytoma. *J Cardiothorac Vasc Anesth*. 2017;31:1427.

Nguyen V, Tiemann D, Park E, Salehi A. Alpha-2 agonists. *Anesthesiol Clin*. 2017;35:233.

Shi R, Tie HT. Dexmedetomidine as a promising prevention strategy for cardiac surgery-associated acute kidney injury: a meta-analysis. *Crit Care*. 2017;21:198.

Zarbock A, Milles K. Novel therapy for renal protection. *Curr Opin Anaesthesiol*. 2015;28:431.

CHAPTER 15

Hypotensive Agents

KEY CONCEPTS

1. Inhaled nitric oxide is a selective pulmonary vasodilator that is used in the treatment of reversible pulmonary hypertension.
2. Acute cyanide toxicity is characterized by metabolic acidosis, cardiac arrhythmias, and increased venous oxygen content (as a result of the inability to utilize oxygen). Another early sign of cyanide toxicity is the acute resistance to the hypotensive effects of increasing doses of sodium nitroprusside (tachyphylaxis).
3. By dilating pulmonary vessels, sodium nitroprusside may prevent the normal vasoconstrictive response of the pulmonary vasculature to hypoxia (hypoxic pulmonary vasoconstriction).
4. Preload reduction makes nitroglycerin an excellent drug for the relief of cardiogenic pulmonary edema.
5. Hydralazine relaxes arteriolar smooth muscle in multiple ways, including dilation of precapillary resistance vessels via increased cyclic guanosine 3′,5′-monophosphate.
6. The body reacts to a hydralazine-induced fall in blood pressure by increasing heart rate, myocardial contractility, and cardiac output. These compensatory responses can be detrimental to patients with coronary artery disease and are minimized by the concurrent administration of a β-adrenergic antagonist.
7. Fenoldopam (infusion rates studied in clinical trials range from 0.01 to 1.6 mcg/kg/min) reduces systolic and diastolic blood pressure in patients with malignant hypertension to an extent comparable to nitroprusside.
8. Dihydropyridine calcium channel blockers preferentially dilate arterial vessels, often preserving or increasing cardiac output.

A multitude of drugs are capable of lowering blood pressure, including volatile anesthetics, sympathetic antagonists and agonists, calcium channel blockers, β-blockers, and angiotensin-converting enzyme inhibitors. Blood pressure is the product of cardiac output and systemic vascular resistance. Agents that lower blood pressure reduce myocardial contractility or produce vasodilatation of the arterial and venous capacitance vessels, or both. This chapter examines agents that may be useful to the anesthesiologist for perioperative control of arterial blood pressure.

As patients age, so too does their vasculature. When a pulse wave is generated by ventricular contraction, it is propagated through the arterial system. At branch points of the aorta, the wave is reflected back toward the heart. In younger patients, the reflected wave tends to augment diastole, improving diastolic pressure. In older patients, the wave arrives sooner, being conducted back by the noncompliant vasculature during late systole, which causes an increase in cardiac workload and a decrease in diastolic pressure (Figure 15–1). Thus, older patients

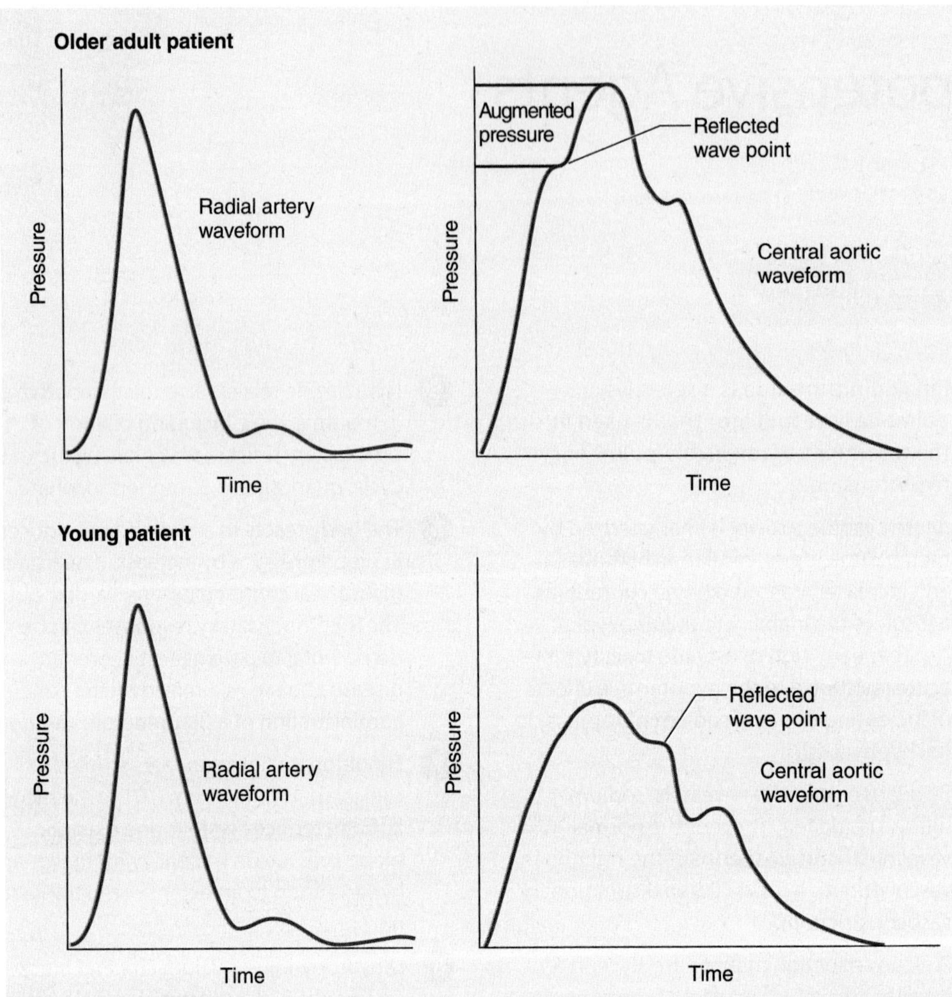

FIGURE 15–1 Illustration of the influence of increased vascular stiffness on peripheral (radial) and central (aortic) pressures. Note the similarity of peripheral radial pressures in individuals with normal (*lower left panel*) and increased (*upper left panel*) vascular stiffness. In young individuals with normal vascular stiffness, central aortic pressures are lower than radial pressures (*lower panels*). In contrast, in older individuals with increased vascular stiffness, central aortic pressures are increased and can approach or equal peripheral pressures as a result of wave reflection and central wave augmentation during systole (*top panels*). (Reproduced with permission from Barodka V, Joshi B, Berkowitz D, et al. Implications of vascular aging. *Anesth Analg.* 2011 May;112(5):1048-1060.)

develop increased systolic pressure and decreased diastolic pressure. Widened pulse pressures (the difference between systolic and diastolic pressures) have been associated with both increased incidence of postoperative kidney dysfunction and increased risk of cerebral events in patients undergoing coronary bypass surgery.

β-Blocker therapy should be maintained perioperatively in patients who are being treated with β-blockers as a part of their routine medical regimen. The American College of Cardiology/American Heart Association guidelines for β-blocker use perioperatively should be followed (see Chapter 14). β-Blockers (esmolol, metoprolol, and others) were previously discussed for the treatment of transient perioperative hypertension and are routinely used during anesthesia. This chapter discusses antihypertensive agents other than adrenergic antagonists that are used perioperatively. Antihypertensive agents are critically important for managing hypertensive emergencies (blood pressure >180/120 mm Hg) with signs of organ injury (eg, encephalopathy). Under most circumstances, mean arterial pressure should be reduced gradually to prevent organ hypoperfusion (eg, 20% decrease in mean arterial pressure or a diastolic blood pressure of 100–110 mm Hg initially). On the other hand, prompt treatment of hypertension is also advisable in patients with acute aortic dissection and following cardiac and intracranial surgery and other procedures where excessive bleeding is a major concern. Perioperative hypertension may be the result of pain, anxiety, hypoxemia, hypercapnia, distended bladder, and failure to continue prescribed antihypertensive medications. These primary etiologies should be considered and addressed when treating perioperative hypertension.

SODIUM NITROPRUSSIDE

Mechanism of Action

Sodium nitroprusside (and other nitrovasodilators) relax both arteriolar and venous smooth muscle. Its primary mechanism of action is shared with other nitrates (eg, hydralazine and nitroglycerin). As nitrovasodilators are metabolized, they release **nitric oxide**, which activates guanylyl cyclase. This enzyme is responsible for the synthesis of cyclic guanosine 3′,5′-monophosphate (cGMP), which controls the phosphorylation of several proteins, including some involved in the control of free intracellular calcium and smooth muscle contraction.

Nitric oxide, a naturally occurring potent vasodilator released by endothelial cells (endothelium-derived relaxing factor), plays an important role in regulating vascular tone throughout the body. Its ultrashort half-life (<5 s) provides nimble endogenous control of regional blood flow. 1 Inhaled nitric oxide is a selective pulmonary vasodilator that is used in the treatment of reversible pulmonary hypertension.

Clinical Uses

Sodium nitroprusside is a potent and reliable antihypertensive. It is usually diluted to a concentration of 100 mcg/mL and administered as a continuous intravenous infusion (0.25–5 mcg/kg/min). Its rapid onset of action (1–2 min) and fleeting duration of action allow precise titration of arterial blood pressure. The potency of this drug requires frequent blood pressure measurements—or, preferably, intra-arterial monitoring—and the use of mechanical infusion pumps. Solutions of sodium nitroprusside must be protected from light because of photodegradation.

Metabolism

After parenteral injection, sodium nitroprusside enters red blood cells, where it receives an electron from the iron (Fe^{2+}) of oxyhemoglobin. This nonenzymatic electron transfer results in an unstable nitroprusside radical and methemoglobin (Hgb Fe^{3+}). The former moiety spontaneously decomposes into five cyanide ions and the active nitroso (N═O) group.

The cyanide ions can be involved in one of three possible reactions: (1) binding to methemoglobin to form **cyanmethemoglobin**; (2) undergoing a reaction in the liver and kidney catalyzed by the enzyme rhodanese (thiosulfate + cyanide → thiocyanate); or (3) binding to tissue cytochrome oxidase, which interferes with normal oxygen utilization (Figure 15–2).

2 The last of these reactions underlies the development of **acute cyanide toxicity**, characterized by metabolic acidosis, cardiac arrhythmias, and increased venous oxygen content (as a result of the inability to utilize oxygen). Another early sign of cyanide toxicity is the acute resistance to the hypotensive effects of increasing doses of sodium nitroprusside (tachyphylaxis). Cyanide toxicity is more likely if the cumulative daily dose of sodium nitroprusside is greater than 500 mcg/kg or if the drug is administered at infusion rates greater than 2 mcg/kg/min for more than a few hours. Patients with cyanide toxicity should be mechanically ventilated with 100% oxygen to maximize oxygen availability. The pharmacological treatment of cyanide toxicity depends on providing alternative binding sites for cyanide ions by administering sodium thiosulfate (150 mg/kg over

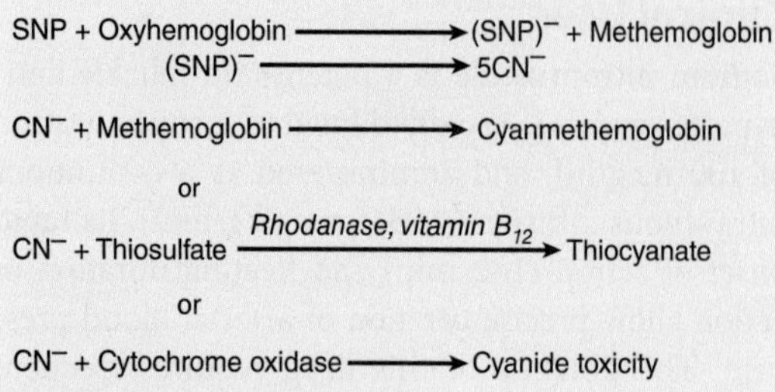

FIGURE 15–2 The metabolism of sodium nitroprusside.

15 min) or 3% sodium nitrite (5 mg/kg over 5 min), which oxidizes hemoglobin to methemoglobin. A methemoglobin concentration of 10% to 20% is the aim of nitrite administration. Caution should be exercised when inducing methemoglobinemia in patients experiencing cyanide toxicity secondary to combustion because carboxyhemoglobinemia from carbon monoxide poisoning might also be present. Additionally, hydroxocobalamin combines with cyanide to form cyanocobalamin (vitamin B_{12}) and likewise can be administered to treat cyanide poisoning. Cyanocobalamin is excreted by the kidney.

Thiocyanate is slowly cleared by the kidney. Accumulation of large amounts of thiocyanate (eg, in patients with kidney failure) may result in a milder toxic reaction that includes thyroid dysfunction, muscle weakness, nausea, hypoxia, and acute toxic psychosis. The risk of cyanide toxicity is not increased by kidney failure, however. Methemoglobinemia from excessive doses of sodium nitroprusside or sodium nitrite can be treated with methylene blue (1–2 mg/kg of a 1% solution over 5 min), which reduces methemoglobin to hemoglobin.

Effects on Organ Systems

The combined dilation of venous and arteriolar vascular beds by sodium nitroprusside results in reductions of preload and afterload. Arterial blood pressure falls due to the decrease in peripheral vascular resistance. Although cardiac output is usually unchanged in normal patients, the reduction in afterload may increase cardiac output in patients with congestive heart failure, mitral regurgitation, or aortic regurgitation. In opposition to any favorable changes in myocardial oxygen requirements are reflex-mediated responses to the fall in arterial blood pressure. These include tachycardia and increased myocardial contractility. In addition, dilation of coronary arterioles by sodium nitroprusside may result in an **intracoronary steal** of blood flow away from ischemic areas that are supplied by arterioles already maximally dilated.

Sodium nitroprusside dilates cerebral vessels and abolishes cerebral autoregulation. Cerebral blood flow is maintained or increases unless arterial blood pressure is markedly reduced. The resulting increase in cerebral blood volume tends to increase intracranial pressure, particularly in patients with reduced intracranial compliance (eg, brain tumors). This intracranial hypertension can be minimized by slow administration of sodium nitroprusside and institution of hypocapnia.

The pulmonary vasculature also dilates in response to sodium nitroprusside infusion. Reductions in pulmonary artery pressure may decrease the perfusion of some normally ventilated alveoli,
3 increasing physiological dead space. By dilating pulmonary vessels, sodium nitroprusside may prevent the normal vasoconstrictive response of the pulmonary vasculature to hypoxia (hypoxic pulmonary vasoconstriction). Both of these effects tend to mismatch pulmonary ventilation to perfusion, increase venous admixture, and decrease arterial oxygenation.

In response to decreased arterial blood pressure, renin and catecholamines are released during the administration of nitroprusside. Renin release can be inhibited with β-blockers. Normally, kidney function is well maintained during sodium nitroprusside infusion, despite moderate drops in arterial blood pressure and renal perfusion. Sodium nitroprusside has largely been replaced by other agents for acute control of perioperative hypertension.

NITROGLYCERIN

Mechanism of Action

Nitroglycerin relaxes vascular smooth muscle, with venous dilation predominating over arterial dilation. Its mechanism of action is similar to that of sodium nitroprusside: metabolism to nitric oxide, which activates guanylyl cyclase, leading to increased cGMP, decreased intracellular calcium, and vascular smooth muscle relaxation.

Clinical Uses

Nitroglycerin relieves myocardial ischemia, hypertension, and ventricular failure. Like sodium nitroprusside, nitroglycerin is commonly diluted to a concentration of 100 mcg/mL and administered as a continuous intravenous infusion (0.5–5 mcg/kg/min). In the past, glass containers and special intravenous tubing were recommended because of the adsorption of nitroglycerin to polyvinylchloride, but these are now rarely used. Nitroglycerin can also be administered by a sublingual (peak effect in 4 min) or transdermal (sustained release for 24 h) route.

Metabolism

Nitroglycerin undergoes rapid reductive hydrolysis in the liver and blood by glutathione-organic nitrate reductase. One metabolic product is nitrite, which can convert hemoglobin to methemoglobin. Significant methemoglobinemia is rare and can be treated with intravenous methylene blue (1–2 mg/kg over 5 min).

Nitroglycerin reduces myocardial oxygen demand and increases myocardial oxygen supply by several mechanisms:

- The pooling of blood in the large-capacitance vessels reduces the effective circulating blood volume and preload. The accompanying decrease in ventricular end-diastolic pressure reduces myocardial oxygen demand and increases endocardial perfusion.
- Any afterload reduction from arteriolar dilation will decrease both end-systolic pressure and oxygen demand. Of course, a fall in diastolic pressure may lower coronary perfusion pressure and actually decrease myocardial oxygen supply.
- Nitroglycerin redistributes coronary blood flow to ischemic areas of the subendocardium.
- Coronary artery spasm may be relieved.

The beneficial effect of nitroglycerin in patients with coronary artery disease contrasts with the coronary steal phenomenon seen with sodium nitroprusside.

4 Preload reduction makes nitroglycerin an excellent drug for the relief of cardiogenic pulmonary edema. Heart rate is unchanged or minimally increased. Rebound hypertension is less likely after discontinuation of nitroglycerin than following discontinuation of sodium nitroprusside. The prophylactic administration of low-dose nitroglycerin to high-risk patients undergoing surgery and anesthesia has no proven benefit.

The effects of nitroglycerin on cerebral blood flow and intracranial pressure are similar to those of sodium nitroprusside. Headache from dilation of cerebral vessels is a common side effect of nitroglycerin. In addition to the dilating effects on the pulmonary vasculature (previously described for sodium nitroprusside), nitroglycerin relaxes bronchial smooth muscle.

Nitroglycerin (50–100 mcg boluses) has been demonstrated to be an effective (but transient) uterine relaxant that can be beneficial during certain obstetrical procedures if the placenta is still present in the uterus (eg, retained placenta, uterine inversion, uterine tetany, breech extraction, and external version of the second twin). Nitroglycerin therapy has been shown to diminish platelet aggregation, but it is rarely the cause of excessive bleeding.

HYDRALAZINE

5 Hydralazine relaxes arteriolar smooth muscle in multiple ways, including dilation of precapillary resistance vessels via increased cGMP.

Hypertension during surgery or during recovery is sometimes controlled with an intravenous dose of 5 to 20 mg of hydralazine. The onset of action is within 15 min, and the antihypertensive effect usually lasts 2 to 4 h. The delayed onset and prolonged duration have made this agent much less attractive than others for perioperative use. Hydralazine can be used to control pregnancy-induced hypertension.

Hydralazine undergoes acetylation and hydroxylation in the liver.

Effects on Organ Systems

The lowering of peripheral vascular resistance causes
6 a drop in arterial blood pressure. The body reacts to a hydralazine-induced fall in blood pressure by increasing heart rate, myocardial contractility, and

cardiac output. These compensatory responses can be detrimental to patients with coronary artery disease and are minimized by the concurrent administration of a β-adrenergic antagonist. Conversely, the decline in afterload often proves beneficial to patients with congestive heart failure.

Hydralazine is a potent cerebral vasodilator and inhibitor of cerebral blood flow autoregulation. Unless blood pressure is markedly reduced, cerebral blood flow and intracranial pressure will rise.

Renal blood flow is usually maintained or increased by hydralazine.

FENOLDOPAM

Mechanism of Action

Fenoldopam causes rapid vasodilation by selectively activating D_1-dopamine receptors. The R-isomer is responsible for the racemic mixture's biological activity due to its much greater receptor affinity compared with the S-isomer.

Clinical Uses

7 Fenoldopam (infusion rates studied in clinical trials range from 0.01 to 1.6 mcg/kg/min) reduces systolic and diastolic blood pressure in patients with malignant hypertension to an extent comparable to nitroprusside. Side effects include headache, flushing, nausea, tachycardia, hypokalemia, and hypotension. The onset of the hypotensive effect occurs within 15 min, and discontinuation of an infusion quickly reverses this effect without rebound hypertension. Some degree of tolerance may develop 48 h after the infusion. Studies are mixed regarding fenoldopam's ability to "protect" and "maintain" kidney function in perioperative patients with hypertension who are at risk for perioperative kidney injury.

Metabolism

Fenoldopam undergoes conjugation without participation of the cytochrome P-450 enzymes, and its metabolites are inactive. Clearance of fenoldopam remains unaltered despite the presence of kidney or hepatic failure, and no dosage adjustments are necessary for these patients.

Effects on Organ Systems

Fenoldopam decreases systolic and diastolic blood pressure. Heart rate typically increases. Low initial doses (0.03–0.1 mcg/kg/min) titrated slowly have been associated with less reflex tachycardia than higher doses. Tachycardia decreases over time but remains substantial at higher doses.

Fenoldopam can lead to rises in intraocular pressure and should be administered with caution or avoided in patients with a history of glaucoma or intraocular hypertension.

As would be expected from a D_1-dopamine receptor agonist, fenoldopam markedly increases kidney blood flow. Despite a drop in arterial blood pressure, the glomerular filtration rate is well maintained. Fenoldopam increases urinary flow rate, urinary sodium extraction, and creatinine clearance compared with sodium nitroprusside.

CALCIUM CHANNEL BLOCKERS

8 Dihydropyridine calcium channel blockers (nicardipine, clevidipine) are arterial selective vasodilators routinely used for perioperative blood pressure control in patients undergoing cardiothoracic surgery. Clevidipine, prepared as a lipid emulsion, has a short half-life secondary to rapid metabolism by blood esterases, which facilitates its rapid titration. Clevidipine is infused initially at a rate of 1 to 2 mg/h, with the dose doubled until the desired effect is obtained, up to 16 mg/h. Because of its formulation as a lipid emulsion, it is contraindicated in patients with soy or egg allergies and those with impaired lipid metabolism. Unlike verapamil and diltiazem, the dihydropyridine calcium channel blockers have minimal effects on cardiac conduction and ventricular contractility. These calcium channel blockers bind to the L-type calcium channel and impair calcium entry into the vascular smooth muscle. L-type receptors are more prevalent on arterial than venous capacitance vessels. Consequently, cardiac filling and preload are less affected by these agents than by nitrates, which might dilate both arterial and venous systems. With preload maintained, cardiac output often increases when vascular

tone is reduced by the use of dihydropyridine calcium blockers. Nicardipine infusion is titrated to effect (5–15 mg/h).

Another intravenous agent that can produce hypotension perioperatively is the intravenous angiotensin-converting enzyme inhibitor enalaprilat (0.625–1.25 mg). The role of enalaprilat as a nondirect-acting agent in the acute treatment of a hypertensive crisis is limited.

INODILATORS

Milrinone is a phosphodiesterase inhibitor that is frequently employed in the treatment of heart failure. Milrinone increases cAMP concentration, resulting in an increased intracellular calcium concentration. In addition to improving myocardial contractility, milrinone is a systemic vasodilator. The perioperative use of milrinone is discussed in greater detail in Chapter 22. Agents that work very similarly to milrinone include enoximone, olprinone, and inamrinone.

Levosimendan is a calcium-sensitizing agent that makes myofibrillar proteins more sensitive to intracellular calcium, resulting in increased myocardial contractility. Levosimendan also produces systemic vasodilation.

These inodilators are primarily employed to improve cardiac function through the combination of increased contractility and vasodilation.

CASE DISCUSSION

Controlled Hypotension

A 59-year-old patient is scheduled for total hip arthroplasty under general anesthesia. The surgeon requests a controlled hypotensive technique.

What is controlled hypotension, and what are its advantages?

Controlled hypotension is the elective lowering of arterial blood pressure. The primary advantages of this technique are minimization of surgical blood loss and better surgical visualization.

How is controlled hypotension achieved?

The primary methods of electively lowering blood pressure are the use of hypotensive anesthetic techniques (eg, neuraxial anesthesia) and the administration of hypotensive drugs. Elevation of the surgical site can selectively reduce the blood pressure at the wound. During general anesthesia, the increase in intrathoracic pressure that accompanies positive-pressure ventilation impedes venous return to the heart, lowering cardiac output and mean arterial pressure. Numerous pharmacological agents effectively lower blood pressure, including volatile anesthetics, spinal and epidural anesthesia, sympathetic antagonists, calcium channel blockers, and the peripheral vasodilators discussed in this chapter.

Which surgical procedures might benefit most from a controlled hypotensive technique?

Controlled hypotension has been successfully used during cerebral aneurysm repair, brain tumor resection, total hip arthroplasty, radical neck dissection, radical cystectomy, major spine surgery, and other operations associated with significant blood loss.

What are some relative contraindications to controlled hypotension?

Some patients have predisposing illnesses that decrease the margin of safety for adequate organ perfusion: severe anemia, hypovolemia, atherosclerotic cardiovascular disease, renal or hepatic insufficiency, cerebrovascular disease, or uncontrolled glaucoma.

What are the possible complications of controlled hypotension?

As the preceding list of contraindications suggests, the risks of low arterial blood pressure include cerebral thrombosis, hemiplegia (due to decreased spinal cord perfusion), acute tubular necrosis, massive hepatic necrosis, myocardial infarction, cardiac arrest, and blindness (from retinal artery thrombosis or ischemic optic neuropathy). These complications are more likely in patients with coexisting anemia.

Consequently, the use of induced or controlled hypotension continues to decline. Patients requiring beach chair positioning for shoulder surgery or sitting position are at particular risk for cerebral hypoperfusion and perioperative cerebral infarction.

What is a safe level of hypotension?

This depends on the patient. Healthy young individuals may tolerate mean arterial pressures as low as 50 to 60 mm Hg without complications. On the other hand, chronically hypertensive patients have altered autoregulation of cerebral blood flow and may tolerate a mean arterial pressure of no more than 20% to 30% lower than baseline. Patients with a history of transient ischemic attacks may not tolerate any decline in cerebral perfusion. Recent studies suggest that the lower limit of cerebral autoregulation may be at a much higher mean arterial pressure than long has been assumed. Consequently, the use of induced or controlled hypotension in patient management continues to decline. The risks and benefits of controlled hypotension should be discussed with the patient, and the risks should likewise be reviewed with the surgeon when this technique is requested.

What special monitoring is indicated during controlled hypotension?

The intraarterial blood pressure monitoring transducer is correctly positioned and zeroed at the level of the external auditory meatus (at the level of the circle of Willis) to determine mean arterial pressure at the brain. Likewise, cerebral oximetry can be employed if hypotensive anesthesia techniques are to be considered.

SUGGESTED READINGS

Espinosa A, Ripollés-Melchor J, Casans-Francés R, et al. Evidence Anesthesia Review Group. Perioperative use of clevidipine: a systematic review and meta-analysis. *PLoS One.* 2016;11:e0150625.

Faisal SA, Apatov DA, Ramakrishna H, Weiner MM. Levosimendan in cardiac surgery: evaluating the evidence. *J Cardiothorac Vasc Anesth.* 2019;33:1146.

Gillies MA, Kakar V, Parker RJ, Honoré PM, Ostermann M. Fenoldopam to prevent acute kidney injury after major surgery—a systematic review and meta-analysis. *Crit Care.* 2015;19:449.

Henretig FM, Kirk MA, McKay CA Jr. Hazardous chemical emergencies and poisonings. *N Engl J Med.* 2019;380:1638.

Hoshijima H, Denawa Y, Mihara T, et al. Efficacy of prophylactic doses of intravenous nitroglycerin in preventing myocardial ischemia under general anesthesia: a systematic review and meta-analysis with trial sequential analysis. *J Clin Anesth.* 2017;40:16.

Hottinger DG, Beebe DS, Kozhimannil T, Prielipp RC, Belani KG. Sodium nitroprusside in 2014: a clinical concepts review. *J Anaesthesiol Clin Pharmacol.* 2014;30:462.

Jain A, Elgendy IY, Al-Ani M, Agarwal N, Pepine CJ. Advancements in pharmacotherapy for angina. *Expert Opin Pharmacother.* 2017;18:457.

Moerman AT, De Hert SG, Jacobs TF, et al. Cerebral oxygen desaturation during beach chair position. *Eur J Anaesthesiol.* 2012;29:82.

Oren O, Goldberg S. Heart failure with preserved ejection fraction: diagnosis and management. *Am J Med.* 2017;130:510.

Pilkington SA, Taboada D, Martinez G. Pulmonary hypertension and its management in patients undergoing non-cardiac surgery. *Anaesthesia.* 2015;70:56.

Ungvari Z, Tarantini S, Donato AJ, Galvan V, Csiszar A. Mechanisms of vascular aging. *Circ Res.* 2018;123:849.

Zhao N, Xu J, Singh B, et al. Nitrates for the prevention of cardiac morbidity and mortality in patients undergoing non-cardiac surgery. *Cochrane Database Syst Rev.* 2016;(8):CD010726.

CHAPTER 16

Local Anesthetics

KEY CONCEPTS

1. Voltage-gated sodium (Na) channels are membrane-associated proteins that comprise one large α subunit, through which Na ions pass, and one or two smaller β subunits. Na channels exist in (at least) three states—*resting* (nonconducting), *open* (conducting), and *inactivated* (nonconducting). Local anesthetics bind and inhibit a specific region of the α subunit, preventing channel activation and the Na influx associated with membrane depolarization.

2. The sensitivity of nerve fibers to inhibition by local anesthetics is influenced by axonal diameter, myelination, and other factors.

3. Clinical local anesthetic potency correlates with octanol solubility and the ability of the local anesthetic molecule to permeate lipid membranes. Potency is increased by adding large alkyl groups to a parent molecule. There is no clinical measurement of local anesthetic potency that is analogous to the minimum alveolar concentration (MAC) of inhalation anesthetics.

4. Onset of action depends on many factors, including lipid solubility and the relative concentration of the nonionized, more lipid-soluble free-base form (B) and the ionized, more water-soluble form (BH^+), expressed by the pK_a. The pK_a is the pH at which there is an equal fraction of ionized and nonionized drug. Less potent, less lipid-soluble agents (eg, lidocaine or mepivacaine) generally have a faster onset than more potent, more lipid-soluble agents (eg, ropivacaine or bupivacaine).

5. Duration of action correlates with potency and lipid solubility. Highly lipid-soluble local anesthetics have a longer duration of action, presumably because they more slowly diffuse from a lipid-rich environment to the aqueous bloodstream.

6. In regional anesthesia, local anesthetics are typically applied close to their intended site of action; thus, their pharmacokinetic profiles in blood are important determinants of elimination and toxicity and have very little to do with the duration of their desired clinical effect.

7. The rates of local anesthetic systemic absorption and the rise of local anesthetic concentrations in blood are related to the vascularity of the site of injection and generally follow this rank order: intravenous (or intraarterial) > tracheal > intercostal > paracervical > epidural > brachial plexus > sciatic > subcutaneous.

8. Ester local anesthetics are metabolized predominantly by pseudocholinesterase. Amide local anesthetics are metabolized (*N*-dealkylation and hydroxylation) by microsomal P-450 enzymes in the liver.

—Continued next page

Continued—

9 In awake patients, rising local anesthetic concentrations in the central nervous system produce the premonitory signs of local anesthetic intoxication.

10 Major cardiovascular toxicity usually requires about three times the local anesthetic concentration in blood as that required to produce seizures.

11 Unintended intravascular injection of bupivacaine during regional anesthesia may produce severe cardiovascular toxicity, including left ventricular depression, atrioventricular heart block, and life-threatening arrhythmias such as ventricular tachycardia and fibrillation.

12 True hypersensitivity reactions (due to IgG or IgE antibodies) to local anesthetics—as distinct from systemic toxicity caused by excessive plasma concentrations—are uncommon. Esters appear more likely to induce an allergic reaction, especially if the compound is a derivative (eg, procaine or benzocaine) of *p*-aminobenzoic acid, a known allergen.

Local and regional anesthesia and analgesia techniques depend on a group of drugs—local anesthetics—that transiently inhibit some or all of sensory, motor, or autonomic nerve function when the drugs are applied near neural tissue. This chapter describes the mechanism of action, structure–activity relationships, and the clinical pharmacology of local anesthetic drugs. The more commonly used regional anesthetic techniques are presented elsewhere (see Chapters 45 and 46).

MECHANISMS OF LOCAL ANESTHETIC ACTION

Neurons (and all other living cells) maintain a resting membrane potential of −60 to −70 mV. The electrogenic, energy-consuming sodium–potassium pump (Na^+-K^+-ATPase) couples the transport of three sodium (Na) ions out of the cell for every two potassium (K) ions it moves into the cell. This creates concentration gradients that favor the movement of K ions from an intracellular to an extracellular location and the movement of Na ions in the opposite direction. The cell membrane is normally much more "leaky" to K ions than to Na ions, so a relative excess of negatively charged ions (anions) accumulates intracellularly. The combined effects of Na^+-K^+-ATPase and K ion leak account for the negative resting membrane potential.

Excitable cells (eg, neurons or myocytes) have the unusual capability of generating **action potentials**. Membrane-associated, voltage-gated Na channels in peripheral nerve axons can produce and transmit membrane depolarizations following chemical, mechanical, or electrical stimuli. Activation of voltage-gated Na channels causes a very brief (roughly 1 ms) change in the conformation of the channels, allowing an influx of Na ions and generating an action potential (Figure 16–1). The increase in Na permeability causes temporary depolarization of the membrane potential to +35 mV. The Na current is brief and terminated by the inactivation of voltage-gated Na channels, which do not conduct Na ions. When there is no Na ion flux, the membrane returns to its resting potential. When a stimulus is sufficient to depolarize a patch of membrane, the signal can be transmitted as a wave of depolarization along the nerve membrane (an impulse). Baseline concentration gradients are maintained by the sodium–potassium pump, and only a minuscule number of Na ions pass into the cell during an action potential.

1 The previously mentioned voltage-gated Na channels are membrane-associated proteins comprising one large α subunit, through which Na ions pass, and one or two smaller β subunits.

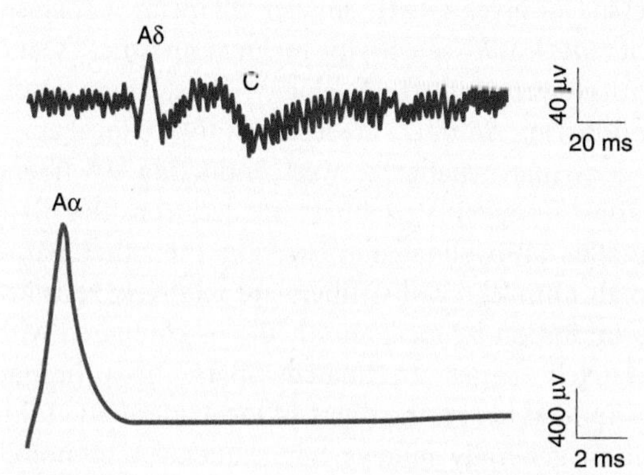

FIGURE 16-1 Compound Aα, Aδ, and C fiber action potentials recorded after supramaximal stimulation of a rat sciatic nerve. Note the differing time scale of the recordings. In peripheral nerves, Aδ and C fibers have much slower conduction velocities, and their compound action potentials are longer and of less amplitude when compared with those from Aα fibers. (Reproduced with permission from Butterworth JF 4th, Strichartz GR. The alpha2-adrenergic agonists clonidine and guanfacine produce tonic and phasic block of conduction in rat sciatic nerve fibers, *Anesth Analg.* 1993 Feb;76(2):295-301.)

Na channels exist in (at least) three states—*resting* (nonconducting), *open* (conducting), and *inactivated* (nonconducting) (Figure 16–2). When local anesthetics bind a specific region of the α subunit, they prevent channel activation and Na influx through the individual channels. Local anesthetic binding to Na channels does not alter the resting membrane potential. With increasing local anesthetic concentrations, an increasing fraction of the Na channels in the membrane bind a local anesthetic molecule and cannot conduct Na ions. As a consequence of more channels binding a local anesthetic, the threshold for excitation and impulse conduction in the nerve increases, the rate of rise and the magnitude of the action potential decreases, and impulse conduction velocity slows. At great enough local anesthetic concentrations (when a sufficient fraction of Na channels has bound a local anesthetic), action potentials can no longer be generated, and impulse propagation is abolished. Local anesthetics have a greater affinity for the Na channel in the open or inactivated state than in the resting state. Depolarizations lead to open and inactivated

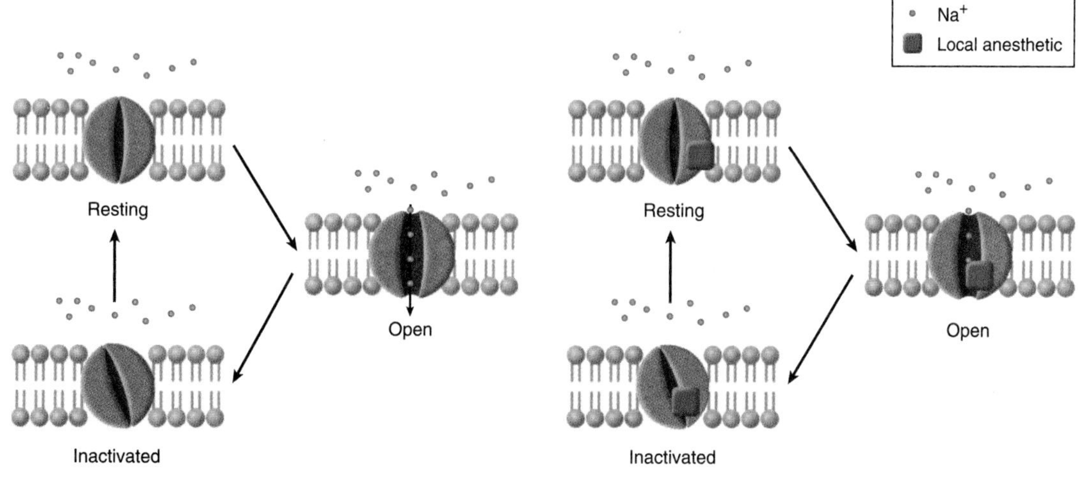

FIGURE 16–2 Voltage-gated sodium (Na_v) channels exist in at least three states—resting, open (activated), and inactivated. Resting Na_v channels activate and open when they are depolarized, briefly allowing Na ions to pass into the cell down their concentration gradient, then rapidly inactivate. Inactivated Na_v channels return to the resting state as the cell membrane repolarizes. In the figure, Na ions are shown on the extracellular side of the cell membrane. Extracellular Na ions conduct only through open Na_v channels that have not bound a local anesthetic molecule. The Na_v channel binding site for local anesthetics is nearer to the cytoplasmic than the extracellular side of the channel.

channels; therefore, depolarization favors local anesthetic binding. The fraction of Na channels that bind a local anesthetic increases with frequent depolarization (eg, during trains of impulses). This phenomenon is termed *use-dependent block*. Put another way, local anesthetic inhibition of Na channels is both voltage (membrane potential) and frequency dependent. Local anesthetic binding is greater when nerve fibers are frequently depolarizing than with infrequent depolarizations.

Local anesthetics may also bind and inhibit calcium (Ca), K, transient receptor potential vanilloid-1 (TRPV1), and many other channels and receptors. Conversely, other classes of drugs, notably tricyclic antidepressants (amitriptyline), meperidine, volatile anesthetics, Ca channel blockers, α_2-receptor agonists, and nerve toxins may also inhibit Na channels. Tetrodotoxin and saxitoxin are poisons that specifically bind Na channels at a site on the exterior of the plasma membrane. Human studies are underway with similar toxins to determine whether they might provide effective, prolonged analgesia.

2 Sensitivity of nerve fibers to inhibition by local anesthetics is influenced by axonal diameter, myelination, and other factors. Table 16–1 lists the most commonly used classification for nerve fibers. In comparing nerve fibers of the same type (myelinated versus unmyelinated), smaller diameter associates with increased sensitivity to local anesthetics and with slower conduction velocity. Thus, larger, faster-conducting Aα fibers are less sensitive to local anesthetics than smaller, slower-conducting Aδ fibers. Larger unmyelinated fibers are less sensitive than smaller unmyelinated fibers. On the other hand, small unmyelinated C fibers are relatively resistant to inhibition by local anesthetics as compared with relatively larger myelinated fibers. In a human peripheral nerve, the onset of local anesthetic inhibition generally follows this sequence: autonomic before sensory before motor. But at steady state, if sensory anesthesia is present, usually all modalities are inhibited.

STRUCTURE–ACTIVITY RELATIONSHIPS

Local anesthetics consist of a lipophilic group (usually an aromatic benzene ring) separated from a hydrophilic group (usually a tertiary amine) by an intermediate chain that includes an ester or amide linkage. The nature of the intermediate chain is the basis of the classification of local anesthetics as either esters or amides (Table 16–2). Articaine, a

TABLE 16–1 Nerve fiber classification.[1]

Fiber Type	Modality Served	Diameter (mm)	Conduction (m/s)	Myelinated?
Aα	Motor efferent	12–20	70–120	Yes
Aα	Proprioception	12–20	70–120	Yes
Aβ	Touch, pressure	5–12	30–70	Yes
Aγ	Motor efferent (muscle spindle)	3–6	15–30	Yes
Aδ	Pain Temperature Touch	2–5	12–30	Yes
B	Preganglionic autonomic fibers	<3	3–14	Some
C Dorsal root	Pain Temperature	0.4–1.2	0.5–2	No
C Sympathetic	Postganglionic sympathetic fibers	0.3–1.3	0.7–2.3	No

[1]An alternative numerical system is sometimes used to classify sensory fibers.

TABLE 16–2 Physicochemical properties of local anesthetics.

Generic (Proprietary)	Structure	Relative Lipid Solubility of Unchanged Local Anesthetic	pK_a	Protein Binding (%)
Amides				
Bupivacaine (Marcaine, Sensorcaine)	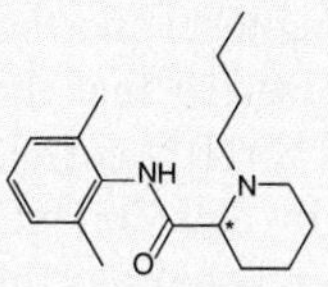	8	8.2	96
Etidocaine (Duranest)	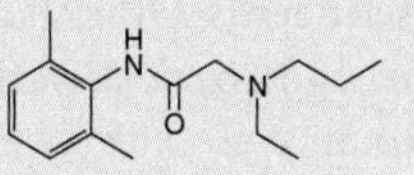	16	8.1	94
Lidocaine (Xylocaine)	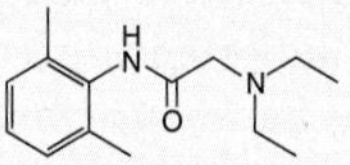	1	8.2	64
Mepivacaine (Carbocaine)	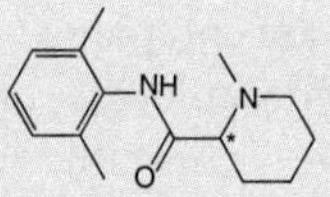	0.3	7.9	78
Prilocaine (Citanest)	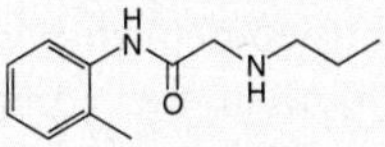	0.4	8.0	53
Ropivacaine (Naropin)	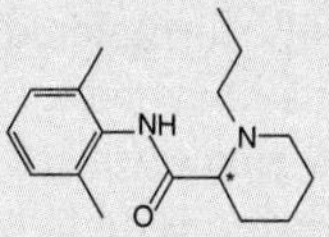	2.5	8.2	94
Esters				
Chloroprocaine (Nesacaine)	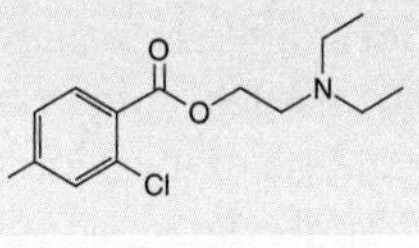	2.3	9.1	NA[1]
Cocaine	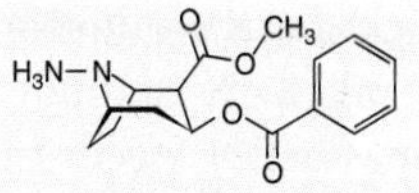	NA	8.7	91
Procaine (Novocaine)	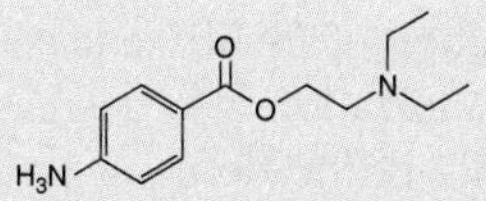	0.3	9.1	NA
Tetracaine (Pontocaine)	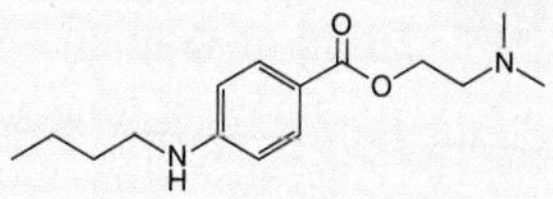	12	8.6	76

*Carbon atom responsible for optical isomerism.

[1]NA, not available.

popular local anesthetic for dentistry in several European countries, is an amide, but it contains a thiophene ring rather than a benzene ring. Local anesthetics are weak bases that at physiological pH usually carry a positive charge at the tertiary amine group. Physicochemical properties of local anesthetics depend on the substitutions in the aromatic ring, the type of linkage in the intermediate chain, and the alkyl groups attached to the amine nitrogen.

3 Clinical local anesthetic potency correlates with octanol solubility and the ability of the local anesthetic molecule to permeate lipid membranes. Potency is increased by adding large alkyl groups to a parent molecule (compare tetracaine with procaine or bupivacaine with mepivacaine). There is no clinical measurement of local anesthetic potency that is analogous to the minimum alveolar concentration (MAC) of inhalation anesthetics. The minimum concentration of local anesthetic that will block nerve impulse conduction is affected by several factors, including fiber size, type, and myelination; pH (an acidic environment antagonizes clinical nerve block); frequency of nerve stimulation; and electrolyte concentrations (hypokalemia and hypercalcemia antagonize blockade).

4 Onset of local anesthetic action depends on many factors, including lipid solubility and the relative concentration of the nonionized, more lipid-soluble free-base form (B) and the ionized water-soluble form (BH^+), expressed by the pK_a. The pK_a is the pH at which there is an equal fraction of ionized and nonionized drug. Less potent, less lipid-soluble agents (eg, lidocaine or mepivacaine) generally have a faster onset than more potent, more lipid-soluble agents (eg, ropivacaine or bupivacaine).

Local anesthetics with a pK_a closest to physiological pH will have (at physiological pH) a greater fraction of nonionized base that more readily permeates the nerve cell membrane, generally facilitating a more rapid onset of action. It is the lipid-soluble free-base form that more readily diffuses across the neural sheath (epineurium) and through the nerve membrane. Curiously, once the local anesthetic molecule gains access to the cytoplasmic side of the Na channel, it is the charged cation (rather than the nonionized base) that more avidly binds the Na channel. For instance, the pK_a of lidocaine exceeds physiological pH. Thus, at physiological pH (7.40), more than half the lidocaine will exist as the charged cation form (BH^+).

The importance of pK_a in understanding differences among local anesthetics is often overstated. It has been asserted that the onset of action of local anesthetics directly correlates with pK_a. This is not supported by data; in fact, the agent of fastest onset (2-chloroprocaine) has the greatest pK_a of all clinically used agents. Other factors, such as ease of diffusion through connective tissue, can affect the onset of action in vivo. Moreover, not all local anesthetics exist in a charged form (eg, benzocaine).

The importance of the ionized and nonionized forms has many clinical implications for those agents that exist in both forms. Local anesthetic solutions are prepared commercially as water-soluble hydrochloride salts (pH 6–7). Because epinephrine is unstable in alkaline environments, commercially formulated local anesthetic solutions containing epinephrine are generally more acidic (pH 4–5) than the comparable "plain" solutions lacking epinephrine. As a direct consequence, these commercially formulated, epinephrine-containing preparations may have a lower fraction of free base and a slower onset than solutions to which the epinephrine is added by the clinician immediately prior to use. Similarly, the extracellular base-to-cation ratio is decreased and onset is delayed when local anesthetics are injected into acidic (eg, infected) tissues. Some researchers have found that alkalinization of local anesthetic solutions (particularly commercially prepared, epinephrine-containing ones) by the addition of sodium bicarbonate (eg, 1 mL 8.4% sodium bicarbonate per 10 mL local anesthetic) speeds the onset and improves the quality of the block, presumably by increasing the fraction of free-base local anesthetic. Interestingly, alkalinization also decreases pain during subcutaneous infiltration.

5 Duration of action correlates with potency and lipid solubility. Highly lipid-soluble local anesthetics have a longer duration of action, presumably because they more slowly diffuse from a lipid-rich environment to the aqueous bloodstream. Lipid solubility of local anesthetics is correlated with

plasma protein binding. In blood, local anesthetics are mostly bound by α_1-acid glycoprotein and, to a lesser extent, to albumin. Sustained-release systems using liposomes or microspheres can significantly prolong local anesthetic duration of action. However, the clinical superiority of liposomal bupivacaine relative to aqueous bupivacaine is currently controversial.

Differential block of sensory but not motor function would be desirable. Unfortunately, only bupivacaine and ropivacaine display *some* clinically useful selectivity (mostly during the onset and offset of block) for sensory nerves; however, the concentrations required for surgical anesthesia almost always result in some motor blockade.

CLINICAL PHARMACOLOGY

Pharmacokinetics

6 In regional anesthesia, local anesthetics are typically applied close to their intended site of action; thus, their pharmacokinetic profiles in blood are important determinants of elimination and toxicity and have very little to do with the duration of their desired clinical effect.

A. Absorption

Absorption after topical application depends on the site. Most mucous membranes (eg, tracheal or oropharyngeal mucosa) provide a minimal barrier to local anesthetic penetration, leading to a rapid onset of action. Intact skin, on the other hand, requires topical application of an increased concentration of lipid-soluble local anesthetic base to ensure permeation and analgesia. EMLA™ (Eutectic Mixture of Local Anesthetics) cream was formulated to overcome the obstacles presented by intact skin. It consists of a mixture of lidocaine and prilocaine bases in an emulsion. Depth of analgesia (usually <0.5 cm), duration of action (usually <2 h), and amount of drug absorbed depend on application time, dermal blood flow, and total dose administered. Typically, 1 to 2 g of cream is applied per 10-cm^2 area of skin. Dermal analgesia sufficient for inserting an intravenous catheter requires about 1 h under an occlusive dressing. EMLA cream should not be used on mucous membranes, broken skin, infants younger than 1 month of age, or patients with a contraindication to either lidocaine or prilocaine.

Systemic absorption of injected local anesthetics depends on blood flow, which is determined by the following factors.

7 **1. Site of injection**—The rates of local anesthetic systemic absorption and rise of local anesthetic concentrations in blood are related to the vascularity of the site of injection and generally follow this rank order: intravenous (or intraarterial) > tracheal (transmucosal) > intercostal > paracervical > epidural > brachial plexus > sciatic > subcutaneous.

2. Presence of additives—The addition of epinephrine causes vasoconstriction at the site of administration, leading to some or all of the following: reduced peak local anesthetic concentration in blood, facilitated neuronal uptake, enhanced quality of analgesia, prolonged duration of analgesia, and reduced toxic side effects. Vasoconstrictors have more pronounced effects on shorter-acting than on longer-acting agents. For example, the addition of epinephrine to lidocaine usually extends the duration of anesthesia by at least 50%, but epinephrine has a limited effect on the duration of bupivacaine peripheral nerve blocks. Epinephrine and clonidine may also augment analgesia through the activation of α_2-adrenergic receptors. Coadministration of dexamethasone or other steroids with local anesthetics can prolong blocks by up to 50%. Mixtures of local anesthetics (eg, ropivacaine and mepivacaine) produce nerve blocks with onset and duration that are intermediate between the two parent compounds.

3. Local anesthetic agent—More lipid-soluble local anesthetics that are highly tissue bound are also more slowly absorbed than less lipid-soluble agents. The agents also vary in their intrinsic vasodilator properties.

B. Distribution

Distribution depends on organ uptake, which is determined by the following factors.

1. Tissue perfusion—The highly perfused organs (brain, lung, liver, kidney, and heart) are responsible for the initial rapid removal of local anesthetics from blood, which is followed by a slower redistribution to a wider range of tissues. In particular, the lung extracts significant amounts of local anesthetic during the "first pass"; consequently, patients with right-to-left cardiac shunts are more susceptible to toxic side effects of lidocaine injected as an antiarrhythmic agent.

2. Tissue/blood partition coefficient—Increasing lipid solubility is associated with greater plasma protein binding and also greater tissue uptake of local anesthetics from an aqueous compartment.

3. Tissue mass—Muscle provides the greatest reservoir for the distribution of local anesthetic agents in the bloodstream because of its large mass.

C. Biotransformation and Excretion

The biotransformation and excretion of local anesthetics are defined by their chemical structure. For all compounds, very little nonmetabolized local anesthetic is excreted by the kidneys.

8 **1. Esters**—Ester local anesthetics are predominantly metabolized by pseudocholinesterase (also termed butyrylcholinesterase). Ester hydrolysis is rapid, and the water-soluble metabolites are excreted in the urine. Procaine and benzocaine are metabolized to *p*-aminobenzoic acid (PABA), which has been associated with rare anaphylactic reactions. Patients with genetically deficient pseudocholinesterase would theoretically be at increased risk for toxic side effects from ester local anesthetics, as metabolism is slower, but clinical evidence for this is lacking, most likely because alternative metabolic pathways are available in the liver. In contrast to other ester anesthetics, cocaine is primarily metabolized (ester hydrolysis) in the liver.

2. Amides—Amide local anesthetics are metabolized (*N*-dealkylation and hydroxylation) by microsomal P-450 enzymes in the liver. The rate of amide metabolism depends on the specific agent (prilocaine > lidocaine > mepivacaine > ropivacaine > bupivacaine) but is consistently slower than ester hydrolysis of ester local anesthetics. Decreases in hepatic function (eg, with cirrhosis) or in liver blood flow (eg, congestive heart failure, β-blockers, or H_2-receptor blockers) will reduce the rate of amide metabolism and potentially predispose patients to have greater blood concentrations and a greater risk of systemic toxicity. Water-soluble local anesthetic metabolites are dependent on renal clearance.

Prilocaine is the only local anesthetic that is metabolized to *o*-toluidine, which produces methemoglobinemia in a dose-dependent fashion. Classical teaching was that a defined dose of prilocaine (in the range of 10 mg/kg) must be exceeded to produce clinically consequential methemoglobinemia; however, recent studies have shown that younger, healthier patients develop medically important methemoglobinemia after lower doses of prilocaine (and at lower doses than needed in older, sicker patients). Prilocaine currently has limited use in North America but is more commonly used in other regions. **Benzocaine, a common ingredient in topical local anesthetic sprays, can also cause dangerous levels of methemoglobinemia**. For this reason, many hospitals no longer permit benzocaine spray during endoscopic procedures. Treatment of medically important methemoglobinemia includes intravenous methylene blue (1–2 mg/kg of a 1% solution over 5 min). Methylene blue reduces methemoglobin (Fe^{3+}) to hemoglobin (Fe^{2+}).

Effects on Organ Systems

Because voltage-gated Na channels underlie action potentials in neurons throughout the body as well as impulse generation and conduction in the heart, it is not surprising that increased circulating concentrations of local anesthetics could produce systemic toxicity. Although organ system effects are discussed for these drugs as a group, individual drugs differ.

Potency at most toxic side effects correlates with local anesthetic potency at nerve blocks. "Maximum safe doses" are listed in Table 16–3, but it must be recognized that the maximum safe dose depends on the patient, the specific nerve block, the rate of injection, and a long list of other factors. In other words, tables of purported maximal safe doses are nearly nonsensical. Mixtures of local anesthetics should be considered to have additive toxic effects; therefore, injecting a solution combining 50% of a toxic dose of lidocaine and 50% of a toxic dose of bupivacaine likely will produce toxic effects.

TABLE 16–3 Clinical use of local anesthetic agents.

Agent	Techniques	Concentrations Available	Maximum Dose (mg/kg)	Typical Duration of Nerve Blocks[1]
Esters				
Benzocaine	Topical[2]	20%	NA[3]	NA
Chloroprocaine	Epidural, infiltration, peripheral nerve block, spinal[4]	1%, 2%, 3%	12	Short
Cocaine	Topical	4%, 10%	3	NA
Procaine	Spinal, local infiltration	1%, 2%, 10%	12	Short
Tetracaine (amethocaine)	Spinal, topical (eye)	0.2%, 0.3%, 0.5%, 1%, 2%	3	Long
Amides				
Bupivacaine	Epidural, spinal, infiltration, peripheral nerve block	0.25%, 0.5%, 0.75%	3	Long
Lidocaine (lignocaine)	Epidural, spinal, infiltration, peripheral nerve block, intravenous regional, topical	0.5%, 1%, 1.5%, 2%, 4%, 5%	4.5 7 (with epinephrine)	Medium
Mepivacaine	Epidural, infiltration, peripheral nerve block, spinal	1%, 1.5%, 2%, 3%	4.5 7 (with epinephrine)	Medium
Prilocaine	EMLA (topical), epidural, intravenous regional (outside North America)	0.5%, 2%, 3%, 4%	8	Medium
Ropivacaine	Epidural, spinal, infiltration, peripheral nerve block	0.2%, 0.5%, 0.75%, 1%	3	Long

[1]Wide variation depending on concentration, location, technique, and whether combined with a vasoconstrictor (epinephrine). Generally, the shortest duration is with spinal anesthesia and the longest with peripheral nerve blocks.

[2]No longer recommended for topical anesthesia.

[3]NA, not applicable or not defined.

[4]Recent literature describes this agent for short-duration spinal anesthesia.

A. Neurological

9 The central nervous system is vulnerable to local anesthetic systemic toxicity (LAST); fortunately, there are premonitory signs and symptoms of increasing local anesthetic concentrations in blood in awake patients. Such symptoms include circumoral numbness, tongue paresthesia, dizziness, tinnitus, blurred vision, and a feeling of impending doom. Such signs include restlessness, agitation, nervousness, and garrulousness. Muscle twitching precedes tonic–clonic seizures. Still higher blood concentrations may produce central nervous system depression (eg, coma and respiratory arrest). The excitatory reactions are thought to be the result of selective blockade of inhibitory pathways. Potent, highly lipid-soluble local anesthetics produce seizures at lower blood concentrations than less potent agents. Benzodiazepines, propofol, and hyperventilation raise the threshold of local anesthetic-induced seizures. Both respiratory and metabolic acidosis reduce the seizure threshold. Propofol (0.5–2 mg/kg) quickly and reliably terminates seizure activity (as do comparable doses of benzodiazepines or barbiturates). Some clinicians use intravenous lipid to terminate

local anesthetic-induced seizures (see below). Maintaining a clear airway with adequate ventilation and oxygenation is most important.

Infused local anesthetics have a variety of actions. Lidocaine infusions are used to inhibit ventricular arrhythmias. Systemically administered local anesthetics such as lidocaine (1.5 mg/kg) can decrease cerebral blood flow and attenuate the rise in intracranial pressure that may accompany intubation in patients with decreased intracranial compliance. Infusions of lidocaine and procaine have been used to supplement general anesthetic techniques, as they are capable of reducing the MAC of volatile anesthetics by up to 40%. Infusions of lidocaine inhibit inflammation and reduce postoperative pain. In some studies, infused lidocaine reduced postoperative opioid requirements sufficiently to reduce length of stay after surgery.

Cocaine stimulates the central nervous system and at moderate doses usually causes a sense of euphoria. An overdose is heralded by restlessness, emesis, tremors, convulsions, arrhythmias, respiratory failure, and cardiac arrest.

In the past, unintentional injection of large volumes of chloroprocaine into the subarachnoid space (during attempts at epidural anesthesia) produced total spinal anesthesia, marked hypotension, and prolonged neurological deficits. The cause of this neural toxicity may be a combination of the low pH of chloroprocaine and a preservative, sodium bisulfite. Chloroprocaine has also been occasionally associated with unexplained severe back pain following epidural administration. Chloroprocaine is available in a preservative (bisulfite)-free formulation that has been used safely and successfully for many thousands of brief spinal anesthetics, providing strong evidence that the compound itself has minimal direct neurotoxicity

Administration of 5% lidocaine has been associated with neurotoxicity (cauda equina syndrome) after use in continuous spinal anesthesia. This may be due to pooling of drug around the cauda equina. In animal experiments, undiluted 5% lidocaine can produce permanent neuronal damage. Transient neurological symptoms (including dysesthesias, burning pain, and aching in the lower extremities and buttocks) have been reported following spinal anesthesia with a variety of local anesthetic agents, but most commonly after use of lidocaine 5% for male outpatients undergoing surgery in the lithotomy position. These symptoms (sometimes referred to as "radicular irritation") typically resolve within 4 weeks. Many clinicians have abandoned lidocaine and substituted 2-chloroprocaine, mepivacaine, or small doses of bupivacaine for spinal anesthesia in the hope of avoiding these transient symptoms.

B. Respiratory

Lidocaine depresses the ventilatory response to low PaO_2 (hypoxic drive). Apnea can result from phrenic and intercostal nerve paralysis (eg, from "high" spinals) or depression of the medullary respiratory center following direct exposure to local anesthetic agents (eg, after retrobulbar blocks; see Chapter 36). However, apnea after administration of a "high" spinal or epidural anesthetic is nearly always the result of hypotension and brain ischemia rather than phrenic block. Local anesthetics relax bronchial smooth muscle. Intravenous lidocaine (1.5 mg/kg) may block the reflex bronchoconstriction sometimes associated with intubation.

C. Cardiovascular

Signs of cardiovascular stimulation (tachycardia and hypertension) may occur with local anesthetic concentrations that produce central nervous system excitation or from injection or absorption of epinephrine (often compounded with local anesthetics). Myocardial contractility and conduction velocity are also depressed at higher blood concentrations. All local anesthetics depress myocardial automaticity (spontaneous phase IV depolarization). These effects result from direct actions on cardiac muscle membrane (ie, cardiac Na channel inhibition) and in intact organisms from inhibition of the autonomic nervous system. At low concentrations, all local anesthetics inhibit nitric oxide, causing vasoconstriction. All local anesthetics except cocaine produce smooth muscle relaxation and arterial vasodilation at higher concentrations, including arteriolar vasodilation. At increased blood concentrations, the combination of arrhythmias, heart block, depression of ventricular contractility, and

10 hypotension may culminate in cardiac arrest. Major cardiovascular toxicity usually requires about three times the local anesthetic concentration in blood as that required to produce seizures. Cardiac arrhythmias or circulatory collapse are the usual presenting signs of cardiac LAST during general anesthesia.

The hypertension associated with laryngoscopy and intubation is often attenuated by intravenous administration of lidocaine (1.5 mg/kg) 1–3 min prior to instrumentation. Overdoses of lidocaine can lead to marked left ventricular contractile dysfunction.

11 Unintended intravascular injection of bupivacaine during regional anesthesia may produce severe cardiovascular LAST, including left ventricular depression, atrioventricular heart block, and life-threatening arrhythmias such as ventricular tachycardia and fibrillation. Pregnancy, hypoxemia, and respiratory acidosis are predisposing risk factors. Young children may also be at increased risk of toxicity. Multiple studies have demonstrated that bupivacaine is associated with more pronounced changes in conduction and a greater risk of arrhythmias than comparable doses of lidocaine. Mepivacaine, ropivacaine, and bupivacaine each have a chiral carbon and therefore can exist in either of two optical isomers (enantiomers). The R(+) optical isomer of bupivacaine blocks more avidly and dissociates more slowly from cardiac Na channels than does the S(−) optical isomer (levobupivacaine or ropivacaine). Resuscitation from bupivacaine-induced cardiac toxicity is often difficult and resistant to standard resuscitation drugs. Multiple clinical reports suggest that bolus administration of nutritional lipid emulsions at 1.5 mL/kg can resuscitate bupivacaine-intoxicated patients who do not respond to standard therapy. We advocate that lipid be a first-line treatment for cardiovascular LAST. We are concerned that case reports indicate persisting delayed use of this nearly risk-free treatment despite an American Society of Regional Anesthesia and Pain Medicine (ASRA) guideline on LAST being available in print, online, and in a mobile app.

Ropivacaine shares many physicochemical properties with bupivacaine. Onset time and duration of action are similar, but ropivacaine produces less motor block when injected at the same volume and concentration as bupivacaine (which may reflect an overall lower potency as compared with bupivacaine). Ropivacaine appears to have a greater therapeutic index than racemic bupivacaine. This improved safety profile likely reflects its formulation as a pure S(−) isomer—that is, having no R(+) isomer—as opposed to racemic bupivacaine. Levobupivacaine, the S(−) isomer of bupivacaine, was reported to have less risk of LAST than the racemic mixture, but it is no longer available in the United States.

Cocaine's cardiovascular reactions are unlike those of any other local anesthetic. Cocaine inhibits the normal reuptake of norepinephrine by adrenergic nerve terminals, thereby potentiating the effects of adrenergic stimulation. Cardiovascular responses to cocaine include hypertension and ventricular ectopy. Initial treatment of systemic cocaine toxicity should include benzodiazepines to reduce the central stimulation. Cocaine-induced arrhythmias have been successfully treated with α-adrenergic antagonists and amiodarone. Cocaine produces vasoconstriction when applied topically and is a useful agent to reduce pain and bleeding related to nasal intubation in awake patients.

D. Immunological

12 True hypersensitivity reactions (due to IgG or IgE antibodies) to local anesthetics—as distinct from LAST caused by excessive plasma concentrations—are uncommon. Esters appear more likely to induce an allergic reaction, especially if the compound is a derivative (eg, procaine or benzocaine) of PABA, a known allergen. Commercial multidose preparations of amides often contain **methylparaben**, which has a chemical structure vaguely similar to that of PABA. As a consequence, generations of anesthesiologists have speculated whether this preservative may be responsible for most of the apparent allergic responses to amide agents, particularly when skin testing fails to confirm true allergy to the local anesthetic.

E. Musculoskeletal

When directly injected into skeletal muscle either intentionally (eg, trigger-point injection treatment of myofascial pain) or unintentionally, local anesthetics are mildly myotoxic. Regeneration usually occurs within 4 weeks after the injection. Compounding the local anesthetic with steroid or epinephrine worsens myonecrosis. When infused into joints for prolonged periods, local anesthetics can produce severe chondromalacia.

F. Hematological

Lidocaine mildly depresses normal blood coagulation (reduced thrombosis and decreased platelet aggregation) and enhances fibrinolysis of whole blood as measured by thromboelastography. These actions could contribute to the lower incidence of thromboembolic events in patients receiving epidural anesthetics in older studies of patients not receiving prophylaxis against deep vein thrombosis.

Drug Interactions

Local anesthetics potentiate nondepolarizing muscle relaxant blockade in laboratory experiments, but this likely has no clinical importance.

As noted earlier, both succinylcholine and ester local anesthetics depend on pseudocholinesterase for metabolism. There is no evidence that this potential competition between ester local anesthetics and succinylcholine for the enzyme has any clinical importance. Dibucaine, an amide local anesthetic, inhibits pseudocholinesterase, and the extent of inhibition by dibucaine defines one form of genetically abnormal pseudocholinesterases (see Chapter 11). Pseudocholinesterase inhibitors (eg, organophosphate poisons) can prolong the metabolism of ester local anesthetics (see Table 11–2).

As noted earlier, drugs that decrease hepatic blood flow (eg, H_2-receptor blockers and β-blockers) decrease amide local anesthetic clearance. Opioids potentiate analgesia produced by epidural and spinal local anesthetics. Similarly, α_2-adrenergic agonists (eg, clonidine) potentiate local anesthetic analgesia produced after epidural or peripheral nerve block injections. Epidural chloroprocaine may interfere with the analgesic actions of neuraxial morphine, notably after cesarean delivery.

CASE DISCUSSION

Local Anesthetic Overdose

An 18-year-old woman in the active stage of labor requests an epidural anesthetic. Immediately following injection of 2 mL and 5 mL test doses of 1.5% lidocaine with 1:200,000 epinephrine through the epidural catheter, the patient reports lip numbness and becomes very apprehensive. Her heart rate has increased from 85 to 105 beats/min.

What is your presumptive diagnosis?

Circumoral numbness and apprehension immediately following administration of lidocaine suggest an intravascular injection of local anesthetic. Abrupt tachycardia strongly suggests intravascular injection of epinephrine. Typically, these symptoms and signs after relatively small test doses will not be followed by a seizure.

What measures should be immediately undertaken?

The patient should receive supplemental oxygen. She should be closely observed for a possible (but unlikely) seizure and be reassured that the symptoms and signs will soon lapse.

What treatment should be initiated for a generalized seizure?

The laboring patient is always considered to be at increased risk for aspiration (see Chapter 41); therefore, the airway should be protected by immediate administration of succinylcholine and tracheal intubation (see Case Discussion, Chapter 17). The succinylcholine will eliminate tonic–clonic activity but will not address the underlying cerebral hyperexcitability. We favor administering an anticonvulsant such as midazolam (1–2 mg) or propofol (20–50 mg) with or before succinylcholine. Thus, wherever conduction anesthetics are administered, resuscitation drugs and equipment must be available just as for a general anesthetic.

What could have been expected if a large dose of bupivacaine (eg, 15 mL 0.5% bupivacaine)—instead of lidocaine—had been given intravascularly?

When administered at "comparably anesthetizing" doses, bupivacaine is more likely to produce cardiac LAST than lidocaine. Acute acidosis (nearly universal after a seizure) tends to potentiate LAST. Ventricular arrhythmias and conduction disturbances may lead to cardiac arrest and death. Cardiac Na channels more slowly unbind bupivacaine than lidocaine. Amiodarone may be given as treatment for LAST-induced ventricular tachyarrhythmias, but we favor immediate administration of lipid emulsion with the onset of seizures and most certainly at the first signs of cardiac toxicity from bupivacaine. Vasopressors may be required. We recommend incremental small (0.5-1 mcg/kg) doses of epinephrine. The reason for the apparent greater susceptibility to local anesthetic cardiotoxicity during pregnancy is unclear. Although the total dose (regardless of concentration) of local anesthetic determines toxicity, the U.S. Food and Drug Administration recommends against the use of 0.75% bupivacaine in pregnant and older adult patients, and in any case this concentration is not needed.

What could have prevented the toxic reaction described?

The risk from accidental intravascular injections during attempted epidural anesthesia is reduced by using test doses and administering the local anesthetic dose in smaller, safer aliquots ("every dose is a test dose"). Finally, one should administer only the minimum required dose for a given regional anesthetic.

SUGGESTED READINGS

Brunton LL, Knollmann BC, Hilal-Dandan R, eds. *Goodman and Gilman's The Pharmacological Basis of Therapeutics*. 13th ed. McGraw-Hill; 2018.

Cousins MJ, Carr DB, Horlocker TT, Bridenbaugh PO, eds. *Cousins & Bridenbaugh's Neural Blockade in Clinical Anesthesia and Pain Medicine*. 4th ed. Lippincott, Williams & Wilkins; 2009.

El-Boghdadly K, Chin KJ. Local anesthetic systemic toxicity: continuing professional development. *Can J Anaesth*. 2016;63:330.

Hadzic A, ed. *Textbook of Regional Anesthesia and Acute Pain Management*. McGraw-Hill; 2016. Includes discussions of the selection of local anesthetic agents.

Hussain N, Brull R, Sheehy B, et al. Perineural liposomal bupivacaine is not superior to nonliposomal bupivacaine for peripheral nerve block analgesia. *Anesthesiology*. 2021;134:147.

Kirksey MA, Haskins SC, Cheng J, Liu SS. Local anesthetic peripheral nerve block adjuvants for prolongation of analgesia: a systematic qualitative review. *PLoS One*. 2015;10:e0137312.

Liu SS, Ortolan S, Sandoval MV, et al. Cardiac arrest and seizures caused by local anesthetic systemic toxicity after peripheral nerve blocks: should we still fear the reaper? *Reg Anesth Pain Med*. 2016;41:5.

Matsen FA 3rd, Papadonikolakis A. Published evidence demonstrating the causation of glenohumeral chondrolysis by postoperative infusion of local anesthetic via a pain pump. *J Bone Joint Surg Am*. 2013;95:1126.

Neal JM, Barrington MJ, Fettiplace MR, et al. The Third American Society of Regional Anesthesia and Pain Medicine practice advisory on local anesthetic systemic toxicity: executive summary 2017. *Reg Anesth Pain Med*. 2018;43:113.

Neal JM, Woodward CM, Harrison TK. The American Society of Regional Anesthesia and Pain Medicine Checklist for managing local anesthetic systemic toxicity: 2017 version. *Reg Anesth Pain Med*. 2018;43:150.

Vasques F, Behr AU, Weinberg G, Ori C, Di Gregorio G. A review of local anesthetic systemic toxicity cases since publication of the American Society of Regional Anesthesia recommendations: to whom it may concern. *Reg Anesth Pain Med*. 2015;40:698.

WEBSITES

This website provides up-to-date information about the use of lipid for rescue from local anesthetic toxicity. http://www.lipidrescue.org

The American Society of Regional Anesthesia and Pain Medicine (ASRA) website provides access to all ASRA guidelines (all of which are related to local anesthetics, regional anesthesia, or pain medicine). http://www.asra.com

CHAPTER

17

Adjuncts to Anesthesia

KEY CONCEPTS

1. Diphenhydramine is one of a diverse group of drugs that competitively blocks H_1 receptors. Many drugs with H_1-receptor antagonist properties have considerable antimuscarinic, or atropine-like, activity (eg, dry mouth) or antiserotonergic activity (antiemetic).
2. H_2 blockers reduce the perioperative risk of aspiration pneumonia by decreasing gastric fluid volume and raising the pH of gastric contents.
3. Metoclopramide increases lower esophageal sphincter tone, speeds gastric emptying, and lowers gastric fluid volume by enhancing the stimulatory effects of acetylcholine on intestinal smooth muscle.
4. Ondansetron, granisetron, tropisetron, and dolasetron selectively block serotonin 5-HT_3 receptors, with little or no effect on dopamine receptors. Located peripherally and centrally, 5-HT_3 receptors appear to play an important role in the initiation of the vomiting reflex.
5. Ketorolac is a parenteral nonsteroidal anti-inflammatory drug that provides analgesia by inhibiting prostaglandin synthesis.
6. Clonidine is a commonly used antihypertensive agent, but in anesthesia, it is used as an adjunct for epidural, caudal, and peripheral nerve block anesthesia and analgesia. It is often used in the management of patients with chronic neuropathic pain to increase the efficacy of epidural opioid infusions.
7. Dexmedetomidine is a parenteral selective α_2-agonist with sedative properties. It appears to be more selective for the α_2-receptor than clonidine.
8. Selective activation of carotid chemoreceptors by low doses of doxapram stimulates hypoxic drive, producing an increase in tidal volume and a slight increase in respiratory rate. Doxapram is not a specific reversal agent and should not replace standard supportive therapy (ie, mechanical ventilation).
9. Naloxone reverses the agonist activity associated with endogenous or exogenous opioid compounds.
10. Flumazenil is useful in the reversal of benzodiazepine sedation and the treatment of benzodiazepine overdose.
11. Aspiration does not necessarily result in aspiration pneumonia. The seriousness of the lung damage depends on the volume and composition of the aspirate. Patients are at risk if their gastric volume is greater than 25 mL (0.4 mL/kg) and their gastric pH is less than 2.5.

Many drugs are routinely administered perioperatively to protect against aspiration pneumonitis, to prevent or reduce the incidence of perianesthetic nausea and vomiting, or to reverse respiratory depression secondary to narcotics or benzodiazepines. This chapter discusses these agents along with other unique classes of drugs that are often administered as adjuvants during anesthesia or analgesia. Additionally, many nonanesthetic agents are increasingly prescribed perioperatively to provide for enhanced recovery following surgery (see Chapter 48).

Aspiration

Aspiration of gastric contents is a rare and potentially fatal event that can complicate anesthesia. Based on an animal study, it is often stated that aspiration of 25 mL of volume at a pH of less than 2.5 will be sufficient to produce aspiration pneumonia. Many factors place patients at risk for aspiration, including "full" stomach, intestinal obstruction, hiatal hernia, obesity, pregnancy, reflux disease, emergency surgery, and inadequate depth of anesthesia.

Many approaches are employed to reduce the potential for aspiration perioperatively. Many of these interventions, such as the application of cricoid pressure (Sellick maneuver) and rapid sequence induction, may only offer limited protection. Cricoid pressure can be applied incorrectly and fail to occlude the esophagus. Whether it has *any* beneficial effect on outcomes even when it is applied correctly remains unproven. Anesthetic agents can decrease lower esophageal sphincter tone and decrease or obliterate the gag reflex, theoretically increasing the risk for passive aspiration. Additionally, inadequately anesthetized patients can vomit; if the airway is unprotected, aspiration of gastric contents may occur. Different combinations of premedications have been advocated to reduce gastric volume, increase gastric pH, or augment lower esophageal sphincter tone. These agents include antihistamines, antacids, and metoclopramide.

HISTAMINE-RECEPTOR ANTAGONISTS

Histamine Physiology

Histamine is found in the central nervous system, in the gastric mucosa, and in other peripheral tissues. It is synthesized by decarboxylation of the amino acid histidine. Histaminergic neurons are primarily located in the posterior hypothalamus but have wide projections in the brain. Histamine also normally plays a major role in the secretion of hydrochloric acid by parietal cells in the stomach (Figure 17–1). The greatest concentrations of histamine are found in the storage granules of circulating basophils and mast cells. Basophils are circulating leukocytes that mediate allergic reactions. Mast cells tend to be concentrated in connective tissue just beneath epithelial (mucosal) surfaces, as well as in the lungs and gastrointestinal tract. Histamine release (degranulation) from these cells can be triggered by chemical, mechanical, or immunological stimulation

Multiple receptors (H_1–H_4) mediate the effects of histamine. The H_1 receptor activates phospholipase C, whereas the H_2 receptor increases intracellular cyclic adenosine monophosphate (cAMP).

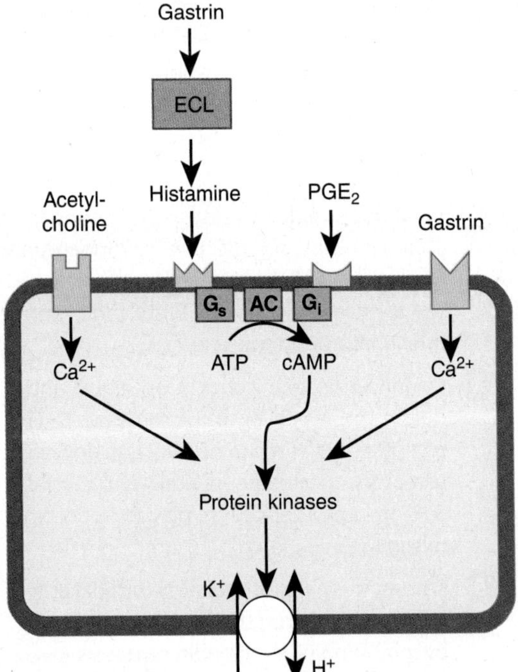

FIGURE 17–1 Secretion of hydrochloric acid is normally mediated by gastrin-induced histamine release from enterochromaffin-like cells (ECL) in the stomach. Note that acid secretion by gastric parietal cells can also be increased indirectly by acetylcholine (AC) via stimulation of M_3 receptors and directly by gastrin through an increase in intracellular Ca^{2+} concentration. Prostaglandin E_2 (PGE_2) can inhibit acid secretion by decreasing cyclic adenosine monophosphate (cAMP) activity. ATP, adenosine triphosphate; G_i, G inhibitory protein; G_s, G stimulatory protein.

The H_3 receptor is primarily located on histamine-secreting cells and mediates negative feedback, inhibiting the synthesis and release of additional histamine. The H_4 receptors are present on hematopoietic cells, mast cells, and eosinophils and are active in allergy and inflammation. Histamine-*N*-methyltransferase metabolizes histamine to inactive metabolites that are excreted in the urine.

A. Cardiovascular

Histamine reduces arterial blood pressure but increases heart rate and myocardial contractility. H_1-Receptor stimulation increases capillary permeability and enhances ventricular irritability, whereas H_2-receptor stimulation increases heart rate and increases contractility. Both types of receptors mediate peripheral arteriolar dilation and some coronary vasodilation.

B. Respiratory

Histamine constricts bronchiolar smooth muscle via the H_1 receptor. H_2-Receptor stimulation may produce mild bronchodilation. Histamine has variable effects on the pulmonary vasculature; the H_1 receptor appears to mediate some pulmonary vasodilation, whereas the H_2 receptor may be responsible for histamine-mediated pulmonary vasoconstriction.

C. Gastrointestinal

Activation of H_2 receptors in parietal cells increases gastric acid secretion. Stimulation of H_1 receptors leads to contraction of intestinal smooth muscle.

D. Dermal

The classic wheal-and-flare response of the skin to histamine results from increased capillary permeability and vasodilation, primarily via H_1-receptor activation.

E. Immunological

Histamine is a major mediator of type 1 hypersensitivity reactions. H_1-Receptor stimulation attracts leukocytes and induces the synthesis of prostaglandin. In contrast, the H_2 receptor appears to activate suppressor T lymphocytes.

1. H_1-Receptor Antagonists

Mechanism of Action

1 Diphenhydramine is one of a diverse group of drugs that competitively blocks H_1 receptors (Table 17–1). Many drugs with H_1-receptor antagonist properties have considerable antimuscarinic, or

TABLE 17–1 Properties of commonly used H_1-receptor antagonists.[1]

Drug	Route	Dose (mg)	Duration (h)	Sedation	Antiemesis
Diphenhydramine (Benadryl)	PO, IM, IV	25–50	3–6	+++	++
Dimenhydrinate (Dramamine)	PO, IM, IV	50–100	3–6	+++	++
Chlorpheniramine (Chlor-Trimeton)	PO IM, IV	2–12 5–20	4–8	++	0
Hydroxyzine (Atarax, Vistaril)	PO, IM	25–100	4–12	+++	++
Promethazine (Phenergan)	PO, IM, IV	12.5–50	4–12	+++	+++
Cetirizine (Zyrtec)	PO	5–10	24	+	
Cyproheptadine (Periactin)	PO	4	6–8	++	
Fexofenadine (Allegra)	PO	30–60	12	0	
Meclizine (Antivert)	PO	12.5–50	8–24	+	
Loratadine (Claritin)	PO	10	24	0	

[1]0, no effect; ++, moderate activity; +++, marked activity; IM, intramuscular, IV, intravenous, PO, oral.

atropine-like, activity (eg, dry mouth) or antiserotonergic activity (antiemetic). Promethazine is a phenothiazine derivative with H_1-receptor antagonist activity as well as antidopaminergic and α-adrenergic–blocking properties.

Clinical Uses

Like other H_1-receptor antagonists, diphenhydramine has a multitude of therapeutic uses: suppression of allergic reactions and symptoms of upper respiratory tract infections (eg, urticaria, rhinitis, conjunctivitis); vertigo, nausea, and vomiting (eg, motion sickness, Ménière disease); sedation; suppression of cough; and dyskinesia (eg, parkinsonism, drug-induced extrapyramidal side effects). Some of these actions are predictable from an understanding of histamine physiology, whereas others are the result of the drugs' antimuscarinic and antiserotonergic effects (see Table 17–1). Although H_1 blockers prevent bronchoconstriction from histamine, they are ineffective in treating bronchial asthma, which is primarily due to other mediators. Likewise, H_1 blockers will not completely prevent the hypotensive effect of histamine unless an H_2 blocker is administered concomitantly.

Although many H_1 blockers cause significant sedation, ventilatory drive is usually unaffected in the absence of other sedative medications. Promethazine and hydroxyzine were often combined with opioids to potentiate analgesia. Newer (second-generation) antihistamines tend to produce little or no sedation because of limited penetration across the blood–brain barrier. This group of drugs is used primarily for allergic rhinitis and urticaria. They include loratadine, fexofenadine, and cetirizine. Many preparations for allergic rhinitis often also contain vasoconstrictors such as pseudoephedrine. Meclizine and dimenhydrinate are used primarily as an antiemetic, particularly for motion sickness, and in the management of vertigo. Cyproheptadine, which also has significant serotonin antagonist activity, has been used in the management of Cushing disease, carcinoid syndrome, and vascular (cluster) headaches.

Dosage

The usual adult dose of diphenhydramine is 25 to 50 mg (0.5–1.5 mg/kg) orally, intramuscularly, or intravenously every 3 to 6 h. The doses of other H_1-receptor antagonists are listed in Table 17–1.

Drug Interactions

The sedative effects of H_1-receptor antagonists can potentiate other central nervous system depressants such as barbiturates, benzodiazepines, and opioids.

2. H_2-Receptor Antagonists

Mechanism of Action

H_2-Receptor antagonists include cimetidine, famotidine, nizatidine, and ranitidine (Table 17–2). These agents competitively inhibit histamine binding to H_2 receptors, thereby reducing gastric acid output and raising gastric pH.

Clinical Uses

All H_2-receptor antagonists are equally effective in the treatment of peptic duodenal and gastric ulcers, hypersecretory states (Zollinger–Ellison syndrome), and gastroesophageal reflux disease (GERD). Intravenous preparations have been used to prevent stress ulceration in critically ill patients. Duodenal and gastric ulcers are usually associated with *Helicobacter pylori* infection, which is treated with various combinations of a proton pump inhibitor, bismuth, and antibiotics.

2 By decreasing gastric fluid volume and hydrogen ion content, H_2 blockers reduce the perioperative risk of aspiration pneumonia. These drugs affect the pH of only those gastric secretions that occur after their administration.

The combination of H_1- and H_2-receptor antagonists provides some protection against drug-induced allergic reactions (eg, intravenous radiocontrast, chymopapain injection for lumbar disk disease, protamine, vital blue dyes used for sentinel node biopsy). Although pretreatment with these agents does not reduce histamine release, it may decrease subsequent hypotension.

Side Effects

Rapid intravenous injection of cimetidine or ranitidine has been rarely associated with hypotension, bradycardia, arrhythmias, and cardiac arrest. H_2-Receptor antagonists change the gastric flora by

TABLE 17–2 Pharmacology of aspiration pneumonia prophylaxis.[1]

Drug	Route	Dose	Onset	Duration	Acidity	Volume	LES Tone
Cimetidine (Tagamet)	PO IV	300–800 mg 300 mg	1–2 h	4–8 h	↓↓↓	↓↓	0
Ranitidine (Zantac)	PO IV	150–300 mg 50 mg	1–2 h	10–12 h	↓↓↓	↓↓	0
Famotidine (Pepcid)	PO IV	20–40 mg 20 mg	1–2 h	10–12 h	↓↓↓	↓↓	0
Nizatidine (Axid)	PO	150–300 mg	0.5–1 h	10–12 h	↓↓↓	↓↓	0
Nonparticulate antacids (Bicitra, Polycitra)	PO	15–30 mL	5–10 min	30–60 min	↓↓↓	↑	0
Metoclopramide (Reglan)	IV PO	10 mg 10–15 mg	1–3 min	1–2 h 30–60 min[2]	0	↓↓	↑↑

[1]0, no effect; ↓↓, moderate decrease; ↓↓↓, marked decrease; ↑, slight increase; ↑↑, moderate increase; IM, intramuscular, IV, intravenous, LES, lower esophageal sphincter; PO, oral.

[2]Oral metoclopramide has a quite variable onset of action and duration of action.

virtue of their pH effects. Cimetidine is now much less commonly used because of its many side effects, including hepatotoxicity, interstitial nephritis, granulocytopenia, thrombocytopenia, and occasional gynecomastia and impotence in men. Finally, it has been associated with mental status changes, including lethargy, hallucinations, and seizures, particularly in older adult patients. In contrast, ranitidine, nizatidine, and famotidine do not affect androgen receptors and penetrate the blood–brain barrier poorly.

Dosage

As a premedication to reduce the risk of aspiration pneumonia, H_2-receptor antagonists should be administered at bedtime and again at least 2 h before surgery. Because all four drugs are eliminated primarily by the kidneys, the dose should be reduced in patients with significant renal dysfunction.

Drug Interactions

Cimetidine may reduce hepatic blood flow and bind to the cytochrome P-450 mixed-function oxidases, slowing the metabolism of a multitude of drugs, including lidocaine, propranolol, diazepam, theophylline, phenobarbital, warfarin, and phenytoin. Ranitidine is a weak inhibitor of the cytochrome P-450 system, and no significant drug interactions have been demonstrated. Famotidine and nizatidine do not appear to affect the cytochrome P-450 system.

ANTACIDS

Mechanism of Action

Antacids neutralize the acidity of gastric fluid by providing a base (usually hydroxide, carbonate, bicarbonate, citrate, or trisilicate) that reacts with hydrogen ions to form water.

Clinical Uses

Common uses of antacids include the treatment of peptic ulcers and GERD. In anesthesiology, antacids provide protection against the harmful effects of aspiration pneumonia by raising the pH of gastric contents. Unlike H_2-receptor antagonists, antacids have an immediate effect. Unfortunately, they increase intragastric volume. Aspiration of particulate antacids (aluminum or magnesium hydroxide) produces abnormalities in lung function comparable to those that occur following acid aspiration. Nonparticulate antacids (sodium citrate or sodium bicarbonate) are much less damaging to lung alveoli if aspirated. Furthermore, nonparticulate antacids mix with gastric contents better than particulate solutions. Timing is critical, as nonparticulate antacids lose their effectiveness 30 to 60 min after ingestion.

Dosage

The usual adult dose of a 0.3 M solution of sodium citrate—Bicitra (sodium citrate and citric acid) or Polycitra (sodium citrate, potassium citrate, and citric acid)—is 15 to 30 mL orally, 15 to 30 min prior to induction (see Table 17–2).

Drug Interactions

Because antacids alter gastric and urinary pH, they change the absorption and elimination of many drugs. The rate of absorption of digoxin, cimetidine, and ranitidine is slowed, whereas the rate of phenobarbital elimination is quickened.

METOCLOPRAMIDE

Mechanism of Action

Metoclopramide acts peripherally as a cholinomimetic (ie, facilitates acetylcholine transmission at selective muscarinic receptors) and centrally as a dopamine receptor antagonist. Its action as a prokinetic agent in the upper gastrointestinal (GI) tract is not dependent on vagal innervation but is abolished by anticholinergic agents. It does not stimulate secretions.

Clinical Uses

3 By enhancing the stimulatory effects of acetylcholine on intestinal smooth muscle, metoclopramide increases lower esophageal sphincter tone, speeds gastric emptying, and lowers gastric fluid volume (see Table 17–2). These properties account for its efficacy in the treatment of patients with diabetic gastroparesis and GERD, as well as prophylaxis for those at risk for aspiration pneumonia. Metoclopramide does not affect the secretion of gastric acid or the pH of gastric fluid.

Metoclopramide produces an antiemetic effect by blocking dopamine receptors in the chemoreceptor trigger zone of the central nervous system. However, at doses used clinically during the perioperative period, the drug's ability to reduce postoperative nausea and vomiting is negligible.

Side Effects

Rapid intravenous injection may cause abdominal cramping, and metoclopramide is contraindicated in patients with complete intestinal obstruction. It can induce a hypertensive crisis in patients with pheochromocytoma by releasing catecholamines from the tumor. Sedation, nervousness, and extrapyramidal signs from dopamine antagonism (eg, akathisia) are uncommon and reversible. Nonetheless, metoclopramide is best avoided in patients with Parkinson disease. Prolonged treatment with metoclopramide can lead to tardive dyskinesia. Metoclopramide-induced increases in aldosterone and prolactin secretion are probably inconsequential during short-term therapy. Metoclopramide may rarely result in hypotension and arrhythmias.

Dosage

An adult dose of 10 to 15 mg of metoclopramide (0.25 mg/kg) is effective orally, intramuscularly, or intravenously (injected over 5 min). Larger doses (1–2 mg/kg) have been used to prevent emesis during chemotherapy. The onset of action is much more rapid following parenteral (3–5 min) than oral (30–60 min) administration. Because metoclopramide is excreted in the urine, its dose should be decreased in patients with kidney dysfunction.

Drug Interactions

Antimuscarinic drugs (eg, atropine, glycopyrrolate) block the GI effects of metoclopramide. Metoclopramide decreases the absorption of orally administered cimetidine. Concurrent use of phenothiazines or butyrophenones (droperidol) increases the likelihood of extrapyramidal side effects.

PROTON PUMP INHIBITORS

Mechanism of Action

These agents, including omeprazole (Prilosec), lansoprazole (Prevacid), rabeprazole (Aciphex), esomeprazole (Nexium), and pantoprazole (Protonix), bind to the proton pump of parietal cells in the gastric mucosa and inhibit secretion of hydrogen ions.

Clinical Uses

Proton pump inhibitors (PPIs) are indicated for the treatment of peptic ulcer, GERD, and Zollinger–Ellison syndrome. They may promote healing of peptic ulcers and erosive GERD more quickly than H_2-receptor blockers. There are ongoing questions regarding the safety of PPIs in patients taking clopidogrel (Plavix). These concerns relate to inadequate antiplatelet therapy when these drugs are combined due to inadequate activation of clopidogrel by hepatic enzyme CYP2C19, which is inhibited to varying degrees by PPIs.

Side Effects

PPIs are generally well tolerated, causing few side effects. Adverse side effects primarily involve the GI system (nausea, abdominal pain, constipation, diarrhea). On rare occasions, these drugs have been associated with myalgias, anaphylaxis, angioedema, and severe dermatological reactions. Long-term use of PPIs has also been associated with gastric enterochromaffin-like cell hyperplasia and an increased risk of pneumonia secondary to bacterial colonization in the higher-pH environment.

Dosage

Recommended oral doses for adults are omeprazole, 20 mg; lansoprazole, 15 mg; rabeprazole, 20 mg; and pantoprazole, 40 mg. Because these drugs are primarily eliminated by the liver, repeat doses should be decreased in patients with severe liver impairment.

Drug Interactions

PPIs can interfere with hepatic P-450 enzymes, potentially decreasing the clearance of diazepam, warfarin, and phenytoin. Concurrent administration can decrease clopidogrel (Plavix) effectiveness, as the latter medication is dependent on hepatic enzymes for activation.

Postoperative Nausea & Vomiting

Without any prophylaxis, postoperative nausea and vomiting (PONV) occurs in approximately 30% or more of the general surgical population and up to 70% to 80% in patients with predisposing risk factors. The Society for Ambulatory Anesthesia (SAMBA) provides extensive guidelines for the management of PONV. Table 17–3 identifies risks factors for PONV and scores the evidence for assessing risk. When PONV risk is sufficiently great, prophylactic antiemetic medications are administered, and strategies to reduce its incidence are initiated. Risk reduction strategies include:

- Avoidance of general anesthesia by the use of regional anesthesia
- Use of propofol for the induction and maintenance of anesthesia

TABLE 17–3 Risk factors for PONV.

Evidence	Risk factors
Positive overall	Female sex (B1) History of PONV or motion sickness (B1) Nonsmoking (B1) Younger age (B1) General versus regional anesthesia (A1) Use of volatile anesthetics and nitrous oxide (A1) Postoperative opioids (A1) Duration of anesthesia (B1) Type of surgery (cholecystectomy, laparoscopic, gynecological) (B1)
Conflicting	ASA physical status (B1) Menstrual cycle (B1) Level of anesthetist's experience (B1) Muscle relaxant antagonists (A2)
Disproven or of limited clinical relevance	BMI (B1) Anxiety (B1) Nasogastric tube (A1) Supplemental oxygen (A1) Perioperative fasting (A2) Migraine (B1)

[1]ASA, American Society of Anesthesiologists; BMI, body mass index; MO, motion sickness; PONV, postoperative nausea and vomiting.

[2]Risk assessment scoring: A1, randomized trials with supportive meta-analyses; A2, randomized trials but of insufficient number for a meta-analysis; B1, observational studies such as case control or cohort designs.

Reproduced with permission from Gan TJ, Diemunsch P, Habib AS, et al. Consensus guidelines for the management of postoperative nausea and vomiting. *Anesth Analg.* 2014 Jan;118(1):85-113.

Risk factors	Points
Female gender	1
Nonsmoker	1
History of PONV	1
Postoperative opioids	1
Sum =	0 ... 4

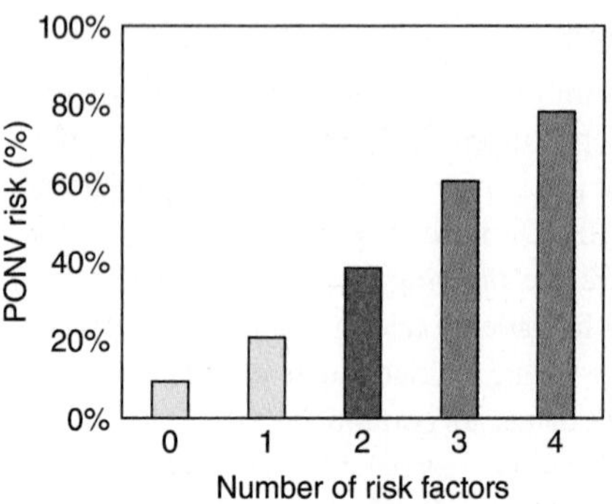

FIGURE 17–2 Risk score for PONV in adults. Simplified risk score from Apfel et al to predict the patient's risk for PONV. When 0, 1, 2, 3, and 4 of the risk factors are present, the corresponding risk for PONV is about 10%, 20%, 40%, 60%, and 80%, respectively. PONV, postoperative nausea and vomiting. (Reproduced with permission from Gan TJ, Diemunsch P, Habib A, et al. Consensus guidelines for the management of postoperative nausea and vomiting, *Anesth Analg.* 2014 Jan;118(1):85-113.)

- Avoidance of nitrous oxide in surgeries lasting over 1 hour
- Avoidance of volatile anesthetics
- Minimization of intraoperative and postoperative opioids
- Adequate hydration
- Use of sugammadex instead of neostigmine for the reversal of neuromuscular blockade

The Apfel score provides a simplified assessment tool to predict the risk of PONV (Figures 17–2 and 17–3). (Obesity, anxiety, and reversal of neuromuscular blockade are not independent risk factors for PONV.)

Drugs used in the prophylaxis and treatment of PONV include 5-HT_3 antagonists, butyrophenones, dexamethasone, neurokinin-1 receptor antagonists (aprepitant); antihistamines and transdermal scopolamine may also be used. At-risk patients often benefit from several prophylactic measures. Because all drugs have adverse effects, the guideline algorithm can be used to help guide PONV prophylaxis and therapy (Figure 17–4).

Risk factors	Points
Surgery ≥ 30 min.	1
Age ≥ 3 years	1
Strabismus surgery	1
History of POV or PONV in relatives	1
Sum =	0 ... 4

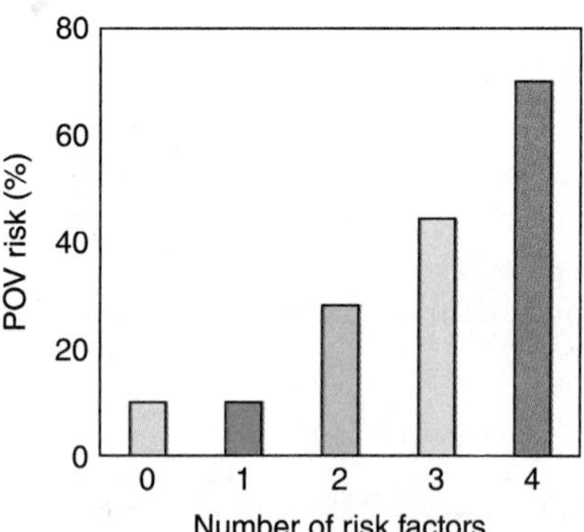

FIGURE 17–3 Simplified risk score for POV in children. Simplified risk score from Eberhart et al to predict the risk for POV in children. When 0, 1, 2, 3, or 4 of the depicted independent predictors are present, the corresponding risk for PONV is approximately 10%, 10%, 30%, 50%, or 70%, respectively. POV, postoperative vomiting; PONV, postoperative nausea and vomiting. (Reproduced with permission from Gan TJ, Diemunsch P, Habib A, et al. Consensus guidelines for the management of postoperative nausea and vomiting. *Anesth Analg.* 2014 Jan;118(1):85-113.)

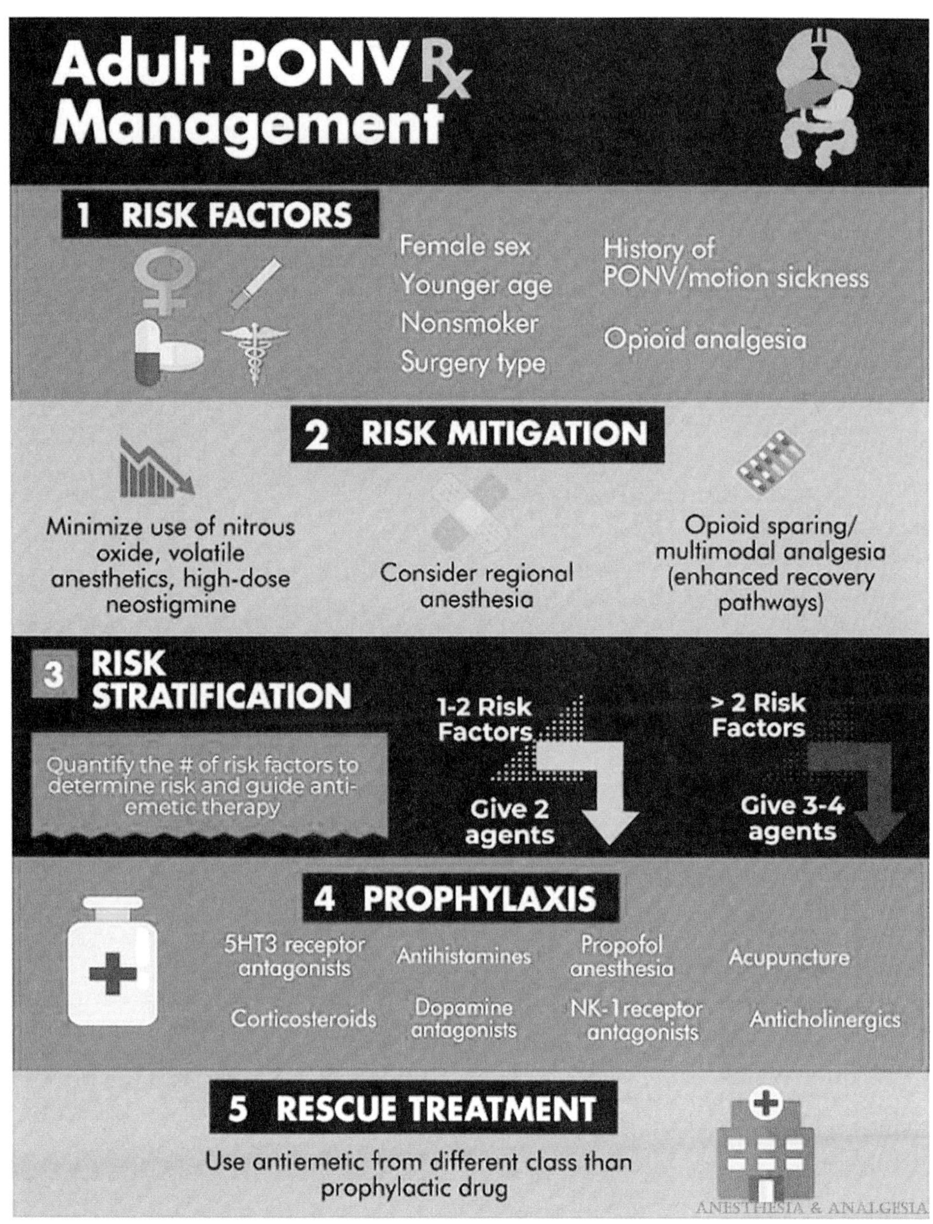

A

FIGURE 17–4A Algorithm for PONV management in adults. Summary of recommendations for PONV management in adults, including risk identification, stratified prophylaxis, and treatment of established postoperative nausea and vomiting. Note that two antiemetics are now recommended for PONV prophylaxis in patients with one to two risk factors. 5-HT3, 5-hydroxytryptamine 3; PONV, postoperative nausea and vomiting. (Used with permission of the American Society for Enhanced Recovery, from Gan TJ, Belani KG, Bergese S, et al: Fourth Consensus Guidelines for the Management of Postoperative Nausea and Vomiting, *Anesth Analg*. 2020 Aug;131(2):411-448.)

Pediatric POV/PONV Management ℞

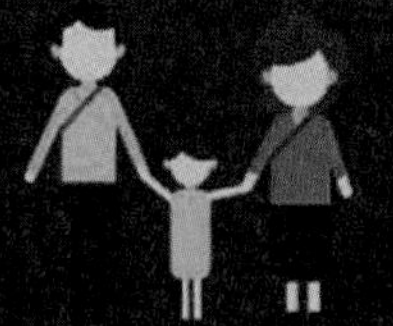

Preoperative
- Age ≥ 3 years
- History of POV/PONV/motion sickness
- Family history of POV/PONV
- Postpubertal female

Intraoperative
- Strabismus surgery
- Adenotonsillectomy
- Otoplasty
- Surgery ≥ 30 mins
- Volatile anesthetics
- Anticholinesterases

1 RISK FACTORS

Postoperative
- Long-acting opioids

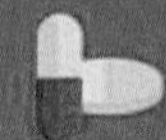

2 RISK STRATIFICATION

*Consider multimodal analgesia to minimize opioid use

No Risk Factors → LOW RISK

1-2 Risk Factors → MEDIUM RISK

≥3 Risk Factors → HIGH RISK

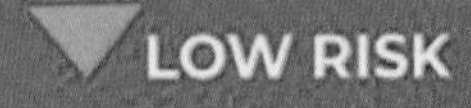

3 PROPHYLAXIS

LOW RISK: None or 5HT3 antagonist or dexamethasone

MEDIUM RISK: 5HT3 antagonist + dexamethasone

HIGH RISK: 5HT3 antagonist + dexamethasone + consider TIVA

4 RESCUE TREATMENT

Use antiemetic from different class than prophylactic drug – droperidol, promethazine, dimenhydrinate, metoclopramide; May also consider accupuncture/accupressure

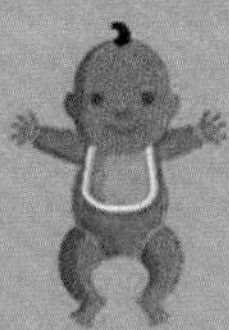

ANESTHESIA & ANALGESIA

B

FIGURE 17–4B Algorithm for POV/PONV management in children. Summary of recommendations for POV/PONV management in children, including risk identification, risk-stratified prophylaxis, and treatment of established postoperative vomiting. 5-HT3, 5-hydroxytryptamine 3; PONV, postoperative nausea and vomiting; POV, postoperative vomiting; TIVA, total intravenous anesthesia. (Used with permission of the American Society for Enhanced Recovery, from Gan TJ, Belani KG, Bergese S, et al: Fourth Consensus Guidelines for the Management of Postoperative Nausea and Vomiting, *Anesth Analg.* 2020 Aug;131(2):411-448.)

5-HT_3 RECEPTOR ANTAGONISTS

Serotonin Physiology

Serotonin, 5-hydroxytryptamine (5-HT), is present in large quantities in platelets and the GI tract (enterochromaffin cells and the myenteric plexus). It is also an important neurotransmitter in multiple areas of the central nervous system. Serotonin is formed by hydroxylation and decarboxylation of tryptophan. Monoamine oxidase inactivates serotonin into 5-hydroxyindoleacetic acid (5-HIAA). The physiology of serotonin is very complex because there are at least seven receptor types, most with multiple subtypes. The 5-HT_3 receptor mediates vomiting and is found in the GI tract and the brain (area postrema). The 5-HT_{2A} receptors are responsible for smooth muscle contraction and platelet aggregation, the 5-HT_4 receptors in the GI tract mediate secretion and peristalsis, and the 5-HT_6 and 5-HT_7 receptors are located primarily in the limbic system, where they appear to play a role in depression. All except the 5-HT_3 receptor are coupled to G proteins and affect either adenylyl cyclase or phospholipase C; effects of the 5-HT_3 receptor are mediated via an ion channel.

A. Cardiovascular

Except in the heart and skeletal muscle, serotonin is a powerful vasoconstrictor of arterioles and veins. Its vasodilator effect in the heart is endothelium dependent. When the myocardial endothelium is damaged following injury, serotonin produces vasoconstriction. The pulmonary and kidney vasculatures are very sensitive to the arterial vasoconstrictive effects of serotonin. Modest and transient increases in cardiac contractility and heart rate may occur immediately following serotonin release; reflex bradycardia often follows. Vasodilation in skeletal muscle can subsequently cause hypotension. Excessive serotonin can produce *serotonin syndrome*, characterized by hypertension, hyperthermia, and agitation.

B. Respiratory

Contraction of smooth muscle increases airway resistance. Bronchoconstriction from released serotonin is often a prominent feature of carcinoid syndrome

C. Gastrointestinal

Direct smooth muscle contraction (via 5-HT_2 receptors) and serotonin-induced release of acetylcholine in the myenteric plexus (via 5-HT_3 receptors) greatly augment peristalsis. Secretions are unaffected.

D. Hematological

Activation of 5-HT_2 receptors causes platelet aggregation.

Mechanism of Action

4 Ondansetron, granisetron, tropisetron, ramosetron, palonosetron, and dolasetron selectively block serotonin 5-HT_3 receptors, with little or no effect on dopamine receptors. 5-HT_3 receptors, which are located peripherally (abdominal vagal afferents) and centrally (chemoreceptor trigger zone of the area postrema and the nucleus tractus solitarius), appear to play an important role in the initiation of the vomiting reflex. The 5-HT_3 receptors of the chemoreceptor trigger zone in the area postrema reside outside the blood–brain barrier (Figure 17–5). The chemoreceptor trigger zone is activated by substances such as anesthetics and opioids and signals the nucleus tractus solitarius, resulting in PONV. Emetogenic stimuli from the GI tract similarly stimulate the development of PONV.

Clinical Uses

5-HT_3-Receptor antagonists are generally administered at the end of surgery. All these agents are effective antiemetics in the postoperative period. Palonosetron has an extended duration of action and may reduce the incidence of postdischarge nausea and vomiting (PDNV). SAMBA guidelines suggest risk factors for PDNV, including:

- Female sex
- History of PONV
- Age 50 years or younger
- Use of opioids in the postanesthesia care unit (PACU)
- Nausea in the PACU

Side Effects

5-HT_3-Receptor antagonists are essentially devoid of serious side effects, even in amounts several times

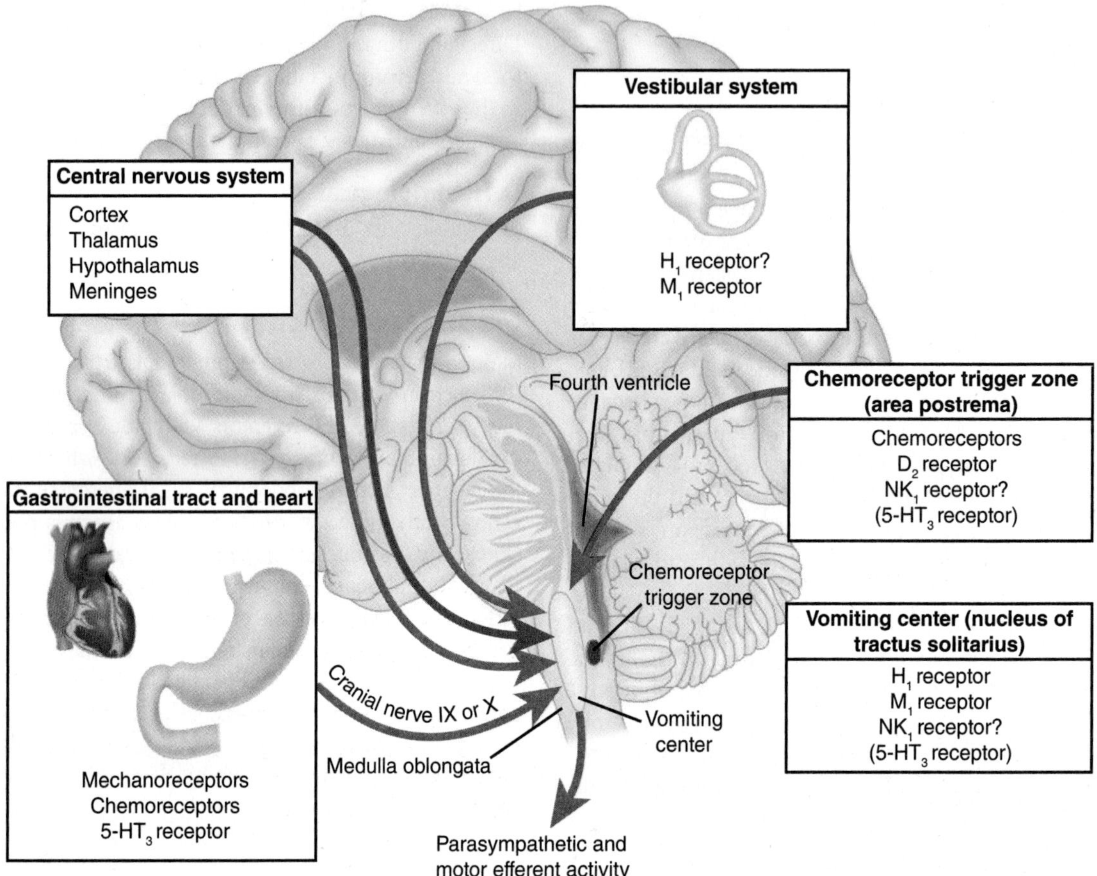

FIGURE 17–5 Neurological pathways involved in the pathogenesis of nausea and vomiting (see text). (Reproduced with permission from Krakauer EL, Zhu AX, Bounds BC, et al. Case records of the Massachusetts General Hospital. Weekly clinicopathological exercises. Case 6-2005. A 58-year-old man with esophageal cancer and nausea, vomiting, and intractable hiccups, *N Engl J Med.* 2005 Feb 24;352(8):817-825.)

the recommended dose. They do not appear to cause sedation, extrapyramidal signs, or respiratory depression. The most commonly reported side effect is headache. These drugs can slightly prolong the QT interval on the electrocardiogram. This effect may be more frequent with dolasetron (no longer available in the United States) and less likely with palonosetron. Nonetheless, these drugs should be used cautiously in patients who are taking antiarrhythmic drugs or who have a prolonged QT interval.

Ondansetron undergoes extensive metabolism in the liver via hydroxylation and conjugation by cytochrome P-450 enzymes. Liver failure impairs clearance several-fold, and the dose should be reduced accordingly.

BUTYROPHENONES

Droperidol (0.625–1.25 mg) was previously used routinely for PONV prophylaxis. Given at the end of the procedure, it blocks dopamine receptors that contribute to the development of PONV. Despite its effectiveness, many practitioners no longer routinely administer this medication because of a U.S. Food and Drug Administration (FDA) black box warning related to concerns that doses described in the product labeling ("package insert") may lead to QT prolongation and development of *torsades des pointes* arrhythmia. However, the doses relevant to the FDA warning, as acknowledged by the FDA, were those used for neurolept anesthesia (5–15 mg), not the much smaller doses employed for PONV. Cardiac monitoring is warranted when large doses of the drug are used. There is no evidence that the use of droperidol at the doses routinely employed for PONV management increases the risk of sudden cardiac death in the perioperative population.

As with other drugs that antagonize dopamine, droperidol use in patients with Parkinson disease and in other patients manifesting extrapyramidal signs should be carefully considered.

The phenothiazine prochlorperazine (Compazine), which affects multiple receptors (histaminergic, dopaminergic, muscarinic), may be used for PONV management. It may cause extrapyramidal and anticholinergic side effects. Promethazine (Phenergan) works primarily as an anticholinergic agent and antihistamine and likewise can be used to treat PONV. As with other agents of this class, anticholinergic effects (sedation, delirium, confusion, vision changes) can complicate the postoperative period.

Amisulpride (5–10 mg IV) is a dopamine (D_2) receptor antagonist that has antiemetic properties without apparent significant QT prolongation and with minimal increase in serum prolactin concentration.

DEXAMETHASONE

Dexamethasone (Decadron) in doses as small as 4 mg has been shown to be as effective as ondansetron in reducing the incidence of PONV. Dexamethasone should be given at induction as opposed to the end of surgery, and its mechanism of action is unclear. It may provide analgesic and mild euphoric effects. Dexamethasone can increase postoperative blood glucose concentration, and some practitioners have suggested that dexamethasone could increase the risk of postoperative infection. Nonetheless, most studies have not demonstrated any increase in wound infections or increased risk of cancer recurrence following dexamethasone administration for PONV prophylaxis.

NEUROKININ-1 RECEPTOR ANTAGONIST

Substance P is a neuropeptide that interacts with neurokinin-1 (NK_1) receptors. NK_1 antagonists inhibit substance P at central and peripheral receptors. Aprepitant, an NK_1 antagonist, has been found to reduce PONV perioperatively and is additive with ondansetron for this indication.

OTHER PONV STRATEGIES

Several other agents and techniques have been employed to reduce the incidence of PONV. Transdermal scopolamine has been used effectively, though it may produce anticholinergic side effects (confusion, blurred vision, dry mouth, urinary retention). Acupuncture, acupressure, and transcutaneous electrical stimulation of the P6 acupuncture point can reduce PONV incidence and medication requirements.

As no single agent will both treat and prevent PONV, perioperative management centers on identifying patients at greatest risk so that prophylaxis, often with multiple agents, may be initiated. Since systemic opioid administration is associated with PONV, *opioid-sparing* strategies (eg, use of regional anesthetics and nonopioid analgesics) can markedly reduce the risk of PONV.

Other Drugs Used as Adjuvants to Anesthesia

KETOROLAC

Mechanism of Action

5 Ketorolac is a parenteral nonsteroidal anti-inflammatory drug (NSAID) that provides analgesia by inhibiting prostaglandin synthesis. A peripherally acting drug, it has become a popular alternative to opioids for postoperative analgesia because of its minimal central nervous system side effects.

Clinical Uses

Ketorolac is indicated for the short-term (<5 days) management of pain and appears to be particularly useful in the immediate postoperative period. A standard dose of ketorolac provides analgesia equivalent to 6 to 12 mg of morphine administered by the same route. Its time to onset is also similar to morphine, but ketorolac has a longer duration of action (6–8 h).

Ketorolac does not cause respiratory depression, sedation, nausea, or vomiting. In fact, ketorolac does not cross the blood–brain barrier to any significant degree. Numerous studies have shown that oral and parenteral NSAIDs have an opioid-sparing effect. They may be most beneficial in patients at increased risk for postoperative respiratory depression or emesis.

Side Effects

As with other NSAIDs, ketorolac inhibits platelet aggregation and prolongs bleeding time. It and other NSAIDs should therefore be used with caution in patients at risk for postoperative hemorrhage. Long-term administration may lead to renal toxicity (eg, papillary necrosis) or GI tract ulceration with bleeding and perforation. Because ketorolac depends on kidney elimination, it should not be given to patients with kidney disease. Ketorolac is contraindicated in patients allergic to aspirin or NSAIDs. Patients with asthma have an increased incidence of aspirin sensitivity (approximately 10%), particularly if they also have a history of nasal polyps (approximately 20%).

Dosage

Ketorolac has been approved for administration as either a 60 mg intramuscular or 30 mg intravenous loading dose; a maintenance dose of 15 to 30 mg every 6 h is recommended. Older adult patients clear ketorolac more slowly and should receive reduced doses.

Drug Interactions

Aspirin decreases the protein binding of ketorolac, increasing the amount of active unbound drug. Ketorolac does not affect the minimum alveolar concentration of inhalation anesthetic agents, and its administration does not alter the hemodynamics of anesthetized patients. It decreases the postoperative requirement for opioid analgesics.

Other NSAID Adjuvant Drugs

Other NSAID agents are used perioperatively. Ketorolac and other NSAIDs inhibit cyclooxygenase (COX) isoenzymes. COX-1 maintains gastric mucosa and stimulates platelet aggregation. COX-2 is expressed during inflammation. Diclofenac and ibuprofen are now available for intravenous administration. Whereas ketorolac, diclofenac, and ibuprofen are nonselective COX inhibitors, other agents such as celecoxib are specific for COX-2. COX-2 inhibitors spare both the gastric mucosa and platelet function. However, their use is associated with an increased risk of hypertension, stroke, and cardiovascular events. Indeed, the FDA warns that all non-aspirin nonsteroidal anti-inflammatory drugs increase the risk of myocardial infarction or stroke.

Intravenous acetaminophen (Ofirmev) is available for perioperative use in the United States. Acetaminophen is a centrally acting analgesic with likely central COX inhibition and with weak peripheral COX effects. Its exact mechanism of action remains controversial; nevertheless, it does not cause gastric irritation and clotting abnormalities. A maximal adult (>50 kg weight) dose of 1 g is infused to a maximum total dose of 4 g/d. Patients weighing 50 kg or less should receive a maximal dose of 15 mg/kg and a maximal total dose of 75 mg/kg/d. Hepatoxicity is a known risk of overdosage, and the drug should be used with caution in patients with hepatic disease or undergoing hepatic surgery. Oral and rectal acetaminophen is as effective as the intravenous form and orders of magnitude less expensive.

CLONIDINE

Mechanism of Action

Clonidine is an imidazoline derivative with predominantly α_2-adrenergic agonist activity. It is highly lipid soluble and readily penetrates the blood–brain barrier and the placenta. Studies indicate that the binding of clonidine to receptors is highest in the rostral ventrolateral medulla in the brainstem (the final common pathway for sympathetic outflow), where it activates inhibitory neurons. The overall effect is to decrease sympathetic activity, enhance parasympathetic tone, and reduce circulating catecholamines. There is also evidence that some of clonidine's antihypertensive action may occur via binding to a nonadrenergic (imidazoline) receptor. In contrast, its analgesic effects, particularly in the spinal cord, are mediated entirely via pre- and possibly postsynaptic α_2-adrenergic receptors that block nociceptive transmission. Clonidine also has local anesthetic effects when applied to peripheral nerves and is frequently added to local anesthetic solutions to increase duration of action.

Clinical Uses

6 Clonidine is a commonly used antihypertensive agent that reduces sympathetic tone, decreasing systemic vascular resistance, heart rate, and blood pressure. In anesthesia, clonidine is used as an adjunct for epidural, caudal, and peripheral nerve block anesthesia and analgesia. It is often used in the management of patients with chronic neuropathic pain to increase the efficacy of epidural opioid infusions. When given epidurally, the analgesic effect of clonidine is segmental, being localized to the level at which it is injected or infused. When added to local anesthetics of intermediate duration (eg, mepivacaine or lidocaine) administered for epidural or peripheral nerve block, clonidine will markedly prolong both the anesthetic and analgesic effects.

Off-label/investigational uses of clonidine include serving as an adjunct in premedication, control of withdrawal syndromes (nicotine, opioids, alcohol, and vasomotor symptoms of menopause), and treatment of glaucoma as well as various psychiatric disorders. Systemic clonidine administration has been shown not to reduce opioid usage following noncardiac surgery in some studies.

Side Effects

Sedation, dizziness, bradycardia, and dry mouth are common side effects. Less commonly, orthostatic hypotension, nausea, and diarrhea may be observed. Abrupt discontinuation of clonidine following long-term administration (>1 month) can produce a withdrawal phenomenon characterized by rebound hypertension, agitation, and sympathetic overactivity.

Dosage

Epidural clonidine is usually started at 30 mcg/h in a mixture with an opioid or a local anesthetic. Oral clonidine is readily absorbed, has a 30 to 60 min onset, and lasts 6 to 12 h. In the initial treatment of hypertension, 0.1 mg can be given two times a day and adjusted until the blood pressure is controlled. The maintenance dose typically ranges from 0.1 to 0.3 mg twice daily. Transdermal preparations of clonidine can also be used for maintenance therapy. They are available as 0.1, 0.2, and 0.3 mg/d patches that are replaced every 7 days. Clonidine is metabolized by the liver and excreted by the kidney. Dosages should be reduced for patients with kidney disease.

Drug Interactions

Clonidine enhances and prolongs sensory and motor blockade from local anesthetics. Additive effects with hypnotic agents, general anesthetics, and sedatives can potentiate sedation, hypotension, and bradycardia. The drug should be used cautiously, if at all, in patients who take β-adrenergic blockers and in those with significant cardiac conduction system abnormalities. Lastly, clonidine can mask the symptoms of hypoglycemia in patients with diabetes.

DEXMEDETOMIDINE

Mechanism of Action

7 Dexmedetomidine is a parenteral selective α_2 agonist with sedative properties. It appears to be more selective for the α_2 receptor than clonidine. At higher doses, it loses its selectivity and also stimulates α_1-adrenergic receptors.

Clinical Uses

Dexmedetomidine causes dose-dependent sedation, anxiolysis, some analgesia, and blunting of the sympathetic response to surgery and to other stress. Most importantly, it has an opioid-sparing effect and does not significantly depress respiratory drive;

excessive sedation, however, may cause airway obstruction. The drug can be used for short-term (<24 h) intravenous sedation of mechanically ventilated patients. Discontinuation after more prolonged use can potentially cause a withdrawal phenomenon similar to that of clonidine. It is also used for intraoperative sedation and as an adjunct to general and regional anesthetics. Dexmedetomidine has been suggested as having neuroprotective effects, including protecting the brain from the toxic effects of anesthetic agents. Supplemental dexmedetomidine administration may decrease the incidence of delirium following cardiac surgery. Moreover, some have indicated that dexmedetomidine may have "renoprotective" qualities. Additional studies are needed to evaluate these claims more fully.

Side Effects

The principal side effects are bradycardia, heart block, and hypotension. It may also cause nausea.

Dosage

The recommended initial loading dose is 1 mcg/kg intravenously over 10 min with a maintenance infusion rate of 0.2 to 0.7 mcg/kg/h. Dexmedetomidine has a rapid onset and terminal half-life of 2 h. The drug is metabolized in the liver, and its metabolites are eliminated in the urine. Dosage should be reduced in patients with liver or kidney disease.

Drug Interactions

Caution should be used when dexmedetomidine is administered with vasodilators, cardiac depressants, and drugs that decrease heart rate. Reduced requirements of hypnotics/anesthetic agents should prevent excessive hypotension.

GABAPENTIN & PREGABALIN

Gabapentin was initially employed as an anticonvulsant. Gabapentin and pregabalin act by blocking voltage-gated calcium channels, resulting in a diminished release of glutamate. Various studies have demonstrated that both drugs may reduce perioperative opioid consumption when included in multimodal pain management, while other reports have questioned the utility of perioperative gabapentinoids. Gabapentin may be given to adults as a 600-mg preemptive dose prior to surgery and continued postoperatively (1200 mg/d in divided doses). These agents are also commonly used for the management of chronic (particularly neuropathic) pain syndromes.

CAPSAICIN

Capsaicin is a TRPV1-receptor agonist. It depletes substance P and inhibits pain signal transmission. Infiltration of capsaicin in surgical wounds reduces opioid consumption and improves perioperative analgesia.

DOXAPRAM

Mechanism of Action

Doxapram is a peripheral and central nervous system stimulant. Selective activation of carotid chemoreceptors by low doses of doxapram stimulates hypoxic drive, producing an increase in tidal volume and a slight increase in respiratory rate. At larger doses, respiratory centers in the medulla are stimulated.

8

Clinical Uses

Doxapram is not a specific reversal agent and should not replace standard supportive therapy (ie, mechanical ventilation). Drug-induced respiratory and central nervous system depression, including that seen immediately postoperatively, can be *temporarily* overcome. Doxapram will not reverse paralysis caused by muscle relaxants and will not alleviate airway obstruction.

Side Effects

Stimulation of the central nervous system leads to a variety of possible side effects: changes in mental status (confusion, dizziness, seizures), cardiac abnormalities (tachycardia, dysrhythmias, hypertension), and pulmonary dysfunction (wheezing, tachypnea). Doxapram's association with vomiting and laryngospasm are of particular concern to the anesthesia provider in the postoperative period. Doxapram should not be used in patients with a history of epilepsy, cerebrovascular disease, acute head injury, coronary artery disease, hypertension, or bronchial asthma.

Dosage

Bolus intravenous administration (0.5–1 mg/kg) results in transient increases in minute ventilation (the onset of action is 1 min; the duration of action is 5–12 min). Continuous intravenous infusions (1–3 mg/min) provide longer-lasting effects (the maximum dose is 4 mg/kg).

Drug Interactions

The sympathetic stimulation produced by doxapram may exaggerate the cardiovascular effects of monoamine oxidase inhibitors or adrenergic agents.

NALOXONE

Mechanism of Action

Naloxone is a competitive opioid receptor antagonist. Its affinity for opioid μ receptors appears to be much greater than for opioid κ or δ receptors. Naloxone has no significant agonist activity.

Clinical Uses

9 Naloxone reverses the agonist activity associated with endogenous (enkephalins, endorphins) or exogenous opioid compounds. A dramatic example is the reversal of unconsciousness that occurs in a patient with opioid overdose who receives naloxone. Thus, naloxone is widely available for first responders and relatives of those who abuse opioids. Perioperative respiratory depression caused by opioids is rapidly antagonized (1–2 min). Some degree of opioid analgesia can often be spared if the dose of naloxone is limited to the minimum required to maintain adequate ventilation (40–80 mcg intravenously in adults, repeated as needed). Small doses of intravenous naloxone reverse the side effects of spinal or epidural opioids without necessarily reversing the analgesia.

Side Effects

Abrupt, complete reversal of opioid analgesia can result in a surge of sympathetic stimulation (tachycardia, ventricular irritability, hypertension, pulmonary edema) caused by severe, acute pain and an acute withdrawal syndrome in patients who are opioid dependent.

Dosage

In postoperative patients experiencing respiratory depression from excessive opioid administration, intravenous naloxone (0.4 mg/mL vial diluted in 9 mL saline to 0.04 mg/mL) can be titrated in increments of 40 to 80 mcg every 3 to 5 min until adequate ventilation and alertness are achieved. Doses in excess of 200 mcg are rarely needed. The brief duration of action of intravenous naloxone (30–45 min) is due to rapid redistribution from the central nervous system. A more prolonged effect will be necessary to prevent the recurrence of respiratory depression from longer-acting opioids. Therefore, intramuscular naloxone (twice the required intravenous dose) or a continuous naloxone infusion is recommended. Naloxone may precipitate symptoms of withdrawal in infants of opioid-exposed mothers.

Drug Interactions

The effect of naloxone on nonopioid anesthetic agents such as nitrous oxide or clonidine is insignificant.

NALTREXONE

Naltrexone is also a pure opioid antagonist with a high affinity for the μ receptor, but it has a significantly longer half-life than naloxone. Naltrexone is used orally for maintenance treatment of addiction. Chapter 48 reviews the use of the peripherally acting opioid receptor antagonists alvimopan and methylnaltrexone in the management and prevention of postoperative ileus as an element of enhanced perioperative recovery.

FLUMAZENIL

Mechanism of Action

Flumazenil, an imidazobenzodiazepine, is a specific and competitive antagonist of benzodiazepines at benzodiazepine receptors.

Clinical Uses

10 Flumazenil is useful in the reversal of benzodiazepine sedation and the treatment of benzodiazepine overdose. Although it promptly (onset <1 min) reverses the hypnotic effects of benzodiazepines, amnesia has proved to be less reliably prevented. Some evidence of respiratory depression may linger despite an alert and awake appearance. Specifically, tidal volume and minute ventilation return to normal, but the slope of the carbon dioxide response curve remains depressed. Effects in older adult patients appear to be particularly difficult to reverse fully, and these patients are more prone to relapse of sedation.

Side Effects & Drug Interactions

Rapid administration of flumazenil may cause anxiety reactions in previously sedated patients and symptoms of withdrawal in those on long-term benzodiazepine therapy. Flumazenil reversal has been associated with increases in intracranial pressure in patients with head injuries and abnormal intracranial compliance. Flumazenil may induce seizure activity if benzodiazepines have been given as anticonvulsants or in conjunction with an overdose of tricyclic antidepressants. Flumazenil reversal following a midazolam–ketamine anesthetic technique may increase the incidence of emergence dysphoria and hallucinations. Nausea and vomiting are not uncommon following the administration of flumazenil. The reversal effect of flumazenil is based on its strong antagonist affinity for benzodiazepine receptors. Flumazenil does not affect the minimum alveolar concentration of inhalation anesthetics.

Dosage

Gradual titration of flumazenil is usually accomplished by intravenous administration of 0.2 mg/min until reaching the desired degree of reversal. The usual total dose is 0.6 to 1.0 mg. Because of flumazenil's rapid hepatic clearance, repeat doses may be required after 1 to 2 h to avoid re-sedation and premature recovery room or outpatient discharge. Liver failure prolongs the clearance of flumazenil and benzodiazepines.

NONADRENERGIC VASOCONSTRICTORS

Intravenous vasopressin is used as a vasoconstrictor to treat vasoplegia following cardiac surgery, as well as in the intensive care unit as a therapy for patients with vasodilatory shock. Infusions of angiotensin II are increasingly employed as perioperative vasoconstrictors. These agents are discussed in greater detail in Chapter 57.

CASE DISCUSSION

Management of Patients at Risk for Aspiration Pneumonia

A 58-year-old patient is scheduled for elective laparoscopic cholecystectomy. The patient's history reveals a persistent problem with heartburn and passive regurgitation of gastric contents into the pharynx. The patient has been told by an internist that these symptoms are due to a hiatal hernia.

Why would a history of hiatal hernia concern the anesthesiologist?

Perioperative aspiration of gastric contents (Mendelson syndrome) is a potentially fatal complication of anesthesia. Hiatal hernia is commonly associated with symptomatic GERD, which is considered a predisposing factor for aspiration. Mild or occasional heartburn may not significantly increase the risk of aspiration. In contrast, symptoms related to passive reflux of gastric fluid, such as acid taste or sensation of refluxing liquid into the mouth, should alert the clinician to a high risk of pulmonary aspiration. Paroxysms of coughing or wheezing, particularly at night or when the patient is flat, may be indicative of chronic aspiration. Aspiration can occur on induction, during maintenance, or upon emergence from anesthesia.

Which patients are predisposed to aspiration?

Patients with altered airway reflexes (eg, drug intoxication, general anesthesia, encephalopathy, neuromuscular disease) or abnormal pharyngeal or esophageal anatomy (eg, large hiatal hernia,

Zenker diverticulum, scleroderma, pregnancy, obesity, history of esophagectomy) are prone to pulmonary aspiration.

Does aspiration consistently result in aspiration pneumonia?

Not necessarily. The seriousness of the lung
11 damage depends on the volume and composition of the aspirate. Traditionally, patients are considered to be at risk if their gastric volume is greater than 25 mL (0.4 mL/kg) and their gastric pH is less than 2.5. Some investigators believe that controlling acidity is more important than volume and that the criteria should be revised to a pH less than 3.5 with a volume greater than 50 mL.

Patients who have eaten immediately prior to emergency surgery are obviously at risk. Traditionally, "NPO after midnight" implied a preoperative fast of at least 6 h. Current opinion allows clear liquids until 2 h before induction of anesthesia. According to the American Society of Anesthesiologists (ASA) guideline, breast milk is permitted up to 4 h before anesthesia. Infant formula, nonhuman milk, and a light meal are permitted up to 6 h before induction. Patients consuming a heavy meal including meat, fats, and fried foods should fast for 8 h. Certain patient populations are particularly likely to have large volumes of acidic gastric fluid: patients with an acute abdomen or peptic ulcer disease, children, older adults, patients with diabetes, pregnant women, and obese patients. Furthermore, pain, anxiety, or opioids may delay gastric emptying. Note that pregnancy and obesity place patients in double jeopardy by increasing the chance of aspiration (increased intraabdominal pressure and distortion of the lower esophageal sphincter) and the risk of aspiration pneumonia (increased acidity and volume of gastric contents). Aspiration is more common in patients undergoing esophageal, upper abdominal, or emergency laparoscopic surgery.

Which drugs lower the risk of aspiration pneumonia?

H_2-Receptor antagonists decrease gastric acid secretion. Although they will not affect gastric contents already in the stomach, they will inhibit further acid production. Both gastric pH and volume are affected. In addition, the long duration of action of ranitidine and famotidine may provide protection in the recovery room.

Metoclopramide shortens gastric emptying time and increases lower esophageal sphincter tone. It does not affect gastric pH, and it cannot clear large volumes of food in a few hours. Nonetheless, metoclopramide with ranitidine is a good combination for most at-risk patients. Antacids usually raise gastric fluid pH, but at the same time, they increase gastric volume. Although antacid administration technically removes a patient from the at-risk category, aspiration of a substantial volume of particulate matter will lead to serious physiological damage. For this reason, clear antacids (eg, sodium citrate) are employed. In contrast to H_2 antagonists, antacids are immediately effective and alter the acidity of existing gastric contents. Thus, they are useful in emergency situations and in patients who have recently eaten.

Anticholinergic drugs, particularly glycopyrrolate, decrease gastric secretions if large doses are administered; however, lower esophageal sphincter tone is reduced. Overall, anticholinergic drugs do not reliably reduce the risk of aspiration pneumonia and can reverse the protective effects of metoclopramide. Proton pump inhibitors are generally as effective as H_2 antagonists.

The ASA guideline recommends that prophylaxis against gastric content aspiration be undertaken only in at-risk patients.

What anesthetic techniques are used in full-stomach patients?

If the full stomach is due to recent food intake and the surgical procedure is elective, the operation should be postponed. If the risk factor is not reversible (eg, large hiatal hernia) or the case is an emergency, proper anesthetic technique can minimize the risk of aspiration pneumonia. Regional anesthesia with minimal sedation should be considered in patients at increased risk for aspiration pneumonia. If local anesthetic techniques are impractical, the patient's airway must be protected.

As in every anesthetic case, the availability of suction must be confirmed before induction. A rapid-sequence induction (or, depending upon airway examination, an awake intubation) is indicated.

How does a rapid-sequence induction differ from a routine induction?

- The patient is always preoxygenated prior to induction. Patients with lung disease require 3 to 5 min of preoxygenation.
- A wide assortment of blades, video laryngoscopes, intubation bougies, and endotracheal tubes are prepared in advance and immediately available.
- An assistant may apply firm pressure over the cricoid cartilage prior to induction (Sellick maneuver). Because the cricoid cartilage forms an uninterrupted and incompressible ring, pressure over it is transmitted to underlying tissue. The esophagus is collapsed, and passively regurgitated gastric fluid cannot reach the hypopharynx. Excessive cricoid pressure (beyond what can be tolerated by a conscious person) applied during active regurgitation has been associated with rupture of the posterior wall of the esophagus. The effectiveness of the Sellick maneuver has been questioned.
- A propofol induction dose is given as a bolus. Obviously, this dose must be modified if there is any indication that the patient's cardiovascular system is unstable. Other rapid-acting induction agents can be substituted (eg, etomidate, ketamine, methohexital).
- Succinylcholine (1.5 mg/kg) or rocuronium (0.9–1.2 mg/kg) is administered immediately following the induction dose, even if the patient has not yet lost consciousness.
- The patient is not ventilated with a bag and mask to avoid filling the stomach with gas and thereby increasing the risk of emesis. Once muscle response to nerve stimulation has disappeared, the patient is rapidly intubated. Cricoid pressure, if used, should be maintained until the endotracheal tube cuff is inflated and tube position is confirmed. A modification of the classic rapid-sequence induction allows gentle ventilation as long as cricoid pressure is maintained.
- If the intubation proves difficult, cricoid pressure is maintained, and the patient is gently ventilated with oxygen until another intubation attempt can be performed. If intubation is still unsuccessful, spontaneous ventilation should be allowed to return, and an awake intubation should be performed. Sugammadex can be administered to reverse rocuronium-induced muscle relaxation.
- After surgery, the patient should remain intubated until airway reflexes and consciousness have returned.

What are the relative contraindications to rapid-sequence inductions?

Rapid-sequence inductions are often associated with increases in intracranial pressure, arterial blood pressure, and heart rate.

Describe the pathophysiology and clinical findings associated with aspiration pneumonia.

The pathophysiological changes depend on the composition of the aspirate. Acid solutions cause atelectasis, alveolar edema, and loss of surfactant. Particulate aspirate will also result in small-airway obstruction and alveolar necrosis. Granulomas may form around food or antacid particles. The earliest physiological change following aspiration is intrapulmonary shunting, resulting in hypoxia. Other changes may include pulmonary edema, pulmonary hypertension, and hypercapnia.

Wheezing, rhonchi, tachycardia, and tachypnea are common physical findings. Decreased lung compliance can make ventilation difficult. Hypotension signals significant fluid shifts into the alveoli and is associated with massive lung injury. Chest roentgenography may not demonstrate diffuse bilateral infiltrates for several hours after the event. Arterial blood gases reveal hypoxemia, hypercapnia, and respiratory acidosis.

What is the treatment for aspiration pneumonia?

As soon as regurgitation is suspected, the patient should be placed in a head-down position so that gastric contents drain out of the mouth instead of into the trachea. The pharynx and, if possible, the trachea should be thoroughly suctioned. The mainstay of therapy in patients who subsequently become hypoxic is positive-pressure ventilation. Intubation and the institution of positive end-expiratory pressure, or noninvasive ventilation, may be required. Bronchoscopy and pulmonary lavage are usually indicated when particulate aspiration has occurred. Use of corticosteroids is generally not recommended, and antibiotics are administered depending upon culture results.

GUIDELINES

Gan TJ, Belani K, Bergtese S. Fourth consensus guidelines for the management of postoperative nausea and vomiting. *Anesth Analg.* 2020;131:411.

Practice guidelines for preoperative fasting and the use of pharmacologic agents to reduce the risk of pulmonary aspiration: application to healthy patients undergoing elective procedures: an updated report by the American Society of Anesthesiologists Task Force on Preoperative Fasting and the Use of Pharmacologic Agents to Reduce the Risk of Pulmonary Aspiration. *Anesthesiology.* 2017;126:376.

SUGGESTED READINGS

Alam A, Suen KC, Hana Z, Sanders RD, Maze M, Ma D. Neuroprotection and neurotoxicity in the developing brain: an update on the effects of dexmedetomidine and xenon. *Neurotoxicol Teratol.* 2017;60:102.

Dahl J, Nielsen V, Wetterslev L, et al. Postoperative effects of paracetamol, NSAIDs, glucocorticoids, gabapentinoids, and their combinations: a topical review. *Acta Anaesthesiol Scand.* 2014;58:1165.

Doleman B, Read D, Lund JN, Williams JP. Preventive acetaminophen reduces postoperative opioid consumption, vomiting, and pain scores after surgery: systematic review and meta-analysis. *Reg Anesth Pain Med.* 2015;40:706.

Fabritius M, Geisler A, Petersen P, et al. Gabapentin for postoperative pain management—a systemic review with meta-analyses and trial sequential analyses. *Acta Anaesthesiol Scand.* 2016;60:1188.

Fathi M, Massoudi N, Nooraee N, Beheshti Monfared R. The effects of doxapram on time to tracheal extubation and early recovery in young morbidly obese patients scheduled for bariatric surgery: a randomised controlled trial. *Eur J Anaesthesiol.* 2020;37:457.

Gan TJ, Kranke P, Minkowitz HS, et al. Intravenous amisulpride for the prevention of postoperative nausea and vomiting: two concurrent, randomized, double-blind, placebo-controlled trials. *Anesthesiology.* 2017;126:268.

Kaye A, Ali S, Urman R. Perioperative analgesia: ever-changing technology and pharmacology. *Best Pract Res Clin Anaesthesiol.* 2014;28:3.

Kelly CJ, Walker RW. Perioperative pulmonary aspiration is infrequent and low risk in pediatric anesthetic practice. *Paediatr Anaesth.* 2015;25:36.

Kiski D, Malec E, Schmidt C. Use of dexmedetomidine in pediatric cardiac anesthesia. *Curr Opin Anaesthesiol.* 2019;32:334.

Lee A, Ryo J. Aspiration pneumonia and related syndromes. *Mayo Clin Proc.* 2018;93:752.

Likhvantsev VV, Landoni G, Grebenchikov OA, et al. Perioperative dexmedetomidine supplement decreases delirium incidence after adult cardiac surgery: a randomized, double-blind, controlled study. *J Cardiothorac Vasc Anesth.* 2021;35:449.

Obara I, Telezhkin V, Alrashdi I, Chazot PL. Histamine, histamine receptors, and neuropathic pain relief. *Br J Pharmacol.* 2020;177:580.

Priebe HJ. Evidence no longer supports use of cricoid pressure. *Br J Anaesth.* 2016;117:537.

Sanchez Munoz MC, De Kock M, Forget P. What is the place of clonidine in anesthesia? Systematic review and meta-analyses of randomized controlled trials. *J Clin Anesth.* 2017;38:140.

Vaezi MF, Yang YX, Howden CW. Complications of proton pump inhibitor therapy. *Gastroenterology.* 2017;153:35.

CHAPTER 18

Preoperative Assessment, Premedication, & Perioperative Documentation

KEY CONCEPTS

1. The cornerstones of an effective preoperative or preprocedure evaluation are the history and physical examination, which should include a complete and up-to-date listing of all medications taken by the patient in the recent past, all pertinent allergies, and responses and reactions to previous anesthetics.

2. The anesthesiologist should not be expected to provide the risk-versus-benefit discussion for the proposed surgery or procedure; this is the responsibility and purview of the responsible surgeon or "proceduralist."

3. By convention, physicians in many countries use the American Society of Anesthesiologists' classification to identify relative risk prior to conscious sedation and surgical anesthesia.

4. In general, the indications for cardiovascular investigations are the same in elective surgical patients as in any other patient with a similar medical condition.

5. Adequacy of long-term blood glucose control can be easily and rapidly assessed by measurement of hemoglobin A1c.

6. In patients deemed at high risk for thrombosis (eg, those with certain mechanical heart valve implants or with atrial fibrillation and a prior thromboembolic stroke), chronic anticoagulants should be replaced by intramuscular low-molecular-weight heparins or by intravenous unfractionated heparin.

7. Current guidelines recommend postponing all but mandatory emergency surgery until at least 1 month after any coronary intervention and suggest that treatment options *other* than a drug-eluting stent (which will require prolonged dual antiplatelet therapy) be used in patients expected to undergo a surgical procedure within 12 months after the intervention.

8. There are no good data to support restricting fluid intake (of any kind or any amount) more than 2 h before induction of general anesthesia in healthy patients undergoing elective procedures; moreover, there is strong evidence that nondiabetic patients who drink fluids containing carbohydrates and protein up to 2 h before induction of anesthesia experience less perioperative nausea and dehydration than those who are fasted longer.

—Continued next page

Continued—

9 To be valuable, preoperative testing must discriminate: There must be an avoidable increased perioperative risk when the results are abnormal (and the risk will remain unknown if the test is not performed), and when testing fails to detect the abnormality (or it has been corrected), there must be reduced risk.

10 The utility of a test depends on its sensitivity and specificity. Sensitive tests have a low rate of false-negative results and rarely fail to identify an abnormality when one is present, whereas specific tests have a low rate of false-positive results and rarely identify an abnormality when one is not present.

11 Premedication should be given purposefully, not as a mindless routine.

12 Incomplete, inaccurate, or illegible records unnecessarily complicate defending a physician against otherwise unjustified allegations of malpractice.

PREOPERATIVE EVALUATION

1 The cornerstones of an effective preoperative or preprocedure evaluation are the medical history and physical examination, which should include a complete and up-to-date listing of all medications taken by the patient in the recent past, all pertinent allergies, and responses and reactions to previous anesthetics. Additionally, this evaluation may include diagnostic tests, imaging procedures, or consultations from other physicians when indicated. A patient's initial contact with a perioperative surgical home or enhanced recovery after surgery (ERAS) program ideally will occur at the time of the preoperative evaluation visit. An enhanced recovery may require "prehabilitation" with smoking cessation and one or more of the following: nutritional supplementation, an exercise regimen, and adjustment of medications. The preoperative evaluation will often guide the anesthetic plan. Inadequate preoperative planning and incomplete patient preparation lead to avoidable delays, cancellations, complications, and costs.

The preoperative evaluation serves multiple purposes. One purpose is to identify those patients whose outcomes likely will be improved by implementation of a specific medical treatment (which rarely may require that planned surgery be rescheduled). For example, a 60-year-old patient scheduled for elective total hip arthroplasty who also has unstable angina from left main coronary artery disease would more likely survive if coronary artery bypass grafting is performed before rather than after the elective orthopedic procedure. Another purpose of the preoperative evaluation is to identify patients whose condition is so poor that the proposed surgery might only hasten death without improving the quality of life. For example, a patient with severe chronic lung disease, end-stage kidney disease, liver failure, and chronic heart failure likely would not survive to derive benefit from an 8-h, complex, multilevel spinal fusion with instrumentation. A patient's preoperative evaluation can uncover findings that will change the anesthetic plan (Table 18–1). For example, the anesthetic plan may need to be adjusted for a patient whose trachea appears difficult to intubate, one with a family history of malignant hyperthermia, or one with an infection near where a proposed regional anesthetic would be administered.

Another purpose of the preoperative evaluation is to provide the patient with an estimate of anesthetic risk. 2 However, the anesthesiologist should not be expected to provide the risk-versus-benefit discussion for the proposed surgery or procedure; this is the responsibility and purview of the responsible surgeon or "proceduralist." For example, a discussion of the risks and benefits of robot-assisted laparoscopic prostatectomy versus "open" prostatectomy, radiation therapy, or "watchful waiting" requires detailed knowledge of the current

TABLE 18–1 The anesthetic plan.

Will sedative-hypnotic premedication be useful?
What type(s) of anesthesia will be employed?
General[1]
Airway management
Induction drugs
Maintenance drugs
Regional
Technique(s)
Agent(s)
Sedation and monitored anesthesia care
Supplemental oxygen
Specific sedative drugs
Are there special intraoperative management issues?
Nonstandard monitors
Positions other than supine
Relative or absolute contraindications to specific anesthetic drugs
Fluid management
Special techniques
Site (anesthetizing location) concerns
How will the patient be managed postoperatively?
Management of acute pain
Intensive care
Postoperative ventilation
Hemodynamic monitoring

[1]Including need for (or need for avoidance of) muscle relaxation.

medical literature and the capabilities of an individual urologist. Finally, the preoperative evaluation presents an opportunity for the anesthesiologist to describe the proposed anesthetic plan in the context of the overall surgical and postoperative plan, provide the patient with psychological support, and obtain informed consent from the patient.

By convention, physicians in many countries use the American Society of Anesthesiologists' (ASA) physical status classification to define relative risk prior to conscious sedation or surgical anesthesia (Table 18–2). The ASA physical status classification has many advantages: it is time tested, simple, and reproducible, and, most importantly, it has been shown to be strongly associated with perioperative risk. However, many other risk assessment tools are available, particularly in the area of cardiovascular risk assessment (see Chapter 21).

TABLE 18–2 American Society of Anesthesiologists' physical status classification of patients.

Class	Definition
1	Normal healthy patient
2	Patient with mild systemic disease (no functional limitations)
3	Patient with severe systemic disease (some functional limitations)
4	Patient with severe systemic disease that is a constant threat to life (functionality incapacitated)
5	Moribund patient who is not expected to survive without the operation
6	Brain-dead patient whose organs are being removed for donor purposes
E	If the procedure is an emergency, the physical status is followed by "E" (eg, "2E")

Data from Committee on Standards and Practice Parameters, Apfelbaum JL, Connis RT, et al. Practice advisory for preanesthesia evaluation: An updated report by the American Society of Anesthesiologists Task Force on Preanesthesia Evaluation. *Anesthesiology.* 2012 Mar;116(3):522–538.

Elements of the Preoperative History

Patients presenting for elective surgery and anesthesia typically require the recording of a focused medical history that emphasizes abnormalities of exercise tolerance; nutritional and functional status; cardiac, pulmonary, endocrine, kidney, or liver function; electrolytes or metabolism; and anatomic issues relevant to airway management or regional anesthesia. How the patient responded to and recovered from previous anesthetics can be helpful. The ASA and other societies publish and periodically update general guidelines for preoperative assessment (see Guidelines at end of chapter).

A. Cardiovascular Issues

Guidelines for preoperative cardiac assessment are regularly updated and available from the American College of Cardiology/American Heart Association and from the European Society of Cardiology (see Guidelines). A more complete discussion of cardiovascular assessment is provided in Chapter 21. The focus of preoperative cardiac assessment should be

on determining whether the patient would benefit from further cardiac evaluation or interventions prior to the scheduled surgery. However, the same approach is not appropriate for all patients. The prudent approach to a patient undergoing elective knee arthroplasty will differ from that for a patient needing resection of pancreatic cancer, given the benign results of a delay in the former procedure and the possible deadly effects of a delay in the latter
4 procedure. In general, the indications for cardiovascular investigations are the same in elective surgical patients as in any other patient with a similar medical condition. Put another way, the fact that a patient is scheduled to undergo elective surgery does not change the indications for testing to diagnose coronary artery disease.

B. Pulmonary Issues

Perioperative pulmonary complications, most notably postoperative respiratory depression and respiratory failure, are vexing problems associated with obesity and obstructive sleep apnea. A guideline developed by the American College of Physicians identifies patients 60 years of age or older and those with chronic obstructive lung disease, with markedly reduced exercise tolerance, with functional dependence, or with heart failure as potentially requiring preoperative and postoperative interventions to avoid respiratory complications. Additionally, the risk of postoperative respiratory complications is also associated with the following: ASA physical status 3 and 4, cigarette smoking, surgeries lasting longer than 4 h, certain types of surgery (abdominal, thoracic, aortic aneurysm, head and neck, emergency surgery), and general anesthesia (compared with cases in which general anesthesia was not used).

Efforts at prevention of respiratory complications in patients at risk should include cessation of cigarette smoking several weeks before surgery and lung expansion techniques (eg, incentive spirometry) after surgery. Patients with asthma, particularly those receiving suboptimal medical management, have an increased risk for bronchospasm during airway manipulation. Appropriate use of analgesia and monitoring are key strategies for avoiding postoperative respiratory depression in patients with obstructive sleep apnea. Further discussion of this topic appears in Chapter 44.

C. Endocrine and Metabolic Issues

The appropriate target blood glucose concentration has been the subject of several celebrated clinical trials. "Tight" control of blood glucose, with a target concentration in the "normal" range, was shown to improve outcomes in ambulatory patients with type 1 diabetes mellitus. Other more recent trials conducted in subjects with critical illness have shown that blood glucose should not be so tightly controlled.

The usual practice is to obtain a blood glucose measurement in patients with diabetes on the morning of elective surgery. Unfortunately, many patients with diabetes who present for elective surgery do not maintain blood glucose within the desired range. Other patients, who may be unaware that they have type 2 diabetes, present with blood glucose measurements
5 above the normal range. The adequacy of long-term blood glucose control can be easily and rapidly assessed by measurement of hemoglobin A1c. In patients with abnormally elevated hemoglobin A1c, referral to a diabetology service for education about the disease and adjustment of diet and medications to improve metabolic control may be beneficial. Elective surgery should be delayed in patients presenting with marked hyperglycemia; in an otherwise well-managed patient with type 1 diabetes, this delay might consist only of rearranging the order of scheduled cases to allow insulin infusion to bring the blood glucose concentration closer to the normal range before surgery. A more complete discussion of diabetes mellitus and other perioperative endocrine concerns is provided in Chapter 35.

D. Coagulation Issues

Three important coagulation issues that must be addressed during the preoperative evaluation are (1) how to manage patients who are taking warfarin or new oral anticoagulants (eg, rivaroxaban, apixaban, dabigatran); (2) how to manage patients with coronary artery disease who are taking clopidogrel or related agents; and (3) whether one can safely provide neuraxial anesthesia to patients who either are currently receiving anticoagulants or who will receive anticoagulation perioperatively. In the first circumstance, most patients undergoing anything more involved than minor surgery will

require discontinuation of anticoagulation in advance of surgery to avoid excessive blood loss. The key issues to be addressed are how far in advance the drug should be discontinued and whether the patient will require "bridging" therapy with another, shorter-acting,
6 agent. In patients deemed at high risk for thrombosis (eg, those with certain mechanical heart valve implants or with atrial fibrillation and a prior thromboembolic stroke), chronic anticoagulants should be bridged with intramuscular low molecular weight heparins (eg, enoxaparin) or by intravenous unfractionated heparin. The prescribing physician and surgeon may need to be consulted regarding discontinuation of these agents and whether bridging will be required. In patients with a high risk of thrombosis who receive bridging therapy, the risk of death from excessive bleeding is an order of magnitude lower than the risk of death or disability from stroke if the bridging therapy is omitted. Patients at lower risk for thrombosis may have their anticoagulant drug discontinued preoperatively and then reinitiated after successful surgery. In general, the indications for bridging are becoming more restricted.

Clopidogrel and similar agents are often administered with aspirin (so-called dual antiplatelet therapy) to patients with coronary artery disease who have received intracoronary stenting. Immediately after stenting, such patients are at increased risk of acute myocardial infarction if these agents are abruptly dis-
7 continued. Therefore, current guidelines recommend postponing all but mandatory surgery until at least 1 month after any coronary intervention and suggest that treatment options *other* than a drug-eluting stent (which will require prolonged dual antiplatelet therapy) be used in patients expected to undergo a surgical procedure within 12 months after the intervention (eg, a patient with coronary disease who also has resectable colon cancer). As the drugs, treatment options, and consensus guidelines are updated frequently, when we are in doubt we consult with a cardiologist when patients receiving these agents require a surgical procedure.

The third issue—when it may be safe to perform regional (particularly neuraxial) anesthesia in patients who are or will be receiving anticoagulation therapy—has also been the subject of debate. The American Society of Regional Anesthesia and Pain Medicine publishes a regularly updated consensus guideline on this topic, and other prominent societies (eg, the European Society of Anaesthesiologists) also provide guidance on this topic (see Chapter 45).

E. Gastrointestinal Issues

Since Mendelson's 1946 report, aspiration of gastric contents has been recognized as a potentially disastrous pulmonary complication of surgical anesthesia. It has also been long recognized that the risk of aspiration is increased in certain groups of patients: pregnant women in the second and third trimesters, those whose stomachs have not emptied after a recent meal, and those with serious gastroesophageal reflux disease (GERD).

Although there is consensus that pregnant women and those who have recently (within 6 h) consumed a full meal should be treated as if they have "full" stomachs, there is less consensus as to the necessary period of time in which patients must fast before elective surgery. Proof of the lack of consensus is the fact that the ASA's guideline on this topic was voted down by the ASA House of Delegates several years in a row before it was presented in a form that received majority approval. The guideline as approved is more permissive of fluid intake than many anesthesiologists would prefer, and many medical centers have policies that are more restrictive
8 than the ASA guideline on this topic. The truth is that there are no good data to support restricting fluid intake (of any kind or any amount) more than 2 h before induction of general anesthesia in healthy patients undergoing elective (other than gastric) procedures; moreover, there is strong evidence that nondiabetic patients who drink fluids containing carbohydrates and protein up to 2 h before induction of anesthesia experience less perioperative nausea and dehydration than those who are fasted longer.

Patients claiming a history of GERD present vexing problems. Some of these patients will be at increased risk for aspiration; others may carry this "self-diagnosis" based on advertisements or internet searches, or may have been given this diagnosis by a physician who did not follow the standard diagnostic criteria. Our approach is to treat patients who have only occasional symptoms like any other patient without GERD and to treat patients with consistent symptoms (multiple times per week) with medications (eg, nonparticulate antacids such as sodium citrate) and techniques (eg, tracheal intubation rather than laryngeal mask airway) as if they were at increased risk for aspiration.

Elements of the Preoperative Physical Examination

The preoperative history and physical examination complement one another: The physical examination may detect abnormalities not apparent from the history, and the history helps focus the physical examination. Examination of healthy asymptomatic patients should include measurement of vital signs (blood pressure, heart rate, respiratory rate, and temperature) and examination of the airway, heart, and lungs using standard techniques of inspection, palpation, percussion, and auscultation. Before administering regional anesthetics or inserting invasive monitors, one should examine the relevant anatomy; infection or anatomic abnormalities near the site may contraindicate the planned procedure (see Chapters 5, 45, and 46). An abbreviated, focused neurological examination serves to document whether any neurological deficits may be present *before* a regional anesthesia procedure is performed.

The anesthesiologist must examine the patient's airway before every anesthetic is administered. Any loose or chipped teeth, caps, bridges, or dentures should be noted. Poor fit of the anesthesia mask should be expected in edentulous patients and those with significant facial abnormalities. Micrognathia (a short distance between the chin and the hyoid bone), prominent upper incisors, a large tongue, limited range of motion of the temporomandibular joint or cervical spine, or a short or thick neck suggest that difficulty may be encountered in direct laryngoscopy for tracheal intubation (see Chapter 19). The Mallampati score is often recorded.

Preoperative Laboratory Testing

Routine laboratory testing is not recommended for fit and asymptomatic patients. "Routine" testing rarely alters perioperative management; moreover, inconsequential abnormal values may trigger further unnecessary testing, delays, and costs. Nonetheless, despite no evidence of benefit, some physicians request blood tests, an electrocardiogram, and a chest radiograph for all patients, perhaps in the misplaced hope of reducing their exposure to litigation.

Ideally, testing should be guided by the history
9 and physical examination. To be valuable, preoperative testing must discriminate: There must be an avoidable increased perioperative risk when the results are abnormal (and the risk will remain unknown if the test is not performed), and when testing fails to detect the abnormality (or it has been corrected), there must be reduced risk. Useful tests have a low rate of false-positive and false-negative
10 results (Table 18–3). **The utility of a test depends on its sensitivity and specificity. Sensitive tests have a low rate of false-negative results and rarely fail to identify an abnormality when one is present, whereas specific tests have a low rate of false-positive results and rarely identify an abnormality when one is not present.**

The prevalence of a disease or of an abnormal test result varies with the population tested. Testing

TABLE 18–3 Calculation of sensitivity and specificity based on presence or absence of disease in the population being tested.

True positives (TP) have both a positive test and the disease for which they are being tested

False positives (FP) have a positive test but do not have the disease

True negatives (TN) have a negative test and do not have the disease for which they are being tested

False negatives (FN) have a negative test but do have the disease

$$\text{Sensitivity} = TP/(TP + FN)$$

$$\text{Specificity} = TN/(TN + FP)$$

The predictive value of a positive test (PV+) indicates the likelihood that the patient has the disease if they test positive.

$$(PV+) = TP/(TP + FP)$$

The predictive value of a negative test (PV–) indicates the likelihood that the patient is free of the disease if they test negative

$$(PV-) = TN/(TN + FN)$$

is therefore most effective when sensitive and specific tests are used in patients in whom the abnormality will be detected frequently enough to justify the expense and inconvenience of the test procedure. Accordingly, laboratory testing should be based on the history and physical examination and the nature of the proposed surgery or procedure. Thus, a baseline hemoglobin or hematocrit measurement is desirable in any patient about to undergo a procedure in which extensive blood loss and transfusion are likely, particularly when there is sufficient time to correct anemia preoperatively (eg, with iron supplements).

Testing fertile women for pregnancy is controversial (but done routinely in many centers) and should not be done without the permission of the patient; pregnancy testing involves detection of chorionic gonadotropin in urine or serum. Routine testing for HIV and routine coagulation studies are not indicated. Urinalysis is not cost-effective in asymptomatic healthy patients; nevertheless, a preoperative urinalysis is required by state law in at least one U.S. jurisdiction.

PREMEDICATION

A classic study showed that a preoperative visit from an anesthesiologist resulted in greater reduction in patient anxiety than preoperative sedative drugs. Yet, there was a time when virtually every patient received premedication before arriving in the preoperative area in anticipation of surgery. The belief was that all patients benefitted from preoperative sedation and anticholinergics, often combined with an opioid. With the transition to outpatient surgery and "same-day" hospital admission, preoperative sedative-hypnotics or opioids are now almost never administered before patients arrive in the preoperative holding area for elective surgery. Children, especially those aged 2 to 10 years who (along with their parents) likely will experience separation anxiety may benefit from premedication administered in the preoperative holding area. This topic is discussed in Chapter 42. Oral or intravenous midazolam or nasal dexmedetomidine are common methods. Adults often receive intravenous midazolam (1–5 mg) once an intravenous line has been established. If a painful procedure (eg, regional block or a central venous line) will be performed while the patient remains awake, small doses of opioid (typically fentanyl) will often be given. Patients who will undergo airway surgery or extensive airway manipulations benefit from preoperative administration of an anticholinergic agent (glycopyrrolate or atropine) to reduce airway secretions before and during surgery. Patients who are expected to have significant amounts of postoperative pain will often be given "multimodal" analgesia, including various combinations of nonsteroidal anti-inflammatory drugs, acetaminophen, gabapentinoids, and anti-nausea drugs in the preoperative
11 holding area. The fundamental message here is that premedication should be given purposefully, not as a mindless routine.

DOCUMENTATION

Physicians should provide high-quality, safe, and cost-efficient medical care and document what they have done. Adequate documentation provides guidance to those who will encounter the patient in the future. It permits others to assess the quality of the care that was given. Without proper documentation, a physician will not be paid for his or her services; incomplete documentation may not justify the otherwise appropriate "full" payment. Incomplete documentation may render it difficult for a hospital system to recover its costs and may incorrectly lead to the conclusion that a patient's hospitalization was unnecessary or inappropriately prolonged. Finally, inadequate and disorganized documentation provide limited support for a potential defense case should a claim for medical malpractice be filed.

Preoperative Assessment Note

The preoperative assessment note should appear in the patient's permanent medical record and should describe pertinent findings, including the medical and surgical history, anesthetic history, current medications and allergies (and whether medications were taken on the day of surgery), physical examination, ASA physical status, pertinent laboratory and imaging results, electrocardiograms, and recommendations of any consultants. A comment is particularly important when a consultant's recommendation will not be followed.

The preoperative note should identify the anesthetic plan, indicating whether regional or general anesthesia (or sedation) will be used, and whether invasive monitoring or other advanced techniques will be employed. It should include a statement regarding the informed consent discussion with the patient (or guardian). Documentation of the informed consent discussion may take the form of a narrative indicating that the plan, alternative plans, and their advantages and disadvantages (including their relative risks) were presented, understood, and accepted by the patient. Some centers include consent for anesthesia within the consent for surgery (or the procedure). Alternatively, the patient may be asked to read and sign a separate anesthesia consent form that contains the same information.

In the United States, the Joint Commission (TJC) requires an immediate preanesthetic "reevaluation" to determine whether the patient's status has changed in the time since the preoperative evaluation was performed. This reevaluation might include a review of the medical record to search for any new laboratory results or consultation reports if the patient was last seen on another date. However, even when the elapsed time is less than a minute, the bureaucracy will not be denied: the "box" must be checked to document that there has been no interval change.

Intraoperative Anesthesia Record

The intraoperative anesthesia record serves many purposes. It functions as documentation of intraoperative monitoring, a reference for future anesthetics for that patient, and a source of data for quality assurance and billing. This record should be terse, pertinent, and accurate. Increasingly, parts of the anesthesia record are generated automatically and recorded electronically. Such anesthesia information management systems (commonly abbreviated AIMS) have many theoretical and practical advantages over the traditional paper record but also introduce all the common pitfalls of computerization, including the potential for unrecognized recording of artefactual data, the possibility that practitioners will find attending to the computer more interesting than attending to the patient, the inevitable occurrence of device and software shutdowns, and increased cost. Regardless of whether the record is on paper or electronic, it should document the anesthetic care in the operating room by including the following elements:

- That there has been a preoperative check of the anesthesia machine and other relevant equipment
- That there has been a reevaluation of the patient immediately prior to induction of anesthesia (a TJC requirement)
- Time of administration, dosage, and route of drugs given intraoperatively
- Intraoperative estimates of blood loss and urinary output
- Results of laboratory tests obtained during the operation (when there is an AIMS linked to an electronic medical record, such testing may be recorded elsewhere)
- Intravenous fluids and any blood products administered
- Pertinent procedure notes (eg, for tracheal intubation or insertion of invasive monitors)
- Any specialized intraoperative techniques such as hypotensive anesthesia, one-lung ventilation, high-frequency jet ventilation, or cardiopulmonary bypass
- Timing and conduct of intraoperative events such as induction, positioning, surgical incision, and extubation
- Unusual events or complications (eg, arrhythmias, cardiac arrest)
- Condition of the patient at the time of "handoff" to the postanesthesia or intensive care unit nurse

By tradition and convention (and, in the United States, according to practice guidelines) arterial blood pressure and heart rate are recorded graphically at no less than 5 min intervals. Data from other monitors are also usually entered graphically, whereas descriptions of techniques or complications are described in text.

Unfortunately, the conventional, handwritten anesthetic record is ill suited for documenting critical incidents, such as a cardiac arrest. In such cases, a separate text note inserted in the patient's medical record may be necessary. Careful recording of the timing of events is needed to avoid discrepancies between multiple simultaneous records (anesthesia record, nurses' notes, cardiopulmonary resuscitation record, and other physicians' entries in the medical record). Such discrepancies are frequently targeted by malpractice attorneys as evidence of
12 incompetence, inaccuracy, or deceit. Incomplete, inaccurate, or illegible records unnecessarily complicate defending a physician against otherwise unjustified allegations of malpractice.

Postoperative Notes

After accompanying the patient to the postanesthesia care unit (PACU), the anesthesia provider should remain with the patient until normal vital signs have been measured and the patient's condition is deemed stable. An unstable patient may require being "handed off" to another physician. Before discharge from the PACU, a note should be written by an anesthesiologist to document the patient's recovery from anesthesia, any apparent anesthesia-related complications, the immediate postoperative condition of the patient, and the patient's disposition (discharge to an outpatient area, an inpatient ward, an intensive care unit, or home). In the United States, as of 2009, the Centers for Medicare and Medicaid Services require that certain elements be included in all postoperative notes (Table 18–4). Recovery from anesthesia should be assessed at least once within 48 h after discharge from the PACU in all inpatients. Postoperative notes should document the general condition of the patient, the presence or absence of any anesthesia-related complications, and any measures undertaken to treat such complications. The anesthesiologist's involvement with the patient may continue through the early stages of postoperative recovery when the anesthesiologist is involved in a functioning perioperative surgical home or is providing treatment of postoperative pain (see Chapters 48, 59).

TABLE 18–4 Elements required by the Center for Medicare and Medicaid Services in all postoperative notes.

Respiratory function, including respiratory rate, airway patency, and oxygen saturation
Cardiovascular function, including pulse rate and blood pressure
Mental status
Temperature
Pain
Nausea and vomiting
Postoperative hydration

Data from the Centers for Medicare and Medicaid Services (CMS). *Revised Anesthesia Services Interpretive Guidelines*. issued December 30, 2009.

CASE DISCUSSION

Medical Malpractice (also see Chapter 54)

A healthy 45-year-old man has a cardiac arrest during an elective laparoscopic cholecystectomy. Although cardiopulmonary resuscitation is successful, the patient is left with permanent neuropsychological deficits that preclude his return to work. One year later, the patient files a complaint against the anesthesiologist, surgeon, and hospital.

What four elements must be proved by the plaintiff (patient) to establish negligence on the part of the defendant (physician or hospital)?

1. *Duty:* Once a physician establishes a professional relationship with a patient, the physician owes that patient certain obligations, such as adhering to the "standard of care."
2. *Breach of Duty:* If these obligations are not fulfilled, the physician has breached his or her duty to the patient.
3. *Injury:* An injury must result. The injury may result in general damages (eg, pain and suffering) or special damages (eg, loss of income).
4. *Causation:* The plaintiff must demonstrate that the breach of duty was the *proximate cause* of the injury. Had it not been for the breach of duty, the injury would not have occurred.

How is the standard of care defined and established?

Individual physicians are expected to perform as any prudent and reasonable physician would in similar circumstances. This does not mandate "best" care or optimal care, only care that would meet the minimum standard of a prudent and reasonable physician. As a specialist, the anesthesiologist is held to a higher standard of knowledge and skill with respect to the subject matter of anesthesia than would a general practitioner or a physician in another specialty. Expert witnesses usually provide testimony to define the standard of care in legal proceedings. Medical malpractice cases are governed by the laws of the state or jurisdiction in which the event took place, and these may differ from state to state. For example, some states require that an expert witness have practiced medicine recently in the state or an immediately adjacent state; others have no "residence" requirement for expert witnesses. The specific circumstances pertaining to each individual case are taken into account. The law recognizes that there are differences of opinion and varying schools of thought within the medical profession.

How is causation determined?

It is usually the plaintiff who bears the burden of proving that the injury would not have occurred "but for" the negligence of the physician, or that the physician's action was a "substantial factor" in causing the injury. An exception is the doctrine of *res ipsa loquitur* ("the thing speaks for itself"), which permits a finding of negligence based solely on the evidence. For example, if a set of keys were visualized inside a patient on a chest radiograph after a thoracotomy, the doctrine of *res ipsa loquitur* would apply. *Res ipsa loquitur* could not be used in the case under discussion because the plaintiff would have to establish that cardiac arrest could not occur in the absence of negligence and that cardiac arrest could not have been due to something outside the control of the anesthesiologist. An important concept is that causation in civil cases in the United States need only be established by a preponderance of the evidence ("more likely than not")—as opposed to criminal cases, in which all elements of a charged offense must be proved "beyond a reasonable doubt."

What factors influence the likelihood of a malpractice suit?

1. *The Physician–Patient Relationship:* This is particularly important for the anesthesiologist, who usually does not meet the patient until immediately before the anesthetic is administered. Another problem is that the patient is unconscious while under the anesthesiologist's care. Thus, the preoperative and postoperative visits with the patient are often the only opportunities to establish a good relationship with the patient. Family members should also be included during these meetings with patients (provided the patient does not object), particularly during the postoperative visit if there has been an intraoperative complication.
2. *Adequacy of Informed Consent:* Rendering care to a competent patient who does not consent constitutes assault and battery. Consent is not enough, however. The patient should be informed of the contemplated procedure, including its reasonably anticipated risks, its possible benefits, and the therapeutic alternatives. The physician may be liable for a complication—even if it is not due to the negligent performance of a procedure—if a jury is convinced that a reasonable person would have refused treatment if properly informed of the possibility of the complication. This does not mean, of course, that a documented consent relieves from liability physicians who violate the standard of care.
3. *Quality of Documentation:* Careful documentation of the perioperative visits, informed consent, consultations with other specialists, intraoperative events, and postoperative care is essential. The viewpoint of many courts and juries, reinforced by plaintiff's attorneys, is that "if it isn't written down, it wasn't done." It goes without saying that medical records should never be intentionally destroyed or altered.

GUIDELINES

http://www.asahq.org/

https://www.asra.com/

Fleisher LA, Fleischmann KE, Auerbach AD, et al. American College of Cardiology; American Heart Association. ACC/AHA guideline on perioperative cardiovascular evaluation and management of patients undergoing noncardiac surgery: a report of the American College of Cardiology/American Heart Association Task Force on practice guidelines. *J Am Coll Cardiol.* 2014;64:e77.

Guarracino F, Baldassarri R, Priebe HJ. Revised ESC/ESA Guidelines on non-cardiac surgery: cardiovascular assessment and management. Implications for preoperative clinical evaluation. *Minerva Anestesiol.* 2015;81:226.

Horlocker TT, Vandermeulen E, Kopp SL, Gogarten W, Leffert LR, Benzon HT. Regional anesthesia in the patient receiving antithrombotic or thrombolytic therapy: American Society of Regional Anesthesia and Pain Medicine Evidence-Based Guidelines (Fourth Edition). *Reg Anesth Pain Med.* 2018;43:263.

Lambert E, Carey S. Practice guideline recommendations on perioperative fasting: a systematic review. *JPEN J Parenter Enteral Nutr.* 2015;pii:0148607114567713.

Practice guidelines for preoperative fasting and the use of pharmacologic agents to reduce the risk of pulmonary aspiration: application to healthy patients undergoing elective procedures: an updated report by the American Society of Anesthesiologists task force on preoperative fasting and the use of pharmacologic agents to reduce the risk of pulmonary aspiration. *Anesthesiology.* 2017;126:376.

SUGGESTED READINGS

Ayoub K, Nairooz R, Almomani A, et al. Perioperative heparin bridging in atrial fibrillation patients requiring temporary interruption of anticoagulation: evidence from meta-analysis. *J Stroke Cerebrovasc Dis.* 2016;pii:S1052.

Bierle DM, Raslau D, Regan DW, Sundsted KK, Mauck KF. Preoperative evaluation before noncardiac surgery. *Mayo Clin Proc.* 2020;95:807.

Centers for Medicare & Medicaid Services (CMS). CMS Manual System. Pub 100-07 State Operations Provider Certification. DHHS. Available at: http://www.kdheks.gov/bhfr/download/Appendix_L.pdf (accessed December 16, 2017).

Doherty JU, Gluckman TJ, Hucker WJ, et al. 2017 ACC Expert consensus decision pathway for periprocedural management of anticoagulation in patients with nonvalvular atrial fibrillation: a report of the American College of Cardiology Clinical Expert Consensus Document Task Force. *J Am Coll Cardiol.* 2017;69:871.

Douketis JD, Spyropoulos AC, Kaatz S, et al; BRIDGE Investigators. Perioperative bridging anticoagulation in patients with atrial fibrillation. *N Engl J Med.* 2015;373:823.

Egbert LD, Battit G, Turndorf H, Beecher HK. The value of the preoperative visit by an anesthetist. A study of doctor-patient rapport. *JAMA.* 1963;185:553.

Friedrich S, Meybohm P, Kranke P. Nulla Per Os (NPO) guidelines: time to revisit? *Curr Opin Anaesthesiol.* 2020;33:740.

Jeong BH, Shin B, Eom JS, et al. Development of a prediction rule for estimating postoperative pulmonary complications. *PLoS One.* 2014;9:e113656.

Mendelson CL. The aspiration of stomach contents into the lungs during obstetric anesthesia. *Am J Obstet Gynecol.* 1946;52:191.

Williams DGA, Molinger J, Wischmeyer PE. The malnourished surgery patient: a silent epidemic in perioperative outcomes? *Curr Opin Anaesthesiol.* 2019;32:405.

CHAPTER

19

Airway Management

KEY CONCEPTS

1. Improper face mask technique can result in continued deflation of the anesthesia reservoir bag despite the adjustable pressure-limiting valve being closed, usually indicating a substantial leak around the mask. In contrast, the generation of high breathing circuit pressures with minimal chest movement and breath sounds implies an obstructed airway or obstructed tubing.
2. The laryngeal mask airway partially protects the larynx from pharyngeal secretions but not gastric regurgitation.
3. After insertion of an endotracheal tube (ETT), the cuff is inflated with the least amount of air necessary to create a seal during positive-pressure ventilation to minimize the pressure transmitted to the tracheal mucosa.
4. Although the persistent detection of carbon dioxide (CO_2) by a capnograph is the best confirmation of tracheal placement of an ETT, it cannot exclude bronchial intubation. The earliest evidence of bronchial intubation often is an increase in peak inspiratory pressure.
5. After intubation, the cuff of an ETT should not be felt above the level of the cricoid cartilage because a prolonged intralaryngeal location may result in postoperative hoarseness and increases the risk of accidental extubation.
6. Unrecognized esophageal intubation can produce catastrophic results. Prevention of this complication depends on direct visualization of the tip of the ETT passing through the vocal cords, careful auscultation for the presence of bilateral breath sounds and the absence of gastric gurgling while ventilating through the ETT, analysis of exhaled gas for the presence of CO_2 (the most reliable automated method), chest radiography, airway ultrasonography, or use of fiberoptic bronchoscopy.
7. Clues to the diagnosis of bronchial intubation include unilateral breath sounds, unexpected hypoxia with pulse oximetry (unreliable with high inspired oxygen concentrations), inability to palpate the ETT cuff in the sternal notch during cuff inflation, and decreased breathing bag compliance (high peak inspiratory pressures).
8. The large negative intrathoracic pressures generated by a struggling patient in laryngospasm can result in the development of negative-pressure pulmonary edema, particularly in healthy patients.

Expert airway management is an essential skill in anesthetic practice. This chapter reviews the anatomy of the upper respiratory tract, describes necessary airway equipment, presents various management techniques, and discusses complications of laryngoscopy, intubation, and extubation. Patient safety requires a thorough understanding of each of these topics.

ANATOMY

The upper airway consists of the nose, mouth, pharynx, larynx, trachea, and mainstem bronchi. The mouth and pharynx are also a part of the upper gastrointestinal tract. The laryngeal structures in part serve to prevent aspiration into the trachea.

There are two openings to the human airway: the nose, which leads to the nasopharynx, and the mouth, which leads to the oropharynx. These passages are separated anteriorly by the palate, but they join posteriorly in the pharynx (Figure 19–1). The pharynx is a U-shaped fibromuscular structure that extends from the base of the skull to the cricoid cartilage at the entrance to the esophagus. It opens anteriorly into the nasal cavity, the mouth, the larynx, and the nasopharynx, oropharynx, and laryngopharynx, respectively. At the base of the tongue, the epiglottis functionally separates the oropharynx from the laryngopharynx (or hypopharynx).

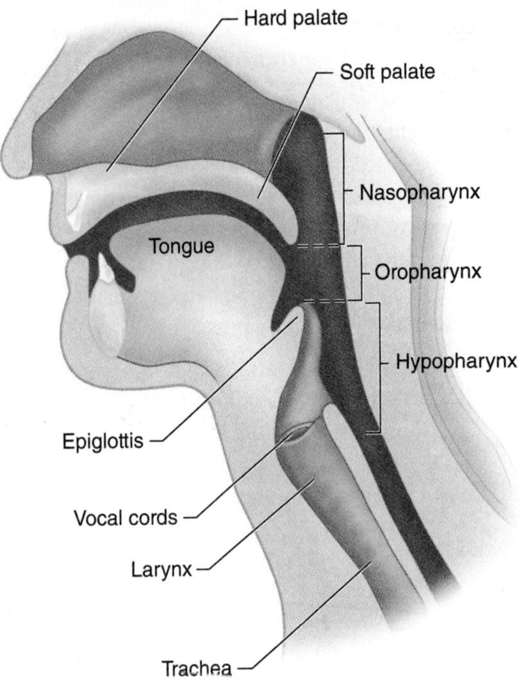

FIGURE 19–1 Anatomy of the airway.

The epiglottis prevents aspiration by covering the glottis—the opening of the larynx—during swallowing. The larynx is a cartilaginous skeleton held together by ligaments and muscle. The larynx is composed of nine cartilages (Figure 19–2): thyroid, cricoid, epiglottic, and (in pairs) arytenoid, corniculate, and cuneiform. The thyroid cartilage shields the conus elasticus, which forms the vocal cords.

The sensory supply to the upper airway is derived from the cranial nerves (Figure 19–3). The mucous membranes of the nose are innervated by the ophthalmic division (V_1) of the trigeminal nerve anteriorly (anterior ethmoidal nerve) and by the maxillary division (V_2) posteriorly (sphenopalatine nerves). The palatine nerves provide sensory fibers from the trigeminal nerve (V_2) to the superior and inferior surfaces of the hard and soft palate. The **olfactory nerve** (cranial nerve I) innervates the nasal mucosa to provide the sense of smell. The lingual nerve (a branch of the mandibular division [V_3] of the trigeminal nerve) and the **glossopharyngeal nerve** (cranial nerve IX) provide general sensation to the anterior two-thirds and posterior one-third of the tongue, respectively. Branches of the **facial nerve** (VII) and glossopharyngeal nerve provide the sensation of taste to those areas, respectively. The **glossopharyngeal nerve** also innervates the roof of the pharynx, the tonsils, and the undersurface of the soft palate. The **vagus nerve** (cranial nerve X) provides sensation to the airway below the epiglottis. The superior laryngeal branch of the vagus divides into an external (motor) nerve and an internal (sensory) laryngeal nerve that provide sensory supply to the larynx between the epiglottis and the vocal cords. Another branch of the vagus, the **recurrent laryngeal nerve**, innervates the larynx below the vocal cords and the trachea.

The muscles of the larynx are innervated by the recurrent laryngeal nerve, with the exception of the cricothyroid muscle, which is innervated by the external (motor) laryngeal nerve, a branch of the superior laryngeal nerve. The posterior cricoarytenoid muscles abduct the vocal cords, whereas the lateral cricoarytenoid muscles are the principal adductors.

Phonation involves complex simultaneous actions by several laryngeal muscles. Damage to the motor nerves innervating the larynx leads to a

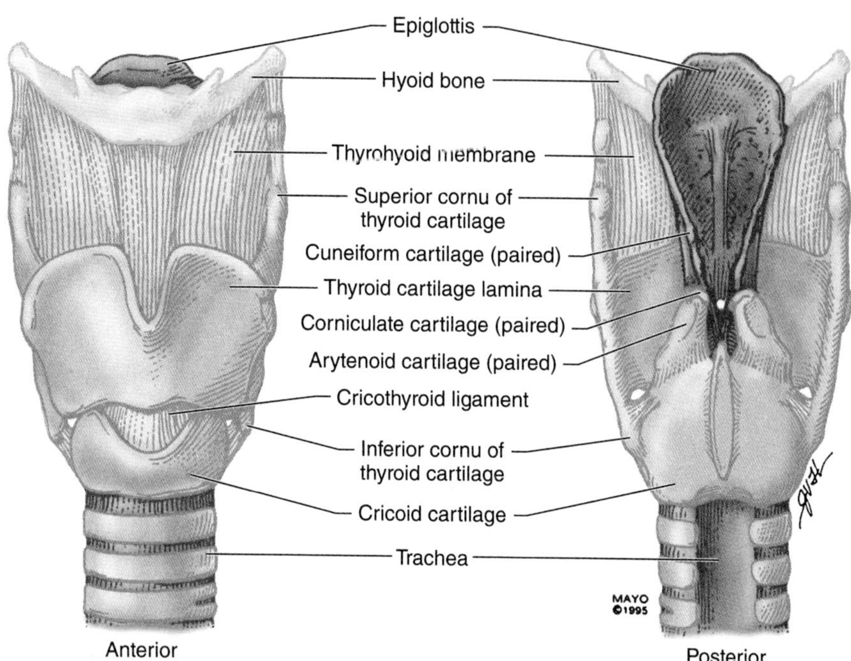

FIGURE 19–2 Cartilaginous structures comprising the larynx. (Used with permission of Mayo Foundation for Medical Education and Research, all rights reserved.)

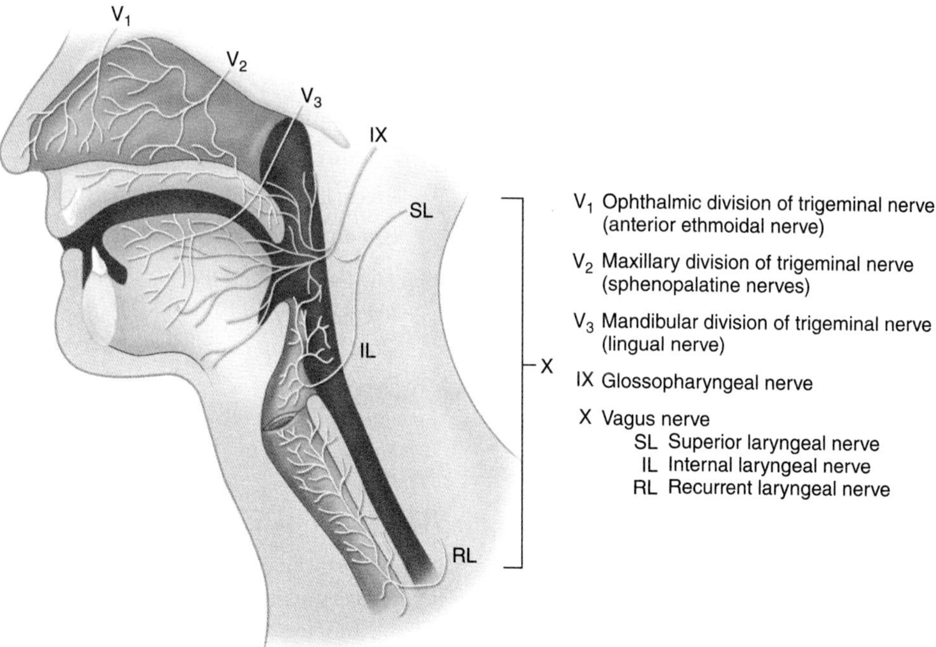

FIGURE 19–3 Sensory nerve supply of the airway.

TABLE 19–1 The effects of laryngeal nerve injury on the voice.

Nerve	Effect of Nerve Injury
Superior laryngeal nerve	
Unilateral	Minimal effects
Bilateral	Hoarseness, tiring of voice
Recurrent laryngeal nerve	
Unilateral	Hoarseness
Bilateral	
Acute	Stridor, respiratory distress
Chronic	Aphonia
Vagus nerve	
Unilateral	Hoarseness
Bilateral	Aphonia

spectrum of speech disorders (Table 19–1). Unilateral denervation of a cricothyroid muscle causes very subtle clinical findings. Bilateral palsy of the superior laryngeal nerve may result in hoarseness or easy tiring of the voice, but airway control is not jeopardized.

Unilateral injury to a recurrent laryngeal nerve results in paralysis of the ipsilateral vocal cord, degrading voice quality. Assuming that the superior laryngeal nerves are intact, *acute* bilateral recurrent laryngeal nerve palsy can result in stridor and respiratory distress because of the remaining unopposed tension of the cricothyroid muscles. Airway problems are less frequent in *chronic* bilateral recurrent laryngeal nerve loss because of the development of various compensatory mechanisms (eg, atrophy of the laryngeal musculature).

Bilateral injury to the vagus nerve affects both the superior and the recurrent laryngeal nerves. Thus, bilateral vagal denervation produces flaccid, midpositioned vocal cords similar to those seen after administration of succinylcholine. Although phonation is severely impaired in these patients, airway control is rarely a problem.

The blood supply of the larynx is derived from branches of the thyroid arteries. The cricothyroid artery arises from the superior thyroid artery itself, the first branch given off from the external carotid artery, and crosses the upper cricothyroid membrane, which extends from the cricoid cartilage to the thyroid cartilage. The superior thyroid artery is found along the lateral edge of the cricothyroid membrane.

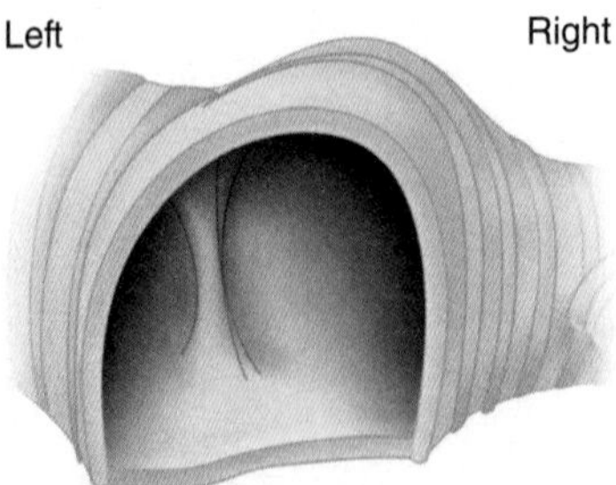

FIGURE 19–4 Carina.

The trachea begins beneath the cricoid cartilage and extends to the carina, the point at which the right and left mainstem bronchi divide (Figure 19–4). Anteriorly, the trachea consists of cartilaginous rings; posteriorly, the trachea is membranous.

ROUTINE AIRWAY MANAGEMENT

Routine airway management associated with general anesthesia consists of:

- Preanesthetic airway assessment
- Preparation and equipment check
- Patient positioning
- Preoxygenation (denitrogenation)
- Bag and mask ventilation
- Tracheal intubation or placement of a laryngeal mask airway (if indicated)
- Confirmation of proper tube or airway placement
- Extubation

AIRWAY ASSESSMENT

A preanesthetic airway assessment is mandatory before every anesthetic procedure. Several anatomical and functional maneuvers can be performed to estimate the difficulty of tracheal intubation; successful ventilation (with or without intubation) must

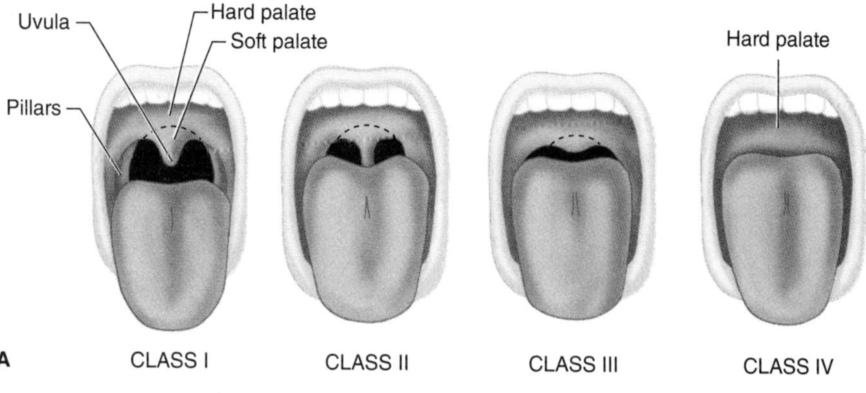

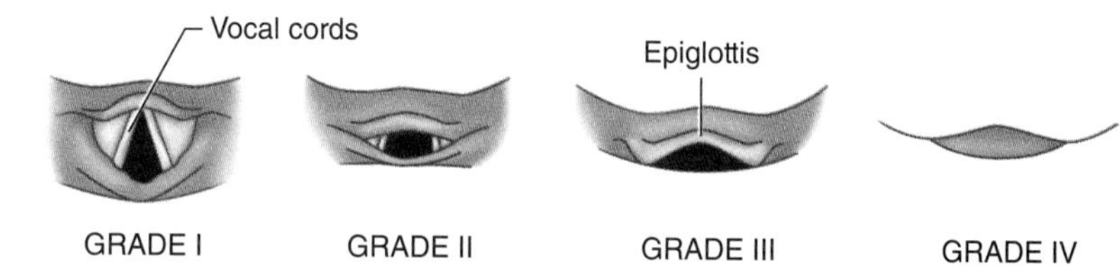

FIGURE 19–5 **A**: Mallampati classification of oral opening. **B**: Grading of the laryngeal view. A difficult orotracheal intubation (grade III or IV) may be predicted by the inability to visualize certain pharyngeal structures (class III or IV) during the preoperative examination of a seated patient. (Reproduced with permission from Mallampati SR, Gatt SP, Gugino LD, et al. A clinical sign to predict difficult tracheal intubation: A prospective study. *Can Anaesth Soc J*. 1985 Jul;32(4):429-434.)

be achieved by the anesthetist if mortality and morbidity are to be avoided. Assessments include:

- Mouth opening: an incisor distance of 3 cm or greater is desirable in an adult.
- Mallampati classification: a frequently performed test that examines the size of the tongue in relation to the oral cavity. The more the tongue obstructs the view of the pharyngeal structures, the more difficult intubation may be (Figure 19–5).
    - Class I: The entire palatal arch, including the bilateral faucial pillars, is visible down to the bases of the pillars.
    - Class II: The upper part of the faucial pillars and most of the uvula are visible.
    - Class III: Only the soft and hard palates are visible.
    - Class IV: Only the hard palate is visible.
- Thyromental distance: This is the distance between the mentum (chin) and the superior thyroid notch. A distance greater than three fingerbreadths is desirable.
- Neck circumference: A neck circumference of greater than 17 inches is associated with difficulties in visualization of the glottic opening.
- Upper lip bite test: The upper lip bite test is performed by having patients bite their upper lip with their lower incisors. The inability to bite the upper lip predicts a difficult intubation, while the ability to bite beyond the lower border of the upper lip suggests a potentially easier intubation.

Although the presence of these examination findings may not be particularly sensitive for detecting a difficult intubation, the absence of these findings is predictive for relative ease of intubation. Nevertheless, any patient's airway may be found to be surprisingly

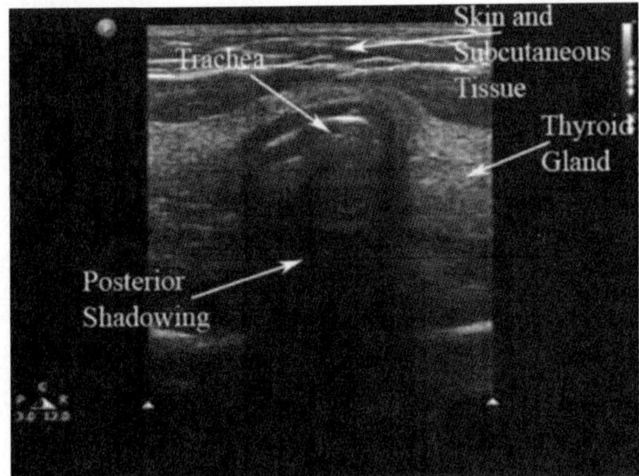

FIGURE 19–6 A transverse view of the trachea with landmarks. The anechoic area posterior to the trachea represents shadowing resulting from an attenuation of the ultrasound beam through the dense cartilage of the rings. (Reproduced with permission from Carmody KA, Moore CL, Feller-Kopman D. *Handbook of Critical Care and Emergency Ultrasound.* New York, NY: McGraw Hill; 2011.)

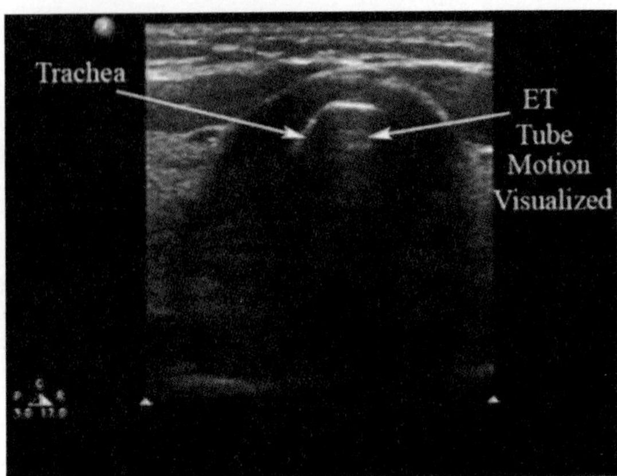

FIGURE 19–7 The trachea during intubation as the tube passes underneath the probe. The *arrow* points to a subtle area of increased echogenicity just distal to the tracheal cartilage. This area is where movement is most often visualized in real time during intubation. (Reproduced with permission from Carmody KA, Moore CL, Feller-Kopman D. *Handbook of Critical Care and Emergency Ultrasound.* New York, NY: McGraw Hill; 2011.)

difficult in spite of assuring bedside airway screening tests, and the anesthetist must always be prepared to address an unexpectedly difficult airway.

Increasingly, patients present with morbid obesity and body mass indices of 30 kg/m^2 or greater. Although some morbidly obese patients have relatively normal head and neck anatomy, others have much redundant pharyngeal tissue and increased neck circumference. Not only may these patients prove to be difficult to intubate, but routine ventilation with bag and mask also may be problematic.

Ultrasound examination of the airway can assist in airway assessment and management (Figures 19–6 through 19–8). Ultrasound can be used as an adjunct to confirm ETT placement as well as to assist in the identification of the cricothyroid membrane during an emergency cricothyroidotomy.

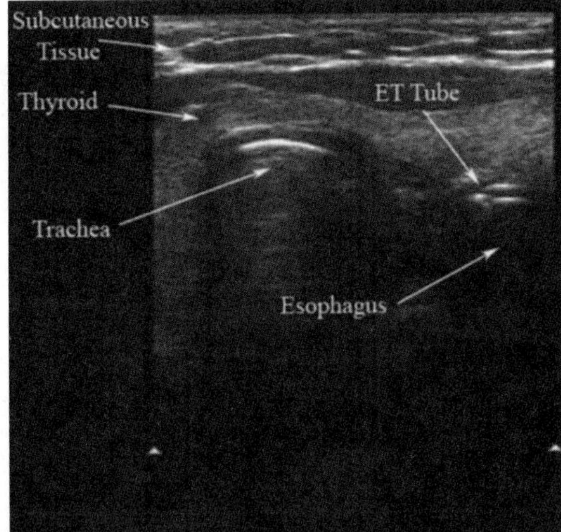

FIGURE 19–8 A transverse view of the trachea and esophagus during esophageal intubation. In this image, the esophagus is visualized posterior and lateral to the trachea. Two parallel echogenic lines are seen in the proximal esophagus, representing the inner and outer walls of the endotracheal (ET) tube as it passes through the lumen of the esophagus. (Reproduced with permission from Carmody KA, Moore CL, Feller-Kopman D. *Handbook of Critical Care and Emergency Ultrasound.* New York, NY: McGraw Hill; 2011.)

EQUIPMENT

The following equipment should be routinely available for airway management:

- An oxygen source
- Equipment for bag and mask ventilation
- Laryngoscopes (direct and video)

- Several ETTs of different sizes with available stylets and bougies
- Other (not ETT) airway devices (eg, oral, nasal, supraglottic airways)
- Suction
- Pulse oximetry and CO_2 detection (preferably waveform capnometry)
- Stethoscope
- Tape
- Blood pressure and electrocardiography (ECG) monitors
- Intravenous access

A flexible fiberoptic bronchoscope should be immediately available when difficult intubation is anticipated but need not be present during all routine intubations.

Oral & Nasal Airways

Loss of upper airway muscle tone (eg, weakness of the genioglossus muscle) in anesthetized patients allows the tongue and epiglottis to fall back against the posterior wall of the pharynx. Repositioning the head, lifting the jaw, or performing the jaw-thrust maneuver are the preferred techniques for opening the airway. To maintain the opening, the anesthesia provider can insert an artificial airway through the mouth or nose to maintain an air passage between the tongue and the posterior pharyngeal wall (Figure 19–9). Awake or lightly anesthetized patients with intact laryngeal reflexes may cough or even develop laryngospasm during airway insertion. Placement of an oral airway is sometimes facilitated by suppressing airway reflexes and depressing the tongue with a tongue blade. Adult oral airways typically come in small (80 mm [Guedel No. 3]), medium (90 mm [Guedel No. 4]), and large (100 mm [Guedel No. 5]) sizes.

The length of a nasal airway can be estimated as the distance from the nares to the meatus of the ear and should be approximately 2 to 4 cm longer than oral airways. Because of the risk of epistaxis, nasal airways should be inserted with caution, if at all, in anticoagulated or thrombocytopenic patients. The risk of epistaxis can be lessened by advance preparation of the nasal mucosa with a vasoconstrictive nasal spray containing phenylephrine or oxymetazoline hydrochloride. Also, nasal airways (and nasogastric tubes) should be used with caution in patients with basilar skull fractures because there has been a case report of a nasogastric tube entering the cranial vault. All tubes inserted through the nose (eg, nasal airways, nasogastric catheters, nasotracheal tubes) should be lubricated before being advanced along the floor of the nasal passage.

Face Mask Design & Technique

The use of a face mask can facilitate the delivery of oxygen or an anesthetic gas from a breathing system to a patient by creating an airtight seal with the

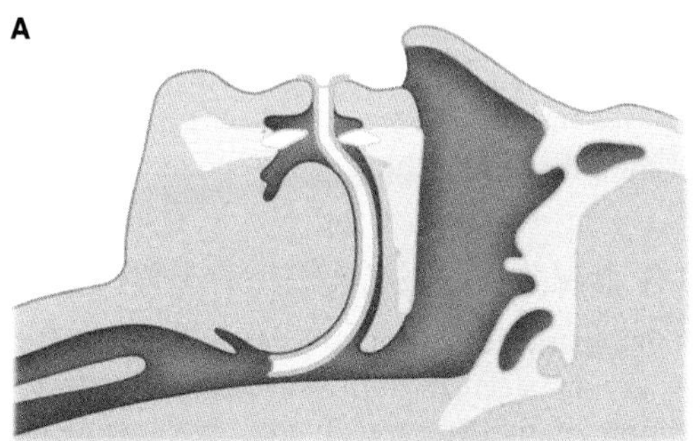

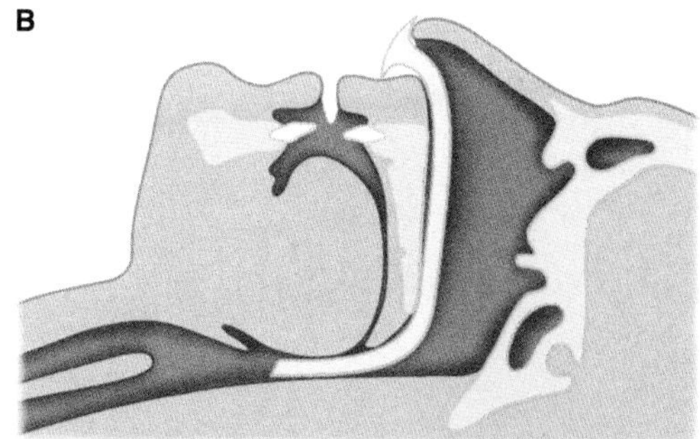

FIGURE 19–9 **A**: The oropharyngeal airway in place. The airway follows the curvature of the tongue, pulling it and the epiglottis away from the posterior pharyngeal wall and providing a channel for air passage. **B**: The nasopharyngeal airway in place. The airway passes through the nose and extends to just above the epiglottis. (Modified with permission from Dorsch JA, Dorsch SE. Face masks and airways. In: *Understanding Anesthesia Equipment*. 4th ed. Philadelphia, PA: Lippincott Williams & Wilkins; 1999.)

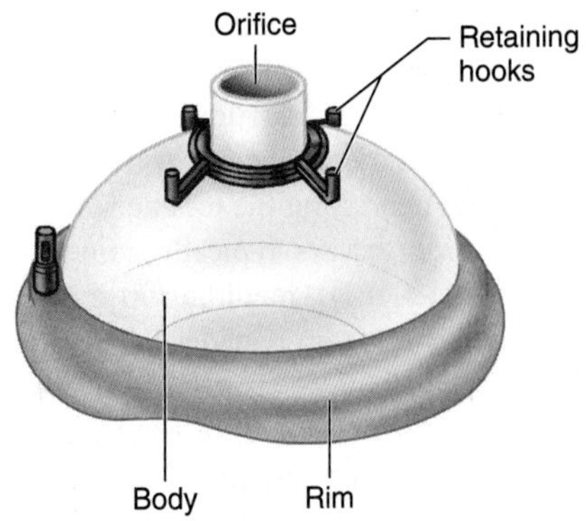

FIGURE 19–10 Clear adult face mask.

patient's face (Figure 19–10). The rim of the mask is contoured and conforms to a variety of facial features. The mask's 22-mm orifice attaches to the breathing circuit of the anesthesia machine through a right-angle connector. Several mask designs are available. Transparent masks allow observation of exhaled humidified gas and immediate recognition of vomitus. Retaining hooks surrounding the orifice can be attached to a head strap so that the mask does not have to be continually held in place. Some pediatric masks are specially designed to minimize apparatus dead space (Figure 19–11).

POSITIONING

When manipulating the airway, correct patient positioning is very helpful. Relative alignment of the oral and pharyngeal axes is achieved by having the patient in the "sniffing" position. When cervical spine pathology is suspected, the head must be kept in a neutral position with in-line stabilization of the neck during

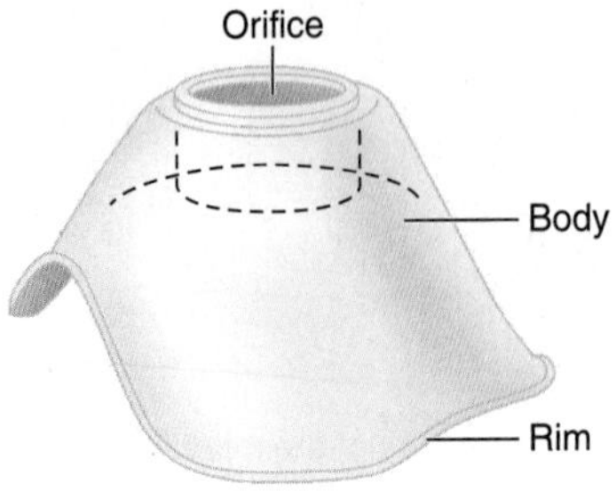

FIGURE 19–11 The Rendell–Baker–Soucek pediatric face mask has a shallow body and minimal dead space.

airway management unless relevant radiographs have been reviewed and cleared by an appropriate specialist. Patients with morbid obesity should be positioned on a 30° upward ramp (see Figure 41–2), as the functional residual capacity (FRC) of obese patients deteriorates in the supine position, leading to more rapid deoxygenation should ventilation be impaired.

PREOXYGENATION

When possible, preoxygenation with face mask oxygen should precede all airway management interventions. Oxygen is delivered by mask for several minutes prior to anesthetic induction. In this way, the patient's oxygen reserve in the functional residual capacity is purged of nitrogen. Up to 90% of the normal FRC of 2 L can be filled with oxygen after preoxygenation. Considering the normal oxygen demand of 200 to 250 mL/min, the preoxygenated patient may add a 5- to 8-min oxygen reserve. Increasing the duration of apnea without desaturation improves safety if ventilation following anesthetic induction is delayed. Conditions that increase oxygen demand (eg, sepsis, pregnancy) and decrease FRC (eg, morbid obesity, pregnancy, ascites) reduce the duration of the apneic period before desaturation ensues. Assuming a patent air passage is present, oxygen insufflated into the pharynx may increase the duration of apnea tolerated by the patient. Because oxygen enters the blood from the FRC at a rate faster than CO_2 leaves the blood, a negative pressure is generated in the alveolus, drawing oxygen into the lung (*apneic oxygenation*). With a flow of 100% oxygen and a patent airway, arterial saturation can be maintained for a longer period despite no ventilation, permitting multiple airway interventions should a difficult airway be encountered.

BAG AND MASK VENTILATION

Bag and mask ventilation (BMV) is the first step in airway management in most situations, with the exception of patients undergoing rapid sequence intubation or elective awake intubation. Rapid sequence inductions avoid BMV to minimize stomach inflation and reduce the potential for the aspiration of gastric contents in nonfasted patients and those with delayed gastric emptying. In emergency situations, BMV may precede attempts at intubation to oxygenate the patient, with the understanding that there is an implicit risk of aspiration.

1 Effective mask ventilation requires both a gas-tight mask fit and a patent airway. Improper face mask technique can result in continued deflation of the anesthesia reservoir bag despite the adjustable pressure-limiting valve being closed, usually indicating a substantial leak around the mask. In contrast, the generation of high breathing circuit pressures with minimal chest movement and breath sounds implies an obstructed airway or obstructed tubing.

If the mask is held with the left hand, the right hand can be used to generate positive-pressure ventilation by squeezing the breathing bag. The mask is held against the face by downward pressure on the mask exerted by the left thumb and index finger (Figure 19–12). The middle and ring finger grasp the mandible to facilitate extension of the atlanto-occipital joint. This is a maneuver that is easier to teach with a mannequin or patient than to describe. Finger pressure should be placed on the bony mandible and not on the nearby soft tissues. The little finger is placed under the angle of the jaw and used to lift the jaw anteriorly, the most important maneuver to open the airway.

In difficult situations, two hands may be needed to provide adequate jaw thrust and create a mask seal. Therefore, an assistant may be needed to squeeze the bag, or the anesthesia machine's ventilator can be used. In such cases, the thumbs hold the mask down, and the fingertips or knuckles displace the jaw forward (Figure 19–13). Obstruction during expiration may be due to excessive downward pressure from the mask or from a ball-valve effect of the jaw thrust. The former can be relieved by decreasing the pressure on the mask, and the latter by releasing the jaw thrust during this phase of the respiratory cycle. Positive-pressure ventilation using a mask should normally be limited to 20 cm of H_2O to avoid stomach inflation. Even when BMV is successful, an oral or nasopharyngeal airway may be utilized to minimize airway pressure and the amount of stomach insufflation.

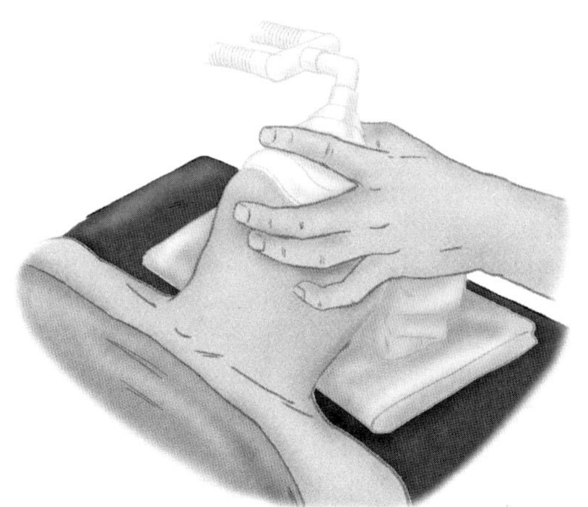

FIGURE 19–12 One-handed face mask technique.

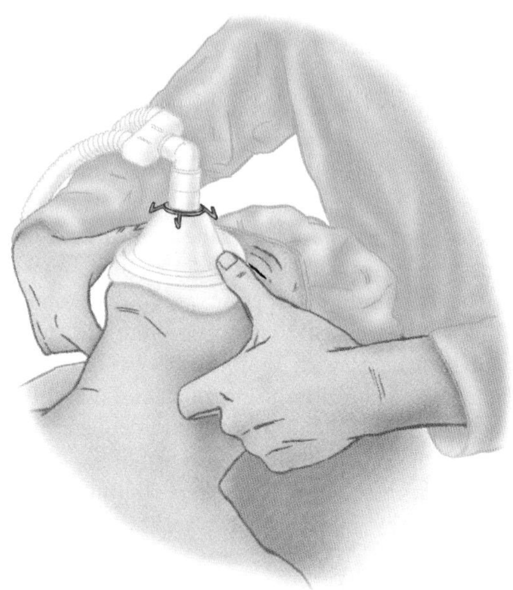

FIGURE 19–13 A difficult airway can often be managed with a two-handed technique.

Most patients' airways can be maintained with a face mask and an oral or nasal airway. Mask ventilation for long periods may result in pressure injury to branches of the trigeminal or facial nerves. Because of the absence of positive airway pressures during spontaneous ventilation, only minimal downward force on the face mask is required to create an adequate seal. If the face mask and mask straps are used for extended periods, the position should be regularly changed to prevent injury. Care should be used to avoid mask or finger contact with the eye, and the eyes should be taped shut as soon as possible to minimize the risk of corneal abrasions.

If the airway is patent, squeezing the bag will result in the rise of the chest. If ventilation is ineffective (no sign of chest rising, no end-tidal CO_2 detected, no condensation in the clear mask), oral or nasal airways can be placed to relieve airway obstruction from lax upper airway muscle tone or redundant pharyngeal tissues. It is often difficult to ventilate patients with morbid obesity, beards, or craniofacial deformities using a bag and mask. It is also frequently difficult to form an adequate mask seal with the cheeks of edentulous patients.

In years past, anesthetics were routinely delivered solely by mask or ETT administration. In recent decades, a variety of supraglottic devices has permitted both airway rescue (when adequate BMV is not possible) and routine anesthetic airway management (when intubation is not necessary).

SUPRAGLOTTIC AIRWAY DEVICES

Supraglottic airway devices (SADs) are used with both spontaneously breathing and ventilated patients during anesthesia. SADs are sometimes employed as conduits to aid endotracheal intubation when both BMV and endotracheal intubation have failed. All SADs consist of a tube connected to a respiratory circuit or breathing bag that is attached to a hypopharyngeal device that seals and directs airflow to the glottis, trachea, and lungs. Additionally, these airway devices occlude the esophagus with varying degrees of effectiveness, reducing gas distention of the stomach. Different sealing devices to prevent airflow from exiting through the mouth are also available. Some are equipped with a port to suction gastric contents. None provide the protection from aspiration pneumonitis offered by a properly sited, cuffed endotracheal tube.

Laryngeal Mask Airway

A laryngeal mask airway (LMA) consists of a wide-bore tube whose proximal end connects to a breathing circuit with a standard 15-mm connector and whose distal end is attached to an elliptical cuff that can be inflated through a pilot tube. The deflated cuff is lubricated and inserted blindly into the hypopharynx so that, once inflated, the cuff forms a low-pressure seal around the entrance to the larynx. This requires anesthetic depth and muscle relaxation slightly greater than that required for the insertion of an oral airway. Although insertion is relatively simple (Figure 19–14), attention to detail will improve the success rate (Table 19–2). An ideally positioned cuff is bordered by the base of the tongue superiorly, the pyriform sinuses laterally, and the upper esophageal sphincter inferiorly. If the esophagus lies within the rim of the cuff, gastric distention and regurgitation become possible. Anatomic variations prevent adequate functioning in some patients. However, if an LMA is not functioning properly after attempts to improve the "fit" of the LMA have failed, most practitioners will try another LMA one size larger or smaller. The shaft can be secured with
2 tape to the skin of the face. The LMA partially protects the larynx from pharyngeal secretions (but *not* gastric regurgitation), and it should remain in place until the patient has regained airway reflexes. This is usually signaled by coughing and mouth opening on command. The LMA is available in many sizes (Table 19–3).

The LMA provides an alternative to ventilation through a face mask or an ETT (Table 19–4). Relative contraindications for the LMA include pharyngeal pathology (eg, abscess), pharyngeal obstruction, aspiration risk (eg, pregnancy, hiatal hernia), or low pulmonary compliance (eg, restrictive airways disease) requiring peak inspiratory pressures greater than 30 cm H_2O. The LMA may be associated with less frequent bronchospasm than an ETT. Although it is clearly not a substitute for endotracheal intubation, the LMA has proven particularly helpful as a lifesaving, temporizing measure in patients with difficult airways (those who cannot be mask ventilated or intubated) because of its ease of insertion and relatively high success rate (95–99%). It has been used as a conduit for an intubating stylet (eg, gum-elastic bougie), ventilating jet stylet, flexible fiberoptic bronchoscope, or small-diameter (6.0 mm) ETT. Several

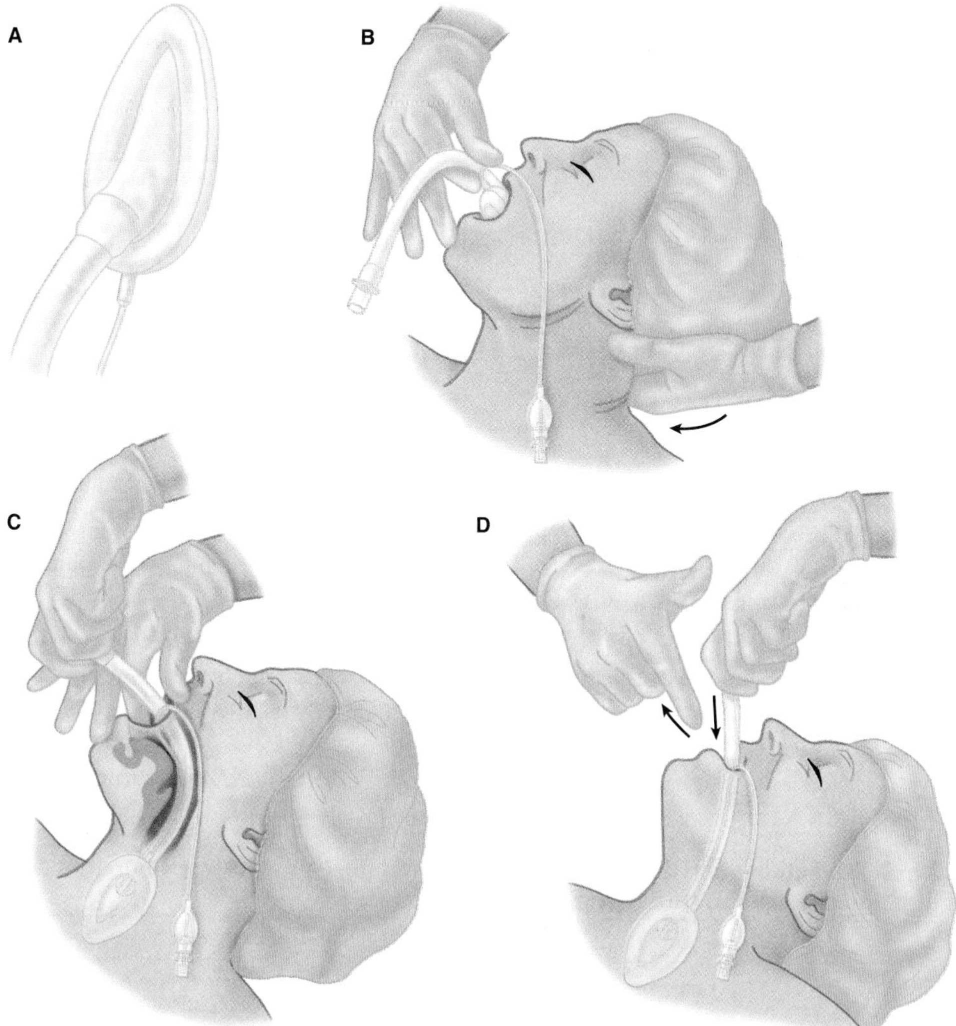

FIGURE 19–14 **A**: The laryngeal mask ready for insertion. The cuff should be deflated tightly, with the rim facing away from the mask aperture. There should be no folds near the tip. **B**: Initial insertion of the laryngeal mask. Under direct vision, the mask tip is pressed upward against the hard palate. The middle finger may be used to push the lower jaw downward. The mask is pressed forward as it is advanced into the pharynx to ensure that the tip remains flattened and avoids the tongue. The jaw should not be held open once the mask is inside the mouth. The nonintubating hand can be used to stabilize the occiput. **C**: By withdrawing the other fingers and with slight pronation of the forearm, it is usually possible to push the mask fully into position in one fluid movement. Note that the neck is kept flexed and the head extended. **D**: The laryngeal mask is grasped with the other hand, and the index finger is withdrawn. The hand holding the tube presses gently downward until resistance is encountered. (Reproduced with permission from LMA North America.)

LMAs are available that have been modified to facilitate placement of a larger ETT, with or without the use of a bronchoscope. Insertion can be performed under topical anesthesia and bilateral superior laryngeal nerve blocks if the airway must be secured while the patient is awake. Some newer supraglottic devices incorporate a channel to facilitate gastric decompression.

TABLE 19–2 Successful insertion of a laryngeal mask airway depends upon attention to several details.

1. Choose the appropriate size (Table 19–3), and check for leaks before insertion.
2. The leading edge of the deflated cuff should be wrinkle free and facing away from the aperture (Figure 19–14A).
3. Lubricate only the back side of the cuff.
4. Ensure adequate anesthesia before attempting insertion.
5. Place the patient's head in sniffing position (Figure 19–14B and Figure 19–26).
6. Use your index finger to guide the cuff along the hard palate and down into the hypopharynx until an increased resistance is felt (Figure 19–14C). The longitudinal black line should always be pointing directly cephalad (ie, facing the patient's upper lip).
7. Inflate with the correct amount of air (Table 19–3).
8. Ensure adequate anesthetic depth during patient positioning.
9. Obstruction after insertion is usually due to a down-folded epiglottis or transient laryngospasm.
10. Avoid pharyngeal suction, cuff deflation, or laryngeal mask removal until the patient is awake (eg, opening mouth on command).

TABLE 19–3 A variety of laryngeal masks with different cuff volumes are available for different sized patients.

Mask Size	Patient Size	Weight (kg)	Cuff Volume (mL)
1	Infant	<6.5	2–4
2	Child	6.5–20	Up to 10
2½	Child	20–30	Up to 15
3	Small adult	>30	Up to 20
4	Normal adult	<70	Up to 30
5	Larger adult	>70	Up to 30

Variations in LMA design include:

- The ProSeal LMA, which permits passage of a gastric tube to decompress the stomach
- The I-Gel, which uses a gel occluder rather than an inflatable cuff
- The Fastrach intubation LMA, which is designed to facilitate endotracheal intubation through the LMA device
- The LMA CTrach, which incorporates a camera to facilitate the passage of an endotracheal tube

TABLE 19–4 Advantages and disadvantages of the laryngeal mask airway compared with face mask ventilation or tracheal intubation.[1]

	Advantages	Disadvantages
Compared with face mask	Hands-free operation Better seal in bearded patients Less cumbersome in ENT surgery Often easier to maintain airway Protects against airway secretions Less facial nerve and eye trauma Less operating room pollution	More invasive More risk of airway trauma Requires new skill Deeper anesthesia required Requires some TMJ mobility N_2O diffusion into cuff Multiple contraindications
Compared with tracheal intubation	Less invasive Very useful in difficult intubations Less tooth and laryngeal trauma Less laryngospasm and bronchospasm Does not require muscle relaxation Does not require neck mobility No risk of esophageal or endobronchial intubation	Increased risk of gastrointestinal aspiration Less safe in prone or jackknife positions Limits maximum PPV Less secure airway Greater risk of gas leak and pollution Can cause gastric distention

[1]ENT, ear, nose, and throat; N_2O, nitrous oxide; PPV, positive-pressure ventilation; TMJ, temporomandibular joint.

Sore throat is common following SAD use. Injuries to the lingual, hypoglossal, and recurrent laryngeal nerves have been reported. Correct device sizing, avoidance of cuff hyperinflation, adequate lubrication, and gentle movement of the jaw during placement may reduce the likelihood of such injuries.

Esophageal–Tracheal Combitube

The esophageal–tracheal Combitube consists of two fused tubes, each with a 15-mm connector on its proximal end (Figure 19–15). The longer blue tube has an occluded distal tip that forces gas to exit through a series of side perforations. The shorter clear tube has an open tip and no side perforations. The Combitube is usually inserted blindly through the mouth and advanced until the two black rings on the shaft lie between the upper and lower teeth. The Combitube has two inflatable cuffs, a 100-mL proximal cuff and a 15-mL distal cuff, both of which should be fully inflated after placement. The distal lumen of the Combitube usually comes to lie in the esophagus approximately 95% of the time so that ventilation through the longer blue tube will force gas out of the side perforations and into the larynx. The shorter, clear tube can be used for gastric decompression. Alternatively, if the Combitube enters the trachea, ventilation through the clear tube will direct gas into the trachea.

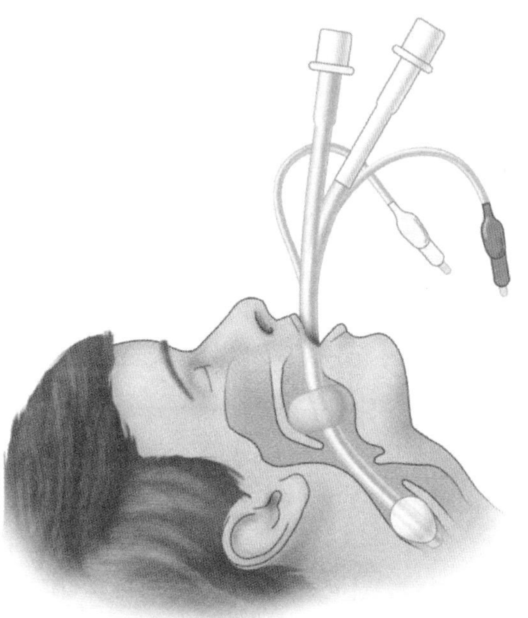

FIGURE 19–15 Combitube.

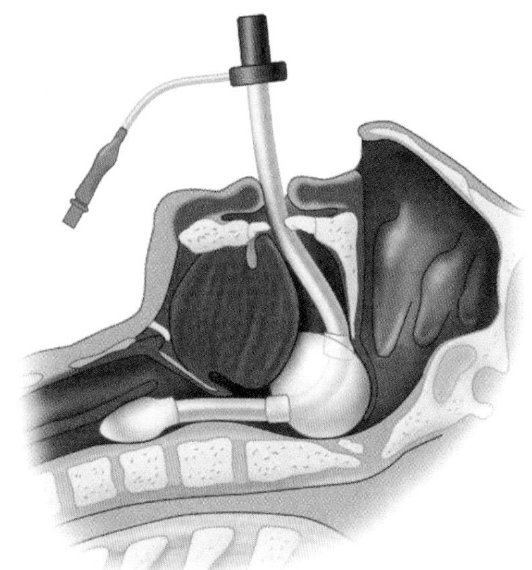

FIGURE 19–16 King laryngeal tube.

King Laryngeal Tube

The King laryngeal tube consists of a tube with a small esophageal balloon and a larger balloon for placement in the hypopharynx (Figure 19–16). Both balloons inflate through one inflation line. The lungs are inflated with gas that exits between the two balloons. A suction port distal to the esophageal balloon is present, permitting decompression of the stomach. If ventilation proves difficult after the King tube is inserted and the cuffs are inflated, the tube is likely inserted too deeply. Slowly withdraw the device until compliance improves.

ENDOTRACHEAL INTUBATION

Endotracheal intubation is employed both for the conduct of general anesthesia and to facilitate the ventilator management of the critically ill.

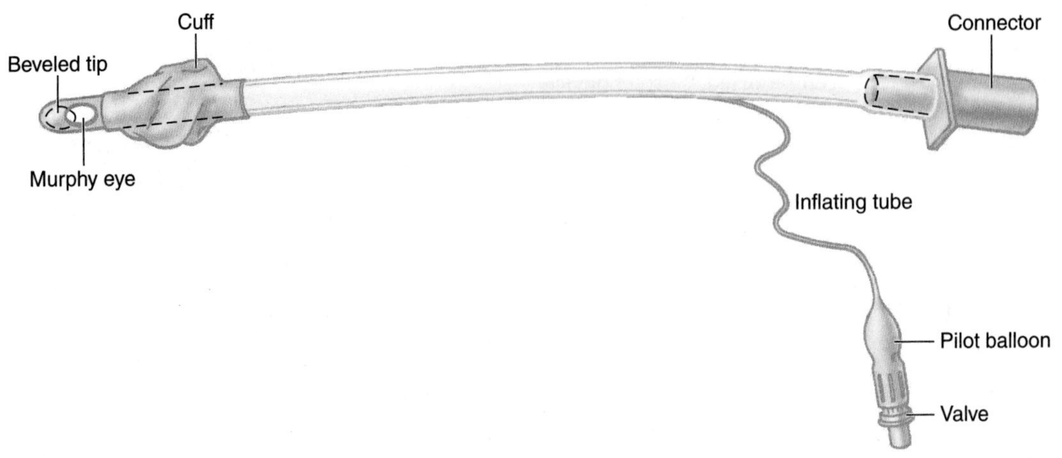

FIGURE 19–17 Murphy endotracheal tube.

Endotracheal Tubes (ETTs)

Standards govern ETT manufacturing (in the United States, American National Standard for Anesthetic Equipment; ANSI Z-79). ETTs are most commonly made from polyvinyl chloride. The shape and rigidity of ETTs can be altered by inserting a stylet. The patient end of the tube is beveled to aid visualization and insertion through the vocal cords. Murphy tubes have a hole (the Murphy eye) to decrease the risk of occlusion should the distal tube opening abut the carina or trachea (Figure 19–17).

Resistance to airflow depends primarily on tube diameter but also on tube length and curvature. ETT size is usually designated in millimeters of internal diameter or, less commonly, in the French scale (external diameter in millimeters multiplied by 3). The choice of tube diameter is always a compromise between maximizing flow with a larger size and minimizing airway trauma with a smaller size (Table 19–5).

Most adult ETTs have a cuff inflation system consisting of a valve, pilot balloon, inflating tube, and cuff (see Figure 19–17). The valve prevents air loss after cuff inflation. The pilot balloon provides a gross indication of cuff inflation. The inflating tube connects the valve to the cuff and is incorporated into the tube's wall. By creating a tracheal seal, ETT cuffs permit positive-pressure ventilation and reduce the likelihood of aspiration. Uncuffed tubes are often used in infants and young children; however, in recent years, cuffed pediatric tubes have been increasingly favored.

There are two major types of cuffs: high pressure (low volume) and low pressure (high volume). High-pressure cuffs are associated with more ischemic damage to the tracheal mucosa and are less suitable for intubations of long duration. Low-pressure cuffs may increase the likelihood of sore throat (larger mucosal contact area), aspiration, spontaneous extubation, and difficult insertion (because of the floppy cuff). Nonetheless, because of their lower incidence of mucosal damage, low-pressure cuffs are most frequently employed.

TABLE 19–5 Oral endotracheal tube size guidelines.

Age	Internal Diameter (mm)	Cut Length (cm)
Full-term infant	3.5	12
Child	$4+\frac{\text{Age}}{4}$	12 + age/2
Adult		
Female	7.0–7.5	24
Male	7.5–9.0	24

Cuff pressure depends on several factors: inflation volume, the diameter of the cuff in relation to the trachea, tracheal and cuff compliance, and intrathoracic pressure (cuff pressures increase with coughing). Cuff pressure may increase during general anesthesia from the diffusion of nitrous oxide from the tracheal mucosa into the ETT cuff.

ETTs have been modified for a variety of specialized applications. Flexible, spiral-wound, wire-reinforced ETTs (armored tubes) resist kinking and may prove valuable in some head and neck surgical procedures or in the prone patient. If an armored tube becomes kinked from extreme pressure (eg, an awake patient biting it), however, the lumen will often remain permanently occluded, and the tube will need replacement. Other specialized tubes include microlaryngeal tubes; double-lumen endotracheal tubes (to facilitate lung isolation and one-lung ventilation); ETTs equipped with bronchial blockers (to facilitate lung isolation and one-lung ventilation); ETTs with an integrated camera to facilitate the proper placement of a double-lumen endotracheal tube or an endobronchial blocker (Ambu VivaSight-DL or Ambu VivaSight-SL, respectively); metal tubes designed for laser airway surgery to reduce fire hazards; ETTs designed to monitor recurrent laryngeal nerve function during thyroid surgery (nerve integrity monitor [NIM] tubes); and preformed curved tubes for nasal and oral intubation in head and neck surgery.

LARYNGOSCOPES

A laryngoscope is an instrument used to examine the larynx and facilitate intubation of the trachea. The handle usually contains batteries to light a bulb on the blade tip (Figure 19–18) or, alternately, a bulb to illuminate a fiberoptic bundle that terminates at the tip of the blade. Laryngoscopes with fiberoptic light bundles in their blades can be made compatible with magnetic resonance imaging. The Macintosh and Miller blades are the most popular curved and straight designs, respectively, in North America. The choice of blade depends on personal preference and patient anatomy. Because no blade is perfect for all situations, the clinician should become proficient with a variety of blade designs (Figure 19–19).

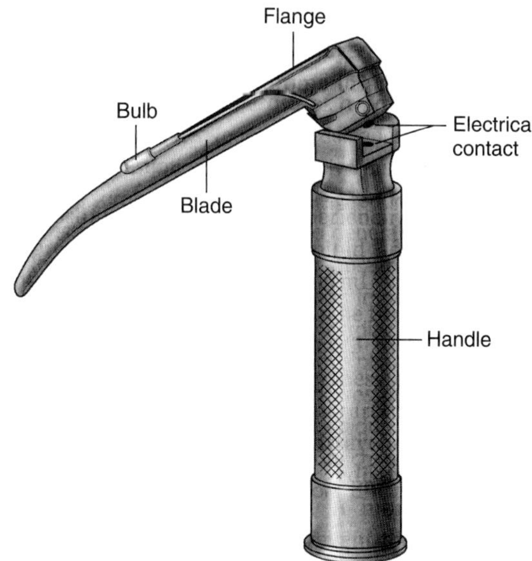

FIGURE 19–18 A rigid laryngoscope.

VIDEO LARYNGOSCOPES

In recent years, video laryngoscopy devices have revolutionized airway management. Successful direct laryngoscopy with a Macintosh or Miller blade requires appropriate alignment of the oral, pharyngeal, and laryngeal structures to visualize the glottis. Various maneuvers, such as the "sniffing" position and external movement of the larynx with cricoid pressure during direct laryngoscopy, are used to improve the view. Video- or optically based laryngoscopes have either a video chip (DCI system, GlideScope, McGrath, Airway) or a lens/mirror (Airtraq) at the tip of the intubation blade to transmit a view of the glottis to the operator. These devices differ in the angulation of the blade, the presence of a channel to guide the tube to the glottis, and the single-use or multiuse nature of the device.

In our opinion, video or indirect laryngoscopy offers minimal advantage to an experienced laryngoscopist who will intubate a patient with a normal airway. However, use in these patients is valuable

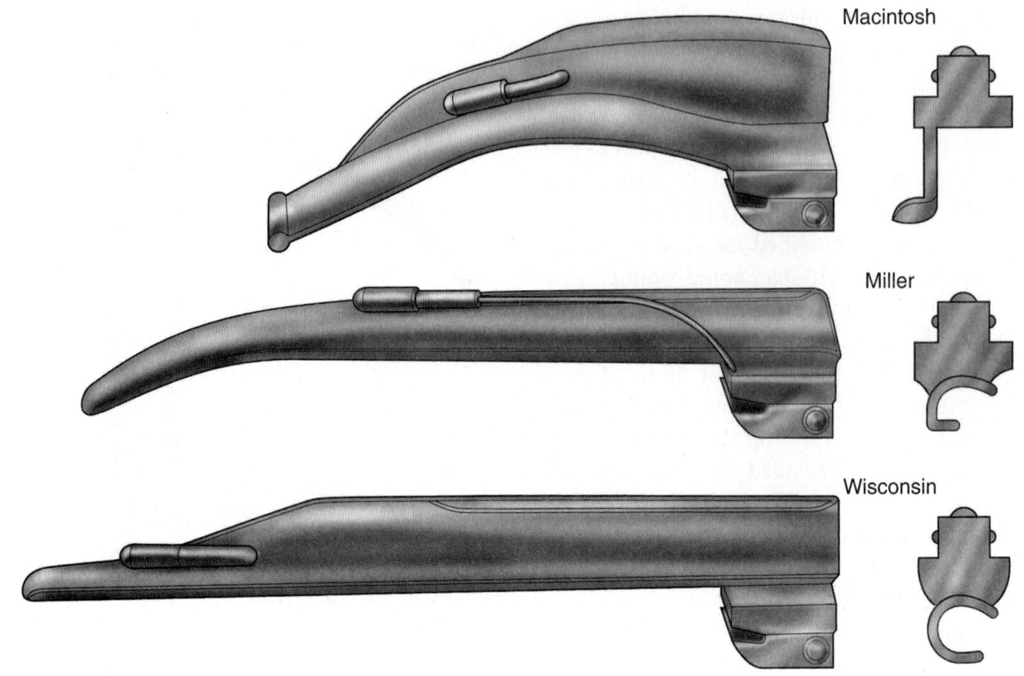

FIGURE 19–19 An assortment of laryngoscope blades.

in training learners because the instructor can see the same image as the learner on the video screen. Additionally, use in uncomplicated airway management patients improves familiarity with the device for times when direct laryngoscopy is not possible. Finally, not every patient needing emergency tracheal intubation will encounter an experienced laryngoscopist!

Indirect laryngoscopes generally improve visualization of laryngeal structures in difficult airways; however, visualization does not always lead to successful intubation. An ETT stylet is recommended when video laryngoscopy is to be performed. Some devices come with stylets designed to facilitate intubation with that particular device. Bending the stylet and ETT in a manner similar to the bend in the curve of the blade often facilitates passage of the ETT into the trachea. Even when the glottic opening is seen clearly, directing the ETT into the trachea can be difficult.

Indirect laryngoscopy may result in less displacement of the cervical spine than direct laryngoscopy; nevertheless, all precautions associated with airway manipulation in a patient with a possible cervical spine fracture should be maintained.

Varieties of indirect laryngoscopes include:

- Various Macintosh and Miller blades in pediatric and adult sizes have video capability in the Storz DCI system. The system can also incorporate an optical intubating stylet (Figure 19–20).

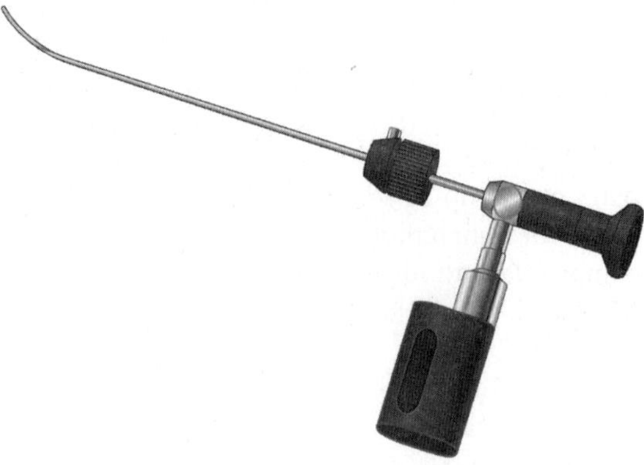

FIGURE 19–20 Optical intubating stylet.

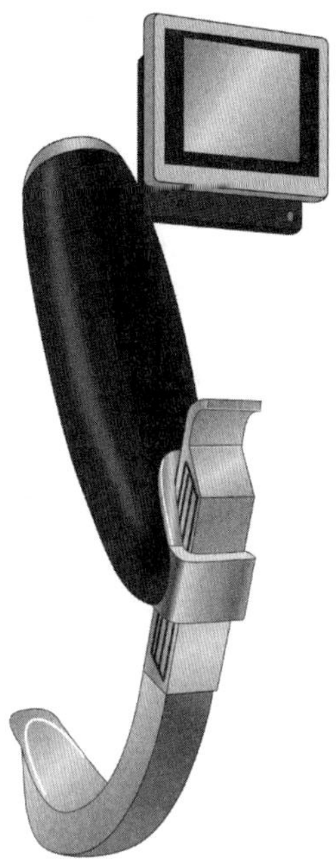

FIGURE 19–21 McGrath laryngoscope.

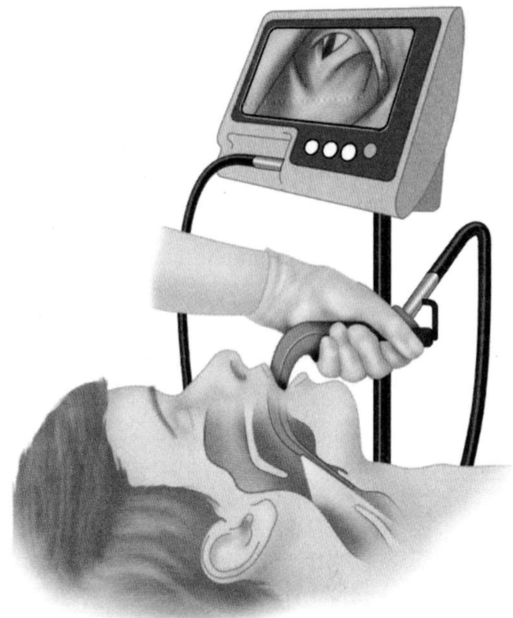

FIGURE 19–22 Glidescope.

The blades are similar to conventional intubation blades, permitting direct laryngoscopy and indirect video laryngoscopy. Assistants and instructors are able to see the view obtained by the operator and adjust their maneuvers accordingly to facilitate intubation or to provide instruction, respectively.

- The McGrath laryngoscope is a portable video laryngoscope with a blade length that can be adjusted to accommodate the airway of a child of age 5 years up to an adult (Figure 19–21). The blade can be disconnected from the handle to facilitate its insertion in morbidly obese patients in whom the space between the upper chest and head is reduced. The blade is inserted midline, with the laryngeal structures viewed at a distance to enhance intubation success.
- The GlideScope comes with disposable adult- and pediatric-sized blades (Figure 19–22). The blade is inserted midline and advanced until glottic structures are identified. The GlideScope has a 60° angle, preventing direct laryngoscopy and necessitating the use of stylet that is similar in shape to the blade.
- Airtraq is a single-use optical laryngoscope available in pediatric and adult sizes (Figure 19–23). The device has a channel to guide the endotracheal tube to the glottis. This device is inserted midline. Success is more likely when the device's tip is not positioned too close to the glottis.

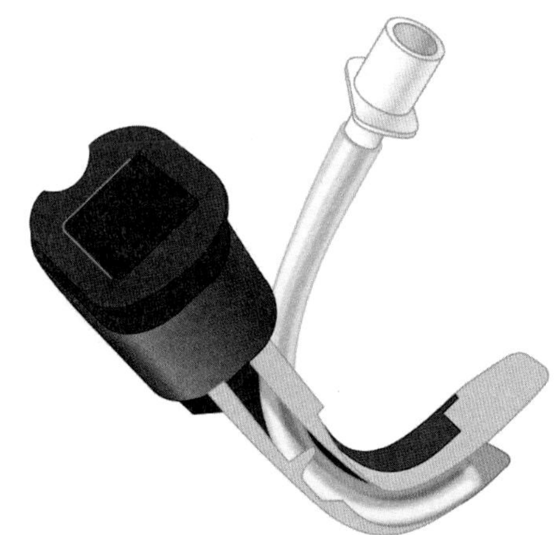

FIGURE 19–23 Airtraq optical laryngoscope.

- Video intubating stylets have a video capability and light source. The stylet is introduced, and the glottis is identified. Intubation with a video stylet may result in less cervical spine movement than with other techniques.

No one device will necessarily ensure successful intubation in every circumstance and with every patient, so the clinician should be fluent with several options.

Flexible Fiberoptic Bronchoscopes

In some situations—for example, patients with unstable cervical spines, poor range of motion of the temporomandibular joint, or certain congenital or acquired upper airway anomalies—laryngoscopy with direct or indirect laryngoscopes may be undesirable or impossible. A flexible fiberoptic bronchoscope (FOB) allows indirect visualization of the larynx in such cases or in any situation in which awake intubation is planned (Figure 19–24). Bronchoscopes are constructed of coated glass fibers that transmit light and images by internal reflection (ie, a light beam becomes trapped within a fiber and exits unchanged at the opposite end). The insertion tube contains two bundles of fibers, each consisting of 10,000 to 15,000 fibers. One bundle transmits light from the light source (light source or incoherent bundle), which is either external to the device or contained within the handle (Figure 19–24B), whereas the other provides a high-resolution image (image or coherent bundle). Directional manipulation of the insertion tube is accomplished with angulation wires. Aspiration channels allow suctioning of secretions, insufflation of oxygen, or instillation of local anesthetic. Aspiration channels can be difficult to clean. If they are not properly cleaned and sterilized, they may promote infection.

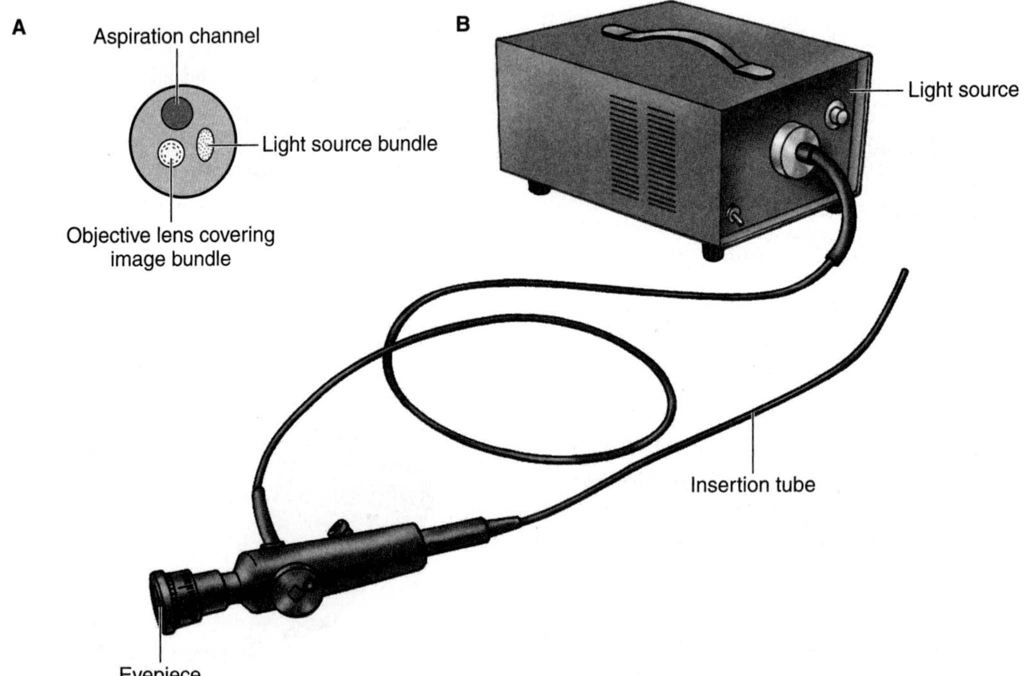

FIGURE 19–24 **A**: Cross-section of a fiberoptic bronchoscope. **B**: A flexible fiberoptic bronchoscope with a fixed light source.

TECHNIQUES OF DIRECT & INDIRECT LARYNGOSCOPY & INTUBATION

Indications for Intubation

Inserting a tube into the trachea has become a routine part of delivering a general anesthetic. Intubation is not a risk-free procedure, and it is not a requirement for all patients receiving general anesthesia. Intubation is indicated to protect the airway in patients who are at risk of aspiration and in those undergoing surgical procedures involving body cavities and the head and neck. It is also indicated in patients who will be positioned so that the airway will be less accessible (eg, those undergoing surgery in the prone position or whose head is rotated away from the anesthesia workstation). Mask ventilation or ventilation with an LMA is usually satisfactory for short minor procedures such as cystoscopy, examination under anesthesia, inguinal hernia repairs, or extremity surgery, and the indications for supraglottic airway devices during anesthesia continues to expand.

Preparation for Direct Laryngoscopy

Preparation for intubation includes checking equipment and properly positioning the patient. The ETT should be examined. The tube's cuff can be tested by inflating the cuff using a syringe. Maintenance of cuff pressure *after detaching the syringe* ensures proper cuff and valve function. Some anesthesiologists cut the ETT to a preset length to decrease dead space, risk of bronchial intubation, or risk of occlusion from tube kinking (see Table 19–5). The connector should be pushed firmly into the tube to decrease the likelihood of disconnection. If a stylet is used, it should be inserted into the ETT, which is then bent to resemble a hockey stick (Figure 19–25). This shape facilitates intubation of an anteriorly positioned larynx. The desired blade is locked onto the laryngoscope handle, and bulb function is tested. The light intensity should remain constant even if the bulb is jiggled. A blinking light signals poor electrical contact, whereas fading indicates depleted batteries. An extra handle, blade, ETT (one size smaller than the anticipated optimal size), stylet, and intubating bougie should be immediately available. A functioning suction unit is mandatory to clear the airway in case of unexpected secretions, blood, or emesis.

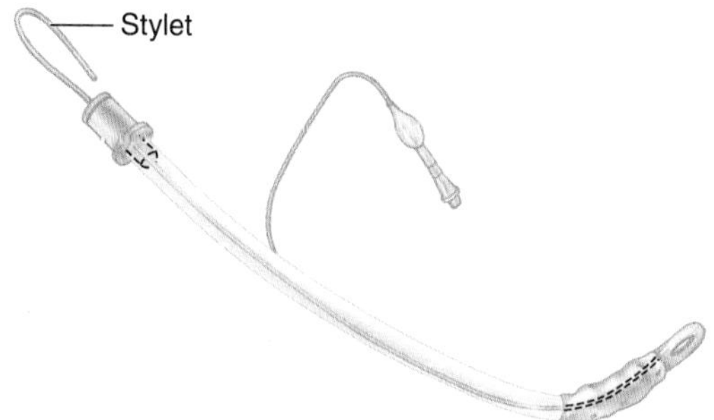

FIGURE 19–25 An endotracheal tube with a stylet bent to resemble a hockey stick.

Adequate glottis exposure during laryngoscopy often depends on correct patient positioning. The patient's head should be level with the anesthesiologist's waist or higher to prevent unnecessary back strain during laryngoscopy.

Direct laryngoscopy displaces pharyngeal soft tissues to create a direct line of vision from the mouth to the glottic opening. Moderate head elevation (5–10 cm above the surgical table) and extension of the atlantooccipital joint place the patient in the desired sniffing position (Figure 19–26). The lower portion of the cervical spine is flexed by resting the head on a pillow or other soft support.

As previously discussed, preparation for induction and intubation also involves routine preoxygenation. Preoxygenation can be omitted in patients who object to the face mask; however, failing to preoxygenate increases the risk of rapid desaturation following apnea, and in this case, preoxygenation can be performed to minimize that risk with BMV after induction of general anesthesia but before the initiation of intubation.

Because general anesthesia abolishes the protective corneal reflex, care must be taken during this period not to injure the patient's eyes by unintentionally abrading the cornea. Thus, the eyes are routinely taped shut as soon as possible, often after applying an ophthalmic ointment, before manipulation of the airway.

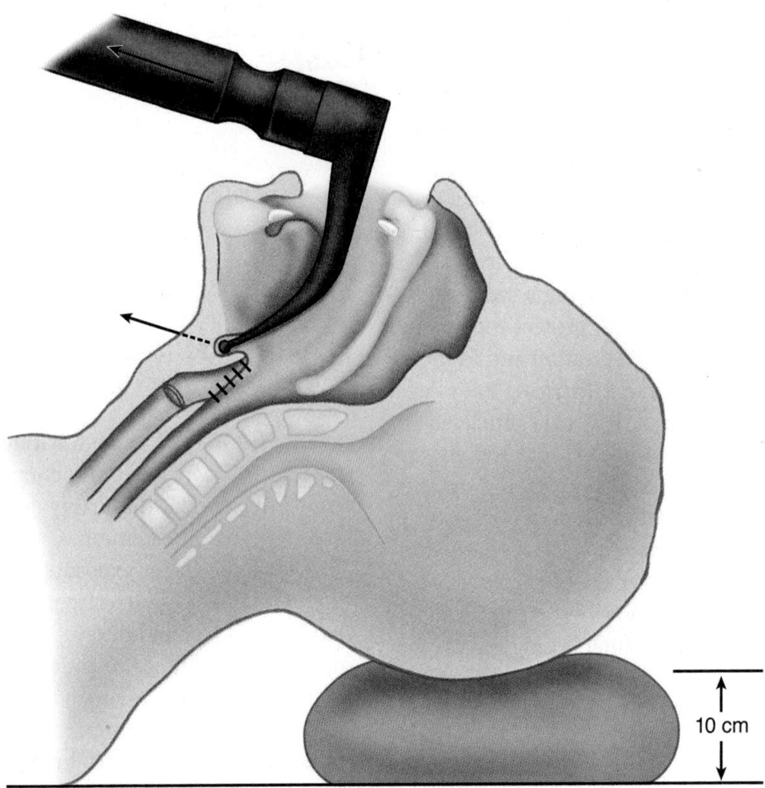

FIGURE 19–26 The sniffing position and intubation with a Macintosh blade. (Modified with permission from Dorsch JA, Dorsch SE. Understanding Anesthesia Equipment: *Construction, Care, and Complications*. Philadelphia, PA: Lippincott Williams & Wilkins, 1991.)

Orotracheal Intubation

The laryngoscope is held in the left hand. With the patient's mouth opened, the blade is introduced into the right side of the oropharynx—with care to avoid the teeth. The tongue is swept to the left and up into the floor of the pharynx by the blade's flange. Successful sweeping of the tongue leftward clears the view for ETT placement. The tip of a curved blade is usually inserted into the vallecula, and the straight blade tip covers the epiglottis. With either blade, the handle is raised up and away from the patient in a plane perpendicular to the patient's mandible to expose the vocal cords (Figure 19–27). One must avoid trapping a lip between the teeth and the blade or directly contacting the teeth with the blade. The ETT is taken with the right hand, and its tip is passed through the abducted vocal cords. The "backward, upward, rightward pressure" (BURP) maneuver applied externally by the intubating anesthetist or by an assistant moves an anteriorly positioned glottis posterior to facilitate visualization of the glottis. The ETT cuff should lie in the upper trachea but beyond the larynx. The laryngoscope is withdrawn, again

3 with care to avoid tooth damage. The cuff is inflated with the least amount of air necessary to create a seal during positive-pressure ventilation to minimize the pressure transmitted to the tracheal mucosa. Overinflation may inhibit capillary blood flow, injuring the trachea. Compressing the pilot balloon with the fingers is *not* a reliable method of determining whether cuff pressure is either sufficient or excessive.

After intubation, the chest and epigastrium are immediately auscultated during hand ventilation, and a capnographic tracing (the definitive test) is monitored to ensure intratracheal location (Figure 19–28). If there is doubt as to whether the tube is in the esophagus or trachea, repeat the laryngoscopy to confirm placement. End-tidal CO_2 will not be produced if there

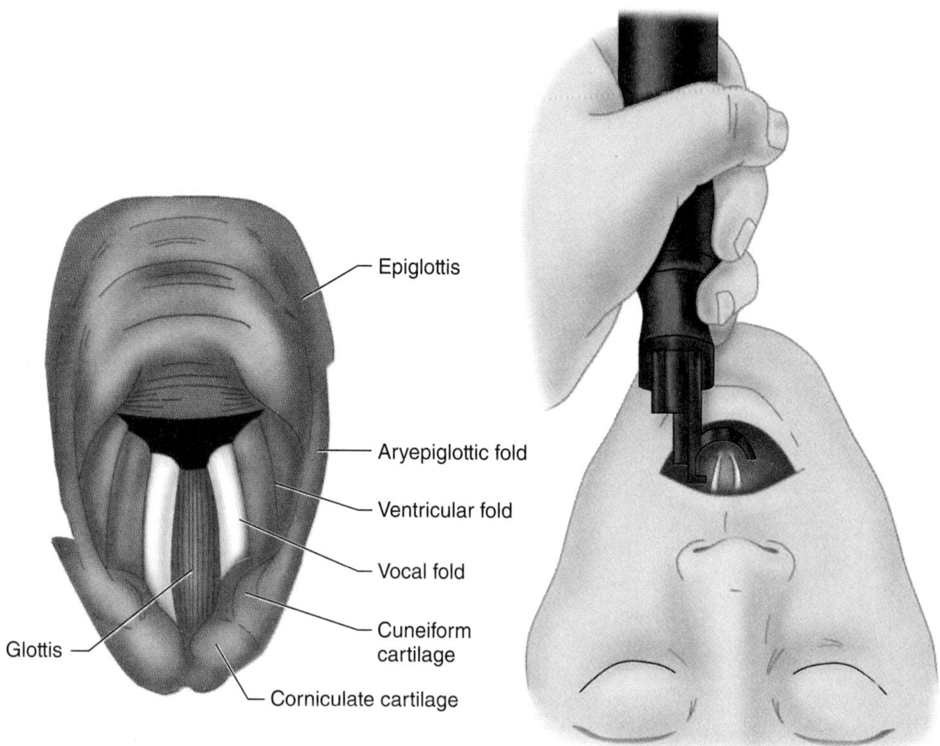

FIGURE 19–27 Typical view of the glottis during laryngoscopy with a curved blade. (Modified with permission from Barash PG. *Clinical Anesthesia.* 4th ed. Philadelphia, PA: Lippincott Williams & Wilkins; 2001.)

is no cardiac output. FOB through the tube and visualization of the tracheal rings and carina will likewise confirm correct placement. Otherwise, the tube is taped or tied to secure its position. **4** Although the persistent detection of CO_2 by a capnograph is the best confirmation of tracheal placement of an ETT, it cannot exclude endobronchial intubation. The earliest evidence of endobronchial intubation often is an increase in peak inspiratory pressure. Proper tube location can be reconfirmed by palpating the cuff in the sternal notch while compressing the pilot balloon with the other hand. **5** The cuff should not be felt above the level of the cricoid cartilage because a prolonged intralaryngeal location may result in postoperative hoarseness and increases the risk of accidental extubation. Tube position can also be documented by chest radiography or point-of-care ultrasound.

The description presented here assumes an unconscious patient. Oral intubation is usually poorly tolerated by awake, fit patients. Awake intubation is facilitated by intravenous sedation, application of a local anesthetic spray in the oropharynx, regional nerve block, and constant reassurance.

A failed intubation should not be followed by identical repeated attempts. Changes must be made to increase the likelihood of success, such as repositioning the patient, decreasing the tube size, adding a stylet, selecting a different blade, using an indirect laryngoscope, attempting a nasal route, and requesting the assistance of another anesthesia provider. If the patient is also difficult to ventilate with a mask, alternative forms of airway management (eg, second-generation supraglottic airway devices, jet ventilation via percutaneous tracheal catheter, cricothyrotomy, tracheostomy) must be immediately pursued. The guidelines developed by the American

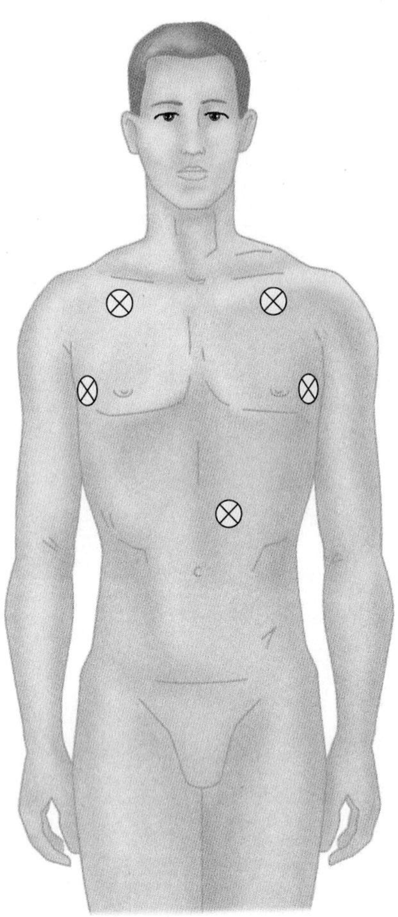

FIGURE 19–28 Sites for auscultation of breath sounds at the apices and over the stomach.

Society of Anesthesiologists for the management of a difficult airway include a treatment plan algorithm for this situation (Figure 19–29).

The Difficult Airway Society (DAS) also provides a useful approach for the management of the unanticipated difficult airway (Figure 19–30A and Figure 19–30B). Various specialty organizations issue guidelines for the management of the difficult airway, and most produce algorithms that discourage the repeated performance of the same failed technique to secure the airway. Rather, these guidelines suggest continually attempting new approaches and proceeding to front-of-neck airway access once it is recognized that a "can't intubate, can't oxygenate" event is in progress.

The combined use of a video laryngoscope and an intubation bougie often can facilitate intubation when the endotracheal tube cannot be directed into the glottis despite good visualization of the laryngeal opening (Figure 19–31). Progression through the DAS plans A to D prevents the anesthetist from unnecessarily repeating the same failed approaches to airway management and maximizes the possibility of preserving patient oxygenation as the airway is secured.

Nasotracheal Intubation

Nasal intubation is similar to oral intubation except that the ETT is advanced through the nose and nasopharynx into the oropharynx before laryngoscopy. The nostril through which the patient breathes most easily is selected in advance and prepared. Phenylephrine (0.5% or 0.25%) or tolazoline nose drops constrict blood vessels and shrink mucous membranes. If the patient is awake, local anesthetic ointment (for the nostril, delivered via an ointment-coated nasopharyngeal airway), spray (for the oropharynx), and nerve blocks can also be utilized.

An ETT lubricated with water-soluble jelly is introduced along the floor of the nose, below the inferior turbinate, *at an angle perpendicular to the face.* The tube's bevel should be directed laterally away from the turbinates. The proximal end of the ETT should be pulled cephalad to ensure that the tube passes along the floor of the nasal cavity. The tube is gradually advanced until its tip can be visualized in the oropharynx. Laryngoscopy, as discussed, reveals the abducted vocal cords. Often, the distal end of the ETT can be pushed into the trachea without difficulty. If difficulty is encountered, the tip of the tube may be directed through the vocal cords with Magill forceps, being careful not to damage the cuff. Nasal passage of ETTs, airways, or nasogastric catheters carries greater risk in patients with severe midfacial trauma because of the risk of intracranial placement (Figure 19–32).

Although less used today, blind nasal intubation of spontaneously breathing patients can be employed. In this technique, after a topical anesthetic is applied to the nostril and pharynx, a breathing tube is passed through the nasopharynx. Using breath sounds as a guide, the anesthetist directs it toward the glottis. When breath sounds are maximal, the anesthetist

American Society of Anesthesiologists®

DIFFICULT AIRWAY ALGORITHM

1. Assess the likelihood and clinical impact of basic management problems:
- **Difficulty with patient cooperation or consent**
- **Difficult mask ventilation**
- **Difficult supraglottic airway placement**
- **Difficult laryngoscopy**
- **Difficult intubation**
- **Difficult surgical airway access**

2. Actively pursue opportunities to deliver supplemental oxygen throughout the process of difficult airway management.

3. Consider the relative merits and feasibility of basic management choices:
- **Awake intubation *vs.* intubation after induction of general anesthesia**
- **Non-invasive technique *vs.* invasive techniques for the initial approach to intubation**
- **Video-assisted laryngoscopy as an initial approach to intubation**
- **Preservation *vs.* ablation of spontaneous ventilation**

4. Develop primary and alternative strategies:

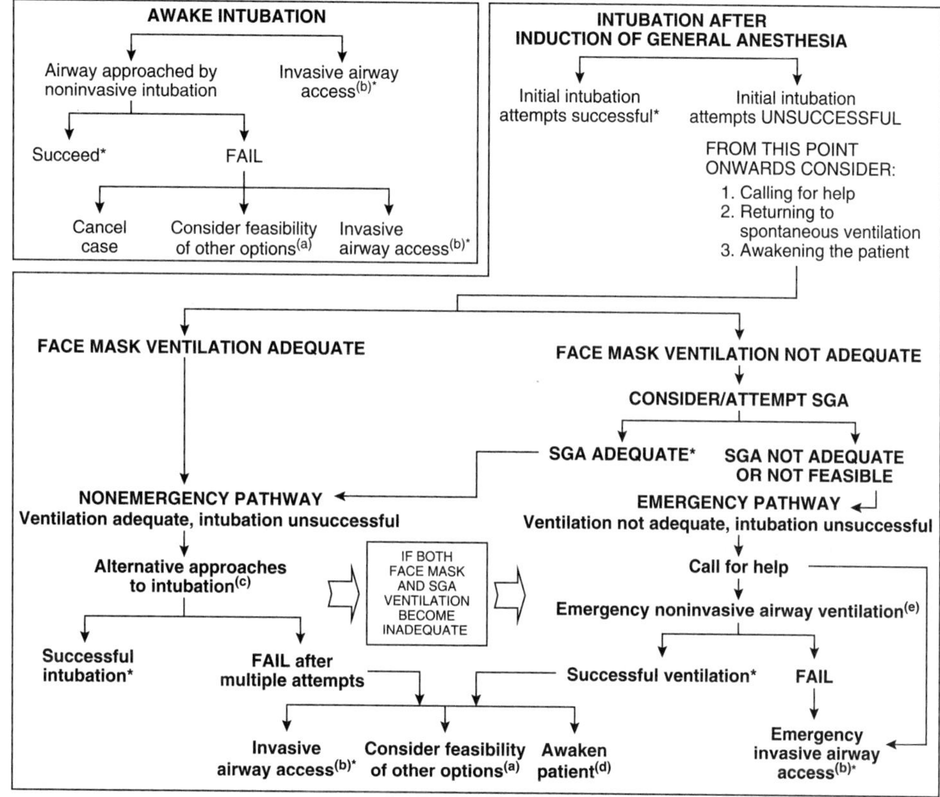

*Confirm ventilation, tracheal intubation, or SGA placement with exhaled CO_2.

FIGURE 19–29 Difficult airway algorithm. Notes: (a) Other options include (but are not limited to): surgery utilizing face mask or supraglottic airway (SGA) anesthesia (eg, laryngeal mask airway [LMA], intubating LMA [ILMA], laryngeal tube), local anesthesia infiltration, or regional nerve blockade. Pursuit of these options usually implies that mask ventilation will not be problematic. Therefore, these options may be of limited value if this step in the algorithm has been reached via the emergency pathway. (b) Invasive airway access includes surgical or percutaneous airway, jet ventilation, and retrograde intubation. (c) Alternative difficult intubation approaches include (but are not limited to) video-assisted laryngoscopy, alternative laryngoscope blades, SGA (eg, LMA, ILMA) as an intubation conduit (with or without fiberoptic guidance), fiberoptic intubation, intubating stylet or tube changer, light wand, and blind oral or nasal intubation. (d) Consider re-preparation of the patient for awake intubation or canceling surgery. (e) Emergency noninvasive airway ventilation consists of an SGA. (Reproduced with permission from American Society of Anesthesiologists Task Force on the Management of the Difficult Airway. Practice guidelines for management of the difficult airway: An updated report by the American Society of Anesthesiologists Task Force on the Management of the Difficult Airway. *Anesthesiology.* 2003 May;98(5):1269-1277.)

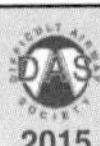

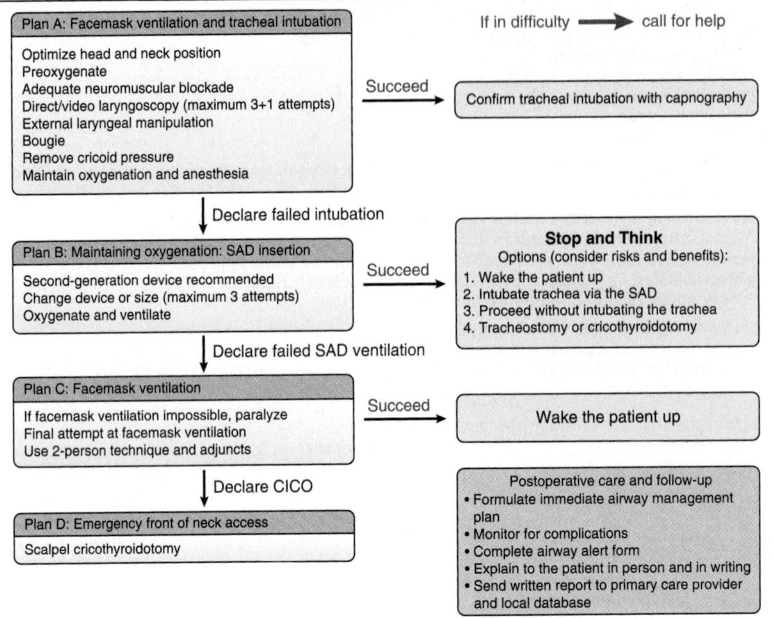

FIGURE 19–30A Difficult Airway Society difficult intubation guidelines: overview. CICO, can't intubate, can't oxygenate; SAD, supraglottic airway device. (Reproduced with permission from Frerk C, Mitchell V, McNarry A, et al. Difficult Airway Society 2015 guidelines for management of unanticipated difficult intubation in adults. *Br J Anaesth.* 2015 Dec;115(6):827-848.)

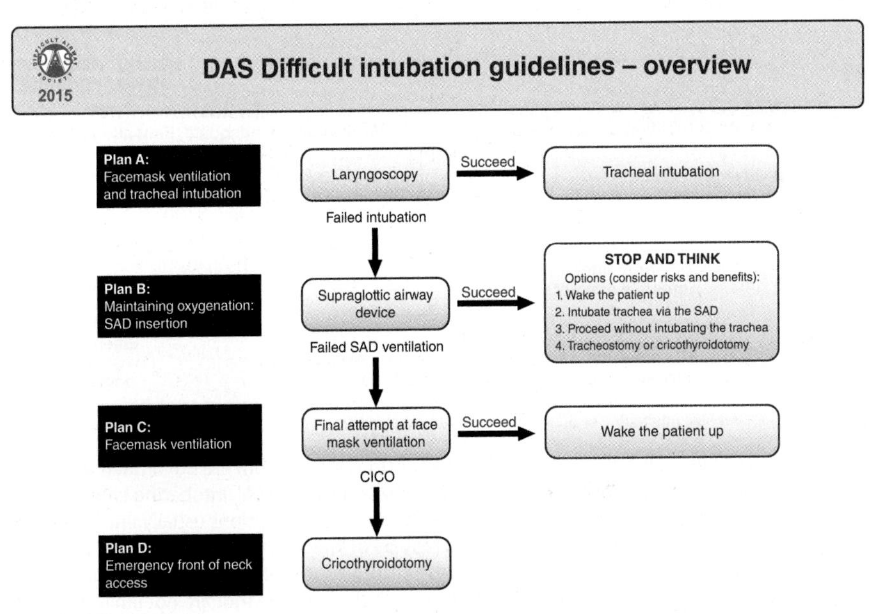

FIGURE 19–30B Overview of Difficult Airway Society (DAS) difficult intubation guidelines. CICO, can't intubate, can't oxygenate; SAD, supraglottic airway device. (Reproduced with permission from Frerk C, Mitchell V, McNarry A, et al. Difficult Airway Society 2015 guidelines for management of unanticipated difficult intubation in adults. *Br J Anaesth.* 2015 Dec;115(6):827-848.)

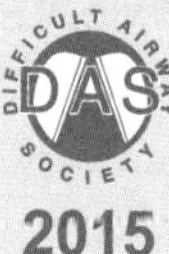

Failed intubation, failed oxygenation in the paralyzed, anesthetized patient

CALL FOR HELP

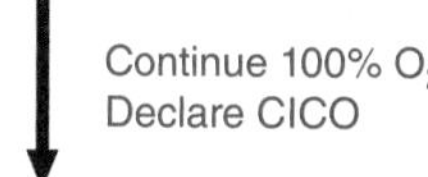

Plan D: Emergency front of neck access

Continue to give oxygen via upper airway
Ensure neuromuscular blockade
Position patient to extend neck

Scalpel cricothyroidotomy

Equipment: 1. Scalpel (number 10 blade)
2. Bougie
3. Tube (cuffed 6-mm ID)

Laryngeal handshake to identify cricothyroid membrane

Palpable cricothyroid membrane
Transverse stab incision through cricothyroid membrane
Turn blade through 90° (sharp edge caudally)
Slide coude tip of bougie along blade into trachea
Railroad lubricated 6-mm cuffed tracheal tube into trachea
Ventilate, inflate cuff, and confirm position with capnography
Secure tube

Impalpable cricothyroid membrane
Make an 8- to 10-cm vertical skin incision, caudad to cephalad
Use blunt dissection with fingers of both hands to separate tissues
Identify and stabilize the larynx
Proceed with technique for palpable cricothyroid membrane as above

Postoperative care and follow-up
- Postpone surgery unless immediately life threatening
- Urgent surgical review of cricothyroidotomy site
- Document and follow up as in main flow chart

This flowchart form 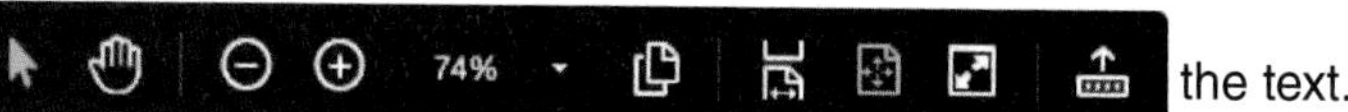 the text.

FIGURE 19–30B *(Continued)*

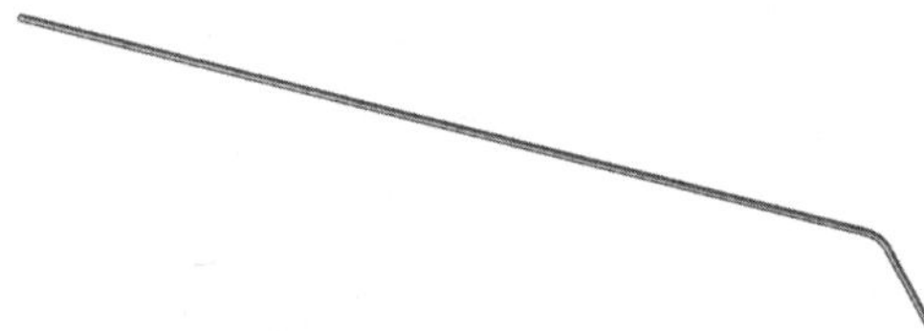

FIGURE 19–31 Bougie.

advances the tube during inspiration in an effort to blindly pass the tube into the trachea.

Flexible Fiberoptic Intubation

Fiberoptic intubation (FOI) is routinely performed in awake or sedated patients with problematic airways. FOI is ideal for:

- A small mouth opening
- Minimizing cervical spine movement in trauma or rheumatoid arthritis
- Upper airway obstruction, such as angioedema or tumor mass
- Facial deformities, facial trauma

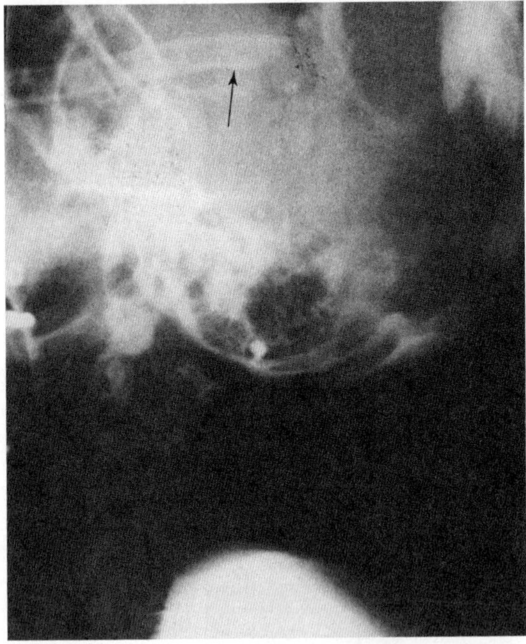

FIGURE 19–32 Radiograph demonstrating a 7.0-mm endotracheal tube placed through the cribriform plate into the cranial vault in a patient with a basilar skull fracture.

FOI can be performed awake or asleep via oral or nasal routes in the following scenarios:

- **Awake FOI**—Predicted inability to ventilate by mask, upper airway obstruction
- **Asleep FOI**—Failed intubation, desire for minimal cervical spine movement in patients who refuse awake intubation, anticipated difficult intubation when ventilation by mask appears easy
- **Oral FOI**—Facial, skull injuries
- **Nasal FOI**—A poor mouth opening

When FOI is considered, careful planning is necessary, as it will otherwise add to the anesthesia time prior to surgery. Patients should be informed of the need for awake intubation as a part of the informed consent process.

The airway is anesthetized with a local anesthetic spray, and patient sedation is provided as tolerated. Dexmedetomidine has the advantage of preserving respiration while providing sedation. Airway anesthesia is discussed in the Case Discussion at the end of this chapter.

If nasal FOI is planned, both nostrils are prepared with vasoconstrictive spray. The nostril through which the patient breathes more easily is identified. Oxygen can be insufflated through the suction port and down the aspiration channel of the FOB to improve oxygenation and blow secretions away from the tip.

Alternatively, a large nasal airway (eg, 36FR) can be inserted in the contralateral nostril. The breathing circuit can be directly connected to the end of this nasal airway to administer 100% oxygen during laryngoscopy. If the patient is unconscious and not breathing spontaneously, the mouth can be closed, and ventilation can be attempted through the single nasal airway. When this technique is used, the adequacy of ventilation and oxygenation should be confirmed by capnography and pulse oximetry. The lubricated shaft of the FOB is introduced into the ETT lumen. It is important to keep the shaft of the bronchoscope relatively straight (Figure 19–33) so that if the head of the bronchoscope is rotated in one direction, the distal end will move to a similar degree and in the same direction. As the tip of

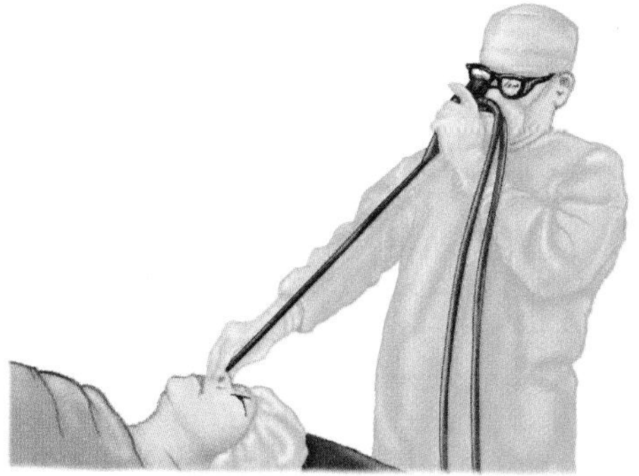

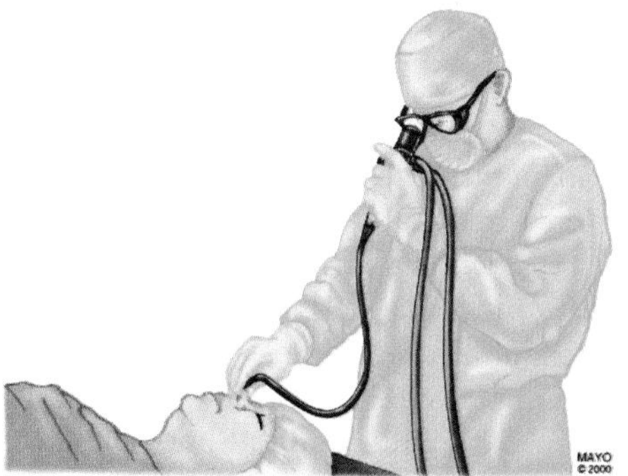

FIGURE 19–33 Correct technique for manipulating a fiberoptic bronchoscope through an endotracheal tube is shown in the top panel; avoid curvature in the bronchoscope, which makes manipulation difficult.

the FOB passes through the distal end of the ETT, the epiglottis or glottis should be visible. The tip of the bronchoscope is manipulated as needed to pass through the abducted cords.

Having an assistant thrust the jaw forward or apply cricoid pressure may improve visualization in difficult cases. Having the assistant grasp the tongue with gauze and pull it forward is very helpful.

Once in the trachea, the FOB is advanced to within sight of the carina. The presence of tracheal rings and the carina is proof of proper positioning. The ETT is pushed off the FOB. The acute angle around the arytenoid cartilage and epiglottis may prevent easy advancement of the tube. The use of an armored tube usually decreases this problem because it has greater lateral flexibility and a more obtusely angled distal end. Proper ETT position is confirmed by viewing the tip of the tube at an appropriate distance (3 cm in adults) above the carina before the FOB is withdrawn.

Oral FOI proceeds similarly, with the aid of various oral airway devices to direct the FOB toward the glottis and to reduce obstruction of the view by the tongue.

SURGICAL AIRWAY TECHNIQUES

Front of neck airways (FONA) airways are required when the "can't intubate, can't oxygenate" scenario presents and may be performed in anticipation of such circumstances in selected patients. The options include surgical tracheostomy, cricothyrotomy, catheter or needle cricothyrotomy, transtracheal catheter with jet ventilation, and retrograde intubation.

Tracheostomy has become an elective surgical procedure, and the other listed techniques are preferred in emergency settings. Surgical cricothyrotomy refers to an incision of the cricothyroid membrane (CTM) and the placement of a breathing tube. More recently, several needle/dilator cricothyrotomy kits have become available. Unlike surgical cricothyrotomy, where a horizontal incision is made across the CTM, these kits utilize the Seldinger catheter/wire/dilator technique. A catheter attached to a syringe is inserted across the CTM (Figure 19–34). When air is aspirated, a guidewire is passed through the catheter into the trachea (Figure 19–35). A dilator is then passed over the guidewire, and a breathing tube is placed (Figure 19–36).

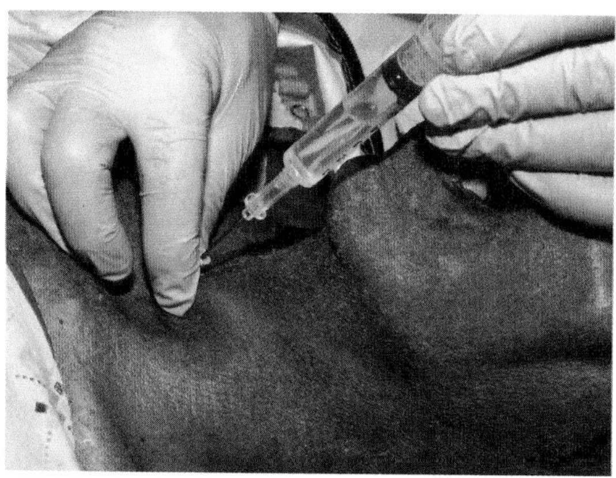

FIGURE 19–34 Cricothyrotomy. Slide catheter into the trachea. (Reproduced with permission from Lawrence B. Stack, MD.)

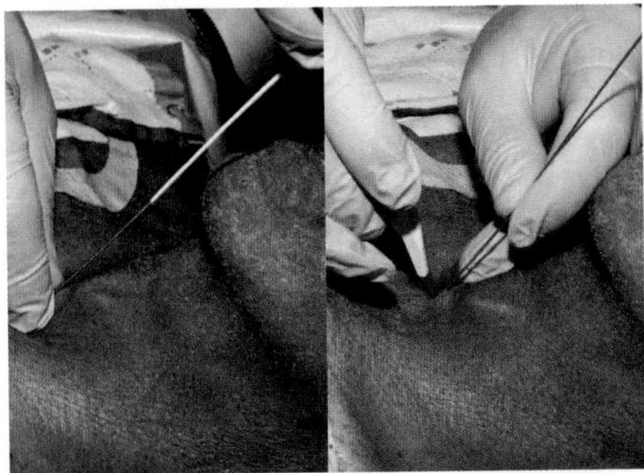

FIGURE 19–35 Cricothyrotomy. Incision at the wire entry site. Remove the catheter, and make an incision at the wire entry site. (Reproduced with permission from Lawrence B. Stack, MD.)

Catheter-based salvage procedures can also be performed. A 16- or 14-gauge intravenous cannula is attached to a syringe and passed through the CTM toward the carina. Air is aspirated. If a jet ventilation system is available, it can be attached. The catheter *must* be secured; otherwise the jet pressure will push the catheter out of the airway, leading to potentially disastrous subcutaneous emphysema. Short (1-s) bursts of oxygen ventilate the patient. Sufficient outflow of expired air must be assured to avoid barotrauma. Patients ventilated in this manner may develop subcutaneous or mediastinal emphysema and may become hypercapnic despite adequate oxygenation. Transtracheal jet ventilation will usually require conversion to a surgical airway or tracheal intubation. Transtracheal jet salvage techniques are increasingly discouraged for airway rescue in favor of scalpel cricothyroidotomy.

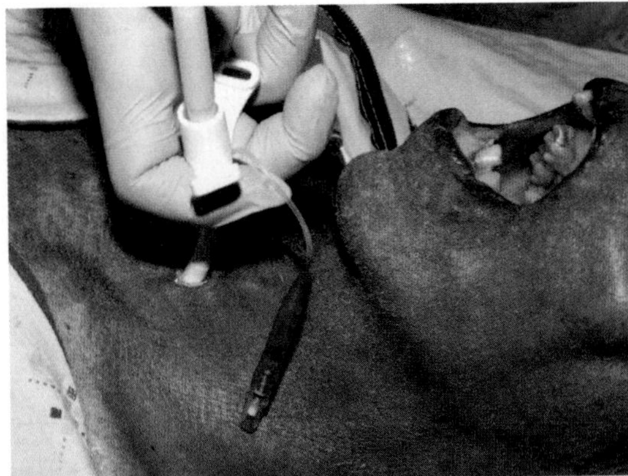

FIGURE 19–36 Cricothyrotomy. Insert tracheostomy tube/introducer. Insert both devices over the wire and into the trachea. (Reproduced with permission from Lawrence B. Stack, MD.)

Should a jet ventilation system not be available, a 3-mL syringe can be attached to the catheter and the syringe plunger removed. A 7.0-mm internal diameter ETT connector can be inserted into the syringe and attached to a breathing circuit or an AMBU bag. As with the jet ventilation system, adequate exhalation must occur to avoid barotraumas.

Retrograde intubation is another approach to secure an airway. A wire is passed via a catheter inserted through the CTM. The wire is angulated cephalad and emerges either through the mouth or nose. The distal end of the wire is secured with a clamp to prevent it from passing through the CTM. The wire can then be threaded into an FOB with a loaded endotracheal tube to facilitate and confirm placement. Conversely, a small endotracheal tube can be guided by the wire into the trachea. Once placed, the wire is removed. In lieu of the wire, an epidural catheter can be passed retrograde through an epidural needle inserted through the CTM.

Difficult Airway Society guidelines suggest performing a cricothyroidotomy utilizing a scalpel, bougie, and small endotracheal tube as the best approach to FONA. Practice simulation of the airway techniques favored in the local care setting is highly recommended so that they are familiar when required in an emergency.

PROBLEMS FOLLOWING INTUBATION

Following apparently successful intubation, several scenarios may develop that require immediate attention. Anesthesia staff *must* confirm that the tube is correctly placed with auscultation of bilateral breath sounds immediately following placement. Measurement of end-tidal CO_2 with a waveform remains the gold standard in this regard, with the caveat that cardiac output must be present for CO_2 production.

Decreases in oxygen saturation can occur following tube placement. This is often secondary to endobronchial intubation, especially in small children and infants. Decreased oxygen saturation perioperatively may be due to inadequate oxygen delivery (oxygen not turned on, patient not ventilated) or to ventilation/perfusion mismatch (almost any form of lung disease). When saturation declines, the patient's chest is auscultated to confirm bilateral breath sounds and listen for wheezes, rhonchi, and rales consistent with lung pathology. The breathing circuit integrity is checked. An intraoperative chest radiograph or point-of-care ultrasound examination may be needed to identify the cause of desaturation. Intraoperative fiberoptic bronchoscopy can also be performed and used to confirm proper tube placement and clear mucous plugs. Bronchodilators and deeper planes of inhalation anesthetics are administered to treat bronchospasm. Obese patients may desaturate secondary to a reduced FRC and atelectasis. Application of positive end-expiratory pressure may improve oxygenation.

Should the end-tidal CO_2 decline suddenly, pulmonary (thrombus) or venous air embolism should be considered. Likewise, other causes of a sudden decline in cardiac output or a leak in the circuit should be considered. A rising end-tidal CO_2 may be secondary to hypoventilation or increased CO_2 production, as occurs with malignant hyperthermia, sepsis, a depleted CO_2 absorber, or breathing circuit malfunction.

Increases in airway pressure may indicate an obstructed or kinked endotracheal tube or reduced pulmonary compliance. The endotracheal tube should be suctioned to confirm that it is patent and the lungs auscultated to assess breath sounds for signs of bronchospasm, pulmonary edema, endobronchial intubation, or pneumothorax. Decreases in airway pressure can occur secondary to leaks in the breathing circuit or inadvertent extubation.

TECHNIQUES OF EXTUBATION

Most often, extubation should be performed when a patient is either deeply anesthetized or awake. In either case, adequate recovery from neuromuscular blocking agents should be established prior to extubation.

Extubation during a light plane of anesthesia (ie, a state between deep and awake) is avoided because of an increased risk of laryngospasm. The distinction between deep and light anesthesia is usually apparent during pharyngeal suctioning: any reaction to suctioning (eg, breath holding, coughing) signals a light plane of anesthesia, whereas no reaction is characteristic of a deep plane. Similarly, eye opening or purposeful movements imply that the patient is sufficiently awake for extubation.

Extubating an awake patient is usually associated with coughing (bucking) on the ETT. This reaction increases the heart rate, central venous pressure, arterial blood pressure, intracranial pressure, intraabdominal pressure, and intraocular pressure. It may also cause wound dehiscence and increased bleeding. The presence of an ETT in an awake asthmatic patient may trigger bronchospasm. Some practitioners attempt to decrease the likelihood of these effects by administering 1.5 mg/kg of intravenous lidocaine 1 to 2 min before suctioning and extubation; however, extubation during deep anesthesia may be preferable in patients who cannot tolerate these effects (provided such patients are not at risk of aspiration or do not have airways that may be difficult to maintain after removal of the ETT).

Regardless of whether the tube is removed when the patient is deeply anesthetized or awake, the patient's pharynx should be thoroughly suctioned before extubation to decrease the potential for aspiration of blood and secretions. In addition, patients should be ventilated with 100% oxygen in case it becomes difficult to establish an airway after the ETT is removed. Just prior to extubation, the ETT is untaped or untied, and its cuff is deflated. The tube is withdrawn in a single smooth motion, and a face mask is applied to deliver oxygen. Oxygen delivery by face mask is maintained during the period of transportation to the postanesthesia care area.

COMPLICATIONS OF LARYNGOSCOPY & INTUBATION

The complications of laryngoscopy and intubation include hypoxia, hypercarbia, dental and airway trauma, tube malpositioning, physiological responses to airway instrumentation, and tube malfunction.

TABLE 19–6 Complications of intubation.

During laryngoscopy and intubation
Malpositioning
Esophageal intubation
Bronchial intubation
Laryngeal cuff position
Airway trauma
Dental damage
Lip, tongue, or mucosal laceration
Sore throat
Dislocated mandible
Retropharyngeal dissection
Physiological reflexes
Hypoxia, hypercarbia
Hypertension, tachycardia
Intracranial hypertension
Intraocular hypertension
Laryngospasm
Tube malfunction
Cuff perforation
While the tube is in place
Malpositioning
Unintentional extubation
Bronchial intubation
Laryngeal cuff position
Airway trauma
Mucosal inflammation and ulceration
Excoriation of nose
Tube malfunction
Fire/explosion
Obstruction
Following extubation
Airway trauma
Edema and stenosis (glottic, subglottic, or tracheal)
Hoarseness (vocal cord granuloma or paralysis)
Laryngeal malfunction and aspiration
Laryngospasm
Negative-pressure pulmonary edema

These complications can occur during laryngoscopy and intubation, while the tube is in place, or following extubation (Table 19–6).

Airway Trauma

Instrumentation with a metal laryngoscope blade and insertion of a stiff ETT often traumatizes delicate airway tissues. Tooth damage is a common cause of (relatively small) malpractice claims against anesthesiologists. Laryngoscopy and intubation can lead to a range of complications from sore throat to tracheal stenosis. Most of these are due to prolonged external pressure on sensitive airway structures. When these pressures exceed the capillary–arteriolar blood pressure (approximately 30 mm Hg), tissue ischemia can lead to a sequence of inflammation, ulceration, granulation, and stenosis. Inflation of an ETT cuff to the minimum pressure that creates a seal during routine positive-pressure ventilation (usually at least 20 mm Hg) reduces tracheal blood flow by 75% at the cuff site. Further cuff inflation or induced hypotension can totally eliminate mucosal blood flow.

Postintubation croup caused by glottic, laryngeal, or tracheal edema is particularly serious in children. The efficacy of corticosteroids (eg, dexamethasone—0.2 mg/kg, up to a maximum of 12 mg) in preventing postextubation airway edema remains controversial, but this approach is often used. Vocal cord paralysis from cuff compression or other trauma to the recurrent laryngeal nerve results in hoarseness and increases the risk of aspiration. The incidence of postoperative hoarseness seems to increase with obesity, multiple intubation attempts, and anesthetics of long duration. Curiously, applying a water-soluble lubricant or a local anesthetic-containing gel to the tip or cuff of the ETT does not decrease the incidence of postoperative sore throat or hoarseness and actually increased the incidence of these complications in some studies. Smaller tubes (size 6.5 in women and size 7.0 in men) are associated with fewer reports of postoperative sore throat. Repeated attempts at laryngoscopy during a difficult intubation may lead to periglottic edema and the inability to ventilate with a face mask, thus turning a difficult situation into a life-threatening one.

Errors of Endotracheal Tube Positioning

6 Unrecognized esophageal intubation can produce catastrophic results. Prevention of this complication depends on direct visualization of the

tip of the ETT passing through the vocal cords, careful auscultation for the presence of bilateral breath sounds, the absence of gastric gurgling detected by auscultation of the stomach while ventilating through the ETT, detection of CO_2 in exhaled gas (the most reliable automated method), chest radiography, airway ultrasonography, or the use of an FOB.

Even though it is confirmed that the tube is in the trachea, it may not be correctly positioned. Overly "deep" insertion usually results in intubation of the right mainstem bronchus because the right bronchus forms a less acute angle with the trachea than the left
7 bronchus. Clues to the diagnosis of bronchial intubation include unilateral breath sounds, unexpected hypoxia with pulse oximetry (unreliable with high inspired oxygen concentrations), inability to palpate the ETT cuff in the sternal notch during cuff inflation, and decreased breathing-bag compliance (high peak inspiratory pressures).

In contrast, inadequate insertion depth will position the cuff in the larynx, predisposing the patient to laryngeal trauma and the risk of the ETT tip moving cephalad into the hypopharynx. Inadequate depth of insertion can be detected by palpating the cuff over the thyroid cartilage. Because no one technique protects against all possibilities for misplacing an ETT, minimal testing should include chest auscultation, routine capnography, and occasionally cuff palpation.

If the patient is repositioned, tube placement must be reconfirmed. Neck extension or lateral rotation most often moves an ETT away from the carina, whereas neck flexion most often moves the tube toward the carina.

At no time should excessive force be employed during intubation. Esophageal intubations can result in esophageal rupture and mediastinitis. Mediastinitis presents as severe sore throat, fever, sepsis, and subcutaneous air, often manifesting as crepitus. Early intervention is necessary to avoid mortality. If esophageal perforation is suspected, consultation with an otolaryngologist or thoracic surgeon is recommended. Vocal cord injury can likewise result from repeated, forceful attempts at endotracheal intubation or excessive pressure of the cuff against the underside of the vocal cords.

Physiological Responses to Airway Instrumentation

Laryngoscopy and tracheal intubation violate the patient's protective airway reflexes and predictably lead to hypertension and tachycardia when performed under "light" planes of general anesthesia. The insertion of an LMA is typically associated with less hemodynamic change. Hemodynamic changes can be attenuated by intravenous administration of propofol, lidocaine, opioids, or β-blockers, or deeper planes of inhalation anesthesia shortly before laryngoscopy. Hypotensive agents, including sodium nitroprusside, nitroglycerin, esmolol, nicardipine, and clevidipine, can attenuate the transient hypertensive response associated with laryngoscopy and intubation. Cardiac arrhythmias—particularly ventricular premature beats—sometimes occur during intubation and may indicate light anesthesia.

Laryngospasm is a forceful involuntary spasm of the laryngeal musculature caused by sensory stimulation of the superior laryngeal nerve. Triggering stimuli include pharyngeal secretions or passing an ETT through the larynx during extubation. Laryngospasm is usually prevented by extubating patients either deeply asleep or fully awake, but it can occur—albeit rarely—in an awake patient. Treatment of laryngospasm includes providing gentle positive-pressure ventilation with an anesthesia bag and mask using 100% oxygen or administering intravenous lidocaine (1–1.5 mg/kg). If laryngospasm persists and hypoxia develops, small doses of succinylcholine (0.25–0.5 mg/kg) may be required (perhaps in combination with small doses of propofol or another anesthetic) to relax the laryngeal muscles
8 and allow controlled ventilation. The large negative intrathoracic pressures generated by a struggling patient during laryngospasm can lead to negative-pressure pulmonary edema, particularly in fit, healthy patients.

Whereas laryngospasm may result from an abnormally sensitive reflex, aspiration can result from depression of laryngeal reflexes following prolonged intubation and general anesthesia.

Bronchospasm is another reflex response to intubation and is most common in asthmatic patients. Bronchospasm can sometimes be a clue to endobronchial intubation. Other pathophysiological effects of intubation include increased intracranial and intraocular pressures.

Endotracheal Tube Malfunction

ETTs do not always function as intended. Polyvinyl chloride tubes may be ignited by cautery or laser in an oxygen/nitrous oxide–enriched environment. Valve or cuff damage is not unusual and should be excluded by careful inspection of the ETT prior to insertion. Obstruction of the ETT can result from kinking, foreign body aspiration, or thick or inspissated secretions in the lumen.

ENDOTRACHEAL INTUBATION OF THE PATIENT WITH COVID-19

At the time of this writing, Covid-19 continues to challenge anesthesia and critical care workers globally. Intubation as an aerosol-generating procedure places anesthesia staff and others in the immediate vicinity at risk for infection. Various organizations continue to provide recommendations for effective infection control during intubation. Proper donning and doffing of personal protective equipment is critical and should be practiced well in advance of the need to actually intubate a patient with Covid-19. Initial recommendations aimed at early intubation appear to have given way to greater use of supplemental oxygen and awake proning in patients with respiratory compromise, potentially reducing the number of patients requiring intubation. Early guidelines suggested using video rather than direct laryngoscopy, avoiding awake intubation when possible, and using rapid sequence intubation to avoid bag-mask ventilation. These guidelines will almost certainly evolve. Readers should visit their country's official disease control agency website for current guidance.

CASE DISCUSSION

Evaluation & Management of a Difficult Airway

A 47-year-old man with a long history of tobacco and alcohol use presents for emergency drainage of a right-sided submandibular abscess.

What are some important anesthetic considerations during the preoperative evaluation of a patient with an abnormal airway?

Induction of general anesthesia followed by direct laryngoscopy and oral intubation is dangerous, if not impossible, in several situations (Table 19–7). To determine the optimal intubation technique, the anesthesia provider must elicit an airway history and carefully examine the patient's head and neck. Any available prior anesthesia records should be reviewed for previous problems in airway management. If a facial deformity is severe enough to preclude a good

TABLE 19–7 Conditions associated with difficult intubations.

Tumors
Cystic hygroma
Hemangioma
Hematoma[1]
Infections
Submandibular abscess
Peritonsillar abscess
Epiglottitis
Congenital anomalies
Pierre Robin syndrome
Treacher Collins syndrome
Laryngeal atresia
Goldenhar syndrome
Craniofacial dysostosis
Foreign body
Trauma
Laryngeal fracture
Mandibular or maxillary fracture
Inhalation burn
Cervical spine injury
Obesity
Inadequate neck extension
Rheumatoid arthritis[2]
Ankylosing spondylitis
Halo traction
Anatomic variations
Micrognathia
Prognathism
Large tongue
Arched palate
Short neck
Prominent upper incisors

[1]Can occur postoperatively in patients who have had any neck surgery.
[2]Also affects arytenoids, making them immobile.

mask seal, positive-pressure ventilation may be impossible. Furthermore, patients with hypopharyngeal disease are more dependent on awake muscle tone to maintain airway patency. These two groups of patients should generally not be allowed to become apneic—including induction of anesthesia, sedation, or muscle paralysis—until their airway is secured.

If there is an abnormal limitation of the temporomandibular joint that may not improve with muscle paralysis, a nasal approach with an FOB should be considered. Infection confined to the floor of the mouth usually does not preclude nasal intubation. If the hypopharynx is involved to the level of the hyoid bone, however, any translaryngeal attempt will be difficult. Other clues to a potentially difficult laryngoscopy include limited neck extension (<35°), a distance between the tip of the patient's mandible and hyoid bone of less than 7 cm, a sternomental distance of less than 12.5 cm with the head fully extended and the mouth closed, and a poorly visualized uvula during voluntary tongue protrusion. It must be stressed that no airway examination technique is foolproof and that signs of a difficult airway may be subtle. The anesthesia provider must always be prepared for unanticipated difficulties.

The anesthesia provider should also evaluate the patient for signs of airway obstruction (eg, chest retraction, stridor) and hypoxia (agitation, restlessness, anxiety, lethargy). Aspiration pneumonia is more likely if the patient has recently eaten or if pus is draining from an abscess into the mouth. In either case, techniques that ablate laryngeal reflexes (eg, topical anesthesia) should be avoided.

Cervical trauma or disease is a factor that should be evaluated prior to direct laryngoscopy. Cervical arthritis or previous cervical fusion may make it difficult to position the head in the sniffing position. Such patients are candidates for fiberoptic bronchoscopy to secure the airway, as discussed previously. Trauma patients with unstable necks or those whose neck has not yet been "cleared" are also candidates for fiberoptic bronchoscopic tracheal intubation. Alternatively, laryngoscopy with in-line stabilization can be performed (Figure 19–37).

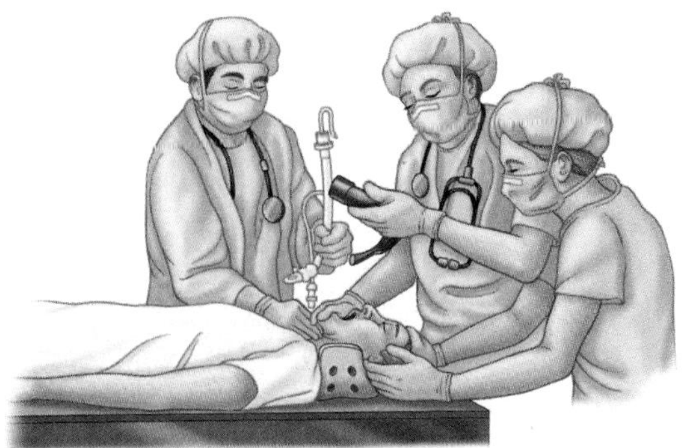

FIGURE 19–37 Technique for airway management of a patient with suspected spinal cord injury. One individual holds the head firmly with the patient on a backboard, with the cervical collar left alone if in place, ensuring that neither the head nor neck moves with direct laryngoscopy. A second person applies cricoid pressure, and the third performs laryngoscopy and intubation.

In the case under discussion, physical examination reveals swelling below the mandible and trismus that limits the patient's ability to open his mouth. Mask fit does not seem to be impaired. CT of the head and neck suggests that the infection has spread along tissue planes and is displacing the airway to the left.

Which intubation technique is indicated?

Oral and nasal intubations can be performed in awake patients. Whether the patient is awake or asleep or whether intubation is to be oral or nasal, it can be performed with direct laryngoscopy, fiberoptic visualization, or video laryngoscopy techniques.

Intubation may be difficult in this patient, however, because of limited mouth opening and distortion/displacement of the glottis. Induction of anesthesia should, therefore, be delayed until after the airway has been secured. Useful alternatives include awake fiberoptic intubation, awake video laryngoscopy, or awake use of optical stylets. The final decision depends on the availability of equipment and the experiences and preferences of the anesthesia caregivers.

Regardless of which alternative is chosen, an emergency surgical airway may be necessary. An experienced team, including a surgeon, should be in the operating room, and all necessary equipment should be available and unwrapped. The neck can be prepped and draped.

What premedication would be appropriate for this patient?

Any loss of consciousness or interference with airway reflexes could result in airway obstruction or aspiration. Glycopyrrolate would be a good choice of premedication because it minimizes upper airway secretions without crossing the blood–brain barrier. Parenteral sedatives should be very carefully titrated. Dexmedetomidine and ketamine could be used as sedatives and preserve respiratory effort. Psychological preparation of the patient, including explaining each step planned in securing the airway, usually improves patient cooperation.

What nerve blocks could be helpful during an awake intubation?

The lingual and some pharyngeal branches of the glossopharyngeal nerve that provide sensation to the posterior third of the tongue and oropharynx are easily blocked by bilateral injection of 2 mL of local anesthetic into the base of the palatoglossal arch (also known as the *anterior tonsillar pillar*) with a 25-gauge spinal needle (Figure 19–38).

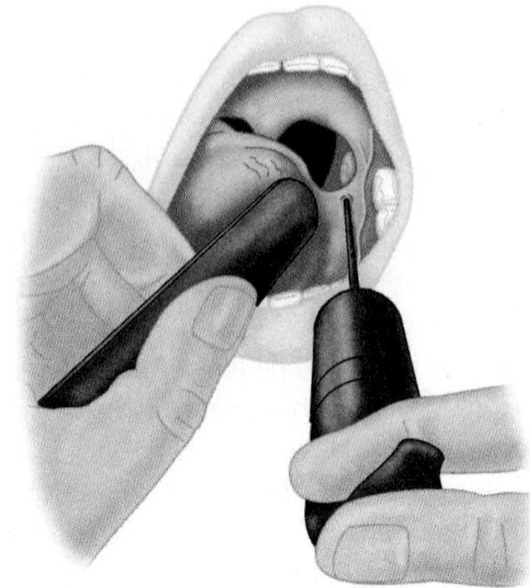

FIGURE 19–38 Nerve block. While the tongue is laterally retracted with a tongue blade, the base of the palatoglossal arch is infiltrated with a local anesthetic to block the lingual and pharyngeal branches of the glossopharyngeal nerve. Note that the lingual branches of the glossopharyngeal nerve are not the same as the lingual nerve, which is a branch of the trigeminal nerve.

Bilateral **superior laryngeal nerve blocks** and a transtracheal block would anesthetize the airway below the epiglottis (Figure 19–39). The hyoid bone is located, and 3 mL of 2% lidocaine is infiltrated 1 cm below each greater cornu, where the internal branch of the superior laryngeal nerves penetrates the thyrohyoid membrane.

A transtracheal block is performed by identifying and penetrating the CTM while the neck is extended. After confirmation of an intratracheal position by aspiration of air, 4 mL of 4% lidocaine is injected into the trachea at end expiration. A deep inhalation and cough immediately following injection distribute the anesthetic throughout the trachea. Although these blocks may allow the awake patient to tolerate intubation better, they also obtund protective cough reflexes, depress the swallowing reflex, and increase the risk of aspiration. Topical anesthesia of the pharynx may induce a transient obstruction from the loss of reflex regulation of airway caliber at the level of the glottis, though this is uncommon.

A simple alternative to all of these is to allow the patient to breath atomized lidocaine for several

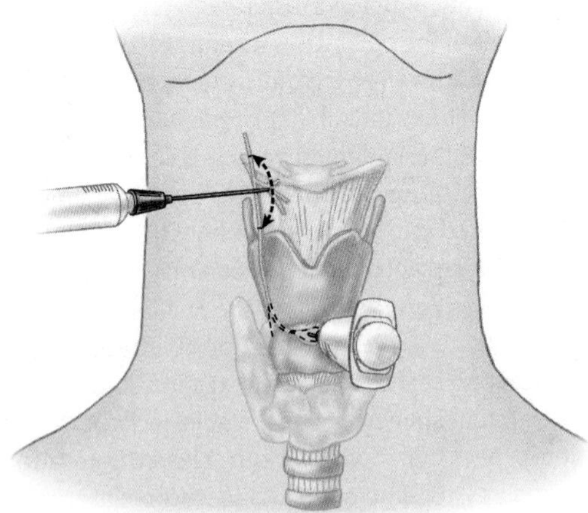

FIGURE 19–39 Superior laryngeal nerve block and transtracheal block.

minutes prior to instrumentation, as is typically done for outpatient bronchoscopy.

Because of this patient's increased risk for aspiration, local anesthesia might best be limited to the nasal passages. Four percent cocaine has no advantages compared with a mixture of 4% lidocaine and 0.25% phenylephrine and can cause cardiovascular side effects. The maximum safe dose of local anesthetic must be calculated and not exceeded. Local anesthetic is applied to the nasal mucosa with cotton-tipped applicators until a nasal airway that has been lubricated with lidocaine jelly can be placed into the naris with minimal discomfort. Benzocaine spray is frequently used to topicalize the airway but can produce methemoglobinemia, and for this reason, we prefer lidocaine.

Why is it necessary to be prepared for a surgical airway?

Laryngospasm is always a potential complication of intubation in the nonparalyzed patient, even if the patient remains awake. Laryngospasm may make positive-pressure mask ventilation impossible. If succinylcholine is administered to break the spasm, the consequent relaxation of pharyngeal muscles may lead to upper airway obstruction and continued inability to ventilate. In this situation, an emergency cricothyrotomy may be lifesaving.

What are some alternative techniques that might be successful?

Other possible strategies include the retrograde passage of a long guidewire or epidural catheter through a needle inserted across the CTM. The catheter is guided cephalad into the pharynx and out through the nose or mouth. An ETT is passed over the catheter, which is withdrawn after the tube has entered the larynx. Variations of this technique include passing the retrograde wire through the suction port of a flexible FOB or the lumen of a reintubation stylet that has been preloaded with an ETT. These thicker shafts help the ETT negotiate the bend into the larynx more easily. Obviously, a vast array of specialized airway equipment exists and must be readily available for the management of difficult airways (Table 19–8). Either of these techniques would have been difficult in the patient described in this case because of the swelling and anatomic distortion of the neck that can accompany a submandibular abscess. In cases such as this one, where unusual airway difficulty is noted in advance, it is extremely important to have skilled assistance immediately available.

TABLE 19–8 Suggested contents of the portable storage unit for difficult airway management.

- Rigid laryngoscope blades of alternate design and size from those routinely used.
- Endotracheal tubes (ETTs) of assorted size.
- ETT guides. Examples include (but are not limited to) semirigid stylets with or without a hollow core for jet ventilation, light wands, and forceps designed to manipulate the distal portion of the ETT.
- Laryngeal mask airways of assorted sizes.
- Fiberoptic intubation equipment and assorted video and indirect laryngoscopes.
- Retrograde intubation equipment.
- At least one device suitable for emergency nonsurgical airway ventilation. Examples include (but are not limited to) transtracheal jet ventilator, hollow jet ventilation stylet, and Combitube.
- Equipment suitable for emergency surgical airway access (eg, cricothyrotomy).
- An exhaled carbon dioxide detector.

[1]The items listed in this table are suggestions. The contents of the portable storage unit should be customized to meet the specific needs, preferences, and skills of the practitioner and health care facility.

Modified with permission from the American Society of Anesthesiologists Task Force on Management of the Difficult Airway. Practice guidelines for management of the difficult airway: A report by the American Society of Anesthesiologists Task Force on Management of the Difficult Airway. *Anesthesiology.* 2003 May;98(5):1269–1277.

What are some approaches when the airway is unexpectedly difficult?

The unexpected difficult airway can present both in elective surgical patients and also in emergency intubations in intensive care units, the emergency department, or general hospital wards. Should video laryngoscopy fail even after attempts with an intubating bougie, an intubating LMA should be attempted (Figure 19–40). If ventilation is adequate, an FOB can be loaded with an ETT and passed through the LMA into the trachea. Correct tube position is confirmed by visualization of the carina.

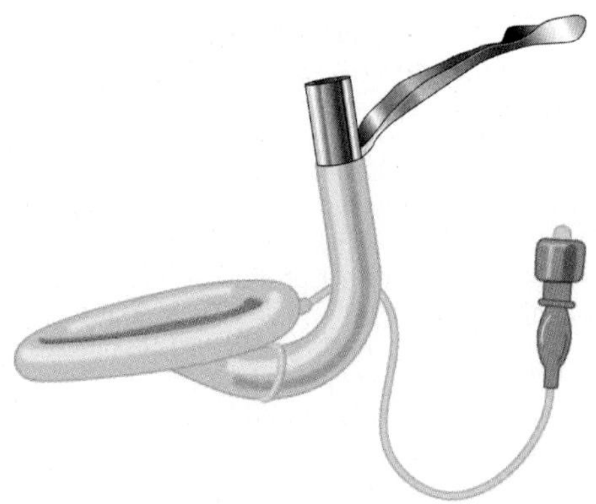

FIGURE 19–40 Intubating laryngeal mask airway.

GUIDELINES

Ahmad I, El-Boghdadly K, Bhagrath R, et al. Difficult Airway Society guidelines for awake tracheal intubation (ATI) in adults. *Anaesthesia*. 2020;75:509.

Apfelbaum J, Hagberg C, Caplan RA, et al. Practice guidelines for management of the difficult airway: an updated report by the American Society of Anesthesiologists Task Force on the Management of the Difficult Airway. *Anesthesiology*. 2013;118:1.

Frerk C, Mitchell V, McNarry A, et al. Difficult Airway Society 2015 guidelines for management of unanticipated difficult intubation in adults. *Br J Anaesth*. 2015;115:827.

Orser BA. Recommendations for Endotracheal Intubation of COVID-19 Patients. *Anesth Analg*. 2020;130:1109.

SUGGESTED READINGS

Ansari U, Malhas L, Mendonca C. Role of ultrasound in emergency front of neck access: a case report and review of literature. *A Pract*. 2019;13:382.

Aziz M, Healy D, Kheterpal S, et al. Routine clinical practice effectiveness of the GlideScope in difficult airway management. *Anesthesiology*. 2011;114:34.

Bercker S, Schmidbauer W, Volk T, et al. A comparison of seal in seven supraglottic airway devices using a cadaver model of elevated esophageal pressure. *Anesth Analg*. 2008;106:445.

Cook TM. A new practical classification of laryngeal view. *Anaesthesia*. 2000;55:274.

Cooper R. Complications associated with the use of the GlideScope video laryngoscope. *Can J Anesth*. 2007;54:54.

Detsky ME, Jivraj N, Adhikari NK, et al. Will this patient be difficult to intubate?: the rational clinical examination systematic review. *JAMA*. 2019;321:493.

Edelman D, Perkins E, Brewster D. Difficult airway management algorithms: a directed review. *Anaesthesia*. 2019;4:1175.

El-Orbany M, Woehlck H, Ramez Salem M. Head and neck position for direct laryngoscopy. *Anesth Analg*. 2011;113:103.

Hagberg C, Johnson S, Pillai D. Effective use of the esophageal tracheal Combitube TN following severe burn injury. *J Clin Anesth*. 2003;15:463.

Houston G, Bourke P, Wilson G, et al. Bonfils intubating fiberscope in normal paediatric airways. *Br J Anaesth*. 2010;105:546.

Kaplan M, Ward D, Hagberg C, et al. Seeing is believing: the importance of video laryngoscopy in teaching and in managing the difficult airway. *Surg Endosc*. 2006;20:S479.

Kristensen MS. Ultrasonography in the management of the airway. *Acta Anaesthesiol Scand*. 2011;55:1155.

Langeron O, Masso E, Huraux C, et al. Prediction of difficult mask ventilation. *Anesthesiology*. 2000;92:1217.

Lewis SR, Butler AR, Parker J, Cook TM, Smith AF. Videolaryngoscopy versus direct laryngoscopy for adult patients requiring tracheal intubation. *Cochrane Database Syst Rev*. 2016;11:CD011136.

Maharaj C, Costello J, McDonnell J, et al. The Airtraq as a rescue airway device following failed direct laryngoscopy: a case series. *Anaesthesia*. 2007;67:598.

Malik M, Maharaj C, Harte B, et al. Comparison of Macintosh, Trueview EVO2, GlideScope, and Airwayscope laryngoscope use in patients with cervical spine immobilization. *Br J Anaesth*. 2008;101:723.

Malik M, Subramanian R, Maharaj C, et al. Randomized controlled trial of the Pentax AWS, GlideScope, and Macintosh laryngoscopes in predicted difficult intubations. *Br J Anaesth*. 2009;103:761.

McNarry AF, Patel A. The evolution of airway management—new concepts and conflicts with traditional practice. *Br J Anaesth*. 2017;119(suppl_1):i154.

Mushambi MC, Athanassoglou V, Kinsella SM. Anticipated difficult airway during obstetric general anaesthesia: narrative literature review and management recommendations. *Anaesthesia*. 2020;75:945.

Noppens R, Möbus S, Heid F, et al. Use of the McGrath Series 5 videolaryngoscope after failed direct laryngoscopy. *Anaesthesia*. 2010;65:716.

Osman A, Sum KM. Role of upper airway ultrasound in airway management. *J Intensive Care*. 2016;4:52.

Patel A, Nouraei SAR. Transnasal humidified rapid insufflation ventilatory exchange (THRIVE): a physiological method of increasing apnoea time in patients with difficult airways. *Anaesthesia.* 2015,70:323.

Robitaille A, Williams S, Trembaly M, et al. Cervical spine motion during tracheal intubation with manual in-line stabilization direct laryngoscopy versus GlideScope video laryngoscopy. *Anesth Analg.* 2008;106:935.

Roth D, Pace NL, Lee A, et al. Airway physical examination tests for detection of difficult airway management in apparently normal adult patients. *Cochrane Database Syst Rev.* 2018;5:CD008874.

Russi C, Hartley M, Buresh C. A pilot study of the King LT supralaryngeal airway use in a rural Iowa EMS system. *Int J Emerg Med.* 2008;1:135.

Tanoubi I, Drolet P, Donati F. Optimizing preoxygenation in adults. *Can J Anesth.* 2009;56:449.

Ting J. Temporomandibular joint dislocation after use of a laryngeal mask airway. *Anaesthesia.* 2006;61:190.

Treki AA, Straker T. Limitations of the videolaryngoscope: an anesthetic management reality. *Int Anesthesiol Clin.* 2017;55:97.

Windpassinger M, Plattner O, Gemeiner J, et al. Pharyngeal oxygen insufflation during AirTraq laryngoscopy slows arterial desaturation in infants. *Anesth Analg.* 2016;122:1153.

CHAPTER 20

Cardiovascular Physiology & Anesthesia

KEY CONCEPTS

1. In contrast to action potentials in axons, the spike in cardiac action potentials is followed by a plateau phase that lasts 0.2 to 0.3 s. Whereas the action potential for skeletal muscle and nerves is due to the abrupt opening of voltage-gated sodium channels in the cell membrane, in cardiac muscle, it is initiated by voltage-gated sodium channels (the spike) and maintained by voltage-gated calcium channels (the plateau).

2. Potent inhalational agents depress sinoatrial (SA) node automaticity. These agents seem to have only modest direct effects on the atrioventricular (AV) node, prolonging conduction time and increasing refractoriness. This combination of effects likely explains the frequent occurrence of junctional tachycardia when an anticholinergic agent is administered for sinus bradycardia during inhalation anesthesia; junctional pacemakers are accelerated more than those in the SA node.

3. Studies suggest that volatile anesthetics depress cardiac contractility by decreasing the entry of Ca^{2+} into cells during depolarization (affecting T- and L-type calcium channels), altering the kinetics of Ca^{2+} release and uptake into the sarcoplasmic reticulum, and decreasing the sensitivity of contractile proteins to calcium.

4. Because the normal cardiac index (CI) has a wide range, it is a relatively insensitive measurement of ventricular performance. Abnormalities in CI therefore usually reflect gross ventricular impairment.

5. In the absence of hypoxia or severe anemia, measurement of mixed venous oxygen tension (or saturation) provides an estimate of the adequacy of cardiac output.

6. Patients with reduced ventricular compliance are most affected by the loss of a normally timed atrial systole.

7. Cardiac output in patients with marked right or left ventricular impairment is very sensitive to acute increases in afterload.

8. The ventricular ejection fraction, the fraction of the end-diastolic ventricular volume ejected, is the most commonly used clinical measurement of systolic function.

9. Left ventricular diastolic function can be assessed clinically by Doppler echocardiography in a transthoracic or transesophageal examination.

10. Because the endocardium is subjected to the greatest intramural pressures during systole, it tends to be most vulnerable to ischemia during decreases in coronary perfusion pressure.

11. The failing heart becomes increasingly dependent on circulating catecholamines. Abrupt withdrawal in sympathetic outflow or decreases in circulating catecholamine levels, such as can occur following induction of anesthesia, may lead to acute cardiac decompensation.

Anesthesiologists must have a thorough understanding of cardiovascular physiology. Anesthetic successes and failures are often directly related to the skill of the practitioner in manipulating cardiovascular physiology. This chapter reviews the physiology of the heart and the systemic circulation and the pathophysiology of heart failure.

The circulatory system consists of the heart, blood vessels, and blood. Its function is to deliver oxygen and nutrients to the tissues and carry away the products of metabolism. The heart propels blood through two vascular systems arranged in series. In the normally low-pressure pulmonary circulation, venous blood flows past the alveolar–capillary membrane, where it takes up oxygen and releases carbon dioxide (CO_2). In the high-pressure systemic circulation, oxygenated arterial blood is pumped to tissues, and the byproducts of metabolism are taken up for elimination by the lungs, kidneys, or liver.

The Heart

The heart can be functionally divided into right and left pumps, each consisting of an atrium and a ventricle. The atria serve as both conduits and priming pumps, whereas the ventricles act as the major pumping chambers. The right ventricle receives systemic venous (deoxygenated) blood and pumps it into the pulmonary circulation, whereas the left ventricle receives pulmonary venous (oxygenated) blood and pumps it into the systemic circulation. Four valves normally ensure unidirectional flow through each chamber. The pumping action of the heart arises from a complex series of electrical and mechanical events. Electrical events precede mechanical ones.

The heart consists of specialized striated muscle in a connective tissue skeleton. Cardiac muscle can be divided into atrial, ventricular, and specialized pacemaker and conducting cells. Electrical activity readily spreads from one atrium to another and from one ventricle to another via specialized conduction pathways. The normal absence of direct connections between the atria and ventricles except through the atrioventricular (AV) node delays ventricular depolarization, enabling the atria to prime the ventricles. Serial low-resistance connections (intercalated disks) between individual myocardial cells allow the rapid and orderly spread of depolarization in each pumping chamber.

CARDIAC ACTION POTENTIALS

At rest, the myocardial cell membrane is minimally permeable to K^+ but almost impermeable to Na^+. Relative to extracellular concentrations, intracellular Na^+ concentration is kept low, and intracellular K^+ concentration is kept high. An electrogenic, membrane-bound Na^+–K^+-adenosine triphosphatase (ATPase) consumes ATP while pumping 2 K^+ intracellularly for every 3 Na^+ extracellularly. The movement of K^+ out of the cell and down its concentration gradient results in a further loss of positive charges from inside the cell. An electrical potential is established across the cell membrane, with the inside of the cell negative with respect to the extracellular environment, because anions do not accompany K^+. Thus, the resting membrane potential represents the balance between two opposing forces: the movement of K^+ down its concentration gradient and the electrical attraction of the negatively charged intracellular space for the positively charged K^+. The relative impermeability of the membrane to calcium also maintains a high extracellular to cytoplasmic calcium gradient.

The normal ventricular cell resting membrane potential is −80 to −90 mV. As with other excitable tissues (nerve, skeletal muscle, and some endocrine cells), when the cell membrane potential becomes less negative and reaches a threshold value, an action potential (depolarization) develops (Figure 20–1 and Table 20–1). The action potential transiently increases the membrane potential of the
1 myocardial cell to +20 mV. In contrast to axonal action potentials, cardiac action potentials include a plateau phase that lasts 0.2 to 0.3 s. Whereas the action potential for skeletal muscle and nerves is due exclusively to the opening of voltage-gated sodium channels, in cardiac muscle, the action potential is initiated by voltage-gated sodium channels (the spike) and maintained primarily by voltage-gated calcium channels (the plateau). In neurons and cardiac cells, voltage-gated sodium channels

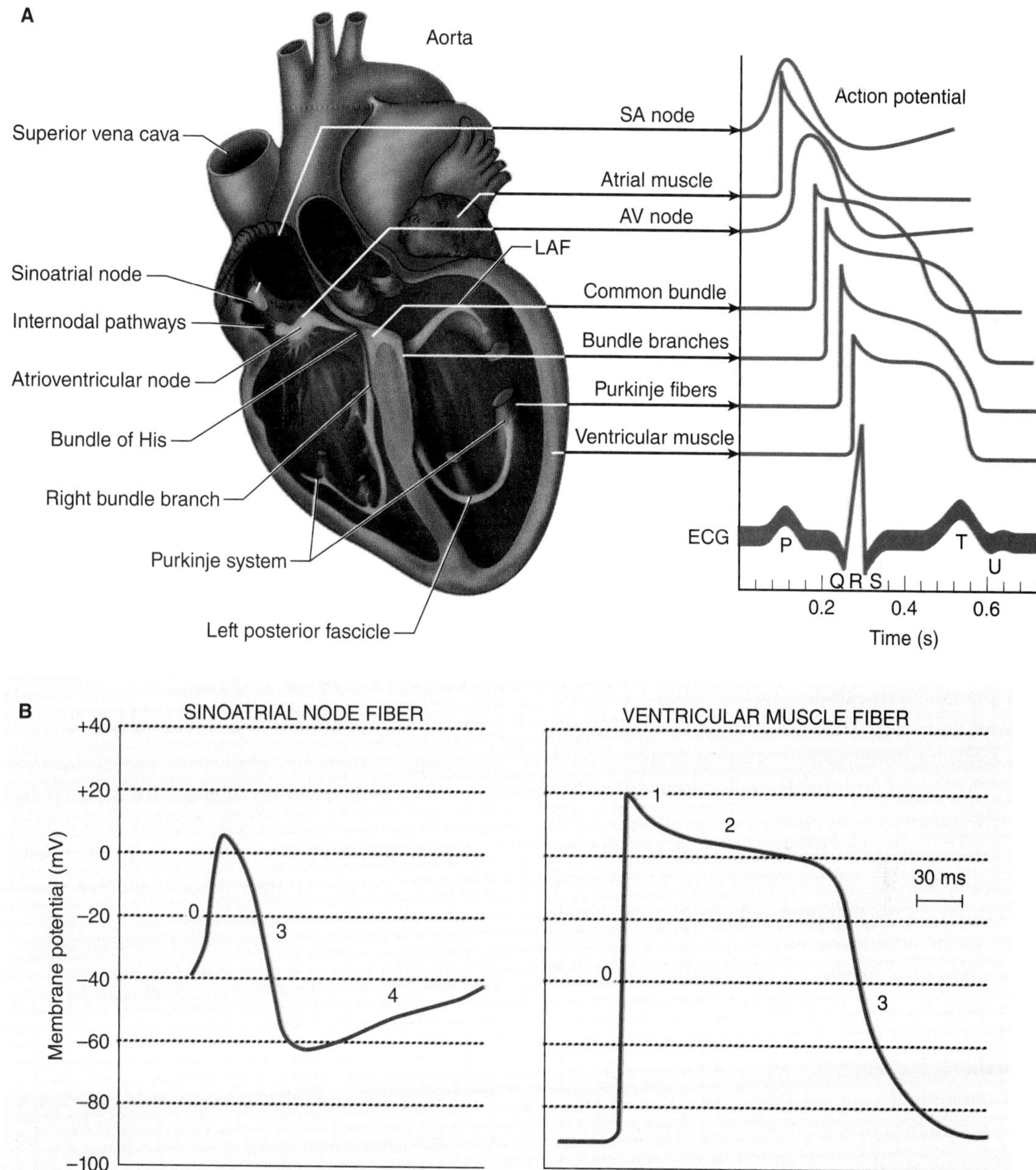

FIGURE 20–1 Cardiac action potentials. **A**: Note the characteristic contours of action potentials recorded from different parts of the heart. AV, atrioventricular; ECG, electrocardiogram; LAF, left anterior fascicle. **B**: Pacemaker cells in the sinoatrial (SA) node lack the same distinct phases as atrial and ventricular muscle cells and display prominent spontaneous diastolic depolarization. See Table 20–1 for an explanation of the different phases of the action potential. (Modified with permission from Barrett KE. *Ganong's Review of Medical Physiology,* 24th ed. New York, NY: McGraw Hill; 2012.)

TABLE 20–1 Cardiac action potential.

Phase	Name	Event	Cellular Ion Movement
0	Upstroke	Activation (opening) of voltage-gated Na^+ channels	Na^+ entry and decreased permeability to K^+
1	Early rapid repolarization	Inactivation of Na^+ channel and transient increase in K^+ permeability	K^+ out (I_{To})
2	Plateau	Activation of slow calcium channels	Ca^{2+} entry
3	Final repolarization	Inactivation of calcium channels and increased permeability to K^+	K^+ out
4	Resting potential	Normal permeability restored (atrial and ventricular cells)	Na^+–K^+-ATPase pumps K^+ in and Na^+ out
	Diastolic repolarization	Intrinsic slow leakage of Ca^{2+} into cells that spontaneously depolarize	Ca^{2+} in

inactivate and cease to conduct within milliseconds of opening. In pacemaker cells, depolarization is initiated by voltage-gated calcium channels rather than by sodium channels. Subsequent termination of calcium channel permeability and activation of several forms of voltage-gated potassium channels restores the membrane potential to its resting value.

Following depolarization, the cells are temporarily refractory to depolarizing stimuli until "phase 4." The *absolute refractory period* is the minimum interval between two maximal stimuli that will result in an action potential. The *relative refractory period* is the additional time beyond the absolute refractory period in which a maximal stimulus, but not a stimulus of normal intensity, will produce a depolarization.

Table 20–2 lists some of the multiple types of ion channels in the cardiac muscle membrane. Some are activated by a change in cell membrane voltage, whereas others open only when bound by ligands. T-type (transient) voltage-gated calcium channels play a role in phase 0 of depolarization. (A more modern nomenclature for voltage-gated calcium channels—Ca_{v1}, Ca_{v2}, Ca_{v3}—is creeping into the scientific literature but remains uncommon in clinical usage.) During the plateau phase (phase 2), Ca^{2+} inflow occurs through slow L-type (long-lasting), voltage-gated calcium channels. Multiple potassium channel forms contribute to repolarization, and a full discussion of cardiac electrophysiology is beyond the focus of this textbook.

INITIATION & CONDUCTION OF THE CARDIAC IMPULSE

The cardiac impulse normally originates in the sinoatrial (SA) node, a group of specialized pacemaker cells in the sulcus terminalis, located at the posterior junction of the right atrium and the superior vena cava. The slow influx of Na^+ through so-called

TABLE 20–2 Cardiac ion channels.

Voltage-gated channels
Na^+
T Ca^{2+}
L Ca^{2+}
K^+
Transient outward
Inward rectifying
Slow (delayed) rectifying
Ligand-gated K^+ channels
Ca^{2+} activated
Na^+ activated
ATP sensitive
Acetylcholine activated
Arachidonic acid activated

ATP, adenosine triphosphate.

Reproduced with permission from Ganong WF. *Review of Medical Physiology*, 21st ed. New York, NY: McGraw Hill; 2003.

hyperpolarization-activated cyclic nucleotide–gated (HCN) channels results in a less negative resting membrane potential (–50 to –60 mV). This has three important consequences: near-constant inactivation of most voltage-gated sodium channels, an action potential that arises primarily from ion movement across the slow calcium channels and with a threshold of –40 mV, and regular spontaneous depolarizations. During each cycle, Na^+ ions passing through HCN channels cause the membrane potential to become progressively less negative; when the threshold potential is reached, calcium channels open, and an action potential develops. Inactivation of L-type calcium channels and activation of potassium channels return the cells in the SA node to their normal resting membrane potential.

The impulse generated at the SA node is normally rapidly conducted across the right atrium, and specialized atrial fibers speed up conduction to both the left atrium and the AV node. The AV node is located in the septal wall of the right atrium, just anterior to the opening of the coronary sinus and above the insertion of the septal leaflet of the tricuspid valve. The normally slower rate of spontaneous depolarization in AV junctional areas (40–60 times/min) allows the faster SA node to control heart rate. Any factor that decreases the rate of SA node depolarization or increases the automaticity of AV junctional areas allows the junctional areas to function as the pacemaker for the heart.

Impulses from the SA node normally arrive at the AV node with a delay of about 0.04 s and "depart" after another 0.11 s. This delay is the result of the slowly conducting small fibers within the AV node that depend on L-type calcium channels for propagation of the action potential. In contrast, conduction of the impulse between adjoining cells in the atria and in the ventricles is due primarily to the activation of sodium channels. The lower fibers of the AV node combine to form the common bundle of His. This specialized group of fibers passes into the interventricular septum before dividing into left and right branches to form the complex network of Purkinje fibers that depolarize both ventricles. In sharp contrast to AV nodal tissue, His–Purkinje fibers have the fastest conduction velocities in the heart, resulting in nearly simultaneous depolarization of the entire endocardium of both ventricles (normally within 0.03 s). Synchronized depolarization of the lateral and septal walls of the left ventricle promotes effective ventricular contraction. When synchronized contraction of the septal and lateral walls is impaired (eg, in patients with heart failure), ventricular function may be improved by biventricular pacing and cardiac resynchronization therapy. The spread of the impulse from the endocardium to the epicardium through ventricular muscle requires an additional 0.03 s. Thus, an impulse arising from the SA node normally requires less than 0.2 s to depolarize the entire heart.

2 Potent inhaled anesthetics depress SA node automaticity. These agents seem to have only modest direct effects on the AV node, prolonging conduction time and increasing refractoriness. This combination of effects likely explains the occurrence of junctional tachycardia when an anticholinergic is administered for sinus bradycardia during inhalation anesthesia; junctional pacemakers are accelerated more than those in the SA node. The electrophysiological effects of volatile agents on Purkinje fibers and ventricular muscle are complex. Both antiarrhythmic and arrhythmogenic properties are described. The former may be due to direct depression of Ca^{2+} influxes, whereas the latter generally involves potentiation of catecholamines, especially with the now seldom-used halothane. Intravenous induction agents have limited electrophysiological effects in usual clinical doses. Opioids, particularly fentanyl and sufentanil, can depress cardiac conduction, increasing the time of AV node conduction and the refractory period and prolonging the duration of the Purkinje fiber action potential.

Local anesthetics have important electrophysiological effects on the heart at blood concentrations that are generally associated with systemic toxicity. In the case of lidocaine, electrophysiological effects at low blood concentrations can be therapeutic. At increased blood concentrations, local anesthetics depress conduction; at extremely high concentrations, they also depress the SA node. The most potent local anesthetics—bupivacaine, etidocaine, and to a lesser degree, ropivacaine—seem to have the most potent effects on the heart, particularly on Purkinje fibers and ventricular muscle. Bupivacaine, like all local anesthetics, preferentially binds open or inactivated sodium channels. Bupivacaine dissociates from them more slowly than less toxic agents. It can cause profound sinus bradycardia and sinus node arrest and malignant ventricular arrhythmias; furthermore, it can depress left ventricular contractility. Twenty percent lipid emulsions have been used to treat local anesthetic cardiac toxicity. The mechanisms of action of this therapy are unclear, though most likely the lipid serves as a reservoir for circulating bupivacaine, decreasing the amount of bupivacaine in the myocardium.

The clinically used calcium channel blockers are organic compounds that block Ca^{2+} influx through L-type but not T-type channels. In a manner reminiscent of local anesthetics and sodium channels, agents such as verapamil and, to a lesser extent, diltiazem preferentially bind the calcium channel in its depolarized inactivated state (use-dependent blockade). Calcium channel blockers are employed perioperatively as antihypertensives and as antiarrhythmics.

MECHANISM OF CONTRACTION

Myocardial cells contract as a result of the interaction of two overlapping, rigid contractile proteins, actin and myosin. Dystrophin, a large intracellular protein, connects actin to the cell membrane (sarcolemma). Cell shortening occurs when the actin and myosin are allowed to interact fully and slide over one another. This interaction is normally prevented by two regulatory proteins, troponin and tropomyosin; troponin is composed of three subunits (troponin I, troponin C, and troponin T). Troponin is attached to actin at regular intervals, whereas tropomyosin lies within the center of the actin structure. An increase in intracellular Ca^{2+} concentration (from about 10^{-7} to 10^{-5} mol/L) promotes contraction as Ca^{2+} ions bind troponin C. The resulting conformational change in these regulatory proteins exposes the active sites on actin that allow interaction with myosin bridges (points of overlapping). The active site on myosin functions as a magnesium-dependent ATPase whose activity is enhanced by the increase in intracellular Ca^{2+} concentration. A series of attachments and disengagements occur as each myosin bridge advances over successive active sites on actin. Adenosine triphosphate (ATP) is consumed during each attachment. Relaxation occurs as Ca^{2+} is actively pumped back into the sarcoplasmic reticulum by a Ca^{2+}–Mg^{2+}-ATPase; the resulting drop in intracellular Ca^{2+} concentration allows the troponin–tropomyosin complex to again prevent the interaction between actin and myosin.

Excitation–Contraction Coupling

The quantity of Ca^{2+} ions required to initiate contraction exceeds that entering the cell through L-type calcium channels during phase 2. The small amount that does enter through slow calcium channels triggers the release of much larger amounts of Ca^{2+} stored intracellularly (calcium-dependent calcium release) within the sarcoplasmic reticulum.

The action potential of muscle cells depolarizes their T systems, tubular extensions of the cell membrane that transverse the cell in close approximation to the muscle fibrils, via L-type voltage-gated calcium channels. This initial increase in intracellular Ca^{2+} triggers an even greater Ca^{2+} inflow across ryanodine receptor 2 (RyR_2). RyRs are nonvoltage-dependent intracellular calcium channels found in the brain, heart, and skeletal muscle. The RyR_2 form is nearly exclusive to the cardiac sarcoplasmic reticulum. The force of contraction is directly dependent on the magnitude of the initial Ca^{2+} influx.

During relaxation, when the L-type channels close, a Ca^{2+}–Mg^{2+}-ATPase actively transports Ca^{2+} back into the sarcoplasmic reticulum. Thus, relaxation of the heart also requires ATP. Ca^{2+} is also extruded extracellularly by an exchange of intracellular Ca^{2+} for extracellular sodium in a 1:3 ratio by the Na^+–Ca^{2+} exchanger in the cell membrane (Figure 20–2).

The quantity of intracellular Ca^{2+} available, its rate of delivery, and its rate of removal determine, respectively, the maximum tension developed, the rate of contraction, and the rate of relaxation. Sympathetic stimulation increases the force of contraction by raising intracellular Ca^{2+} concentration via a β_1-adrenergic receptor-mediated increase in intracellular cyclic adenosine monophosphate

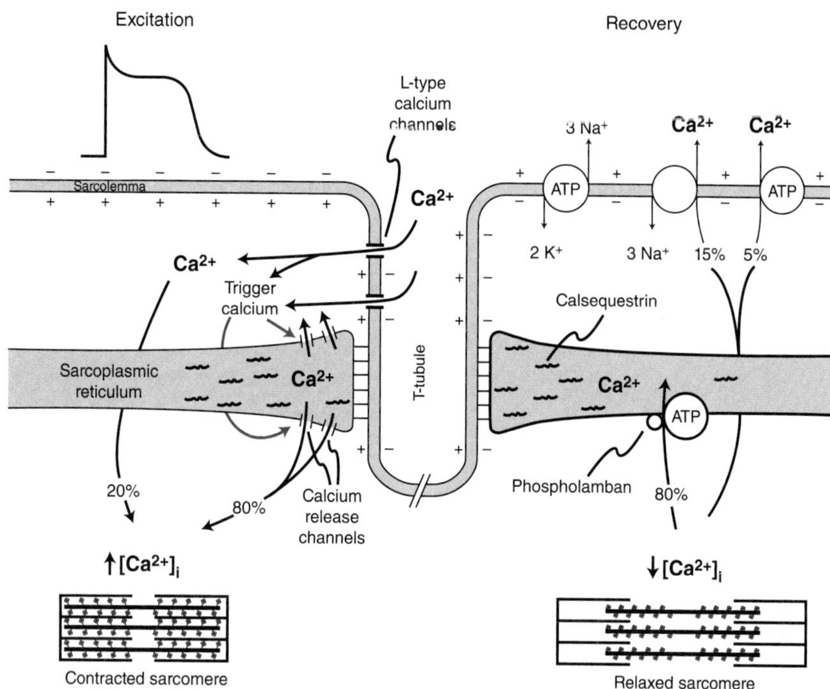

FIGURE 20–2 Excitation–contraction coupling, sarcomere shortening, and relaxation. ATP, adenosine triphosphate. (Reproduced with permission from Mohrman DE, Heller LJ. *Cardiovascular Physiology,* 8th ed. New York, NY: McGraw Hill; 2014.)

(cAMP) through the action of a stimulatory G protein. The increase in cAMP mediates most adrenergic effects on chronotropy, inotropy, and lusitropy (myocardial relaxation) indirectly by activating protein kinase A (PKA). In addition, cAMP has direct effects on exchange proteins directly activated by cAMP (EPACS) that have only recently been described. Phosphodiesterase inhibitors, such as milrinone, increase intracellular cAMP by preventing the breakdown of intracellular cAMP by inhibiting phosphodiesterase 3. Milrinone has lusitropic effects, improving relaxation and diastolic function. Digitalis glycosides increase intracellular Ca^{2+} concentration through inhibition of the membrane-bound Na^+–K^+-ATPase; the resulting small increase in intracellular Na^+ relatively disfavors the normal pumping of Ca^{2+} from the cytoplasm via the Na^+–Ca^{2+} exchange mechanism, increasing the intracellular Ca^{2+} concentration. Glucagon enhances contractility by increasing intracellular cAMP levels via activation of a specific receptor. Levosimendan is a calcium sensitizer that enhances contractility by binding to troponin C. The investigational drug omecamtiv mecarbil is a myosin activator that increases the duration of cardiac muscle contractility. Istaroxime has both inotropic and lusitropic effects, improving both systolic and diastolic function (Table 20–3). Investigations are underway into agents that affect mitochondrial energetics to improve myocardial ATP production and thus myocyte performance.

Release of acetylcholine with vagal stimulation stimulates acetylcholine release from cardiac myocytes. The net effect is to depress contractility through increased cyclic guanosine monophosphate (cGMP) levels and inhibition of adenylyl cyclase; these effects are mediated by an inhibitory G protein. Acidosis inhibits L-type calcium channels and therefore also depresses cardiac contractility by unfavorably altering intracellular Ca^{2+} kinetics (Figure 20–3).

3 Studies suggest that volatile anesthetics depress cardiac contractility by decreasing the entry of Ca^{2+} into cells during depolarization (affecting T- and L-type calcium channels), altering the

TABLE 20–3 Inotropic drugs: Mechanisms and outcomes.

Drug	Mechanism
Digoxin	Na–K pump inhibitor, raises SR calcium
Dopamine	Dose-dependent D_1, α_1-, and β_1-adrendergic receptor agonist
Norepinephrine	β_1- and α_1-adrenergic receptor agonist
Dobutamine	β_1- and β_2-adrenergic receptor agonist
Milrinone	PDE inhibitor, raises SR calcium
Levosimendan	Myofilament calcium sensitizer, PDE-3 inhibitor
Omecamtiv mecarbil	Potentiates the effects of myosin on actin to prolong systole
Istaroxime	Na–K pump inhibitor, PDE inhibitor
SERCA2a gene therapy	Restoration of SERCA2a to improve calcium release and reuptake from the SR

PDE, phosphodiesterase; SERCA, sarco/endoplasmic reticulum Ca^{2+}–ATPase; SR, sarcoplasmic reticulum.

Modified with permission from Francis GS, Bartos JA, Adatya S et al. Inotropes. *J Am Coll Cardiol.* 2014 May 27;63:2069-2078.

kinetics of Ca^{2+} release and uptake into the sarcoplasmic reticulum, and decreasing the sensitivity of contractile proteins to Ca^{2+}. Inhalational anesthetics appear to have minimal effect upon early diastolic relaxation in subjects without known diastolic dysfunction. However, they do decrease atrial function, perhaps resulting in reduced late diastolic filling. Anesthetic-induced cardiac depression is potentiated by hypocalcemia, β-adrenergic blockade, and calcium channel blockers. Nitrous oxide also produces concentration-dependent decreases in contractility by reducing the availability of intracellular Ca^{2+} during contraction. The mechanisms of direct cardiac depression from intravenous anesthetics are not well established but presumably involve similar actions. Of all the typical intravenous induction agents, ketamine seems to have the least depressant effect on contractility due to its central nervous system excitatory effects.

INNERVATION OF THE HEART

Parasympathetic fibers innervate the atria and conducting tissues. Acetylcholine acts on specific cardiac muscarinic receptors (M_2) to produce negative chronotropic, dromotropic, and inotropic effects. In contrast, sympathetic fibers are more widely distributed throughout the heart. Cardiac sympathetic fibers originate in the thoracic spinal cord (T1–T4) and travel to the heart initially through the cervical (stellate) ganglia and from the ganglia as the cardiac nerves. Norepinephrine release at the heart causes positive chronotropic, dromotropic, and inotropic effects primarily through activation of β_1-adrenergic receptors. β_2-Adrenergic receptors are normally fewer in number and are found primarily in the atria; activation increases heart rate and, to a lesser extent, contractility. The relative fraction of β_2- to β_1-adrenergic receptors increases in heart failure.

Cardiac autonomic innervation has *sidedness* because the right sympathetic and right vagus nerves primarily affect the SA node, whereas the left sympathetic and vagus nerves principally affect the AV node. Vagal effects frequently have a very rapid onset and resolution, whereas sympathetic influences generally have a more gradual onset and dissipation. Sinus arrhythmia is a cyclic variation in heart rate that corresponds to respiration (increasing with inspiration and decreasing during expiration); it is due to cyclic changes in vagal tone.

THE CARDIAC CYCLE

The cardiac cycle can be defined by both electrical and mechanical events (Figure 20–4). *Systole* refers to contraction, and *diastole* refers to relaxation. Most diastolic ventricular filling occurs passively before atrial contraction. Contraction of the atria normally contributes 20% to 30% of ventricular filling. **Three waves can generally be identified on atrial or central venous pressure tracings** (see Figure 20–4). The *a* wave is due to atrial systole. The *c* wave coincides with ventricular contraction and is said to be caused by bulging of the AV valve into the

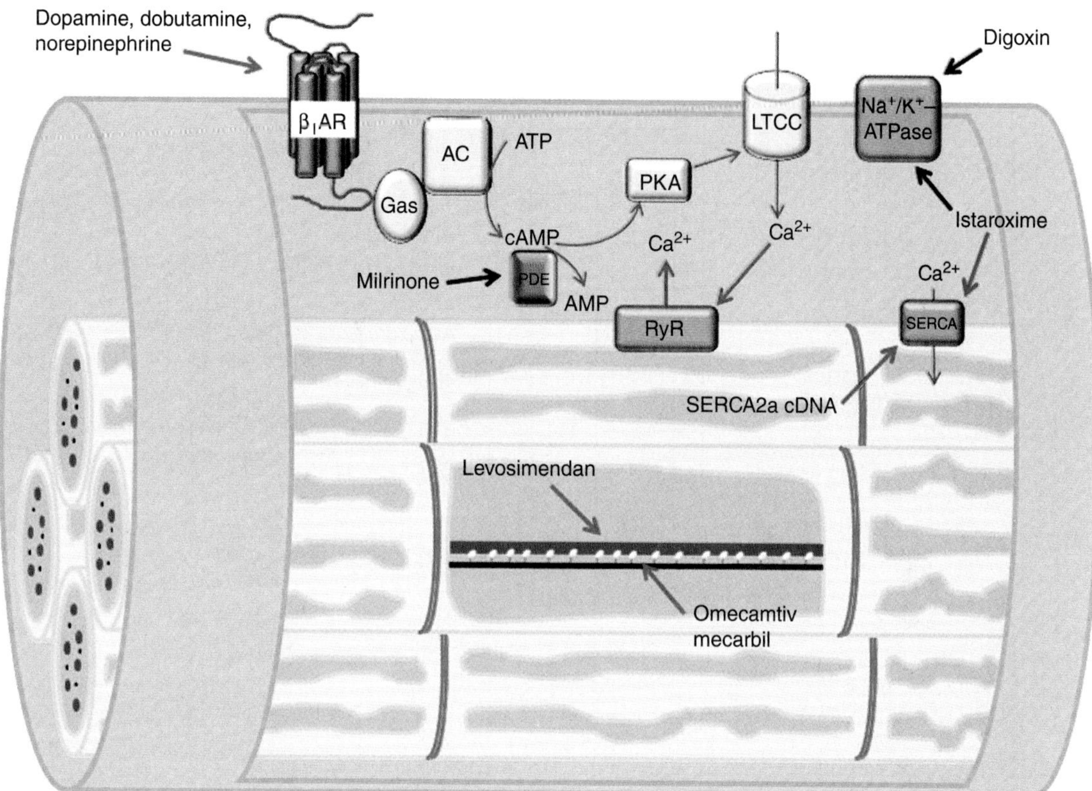

FIGURE 20–3 Diagram of intracellular signaling cascades within cardiomyocytes altered by inotropes dopamine, dobutamine, and norepinephrine that activate the β_1-adrenergic receptor, which activates the G protein Gas, which in turn, activates adenylyl cyclase. Adenylyl cyclase converts ATP to cAMP when activated. cAMP can activate PKA, which then phosphorylates the L-type calcium channel, among other targets. cAMP is converted to AMP by PDE. Milrinone inhibits PDE-3, thereby increasing the effective concentration of cAMP. Calcium influx through the L-type calcium channel induces activation of ryanodine receptors, leading to calcium-induced Ca^{2+} release. Free intracellular Ca^{2+} interacts with troponin C, which changes the binding properties of tropomyosin and allows the interaction between actin and myosin. Levosimendan potentiates the interaction between troponin and calcium. It may also have PDE-3 inhibitor activity. Omecamtiv mecarbil increases the rate of ATP turnover and slows the rate of ADP release, thereby increasing the number of myosin molecules bound to actin at any given time. SERCA is responsible for the uptake of calcium into the sarcoplasmic reticulum while the Na^+–K^+-ATPase participates in resetting the membrane potential of the cell. Istaroxime inhibits Na^+–K^+-ATPase while also potentiating SERCA. Digoxin inhibits the Na^+–K^+-ATPase. *Red arrows* denote agonists, whereas *black arrows* signify antagonists. AC, adenylyl cyclase; ADP, adenosine diphosphate; ATP, adenosine triphosphate; β_1AR, β_1-adrenergic receptor; cAMP, cyclic adenosine monophosphate; LTCC, L-type calcium channel; PDE, phosphodiesterase; PKA, protein kinase A; RyR, ryanodine receptor; SERCA, sarco/endoplasmic reticulum Ca^{2+}–ATPase. (Reproduced with permission from Francis GS, Bartos JA, Adatya S, et al. Inotropes. *J Am Coll Cardiol.* 2014 May 27;63:2069-2078.)

atrium. The *v* wave is the result of pressure buildup from venous return before the AV valve opens again. The *x* descent is the decline in pressure between the *c* and *v* waves and is thought to be due to a pulling down of the atrium by ventricular contraction. Incompetence of the AV valve on either side of the heart abolishes the *x* descent on that side, resulting in a prominent *cv* wave. The *y* descent follows the *v* wave and represents the decline in atrial pressure as the AV valve opens. The notch in the aortic pressure tracing is referred to as the *incisura* and is said to represent the brief pressure change from transient

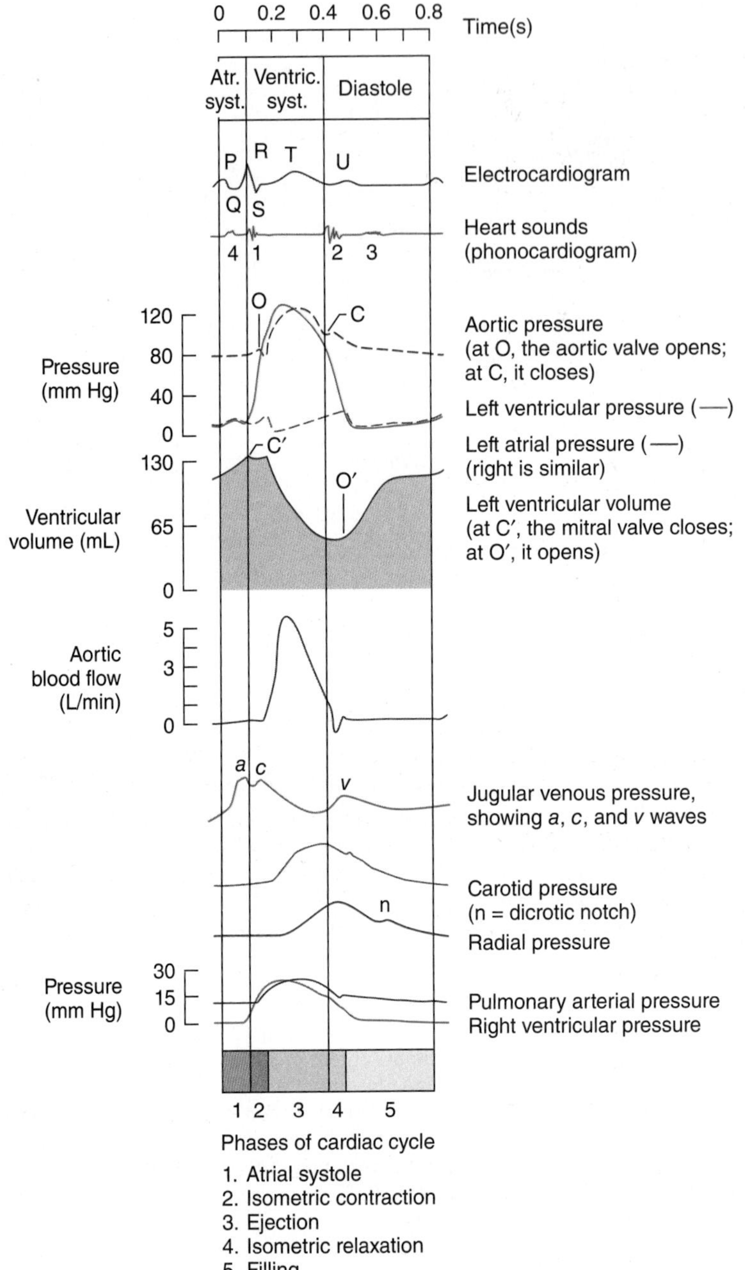

FIGURE 20–4 The normal cardiac cycle. Note the correspondence between electrical and mechanical events. Atr. syst., atrial systole; Ventric. Syst., ventricular systole. (Modified with permission from Barrett KE. *Ganong's Review of Medical Physiology*, 25th ed. New York, NY: McGraw Hill; 2016.)

backflow of blood into the left ventricle just before aortic valve closure.

DETERMINANTS OF VENTRICULAR PERFORMANCE

Discussions of ventricular function usually refer to the left ventricle, but the same concepts apply to the right ventricle. Although the ventricles are often thought of as functioning separately, they are interdependent. Moreover, factors affecting systolic and diastolic functions can be differentiated: Systolic function involves ventricular ejection, whereas diastolic function is related to ventricular filling.

Ventricular systolic function is often (erroneously) equated with cardiac output, which can be defined as the volume of blood pumped by the heart per minute. Because the two ventricles function in series, their outputs are normally equal. Cardiac output (CO) is expressed by the following equation:

$$CO = SV \times HR$$

where SV is the stroke volume (the volume pumped per contraction) and HR is heart rate. To compensate for variations in body size, CO is often expressed in terms of total body surface area:

$$CI = \frac{CO}{BSA}$$

where CI is the cardiac index and BSA is body surface area. BSA is usually obtained from nomograms based on height and weight. Normal CI is 2.5 to 4.2
4 L/min/m^2. Because the normal CI has a wide range, it is a relatively insensitive measurement of ventricular performance. Abnormalities in CI therefore usually reflect gross ventricular impairment. A more accurate assessment can be obtained if the response of the cardiac output to exercise is evaluated. Under these conditions, failure of the cardiac output to increase and keep up with oxygen consumption is reflected by a decreasing mixed venous oxygen saturation. A decrease in mixed venous oxygen saturation in response to increased demand
5 usually reflects inadequate tissue perfusion. Thus, in the absence of hypoxia or severe anemia, measurement of mixed venous oxygen tension (or saturation) provides an estimate of the adequacy of cardiac output.

1. Heart Rate

When stroke volume remains constant, cardiac output is directly proportional to heart rate. Heart rate is an intrinsic function of the SA node (spontaneous depolarization) but is modified by autonomic, humoral, and local factors. The normal intrinsic rate of the SA node in young adults is about 90 to 100 beats/min, but it decreases with age based on the following formula:

$$\text{Normal intrinsic heart rate} = 118 \text{ beats/min} - (0.57 \times \text{Age})$$

Enhanced vagal activity slows the heart rate via stimulation of M_2 cholinergic receptors, whereas enhanced sympathetic activity increases the heart rate mainly through activation of β_1-adrenergic receptors and, to a lesser extent, β_2-adrenergic receptors (see above).

2. Stroke Volume

Stroke volume is normally determined by three major factors: preload, afterload, and contractility. This is analogous to laboratory observations on skeletal muscle preparations. Preload is muscle length prior to contraction, whereas afterload is the tension against which the muscle must contract. Contractility is an intrinsic property of the muscle that is related to the force of contraction but is independent of both preload and afterload. Because the heart is a three-dimensional multichambered pump, both ventricular geometric form and valvular dysfunction can also affect stroke volume (Table 20–4).

Preload

Ventricular preload is end-diastolic volume, which is generally dependent on ventricular filling. The relationship between cardiac output and left ventricular end-diastolic volume was first described by

TABLE 20–4 Major factors affecting cardiac stroke volume.

Preload
Afterload
Contractility
Wall motion abnormalities
Valvular dysfunction

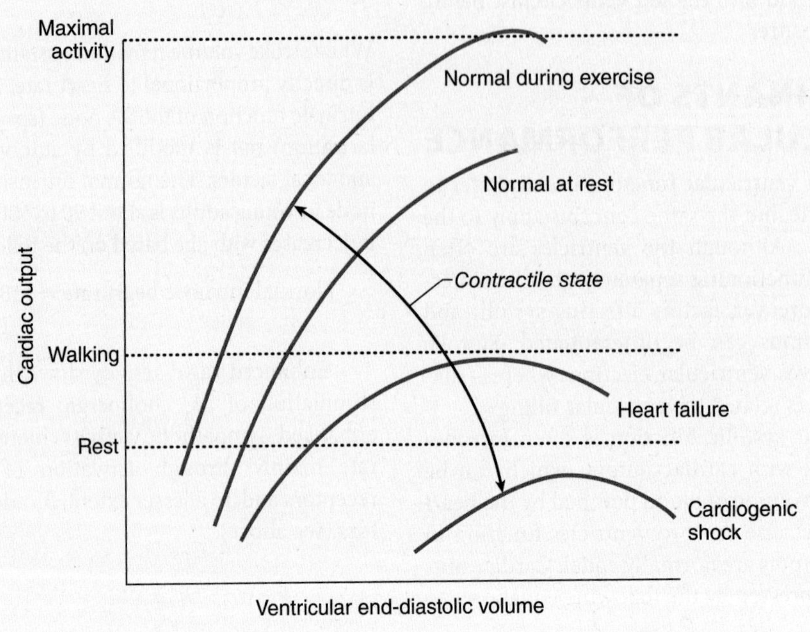

FIGURE 20–5 Starling's law of the heart. (Reproduced with permission from Braunwald E, Ross J, Sonnenblick EH. Mechanisms of contraction of the normal and failing heart. *N Engl J Med.* 1967 Oct 12;277(15):794-800.)

Starling (Figure 20–5). Note that when the heart rate and contractility remain constant, cardiac output increases with increasing preload until excessive end-diastolic volumes are reached. At that point, cardiac output does not appreciably change—or may even decrease. Excessive distention of either ventricle can lead to dilation and incompetence of the AV valves.

A. Determinants of Ventricular Filling

Ventricular filling can be influenced by a variety of factors (Table 20–5), of which the most important is venous return. The heart cannot pump what the heart does not receive; therefore, venous return normally equals cardiac output. Because most of the other factors affecting venous return are usually fixed, vascular capacity is normally its major determinant. Increases in metabolic activity reduce vascular capacity, so venous return to the heart and cardiac output increase as the volume of venous capacitance vessels decreases. Changes in blood volume and vascular capacity are important causes of intraoperative and postoperative changes in ventricular filling and cardiac output. Any factor that alters the normally small venous pressure gradient favoring blood return to the heart also affects cardiac filling. Such factors include changes in intrathoracic pressure (positive-pressure ventilation or thoracotomy), posture (positioning during surgery), and pericardial pressure (pericardial disease).

The most important determinant of right ventricular preload is venous return. **In the absence of significant pulmonary or right ventricular**

TABLE 20–5 Factors affecting ventricular preload.

Blood volume
Distribution of blood volume
Posture
Intrathoracic pressure
Pericardial pressure
Venous tone
Rhythm (atrial contraction)
Heart rate

dysfunction, venous return is also the major determinant of left ventricular preload.

Both heart rate and rhythm can affect ventricular preload. Increases in heart rate are associated with proportionately greater reductions in diastole than systole. Ventricular filling therefore progressively becomes impaired at increased heart rates (>120 beats/min in adults). Absent (atrial fibrillation), ineffective (atrial flutter), or altered timing of atrial contraction (low atrial or junctional rhythms) can also reduce ventricular filling by 20% to 30%. 6 Patients with reduced ventricular compliance are more affected by the loss of a normally timed atrial systole than are those with normal ventricular compliance.

B. Diastolic Function and Ventricular Compliance

Left ventricular end-diastolic pressure (LVEDP) can be used as a measure of preload only if the relationship between ventricular volume and pressure (ventricular compliance) is constant. However, ventricular compliance is normally nonlinear (Figure 20–6). Impaired diastolic function reduces ventricular compliance. Therefore, the same LVEDP that corresponds to a normal preload in a normal patient may correspond to a decreased preload in a patient with impaired diastolic function. Many factors are known to influence ventricular diastolic function and compliance. Nonetheless, measurement of LVEDP or other pressures approximating LVEDP (such as pulmonary artery occlusion pressure) are potential means of estimating left ventricular preload. Changes in central venous pressure can be used as a rough index for changes in right and left ventricular preload in most normal individuals.

Factors affecting ventricular compliance can be separated into those related to the rate of relaxation (early diastolic compliance) and passive stiffness of the ventricles (late diastolic compliance). Left ventricular hypertrophy (from hypertension or aortic valve stenosis), ischemia, and asynchrony reduce early compliance; hypertrophy and fibrosis reduce late compliance. Extrinsic factors (such as pericardial disease, excessive distention of the contralateral ventricle, increased airway or pleural pressure, tumors, and surgical compression) can also reduce ventricular compliance. Because of its normally thinner wall, the right ventricle is more compliant than the left.

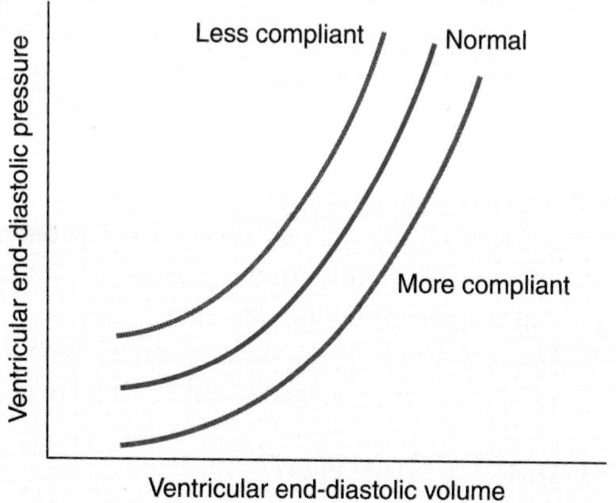

FIGURE 20–6 Normal and abnormal ventricular compliance.

Afterload

Afterload for the intact heart is commonly equated with either ventricular wall tension during systole or arterial impedance to ejection. Wall tension may be thought of as the pressure the ventricle must overcome to reduce its cavity volume. If the ventricle is assumed to be spherical, ventricular wall tension can be expressed by Laplace's law:

$$\text{Circumferential stress} = \frac{P \times R}{2 \times H}$$

where P is intraventricular pressure, R is the ventricular radius, and H is wall thickness. Although the normal ventricle is usually ellipsoidal, this relationship is still useful. The larger the ventricular radius, the greater the wall tension required to develop the same ventricular pressure. Conversely, an increase in wall thickness reduces ventricular wall tension.

Systolic intraventricular pressure is dependent on the force of ventricular contraction; the viscoelastic properties of the aorta, its proximal branches, and blood (viscosity and density); and **systemic vascular resistance (SVR).** Arteriolar tone is the primary determinant of SVR. Because viscoelastic properties are generally fixed in any given patient, left ventricular afterload is usually equated clinically with SVR, which is calculated by the following equation:

$$SVR = 80 \times \frac{MAP - CVP}{CO}$$

where MAP is mean arterial pressure in millimeters of mercury, CVP is central venous pressure in millimeters of mercury, and CO is cardiac output in liters per minute. Normal SVR is 900–1500 dyn · s cm^{-5}. Systolic blood pressure may also be used as an approximation of left ventricular afterload in the absence of chronic changes in the size, shape, or thickness of the ventricular wall or acute changes in systemic vascular resistance. Some clinicians prefer to use CI instead of CO in calculating a systemic vascular resistance index (SVRI) so that SVRI = SVR × BSA (body surface area).

Right ventricular afterload is mainly dependent on pulmonary vascular resistance (PVR) and is expressed by the following equation:

$$PVR = 80 \times \frac{PAP - LAP}{CO}$$

where PAP is mean pulmonary artery pressure and LAP is left atrial pressure. In practice, pulmonary capillary wedge pressure (PCWP) can be substituted as an approximation for LAP. Normal PVR is 50 to 150 dyn · s cm^{-5}.

Cardiac output declines in response to large increases in afterload on the left ventricle; however, small increases or decreases in afterload may have no effect on cardiac output. Because of its thinner wall, the right ventricle is more sensitive to changes
7 in afterload than is the left ventricle. Cardiac output in patients with marked right or left ventricular impairment is very sensitive to acute increases in afterload. The latter is particularly true in the presence of drug- or ischemia-induced myocardial depression or chronic heart failure.

Contractility

Cardiac contractility (inotropy) is the intrinsic ability of the myocardium to pump in the absence of changes in preload or afterload. Contractility is related to the rate of myocardial muscle shortening, which is, in turn, dependent on the intracellular Ca^{2+} concentration during systole.

Contractility can be altered by neural, humoral, or pharmacological influences. Sympathetic nervous system activity normally has the most important effect on contractility. Sympathetic fibers innervate atrial and ventricular muscle, as well as nodal tissues. In addition to its positive chronotropic effect, norepinephrine release also enhances contractility primarily via β_1-receptor activation. α-Adrenergic receptors are also present in the myocardium but seem to have only minor positive inotropic and chronotropic effects that are overwhelmed by the vascular actions of α-adrenergic agonists when these drugs are administered systemically. Sympathomimetic drugs and secretion of epinephrine from the adrenal glands similarly increase contractility via β_1-receptor activation.

Myocardial contractility is depressed by hypoxia, acidosis, depletion of catecholamine stores within the heart, and loss of functioning muscle mass as a result of ischemia or infarction. At large enough doses, most anesthetics and antiarrhythmic agents are negative inotropes (ie, they decrease contractility).

Wall Motion Abnormalities

Regional wall motion abnormalities cause a breakdown of the analogy between the intact heart and skeletal muscle preparations. Such abnormalities may be due to ischemia, scarring, hypertrophy, or altered conduction. When the ventricular cavity does not collapse symmetrically or fully, emptying becomes impaired. Hypokinesis (decreased contraction), akinesis (failure to contract), and dyskinesis (paradoxical bulging) during systole reflect increasing degrees of contraction abnormalities. Although contractility may be normal or even enhanced in some areas, abnormalities in other areas of the ventricle can impair emptying and reduce stroke volume. The severity of the impairment depends on the size and number of abnormally contracting areas.

Valvular Dysfunction

Valvular dysfunction can involve any one of the four valves in the heart and can include stenosis, regurgitation (incompetence), or both. Stenosis of an AV valve (tricuspid or mitral) reduces stroke volume primarily by decreasing ventricular preload, whereas stenosis of a semilunar valve (pulmonary or aortic) reduces stroke volume primarily by increasing ventricular afterload. In contrast, valvular regurgitation can reduce stroke volume without changes in preload, afterload, or contractility and without wall motion abnormalities. The effective stroke volume is reduced by the regurgitant volume with every contraction. When an AV valve is incompetent, a significant part of the ventricular end-diastolic volume can flow backward into the atrium during systole; the stroke volume is reduced by the regurgitant volume. Similarly, when a semilunar valve is incompetent, a fraction of end-diastolic volume arises from backward flow into the ventricle during diastole.

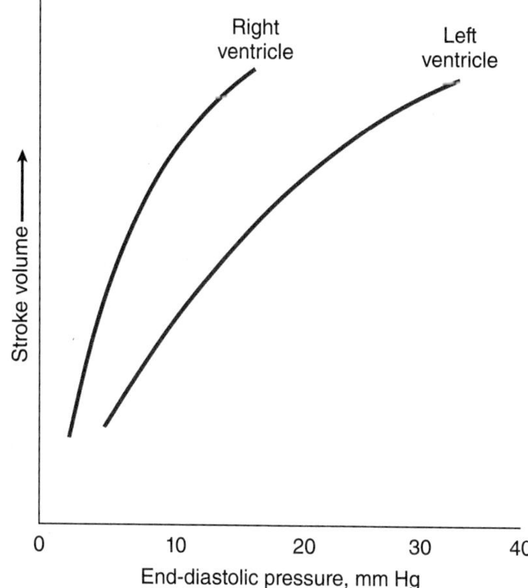

FIGURE 20–7 Function curves for the left and right ventricles.

ASSESSMENT OF VENTRICULAR FUNCTION

1. Ventricular Function Curves

Plotting cardiac output or stroke volume against preload can be useful in evaluating pathological states and understanding drug therapy. Normal right and left ventricular function curves are shown in Figure 20–7.

Ventricular pressure–volume diagrams dissociate contractility from both preload and afterload. Two points are identified on such diagrams: the end-systolic point (ESP) and the end-diastolic point (EDP) (Figure 20–8). ESP is reflective of systolic function, whereas EDP is more reflective of diastolic function. For any given contractile state, all ESPs are on the same line (ie, the relationship between end-systolic volume and end-systolic pressure is fixed). Figure 20–9 describes the events occurring in the left ventricle during each cardiac cycle.

2. Assessment of Systolic Function

The change in ventricular pressure over time during systole (*dP/dt*) is defined by the first derivative of the ventricular pressure curve and can be used as a measure of contractility. Contractility is directly proportional to *dP/dt*, but accurate measurement of this value requires a high-fidelity (Millar) ventricular catheter. Ventricular systolic function is routinely estimated using echocardiography.

Ejection Fraction

8 The ventricular ejection fraction (EF), the fraction of the end-diastolic ventricular volume ejected, is the most commonly used clinical measurement of systolic function. EF can be calculated by the following equation:

$$EF = \frac{EDV - ESV}{EDV}$$

where EDV is left ventricular diastolic volume and ESV is end-systolic volume. Normal EF is approximately 0.67 ± 0.08. Measurements can be made preoperatively from cardiac catheterization, radionucleotide studies, or transthoracic (TTE) or transesophageal echocardiography (TEE). Pulmonary artery catheters with fast-response thermistors allow measurement of the right ventricular EF. Unfortunately, when pulmonary vascular resistance increases, decreases in right ventricular EF may

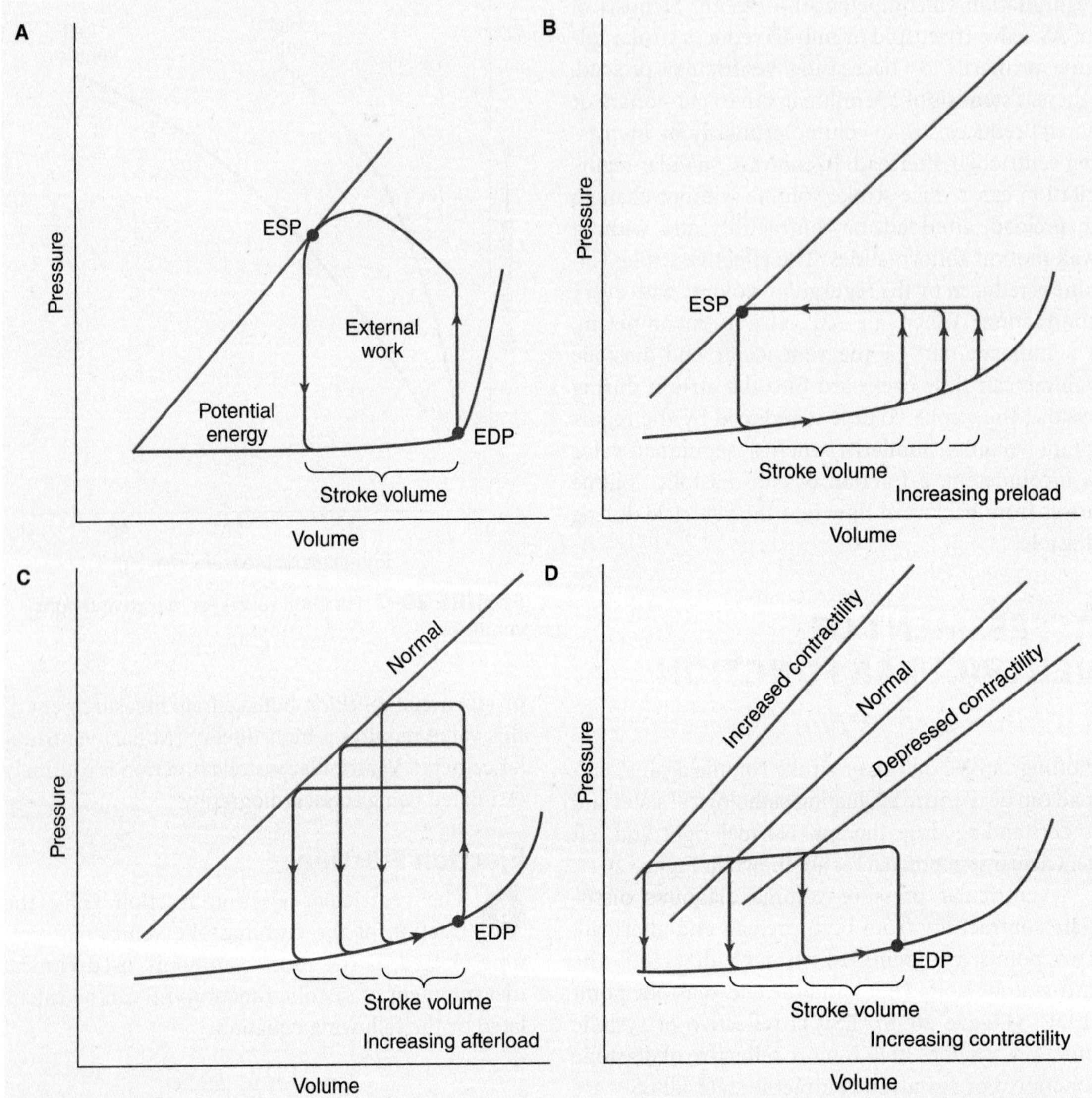

FIGURE 20–8 Ventricular pressure–volume diagrams. **A**: A single ventricular contraction. Note that stroke volume represents a change in volume on the x-axis (difference between end-systolic volume and end-diastolic volume). Note also that the circumscribed area represents external work performed by the ventricle. **B**: Increasing preload with constant contractility and afterload. **C**: Increasing afterload with constant preload and contractility. **D**: Increasing contractility with constant preload and afterload. EDP, end-diastolic point; ESP, end-systolic point.

reflect afterload rather than contractility. Left ventricular EF is not an accurate measure of ventricular contractility in the presence of mitral insufficiency.

Myocardial deformation analysis provides another measure to quantify ventricular function by assessing the movement of speckles from echocardiographic images. Deformation of the heart occurs along three dimensions: circumferential, radial, and longitudinal (Figure 20–10). Strain is a measure of the change of length between two

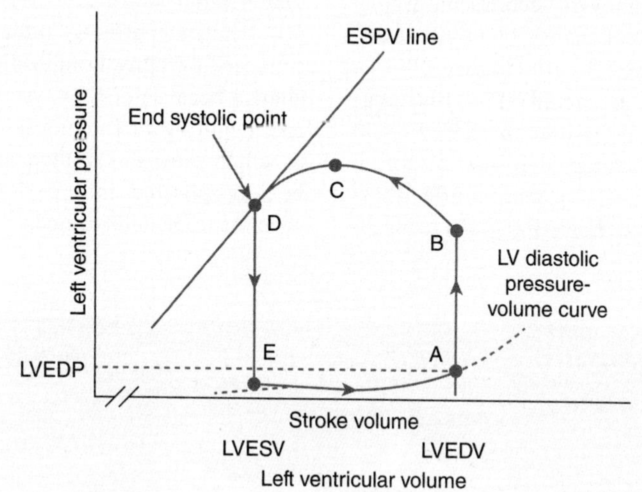

FIGURE 20–9 The pressure–volume loop depicts graphically the hemodynamic changes in the left ventricle during a heartbeat and the ejection of one stroke volume (SV). Segment A–B occurs at the beginning of systole after the mitral valve closes. Point A: The left ventricular end-diastolic pressure is noted on the graph at the end of diastolic filling. Pressure in the ventricle gradually builds until point B is reached, when the aortic valve opens, and blood is ejected from the ventricle. The aortic valve closes when ejection is complete at end systole. The line at point D identifies end systole. Moving the slope of this line to the reader's right represents a shift to a less contractile state. Moving the slope to the left reflects a more highly contractile ventricle. Segment D–E represents isovolumetric relaxation. Once pressure in the ventricle is reduced, the mitral valve opens again (point E), and diastolic filling resumes in preparation for the heart's next systole. Point C reflects peak systolic pressure. ESPV, end-systolic pressure–volume; LVEDP, left ventricular end-diastolic pressure; LVEDV, left ventricular end-diastolic volume. (Reproduced with permission from Hoffman WJ, Wasnick JD. *Postoperative Critical Care of the Massachusetts General Hospital*, 2nd ed. Boston, MA: Little, Brown and Company; 1992.)

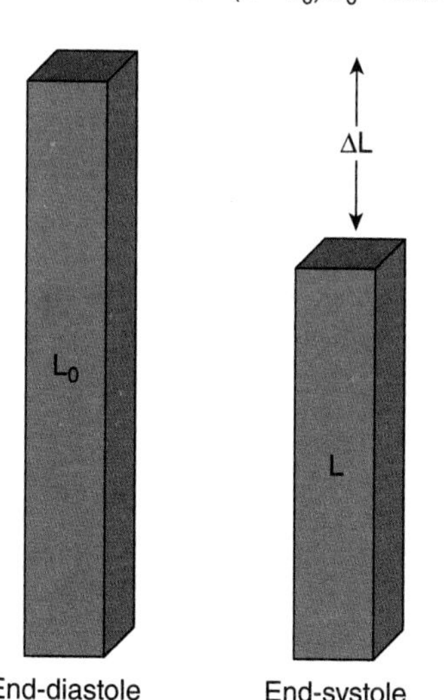

FIGURE 20–10 Strain describes the fractional change of a myocardial segment length compared with its initial length (at end-diastole). ε, myocardial strain; L, length at end-systole; L_0, initial length. (Reproduced with permission from Cleveland Clinic Center for Medical Art & Photography © 2013. All Rights Reserved.)

points. With strain analysis, echocardiography can determine the percent change in length at different points of the myocardium (Figure 20–11). Longitudinal strain is measured at various segments during systole and diastole; the global strain is −21%, reflecting the average deformation for all segments. Normal estimates for strain under anesthesia are not established; however, −19% to −22% longitudinal strain is a normal range established for healthy patients undergoing transthoracic echocardiography. Longitudinal strain is a negative change because during systole the ventricle shortens, resulting in L being less than L_0. The degree to which estimates of myocardial deformation will be incorporated into perioperative management remains to be determined.

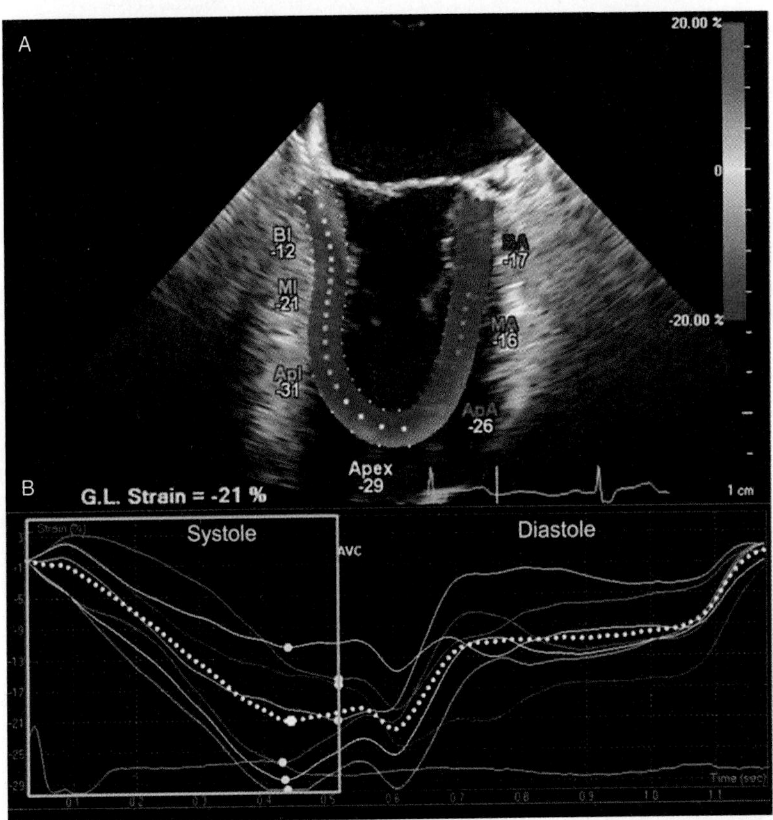

FIGURE 20–11 Longitudinal strain analysis assessed with Cardiac Motion Quantification (CMQ) (Philips Medical Systems, Andover, MA). **A**: Midesophageal two-chamber echocardiographic view depicting the left ventricle, where the myocardial walls are divided into six segments distinguished by color-coded labels and dots. Segmental strain measurements are shown adjacent to each segment. The myocardium is colored in shades of red corresponding to percent longitudinal shortening (strain) measured by the red-to-blue scale on the upper right-hand side. **B**: Longitudinal strain curves, which are color-coded to correspond to myocardial segments in A, with time on the x-axis relative to the cardiac cycle and percent shortening (strain) on the y-axis, demonstrate shortening during systole and returning to baseline at end-diastole. The pink curve, for example, represents the apical anterior wall that experiences peak shortening of −26% during systole (yellow dot identifies peak systolic strain). In contrast, end-systolic strain, measured at the time of aortic valve closure, measures −23%, demonstrating that peak strain may differ from end-systolic strain. The dotted white curve represents global longitudinal strain. ApA, apical anterior; ApI, apical inferior myocardial walls; AVC, aortic valve closure; BA, basal anterior; BI, basal inferior; G.L. Strain, global longitudinal strain; MA, mid anterior; MI, mid inferior. (Reproduced with permission from Cleveland Clinic Center for Medical Art & Photography © 2013. All Rights Reserved.)

3. Assessment of Diastolic Function

9 Left ventricular diastolic function can be assessed clinically by Doppler echocardiography on a transthoracic or transesophageal examination. Flow velocities are measured across the mitral valve during diastole or by interrogation of the motion of the mitral valve annulus (tissue Doppler). Three patterns of diastolic dysfunction are generally recognized based on isovolumetric relaxation time, the ratio of peak early diastolic flow (E) to peak atrial systolic flow (A), and the deceleration time (DT) of E (DT_E) (Figure 20–12). Tissue Doppler is frequently used to distinguish "pseudonormal" from normal diastolic function. Tissue Doppler discerns the velocity of movement of the myocardial tissue during the cardiac cycle. During systole, the mitral annulus moves toward the apex of the heart, away from the echocardiography probe in the esophagus. A negative deflection s' wave is generated, reflecting systolic movement away from the probe. During diastolic filling, the mitral annulus moves toward the transesophageal echocardiography probe, producing a positive e' wave. An e' wave peak velocity of less than 8 cm/s is associated with impaired diastolic function. An E/e' wave ratio that is greater than 15 is consistent with elevated left ventricular end-diastolic pressure (Figures 20–13 and 20-14).

Systemic Circulation

The systemic vasculature can be divided functionally into arteries, arterioles, capillaries, and veins. Arteries are the high-pressure conduits that supply the various organs. Arterioles are the small vessels that directly feed and control blood flow through each capillary bed. Capillaries are thin-walled vessels that allow the exchange of nutrients between blood and tissues. Veins return blood from capillary beds to the heart.

The distribution of blood between the various components of the circulatory system is shown in Table 20–6. Note that most of the blood volume is in the systemic circulation—specifically, within systemic veins. Changes in systemic venous tone allow these vessels to function as a reservoir for blood. Following significant blood or fluid losses, a sympathetically mediated increase in vascular tone reduces the capacity of these vessels and shifts blood

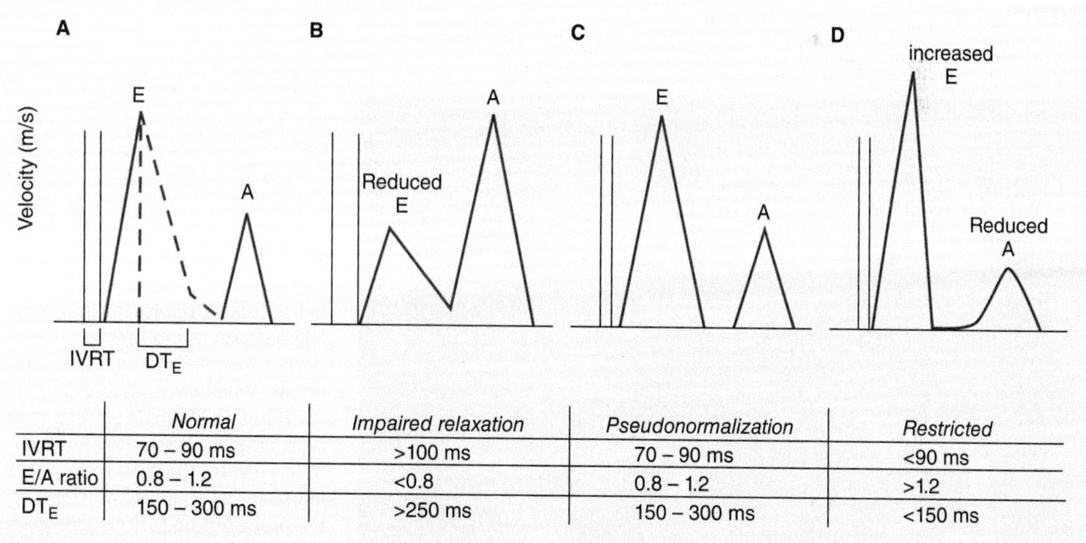

	Normal	Impaired relaxation	Pseudonormalization	Restricted
IVRT	70 – 90 ms	>100 ms	70 – 90 ms	<90 ms
E/A ratio	0.8 – 1.2	<0.8	0.8 – 1.2	>1.2
DT_E	150 – 300 ms	>250 ms	150 – 300 ms	<150 ms

FIGURE 20–12 Doppler echocardiography of diastolic flow across the mitral valve. **A–D** (from left to right) represents the increasing severity of diastolic dysfunction. A, peak atrial systolic flow; DT_E, deceleration time of E; E, early diastolic flow; IVRT, isovolumic relaxation time.

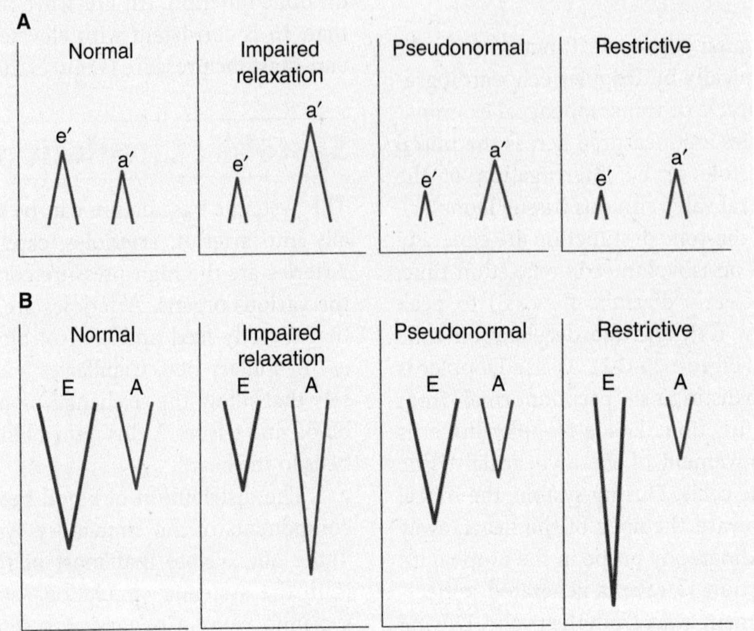

FIGURE 20–13 Tissue Doppler. **A:** Tissue Doppler at the lateral mitral annulus. During diastole, the annulus moves toward the transesophageal examination transducer in the esophagus. Thus the e′ and a′ waves of diastolic filling are positive deflections above the baseline. **B:** When transesophageal examination is used to measure transmitral diastolic inflow, the E and A waves of early and late filling are below the baseline because flow is moving away from the Doppler probe in the esophagus. Tissue Doppler can be used to distinguish normal from pseudonormal diastolic inflow pattern because the e′ wave remains depressed as diastolic dysfunction progresses. (Reproduced with permission from Wasnick JD, Hillel Z, Kramer D, et al. *Cardiac Anesthesia and Transesophageal Echocardiography.* New York, NY: McGraw Hill; 2011.)

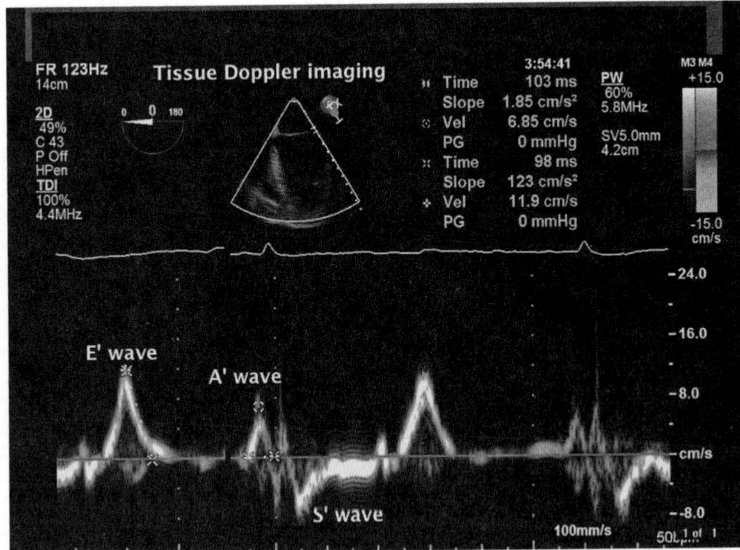

FIGURE 20–14 The E′ wave of early diastolic filling is demonstrated in this tissue Doppler tracing. Early filling occurs as the ventricle relaxes during diastole and the mitral valve opens. The A′ wave reflects the contribution of atrial contraction to diastolic filling. Lastly, the S′ wave demonstrates the movement of the lateral mitral annulus away from the tee probe during systole. (Reproduced with permission from Wasnick JD, Hillel Z, Kramer D, et al. *Cardiac Anesthesia and Transesophageal Echocardiography.* New York, NY: McGraw Hill; 2011.)

TABLE 20–6 Distribution of blood volume.

Heart	7%
Pulmonary circulation	9%
Systemic circulation	
Arterial	15%
Capillary	5%
Venous	64%

into other parts of the vascular system. Conversely, increased capacity (venodilation) allows these vessels to accommodate increases in blood volume. Sympathetic control of vascular tone is an important determinant of venous return to the heart. Reduced venous tone following induction of anesthesia frequently results in pooling of blood, reduced cardiac output, and hypotension.

Many factors influence blood flow in the vascular tree, including metabolic products, endothelium-derived factors, the autonomic nervous system, and circulating hormones.

AUTOREGULATION

Most tissue beds regulate their own blood flow (autoregulation). Arterioles generally dilate in response to reduced perfusion pressure or increased tissue demand. Conversely, arterioles constrict in response to increased pressure or reduced tissue demand. These phenomena are likely due to both an intrinsic response of vascular smooth muscle to stretch and the accumulation of vasodilatory metabolic byproducts. The latter may include K^+, H^+, CO_2, adenosine, and lactate.

ENDOTHELIUM-DERIVED FACTORS

The vascular endothelium is metabolically active in elaborating or modifying substances that play a major role in controlling blood pressure and flow. These include vasodilators (eg, nitric oxide, prostacyclin [PGI_2]), vasoconstrictors (eg, endothelins, thromboxane A_2), anticoagulants (eg, thrombomodulin, protein C), fibrinolytics (eg, tissue plasminogen activator), and factors that inhibit platelet aggregation (eg, nitric oxide, PGI_2). Nitric oxide is synthesized from arginine by nitric oxide synthetase. Nitric oxide binds guanylate cyclase, increasing cGMP levels, and potently produces vasodilation. Endothelially derived vasoconstrictors (endothelins) are released in response to thrombin and epinephrine.

AUTONOMIC CONTROL OF THE SYSTEMIC VASCULATURE

Although the parasympathetic system can exert important influences on the circulation, autonomic control of the vasculature is primarily sympathetic. Sympathetic outflow to the circulation passes out of the spinal cord at all thoracic segments and the first two lumbar segments. These fibers reach blood vessels via specific autonomic nerves or by traveling along spinal nerves. Sympathetic fibers innervate all parts of the vasculature except for capillaries. Their principal function is to regulate vascular tone. Variations of arterial vascular tone serve to regulate blood pressure and the distribution of blood flow to the various organs, whereas variations in venous tone alter vascular capacity, venous pooling, and venous return to the heart.

The vasculature has sympathetic vasoconstrictor and vasodilator fibers, but the former are more important physiologically in most tissue beds. Sympathetic-induced vasoconstriction (via α_1-adrenergic receptors) can be potent in skeletal muscle, kidneys, gut, and skin; it is least active in the brain and heart. The most important vasodilatory fibers are those feeding skeletal muscle, mediating increased blood flow (via β_2-adrenergic receptors) in response to exercise. Vasodepressor (vasovagal) syncope, which can occur following intense emotional strain associated with high sympathetic tone, results from reflex activation of both vagal and sympathetic vasodilator fibers.

Vascular tone and autonomic influences on the heart are controlled by vasomotor centers in the reticular formation of the brainstem. Distinct vasoconstrictor and vasodilator areas have been identified. Vasoconstriction is mediated by the anterolateral areas of the lower pons and upper medulla. They are also responsible for the adrenal secretion of catecholamines, as well as the enhancement of cardiac automaticity and contractility. Vasodilatory areas, which are located in the lower medulla, are also adrenergic. They function by projecting inhibitory fibers upward to the vasoconstrictor areas. Vasomotor output is modified by inputs from throughout the central nervous system, including the hypothalamus, cerebral cortex, and the other areas in the brainstem. Areas in the posterolateral medulla receive input from both the vagal and the glossopharyngeal nerves and play an important role in mediating a variety of circulatory reflexes. The sympathetic system normally maintains some tonic vasoconstriction on the vascular tree. Loss of this tone following induction of anesthesia or sympathectomy frequently contributes to perioperative hypotension.

ARTERIAL BLOOD PRESSURE

Systemic blood flow is pulsatile in large arteries because of the heart's cyclic activity; when the blood reaches the systemic capillaries, flow is continuous. The mean pressure falls to less than 20 mm Hg in the large systemic veins that return blood to the heart. The largest pressure drop, nearly 50%, is across the arterioles, and the arterioles account for the majority of SVR.

MAP is proportionate to the product of SVR × CO. This relationship is based on an analogy to Ohm's law, as applied to the circulation:

$$\text{MAP} - \text{CVP} \approx \text{SVR} \times \text{CO}$$

Because CVP is normally very small compared with MAP, the former can usually be ignored. From this relationship, it is readily apparent that hypotension is the result of a decrease in SVR, CO, or both: For arterial blood pressure to be maintained, a decrease in either SVR or CO must be compensated by an increase in the other. MAP may be estimated by the following formula:

$$\text{MAP} = \text{Diastolic pressure} + \frac{\text{Pulse pressure}}{3}$$

where pulse pressure is the difference between systolic and diastolic blood pressure. Arterial pulse pressure is directly related to stroke volume but is inversely related to the compliance of the arterial tree. Thus, decreases in pulse pressure may be due to a decrease in stroke volume, an increase in SVR, or both. Increased pulse pressure increases shear stress on vessel walls, potentially leading to atherosclerotic plaque rupture and thrombosis or rupture of aneurysms. Increased pulse pressure in patients undergoing cardiac surgery has been associated with adverse renal and neurological outcomes.

Transmission of the arterial pressure wave from large arteries to smaller vessels in the periphery is faster than the actual movement of blood; the pressure wave velocity is 15 times the velocity of blood in the aorta. Moreover, reflections of the propagating waves off arterial walls widen pulse pressure before the pulse wave is completely dampened in very small arteries. Thus, the pulse pressure is generally greater when measured in the femoral or dorsalis pedis arteries than in the aorta.

Control of Arterial Blood Pressure

Arterial blood pressure is regulated by a series of immediate, intermediate, and long-term adjustments that involve complex neural, humoral, and renal mechanisms.

A. Immediate Control

Minute-to-minute control of blood pressure is primarily the function of autonomic nervous system reflexes. Changes in blood pressure are sensed both centrally (in hypothalamic and brainstem areas) and peripherally by specialized sensors (baroreceptors). Decreases in arterial blood pressure result in increased sympathetic tone, increased adrenal secretion of epinephrine, and reduced vagal activity. **The resulting systemic vasoconstriction, increased heart rate, and enhanced cardiac contractility serve to increase blood pressure.**

Peripheral baroreceptors are located at the bifurcation of the common carotid arteries and the aortic arch. Elevations in blood pressure increase baroreceptor discharge, inhibiting systemic vasoconstriction and enhancing vagal tone (**baroreceptor reflex**). Reductions in blood pressure decrease baroreceptor discharge, allowing vasoconstriction and reduction of vagal tone. Carotid baroreceptors send afferent signals to circulatory brainstem centers via the nerve of Hering (a branch of the glossopharyngeal nerve), whereas aortic baroreceptor afferent signals travel along the vagus nerve. Of the two peripheral sensors, the carotid baroreceptor is physiologically more important and serves to minimize changes in blood pressure caused by acute events, such as a change in posture. Carotid baroreceptors sense MAP most effectively between pressures of 80 and 160 mm Hg. Adaptation to acute changes in blood pressure occurs over the course of 1 to 2 days, rendering this reflex ineffective for long-term blood pressure control. All volatile anesthetics depress the normal baroreceptor response. Cardiopulmonary stretch receptors located in the atria, left ventricle, and pulmonary circulation can cause a similar effect.

B. Intermediate Control

In the course of a few minutes, sustained decreases in arterial pressure, together with enhanced sympathetic outflow, activate the renin–angiotensin–aldosterone system, increase secretion of arginine vasopressin (AVP), and alter normal capillary fluid exchange. Both angiotensin II and AVP are potent arteriolar vasoconstrictors. Their immediate action is to increase SVR. In contrast to the formation of angiotensin II, which responds to relatively smaller changes, sufficient AVP secretion to produce vasoconstriction will only occur in response to more marked degrees of hypotension. Angiotensin constricts arterioles via AT_1 receptors. AVP mediates vasoconstriction via V_1 receptors and exerts its antidiuretic effect via V_2 receptors.

Sustained changes in arterial blood pressure can also alter fluid exchange in tissues by their secondary effects on capillary pressures. Hypertension increases interstitial movement of intravascular fluid, whereas hypotension increases reabsorption of interstitial fluid. Such compensatory changes in intravascular volume can reduce fluctuations in blood pressure, particularly in the absence of adequate renal function (see below).

C. Long-Term Control

The effects of slower renal mechanisms become apparent within hours of sustained changes in arterial pressure. As a result, the kidneys alter total body sodium and water balance to restore blood pressure to normal. Hypotension results in sodium (and water) retention, whereas hypertension generally increases sodium excretion and water loss in normal individuals.

ANATOMY & PHYSIOLOGY OF THE CORONARY CIRCULATION

1. Anatomy

Myocardial blood supply is derived entirely from the right and left coronary arteries (Figure 20–15). Blood flows from epicardial to endocardial vessels. After perfusing the myocardium, blood returns to the right atrium via the coronary sinus and the anterior cardiac veins. A small amount of blood returns directly into the chambers of the heart by way of the thebesian veins.

The right coronary artery (RCA) normally supplies the right atrium, most of the right ventricle, and a variable portion of the left ventricle (inferior wall). In 85% of persons, the RCA gives rise to the posterior descending artery (PDA), which supplies the superior–posterior interventricular septum and inferior wall—a right dominant circulation; in the remaining 15% of persons, the PDA is a branch of the left coronary artery—a left dominant circulation.

The left coronary artery normally supplies the left atrium and most of the interventricular septum and left ventricle (septal, anterior, and lateral walls). After a short course, the left main coronary artery bifurcates into the left anterior descending artery (LAD) and the circumflex artery (CX); the LAD supplies the septum and anterior wall, and the CX supplies the lateral wall. In a left dominant circulation, the CX wraps around the AV groove and continues down as the PDA to also supply most of the posterior septum and inferior wall.

The arterial supply to the SA node may be derived from either the RCA (60% of individuals) or the LAD (the remaining 40%). The AV node is usually supplied by the RCA (85–90%) or, less frequently, by the CX (10–15%); the bundle of His has a dual blood supply derived from the PDA and LAD. The anterior papillary muscle of the mitral valve also has a dual blood supply that is fed by diagonal branches of the LAD and marginal branches of the CX. In contrast, the posterior papillary of the

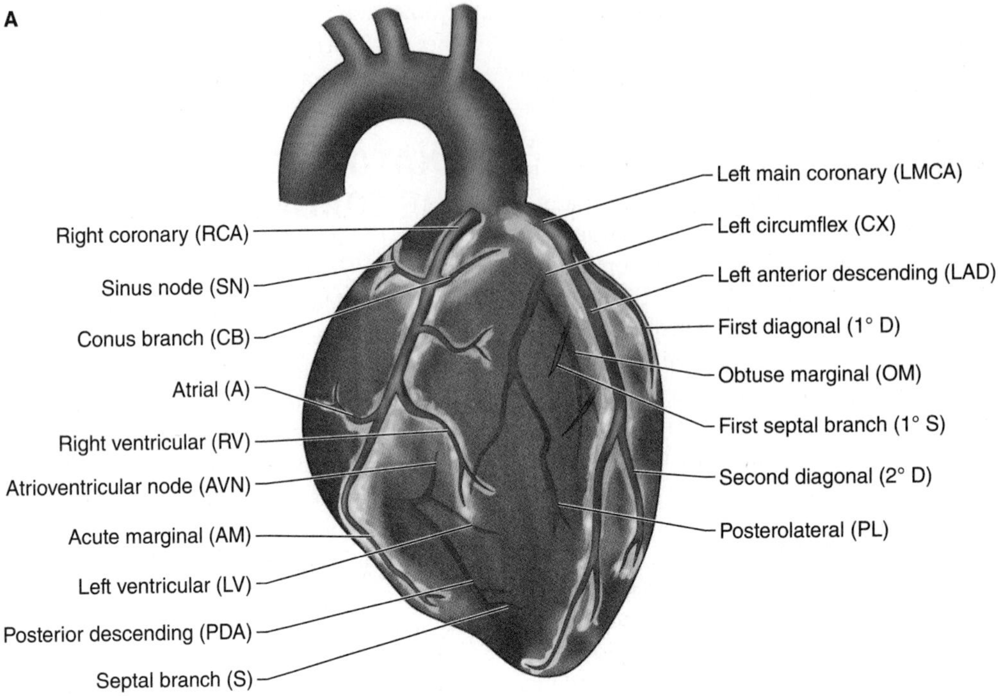

A
Left main coronary (LMCA)
Right coronary (RCA)
Left circumflex (CX)
Sinus node (SN)
Left anterior descending (LAD)
Conus branch (CB)
First diagonal (1° D)
Obtuse marginal (OM)
Atrial (A)
First septal branch (1° S)
Right ventricular (RV)
Second diagonal (2° D)
Atrioventricular node (AVN)
Posterolateral (PL)
Acute marginal (AM)
Left ventricular (LV)
Posterior descending (PDA)
Septal branch (S)

B
SN
CB
RCA
LMCA
CX
RV
LAD
AVN
1° D
OM
AM
2° D
PD
PL
LV

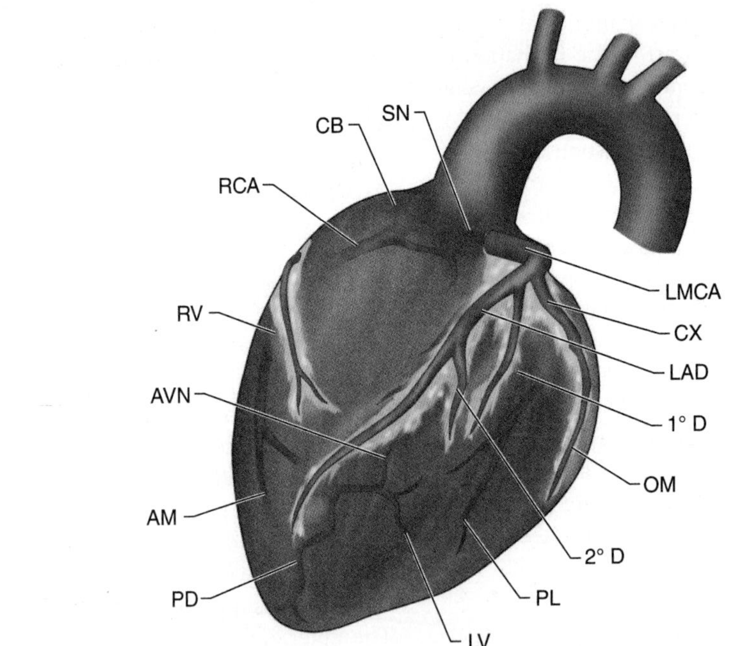

FIGURE 20–15 Anatomy of the coronary arteries in a patient with a right dominant circulation. **A**: Right anterior oblique view. **B**: Left anterior oblique view.

mitral valve is usually supplied only by the PDA and is therefore much more vulnerable to ischemic dysfunction.

2. Determinants of Coronary Perfusion

Coronary perfusion is unique in that it is intermittent rather than continuous, as it is in other organs. During contraction, intramyocardial pressures in the left ventricle approach systemic arterial pressure. The force of left ventricular contraction almost completely occludes the intramyocardial part of the coronary arteries. **Coronary perfusion pressure is usually determined by the difference between aortic pressure and ventricular pressure.** The left ventricle is perfused almost entirely during diastole. In contrast, the right ventricle is perfused during both systole and diastole (Figure 20–16). Moreover, as a determinant of left heart myocardial blood flow, arterial diastolic pressure is more important than MAP. Therefore, left coronary artery perfusion pressure is determined by the difference between arterial diastolic pressure and left ventricular end-diastolic pressure (LVEDP).

Coronary perfusion pressure = Arterial diastolic pressure − LVEDP

Decreases in aortic pressure or increases in ventricular end-diastolic pressure can reduce coronary perfusion pressure. Increases in heart rate also decrease coronary perfusion because of the disproportionately greater reduction in diastolic time as

10 heart rate increases (Figure 20–17). Because the endocardium is subjected to the greatest intramural pressures during systole, it tends to be most vulnerable to ischemia during decreases in coronary perfusion pressure.

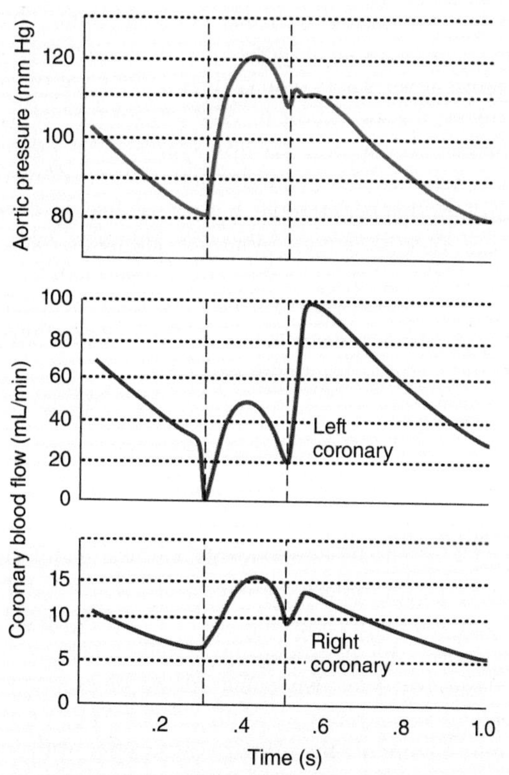

FIGURE 20–16 Coronary blood flow during the cardiac cycle. (Modified with permission from Berne RM, Levy MD, Pappao A, et al. *Cardiovascular Physiology,* 10th ed. Philadelphia, PA: Mosby; 2013.)

Control of Coronary Blood Flow

Coronary blood flow normally parallels myocardial metabolic demand. In the average adult man, coronary blood flow is approximately 250 mL/min at rest. The myocardium regulates its own blood flow closely between perfusion pressures of 50 and 120 mm Hg. Beyond this range, blood flow becomes increasingly pressure dependent.

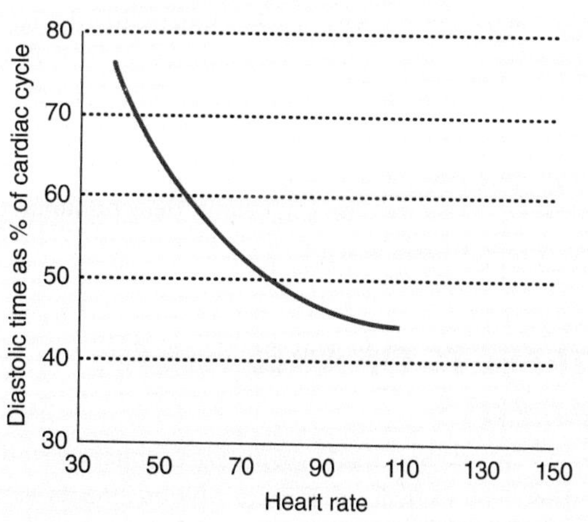

FIGURE 20–17 The relationship between diastolic time and heart rate.

Under normal conditions, changes in blood flow are entirely due to variations in coronary arterial tone (resistance) in response to metabolic demand. Hypoxia—either directly or indirectly through the release of adenosine—causes coronary vasodilation. Autonomic influences are generally weak. Both α_1- and β_2-adrenergic receptors are present in the coronary arteries. The α_1-receptors are primarily located on larger epicardial vessels, whereas the β_2-receptors are mainly found on the smaller intramuscular and subendocardial vessels. Sympathetic stimulation generally increases myocardial blood flow because of an increase in metabolic demand and a predominance of β_2-receptor activation. Parasympathetic effects on the coronary vasculature are generally minor and weakly vasodilatory.

TABLE 20–7 Factors affecting myocardial oxygen supply–demand balance.

Supply
Heart rate (diastolic filling time)
Coronary perfusion pressure
Aortic diastolic blood pressure
Ventricular end-diastolic pressure
Arterial oxygen content
Arterial oxygen tension
Hemoglobin concentration
Coronary vessel diameter
Demand
Basal metabolic requirements
Heart rate
Wall tension
Preload (ventricular radius)
Afterload
Contractility

3. Myocardial Oxygen Balance

Myocardial oxygen demand is usually the most important determinant of myocardial blood flow. Relative contributions to oxygen requirements include basal requirements (20%), electrical activity (1%), volume work (15%), and pressure work (64%). The myocardium usually extracts 65% of the oxygen in arterial blood, compared with 25% in most other tissues. Coronary sinus oxygen saturation is usually 30%. Therefore, the myocardium (unlike other tissues) cannot compensate for reductions in blood flow by extracting more oxygen from hemoglobin. Any increases in myocardial metabolic demand must be met by an increase in coronary blood flow. Table 20–7 lists the most important factors in myocardial oxygen demand and supply. Note that the heart rate and, to a lesser extent, ventricular end-diastolic pressure are important determinants of both supply and demand.

EFFECTS OF ANESTHETIC AGENTS

Most volatile anesthetic agents are coronary vasodilators. Their effect on coronary blood flow is variable because of their direct vasodilating properties, reduction of myocardial metabolic requirements, and effects on arterial blood pressure.

Volatile agents exert beneficial effects in experimental myocardial ischemia and infarction. They reduce myocardial oxygen requirements and protect against reperfusion injury; these effects are mediated by the activation of ATP-sensitive K^+ (K_{ATP}) channels. Some evidence also suggests that volatile anesthetics enhance recovery of the "stunned" myocardium (hypocontractile, but recoverable, myocardium after ischemia). Moreover, although volatile anesthetics decrease myocardial contractility, at moderate doses they can be potentially beneficial in patients with heart failure because most of them decrease preload and afterload.

The Pathophysiology of Heart Failure

Systolic heart failure occurs when the heart is unable to pump a sufficient amount of blood to meet the body's metabolic requirements. Clinical manifestations usually reflect the effects of the low cardiac output on tissues (eg, fatigue, dyspnea, oxygen debt, acidosis), the damming-up of blood behind the failing ventricle (dependent edema or pulmonary venous congestion), or both. The left ventricle is most commonly the primary cause, often with secondary involvement of the right ventricle. Isolated right ventricular failure can occur in the setting of advanced disease of the lung parenchyma or pulmonary vasculature. Left ventricular failure is most commonly the result of myocardial dysfunction, usually from coronary artery disease, but it may also be the result of viral disease, toxins, untreated hypertension, valvular dysfunction, arrhythmias, or pericardial disease.

Diastolic dysfunction can be present in the absence of signs or symptoms of heart failure, as for example in patients with hypertension or aortic valve stenosis. Symptoms arising from diastolic dysfunction are the result of atrial hypertension and pulmonary congestion (Figure 20–18). Failure of the heart to relax during diastole leads to elevated left ventricular end-diastolic pressure, which is transmitted to the left atrium and pulmonary vasculature. Common causes of diastolic dysfunction include hypertension, coronary artery disease, hypertrophic cardiomyopathy, valvular heart disease, and pericardial disease. Diastolic dysfunction is not the same as diastolic heart failure. In a patient with systolic heart failure, the heart compensates by dilating, which leads to an increase in end-diastolic ventricular volume in an attempt to preserve the stroke volume. In a patient with diastolic failure, poor ventricular relaxation leads to a higher LVEDP than would be noted in a patient without diastolic dysfunction for the same end-diastolic volume.

Diastolic dysfunction is diagnosed echocardiographically. Placing the pulse wave Doppler sample gate at the tips of the mitral valve during left ventricular filling will produce the characteristic diastolic flow pattern (see Figure 20–13). In patients with normal diastolic function, the ratio between the peak velocities of the early (E) and the atrial (A) waves is from 0.8 to 2. In the early stages of diastolic dysfunction, the primary abnormality is impaired relaxation. When left ventricular relaxation is delayed, the initial pressure gradient between the left atrium and the left ventricle is reduced, resulting in a decline in early filling and, consequently, a reduced peak E wave velocity. The A wave velocity is increased relative to the E wave, and the E/A ratio is reduced. As diastolic dysfunction advances, the left atrial pressure increases, restoring the gradient between the left atrium and left ventricle with an apparent restoration of the normal E/A ratio. This pattern is characterized as *pseudonormalized*. Using the E/A ratio alone cannot distinguish between a normal and pseudonormalized pattern of diastolic inflow. As diastolic dysfunction worsens further, a restrictive pattern is obtained. In this scenario, the left ventricle is so stiff that pressure builds in the left atrium, resulting in a dramatic peak of early filling and a prominent, tall, narrow E wave. Because the ventricle is so poorly compliant, the atrial contraction contributes little to filling, resulting in a diminished A wave and an E/A ratio greater than 2:1.

Doppler patterns of pulmonary venous flow have been used to distinguish between a pseudonormalized and normal E/A ratio. Currently, most echocardiographers use tissue Doppler to examine

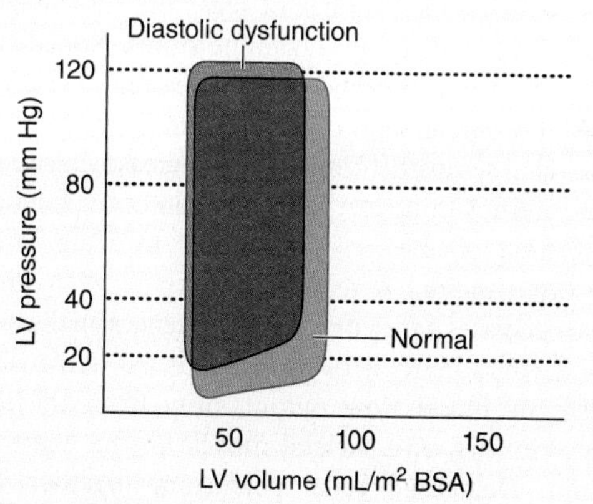

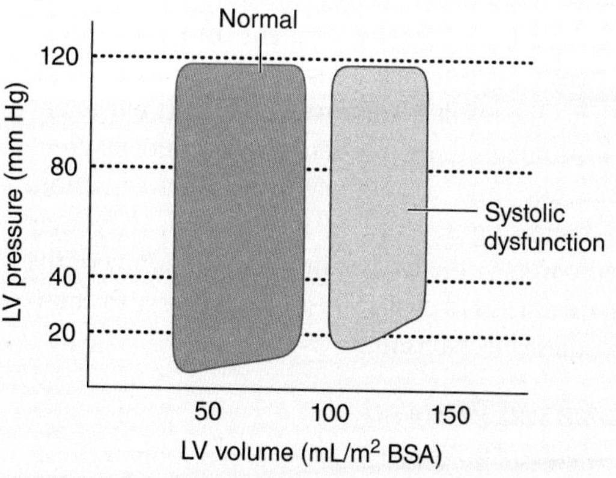

FIGURE 20–18 Ventricular pressure–volume relationships in isolated systolic and diastolic dysfunction. LV, left ventricular.

the movement of the lateral annulus of the mitral valve during ventricular filling (see Figure 20–13). Tissue Doppler allows the echocardiographer to determine both the velocity and the direction of the movement of the heart. During systole, the heart contracts toward the apex, away from a TEE transducer in the esophagus. This motion produces the s' wave of systole. During early and late diastolic filling, the heart moves toward the transducer producing the e' and a' waves. Like the inflow patterns achieved with pulse wave Doppler, characteristic patterns of diastolic dysfunction are reflected in the tissue Doppler trace. An e' wave less than 8 cm/s is consistent with diastolic dysfunction. Of note, the tissue Doppler trace does not produce a pseudonormalized pattern, permitting the echocardiographer to readily distinguish between normal and abnormal diastolic function.

Cardiac output *may* be reduced at rest with heart failure, but the key point is that the heart is incapable of appropriately *increasing* cardiac output and oxygen delivery in response to demand. Inadequate oxygen delivery to tissues is reflected by a low mixed venous oxygen tension and an increase in the arteriovenous oxygen content difference. In compensated heart failure, the arteriovenous difference may be normal at rest, but it rapidly widens during stress or exercise.

COMPENSATORY MECHANISMS

Compensatory mechanisms generally present in patients with heart failure include activation of the sympathetic nervous system and the renin–angiotensin–aldosterone system and increased release of AVP. One result is increased preload (fluid retention). Although these mechanisms can initially compensate for mild to moderate cardiac dysfunction, with increasing severity of dysfunction, they may actually worsen the cardiac impairment. Many of the drug treatments of chronic heart failure serve to counteract these mechanisms.

Increased Preload

An increase in ventricular size not only reflects an inability to keep up with an increased circulating blood volume, but it also serves to increase stroke volume by moving the heart up the Starling curve (see Figure 20–5). Even when EF is reduced, an increase in ventricular end-diastolic volume can maintain a normal stroke volume. Worsening venous congestion caused by the pooling of blood behind the failing ventricle and excessive ventricular dilation can rapidly lead to clinical deterioration. Left ventricular failure results in pulmonary vascular congestion and progressive transudation of fluid, first into the pulmonary interstitium and then into the alveoli (pulmonary edema). Right ventricular failure leads to systemic venous hypertension, which results in peripheral edema, hepatic congestion and dysfunction, and ascites. Dilation of the annulus of either the mitral or tricuspid valves from ventricular dilation leads to valvular regurgitation, further impairing ventricular output.

Increased Sympathetic Tone

Sympathetic activation increases the release of norepinephrine from nerve endings in the heart and secretion of epinephrine from the adrenal glands into the circulation. Although enhanced sympathetic outflow can initially maintain cardiac output by increasing heart rate and contractility, worsening ventricular function elicits increasing degrees of vasoconstriction in an effort to maintain arterial blood pressure. The associated increase in afterload, however, reduces cardiac output and exacerbates ventricular failure.

Chronic sympathetic activation in patients with heart failure eventually decreases the response of adrenergic receptors to catecholamines (receptor uncoupling), the number of receptors (downregulation), and cardiac catecholamine stores. Nonetheless,
11 the failing heart becomes increasingly dependent on circulating catecholamines. Abrupt withdrawal in sympathetic outflow or decreases in circulating catecholamine levels, such as can occur following induction of anesthesia, may lead to acute cardiac decompensation. A reduced density of M_2 receptors also decreases parasympathetic influences on the heart.

Sympathetic activation tends to redistribute systemic blood flow output away from the skin, gut, kidneys, and skeletal muscle to the heart and brain. Decreased renal perfusion, together with β_1-adrenergic activity at the juxtaglomerular apparatus, activates the renin–angiotensin–aldosterone axis, which leads to sodium retention and interstitial edema. Moreover, vasoconstriction secondary to elevated angiotensin II levels increases left ventricular afterload and causes further deterioration of systolic function. The latter partially accounts for the efficacy of angiotensin-converting enzyme (ACE) inhibitors and angiotensin receptor blockers in heart failure. Outcomes in heart failure are improved by the administration of ACE inhibitors (or angiotensin receptor blockers), certain long-acting β-blockers (carvedilol or extended-release metoprolol), and aldosterone inhibitors (spironolactone or eplerenone). All these drugs tend to slow the process of "cardiac remodeling," in which contractile tissue is replaced by connective tissue. Patients with more advanced heart failure may benefit from biventricular pacing.

Circulating AVP levels are often markedly increased in patients with severe heart failure. Increased AVP increases ventricular afterload and leads to a defect in free water clearance that results in hyponatremia.

Brain natriuretic peptide (BNP) is produced in the heart in response to myocyte distention. Elevated BNP concentration (>500 pg/mL) usually indicates heart failure, and measurement of BNP concentration can be used to distinguish between heart failure and lung disease as a cause of dyspnea. Recombinant BNP was developed as a vasodilator and inhibitor of the renin–angiotensin–aldosterone system for use in patients with severe decompensated heart failure, but outcomes were not improved with its use.

Ventricular Hypertrophy

Ventricular hypertrophy can occur with or without dilation, depending on the type of stress imposed on the ventricle. When the heart is subjected to either pressure or volume overload, the initial response is to increase sarcomere length and optimally overlap actin and myosin. With time, ventricular muscle mass begins to increase in response to the abnormal stress.

In the volume-overloaded ventricle, the problem is an increase in diastolic wall stress. The increase in ventricular muscle mass is sufficient only to compensate for the increase in diameter: The ratio of the ventricular radius to wall thickness is unchanged. Sarcomeres replicate mainly in series, resulting in eccentric hypertrophy. Although ventricular EF remains depressed, the increase in end-diastolic volume can maintain normal at-rest stroke volume (and cardiac output).

The problem in a pressure-overloaded ventricle (as in untreated hypertension or aortic valve stenosis) is an increase in systolic wall stress. In this case, sarcomeres mainly replicate in parallel, resulting in concentric hypertrophy. The hypertrophy is such that the ratio of myocardial wall thickness to ventricular radius increases. As can be seen from the law of Laplace, systolic wall stress can then be normalized. Ventricular hypertrophy, particularly that caused by pressure overload, usually results in progressive diastolic dysfunction. The most common reasons for isolated left ventricular hypertrophy are hypertension and aortic stenosis.

CASE DISCUSSION

A Patient With a Short P–R Interval

A 38-year-old man is scheduled for endoscopic sinus surgery following a recent onset of headaches. He gives a history of having passed out at least once during one of these headaches. A preoperative electrocardiogram (ECG) is normal, except for a P–R interval of 0.116 s with normal P-wave morphology.

What is the significance of the short P–R interval?

The P–R interval, which is measured from the beginning of atrial depolarization (P wave) to the beginning of ventricular depolarization (QRS complex), usually represents the time required for depolarization of both atria, the AV node, and the His–Purkinje system. Although the P–R interval can vary with heart rate, it is normally 0.12 to 0.2 s in duration.

What is preexcitation?

Preexcitation usually refers to early depolarization of the ventricles by an abnormal conduction pathway from the atria. Rarely, more than one such pathway is present. The most common form of preexcitation is due to the presence of an accessory pathway (bundle of Kent) that connects one of the atria with one of the ventricles. This abnormal connection between the atria and ventricles allows electrical impulses to bypass the AV node (hence the term *bypass tract*). The ability to conduct impulses along the bypass tract can be quite variable and may be only intermittent or rate dependent. Bypass tracts can conduct in both directions, retrograde only (ventricle to atrium) or, rarely, anterograde only (atrium to ventricle). The name Wolff–Parkinson–White (WPW) syndrome is often applied to ventricular preexcitation associated with tachyarrhythmias.

How does preexcitation shorten the P–R interval?

In patients with preexcitation, the normal cardiac impulse originating from the SA node is conducted simultaneously through the normal (AV nodal) and anomalous (bypass tract) pathways. Because conduction is more rapid in the anomalous pathway than in the AV nodal pathway, the cardiac impulse rapidly reaches and depolarizes the area of the ventricles where the bypass tract ends. This early depolarization of the ventricle is reflected by a short P–R interval and a slurred initial deflection (δ wave) in the QRS complex. The spread of the anomalous impulse to the rest of the ventricle is delayed because it must be conducted by ordinary ventricular muscle, not by the much faster Purkinje system. The remainder of the ventricle is then depolarized by the normal impulse from the AV node as it catches up with the preexcitation front. Although the P–R interval is shortened, the resulting QRS is slightly prolonged and represents a fusion complex of normal and abnormal ventricular depolarizations.

The P–R interval in patients with preexcitation depends on relative conduction times between the AV nodal pathway and the bypass pathway. If conduction through the former is fast, preexcitation (and the δ wave) is less prominent, and QRS will be relatively normal. If conduction is delayed in the AV nodal pathway, preexcitation is more prominent, and more of the ventricle will be depolarized by the abnormally conducted impulse. When the AV nodal pathway is completely blocked, the entire ventricle is depolarized by the bypass pathway, resulting in a very short P–R interval, a very prominent δ wave, and a wide, bizarre QRS complex. Other factors that can affect the degree of preexcitation include interatrial conduction time, the distance of the atrial end of the bypass tract from the SA node, and autonomic tone. The P–R interval is often normal or only slightly shortened with a left lateral bypass tract (the most common location). Preexcitation may be more apparent at fast heart rates because conduction slows through the AV node with increasing heart rates. Secondary ST-segment and T-wave changes are also common because of abnormal ventricular repolarization.

What is the clinical significance of preexcitation?

Preexcitation occurs in approximately 0.3% of the general population. Up to 50% of affected persons develop paroxysmal tachyarrhythmias, typically paroxysmal supraventricular tachycardia (PSVT). Although most patients are otherwise normal, preexcitation can be associated with other cardiac anomalies, including Ebstein anomaly, mitral valve prolapse, and cardiomyopathies. Depending on its conductive properties, the bypass tract in some patients may predispose them to tachyarrhythmias and even sudden death. Tachyarrhythmias include PSVT, atrial fibrillation, and, less commonly, atrial flutter. Ventricular fibrillation can be precipitated by a critically timed premature atrial beat that travels down the bypass tract and catches the ventricle at a vulnerable period. Alternatively, very rapid conduction of impulses into the ventricles by the bypass tract during atrial fibrillation can rapidly lead to myocardial ischemia, hypoperfusion, and hypoxia and culminate in ventricular fibrillation.

Recognition of the preexcitation phenomenon is also important because its QRS morphology on the surface ECG can mimic bundle branch block, right ventricular hypertrophy, ischemia, myocardial infarction, and ventricular tachycardia (during atrial fibrillation).

What is the significance of the history of syncope in this patient?

This patient should be evaluated preoperatively with electrophysiological studies and may possibly require curative radiofrequency ablation of the bypass tract and antiarrhythmic drug therapy. Such studies can identify the location of the bypass tracts, reasonably predict the potential for malignant arrhythmias by programmed pacing, and assess the efficacy of antiarrhythmic therapy if curative ablation is not possible. Ablation is reported to be curative in over 90% of patients. A history of syncope may be ominous because it may indicate the ability to conduct impulses very rapidly through the bypass tract, leading to systemic hypoperfusion and perhaps predisposing the patient to sudden death.

How do tachyarrhythmias generally develop?

Tachyarrhythmias develop as a result of either abnormal impulse formation or abnormal impulse propagation (reentry). Abnormal impulses result from enhanced automaticity, abnormal automaticity, or triggered activity. Usually, only cells of the SA node, specialized atrial conduction pathways, AV nodal junctional areas, and the His–Purkinje system depolarize spontaneously. Because diastolic repolarization (phase 4) is fastest in the SA node, other areas of automaticity are suppressed. Enhanced or abnormal automaticity in other areas, however, can usurp pacemaker function from the SA node and lead to tachyarrhythmias. Triggered activity is the result of either early after-depolarizations (phase 2 or 3) or delayed after-depolarizations (after phase 3). It consists of small-amplitude depolarizations that can follow action potentials under some conditions in atrial, ventricular, and His–Purkinje tissue. If these after-depolarizations reach threshold potential, they can result in an extrasystole or repetitive, sustained tachyarrhythmias. Factors that can promote the formation of abnormal impulses include increased catecholamine levels, electrolyte disorders (hyperkalemia, hypokalemia, hypercalcemia), ischemia, hypoxia, mechanical stretch, and drug toxicity (particularly digoxin).

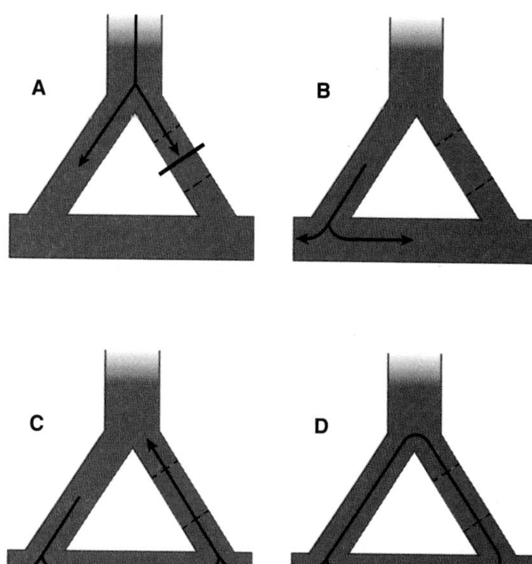

FIGURE 20–19 A–D: The mechanism of reentry. See text for description.

The most common mechanism for tachyarrhythmias is reentry. Four conditions are necessary to initiate and sustain reentry (Figure 20–19): (1) two areas in the myocardium that differ in conductivity or refractoriness and that can form a closed electrical loop; (2) unidirectional block in one pathway (see Figure 20–19A and B); (3) slow conduction or sufficient length in the circuit to allow recovery of the conduction block in the first pathway (see Figure 20–19C); and (4) excitation of the initially blocked pathway to complete the loop (see Figure 20–19D). Reentry is usually precipitated by a premature cardiac impulse.

What is the mechanism of PSVT in patients with WPW syndrome?

If the bypass tract is refractory during anterograde conduction of a cardiac impulse, as during a critically timed atrial premature contraction (APC), and the impulse is conducted by the AV node, the same impulse can be conducted retrograde from the ventricle back into the atria via the bypass tract. The retrograde impulse can then depolarize the atrium and travel down the AV nodal pathway again, establishing a continuous repetitive circuit (circus movement). The impulse reciprocates between the atria and ventricles, and conduction alternates between the AV nodal pathway and the bypass tract. The term *concealed conduction* is often applied because the absence of preexcitation during this arrhythmia results in a normal QRS that lacks a δ wave.

The circus movement less commonly involves anterograde conduction through the bypass tract and retrograde conduction through the AV nodal pathway. In such instances, the QRS has a δ wave and is completely abnormal; the arrhythmia can be mistaken for ventricular tachycardia.

What other mechanisms may be responsible for PSVT?

In addition to the WPW syndrome, PSVT can be caused by AV reentrant tachycardia, AV nodal reentrant tachycardia, and SA node and atrial reentrant tachycardias. Patients with AV reentrant tachycardia have an extranodal bypass tract similar to patients with WPW syndrome, but the bypass tract conducts only retrograde; preexcitation and a δ wave are absent

Functional differences in conduction and refractoriness may occur within the AV node, SA node, or atria; a large bypass tract is not necessary. Thus, the circus movement may occur on a smaller scale within the AV node, SA node, or atria, respectively.

How does atrial fibrillation in patients with WPW syndrome differ from the arrhythmia in other patients?

Atrial fibrillation can occur when a cardiac impulse is conducted rapidly retrograde up into the atria and arrives to find different parts of the atria out of phase in recovery from the impulse. Once atrial fibrillation is established, conduction into the ventricles most commonly occurs through the bypass tract only; because of the accessory pathway's ability to conduct very rapidly (unlike the AV nodal pathway), the ventricular rate is typically very rapid (180–300 beats/min). The majority of QRS complexes are abnormal, but periodic conduction of an impulse through the AV nodal pathway results in occasional normal-looking QRS complexes. Less commonly, impulses during atrial fibrillation are conducted mainly through the AV nodal pathway (resulting in mostly normal QRS complexes) or through both the bypass tract and the AV nodal pathway (resulting in a mixture of normal, fusion, and abnormal QRS complexes). As stated previously, atrial fibrillation in patients with WPW syndrome is a very dangerous arrhythmia.

What anesthetic agents can safely be used in patients with preexcitation?

Few data are available comparing the use of different anesthetic agents or techniques in patients with preexcitation. Almost all the volatile and intravenous agents have been used. Volatile anesthetics increase antegrade refractoriness in both normal and accessory pathways. Propofol, opioids, and benzodiazepines seem to have little direct electrophysiological effects but can alter autonomic tone, generally reducing sympathetic outflow. Factors that tend to cause sympathetic stimulation and increased cardiac automaticity are undesirable. Light anesthesia, hypercapnia, acidosis, and even transient hypoxia will activate the sympathetic system and are to be avoided. When patients with preexcitation are anesthetized for electrophysiological study and surgical ablation, opioids, propofol, and benzodiazepines may be the agents least likely to alter conduction characteristics.

How are antiarrhythmic agents selected for tachyarrhythmias?

Most antiarrhythmic agents act by altering myocardial cell conduction (phase 0), repolarization (phase 3), or automaticity (phase 4). Prolongation of repolarization increases the refractoriness of cells. Many antiarrhythmic drugs also exert direct or indirect autonomic effects. Although antiarrhythmic agents are generally classified according to broad mechanisms of action or electrophysiological effects (Table 20–8), the most commonly

TABLE 20–8 Summary of antiarrhythmic drugs.

Subclass, Drug	Mechanism of Action	Effects	Clinical Applications	Route, Pharmacokinetics, Toxicities, Interactions
CLASS 1A				
Procainamide	I_{Na} (primary) and I_{Kr} (secondary) blockade	Slows conduction velocity and pacemaker rate Prolongs action potential duration and dissociates from I_{Na} channel with intermediate kinetics Direct depressant effects on sinoatrial (SA) and atrioventricular (AV) nodes	Most atrial and ventricular arrhythmias Drug of second choice for most sustained ventricular arrhythmias associated with acute myocardial infarction	Oral, IV, IM Eliminated by hepatic metabolism to *N*-acetylprocainamide (NAPA) and renal elimination NAPA implicated in torsades de pointes in patients with renal failure *Toxicity:* Hypotension. Long-term therapy produces reversible lupus-related symptoms
Quinidine: Similar to procainamide but more toxic (cinchonism, torsades de pointes); rarely used in arrhythmias *Disopyramide: Similar to procainamide but significant antimuscarinic effects; may precipitate heart failure; not commonly used*				
CLASS 1B				
Lidocaine	Sodium channel (I_{Na}) blockade	Blocks activated and inactivated channels with fast kinetics Does not prolong and may shorten action potential	Terminates ventricular tachycardias and prevents ventricular fibrillation after cardioversion	IV First-pass hepatic metabolism Reduce dose in patients with heart failure or liver disease *Toxicity:* Neurological symptoms
Mexiletine: Orally active congener of lidocaine; used in ventricular arrhythmias, chronic pain syndromes				
CLASS 1C				
Flecainide	Sodium channel (I_{Na}) blockade	Dissociates from channel with slow kinetics No change in action potential duration	Supraventricular arrhythmias in patients with normal heart Do not use in ischemic conditions (post myocardial infarction)	Oral Hepatic and kidney metabolism Half-life ~ 20 h *Toxicity:* Proarrhythmic
Propafenone: Orally active, weak β-blocking activity; supraventricular arrhythmias; hepatic metabolism *Moricizine: Phenothiazine derivative, orally active; ventricular arrhythmias, proarrhythmic. Withdrawn in the United States.*				
CLASS 2				
Propranolol	β-Adrenoceptor blockade	Direct membrane effects (sodium channel block) and prolongation of action potential duration Slows SA node automaticity and AV nodal conduction velocity	Atrial arrhythmias and prevention of recurrent infarction and sudden death	Oral, parenteral Duration 4–6 h *Toxicity:* Asthma, AV blockade, acute heart failure *Interactions:* With other cardiac depressants and hypotensive drugs
Esmolol: Short-acting, IV only; used for intraoperative and other acute arrhythmias				

(*continued*)

TABLE 20–8 Summary of antiarrhythmic drugs. (Continued)

Subclass, Drug	Mechanism of Action	Effects	Clinical Applications	Route, Pharmacokinetics, Toxicities, Interactions
CLASS 3				
Amiodarone	Blocks I_{Kr}, I_{Na}, $I_{Ca\text{-}L}$ channels, β-adrenoceptors	Prolongs action potential duration and QT interval Slows heart rate and AV node conduction Low incidence of torsades de pointes	Serious ventricular arrhythmias and supraventricular arrhythmias	Oral, IV Variable absorption and tissue accumulation • hepatic metabolism, elimination complex and slow *Toxicity:* Bradycardia and heart block in diseased heart, peripheral vasodilation, pulmonary and hepatic toxicity Hyper- or hypothyroidism *Interactions:* Many, based on CYP metabolism
Dofetilide	I_{Kr} block	Prolongs action potential, effective refractory period	Maintenance or restoration of sinus rhythm in atrial fibrillation	Oral Renal excretion *Toxicity:* Torsades de pointes (initiate in hospital) *Interactions:* Additive with other QT-prolonging drugs
Sotalol: β-Adrenergic and I_{Kr} blocker, direct action potential prolongation properties, use for ventricular arrhythmias, atrial fibrillation *Ibutilide: Potassium channel blocker, may activate inward current; IV use for conversion in atrial flutter and fibrillation* *Dronedarone: Amiodarone derivative; multichannel actions, reduces mortality in patients with atrial fibrillation* *Vernakalant: Investigational in the United States, multichannel actions in atria, prolongs atrial refractoriness, effective in atrial fibrillation*				
CLASS 4				
Verapamil	Calcium channel ($I_{Ca\text{-}L}$ type) blockade	Slows SA node automaticity and AV nodal conduction velocity Decreases cardiac contractility Reduces blood pressure	Supraventricular tachycardias, hypertension, angina	Oral, IV Hepatic metabolism Caution in patients with hepatic dysfunction
Diltiazem: Equivalent to verapamil				
MISCELLANEOUS				
Adenosine	Activates inward rectifier I_K • blocks I_{Ca}	Very brief, usually complete AV blockade	Paroxysmal supraventricular tachycardias	IV only Duration 10–15 s *Toxicity:* Flushing, chest tightness, dizziness *Interactions:* Minimal

(*continued*)

TABLE 20–8 Summary of antiarrhythmic drugs. (Continued)

Subclass, Drug	Mechanism of Action	Effects	Clinical Applications	Route, Pharmacokinetics, Toxicities, Interactions
Magnesium	Poorly understood • interacts with Na^+–K^+–ATPase, K^+, and Ca^{2+} channels	Normalizes or increases plasma Mg^{2+}	Torsades de pointes • digitalis-induced arrhythmias	IV Duration dependent on dosage *Toxicity:* Muscle weakness in overdose
Potassium	Increases K^+ permeability, K^+ currents	Slows ectopic pacemakers • slows conduction velocity in heart	Digitalis-induced arrhythmias • arrhythmias associated with hypokalemia	Oral, IV *Toxicity:* Reentrant arrhythmias, fibrillation or arrest in overdose

Data from Trevor AJ, Katzung BG, Kruidering-Hall M. *Katzung & Trevor's Pharmacology Examination and Board Review,* 11th ed. New York, NY: McGraw Hill; 2015.

used classification system is not perfect because some agents have more than one mechanism of action.

The selection of an antiarrhythmic agent generally depends on whether the arrhythmia is ventricular or supraventricular and whether acute control or chronic therapy is required. Intravenous agents are usually employed in the acute management of arrhythmias, whereas oral agents are reserved for chronic therapy (Table 20–9).

Which agents are most useful for tachyarrhythmias in patients with WPW syndrome?

Cardioversion is the treatment of choice in hemodynamically compromised patients. Small doses of phenylephrine (100 mcg), together with vagal maneuvers (carotid massage if not contraindicated by carotid occlusive disease), help support arterial blood pressure and may terminate the arrhythmia. The most useful pharmacological agents are class Ia drugs (eg, procainamide). Procainamide increases the refractory period and decreases conduction in the accessory pathway. Moreover, class Ia drugs frequently terminate and can suppress the recurrence of PSVT and atrial fibrillation. Amiodarone is not recommended. Adenosine, verapamil, and digoxin are contraindicated during atrial fibrillation or flutter in these patients because they can dangerously accelerate the ventricular response. Both types of agents decrease conduction through the AV node, favoring the conduction of impulses down the accessory pathway. The bypass tract is capable of conducting impulses into the ventricles much faster than the AV nodal pathway. Digoxin may also increase the ventricular response by shortening the refractory period and increasing conduction in accessory pathways. Although verapamil can terminate PSVT, its use in this setting may be hazardous because patients can subsequently develop atrial fibrillation or flutter. Moreover, atrial fibrillation may not be readily distinguishable from ventricular tachycardia in these patients if wide QRS tachycardia develops.

TABLE 20–9 Clinical pharmacological properties of antiarrhythmic drugs.

Drug	Effect on SA Nodal Rate	Effect on AV Nodal Refractory Period	PR Interval	QRS Duration	QT Interval	Usefulness in Arrhythmias: Supraventricular	Usefulness in Arrhythmias: Ventricular	Half-Life
Adenosine	↓↑	↑↑↑	↑↑↑	0	0	++++	?	<10 s
Amiodarone	↓↓[1]	↑↑	Variable	↑	↑↑↑↑	+++	+++	(weeks)
Diltiazem	↑↓	↑↑	↑	0	0	+++	–	4–8 h
Disopyramide	↑↓[1,2]	↑↓[2]	↑↓[2]	↑↑	↑↑	+	+++	7–8 h
Dofetilide	↓(?)	0	0	0	↑↑	++	None	7 h
Dronedarone					↑	+++	–	24 h
Esmolol	↓↓	↑↑	↑↑	0	0	+	+	10 min
Flecainide	None,↓	↑	↑	↑↑↑	0	+[3]	++++	20 h
Ibutilide	↓(?)	0	0	0	↑↑	++	?	6 h
Lidocaine	None[1]	None	0	0	0	None[4]	+++	1–2 h
Mexiletine	None[1]	None	0	0	0	None	+++	8–20 h
Procainamide	↓[1]	↑↓[2]	↑↓[2]	↑↑	↑↑	+	+++	3–4 h
Propafenone	0, ↓	↑	↑	↑↑↑	0	+	+++	5–7 h
Propranolol	↓↓	↑↑	↑↑	0	0	+	+	5 h
Quinidine	↑↓[1,2]	↑↓[2]	↑↓[2]	↑↑	↑↑	+	+++	6 h
Sotalol	↓↓	↑↑	↑↑	0	↑↑↑	+++	+++	7–12 h
Verapamil	↓↓	↑↑	↑↑	0	0	+++	–	7 h
Vernakalant		↑	↑			+++	–	2 h

[1]May suppress diseased sinus nodes.

[2]Anticholinergic effect and direct depressant action.

[3]Especially in Wolff–Parkinson–White syndrome.

[4]May be effective in atrial arrhythmias caused by digitalis.

Data from Trevor AJ, Katzung BG, Kruidering-Hall M. *Katzung & Trevor's Pharmacology Examination and Board Review,* 11th ed. New York, NY: McGraw Hill; 2015.

SUGGESTED READINGS

Benson MJ, Silverton N, Morrissey C, Zimmerman J. Strain imaging: an everyday tool for the perioperative echocardiographer. *J Cardiothorac Vasc Anesth.* 2020;34:2707.

Bollinger D, Seeberger M, Kasper J, et al. Different effects of sevoflurane, desflurane, and isoflurane on early and late left ventricular diastolic function in young healthy adults. *Br J Anaesth.* 2010;104:547.

Colson P, Ryckwaert F, Coriat P. Renin angiotensin system antagonists and anesthesia. *Anesth Analg.* 1999;89:1143.

Combes A, Price S, Slutsky AS, Brodie D. Temporary circulatory support for cardiogenic shock. *Lancet.* 2020;396:199.

de Baaij JH, Hoenderop JG, Bindels RJ. Magnesium in man: implications for health and disease. *Physiol Rev.* 2015;95:1.

De Hert S. Physiology of hemodynamic homeostasis. *Best Pract Res Clin Anesthesiol.* 2012;26:409.

Duncan A, Alfirevic A, Sessler D, Popovic Z, Thomas J. Perioperative assessment of myocardial deformation. *Anesth Analg.* 2014;118:525.

Epstein AE, Olshansky B, Naccarelli GV, et al. Practical management guide for clinicians who treat patients with amiodarone. *Am J Med.* 2016;129:468.

Forrest P. Anaesthesia and right ventricular failure. *Anaesth Intensive Care.* 2009;37:370.

Francis G, Barots J, Adatya S. Inotropes. *J Am Coll Cardiol.* 2014;63:2069.

Harjola VP, Mebazaa A, Čelutkienė J, et al. Contemporary management of acute right ventricular failure: a statement from the heart failure association and the Working Group on Pulmonary Circulation and Right Ventricular Function of the European Society of Cardiology. *Eur J Heart Fail.* 2016;18:226.

Jacobsohn E, Chorn R, O'Connor M. The role of the vasculature in regulating venous return and cardiac output: historical and graphical approach. *Can J Anaesth.* 1997;44:849.

Obokata M, Reddy YNV, Borlaug BA. Diastolic dysfunction and heart failure with preserved ejection fraction: understanding mechanisms by using noninvasive methods. *JACC Cardiovasc Imaging.* 2020;13(1 Pt 2):245.

Psotka MA, Gottlieb SS, Francis GS, et al. Cardiac calcitropes, myotropes, and mitotropes: JACC review topic of the week. *J Am Coll Cardiol.* 2019;73:2345.

Saw EL, Kakinuma Y, Fronius M, Katare R. The non-neuronal cholinergic system in the heart: a comprehensive review. *J Mol Cell Cardiol.* 2018;125:129.

Sharkey A, Mahmood F, Matyal R. Diastolic dysfunction—what an anesthesiologist needs to know? *Best Pract Res Clin Anaesthesiol.* 2019;33:221.

Shi WY, Li S, Collins N, et al. Peri-operative levosimendan in patients undergoing cardiac surgery: an overview of the evidence. *Heart Lung Circ.* 2015;24:667.

Thandavarayan RA, Chitturi KR, Guha A. Pathophysiology of acute and chronic right heart failure. *Cardiol Clin.* 2020;38:149.

Vistisen ST, Enevoldsen JN, Greisen J, Juhl-Olsen P. What the anaesthesiologist needs to know about heart-lung interactions. *Best Pract Res Clin Anaesthesiol.* 2019;33:165.

Woods J, Monteiro P, Rhodes A. Right ventricular dysfunction. *Curr Opin Crit Care.* 2007;13:535.

C H A P T E R

21

Anesthesia for Patients with Cardiovascular Disease

KEY CONCEPTS

1. Cardiovascular complications are estimated to account for 25% to 50% of deaths following noncardiac surgery. Perioperative myocardial infarction (MI), pulmonary edema, systolic and diastolic heart failure, arrhythmias, stroke, and thromboembolism are the most common diagnoses in patients with preexisting cardiovascular disease.
2. Regardless of the level of preoperative blood pressure control, many patients with hypertension display an accentuated hypotensive response to induction of anesthesia, followed by an exaggerated hypertensive response to intubation.
3. Patients with extensive coronary artery disease, a history of MI, or ventricular dysfunction are at risk of adverse cardiovascular complications.
4. The sudden withdrawal of antianginal medication perioperatively—particularly β-blockers—can precipitate a sudden, rebound increase in ischemic episodes.
5. The overwhelming priority in managing patients with ischemic heart disease is maintaining a favorable myocardial supply–demand relationship. Autonomic-mediated increases in heart rate and blood pressure should be controlled with deeper planes of general anesthesia or adrenergic blockade, vasodilators, or a combination of these.
6. Intraarterial pressure monitoring is reasonable in most patients with severe coronary artery disease and major or multiple cardiac risk factors who are undergoing any but the most minor procedures. Central venous (or rarely pulmonary artery) pressure can be monitored during prolonged or complicated procedures involving large fluid shifts or blood loss.
7. The principal hemodynamic goals in managing mitral stenosis are to maintain a sinus rhythm (if present preoperatively) and to avoid tachycardia, large increases in cardiac output, and both hypovolemia and fluid overload by judicious administration of intravenous fluids.
8. Anesthetic management of mitral regurgitation should be tailored to the severity of regurgitation as well as the underlying left ventricular function. Factors that exacerbate the regurgitation, such as slow heart rates and acute increases in afterload, should be avoided.
9. Maintenance of normal sinus rhythm, heart rate, vascular resistance, and intravascular volume is critical in patients with aortic stenosis. Loss of a normally timed atrial systole often leads to rapid deterioration, particularly when associated with tachycardia.

—Continued next page

Continued—

10 Bradycardia and increases in systemic vascular resistance (SVR) increase the regurgitant volume in patients with aortic regurgitation, whereas tachycardia can contribute to myocardial ischemia. Excessive myocardial depression should also be avoided. The compensatory increase in cardiac preload should be maintained, but excessive fluid replacement can readily result in pulmonary edema.

11 In patients with congenital heart disease, an increase in SVR relative to pulmonary vascular resistance (PVR) favors left-to-right shunting, whereas an increase in PVR relative to SVR favors right-to-left shunting.

12 The presence of shunt flow between the right and left hearts, regardless of the direction of blood flow, mandates the meticulous exclusion of air bubbles or particulate material from intravenous fluids to prevent paradoxical embolism into the cerebral or coronary circulations.

13 The goals of anesthetic management in patients with tetralogy of Fallot should be to maintain intravascular volume and SVR. Increases in PVR, such as might occur from acidosis or excessive airway pressures, should be avoided. The right-to-left shunting tends to slow the uptake of inhalation anesthetics; in contrast, it may accelerate the onset of intravenous agents.

14 The transplanted heart is totally denervated, so direct autonomic influences are absent. Moreover, the absence of reflex increases in heart rate can make patients particularly sensitive to rapid vasodilation. Indirect vasopressors, such as ephedrine, are less effective than direct-acting agents because of the absence of catecholamine stores in myocardial neurons.

Cardiovascular diseases—particularly hypertensive, ischemic, congenital, and valvular heart disease—are among the medical illnesses most frequently encountered in anesthetic practice and are a major cause of perioperative morbidity and mortality. The neuroendocrine response to surgical stimulation and the circulatory effects of anesthetic agents, endotracheal intubation, positive-pressure ventilation, blood loss, fluid shifts, and alterations in body temperature impose additional burdens on an often already compromised cardiovascular system. Most anesthetic agents cause cardiac depression, vasodilation, or both. Even anesthetics that have no direct circulatory effects may cause apparent circulatory depression in severely compromised patients who are dependent on the enhanced sympathetic activity characteristic of heart failure or acute blood loss. Decreased sympathetic activity as a consequence of the anesthetized state can lead to acute circulatory collapse.

Anesthetic management of patients with cardiovascular disease requires a thorough knowledge of normal cardiac physiology, the circulatory effects of the various anesthetic agents, and the pathophysiology and treatment of these diseases. The same principles used in treating cardiovascular diseases in patients not undergoing surgery should be used perioperatively. In most instances, the choice of anesthetic agent is not terribly important; on the other hand, knowing how the agent is used, understanding the underlying pathophysiology, and understanding how the two interact are critical.

Patients with severe cardiovascular illnesses commonly undergo both cardiac and noncardiac surgery. The American College of Cardiology (ACC) has collaborated with the American Heart Association (AHA) in issuing numerous guidelines related to the management of patients with heart disease, and many of their recommendations are relevant to patients undergoing sedation or anesthesia. Because guidelines change as new evidence becomes available, readers are advised to review the AHA website for current evidence-based indications for the management of heart disease. Other jurisdictions likewise issue copious guidelines: readers are reminded to familiarize themselves with the guidelines that apply in their localities.

Perioperative Cardiovascular Evaluation and Preparation for Noncardiac Surgery

The prevalence of acquired cardiovascular disease increases with advancing age. Moreover, the number of patients older than 65 years of age is expected to increase dramatically over the next two decades.
1 Cardiovascular complications are estimated to account for 25% to 50% of deaths following noncardiac surgery. Perioperative myocardial infarction (MI), pulmonary edema, systolic and diastolic heart failure, arrhythmias, stroke, and thromboembolism are the most common diagnoses in patients with preexisting cardiovascular disease. The relatively high prevalence of cardiovascular disorders in surgical patients has given rise to attempts to define *cardiac risk* or the likelihood of intraoperative or postoperative fatal or life-threatening cardiac complications.

The ACC/AHA Task Force Report guidelines state that the patient's medical history is critical in determining the requirements for preoperative cardiac evaluation and that certain conditions (eg, unstable coronary syndromes and decompensated heart failure) warrant cardiology intervention prior to all but emergency procedures. The preoperative history should also address any past procedures, such as cardioverter defibrillator implants, coronary stents, and other interventions. Additionally, the patient's ability to perform the tasks of daily living should be assessed as a guide to determine functional capacity. A patient with a history of cardiac disease and advanced age, but good exercise tolerance, will likely have a lower perioperative risk than a similar individual with dyspnea after minimal physical activity (Table 21–1).

The patient should be queried about other disease processes that frequently accompany heart disease. Cardiac patients often present with obstructive pulmonary disease, reduced kidney function, and diabetes mellitus.

A physical examination should be performed on all patients, and the heart and lungs should be

TABLE 21–1 Estimated energy requirements for various activities.

	Can you ...		Can you ...
1 MET	Take care of yourself?	4 METs	Climb a flight of stairs or walk up a hill?
	Eat, dress, or use the toilet?		Walk on level ground at 4 mph (6.4 kph)?
	Walk indoors around the house?		Run a short distance?
	Walk a block or 2 on level ground at 2 to 3 mph (3.2 to 4.8 kph)?		Do heavy work around the house like scrubbing floors or lifting or moving heavy furniture?
4 METs	Do light work around the house like dusting or washing dishes?		Participate in moderate recreational activities like golf, bowling, dancing, doubles tennis, or throwing a baseball or football?
		Greater than 10 METs	Participate in strenuous sports like swimming, singles tennis, football, basketball, or skiing?

kph, kilometers per hour; MET, metabolic equivalent; mph, miles per hour.

Modified with permission from Hlatky MA, Boineau RE, Higginbotham MB, et al. A brief self-administered questionnaire to determine functional capacity (the Duke Activity Status Index). *Am J Cardiol.* 1989 Sep 15;64(10):651-654.

auscultated. The physical examination is especially useful in patients with certain conditions. For example, if a harsh systolic murmur suggestive of aortic stenosis is detected in a candidate for elective surgery, additional ultrasound evaluation will likely be warranted as aortic stenosis substantially increases risks in patients undergoing noncardiac surgery.

The following conditions are associated with increased risk:

- Ischemic heart disease (history of MI, evidence on electrocardiogram [ECG], chest pain)
- Congestive heart failure (dyspnea, pulmonary edema)
- Cerebral vascular disease (stroke)
- High-risk surgery (vascular, thoracic)
- Diabetes mellitus
- Preoperative creatinine greater than 2 mg/dL

The ACC/AHA guidelines identify conditions that are a major cardiac risk and warrant intensive management prior to all but emergency surgery. These conditions include unstable coronary syndromes (recent MI, unstable angina), decompensated heart failure, significant arrhythmias, and severe valvular heart disease. The ACC/AHA guidelines identify an MI within 7 days, or one within 1 month with myocardium at risk for ischemia, as "active" cardiac conditions. On the other hand, evidence of past MI with no myocardium thought at ischemic risk is considered a low risk for perioperative infarction after noncardiac surgery. The ACC/AHA guidelines classify recommendations into four categories: class I (benefit >>> risk), class IIa (benefit >> risk), class IIb (benefit ≥ risk), and class III (no benefit or harm). Additionally, they grade the strength of the evidence upon which the recommendations are based as A (multiple randomized trials), B (limited trials, nonrandomized studies), and C (consensus of experts, case studies).

Class I recommendations are as follows:

- Patients who have a need for emergency noncardiac surgery should proceed to the operating room with perioperative surveillance and postoperative risk factor management
- Patients with active cardiac conditions should be evaluated by a cardiologist and treated according to ACC/AHA guidelines
- Patients undergoing low-risk procedures should proceed to surgery
- Patients with poor exercise tolerance (<4 metabolic equivalents [METs]) and no known risk factors should proceed to surgery

The ACC/AHA guidelines use an algorithmic approach to discern risks of major adverse cardiac events (MACE; eg, perioperative death or myocardial infarction). Risks accrue secondary to the nature of surgery and because of patient characteristics. The ACC/AHA suggests various risk calculators that are available online (eg, American College of Surgeons risk calculator, www.surgicalriskcalculator.com) to estimate patient risk of perioperative major adverse cardiac events (Figure 21–1).

The ACC/AHA guidelines also provide specific recommendations regarding various preexistent cardiac conditions (eg, heart failure, valvular heart disease, arrhythmias) likely to be encountered perioperatively. Recommendations regarding supplemental preoperative evaluation are presented in Table 21–2.

CORONARY ARTERY DISEASE

The ACC/AHA guidelines suggest that 60 days or more should elapse after an MI not treated with a coronary intervention before noncardiac surgery. Moreover, an MI within 6 months of surgery is associated with increased perioperative mortality. Increased patient age and frailty are likewise associated with greater risk for acute coronary syndromes and stroke. Recently, studies have found a surprising number of asymptomatic patients with elevated levels of troponin after surgery. Such findings are indicative of myocardial injury despite there being no other evidence suggestive of MI. Nevertheless, these patients are at considerably increased risk. Which patients should undergo troponin testing and what should be done for the patients who test "positive" remain controversial.

HYPERTENSION

Patients with hypertension frequently present for elective surgical procedures. Some will have been effectively managed, but unfortunately, many others will not have been. Hypertension is a leading cause of death and disability in most Western societies and the most prevalent preoperative medical abnormality in surgical patients, with an overall prevalence of 20% to 25%. Long-standing uncontrolled hypertension accelerates atherosclerosis and hypertensive organ damage. Hypertension is a major risk factor for cardiac, cerebral, kidney, and vascular disease. **Complications of hypertension include MI, congestive heart failure, stroke, kidney failure, peripheral occlusive disease, and aortic dissection**. The presence of concentric left ventricular hypertrophy (LVH) in hypertensive patients may be an important predictor of cardiac mortality. However, systolic blood pressures below 180 mm Hg and diastolic pressures below 110 mm Hg have not been associated with increased perioperative risks. When patients present with systolic blood pressures greater than 180 mm Hg and diastolic pressures greater than 110 mm Hg, anesthesiologists face the dilemma of delaying surgery to allow optimization of oral antihypertensive therapy but adding the risk of a surgical delay versus proceeding with surgery and achieving blood pressure control with rapidly acting intravenous agents. The incidence of adverse cardiac events in patients treated and operated upon may be similar to that in patients delayed to allow for better long-term blood pressure control. Of note, patients with preoperative hypertension are more likely than others to develop intraoperative hypotension.

Blood pressure measurements are affected by many variables, including posture, time of day, emotional state, recent activity, and drug intake, as well as the equipment and technique used. A diagnosis of hypertension cannot be made with one preoperative reading but requires confirmation by a history of consistently elevated measurements. Although preoperative anxiety or pain may produce some degree of hypertension in normal patients, patients with a history of hypertension generally exhibit greater preoperative elevations in blood pressure.

Epidemiological studies demonstrate a direct and continuous correlation between both diastolic and systolic blood pressures and mortality rates. The definition of systemic hypertension is arbitrary and varies depending upon which management guideline is employed. According to the 2017 ACC guideline, normal blood pressure in adults is a systolic blood pressure less than 120 mm Hg and a diastolic pressure less than 80 mm Hg. Elevated blood pressure constitutes a systolic pressure between 120 and 129 mm Hg, with the diastolic pressure below 80 mm Hg. Hypertension in this definition includes two stages. Stage 1 hypertension exists when the systolic blood pressure is between 130 and 139 mm Hg and the diastolic pressure is between 80 and 89 mm Hg. Stage 2 hypertension is a pressure greater than 140 mm Hg systolic and greater than 90 mm Hg diastolic. If nonpharmacologic interventions (eg, diet, weight loss) fail to correct blood pressure, oral antihypertensive therapy with a primary agent (eg, thiazides, angiotensin-converting enzyme [ACE] inhibitors, angiotensin II receptor blockers [ARBs], calcium channel blockers). Additional secondary agents (eg, β-blockers) may also be required to achieve blood pressure control. A hypertensive urgency reflects blood pressure greater than 180/120 mm Hg without signs of organ injury (eg, hypertensive encephalopathy, heart failure). A hypertensive emergency is characterized by severe hypertension (>180/120 mm Hg) often associated with papilledema, encephalopathy, or other organ injury.

Pathophysiology

Hypertension can be either idiopathic (essential) or, less commonly, secondary to other medical conditions such as kidney disease, renal artery stenosis, primary hyperaldosteronism, Cushing disease, acromegaly, pheochromocytoma, pregnancy, or estrogen therapy. Essential hypertension accounts for 80% to 95% of cases and may be associated with an abnormal baseline elevation of cardiac output, systemic vascular resistance (SVR), or both. An evolving pattern is commonly seen over the course of the disease, where cardiac output returns to (or remains) normal but SVR becomes abnormally high. The chronic increase in cardiac afterload results in

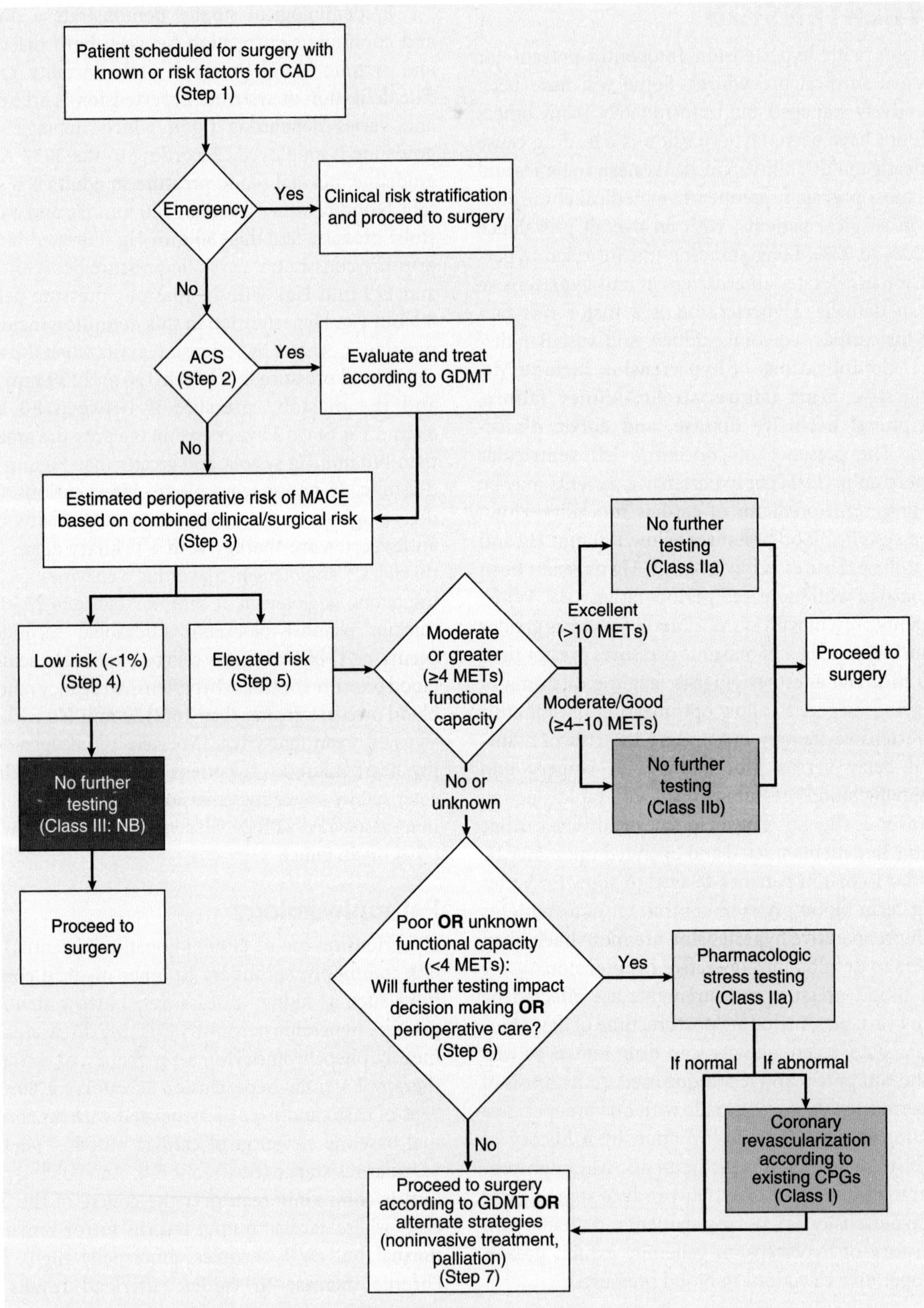

Patient scheduled for surgery with known or risk factors for CAD (Step 1)
Emergency
Yes
Clinical risk stratification and proceed to surgery
No
ACS (Step 2)
Yes
Evaluate and treat according to GDMT
No
Estimated perioperative risk of MACE based on combined clinical/surgical risk (Step 3)
Low risk (<1%) (Step 4)
Elevated risk (Step 5)
No further testing (Class III: NB)
Proceed to surgery
Moderate or greater (≥4 METs) functional capacity
Excellent (>10 METs)
Moderate/Good (≥4–10 METs)
No further testing (Class IIa)
No further testing (Class IIb)
Proceed to surgery
No or unknown
Poor OR unknown functional capacity (<4 METs): Will further testing impact decision making OR perioperative care? (Step 6)
Yes
Pharmacologic stress testing (Class IIa)
If normal
If abnormal
Coronary revascularization according to existing CPGs (Class I)
No
Proceed to surgery according to GDMT OR alternate strategies (noninvasive treatment, palliation) (Step 7)

concentric left ventricular hypertrophy and altered diastolic function. Hypertension also alters cerebral autoregulation, such that normal cerebral blood flow is maintained in the face of high blood pressures; autoregulation limits may be in the range of mean blood pressures of 110 to 180 mm Hg.

The mechanisms responsible for the changes observed in hypertensive patients seem to involve vascular hypertrophy, hyperinsulinemia, abnormal increases in intracellular calcium, and increased intracellular sodium concentrations in vascular smooth muscle and renal tubular cells. Sympathetic nervous system overactivity and enhanced responses to sympathetic agonists are present in some patients. Hypertensive patients sometimes display an exaggerated response to vasopressors and vasodilators. Overactivity of the renin–angiotensin–aldosterone system seems to play an important role in patients with accelerated hypertension.

Long-Term Treatment

Effective drug therapy reduces the progression of hypertension and the incidence of stroke, congestive heart failure, coronary artery disease (CAD), and kidney damage. Effective treatment can also delay and sometimes reverse concomitant pathophysiological changes, such as left ventricular hypertrophy and altered cerebral autoregulation.

Some patients with stage 1 hypertension require only single-drug therapy, which may consist of a

FIGURE 21–1 Stepwise approach to perioperative cardiac assessment for coronary artery disease (CAD). Colors correspond to the following classes of recommendations: class I, green; class IIa, yellow; class IIb, orange; class III, red. *Step 1:* In patients scheduled for surgery with risk factors for or known CAD, determine the urgency of surgery. If an emergency, then determine the clinical risk factors that may influence perioperative management and proceed to surgery with appropriate monitoring and management strategies based on the clinical assessment (see Section 2.1 of the ACC/AHA guidelines for more information on CAD). (For patients with symptomatic heart failure [HF], valvular heart disease [VHD], or arrhythmias, see Sections 2.2, 2.4, and 2.5 of the guidelines for information on evaluation and management.) *Step 2:* If the surgery is urgent or elective, determine if the patient has an acute coronary syndrome (ACS). If yes, then refer the patient for cardiology evaluation and management according to guideline-directed medical therapy (GDMT) according to the UA/NSTEMI and STEMI clinical practice guidelines (CPGs). *Step 3:* If the patient has risk factors for stable CAD, then estimate the perioperative risk of a major adverse cardiac event (MACE) on the basis of the combined clinical/surgical risk. This estimate can use the American College of Surgeons NSQIP risk calculator (http://www.surgicalriskcalculator.com) or incorporate the Revised Cardiac Risk Index (RCRI) with an estimation of surgical risk. For example, a patient undergoing very low-risk surgery (eg, ophthalmologic surgery), even with multiple risk factors, would have a low risk of MACE, whereas a patient undergoing major vascular surgery with few risk factors would have an elevated risk of MACE (see Section 3 of the ACC/AHA guidelines). *Step 4:* If the patient has a low risk of MACE (<1%), then no further testing is needed, and the patient may proceed to surgery (see Section 3 of the guidelines). *Step 5:* If the patient is at elevated risk of MACE, then determine functional capacity with an objective measure or scale such as the Duke Activity Status Index (DASI). If the patient has moderate, good, or excellent functional capacity (>4 METs), then proceed to surgery without further evaluation (see Section 4.1 of the ACC/AHA guidelines). *Step 6:* If the patient has poor (<4 METs) or unknown functional capacity, then the clinician should consult with the patient and perioperative team to determine whether further testing will impact patient decision making (eg, decision to perform original surgery or willingness to undergo coronary artery bypass graft or percutaneous coronary intervention, depending on the results of the test) or perioperative care. If yes, then pharmacological stress testing is appropriate. In those patients with unknown functional capacity, exercise stress testing may be reasonable to perform. If the stress test is abnormal, consider coronary angiography and revascularization depending on the extent of the abnormal test. The patient can then proceed to surgery with GDMT or consider alternative strategies, such as noninvasive treatment of the indication for surgery (eg, radiation therapy for cancer) or palliation. If the test is normal, proceed to surgery according to GDMT (see Section 5.3 of the guidelines). *Step 7:* If testing will not impact decision making or care, then proceed to surgery according to GDMT or consider alternative strategies, such as noninvasive treatment of the indication for surgery (eg, radiation therapy for cancer) or palliation. MET, metabolic equivalent; NB, No Benefit; NSQIP, National Surgical Quality Improvement Program; STEMI, ST-elevation myocardial infarction; UA/NSTEMI, unstable angina/non–ST-elevation myocardial infarction. (Reproduced with permission from Fleisher LA, Fleischman KE, Auerbach AD, et al. 2014 ACC/AHA guideline on perioperative cardiovascular evaluation and management of patients undergoing noncardiac surgery: A report of the American College of Cardiology/American Heart Association Task Force on practice guidelines. *J Am Coll Cardiol.* 2014 Dec 9;64(22):e77-e137.)

TABLE 21–2 Summary of recommendations for supplemental preoperative evaluation.

Recommendations	COR[2]	LOE
The 12-lead ECG		
Preoperative resting 12-lead ECG is reasonable for patients with known coronary heart disease or other significant structural heart disease, except for low-risk surgery	IIa	B
Preoperative resting 12-lead ECG may be considered for asymptomatic patients, except for low-risk surgery	IIb	B
Routine preoperative resting 12-lead ECG is not useful for asymptomatic patients undergoing low-risk surgical procedures	III: No Benefit	B
Assessment of LV function		
It is reasonable for patients with dyspnea of unknown origin to undergo preoperative evaluation of LV function	IIa	C
It is reasonable for patients with HF with worsening dyspnea or other change in clinical status to undergo preoperative evaluation of LV function	IIa	C
Reassessment of LV function in clinically stable patients may be considered	IIb	C
Routine preoperative evaluation of LV function is not recommended	III: No Benefit	B
Exercise stress testing for myocardial ischemia and functional capacity		
For patients with elevated risk and excellent functional capacity, it is reasonable to forgo further exercise testing and preceed to surgery	IIa	B
For patients with elevated risk and unknown functional capacity it may be reasonable to perform exercise testing to assess for functional capacity if it will change management	IIb	B
For patients with elevated risk and moderate to good functional capacity, it may be reasonable to forgo further exercise testing and proceed to surgery	IIb	B
For patients with elevated risk and poor or unknown functional capacity, it may be reasonable to perform exercise testing with cardiac imaging to assess for myocardial ischemia	IIb	C
Routine screening with noninvasive stress testing is not useful for low-risk noncardiac surgery	III: No Benefit	B
Cardiopulmonary exercise testing		
Cardiopulmonary exercise testing may be considered for patients undergoing elevated risk procedures	IIb	B
Noninvasive pharmacological stress testing before noncardiac surgery		
It is reasonable for patients at elevated risk for noncardiac surgery with poor functional capacity to undergo either DSE or MPI if it will change management	IIa	B
Routine screening with noninvasive stress testing is not useful for low-risk noncardiac surgery	III: No Benefit	B
Preoperative coronary angiography		
Routine preoperative coronary angiography is not recommended	III: No Benefit	C

COR, class of recommendation; DSE, dobutamine stress echocardiogram; ECG, electrocardiogram, HF, heart failure; LF, left ventricular; LOE, level of evidence; MPI, myocardial perfusion imaging.

Reproduced with permission from Fleisher LA, Fleischman KE, Auerbach AD, et al. 2014 ACC/AHA guideline on perioperative cardiovascular evaluation and management of patients undergoing noncardiac surgery: A report of the American College of Cardiology/American Heart Association Task Force on practice guidelines. *J Am Coll Cardiol.* 2014 Dec 9;64(22):e77-e137.

thiazide diuretic, angiotensin-converting enzyme (ACE) inhibitor, angiotensin-receptor blocker (ARB), or calcium channel blocker, though guidelines and outcome studies favor the first three options. Concomitant illnesses should guide drug selection. Patients with moderate to severe hypertension often require two or three drugs for control. The combination of a diuretic with a β-adrenergic blocker and an ACE inhibitor is often effective when single-drug therapy is not. As previously noted, ACE inhibitors (or ARBs) prolong survival in patients with congestive heart failure, left ventricular dysfunction, or prior MI. Familiarity with the names, mechanisms of action, and side effects of commonly used antihypertensive agents is important for anesthesia providers (Table 21–3).

PREOPERATIVE MANAGEMENT

A recurring question in anesthetic practice is the degree of preoperative hypertension that is acceptable for patients scheduled for elective surgery. Except for optimally controlled patients, most hypertensive patients present to the operating room with some degree of hypertension. Although data suggest that even moderate preoperative hypertension (diastolic pressure >90–110 mm Hg) is not clearly statistically associated with *postoperative* complications, other data indicate that the untreated or poorly controlled hypertensive patient is more apt to experience *intraoperative* episodes of myocardial ischemia, arrhythmias, or hemodynamic instability. Careful intraoperative adjustments in anesthetic depth and the use of vasoactive drugs should reduce the incidence of postoperative complications referable to poor preoperative control of hypertension.

Although patients should ideally undergo elective surgery only when rendered normotensive, accomplishing this over the short term is not always feasible or even desirable because hypertensive patients have altered cerebral autoregulation. Excessive reductions in blood pressure can compromise cerebral perfusion. Moreover, the decision to delay or to proceed with surgery should be individualized, based on the severity of the preoperative blood pressure elevation; the likelihood of coexisting myocardial ischemia, ventricular dysfunction, or cerebrovascular or renal complications; and the nature and urgency of the procedure. With rare exceptions, antihypertensive drug therapy should be continued up to the time of surgery. Some clinicians withhold ACE inhibitors and ARBs on the morning of surgery because of their association with an increased incidence of intraoperative hypotension; however, withholding these agents increases the risk of marked perioperative hypertension and the need for parenteral antihypertensive agents. It also requires the surgical team to remember to restart the medication after surgery. The decision to delay elective surgical procedures in patients with sustained preoperative diastolic blood pressures higher than 110 mm Hg should be made when the perceived benefits of delayed surgery exceed the risks. Unfortunately, there are few appropriate studies to guide the decision-making.

History

The preoperative history should address the severity and duration of the hypertension, the drug therapy currently prescribed, and the presence or absence of hypertensive complications. Symptoms of myocardial ischemia, ventricular failure, impaired cerebral perfusion, or peripheral vascular disease should be elicited, as well as the patient's record of compliance with the drug regimen. The patient should be questioned regarding chest pain, exercise tolerance, shortness of breath (particularly at night), dependent edema, postural lightheadedness, syncope, episodic visual disturbances or episodic neurological symptoms, and claudication. Adverse effects of current antihypertensive drug therapy (Table 21–4) should also be identified.

Physical Examination & Laboratory Evaluation

Ophthalmoscopy is useful in hypertensive patients. Visible changes in the retinal vasculature usually parallel the severity and progression of arteriosclerosis and hypertensive damage in other organs. An S_4 cardiac gallop is common in patients with LVH. Other physical findings, such as pulmonary rales and an S_3 cardiac gallop, are late findings and indicate congestive heart failure. Blood pressure can be measured in both the supine and standing positions. Orthostatic changes may be due to volume depletion, excessive vasodilation, or sympatholytic drug therapy. Preoperative administration of a carbohydrate drink the night before and on the morning of surgery can promote hemodynamic stability after induction of anesthesia. Although asymptomatic carotid bruits are usually hemodynamically insignificant, they may be reflective of atherosclerotic vascular disease

TABLE 21–3 Summary of drugs used in hypertension.

Subclass, Drug	Mechanism of Action	Effects	Clinical Applications	Pharmacokinetics, Toxicities, Interactions
DIURETICS				
Thiazides: hydrochlorothiazide, chlorthalidone	Block Na/Cl transporter in renal distal convoluted tubule	Reduce blood volume and poorly understood vascular effects	Hypertension, mild heart failure	
Loop diuretics: furosemide	Block Na/K/Cl transporter in renal loop of Henle	Like thiazides; greater efficacy	Severe hypertension, heart failure	
Spironolactone, eplerenone	Block aldosterone receptor in renal collecting tubule	Increase Na and decrease K excretion Poorly understood reduction in heart failure mortality	Aldosteronism, heart failure, hypertension	
SYMPATHOPLEGICS, CENTRALLY ACTING				
Clonidine, methyldopa	Activate α_2-adrenoceptors	Reduce central sympathetic outflow Reduce norepinephrine release from noradrenergic nerve endings	Hypertension Clonidine also used in withdrawal from abused drugs	Oral; clonidine also as patch *Toxicity:* sedation; methyldopa hemolytic anemia
SYMPATHETIC NERVE TERMINAL BLOCKERS				
Reserpine	Blocks vesicular amine transporter in noradrenergic nerves and depletes transmitter stores	Reduces all sympathetic effects, especially cardiovascular, and reduces blood pressure	Hypertension but rarely used	Oral; long duration (days) *Toxicity:* Psychiatric depression, gastrointestinal disturbances
Guanethidine	Interferes with amine release and replaces norepinephrine in vesicles	Same as reserpine	Same as reserpine	Severe orthostatic hypotension, sexual dysfunction
α-BLOCKERS				
Prazosin Terazosin Doxazosin	Selectively block α_1-adrenoceptors	Prevent sympathetic vasoconstriction Reduce prostatic smooth muscle tone	Hypertension Benign prostatic hyperplasia	Oral *Toxicity:* Orthostatic hypotension
β-BLOCKERS				
Metoprolol, others Carvedilol Nebivolol	Block β_1-receptors; carvedilol also blocks α-receptors; nebivolol also releases nitric oxide	Prevent sympathetic cardiac stimulation Reduce renin secretion	Hypertension, heart failure, coronary disease	
Propranolol: Nonselective prototype β-blocker *Metoprolol and atenolol: Very widely used β_1-selective blockers*				

(*continued*)

TABLE 21–3 Summary of drugs used in hypertension. (Continued)

Subclass, Drug	Mechanism of Action	Effects	Clinical Applications	Pharmacokinetics, Toxicities, Interactions
VASODILATORS				
Verapamil Diltiazem	Nonselective block of L-type calcium channels	Reduce cardiac rate and output Reduce vascular resistance	Hypertension, angina, arrhythmias	
Nifedipine, amlodipine, other dihydropyridines	Block vascular calcium channels > cardiac calcium channels	Reduce vascular resistance	Hypertension, angina	
Hydralazine Minoxidil	Causes nitric oxide release Metabolite opens K channels in vascular smooth muscle	Vasodilation Reduces vascular resistance Arterioles more sensitive than veins Reflex tachycardia	Hypertension Minoxidil also used to treat hair loss	Oral *Toxicity:* Angina, tachycardia Hydralazine: Lupus-like syndrome Minoxidil: Hypertrichosis
PARENTERAL AGENTS				
Nitroprusside Fenoldopam Diazoxide Labetalol	Releases nitric oxide Activates D_1 receptors Opens K channels α-, β-blocker	Powerful vasodilation	Hypertensive emergencies	Parenteral; short duration *Toxicity:* Excessive hypotension, shock
ANGIOTENSIN-CONVERTING ENZYME (ACE) INHIBITORS				
Captopril, many others	Inhibit angiotensin-converting enzyme	Reduce angiotensin II levels Reduce vasoconstriction and aldosterone secretion Increase bradykinin	Hypertension, heart failure Diabetes	Oral *Toxicity:* Cough, angioedema, hyperkalemia, renal impairment Teratogenic
ANGIOTENSIN RECEPTOR BLOCKERS (ARBs)				
Losartan, many others	Block AT_1 angiotensin receptors	Same as ACE inhibitors but no increase in bradykinin	Hypertension, heart failure	Oral *Toxicity:* Same as ACE inhibitors but less cough
RENIN INHIBITOR				
Aliskiren	Inhibits enzyme activity of renin	Reduces angiotensin I and II and aldosterone	Hypertension	Oral *Toxicity:* Hyperkalemia, renal impairment Potential teratogen

that may affect coronary circulation. When a bruit is detected, further workup should be guided by the urgency of the scheduled surgery and the likelihood that further investigations, if diagnostic, would result in a change in therapy. Doppler studies of the carotid arteries can be used to define the extent of carotid disease.

The ECG is often normal, but in patients with a long history of hypertension, it may show evidence of ischemia, conduction abnormalities, an old

TABLE 21–4 Adverse effects of long-term antihypertensive therapy.

Class	Adverse Effects
Diuretics	
Thiazide	Hypokalemia, hyponatremia, hyperglycemia, hyperuricemia, hypomagnesemia, hyperlipidemia, hypercalcemia
Loop	Hypokalemia, hyperglycemia, hypocalcemia, hypomagnesemia, metabolic alkalosis
Potassium sparing	Hyperkalemia
Sympatholytics	
β-Adrenergic blockers	Bradycardia, conduction blockade, myocardial depression, enhanced bronchial tone, sedation, fatigue, depression
α-Adrenergic blockers	Postural hypertension, tachycardia, fluid retention
Central α_2-agonists	Postural hypotension, sedation, dry mouth, depression, decreased anesthetic requirements, bradycardia, rebound hypertension, positive Coombs test and hemolytic anemia (methyldopa), hepatitis (methyldopa)
Ganglionic blockers	Postural hypotension, diarrhea, fluid retention, depression (reserpine)
Vasodilators	
Calcium channels blockers	Cardiac depression, bradycardia, conduction blockade (verapamil, diltiazem), peripheral edema (nifedipine), tachycardia (nifedipine), enhanced neuromuscular nondepolarizing blockade
ACE inhibitors[1]	Cough, angioedema, reflex tachycardia, fluid retention, renal dysfunction, hyperkalemia, bone marrow depression (captopril)
Angiotensin-receptor antagonists	Hypotension, kidney failure in bilateral renal artery stenosis, hyperkalemia
Direct vasodilators	Reflex tachycardia, fluid retention, headache, systemic lupus erythematosus-like syndrome (hydralazine), pleural or pericardial effusion (minoxidil)

[1]ACE, angiotensin-converting enzyme.

infarction, or LVH or strain. A normal ECG does not exclude CAD or LVH. Similarly, a normal heart size on a chest radiograph does not exclude ventricular hypertrophy. Echocardiography is a sensitive test for LVH and can be used to evaluate ventricular systolic and diastolic functions in patients with symptoms of heart failure. Chest radiographs are rarely useful in an asymptomatic patient but may show frank cardiomegaly or pulmonary vascular congestion.

Kidney function is typically evaluated by measurement of serum creatinine levels. Serum electrolyte levels (K) should be determined in patients taking diuretics or digoxin or those with kidney impairment. Mild to moderate hypokalemia (3–3.5 mEq/L) is often seen in patients taking diuretics, but it does not have adverse outcome effects. Potassium replacement should be undertaken only in patients who are symptomatic or who are also taking digoxin. Hypomagnesemia is often present and may be a cause of perioperative arrhythmias. Hyperkalemia may be encountered in patients who are taking potassium-sparing diuretics or ACE inhibitors, particularly those with impaired kidney function.

Premedication

Mild to moderate preoperative "white coat" hypertension often resolves following administration of an anxiolytic agent such as midazolam.

INTRAOPERATIVE MANAGEMENT

Objectives

The anesthetic for a hypertensive patient should maintain an appropriately stable blood pressure range. Patients with borderline hypertension may be treated as normotensive patients. Those with long-standing or poorly controlled hypertension, however, have altered autoregulation of cerebral blood flow; higher than normal mean blood pressures may be required to maintain adequate cerebral blood flow. Hypertension, particularly in association with tachycardia, can precipitate or exacerbate myocardial ischemia, ventricular dysfunction, or both. Arterial blood pressure should generally be kept within 20% of preoperative levels.

Monitoring

Most hypertensive patients do not require special intraoperative monitors. Direct intraarterial pressure monitoring should be reserved for patients with wide swings in blood pressure and those undergoing major surgical procedures associated with rapid or marked changes in cardiac preload or afterload. Electrocardiographic monitoring should focus on detecting signs of ischemia. Urinary output should generally be monitored with an indwelling urinary catheter in patients with a preexisting kidney impairment who are undergoing procedures expected to last more than 2 h. Ventricular compliance (see Chapter 20) is typically reduced in patients with ventricular hypertrophy. Excessive intravenous fluid administration in patients with decreased ventricular compliance can also result in elevated pulmonary arterial pressures and pulmonary congestion.

Induction

Induction of anesthesia and endotracheal intubation are often associated with hemodynamic instability
2 in hypertensive patients. Regardless of the level of preoperative blood pressure control, many patients with hypertension display an accentuated hypotensive response to induction of anesthesia, followed by an exaggerated hypertensive response to intubation. Many, if not most, antihypertensive agents and general anesthetics are vasodilators, cardiac depressants, or both. In addition, many hypertensive patients present for surgery in a volume-depleted state. Sympatholytic agents attenuate the normal protective circulatory reflexes, reducing sympathetic tone and allowing unopposed vagal activity.

Hypertensive patients may exhibit severe hypertension during airway manipulation. One of several techniques may be used before intubation to attenuate the hypertensive response:

- Deepening anesthesia with a potent volatile agent
- Administering a bolus of an opioid (fentanyl, 2.5–5 mcg/kg; alfentanil, 15–25 mcg/kg; sufentanil, 0.5–1.0 mcg/kg; or remifentanil, 0.5–1 mcg/kg)
- Administering lidocaine, 1.5 mg/kg intravenously, intratracheally, or topically in the airway
- Achieving β-adrenergic blockade with esmolol, 0.3–1.5 mg/kg; metoprolol 1–5 mg; or labetalol, 5–20 mg

Choice of Anesthetic Agents

A. Induction Agents

The superiority of any one agent or technique over another has not been established. Propofol, barbiturates, benzodiazepines, and etomidate are equally safe for inducing general anesthesia in most hypertensive patients. Ketamine by itself can precipitate marked hypertension; however, it is almost never used as a single agent. When administered with a small dose of another agent, such as a benzodiazepine or propofol, ketamine's sympathetic stimulating properties can be blunted or eliminated.

B. Maintenance Agents

General anesthesia may be safely maintained with volatile or intravenous agents. Regardless of the primary maintenance technique, the addition of a volatile agent or intravenous vasodilator generally allows convenient intraoperative blood pressure control.

C. Vasopressors

Should hypotension develop, a small dose of a direct-acting agent, such as phenylephrine (25–50 mcg), may be beneficial. Patients taking sympatholytics preoperatively may exhibit a decreased response to ephedrine. Vasopressin as a bolus or infusion, or a norepinephrine infusion, can also be employed to restore vascular tone in the hypotensive patient.

TABLE 21–5 Parenteral agents for the acute treatment of hypertension.

Agent	Dosage Range	Onset	Duration
Nitroprusside	0.5–10 mcg/kg/min	30–60 (s)	1–5 min
Nitroglycerin	0.5–10 mcg/kg/min	1 min	3–5 min
Esmolol	0.5 mg/kg over 1 min; 50–300 mcg/kg/min	1 min	12–20 min
Labetalol	5–20 mg	1–2 min	4–8 h
Metoprolol	2.5–5 mg	1–5 min	5–8 h
Hydralazine	5–20 mg	5–20 min	4–8 h
Clevidipine	1–32 mg/h	1–3 min	5–15 min
Nicardipine	5–15 mg/h	1–5 min	3–4 h
Enalaprilat	0.625–1.25 mg	6–15 min	4–6 h
Fenoldopam	0.1–1.6 mg/kg/min	5 min	5 min

Intraoperative Hypertension

Intraoperative hypertension not responding to an increase in anesthetic depth (particularly with a volatile agent) can be treated with a variety of parenteral agents (Table 21–5). Readily reversible causes—such as inadequate anesthetic depth, hypoxemia, or hypercapnia—should always be excluded before initiating antihypertensive therapy. The selection of a hypotensive agent depends on the severity, acuteness, and cause of hypertension; the baseline ventricular function; the heart rate; and the presence of bronchospastic pulmonary disease. β-Adrenergic blockade alone or as a supplement is a good choice for a patient with good ventricular function and an elevated heart rate but is relatively contraindicated in a patient with reactive airway disease. Metoprolol, esmolol, or labetalol are often used intraoperatively. Nicardipine or clevidipine may be preferable to β-blockers for patients with bronchospastic disease. Nitroprusside remains the most rapid and effective agent for the intraoperative treatment of moderate to severe hypertension, but it has been largely supplanted by other agents. Nitroglycerin may be less effective, but it is also useful in treating or preventing myocardial ischemia. Fenoldopam, a dopaminergic agonist, is also a useful hypotensive agent; furthermore, it increases renal blood flow. Hydralazine provides sustained blood pressure control but has a delayed onset and can cause reflex tachycardia. Reflex tachycardia is not seen with labetalol because of its combined α- and β-adrenergic blockade.

POSTOPERATIVE MANAGEMENT

Postoperative hypertension is common and should be anticipated in patients who have poorly controlled baseline blood pressure. Close blood pressure monitoring should be continued in both the postanesthesia care unit and the early postoperative period. Postoperatively, marked sustained elevations in blood pressure can contribute to the formation of wound hematomas and the disruption of vascular suture lines.

Hypertension in the recovery period is often multifactorial and accentuated by respiratory abnormalities, anxiety and pain, volume overload, bladder distention, or any combination of these. Contributing causes should be corrected and parenteral antihypertensive agents given if necessary. Intravenous labetalol is particularly useful in controlling hypertension and tachycardia, whereas vasodilators are useful in controlling blood pressure in the setting of a slow heart rate. When the patient resumes oral intake, preoperative antihypertensive medications should be restarted.

ISCHEMIC HEART DISEASE

Preoperative Considerations

Myocardial ischemia results from metabolic oxygen demand that exceeds the oxygen supply. Ischemia can therefore result from increased myocardial metabolic demand, reduced myocardial oxygen delivery, or a combination of both. Common causes include coronary arterial atherosclerosis, thrombosis, or vasospasm; severe hypertension or tachycardia (particularly in the presence of ventricular hypertrophy); severe hypotension, hypoxemia, or anemia; and severe aortic stenosis or regurgitation.

By far, the most common cause of myocardial ischemia is atherosclerosis of the coronary arteries. CAD is responsible for about 25% of all deaths in Western societies and is a major cause of perioperative morbidity and mortality. The overall incidence of CAD in surgical patients is estimated to be between 5% and 10%. Major preoperative risk factors for CAD include hyperlipidemia, hypertension, diabetes, cigarette smoking, increasing age, male sex, and a positive family history. Other risk factors include obesity, a history of cerebrovascular or peripheral vascular disease, menopause, use of high-estrogen oral contraceptives by women who smoke, and a sedentary lifestyle.

CAD may be manifested by symptoms, characteristic electrocardiographic or echocardiographic findings, or biochemical evidence of myocardial infarction; symptoms (usually angina) or characteristic echocardiographic or electrocardiographic findings of ischemia; or arrhythmias (including sudden death), symptoms (orthopnea, dyspnea on exertion), signs (rales, dependent edema, shock), or echocardiographic changes suggestive of ventricular dysfunction. An ambulatory patient presenting with risk factors for CAD and new symptoms would normally undergo some form of cardiac stress testing to confirm the suspected diagnosis.

Unstable Angina

Unstable angina is defined as (1) an abrupt increase in severity, frequency (more than three episodes per day), or duration of anginal attacks (crescendo angina); (2) angina at rest; or (3) new onset of angina (within the past 2 months) with severe or frequent episodes (more than three per day). Unstable angina may occur following MI or be precipitated by major surgery or by noncardiac medical conditions, including severe anemia, fever, infections, thyrotoxicosis, hypoxemia, and emotional distress in previously stable patients.

Unstable angina, particularly when it is associated with significant ST-segment changes at rest, usually reflects severe underlying coronary disease and may be followed by MI. Plaque disruption with platelet aggregates or thrombi and vasospasm are frequent pathological correlates. Critical stenosis in one or more major coronary arteries is present in more than 80% of patients with these symptoms. Patients with unstable angina require evaluation and treatment, which may include some form of coronary intervention.

Chronic Stable Angina

Anginal chest pains are most often substernal, exertional, radiating to the neck or arm, and relieved by rest or nitroglycerin. Variations are common, including epigastric, back, or neck pain or transient shortness of breath from ventricular dysfunction (anginal equivalent). Nonexertional ischemia and silent (asymptomatic) ischemia are fairly common occurrences, particularly following surgery. Patients with diabetes have an increased incidence of silent ischemia.

Symptoms are generally absent until the atherosclerotic lesions cause 50% to 75% occlusion of the coronary circulation. When a stenotic segment reaches 70% occlusion, maximum compensatory dilation is usually present distally: blood flow may be adequate at rest but inadequate with increased metabolic demand. An extensive collateral blood supply allows some patients to remain relatively asymptomatic despite severe disease. Coronary vasospasm is also a cause of transient transmural ischemia in some patients; most vasospastic episodes occur at

TABLE 21–6 Comparison of antianginal agents.[1]

		Calcium Channel Blockers			
Cardiac Parameter	**Nitrates**	**Verapamil**	**Nifedipine Nicardipine Nimodipine**	**Diltiazem**	**β-Blockers**
Preload	↓↓	—	—	—	—/↑
Afterload	↓	↓	↓↓	↓	—/↓
Contractility	—	↓↓	—	↓	↓↓↓
SA node automaticity	↑/—	↓↓	↑/—	↓↓	↓↓↓
AV conduction	—	↓↓↓	—	↓↓	↓↓↓
Vasodilatation					
Coronary	↑	↑↑	↑↑↑	↑↑	—/↓
Systemic	↑↑	↑	↑↑	↑	—/↓

[1]AV, atrioventricular; SA, sinoatrial; ↑, increases; —, no change; ↓, decreases.

preexisting stenotic lesions in epicardial vessels and may be precipitated by a variety of factors, including emotional upset and hyperventilation (Prinzmetal angina). Coronary spasm is more often observed in patients who have angina with varying levels of activity or emotional stress (variable-threshold); it is less common with classic exertional (fixed-threshold) angina.

The overall prognosis of patients with CAD is related to both the number and severity of coronary obstructions as well as to the extent of ventricular dysfunction.

Treatment of Ischemic Heart Disease

The general approach in treating patients with ischemic heart disease is five-fold:

- Correction of risk factors, with the hope of slowing disease progression
- Modification of the patient's lifestyle to reduce stress and improve exercise tolerance
- Correction of complicating medical conditions that can exacerbate ischemia (ie, hypertension, anemia, hypoxemia, hyperthyroidism, fever, infection, adverse drug effects)
- Pharmacological manipulation of the myocardial oxygen supply–demand relationship
- Anticoagulation
- Correction of coronary lesions by percutaneous coronary intervention (angioplasty [with or without stenting] or atherectomy) or coronary artery bypass surgery

The most commonly used pharmacological agents for stable ischemic heart disease are nitrates, β-blockers, calcium channel blockers, and platelet inhibitors. Those drugs with circulatory effects are compared in Table 21–6.

A. β-Adrenergic Blocking Agents

These drugs are first-line agents for patients with stable ischemic heart disease. They decrease myocardial oxygen demand by reducing heart rate and contractility and, in some cases, afterload (via their antihypertensive effect). In contrast to other agents, they increase survival in patients with impaired left ventricular function, increase survival after MI, and reduce the likelihood of a subsequent infarction. Optimal blockade results in a resting heart rate between 50 and 60 beats/min and prevents appreciable increases with exercise (<20 beats/min increase during exercise). Available agents differ in receptor selectivity, intrinsic sympathomimetic (partial agonist) activity, and membrane-stabilizing properties (Table 21–7). Membrane stabilization results in

TABLE 21–7 Comparison of β-adrenergic blocking agents.

Agent	β_1-Receptor Selectivity	Half-Life	Sympathomimetic	α-Receptor Blockade	Membrane Stabilizing
Acebutolol	+	2–4 h	+		+
Atenolol	++	5–9 h			
Betaxolol	++	14–22 h			
Esmolol	++	9 min			
Metoprolol	++	3–4 h			±
Bisoprolol	+	9–12 h			
Oxprenolol		1–2 h	+		+
Alprenolol		2–3 h	+		+
Pindolol		3–4 h	++		±
Penbutolol		5 h	+		+
Carteolol		6 h	+		
Labetalol		4–8 h		+	±
Propranolol		3–6 h			++
Timolol		3–5 h			
Sotalol[1]		5–13 h			
Nadolol		10–24 h			
Carvedilol		6–8 h		+	±

[1]Also possesses unique antiarrhythmic properties.

antiarrhythmic activity. Agents with intrinsic sympathomimetic properties are better tolerated by patients with mild to moderate ventricular dysfunction. Certain β-blockers (bisoprolol, carvedilol, extended-duration metoprolol) improve survival in patients with chronic heart failure. Blockade of β_2-adrenergic receptors also can mask hypoglycemic symptoms in patients with diabetes, delay metabolic recovery from hypoglycemia, and impair the handling of large potassium loads. Cardioselective (β_1-receptor-specific) agents, though generally better tolerated than nonselective agents in patients with reactive airways, must still be used cautiously in such patients. The selectivity of cardioselective agents tends to be dose dependent. Patients on long-standing β-blocker therapy should have these agents continued perioperatively. Acute β-blocker withdrawal in the perioperative period places patients at a markedly increased risk of cardiac morbidity and mortality.

B. Calcium Channel Blockers

These agents are chosen when a patient cannot take a β-blocker or when treatment with a β-blocker is insufficient. The effects and uses of the most commonly used calcium channel blockers are shown in Table 21–8. Calcium channel blockers reduce myocardial oxygen demand by decreasing cardiac afterload and augment myocardial oxygen supply via coronary vasodilation. Verapamil and diltiazem also reduce demand by slowing the heart rate.

TABLE 21–8 Comparison of calcium channel blockers.

				Clinical Use			
Agent	**Route**	**Dosage[1]**	**Half-life**	***Angina***	***Hypertension***	***Cerebral Vasospasm***	***Supraventricular Tachycardia***
Verapamil	PO	40–240 mg	5 h	+	+		+
	IV	5–15 mg	5 h	+			+
Nifedipine	PO	30–180 mg	2 h	+	+		
	SL	10 mg	2 h	+	+		
Diltiazem	PO	30–60 mg	4 h	+	+		+
	IV	0.25–0.35 mg/kg	4 h	+			+
Nicardipine	PO	60–120 mg	2–4 h	+	+		
	IV	5 mg/hr	2–4 h	+	+		
Nimodipine	PO	240 mg	2 h			+	
Bepridil[2]	PO	200–400 mg	24 h	+	+		
Isradipine	PO	2.5–5.0 mg	8 h		+		
Felodipine	PO	5–20 mg	9 h		+		
Amlodipine	PO	2.5–10 mg	30–50 h	+	+		

[1]Total oral dose per day divided into three doses unless otherwise stated.
[2]Also possesses antiarrhythmic properties.

Nifedipine's potent effects on systemic blood pressure may precipitate hypotension, reflex tachycardia, or both. Its tendency to decrease afterload generally offsets any negative inotropic effect. Long-acting verapamil, diltiazem, amlodipine, or felodipine are preferred. Nicardipine and clevidipine generally have the same effects as nifedipine but are shorter acting, and clevidipine is particularly useful as a vasodilator infusion. Nimodipine is primarily used in preventing cerebral vasospasm following subarachnoid hemorrhage.

All calcium channel blockers potentiate depolarizing and nondepolarizing neuromuscular blocking agents and the circulatory effects of volatile agents. Verapamil and diltiazem can potentiate depression of cardiac contractility and conduction in the atrioventricular (AV) node by volatile anesthetics. Nifedipine and similar agents can potentiate systemic vasodilation by volatile and intravenous agents.

C. Nitrates

Nitrates decrease venous and arteriolar tone, increase vascular capacitance, and reduce ventricular wall tension. These effects tend to reduce myocardial oxygen demand. Prominent venodilation makes nitrates excellent agents when congestive heart failure is also present.

Additionally, nitrates dilate the coronary arteries. Even minor degrees of dilation at stenotic sites may be sufficient to increase blood flow because flow is directly related to the fourth power of the radius. Nitrate-induced coronary vasodilation preferentially increases subendocardial blood flow in ischemic areas. This favorable redistribution of coronary blood flow to ischemic areas may be dependent on the presence of collaterals in the coronary circulation.

Nitrates can be used for both the treatment of acute ischemia and prophylaxis against frequent anginal episodes.

D. Anticoagulants

Chronic aspirin therapy reduces coronary events in patients with CAD and prevents coronary and ischemic cerebral events in at-risk patients. Other platelet antagonists are generally also included in patients who have undergone percutaneous coronary stenting. Careful review of anticoagulant/antiplatelet medications is a mandatory element of preanesthetic assessment, especially if neuraxial anesthesia is being considered (see Chapter 45).

E. Other Agents and Other Treatments

ACE inhibitors prolong survival in patients with congestive heart failure or left ventricular dysfunction. Antiarrhythmic therapy in patients with complex ventricular ectopy who have significant CAD and left ventricular dysfunction should be guided by an electrophysiological study. Patients with inducible sustained ventricular tachycardia (VT) or ventricular fibrillation are candidates for an automatic internal cardioverter-defibrillator (ICD). Treatment of ventricular ectopy (with the exception of sustained VT) in patients with good ventricular function does not improve survival and may increase mortality. In contrast, ICDs have been shown to improve survival in patients with advanced cardiomyopathy (ejection fraction <30%), even in the absence of demonstrable arrhythmias.

F. Combination Therapy

Moderate to severe angina frequently requires combination therapy with two or more classes of agents. Patients with ventricular dysfunction may not tolerate the combined negative inotropic effect of a β-blocker and a calcium channel blocker together; an ACE inhibitor or ARB is better tolerated and seems to improve survival. Similarly, the additive effect of a β-blocker and a calcium channel blocker on the AV node may precipitate heart block in susceptible patients.

PREOPERATIVE MANAGEMENT

The importance of ischemic heart disease—particularly a history of MI—as a risk factor for perioperative morbidity and mortality is reviewed earlier in this chapter. Most studies confirm that perioperative outcome is related to disease severity, ventricular function, and the type of surgery to be undertaken. 3 Patients with extensive (three-vessel or left main) CAD, a recent history of MI, or ventricular dysfunction are at greatest risk of cardiovascular complications. As previously mentioned, current guidelines recommend revascularization only when such treatment would be indicated irrespective of the patient's need for surgery.

Chronic stable (mild to moderate) angina does not seem to increase perioperative risk substantially. Similarly, a history of prior coronary artery bypass surgery or coronary angioplasty alone does not seem to substantially increase perioperative risk. In some studies, maintenance of chronic β-receptor blockers in the perioperative period has been shown to reduce perioperative mortality and the incidence of postoperative cardiovascular complications; however, other studies have shown an increase in stroke and death following preoperative introduction of β-blockers to at-risk patients. Consequently, acutely initiating therapy with β-blockers in at-risk patients who will undergo surgery is no longer recommended. Like β-blockers, statins should be continued perioperatively in patients so routinely treated because acute perioperative withdrawal of statins is associated with adverse outcomes. The ACC/AHA 2014 recommendations are summarized in a set of useful guidelines that also provide guidance on the timing of surgery following percutaneous coronary interventions and the deployment of coronary stents (Table 21–9).

History

The most important symptoms to elicit include chest pain, dyspnea, poor exercise tolerance, syncope, or near syncope. The relationship between symptoms and activity level should be established. Activity should be described in terms of everyday tasks, such as walking or climbing stairs. Patients

TABLE 21–9 Summary of recommendations for perioperative therapy.

Recommendations	COR[1]	LOE
Coronary revascularization before noncardiac surgery		
Revascularization before noncardiac surgery is recommended when indicated by existing CPGs	I	C
Coronary revascularization is not recommended before noncardiac surgery exclusively to reduce perioperative cardiac events	III: No Benefit	B
Timing of elective noncardiac surgery in patients with previous PCI		
Noncardiac surgery should be delayed after PCI	I	C: 14 d after balloon angioplasty B: 30 d after BMS implantation
Noncardiac surgery should optimally be delayed 365 d after DES implantation	I	B
A consensus decision as to the relative risks of discontinuation or continuation of antiplatelet therapy can be useful	IIa	C
Elective noncardiac surgery after DES implantation may be considered after 180 d	IIb[2]	B
Elective noncardiac surgery should not be performed in patients in whom DAPT will need to be discontinued perioperatively within 30 d after BMS implantation or within 12 mo after DES implantation	III: Harm	B
Elective noncardiac surgery should not be performed within 14 d of balloon angioplasty in patients in whom aspirin will need to be discontinued perioperatively	III: Harm	C
Perioperative-β-blocker therapy		
Continue-β-blockers in patients who are on β-blockers chronically	I	B[SR4]
Guide management of β-blockers after surgery by clinical circumstances	IIa	B[SR4]
In patients with intermediate- or high-risk preoperative tests, it may be reasonable to begin β-blockers	IIb	C[SR4]
In patients with ≥3 RCRI factors, it may be reasonable to begin β-blockers before surgery	IIb	B[SR4]
Initiating β-blockers in the perioperative setting as an approach to reduce perioperative risk is of uncertain benefit in those with a long-term indication but no other RCRI risk factors	IIb	B[SR4]
It may be reasonable to begin perioperative β-blockers long enough in advance to assess safety and tolerability, preferably >1 d before surgery	IIb	B[SR4]
β-blocker therapy should not be started on the day of surgery	III: Harm	B[SR4]
Preoperative statin therapy		
Continue statins in patients currently taking statins	I	B
Perioperative initiation of statin use is reasonable in patients undergoing vascular surgery	IIa	B
Perioperative initiation of statins may be considered in patients with a clinical risk factor who are undergoing elevated-risk procedures	IIb	C
α_2-Agonists		
α_2-Agonists are not recommended for prevention of cardiac events	III: No Benefit	B

(*continued*)

TABLE 21–9 Summary of recommendations for perioperative therapy. (Continued)

Recommendations	COR[1]	LOE
ACE inhibitors		
Continuation of ACE inhibitors or ARBs is reasonable perioperatively	IIa	B
If ACE inhibitors or ARBs are held before surgery, it is reasonable to restart as soon as clinically feasible postoperatively	IIa	C
Antiplatelet agents		
Continue DAPT in patients undergoing urgent noncardiac surgery during the first 4 to 6 wk after BMS or DES implantation, unless the risk of bleeding outweighs the benefit of stent thrombosis prevention	I	C
In patients with stents undergoing surgery that requires discontinuation $P2Y_{12}$ inhibitors, continue aspirin and restart the $P2Y_{12}$ platelet receptor-inhibitor as soon as possible after surgery	I	C
Management of perioperative antiplatelet therapy should be determined by consensus of treating clinicians and the patient	I	C
In patients undergoing nonemergency/nonurgent noncardiac surgery without prior coronary stenting, it may be reasonable to continue aspirin when the risk of increased cardiac events outweighs the risk of increased bleeding	IIb	B
Initiation or continuation of aspirin is not beneficial in patients undergoing elective noncardiac noncarotid surgery who have not had previous coronary stenting	III: No Benefit	B C: If risk of ischemic events outweighs risk of surgical bleeding
Perioperative management of patients with CIEDs		
Patients with ICDs should be on a cardiac monitor continuously during the entire period of inactivation, and external defibrillation equipment should be available. Ensure that ICDs are reprogrammed to active therapy	I	C

[1]ACE, angiotensin-converting enzyme; ARB, angiotensin receptor blocker; BMS, bare metal stent; CIED, cardiovascular implantable electronic device; COR, class of recommendation; CPG, clinical practice guidelines; DAPT, dual antiplatelet therapy; DES, drug-eluting stent; ERC, Evidence Review Committee; ICD, implantable cardioverter-defibrillator; LOE, level of evidence; PCI, percutaneous coronary intervention; RCRI, Revised Cardiac Risk Index; SR, systematic review.

[2]Because of new evidence, this is a new recommendation since the publication of the 2011 PCI CPG.

[3]These recommendations have been designated with an [SR] to emphasize the rigor of support from the ERC's systemic review.

Reproduced with permission from Fleisher LA, Fleischman KE, Auerbach AD, et al. 2014 ACC/AHA guideline on perioperative cardiovascular evaluation and management of patients undergoing noncardiac surgery: A report of the American College of Cardiology/American Heart Association Task Force on practice guidelines. *J Am Coll Cardiol.* 2014 Dec 9;64(22):e77-e137.

may be relatively asymptomatic despite severe CAD if they have a sedentary lifestyle. Patients with diabetes are particularly prone to silent ischemia. Easy fatigability or shortness of breath suggests impaired ventricular function.

A history of unstable angina or MI should include the time of its occurrence and whether it was complicated by arrhythmias, conduction disturbances, or heart failure. Arrhythmias and conduction abnormalities are more common in patients with previous infarction and in those with poor ventricular function. This latter group of patients will often have ICDs.

Physical Examination & Routine Laboratory Evaluation

Evaluation of patients with CAD is similar to that of patients with hypertension. Laboratory evaluation in patients who have a history compatible with recent unstable angina and are undergoing emergency procedures should include cardiac enzymes. Normal serum levels of troponins, creatine kinase (MB isoenzyme), and lactate dehydrogenase (type 1 isoenzyme) are useful in excluding MI. Measures of brain natriuretic peptide (BNP) or its prohormone can be useful to identify patients with ventricular dysfunction and to screen for perioperative risk.

The baseline ECG is normal in 25% to 50% of patients with CAD but no prior MI. Electrocardiographic evidence of ischemia often becomes apparent only during angina. The most common baseline abnormalities are nonspecific ST-segment and T-wave changes. Prior infarction may be manifested by Q waves or loss of R waves in the leads closest to the infarct. First-degree AV block, bundle-branch block, or hemiblock may be present. Persistent ST-segment elevation following MI may be indicative of a left ventricular aneurysm. A long rate-corrected QT interval (QT_c >0.44 s) may reflect the underlying ischemia, drug toxicity (usually class Ia antiarrhythmic agents, antidepressants, or phenothiazines), electrolyte abnormalities (hypokalemia or hypomagnesemia), autonomic dysfunction, mitral valve prolapse, or, less commonly, a congenital abnormality. Patients with a long QT interval are at risk of developing ventricular arrhythmias—particularly polymorphic VT (torsades de pointes), which can lead to ventricular fibrillation. The long QT interval reflects nonuniform prolongation of ventricular repolarization and predisposes patients to reentry phenomena. In contrast to polymorphic ventricular arrhythmias with a normal QT interval, which respond to conventional antiarrhythmics, polymorphic tachyarrhythmias with a long QT interval generally respond best to pacing or magnesium salts.

The chest radiograph can be used to exclude cardiomegaly or pulmonary vascular congestion secondary to ventricular dysfunction.

Specialized Studies

A. Holter Monitoring

Continuous ambulatory electrocardiographic (Holter) monitoring is useful in evaluating arrhythmias, antiarrhythmic drug therapy, and severity and frequency of ischemic episodes. Silent (asymptomatic) ischemic episodes are frequently found in patients with CAD. Frequent ischemic episodes on preoperative Holter monitoring correlate well with intraoperative and postoperative ischemia. Holter monitoring showing no ischemic episodes has an excellent negative predictive value for postoperative cardiac complications.

B. Exercise Electrocardiography

The usefulness of this test without associated cardiac imaging is limited in patients with baseline ST-segment abnormalities and those who are unable to increase their heart rate (>85% of maximal predicted) because of fatigue, dyspnea, or drug therapy. Overall sensitivity is 65%, and specificity is 90%. Exercise testing is most sensitive (85%) in patients with three-vessel or left main CAD. Disease that is limited to the left circumflex artery may also be missed because ischemia in its distribution may not be evident on the standard surface ECG. A normal test does not necessarily exclude CAD but suggests that severe disease is not likely. The degree of ST-segment depression, its severity and configuration, the time of onset in the test, and the time required for resolution are important findings. A myocardial ischemic response at low levels of exercise is associated with a significantly increased risk of perioperative complications and long-term cardiac events. Other significant findings include changes in blood pressure and the occurrence of arrhythmias. Exercise-induced ventricular ectopy frequently indicates severe CAD associated with ventricular dysfunction. The ischemia presumably leads to electrical instability in myocardial cells. Given that risk seems to be associated with the extent of potentially ischemic myocardium, testing often includes perfusion scans or echocardiographic assessments; however, in ambulatory patients, exercise ECG testing alone is useful because it estimates functional capacity and detects myocardial ischemia.

C. Myocardial Perfusions Scans and Other Imaging Techniques

Myocardial perfusion imaging using thallium-201 or technetium-99m is used in evaluating patients who cannot exercise (eg, peripheral vascular disease) or who have underlying ECG abnormalities that preclude interpretation during exercise (eg, left bundle-branch block). If the patient cannot exercise, images are obtained before and after injection of an intravenous coronary dilator (eg, dipyridamole or adenosine) to produce a hyperemic response similar to exercise. Myocardial perfusion studies following exercise or injection of dipyridamole or adenosine have a high sensitivity but only fairly good specificity for CAD. They are best for detecting two- or three-vessel disease. These scans can locate and quantitate areas of ischemia or scarring and differentiate between the two. Perfusion defects that fill in on the redistribution phase represent ischemia, not previous infarction. The negative predictive value of a normal perfusion scan is approximately 99%.

Magnetic resonance imaging, positron emission tomography, and computed tomography scans are increasingly being used to define coronary artery anatomy and determine myocardial viability.

D. Echocardiography

This technology provides information about both regional and global ventricular function and may be carried out at rest, following exercise, or with administration of dobutamine. Detectable regional wall motion abnormalities and the derived left ventricular ejection fraction correlate well with angiographic findings. Moreover, dobutamine stress echocardiography seems to be a reliable predictor of adverse cardiac complications in patients who cannot exercise. New or worsening wall motion abnormalities following dobutamine infusion are indicative of significant ischemia. Patients with an ejection fraction of less than 50% tend to have more severe disease and increased perioperative morbidity. Dobutamine stress echocardiography, however, may not be reliable in patients with left bundle-branch block because septal motion may be abnormal, even in the absence of left anterior descending CAD in some patients.

E. Coronary Angiography

Coronary angiography remains the definitive way to evaluate CAD and is associated with a low complication rate (<1%). The location and severity of occlusions can be defined, and coronary vasospasm may also be observed on angiography. In evaluating fixed stenotic lesions, occlusions greater than 50% to 75% are generally considered significant. The severity of disease is often expressed according to the number of major coronary vessels affected (one-, two-, or three-vessel disease). Significant stenosis of the left main coronary artery is of great concern because disruption of flow in this vessel will have adverse effects on almost the entire left ventricle.

Ventriculography, measurement of the ejection fraction, and measurement of intracardiac pressures also provide important information. Indicators of significant ventricular dysfunction include an ejection fraction less than 50%, a left ventricular end-diastolic pressure greater than 18 mm Hg, a cardiac index less than 2.2 L/min/m^2, and marked or multiple wall motion abnormalities.

Premedication

Allaying fear, anxiety, and pain preoperatively are desirable goals in patients with CAD. Satisfactory premedication minimizes sympathetic activation, which adversely affects the myocardial oxygen supply–demand balance. Overmedication is equally detrimental and should be avoided because it may result in hypoxemia, respiratory acidosis, or hypotension. Most clinicians now limit premedication to small doses of intravenous midazolam (or the equivalent) given immediately before invasive procedures or before transporting the patient to the operating theater.

Preoperative medications should generally be continued until the time of surgery. The sudden withdrawal of antianginal medication perioperatively—particularly β-blockers—can precipitate a sudden, rebound increase in ischemic episodes. Statins should also be continued in the perioperative period. Prophylactic administration of nitrates intravenously or transdermally to patients with CAD in the perioperative period provides no benefit to patients not previously on long-term nitrate therapy and without evidence of ongoing ischemia. Transdermal absorption of nitroglycerin may be erratic in the perioperative period.

4

INTRAOPERATIVE MANAGEMENT

The intraoperative period is regularly associated with factors and events that can adversely affect the myocardial oxygen demand–supply relationship. Activation of the sympathetic system plays a major role. Hypertension and enhanced contractility increase myocardial oxygen demand, whereas tachycardia increases demand and reduces supply. Although myocardial ischemia is commonly associated with tachycardia, ischemia can occur in the absence of any apparent hemodynamic derangement.

Objectives

5 The overwhelming priority in managing patients with ischemic heart disease is maintaining a favorable myocardial supply–demand relationship. Autonomic-mediated increases in heart rate and blood pressure should be controlled with deeper planes of general anesthesia, adrenergic blockade, vasodilators, or a combination of these. Excessive reductions in coronary perfusion pressure or arterial oxygen content must be avoided. Higher diastolic pressures may be preferable in patients with high-grade coronary occlusions. Excessive increases—such as those caused by fluid overload—in left ventricular end-diastolic pressure should be avoided because they increase ventricular wall tension (afterload) and can reduce subendocardial perfusion (see Chapter 20). Transfusion carries its own risks, and consequently there is no set transfusion trigger in patients with CAD; however, most clinicians are reluctant to have hemoglobin levels fall below 7 g/dL. Anemia can lead to tachycardia, worsening the balance between myocardial oxygen supply and demand. The ACC/AHA recommendations for the anesthetic management of the patient with CAD disease for noncardiac surgery are summarized in Table 21–10

TABLE 21–10 Summary of recommendations for anesthetic consideration and intraoperative management.

Recommendations	COR[2]	LOE
Volatile general anesthesia versus total intravenous anesthesia		
Use of either a volatile anesthetic agent or total intravenous anesthesia is reasonable for patients undergoing noncardiac surgery	IIa	A
Perioperative pain management		
Neuraxial anesthesia for *postoperative* pain relief can be effective to reduce MI in patients undergoing abdominal aortic surgery	IIa	B
Preoperative epidural analgesia may be considered to decrease the incidence of *preoperative* cardiac events in patients with hip fracture	IIb	B
Prophylactic intraoperative nitroglycerin		
Prophylactic intravenous nitroglycerin is not effective in reducing myocardial ischemia in patients undergoing noncardiac surgery	III: No Benefit	B
Intraoperative monitoring techniques		
Emergency use of perioperative TEE in patients with hemodynamic instability is reasonable in patients undergoing noncardiac surgery if expertise is readily available	IIa	C
Routine use of intraoperative TEE during noncardiac surgery is not recommended	III: No Benefit	C
Maintenance of body temperature		
Maintenance of normothermia may be reasonable to reduce perioperative cardiac events	IIb	B
Hemodynamic assist devices		
Use of hemodynamic assist devices may be considered when urgent or emergency noncardiac surgery is required in the setting of acute severe cardiac dysfunction	IIb	C
Perioperative use of pulmonary artery catheters		
Use of pulmonary artery catheterization may be considered when underlying medical conditions that significantly affect hemodynamics cannot be corrected before surgery	IIb	C
Routine use of pulmonary artery catheterization is not recommended	III: No Benefit	A

COR, class of recommendation; LOE, level of evidence; MI, myocardial infarction; TEE, transesophageal echocardiogram.

Reproduced with permission from Fleisher LA, Fleischman KE, Auerbach AD, et al. 2014 ACC/AHA guideline on perioperative cardiovascular evaluation and management of patients undergoing noncardiac surgery: A report of the American College of Cardiology/American Heart Association Task Force on practice guidelines. *J Am Coll Cardiol.* 2014 Dec 9;64(22):e77-e137.

MONITORING

6 Intraarterial pressure monitoring is reasonable in most patients with severe CAD and major or multiple cardiac risk factors who are undergoing any but the most minor procedures. Central venous (or rarely pulmonary artery) pressure can be monitored during prolonged or complicated procedures involving large fluid shifts or blood loss. Noninvasive methods of cardiac output determination and volume assessment have been previously discussed in this text and we recommend them. Transesophageal echocardiography (TEE) and transthoracic echocardiography (TTE) provide valuable information, both qualitative and quantitative, on contractility and ventricular chamber size (preload) perioperatively.

A. Electrocardiography

Early ischemic changes are subtle and involve changes in T-wave morphology, including inversion, tenting, or both (Figure 21–2). More obvious ischemia may be seen in the form of progressive ST-segment depression. Down-sloping and horizontal ST depressions are of greater specificity for ischemia than is up-sloping depression. New ST-segment elevations are rare during noncardiac surgery and are indicative of severe ischemia, vasospasm, or infarction.

It should be noted that an isolated minor ST elevation in the mid-precordial leads (V_3 and V_4) can be a normal variant in young patients. Ischemia may also present as an unexplained intraoperative atrial or ventricular arrhythmia or the onset of a new

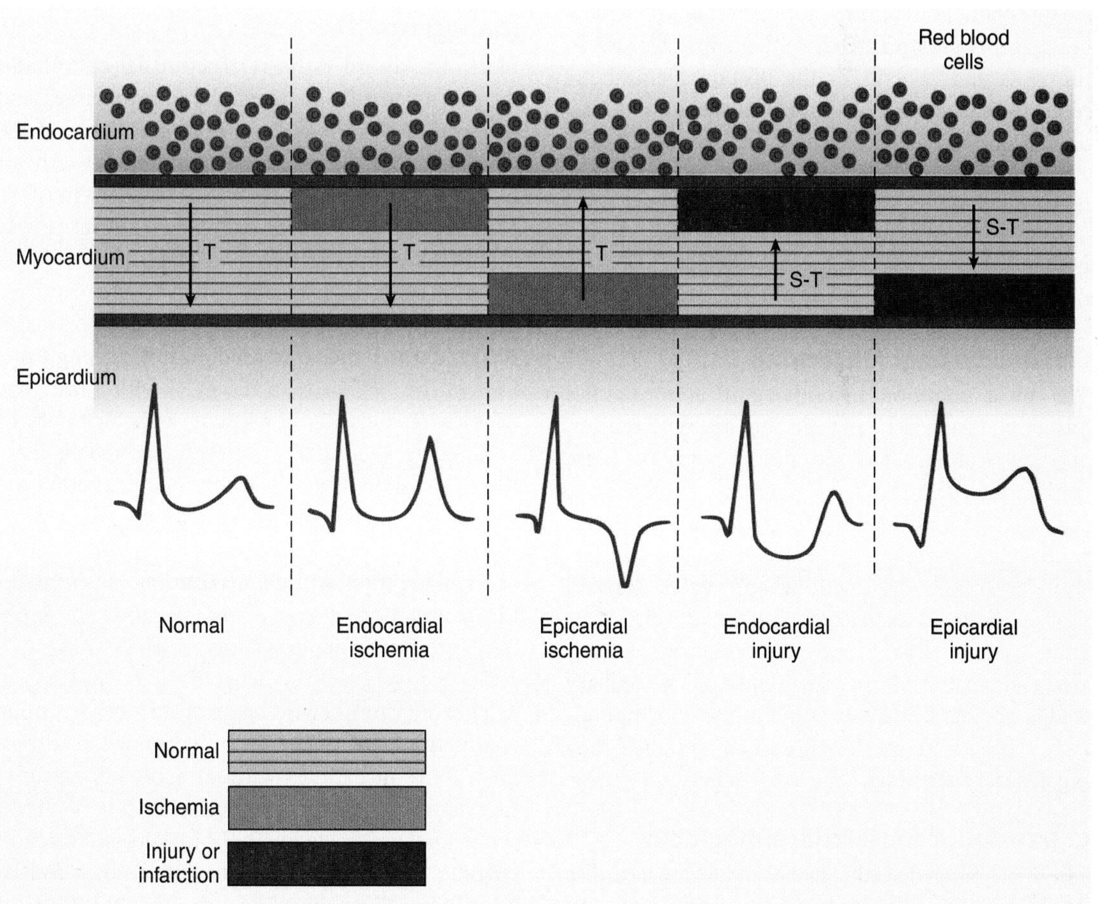

FIGURE 21–2 Electrocardiographic signs of ischemia. Patterns of ischemia and injury. (Data from Schamroth L. The 12 Lead *Electrocardiogram*. Oxford, UK: Blackwell; 1989.)

conduction abnormality. The sensitivity of the ECG in detecting ischemia is related to the number of leads monitored. Studies suggest that the V_5, V_4, II, V_2, and V_3 leads (in order of decreasing sensitivity) are most useful. Ideally, at least two leads should be monitored simultaneously. Usually, lead II is monitored for inferior wall ischemia and arrhythmias, and V_5 is monitored for anterior wall ischemia. When only one lead can be monitored, a modified V_5 lead provides the greatest sensitivity.

The increasing number of individuals treated with drug-eluting stents can be problematic perioperatively, especially when antiplatelet therapy must be discontinued (eg, emergency spinal surgery). Such patients are at very increased risk of thrombosis and perioperative MI. Anesthesia providers should never for nonsurgical reasons (eg, desire to perform a spinal anesthetic) discontinue antiplatelet or antithrombotic agents perioperatively without first discussing the risks and benefits of the proposed anesthetic requiring suspension of antiplatelet therapy with the patient and his or her cardiologist. The ACC/AHA 2016 focused guidelines offer updated recommendations on the approach of bringing patients to surgery following percutaneous coronary interventions and the type of interventions suggested when subsequent surgery is expected (Figure 21–3).

B. Hemodynamic Monitoring

The most common hemodynamic abnormalities observed during ischemic episodes are hypertension and tachycardia. They are almost always a cause (rather than the result) of ischemia. Hypotension is a late and ominous manifestation of progressive ventricular dysfunction. TEE will readily demonstrate ventricular dysfunctional and ventricular wall motion changes associated with myocardial ischemia. Ischemia is frequently, but not always, associated with an abrupt increase in pulmonary capillary wedge pressure; however, it is now rare for pulmonary capillary wedge pressure to be measured during general anesthesia.

C. Transesophageal Echocardiography

TEE is helpful in detecting global and regional cardiac dysfunction, as well as valvular function, in surgical patients. Moreover, detection of new regional wall motion abnormalities is a more sensitive and earlier indication of myocardial ischemia than the ECG. In animal studies in which coronary blood flow is gradually reduced, regional wall motion abnormalities develop before the ECG changes. Although the occurrence of new intraoperative abnormalities correlates with postoperative MIs in some studies, not all such abnormalities are necessarily ischemic. Both regional and global abnormalities can be caused by changes in heart rate, altered conduction, preload, afterload, or drug-induced changes in contractility. Decreased systolic wall thickening may be a more reliable index for ischemia than endocardial wall motion alone.

Arrhythmias, Pacemakers, & Internal Cardioverter-Defibrillator Management

Electrolyte disorders, heart structure defects, inflammation, myocardial ischemia, cardiomyopathies, and conduction abnormalities can all contribute to the development of perioperative arrhythmias and heart block. Consequently, anesthesia providers must be prepared to treat both chronic and new-onset cardiac rhythm abnormalities.

Supraventricular tachycardias (SVTs) can have hemodynamic consequences secondary to loss of AV synchrony and decreased diastolic filling time. Loss of the “P” wave on the ECG with a fast ventricular response is consistent with SVTs. Most SVTs occur secondary to a reentrant mechanism. Reentrant arrhythmias occur when conduction tissues in the heart depolarize or repolarize at varying rates. In this manner, a self-perpetuating loop of repolarization and depolarization can occur in the conduction pathways or AV node, or both. SVTs producing hemodynamic collapse are treated perioperatively with synchronized cardioversion. Adenosine can likewise be given to slow AV node conduction and potentially disrupt the reentrant loop. SVTs in patients without accessory conduction bundles (Wolff–Parkinson–White [WPW] syndrome) are treated with β-blockers and calcium channel blockers. In patients with known WPW, procainamide or ibutilide can be used to treat SVTs. Use of intravenous amiodarone, adenosine,

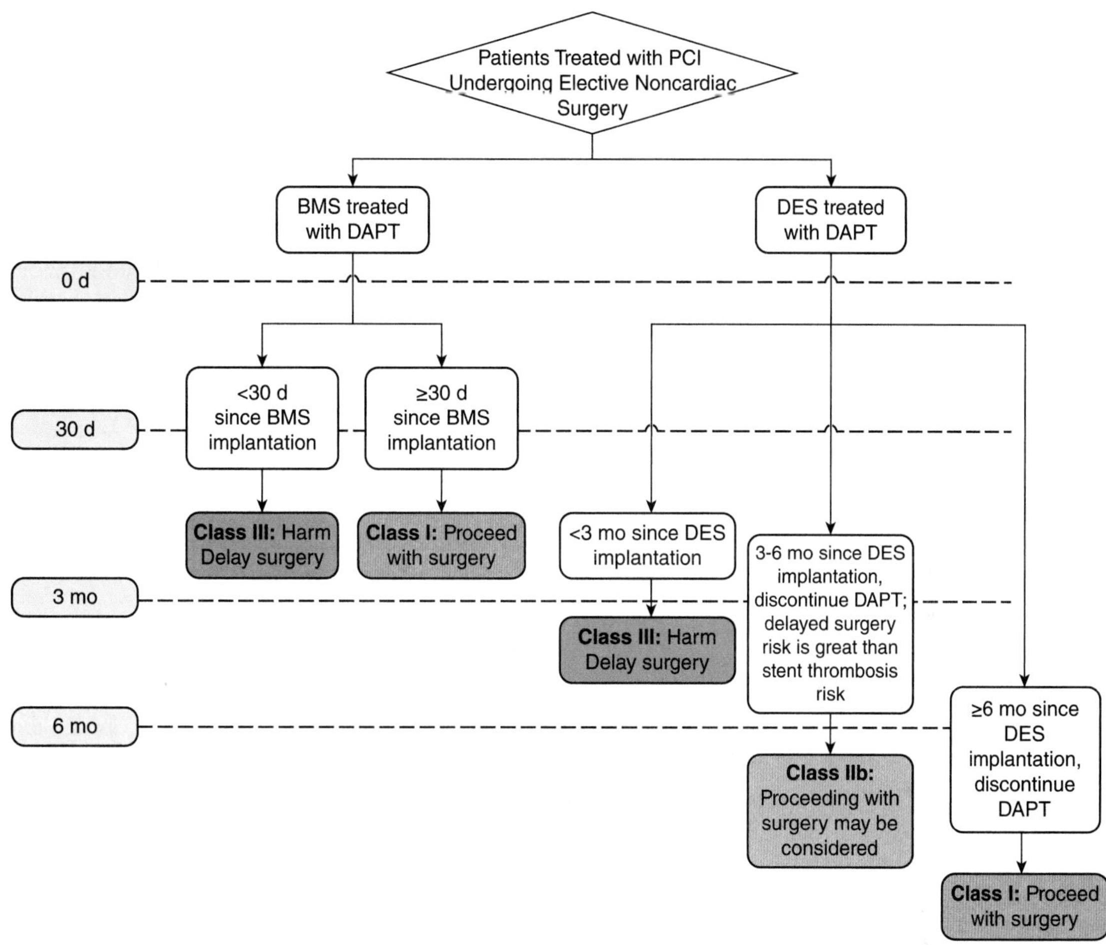

FIGURE 21–3 Treatment algorithm for the timing of elective noncardiac surgery in patients with coronary stents. BMS, bare metal stent; DAPT, dual antiplatelet therapy; DES, drug-eluting stent; PCI, percutaneous coronary intervention. (Reproduced with permission from Levine GN, Bates ER, Bittl JA, et.al. 2016 ACC/AHA guideline focused update on duration of dual antiplatelet therapy in patients with coronary artyer disease: a report of the American College of Cardiology/American Heart Association Task Force on Clinical Practice Guidelines, *Circulation.* 2016 Sep 6;134(10):e123-e155.)

digoxin, or non-dihydropyridine calcium channel antagonists is considered a class III recommendation by the AHA/ACC as these agents may harmfully increase the ventricular response in patients with preexcitation syndromes such as WPW. At times, SVTs manifest with a broad QRS complex and seem to be similar to VTs. Such rhythms, when they present, should be treated like VT until proven otherwise.

Atrial fibrillation (AF) can complicate the perioperative period (Figure 21–4). Up to 35% of cardiac surgery patients develop postoperative AF.

The ACC/AHA guidelines recommend anticoagulant therapy in patients with long-standing AF to prevent thromboembolic ischemic stroke. Consequently, many patients with AF will present to the operating room on some form of antithrombotic therapy (eg, warfarin, direct thrombin, factor Xa inhibitors). Patients may require discontinuation of oral anticoagulation therapy prior to invasive procedures. Bridging with heparin is often utilized in patients at high risk for thromboembolism (eg, patients with mechanical heart valves).

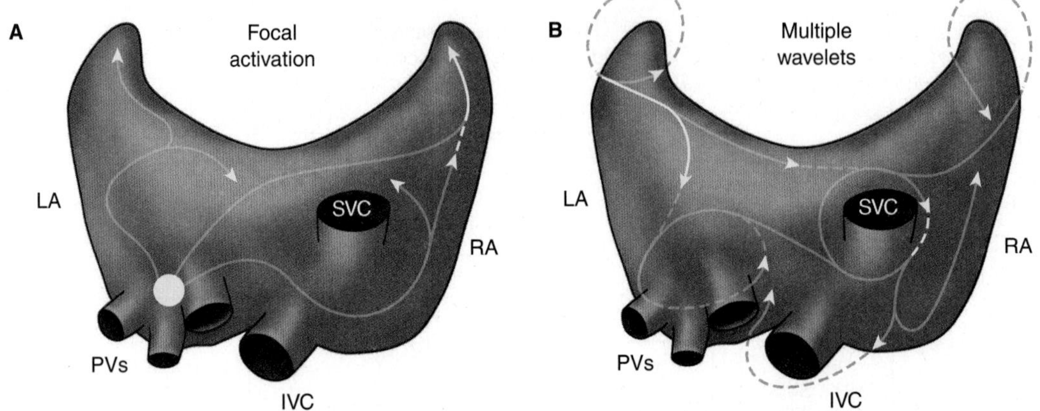

FIGURE 21–4 Posterior view of principal electrophysiological mechanisms of atrial fibrillation. **A**: Focal activation. The initiating focus (indicated by the dot) often lies within the region of the pulmonary veins. The resulting wavelets represent fibrillatory conduction, as in multiple-wavelet reentry. **B**: Multiple-wavelet reentry. Wavelets (*arrows*) randomly reenter tissue previously activated by the same or another wavelet. The routes the wavelets travel vary. ICV, inferior vena cava; LA, left atrium; PV, pulmonary vein; RA, right atrium; SCV, superior vena cava. (Reproduced with permission from Konings KT, Kirchhof CJ, Smeets JR, et al. High-density mapping of electrically induced atrial fibrillation in humans. *Circulation.* 1994 Apr;89(4):1665-1680.)

When AF develops perioperatively, rate control with β-blockers can often be instituted. Chemical cardioversion can be attempted with amiodarone or procainamide. Of note, if the duration of AF is greater than 48 hours, or unknown, ACC/AHA guidelines recommend anticoagulation for 3 weeks prior to, and 4 weeks following, either electrical or chemical cardioversion. Additionally, TEE can be performed to rule out the presence of left atrial or left atrial appendage thrombus.

Should AF develop postoperatively, ventricular rate response can be controlled with AV nodal blocking agents unless contraindicated. Should AF result in hemodynamic instability, synchronized cardioversion should be attempted. Patients at high risk of AF following cardiac surgery can be treated with prophylactic amiodarone. Many centers routinely administer β-blockers or amiodarone to all patients undergoing coronary artery surgery to reduce the risk of new onset AF.

AF is most frequently associated with loss of atrial muscle and the development of fibrosis. Fibrosis may contribute to reentrant mechanisms of AF as depolarization/repolarization becomes nonhomogeneous. AF may also develop from a focal source often located in the pulmonary veins. In patients with an accessory bundle, AF can produce rapid ventricular responses and hemodynamic collapse. Drugs that slow conduction across the AV node (eg, digitalis, verapamil, diltiazem) do not slow conduction across the accessory pathway, potentially leading to hemodynamic collapse. The ACC/AHA guidelines likewise recommend caution in the use of β-blockers for AF in patients with preexcitation syndromes.

Ventricular arrhythmias have been the subject of much review by the AHA (Table 21–11). Ventricular premature contractions (VPCs) can appear perioperatively secondary to electrolyte abnormalities (hypokalemia, hypomagnesemia, hypocalcemia), acidosis, ischemia, embolic phenomenon, mechanical irritation of the heart from central lines, cardiac manipulation, and drug effects. Correction of the underlying source of any arrhythmia should be addressed. Patients can likewise present with VPCs secondary to various cardiomyopathies.

The incidence of sudden cardiac death (SCD) is estimated at 1 to 2 out of 1000 people per year. Consequently, some patients will experience an unexpected death in the perioperative period. All anesthesia providers must be prepared to resuscitate and manage patients with ventricular arrhythmias, including nonsustained and sustained VT and ventricular fibrillation.

TABLE 21–11 Classification of ventricular arrhythmias.

Classification by Clinical Presentation		
Hemodynamically stable	Asymptomatic	The absence of symptoms that could result from an arrhythmia.
	Minimal symptoms, eg, palpitations	Patient reports palpitations felt in either the chest, throat, or neck as described by the following: • Heartbeat sensations that feel like pounding or racing • An unpleasant awareness of heartbeat • Feeling skipped beats or a pause
Hemodynamically unstable	Presyncope	Patient reports presyncope as described by the following: • Dizziness • Lightheadedness • Feeling faint • "Graying out"
	Syncope	Sudden loss of consciousness with loss of postural tone, not related to anesthesia, with spontaneous recovery as reported by the patient or observer. Patient may experience syncope when supine.
	Sudden cardiac death	Death from an unexpected circulatory arrest, usually due to a cardiac arrhythmia occurring within an hour of the onset of symptoms.
	Sudden cardiac arrest	Death from an unexpected circulatory arrest, usually due to a cardiac arrhythmia occurring within an hour of the onset of symptoms, in whom medical intervention (eg, defibrillation) reverses the event.
Classification by Electrocardiography		
Nonsustained VT		Three or more beats in duration, terminating spontaneously in <30 s. VT is a cardiac arrhythmia of three or more consecutive complexes in duration emanating from the ventricles at a rate of >100 bpm (cycle length <600 ms)
	Monomorphic	Nonsustained VT with a single QRS morphology.
	Polymorphic	Nonsustained VT with a changing QRS morphology at cycle length between 600 and 180 ms.
Sustained VT		VT >30 s in duration and/or requiring termination due to hemodynamic compromise in <30 s.
	Monomorphic	Sustained VT with a stable single QRS morphology.
	Polymorphic	Sustained VT with a changing or multiform QRS morphology at cycle length between 600 and 180 ms.
Bundle-branch reentrant tachycardia		VT due to reentry involving the His-Purkinje system, usually with LBBB morphology; this usually occurs in the setting of cardiomyopathy.
Bidirectional VT		VT with a beat-to-beat alternans in the QRS frontal plane axis, often associated with digitalis toxicity.
Torsades de pointes		Characterized by VT associated with a long QT or QTc, and electrocardiographically characterized by twisting of the peaks of the QRS complexes around the isoelectric line during the arrhythmia: "Typical," initiated following "short-long-short" coupling intervals. Short coupled variant initiated by normal-short coupling.
Ventricular flutter		A regular (cycle length variability ≤30 ms) ventricular arrhythmia approximately 300 bpm (cycle length 200 ms) with a monomorphic appearance; no isoelectric interval between successive QRS complexes.

(continued)

TABLE 21–11 Classification of ventricular arrhythmias. (Continued)

Ventricular fibrillation	Rapid, usually more than 300 bpm/200 ms (cycle length ≤180 ms), grossly irregular ventricular rhythm with marked variability in QRS cycle length, morphology, and amplitude.
Classification by Disease Entity	
Chronic coronary heart disease	
Heart failure	
Congenital heart disease	
Neurological disorders	
Structurally normal hearts	
Sudden infant death syndrome	
Cardiomyopathies:	
Dilated cardiomyopathy	
Hypertrophic cardiomyopathy	
Arrhythmogenic right ventricular cardiomyopathy	

LBBB, left bundle-branch block; VT, ventricular tachycardia.

Reproduced with permission from Zipes DP, Camm AJ, Borggrefe M, et al. ACC/AHA/ESC 2006 guidelines for management of patients with ventricular arrhythmias and the prevention of sudden cardiac death—executive summary. *Circulation*. 2006 Sep 5;114(10):1088-1132.

Nonsustained VT is a short run of ventricular ectopy that lasts less than 30 s and spontaneously terminates, whereas sustained VT persists longer than 30 s. VT is either monomorphic or polymorphic, depending on the QRS complex. If the QRS complex morphology changes, it is designated as polymorphic VT. Torsades des pointes is a form of VT associated with a prolonged QT interval, producing a sine wave–like VT pattern on the ECG. Ventricular fibrillation requires immediate resuscitative efforts and defibrillation.

Patients presenting with ventricular ectopy and nonsustained runs of VT routinely undergo investigation prior to surgery; however, patients with such rhythm abnormalities may not be at greater risk for nonfatal MI or cardiac death perioperatively. Supraventricular and ventricular arrhythmias constitute active cardiac conditions that warrant evaluation and treatment prior to elective noncardiac surgery. Electrophysiological studies are undertaken to determine the possibility for catheter-mediated ablation of VTs.

Should VT present perioperatively, cardioversion is recommended whenever hemodynamic compromise occurs. Otherwise, treatment with amiodarone or procainamide can be attempted. At all times, therapy should also be directed at identifying any causative sources of the arrhythmia. β-Blockers are useful in the treatment of VT, especially if ischemia is a suspected causative factor in the development of rhythm. The use of β-blockers following MI has reduced the incidence of post-MI ventricular fibrillation.

Torsades des pointes is associated with conditions that lengthen the QT interval. If the arrhythmia develops in association with pauses, pacing can be effective. Likewise, some patients may benefit from isoproterenol infusions if they develop pause-dependent torsades des pointes. Magnesium sulfate may be useful in patients with long QT syndrome and episodes of torsades.

Perioperative ventricular fibrillation requires defibrillation and the use of resuscitation algorithms. Amiodarone can be used to stabilize the rhythm following successful defibrillation.

ICDs are recommended in patients with a history of survived SCD, decreased ventricular function following MI, and left ventricular ejection fractions less than 35%. Additionally, ICDs are used to treat potential sudden cardiac death in patients with dilated, hypertrophic, arrhythmogenic right ventricular and genetic cardiomyopathies. ICDs usually have a biventricular pacing function that improves the effectiveness of left ventricular contraction. Patients with heart failure frequently have a widened QRS complex greater than 120 ms. In such patients, ventricular systole is less efficient as the lateral and septal left ventricular walls do not effectively contract because of the conduction delay. Cardiac resynchronization therapy has been shown to improve functional status in patients with heart failure.

Anesthetic management for the placement of ICDs and other electrophysiological procedures (eg, catheter ablation) depends on the patient's underlying conditions. Many patients present with systolic and diastolic heart failure and depend on sympathetic tone to maintain blood pressure. Some patients tolerate ICD placement using deep sedation rather than general anesthesia. However, catheter-based electrophysiological studies can be quite time consuming, and patients can develop atelectasis and airway obstruction. Thus, general anesthesia is often used in the electrophysiology laboratory. Should the patient's blood pressure suddenly decline during electrophysiologic studies, development of pericardial tamponade should be suspected. Emergency drainage of tamponade may be necessary.

Many patients present to surgery with ICDs in place. Published guidelines of the American Society of Anesthesiologists can provide assistance in the management of such patients. Management is a three-step process, as follows:

1. *Preoperative.* Identify the type of device and determine if it is used for antibradycardia functions. Consult with the patient's cardiologist preoperatively as to the device's function and use history.
2. *Intraoperative.* Determine what electromagnetic interference is likely to present intraoperatively, and advise the use of bipolar electrocautery where possible. Assure the availability of temporary pacing and defibrillation equipment, and apply pads as necessary. Patients who are pacemaker dependent can be programmed to an asynchronous mode to mitigate electrical interference. Magnet application to ICDs may disable the antitachycardia function but not convert to an asynchronous pacemaker. Consultation with the patient's cardiologist and interrogation of the device is typically necessary. Most patients will carry a card on which the device model and manufacturer are provided. A telephone call to the device manufacturer can provide information about device performance and the best method for managing the device (eg, reprogramming or applying a magnet) prior to surgery. A large number of ICD models are in use; however, most suspend their antitachycardia function in response to a magnet.
3. *Postoperative.* The device must be interrogated to ensure that therapeutic functions have been restored. Patients should be continuously monitored until the antitachycardia functions of the device are restored and its function has been confirmed.

ICDs are particularly problematic intraoperatively when electrocautery is used because the device may (1) interpret cautery as ventricular fibrillation; (2) inhibit pacemaker function due to cautery artifact; (3) increase the pacing rate due to activation of a rate-responsive sensor; or (4) temporarily or permanently reset to a backup or reset mode. Use of bipolar cautery, placement of the grounding pad far from the ICD device, and limiting use of the cautery to only short bursts help reduce the likelihood of problems but will not eliminate them.

When there is greater risk of stray currents from the cautery, the ICD device should have the defibrillator function programmed off immediately before surgery and reprogrammed back on immediately afterward. External defibrillation pads should be applied and remain attached to a defibrillator machine intraoperatively. Careful monitoring of the arterial pulse with pulse oximetry or an arterial waveform is necessary to ensure that the pacemaker is not inhibited and that there is arterial perfusion during episodes of ECG artifact from surgical cautery.

HEART FAILURE

An increasing number of patients present for surgery with either systolic or diastolic heart failure. Heart failure may be secondary to ischemia, valvular heart disease, infectious agents, or many forms of cardiomyopathy. Patients may experience heart failure symptoms with a preserved or reduced ejection fraction. Most patients with heart failure seek medical attention because of dyspnea and fatigue. Symptoms worsen as heart failure progresses over time (Figure 21–5). Patients usually undergo echocardiography so the clinician can diagnose structural heart defects, detect signs of cardiac "remodeling," determine the left ventricular ejection fraction, and assess the heart's diastolic function. Laboratory evaluations of concentration of BNP are likewise obtained to distinguish heart failure from other causes of dyspnea. BNP is released from the heart, and its elevation is associated with impaired ventricular function.

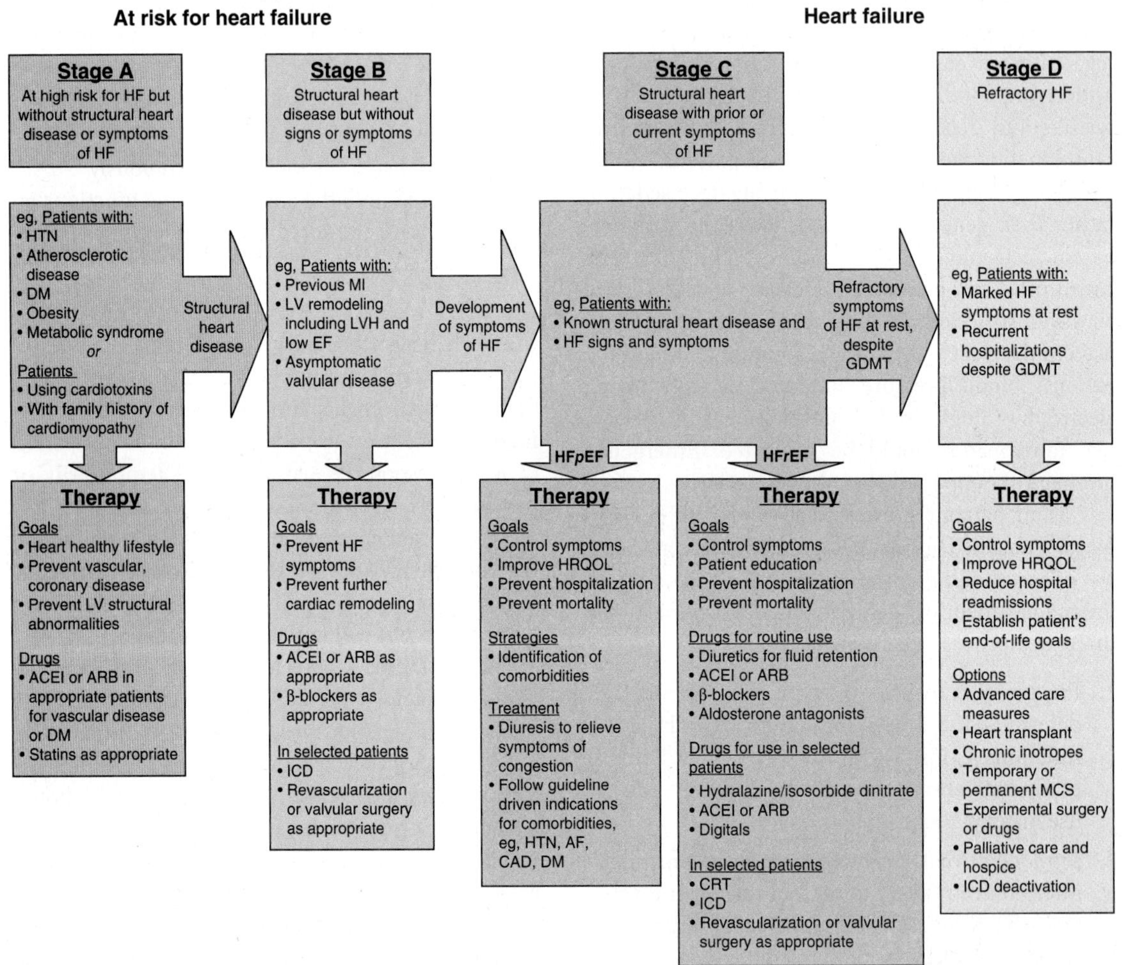

FIGURE 21–5 Stages in the development of heart failure and recommended therapy by stage. ACEI, angiotensin-converting enzyme inhibitor; AF, atrial fibrillation; ARB, angiotensin-receptor blocker; CAD, coronary artery disease; CRT, cardiac resynchronization therapy; DM, diabetes mellitus; EF, ejection fraction; GDMT, guideline-directed medical therapy; HF, heart failure; HFpEF, heart failure with preserved ejection fraction; HFrEF, heart failure with reduced ejection fraction; HRQOL, health-related quality of life; HTN, hypertension; ICD, implantable cardioverter-defibrillator; LV, left ventricular; LVH, left ventricular hypertrophy; MCS, mechanical circulatory support; MI, myocardial infarction. (Reproduced with permission from Yancy C, Jessup M, Bozkurt B, et al. 2013 ACCF/AHA guideline for the management of heart failure: A report of the American College of Cardiology Foundation/American Heart Association Task Force on Practice Guidelines. *J Am Coll Cardiol.* 2013 Oct 15;62(16):e147-e239.)

The body attempts to compensate for LV systolic failure through activation of the sympathetic and renin–angiotensin–aldosterone system. Consequently, patients experience salt retention, volume expansion, sympathetic stimulation, and vasoconstriction. The heart dilates to maintain stroke volume in spite of decreased contractility. Over time, compensatory mechanisms fail and contribute to the manifestations associated with heart failure (eg, dyspnea, dependent edema, tachycardia, decreased tissue perfusion). Patients with systolic heart failure are likely to present to surgery having been previously treated with diuretics, β-blockers, ACE inhibitors or ARBs, and possibly aldosterone antagonists. Electrolytes must be measured as diuretics frequently lead to hypokalemia. ARB or ACE inhibitor use may contribute to hypotension in the surgical patient with heart failure. ACE inhibitors are rarely associated with angioedema requiring emergency airway management.

Myocardial relaxation is a dynamic, not passive, process. The heart with preserved diastolic function accommodates volume during diastole, with minimal increases in left ventricular end-diastolic pressure. Conversely, the heart with diastolic dysfunction relaxes poorly and produces increased left ventricular end-diastolic pressure. The increased left ventricular end-diastolic pressure is transmitted to the left atrium and pulmonary vasculature, resulting in symptoms of congestion. Patients with any form of heart failure have an increased risk of perioperative morbidity.

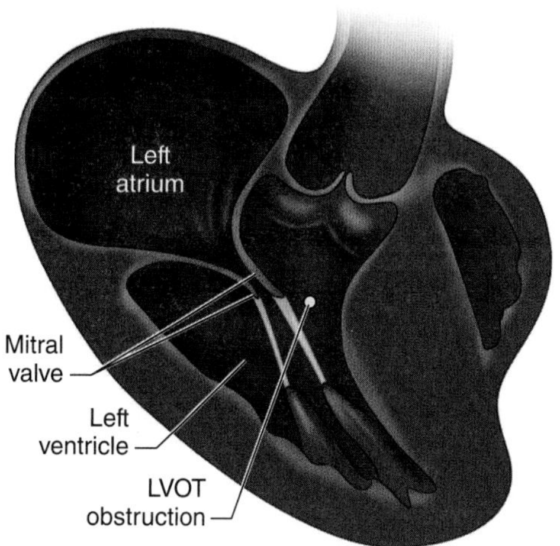

FIGURE 21–6 The midesophageal long axis view is shown. As a consequence of the hypertrophied interventricular septum, flow patterns within the heart are altered so that the anterior leaflet of the mitral valve is drawn during ventricular systole into the left ventricular outflow tract (LVOT), producing obstruction. This is known as *systolic anterior motion of the mitral valve*. (Reproduced with permission from Wasnick J, Hillel Z, Kramer D, et al. Cardiac Anesthesia & Transesophageal *Echocardiography*. New York, NY: McGraw Hill; 2011.)

HYPERTROPHIC CARDIOMYOPATHY

Hypertrophic cardiomyopathy (HCM) is an autosomal dominant trait that affects 1 in 500 adults. Many patients are unaware of the condition, and some will present with sudden cardiac death as the initial manifestation. Symptoms include dyspnea, exercise intolerance, palpitations, and chest pain. Clinically, HCM is detected by the murmur of dynamic left ventricular outflow tract (LVOT) obstruction in late systole. Symptomatic patients frequently have a thickened intraventricular septum of 20 to 30 mm. A variety of genetic variants have been identified as causative. The myocardium of the intraventricular septum is abnormal, and many patients can develop diastolic dysfunction without pronounced dynamic obstructive gradients. During systole, the anterior leaflet of the mitral valve abuts the intraventricular septum (Figure 21–6), producing obstruction and a late systolic murmur.

Perioperative management is aimed at minimizing the degree of LVOT obstruction. This is accomplished by maintaining adequate intravascular volume, avoiding vasodilatation, and reducing myocardial contractility through the use of β-blockers.

Valvular Heart Disease

1. General Evaluation of Patients

Regardless of the lesion or its cause, preoperative evaluation should be primarily concerned with determining the identity and severity of the lesion and its hemodynamic significance, ventricular function, and the presence of any secondary effects on pulmonary, kidney, or hepatic function. Concomitant CAD should not be overlooked, particularly in older patients and those with known risk factors (see earlier discussion). Myocardial ischemia may occur in the absence of significant coronary occlusion in patients with severe aortic stenosis or regurgitation.

History

One should evaluate exercise tolerance, fatigability, pedal edema, and shortness of breath in general (dyspnea), when lying flat (orthopnea), or at night (paroxysmal nocturnal dyspnea). Patients should also be questioned about chest pains and neurological symptoms. Some valvular lesions are associated with thromboembolic phenomena. Prior procedures, such as valvotomy or valve replacement and their effects, should also be well documented.

Medications commonly used by valvular heart disease patients include diuretics, vasodilators, ACE inhibitors, β-blockers, antiarrhythmics, and anticoagulants. Preoperative vasodilator therapy may be used to decrease preload, afterload, or both. Excessive vasodilation worsens exercise tolerance and is often first manifested as postural (orthostatic) hypotension.

Physical Examination

The most important signs to identify on physical examination are those of congestive heart failure. Left-sided (S_3 gallop or pulmonary rales) and right-sided (jugular venous distention, hepatojugular reflux, hepatosplenomegaly, pedal edema) signs may be present. Auscultatory findings may suggest valvular dysfunction, but echocardiographic studies are more reliable. The ACC/AHA guidelines recommend that transthoracic echocardiography be performed as a class I indication in the initial evaluation of patients suspected of having valvular heart disease. Moreover, the ACC/AHA suggest that any change in symptoms or physical examination findings warrants a repeat transthoracic echocardiography examination. Neurological deficits, usually secondary to embolic phenomena, should be documented.

Laboratory Evaluation

In addition to the laboratory studies discussed for patients with hypertension and CAD, liver function tests are useful in assessing hepatic dysfunction caused by passive hepatic congestion in patients with severe or chronic right-sided failure. Adequate reversal of warfarin or heparin anticoagulation may be documented with a prothrombin time and international normalized ratio (INR) or partial thromboplastin time, respectively, prior to surgery.

Electrocardiographic findings are generally nonspecific. The chest radiograph is useful to assess cardiac size and pulmonary vascular congestion.

Special Studies

Echocardiography, imaging studies, and cardiac catheterization should only be obtained if the results will change therapy or outcomes. In many instances, noninvasive studies obviate the need for cardiac catheterization, unless there are concerns about CAD. When advanced imaging procedures are performed, they generally address the following questions:

- Which valvular abnormality is most important hemodynamically?
- What is the severity of an identified lesion?
- What degree of ventricular impairment is present?
- What is the hemodynamic significance of other identified abnormalities?
- Is there any evidence of CAD?

The ACC/AHA have prepared detailed guidelines to assist in the management of patients with valvular heart disease. Although the evaluation of the patient with a heart murmur generally rests with the cardiologist, anesthesia providers will on occasion discover a previously undetected murmur on preanesthetic examination. In particular, anesthetists are concerned that undiagnosed, critical aortic stenosis might be present, which could lead to hemodynamic collapse with either regional or general anesthesia. In the past, most valvular heart diseases were a consequence of rheumatic heart disease; however, with an aging surgical population, increasing numbers of patients have degenerative valve problems. More than one in eight patients older than age 75 years may manifest at least one form of moderate to severe valvular heart disease.

A study conducted in the Netherlands reported that the prevalence of aortic stenosis was 2.4% in patients older than age 60 years who were scheduled for elective surgery.

Murmurs occur as a consequence of the accelerated blood flow through narrowed openings in stenotic and regurgitant lesions. When new murmurs are detected in a preoperative evaluation, consultation with the patient's personal physician is helpful to determine the need for echocardiographic evaluation. In many centers, immediate echocardiographic evaluation can be performed in the preoperative area, often by a member of the anesthesia department.

2. Specific Valvular Disorders

MITRAL STENOSIS

Preoperative Considerations

Mitral stenosis almost always occurs as a delayed complication of rheumatic fever. However, mitral stenosis can also occur in dialysis-dependent patients. Two-thirds of patients with mitral stenosis are female. The stenotic process is estimated to begin after a minimum of 2 years following rheumatic heart disease and results from progressive fusion and calcification of the valve leaflets. Symptoms generally develop after 20 to 30 years, when the mitral valve orifice is reduced from its normal 4 to 6 cm^2 opening to less than 1.5 cm^2. Less than 50% of patients have isolated mitral stenosis; the remaining patients also have mitral regurgitation, and up to 25% of patients also have rheumatic involvement of the aortic valve (stenosis or regurgitation).

Pathophysiology

The rheumatic process causes the valve leaflets to thicken, calcify, and become funnel shaped; annular calcification may also be present. The mitral commissures fuse, the chordae tendineae fuse and shorten, and the valve cusps become rigid; as a result, the valve leaflets typically display bowing or doming during diastole on echocardiography.

Significant restriction of blood flow through the mitral valve results in a transvalvular pressure gradient that depends on cardiac output, heart rate (diastolic time), and cardiac rhythm. Increases in either cardiac output or heart rate (decreased diastolic time) necessitate higher flows across the valve and result in higher transvalvular pressure gradients. The left atrium is often markedly dilated, promoting SVTs, particularly AF. Blood flow stasis in the atrium promotes the formation of thrombi, usually in the left atrial appendage. Loss of normal atrial systole with AF (which is usually responsible for 20–30% of ventricular filling) necessitates even higher diastolic flow across the valve to maintain the same cardiac output and increases the transvalvular gradient.

Acute elevations in left atrial pressure are rapidly transmitted back to the pulmonary capillaries. If mean pulmonary capillary pressure acutely and significantly rises, transudation of capillary fluid may result in pulmonary edema. Chronic elevations in pulmonary capillary pressure are partially compensated by increases in pulmonary lymph flow but eventually result in pulmonary vascular changes, leading to irreversible increases in pulmonary vascular resistance (PVR) and pulmonary hypertension. Reduced lung compliance and a secondary increase in the work of breathing contribute to chronic dyspnea. Right ventricular failure is frequently precipitated by acute or chronic elevations in right ventricular afterload. Marked dilation of the right ventricle can result in tricuspid or pulmonary valve regurgitation.

Embolic events are common in patients with mitral stenosis and AF. Dislodgment of clots from the left atrium results in systemic emboli, commonly to the cerebral circulation. Patients also have an increased incidence of pulmonary emboli, pulmonary infarction, hemoptysis, and recurrent bronchitis. Chest pain occurs in 10% to 15% of patients with mitral stenosis, even in the absence of CAD; its cause often remains unexplained but may be emboli in the coronary circulation or acute right ventricular pressure overload. Patients may develop hoarseness as a result of compression of the left recurrent laryngeal nerve by the enlarged left atrium.

Left ventricular function is preserved in most patients with pure mitral stenosis (Figure 21–7); however, impaired left ventricular function may be encountered in up to 25% of patients and presumably

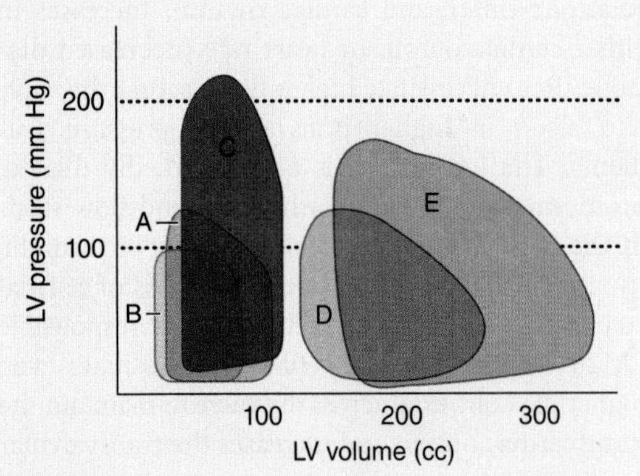

FIGURE 21–7 Pressure–volume loops in patients with valvular heart disease. A, normal; B, mitral stenosis; C, aortic stenosis; D, mitral regurgitation (chronic); E, aortic regurgitation (chronic). LV, left ventricular. (Reproduced with permission from Jackson JM, Thomas SJ, Lowenstein E. Anesthetic management of patients with valvular heart disease. *Semin Anesth.* 1982;1:239.)

represents residual damage from rheumatic myocarditis or coexistent hypertensive or ischemic heart disease.

The left ventricle is chronically underloaded in the patient with mitral stenosis, and stroke volume may be reduced. At the same time, the left atrium, right ventricle, and right atrium are frequently dilated and dysfunctional. Vasodilation that occurs following both neuraxial and general anesthesia can lead to peripheral venous blood pooling and inadequate volume delivery to the left ventricle. This can precipitate hemodynamic collapse.

Treatment

The time from onset of symptoms to incapacitation averages 5 to 10 years. At that stage, most patients die within 2 to 5 years. Surgical correction is therefore usually undertaken once significant symptoms develop. Percutaneous transseptal balloon valvuloplasty may be used in selected young or pregnant patients, as well as older patients who are poor surgical candidates. Medical management is primarily supportive and includes limitation of physical activity, sodium restriction, and diuretics. Small doses of a β-adrenergic blocking drug may also be useful in controlling heart rate in patients with mild to moderate symptoms. Patients with a history of emboli and those at high risk (age older than 40 years; a large atrium with chronic atrial fibrillation) are usually anticoagulated.

Anesthetic Management

A. Objectives

7 The principal hemodynamic goals are to maintain a sinus rhythm (if present preoperatively) and to avoid tachycardia, large increases in cardiac output, and both hypovolemia and fluid overload by judicious administration of intravenous fluids.

B. Monitoring

Invasive hemodynamic monitoring is often used for major surgical procedures, particularly those associated with large fluid shifts. TEE and noninvasive cardiac output monitors can also be used to help guide perioperative management. Overzealous fluid replacement readily precipitates pulmonary edema in patients with severe disease. Pulmonary capillary wedge pressure measurements in the presence of mitral stenosis reflect the transvalvular gradient and not necessarily left ventricular end-diastolic pressure. Prominent *a* waves and a decreased *y* descent are typically present on the pulmonary capillary wedge pressure waveform in patients who are in sinus rhythm. A prominent *cv* wave on the central venous pressure waveform is usually indicative of secondary tricuspid regurgitation. The ECG typically shows a notched P wave in patients who are in sinus rhythm.

C. Choice of Agents

Patients may be very sensitive to the vasodilating effects of spinal and epidural anesthesia. In theory, epidural anesthesia may be easier to manage than spinal anesthesia because of the more gradual onset of sympathetic blockade. There is no "ideal" general anesthetic, and agents should be employed to achieve the desired effects of permitting sufficient diastolic time to adequately load the left ventricle. Vasopressors are often needed to maintain vascular tone following anesthetic induction.

Intraoperative tachycardia may be controlled by deepening anesthesia with an opioid (excluding meperidine) or β-blocker (esmolol or metoprolol). In the presence of atrial fibrillation, ventricular rate should be controlled. **Marked hemodynamic**

deterioration from sudden SVT necessitates cardioversion. Phenylephrine is preferred over ephedrine as a vasopressor because the former lacks β-adrenergic agonist activity. Vasopressin or norepinephrine can also be employed to restore vascular tone should hypotension develop secondary to anesthetic induction.

MITRAL REGURGITATION

Preoperative Considerations

Mitral regurgitation can develop acutely or insidiously as a result of a large number of disorders. Chronic mitral regurgitation is usually the result of rheumatic fever (often with concomitant mitral stenosis); congenital or developmental abnormalities of the valve apparatus; or dilation, destruction, or calcification of the mitral annulus. Acute mitral regurgitation is usually due to myocardial ischemia or infarction (papillary muscle dysfunction or rupture of a chorda tendinea), infective endocarditis, or chest trauma. The ACC/AHA indicates that primary mitral regurgitation is present when one or more of the components of the mitral valve apparatus contribute to valvular incompetence. Correction of the structure of the mitral valve corrects the underlying disease process. In contrast, the ACC/AHA describes secondary mitral regurgitation as present when ventricular dilation prevents coaptation of the mitral valve leaflets. In this instance, repair of the valve is not curative according to the ACC/AHA's valvular heart disease guidelines because the underlying disease process likewise must be addressed in addition to restoration of valvular competency.

Pathophysiology

The principal derangement is a reduction in forward stroke volume due to backward flow of blood into the left atrium during systole. The left ventricle compensates by dilating and increasing end-diastolic volume (see Figure 21–7). Regurgitation through the mitral valve initially maintains a normal end-systolic volume in spite of an increased end-diastolic volume. However, as the disease progresses, the end-systolic volume increases. By increasing end-diastolic volume, the volume-overloaded left ventricle can maintain a normal cardiac output despite blood being ejected retrograde into the atrium. With time, patients with chronic mitral regurgitation eventually develop eccentric left ventricular hypertrophy and progressive impairment in contractility. In patients with severe mitral regurgitation, the regurgitant volume may exceed the forward stroke volume. In time, wall stress increases, resulting in an increased demand for myocardial oxygen supply.

The regurgitant volume passing through the mitral valve is dependent on the size of the mitral valve orifice (which can vary with ventricular cavity size), the heart rate (systolic time), and the left ventricular–left atrial pressure gradient during systole. The last factor is affected by the relative resistances of the two outflow paths from the left ventricle, namely, SVR and left atrial compliance. Thus, a decrease in SVR or an increase in mean left atrial pressure will reduce the regurgitant volume. Atrial compliance also determines the predominant clinical manifestations. Patients with normal or reduced atrial compliance (acute mitral regurgitation) have primarily pulmonary vascular congestion and edema. Patients with increased atrial compliance (long-standing mitral regurgitation resulting in a large dilated left atrium) primarily show signs of a reduced cardiac output. Most patients are between the two extremes and exhibit symptoms of both pulmonary congestion and low cardiac output. Patients with a regurgitant fraction of less than 30% of the total stroke volume generally have mild symptoms. Regurgitant fractions of 30% to 60% generally cause moderate symptoms, whereas fractions greater than 60% are associated with severe disease.

Echocardiography, particularly TEE, is useful in delineating the underlying pathophysiology of mitral regurgitation and guiding treatment. Mitral valve leaflet motion is often described as normal, prolapsing, or restrictive (Figure 21–8). Excessive motion or prolapse is defined by systolic movement of a leaflet beyond the plane of the mitral valve and into the left atrium (see later section on mitral valve prolapse).

Treatment

Reduction of SVR increases forward stroke volume and decreases the regurgitant volume. Surgical

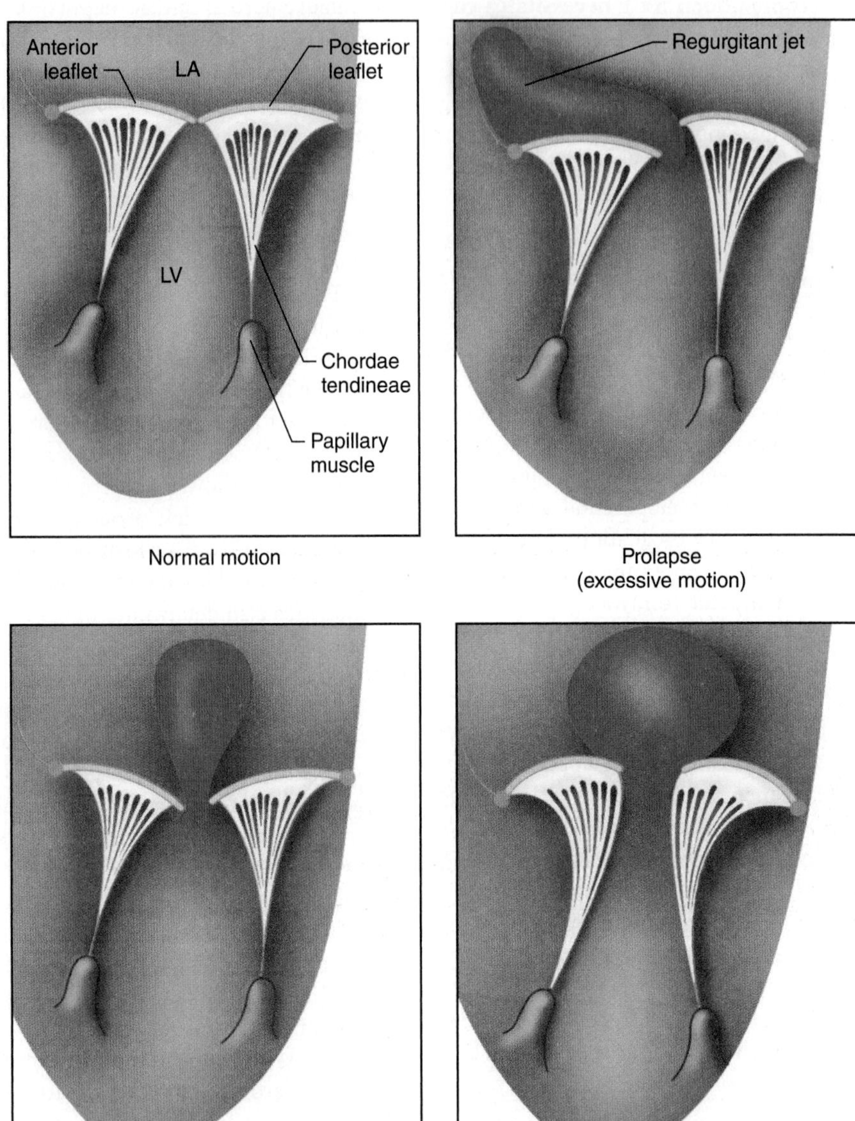

FIGURE 21–8 Classification of mitral valve leaflet motion (as seen from transesophageal echocardiography). Note that with prolapse, the free edge of the leaflet(s) extends beyond the plane of the mitral annulus, producing an eccentric jet. With restricted motion, the leaflets fail to coapt, resulting in a central jet. LA, left atrium; LV, left ventricle.

treatment is usually reserved for patients with moderate to severe symptoms. Valvuloplasty or valve repair are performed whenever possible to avoid the problems associated with valve replacement (eg, thromboembolism, hemorrhage, prosthetic failure). Catheter-mediated valve repairs are continually being refined, potentially reducing the need for "open" surgery. Anesthesiologists skilled in advanced perioperative echocardiography assist in correctly identifying the leaflet(s) to be repaired and determining the repair's success. Three-dimensional echocardiography is increasingly employed to assist in the assessment of the mitral valve (see Figure 5–31).

Anesthetic Management

A. Objectives

8 Anesthetic management should be tailored to the severity of mitral regurgitation as well as the underlying left ventricular function. Factors that exacerbate the regurgitation, such as slow heart rates and acute increases in afterload, should be avoided. Bradycardia can increase the regurgitant volume by increasing left ventricular end-diastolic volume and acutely dilating the mitral annulus. The heart rate should ideally be kept between 80 and 100 beats/min. Acute increases in left ventricular afterload, such as with endotracheal intubation and surgical stimulation under "light" anesthesia, should be treated rapidly.

B. Monitoring

Monitors are based on the severity of ventricular dysfunction as well as the procedure. Color-flow Doppler TEE can be invaluable in quantitating the severity of the regurgitation and guiding therapeutic interventions in patients with severe mitral regurgitation. Doppler echocardiography identifies the acceleration of blood as it is ejected through the regurgitant orifice during systole from the left ventricle into the left atrium (Figure 21–9).

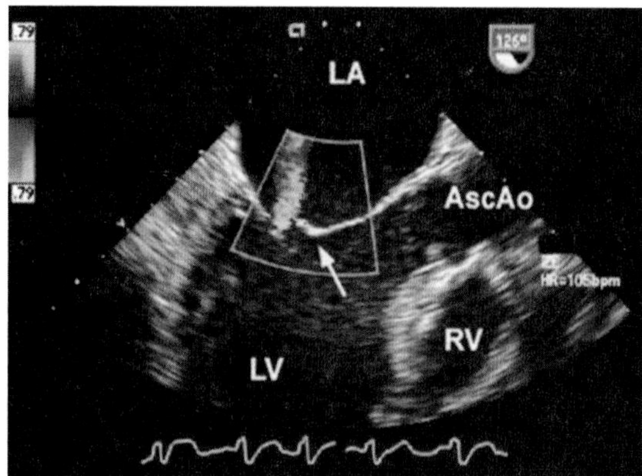

FIGURE 21–9 Transesophageal echocardiography using color-flow Doppler demonstrates mitral regurgitation. The left atrium (LA), left ventricle (LV), right ventricle (RV), and ascending aorta (AscAo) are shown. The *arrow* indicates a jet of mitral regurgitation. (Reproduced with permission from Mathew JP, Swaminathan M, Ayoub CM. *Clinical Manual and Review of Transesophageal Echocardiography*, 2nd ed. New York, NY: McGraw Hill; 2010.)

C. Choice of Agents

Patients with relatively well-preserved ventricular function tend to do well with most anesthetic techniques. Spinal and epidural anesthesia are well tolerated, provided bradycardia is avoided. Patients with compromised ventricular function can likewise be managed with a variety of anesthetic agents and techniques. Invasive monitoring (arterial line, TEE) can be used to guide perioperative management in patients with severe mitral regurgitation and poor ventricular function. Inodilators such as milrinone may be employed to improve ventricular function and reduce systemic resistance in patients with poor ventricular function and severe mitral regurgitation to promote forward, as opposed to regurgitant, blood flow.

MITRAL VALVE PROLAPSE

Preoperative Considerations

Mitral valve prolapse (Barlow syndrome) is classically characterized by a midsystolic click, with or without a late apical systolic murmur on auscultation. It is a relatively common abnormality that is present in up to 1% to 2.5% of the general population. The diagnosis is suggested by auscultatory findings and confirmed by echocardiography, which shows systolic prolapse of mitral valve leaflets into the left atrium. Patients with the murmur often have some element of mitral regurgitation. The posterior mitral leaflet is more commonly affected than the anterior leaflet. The mitral annulus may also be dilated. Pathologically, most patients have redundancy or some myxomatous degeneration of the valve leaflets. Most cases of mitral valve prolapse are sporadic or familial, affecting otherwise normal persons. A high incidence of mitral valve prolapse is found in patients with connective tissue disorders (particularly Marfan syndrome).

The overwhelming majority of patients with mitral valve prolapse are asymptomatic, but in a small percentage of patients, the myxomatous degeneration is progressive. Manifestations, when they occur, can include chest pains, arrhythmias, embolic events, florid mitral regurgitation, infective endocarditis, and, rarely, sudden death. The diagnosis can be made preoperatively by auscultation of the characteristic click but must be confirmed by echocardiography. The prolapse is accentuated by maneuvers that decrease ventricular volume (preload). Both atrial and ventricular arrhythmias are common. Although bradyarrhythmias have been reported, paroxysmal supraventricular tachycardia is the most commonly encountered sustained arrhythmia. An increased incidence of abnormal AV bypass tracts is reported in patients with mitral valve prolapse.

Most patients have a normal life span. About 15% develop progressive mitral regurgitation. A smaller percentage develops embolic phenomena or infective endocarditis. Patients with both a click and a systolic murmur seem to be at greater risk of developing complications. Anticoagulation or antiplatelet agents may be used for patients with a history of emboli, whereas β-adrenergic blocking drugs are commonly used for arrhythmias.

Anesthetic Management

The management of these patients is based on their clinical course. Most patients are asymptomatic and do not require special care. Ventricular arrhythmias may occur intraoperatively, particularly following sympathetic stimulation, and will generally respond to lidocaine or β-adrenergic blocking agents. Mitral regurgitation caused by prolapse is generally exacerbated by decreases in ventricular size. Hypovolemia and factors that increase ventricular emptying or decrease afterload should be avoided. Vasopressors with pure α-adrenergic agonist activity (such as phenylephrine) may be preferable to those that are primarily β-adrenergic agonists.

AORTIC STENOSIS

Preoperative Considerations

Valvular aortic stenosis is the most common cause of obstruction to left ventricular outflow. Left ventricular outflow obstruction is less commonly due to hypertrophic cardiomyopathy, discrete congenital subvalvular stenosis, or, rarely, supravalvular stenosis. Valvular aortic stenosis is typically congenital, rheumatic, or degenerative. Abnormalities in the number of cusps (most commonly a bicuspid valve) or their architecture produce turbulence that traumatizes the valve and eventually leads to stenosis. Rheumatic aortic stenosis is rarely isolated; it is more commonly associated with aortic regurgitation or mitral valve disease. In the most common degenerative form, calcific aortic stenosis, wear and tear results in the buildup of calcium deposits on normal cusps, preventing them from opening completely (Figure 21–10).

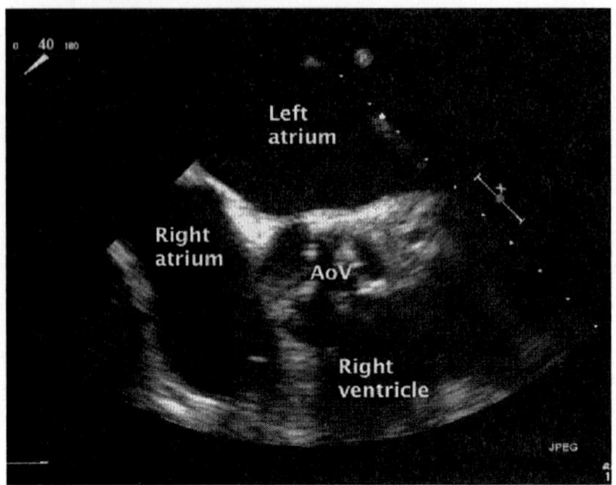

FIGURE 21–10 A stenotic aortic valve is clearly seen in this midesophageal short-axis aortic valve view. Calcification of the aortic valve is usually associated with senile degeneration. However, congenitally abnormal (bicuspid) and rheumatic presentations also occur. (Reproduced with permission from Wasnick J, Hillel Z, Kramer D, et al. *Cardiac Anesthesia & Transesophageal Echocardiography.* New York, NY: McGraw Hill; 2011.)

Pathophysiology

Left ventricular outflow obstruction caused by valvular aortic stenosis is almost always gradual, allowing the ventricle, at least initially, to compensate and maintain stroke volume. Concentric left ventricular hypertrophy enables the ventricle to maintain stroke volume by generating the needed transvalvular pressure gradient and reducing ventricular wall stress.

Critical aortic stenosis is said to exist when the aortic valve orifice is reduced to 0.5 to 0.7 cm^2

(normal is 2.5–3.5 cm^2). With this degree of stenosis, patients generally have a transvalvular gradient of approximately 50 mm Hg at rest (with a normal cardiac output) and are unable to increase cardiac output in response to exertion. Moreover, further increases in the transvalvular gradient do not significantly increase stroke volume. With long-standing aortic stenosis, myocardial contractility progressively deteriorates, compromising left ventricular function.

Classically, patients with advanced (end-stage) aortic stenosis have the triad of heart failure, angina, and syncope. Initial diagnosis in the modern era is usually made earlier in the course of the disease when the more typical complaints are exercise-induced dyspnea, vertigo, or angina. A prominent feature of aortic stenosis is a decrease in left ventricular compliance as a result of hypertrophy. Diastolic dysfunction as a result of an increase in ventricular muscle mass, fibrosis, or myocardial ischemia is to be expected. In contrast to left ventricular end-diastolic volume, which remains normal until very late in the disease, left ventricular end-diastolic pressure is elevated early in the disease. The decreased diastolic pressure gradient between the left atrium and left ventricle impairs ventricular filling, which becomes quite dependent on a normal atrial contraction. Loss of atrial systole can precipitate congestive heart failure or hypotension in patients with aortic stenosis. Cardiac output may be normal in symptomatic patients at rest, but characteristically, it does not appropriately increase with exertion. Patients may experience angina even in the absence of CAD. Myocardial oxygen demand increases because of ventricular hypertrophy, whereas myocardial oxygen supply decreases as a result of the marked compression of intramyocardial coronary vessels caused by high intracavitary systolic pressures (up to 300 mm Hg). Exertional syncope or near-syncope is thought to be due to an inability to tolerate the vasodilation in muscle tissue during exertion. Arrhythmias leading to severe hypoperfusion may also account for syncope and sudden death in some patients.

Treatment

Once symptoms develop, most patients will die within a few years without valve replacement. Catheter-delivered aortic valves are increasingly being perfected and deployed in the treatment of aortic valve disease to an ever-expanding number of patients. Surgical replacement of the stenotic aortic valve is also undertaken in younger patients who require a mechanical valve.

Anesthetic Management

A. Objectives

9 Maintenance of normal sinus rhythm, heart rate, vascular resistance, and intravascular volume is critical in patients with aortic stenosis. Loss of a normally timed atrial systole often leads to rapid deterioration, particularly when associated with tachycardia. The combination of the two (AF with rapid ventricular response) seriously impairs ventricular filling and necessitates immediate cardioversion. The reduced ventricular compliance also makes the patient very sensitive to abrupt changes in intravascular volume. Many patients behave as though they have a fixed stroke volume in spite of adequate hydration; under these conditions, cardiac output becomes very rate dependent. Extreme bradycardia (<50 beats/min) is therefore poorly tolerated. Heart rates between 60 and 90 beats/min are optimal in most patients.

B. Monitoring

Monitoring for ischemia is complicated by baseline ST-segment and T-wave abnormalities often seen in the aortic stenosis patient. Intraarterial pressure monitoring is desirable in patients with severe aortic stenosis as many of these patients do not tolerate even brief episodes of hypotension. Vasodilators should be used cautiously, if at all, because patients are often very sensitive to these agents. TEE is useful in these patients for monitoring ischemia, ventricular preload, contractility, valvular function, and the effects of therapeutic interventions.

C. Choice of Agents

Patients with mild to moderate aortic stenosis (generally asymptomatic) may tolerate spinal or epidural anesthesia. These techniques should be employed very cautiously, however, because hypotension readily occurs as a result of reductions in preload, afterload, or both. A vasoconstrictor medication must be immediately available. Epidural anesthesia may be preferable to single-shot spinal anesthesia because of its slower onset of hypotension, which allows more timely correction. In theory, continuous spinal catheters can similarly be used to gradually increase the level of block and slow the onset of hypotension.

In the patient with severe aortic stenosis, the choice of anesthetic agents and techniques is less important than effective management of their hemodynamic effects. Most general anesthetics can produce both vasodilation and hypotension, which require treatment after induction. If a volatile agent is used, the concentration should be controlled to avoid excessive vasodilation, myocardial depression, or loss of normal atrial systole. Significant tachycardia and severe hypertension, which can precipitate ischemia, should be treated immediately by increasing anesthetic depth or administration of a β-adrenergic blocking agent. Most patients with aortic stenosis tolerate moderate hypertension and are sensitive to vasodilators. The use of vasoconstrictors (eg, vasopressin, phenylephrine, norepinephrine) is often necessary to preserve systemic blood pressure in the anesthetized aortic stenosis patient. Moreover, because of an already precarious myocardial oxygen demand–supply balance, aortic stenosis patients tolerate even mild degrees of hypotension poorly. Intraoperative SVTs with hemodynamic compromise should be treated with immediate synchronized cardioversion. Frequent ventricular ectopy (which often reflects ischemia) is usually poorly tolerated hemodynamically and should be treated.

AORTIC REGURGITATION

Preoperative Considerations

Aortic regurgitation usually develops slowly and is progressive (chronic), but it can also develop quickly (acute). Chronic aortic regurgitation may be caused by abnormalities of the aortic valve, the aortic root, or both. Abnormalities in the valve are usually congenital (bicuspid valve) or due to rheumatic fever. Diseases affecting the ascending aorta cause regurgitation by dilating the aortic annulus; they include syphilis, annuloaortic ectasia, cystic medial necrosis (with or without Marfan syndrome), ankylosing spondylitis, rheumatoid and psoriatic arthritis, and a variety of other connective tissue disorders. Acute aortic insufficiency most commonly follows infective endocarditis, trauma, or aortic dissection.

Pathophysiology

Regardless of the cause, aortic regurgitation produces volume overload of the left ventricle. The effective forward stroke volume is reduced because of the backward (regurgitant) flow of blood into the left ventricle during diastole. Systemic arterial diastolic pressure and SVR are typically low. The decrease in cardiac afterload helps facilitate ventricular ejection. Total stroke volume is the sum of the effective stroke volume and the regurgitant volume. The regurgitant volume depends on the heart rate (diastolic time) and the diastolic pressure gradient across the aortic valve (diastolic aortic pressure minus left ventricular end-diastolic pressure). Slow heart rates increase regurgitation because of the associated disproportionate increase in diastolic time, whereas increases in diastolic arterial pressure favor regurgitant volume by increasing the pressure gradient for backward flow.

With chronic aortic regurgitation, the left ventricle progressively dilates and undergoes eccentric hypertrophy. Patients with severe aortic regurgitation have the largest end-diastolic volumes of any heart disease. The resulting increase in end-diastolic volume maintains an effective stroke volume. Any increase in the regurgitant volume is compensated by an increase in end-diastolic volume. Left ventricular end-diastolic pressure is usually normal or only slightly elevated because ventricular compliance initially increases. Eventually, as ventricular function deteriorates, the ejection fraction declines, and impaired ventricular emptying is manifested as gradual increases in left ventricular end-diastolic pressure and end-systolic volume.

Sudden incompetence of the aortic valve does not allow compensatory dilation or hypertrophy of the left ventricle. Effective stroke volume rapidly declines because the normal-sized ventricle is unable to accommodate a sudden large regurgitant volume. The sudden rise in left ventricular end-diastolic pressure is transmitted back to the pulmonary circulation and causes acute pulmonary venous congestion.

Acute aortic regurgitation typically presents as the sudden onset of pulmonary edema and hypotension, whereas chronic regurgitation ultimately manifests as congestive heart failure. Symptoms are generally nil or minimal in the chronic form when the regurgitant volume remains under 40% of stroke volume but become severe when it exceeds 60%. Angina can occur even in the absence of coronary disease. The myocardial oxygen demand is increased from muscle hypertrophy and dilation; the myocardial blood supply is reduced by low diastolic pressures in the aorta as a result of the regurgitation, and peak myocardial blood flow occurs in systole rather than diastole.

Treatment

Most patients with chronic aortic regurgitation remain asymptomatic for 10 or more years. Once significant symptoms develop, the expected survival time is about 5 years without valve replacement. Diuretics and afterload reduction, particularly with ACE inhibitors, generally benefit patients with advanced chronic aortic regurgitation. The decrease in arterial blood pressure reduces the diastolic gradient for regurgitation. Patients with chronic aortic regurgitation should receive valve replacement before irreversible ventricular dysfunction occurs. Patients with acute aortic regurgitation typically require intravenous inotropic and vasodilator therapy. Early intervention is indicated in patients with acute aortic regurgitation; medical management alone is associated with a high mortality rate.

Anesthetic Management

A. Objectives

The heart rate should be maintained toward the upper limits of normal (80–100 beats/min). Bradycardia
10 and increases in SVR increase the regurgitant volume in patients with aortic regurgitation, whereas tachycardia can contribute to myocardial ischemia. Excessive myocardial depression should also be avoided. The compensatory increase in cardiac preload should be maintained, but overzealous fluid replacement can readily result in pulmonary edema.

B. Monitoring

Invasive hemodynamic monitoring should be employed in patients with acute aortic regurgitation or those with severe chronic regurgitation. Premature closure of the mitral valve often occurs during acute aortic regurgitation and may cause pulmonary capillary wedge pressure to give a falsely high estimate of left ventricular end-diastolic pressure. The arterial pressure wave in patients with aortic regurgitation characteristically has a very wide pulse pressure. *Pulsus bisferiens* may also be present in patients with moderate to severe aortic insufficiency and is thought to result from the rapid ejection of a large stroke volume. Color-flow Doppler TEE is invaluable in quantitating the severity of the regurgitation and guiding therapeutic interventions (Figure 21–11).

Severe aortic regurgitation rapidly raises left ventricular pressure during diastole. Echocardiography can also detect reversal of blood flow in the aorta during diastole in patients with severe aortic regurgitation. The more severe the regurgitation, the further distal in the aorta that diastolic flow reversal is identified.

C. Choice of Agents

Most patients with aortic insufficiency tolerate spinal and epidural anesthesia well, provided intravascular

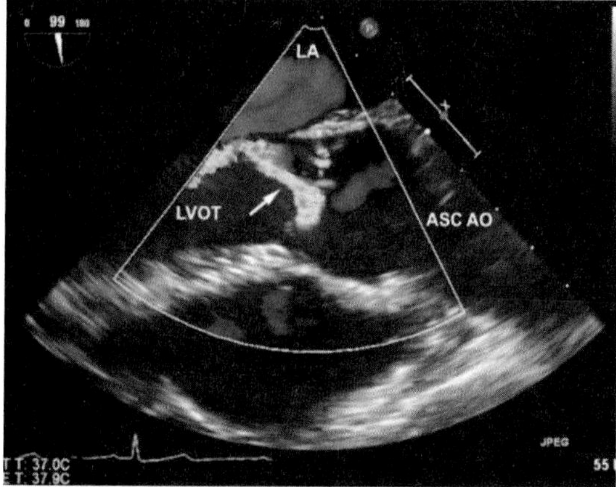

FIGURE 21–11 Transesophageal echocardiography using color-flow Doppler demonstrates aortic regurgitation. The left ventricular outflow tract (LVOT), left atrium (LA), and ascending aorta (ASCAO) are seen. The *arrow* demonstrates an eccentrically directed jet of aortic regurgitation. (Reproduced with permission from Mathew JP, Swaminathan M, Ayoub CM. *Clinical Manual and Review of Transesophageal Echocardiography,* 2nd ed. New York, NY: McGraw Hill; 2010.)

volume is maintained. When general anesthesia is required, inhalational agents may be ideal because of the associated vasodilation. Phenylephrine (25–50 mcg) or norepinephrine can be used to treat hypotension secondary to excessive anesthetic-induced vasodilatation; however, large doses of either drug may increase SVR (and arterial diastolic pressure) sufficiently to worsen the regurgitation.

TRICUSPID REGURGITATION

Preoperative Considerations

Most patients have trace to mild tricuspid regurgitation on echocardiography; the regurgitant volume in these cases is almost always trivial. Clinically significant tricuspid regurgitation, however, is most commonly due to dilation of the right ventricle from pulmonary hypertension that is associated with chronic left ventricular failure. Tricuspid regurgitation can also follow infective endocarditis, rheumatic fever, carcinoid syndrome, or chest trauma or may be due to Ebstein anomaly (downward displacement of the valve because of abnormal attachment of the valve leaflets).

Pathophysiology

Chronic left ventricular failure often leads to sustained increases in pulmonary vascular pressures. The chronic increase in afterload causes progressive dilation of the thin-walled right ventricle, and excessive dilation of the tricuspid annulus eventually results in regurgitation. An increase in end-diastolic volume allows the right ventricle to compensate for the regurgitant volume and maintain an effective forward flow. Because the right atrium and the vena cava are compliant and can usually accommodate the volume overload, mean right atrial and central venous pressures are generally only slightly elevated. Acute or marked elevations in pulmonary artery pressures increase the regurgitant volume and are reflected by an increase in central venous pressure. Moreover, sudden marked increases in right ventricular afterload sharply reduce the effective right ventricular output, reduce left ventricular preload, and can precipitate systemic hypotension.

Chronic venous hypertension leads to passive congestion of the liver and progressive hepatic dysfunction. Severe right ventricular failure with underloading of the left heart may also produce right-to-left shunting through a patent foramen ovale, which can result in marked hypoxemia.

The normal right ventricle does not extend to the apex of the heart when visualized using echocardiography. As the right heart dilates, it acquires a more spherical shape, the right ventricle extends to the apex of the heart, and the interventricular septum is flattened. These changes can impair left heart function.

Treatment

Tricuspid regurgitation is generally well tolerated by most patients. Because the underlying disorder is generally more important than the tricuspid regurgitation itself, treatment is aimed at the underlying disease process. Recent studies suggest that correction of significant tricuspid regurgitation with annuloplasty is beneficial when patients with moderate to severe tricuspid regurgitation are brought to surgery for replacement of another valve.

Anesthetic Management

A. Objectives

Hemodynamic goals should be directed primarily toward the underlying disorder. Hypovolemia and factors that increase right ventricular afterload, such as hypoxia and acidosis, should be avoided to maintain effective right ventricular stroke volume and left ventricular preload. Positive end-expiratory pressure and high mean airway pressures may also be undesirable during mechanical ventilation because they reduce venous return and increase right ventricular afterload.

B. Monitoring

Invasive monitoring may be useful. Pulmonary artery catheterization is rarely used and often not feasible; rarely a large regurgitant flow may make passage of a pulmonary artery catheter across the tricuspid valve difficult. Increasing central venous pressure implies worsening right ventricular dysfunction. The x descent is absent, and a prominent cv wave is usually present on the central venous pressure waveform. Thermodilution cardiac output measurements are falsely elevated because of the tricuspid regurgitation. Color-flow Doppler TEE is useful in evaluating the severity of the regurgitation and other associated abnormalities.

C. Choice of Agents

The selection of anesthetic agents should be based on the underlying disorder. Most patients tolerate spinal and epidural anesthesia well. Coagulopathy secondary to hepatic dysfunction should be excluded prior to any regional technique.

ENDOCARDITIS PROPHYLAXIS

The ACC/AHA guidelines regarding prophylactic antibiotic regimens in patients with prosthetic heart valves and other structural heart abnormalities have dramatically changed in recent years, decreasing the number of indications for antibiotic administration. The risk of antibiotic administration is often considered greater than the potential for developing perioperative endocarditis. At present, the ACC/AHA guidelines suggest the use of endocarditis prophylaxis in the highest risk patients undergoing dental procedures involving gingival manipulation or perforation of the oral mucosa (class IIa); see Table 21–12. Such conditions include:

TABLE 21–12 Regimens for a dental procedure.

		Regimen: Single Dose 30–60 min Before Procedure	
Situation	**Agent**	**Adults**	**Children**
Oral	Amoxicillin	2 g	50 mg/kg
Unable to take oral medication	Ampicillin	2 g IM or IV[2]	50 mg/kg IM or IV
	OR		
	Cefazolin or ceftriaxone	1 g IM or IV	50 mg/kg IM or IV
Allergic to penicillins or ampicillin—oral	Cephalexin[3,4]	2 g	50 mg/kg
	OR		
	Clindamycin	600 mg	20 mg/kg
	OR		
	Azithromycin or clarithromycin	500 mg	15 mg/kg
Allergic to penicillins or ampicillin and unable to take oral medication	Cefazolin or ceftriaxone	1 g IM or IV	50 mg/kg IM or IV
	OR		
	Clindamycin	600 mg IM or IV	20 mg/kg IM or IV

[1]IM, intramuscular; IV, intravenous.

[2]Or use other first- or second-generation oral cephalosporin in equivalent adult or pediatric dosage.

[3]Cephalosporins should not be used in an individual with a history of anaphylaxis, angioedema, or urticaria with penicillins or ampicillin.

Reproduced with permission from Nishimura RA, Carabello BA, Faxon DP, et al. ACC/AHA 2008 guideline update on valvular heart disease: Focused update on infective endocarditis prophylaxis. *J Am Coll Cardiol.* 2008 Aug 19;52(8):676-685.

- Patients with prosthetic cardiac valves or prosthetic heart materials
- Patients with a history of endocarditis
- Patients with congenital heart disease that is either partially repaired or unrepaired
- Patients with congenital heart disease with residual defects following repair
- Patients with congenital heart disease within 6 months of a complete repair, whether catheter-based or surgical
- Cardiac transplant patients with structurally abnormal valves

Class III recommendations indicate that prophylaxis is not necessary for nondental procedures, including TEE and esophagogastroduodenoscopy, except in the presence of an active infection.

Endocarditis is believed to occur in areas of cardiac endothelial damage, where in cases of bacteremia, bacteria can be deposited and multiply. Areas of increased myocardial blood flow velocity lead to damaged endothelium, providing a locus for bacterial adherence and growth. Guidelines are ever changing and not considered to be "standard of care." Nevertheless, deviation from guidelines often requires explanation as being outside of "evidence-based" practice. Review of the ACC/AHA guidelines is recommended when such high-risk patients are encountered.

ANTICOAGULATION

Patients with mechanical prosthetic heart valves require anticoagulation, which is currently accomplished with warfarin. Aspirin is also indicated in this population, as well as in patients with bioprosthetic valves, to prevent thrombus formation. Warfarin is sometimes also used initially for mitral bioprosthetic valves.

Patients with prosthetic valves often present for noncardiac surgery that will require temporary discontinuation of anticoagulation. The ACC/AHA guidelines indicate that patients at low risk of thrombosis, such as those with bileaflet mechanical valves in the aortic position with no additional problems (eg, no AF or hypercoagulable state) can discontinue warfarin 48 to 72 hours preoperatively so that the INR falls below 1.5. In patients at greater risk of thrombosis, warfarin should be discontinued and heparin, either unfractionated or low molecular weight, started when the INR falls below 2.0. Heparin can be discontinued 4 to 6 hours prior to surgery and then restarted as soon as surgical bleeding permits, until the patient can be restarted on warfarin therapy. Fresh frozen plasma or prothrombin complex concentrates may be given, if needed, in an emergency situation to interrupt warfarin therapy. Anesthesia providers should always consult with the patient's surgeon and the physician responsible for prescribing the anticoagulation before adjusting anticoagulation or antiplatelet regimens perioperatively.

Congenital Heart Disease

Preoperative Considerations

Congenital heart disease encompasses a seemingly endless list of abnormalities that may be detected in infancy, early childhood, or, less commonly, adulthood. The incidence of congenital heart disease in all live births approaches 1%. The natural history of some defects is such that patients often survive to adulthood (Table 21–13). Moreover, the number of surviving adults with corrected or palliated congenital heart disease is steadily increasing with advances in surgical and medical treatment. Patients with congenital heart disease may therefore be encountered during noncardiac surgery and obstetric deliveries. Knowledge of the anatomy of the original heart structure defect and of any corrective repairs is essential prior to anesthetizing the patient with congenital heart disease.

TABLE 21–13 Common congenital heart defects in which patients typically survive to adulthood without treatment.

Bicuspid aortic valve
Coarctation of the aorta
Pulmonic valve stenosis
Ostium secundum atrial septal defect
Ventricular septal defect
Patent ductus arteriosus

TABLE 21–14 Classification of congenital heart disease.

Lesions causing outflow obstruction
Left ventricle
Coarctation of the aorta
Aortic stenosis
Right ventricle
Pulmonic valve stenosis
Lesions causing left-to-right shunting
Ventricular septal defect
Patent ductus arteriosus
Atrial septal defect
Endocardial cushion defect
Partial anomalous pulmonary venous return
Lesions causing right-to-left shunting
With decreased pulmonary blood flow
Tetralogy of Fallot
Pulmonary atresia
Tricuspid atresia
With increased pulmonary blood flow
Transposition of the great vessels
Truncus arteriosus
Single ventricle
Double-outlet right ventricle
Total anomalous pulmonary venous return
Hypoplastic left heart

The complex nature and varying pathophysiology of congenital heart defects make classification difficult. A commonly used scheme is presented in Table 21–14. Most patients present with cyanosis, congestive heart failure, or an asymptomatic abnormality. Cyanosis is typically the result of an abnormal intracardiac communication that allows unoxygenated blood to reach the systemic arterial circulation (right-to-left shunting). Congestive heart failure is most prominent with defects that either obstruct left ventricular outflow or markedly increase pulmonary blood flow. The latter is usually due to an abnormal intracardiac communication that returns oxygenated blood to the right heart (left-to-right shunting). Whereas right-to-left shunts generally decrease pulmonary blood flow, some complex lesions increase pulmonary blood flow—even in the presence of right-to-left shunting. In many cases, more than one lesion is present. Survival prior to surgical correction with some anomalies (eg, transposition, total anomalous venous return, pulmonary atresia) depends on the simultaneous presence of another shunting lesion (eg, patent ductus arteriosus, patent foramen ovale, ventricular septal defect). Chronic hypoxemia in patients with cyanotic heart disease typically results in erythrocytosis. This increase in red cell mass, which is due to increased erythropoietin secretion from the kidneys, serves to restore tissue oxygen concentration to normal. Unfortunately, blood viscosity can also rise to the point at which it may interfere with oxygen delivery. When tissue oxygenation is restored to normal, the hematocrit is stable (usually <65%), and symptoms of hyperviscosity syndrome are absent, the patient is said to have *compensated erythrocytosis.* Patients with uncompensated erythrocytosis do not establish this equilibrium; they have symptoms of hyperviscosity and may be at risk of thrombotic complications, particularly stroke. The risk of stroke is aggravated by dehydration. Children younger than age 4 years seem to be at greatest risk of stroke. Phlebotomy is generally not recommended if symptoms of hyperviscosity are absent and the hematocrit is less than 65%.

Coagulation abnormalities are common in patients with cyanotic heart disease. Platelet counts tend to be low-normal, and many patients have defects in the coagulation cascade. Hyperuricemia often occurs because of increased urate reabsorption secondary to renal hypoperfusion and can result in progressively impaired kidney function.

Preoperative echocardiography is invaluable in defining the anatomy of the defect(s) and to confirm or exclude the existence of other lesions or complications, their physiological significance, and the effects of any therapeutic interventions.

Anesthetic Management

This population of patients includes four groups: (1) those who have undergone corrective cardiac surgery and require no further operations, (2) those who have had only palliative surgery, (3) those who have not yet undergone any cardiac surgery, and (4) those whose conditions are inoperable and may be awaiting cardiac transplantation. Although the management of the first group of patients may be the same as that of normal patients (except for consideration of prophylactic antibiotic therapy), the care of others requires familiarity with the complex

TABLE 21–15 Common problems in survivors of surgery for congenital heart defects.

Arrhythmias
Hypoxemia
Pulmonary hypertension
Existing shunts
Paradoxical embolism
Bacterial endocarditis

pathophysiology of these defects (Tables 21–15 and 21–16).

For the purpose of anesthetic management, congenital heart defects may be divided into obstructive lesions, predominantly left-to-right shunts, or predominantly right-to-left shunts. Shunts can also be bidirectional and may reverse under certain conditions.

1. Obstructive Lesions

Pulmonic Stenosis

Pulmonary valve stenosis obstructs right ventricular outflow and causes concentric right ventricular hypertrophy. Severe obstruction presents in the neonatal period, whereas lesser degrees of obstruction may go undetected until adulthood. The valve is usually deformed and is either bicuspid or tricuspid. Valve leaflets are often partially fused and display systolic doming on echocardiography. The right ventricle undergoes hypertrophy, and poststenotic dilation of the pulmonary artery is often present. Symptoms are those of right ventricular heart failure. Symptomatic patients readily develop fatigue, dyspnea, and peripheral cyanosis with exertion as a result of the limited pulmonary blood flow and increased oxygen extraction by tissues. With severe stenosis, the pulmonic valve gradient exceeds 60 to 80 mm Hg, depending on the age of the patient. Right-to-left shunting may also occur in the presence of a patent foramen ovale or atrial septal defect. Cardiac output is very dependent on an elevated heart rate, but excessive increases in the latter can compromise ventricular filling. Percutaneous balloon valvuloplasty is generally considered the initial treatment of choice in most patients with symptomatic pulmonic stenosis. Anesthetic management for patients undergoing surgery should maintain a normal or slightly high heart rate, augment preload, and avoid factors that increase PVR (such as hypoxemia or hypercarbia).

TABLE 21–16 Congenital cardiac lesions and perioperative risk for noncardiac surgery.

High risk
Pulmonary hypertension, primary or secondary
Cyanotic congenital heart disease
New York Heart Association class III or IV
Severe systemic ventricular dysfunction (ejection fraction less than 35%)
Severe left-sided heart obstructive lesions
Moderate risk
Prosthetic valve or conduit
Intracardiac shunt
Moderate left-sided heart obstruction
Moderate systemic ventricular dysfunction

Reproduced with permission from Warnes C, Williams R, Bashore T, et al. ACC/AHA 2008 guidelines for the management of adults with congenital heart disease. *Circulation*. 2008 Dec 2;118(23):2395-2451.

2. Predominantly Left-to-Right (Simple) Shunts

Simple shunts are isolated abnormal communications between the right and left sides of the heart. Because pressures are normally higher on the left side of the heart, blood usually flows across from left to right, and blood flow through the right heart and the lungs increases. Depending on the size and location of the communication, the right ventricle may also be subjected to the higher left-sided pressures, resulting in both pressure and volume overload. Right ventricular afterload is normally 5% that of the left ventricle, so even small left-to-right pressure gradients can produce large increases in pulmonary blood flow. The ratio of pulmonary (Qp) to systemic (Qs) blood flow is useful to determine the directionality of the shunt.

A ratio greater than 1 usually indicates a left-to-right shunt, whereas a ratio less than 1 indicates a right-to-left shunt. A ratio of 1 indicates either no shunting or a bidirectional shunt of equal opposing magnitudes.

Large increases in pulmonary blood flow produce pulmonary vascular congestion and increase extravascular lung water. The latter interferes with gas exchange, decreases lung compliance, and increases the work of breathing. Left atrial distention also compresses the left bronchus, whereas distention of pulmonary vessels compresses smaller bronchi.

Over the course of several years, chronic increases in pulmonary blood flow produce vascular changes that irreversibly increase PVR. Elevation of right ventricular afterload produces hypertrophy and progressively raises right-sided cardiac pressures. With advanced disease, the pressures within the right heart can exceed those within the left heart. Under these conditions, the intracardiac shunt reverses and becomes a right-to-left shunt (Eisenmenger syndrome).

When a communication is small, shunt flow depends primarily on the size of the communication (restrictive shunt). When the communication is large (nonrestrictive shunt), shunt flow depends on
11 the relative balance between PVR and SVR. An increase in SVR relative to PVR favors left-to-right shunting, whereas an increase in PVR relative to SVR favors right-to-left shunting. Common chamber lesions (eg, single atrium, single ventricle, truncus arteriosus) represent the extreme form of nonrestrictive shunts; shunt flow with these lesions is bidirectional and totally dependent on relative changes in the ventricular afterload.

12 The presence of shunt flow between the right and left hearts, regardless of the direction of blood flow, mandates the meticulous exclusion of air bubbles and particulate material from intravenous fluids to prevent paradoxical embolism into the cerebral or coronary circulations.

Atrial Septal Defects

Ostium secundum atrial septal defects (ASDs) are the most common form and usually occur as isolated lesions in the area of the fossa ovalis. The defect is sometimes associated with partial anomalous pulmonary venous return, most commonly of the right upper pulmonary vein. A secundum ASD may result in single or multiple (fenestrated) openings between the atria. The less common sinus venosus and ostium primum ASDs are typically associated with other cardiac abnormalities. Sinus venosus defects are located in the upper interatrial septum close to the superior vena cava; one or more of the right pulmonary veins often abnormally drains into the superior vena cava. In contrast, ostium primum ASDs are located in the lower interatrial septum and overlie the mitral and tricuspid valves; most patients also have a cleft in the anterior leaflet of the mitral valve, and some have an abnormal septal leaflet in the tricuspid valve.

Most children with ASDs are minimally symptomatic; some have recurrent pulmonary infections. Congestive heart failure and pulmonary hypertension are more commonly encountered in adults with ASDs. Patients with ostium primum defects often have large shunts and may also develop significant mitral regurgitation. In the absence of heart failure, anesthetic responses to inhalation and intravenous agents are generally not significantly altered in patients with ASDs. **Large increases in SVR should be avoided because they may worsen left-to-right shunting**.

Ventricular Septal Defects

Ventricular septal defect (VSD) is a common congenital heart defect, accounting for up to 25% to 35% of congenital heart disease. The defect is most frequently found in the membranous part of the interventricular septum (membranous or infracristal VSD) in a posterior position and anterior to the septal leaflet of the tricuspid valve. Muscular VSDs are the next most frequent type and are located in the mid or apical portion of the interventricular septum, where there may be a single defect or multiple openings (resembling Swiss cheese). Defects in the subpulmonary (supracristal) septum are often associated with aortic regurgitation because the right coronary cusp can prolapse into the VSD. Septal defects at the ventricular inlet are usually similar in development and location to AV septal defects (see the following section).

The resulting functional abnormality of a VSD is dependent on the size of the defect, PVR, and the presence or absence of other abnormalities. Small VSDs, particularly of the muscular type, may close during childhood. Restrictive defects are associated with only small left-to-right shunts. Patients with small VSDs are treated medically and followed with electrocardiography (for signs of right ventricular hypertrophy) and echocardiography. Surgical closure is usually undertaken in patients with large VSDs before pulmonary vascular disease and Eisenmenger physiology develop. In the absence of heart failure, anesthetic responses to inhalation and intravenous agents are generally not significantly altered. Similarly, increases in SVR worsen left-to-right shunting. **When right-to-left shunting is present, abrupt increases in PVR or decreases in SVR are poorly tolerated.**

Atrioventricular Septal Defects

Endocardial cushion (AV canal) defects produce contiguous atrial and ventricular septal defects, often with very abnormal AV valves. This is a common lesion in patients with Down syndrome. The defect can produce large shunts both at the atrial and ventricular levels. Mitral and tricuspid regurgitation exacerbate the volume overload on the ventricles. Initially, shunting is predominately left to right; however, with increasing pulmonary hypertension, Eisenmenger syndrome with obvious cyanosis develops.

Patent Ductus Arteriosus

Persistence of the communication between the main pulmonary artery and the aorta can produce restrictive or nonrestrictive left-to-right shunts. This abnormality is commonly responsible for the cardiopulmonary deterioration of premature infants and occasionally presents later in life when it can be corrected thoracoscopically. Anesthetic goals should be similar to atrial and ventricular septal defects.

Partial Anomalous Venous Return

This defect is present when one or more pulmonary veins drains into the right side of the heart; the anomalous veins are usually from the right lung. Possible anomalous entry sites include the right atrium, the superior or inferior vena cava, and the coronary sinus. The resulting abnormality produces a variable amount of left-to-right shunting. The clinical course and prognosis are usually excellent and similar to that of a secundum ASD. Obstructed total anomalous pulmonary venous return is corrected as emergency surgery immediately after birth.

3. Predominantly Right-to-Left (Complex) Shunts

Lesions within this group (some also called ***mixing lesions***) often produce both ventricular outflow obstruction and shunting. The obstruction favors shunt flow toward the unobstructed side. When the obstruction is relatively mild, the amount of shunting is affected by the ratio of SVR to PVR, but increasing degrees of obstruction fix the direction and magnitude of the shunt. Atresia of any one of the cardiac valves represents the extreme form of obstruction. Shunting occurs proximal to the atretic valve and is completely fixed; survival depends on another distal shunt (usually a patent ductus arteriosus [PDA], patent foramen ovale, ASD, or VSD), where blood flows in the opposite direction. This group of defects may also be divided according to whether they increase or decrease pulmonary blood flow.

Tetralogy of Fallot

This anomaly classically includes right ventricular outflow obstruction, right ventricular hypertrophy, and a VSD with an overriding aorta. Right ventricular obstruction in most patients is due to infundibular stenosis, which is due to hypertrophy of the subpulmonic muscle (crista ventricularis). At least 20% to 25% of patients also have pulmonic stenosis, and a small percentage of patients has some element of supravalvular obstruction. The pulmonic valve is often bicuspid, or, less commonly, atretic. Infundibular obstruction may be increased by sympathetic tone and is therefore dynamic; this obstruction is likely responsible for the hypercyanotic spells observed in very young patients. **The combination of right ventricular outflow obstruction and a VSD results in ejection of unoxygenated right ventricular blood, as well as oxygenated left ventricular blood into the aorta**. The right-to-left shunting across the VSD has both fixed and variable components. The fixed component is determined by the severity of the right ventricular obstruction, whereas the variable component depends on SVR and PVR.

Surgical palliation with a left-to-right systemic shunt or complete correction is usually undertaken. For the former, a modified Blalock–Thomas–Taussig (systemic–pulmonary artery) shunt is most often used to increase pulmonary blood flow. In this procedure, a synthetic graft is anastomosed between a subclavian artery and an ipsilateral pulmonary artery. Complete correction involves closure of the VSD, removal of obstructing infundibular muscle, and pulmonic valvulotomy or valvuloplasty, when necessary.

13 The goals of anesthetic management in patients with tetralogy of Fallot should be to maintain intravascular volume and SVR. Increases in PVR, such as might occur from acidosis or excessive airway pressures, should be avoided. **Ketamine (intramuscular or intravenous) is a commonly used induction agent because it maintains or increases SVR and therefore does not aggravate the right-to-left shunting.** Patients with milder degrees of shunting generally tolerate inhalation induction. The right-to-left shunting tends to slow the uptake of inhalation anesthetics; in contrast, it may accelerate the onset of intravenous agents. Oxygenation often improves following induction of anesthesia. Muscle relaxants that release histamine should be avoided. Hypercyanotic spells may be treated with intravenous fluid and phenylephrine (5 mcg/kg). β-Blockers (eg, propranolol) may also be effective in relieving infundibular spasm.

Tricuspid Atresia

With tricuspid atresia, blood can flow out of the right atrium only via a patent foramen ovale (or an ASD). Moreover, a PDA (or VSD) is necessary for blood to flow from the left ventricle into the pulmonary circulation. Cyanosis is usually evident at birth, and its severity depends on the amount of pulmonary blood flow that is achieved. Early survival is dependent on prostaglandin E_1 infusion (to maintain PDA patency), with or without a percutaneous balloon atrial septostomy. Severe cyanosis requires a modified Blalock–Thomas–Taussig shunt early in life. The preferred surgical management is a modified Fontan procedure, in which the venous drainage is directed to the pulmonary circulation. In some centers, a superior vena cava to the main pulmonary artery (bidirectional Glenn) shunt may be employed before or instead of a Fontan procedure. With both procedures, blood from the systemic veins flows through the pulmonary circulation to the left atrium without the assistance of the right ventricle. Success of the procedure depends on a high systemic venous pressure and maintaining both low PVR and low left atrial pressure. Heart transplantation may be necessary for a failed Fontan procedure.

Transposition of the Great Arteries

In patients with transposition of the great arteries, pulmonary and systemic venous return flows normally back to the right and left atrium, respectively, but the aorta arises from the right ventricle, and the pulmonary artery arises from the left ventricle. Thus, deoxygenated blood returns back into the systemic circulation, and oxygenated blood returns back to the lungs. Survival is possible only through mixing of oxygenated and deoxygenated blood across the foramen ovale and a PDA. The presence of a VSD increases mixing and reduces the level of hypoxemia. Prostaglandin E_1 infusion is usually necessary. Corrective surgical treatment involves an arterial switch procedure in which the aorta is divided and reanastomosed to the left ventricle, and the pulmonary artery is divided and reanastomosed to the right ventricle. The coronary arteries must also be reimplanted into the old pulmonary artery root. A VSD, if present, is closed. Less commonly, an atrial switch (Senning) procedure may be carried out if an arterial switch is not possible. In this latter procedure, an intraatrial baffle is created from the atrial wall, and blood from the pulmonary veins flows across an ASD to the right ventricle, from which it is ejected into the systemic circulation.

Transposition of the great vessels may occur with a VSD and pulmonic stenosis. This combination of defects mimics tetralogy of Fallot; however, the obstruction affects the left ventricle, not the right ventricle. Corrective surgery involves performing patch closure of the VSD, directing left ventricular outflow into the aorta, ligating the proximal pulmonary artery, and connecting the right ventricular outflow to the pulmonary artery with a valved conduit (Rastelli procedure).

Truncus Arteriosus

With a truncus arteriosus defect, a single arterial trunk supplies the pulmonary and systemic circulation. Both ventricles eject into the truncus as it always overrides a VSD. As PVR gradually decreases after birth, pulmonary blood flow increases greatly, resulting in heart failure. If left untreated, PVR increases, and cyanosis develops again, along with Eisenmenger physiology. Surgical correction closes the VSD, separates the pulmonary artery from the truncus, and connects the right ventricle to the pulmonary artery with a conduit (Rastelli repair).

Hypoplastic Left Heart Syndrome

This syndrome describes a group of defects characterized by aortic valve atresia and marked underdevelopment of the left ventricle. The right ventricle is the main pumping chamber for both systemic and pulmonary circulations. It ejects normally into the pulmonary artery, and all (or nearly all) blood flow entering the aorta is usually derived from a PDA. Surgical treatment includes both the Norwood repair and a hybrid approach to palliation. In the Norwood repair, a new aorta is created from the hypoplastic aorta and the main pulmonary artery. Pulmonary blood flow is delivered via a Blalock–Thomas–Taussig shunt. The right ventricle becomes the heart's systemic pumping ventricle. A hybrid approach has also been advocated for the palliation of hypoplastic left heart syndrome. In this approach, the pulmonary arteries are banded to reduce pulmonary blood flow, and the PDA is stented to provide for systemic blood flow.

The Patient with a Transplanted Heart

Preoperative Considerations

The number of patients with cardiac transplants is increasing because of both the increasing frequency of transplantation and improved posttransplant survival rates. These patients may present to the operating room early in the postoperative period for mediastinal exploration or retransplantation, or they may appear later for incision and drainage of infections, orthopedic surgery, or unrelated procedures.

14 The transplanted heart is totally denervated, so direct autonomic influences are absent. Cardiac impulse formation and conduction are normal, but the absence of vagal influences causes a relatively high resting heart rate (100–120 beats/min). Although sympathetic fibers are similarly interrupted, the response to circulating catecholamines is normal or even enhanced because of denervation sensitivity (increased receptor density). Cardiac output tends to be low-normal and increases relatively slowly in response to exercise because the response is dependent on an increase in circulating catecholamines. Because the Starling relationship between end-diastolic volume and cardiac output is normal, the transplanted heart is also often said to be preload dependent. Coronary autoregulation is preserved.

Preoperative evaluation should focus on evaluating the functional status of the transplanted heart and detecting complications of immunosuppression. Rejection may be heralded by arrhythmias (in the first 6 months) or decreased exercise tolerance from a progressive deterioration of myocardial performance. Periodic echocardiographic evaluations are commonly used to monitor for rejection, but the most reliable technique is endomyocardial biopsy. Accelerated atherosclerosis in the graft is a very common and serious problem that limits the life of the transplant. Moreover, myocardial ischemia and infarction are almost always silent because of the denervation. Because of this, patients must undergo periodic evaluations, including angiography, for assessment of coronary atherosclerosis.

Immunosuppressive therapy may include cyclosporine, tacrolimus, and prednisone. Important side effects include nephrotoxicity, bone marrow suppression, hepatotoxicity, opportunistic infections, and osteoporosis. Hypertension and fluid retention are common and typically require treatment with a diuretic and an ACE inhibitor.

Anesthetic Management

Almost all anesthetic techniques, including regional anesthesia, have been used successfully for transplanted patients. The preload-dependent function of the graft makes maintenance of a normal or high cardiac preload desirable. Moreover, the absence of reflex increases in heart rate can make patients particularly sensitive to rapid vasodilation. Indirect vasopressors, such as ephedrine, are less effective than direct-acting agents because of the absence of catecholamine stores in myocardial neurons. Isoproterenol (now rarely available) or epinephrine infusions should be readily available to increase the heart rate if necessary. β-Blockers should be used only with extreme caution in these patients.

Electrocardiographic monitoring for ischemia is necessary. The ECG usually demonstrates two sets of P waves, one representing the recipient's own sinoatrial (SA) node (which is left intact) and the other representing the donor's SA node. The recipient's SA node may still be affected by autonomic influences, but it does not affect cardiac function. Direct arterial pressure monitoring should be used for major operations; strict asepsis should be observed during placement.

In a recently transplanted patient, the right ventricle of the transplanted heart may not be able to overcome the resistance of the pulmonary vasculature. Right ventricular failure can occur perioperatively, requiring the use of inhaled nitric oxide, inotropes, and, at times, right ventricular assist devices.

Because the number of transplantable hearts is limited, patients are increasingly treated with left ventricular assist devices (LVADs). LVADs drain blood from the apex of the left ventricular and in a nonpulsatile manner pump oxygenated blood into the aorta, restoring blood delivery to the tissues (Figure 21–12). Patients require anticoagulation to prevent pump thrombosis. Maintenance of right heart function is essential to adequately supply the left side of the heart with sufficient blood for the device to eject. Hypovolemia, pulmonary hypertension, and right heart failure can lead to inadequate loading of the left heart, resulting in reduced LVAD pump flows. LVAD patients presenting for noncardiac procedures are routinely managed by cardiac anesthesiologists familiar with LVAD operations and skilled in advanced perioperative echocardiography.

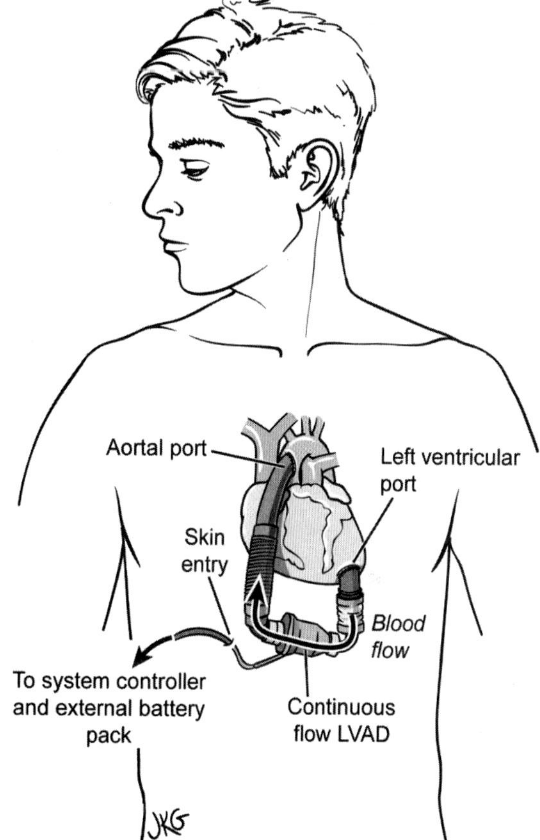

FIGURE 21–12 Schematic of an implanted left ventricular assist device (LVAD). (Reproduced with permission from Wasnick J, Hillel Z, Kramer D, et al. *Cardiac Anesthesia & Transesophageal Echocardiography.* New York, NY: McGraw Hill; 2011.)

CASE DISCUSSION

Hip Fracture in an Older Adult Woman Who Fell

A 71-year-old patient presents for open reduction and internal fixation of a left hip fracture. She gives a history of two episodes of lightheadedness several days prior to her fall today. When questioned about her fall, she can only recall standing in her bathroom while brushing her teeth and then awakening on the floor with hip pain. The preoperative ECG shows a sinus rhythm with a P–R interval of 220 ms and a right bundle-branch block (RBBB) pattern.

Why should the anesthesiologist be concerned about a history of syncope?

A history of syncope in older adult patients should always raise the possibility of arrhythmias and underlying organic heart disease. Although arrhythmias can occur in the absence of organic heart disease, the two are commonly related. Cardiac syncope usually results from an abrupt arrhythmia that suddenly compromises cardiac output and impairs cerebral perfusion. Lightheadedness and presyncope may reflect lesser degrees of cerebral impairment. Both bradyarrhythmias and tachyarrhythmias (see Chapter 20) can produce syncope. Table 21–17 lists other cardiac and noncardiac causes of syncope.

How do bradyarrhythmias commonly arise?

Bradyarrhythmias may arise from either SA node dysfunction or abnormal AV conduction of the cardiac impulse. A delay or block of the impulse can occur anywhere between the SA node and the distal His-Purkinje system. Reversible abnormalities may be due to abnormal vagal tone, electrolyte abnormalities, drug toxicity, hypothermia, or myocardial ischemia. Irreversible abnormalities, which initially may be only intermittent before they become permanent, reflect either isolated conduction system abnormalities or underlying heart disease (most commonly hypertensive, coronary artery, or valvular heart disease).

What is the pathophysiology of sinus node dysfunction?

Patients with sinus node dysfunction may have a normal baseline 12-lead ECG but abrupt pauses in SA node activity (sinus arrest) or intermittent block of conduction of the SA impulse to the surrounding tissue (exit block). Symptoms are usually present when pauses are prolonged (>3 s) or the effective ventricular rate is less than 40 beats/min. Patients may experience intermittent dizziness, syncope, confusion, fatigue, or shortness of breath. Symptomatic SA node dysfunction, or sick sinus syndrome, is often unmasked by β-adrenergic blocking agents, calcium channel blockers, digoxin, or quinidine. The term *tachycardia–bradycardia syndrome* is often used when patients experience paroxysmal tachyarrhythmias (usually atrial flutter or fibrillation) followed by sinus pauses or bradycardia. The latter, bradycardia, probably represents failure of the SA node to recover normal automaticity following suppression by the tachyarrhythmia.

TABLE 21–17 Causes of syncope.

Cardiac
Arrhythmias
Tachyarrhythmias (usually >180 beats/min)
Bradyarrhythmias (usually <40 beats/min)
Impairment of left ventricular ejection
Aortic stenosis
Hypertrophic cardiomyopathy
Massive myocardial infarction
Atrial myxoma
Impairment of right ventricular output
Tetralogy of Fallot
Primary pulmonary hypertension
Pulmonary embolism
Pulmonic valve stenosis
Biventricular impairment
Cardiac tamponade
Massive myocardial infarction
Noncardiac
Accentuated reflexes
Vasodepressor reflex (ie, vasovagal syncope)
Carotid sinus hypersensitivity
Neuralgias
Postural hypotension
Hypovolemia
Sympathectomy
Autonomic dysfunction
Sustained Valsalva maneuver
Cerebrovascular disease
Seizures
Metabolic
Hypoxia
Marked hypocapnia
Hypoglycemia

How are AV conduction abnormalities manifested on the surface 12-lead ECG?

AV conduction abnormalities are usually manifested by abnormal ventricular depolarization (bundle-branch block), prolongation of the P–R interval (first-degree AV block), failure of some atrial impulses to depolarize the ventricles (second-degree

AV block), or AV dissociation (third-degree AV block; also called *complete heart block*).

What determines the significance of these conduction abnormalities?

The significance of a conduction system abnormality depends on its location, its likelihood for progression to complete heart block, and the likelihood that a more distal pacemaker site will be able to maintain a stable and adequate escape rhythm (>40 beats/min). The His bundle is normally the lowest area in the conduction system that can maintain a stable rhythm (usually 40–60 beats/min). When conduction fails anywhere above it, a normal His bundle can take over the pacemaker function of the heart and maintain a normal QRS complex, unless a distal intraventricular conduction defect is present. When the escape rhythm arises farther down the His-Purkinje system, the rhythm is usually slower (<40 beats/min) and is often unstable; it results in a wide QRS complex.

What is the significance of isolated bundle-branch block with a normal P–R interval?

A conduction delay or block in the right bundle-branch results in a typical RBBB QRS pattern on the surface ECG (M-shape or rSR′ in V_1) and may represent a congenital abnormality or underlying organic heart disease. In contrast, a delay or block in the main left bundle-branch results in a left bundle-branch block (LBBB) QRS pattern (wide R with a delayed upstroke in V_5) and nearly always represents underlying heart disease. The term *hemiblock* is often used if only one of the two fascicles of the left bundle-branch is blocked (left anterior or left posterior hemiblock). When the P–R interval is normal—and in the absence of an acute MI—a conduction block in either the left or right bundle rarely leads to complete heart block.

Can the site of an AV block always be determined from a 12-lead ECG?

No. A first-degree AV block (P–R interval >200 ms) can reflect abnormal conduction anywhere between the atria and the distal His-Purkinje system. Mobitz type I second-degree AV block, which is characterized by progressive lengthening of the P–R interval before a P wave is not conducted (a QRS does not follow the P wave), is usually due to a block in the AV node itself and can be caused by digitalis toxicity or myocardial ischemia; progression to a third-degree AV block is uncommon.

In patients with Mobitz type II second-degree AV block, atrial impulses are periodically not conducted into the ventricle without progressive prolongation of the P–R interval. The conduction block is nearly always in or below the His bundle and frequently progresses to complete (third-degree) AV block, particularly following an acute anteroseptal MI. The QRS is typically wide.

In patients with a third-degree AV block, the atrial rate and ventricular depolarization rates are independent (AV dissociation) because atrial impulses completely fail to reach the ventricles. If the site of the block is in the AV node, a stable His bundle rhythm will result in a normal QRS complex, and the ventricular rate will often increase following administration of atropine. If the block involves the His bundle, the origin of the ventricular rhythm is more distal, resulting in wide QRS complexes. A wide QRS complex does not necessarily exclude a normal His bundle as it may represent a more distal block in one of the bundle branches.

Can AV dissociation occur in the absence of AV block?

Yes. AV dissociation may occur during anesthesia with volatile agents in the absence of AV block and results from sinus bradycardia or an accelerated AV junctional rhythm. During isorhythmic dissociation, the atria and ventricles beat independently at nearly the same rate. The P wave often just precedes or follows the QRS complex, and their relationship is generally maintained. In contrast, interference AV dissociation results from a junctional rhythm that is faster than the sinus rate—such that sinus impulses always find the AV node refractory.

How do bifascicular and trifascicular blocks present?

A bifascicular block exists when two of the three major His bundle-branches (right, left anterior, or left posterior) are partially or completely blocked. If one fascicle is completely blocked and the others are only partially blocked, a bundle-branch block pattern will be associated with either first-degree or second-degree AV block. If all three are affected, a trifascicular block is said to exist. A delay or partial block in all three fascicles results in either a prolonged P–R interval (first-degree AV block) or alternating LBBB and RBBB. Complete block in all three fascicles results in third-degree AV block.

What is the significance of the electrocardiographic findings in this patient?

The electrocardiographic findings (first-degree AV block plus RBBB) suggest a bifascicular block. Extensive disease of the conduction system is likely. Moreover, the patient's syncopal and near-syncopal episodes suggest that she may be at risk of life-threatening bradyarrhythmias (third-degree AV block). Intracardiac electrocardiographic recordings would be necessary to confirm the site of the conduction delay.

What is appropriate management for this patient?

Cardiac evaluation is required because of the symptomatic bifascicular block. However, hip fractures must be repaired promptly. For such emergency surgery, a temporary transvenous pacing catheter or a transcutaneous pacemaker is indicated prior to induction of general or regional anesthesia. If the patient required surgery that could be postponed 24 to 48 h, continuous electrocardiographic monitoring, echocardiography, serial 12-lead ECGs, and measurements of cardiac biomarkers can be obtained to exclude myocardial ischemia or infarction, valvular heart disease, or congestive heart failure, in addition to other pathological conditions that might adversely affect the patient's surgical outcome.

What are general perioperative indications for temporary pacing?

Suggested indications include any documented symptomatic bradyarrhythmia, second-degree (type II) AV block, or third-degree AV block and refractory supraventricular tachyarrhythmias. The first three indications generally require ventricular pacing, whereas the fourth requires atrial pacing electrodes and a programmable rapid atrial pulse generator.

How can temporary cardiac pacing be established?

Pacing can be established by transvenous, transcutaneous, epicardial, or transesophageal electrodes. The most reliable method is generally via a transvenous pacing electrode in the form of a pacing wire or a balloon-tipped pacing catheter. A pacing wire should always be positioned fluoroscopically, but a flow-directed pacing catheter can also be placed in the right ventricle under pressure monitoring. If the patient has a rhythm, an intracardiac electrocardiographic recording showing ST-segment elevation when the electrode comes in contact with the right ventricular endocardium confirms placement of either type of electrode. Transcutaneous ventricular pacing is also possible via large stimulating adhesive pads placed on the chest and should be used whenever transvenous pacing is not readily available. Epicardial electrodes are usually used during cardiac surgery. Pacing the left atrium via an esophageal electrode is a simple, relatively noninvasive technique, but it is useful only for symptomatic sinus bradycardias and for terminating some supraventricular tachyarrhythmias.

Once positioned, the pacing electrodes are attached to an electrical pulse generator that periodically delivers an impulse at a set rate and magnitude. Most pacemaker generators can also sense the heart's spontaneous (usually ventricular) electrical activity: When activity is detected, the generator suppresses its next impulse. By altering the generator's sensing threshold, the pacemaker generator can function in a fixed (asynchronous) mode or in a demand mode (by increasing sensitivity). The lowest current through the electrode that can depolarize the myocardium is called the *threshold current* (usually <2 mA for transvenous electrodes).

What is AV sequential pacing?

Ventricular pacing often reduces cardiac output because the atrial contribution to ventricular filling is lost. When the AV conducting system is diseased, atrial contraction can still be maintained by sequential stimulation by separate atrial and ventricular electrodes. The P–R interval can be varied by adjusting the delay between the atrial and ventricular impulses (usually set at 150–200 ms).

How are pacemakers classified?

Pacemakers are categorized by a five-letter code, according to the chambers paced, chambers sensed, response to sensing, programmability, and arrhythmia function (Table 21–18). The two most commonly used pacing modes are VVI and DDD (the last two letters are frequently omitted).

If a pacemaker is placed in this patient, how can its function be evaluated?

If the patient's underlying rhythm is slower than the rate of a demand pacemaker, pacing spikes should be seen on the ECG. The spike rate should be identical to the programmed (permanent pacemaker—usually 72/min) or set (temporary) pacemaker rate; a slower rate may indicate a low battery. Every pacing spike should be followed by a QRS complex (100% capture). Moreover, every impulse should be followed by a palpable arterial pulse. If the patient has a temporary pacemaker, the escape rhythm can be established by temporarily slowing the pacing rate.

When the patient's heart rate is faster than the set pacemaker rate, pacing spikes should not be observed if the generator is sensing properly. In this instance, ventricular capture cannot be evaluated unless the pacemaker rate increases or the spontaneous heart rate decreases.

What intraoperative conditions may cause the pacemaker to malfunction?

Electrical interference from surgical electrocautery units can be interpreted as myocardial electrical activity and can suppress the pacemaker generator. Problems with electrocautery may be minimized by limiting its use to short bursts, limiting its power output, placing its grounding plate as far from the pacemaker generator as possible, and using bipolar cautery. Moreover, continuous monitoring of an arterial pulse wave (pressure, plethysmogram, or oximetry signal) is mandatory to ensure continuous perfusion during electrocautery.

Both hypokalemia and hyperkalemia can alter the pacing electrodes' threshold for depolarizing the myocardium and can result in failure of the pacing impulse to depolarize the ventricle. Myocardial ischemia, infarction, or scarring can also increase the electrodes' threshold and cause failure of ventricular capture.

What are appropriate measures if a pacemaker fails intraoperatively?

If a temporary pacemaker fails intraoperatively, the inspired oxygen concentration should be increased to 100%. All connections and the generator battery should be checked. Most units have a battery-level indicator and a light that flashes with every impulse. The generator should be set into the asynchronous mode, and the ventricular output should be set on maximum. Failure of a temporary transvenous electrode to capture the ventricle

TABLE 21–18 Classification of pacemakers.

Chamber Paced	Chamber Sensed	Response to Sensing	Programmability	Antitachyarrhythmia Function
O = none	O = none	O = none	O = none	O = none
A = atrium	A = atrium	T = triggered	P = simple	P = pacing
V = ventricle	V = ventricle	I = inhibited	M = multi-programmable	S = shock
D = dual (atrium and ventricle)	D = dual (atrium and ventricle)	D = dual (triggered and inhibited)	C = communicating R = rate modulation	D = dual (pacing and shock)

is usually due to displacement of the electrode away from the ventricular endocardium; careful slow advancement of the catheter or wire while pacing often results in capture. Pharmacological management (atropine, isoproterenol, or epinephrine) may be useful until the problem is resolved. If an adequate arterial blood pressure cannot be maintained with adrenergic agonists, cardiopulmonary resuscitation should be instituted until another pacing electrode is placed or a new generator box is obtained. Transcutaneous pacing can be employed.

If a permanent pacemaker malfunctions (as with electrocautery), it should generally be converted to an asynchronous mode. Some units will automatically reprogram themselves to the asynchronous mode if malfunction is detected. Other pacemaker units must be reprogrammed by placing either an external magnet or, preferably, a programming device over the generator. The effect of an external magnet on some pacemakers—particularly during electrocautery—may be unpredictable and should generally be determined prior to surgery.

Which anesthetic agents are appropriate for patients with pacemakers?

All anesthetic agents have been safely used in patients who already have pacemakers. Even volatile agents seem to have no effect on pacing electrode thresholds. Local anesthesia with moderate to deep intravenous sedation is usually used for placement of permanent pacemakers.

GUIDELINES

Fleisher L, Fleischman K, Auerbach A, et al. 2014 ACC/AHA guideline on perioperative cardiovascular evaluation and management of patients undergoing noncardiac surgery: a report of the American College of Cardiology Guidelines. *J Am Coll Cardiol.* 2014;64:e77.

Duceppe E, Parlow J, MacDonald P, et al. Canadian Cardiovascular Society guidelines on perioperative cardiac risk assessment and management for patients who undergo noncardiac surgery. *Can J Cardiol.* 2017;33:17.

James PA, Oparil S, Carter BL, et al. 2014 evidence based guidelines for the management of high blood pressure in adults: report from the panel members appointed to the Eight Joint National Committee (JNC8). *JAMA.* 2014;311:507.

January C, Wann L, Alpert J, et al. 2014 AHA/ACC/HRS guideline for the management of patients with atrial fibrillation: a report of the American College of Cardiology/American Heart Association Task Force on Practice Guidelines and the Heart Rhythm Society. *J Am Coll Cardiol.* 2014;64:e1.

January CT, Wann LS, Calkins H, et al. 2019 AHA/ACC/HRS focused update of the 2014 AHA/ACC/HRS guideline for the management of patients with atrial fibrillation: a report of the American College of Cardiology/American Heart Association task force on clinical practice guidelines and the Heart Rhythm Society in collaboration with the Society of Thoracic Surgeons. *Circulation.* 2019;140:e125.

Fellahi JL, Godier A, Benchetrit D, et al. Perioperative management of patients with coronary artery disease undergoing non-cardiac surgery: summary from the French Society of Anaesthesia and Intensive Care Medicine 2017 convention. *Anaesth Crit Care Pain Med.* 2018;37:367.

Kusumoto FM, Schoenfeld MH, Barrett C, et al. 2018 ACC/AHA/HRS guideline on the evaluation and management of patients with bradycardia and cardiac conduction delay: executive summary: a report of the American College of Cardiology/American Heart Association task force on clinical practice guidelines, and the Heart Rhythm Society. *J Am Coll Cardiol.* 2019;74:932.

Levine GN, Bates ER, Bittl JA, et al. 2016 ACC/AHA guideline focused update on duration of dual antiplatelet therapy in patients with coronary artery disease: a report of the American College of Cardiology/American Heart Association task force on clinical practice guidelines: an update of the 2011 ACCF/AHA/SCAI guideline for percutaneous coronary intervention, 2011 ACCF/AHA guideline for coronary artery bypass graft surgery, 2012 ACC/AHA/ACP/AATS/PCNA/SCAI/STS guideline for the diagnosis and management of patients with stable ischemic heart disease, 2013 ACCF/AHA guideline for the management of ST-elevation myocardial infarction, 2014 AHA/ACC guideline for the management of patients with non-ST-elevation acute coronary syndromes, and 2014 ACC/AHA guideline on perioperative cardiovascular evaluation and management of patients undergoing noncardiac surgery. *Circulation.* 2016;134:e123.

Nishimura R, Otto C, Bonow R, et al. 2014 AHA/ACC guideline for the management of patients with valvular heart disease: a report of the American College of Cardiology/American Heart Association Task Force on Practice Guidelines. *Circulation*. 2014;129:e1.

Strickberger S, Conti J, Daoud E, et al. Patient selection for cardiac resynchronization therapy: from the Council of Clinical Cardiology Subcommittee on Electrocardiography and Arrhythmias and the Quality of Care and Outcomes Research Interdisciplinary Working Group in collaboration with the Heart Rhythm Society. *Circulation*. 2005;111:2146.

Warnes C, Williams R, Bashore T, et al. ACC/AHA 2008 guidelines for the management of adults with congenital heart disease: a report of the American College of Cardiology/American Heart Association Task Force on Practice Guidelines (writing committee to develop guidelines on the management of adults with congenital heart disease). *Circulation*. 2008;118:e714.

Wijeysundera DN, Duncan D, Nkonde-Price C, et al. Perioperative beta blockade in noncardiac surgery: a systematic review for the 2014 ACC/AHA guideline on perioperative cardiovascular evaluation and management of patients undergoing noncardiac surgery: a report of the American College of Cardiology/American Heart Association Task Force on practice guidelines. *J Am Coll Cardiol*. 2014;64:2406.

Yancy C, Jessup M, Bozkurt B, et al. 2013 ACCF/AHA guideline for the management of heart failure: a report of the American College of Cardiology Foundation/American Heart Association Task Force on Practice Guidelines. *J Am Coll Cardiol*. 2013;62:e147.

Yancy CW, Jessup M, Bozkurt B, et al. 2017 ACC/AHA/HFSA focused update of the 2013 ACCF/AHA guideline for the management of heart failure: a report of the American College of Cardiology/American Heart Association Task Force on Clinical Practice Guidelines and the Heart Failure Society of America. *Circulation*. 2017;136:e137.

Zipes D, Camm A, Borggrefe M, et al. ACC/AHA/ESC 2006 guidelines for management of patients with ventricular arrhythmias and the prevention of sudden cardiac death—executive summary. *Circulation*. 2006;114:1088.

SUGGESTED READINGS

Atlee JL, Bernstein AD. Cardiac rhythm management devices (part I). Indications, device selection, and function. *Anesthesiology*. 2001;95:1265.

Atlee JL, Bernstein AD. Cardiac rhythm management devices (part II). Perioperative management. *Anesthesiology*. 2001;95:1492.

Baehner T, Ellerkmann RK. Anesthesia in adults with congenital heart disease. *Curr Opin Anaesthesiol*. 2017;30:418.

Bonow RO, Mann DL, Zipes DP, Libby P. *Braunwald's Heart Disease*. 11th ed. Elsevier; 2021.

Chung M. Perioperative management of the patient with a left ventricular assist device for noncardiac surgery. *Anesth Analg*. 2018;126:1839.

Colquhoun AD, Zuelzer W, Butterworth JF 4th. Improving the management of hip fractures in the elderly: a role for the perioperative surgical home? *Anesthesiology*. 2014;121:1144.

Dalia AA, Cronin B, Stone ME, et al. Anesthetic management of patients with continuous-flow left ventricular assist devices undergoing noncardiac surgery: an update for anesthesiologists. *J Cardiothorac Vasc Anesth*. 2018;32:1001.

Fleisher L. Preoperative assessment of the patient with cardiac disease undergoing noncardiac surgery. *Anesthesiology Clin*. 2016;34:59.

Jain P, Patel P, Fabbro M. Hypertrophic cardiomyopathy and let ventricular outflow tract obstruction: expecting the unexpected. *J Cardiothorac Vasc Anesth*. 2018;32:467.

James PA, Oparil S, Carter BL, et al. 2014 evidence based guidelines for the management of high blood pressure in adults: report from the panel members appointed to the Eight Joint National Committee (JNC8). *JAMA*. 2014;311:507.

Nguyen L, Banks DA. Anesthetic management of the patient undergoing heart transplantation. *Best Pract Res Clin Anaesthesiol*. 2017;31:189.

Otto CM. *Textbook of Clinical Echocardiography*. 6th ed. Elsevier; 2021.

Park KW. Preoperative cardiac evaluation. *Anesth Clin North Am*. 2004;22:199.

Pilkington M, Egan JC. Noncardiac surgery in the congenital heart patient. *Semin Pediatr Surg*. 2019;28:11.

Sanders RD, Hughes F, Shaw A, et al; Perioperative Quality Initiative-3 Workgroup; POQI chairs; Physiology group; Preoperative blood pressure group; Intraoperative blood pressure group; Postoperative blood pressure group. Perioperative Quality Initiative consensus statement on preoperative blood pressure, risk and outcomes for elective surgery. *Br J Anaesth*. 2019;122:552.

Smit-Fun V, Buhre WF. The patient with chronic heart failure undergoing surgery. *Curr Opin Anaesthesiol*. 2016;29:391.

Sessler DI, Bloomstone JA, Aronson S, et al; Perioperative Quality Initiative-3 workgroup; POQI chairs, Miller TE, Mythen MG, Grocott MP, Edwards MR; Physiology group; Preoperative blood pressure group; Intraoperative blood pressure group; Postoperative blood pressure group. Perioperative Quality Initiative consensus statement on intraoperative blood pressure, risk and outcomes for elective surgery. *Br J Anaesth.* 2019;122:563.

Tickoo M, Bardia A. Anesthesia at the edge of life: mechanical circulatory support. *Anesthesiol Clin.* 2020;38:19.

Wasnick J, Hillel Z, Nicoara A. *Cardiac Anesthesia and Transesophageal Echocardiography.* 2nd ed. McGraw-Hill; 2019.

Wise-Faberowski L, Asija R, McElhinney DB. Tetralogy of Fallot: everything you wanted to know but were afraid to ask. *Paediatr Anaesth.* 2019;29:475.

CHAPTER 22

Anesthesia for Cardiovascular Surgery

Nirvik Pal, MD

KEY CONCEPTS

1. Cardiopulmonary bypass (CPB) diverts venous blood away from the heart (most often via one or more cannulas in the right atrium), adds oxygen, removes carbon dioxide (CO_2), and returns the blood through a cannula in a large artery (usually the ascending aorta or a femoral artery). As a result, nearly all blood bypasses the heart and lungs.
2. The fluid level in the reservoir is critical. If a "roller" pump is used and the reservoir is allowed to empty, air can enter the main pump and be propelled into the patient, where it may cause organ damage or fatality.
3. Initiation of CPB is associated with a variable increase in stress hormones and systemic inflammation.
4. Establishing the adequacy of the patient's preoperative cardiac function should be based on exercise (activity) tolerance, measurements of myocardial contractility such as ejection fraction, severity and location of coronary stenoses, ventricular wall motion abnormalities, cardiac end-diastolic pressures, cardiac output, and valvular areas and gradients.
5. Blood should be immediately available for transfusion if the patient has had previous cardiac surgery (a "redo"); when there has been a previous sternotomy, the right ventricle or coronary grafts may be adherent to the sternum and may be accidentally entered during the repeat sternotomy.
6. Transesophageal echocardiography (TEE) provides valuable information about cardiac anatomy and function during surgery. Two-dimensional, multiplane TEE can detect regional and global ventricular abnormalities, chamber dimensions, valvular anatomy, and the presence of intracardiac air.
7. Anesthetic dose requirements are variable. Severely compromised patients should be given anesthetic agents in incremental, small doses. Patient tolerance of inhaled anesthetics generally declines with declining ventricular function.
8. Anticoagulation must be established before CPB to prevent acute disseminated intravascular coagulation and the formation of clots in the CPB pump.
9. Antifibrinolytic therapy may be particularly useful for patients who are undergoing a repeat operation; who refuse blood products, such as Jehovah's Witnesses; who are at high risk for postoperative bleeding because of recent administration of glycoprotein IIb/IIIa inhibitors (abciximab, eptifibatide, or tirofiban); who have preexisting coagulopathy; or who are undergoing long and complicated procedures.
10. Hypotension from impaired ventricular filling may occur during manipulation of the venae cavae and the heart.

—Continued next page

Continued—

11 Hypothermia (<34°C) potentiates general anesthetic potency, but failure to give anesthetic agents, particularly during rewarming on CPB, may result in awareness and recall.

12 Protamine administration can result in a number of adverse hemodynamic effects, some of which are immunological in origin. Protamine given slowly (5–10 min) usually has few effects; when given more rapidly, it produces a fairly consistent vasodilation that is easily treated with blood from the pump oxygenator and small doses of phenylephrine. Catastrophic protamine reactions often include myocardial depression and marked pulmonary hypertension. Patients with diabetes who were previously maintained on protamine-containing insulin (such as NPH) may be at increased risk for adverse reactions to protamine.

13 Persistent bleeding often follows prolonged durations of bypass (>2 h) and in most instances has multiple causes. Inadequate surgical control of bleeding sites, incomplete reversal of heparin, thrombocytopenia, platelet dysfunction, hypothermia-induced coagulation defects, undiagnosed preoperative hemostatic defects, or newly acquired factor deficiency or hypofibrinogenemia may be responsible.

14 Chest tube drainage in the first 2 h of more than 250 to 300 mL/h (10 mL/kg/h)—in the absence of a hemostatic defect—is excessive and may require surgical reexploration. Intrathoracic bleeding at a site not adequately drained may cause cardiac tamponade, requiring immediate reopening of the chest.

15 Factors known to increase pulmonary vascular resistance (PVR), such as acidosis, hypercapnia, hypoxia, enhanced sympathetic tone, and high mean airway pressures, are to be avoided for patients with right-to-left shunting; hyperventilation (hypocapnia) with 100% oxygen is usually effective in lowering PVR. Conversely, patients with left-to-right shunting may benefit from systemic vasodilation and increases in PVR.

16 Induction of general anesthesia in patients with cardiac tamponade can precipitate severe hypotension and cardiac arrest.

17 The sudden increase in left ventricular afterload after application of the aortic cross-clamp during aortic surgery may precipitate acute left ventricular failure and myocardial ischemia, particularly in patients with underlying ventricular dysfunction or coronary disease. The period of greatest hemodynamic instability follows the release of the aortic cross-clamp; the abrupt decrease in afterload together with bleeding and the release of vasodilating acid metabolites from the ischemic lower body can precipitate severe systemic hypotension.

18 The emphasis of anesthetic management during carotid surgery is on maintaining adequate perfusion to the brain and heart.

To provide anesthesia for cardiovascular surgery, one will ideally have an understanding of circulatory physiology, pharmacology, and pathophysiology; cardiopulmonary bypass (CPB) pumps, filters, and circuitry; transesophageal echocardiography (TEE); and techniques of myocardial preservation. Because surgical manipulations of the heart and great vessels will often have a profound impact on circulatory function, the anesthesia provider must understand the rationale behind the surgical techniques and follow the progress of the surgery closely so that they can anticipate potential problems associated with each sequential step of the procedure.

This chapter presents an overview of anesthesia for cardiovascular surgery and of the principles, techniques, and physiology of CPB. Surgery on the aorta, the carotid arteries, and the pericardium presents special problems, which are also discussed herein.

Cardiopulmonary Bypass

1 CPB diverts venous blood away from the heart (most often via one or more cannulae in the right atrium), adds oxygen, removes carbon dioxide (CO_2), and returns the blood through a cannula in a large artery (usually the ascending aorta or a femoral artery). As a result, nearly all blood bypasses the heart and lungs. When CPB is fully established, it provides both artificial ventilation and circulation via the systemic vasculature. CPB provides distinctly nonphysiological conditions because mean arterial pressure is usually less than normal and blood flow is usually nonpulsatile. Varying degrees of systemic hypothermia may be employed to minimize organ damage during this stressful period. Topical hypothermia (bathing the heart in an ice-slush solution) and cardioplegia (a chemical solution for arresting myocardial electrical activity given via the coronary arteries or coronary sinus) may also be used to protect the heart.

The operation of the CPB machine is a complex task requiring the attention of a specialized, certified perfusionist. Optimal results with CPB demand close cooperation and clear, continuing communication among the surgeon, anesthesiologist, and perfusionist.

BASIC CIRCUIT

The typical CPB machine has six basic components: a venous reservoir, an oxygenator, a heat exchanger, a main pump, an arterial filter, tubing that conducts venous blood to the venous reservoir, and tubing that conducts oxygenated blood back to the patient (Figure 22–1). Modern CPB machines use a single disposable unit that includes the reservoir, oxygenator, and heat exchanger. Most machines also have separate accessory pumps that can be used for blood salvage (cardiotomy suction), venting (draining) the left ventricle, and administration of cardioplegia solutions. A number of other filters, alarms, and in-line pressure, oxygen-saturation, and temperature monitors are also typically used.

Prior to use, the CPB circuit must be primed with fluid (typically 1200–1800 mL for adults) that

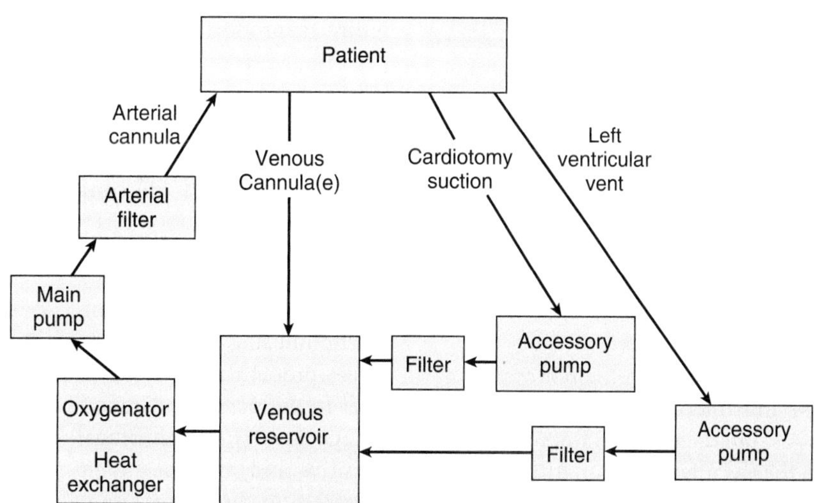

FIGURE 22–1 The basic design of cardiopulmonary bypass machines.

is devoid of bubbles. A balanced salt solution, such as lactated Ringer solution, is generally used, but other components are frequently added, including colloid (albumin or starch), mannitol (to promote diuresis), heparin (500–5000 units), and bicarbonate. At the onset of bypass in adults, when using a crystalloid priming solution, hemodilution typically decreases the hematocrit to about 22% to 27%. Blood is included in priming solutions for smaller children and severely anemic adults to prevent excessive hemodilution.

Reservoir

The reservoir of the CPB machine receives blood from the patient via one or two venous cannulae placed in the right atrium, the superior or inferior vena cava, or a femoral vein. Blood returns to the reservoir by gravity drainage with most circuits. The driving force for flow into the pump reservoir is directly related to the difference in height between the supine patient and the reservoir and is inversely proportional to the resistance of the cannulae and tubing. An appropriately primed CPB machine draws in blood like a siphon. Air entrained in the venous line can produce an air lock that may prevent blood flow. With some circuits (eg, use of an unusually small venous cannula), assisted venous drainage may be required; a regulated vacuum together with a hard shell venous reservoir or centrifugal pump (see below) is used in

2 such instances. The fluid level in the reservoir is critical. If a "roller" pump is used and the reservoir is allowed to empty, air can enter the main pump and be propelled into the patient, where it may cause organ damage or fatality. A low reservoir level alarm is typically present. Centrifugal pumps will not pump air but have the disadvantage of not impelling a well-defined volume with each revolution of the head (unlike roller pumps).

Oxygenator

Blood is drained by gravity from the bottom of the venous reservoir into the oxygenator, which contains a blood–gas interface that allows blood to equilibrate with the gas mixture (primarily oxygen). A volatile anesthetic is frequently added to the oxygenator gas mixture. The blood–gas interface in a modern, membrane-type oxygenator is a very thin, gas-permeable silicone membrane. Arterial CO_2 tension during CPB is dependent on total gas flow past the oxygenator. A membrane oxygenator permits the perfusionist to have independent control of PaO_2 and $PaCO_2$ by varying the inspired oxygen concentration and the gas flow rate.

Heat Exchanger

Blood from the oxygenator enters the heat exchanger and can either be cooled or warmed, depending on the temperature of the water flowing through the exchanger; heat transfer occurs by conduction. Because gas solubility decreases as blood temperature rises, a filter or trap is built into the unit to catch any bubbles that may form during rewarming.

Main Pump

Modern CPB machines use either an electrically driven double-arm roller (positive displacement) or a centrifugal pump to propel blood through the CPB circuit.

A. Roller Pumps

Roller pumps produce flow by compressing large-bore tubing in the main pumping chamber as the roller heads turn. Subtotal occlusion of the tubing prevents excessive red cell trauma. The rollers pump blood regardless of the resistance encountered and produce a nearly continuous nonpulsatile flow. Flow is directly proportional to the number of revolutions per minute. In some pumps, an emergency backup battery provides power in case of an electrical power failure. All roller pumps have a hand crank to allow manual pumping, but those who have hand-cranked a roller pump head will confirm that this is not a good long-term solution to an electric power failure.

B. Centrifugal Pumps

Centrifugal pumps consist of a series of cones in a plastic housing. As the cones spin, the centrifugal forces propel the blood from the centrally located inlet to the periphery. In contrast to roller pumps, blood flow with centrifugal pumps is pressure sensitive and must be monitored by a flowmeter. Increases in distal pressure will decrease flow and must be compensated for by increasing the pump speed. Because these pumps are nonocclusive, they are less traumatic to blood than roller pumps. Unlike roller pumps, which are placed after the oxygenator (see Figure 22–1), centrifugal pumps are normally located between the venous reservoir and the oxygenator. Centrifugal (unlike roller) pumps cannot pump air into the patient.

C. Pulsatile Flow

Pulsatile blood flow is possible with some roller pumps. Pulsations can be produced by instantaneous variations in the rate of rotation of the roller heads; they can also be added after flow is generated. Pulsatile flow is not available with centrifugal pumps. Although there is no consensus and the data are contradictory, some clinicians believe that pulsatile flow improves tissue perfusion, enhances oxygen extraction, attenuates the release of stress hormones, and results in lower systemic vascular resistance during CPB.

Arterial Filter

Particulate matter (eg, thrombi, fat globules, tissue debris) may enter the CPB circuit via the cardiotomy suction line. A final, in-line, arterial filter (that passes particles smaller than 27–40 μm) helps to reduce systemic embolism. Once filtered, the propelled blood returns to the patient, usually via a cannula in the ascending aorta or, less commonly, in the femoral artery. A competent aortic valve prevents blood from regurgitating into the left ventricle.

Arterial inflow pressure is measured before the filter so as to detect filter clogging. The filter is always in parallel with a (normally clamped) bypass limb. The filter is also designed to trap gas bubbles, which can be bled out through a built-in stopcock.

Accessory Pumps & Devices

A. Cardiotomy Suction

The cardiotomy suction pump aspirates blood from the surgical field during CPB and returns it directly to the main pump reservoir. This is a potential portal for fat and other debris to enter the pump and embolize to organs. A red cell salvage suction device may also be used to aspirate blood from the surgical field, in which case blood is returned to a separate reservoir. When sufficient blood has accumulated (or at the end of the procedure), the salvaged blood is centrifuged, washed, and returned to the patient. Excessive suction pressure can theoretically contribute to red cell trauma. Extensive use of cell salvage suction (instead of cardiotomy suction) during bypass will deplete CPB circuit volume when blood loss is brisk. The high negative pressure of ordinary wall suction devices produces excessive red cell trauma, precluding blood salvage from that source.

B. Left Ventricular Vent

Over time, even with "total" CPB, blood reaccumulates in the left ventricle as a result of residual pulmonary flow via the bronchial arteries (which arise directly from the aorta or the intercostal arteries) or thebesian vessels (see Chapter 20), or sometimes as a result of aortic valvular regurgitation. Aortic regurgitation can occur as a result of either structural valvular abnormalities or surgical manipulation of the heart. Distention of the left ventricle compromises myocardial preservation (see below) and requires decompression (venting). Surgeons may "vent" the left ventricle by inserting a catheter via the right superior pulmonary vein, through the left atrium, and across the mitral valve into the left ventricle, or by inserting a catheter in the left ventricular apex or across the aortic valve. The blood aspirated by the vent pump normally passes through a filter before being returned to the venous reservoir.

C. Cardioplegia Pump

Cardioplegic solutions are most often administered via an accessory pump on the CPB machine. This technique allows optimal control over the infusion pressure, rate, and temperature. A separate heat exchanger ensures control of the temperature of the cardioplegia solution. Less commonly, cardioplegic solutions may be infused from a pressurized cold intravenous fluid bag.

D. Ultrafiltration

Ultrafiltration can be used during CPB to increase the patient's hematocrit without transfusion. Ultrafilters consist of hollow capillary fibers that can function as membranes, allowing separation of the aqueous phase of blood from its cellular and proteinaceous elements. Blood can be diverted to pass through the fibers either from the arterial side of the main pump or from the venous reservoir using an accessory pump. Hydrostatic pressure forces water and electrolytes across the fiber membrane.

SYSTEMIC HYPOTHERMIA

Intentional hypothermia is often used following the initiation of CPB. Core body temperature may be reduced to 20°C to 32°C. In recent years, so-called tepid bypass has been used; this may be accomplished by allowing the patient's temperature to "drift" downward to 30°C to 35°C. Metabolic oxygen requirements are generally halved with each reduction of 10°C in body temperature. Some of the adverse effects of hypothermia include platelet dysfunction, coagulopathy, and depression of myocardial contractility. At the end of the surgical procedure, rewarming via the heat exchanger restores normal body temperature.

For complex repairs, profound hypothermia to temperatures of 15°C to 18°C allows total circulatory arrest for durations of as long as 60 min. During that time, both the heart and the CPB machine are stopped.

MYOCARDIAL PRESERVATION

Optimal results in cardiac surgery require an expeditious and complete surgical repair with minimal physical trauma to the heart. Several techniques are used to prevent myocardial damage during CPB. Nearly all patients sustain at least minimal myocardial injury during cardiac surgery. With good preservation techniques, however, most of the injury is reversible. Myocardial injury can be related to hemodynamic instability before or after CPB, or surgical technique, but it most commonly appears to be related to incomplete myocardial preservation during CPB. Injury related to hemodynamic instability results from an imbalance between oxygen demand and supply, producing cell ischemia. Reperfusion following a period of ischemia may produce excess oxygen-derived free radicals, intracellular calcium overload, abnormal endothelial–leukocyte interactions, and myocardial cellular edema. Patients at greatest risk are those with poor preoperative ventricular function (see Table 21–13), ventricular hypertrophy, diffuse severe coronary artery disease, or a combination of these. Inadequate myocardial preservation is usually manifested at the end of bypass as a reduced cardiac output, worsened ventricular function as assessed by TEE, or cardiac arrhythmias. Electrocardiographic signs of myocardial ischemia are often difficult to detect because of the frequent use of electrical pacing. Myocardial "stunning," resulting from ischemia and reperfusion, produces systolic and diastolic dysfunction that is reversible with time. The stunned myocardium usually responds to positive inotropic drugs. Myocardial necrosis, on the other hand, produces irreversible injury.

Aortic cross-clamping during CPB completely excludes the coronary arteries from the bypass machine flow to the body, halting coronary blood flow. Although it is difficult to estimate a safe time period for cross-clamping or CPB duration because of differing vulnerabilities among patients and differing techniques for myocardial preservation, CPB times longer than 120 min (while often unavoidable) increase risk. Myocardial ischemia during bypass may occur not only during aortic clamping but also after release of the cross-clamp. Low arterial pressures, obstruction of the bypass graft ostium, coronary artery embolism (from thrombi, platelets, air, fat, or atheromatous debris), reperfusion injury, coronary artery or bypass graft vasospasm, kinking of excessively long or short bypass grafts, and contortion of the heart—causing compression or kinking of the coronary vessels—are all possible causes. Myocardium distal to a high-grade coronary artery obstruction is at greatest risk.

Ischemia causes depletion of high-energy phosphate compounds and accumulation of intracellular calcium. When coronary blood flow ceases, anaerobic metabolism becomes the principal source of cellular energy, and fatty acid oxidation is impaired. Unfortunately, these high-energy phosphate stores are rapidly depleted, producing progressive acidosis.

Cardioplegic solutions maintain normal cellular integrity and function during CPB by reducing energy expenditure and preserving the availability of high-energy phosphate compounds. Although measures directed at increasing or replenishing energy substrates in the form of glucose or glutamate/aspartate infusions are used, the emphasis of myocardial preservation is on reducing cellular energy requirements to minimal levels. This is accomplished initially by the use of potassium cardioplegia (described below). The initial dose of cardioplegic solution may be hypothermic or may start warm ("hot shot") and progress to cold. Maintenance of myocardial protection may be facilitated by systemic and topical cardiac hypothermia (ice slush). Myocardial hypothermia reduces basal metabolic oxygen consumption, and potassium cardioplegia minimizes energy expenditure by arresting both electrical and mechanical activity. Myocardial temperature is often monitored directly; 10°C to 15°C is usually considered desirable. As mentioned previously, cardioplegic solutions can be administered either antegrade through a catheter placed in the proximal aorta between the aortic clamp and the aortic valve or retrograde through a catheter placed through the right atrium into the coronary sinus.

Ventricular fibrillation and distention (previously discussed) are important causes of myocardial damage. Ventricular fibrillation can dangerously increase myocardial oxygen demand, whereas distention not only increases oxygen demand but also reduces oxygen supply by interfering with subendocardial blood flow. The combination of the two is particularly bad. Other factors that might contribute to perioperative myocardial damage include the use of excessive doses of positive inotropes or calcium salts. In open-heart procedures, de-airing of cardiac chambers and venting before and during initial cardiac ejection are critically important in preventing cerebral air embolism (and strokes—see later discussion) or coronary air embolism. Removing air from coronary grafts during bypass procedures is similarly important. Depending on the amount and the location of coronary emboli, even small air bubbles can cause varying degrees of ventricular dysfunction at the end of CPB. Air emboli may preferentially find their way into the right (versus left) coronary ostium because of its superior location on the aortic root in the supine patient.

Potassium Cardioplegia

The most widely used method of arresting myocardial electrical activity is the administration of potassium-rich crystalloid or blood–crystalloid solutions. Following initiation of CPB and aortic cross-clamping, the coronary circulation is perfused intermittently with (usually cold) cardioplegic solutions. The resulting increase in extracellular potassium concentration reduces transmembrane potential. Eventually, the heart is arrested in diastole. Usually, cold cardioplegia must be repeated at intervals (about every 30 min) because of gradual washout and rewarming of the myocardium. The heart is subject to warming by contact with blood in the adjacent descending aorta and by contact with warmer ambient air in the surgical theater. Moreover, multiple doses of cardioplegia solutions may improve myocardial preservation by preventing an excessive accumulation of metabolites that inhibit anaerobic metabolism.

Although the exact recipe varies from center to center, the essential ingredient of the induction dose of cardioplegic solution is the same: an elevated potassium (10–40 mEq/L) concentration in the initial dose. Potassium concentration is kept below 40 mEq/L because higher levels can be associated with an excessive potassium load and excessive potassium concentrations at the end of termination of bypass perfusion. Sodium concentration in cardioplegic solutions is usually less than in plasma (<140 mEq/L) because ischemia tends to increase intracellular sodium content. A small amount of calcium (0.7–1.2 mmol/L) is needed to maintain cellular integrity, whereas magnesium (1.5–15 mmol/L) is usually added to control excessive intracellular influxes of calcium. A buffer—most commonly bicarbonate—is necessary to prevent excessive buildup of acid metabolites; in fact, alkalotic perfusates are reported to produce better myocardial preservation. Alternative buffers include histidine and tromethamine (also known as THAM). Other components may include hypertonic agents to control cellular edema (mannitol) and agents thought to have membrane-stabilizing effects (lidocaine or glucocorticoids). Energy substrates are provided as glucose, glutamate, or aspartate. Blood (rather than crystalloid) is commonly used as a vehicle for delivering cardioplegia in North America. Evidence suggests that some high-risk patients may benefit from blood cardioplegia. Certainly, oxygenated blood cardioplegia may contain more oxygen than crystalloid cardioplegia.

Because cardioplegia may not reach areas distal to high-grade coronary obstructions (the areas that need cardioplegia most), many surgeons administer retrograde cardioplegia through a coronary sinus catheter. Some centers have reported that the combination of antegrade plus retrograde cardioplegia is superior to either technique alone. Others have suggested that continuous warm blood cardioplegia is superior to intermittent hypothermic cardioplegia for myocardial preservation, but many surgeons avoid continuous cardioplegia so that they can operate in a "bloodless" surgical field. Cardiac surgery performed with true normothermia (rather than tepid bypass) raises additional concerns about loss of the potentially protective effects of systemic hypothermia against cerebral injury.

As discussed previously, following prolonged myocardial ischemic times (cross-clamp times), myocardial reperfusion can lead to the rapid accumulation of intracellular calcium, extensive cell injury, and, potentially, necrosis. Ischemia–reperfusion injury has been attributed to accumulation of oxygen-derived free radicals. Free radical scavengers, such as mannitol, may help decrease reperfusion injury and are typical constituents of cardioplegic solutions and bypass "priming" solutions. Several steps may help limit reperfusion injury before unclamping of the aorta. Just prior to reperfusion, the heart may be perfused by a reduced potassium cardioplegic solution that serves to wash out accumulated metabolic byproducts. Alternatively, a "hot shot" or warm blood cardioplegic solution may be administered to wash out byproducts and replenish metabolic substrates. Hypercalcemia should be avoided in the immediate reperfusion period. Reperfusion pressures should be controlled closely because of altered coronary autoregulation. Systemic perfusion pressure is reduced just prior to clamp release; it is then brought up initially to about 40 mm Hg before gradually being increased and maintained at about 70 mm Hg. To further minimize metabolic requirement, the heart should have the opportunity to recover and resume contracting in an empty state for some additional time (5–10 min), and acidosis and hypoxemia should be corrected before attempting to wean the patient from CPB.

Inadequate myocardial protection or inadequate washout and recovery from cardioplegia can result in asystole, conduction blocks, or a poorly contracting heart at the end of bypass. Excessive volumes of hyperkalemic cardioplegic solutions may produce persisting systemic hyperkalemia. Although calcium salt administration partially offsets hyperkalemia, excessive calcium can promote and enhance myocardial damage. In the usual patient, myocardial performance improves with time as the contents of the cardioplegia are cleared from the heart.

PHYSIOLOGICAL EFFECTS OF CARDIOPULMONARY BYPASS

Hormonal, Humoral, & Immunological Responses

3 Initiation of CPB is associated with increases in stress hormone levels and systemic inflammation that are variously influenced by the depth of anesthesia, blood pressure, the type of surgical repair, or the presence of pulsatile CPB. Elevated concentrations of catecholamines, cortisol, arginine vasopressin, and angiotensin are observed.

Multiple humoral systems are activated, including complement, coagulation, fibrinolysis, and the kallikrein system. Contact of blood with the internal surfaces of the CPB system activates the complement cascade via both the alternate pathway (C3) and the classical pathway. The latter also activates the coagulation cascade, platelets, plasminogen, and kallikrein. Mechanical trauma from blood contact with the CPB apparatus activates platelets and leukocytes. Increased amounts of oxygen-derived free radicals are generated. A systemic inflammatory response similar to that seen with sepsis and trauma can develop.

CPB alters and depletes glycoprotein receptors on the surface of platelets. The resulting platelet dysfunction likely increases perioperative bleeding and potentiates other coagulation abnormalities that may arise.

The inflammatory response to CPB can be attenuated. Leukocyte depletion reduces inflammation and may reduce complications. Leukocyte-depleted blood cardioplegia has been shown to improve myocardial preservation in some studies. Hemofiltration (ultrafiltration) during CPB, which presumably removes inflammatory cytokines, appears beneficial to pediatric patients. Administration of free radical scavengers such as high-dose vitamins C and E and mannitol has improved outcomes in some studies but remains investigational. Systemic corticosteroids before and during CPB can modulate the inflammatory response during CPB. Whether there is an outcome benefit to the routine use of systemic corticosteroids or statins in patients undergoing CPB remains controversial.

A once-promising agent, aprotinin, a protease inhibitor, reduced inflammation and surgical bleeding following CPB. Unfortunately, as its use expanded beyond its labeled indications, it increased mortality. It is no longer available in North America.

CPB Effects on Pharmacokinetics

Plasma and serum concentrations of most water-soluble drugs (eg, nondepolarizing muscle relaxants) abruptly decrease at the onset of CPB, but the change can be inconsequential for most lipid-soluble drugs (eg, fentanyl and sufentanil). The effects of CPB are complex because of the sudden increase in volume of distribution with hemodilution, decreased protein binding, and changes in perfusion and redistribution between peripheral and central compartments. Some drugs (eg, opioids) bind CPB components, but this has inconsequential effects on blood concentrations. Heparin causes the release and activation of lipoprotein lipase, which hydrolyzes plasma triglycerides into free fatty acids. Free fatty acids can competitively inhibit drug binding to plasma proteins and bind free calcium ions. Constant infusion of a drug during CPB, even if adjusted to maintain a constant "effect site" concentration (such "target-controlled infusion" devices use pharmacokinetic data from patients *not* undergoing CPB), generally causes progressively increasing blood concentrations due to reduced hepatic and renal perfusion (reduced elimination) and hypothermia (reduced metabolism). Target-controlled infusions of propofol may be the sole exception.

Anesthetic Management of Cardiac Surgery

ADULT PATIENTS

The preoperative evaluation and anesthetic management of common cardiovascular diseases are discussed in Chapter 21. The same principles apply whether these patients are undergoing cardiac or noncardiac surgery. An important distinction is that patients undergoing cardiac procedures will by

4 definition have advanced disease. Establishing the adequacy of the patient's preoperative cardiac function should be based on exercise tolerance, measurements of left ventricular ejection fraction, location and severity of coronary stenoses, ventricular wall motion abnormalities, cardiac end-diastolic pressures, cardiac output, and valvular function, areas, and gradients. Fortunately, unlike noncardiac surgery, the purpose of cardiac surgery is to improve cardiac function, and it is successful in most patients. These patients have usually been extensively evaluated before surgical repair. The anesthetic preoperative evaluation should also focus on pulmonary, neurological, and kidney function as preoperative impairment of these organ systems predisposes patients to myriad postoperative complications.

1. Preinduction Period

Premedication

Only a rare patient would not regard the prospect of heart surgery as frightening; thus, relatively "heavy" premedication was often prescribed in the past (see Chapter 21). Benzodiazepine sedative-hypnotics (diazepam, 5–10 mg orally), alone or in combination with an opioid (morphine, 5–10 mg intramuscularly or hydromorphone, 1–2 mg intramuscularly), were typically prescribed. But in current practice, most patients receive no anesthetic premedication until they arrive in the surgical unit; at that time, many will receive small doses of intravenous midazolam. Longer-acting premedicant agents (eg, lorazepam) are avoided to permit fast-tracking of patients through their enhanced recovery.

Preparation

The wisest practitioners of cardiac anesthesia formulate a simple anesthetic plan that includes adequate preparations for contingencies. In an emergency, one cannot wait for an assistant to search for drugs and equipment. Preparation, organization, and attention to detail permit one to deal more efficiently with unexpected intraoperative problems. The anesthesia machine, monitors, infusion pumps, and blood warmer should all be checked before the patient arrives. Drugs—including anesthetic and vasoactive agents—should be immediately available. We insist on having one vasoconstrictor and one vasodilator infusion immediately available before the start of the procedure.

Venous Access

Cardiac surgery is sometimes associated with large and rapid blood loss and the need for multiple drug infusions. Thus, we prefer to have two or more large-bore (16-gauge or larger) intravenous catheters in each patient. One of these should be in a large central vein, usually an internal or external jugular or subclavian vein. Studies show no benefit from placing either central venous or pulmonary arterial catheters in awake (versus anesthetized) patients undergoing cardiovascular surgery.

Drug infusions should ideally be given into a central catheter, preferably directly into the catheter or into the injection port closest to the catheter (to minimize dead space). Multilumen central venous catheters and multilumen introducer sheaths allow for multiple drug infusions with simultaneous measurement of vascular pressures. One intravenous port should be reserved for drug infusions; drug and fluid boluses should be administered through another site.

5 Blood should be immediately available for transfusion if the patient has had previous cardiac surgery (a "redo"); when there has been a previous sternotomy, the right ventricle or any coronary grafts may be adherent to the sternum and may be accidentally cut or torn during the repeat sternotomy.

Monitoring

A. Electrocardiography

The electrocardiogram (ECG) is continuously monitored with two leads, usually leads II and V_5. Baseline tracings of all leads may be recorded for future reference. Computerized ST-segment analysis and the use of TEE have greatly improved the detection of ischemic episodes.

B. Arterial Blood Pressure

In addition to all basic monitoring, arterial cannulation is always performed either prior to or immediately after induction of anesthesia. Radial arterial catheters may occasionally give falsely low readings following sternal retraction as a result of compression of the subclavian artery between the clavicle and the first rib. They may also provide falsely low values early after CPB due to the opening of atrioventricular shunts in the hand during rewarming. The radial artery on the side of a previous brachial artery cutdown should be avoided because its use is associated with a greater incidence of arterial thrombosis and wave distortion. Obviously, if a radial artery will be harvested for a coronary bypass conduit, it cannot be used as a site for arterial pressure monitoring. Other useful catheterization sites include the brachial, femoral, and axillary arteries. A backup manual or automatic blood pressure cuff should also be used.

C. Central Venous and Pulmonary Artery Pressure

An isolated measurement of central venous pressure (CVP) is not terribly useful for diagnosis of hypovolemia, but CVP has been customarily monitored in nearly all patients undergoing cardiac surgery. We find it useful as an indicator of trends. The pulmonary artery occlusion pressure provides a better measure of left ventricular filling pressure. Pulmonary artery catheterization has declined precipitously in nearly all circumstances due to minimal evidence of a positive effect on patient outcomes. In theory, the decision about whether to use a pulmonary artery catheter should be based on the patient and the procedure; however, in most centers, it is the preferences of the anesthetic, surgical, and critical care teams that matter most. In many centers, either every or almost no cardiac surgery patient receives pulmonary artery catheterization. In general, pulmonary artery catheterization has been most often used in patients with reduced ventricular function, pulmonary hypertension, or those undergoing cardiac transplant or other complicated procedures. The most useful data are pulmonary artery pressures, the pulmonary artery occlusion ("wedge") pressure, and thermodilution cardiac outputs. Specialized catheters provide extra infusion ports, continuous measurements of mixed venous oxygen saturation and cardiac output, and the capability for right ventricular or atrioventricular sequential pacing. Given the risk associated with placing any pulmonary artery catheter, some clinicians opine that it makes sense to insert only those devices that offer these advanced capabilities. Intraoperatively and postoperatively, when pulmonary artery occlusion pressure measurements are not available, left ventricular filling pressures can be measured with a left atrial pressure line inserted by the surgeon during bypass.

The right internal jugular vein is a preferred approach for intraoperative central venous cannulation, given the "straight shot" from the vein to the right atrium. Catheters placed through the other sites, particularly in the left internal and external jugular veins, are less easily passed into the superior vena cava than those placed through the right internal jugular vein.

Pulmonary artery catheters migrate distally during CPB and may spontaneously wedge without balloon inflation. Inflation of the balloon under these conditions can rupture a pulmonary artery, causing lethal hemorrhage. Pulmonary artery catheters should be routinely retracted 2 to 3 cm during CPB and the balloon subsequently inflated slowly. Whenever the catheter wedges with less than 1.5 mL of air in the balloon, it should be withdrawn farther.

D. Urinary Output

Once the patient is anesthetized, an indwelling urinary catheter is inserted to monitor the output. Bladder temperature is often monitored as a measure of core temperature but may not track core temperature well with reduced urinary flow. The sudden appearance of reddish urine may indicate excessive red cell hemolysis caused by CPB or a transfusion reaction.

E. Temperature

Multiple temperature monitors are usually placed once the patient is anesthetized. Bladder (or rectal), esophageal, and pulmonary artery (blood) temperatures are often simultaneously monitored. During cooling and rewarming, bladder and rectal readings are generally taken to represent an average body temperature, whereas esophageal represents core temperature. Pulmonary artery temperature provides an accurate estimate of blood temperature, which should be the same as core temperature in the absence of active cooling or warming. Nasopharyngeal and tympanic probes may most closely approximate brain temperature. Myocardial temperature is often measured directly during instillation of cardioplegia.

F. Laboratory Parameters

Laboratory testing is required during cardiac surgery. Blood gases, hemoglobin, potassium, ionized calcium, and glucose measurements should be immediately available. The **activated clotting time (ACT)** approximates the Lee–White clotting time and is used to monitor heparin anticoagulation and its reversal with protamine. Some centers routinely use thromboelastography (TEG) to identify causes of bleeding after CPB.

G. Surgical Field

One of the most important forms of intraoperative monitoring is continual inspection of the surgical field. Once the sternum is opened, lung expansion can be observed through the pleura. When the pericardium is opened, the heart (primarily the right ventricle) is visible; thus, cardiac rhythm, volume, and contractility can often be judged visually. Blood loss and surgical maneuvers must be closely watched and related to changes in hemodynamics and rhythm.

H. Transesophageal Echocardiography

6 TEE provides valuable information about cardiac anatomy and function during surgery. Two-dimensional, multiplane TEE can detect regional and global ventricular abnormalities, chamber dimensions, valvular anatomy, and the presence of intracardiac air. TEE can also be helpful in confirming cannulation of the coronary sinus for cardioplegia. Multiple views should be obtained from the upper esophagus, mid-esophagus, and transgastric positions in the transverse, sagittal, and in-between planes (Figure 22–2). The two views most commonly used for monitoring during cardiac

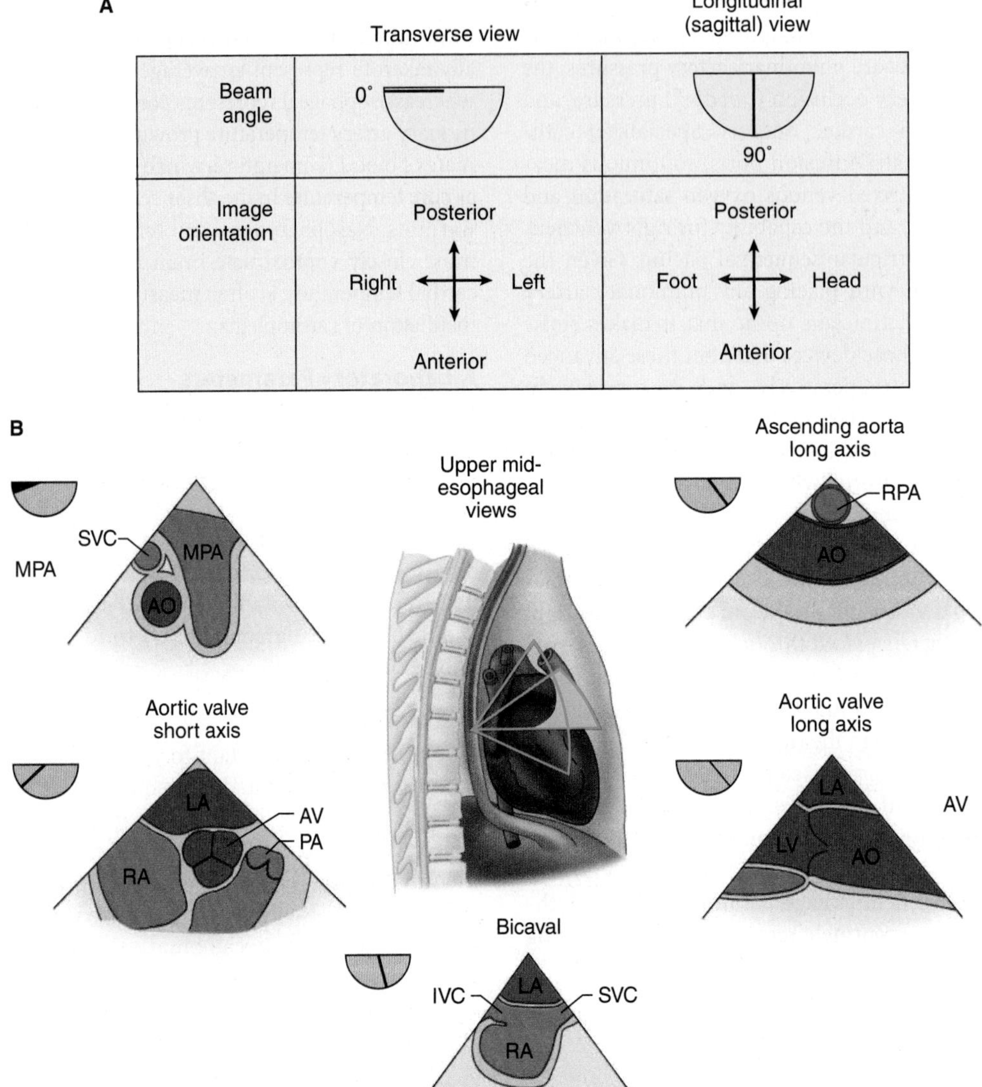

FIGURE 22–2 Useful views during transesophageal echocardiography. **A**: The relationship between the angle of the ultrasound beam and image orientation relative to the patient. **B–D**: Echocardiographic views from the upper mid-esophagus, lower mid-esophagus, and transgastric position (**C**). Note that different views can be obtained in each position as the tip of the probe is tilted either upward (anteflexion) or backward (retroflexion) and the angle of the beam is changed from 0° to 180°. The angle of the beam is shown in the upper left-hand corner of each image. The probe is also rotated clockwise or counterclockwise to optimize viewing of the various structures. AO, aorta; AV, aortic valve; CS, coronary sinus; IVC, inferior vena cava; LA, left atrium; LAA, left atrial appendage; LUPV, left upper pulmonary vein; LV, left ventricle; MPA, main pulmonary artery; MV, mitral valve; PA, pulmonary artery; RA, right atrium; RPA, right pulmonary artery; RV, right ventricle; SVC, superior vena cava.

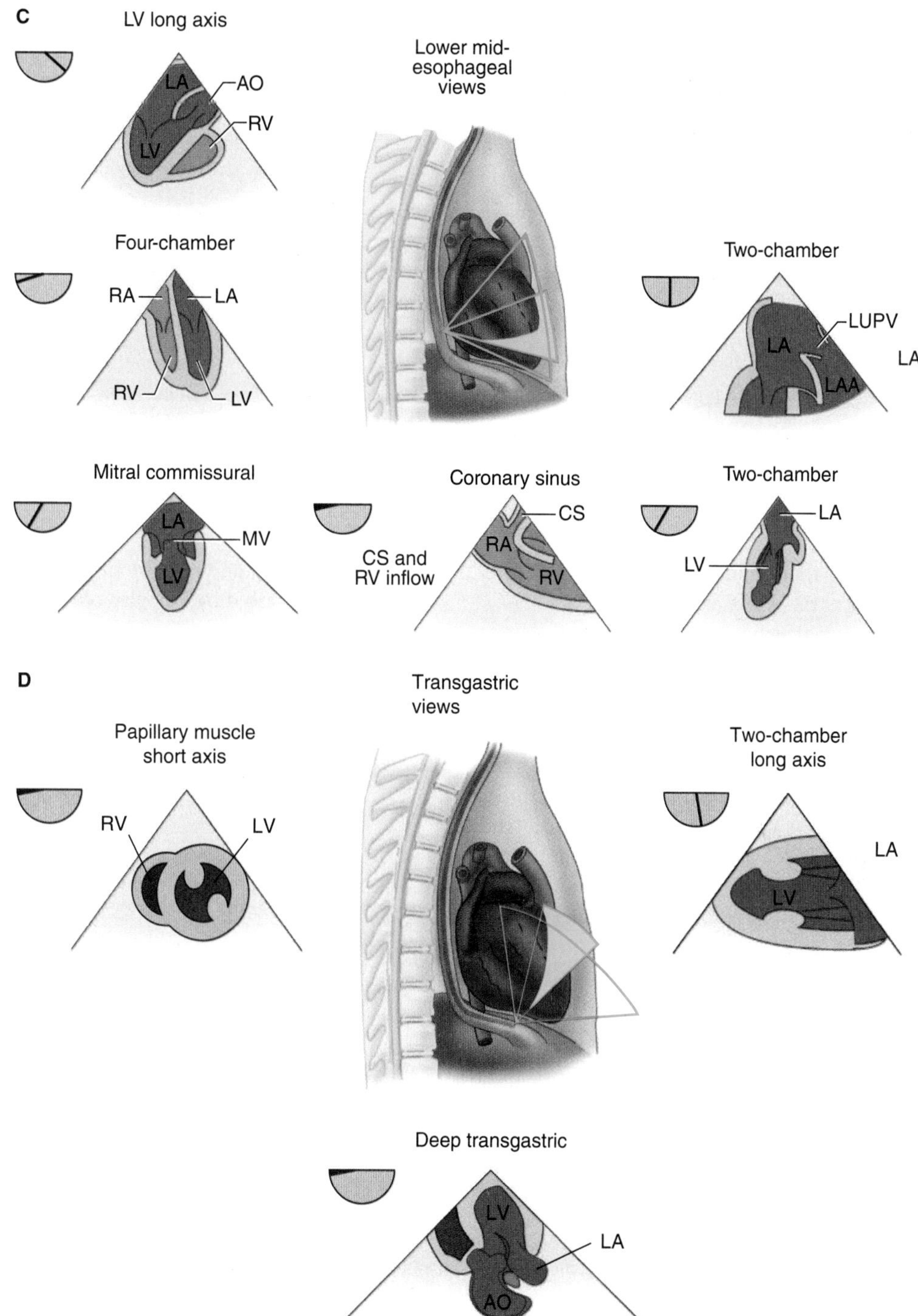

FIGURE 22–2 *(Continued)*

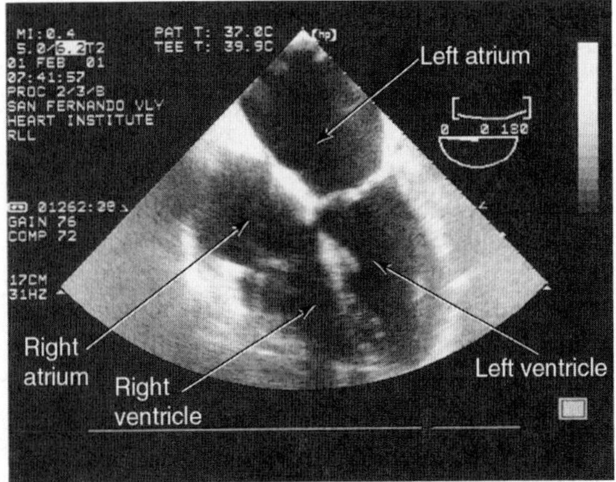

FIGURE 22–3 Transesophageal echocardiogram of the mid-esophageal four-chamber view, showing the right and left atria and ventricles.

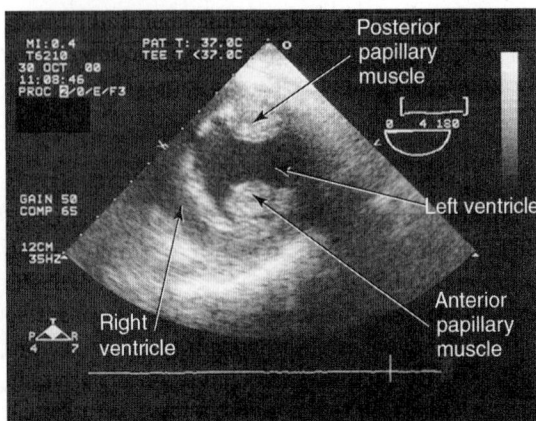

FIGURE 22–4 Transesophageal echocardiogram at the lower esophageal/transgastric level looking up at the left ventricle at the level of the papillary muscles.

surgery are the four-chamber view (Figure 22–3) and the transgastric (short-axis) view (Figure 22–4). Three-dimensional echocardiography offers better visualization of complex anatomic features, particularly of cardiac valves. The following represent the most important applications of intraoperative TEE.

1. Assessment of valvular function—Valvular morphology can be assessed by multiplane and three-dimensional TEE. Pressure gradients, area and severity of stenosis, and severity of valvular regurgitation can be assessed by Doppler echocardiography and color-flow imaging (Figure 22–5). Colors are usually adjusted so that flow toward the probe is red and flow in the opposite direction is blue. TEE also can detect prosthetic valve dysfunction in the forms of obstruction, regurgitation, paravalvular leak, or vegetations from endocarditis. The TEE images in the upper mid-esophagus at 40° to 60° and 110° to 130°

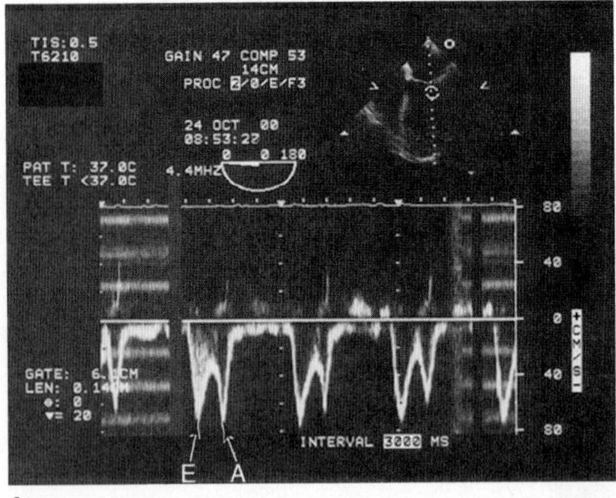

A

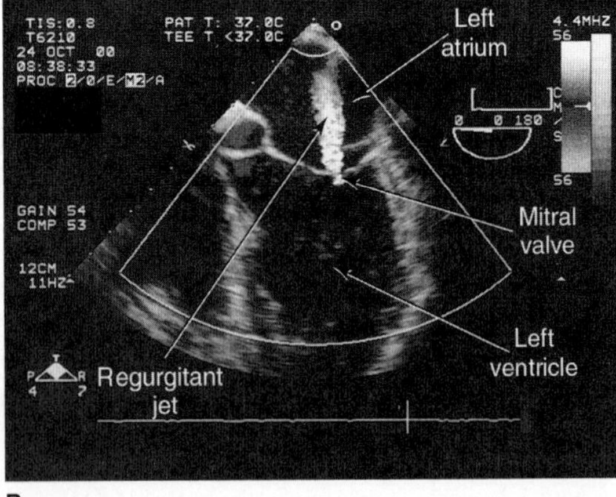

B

FIGURE 22–5 Transesophageal echocardiography Doppler and color-flow imaging. **A**: Pulse-wave Doppler recording of mitral valve inflow showing two phases, E (early filling) and A (atrial filling). **B**: Color-flow imaging demonstrates backward flow (regurgitant jet) across the mitral valve during systole (mitral regurgitation).

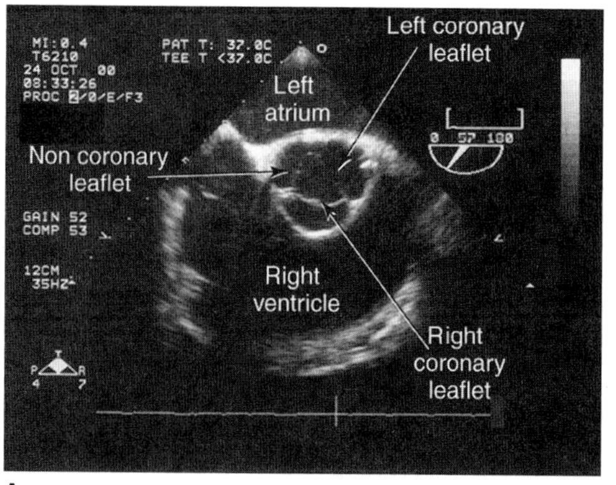

A

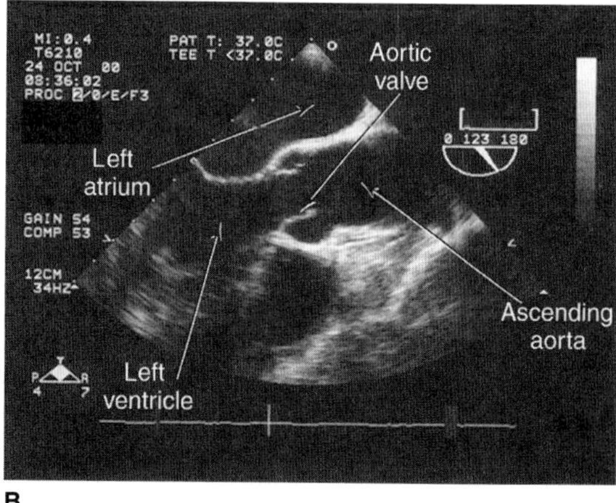

B

FIGURE 22–6 Two views of the aortic valve. **A**: Between 40° and 60°, all three leaflets are usually visualized. **B**: Between 110° and 130°, the left ventricular outflow, aortic valve, and ascending aorta are clearly visualized.

are useful for examining the aortic valve and ascending aorta (Figure 22–6). The diameter of the aortic valve annulus can be estimated accurately. Doppler flow across the aortic valve must be measured looking up from the deep transgastric view (Figure 22–7). The anatomic features of the mitral valve relevant to TEE are shown in Figure 22–8. The mitral valve is examined from the mid-esophageal position, looking at the mitral valve apparatus with and without color in the 0° through 180° views (Figure 22–9). TEE is an invaluable aid to guide and assess the completeness of mitral valve repair surgery. The commissural view (at about 60°) is particularly helpful because it cuts across many scallops of the mitral valve.

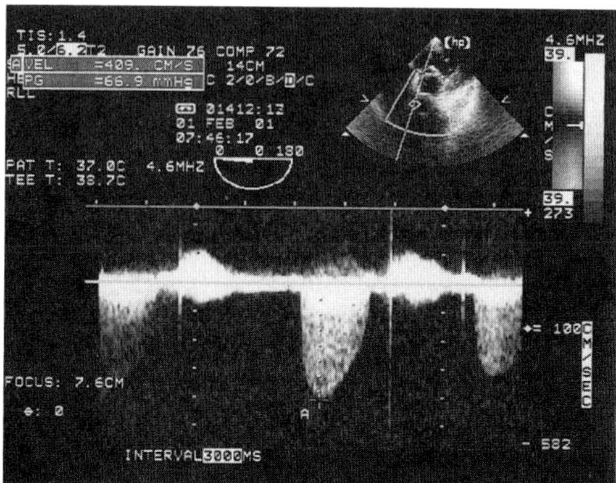

FIGURE 22–7 Transesophageal echocardiographic recording of continuous-wave Doppler from the transgastric view looking up at the aortic valve, demonstrating severe aortic stenosis. Peak velocity of 409 cm/s indicates a gradient of 66.9 mm Hg.

2. Assessment of ventricular function—Ventricular function can be estimated using ejection fraction (often calculated using the Simpson method of disks) and left ventricular end-diastolic volume; diastolic function (ie, looking for abnormal relaxation and restrictive diastolic patterns by checking mitral flow velocity or by measuring movements of the mitral valve annulus using tissue Doppler techniques); and regional systolic function (by assessing wall motion and thickening abnormalities). Regional wall abnormalities from myocardial ischemia often appear before ECG changes. Regional wall motion abnormalities can be classified into three categories based on severity (Figure 22–10): hypokinesis (reduced wall motion), akinesis (no wall motion), and dyskinesis (paradoxical wall motion). The location of a regional wall motion abnormality can indicate which coronary artery is experiencing reduced flow. The left ventricular myocardium is supplied by three major arteries: the left anterior descending artery, the left circumflex artery, and the right coronary artery (Figure 22–11). The approximate areas of distribution of these arteries on echocardiographic

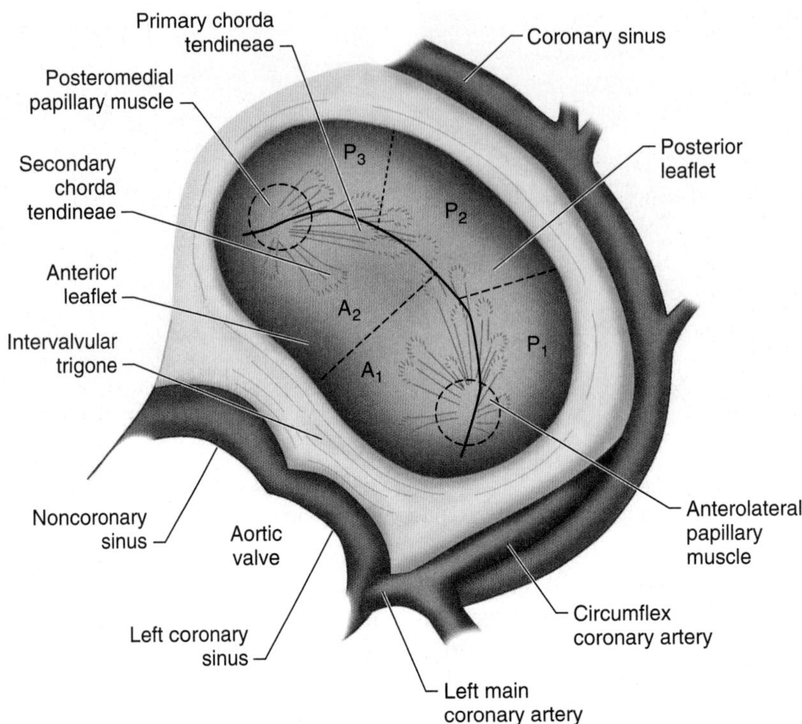

FIGURE 22–8 The anatomy of the mitral valve and its anatomic relationships to the aortic valve and left circumflex coronary artery. The posterior leaflet has three scallops, P_1, P_2, and P_3. The anterior leaflet is usually divided into A_1 and A_2 regions; in some classifications the anterior leaflet is divided into three areas (A_1, A_2, A_3), corresponding to the opposing corresponding areas of the posterior leaflet.

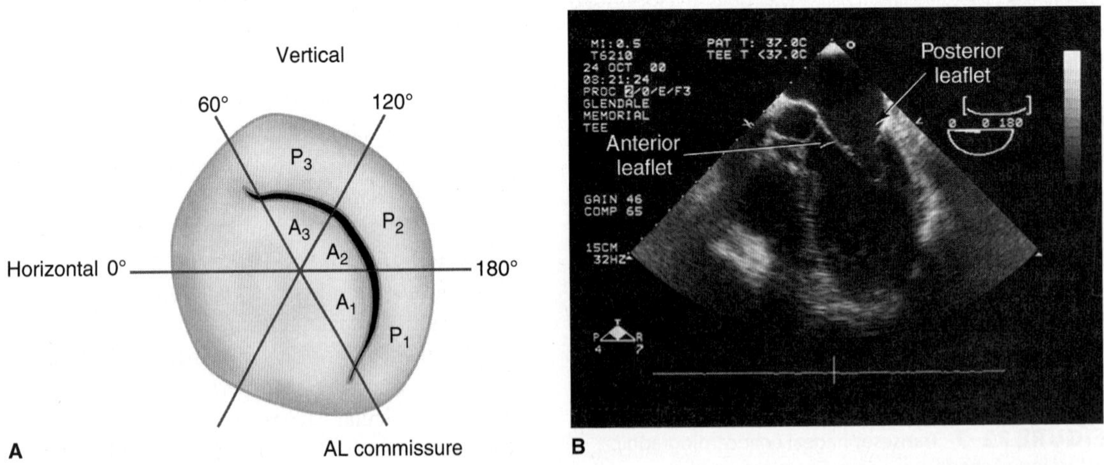

FIGURE 22–9 Multiplane imaging cuts across different segments of the mitral valve apparatus between 0° and 180° (**A**). Images of the mitral valve at 0°, 71°, and 142° (**B**, **C**, and **D**, respectively).

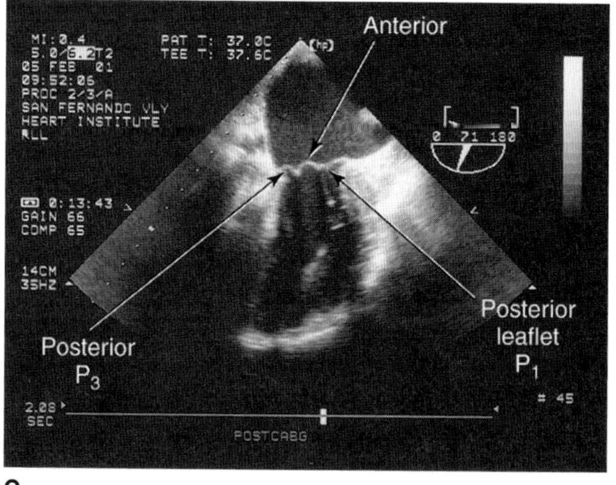

C

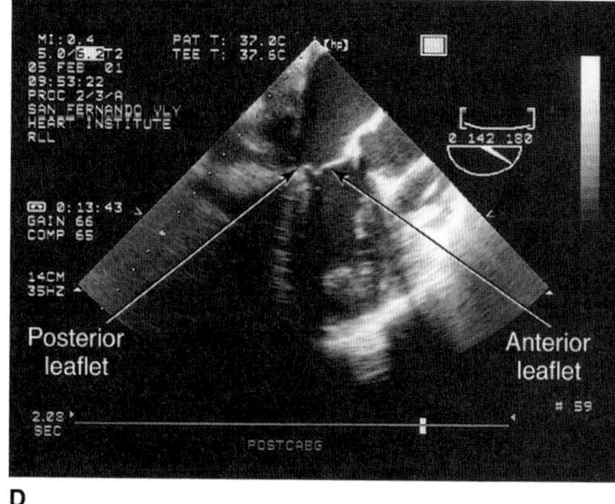

D

FIGURE 22–9 *(Continued)*

views are shown in Figure 22–12. Increasingly it is recognized that areas classically presented as the distribution of the circumflex artery may receive blood flow from the right coronary artery or the left anterior descending artery. The ventricular short-axis mid-view at the mid-papillary muscle level contains all three blood supplies from the major coronary arteries.

3. Assessment of other cardiac structures and abnormalities—In adults undergoing elective cardiac surgery, we have used TEE to diagnose previously undetected congenital defects such as an atrial or ventricular septal defect; pericardial effusions and constrictive pericarditis; and cardiac tumors. Doppler color-flow imaging delineates l intracardiac blood flows and shunts. TEE can assess the extent of myomectomy in patients with hypertrophic cardiomyopathy (idiopathic hypertrophic subaortic stenosis). Upper-, mid-, and lower-esophageal views are valuable in diagnosing aortic disease processes such as dissection, aneurysm, and atheroma (Figure 22–13). The extent of dissections in the ascending and descending aorta can be accurately defined; however, airway structures prevent complete visualization of the aortic arch with TEE. Protruding atheromas in the ascending aorta increase the risk of postoperative stroke and

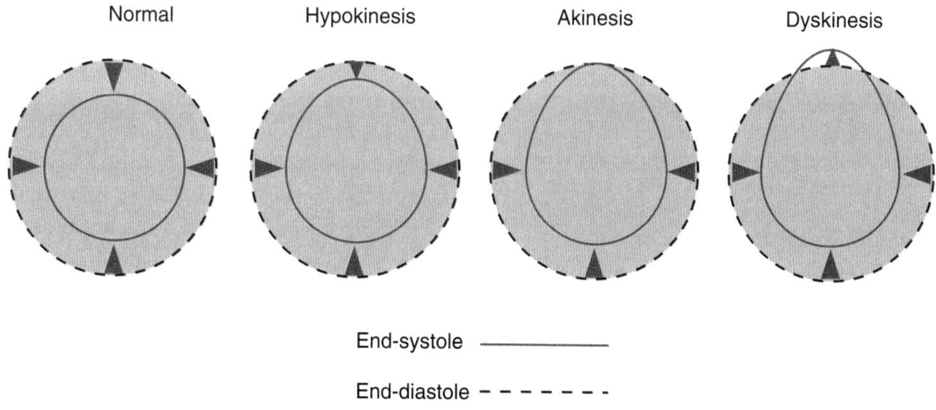

FIGURE 22–10 Classification of regional wall motion abnormalities.

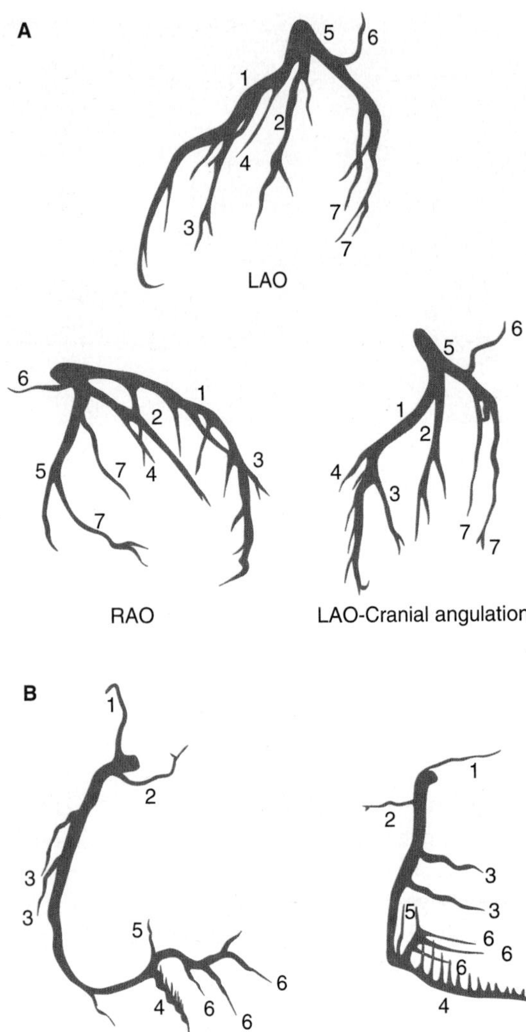

FIGURE 22–11 Standard angiographic views of the left (**A**) and right (**B**) coronary arteries. Note the left main coronary artery quickly divides into the left anterior descending and the left circumflex arteries. **A**: (1) Left anterior descending artery with septal branches; (2) ramus medianus; (3) diagonal artery; (4) first septal branch; (5) left circumflex artery; (6) left atrial circumflex artery; (7) obtuse marginal artery. **B**: (1) Conus artery; (2) sinoatrial node artery; (3) acute marginal artery; (4) posterior descending artery with septal branches; (5) atrioventricular node artery; (6) posterior left ventricular artery. LAO, left anterior oblique; RAO, right anterior oblique.

may prompt the use of epiaortic scanning to identify an atheroma-free cannulation site or a change in cannulation site.

4. Examination for residual air—Air is introduced into the cardiac chambers during all "open" heart procedures, such as valve surgery. Residual amounts of air often remain in the left ventricular apex even after the best de-airing maneuvers. TEE is helpful in defining the volume of residual air to determine whether additional surgical maneuvers need to be undertaken to help avoid cerebral or coronary embolism.

I. Electroencephalography

Computer-processed electroencephalographic (EEG) recordings can be used to assess anesthetic depth during cardiac surgery, and either the processed or "raw" EEG can be used to ensure complete drug-induced electrical silence (hoping for brain protection) prior to circulatory arrest. The usual one- or two-channel recordings are generally not useful in detecting neurological insults during CPB. Most strokes and persisting neurobehavioral deficits associated with CPB are not heralded by changes in the EEG. Progressive hypothermia (or progressively deepened anesthesia) is typically associated with EEG slowing, burst suppression, and, finally, an isoelectric recording. Artifacts from the CPB roller pump may be seen on the raw EEG (due to piezoelectric effects from compression of the pump tubing) but can usually be identified as such by computer processing.

J. Transcranial or Carotid Doppler

Transcranial Doppler (TCD) provides noninvasive measurements of blood flow velocity in the middle cerebral artery, which is interrogated through the temporal bone. TCD and carotid Doppler are useful for detecting cerebral emboli. Increased numbers of emboli detected by TCD or carotid Doppler have been associated with an increased risk of postoperative neurobehavioral dysfunction.

K. Near-Infrared Cerebral Oximetry (NIRS)

Cerebral oximetry (see Chapter 6) is increasingly employed during cardiac surgery. A baseline value

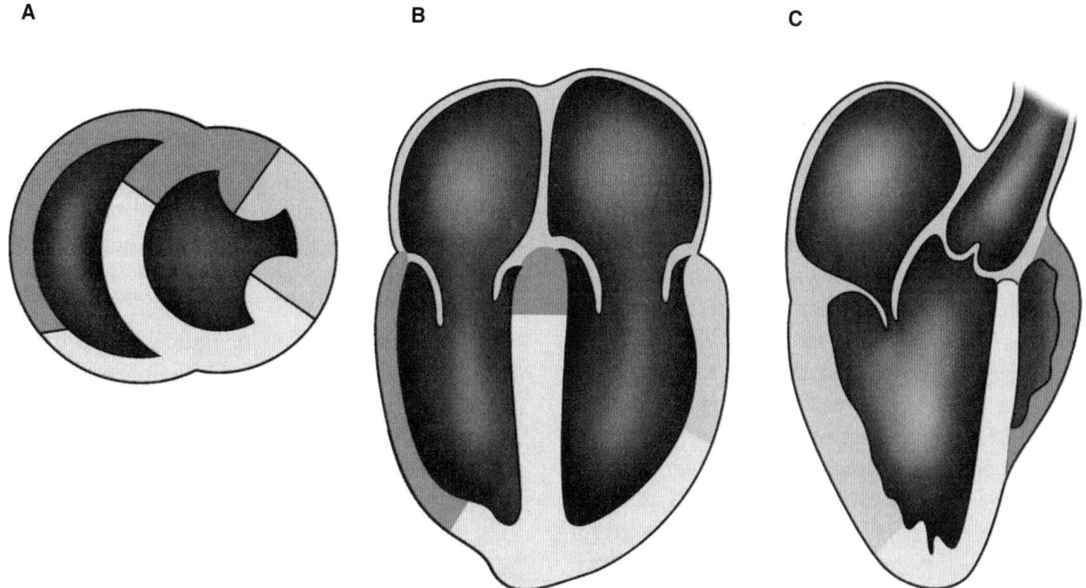

FIGURE 22–12 Coronary artery supply of the left and right ventricles in three views: the short-axis view (**A**), the four-chamber view (**B**), and the three-chamber view (**C**). Green, right coronary artery; blue, left anterior descending artery; pink, left circumflex artery.

is established for each patient prior to preoxygenation. Decreased cerebral oxygen saturation may be seen when oxygen delivery is impaired secondary to decreased $PaCO_2$ tension, anemia, decreased arterial oxygen saturation, and diminished cardiac output.

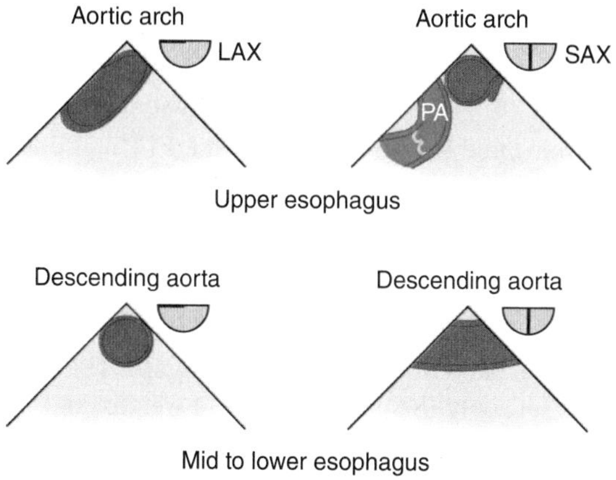

Aortic arch
LAX
Aortic arch
SAX
PA
Upper esophagus
Descending aorta
Descending aorta
Mid to lower esophagus

FIGURE 22–13 Upper esophageal views of the aortic arch and descending aorta. The ascending aorta can be visualized in the upper mid-esophagus at 110° to 130° with anteflexion at the aortic valve level (see Figures 22–2B and 22–6B). LAX, long axis; PA, pulmonary artery; SAX, short axis.

Induction of Anesthesia

Cardiac operations usually require general anesthesia, endotracheal intubation, and controlled ventilation. Some centers have used thoracic epidural anesthesia alone for minimally invasive surgery without CPB or combined thoracic epidural with light general endotracheal anesthesia for other forms of cardiac surgery. These techniques have never been popular in North America due to concerns about the risk of spinal hematomas following heparinization, the associated medical–legal consequences, and the limited evidence of an outcome benefit. Some centers use a single intrathecal opioid injection to provide postoperative analgesia.

Induction of general anesthesia should be performed in a smooth, controlled (but not necessarily "slow") fashion—often referred to as a "cardiac induction" when it is used for other types of surgery. The principles are discussed in Chapter 21. The selection of anesthetic agents is generally less important than the

way they are used. Indeed, studies have failed to show differences in long-term outcomes with various anes-
7 thetic techniques. Anesthetic dose requirements are variable. Severely compromised patients should be given anesthetic agents in incremental, small doses. Patient tolerance of inhaled anesthetics generally declines with declining ventricular function. Blood pressure and heart rate are continuously evaluated following unconsciousness, insertion of an oral airway, urinary catheterization, and tracheal intubation. A sudden increase in heart rate or blood pressure may indicate light anesthesia and the need for more anesthetic prior to the next challenge, whereas a decrease or no change suggests that the patient is ready for the subsequent stimulus. Reductions in blood pressure greater than 20% generally call for administration of a vasopressor (as described later). A series of challenges may be used to judge when anesthetic depth will allow intubation without a marked hypertensive response, while also avoiding hypotension from excessive anesthetic depth.

The period following intubation is often characterized by a gradual decrease in blood pressure resulting from the anesthetized state (often associated with vasodilation and decreased sympathetic tone) and a lack of surgical stimulation. Patients will usually respond to fluid boluses or a vasoconstrictor. Nevertheless, the administration of large amounts of intravenous fluids prior to the bypass may serve to accentuate the hemodilution associated with CPB (as described below). Small doses of phenylephrine (25–100 mcg), ephedrine (5–10 mg), or infusions of phenylephrine or norepinephrine may be useful to avoid excessive hypotension. Following intubation and institution of controlled ventilation, arterial blood gases, hematocrit, serum potassium, and glucose concentrations are measured. The baseline ACT (normal <130 s) is best measured after skin incision.

Choice of Anesthetic Agents

Anesthetic techniques for cardiac surgery have evolved over the years. Successful techniques range from primarily inhalation anesthesia to high-dose opioid totally intravenous techniques. In recent years, total intravenous anesthesia techniques with short-acting agents or combinations of intravenous and volatile agents have become most popular.

A. "High-Dose" Opioid Anesthesia

This technique was originally developed to circumvent the myocardial depression associated with older volatile anesthetics, particularly halothane. But pure, high-dose opioid anesthesia (eg, fentanyl, 50–100 mcg/kg, or sufentanil, 15–25 mcg/kg) produces prolonged postoperative respiratory depression (12–24 h), is associated with an unacceptably increased incidence of patient awareness (recall) during surgery, and often fails to control the hypertensive response to stimulation in patients with preserved left ventricular function. Other undesirable effects include skeletal muscle rigidity during induction and prolonged postoperative ileus. Moreover, simultaneous administration of benzodiazepines with large doses of opioids can produce hypotension and myocardial depression. Patients anesthetized with sufentanil and other shorter acting agents generally regain consciousness and can be extubated sooner than those anesthetized with comparable doses of fentanyl.

B. Total Intravenous Anesthesia (TIVA)

The drive for cost containment in cardiac surgery was a major impetus for the development of anesthesia techniques with short-acting agents. Although the drugs themselves may be costly, large economic benefits result from earlier extubation, decreased intensive care unit (ICU) stays, earlier ambulation, and earlier hospital discharge ("fast-track" management). One technique employs induction with propofol (0.5–1.5 mg/kg followed by 25–100 mcg/kg/min) and modest doses of fentanyl (total doses of 5–7 mcg/kg) or remifentanil (0–1 mcg/kg bolus followed by 0.25–1 mcg/kg/min). Target-controlled infusion (TCI) employs software and hardware (computerized infusion pump) to deliver a drug and achieve a set concentration at the effect site based on pharmacokinetic modeling. For propofol, the clinician sets only the patient's age and weight, and the desired blood concentration on the Diprifusor™, a TCI device widely available in countries outside North America. During cardiac surgery, a target propofol concentration of 1.5 to 2 mcg/mL is often used. When remifentanil (rather than a longer persisting agent) is used during anesthesia, one must anticipate the need for postoperative analgesia after its discontinuation.

C. Mixed Intravenous/Inhalation Anesthesia

Selection of anesthetic agents is oriented to convenience and hemodynamic stability, as well as to early extubation (1–6 h). Incremental doses of propofol (0.5–1.5 mg/kg) or etomidate (0.1–0.3 mg/kg) are often used for induction. Induction usually follows sedation with small doses of midazolam (0.05 mg/kg). Renewed interest in volatile agents came about following studies demonstrating the protective effects of volatile agents on ischemic myocardium and the utility of these agents for fast-track recovery of cardiac patients. Opioids are given in small doses together with a volatile agent (0.5–1.5 minimum alveolar concentration [MAC]) to maintain anesthesia and to blunt the sympathetic response to stimulation. The opioid may be given by intermittent bolus injections, by continuous infusion, or both (Table 22–1). To facilitate fast-track management, typical total doses of fentanyl and sufentanil generally do not exceed 15 and 5 mcg/kg, respectively, and some clinicians combine smaller doses of fentanyl or sufentanil with an analgesic dose of hydromorphone or morphine administered toward the end of CPB. Some clinicians also administer propofol in a low-dose infusion (25–50 mcg/kg/min) or TCI (1.5–2.0 mcg/mL) for maintenance. The major advantage of volatile agents or infusions of remifentanil or propofol is the ability to change the anesthetic concentration and depth rapidly. Isoflurane and sevoflurane are the most commonly used volatile anesthetics. Early laboratory reports that isoflurane might induce intracoronary "steal" have been overshadowed by more recent reports that it produces myocardial protection. Nitrous oxide is generally not used. Nitrous is particularly disadvantageous during the time interval between cannulation and decannulation because of its tendency to expand any intravascular air bubbles that may form. Moreover, it cannot be given conveniently during CPB.

TABLE 22–1 Opioid dosing compatible with early extubation after cardiac surgery.

Opioid	Loading Dose (mcg/kg)	Maintenance Infusion	Boluses (mcg/kg)
Fentanyl	1–5	1–3 mcg/kg/h	0.5–1
Sufentanil	0.25–1.25	0.25–0.75 mcg/kg/h	0.125–0.25
Remifentanil	0.5–1	0.1–1 mcg/kg/min	0.25–1

D. Other Techniques

The combination of ketamine with midazolam (or propofol) for induction and maintenance of anesthesia is a useful technique, particularly in frail patients with hemodynamic compromise. It is associated with stable hemodynamics, reliable amnesia and analgesia, minimal postoperative respiratory depression, and rare (if any) psychotomimetic side effects. For induction, ketamine, 1 to 2 mg/kg, with midazolam, 0.05 to 0.1 mg/kg, is given as a slow intravenous bolus. Anesthesia can then be maintained by infusion of ketamine, 1.3 to 1.5 mg/kg/h (or propofol in appropriate doses), and midazolam, 0.065 to 0.075 mg/kg/h, or more easily with an inhaled agent. Hypertension following intubation or surgical stimulation can be treated with propofol, opioids, β-blockers, or a volatile agent.

E. Muscle Relaxants

Muscle relaxation is helpful for intubation, to facilitate sternal retraction, and to prevent patient movement and shivering. Unless airway difficulties are expected, intubation may be accomplished after administration of a nondepolarizing muscle relaxant. Modern, shorter acting agents such as rocuronium, vecuronium, and cisatracurium have almost no hemodynamic side effects of their own. Vecuronium, however, has been reported to markedly enhance bradycardia associated with large doses of opioids, particularly sufentanil. Because of its vagolytic effects, pancuronium was often used to counteract bradycardia in patients taking β-blockers. Succinylcholine remains appropriate for endotracheal intubation, particularly for rapid sequence induction. Some clinicians prefer succinylcholine to minimize the time during which one's hands are occupied with bag and mask ventilation. Judicious dosing, appropriate use of a peripheral nerve stimulator, and reversal (if needed) allow fast-tracking with any of these agents.

2. Prebypass Period

Following induction and intubation, the anesthetic course is typically characterized by an initial period of minimal stimulation (skin preparation and draping) that is frequently associated with hypotension, followed by discrete periods of intense stimulation that can produce tachycardia and hypertension. These periods of intense stimulation include the skin incision, sternotomy and sternal retraction, opening the pericardium, and, sometimes, aortic dissection. The anesthetic agent should be adjusted appropriately in anticipation of these events. Accentuated vagal responses with marked bradycardia and hypotension may occasionally be seen during sternal retraction or opening of the pericardium, perhaps more common in patients who have been taking β-adrenergic blocking agents.

Myocardial ischemia in the prebypass period is not always associated with hemodynamic perturbations. Prophylactic infusion of nitroglycerin (1–2 mcg/kg/min) has been studied many times and continues to be used in some centers, but it has never been shown to reduce the incidence of ischemia or to improve outcomes.

Anticoagulation

8 Anticoagulation must be established before CPB to prevent the formation of clots in the CPB pump. In most centers, the adequacy of anticoagulation will be confirmed by measuring the ACT. An ACT longer than 400 to 480 s is considered adequate. Heparin, 300 to 400 units/kg, is usually given before aortic cannulation. Some surgeons prefer to administer the heparin themselves directly into the right atrium. If heparin is administered by the anesthesiologist, it should be given through a reliable (usually central) intravenous line, and the ACT should be measured 3 to 5 min later. If the ACT is less than 400 s, additional heparin (100 units/kg) is given. Some drugs (eg, aprotinin) prolong the celite-activated ACT but not the kaolin-activated ACT. Heparin concentration assays (see Reversal of Anticoagulation, later) measure heparin levels and not heparin effect; these assays are therefore not reliable for measuring the degree of anticoagulation but can be used as an adjunct. A whole blood heparin concentration of 3 to 4 units/mL is usually sufficient for CPB. The high-dose thrombin time (HiTT) is more complicated to perform than a kaolin-ACT, cannot provide a preheparin control, and cannot assess the adequacy of heparin reversal by protamine.

Resistance to heparin is occasionally encountered; many such patients have antithrombin III deficiency (acquired or congenital). Antithrombin III is a circulating serine protease that irreversibly binds and inactivates thrombin (as well as the activated forms of factors X, XI, XII, and XIII). When heparin complexes with antithrombin III, the anticoagulant activity of antithrombin III is enhanced 1000-fold. Patients with antithrombin III deficiency will achieve adequate heparin anticoagulation following infusion of antithrombin III (or 1 unit of fresh frozen plasma). Milder forms of heparin resistance can be managed by the administration of a modestly larger than normal dose of heparin.

Patients with a history of heparin-induced thrombocytopenia (HIT) require special consideration. These patients produce heparin-dependent (platelet factor 4) antibodies that agglutinate platelets and produce thrombocytopenia, sometimes associated with thromboembolism. If the history of HIT is remote and antibodies can no longer be demonstrated, heparin may safely be used for CPB. When significant antibody titers are detected, alternative anticoagulants may be considered.

Bleeding Prophylaxis

Bleeding prophylaxis with antifibrinolytic agents may be initiated before or after anticoagulation. Some clinicians prefer to administer antifibrinolytic agents after heparinization to reduce the possible incidence of thrombotic complications; others fear that delayed administration may reduce antifibrinolytic
9 efficacy. Antifibrinolytic therapy may be particularly useful for patients who are undergoing a repeat operation; who refuse blood products (such as Jehovah's Witnesses); who are at high risk for postoperative bleeding because of recent administration of glycoprotein IIb/IIIa inhibitors, who have preexisting coagulopathy, or who are undergoing long and complicated procedures. The antiplatelet effect of abciximab typically lasts 24 to 48 h; those of eptifibatide and tirofiban are 2 to 4 h and 4 to 8 h, respectively. The frequent combination of aspirin and the adenosine diphosphate receptor antagonist clopidogrel (Plavix) is also associated with excessive bleeding.

The antifibrinolytic agents currently available, ε-aminocaproic acid and tranexamic acid, do not affect the ACT and only rarely induce allergic reactions. ε-Aminocaproic acid is usually administered as a 50- to 75-mg/kg loading dose followed by a 20- to 25-mg/kg/h maintenance infusion (some clinicians use a standard 5- to 10-g loading dose followed by 1 g/h). Tranexamic acid is often dosed at 10 mg/kg followed by 1 mg/kg/h, though pharmacokinetic studies suggest that larger doses may more reliably maintain effective blood concentrations. Intraoperative collection of platelet-rich plasma by pheresis prior to CPB is employed by some centers; reinfusion following bypass may decrease bleeding and reduce transfusion requirements.

Cannulation

Placement of venous and arterial cannulas for CPB is a critical time. *After heparinization*, aortic cannulation is usually done first because of the hemodynamic problems sometimes associated with venous cannulation and to allow convenient and rapid transfusion from the pump oxygenator. The inflow cannula is most often placed in the ascending aorta. The systemic arterial pressure is customarily reduced to 90 to 100 mm Hg systolic during placement of the aortic cannula to reduce the likelihood of dissection. Air bubbles should be absent from the arterial cannula and inflow line, and adequacy of the connection between the arterial inflow line and the patient must be demonstrated before bypass is initiated. Failure to remove all air bubbles will result in air emboli, possibly into the coronary or cerebral circulations. The small distal opening of most arterial cannulas produces a jet stream that, when not positioned properly, can cause aortic dissection or preferential flow of blood to the innominate artery. Some clinicians routinely put the patient in a "head down" position during aortic cannulation to decrease the likelihood of cerebral emboli.

One or two venous cannulas are placed in the right atrium, usually through the right atrial appendage. One cannula is usually adequate for most coronary artery bypass and aortic valve operations. The single cannula used often has two portals (two-stage); when it is properly positioned, one opening is in the right atrium, and the other is in the inferior vena cava.

Separate cannulas in the superior and inferior venae cavae are used for other forms of open-heart procedures (other forms of valve surgery and
10 congenital repairs). Hypotension from impaired ventricular filling may occur during manipulation of the venae cavae and the heart. Venous cannulation also frequently precipitates atrial or, less commonly, ventricular arrhythmias. Premature atrial contractions and transient bursts of a supraventricular tachycardia are common and need no treatment if they are not sustained. Sustained paroxysmal atrial tachycardia or atrial fibrillation frequently leads to hemodynamic deterioration, which may be treated pharmacologically, electrically, or by immediate initiation of bypass (provided that full anticoagulation has been confirmed). Malpositioning of the venous cannulas can interfere with venous return or impede venous drainage from the head and neck (superior vena cava syndrome). Upon initiation of CPB, the former is manifested as inadequate volume in the venous reservoir, whereas the latter produces engorgement of the head and neck.

3. Bypass Period

Initiation

Once the cannulas are properly placed and secured, the ACT is acceptable, and the perfusionist is ready, CPB is initiated. The main CPB pump is started, and with satisfactory arterial inflow, the venous cannula(s) is unclamped. Establishing the adequacy of venous return to the pump reservoir is critical. Normally, the reservoir level rises, and CPB pump flow is gradually increased. If venous return is poor, the level of blood in the reservoir will decline; the cannulae should be checked for proper placement and for forgotten clamps, kinks, or air locks. CPB pump flow should be slowed until the problem is resolved. Adding volume (blood or colloid) to the reservoir may be necessary. With full CPB and unimpeded venous drainage, the heart should empty; failure to empty or progressive distention may result from malpositioning of the venous cannula or aortic insufficiency. In the rare case of unexpected severe aortic insufficiency that limits the extent of peripheral perfusion, immediate aortic cross-clamping (and cardioplegia) may be necessary.

Flow & Pressure

Systemic mean arterial pressure is closely monitored as pump flow is gradually increased to 2 to

2.5 L/min/m^2. At the onset of CPB, systemic arterial pressure usually decreases abruptly. Initial mean systemic arterial (radial) pressures of 30 to 40 mm Hg are not unusual. This decrease is usually attributed to abrupt hemodilution, which reduces blood viscosity and effectively lowers SVR. It is often treated with increased flow and vasopressors.

Persistent and excessive hypotension (<30 mm Hg) should prompt a search for unrecognized aortic dissection. If dissection is present, CPB must be temporarily stopped until a cannula can be placed distally in the "true" aortic lumen. Other possible causes for hypotension include inadequate pump flow from poor venous return or a pump malfunction, or pressure transducer error. Factitious hypertension has been reported when the right radial artery is used for monitoring and the aortic cannula is directed toward the innominate artery.

The relationship between pump flow, SVR, and mean systemic arterial blood pressure may be conceptualized as follows:

$$\text{Mean arterial pressure} = \text{Pump flow} \cdot \text{SVR}$$

Consequently, with a constant SVR, mean arterial pressure is proportional to pump flow. Similarly, at any given pump flow, mean arterial pressure is proportional to SVR. To maintain both adequate arterial pressures and blood flows, one can manipulate pump flow and SVR. Most centers strive for blood flows of 2 to 2.5 L/min/m^2 (50–60 mL/kg/min) and mean arterial pressures between 65 and 80 mm Hg in adults. Metabolic flow requirements decline with decreasing core body temperature. Evidence also suggests that during deep hypothermia (20–25°C), mean blood pressures as low as 30 mm Hg may still be consistent with adequate cerebral oxygen delivery. Moderately decreased SVR can be increased with phenylephrine or norepinephrine.

Increased mean arterial pressures (>110 mm Hg) are deleterious and may promote aortic dissection or cerebral hemorrhage. Generally, when mean arterial pressure exceeds 100 mm Hg, hypertension is treated by decreasing pump flow, increasing the concentration of a volatile agent to the oxygenator inflow gas, or infusing a vasodilator such as clevidipine, nicardipine, or nitroprusside.

Monitoring

Additional monitoring during CPB includes the pump flow rate, venous reservoir level, arterial inflow line pressure (as noted earlier), blood (perfusate and venous) and myocardial temperatures, and in-line (arterial and venous) oxygen saturations. In-line pH, CO_2 tension, and oxygen tension sensors are often used. Blood gas tensions and pH should be confirmed by direct measurements. In the absence of hypoxemia, low venous oxygen saturations (<70%), a progressive metabolic acidosis, or reduced urinary output may indicate inadequate CPB flow rates.

During bypass, arterial inflow line pressure is almost always greater than the systemic arterial pressure recorded from a radial artery or even an aortic catheter. The difference in pressure represents the pressure drop across the arterial filter, the arterial tubing, and the narrow opening of the aortic cannula. Nonetheless, monitoring this pressure is important for detecting problems with an arterial inflow line. Inflow pressures should remain below 300 mm Hg; higher pressures may indicate a clogged arterial filter, obstruction of the arterial tubing or cannula, or aortic dissection.

Serial ACT, hematocrit, and potassium measurements are performed during CPB. Blood glucose should be checked even in patients without a history of diabetes. The ACT is measured immediately after bypass and then every 20 to 30 min thereafter. Cooling generally increases the half-life of heparin and prolongs its effect. Some centers calculate a heparin dose–response curve to guide the calculation of heparin dosing and protamine reversal (Figure 22–14). The hematocrit is usually not allowed to fall much below 20%. Red cell transfusions into the pump reservoir may be necessary. Marked increases in serum potassium concentrations (secondary to cardioplegia) are usually treated with a furosemide-induced diuresis.

Hypothermia & Cardioplegia

Moderate (26–32°C) or deep (≤25°C) hypothermia (possibly with circulatory arrest) is used routinely for procedures involving the aortic root and great vessels. The lower the temperature, the longer the

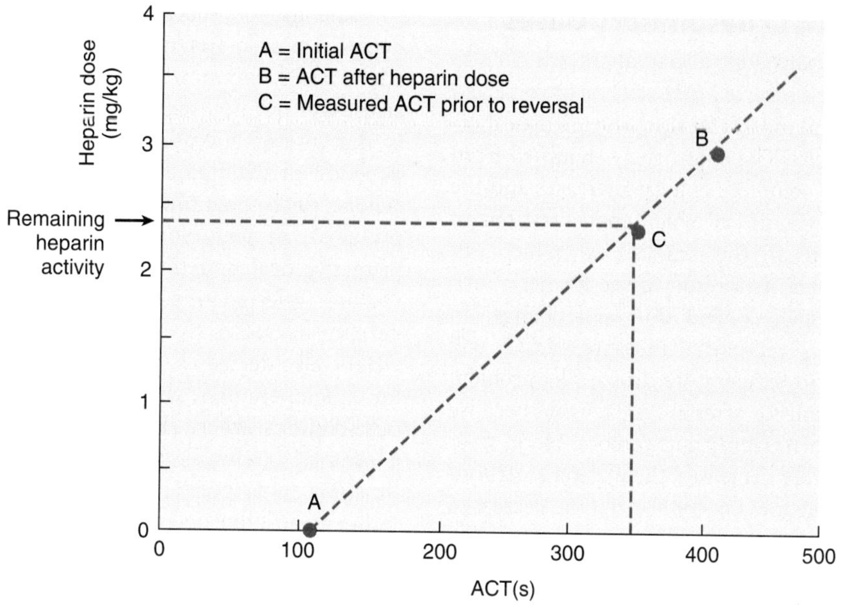

FIGURE 22–14 Heparin dose–response curve; activated clotting time (ACT) in seconds versus total heparin dose in milligrams per kilogram. (1) Plot the initial ACT on the *x*-axis (point A). (2) Plot the ACT after heparinization (point B). (3) Draw the line defined by these two points. (4) If additional anticoagulation is needed, find the desired ACT on that line. The amount of additional heparin needed is the difference on the *y*-axis between the present ACT and the desired ACT (point C). (5) If the third point does not lie on the original line, a new line is drawn originating from the baseline ACT and passing midway between the other two points. (6) For reversal of anticoagulation, the protamine dose is based on the remaining heparin activity, estimated to be the heparin dose corresponding to the latest ACT on the dose–response line.

time required to cool or rewarm. Lower temperatures, however, permit lower CPB flows to be used safely. At a temperature of 20°C, flows as low as 1.2 L/min/m^2 may be adequate.

Hypothermia produces characteristic changes in the ECG such as the Osborne wave, a positive deflection between the QRS and ST segments. Ventricular fibrillation often occurs as the heart is cooled below 28°C to 29°C. Cardioplegia should be established immediately, as ventricular fibrillation consumes high-energy phosphates at a greater rate than slower rhythms. Cardioplegia is achieved by cross-clamping the ascending aorta proximal to the aortic inflow cannula and (as previously described) infusing cardioplegia solution through a small catheter proximal to the cross-clamp, directly into the coronary ostia if the aorta is opened (eg, for aortic valve replacement), or retrograde through the coronary sinus.

Ventilation

Ventilation of the lungs is discontinued when adequate pump flows are reached and the heart stops ejecting blood. Following institution of full CPB, ventricular ejection continues briefly until the left ventricular volume reaches a critically low level. Discontinuing ventilation when there is any remaining pulmonary blood flow acts as a right-to-left shunt that can promote hypoxemia. The importance of this mechanism depends on the relative ratio of remaining pulmonary blood flow to pump flow. Once ventilation is stopped, most centers either stop all gas flow or maintain a very reduced oxygen flow in the anesthesia circuit with a small amount of continuous positive airway pressure (CPAP) (5 cm H_2O) in the hope of preventing postoperative pulmonary dysfunction. Ventilation is resumed at the conclusion of CPB in anticipation of the heart beginning to eject blood.

Management of Respiratory Gases

There formerly was controversy about whether to use temperature-corrected (pH stat) or uncorrected (α-stat) arterial blood gas tensions during hypothermic CPB in adults. The controversy stemmed from the fact that the solubility of a gas increases and the neutral pH (ie, the pH at which concentrations of H^+ and OH^- ions are the same) of water increases with hypothermia. As a result of the former effect, although total CO_2 content does not change (in a closed system), the partial pressure of CO_2 will decrease as blood temperature drops. The problem is most significant for arterial CO_2 tension because of its effect on arterial pH and cerebral blood flow. As the temperature decreases, the plasma bicarbonate concentration does not change, but the decreased arterial CO_2 tension increases pH to what would be alkalotic values at normothermia. Blood with a CO_2 tension of 40 mm Hg and a pH of 7.40 at 37°C, when cooled to 25°C, will have a CO_2 tension of about 23 mm Hg and a pH of 7.60, yet will have an unchanged ratio of H^+ to OH^- ions.

Regardless of the patient's temperature, all blood samples are heated to 37°C by blood gas analyzers before measuring gas tensions. If a temperature-corrected reading is desired, a table or a program in the blood gas analyzer can be used to estimate what the gas tension and pH would have been had they been measured at the patient's temperature. The practice of temperature correcting gas tensions with the goal of maintaining a constant CO_2 tension of 40 mm Hg and a constant pH of 7.40 during hypothermia is referred to as **pH-stat management**. During hypothermic CPB, pH-stat management, which may require adding CO_2 to the oxygenator gas inflow to maintain a constant $PaCO_2$, increases total blood CO_2 content. Under these conditions, cerebral blood flow increases (due to increased CO_2 tension relative to α-stat management) more than is required based on oxygen consumption. Increased cerebral blood flow is useful to increase the uniformity of brain cooling prior to deep hypothermic circulatory arrest. On the other hand, increased cerebral blood flow can also direct a greater fraction of atheromatous arterial emboli to the brain—a greater concern than uniformity of brain cooling during most cardiac surgery in adults.

The use of uncorrected gas tensions during hypothermia—**α-stat management**—is the rule in adults and is common in children when circulatory arrest will not be used. The basis of this approach is that preservation of normal protein function depends on maintaining a constant state of intracellular electroneutrality (the balance of charges on proteins). At physiological pH, these charges are primarily located on the imidazole rings of histidine residues (referred to as *α residues*). Moreover, as temperature decreases, K_w—the dissociation constant for water—also decreases (pK_w increases). Therefore, at lower temperatures, the electroneutrality of aqueous solutions, where $[H^+] = [OH^-]$, corresponds to a lower $[H^+]$ (a higher pH). Hypothermic "alkalosis" thus does not necessarily reflect $[OH^-] > [H^+]$ but rather an absolute decrease in both $[H^+]$ and $[OH^-]$. Hypothermic CPB with α-stat management does not require the addition of CO_2 to the oxygenator: The total CO_2 content of blood and the electroneutrality are unchanged. In contrast to pH-stat management, α-stat management appears to preserve cerebral autoregulation of blood flow. Despite the theoretical and observed differences, in most studies, comparisons between the two techniques fail to reveal appreciable differences in patient outcomes except when used prior to circulatory arrest.

Anesthesia

11 Hypothermia (<34°C) potentiates general anesthetic potency, but failure to give anesthetic agents, particularly during rewarming on CPB, may result in awareness and recall. Light anesthesia may associate with patient movement if muscle paralysis is allowed to wear off. Consequently, additional doses of anesthetic agents may be necessary during CPB. Reduced concentrations of a volatile agent (eg, 0.5–0.75% isoflurane) are often administered via the oxygenator. The volatile agent concentration may need to be reduced to a value that does not depress contractility immediately prior to termination of bypass if residual myocardial depression is apparent. Those relying on opioids and benzodiazepines for anesthesia during CPB may need to administer additional doses of these agents or commence a propofol infusion during rewarming. Some clinicians routinely administer midazolam when

rewarming is initiated. Alternatively, a propofol, opioid, or ketamine–midazolam infusion may be continued throughout CPB. Sweating during rewarming is common and usually indicates a hypothalamic response to perfusion with warm blood (rather than "light" anesthesia). During rewarming, inflow blood temperature should not exceed core temperature by more than 2°C.

Cerebral Protection

The incidence of neurobehavioral deficits after CPB varies widely, depending on how long after surgery the examination is performed and the criteria for diagnosis. In the first week after surgery, the incidence may be as great as 80%. Fortunately, most of these early deficits are transient. Neurobehavioral deficits or strokes detectable 8 weeks or more after operation are less common, with incidences of 20% to 25% and 2% to 6%, respectively. Factors that have been associated with adverse neurological or neurobehavioral sequelae include increased numbers of cerebral emboli, combined intracardiac (valvular) and coronary procedures, advanced age, and preexisting cerebrovascular disease.

During open-heart procedures, de-airing of cardiac chambers, assumption of a head-down position, and venting before and during initial cardiac ejection are important in preventing gas emboli. Many centers fill the surgical field with CO_2, a gas that if entrained and embolized will more rapidly be reabsorbed. TEE can detect residual air within the heart and the need for further de-airing procedures. During coronary bypass procedures, minimizing the amount of aortic manipulation, the number of aortic clampings, and the number of graft sites on the surface of the aorta and using sutureless proximal anastomotic devices may help reduce atheromatous emboli. Gentle palpation of the aorta, TEE, and especially epiaortic echocardiography can help identify high-risk patients and guide management. Epiaortic echocardiography is the most sensitive and specific technique.

The relative contributions of emboli versus cerebral hypoperfusion in causing neurological deficits remain unclear. The data are controversial and sparse that prophylactic drug infusions immediately before and during intracardiac (open ventricle) procedures will decrease the incidence and severity of neurological deficits. Prior to circulatory arrest with very deep hypothermia, some clinicians administer a corticosteroid (methylprednisolone, 30 mg/kg, or the equivalent dose of dexamethasone) and mannitol (0.5 g/kg). The head is also covered with ice bags (avoiding the eyes). Surface cooling delays rewarming and may also facilitate adequacy of brain cooling. A long list of drugs has failed to improve cerebral outcomes after heart surgery. Human studies during cardiac surgery have not shown improved neurobehavioral outcomes with prophylactic administration of calcium channel blockers (nimodipine), *N*-methyl-D-aspartate (NMDA) antagonists (remacemide), free radical scavengers (pegorgotein), sedative-hypnotics (thiopental, propofol, clomethiazole), or lazaroids (tirilazad).

4. Termination of CPB

Discontinuation of bypass is accomplished by a series of necessary procedures and conditions, the first of which is adequate rewarming. The surgeon's decision about when to rewarm is important; adequate rewarming requires time, but rewarming too soon removes the protective effects of hypothermia. Rapid rewarming often results in large temperature gradients between well-perfused organs and peripheral vasoconstricted tissues; subsequent equilibration following separation from CPB decreases core temperature again. An excessive gradient between the infusate temperature and the patient's core temperature can result in deleterious brain hyperthermia. Infusion of a vasodilator drug (eg, isoflurane) allows greater pump flows and often speeds the rewarming process. Allowing some minimal ventricular ejection may also speed rewarming. Excessively rapid rewarming, however, can result in the formation of gas bubbles in the bloodstream as the solubility of gases rapidly decreases. If the heart fibrillates during rewarming, direct electrical defibrillation (5–10 J) may be necessary. Administration of lidocaine, 100 to 200 mg, and magnesium sulfate, 1 to 2 g, prior to removal of aortic cross-clamping is a common protocol and may decrease the likelihood of fibrillation. Many clinicians advocate a head-down position while intracardiac air is being evacuated to decrease the likelihood of cerebral emboli. Lung inflation facilitates expulsion of air in the left atrium and ventricle by compressing pulmonary vessels and returning blood into the left heart. TEE is useful in detecting residual intracardiac air. Initial reinflation of the lungs requires greater than normal airway pressure and should generally be done under direct visualization of the surgical field. Excessive lung expansion can interfere with internal mammary artery grafts and surgical visualization.

General guidelines for separation from CPB include the following:

- The core body temperature should be at least 37°C.
- A stable rhythm must be present. Pacing is often used and confers the benefit of a properly timed atrial systole. Persisting atrioventricular block should prompt measurement of serum potassium concentration. If hyperkalemia is present, it can be treated with calcium, $NaHCO_3$, furosemide, or glucose and insulin.
- The heart rate must be adequate (generally 80–100 beats/min). Slow heart rates are generally treated by pacing. Many inotropic agents will also increase heart rate. Supraventricular tachycardias generally require cardioversion.
- Laboratory values must be within acceptable limits. Significant acidosis (pH <7.20), hypocalcemia (ionized), and hyperkalemia (>5.5 mEq/L) should be treated; ideally, the hematocrit should exceed 22%; however, a hematocrit <22% should not by itself trigger transfusion of red blood cells at this time. When CPB reservoir volume and flow are adequate, ultrafiltration may be used to increase the hematocrit.
- Adequate ventilation with 100% oxygen must have been resumed.
- All monitors should be rechecked for proper function and recalibrated if necessary.

Weaning from CPB

CPB should be discontinued as systemic arterial pressure, ventricular volumes and filling pressures, and cardiac function (on TEE) are assessed. Central aortic pressure can be measured directly and compared with the radial artery pressure and cuff pressure if there is concern about radial artery hypotension. A reversal of the normal systolic pressure gradient, with aortic pressure normally being greater than radial pressure, is often seen immediately after discontinuation of CPB. Radial artery hypotension has been attributed to opening of arteriovenous connections in the hand as a consequence of rewarming. Central aortic root pressure can also be estimated by palpation by an experienced surgeon. Right ventricular volume and contractility can be estimated visually, whereas filling pressures are measured directly by central venous, pulmonary artery, or left atrial catheters. Cardiac output can be measured by thermodilution with a pulmonary artery catheter or with TEE. In addition, TEE can define adequacy of end-diastolic volumes, right and left ventricular contractility, and valvular function.

Weaning is typically accomplished by progressively clamping the venous return line (tubing). As the beating heart fills, ventricular ejection resumes. Pump flow is gradually decreased as arterial pressure rises. Once the venous line is completely occluded and systolic arterial pressure is judged to be adequate (>80–90 mm Hg), pump flow is stopped, and the patient is evaluated. **Some surgeons wean by clamping the venous line and then progressively "filling" the patient with arterial inflow.**

Most patients fall into one of four groups when coming off bypass (Table 22–2). Patients with good ventricular function are usually quick to develop good blood pressure and cardiac output and can be separated from CPB immediately. Hyperdynamic patients can also be rapidly weaned. These patients emerge from CPB with a very low SVR, demonstrating good contractility and adequate volume, but have low arterial pressure; their hematocrit is often reduced (<22%). Diuresis (off CPB), red blood cell transfusions, and vasoconstrictors increase arterial blood pressure.

Hypovolemic patients include those with normal ventricular function and those with varying degrees of impairment. Those with preserved myocardial function quickly respond to infusion of blood via the aortic cannula. Blood pressure and

TABLE 22–2 Post-CPB hemodynamic subgroups.[1]

	Group I: Vigorous	Group II: Hypovolemic	Group IIIA: LV Pump Failure	Group IIIB: RV Failure	Group IV: Vasodilated (Hyperdynamic)
Blood pressure	Normal	Low	Low	Low	Low
Central venous pressure	Normal	Low	Normal or high	High	Normal or low
Pulmonary wedge pressure	Normal	Low	High	Normal or high	Normal or low
TEE findings	Normal	Underfilled RV/LV	Reduced LV performance	Dilated RV	Normal or underfilled RV/LV
Cardiac output	Normal	Low	Low	Low	High
Systemic vascular resistance	Normal	Low, normal, or high	Low, normal or high	Normal or high	Low
Treatment	None	Volume	Inotrope; IABP, LVAD	Inotrope, pulmonary vasodilator; RVAD	Vasoconstrictor, volume

[1]CPB, cardiopulmonary bypass; IABP, intraaortic balloon pump; LV, left ventricular; LVAD, left ventricular assist device; RV, right ventricular; RVAD, right ventricular assist device; TEE, transesophageal echocardiography.

cardiac output rise with each bolus, and the increase becomes progressively more sustained. Most of these patients maintain good blood pressure and cardiac output with an estimated left ventricular filling pressure below 10 to 15 mm Hg. Ventricular impairment should be suspected (when TEE is not available) in apparently hypovolemic patients whose filling pressures rise during volume infusion without appropriate improvement in blood pressure or cardiac output. Ventricular dysfunction is easily diagnosed by TEE.

Patients with heart failure emerge from CPB with a sluggish, poorly contracting heart that progressively distends. In such cases, CPB may need to be reinstituted while inotropic therapy is initiated; alternatively, if the patient is less unstable, a positive inotrope (epinephrine, dopamine, dobutamine) can be administered while the patient is observed for improvement. If the patient does not respond to reasonable doses of one of these three agents, milrinone can be added. In patients with poor preoperative ventricular function (or in other patients who are suspected to require intensive inotropic support), milrinone may be administered as the first-line agent prior to separation from CPB. If SVR is increased (when cardiac output is decreased), afterload reduction with nitroprusside, clevidipine, or milrinone can be tried. All patients with low cardiac output syndrome should be evaluated for unrecognized ischemia (kinked grafts or coronary vasospasm), valvular dysfunction, shunting, or right ventricular failure. TEE will facilitate the diagnosis in these cases.

If drug therapies fail, **intraaortic balloon pump** (IABP) counterpulsation may be initiated while the heart is "rested" on CPB. The efficacy of IABP depends on proper timing of inflation and deflation of the balloon (Figure 22–15). **The balloon should inflate just after the dicrotic notch is seen on the intraaortic pressure tracing (indicating closure of the aortic valve) to augment diastolic blood pressure and coronary flow.** Inflation too early (before aortic valve closure) increases afterload and exacerbates aortic regurgitation, whereas delayed inflation reduces diastolic augmentation. Balloon deflation should be timed just prior to left ventricular ejection to avoid increasing afterload. Early deflation makes diastolic augmentation and afterload reduction less effective. Use of a left or right ventricular assist device (LVAD or RVAD, respectively) may be necessary for

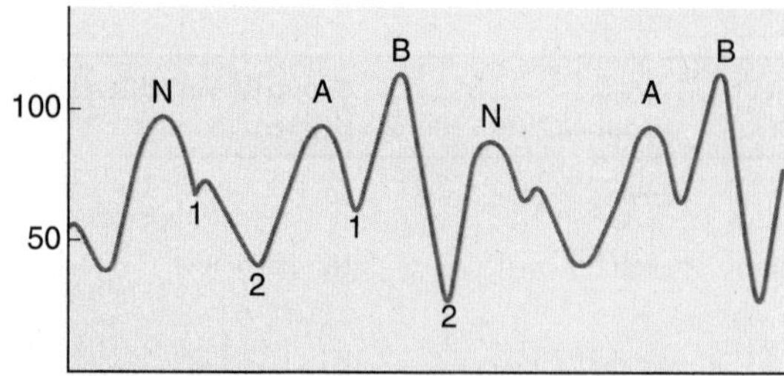

FIGURE 22–15 A central arterial waveform during 1:2 intraaortic balloon pump counterpulsation. Ideally the balloon, which is positioned in the descending aorta just distal to the left subclavian artery, should inflate at the dicrotic notch (1) and be completely deflated just as the left ventricle begins to eject (2). Note the lower end-diastolic pressures after balloon augmentation and slightly lower systolic pressure in the following beat. A, augmented beat; B, balloon augmentation; N, nonaugmented beat.

patients with refractory pump failure. If myocardial stunning is a major contributor or there are areas of hibernating myocardium, a delayed improvement in contractile function may allow complete weaning from all drugs and support devices only after 12 to 48 h of therapy. Ventricular assist devices can be used as a bridge to cardiac transplantation.

Many clinicians do not routinely administer positive inotropes to all patients separating from CPB because these agents increase myocardial oxygen demand. The routine use of calcium similarly may worsen ischemic injury and may contribute to coronary spasm (particularly in patients who were taking calcium channel blockers preoperatively). Nevertheless, there are centers that administer calcium salts or a positive inotrope (eg, dobutamine), or both, to every patient at the conclusion of CPB. Commonly used positive inotropes and vasopressors are listed in Table 22–3. Epinephrine, dopamine, and dobutamine are the most commonly used agents. Epinephrine is the most potent inotrope and is often effective in increasing both cardiac output and systemic blood pressure when other agents have failed. In lower doses, it has predominantly β-agonist activity. Dobutamine, unlike dopamine, does not increase filling pressures and *may*

TABLE 22–3 Vasopressors and inotropic agents.[1]

			Adrenergic Activity			Phosphodiesterase Inhibition
	Bolus	**Infusion**	**α**	**β**	**Indirect**	
Epinephrine	2–10 mcg	0.01–0.03 mcg/kg/min	+	+++	0	0
		0.04–0.1 mcg/kg/min	++	+++	0	0
		>0.1 mcg/kg/min	+++	+++	0	0
Norepinephrine		0.01–0.1 mcg/kg/min	+++	++	0	0
Isoproterenol	1–4 mcg	0.01–0.1 mcg/kg/min	0	+++	0	0
Dobutamine		2–20 mcg/kg/min	0	++	0	0
Dopamine		2–10 mcg/kg/min	+	++	+	0
		10–20 mcg/kg/min	++	++	+	0
Ephedrine	5–25 mg		+	++	+	0
Phenylephrine	50–200 mcg	10–50 mcg/min	+++	0	0	0
Inamrinone	0.5–1.5 mg/kg	5–10 mcg/kg/min	0	0	0	+++
Milrinone	50 mcg/kg	0.375–0.75 mcg/kg/min	0	0	0	+++
Vasopressin	1–2 units	2–8 units/h	0	0	0	0

[1]+, mild activity; ++, moderate activity; +++, marked activity.

be associated with less tachycardia than dopamine; unfortunately, cardiac output often increases without significant changes in blood pressure. On the other hand, dopamine is sometimes more effective in increasing blood pressure than in increasing cardiac output. Interestingly, when infused to increase SV by the same amount, epinephrine is associated with equal (and perhaps less) increase in heart rate than dobutamine. Inamrinone, enoximone, milrinone, and olprinone are selective phosphodiesterase inhibitors and inotropes with arterial and venous dilator properties. Only inamrinone and milrinone are available in North America, and the latter is much more commonly used. In studies of patients with chronic heart failure, inamrinone and milrinone, unlike other inotropes, did not appreciably increase myocardial oxygen consumption. The combination of an 49nodilators (usually milrinone) and a β-adrenergic agonist results in at least additive (and possibly synergistic) inotropic effects. Norepinephrine is useful for increasing SVR but may compromise splanchnic and renal blood flow at increased doses. Some clinicians use norepinephrine in combination with phosphodiesterase inhibitors to prevent excessive reductions in systemic arterial pressure. Arginine vasopressin may be used in patients with refractory low SVR and resistance to norepinephrine. There are experimental reports in which doses of methylene blue or vitamin C have successfully counteracted vasodilation that could not be overcome with norepinephrine, vasopressin, or both. Inhaled nitric oxide and prostaglandin E_1 (or even inhaled milrinone) may also be helpful for refractory pulmonary hypertension and right ventricular failure (Table 22–4); nitric oxide has the added advantage of not decreasing systemic arterial pressure. Studies have not confirmed outcome benefits to the use of thyroid hormone (T_3) or glucose–insulin–potassium infusions for vasoactive/inotropic support after CPB.

5. Postbypass Period

Following CPB, bleeding is controlled, bypass cannulas are removed, anticoagulation is reversed, and the chest is closed. Systolic arterial pressure is generally maintained at less than 140 mm Hg to minimize bleeding. Checking for bleeding, particularly from the posterior surface of the heart, requires lifting the heart, which can cause periods of precipitous hypotension. Some surgeons will need to be informed of the extent and duration of the hypotension; others have greater situational awareness. The atrial cannula(e) is removed before the aortic cannula in case the latter must be used to rapidly administer volume to the patient. Most patients need additional volume after the termination of bypass. Administration of blood, colloids, and crystalloid is guided by observation of the left ventricle on TEE, filling pressures, and the postbypass hematocrit. A final hematocrit of 25% or greater is desirable. Blood remaining in the CPB reservoir can be transfused via the aortic cannula, or it can be washed and processed by a cell-saver device and given intravenously. Frequent ventricular ectopy may reflect electrolyte disturbances or residual ischemia and usually should be treated with amiodarone; hypokalemia or hypomagnesemia should be corrected. Ventricular arrhythmias in this setting can rapidly deteriorate into ventricular tachycardia and fibrillation.

TABLE 22–4 Vasodilators.

Drug	Dosage
Clevidipine	1–16 mg/h
Fenoldopam	0.03–0.6 mcg/kg/min
Nicardipine	2.5–10 mg/h
Nitric oxide	10–60 ppm (inhaled)
Nitroglycerin	0.5–10 mcg/kg/min
Nitroprusside	0.5–10 mcg/kg/min
Prostaglandin E_1	0.01–0.2 mcg/kg/min

Reversal of Anticoagulation

Once hemostasis is judged acceptable and the patient remains hemodynamically stable, heparin is reversed with protamine. **Protamine** is a highly positively charged protein that binds and effectively inactivates heparin (a highly negatively charged polysaccharide). Heparin–protamine complexes are then removed by the reticuloendothelial system. Protamine can be dosed in varying ways, but the results of all techniques should be checked for adequacy by repeating the ACT 3 to 5 min after completion of the protamine infusion. Additional incremental doses of protamine may be necessary.

One dosing technique bases the protamine dose on the amount of heparin initially required to produce the desired ACT; the protamine is then given in a ratio of 1 to 1.3 mg of protamine per 100 units of heparin. A still simpler approach is to give adult patients a defined dose (eg, 3–4 mg/kg) then check for adequacy of reversal. Another approach calculates the protamine dose based on the heparin dose–response curve (see Figure 22–14). Automated heparin–protamine titration assays measure residual heparin concentration and can be used to calculate the protamine dose. The justification for using this methodology is the observation that when protamine is given in excess it may have anticoagulant activity, though this has never been demonstrated in humans. This approach also assumes that administered protamine remains in circulation for a prolonged time (which has been proven false in studies of volunteers and in patients undergoing cardiac surgery). Premeasured amounts of protamine are added in varying quantities to several wells, each containing a blood sample, to accomplish the heparin–protamine titration. The well whose protamine concentration best matches the heparin concentration will clot first. Clotting will be prolonged in wells containing either too much or too little protamine. The protamine dose can then be estimated by multiplying the concentration in the tube that clots first by the patient's calculated blood volume. Supplemental protamine (50–100 mg) may be considered after administration of unwashed blood remaining in the pump reservoir after CPB because that blood contains heparin.

12 Protamine administration can result in a number of adverse hemodynamic effects, some of which are immunological in origin. Protamine given slowly (over 5–10 min) usually has few effects; when given more rapidly, it produces a consistent vasodilation that is easily treated with blood from the pump oxygenator and small doses of a vasoconstrictor. Rare catastrophic protamine reactions often include myocardial depression and marked pulmonary hypertension. Patients with diabetes who were previously maintained on protamine-containing insulin (such as NPH) may be at increased risk for adverse reactions to protamine.

Persistent Bleeding

13 Persistent bleeding often follows prolonged durations of bypass (>2 h) and in most instances has multiple causes. Inadequate surgical control of bleeding sites, incomplete reversal of heparin, thrombocytopenia, platelet dysfunction, hypothermia-induced coagulation defects, and undiagnosed preoperative hemostatic defects, or newly acquired factor or fibrinogen deficiencies may be responsible. The absence (or loss) of clot formation may be noted in the surgical field. Normally, the ACT should return to baseline following administration of protamine; additional doses of protamine (25–50 mg) may be necessary. Reheparinization (heparin rebound) after apparent adequate reversal is poorly understood but often attributed to redistribution of peripherally bound heparin to the central compartment and the short persistence of protamine in blood. Hypothermia (<35°C) accentuates hemostatic defects and should be corrected. The administration of platelets and coagulation factors should be guided by additional coagulation studies, but empiric therapy may be necessary when such tests are not readily or promptly available when treating massive, catastrophic bleeding. On the other hand, there can be abnormalities in multiple tests of coagulation when there is no excessive bleeding, so the true diagnostic specificity and reliability of these tests are often overstated.

If diffuse oozing continues despite adequate surgical hemostasis and the ACT is normal or the heparin–protamine titration assay shows no residual heparin, thrombocytopenia or platelet dysfunction is most likely. Comparison of a conventional ACT with an ACT measured in the presence of heparinase (an enzyme that cleaves and inactivates heparin) can confirm that no residual heparin requiring protamine reversal remains present if both tests provide the same result. Platelet defects are recognized complications of CPB, which may necessitate platelet transfusion. Significant depletion of coagulation factors during CPB, typically factors V and VIII, is less commonly responsible for bleeding; if present, it can be treated with fresh frozen plasma. Both the prothrombin time and the partial thromboplastin time are usually prolonged in such instances. Hypofibrinogenemia (fibrinogen level <100 mg/dL or a prolonged thrombin time without residual heparin) should be treated with cryoprecipitate. Desmopressin (DDAVP), 0.3 mcg/kg (intravenously over 20 min), can increase the activity of factors VIII and XII and the von Willebrand factor by releasing them from the vascular endothelium. DDAVP may reverse qualitative platelet defects in some patients, but it is not recommended for routine use. Accelerated fibrinolysis may occasionally be encountered following CPB and should be treated with ε-aminocaproic acid or tranexamic acid if one or the other of these agents has not already been given; the diagnosis should be confirmed by elevated fibrin degradation products (≥32 mg/mL), or evidence of clot lysis on thromboelastography. Increasingly, factor VII concentrate or prothrombin complex concentrate are administered as a "last resort" in the setting of coagulopathic bleeding following cardiac surgery.

Anesthesia

Unless a continuous intravenous infusion technique is used, additional anesthetic agents are necessary following CPB; the choice may be determined by the hemodynamic response of the patient following CPB. We have found that most patients tolerate modest doses of isoflurane or a propofol infusion. Patients with hypertension that is unresponsive to adequate anesthesia with opioids and either a volatile agent or propofol (or all) should receive a vasodilator (see Table 22–4). Fenoldopam may be used and has the added benefit of increasing renal blood flow, which might possibly improve kidney function in the early postoperative period.

It is common for an opioid (morphine 10 mg or hydromorphone 2 mg) and either propofol or dexmedetomidine to be given to provide analgesia and sedation during transfer to the ICU and analgesia, anticipating discontinuation of the propofol or dexmedetomidine during emergence in the ICU.

Transportation

Transporting patients with critical illness from the operating room to the ICU is consistently nerve-wracking and occasionally hazardous, complicated by the possibilities of monitor failure, unintended drug overdosage or interruption of drug infusions, or hemodynamic instability en route. Portable monitoring equipment, infusion pumps, and a full oxygen cylinder with a self-inflating bag for ventilation should be readied before the end of the operation. Minimum monitoring during transportation includes the ECG, arterial blood pressure, and pulse oximetry. A spare endotracheal tube, laryngoscope, succinylcholine, and emergency resuscitation drugs should also accompany the patient. Upon the patient's arrival in the ICU, the endotracheal tube should be attached to the ventilator, breath sounds should be checked, and an orderly transfer of monitors and infusions should follow. The handoff to the ICU staff should include a brief summary of the procedure, intraoperative problems, current drug therapy, and any expected difficulties. Many centers insist on a standard protocol for the "handoff," and we strongly recommend this practice.

6. Postoperative Period

Depending on the patient, the type of surgery, and local practices, patients may be mechanically ventilated for 1 to 12 h postoperatively. Sedation may be maintained with a propofol or dexmedetomidine infusion. The emphasis in the first few postoperative hours should be on maintaining hemodynamic stability and monitoring for excessive postoperative
14 bleeding. Chest tube drainage in the first 2 h of more than 250 to 300 mL/h (10 mL/kg/h)—in the absence of a hemostatic defect—is excessive and may require surgical reexploration. Subsequent drainage that exceeds 100 mL/h is also worrisome. Intrathoracic bleeding at a site not adequately drained may cause cardiac tamponade, requiring immediate reentry of the chest.

Hypertension despite analgesia and sedation is a common postoperative problem and should generally be treated promptly so as not to exacerbate bleeding or myocardial ischemia. Vasodilator or esmolol infusions are generally used. Fluid replacement may be guided by filling pressures, echocardiography, or by responses to treatment. Most patients present with relative hypovolemia for several hours after an operation. Hypokalemia (from intraoperative diuretics) often develops and requires replacement. Postoperative hypomagnesemia should be expected in patients who receive no magnesium supplementation intraoperatively.

Extubation should be considered only when muscle paralysis has worn off (or been reversed) and the patient is hemodynamically stable. Caution should be exercised in obese and older adult patients and those with underlying pulmonary disease. Cardiothoracic procedures are typically associated with marked decreases in functional residual capacity and postoperative diaphragmatic dysfunction.

Off-Pump Coronary Artery Bypass Surgery

The development of advanced epicardial stabilizing devices, such as the Octopus (Figure 22–16), facilitated coronary artery bypass grafting without the use of CPB, also known as *off-pump coronary artery bypass* (OPCAB). This type of retractor uses suction to stabilize and lift the anastomotic site rather than compress it down, which allows for greater hemodynamic stability. Full (CPB) dose heparinization is usually given, and the CPB machine is usually immediately available if needed.

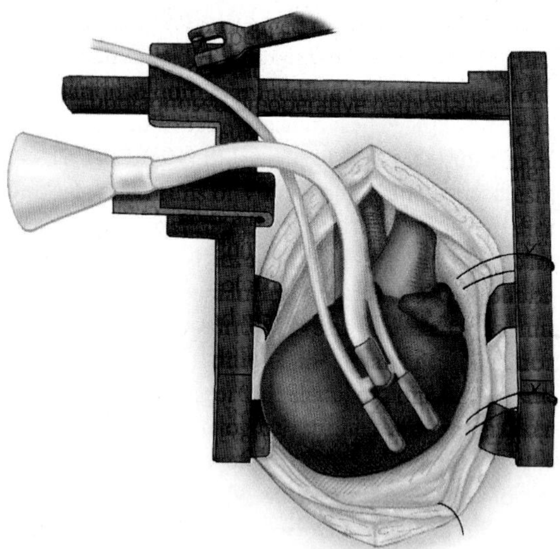

FIGURE 22–16 Schematic illustration of the Octopus retractor for off-pump coronary artery bypass surgery.

Intravenous fluid loading together with intermittent or continuous infusion of a vasopressor may be necessary while the distal anastomoses are sewn. In contrast, a vasodilator may be required to reduce the systolic pressure to 90 to 100 mm Hg during partial clamping of the aorta for the proximal anastomosis. Intravenous nitroglycerin is often used because of its ability to ameliorate myocardial ischemia.

Although OPCAB was initially proposed for "simple" one- or two-vessel bypass grafting in patients with good left ventricular function, it may be the sicker, older patients who benefit most from avoidance of CPB. The surgeon may use an intraluminal shunt to maintain coronary blood flow during sewing of distal anastomoses. Volatile anesthetic agents and morphine provide myocardial protection during prolonged periods of ischemia. Maintenance of anesthesia with a volatile agent may therefore be desirable. When the surgeon is skillful, long-term graft patency may be comparable to procedures done with CPB. Patients with extensive coronary disease, particularly those with poor target vessels, may not be good candidates. OPCAB may decrease the incidence of postoperative neurological complications and the need for transfusion relative to conventional coronary bypass with CPB.

PERCUTANEOUS VALVE REPLACEMENT

Advances in technology now permit percutaneous aortic valve replacements. Catheter-delivered aortic valve replacements are increasingly routine. Patients are taken to a hybrid operating room where the valve is deployed under angiographic guidance. During deployment, rapid ventricular pacing is initiated to impede ventricular ejection. Both general anesthesia and sedation have been successfully used in this patient population. Choice of anesthetic technique is dependent upon both patient and practitioner characteristics. In patients managed with general anesthesia, transesophageal echocardiography is performed during the procedure to assess the integrity of the deployed prosthetic aortic valve (eg, to rule out perivalvular leaks) and to ensure that the adjacent mitral valve has not been injured in the process.

Currently, catheter-based repairs of the mitral valve are similarly undertaken. The anterior and posterior mitral valve leaflets can be clipped together to reduce mitral regurgitation. With a trans-septal punction, clips are introduced into the left atrium and positioned to bring the anterior and posterior leaflets together. A double orifice mitral valve is then created with the intention of reducing the severity of mitral regurgitation. TEE is employed to both assess the success of the repair in reducing mitral regurgitation and to also confirm that iatrogenic mitral stenosis has not been created. Cardiac anesthesiologists with advanced echocardiography skills are routinely required to anesthetize patients for catheter-based procedures.

PEDIATRIC PATIENTS

Cardiovascular function in infants and young children differs from that in adults. Stroke volume is relatively fixed, so cardiac output is primarily dependent on heart rate. The immature hearts of neonates and infants often are less forgiving of pressure or volume overload. Furthermore, the functions of both ventricles are more interdependent, so failure of one ventricle often precipitates failure of the other (**biventricular heart failure**). The transition of the neonate from the fetal to the adult circulation is discussed in Chapter 40.

Preoperative Evaluation

The potentially complex nature of congenital heart defects and their operative repair demand close communication among the anesthesiologist, perfusionist, and surgeon. In children, the focus should include the exact anatomic abnormality and its physiological consequences, whether there has been any previous palliation or correction, and whether there are any other congenital malformations. The hemodynamic significance of the lesion and the planned surgical correction must be clearly understood. Heart failure and pulmonary infections should be treated. Prostaglandin E_1 infusion (0.05–0.1 mcg/kg/min) is used preoperatively to prevent closure of the ductus arteriosus in infants dependent on ductal flow for survival. True pediatric cardiac surgical emergencies are rare: correction of total anomalous pulmonary venous return, excessive postoperative bleeding, or institution of extracorporeal membrane oxygenation (ECMO).

Assessment of disease severity relies on both clinical and laboratory evaluation. Deterioration in infants may be manifested by increasing tachypnea, cyanosis, or sweating, particularly during feeding. Older children may report easy fatigability. In infants, bodyweight is generally a good indication of disease severity, with the sickest children showing failure to thrive and reduced weight relative to expectations for age. Signs of congestive heart failure include failure to thrive, tachycardia, an S_3 gallop, weak pulses, tachypnea, rales, and hepatomegaly. Cyanosis may be noted, but hypoxemia is best assessed using pulse oximetry, measurements of arterial blood gases, and the hematocrit. In the absence of iron deficiency, the degree of polycythemia is related to the severity and duration of hypoxemia. Clubbing of the fingers is frequent in children with cyanotic defects. The evaluation should also search for other congenital abnormalities, which are present in up to 30% of patients with congenital heart disease.

The results of echocardiography, heart catheterization, electrocardiography, and chest radiography should be reviewed. Laboratory evaluation typically includes a complete blood count (with platelet count), coagulation studies, electrolytes, blood urea nitrogen, and serum creatinine. Measurements of ionized calcium and glucose are also useful in neonates and critically ill children.

Preinduction Period

A. Fasting

Fasting requirements vary according to the patient's age and current guidelines. A preoperative intravenous infusion that provides maintenance fluid requirements should be used in patients susceptible to dehydration, in those with severe polycythemia, and when excessive delays occur prior to surgery.

B. Premedication

Premedication varies according to age and cardiac and pulmonary reserves. Atropine, 0.02 mg/kg intramuscularly (minimum dose, 0.15 mg), has by tradition been given to pediatric cardiac patients to counteract enhanced vagal tone. Neonates and infants younger than 6 months of age may receive no premedication or be given only atropine. Sedation is desirable in older patients, particularly those with cyanotic lesions (tetralogy of Fallot), as agitation and crying worsen right-to-left shunting. Patients older than 1 year may be given midazolam orally (0.5–0.6 mg/kg) or intramuscularly (0.08 mg/kg).

Induction of Anesthesia

A. Hemodynamic Anesthetic Goals

1. Obstructive lesions—Anesthetic management should strive to avoid hypovolemia, bradycardia, tachycardia, and myocardial depression. The optimal heart rate should be selected according to age; slow rates decrease cardiac output, whereas fast rates may impair ventricular filling. Mild cardiac depression may be desirable in some hyperdynamic patients, such as those with coarctation of the aorta.

2. Shunts—A favorable ratio of pulmonary vascular resistance (PVR) to SVR should be maintained in the
15 presence of shunting. Factors known to increase PVR, such as acidosis, hypercapnia, hypoxia, enhanced sympathetic tone, and high mean airway pressures, are to be avoided in patients with right-to-left shunting; hyperventilation (hypocapnia) with 100% oxygen is usually effective in lowering PVR. Systemic vasodilation also worsens right-to-left shunting and should be avoided; phenylephrine may be used to raise SVR. Inhaled nitric oxide has no effect on systemic arterial pressure. Conversely, patients with left-to-right shunting may benefit from systemic vasodilation, increases in PVR, and avoidance of hyperventilation.

B. Monitoring

Standard intraoperative monitors are generally used, but they may be first applied during the course of an inhaled induction in some patients. A large discrepancy between end-tidal and arterial CO_2 tensions should be anticipated in patients with large right-to-left shunts because of increased dead space. Following induction, intraarterial and central venous pressure monitoring are employed for most thoracotomies and all procedures employing CPB. We recommend sonographic guidance for these cannulations. A 22- or 24-gauge catheter is used to enter the radial artery; 24-gauge catheters may be more appropriate for small neonates and premature infants. A cutdown may be necessary in some instances. The internal jugular or subclavian vein is generally used for central venous cannulation; if this approach is unsuccessful, a right atrial catheter may be placed intraoperatively by the surgeon. TEE is invaluable for assessing the surgical repair following CPB. Ever smaller probes are yielding better resolution as the technology advances. Probes are currently available for patients as small as 3 kg. Intraoperative epicardial echocardiography is commonly used either in addition to or instead of TEE.

C. Venous Access

Venous access is desirable but not always necessary for induction. Agitation and crying are particularly undesirable in patients with cyanotic lesions and can increase right-to-left shunting. Intravenous access can be established after induction but before intubation in most patients. Subsequently, at least two intravenous fluid infusion portals are required; one is typically via a central venous catheter. Caution is necessary to avoid even the smallest air bubbles. Shunting lesions allow the passage of venous air into the arterial circulation; paradoxical embolism can occur through the foramen ovale even in patients without obvious right-to-left shunting. Aspiration prior to each injection prevents dislodgment of any trapped air at stopcock injection ports.

D. Route of Induction

To a major extent, the effect of premedication and the presence of venous access determine the induction technique.

1. Intravenous—Propofol (2–3 mg/kg), ketamine (1–2 mg/kg), fentanyl (25–50 mcg/kg), or sufentanil (5–15 mcg/kg) can be used for intravenous induction. A pure opioid technique may be suitable for critically ill patients when postoperative ventilation is planned. Intravenous agents' onset of action may be more rapid in patients with right-to-left shunting; drug boluses should be given slowly to avoid transiently high arterial blood levels. In contrast, recirculation in patients with large left-to-right shunts dilutes arterial blood concentration and can delay the appearance of intravenous agents' clinical effects.

2. Intramuscular—Ketamine, 4 to 10 mg/kg, is most commonly used, and onset of anesthesia is within 5 min. Coadministration with atropine helps prevent excessive secretions. Ketamine is a good choice for agitated and uncooperative patients as well as patients with decreased cardiac reserve. Its safety with cyanotic lesions (particularly in patients with tetralogy of Fallot) is well established. Ketamine does not appear to increase PVR in children.

3. Inhalation—Sevoflurane is the most commonly used volatile agent. The technique is the same as for noncardiac surgery, except for greater concerns about avoiding excessive anesthetic doses. Sevoflurane is particularly suitable for patients with good cardiac reserve. Nitrous oxide is not often used other than to speed loss of consciousness with inhalation inductions. The uptake of inhalation agents may be slowed in patients with right-to-left shunts; in contrast, no significant effect on uptake is generally observed with left-to-right shunting. Intubation is facilitated by a nondepolarizing agent (rocuronium, 1.2 mg/kg, or vecuronium, 0.1 mg/kg) or, much less commonly, succinylcholine, 1.5 to 2 mg/kg.

Maintenance Anesthesia

Following induction, opioids or inhalation anesthetics are used for maintenance. Fentanyl and sufentanil are the most commonly used intravenous agents, and isoflurane and sevoflurane are the most commonly used inhalation agents. Some clinicians choose the anesthetic according to the patient's hemodynamic responses. Isoflurane and sevoflurane may be more suitable than halothane (the most commonly used inhaled agent in years past) for most patients; in equivalent anesthetic doses, halothane causes more myocardial depression, more slowing of the heart rate, but less vasodilation than sevoflurane or isoflurane. However, one can make a sound theoretical argument in favor of halothane over sevoflurane for patients with tetralogy of Fallot (and similarly obstructive lesions such as hypertrophic subaortic stenosis), where myocardial depression is preferred over vasodilation.

Cardiopulmonary Bypass

The circuit and technique used are similar to those used for adults. Because the smallest circuit volume used is still about three times an infant's blood volume, blood is used to prime the circuit for neonates and infants to prevent excessive hemodilution. CPB may be complicated by intracardiac and extracardiac shunts and a very compliant arterial system (in very young patients); both tend to lower mean arterial pressure (20–50 mm Hg) and can impair systemic perfusion. High flow rates (up to 200 mL/kg/min) may be necessary to ensure adequate perfusion in very young patients. As noted previously, some evidence suggests that pH-stat management during CPB may be associated with better neurological outcomes in children who will undergo circulatory arrest. Weaning from CPB is generally not a problem in pediatric patients if the surgical repair is adequate; primary pump failure is unusual. Difficulty in weaning should prompt the surgeon to check the repair and search for undiagnosed and uncorrected lesions. Intraoperative echocardiography, together with measurement of the pressure and oxygen saturation within the various chambers, may reveal the problem. Inotropic support may be provided by any of the agents used for adults. Calcium salts are more often useful in critically ill young patients than in adults as children more often have impaired calcium homeostasis; ionized calcium measurements are invaluable in such cases. Close monitoring of glucose is required because both hyperglycemia and hypoglycemia may be observed. Dopamine and epinephrine are the most commonly used inotropes in pediatric patients. Adding a phosphodiesterase inhibitor is also useful when PVR or SVR is increased. Hypocapnia, systemic alkalosis, and a high inspired oxygen concentration should also be used to decrease PVR in patients with pulmonary hypertension; additional pharmacological adjuncts may include prostaglandin E_1 (0.05–0.1 mcg/kg/min) or prostacyclin (1–40 mcg/kg/min). Inhaled nitric oxide may also be helpful for refractory pulmonary hypertension.

Children appear to have an intense inflammatory response during CPB that may be related to their blood being exposed to very large artificial surfaces relative to their size. Corticosteroids are often given to suppress this response. Many centers use modified ultrafiltration after weaning from CPB to partially correct the hemodilution but remove inflammatory vasoactive substances (cytokines); the technique takes blood from the aortic cannula and venous reservoir, passes it through an ultrafilter, and returns it to the right atrium.

Surgical correction of complex congenital lesions often requires a period of deep hypothermia with circulatory arrest (DHCA). Following institution of CPB, cooling is accomplished by a combination of surface cooling and a cold perfusate. At a core temperature of 15°C, up to 60 min of complete circulatory arrest may be feasible. Ice packing around the head is used to delay rewarming and promote cooling of the brain. Pharmacological brain protection is often attempted with methylprednisolone, 30 mg/kg, and mannitol, 0.5 g/kg. Following the repair, CPB flow is restarted, and rewarming takes place.

Postbypass Period

Because of the large priming volumes used (often 200–300% of the patient's blood volume), hemostatic defects from dilution of clotting factors and platelets are commonly seen after CPB in infants; in addition to heparin reversal, administration of fresh frozen plasma and platelets is often necessary.

Patients undergoing extensive or complicated procedures will often remain intubated. Extubation may be considered when the postoperative team is prepared for "fresh postops" who are extubated, and especially for older, relatively healthy patients undergoing simple procedures such as closure of a patent ductus or atrial septal defect or repair of coarctation of the aorta.

Cardiac Transplantation

Preoperative Considerations

Cardiac transplantation is the treatment of choice for patients with end-stage heart disease so severe that they are unlikely to survive the next 6 to 12 months. The procedure is generally associated with 80% to 90% postoperative survival at 1 year and 60% to 90% survival at 5 years. Transplantation improves quality of life, allowing most patients to resume a relatively normal lifestyle. The number of cardiac transplants is limited by the supply of donor hearts, which are obtained from brain-dead patients, most commonly following intracranial hemorrhage or head trauma.

Patients with intractable heart failure have an ejection fraction of less than 20% and fall into New York Heart Association functional class IV (see Chapter 21) and heart failure class D. For most patients, the primary diagnosis is cardiomyopathy. Intractable heart failure may be the result of a severe congenital lesion, ischemic cardiomyopathy, viral cardiomyopathy, peripartum cardiomyopathy, a failed prior transplantation, or valvular heart disease. Medical therapy should include the standard drugs used for heart failure, including angiotensin-converting enzyme inhibitors (or angiotensin receptor blockers, or both) and β blockade (usually with carvedilol). Many will receive electrical pacing with an automatic implanted defibrillator. Other drugs may include diuretics, vasodilators, and even oral inotropes; oral anticoagulation with warfarin may also be necessary. Patients may not be able to survive without intravenous inotropes while awaiting transplantation. Intraaortic balloon counterpulsation, an LVAD, or even a total mechanical heart may also be required for survival while the patient awaits a transplant.

Transplant candidates must not have experienced extensive end-organ damage or have other major systemic illnesses. Reversible kidney and hepatic dysfunction are common because of chronic hypoperfusion and venous congestion. PVR must be normal or at least responsive to oxygen or vasodilators. Irreversible pulmonary vascular disease with a PVR of more than 6 to 8 Wood units (1 Wood unit = 80 dyn·s·cm^{-5}) is a contraindication to cardiac transplantation because right ventricular failure is a major cause of early postoperative mortality. Patients with long-standing pulmonary hypertension may, however, be candidates for combined heart–lung transplantation.

Tissue cross-matching is generally not performed. Donor–recipient compatibility is based on size, ABO blood-group typing, and cytomegalovirus serology. Donor organs from patients with hepatitis B or C or HIV infections are excluded.

ANESTHETIC MANAGEMENT

Proper timing and coordination are necessary between the donor organ retrieval team and the transplant center. Premature induction of anesthesia unnecessarily prolongs the time under anesthesia for the recipient, whereas delayed induction may jeopardize graft function by prolonging the ischemia time of the donor heart.

Patients receive little advance warning of the availability of a suitable organ. Many will have eaten a recent meal and should be considered to have a full stomach. Oral cyclosporine must be given preoperatively. Administration of a clear antacid (sodium citrate), a histamine H_2-receptor blocker, and metoclopramide should be considered. Any sedating premedication may be administered intravenously just prior to induction.

Monitoring is similar to that used for other cardiac procedures. Strict asepsis should be observed during invasive procedures. Use of the right internal jugular vein for central access does not appear to compromise its future use for postoperative endomyocardial biopsies. A pulmonary artery catheter is used in many centers for postbypass management. It need not be placed in the pulmonary artery before CPB.

A rapid sequence induction may be performed. The principal objective of anesthetic management is to maintain organ perfusion until the patient is on CPB. Induction may be carried out with small doses of opioids (fentanyl, 5–10 mcg/kg) with or without etomidate (0.2–0.3 mg/kg). A low-dose ketamine–midazolam technique (as noted earlier) may also be suitable. Sufentanil, 5 mcg/kg, followed by succinylcholine, 1.5 mg/kg, can be used as a rapid-sequence technique. Anesthesia is maintained in a similar fashion as for other cardiac operations. A TEE probe is placed following induction, and antirejection drugs are given.

Sternotomy and cannulation for CPB may be complicated by scarring from prior cardiac operations. Aminocaproic acid or tranexamic acid can be used to decrease postoperative bleeding. CPB is initiated following cannulation of the aorta and both cavae. If a pulmonary artery catheter was placed, it must be completely withdrawn from the heart with its tip in the superior vena cava. It must remain within its sterile, protective sheath if it is to be safely refloated again into the pulmonary artery following CPB. The recipient's heart is then excised, allowing the posterior wall of both atria (with the caval and pulmonary vein openings) to remain. The atria of the donor heart are anastomosed to the recipient's atrial remnants (left side first). The aorta and then the pulmonary artery are anastomosed end to end. The donor heart is then flushed with saline, and intracardiac air is evacuated. Methylprednisolone is given before the aortic cross-clamp is released.

Inotropic support is usually started prior to separation from CPB to counteract bradycardia from sympathetic denervation. Prolonged graft ischemia may result in transient myocardial depression. Slow junctional rhythms are common and may require epicardial pacing. Although the transplanted heart is totally denervated and direct autonomic influences are absent, its response to circulating catecholamines is usually normal. The pulmonary artery catheter can be refloated into position after CPB and is used in conjunction with TEE to evaluate the patient. Right ventricular failure from pulmonary hypertension, a common post-CPB problem, can be treated with hyperventilation, prostaglandin E_1 (0.025–0.2 mcg/kg/min), inhaled nitric oxide (10–60 ppm), milrinone, or a right ventricular assist device (RVAD), if necessary. Bleeding is also a common problem.

Patients will be extubated when they meet criteria, as with other major cardiac operations. The postoperative course may be complicated by acute rejection, renal or hepatic dysfunction, or infections.

Many heart failure patients are treated with "destination" left ventricular assist devices (LVADs), as they do not qualify for heart transplantation. Moreover, there are insufficient donor hearts available to meet the needs of the heart failure population. Perioperative management concerns of the LVAD patient are similar to those of the heart failure patient as both procedures are surgical interventions to treat heart failure. Patients are routinely scheduled for LVAD placement as elective procedures. Such patients are frequently managed with home milrinone inotropic therapy and often are treated with furosemide infusions to promote diuresis while awaiting surgical intervention. Ideally, LVAD placement and heart transplantation occur before deterioration in hepatic and kidney function.

TEE examination is required perioperatively to rule out the presence of a patent foramen ovale or other conditions that could lead to a right-to-left

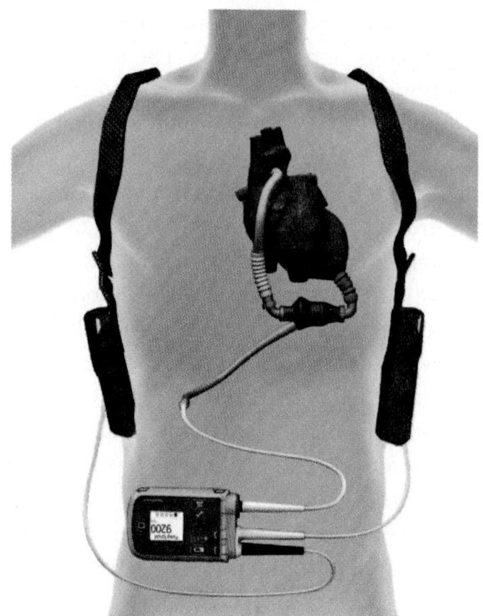

FIGURE 22–17 HeartMate II left ventricular assist device. (HeartMate II and St. Jude Medical are trademarks of St. Jude Medical, LLC or its related companies. Reproduced with permission of St. Jude Medical, ©2018. All rights reserved.)

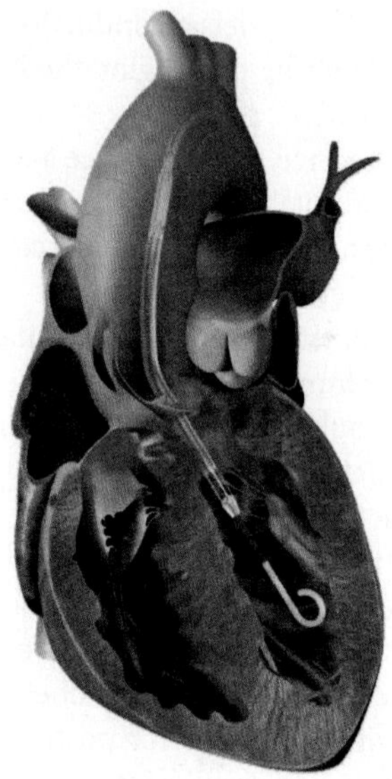

FIGURE 22–18 Impella percutaneous microaxial blood pump. (Reproduced with permission from Abiomed, Inc, Danvers, MA.)

shunt (eg, atrial septal defects) following LVAD placement. When activated, the LVAD drains blood from the left ventricle and in a nonpulsatile manner pumps it into the aorta (Figure 22–17). Left-sided heart pressures decrease. If right-sided pressures are greater than those of the left heart, venous blood will flow across an atrial septal defect or patent foramen ovale into the left atrium, decreasing arterial oxygen saturation.

Additionally, TEE examination is necessary to assess right heart function perioperatively. The right ventricle must sufficiently overcome any pulmonary hypertension to deliver an adequate blood volume to the left heart for the LVAD to pump into the aorta. Should the left heart be inadequately filled, the LVAD device will "suck down" the walls of the left ventricle, resulting in dramatically reduced LVAD pump flow.

A temporary RVAD may be needed perioperatively if right ventricular failure ensues. Pulmonary arterial vasodilators (eg, nitric oxide) are used to reduce pulmonary artery pressure and thus decrease the resistance against which the right ventricle must pump.

Various temporary assist devices are available to transiently support ventricular function. Percutaneous devices can be placed in the cardiac catheterization laboratory to support left ventricular function by pumping blood from the left ventricle and ejecting it past the aortic valve into the aorta. Often these devices are employed during percutaneous coronary artery interventions to support ventricular function. Patients in need of emergency coronary artery bypass surgery following failed percutaneous interventions will routinely present to the operating room supported with a percutaneous ventricular assist device (Figure 22–18).

PERICARDIAL DISEASE

The parietal pericardium is a fibrous membrane surrounding the heart, to which it normally is not adherent. The pericardium encompasses a relatively fixed intrapericardiac volume that includes a small volume of pericardial fluid (20–50 mL in adults), in addition to the heart and blood. As a result, the pericardium normally limits acute dilation of the ventricles and promotes diastolic coupling of the two ventricles (distention of one ventricle interferes with the filling of the other). The latter effect is also due to the interventricular septal wall they share. Moreover, diseases of the pericardium or larger pericardial fluid collections can seriously impair cardiac output.

Pericardial effusions may be due to viral, bacterial, or fungal infections; malignancies; bleeding after cardiac surgery; trauma; uremia; myocardial infarction; aortic dissection; hypersensitivity or autoimmune disorders; drugs; or myxedema.

1. Cardiac Tamponade

Preoperative Considerations

Cardiac tamponade exists when increased pericardial pressure impairs diastolic filling of the heart. Cardiac filling is ultimately related to the diastolic transmural (distending) pressure across each chamber, and any increase in pericardial pressure relative to the pressure within the chamber reduces filling. Pressure is applied equally to each cardiac chamber when the problem is a pericardial fluid collection, or it can be applied "selectively," as, for example, when an isolated pericardial blood clot compresses the left atrium. In general, the thin-walled atria and the right ventricle are more susceptible to pressure-induced abnormalities of filling than the left ventricle.

Pericardial pressure is normally similar to pleural pressure, varying with respiration between –4 and +4 mm Hg. Elevations in pericardial pressure are most commonly due to increases in pericardial fluid volume (as a consequence of effusions or bleeding). The magnitude of the increased pressure depends on both the volume of fluid and the rate of fluid accumulation; sudden increases exceeding 100 to 200 mL precipitously increase pericardial pressure, whereas very slow accumulations up to 1000 mL allow the pericardium to stretch with minimal increases in pericardial pressure.

The principal hemodynamic features of cardiac tamponade include decreased cardiac output from reduced stroke volume with an increase in central venous pressure. In the absence of severe left ventricular dysfunction, equalization of diastolic pressure occurs throughout the heart (right atrial pressure [RAP] = right ventricular end-diastolic pressure [RVEDP] = left atrial pressure [LAP] = left ventricular end-diastolic pressure [LVEDP]).

The central venous pressure waveform is a characteristic of cardiac tamponade. Impairment of both diastolic filling and atrial emptying abolishes the *y* descent; the *x* descent (systolic atrial filling) is normal or even accentuated. Reflex sympathetic activation is a prominent compensatory response in cardiac tamponade. The resulting increases in heart rate and contractility help maintain cardiac output. Arterial vasoconstriction (increased SVR) supports systemic blood pressure, whereas sympathetic activation reduces vascular capacitance, having the effect of an autotransfusion. Because stroke volume remains relatively fixed, cardiac output becomes primarily dependent on heart rate.

Acute cardiac tamponade usually presents as sudden hypotension, tachycardia, and tachypnea. Physical signs include jugular venous distention, a narrowed arterial pulse pressure, and muffled heart sounds. The patient may report an inability to lie flat. A prominent pulsus paradoxus (a cyclic inspiratory decrease in systolic blood pressure of more than 10 mm Hg) is typically present. The latter actually represents an exaggeration of a normal phenomenon related to inspiratory decreases in intrathoracic pressure. (A marked pulsus paradoxus may also be seen with severe airway obstruction or right ventricular infarction.) The heart may appear normal or enlarged on a chest radiograph. Electrocardiographic signs are generally nonspecific and are often limited to decreased voltage in all leads and nonspecific ST-segment and T-wave abnormalities. Electrical alternans (a cyclic alteration in the magnitude of the P waves, QRS complex, and T waves) may be seen with large pericardial effusions and is thought to be due to pendular swinging of the heart within the pericardium. Generalized ST-segment elevation may also be seen in two or three limb leads as well as V_2 to V_6 in the early phase of pericarditis. A friction rub may be heard by auscultation. Echocardiography is invaluable in diagnosing and measuring pericardial effusions and cardiac tamponade, and as a guide for accurate needle insertion for pericardiocentesis. Signs of tamponade include diastolic compression or collapse of the right atrium and right ventricle, leftward displacement of the ventricular septum, and an exaggerated increase in right ventricular size with a reciprocal decrease in left ventricular size during inspiration.

Anesthetic Considerations

Symptomatic cardiac tamponade requires evacuation of the pericardial fluid, either surgically or by pericardiocentesis. The latter is associated with a risk of lacerating the heart or coronary arteries and of pneumothorax. Traumatic postoperative (following thoracotomy) cardiac tamponade is nearly always treated surgically, whereas tamponade from other causes may more often be amenable to pericardiocentesis. Surgical treatment is also often undertaken for large recurrent pericardial effusions (infectious, malignant, autoimmune, uremic, or radiation induced) to prevent tamponade. Simple needle drainage of pericardial fluid may be achieved through a subxiphoid approach, whereas drainage combined with pericardial biopsy or pericardiectomy may be performed via a left anterior thoracotomy or median sternotomy. Drainage and biopsies can also be accomplished through left-sided thoracoscopy.

The anesthetic approach must be tailored to the patient. For the intubated postoperative cardiac patient in extremis, the chest may be reopened immediately in the ICU. For awake, conscious patients who will undergo left thoracotomy or median sternotomy, general anesthesia and endotracheal intubation are necessary. Local anesthesia may be used for patients undergoing simple drainage through a subxiphoid approach or pericardiocentesis. Removal of even a small volume of fluid may be sufficient to greatly improve cardiac output and allow safe induction of general anesthesia. Small doses (10 mg intravenously at a time) of ketamine also provide excellent supplemental analgesia.

16 Induction of general anesthesia in patients with cardiac tamponade can precipitate severe hypotension and cardiac arrest. We find it useful to have an epinephrine infusion available, and we sometimes initiate it before induction.

Large-bore intravenous access is mandatory. Monitoring of intraarterial pressure is useful, but placement of monitors should not delay pericardial drainage if the patient is unstable. The anesthetic technique should maintain an increased sympathetic tone until the tamponade is relieved; in other words, "deep" anesthesia is not the object. Cardiac depression, vasodilation, and slowing of the heart rate should be avoided. Similarly, increases in mean airway pressures can seriously jeopardize venous return. Awake intubation with maintenance of spontaneous ventilation is theoretically desirable but rarely done because coughing, straining, hypoxemia, and respiratory acidosis are detrimental and should be avoided. Thoracoscopy requires one-lung anesthesia.

Ketamine is the agent of choice for induction and maintenance until the tamponade is relieved. Small doses of epinephrine (5–10 mcg) may be useful as a temporary inotrope and chronotrope. Generous intravenous fluid administration is useful in maintaining cardiac output.

2. Constrictive Pericarditis

Preoperative Considerations

Constrictive pericarditis may develop as a sequela of acute or recurrent pericarditis. Pathologically, the pericardium is thickened, fibrotic, and often calcified. The parietal pericardium is typically adherent to the visceral pericardium on the heart, often obliterating the pericardial space. The stiffened parietal pericardium limits diastolic filling of the heart to a fixed and reduced volume. In contrast to acute cardiac tamponade, filling during early diastole is typically accentuated and manifested by a prominent y descent on the central venous pressure waveform.

Patients with constrictive pericarditis display jugular venous distention, hepatomegaly, and often ascites. Liver function may be abnormal. In contrast to acute tamponade, constrictive pericarditis prevents respiratory fluctuations in pericardial pressure; because venous return to the heart does not increase during inspiration, pulsus paradoxus is uncommon. In fact, venous pressure does not fall or may paradoxically rise during inspiration (Kussmaul sign). The chest radiograph will often reveal pericardial calcification. Low QRS voltage and diffuse T-wave abnormalities are usually present on the ECG. Atrial fibrillation and conduction blocks may be present. Echocardiography may be helpful in making the diagnosis.

Anesthetic Considerations

Pericardiectomy is usually reserved for patients with moderate to severe disease. The procedure is usually performed through a median sternotomy. It is complicated by the necessity for extensive manipulations of the heart that interfere with cardiac filling and ejection, induce frequent arrhythmias, and risk cardiac perforation. CPB may be required.

Selection of specific anesthetic agents is less important than avoiding excessive cardiac depression, vasodilation, and bradycardia. Cardiac output is generally rate dependent. Adequate large-bore intravenous access and direct arterial and central venous pressure monitoring are usually employed. Although cardiac function usually improves immediately following pericardiectomy, some patients display a persistently low cardiac output and require temporary postoperative inotropic support.

Anesthetic Management of Vascular Surgery

ANESTHESIA FOR SURGERY ON THE AORTA

Preoperative Considerations

Open surgery on the aorta represents a great challenge for anesthesiologists. Regardless of which part of the vessel is involved, the procedure is complicated by the need to cross-clamp the aorta and by the potential for large intraoperative blood losses. Aortic cross-clamping without CPB acutely increases left ventricular afterload and severely compromises organ perfusion distal to the point of occlusion. Severe hypertension, myocardial ischemia, left ventricular failure, or aortic valve regurgitation may be precipitated. Interruption of blood flow to the spinal cord, kidneys, and intestines can produce paraplegia, kidney failure, or intestinal infarction, respectively. Moreover, emergency aortic surgery is frequently necessary in critically ill patients who are acutely hypovolemic and have a high incidence of coexistent cardiac, renal, and pulmonary disease; hypertension; and diabetes. Advances in surgical techniques now permit many aortic lesions to be managed using stents, thereby avoiding many of the challenges presented by open surgery.

Indications for aortic surgery include aortic dissections, aneurysms, occlusive disease, trauma, and coarctation. Lesions of the ascending aorta lie between the aortic valve and the innominate artery, whereas lesions of the aortic arch lie between the innominate and left subclavian arteries. Disease distal to the left subclavian artery but above the diaphragm involves the descending thoracic aorta; lesions below the diaphragm involve the abdominal aorta.

SPECIFIC LESIONS OF THE AORTA

Aortic Dissection

In an aortic dissection, an intimal tear allows blood to track into the aortic wall (the media), creating a new pathway for blood flow. In many cases, a primary degenerative process called *cystic medial necrosis* predisposes for dissection to occur. Patients with hereditary connective tissue defects such as Marfan syndrome and Ehlers–Danlos syndrome eventually develop cystic medial necrosis and are at risk for aortic dissection. Propagation of the dissection is thought to occur as a result of hemodynamic shear forces acting on the intimal tear; indeed, hypertension is a common finding in patients with aortic dissection. Dissection can also occur from hemorrhage into an atheromatous plaque or at the aortic cannulation site following cardiac surgery.

Dissections may occlude the orifice of any artery arising directly from the aorta; they may extend into the aortic root, producing incompetence of the aortic valve; or they may rupture into the pericardium or pleura, producing cardiac tamponade or hemothorax, respectively. TEE plays an important role in diagnosing and characterizing aortic dissections. Dissections are most commonly of the proximal type (Stanford type A, De Bakey types I and II) involving the ascending aorta. Type II dissections do not extend beyond the innominate artery. Distal dissections (Stanford type B, De Bakey type III) originate beyond the left subclavian artery and propagate only distally. Proximal dissections are nearly always treated surgically, whereas distal dissections may be treated medically. In either case, from the time the diagnosis is suspected, measures to reduce systolic blood pressure (usually to 90–120 mm Hg) and aortic wall stress are initiated. These measures usually include intravenous vasodilators (nicardipine or nitroprusside) and β-adrenergic blockade (esmolol or a longer acting agent). The latter is important in reducing the shear forces related to the rate of rise of aortic pressure (*dP/dt*), which may actually increase with nitroprusside alone.

Aortic Aneurysms

Aneurysms more commonly occur in the abdominal than in the thoracic aorta. The vast majority of aortic aneurysms are due to atherosclerosis; cystic medial necrosis is also an important cause of thoracic aortic aneurysms. Syphilitic aneurysms characteristically involve the ascending aorta. Other etiologies include various connective tissue diseases and trauma. Dilation of the aortic root often produces aortic regurgitation. Expanding aneurysms of the upper thoracic aorta can also cause tracheal or bronchial compression or deviation, hemoptysis, and superior vena cava syndrome. Compression of the left recurrent laryngeal nerve produces hoarseness and left vocal cord paralysis. Distortion of the normal anatomy may also complicate endotracheal or endobronchial intubation or cannulation of the internal jugular and subclavian veins.

The greatest danger from untreated aortic aneurysms is rupture and exsanguination. A pseudoaneurysm forms when the intima and media are ruptured and only adventitia or blood clot forms the outer layer. Acute expansion (from leaking), manifested as sudden severe pain, may herald rupture. The likelihood of catastrophic rupture is related to size. The normal aorta in adults varies from 2 to 3 cm in width (it is wider cephalad). The data are clear for abdominal aortic aneurysms; rupture occurs in 50% of patients within 1 year when an aneurysm is 6 cm or greater in diameter. Elective treatment is generally performed in most patients with aneurysms 5 cm or greater. Most often this is accomplished with an intravascular stent; less often, open surgery and a prosthetic graft are used. The operative mortality rate is about 2% to 5% in good-risk patients and exceeds 50% if leaking or rupture has already occurred. The risks are much less with intravascular stenting, which has become the preferred procedure whenever the anatomy permits.

Occlusive Disease of the Aorta

Atherosclerotic obliteration of the aorta most commonly occurs near the aortic bifurcation (Leriche syndrome). Occlusion results from a combination of atherosclerotic plaque and thrombosis. Atherosclerosis is usually generalized and affects other parts of the arterial system, including the cerebral, coronary, and renal arteries. Treatment may be accomplished by intravascular stenting or by open surgery with an aortobifemoral bypass graft; proximal thromboendarterectomy may also be necessary.

Aortic Trauma

Aortic trauma may be penetrating or nonpenetrating. Both types of injuries can result in massive hemorrhage and require immediate operation. Whereas penetrating injuries are usually obvious, blunt aortic trauma may be easily overlooked if not suspected and the appropriate diagnostic testing performed. Nonpenetrating aortic trauma typically results from sudden high-speed decelerations such as those caused by automobile accidents (eg, in which the driver's chest impacts the steering wheel) and falls. The injury can vary from a partial tear to a complete aortic transection. Because the aortic arch is relatively fixed whereas the descending aorta is relatively mobile, the shear forces are greatest and the site of injury most common just distal to the subclavian artery. The most consistent initial finding is a widened mediastinum on a chest radiograph. Definitive diagnosis can be accomplished with magnetic resonance or computed tomographic imaging or TEE.

Coarctation of the Aorta

This congenital heart defect may be classified according to the position of the narrowed segment relative to the position of the ductus arteriosus. In the *preductal* (infantile) type, the narrowing occurs proximal to the opening of the ductus. This lesion, which is often associated with other congenital heart defects, is recognized in infancy because of a marked difference in perfusion between the upper and lower halves of the body; the lower half is cyanotic. Perfusion to the upper body is derived from the aorta, whereas perfusion to the lower body is primarily from the pulmonary artery. *Postductal* coarctation of the aorta may not be recognized until adulthood. The symptoms and hemodynamic significance of this lesion depend on the severity of the narrowing and the extent of collateral circulation that develops to the lower body (internal mammary, subscapular, and lateral thoracic to intercostal arteries). Hypertension in the upper body, with or without left ventricular failure, is usually present. So-called rib notching may be present on the chest radiograph as a result of dilated collateral intercostal arteries.

ANESTHETIC MANAGEMENT

Surgery on the Ascending Aorta

Surgery on the ascending aorta routinely uses median sternotomy and CPB and may also include DHCA. The conduct of anesthesia is similar to that for cardiac operations involving CPB, but the intraoperative course may be complicated by long aortic cross-clamp times and large intraoperative blood losses. TEE is especially useful. Blood loss can be reduced by administration of ε-aminocaproic acid or tranexamic acid. Concomitant aortic valve replacement and coronary reimplantation are often necessary (Bentall procedure). The radial artery cannulation site should be guided by the possible need for clamping of either the subclavian or innominate arteries during the procedure. Nicardipine or nitroprusside may be used for precise blood pressure control. β-Adrenergic blockade should also be employed in the presence of an aortic dissection. On the other hand, bradycardia worsens aortic regurgitation and should be avoided. The arterial inflow cannula for CPB is placed in a femoral artery for patients with dissections. In the event that sternotomy may rupture an aneurysm, prior establishment of partial CPB (using the femoral artery and femoral vein) should be considered.

Surgery Involving the Aortic Arch

These procedures are usually performed through a median sternotomy with DHCA (following institution of CPB). Additional considerations focus on achieving optimal cerebral protection with systemic and topical hypothermia (as noted earlier). Hypothermia to 15°C, drug infusion to maintain a flat EEG, methylprednisolone or dexamethasone, mannitol, and phenytoin are also commonly administered (but there is vanishingly small evidence for the efficacy of these drug treatments). The necessarily long rewarming periods probably contribute to the larger intraoperative blood losses commonly observed after CPB.

Surgery Involving the Descending Thoracic Aorta

Surgery limited to the descending thoracic aorta may be performed through a left thoracotomy without CPB, with or without (so-called "clamp-and-run" technique) a heparin-impregnated left ventricular apex to femoral artery shunt; or using partial right atrium to femoral artery bypass. Alternatively, stenting may obviate the need for complex open surgery. A thoracoabdominal incision is necessary for lesions that also involve the abdominal aorta. One-lung anesthesia greatly facilitates surgical exposure. Correct positioning of the endobronchial tube (even with fiberoptic bronchoscopy) may be difficult because of distortion of the anatomy. A double-lumen tube or a regular endotracheal tube with a bronchial blocker may be necessary.

The aorta must be cross-clamped above and below the lesion. Acute hypertension develops above the clamp, with hypotension below when there is no shunt or partial bypass. Arterial blood pressure should be monitored from the right radial artery, as clamping of the left subclavian artery may be necessary.
17 The sudden increase in left ventricular afterload after application of the aortic cross-clamp during aortic surgery may precipitate acute left ventricular failure and myocardial ischemia, particularly in patients with underlying ventricular dysfunction

or coronary disease; it can also exacerbate preexisting aortic regurgitation. Cardiac output falls, and left ventricular end-diastolic pressure and volume rise. The magnitude of these changes is inversely related to ventricular function. These effects can be ameliorated by the use of shunting or partial bypass. Moreover, the adverse effects of aortic clamping become less pronounced the more distal on the aorta that the clamp is applied. A vasodilator infusion is often needed to prevent excessive increases in blood pressure. In patients with good ventricular function, increasing anesthetic depth just prior to cross-clamping may also be helpful.

Excessive intraoperative bleeding may occur during these procedures. Prophylaxis with antifibrinolytic agents may be helpful. A blood scavenging device (cell saver) for autotransfusion is routinely used. Adequate venous access and intraoperative monitoring are critical. Multiple large-bore (14-gauge) intravenous catheters (preferably with blood warmers) are useful. Intraoperative TEE is often used. The period of greatest hemodynamic instability follows the release of the aortic cross-clamp; the abrupt decrease in afterload together with bleeding and the release of vasodilating acid metabolites from the ischemic lower body can precipitate severe systemic hypotension and, less commonly, hyperkalemia. Decreasing anesthetic depth, volume loading, and partial or slow release of the cross-clamp are helpful in avoiding severe hypotension. A bolus dose of a vasopressor may be necessary. Sodium bicarbonate is often given prophylactically and for persistent severe metabolic acidosis (pH <7.20) in association with hypotension. Calcium chloride may be necessary when symptomatic hypocalcemia follows massive transfusion of citrated blood products.

A. Paraplegia

Spinal cord ischemia can complicate thoracic aortic cross-clamping. The incidence of transient postoperative deficits and postoperative paraplegia are 11% and 6%, respectively. Increased rates are associated with cross-clamping periods longer than 30 min, extensive surgical dissections, and emergency procedures. The classic deficit is an anterior spinal artery syndrome with loss of motor function and pinprick sensation but preservation of vibration and proprioception. Anatomic variations in spinal cord blood supply are responsible for the unpredictable occurrence and variable nature of deficits. The spinal cord receives its blood supply from the vertebral arteries and from the thoracic and abdominal aorta. One anterior and two posterior arteries descend along the cord. Intercostal arteries feed the anterior and posterior arteries in the upper thoracic aorta. Textbook descriptions suggest that in the lower thoracic and lumbar cord, the anterior spinal artery is supplied by the thoracolumbar artery of Adamkiewicz. The truth is that a single large feeding artery cannot always be identified. When present, this artery has a variable origin from the aorta, arising between T5 and T8 in 15%, between T9 and T12 in 60%, and between L1 and L2 in 25% of individuals; it nearly always arises on the left side. It may be damaged during surgical dissection or occluded by the aortic cross-clamping. Monitoring motor and somatosensory evoked potentials may be useful in preventing paraplegia, but clearly surgical technique and speed are most important.

As noted earlier, the use of a temporary heparin-coated shunt or partial CPB with hypothermia maintains distal perfusion and decreases the incidence of paraplegia, hypertension, and ventricular failure. Partial CPB has the disadvantage of requiring heparinization, which increases blood loss. Using a heparin-coated shunt precludes the need for heparinization. It is usually positioned proximally in the left ventricular apex and distally in a femoral artery. Other therapeutic measures that may be protective of the spinal cord include methylprednisolone, mild hypothermia, mannitol, and drainage of cerebrospinal fluid (CSF) to reduce the CSF pressure. The efficacy of mannitol appears to be related to its ability to lower CSF pressure by decreasing its production. Spinal cord perfusion pressure is mean arterial blood pressure minus CSF pressure; the rise in CSF pressure following experimental cross-clamping of the aorta may explain how a mannitol-induced decrease in CSF pressure could improve spinal cord perfusion pressure during cross-clamping. Any protective effect of drainage of CSF via a lumbar catheter may have a similar mechanism.

The excessive use of vasodilators to control the hypertensive response to cross-clamping may be a contributing factor in spinal cord ischemia because drug actions also occur distal to the cross-clamp. Excessive reduction in blood pressure above the cross-clamp should therefore be avoided to prevent inadequate blood flow and excessive hypotension below it.

B. Kidney Failure

An increased incidence of acute kidney failure following aortic surgery is reported after emergency procedures, prolonged cross-clamping periods, and prolonged hypotension, particularly in patients with preexisting kidney disease. A variety of "cocktails" have been employed in the hope of reducing the risk of kidney failure, including infusion of mannitol (0.5 g/kg) prior to cross-clamping, furosemide, and fenoldopam (or low-dose dopamine); however, there is no convincing evidence that these treatments improve renal outcomes.

Surgery on the Abdominal Aorta

Stents are most often placed via catheters inserted in a femoral artery in awake but sedated patients. When an open technique is chosen, either an anterior transperitoneal or an anterolateral retroperitoneal approach can be used to access the abdominal aorta. Depending on the location of the lesion, the cross-clamp can be applied to the supraceliac, suprarenal, or infrarenal aorta. Heparin is usually administered prior to aortic clamping. Intraarterial blood pressure can be monitored from either upper extremity. In general, the more distally the clamp is applied to the aorta, the less the effect on left ventricular afterload. In fact, occlusion of the infrarenal aorta frequently results in minimal hemodynamic changes. In contrast, release of the clamp usually produces hypotension; the same techniques that were described earlier may be used to counteract the effects of unclamping. The large incision and extensive retroperitoneal surgical dissection increase fluid requirements beyond intraoperative blood loss. Fluid replacement may be guided by monitoring central venous pressure, or better, noninvasive monitors of stroke volume or TEE.

Clamping of the infrarenal aorta nevertheless decreases renal blood flow, which may contribute to postoperative kidney failure. The decrease in renal blood flow is not prevented by epidural anesthesia or blockade of the renin–angiotensin system. Some centers use continuous epidural anesthesia combined with general anesthesia for abdominal aortic surgery. This combined technique decreases the general anesthetic requirement and provides an excellent route for administering postoperative analgesia. Systemic heparinization during surgery introduces concern regarding the risk of paraplegia secondary to an epidural hematoma; however, all credible studies suggest that when the catheter is placed atraumatically well in advance of heparinization and removed after reversal of anticoagulation there is no increased risk of neuraxial hematoma.

Postoperative Considerations

Those undergoing stenting may not require intubation either during or after the procedure. Most patients undergoing open surgery on the ascending aorta, the arch, or the thoracic aorta will remain intubated and ventilated for 1 to 24 h postoperatively. As with cardiac surgery, the initial emphasis in their postoperative care should be on hemodynamic stability and monitoring for postoperative bleeding. Patients undergoing open abdominal aortic surgery may be extubated at the end of the procedure.

NONOPERATING ROOM ANESTHESIA (NORA) FOR CARDIOLOGY

Cardiac Catheterization Laboratory/Suite

Patients presenting with acute coronary syndrome are always a challenge. Interventional cardiology has seen tremendous growth as technology has improved. This growth has resulted in a greater anesthetic challenge: routine surgical revascularizations are less frequent, patients undergoing surgical revascularization are more medically complex, and an increasing number of medically complicated patients now undergo noninvasive cardiac interventions. Complete revascularization is preferred for both acute and chronic coronary syndromes; however, patients with acute coronary syndrome and cardiogenic shock may undergo culprit lesion revascularization followed by complete revascularization at a later date. These patients may need to be supported with temporary mechanical devices such as an intraaortic balloon pump (IABP), extracorporeal membrane oxygenation (ECMO), or any of a variety of new devices, including Tandem Heart (inflow: left atrium through trans-septal puncture; outflow: femoral artery; pump: paracorporeal); Impella (inflow: left ventricle; outflow: aorta; pump: trans-aortic); and Centrimag (inflow: left ventricle and femoral vein; outflow: axillary artery; pump: external). Sometimes there will be a combination of devices like ECMO with Impella (ECMELLA).

Electrophysiology Laboratory/Suite

Atrial fibrillation is the most common sustained arrhythmia in adults. It is associated with increased mortality and morbidities, including stroke, heart failure, and dementia. There is a trend to prefer endocardial ablation rather than medical therapy for atrial fibrillation.

Ablation for atrial fibrillation may be performed with either sedation or general anesthesia with a laryngeal mask airway or endotracheal tube. Neither method has been shown to be superior to the other. Three major complications may arise from ablations: atrioesophageal fistula, atrial perforation leading to tamponade, and phrenic nerve injury. The proceduralist may request spontaneous ventilation to monitor phrenic nerve integrity. An esophageal temperature probe and an esophageal retraction device (placed through an orogastric tube) may be requested.

Interventional TEE

There now are a number of nonsurgical interventions for structural heart disease, and interventional transesophageal echocardiography (iTEE) has been consistently requested. Transcatheter aortic valve replacement (TAVR) has been the most common of these procedures. General endotracheal tube anesthesia with TEE was initially the rule for TAVRs; however, currently, most centers use sedation with transthoracic echocardiography for all but transapical approaches where general anesthesia with TEE remains the method of choice.

Percutaneous interventions are now available for the mitral valve. TEE is vital during percutaneous mitral valve repairs or replacements. Percutaneous closure has become a treatment of choice for residual postsurgical paravalvular leaks after mitral valve replacement. For treatment of persistent atrial fibrillation, left atrial appendage occlusion devices are being used (WatchMan, Amulet, Lariat) for patients who are unable to tolerate anticoagulation. Similar to edge-to-edge mitral valve repair, these procedures involve transseptal puncture guided by TEE and fluoroscopy and then implantation of the device. Atrial septal defects and persistent foramen ovale in adults may be closed percutaneously. TEE is often used for larger defects.

PREGNANCY AND HEART DISEASE

Both acquired and congenital heart disease may present in pregnancy. Of all the developed countries, the United States has the highest maternal mortality rate, and cardiovascular disease is a major contributor. Peripartum cardiomyopathy, pulmonary hypertension, and ischemic heart disease are commonly acquired forms of cardiovascular disease. Patients may present with uncorrected congenital heart disease or sequelae from prior corrective surgeries.

ANESTHESIA FOR CAROTID ARTERY SURGERY

Preoperative Considerations

Ischemic cerebrovascular disease accounts for 80% of strokes; the remaining 20% are due to hemorrhage. Ischemic strokes are usually the result of embolism or (less commonly) thrombosis in one of the blood vessels supplying the brain. Ischemic stroke may follow severe vasospasm after subarachnoid hemorrhage. By convention, a stroke is defined as a neurological deficit that lasts more than 24 h; its pathological correlate is typically focal infarction of the brain. Transient ischemic attacks (TIAs), on the other hand, are neurological deficits that resolve within 24 h; they may be due to a low-flow state at a tightly stenotic lesion or to emboli that arise from an extracranial vessel or the heart. When a stroke is associated with progressive worsening of signs and symptoms, it is frequently termed a *stroke in evolution*. A second distinction is also often made between complete and incomplete strokes, based on whether the territory involved is completely affected or additional brain remains at risk for focal ischemia (eg, hemiplegia vs hemiparesis). The bifurcation of the common carotid artery (the origin of the internal carotid artery) is a common site of atherosclerotic plaques that may lead to TIA or stroke. The mechanism may be embolization of platelet-fibrin or plaque material, stenosis, or complete occlusion. The last may be the result of thrombosis or hemorrhage into a plaque. Symptoms depend on the adequacy of collateral circulation. Emboli distal to regions lacking collateral blood flow are more likely to produce symptoms. Small emboli in the ophthalmic branches can cause transient monocular blindness (amaurosis fugax). Larger emboli usually enter the middle cerebral artery, producing contralateral motor and sensory deficits that primarily affect the arm and face. Aphasia also develops if the dominant hemisphere is affected. Emboli in the anterior cerebral artery territory typically result in contralateral motor and sensory deficits that are worse in the leg. It is common for TIAs or minor strokes to precede a major stroke.

Indications for surgical interventions include TIAs associated with ipsilateral severe carotid stenosis (>70% occlusion), severe ipsilateral stenosis in a patient with a minor (incomplete) stroke, and 30% to 70% occlusion in a patient with ipsilateral symptoms (usually an ulcerated plaque). In the past, carotid endarterectomy was recommended for asymptomatic but significantly stenotic lesions (>60%). Currently, stenting would be the recommendation. Operative mortality for open surgery is 1% to 4% and is primarily due to cardiac complications (myocardial infarction). Perioperative morbidity is 4% to 10% and is principally neurological; patients with preexisting neurological deficits have the greatest risk of perioperative neurological events. **Studies suggest that age greater than 75 years, symptomatic lesions, uncontrolled hypertension, angina, carotid thrombus, and occlusions near the carotid siphon increase operative risk.**

Over the last two decades, the incidence of complications has been greatly reduced. There remains controversy regarding the choice of anesthetic: cervical plexus block with sedation or general endotracheal anesthesia with neuromonitoring.

Preoperative Anesthetic Evaluation & Management

Most patients undergoing carotid endarterectomy are older adults and hypertensive, with generalized arteriosclerosis. Many also have diabetes. Preoperative evaluation and management should focus on defining preexisting neurological deficits as well as optimizing the patient's clinical status in terms of coexisting diseases. Most postoperative neurological deficits appear to be related to surgical technique. Uncontrolled perioperative hyperglycemia can increase morbidity by enhancing ischemic cerebral injury.

Patients should receive their usual cardiac medications on schedule until the time of surgery. Blood pressure and the blood glucose concentration should be controlled. Angina should be stable and controlled, and signs of overt congestive heart failure should be absent. Because most patients are older adults, enhanced sensitivity to premedication should be expected.

General Anesthesia

18 The emphasis of anesthetic management during carotid surgery is on maintaining adequate perfusion to the brain and heart. Traditionally, this is accomplished by close regulation of arterial blood pressure and avoidance of tachycardia. Monitoring of intraarterial pressure is therefore nearly always done. Electrocardiographic monitoring should include the V_5 lead to detect ischemia. Continuous computerized ST-segment analysis is desirable. Carotid endarterectomy is not usually associated with significant blood loss or fluid shifts.

Regardless of the anesthetic agents selected, mean arterial blood pressure should be maintained at—or slightly above—the patient's usual range. Propofol and etomidate are popular choices for induction because they reduce cerebral metabolic rate proportionately more than cerebral blood flow. Small doses of an opioid or β-adrenergic blocker can be used to blunt the hypertensive response to endotracheal intubation. In theory, isoflurane may be the volatile agent of choice because it appears to provide the greatest protection against cerebral ischemia. However, we do not regard the differences in neuroprotection among inhaled agents as clinically important. Some clinicians also prefer remifentanil as the opioid for rapid emergence.

Intraoperative hypertension is common and generally necessitates the use of an intravenous vasodilator. Nitroglycerin is usually a good choice for mild to moderate hypertension because of its beneficial effects on coronary circulation. Marked hypertension requires a more potent agent, such as nicardipine, nitroprusside, or clevidipine. β-Adrenergic blockade facilitates the management of the hypertension and prevents reflex tachycardia from vasodilators, but it should be used cautiously. Hypotension should be treated with vasopressors. Many clinicians consider phenylephrine the vasopressor of choice; if selected, it should be administered in small increments to prevent excessive hypertension.

Pronounced or sustained reflex bradycardia or heart block caused by manipulation of the carotid baroreceptor can be treated with atropine. To prevent this response, some surgeons infiltrate the area of the carotid sinus with lidocaine, but the infiltration itself can induce bradycardia. Arterial CO_2 tension should be maintained in the normal range because hypercapnia can induce intracerebral steal, whereas extreme hypocapnia decreases cerebral perfusion. Ventilation should be adjusted to maintain normocapnia. Maintenance intravenous fluids should consist of glucose-free solutions because of the potentially adverse effects of hyperglycemia, particularly on ischemic neurons. Heparin (5000–7500 units intravenously) is usually administered prior to occlusion of the carotid artery. Some clinicians routinely use a shunt (as noted below). Protamine is usually given to reverse heparin prior to skin closure.

Rapid emergence from anesthesia is desirable because it allows immediate neurological assessment, but the clinician must be prepared to treat hypertension and tachycardia. **Postoperative hypertension may be related to surgical denervation of the ipsilateral carotid baroreceptor. Denervation of the carotid body blunts the ventilatory response to hypoxemia.** Following extubation, patients should be observed closely for the development of a wound hematoma. When an expanding wound hematoma compromises the airway, the initial treatment maneuver may require opening the wound to release the hematoma. Transient postoperative hoarseness and ipsilateral deviation of the tongue may be noted; they are due to intraoperative retraction of the recurrent laryngeal or hypoglossal nerves, respectively.

Monitoring Cerebral Function

When general anesthesia is selected for these patients, near-infrared spectroscopy (NIRS) for cerebral oximetry may be a quick way to address hemispheric desaturation if it were to happen during temporary clamping and assess the need for a shunt. Again, there are equivocal data regarding shunting and outcomes for carotid endarterectomy surgeries. The risk of shunting is embolization, and the risk of not shunting is cerebral hypoxemia.

Some surgeons routinely use a shunt, but this practice may increase the incidence of postoperative neurological deficits; shunt insertion can dislodge and embolize atheromata. Another way to detect the adequacy of the blood supply (through a presumed complete circle of Willis from the contralateral side) is to measure the "stump pressure" in the internal carotid artery cranial to the temporary clamp. If the stump pressure is less than 50 mm Hg, a shunt may need to be considered.

Other centers monitor EEG or somatosensory evoked potentials (SSEPs) to determine whether a shunt is needed. Electrophysiological signs of ischemia after cross-clamping dictate the use of a shunt; changes lasting more than 10 min may be associated with a new postoperative neurological deficit. Although multichannel recordings and computer processing can enhance the sensitivity of the EEG, neither EEG nor SSEP monitoring is sufficiently sensitive or specific to reliably predict the need for shunting or the occurrence of postoperative deficits (see case discussion in Chapter 26). Other techniques, including measurements of regional cerebral blood flow with radioactive xenon-133, transcranial Doppler measurement of middle cerebral artery flow velocity, jugular venous oxygen saturation, and transconjunctival oxygen tension, are also not sufficiently reliable.

Regional Anesthesia

Carotid surgery may be performed under regional anesthesia. Blockade of the superficial cervical plexus effectively blocks the C2 to C4 nerves and allows the patient to remain comfortably awake during surgery. Deep cervical plexus block is not required. A substantial fraction of patients will require administration of local anesthetic by the surgeon into the carotid sheath (whether or not a deep cervical block is performed). The principal advantage of regional anesthesia (and it is a tremendous advantage) is that the patient can be examined intraoperatively; thus, the need for a temporary shunt can be assessed and any new neurological deficits diagnosed immediately during surgery. In fact, an intraoperative neurological examination may be the most reliable method for assessing the adequacy of cerebral perfusion during carotid cross-clamping. The examination minimally consists of level of consciousness, speech, and contralateral handgrip. Experienced clinicians use minimal sedation and "cocktail conversation" with the patient to monitor the neurological status. Some studies also suggest that when compared with general anesthesia, regional anesthesia results in more stable hemodynamics, but outcomes appear similar. Regional anesthesia for carotid surgery requires the cooperation of the surgeon and patient.

Stenting Procedures

These procedures are usually performed in awake, minimally sedated patients. Good intravenous access and invasive arterial pressure monitoring will be required. The operator will often want to communicate with the patient during the procedure. The stent will be introduced and guided by cerebral arteriography. Intraoperative and postoperative blood pressure issues are similar to those with open carotid endarterectomy.

CASE DISCUSSION

A Patient for Cardioversion

A 55-year-old man with new-onset atrial fibrillation is scheduled for elective cardioversion.

What are the indications for an elective cardioversion?

Direct current (DC) cardioversion may be used to terminate supraventricular and ventricular tachyarrhythmias caused by reentry. It is not effective for arrhythmias from enhanced automaticity (multifocal atrial tachycardia) or triggered activity (digitalis toxicity). By simultaneously depolarizing the entire myocardium and possibly prolonging the refractory period, DC cardioversion can terminate atrial fibrillation and flutter, atrioventricular nodal reentry, reciprocating tachycardias from preexcitation syndromes, and ventricular tachycardia or fibrillation.

Specific indications for cardioversion of patients with atrial fibrillation include symptomatic fibrillation, recent onset, and no response to medications. Patients with long-standing fibrillation, a large atrium, chronic obstructive lung disease, congestive heart failure, or mitral regurgitation have a high recurrence rate. A TEE is often performed shortly before cardioversion to rule out left atrial blood clots. Such clots are typically located in the left atrial appendage and can be embolized by the cardioversion procedure or by sinus rhythm.

Emergency cardioversion is indicated for any tachyarrhythmia associated with hypotension, heart failure, or angina.

How is cardioversion performed?

Although the procedure is usually performed by cardiologists, the need for immediate cardioversion may arise in the operating room, ICU, or during cardiopulmonary resuscitation. Anesthesiologists must therefore be familiar with the technique. Following deep sedation or light general anesthesia, DC shock is applied by either self-adhesive pads or 8- to 13-cm paddles. Larger paddles help reduce any shock-induced myocardial necrosis by distributing the current over a wider area. The energy output should be kept at the minimally effective level to prevent myocardial damage. Placement of the electrodes can be anterolateral or anteroposterior. In the first position, one electrode is placed on the right second intercostal space next to the sternum, and the other is placed on the left fifth intercostal space in the midclavicular line. When pads are used for the anteroposterior technique, one is placed anteriorly over the ventricular apex in the fifth intercostal space and the other underneath the patient in the left infrascapular region.

For supraventricular tachycardias, with the notable exception of atrial fibrillation, energy levels of 25 to 50 J can successfully reestablish normal sinus rhythm. Synchronized shocks should be used for all tachyarrhythmias except ventricular fibrillation. Synchronization times the delivery so that it is given during the QRS complex. If the shock occurs in the ST segment or the T wave (unsynchronized), it can precipitate a more serious arrhythmia, including ventricular fibrillation. All medical personnel should stand clear of the patient and the bed during the shock.

Atrial fibrillation usually requires a minimum of 50 to 100 J, and larger energy levels are often used. Hemodynamically stable ventricular tachycardia can often be terminated with 25 to 50 J, but ventricular fibrillation and unstable ventricular tachycardia require 200 to 360 J. Regardless of the arrhythmia, a higher energy level is necessary when the first shock is ineffective.

The cardiologist wants to do the cardioversion in the postanesthesia care unit (PACU). Is this an appropriate place for cardioversion?

Elective cardioversion can be performed in any setting in which full provisions for cardiopulmonary resuscitation, including cardiac pacing capabilities, are immediately available. A physician skilled in airway management should be in attendance. Cardioversions are commonly performed in an ICU, emergency department, PACU, procedure room, or cardiac catheterization suite.

How would you evaluate this patient?

The patient should be fasted, evaluated, and treated as though he were receiving a general anesthetic in the operating room. An ECG is performed immediately before the procedure to confirm that the arrhythmia is still present; another is performed immediately afterward to confirm the new rhythm. Preoperative laboratory values should be within normal limits because metabolic disorders, particularly electrolyte and acid–base abnormalities, may contribute to the arrhythmia. If not corrected preoperatively, they can reinitiate the tachycardia following cardioversion. An antiarrhythmic agent is often started in patients with atrial fibrillation 1 to 2 days prior to the procedure to help maintain normal sinus rhythm. Patients with atrial fibrillation of longer than a few hours duration likely will have been anticoagulated for a sufficient time prior to cardioversion to reduce the likelihood of a left atrial thrombus. Such clots may embolize upon restoration of a sinus rhythm.

What are the minimum monitors and anesthetic equipment required?

Minimum monitoring consists of the ECG, blood pressure, and pulse oximetry. A precordial stethoscope is useful for monitoring breath sounds before and after the procedure. Maintaining continuous verbal contact with the patient may be the best method for assessing whether a sufficient amnestic dose of (usually) propofol has been given.

In addition to a DC defibrillator capable of delivering up to 400 J (synchronized or unsynchronized) and transcutaneous pacing, the minimum equipment should include the following:

- Reliable intravenous access.
- A functional bag-mask device capable of delivering 100% oxygen (see Chapter 3).
- An oxygen source from a wall outlet or a full tank.
- An airway kit with oral and nasal airways and appropriate laryngoscopes and endotracheal tubes.
- A functional suction apparatus.
- An anesthetic drug kit that includes at least one sedative-hypnotic as well as succinylcholine.
- A cart that includes all necessary drugs and equipment for cardiopulmonary resuscitation (see Chapter 55).

What anesthetic techniques would be appropriate?

Premedication is not necessary. Only very brief (1–2 min) light general anesthesia is required. A short-acting agent such as propofol or methohexital is customarily used. Etomidate may be used but may be associated with phonation. Following preoxygenation with 60% to 100% oxygen for 3 to 5 min, the sedative-hypnotic is given in small increments) every 30 to 60 s while maintaining verbal contact with the patient. The shock is delivered when the patient is no longer able to respond verbally; some clinicians use loss of the eyelid reflex as an endpoint. The shock usually arouses the patient. Transient airway obstruction or apnea may be observed, particularly if more than one shock is necessary.

What are the complications of cardioversion?

Complications include transient myocardial depression, postshock arrhythmias, and arterial embolism. Arrhythmias are usually due to inadequate synchronization, but even a properly timed cardioversion can occasionally result in ventricular fibrillation. Most arrhythmias are transient and resolve spontaneously. Although patients may develop ST-segment elevation, serum creatine phosphokinase levels (MB fraction) are usually normal. Embolism of a left-sided clot may be responsible for delayed awakening.

How should the patient be cared for following cardioversion?

Although recovery of consciousness is usually very rapid, patients should be treated like others receiving general anesthesia (see Chapter 56). Recovery also specifically includes monitoring for both recurrence of the arrhythmia and signs of cerebral embolism.

GUIDELINES

American Society of Extracorporeal Technology Standards and Guidelines for Perfusion Practice (11/08/2013). http://www.amsect.org/page/standards-and-guidelines-1117

Authors/Task Force Members, Kunst G, Milojevic M, Boer C, et al; EACTS/EACTA/EBCP Committee Reviewers. 2019 EACTS/EACTA/EBCP guidelines on cardiopulmonary bypass in adult cardiac surgery. *Br J Anaesth.* 2019;123:713.

Hiratzka LF, Bakris GL, Beckman JA, et al. 2010 ACCF/AHA/AATS/ACR/ASA/SCA/SCAI/SIR/STS/SVM Guidelines for the diagnosis and management of patients with thoracic aortic disease: executive summary: a report of the American College of Cardiology Foundation/American Heart Association Task Force on Practice Guidelines, American Association for Thoracic Surgery, American College of Radiology, American Stroke Association, Society of Cardiovascular Anesthesiologists, Society for Cardiovascular Angiography and Interventions, Society of Interventional Radiology, Society of Thoracic Surgeons, and Society for Vascular Medicine. *Anesth Analg.* 2010;111:279.

Nishimura RA, Otto CM, Bonow RO, et al. 2017 AHA/ACC focused update of the 2014 AHA/ACC guideline for the management of patients with valvular heart disease: a report of the American College of Cardiology/American Heart Association task force on clinical practice guidelines. *Circulation.* 2017;135:e1159.

Shore-Lesserson L, Baker RA, Ferraris VA, et al. The Society of Thoracic Surgeons, The Society of Cardiovascular Anesthesiologists, and The American Society of ExtraCorporeal Technology: clinical practice guidelines-anticoagulation during cardiopulmonary bypass. *Anesth Analg.* 2018;126:413.

Wahba A, Milojevic M, Boer C, et al; EACTS/EACTA/EBCP Committee Reviewers. 2019 EACTS/EACTA/EBCP guidelines on cardiopulmonary bypass in adult cardiac surgery. *Eur J Cardiothorac Surg.* 2020;57:210.

Writing Committee Members, Otto CM, Nishimura RA, Bonow RO, et al. 2020 ACC/AHA guideline for the management of patients with valvular heart disease: a report of the American College of Cardiology/American Heart Association joint committee on clinical practice guidelines. *J Am Coll Cardiol.* 2021;77:e25.

See www.guidelines.gov for additional guidelines from multiple organizations related to these topics.

SUGGESTED READINGS

Engelman R, Baker RA, Likosky DS, et al. The Society of Thoracic Surgeons, The Society of Cardiovascular Anesthesiologists, and The American Society of ExtraCorporeal Technology: clinical practice guidelines for cardiopulmonary bypass—temperature management during cardiopulmonary bypass. *J Extra Corpor Technol.* 2015;47:145.

Fedorow CA, Moon MC, Mutch WA, Grocott HP. Lumbar cerebrospinal fluid drainage for thoracoabdominal aortic surgery: rationale and practical considerations for management. *Anesth Analg.* 2010;111:46.

Fudulu D, Benedetto U, Pecchinenda GG, et al. Current outcomes of off-pump versus on-pump coronary artery bypass grafting: evidence from randomized controlled trials. *J Thorac Dis*. 2016;8(suppl 10):S758.

Hessel EA 2nd. What's new in cardiopulmonary bypass. *J Cardiothorac Vasc Anesth*. 2019;33:2296.

Hosseinian L, Weiner M, Levin MA, Fischer GW. Methylene blue: magic bullet for vasoplegia? *Anesth Analg*. 2016;122:194.

Meersch M, Zarbock A. Prevention of cardiac surgery-associated acute kidney injury. *Curr Opin Anaesthesiol*. 2017;30:76.

Parissis H, Lau MC, Parissis M, et al. Current randomized control trials, observational studies and meta-analysis in off-pump coronary surgery. *J Cardiothorac Surg*. 2015;10:185.

Seco M, Edelman JJ, Van Boxtel B, et al. Neurologic injury and protection in adult cardiac and aortic surgery. *J Cardiothorac Vasc Anesth*. 2015;29:185.

Smilowitz NR, Berger JS. Perioperative management to reduce cardiovascular events. *Circulation*. 2016;133:1125.

Wilkey BJ, Weitzel NS. Anesthetic considerations for surgery on the aortic arch. *Semin Cardiothorac Vasc Anesth*. 2016;20:265.

Wong WT, Lai VK, Chee YE, Lee A. Fast-track cardiac care for adult cardiac surgical patients. *Cochrane Database Syst Rev*. 2016;(9):CD003587.

CHAPTER 23

Respiratory Physiology & Anesthesia

KEY CONCEPTS

1. The trachea serves as a conduit for ventilation and for clearance of tracheal and bronchial secretions and has an average length of 10 to 13 cm. The trachea bifurcates at the carina into the right and left mainstem bronchi. The right mainstem bronchus lies in a more linear arrangement with the trachea, whereas the left mainstem bronchus lies in a more angular orientation with the trachea.

2. The periodic exchange of alveolar gas with the fresh gas from the upper airway reoxygenates desaturated blood and eliminates carbon dioxide (CO_2). This exchange is normally brought about by small cyclic pressure gradients established within the airways. During spontaneous ventilation, these gradients are secondary to variations in intrathoracic pressure; during mechanical ventilation, they are produced by intermittent positive pressure in the upper airway.

3. The lung volume at the end of a normal exhalation is called *functional residual capacity* (FRC). At this volume, the inward elastic recoil of the lung approximates the outward elastic recoil of the chest (including resting diaphragmatic tone).

4. Closing capacity is normally well below FRC, but it rises steadily with age. This increase is probably responsible for the normal age-related decline in arterial O_2 tension.

5. Whereas both forced expiratory volume in the first second of exhalation (FEV_1) and forced vital capacity (FVC) are effort dependent, forced midexpiratory flow ($FEF_{25-75\%}$) is more effort independent and may be a more reliable measure of obstruction.

6. Changes in lung mechanics due to general anesthesia occur shortly after induction. The supine position reduces the FRC by 0.8 to 1.0 L, and induction of general anesthesia further reduces the FRC by 0.4 to 0.5 L. FRC reduction is a consequence of alveolar collapse, and compression atelectasis is due to loss of inspiratory muscle tone, change in chest wall rigidity, and upward shift of the diaphragm.

7. Local factors are more important than the autonomic system in influencing pulmonary vascular tone. Hypoxia is a powerful stimulus for pulmonary vasoconstriction (the opposite of its systemic effect).

8. Because alveolar ventilation ($\dot{V}_A$) is normally about 4 L/min and pulmonary capillary perfusion ($\dot{Q}$) is 5 L/min, the overall ratio is about 0.8.

9. Shunting denotes the process whereby desaturated, mixed venous blood from the right heart returns to the left heart without being oxygenated in the lungs. The overall effect of shunting is to decrease (dilute) arterial O_2 content; this type of shunt is referred to as *right-to-left*.

— Continued next page

Continued—

10 General anesthesia commonly increases venous admixture to 5% to 10%, probably as a result of atelectasis and airway collapse in dependent areas of the lung.

11 Note that large increases in $PaCO_2$ (>75 mm Hg) readily produce hypoxia (PaO_2 <60 mm Hg) at room air but not at high inspired O_2 concentrations.

12 The binding of O_2 to hemoglobin seems to be the principal rate-limiting factor in the transfer of O_2 from alveolar gas to blood.

13 The greater the shunt, the less likely the possibility that an increase in the fraction of inspired oxygen (FiO_2) will correct hypoxemia.

14 A rightward shift in the oxygen–hemoglobin dissociation curve lowers O_2 affinity, displaces O_2 from hemoglobin, and makes more O_2 available to tissues; a leftward shift increases hemoglobin's affinity for O_2, reducing its availability to tissues.

15 Bicarbonate represents the largest fraction of CO_2 in blood.

16 Central chemoreceptors are thought to lie on the anterolateral surface of the medulla and respond primarily to changes in cerebrospinal fluid [H^+]. This mechanism is effective in regulating $PaCO_2$ because the blood–brain barrier is permeable to dissolved CO_2 but not to bicarbonate ions.

17 With increasing depth of anesthesia, the slope of the $PaCO_2$/min ventilation curve decreases, and the apneic threshold increases.

The importance of pulmonary physiology to anesthetic practice is obvious. Inhalation anesthetics depend on the lungs for their uptake and elimination. Both inhalation and intravenously administered anesthetics produce prominent respiratory side effects. Moreover, muscle paralysis, unusual positioning during surgery, and techniques such as one-lung anesthesia and cardiopulmonary bypass profoundly alter normal pulmonary physiology.

This chapter reviews the basic pulmonary concepts necessary for understanding and applying anesthetic techniques. Although the pulmonary effects of each of the various anesthetic agents are discussed elsewhere in the book, this chapter also reviews the overall effects of general anesthesia on lung function.

FUNCTIONAL RESPIRATORY ANATOMY

1. Rib Cage & Muscles of Respiration

The rib cage contains the two lungs, each surrounded by its own pleura. The apex of the chest is small, allowing only for entry of the trachea, esophagus, and blood vessels, whereas the base is formed by the diaphragm. Contraction of the diaphragm—the principal pulmonary muscle—causes the base of the thoracic cavity to descend 1.5 to 7 cm and its contents (the lungs) to expand. Diaphragmatic movement normally accounts for 75% of the change in chest volume. Accessory respiratory muscles also increase chest volume (and lung expansion) by their actions on the ribs. Each rib (except for the last two) articulates posteriorly with a vertebra and is angulated downward as it attaches anteriorly to the sternum. Upward and outward rib movement expands the chest.

During normal breathing, the diaphragm and, to a lesser extent, the external intercostal muscles are responsible for inspiration; expiration is generally passive. The sternocleidomastoid, scalene, and pectoralis muscles can be recruited to assist during inspiration. The sternocleidomastoid muscles assist in elevating the rib cage, whereas the scalene muscles prevent inward displacement of the upper ribs during inspiration. The pectoralis muscles can assist chest expansion when the arms are placed on a fixed support. Expiration is normally passive in the supine position but becomes active in the upright position and with increased effort. Exhalation may be facilitated by the abdominal muscles (rectus abdominis, external and internal oblique, transversus) and perhaps by the internal intercostal muscles—aiding the downward movement of the ribs.

Although not usually considered respiratory muscles, some pharyngeal muscles are important in maintaining the patency of the airway. Tonic and reflex inspiratory activity in the genioglossus keeps the tongue away from the posterior pharyngeal wall. Tonic activity in the levator palati, tensor palati, palatopharyngeus, and palatoglossus muscles prevents the soft palate from falling back against the posterior pharynx, particularly in the supine position.

2. Tracheobronchial Tree

1 The trachea serves as a conduit for ventilation and clearance of tracheal and bronchial secretions. The trachea begins at the lower border of the cricoid cartilage, extends to the carina, and has an average length of 10 to 13 cm. It is composed of C-shaped cartilaginous rings, which form the anterior and lateral walls of the trachea and are connected posteriorly by the membranous wall of the trachea. The cricoid cartilage is the narrowest part of the trachea in adults, with an average diameter of 17 mm in men and 13 mm in women.

The tracheal lumen narrows slightly as it progresses toward the carina, where it bifurcates into the right and left mainstem bronchi at the level of the sternal angle. The right mainstem bronchus lies in a more linear arrangement with the trachea, whereas the left mainstem bronchus lies in a more angular orientation with the trachea. The right mainstem bronchus continues as the bronchus intermedius after the take-off of the right upper lobe bronchus. The distance from the tracheal carina to the take-off of the right upper lobe bronchus is an average of 2.0 cm in men and approximately 1.5 cm in women. One in every 250 individuals in the general population may have an abnormal take-off of the right upper lobe bronchus emerging from above the tracheal carina on the right side. The left mainstem bronchus is longer than the right mainstem bronchus and measures an average of 5.0 cm in men and 4.5 cm in women. The left mainstem bronchus divides into the left upper lobe bronchus and the left lower lobe bronchus.

Humidification and filtering of inspired air are functions of the upper airway (nose, mouth, and pharynx). The tracheobronchial tree serves to conduct gas flow to and from the alveoli. Dichotomous division (each branch dividing into two smaller branches), starting with the trachea and ending in alveolar sacs, is estimated to involve 23 divisions, or generations (Figure 23–1). With each generation, the number of airways is approximately doubled. Most alveoli are in alveolar sacs that contain, on average, 17 alveoli. An estimated 300 to 500 million alveoli provide an enormous membrane surface area (50–100 m^2) for gas exchange in the average adult.

Starting in the trachea and ending in the alveoli, the mucosa makes a gradual transition from ciliated columnar to cuboidal and finally to flat alveolar epithelium. Gas exchange can occur only across the flat epithelium, which begins to appear on respiratory bronchioles (generations 17–19). The wall of the airway gradually loses its cartilaginous support (at the bronchioles) and then its smooth muscle. Loss of cartilaginous support causes the patency of smaller airways to become dependent on radial traction by the elastic recoil of the surrounding tissue; as a corollary, airway diameter becomes dependent on total lung volume.

Cilia on the columnar and cuboidal epithelium normally beat in a synchronized fashion, such that mucus produced by the secretory glands lining the airway moves toward the mouth along with any associated bacteria or debris.

Alveoli

Alveolar size is a function of both gravity and lung volume. In the upright position, for example, the largest alveoli are at the pulmonary apex, whereas the smallest tend to be at the base. With inspiration, discrepancies in alveolar size diminish.

Each alveolus is in close contact with a network of pulmonary capillaries. The walls of each alveolus are asymmetrically arranged (Figure 23–2). Gas exchange occurs primarily on the thin side of the

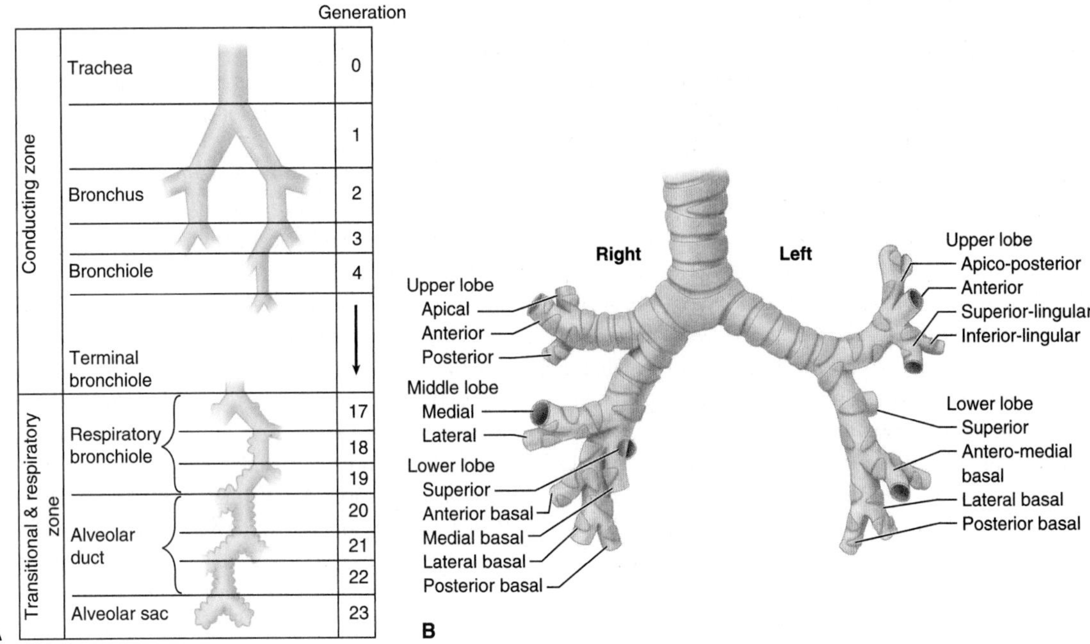

FIGURE 23–1 **A**: Dichotomous division of the airways. **B**: The segmental bronchi. (A, Reproduced with permission from Guyton AC. Textbook of Medical Physiology. 7th ed. Philadelphia, PA: WB Saunders; 1986. B, Reproduced with permission from Minnich DJ, Mathisen DJ. Anatomy of the trachea, carina, and bronchi. *Thorac Surg Clin*. 2007 Nov;17(4):571-585.)

alveolocapillary membrane, which is less than 0.4 μm thick. The thick side (1–2 μm) provides structural support for the alveolus. On the thin side, the alveolar epithelium and capillary endothelium are separated by their respective cellular and basement membranes; on the thick side, where fluid and solute exchange occurs, the pulmonary interstitial space separates alveolar epithelium from capillary endothelium. The pulmonary interstitial space contains mainly elastin, collagen, and nerve fibers.

The pulmonary epithelium contains at least two cell types. Type I pneumocytes are flat and form tight (1-nm) junctions with one another. These tight junctions are important in preventing the passage of large oncotically active molecules such as albumin into the alveolus. Type II pneumocytes, which are more numerous than type I pneumocytes (but because of their size and shape occupy <10% of the alveolar space), are round cells that contain prominent cytoplasmic inclusions (lamellar bodies). The lamellar bodies contain surfactant, an important substance necessary for normal pulmonary mechanics. Unlike type I cells, type II pneumocytes are capable of cell division and can produce type I pneumocytes if the latter are destroyed. Other cell types present in the lower airways include pulmonary alveolar macrophages, mast cells, lymphocytes, and amino precursor uptake and decarboxylation (APUD) cells. Neutrophils are also typically present in smokers and patients with pneumonia or acute lung injury.

3. Pulmonary Circulation & Lymphatics

The lungs are supplied by two circulations, pulmonary and bronchial. The bronchial circulation arises from the thoracic aorta and from intercostal arteries and provides a small amount of blood flow (<4% of the cardiac output), which sustains the metabolic needs of the tracheobronchial tree. Branches of the bronchial arteries supply the wall of the bronchi and follow the airways as far as the terminal bronchioles. Along their courses, the bronchial vessels anastomose with the pulmonary

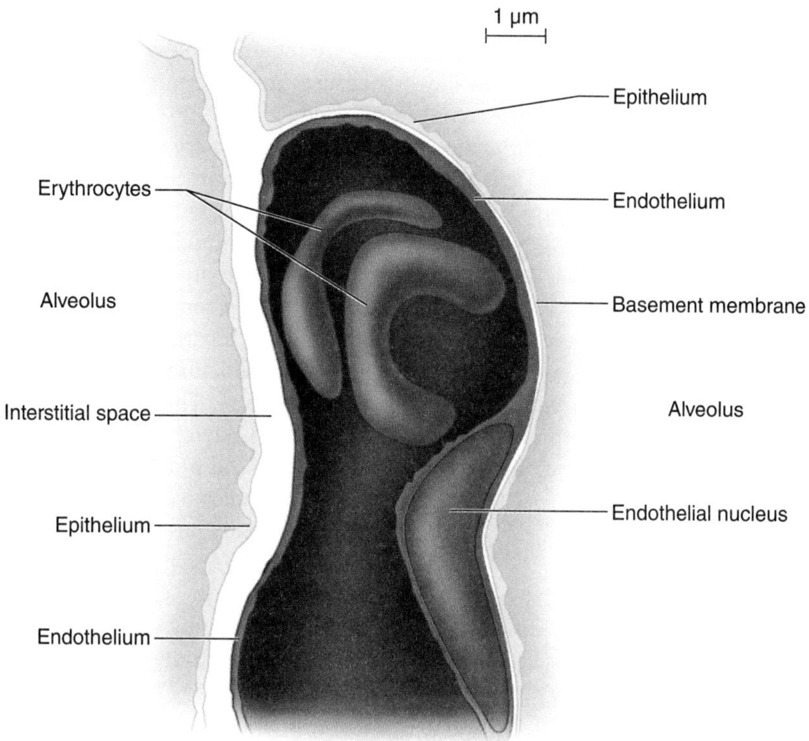

FIGURE 23–2 The pulmonary interstitial space, with a capillary passing between the two alveoli. The capillary is incorporated into the thin (gas-exchanging) side of the alveolus on the right. The interstitial space is incorporated into the thick side of the alveolus on the left. (Reproduced with permission from Nunn JF. *Nunn's Applied Physiology*, 4th ed. Oxford, UK: Butterworth; 2000.)

arterial circulation and continue as far as the alveolar duct. Below that level, lung tissue is supported by a combination of alveolar gas and pulmonary circulation.

The pulmonary circulation normally receives the total output of the right heart via the pulmonary artery, which divides into right and left branches to supply each lung. Deoxygenated blood passes through the pulmonary capillaries, where O_2 is taken up and CO_2 is eliminated. The oxygenated blood is then returned to the left heart by four main pulmonary veins (two from each lung). Pulmonary arteries and veins normally have thinner walls with less smooth muscle than systemic vessels. Although flows through the systemic and pulmonary circulations are equal except in the case of right-to-left or left-to-right shunt, the lower pulmonary vascular resistance results in pulmonary pressures that are less than those in the systemic vessels.

There are connections between the bronchial and pulmonary circulations. Direct pulmonary arteriovenous communications, bypassing the pulmonary capillaries, are normally insignificant but may become important in certain pathological states. The importance of the bronchial circulation in contributing to the normal venous admixture is discussed below.

Pulmonary Capillaries

Pulmonary capillaries are incorporated into the walls of alveoli. The average diameter of these capillaries (about 10 μm) is barely enough to allow passage of a single red cell. Because each capillary network supplies more than one alveolus, blood may pass through several alveoli before reaching the pulmonary veins. Because of the relatively low pressure in the pulmonary circulation, the amount of blood flowing through a given capillary network is affected by both gravity and alveolar size. In the upright position, for example, apical capillaries tend to have reduced flows, whereas basal capillaries have greater flows.

The pulmonary capillary endothelium has relatively large junctions (5 nm wide), allowing the passage of large molecules such as albumin. As a result, pulmonary interstitial fluid is relatively rich in albumin. Circulating macrophages and neutrophils are able to pass through the endothelium, as well as the smaller alveolar epithelial junctions, with relative ease. Pulmonary macrophages are commonly seen in the interstitial space and inside alveoli; they serve to scavenge bacteria and debris.

Pulmonary Lymphatics

Lymphatic channels in the lung originate in the interstitial spaces of large septa and are close to the bronchial arteries. Bronchial lymphatics return fluids, proteins, and various cells that have entered the peribronchovascular interstitium back to the blood circulation. Because of the large endothelial junctions, pulmonary lymph has a relatively high protein content, and total pulmonary lymph flow may be as much as 20 mL/h. Large lymphatic vessels travel upward alongside the airways, forming the tracheobronchial chain of lymph nodes. Lymphatic drainage channels from both lungs communicate along the trachea.

4. Innervation

Motor innervation of the diaphragm, along with sensory innervation of the central diaphragm, is supplied by the phrenic nerves, which arise from the C3–C5 nerve roots. Sensory innervation of the peripheral diaphragm is supplied by the adjacent sixth through eleventh intercostal nerves. Unilateral phrenic nerve block or palsy only modestly reduces most indices of pulmonary function (about 25%) in normal subjects. Although bilateral phrenic nerve palsies produce more severe impairment, accessory muscle activity may maintain adequate ventilation in some patients. Intercostal muscles are innervated by their respective thoracic nerve roots. Complete cervical cord injuries above C5 are incompatible with spontaneous ventilation because both phrenic and intercostal nerves are affected.

The vagus nerves provide sensory innervation to the tracheobronchial tree. Both sympathetic and parasympathetic autonomic innervation of bronchial smooth muscle and secretory glands is present. Vagal activity mediates bronchoconstriction and increases bronchial secretions via muscarinic receptors. Sympathetic activity (T1–T4) mediates bronchodilation and also decreases secretions via β_2-receptors. The nerve supply of the larynx is reviewed in Chapter 19.

Both α- and β-adrenergic receptors are present in the pulmonary vasculature, but the sympathetic system normally has little effect on pulmonary vascular tone. α_1 Activity causes vasoconstriction; β_2 activity mediates vasodilation. Parasympathetic vasodilatory activity seems to be mediated via the release of nitric oxide.

MECHANISMS OF BREATHING

2 The exchange of alveolar gas with the fresh gas from the upper airway reoxygenates desaturated blood and eliminates CO_2. This exchange is normally brought about by small cyclic pressure gradients established within the airways. During spontaneous ventilation, these gradients are secondary to variations in intrathoracic pressure; during mechanical ventilation, they are produced by intermittent positive pressure in the upper airway. During apneic oxygenation, gas exchange depends on the mass movement of gases along concentration gradients.

Spontaneous Ventilation

Normal pressure variations during spontaneous breathing are shown in Figure 23–3. The pressure within alveoli is always greater than the surrounding (intrathoracic) pressure unless the alveoli are collapsed. Alveolar pressure is normally atmospheric (zero for reference) at end-inspiration and end-expiration during spontaneous breathing. By convention, in pulmonary physiology, pleural pressure is

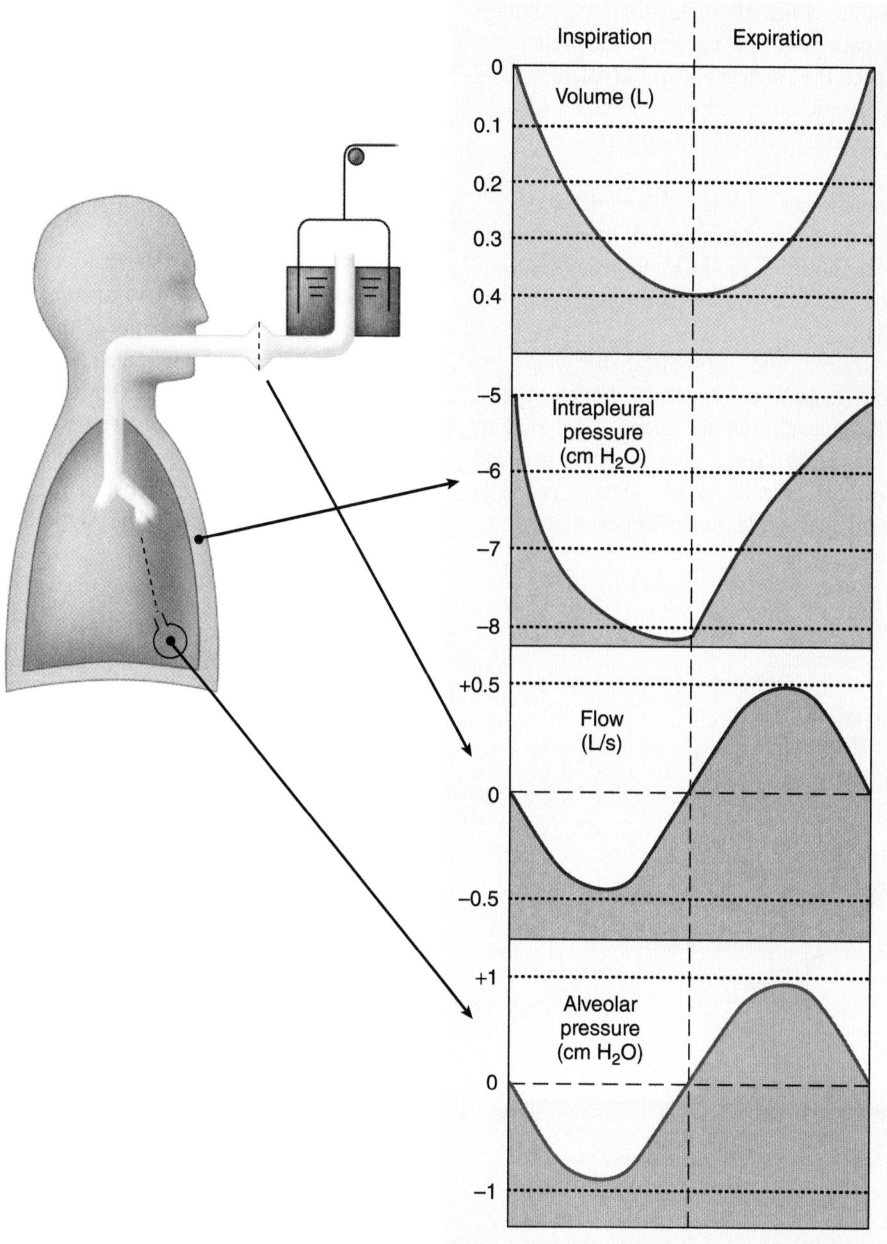

FIGURE 23–3 Changes in intrapleural and alveolar pressures during normal breathing. Note that at end inspiration, volume is maximal, flow is zero, and alveolar pressure is atmospheric. (Adapted with permission from West JB. *Respiratory Physiology: The Essentials,* 6th ed. Philadelphia, PA: Williams & Wilkins; 2000.)

used as a measure of intrathoracic pressure. Although it may not be entirely correct to refer to the pressure in a potential space, the concept allows the calculation of transpulmonary pressure. Transpulmonary pressure, or $P_{transpulmonary}$, is then defined as follows:

$$P_{transpulmonary} = P_{alveolar} - P_{intrapleural}$$

At end-expiration, intrapleural pressure normally averages about –5 cm H_2O, and because alveolar pressure is 0 (no flow), transpulmonary pressure is +5 cm H_2O.

Diaphragmatic and intercostal muscle activation during inspiration expands the chest and decreases intrapleural pressure from –5 cm H_2O to –8 or –9 cm H_2O. As a result, alveolar pressure also decreases, and an alveolar–upper airway gradient is established; gas flows from the upper airway into alveoli (Figure 23–4).

Diaphragmatic relaxation returns intrapleural pressure to –5 cm H_2O during expiration in normal breathing. Now the transpulmonary pressure does not support the new lung volume, and the elastic recoil of the lung causes a reversal of the previous alveolar–upper airway gradient; gas flows out of alveoli, and original lung volume is restored.

Mechanical Ventilation

Most forms of mechanical ventilation intermittently apply positive airway pressure at the upper airway. During inspiration, gas flows into alveoli until the pressure in the alveoli equilibrates with that of the upper airway. During the expiratory phase of the ventilator, the positive upper airway pressure is decreased, reversing the pressure gradient between the upper airway and the alveoli at the start of inspiration, allowing gas flow out of the alveoli.

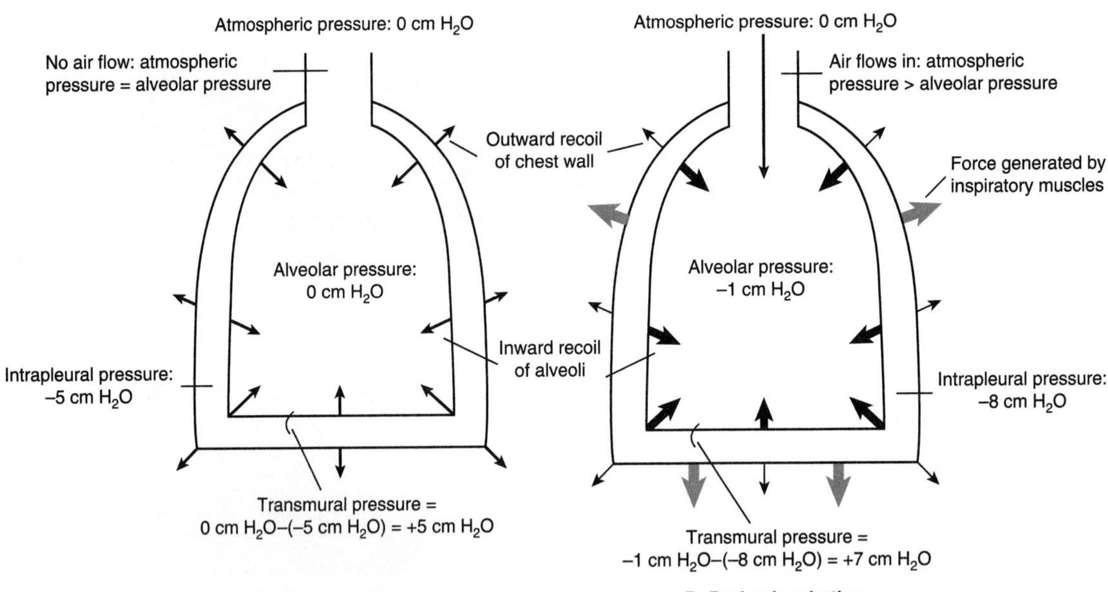

FIGURE 23–4 Representation of the interaction of the lung and chest wall. **A**: At end-expiration, the muscles of respiration are relaxed. The inward elastic recoil of the lung is balanced by the outward elastic recoil of the chest wall. Intrapleural pressure is –5 cm H_2O; alveolar pressure is 0. The transmural pressure difference across the alveolus is therefore 0 cm H_2O –(–5 cm H_2O), or 5 cm H_2O. Since alveolar pressure is equal to atmospheric pressure, no airflow occurs. **B**: During inspiration, contraction of the muscles of inspiration causes intrapleural pressure to become more negative. The transmural pressure difference increases, and the alveoli are distended, decreasing alveolar pressure below atmospheric pressure, which causes air to flow into the alveoli. (Reproduced with permission from Levitzky MG. *Pulmonary Physiology*, 8th ed. New York, NY: McGraw Hill; 2013.)

LUNG MECHANICS

The movement of the lungs is passive and determined by the impedance of the respiratory system, which can be divided into the elastic resistance of tissues and the gas–liquid interface and the nonelastic resistance to gas flow. Elastic resistance governs lung volume and the associated pressures under static conditions (no gas flow). Resistance to gas flow relates to frictional resistance to airflow and tissue deformation.

1. Elastic Resistance

Both the lungs and the chest wall have elastic properties. The chest tends to expand outward, whereas the lungs tend to collapse. When the pleural space is exposed to atmospheric pressure (open pneumothorax), the chest usually expands about 1 L in adults. In contrast, when the pleural space is exposed to atmospheric pressure, the normal lung collapses completely, and all the gas within it is expelled. The recoil properties of the chest wall are due to structural components that resist deformation and chest wall muscle tone. The elastic recoil of the lungs is due to their high content of elastin fibers and, even more importantly, to the surface tension forces acting at the air–fluid interface in alveoli.

Surface Tension Forces

The gas–fluid interface lining the alveoli causes them to behave as bubbles. Surface tension forces tend to reduce the area of the interface and favor alveolar collapse. Laplace's law can be used to quantify these forces:

$$\text{Pressure} = \frac{2 \times \text{Surface tension}}{\text{Radius}}$$

The pressure derived from the equation is that within the alveolus, and it is directly proportional to surface tension. **Fortunately, pulmonary surfactant decreases alveolar surface tension in proportion to its concentration within the alveolus.** As alveoli become smaller, the surfactant within becomes more concentrated, and surface tension is more effectively reduced. Conversely, when alveoli are overdistended, surfactant becomes less concentrated, and surface tension increases. The net effect is to stabilize alveolar size: small alveoli are prevented from getting smaller, whereas large alveoli are prevented from getting larger.

Compliance

Elastic recoil is usually measured in terms of compliance (C), which is defined as the change in volume divided by the change in distending pressure. Compliance measurements can be obtained for either the chest, the lung, or both together. In the supine position, chest wall compliance (CW) is reduced because of the weight of the abdominal contents against the diaphragm. Measurements are usually obtained under static conditions (ie, at equilibrium). Dynamic lung compliance [Cdyn, L], which is measured during rhythmic breathing, is also dependent on airway resistance.) **Lung compliance (CL)** is defined as:

$$\text{CL} = \frac{\text{Change in lung volume}}{\text{Change in transpulmonary pressure}}$$

CL is normally 150 to 200 mL/cm H_2O. A variety of factors, including lung volume, pulmonary blood volume, extravascular lung water, and pathological processes (eg, inflammation and fibrosis), affect CL,

$$\text{CW} = \frac{\text{Change in chest volume}}{\text{Change in transthoracic pressure}}$$

where transthoracic pressure equals atmospheric pressure minus intrapleural pressure.

Normal chest wall compliance is 200 mL/cm H_2O. Total compliance (lung and chest wall together) is 100 mL/cm H_2O and is expressed by the following equation:

$$\frac{1}{C_{\text{total}}} = \frac{1}{\text{CW}} + \frac{1}{\text{CL}}$$

2. Lung Volumes

Lung volumes are important parameters for both respiratory physiology and clinical practice (Table 23–1 and Figure 23–5). The sum of all of the named lung

TABLE 23–1 Lung volumes and capacities.

Measurement	Definition	Average Adult Values (mL)
Tidal volume (V_T)	Each normal breath	500
Inspiratory reserve volume (IRV)	Maximal additional volume that can be inspired above V_T	3000
Expiratory reserve volume (ERV)	Maximal volume that can be expired below V_T	1100
Residual volume (RV)	Volume remaining after maximal exhalation	1200
Total lung capacity (TLC)	RV + ERV + V_T + IRV	5800
Functional residual capacity (FRC)	RV + ERV	2300

volumes equals the maximum to which the lung can be inflated. Lung capacities are clinically useful measurements that represent a combination of two or more volumes.

Functional Residual Capacity

3 The lung volume at the end of a normal exhalation is called functional residual capacity (FRC). At this volume, the inward elastic recoil of the lung approximates the outward elastic recoil of the chest (including resting diaphragmatic tone). Thus, the elastic properties of both chest and lung define the point from which normal breathing takes place. FRC can be measured by nitrogen washout, helium wash-in technique, or body plethysmography. Factors known to alter the FRC include the following:

- **Body habitus:** FRC is directly proportional to height. Obesity, however, can markedly decrease FRC (from reduced chest wall compliance and increased abdominal pressure on the diaphragm). Kyphosis can adversely impact both lung volumes and rib mobility.
- **Sex:** FRC is reduced by about 10% in females compared with males.
- **Increased intraabdominal pressure:** Decreased FRC is associated with laparoscopic procedures, pregnancy, and significant ascites due to increased pressure

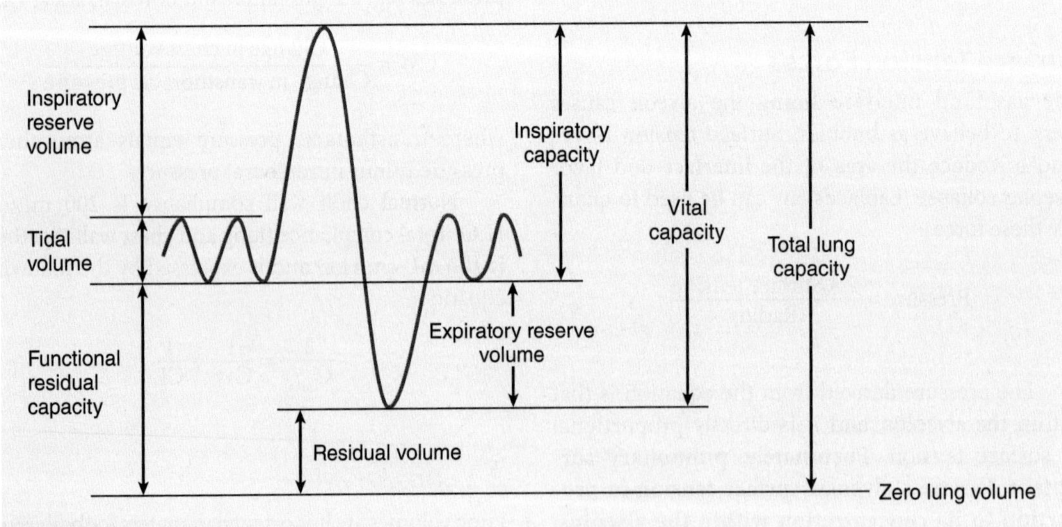

FIGURE 23–5 Spirogram showing static lung volumes. (Reproduced with permission from Lumb A. *Nunn's Applied Respiratory Physiology,* 8th ed. St. Louis, MO: Elsevier; 2017.)

on the diaphragm from the laparoscopy pneumoperitoneum, the gravid uterus, or from ascitic fluid, respectively.

- **Posture:** FRC decreases as a patient is moved from an upright to a supine or prone position. This is the result of reduced chest compliance as the abdominal contents push up against the diaphragm. The greatest change occurs between 0° and 60° of inclination.
- **Lung disease:** Decreased compliance of the lung, chest, or both is characteristic of restrictive pulmonary disorders, all of which are associated with a low FRC.
- **Diaphragmatic tone:** This normally contributes to FRC, and its contribution is evident with unilateral or bilateral phrenic nerve paralysis.

Closing Capacity

As described earlier, small airways lacking cartilaginous support depend on radial traction caused by the elastic recoil of surrounding tissue to keep them open; patency of these airways, particularly in dependent areas of the lung, is highly dependent on lung volume. The volume at which these airways begin to close in dependent areas of the lung is called the **closing capacity**. At lower lung volumes, alveoli in dependent areas continue to be perfused but are no longer ventilated; the resulting **intrapulmonary shunting** of deoxygenated blood (venous admixture) promotes hypoxemia.

Closing capacity is usually measured with 100% oxygen, which is inhaled near residual volume and then exhaled from total lung capacity. Changes in the nitrogen concentration of the exhaled gas following oxygen inhalation are measured. The nitrogen concentration from alveoli at the base of the lungs is lower than that at the apex because any air remaining in the lungs at the residual volume is in the nondependent alveoli. Closing volume is discerned when the concentration of expired nitrogen rises, indicating that the alveoli from the dependent regions of the lung are no longer contributing to the exhaled gas because their airways have closed (Figure 23–6).

Closing capacity is normally well below FRC (Figure 23–7) but rises steadily with age (Figure 23–8). This increase is probably responsible for the normal age-related decline in arterial O_2 tension. For individuals at an average age of 44 years, closing capacity equals FRC in the supine position; by age 66, closing capacity equals or exceeds FRC in the upright position in most individuals. Unlike FRC, closing capacity is unaffected by posture. Closing capacity also approaches or exceeds FRC in morbid obesity.

Vital Capacity

Vital capacity (VC) is the maximum volume of gas that can be exhaled following maximal inspiration. In addition to body habitus, VC is also dependent on respiratory muscle strength and chest–lung compliance. Normal VC is about 60 to 70 mL/kg.

3. Nonelastic Resistances

Airway Resistance to Gas Flow

Gas flow in the lung is a mixture of laminar and turbulent flow. Laminar flow can be thought of as consisting of concentric cylinders of gas flowing at different velocities; velocity is greatest in the center and decreases toward the periphery. During laminar flow,

$$\text{Flow} = \frac{\text{Pressure gradient}}{R_{aw}}$$

where R_{aw} is airway resistance.

$$R_{aw} = \frac{8 \times \text{Length} \times \text{Gas viscosity}}{\pi \times (\text{Radius})^4}$$

Turbulent flow is characterized by random movement of the gas molecules down the air passages. Mathematical description of turbulent flow is considerably more complex:

$$\text{Pressure gradient} \approx \text{Flow}^2 \times \frac{\text{Gas density}}{\text{Radius}^5}$$

Resistance is not constant but increases in proportion to gas flow. Moreover, resistance is directly proportional to gas density and inversely proportional to the fifth power of the radius. As a result, turbulent gas flow is extremely sensitive to airway caliber.

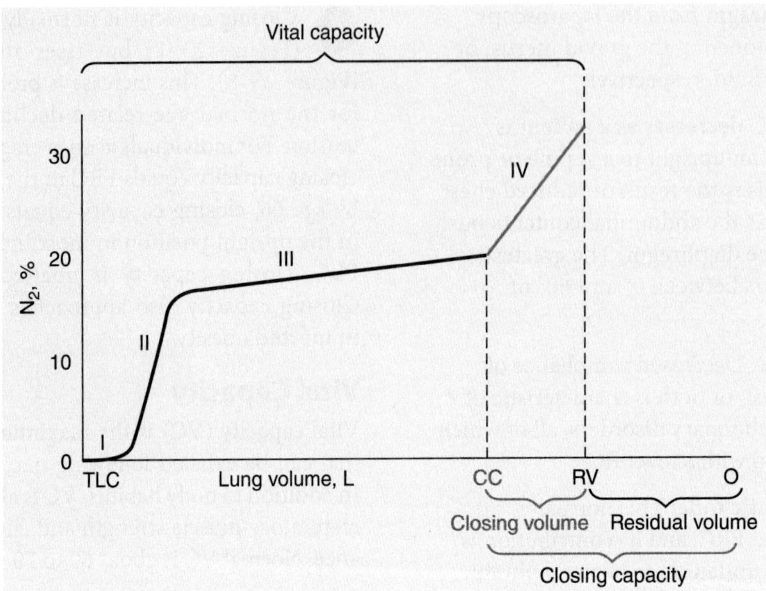

FIGURE 23–6 Expired nitrogen concentration after inhalation of a single breath of 100% oxygen from the residual volume to the total lung capacity. Subject exhales to the residual volume. Phase I: 0% nitrogen from anatomic dead space. Phase II: mixture of gas from anatomic dead space and alveoli. Phase III: "alveolar plateau" gas from alveoli. A steep slope of phase III indicates nonuniform distribution of alveolar gas. Phase IV: closing volume. Take-off point (closing capacity) of phase IV denotes the beginning of airway closure in dependent portions of the lung. (Reproduced with permission from Levitzky MG. *Pulmonary Physiology*, 8th ed. New York, NY: McGraw Hill; 2013.)

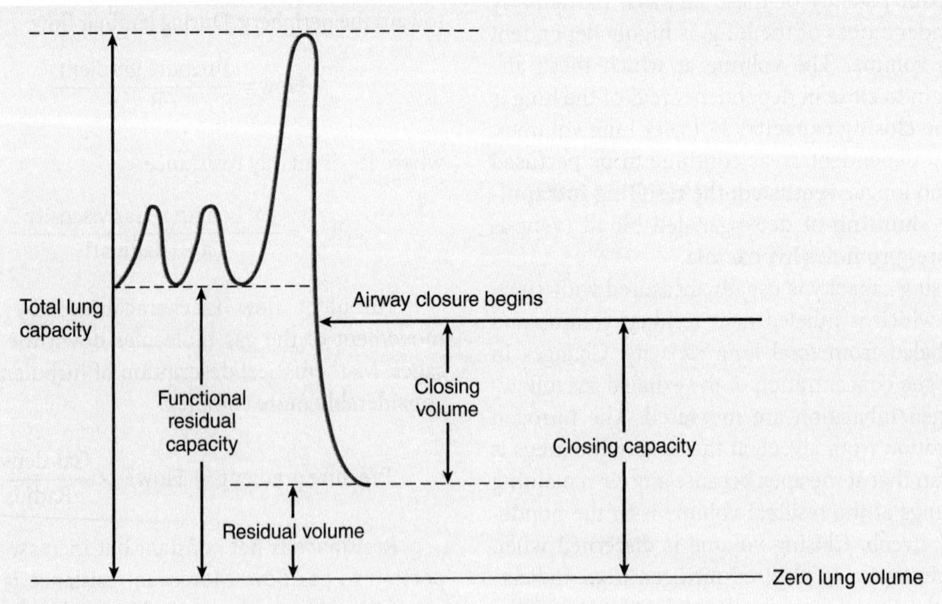

FIGURE 23–7 The relationship between functional residual capacity, closing volume, and closing capacity. (Reproduced with permission from Lumb A. *Nunn's Applied Respiratory Physiology*, 8th ed. St. Louis, MO: Elsevier; 2017.)

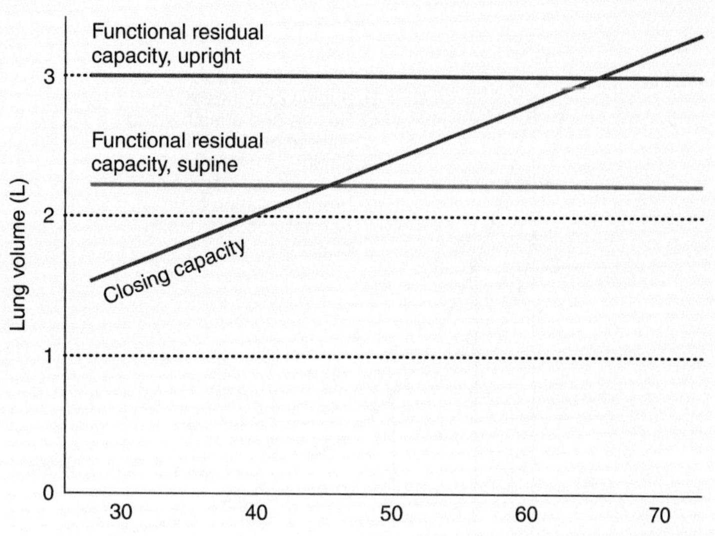

FIGURE 23–8 The effect of age on closing capacity and its relationship to functional residual capacity (FRC). Note that FRC does not change. (Reproduced with permission from Lumb A. *Nunn's Applied Respiratory Physiology,* 8th ed. St. Louis, MO: Elsevier; 2017.)

Turbulence generally occurs at high gas flows, at sharp angles or branching points, and in response to abrupt changes in airway diameter. Whether turbulent or laminar flow occurs can be predicted by the *Reynolds number*, which results from the following equation:

$$\text{Reynolds number} = \frac{\text{Linear velocity} \times \text{Diameter} \times \text{Gas density}}{\text{Gas viscosity}}$$

A low Reynolds number (<1000) is associated with laminar flow, whereas a high value (>1500) produces turbulent flow. Laminar flow normally occurs only distal to small bronchioles (<1 mm). Flow in larger airways is probably turbulent. Of the gases used clinically, only helium has a significantly lower density-to-viscosity ratio, making it useful clinically during severe turbulent flow (as caused by upper airway obstruction). A helium–O_2 mixture is not only less likely to cause turbulent flow in comparison with pure O_2 but also reduces airway resistance when turbulent flow is present.

Normal total airway resistance is about 0.5 to 2 cm H_2O/L/s, with the largest contribution coming from medium-sized bronchi (before the seventh generation). Resistance in large bronchi is low because of their large diameters, whereas resistance in small bronchi is low because of their large total cross-sectional area. The most important causes of increased airway resistance include bronchospasm, secretions, mucosal edema, and volume-related or flow-related airway collapse.

A. Volume-Related Airway Collapse

At low lung volumes, loss of radial traction increases the contribution of small airways to total resistance; airway resistance becomes inversely proportional to lung volume (Figure 23–9). Increasing lung volume up to normal with positive end-expiratory pressure (PEEP) can reduce airway resistance.

B. Flow-Related Airway Collapse

During forced exhalation, reversal of the normal transmural airway pressure can cause collapse of

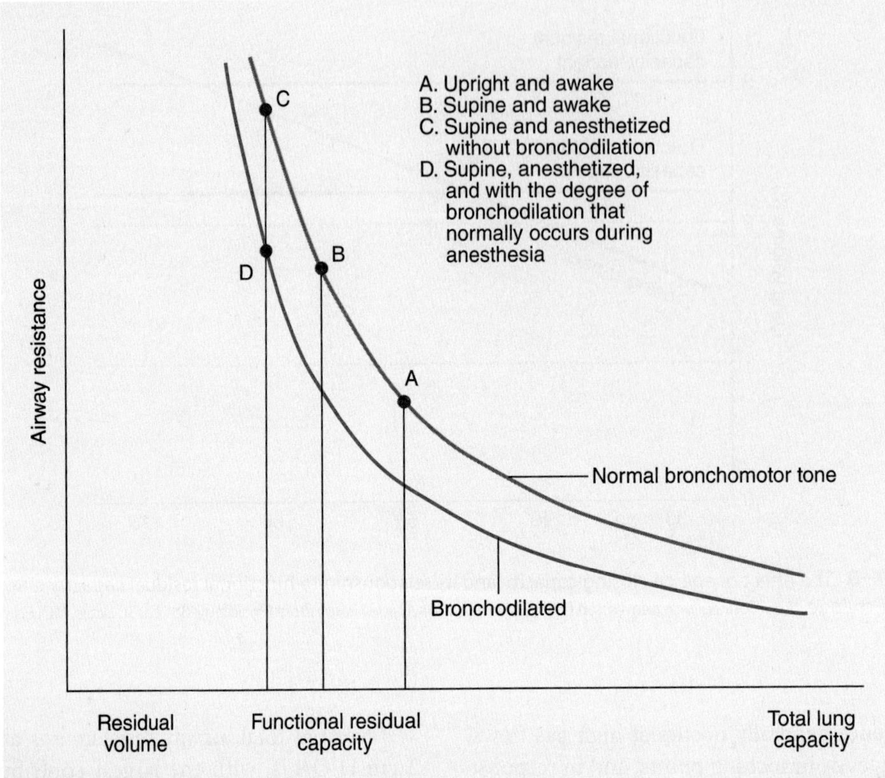

FIGURE 23–9 The relationship between airway resistance and lung volume. (Reproduced with permission from Lumb A. *Nunn's Applied Respiratory Physiology,* 8th ed. St. Louis, MO: Elsevier; 2017.)

these airways (dynamic airway compression). Two contributing factors are responsible: the generation of positive pleural pressure and a large pressure drop across intrathoracic airways as a result of increased airway resistance. The latter is in turn due to high (turbulent) gas flow and the reduced lung volume. The terminal portion of the flow/volume curve is therefore considered to be effort independent (Figure 23–10).

The point along the airways where dynamic compression occurs is called the *equal pressure point*. It is normally beyond the 11th to 13th generation of bronchioles where cartilaginous support is absent (see earlier discussion). The equal pressure point moves toward smaller airways as lung volume decreases. Emphysema and asthma predispose patients to dynamic airway compression. Emphysema destroys the elastic tissues that normally support smaller airways. In patients with asthma, bronchoconstriction and mucosal edema intensify airway collapse and promote reversal of transmural pressure gradients across airways. Patients may terminate exhalation prematurely or purse their lips to increase expiratory resistance at the mouth. Premature termination of exhalation may increase FRC above normal, resulting in air trapping and auto-PEEP.

C. Forced Vital Capacity

Measuring vital capacity as an exhalation that is as forceful and rapid as possible (Figure 23–11) provides important information about airway resistance. The ratio of the forced expiratory volume in the first second of exhalation (FEV_1) to the total forced vital capacity (FVC) is proportional to the degree of airway obstruction. Normally,

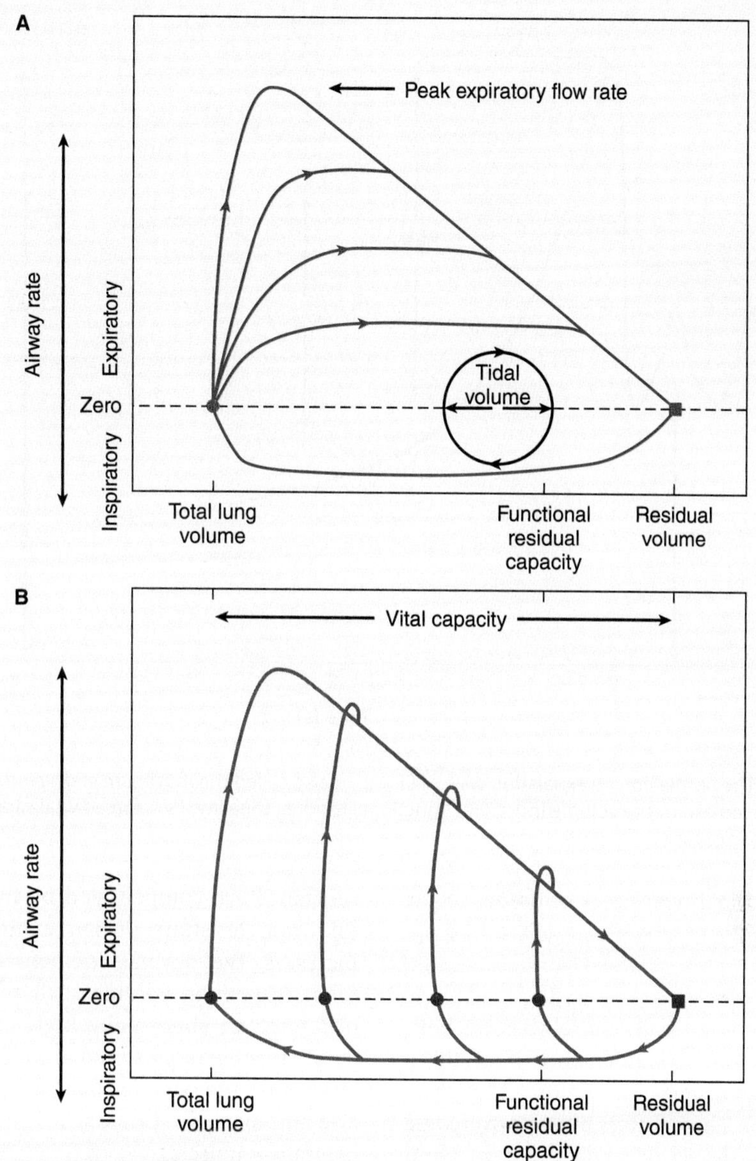

FIGURE 23–10 Gas flow (**A**) during forced exhalation from total lung capacity with varying effort and (**B**) with maximal effort from different lung volumes. Note that regardless of initial lung volume or effort, terminal expiratory flows are effort independent. (Reproduced with permission from Lumb A. *Nunn's Applied Respiratory Physiology,* 8th ed. St. Louis, MO: Elsevier; 2017.)

5 FEV_1/FVC is 80% or greater. Whereas both FEV_1 and FVC are effort dependent, forced midexpiratory flow ($FEF_{25-75\%}$) is more effort independent and may be a more reliable measurement of obstruction.

Tissue Resistance

This component of nonelastic resistance is generally underestimated and often overlooked, but it may account for up to half of total airway resistance. It seems to be primarily due to

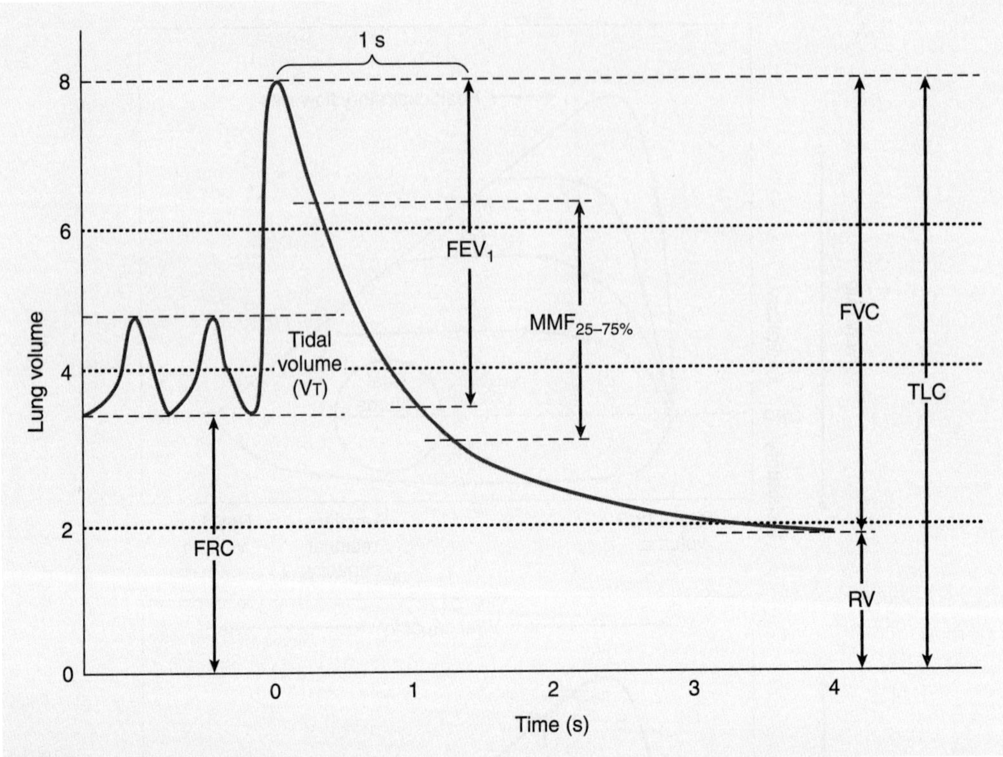

FIGURE 23–11 The normal forced exhalation curve. $FEF_{25-75\%}$ is also called the *maximum midexpiratory flow rate* ($MMF_{25-75\%}$). FEV_1, forced expiratory volume in 1 s; FRC, functional residual capacity; FVC, forced vital capacity; RV, residual volume; TLC, total lung capacity.

viscoelastic (frictional) resistance of tissues to gas flow.

4. Work of Breathing

Because expiration is normally entirely passive, both the inspiratory and the expiratory work of breathing is accomplished by the inspiratory muscles (primarily the diaphragm). Three factors must be overcome during ventilation: the elastic recoil of the chest and lung, frictional resistance to gas flow in the airways, and tissue frictional resistance.

Respiratory work can be expressed as the product of volume and pressure. During inhalation, both inspiratory airway resistance and pulmonary elastic recoil must be overcome; nearly 50% of the energy expended is stored pulmonary elastic recoil. During exhalation, the stored potential energy is released and overcomes expiratory airway resistance. Increases in either inspiratory or expiratory resistance are compensated by increased inspiratory muscle effort. When expiratory resistance increases, the normal compensatory response is to increase lung volume such that VT breathing occurs at an abnormally high FRC. The greater elastic recoil energy stored at a higher lung volume overcomes the added expiratory resistance. Excessive amounts of expiratory resistance also activate expiratory muscles.

Respiratory muscles normally account for only 2% to 3% of O_2 consumption but operate at about 10% efficiency. Ninety percent of the work is dissipated as heat (due to elastic and airflow resistance). In pathological conditions that increase the load on the diaphragm, muscle efficiency usually progressively decreases, and contraction may become uncoordinated with increasing ventilatory effort; moreover, a point may be reached whereby any increase in O_2 uptake (because of augmented

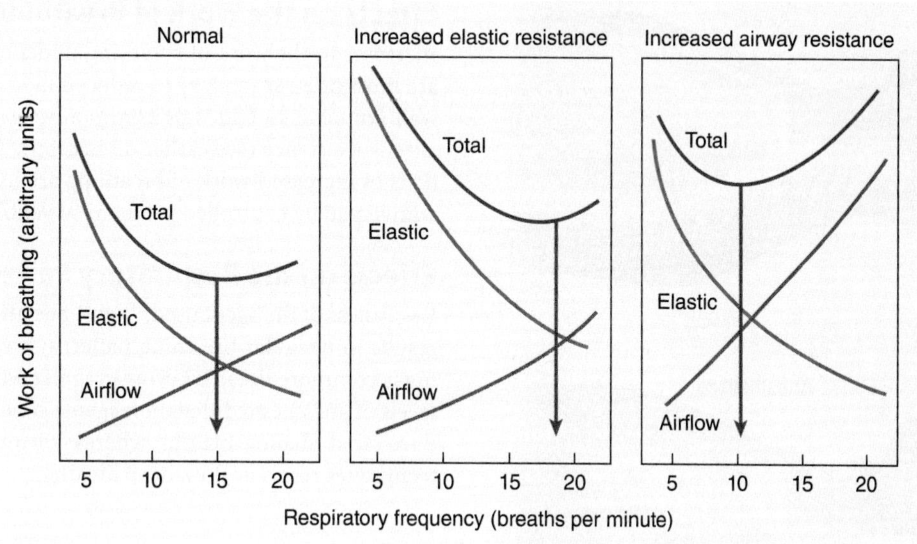

FIGURE 23–12 The work of breathing in relation to respiratory rate for normal individuals, patients with increased elastic resistance, and patients with increased airway resistance. (Reproduced with permission from Lumb A. *Nunn's Applied Respiratory Physiology*, 8th ed. St. Louis, MO: Elsevier; 2017.)

ventilation) is consumed by the respiratory muscles themselves.

The work required to overcome elastic resistance increases as V_T increases, whereas the work required to overcome airflow resistance increases as respiratory rate (and, necessarily, expiratory flow) increases. Faced with either condition, patients minimize the work of breathing by altering the respiratory rate and V_T (Figure 23–12). **Patients with reduced compliance tend to have rapid, shallow breaths, whereas those with increased airflow resistance have a slow, deep breathing pattern.**

5. Effects of Anesthesia on Pulmonary Mechanics

The effects of anesthesia on breathing are complex and relate to changes both in position and anesthetic agent.

Effects on Lung Volumes & Compliance

6 Changes in lung mechanics due to general anesthesia occur shortly after induction. The supine position reduces the FRC by 0.8 to 1.0 L, and induction of general anesthesia further reduces the FRC by 0.4 to 0.5 L. FRC reduction is a consequence of alveolar collapse and compression atelectasis due to loss of inspiratory muscle tone, change in chest wall rigidity, and upward shift of the diaphragm. The mechanisms may be more complex; for example, only the dependent (dorsal) part of the diaphragm in the supine position moves cephalad. Other factors are likely due to a change in intrathoracic volume secondary to increased blood volume in the lung and changes in chest wall shape (Figure 23–13). The higher position of the dorsal diaphragm and changes in the thoracic cavity itself decrease lung volumes. This decrease in FRC is not related to anesthetic depth and may persist for several hours or days after anesthesia. Steep head-down (Trendelenburg) position (>30°) may reduce FRC even further as intrathoracic blood volume increases. In contrast, induction of anesthesia in the sitting position seems to have little effect on FRC. Muscle paralysis does not seem to change FRC significantly in anesthetized patients.

The effects of anesthesia on closing capacity are variable. Both FRC and closing capacity are generally

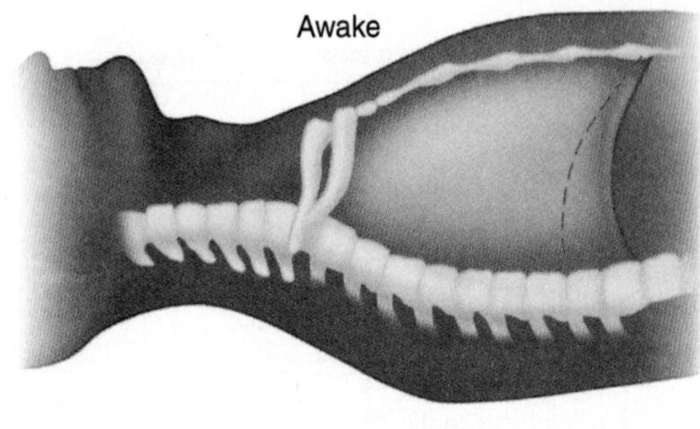

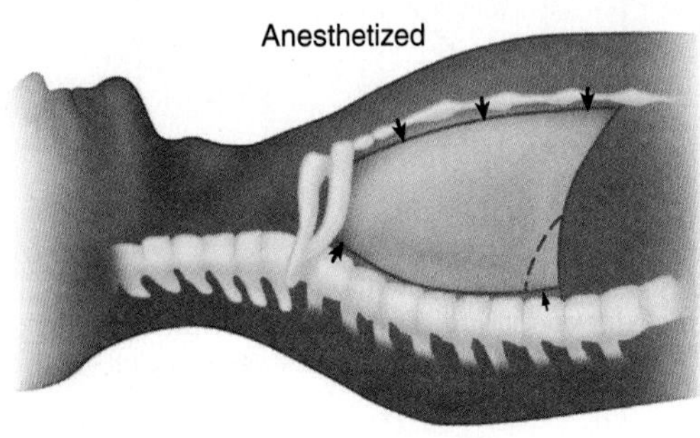

FIGURE 23–13 With induction of anesthesia in the supine position, the abdominal contents exert cephalad pressure on the diaphragm. At end-expiration, the dorsal portion of the diaphragm is more cephalad and the ventral portion is more caudal than when awake, the thoracic spine is more lordotic, and the rib cage moves inward, all secondary to loss of motor tone.

reduced to the same extent under anesthesia. Thus, the risk of increased intrapulmonary shunting under anesthesia is similar to that in the conscious state; it is greatest in obese and older adult patients and in those with underlying pulmonary disease.

Effects on Airway Resistance

The reduction in FRC associated with general anesthesia would be expected to increase airway resistance. Increases in airway resistance are not usually observed, however, because of the bronchodilating properties of the inhalation anesthetics. Increased airway resistance is more commonly due to pathological factors (posterior displacement of the tongue; laryngospasm; bronchoconstriction; or secretions, blood, or tumor in the airway) or equipment problems (small tracheal tubes or connectors, malfunction of valves, or obstruction of the breathing circuit).

Effects on the Work of Breathing

Increases in the work of breathing under anesthesia are most often secondary to reduced lung and chest wall compliance and, less commonly, increases in airway resistance (see earlier discussion). The problems of increased work of breathing are usually circumvented by controlled mechanical ventilation.

Effects on the Respiratory Pattern

Regardless of the agent used, "light" anesthesia often results in irregular breathing patterns; breath holding is common. Breaths become regular with deeper levels of anesthesia. Inhalation agents generally produce rapid, shallow breaths, whereas nitrous–opioid techniques result in slow, deep breaths.

VENTILATION/PERFUSION RELATIONSHIPS

1. Ventilation

Ventilation is usually measured as the sum of all exhaled gas volumes in 1 min (minute ventilation, or $\dot{V}$).

$$\text{Minute ventilation} = \text{Respiratory rate} \times \text{Tidal volume}$$

For the average adult at rest, minute ventilation is about 5 L/min.

Not all of the inspired gas mixture reaches alveoli; some of it remains in the airways and is exhaled without being exchanged with alveolar gases. The part of the V_T not participating in alveolar gas exchange is known as dead space (V_D). Alveolar ventilation ($\dot{V}_A$) is the volume of inspired gases actually taking part in gas exchange in 1 min.

$$\dot{V}_A = \text{Respiratory rate} \times (V_T - V_D)$$

Dead space is actually composed of gases in nonrespiratory airways **(anatomic dead space)** and alveoli that are not perfused **(alveolar dead space)**. The sum of the two components is referred to as **physiological dead space**. In the upright position, dead space is normally about 150 mL for most adults (approximately 2 mL/kg) and is nearly all anatomic. Dead space can be affected by a variety of factors (Table 23–2).

TABLE 23–2 Factors affecting dead space.

Factor	Effect
Posture	
Upright	↑
Supine	↓
Position of airway	
Neck extension	↑
Neck flexion	↓
Age	↑
Artificial airway	↓
Positive-pressure ventilation	↑
Drugs—anticholinergic	↑
Pulmonary perfusion	
Pulmonary emboli	↑
Hypotension	↑
Pulmonary vascular disease	
Emphysema	↑

Because VT in the average adult is approximately 450 mL (6 mL/kg), VD/VT is normally 33%. This ratio can be derived by the Bohr equation:

$$\frac{V_D}{V_T} = \frac{P_ACO_2 - P_ECO_2}{P_ACO_2}$$

where P_ACO_2 is the alveolar CO_2 tension and P_ECO_2 is the mixed expired CO_2 tension. This equation is useful clinically if arterial CO_2 tension ($PaCO_2$) is used to approximate the alveolar concentration and the CO_2 tension in expired air gases is the average measured over several minutes.

Distribution of Ventilation

Regardless of body position, alveolar ventilation is unevenly distributed in the lungs. The right lung receives more ventilation than the left lung (53% vs 47%), and the lower (dependent) areas of both lungs tend to be better ventilated than the upper areas because of a gravitationally induced gradient in intrapleural pressure (transpulmonary pressure). Pleural pressure decreases about 1 cm H_2O (becomes less negative) per 3-cm decrease in lung height. This difference places alveoli from different areas at different points on the pulmonary compliance curve (Figure 23–14). Because of higher transpulmonary pressure, alveoli in upper lung areas are near-maximally inflated and relatively noncompliant, and they undergo little expansion during inspiration. In contrast, the smaller alveoli in dependent areas have lower transpulmonary pressure, are more compliant, and undergo greater expansion during inspiration.

Airway resistance can also contribute to regional differences in pulmonary ventilation. Final alveolar inspiratory volume is solely dependent on compliance only if inspiratory time is unlimited. In reality, inspiratory time is necessarily limited by the respiratory rate and the time necessary for expiration; consequently, an excessively short inspiratory time will prevent alveoli from reaching the expected change in volume. Moreover, alveolar filling follows an exponential function that is dependent on both compliance and airway resistance. Therefore, even with a normal inspiratory time, abnormalities in either compliance or resistance can prevent complete alveolar filling.

Time Constants

Lung inflation can be described mathematically by the time constant, τ.

$$\tau = \text{Total compliance} \times \text{Airway resistance}$$

Regional variations in resistance or compliance not only interfere with alveolar filling but also can cause asynchrony in alveolar filling during inspiration; some alveolar units may continue to fill as others empty.

Variations in time constants within the normal lung can be demonstrated in normal individuals breathing spontaneously during abnormally high respiratory rates. Rapid shallow breathing reverses the normal distribution of ventilation, preferentially favoring upper (nondependent) areas of the lung over the lower areas.

2. Pulmonary Perfusion

Of the approximately 5 L/min of blood flowing through the lungs, only about 70 to 100 mL at any one time are within the pulmonary capillaries undergoing gas exchange. At the alveolar–capillary

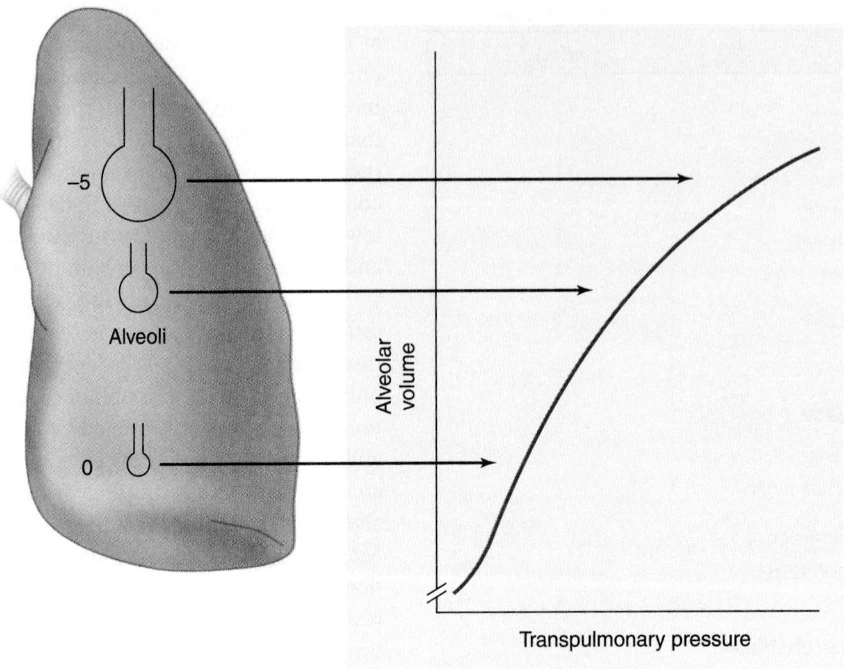

FIGURE 23–14 The effect of gravity on alveolar compliance in the upright position.

membrane, this small volume forms a 50 to 100 m^2-sheet of blood that is approximately one red cell thick. Moreover, to ensure optimal gas exchange, each capillary perfuses more than one alveolus.

Although capillary volume remains relatively constant, total pulmonary blood volume can vary between 500 mL and 1000 mL. Large increases in either cardiac output or blood volume are tolerated with little change in pressure as a result of passive dilation of open vessels and perhaps some recruitment of collapsed pulmonary vessels. Small increases in pulmonary blood volume normally occur during cardiac systole and with each normal (spontaneous) inspiration. A shift in posture from supine to erect decreases pulmonary blood volume (up to 27%); Trendelenburg positioning has the opposite effect. Changes in systemic capacitance also influence pulmonary blood volume: Systemic venoconstriction shifts blood from the systemic to the pulmonary circulation, whereas vasodilation causes a pulmonary-to-systemic redistribution. In this way, the lung acts as a reservoir for the systemic circulation.

7 Local factors are more important than the autonomic system in influencing pulmonary vascular tone. Hypoxia is a powerful stimulus for pulmonary vasoconstriction (the opposite of its systemic effect). Both pulmonary arterial (mixed venous) and alveolar hypoxia induce vasoconstriction, but the latter is a more powerful stimulus. This response seems to be due to either the direct effect of hypoxia on the pulmonary vasculature or increased production of leukotrienes relative to vasodilatory prostaglandins. Inhibition of nitric oxide production may also play a role. Hypoxic pulmonary vasoconstriction is an important physiological mechanism in reducing intrapulmonary shunting and preventing hypoxemia. Hyperoxia has little effect on the pulmonary circulation in normal individuals. Hypercapnia and acidosis have a constrictor effect, whereas hypocapnia causes pulmonary vasodilation, the opposite of what occurs in the systemic circulation.

Distribution of Pulmonary Perfusion

Pulmonary blood flow is not uniform. Regardless of body position, dependent areas of the lung receive greater blood flow than nondependent areas. This pattern is the result of a gravitational gradient of 1 cm H_2O/cm lung height. The normally low pressures in the pulmonary circulation allow gravity to exert a significant influence on blood flow. Also, in vivo perfusion scanning in normal individuals has shown an "onion-like" layering distribution of perfusion, with reduced flow at the periphery of the lung and increased perfusion toward the hilum.

Although the pulmonary perfusion pressure is not uniform across the lung, the alveolar distending pressure is relatively constant. The interplay of these pressures results in the dividing of the lung into four distinct zones (ie, the *West zones*; Figure 23–15). In zone 1 (PA > Pa > Pv), alveolar pressure (PA) is greater than both the arterial pulmonary pressure (Pa) and venous pulmonary pressure (Pv), resulting in obstruction of blood flow and creation of alveolar dead space. West zone 1 is fairly small in a spontaneously breathing individual, but it can enlarge during positive pressure ventilation. In dependent areas of the lungs, Pa progressively increases due to reduced elevation above the heart. In zone 2 (Pa > PA > Pv), Pa is greater than PA, but Pv remains less than both, resulting in blood flow that is dependent on the differential between Pa and PA. The bulk of the lung is described by zone 3 (Pa > Pv > PA), where both Pa and Pv are greater than PA, resulting in blood flow independent of the alveolar pressure. Zone 4, the most dependent part of the lung, is where atelectasis and interstitial pulmonary edema occur, resulting in blood flow that is dependent on the differential between Pa and pulmonary interstitial pressure.

Ventilation/Perfusion Ratios

8 Because alveolar ventilation $\dot{V}_A$ is normally about 4 L/min, and pulmonary capillary perfusion ($\dot{Q}$) is 5 L/min, the overall $\dot{V}/\dot{Q}$ ratio is about

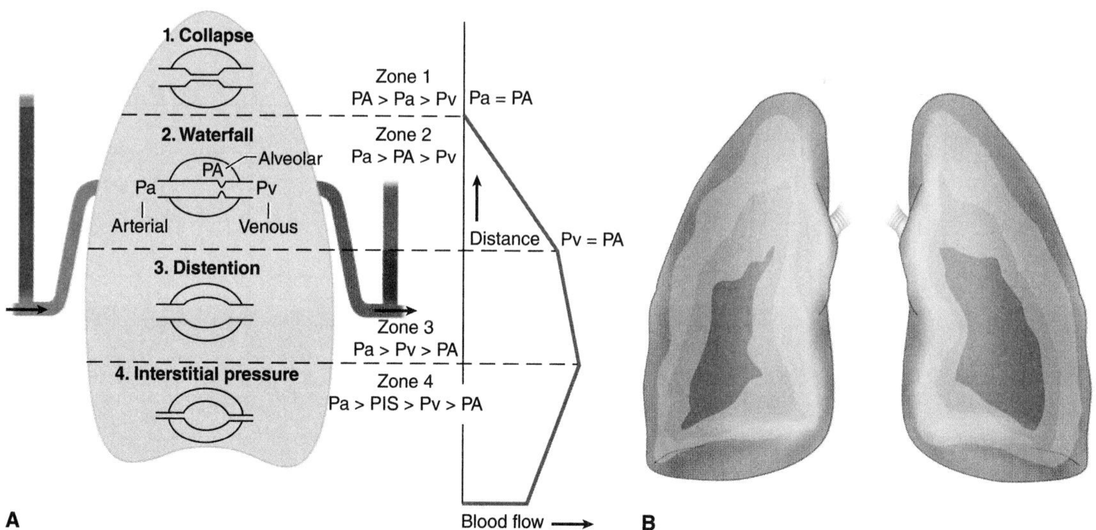

FIGURE 23–15 Pulmonary blood flow distribution relative to the alveolar pressure (PA), the pulmonary arterial pressure (Pa), the pulmonary venous pressure (Pv), and the interstitial pressure (PIS) at various gravitation levels. **A**: Classic West zones of blood flow distribution in the upright position. **B**: In vivo perfusion scanning illustrating central-to-peripheral, in addition to gravitational, blood flow distribution in the upright position. (A, Modified with permission from West JB. Respiratory Physiology: The Essentials, 6th ed. Philadelphia, PA: Williams & Wilkins; 2000. B, Reproduced with permission from Lohser J. Evidence based management of one lung ventilation, *Anesthesiol Clin.* 2008 June;26(2):241-272.)

0.8. $\dot{V}/\dot{Q}$ for individual lung units (each alveolus and its capillary) can range from 0 (no ventilation) to infinity (no perfusion); the former is referred to as *intrapulmonary shunt*, whereas the latter constitutes *alveolar dead space*. $\dot{V}/\dot{Q}$ normally ranges between 0.3 and 3.0; the majority of lung areas, however, are close to 1.0 (Figure 23–16A). Because perfusion increases at a greater rate than ventilation, nondependent (apical) areas tend to have higher $\dot{V}/\dot{Q}$ ratios than do dependent (basal) areas (Figure 23–16B).

The importance of $\dot{V}/\dot{Q}$ ratios relates to the efficiency with which lung units resaturate venous blood with O_2 and eliminate CO_2. **Pulmonary venous blood (the effluent) from areas with low $\dot{V}/\dot{Q}$ ratios has a low O_2 tension and high CO_2 tension—similar to systemic mixed venous blood.** Blood from these units tends to depress arterial O_2 tension and elevate arterial CO_2 tension. Their effect on arterial O_2 tension is much more profound than that on CO_2 tension; in fact, arterial CO_2 tension often decreases from a hypoxemia-induced reflex increase in alveolar ventilation. An appreciable compensatory increase in O_2 uptake cannot take place in remaining areas where $\dot{V}/\dot{Q}$ is normal because pulmonary end-capillary blood is usually already maximally saturated with O_2 (see below).

COVID-19 is associated with increased ventilation–perfusion mismatch, resulting in reduced oxygenation. Alveolar and interstitial damage contribute to impaired ventilation of alveoli. Additionally, prothrombotic effects of COVID-19 contribute to the development of pulmonary emboli, reducing lung perfusion and increasing dead space ventilation.

3. Shunts

9 *Shunting* denotes the process whereby desaturated, mixed venous blood from the right heart returns to the left heart without being oxygenated

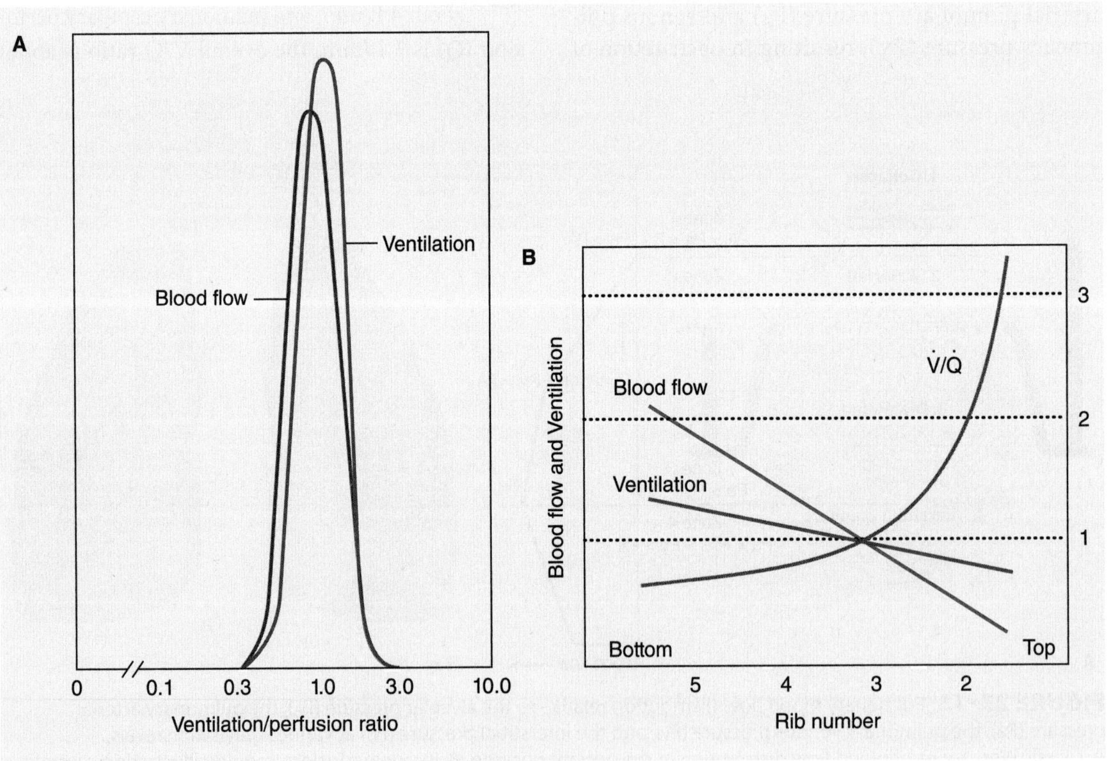

FIGURE 23–16 The distribution of $\dot{V}/\dot{Q}$ ratios for the whole lung (**A**) and according to height (**B**) in the upright position. Note that blood flow increases more rapidly than ventilation in dependent areas. (Reproduced with permission from West JB: Ventilation/Blood Flow and Gas Exchange, 3rd ed. Oxford: Blackwell Science Ltd; 1977.)

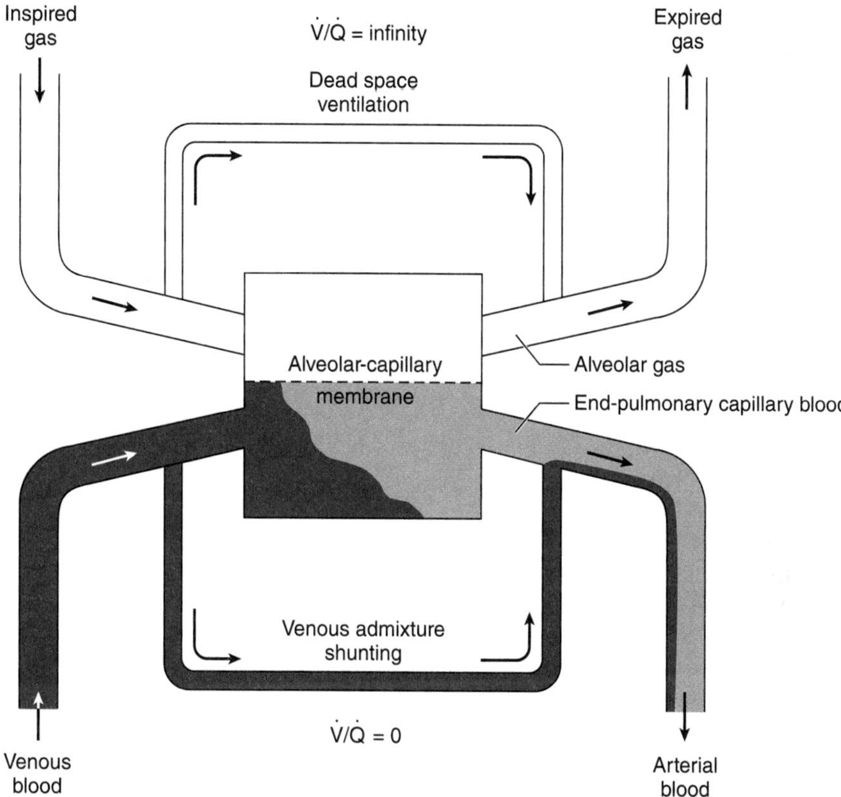

FIGURE 23–17 A three-compartment model of gas exchange in the lungs, showing dead space ventilation, normal alveolar–capillary exchange, and shunting (venous admixture). (Reproduced with permission from Lumb A. *Nunn's Applied Respiratory Physiology*, 8th ed. St. Louis, MO: Elsevier; 2017.)

in the lungs (Figure 23–17). The overall effect of shunting is to decrease (dilute) arterial O_2 content; this type of shunt is referred to as right-to-left. Left-to-right shunts (in the absence of pulmonary congestion) do not produce hypoxemia.

Intrapulmonary shunts are often classified as *absolute* or *relative*. An absolute shunt refers to anatomic shunts and lung units where $\dot{V}/\dot{Q}$ is zero. A relative shunt is an area of the lung with a low $\dot{V}/\dot{Q}$ ratio. Clinically, hypoxemia from a relative shunt can usually be partially corrected by increasing the inspired O_2 concentration; hypoxemia caused by an absolute shunt cannot achieve such correction.

Venous Admixture

Venous admixture is the amount of mixed venous blood that would have to be mixed with pulmonary end-capillary blood to account for the difference in O_2 tension between arterial and pulmonary end-capillary blood. Pulmonary end-capillary blood is considered to have the same concentrations as alveolar gas. Venous admixture is usually expressed as a fraction of total cardiac output $\dot{Q}_S/\dot{Q}_T$. The equation for $\dot{Q}_S/\dot{Q}_T$ may be derived with the law for the conservation of mass for O_2 across the pulmonary bed:

$$\dot{Q}_T \times Ca_{O_2} = (\dot{Q}_S \times C\bar{v}_{O_2}) + (\dot{Q}c' \times Cc'_{O_2})$$

where

$\dot{Q}_S$ = blood flow through the physiologic shunt compartment

Q_T = total cardiac output

$\dot{Q}c'$ = blood flow across normally ventilated pulmonary capillaries

$$\dot{Q}_T = \dot{Q}_{c'} + \dot{Q}_S$$

$Cc'O_2$ = oxygen content of ideal pulmonary end-capillary blood

CaO_2 = arterial oxygen content

$C\bar{v}O_2$ = mixed venous content

The simplified equation is:

$$\dot{Q}_S/\dot{Q}_T = \frac{Cc'O_2 - CaO_2}{Cc'O_2 - C\bar{v}O_2}$$

The formula for calculating the O_2 content of blood is given below.

$\dot{Q}_S/\dot{Q}_T$ can be calculated clinically by obtaining mixed venous and arterial blood gas measurements; the former requires a pulmonary artery catheter. The alveolar gas equation is used to derive pulmonary end-capillary O_2 tension. Pulmonary capillary blood is usually assumed to be 100% saturated for an FiO_2 of 0.21 or greater.

The calculated venous admixture assumes that all shunting is intrapulmonary and due to absolute shunts $\dot{V}/\dot{Q} = 0$. In reality, neither is ever the case; nonetheless, the concept is useful clinically. Normal $\dot{Q}_S/\dot{Q}_T$ is primarily due to communication between deep bronchial veins and pulmonary veins, the thebesian circulation in the heart, and areas of low $\dot{V}/\dot{Q}$ in the lungs (Figure 23–18). The venous admixture in normal individuals (physiological shunt) is typically less than 5%.

4. Effects of Anesthesia on Gas Exchange

Abnormalities in gas exchange during anesthesia are common. They include increased dead space, hypoventilation, and increased intrapulmonary shunting. There is increased scatter of $\dot{V}/\dot{Q}$ ratios. Increases in alveolar dead space are most commonly seen during controlled ventilation but may also
10 occur during spontaneous ventilation. General anesthesia commonly increases venous admixture to 5% to 10%, probably as a result of atelectasis and airway collapse in dependent areas of the lung. Inhalation agents, vasodilators, and inodilators also can inhibit **hypoxic pulmonary vasoconstriction**; for volatile agents, the ED_{50} is about twice the minimum alveolar concentration (MAC). Older adult patients seem to have the largest increases in $\dot{Q}_S/\dot{Q}_T$. Inspired O_2 tensions of 30% to 40% usually prevent hypoxemia, suggesting anesthesia increases relative shunt. PEEP is often effective in reducing venous admixture and preventing hypoxemia during general anesthesia, as long as cardiac output is maintained. Prolonged administration of high inspired O_2 concentrations may be associated with atelectasis formation and increases in absolute shunt. Atelectasis in this situation is known as *resorption atelectasis* and appears in areas with a low $\dot{V}/\dot{Q}$ ratio ventilated at an O_2-inspired concentration close to 100%. Perfusion results in O_2 being transported out of the alveoli at a rate faster than it enters the alveoli, leading to an emptying and collapse of the alveoli.

ALVEOLAR, ARTERIAL, & VENOUS GAS TENSIONS

When dealing with gas mixtures, each gas is considered to contribute separately to total gas pressure, and its partial pressure is directly proportional to its concentration. Air has an O_2 concentration of approximately 21%; therefore, if the barometric pressure is 760 mm Hg (sea level), the partial pressure of O_2 (PO_2) in air is normally 159.6 mm Hg:

$$760 \text{ mm Hg} \times 0.21 = 159.6 \text{ mm Hg}$$

In its general form, the equation may be written as follows:

$$P_{IO_2} = P_B \times FiO_2$$

where P_B = barometric pressure and FiO_2 = the fraction of inspired O_2.

1. Oxygen

Alveolar Oxygen Tension

With every breath, the inspired gas mixture is humidified at 37°C in the upper airway. The inspired tension of O_2 (P_{IO_2}) is therefore reduced by the

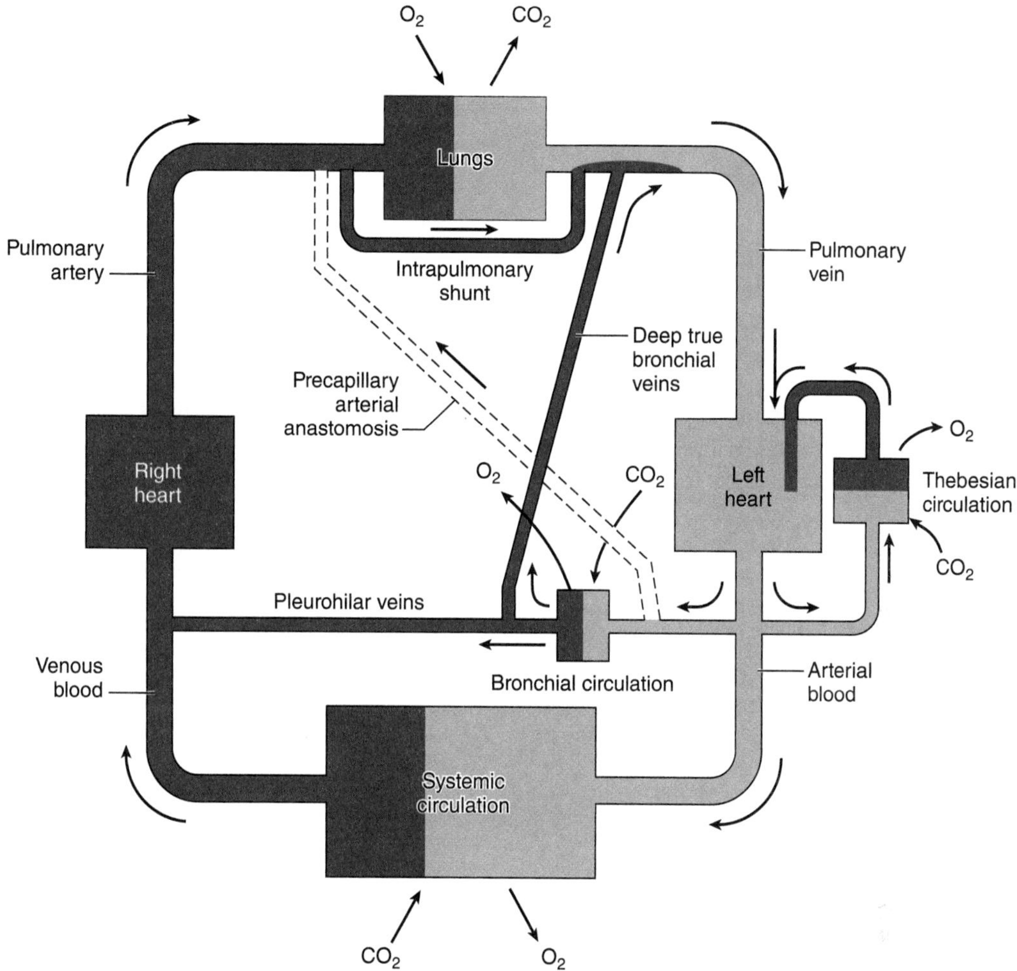

FIGURE 23–18 Components of the normal venous admixture. (Reproduced with permission from Lumb A. *Nunn's Applied Respiratory Physiology*, 8th ed. St. Louis, MO: Elsevier; 2017.)

added water vapor. Water vapor pressure is dependent upon temperature and is 47 mm Hg at 37°C. In humidified air, the normal partial pressure of O_2 at sea level is 150 mm Hg:

$$(760 - 47) \times 0.21 = 150 \text{ mm Hg}$$

The general equation is:

$$P_{IO_2} = (P_B - P_{H_2O}) \times F_{IO_2}$$

where P_{H_2O} = the vapor pressure of water at body temperature.

In alveoli, the inspired gases are mixed with residual alveolar gas from previous breaths, O_2 is taken up, and CO_2 is added. The final alveolar O_2 tension (P_{AO_2}) is therefore dependent on all of these factors and can be estimated by the following equation:

$$P_{AO_2} = P_{IO_2} - \frac{P_{aCO_2}}{R_Q}$$

where P_{aCO_2} = arterial CO_2 tension and RQ = respiratory quotient.

11 RQ is usually not measured. Note that large increases in $PaCO_2$ (>75 mm Hg) readily produce hypoxia (PaO_2 <60 mm Hg) at room air but not at high inspired O_2 concentrations.

Pulmonary End-Capillary Oxygen Tension

For all practical purposes, pulmonary end-capillary O_2 tension ($Pc'O_2$) may be considered identical to PAO_2; the PAO_2–$Pc'O_2$ gradient is normally minute. $Pc'O_2$ is dependent on the rate of O_2 diffusion across the alveolar–capillary membrane, as well as on pulmonary capillary blood volume and transit time. The large capillary surface area in alveoli and the 0.4 to 0.5 μm thickness of the alveolar–capillary membrane greatly facilitate O_2 diffusion. Enhanced O_2 binding to hemoglobin at saturations above 80% also augments O_2 diffusion (see below). Capillary transit time can be estimated by dividing pulmonary capillary blood volume by cardiac output (pulmonary blood flow); thus, normal capillary transit time is 70 mL ÷ 5000 mL/min (0.8 s). Maximum $Pc'O_2$ is usually attained after only 0.3 s, providing a large safety margin.

12 The binding of O_2 to hemoglobin seems to be the principal rate-limiting factor in the transfer of O_2 from alveolar gas to blood. Therefore, pulmonary diffusing capacity reflects not only the capacity and permeability of the alveolar–capillary membrane but also pulmonary blood flow. Moreover, O_2 uptake is normally limited by pulmonary blood flow, not O_2 diffusion across the alveolar-capillary membrane; the latter may become significant during exercise in normal individuals at high altitudes and in patients with extensive destruction of the alveolar–capillary membrane.

O_2 transfer across the alveolar–capillary membrane is expressed as O_2 *diffusing capacity* (DLO_2):

$$DLO_2 = \frac{\text{Oxygen uptake}}{PAO_2 - Pc'O_2}$$

Because $Pc'O_2$ cannot be measured accurately, measurement of carbon monoxide diffusion capacity (DLCO) is used instead to assess gas transfer across the alveolar–capillary membrane. Because carbon monoxide has a very high affinity for hemoglobin, there is little or no carbon monoxide in pulmonary capillary blood, so even when it is administered at a low concentration, Pc′CO can be considered zero. Therefore,

$$DLCO = \frac{\text{Carbon monoxide uptake}}{PACO}$$

Reductions in DLCO imply an impediment in gas transfer across the alveolar–capillary membrane. Such impediments may be due to abnormal $\dot{V}/\dot{Q}$ ratios, extensive destruction of the gas alveolar–capillary membrane, or very short capillary transit times. Abnormalities are accentuated by increases in O_2 consumption and cardiac output, such as occurs during exercise.

Arterial Oxygen Tension

PaO_2 cannot be calculated like PAO_2 but must be measured at room air. The *alveolar-to-arterial O_2 partial pressure gradient* (A–a gradient) is normally less than 15 mm Hg, but it progressively increases with age up to 20 to 30 mm Hg. Arterial O_2 tension can be approximated by the following formula (in mm Hg):

$$PaO_2 = 120 - \frac{\text{Age}}{3}$$

The range is 60 to 100 mm Hg. Decreases are probably the result of a progressive increase in closing capacity relative to FRC (see earlier discussion). Table 23–3 lists the mechanisms of hypoxemia (PaO_2 <60 mm Hg).

The most common mechanism for hypoxemia is an increased alveolar–arterial gradient. The A–a gradient for O_2 depends on the amount of right-to-left shunting, the amount of $\dot{V}/\dot{Q}$ scatter, and the mixed venous O_2 tension (see below). The last depends on cardiac output, O_2 consumption, and hemoglobin concentration.

The A–a gradient for O_2 is directly proportional to shunt but inversely proportional to mixed venous O_2 tension. Figure 23–19 shows the effect
13 of different degrees of shunting on PaO_2. It should also be noted that the greater the shunt, the less likely the possibility that an increase in FiO_2 will correct hypoxemia. Moreover, iso-shunt lines

TABLE 23–3 Mechanisms of hypoxemia.

Low alveolar oxygen tension
Low inspired oxygen tension
Low fractional inspired concentration
High altitude
Alveolar hypoventilation
Diffusion hypoxia
Increased oxygen consumption
Increased alveolar–arterial gradient
Right-to-left shunting
Increased areas of low[1] ratios
Low mixed venous oxygen tension
Decreased cardiac output
Increased oxygen consumption
Decreased hemoglobin concentration

[1] $\dot{V}/\dot{Q}$ ventilation/perfusion.

seem to be most useful for O_2 concentrations between 35% and 100%. Lower O_2 concentrations require modification of iso-shunt lines to account for the effect of $\dot{V}/\dot{Q}$ scatter.

The effect of cardiac output on the A–a gradient (Figure 23–20) is due not only to its secondary effects on mixed venous O_2 tension but also to a direct relationship between cardiac output and intrapulmonary shunting. As can be seen, a low cardiac output tends to accentuate the effect of shunt on PaO_2. A reduction in venous admixture may be observed with low-normal cardiac outputs secondary to accentuated pulmonary vasoconstriction from a lower mixed venous O_2 tension. On the other hand, high cardiac outputs can increase venous admixture by elevating mixed venous O_2 tension, which in turn inhibits hypoxic pulmonary vasoconstriction.

O_2 consumption and hemoglobin concentration can also affect PaO_2 through their secondary effects on mixed venous O_2 tension (below). High O_2 consumption rates and low hemoglobin concentrations can increase the A–a gradient and depress PaO_2.

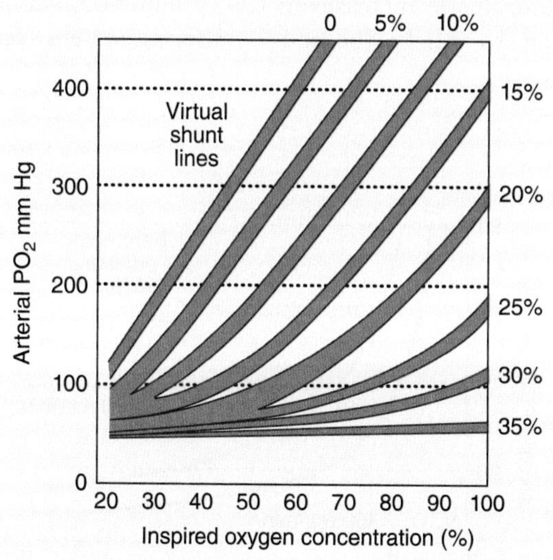

FIGURE 23–19 Iso-shunt curves showing the effect of varying amounts of shunt on PaO_2. Note that there is little benefit in increasing inspired oxygen concentration in patients with very large shunts. (Modified with permission from Benatar SR, Hewlett AM, Nunn JF. The use of isoshunt lines for control of oxygen therapy, *Br J Anaesth*. 1973 July;45(7):711-718.)

Mixed Venous Oxygen Tension

Normal mixed venous O_2 tension $P\bar{v}O_2$ is about 40 mm Hg and represents the overall balance between O_2 consumption and O_2 delivery (Table 23–4). A true mixed venous blood sample contains venous drainage from the superior vena cava, the inferior vena cava, and the heart; it must therefore be obtained from a pulmonary artery catheter.

2. Carbon Dioxide

Carbon dioxide is produced by aerobic metabolism in mitochondria. Therefore, there are gradients for CO_2 tension from mitochondria to cell cytoplasm, extracellular fluid, venous blood, and alveoli, where the CO_2 is finally eliminated.

Mixed Venous Carbon Dioxide Tension

Normal mixed venous CO_2 tension $P\bar{v}CO_2$ is about 46 mm Hg and is the end result of the mixing of blood from tissues of varying metabolic activity. Venous CO_2 tension is lower in tissues with low metabolic activity (eg, skin) but higher in blood from those with relatively high activity (eg, heart).

Alveolar Carbon Dioxide Tension

Alveolar CO_2 tension (P_ACO_2) is generally considered to represent the balance between total

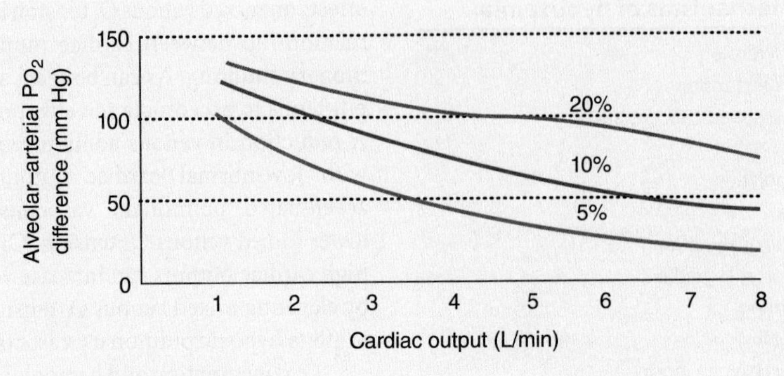

FIGURE 23–20 The effect of cardiac output on the alveolar–arterial PO_2 difference with varying degrees of shunting. $\dot{V}O_2$ = 200 mL/min and PaO_2 = 180 mm Hg.) (Reproduced with permission from Lumb A. *Nunn's Applied Respiratory Physiology,* 8th ed. St. Louis, MO: Elsevier; 2017.)

CO_2 production $\bar{V}CO_2$ and alveolar ventilation (elimination):

$$P_ACO_2 = \frac{\bar{V}CO_2}{\bar{V}_A}$$

where $\dot{V}_A$ is alveolar ventilation (Figure 23–21). During periods of acute hypoventilation or hypoperfusion, body content of carbon dioxide increases. Clinically, P_ACO_2 is more dependent on variations in alveolar ventilation than in CO_2 production, because CO_2 production does not vary appreciably under most circumstances. However, conditions such as malignant hyperthermia can lead to dramatic increases in CO_2 production, which can overwhelm the body's buffering system (see below).

TABLE 23–4 Alterations in mixed venous oxygen tension (and saturation).

Decreased $P\bar{v}O_2$
Increased O_2 consumption
Fever
Shivering
Exercise
Malignant hyperthermia
Thyroid storm
Decreased O_2 delivery
Hypoxia
Decreased cardiac output
Decreased hemoglobin concentration
Abnormal hemoglobin
Increased $P\bar{v}O_2$
Left-to-right shunting
High cardiac output
Impaired tissue uptake
Cyanide poisoning
Decreased oxygen consumption
Hypothermia
Combined mechanisms
Sepsis
Sampling error
Wedged pulmonary artery catheter

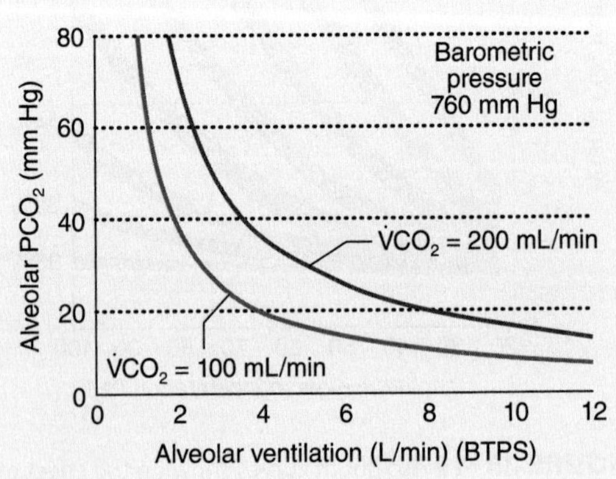

FIGURE 23–21 The effect of alveolar ventilation on alveolar PCO_2 at two rates of CO_2 production. (Reproduced with permission from Lumb A. *Nunn's Applied Respiratory Physiology,* 8th ed. St. Louis, MO: Elsevier; 2017.)

Pulmonary End-Capillary Carbon Dioxide Tension

Pulmonary end-capillary CO_2 tension ($Pc'CO_2$) is virtually identical to P_ACO_2 for the same reasons as those discussed in the section about O_2. In addition, the diffusion rate for CO_2 across the alveolar–capillary membrane is 20 times that of O_2.

Arterial Carbon Dioxide Tension

Arterial CO_2 tension ($PaCO_2$), which is readily measurable, is identical to $Pc'CO_2$, and, necessarily, P_ACO_2. Normal $PaCO_2$ is 38 ± 4 mm Hg (5.1 ± 0.5 kPa); in practice, 40 mm Hg is usually considered normal.

Although low $\dot{V}/\dot{Q}$ ratios tend to increase $PaCO_2$, whereas high $\dot{V}/\dot{Q}$ ratios tend to decrease it, significant arterial-to-alveolar gradients for CO_2 develop only in the presence of marked $\dot{V}/\dot{Q}$ abnormalities (>30% venous admixture); even then, the gradient is relatively small (2–3 mm Hg). Moreover, small increases in the gradient appreciably increase CO_2 output into alveoli with relatively normal $\dot{V}/\dot{Q}$. Even moderate to severe disturbances usually fail to appreciably alter arterial CO_2 because of a reflex increase in ventilation from concomitant hypoxemia.

End-Tidal Carbon Dioxide Tension

Because end-tidal gas is primarily alveolar gas and P_ACO_2 is virtually identical to $PaCO_2$, end-tidal CO_2 tension ($PETCO_2$) is used clinically as an estimate of $PaCO_2$. The P_ACO_2–$PETCO_2$ gradient is normally less than 5 mm Hg and represents the dilution of alveolar gas with CO_2-free gas from nonperfused alveoli (alveolar dead space).

TRANSPORT OF RESPIRATORY GASES IN BLOOD

1. Oxygen

O_2 is carried in blood in two forms: dissolved in solution and in reversible association with hemoglobin.

Dissolved Oxygen

The amount of O_2 dissolved in blood can be derived from **Henry's law**, which states that the concentration of any gas in solution is proportional to its partial pressure. The mathematical expression is as follows:

$$\text{Gas concentration} = \alpha \times \text{Partial pressure}$$

where α = the gas solubility coefficient for a given solution at a given temperature.

The solubility coefficient for O_2 at normal body temperature is 0.003 mL/dL/mm Hg. Even with a PaO_2 of 100 mm Hg, the maximum amount of O_2 dissolved in blood is very small (0.3 mL/dL) compared with that bound to hemoglobin.

Hemoglobin

Hemoglobin is a complex molecule consisting of four heme and four protein subunits. Heme is an iron–porphyrin compound that is an essential part of the O_2-binding sites; only the divalent form (+2 charge) of iron can bind O_2. The normal hemoglobin molecule (hemoglobin A_1) consists of two α and two β chains (subunits); the four subunits are held together by weak bonds between the amino acid residues. Each gram of hemoglobin can theoretically carry up to 1.39 mL of O_2.

Hemoglobin Dissociation Curve

Each hemoglobin molecule binds up to four O_2 molecules. The complex interaction between the hemoglobin subunits results in nonlinear (an elongated S shape) binding with O_2 (Figure 23–22). Hemoglobin saturation is the amount of O_2 bound as a percentage of its total O_2-binding capacity. Four separate chemical reactions are involved in binding each of the four O_2 molecules. The change in molecular conformation induced by the binding of the first three molecules greatly accelerates binding of the fourth O_2 molecule. The last reaction is responsible for the accelerated binding between 25% and 100% saturation. At about 90% saturation, the decrease in available O_2 receptors flattens the curve until full saturation is reached.

Factors Influencing the Hemoglobin Dissociation Curve

Clinically important factors altering O_2 binding include hydrogen ion concentration, CO_2 tension, temperature, and 2,3-diphosphoglycerate (2,3-DPG) concentration. Their effect on hemoglobin–O_2

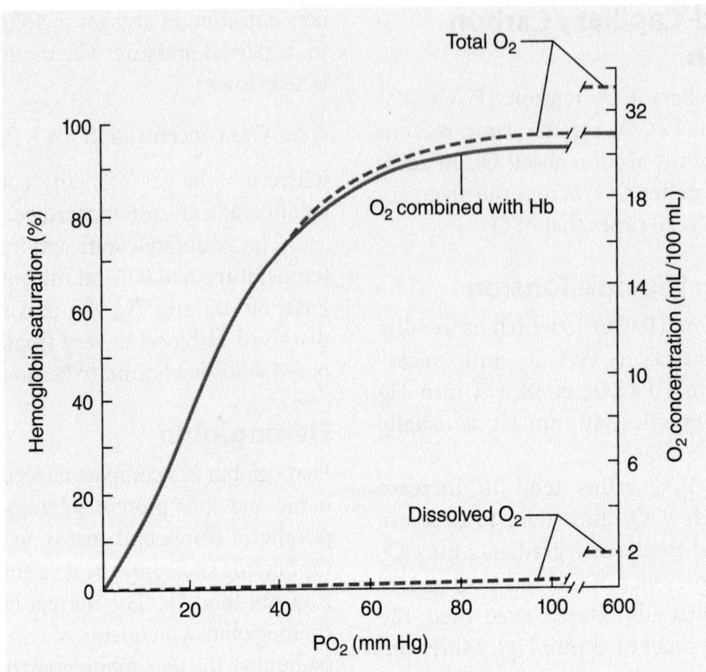

FIGURE 23–22 The normal adult hemoglobin–oxygen dissociation curve. (Modified with permission from West JB. *Respiratory Physiology: The Essentials.* 6th ed. Philadelphia, PA: Williams and Wilkins; 2000.)

interaction can be expressed by P_{50}, the O_2 tension at which hemoglobin is 50% saturated (Figure 23–23). Each factor shifts the dissociation curve either to the right (increasing P_{50}) or to the left (decreasing P_{50}). 14 A rightward shift in the oxygen–hemoglobin dissociation curve lowers O_2 affinity, displaces O_2 from hemoglobin, and makes more O_2 available to tissues; a leftward shift increases hemoglobin's affinity for O_2, reducing its availability to tissues. The normal P_{50} in adults is 26.6 mm Hg.

An increase in blood hydrogen ion concentration reduces O_2 binding to hemoglobin (Bohr effect). Because of the shape of the **hemoglobin dissociation curve**, the effect is more important in venous blood than arterial blood (see Figure 23–23); the net result is the facilitation of O_2 release to tissue with little impairment in O_2 uptake (unless severe hypoxia is present).

The influence of CO_2 tension on hemoglobin's affinity for O_2 is important physiologically and is secondary to the associated rise in hydrogen ion concentration when CO_2 tension increases. The high CO_2 content of venous capillary blood, by decreasing hemoglobin's affinity for O_2, facilitates the release of O_2 to tissues; conversely, the lower CO_2 content in pulmonary capillaries increases hemoglobin's affinity for O_2 again, facilitating O_2 uptake from alveoli.

2,3-DPG is a byproduct of glycolysis and accumulates during anaerobic metabolism. Although its effects on hemoglobin under these conditions are theoretically beneficial, its physiological importance normally seems minor. 2,3-DPG levels may, however, play an important compensatory role in patients with chronic anemia and may significantly affect the O_2-carrying capacity of blood transfusions.

Abnormal Ligands & Abnormal Forms of Hemoglobin

Carbon monoxide, cyanide, sulfur monoxide, and hydrogen sulfide can combine with hemoglobin at O_2-binding sites. Carbon monoxide is particularly potent, having 200 to 300 times the affinity of O_2 for hemoglobin, combining with it to form

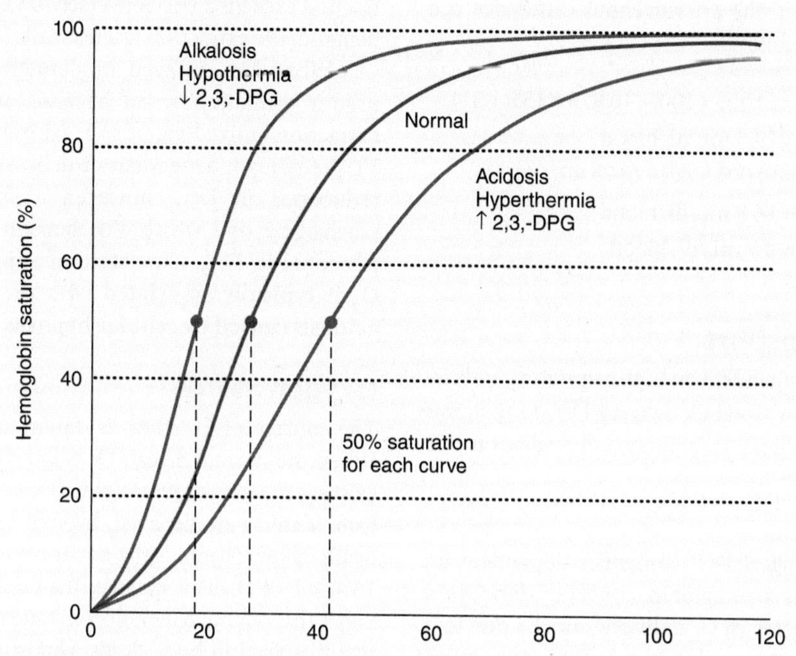

FIGURE 23–23 The effects of changes in acid–base status, body temperature, and 2,3-DPG concentration on the hemoglobin–oxygen dissociation curve.

carboxyhemoglobin. Carbon monoxide decreases hemoglobin's O_2-carrying capacity and impairs the release of O_2 to tissues. Carbon dioxide binds to a different site on heme, allosterically favoring the unloading of O_2. The interaction of nitric oxide with hemoglobin is complex, and some investigators have hypothesized that the transport and delivery of nitric oxide by hemoglobin likely serves to regulate oxygen delivery to tissues.

Methemoglobin results when the iron in heme is oxidized to its trivalent (+3) form. Nitrates, nitrites, sulfonamides, and other drugs can rarely result in significant methemoglobinemia. Methemoglobin cannot combine with O_2 unless reconverted by the enzyme methemoglobin reductase; methemoglobin also shifts the normal hemoglobin saturation curve to the left. Methemoglobinemia, like carbon monoxide poisoning, therefore decreases the O_2-carrying capacity and impairs the release of O_2. Reduction of methemoglobin to normal hemoglobin is facilitated by such agents as methylene blue or ascorbic acid.

Abnormal hemoglobins can also result from variations in the protein subunit composition. Each variant has its own O_2-saturation characteristics. These include fetal hemoglobin, hemoglobin A_2, and sickle hemoglobin, among many others.

Oxygen Content

The total O_2 content of blood is the sum of that in solution plus that carried by hemoglobin. In reality, O_2 binding to hemoglobin never achieves the theoretical maximum, but it is closer to 1.31 mL O_2/dL blood per millimeter of mercury. Total O_2 content is expressed by the following equation:

$$O_2 \text{ content} = ([0.003 \text{ mL } O_2/\text{dL blood per mm Hg}] \times Po_2) + (So_2 \times Hb \times 1.31 \text{ mL/dL blood})$$

where Hb is hemoglobin concentration in g/dL blood, and So_2 is hemoglobin saturation at the given Po_2.

Using this formula and a hemoglobin of 15 g/dL, the normal O_2 content for both arterial and mixed venous blood and the arteriovenous difference can be calculated as follows:

$$\begin{aligned}
Cao_2 &= (0.003 \times 100) + (0.975 \times 15 \times 1.31) \\
&= 19.5 \text{ mL/dL blood} \\
C\overline{v}o_2 &= (0.003 \times 40) + (0.75 \times 15 \times 1.31) \\
&= 14.8 \text{ mL/dL blood} \\
Cao_2 - C\overline{v}o_2 &= 4.7 \text{ mL/dL blood}
\end{aligned}$$

Oxygen Transport

O_2 transport is dependent on both respiratory and circulatory function. Total O_2 delivery $\dot{D}o_2$ to tissues is the product of arterial O_2 content and cardiac output:

$$\dot{D}O_2 = CaO_2 \times \dot{Q}T$$

Note that arterial O_2 content is dependent on PaO_2 as well as hemoglobin concentration. **As a result, deficiencies in O_2 delivery may be due to a low PaO_2, a low hemoglobin concentration, or an inadequate cardiac output.** Normal O_2 delivery can be calculated as follows:

$$\begin{aligned}
O_2 \text{ delivery} &= 20 \text{ mL } O_2\text{/dL blood} \\
&\times 50 \text{ dL blood/min} \\
&= 1000 \text{ mL } O_2\text{/min}
\end{aligned}$$

The Fick equation expresses the relationship between O_2 consumption, O_2 content, and cardiac output:

$$O_2 \text{ consumption} = \dot{V}o_2 = \dot{Q}T \times (Cao_2 - C\overline{v}o_2)$$

Rearranging the equation:

$$Cao_2 = \frac{\dot{V}o_2}{\dot{Q}T} + C\overline{v}o_2$$

Consequently, the arteriovenous difference is a good measure of the overall adequacy of O_2 delivery.

As calculated above, the arteriovenous difference $Cao_2 - C\overline{v}o_2$ is about 5 mL O_2/dL blood (20 mL O_2/dL – 15 mL O_2/dL). Note that the normal extraction fraction for $O_2[(Cao_2 - C\overline{v}o_2)/Cao_2]$ is 5 mL ÷ 20 mL, or 25%; thus, the body normally consumes only 25% of the O_2 carried on hemoglobin. When O_2 demand exceeds supply, the extraction fraction exceeds 25%. Conversely, if O_2 supply exceeds demand, the extraction fraction falls below 25%.

When $\dot{D}o_2$ is even moderately reduced, $\dot{V}o_2$ usually remains normal because of increased O_2 extraction (mixed venous O_2 saturation decreases); $\dot{V}o_2$ remains independent of delivery. With further reductions in $\dot{D}o_2$, however, a critical point is reached beyond which $\dot{V}o_2$ becomes directly proportional to $\dot{D}o_2$. **This state of supply-dependent O_2 is typically associated with progressive lactic acidosis caused by cellular hypoxia.**

Oxygen Stores

The concept of O_2 stores is important in anesthesia. When the normal flux of O_2 is interrupted by apnea, existing O_2 stores are consumed by cellular metabolism; if stores are depleted, hypoxia and eventual cell death follow. Theoretically, adults normally store about 1500 mL of O_2. This includes the O_2 remaining in the lungs, that bound to hemoglobin (and myoglobin), and that dissolved in body fluids. Unfortunately, the high affinity of hemoglobin for O_2 (the affinity of myoglobin is even higher), and the very limited quantity of O_2 in solution, restrict the availability of these stores. The O_2 contained within the lungs at FRC (initial lung volume during apnea), therefore, becomes the most important source of O_2. Apnea in a patient previously breathing room air leaves approximately 480 mL of O_2 in the lungs. (If $FiO_2 = 0.21$ and FRC = 2300 mL, O_2 content = $FiO_2 \times$ FRC.) The metabolic activity of tissues rapidly depletes this reservoir (presumably at a rate equivalent to VO_2); severe hypoxemia usually occurs within 90 sec. The onset of hypoxemia can be delayed by increasing the FiO_2 prior to the apnea. Following ventilation with 100% O_2, FRC contains about 2300 mL of O_2; this delays hypoxemia following apnea for 4 to 5 min. This concept is the basis for preoxygenation (denitrogenation) prior to induction of anesthesia.

2. Carbon Dioxide

Carbon dioxide is transported in blood in three forms: dissolved in solution, as bicarbonate, and with proteins in the form of carbamino compounds (Table 23–5). The sum of all three forms is the total CO_2 content of blood (routinely reported with electrolyte measurements).

TABLE 23–5 Contributions to carbon dioxide transport in 1 L of whole blood.

Form	Plasma	Erythrocytes	Combined	Contribution (%)
Mixed venous whole blood				
Dissolved CO_2	0.76	0.51	1.27	5.5
Bicarbonate	14.41	5.92	20.33	87.2
Carbamino CO_2	Negligible	1.70	1.70	7.3
Total CO_2	15.17	8.13	23.30	
Arterial whole blood				
Dissolved CO_2	0.66	0.44	1.10	5.1
Bicarbonate	13.42	5.88	19.30	89.9
Carbamino CO_2	Negligible	1.10	1.10	5.1
Total CO_2	14.08	7.42	21.50	

Values are expressed in millimoles, except where indicated otherwise.
Data from Nunn JF. *Nunn's Applied Physiology.* 4th ed. Philadelphia, PA: Butterworth; 2000.

Dissolved Carbon Dioxide

Carbon dioxide is more soluble in blood than O_2, with a solubility coefficient of 0.031 mmol/L/mm Hg (0.067 mL/dL/mm Hg) at 37°C.

Bicarbonate

In aqueous solutions, CO_2 slowly combines with water to form carbonic acid and bicarbonate, according to the following reaction:

$$H_2O + CO_2 \leftrightarrow H_2CO_3 \leftrightarrow H^+ + HCO_3^-$$

In plasma, although less than 1% of the dissolved CO_2 undergoes this reaction, the presence of the enzyme **carbonic anhydrase** within erythrocytes and endothelium greatly accelerates the reaction.
15 As a result, bicarbonate represents the largest fraction of the CO_2 in blood (see Table 23–5). Administration of acetazolamide, a carbonic anhydrase inhibitor, can impair CO_2 transport between tissues and alveoli.

On the venous side of systemic capillaries, CO_2 enters red blood cells and is converted to bicarbonate, which diffuses out of red cells into plasma; chloride ions move from plasma into red cells to maintain electrical balance. In the pulmonary capillaries, the reverse occurs: chloride ions move out of red cells as bicarbonate ions reenter them for conversion back to CO_2, which diffuses out into alveoli. This sequence is referred to as the *chloride* or *Hamburger shift*.

Carbamino Compounds

Carbon dioxide can react with amino groups on proteins, as shown by the following equation:

$$R - NH_2 + CO_2 \rightarrow RNH - CO_2^- + H^+$$

At physiological pH, only a small amount of CO_2 is carried in this form, mainly as carbaminohemoglobin. Deoxygenated hemoglobin (deoxyhemoglobin) has a greater affinity (3.5 times) for CO_2 than does oxyhemoglobin. As a result, venous blood carries more CO_2 than does arterial blood (Haldane effect; see Table 23–5). PCO_2 normally has little effect on the fraction of CO_2 carried as carbaminohemoglobin.

Effects of Hemoglobin Buffering on Carbon Dioxide Transport

The buffering action of hemoglobin also accounts for part of the Haldane effect. Hemoglobin can act as a buffer at physiological pH because of its high content of histidine. Moreover, the acid–base behavior of hemoglobin is influenced by its oxygenation state:

$$H^+ + HbO_2 \rightarrow HbH^+ + O_2$$

Removal of O_2 from hemoglobin in tissue capillaries causes the hemoglobin molecule to behave more like a base; by taking up hydrogen ions, hemoglobin shifts the CO_2–bicarbonate equilibrium in favor of greater bicarbonate formation:

$$CO_2 + H_2O + HbO_2 \rightarrow HbH^+ + HCO_3^- + O_2$$

As a direct result, deoxyhemoglobin also increases the amount of CO_2 that is carried in venous blood as bicarbonate. As CO_2 is taken up from tissue and converted to bicarbonate, the total CO_2 content of blood increases (see Table 23–5).

In the lungs, the reverse is true. Oxygenation of hemoglobin favors its action as an acid, and the release of hydrogen ions shifts the equilibrium in favor of greater CO_2 formation:

$$O_2 + HCO_3^- + HbH^+ \rightarrow H_2O + CO_2 + HbO_2$$

Bicarbonate concentration decreases as CO_2 is formed and eliminated, so the total CO_2 content of blood decreases in the lungs. Note that there is a difference between CO_2 content (concentration per liter) of whole blood (see Table 23–5) and plasma (Table 23–6).

Carbon Dioxide Dissociation Curve

A CO_2 dissociation curve can be constructed by plotting the total CO_2 content of blood against PCO_2. The contribution of each form of CO_2 can also be quantified in this manner (Figure 23–24).

TABLE 23–6 Carbon dioxide content of plasma (mmol/L).

	Arterial	Venous
Dissolved CO_2	1.2	1.4
Bicarbonate	24.4	26.2
Carbamino CO_2	Negligible	Negligible
Total CO_2	25.6	27.6

Values are expressed in millimoles, except where indicated otherwise.
Data from Nunn JF. *Nunn's Applied Physiology.* 4th ed. Philadelphia, PA: Butterworth; 2000.

Carbon Dioxide Stores

Carbon dioxide stores in the body are large (approximately 120 L in adults) and primarily in the form of dissolved CO_2 and bicarbonate. When an imbalance occurs between production and elimination, establishing a new CO_2 equilibrium requires 20 to 30 min (compared with less than 4 to 5 min for O_2; see above). Carbon dioxide is stored in the rapid-, intermediate-, and slow-equilibrating compartments. Because of the larger capacity of the intermediate and slow compartments, the rate of rise in arterial CO_2 tension is generally slower than its fall following acute changes in ventilation.

CONTROL OF BREATHING

Spontaneous ventilation is the result of rhythmic neural activity in respiratory centers within the brainstem. This activity regulates respiratory muscles to maintain normal tensions of O_2 and CO_2 in the body. The basic neuronal activity is modified by inputs from other areas in the brain, volitional and autonomic, as well as various central and peripheral receptors (sensors).

1. Central Respiratory Centers

The basic breathing rhythm originates in the medulla. Two medullary groups of neurons are generally recognized: a dorsal respiratory group, which is primarily active during inspiration, and a ventral respiratory group, which is active during inspiration and expiration.

Two pontine areas influence the dorsal (inspiratory) medullary center. A lower pontine (apneustic) center is excitatory, whereas an upper pontine (pneumotaxic) center is inhibitory. The pontine centers appear to fine-tune respiratory rate and rhythm.

2. Central Sensors

The most important of these sensors are chemoreceptors that respond to changes in hydrogen ion
16 concentration. Central chemoreceptors are thought to lie on the anterolateral surface of the medulla and respond primarily to changes in cerebrospinal fluid (CSF) [H^+]. This mechanism is effective in regulating $PaCO_2$ because the blood–brain barrier is permeable to dissolved CO_2 but not to bicarbonate ions. Acute changes in $PaCO_2$ but not

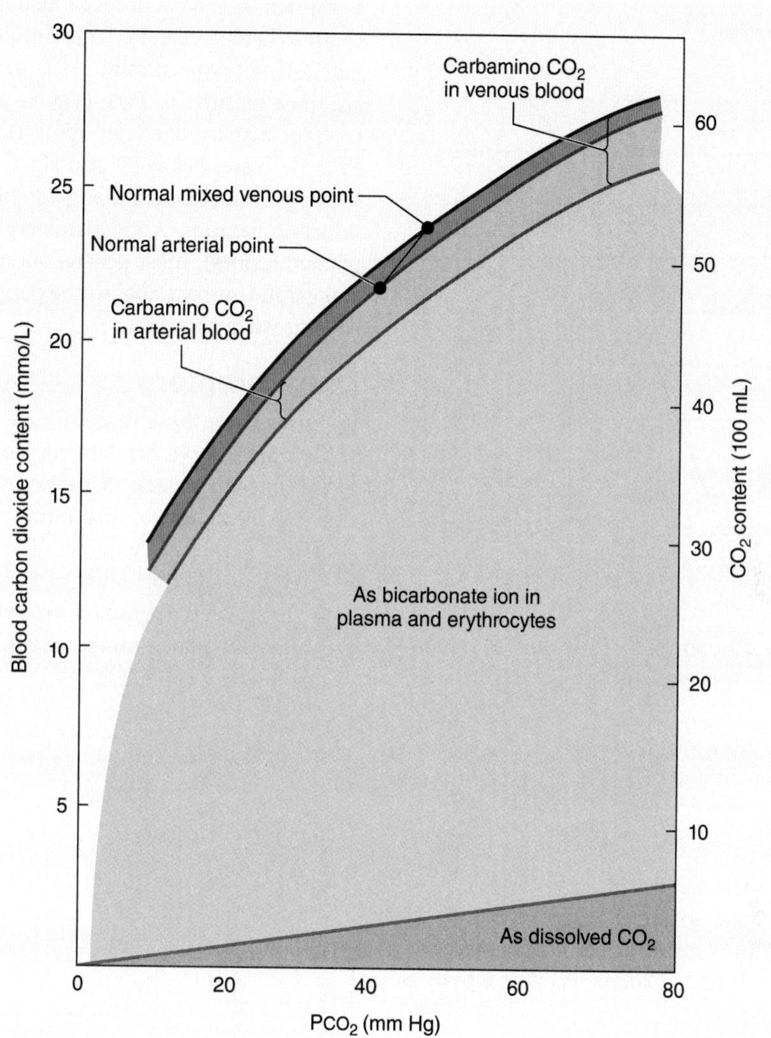

FIGURE 23–24 The CO_2 dissociation curve for whole blood. (Reproduced with permission from Lumb A. *Nunn's Applied Respiratory Physiology,* 8th ed. St. Louis, MO: Elsevier; 2017.)

in arterial $[HCO_3^-]$, are reflected in CSF; thus, a change in CO_2 must result in a change in $[H^+]$:

$$CO_2 + H_2O \leftrightarrow H^+ + HCO_3^-$$

Over the course of a few days, CSF $[HCO_3^-]$ can compensate to match any change in arterial $[HCO_3^-]$.

Increases in $PaCO_2$ elevate CSF hydrogen ion concentration and activate the chemoreceptors. Secondary stimulation of the adjacent respiratory medullary centers increases alveolar ventilation (Figure 23–25) and reduces $PaCO_2$ back to normal. Conversely, decreases in CSF hydrogen ion concentration secondary to reductions in $PaCO_2$ reduce alveolar ventilation and elevate $PaCO_2$. Note that the relationship between $PaCO_2$ and minute volume is nearly linear. Also note that very high arterial $PaCO_2$ tensions depress the ventilatory response (CO_2 narcosis). The $PaCO_2$ at which ventilation is zero (*x*-intercept) is known as the *apneic threshold*. Spontaneous respirations are typically absent under anesthesia when $PaCO_2$ falls below the

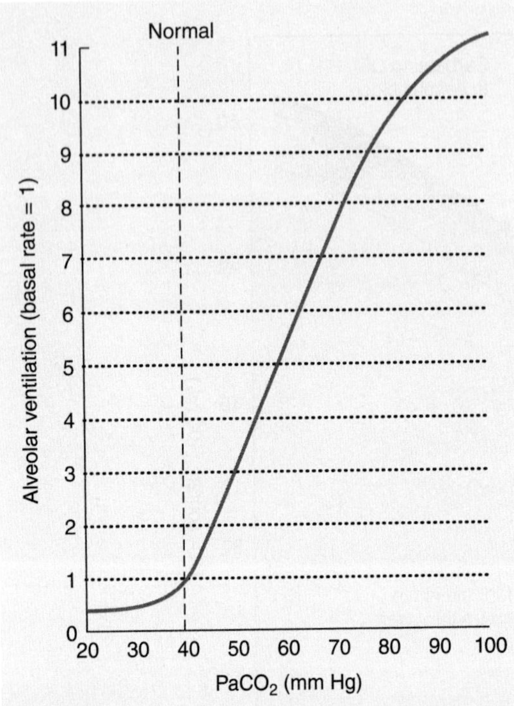

FIGURE 23–25 The normal relationship between $PaCO_2$ and minute ventilation. (Reproduced with permission from Guyton AC. *Textbook of Medical Physiology,* 7th ed. Philadelphia, PA: WB Saunders; 1986.)

apneic threshold. (In the awake state, cortical influences prevent apnea, so apneic thresholds are not ordinarily seen.) In contrast to peripheral chemoreceptors (see below), central chemoreceptor activity is depressed by hypoxia.

3. Peripheral Sensors

Peripheral Chemoreceptors

Peripheral chemoreceptors include the *carotid bodies* (at the bifurcation of the common carotid arteries) and the *aortic bodies* (surrounding the aortic arch). The carotid bodies are the principal peripheral chemoreceptors in humans and are sensitive to changes in PaO_2, $PaCO_2$, pH, and arterial perfusion pressure. They interact with central respiratory centers via the glossopharyngeal nerves, producing reflex increases in alveolar ventilation in response to reductions in PaO_2, arterial perfusion, or elevations in $[H^+]$ and $PaCO_2$. Peripheral chemoreceptors are also stimulated by cyanide, doxapram, and large doses of nicotine. In contrast to central chemoreceptors, which respond primarily to $PaCO_2$ (more specifically, $[H^+]$), the carotid bodies are most sensitive to Pao_2 (Figure 23–26). Note that receptor activity does not appreciably increase until PaO_2 decreases below 50 mm Hg. Cells of the carotid body (glomus cells) are thought to be primarily dopaminergic neurons. Antidopaminergic drugs (such as phenothiazines), most general anesthetics, and bilateral carotid surgery abolish the peripheral ventilatory response to hypoxemia.

Lung Receptors

Impulses from these receptors are carried centrally by the vagus nerve. Stretch receptors are distributed in the smooth muscle of airways; they are responsible for inhibition of inspiration when the lung is inflated to excessive volumes (*Hering–Breuer inflation reflex*) and shortening of exhalation when the lung is deflated (*deflation reflex*). Stretch receptors normally play a minor role in humans. In fact,

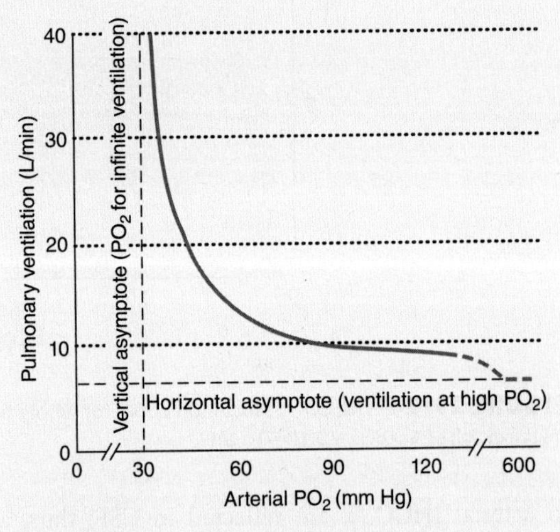

FIGURE 23–26 The relationship between PaO_2 and minute ventilation at rest and with a normal $PaCO_2$. (Data from Weil JV, Byrne-Quinn E, Sodal IE, et al. Hypoxic ventilatory drive in normal man. *J Clin Invest.* 1970;49:1061-1072; Dripps RD, Comroe JH. The effect of the inhalation of high and low oxygen concentration on respiration, pulse rate, ballistocardiogram and arterial oxygen saturation (oximeter) of normal individuals. *Am J Physiol.* 1947;149:277–291; Cormac RS, Cunningham DJC, Gee JBL. The effect of carbon dioxide on the respiratory response to want of oxygen in man. *Q J Exp Physiol.* 1957;42:303-316.)

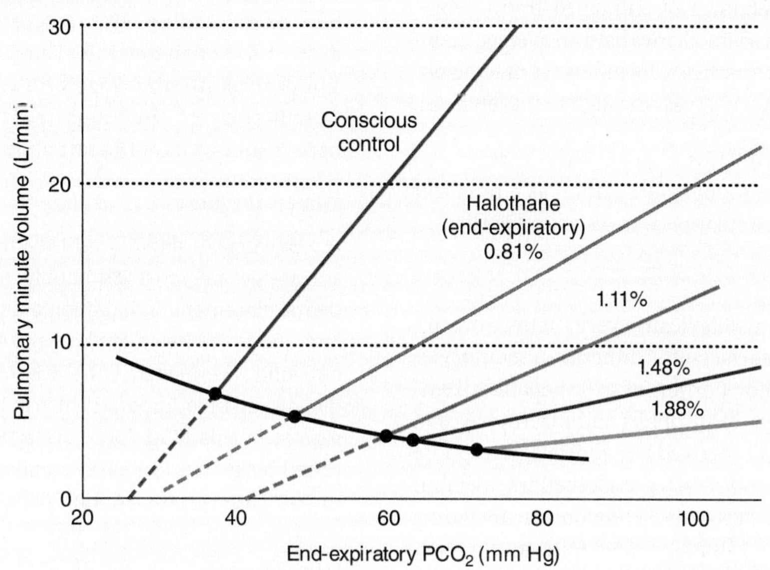

FIGURE 23–27 The effect of volatile agents (halothane) on the $PETCO_2$–ventilation response curve (see text). (Data from Munson ES, Larson CP, Babad AA, et al. The effects of halothane, fluroxene and cyclopropane on ventilation: A comparative study in man. *Anesthesiology.* 1966 Nov-Dec;27(6):716-728.)

bilateral vagal nerve blocks have a minimal effect on the normal respiratory pattern.

Irritant receptors in the tracheobronchial mucosa react to noxious gases, smoke, dust, and cold gases; activation produces reflex increases in respiratory rate, bronchoconstriction, and coughing. *Juxtacapillary (J) receptors* are located in the interstitial space within alveolar walls; these receptors induce dyspnea in response to the expansion of interstitial space volume and various chemical mediators following tissue damage.

Other Receptors

These include various muscle and joint receptors on pulmonary muscles and the chest wall. Input from these sources is probably important during exercise and in pathological conditions associated with decreased lung or chest compliance.

4. Effects of Anesthesia on the Control of Breathing

The most important effect of most general anesthetics on breathing is a tendency to promote hypoventilation. The mechanism is probably dual: central depression of the chemoreceptor and depression of external intercostal muscle activity. The magnitude of the hypoventilation is generally proportional to 17 anesthetic depth. With increasing depth of anesthesia, the slope of the $PaCO_2$/minute ventilation curve decreases, and the apneic threshold increases (Figure 23–27). This effect is at least partially reversed by surgical stimulation.

The peripheral response to hypoxemia is even more sensitive to anesthetics than the central CO_2 response and is nearly abolished by even subanesthetic doses of most inhalation agents (including nitrous oxide) and many intravenous agents.

NONRESPIRATORY FUNCTIONS OF THE LUNG

Filtration & Reservoir Function

A. Filtration

The unique in-series position of the pulmonary capillaries within the circulation allows them to act as a filter for debris in the bloodstream. The high content of heparin and plasminogen activator in the lungs facilitates the breakdown of entrapped fibrin debris. Although pulmonary capillaries have an average diameter of 7 μm, larger particles, including fat macroglobules, have been shown to pass through to the left heart.

B. Reservoir Function

The role of the pulmonary circulation as a reservoir for the systemic circulation was discussed earlier.

Metabolism

The lungs are metabolically very active organs. In addition to surfactant synthesis, pneumocytes account for a major portion of extrahepatic mixed-function oxidation. Neutrophils and macrophages in the lung produce O_2-derived free radicals in response to infection. The pulmonary endothelium metabolizes a variety of vasoactive compounds, including norepinephrine, serotonin, bradykinin, and a variety of prostaglandins and leukotrienes. Histamine and epinephrine are generally not metabolized in the lungs; in fact, the lungs can be a major site of histamine synthesis and release during allergic reactions.

The lungs are also responsible for converting angiotensin I to its physiologically active form, angiotensin II. The enzyme responsible, angiotensin-converting enzyme, is bound on the surface of the pulmonary endothelium.

CASE DISCUSSION

Unilaterally Diminished Breath Sounds During General Anesthesia

A 67-year-old patient is undergoing laparoscopic hemicolectomy under general anesthesia for carcinoma. The history includes an anterior myocardial infarction and heart failure treated with enalapril, carvedilol, furosemide, and spironolactone. Arterial and central venous catheters are placed preoperatively for monitoring during surgery. Following a smooth induction and an atraumatic intubation, anesthesia is maintained with 40% oxygen, sevoflurane, and vecuronium. Thirty minutes into the operation, the surgeon asks for steep Trendelenburg position to facilitate surgical exposure. The pulse oximeter, which had been reading 99% saturation, suddenly drops and remains at 93%. The pulse oximeter's signal strength and waveform are unchanged. Auscultation of the lungs reveals diminished breath sounds over the left lung.

What is the most likely explanation?

Unilaterally diminished breath sounds under anesthesia are most commonly caused by accidental placement or migration of the tracheal tube into one of the two main bronchi. As a result, only one lung is ventilated. Other causes of unilaterally diminished breath sounds (such as pneumothorax, a large mucus plug, lobar atelectasis, or undiagnosed bullae) are less easily diagnosed but are fortunately less common during anesthesia.

The Trendelenburg (head-down) position typically causes the tip of the tracheal tube to advance 1 to 2 cm relative to the carina. In this case, the tube was apparently placed just above the carina with the patient in the supine position, but it migrated into the right bronchus when the Trendelenburg position was imposed. The diagnosis is confirmed by drawing the tube back 1 to 2 cm at a time as the chest is auscultated. Breath sounds will become equal again when the tip of the tube reenters the trachea. Following initial placement, tracheal tubes should be routinely checked for correct positioning by auscultating the chest, ascertaining the depth of tube insertion by the markings on the tube (normally 20–24 cm at the teeth for an adult), and feeling for the cuff in the suprasternal notch. Tube position relative to the carina can also be quickly confirmed with a flexible fiberoptic bronchoscope.

Are tracheal tubes just as likely to enter either main bronchus?

In nearly all cases of unintentional bronchial intubation, the tracheal tube enters the right bronchus because the latter diverges away from the trachea at a less acute angle than does the left bronchus.

Why did hemoglobin saturation decrease?

Failure to ventilate one lung as it continues to be perfused creates a large intrapulmonary shunt. Venous admixture increases and tends to depress

PaO_2 and hemoglobin saturation. If the patient had been ventilated with 100% oxygen, desaturation may not have occurred, and the tube migration may not have been identified.

Does a saturation of 93% exclude bronchial intubation?

No; if both lungs continued to have equal blood flow, venous admixture should have theoretically increased to 50%, resulting in severe hypoxemia and very low hemoglobin saturation. Fortunately, hypoxic pulmonary vasoconstriction is a powerful compensatory response that tends to reduce flow to the hypoxic lung and reduces the expected venous admixture. In fact, if the patient has been receiving a higher inspired O_2 concentration (50–100%), the drop in arterial tension may not be detectable by the pulse oximeter due to the characteristics of the normal hemoglobin saturation curve. For example, bronchial intubation in a patient inspiring 50% O_2 might drop P_{AO_2} from 250 mm Hg to 95 mm Hg; the resulting change in pulse oximeter readings (100–99% to 98–97%) would hardly be noticeable.

Arterial and mixed venous blood gas tensions are obtained with the following results:

PaO_2 = 69 mm Hg; $PaCO_2$ = 42 mm Hg; SaO_2 = 93%; $P\bar{v}O_2$ = 40 mm Hg; and $S\bar{v}O_2$ = 75%. Hemoglobin concentration is 15 g/dL.

What is the calculated venous admixture?

In this case, $Pc'\,O_2 = P_{AO_2} = ([760 - 47] \times 0.4) - 42 = 243$ mm Hg. Therefore, $Cc'_{O_2} = (15 \times 1.31 \times 1.0) + (243 \times 0.003) = 20.4$ mL/dL.

$CaO_2 = (15 \times 1.31 \times 0.93) + (69 \times 0.003) =$ 18.5 mL/dL

$C\bar{v}_{O_2} = (15 \times 1.31 \times 0.75) + (40 \times 0.003) =$ 14.8 mL/dL

$\dot{Q}_S/\dot{Q}_T = (20.4 - 18.5)/(20.4 - 14.8) = 34\%$

How does bronchial intubation affect arterial and end-tidal CO_2 tensions?

$PaCO_2$ is typically not appreciably altered as long as the same minute ventilation is maintained (see One-Lung Ventilation, Chapter 25). Clinically, the $PaCO_2$–$PETCO_2$ gradient often widens, possibly because of increased alveolar dead space (overdistention of the ventilated lung). Thus, $PETCO_2$ may decrease or remain unchanged.

SUGGESTED READINGS

Baumgardner JE, Hedenstierna G. Ventilation/perfusion distributions revisited. *Curr Opin Anaesthesiol.* 2016;29:2.

Hedenstierna G, Edmark L. Effects of anesthesia on the respiratory system. *Best Pract Res Clin Anaesthesiol.* 2015;29:273.

Hedenstierna G, Tokics L, Scaramuzzo G, Rothen HU, Edmark L, Öhrvik J. Oxygenation impairment during anesthesia: influence of age and body weight. *Anesthesiology.* 2019;131:46.

Levitsky MG. *Pulmonary Physiology*. 9th ed. McGraw-Hill Education; 2018.

Lumb AB, Slinger P. Hypoxic pulmonary vasoconstriction: physiology and anesthetic implications. *Anesthesiology*. 2015;122:932.

Mauri T, Spinelli E, Scotti E, et al. Potential for lung recruitment and ventilation-perfusion mismatch in patients with the acute respiratory distress syndrome from coronavirus disease 2019. *Crit Care Med.* 2020;48:1129.

Minnich D, Mathisen D. Anatomy of the trachea, carina, and bronchi. *Thorac Surg Clin.* 2007;17:571.

Warner DO. Diaphragm function during anesthesia: still crazy after all these years. *Anesthesiology.* 2002;97:295.

CHAPTER 24

Anesthesia for Patients with Respiratory Disease

KEY CONCEPTS

1. In a patient with an acute asthma attack, a normal or high $PaCO_2$ indicates that the patient can no longer maintain the work of breathing and is often a sign of impending respiratory failure. A pulsus paradoxus and electrocardiographic signs of right ventricular strain (ST-segment changes, right axis deviation, and right bundle-branch block) are also indicative of severe airway obstruction.

2. Asthmatic patients with active bronchospasm presenting for emergency surgery should be treated aggressively. Supplemental oxygen, aerosolized β_2-agonists, and intravenous glucocorticoids can dramatically improve lung function in a few hours.

3. Intraoperative bronchospasm is usually manifested as wheezing, increasing peak airway pressures (plateau pressure may remain unchanged), decreasing exhaled tidal volumes, or a slowly rising waveform on the capnograph.

4. Other causes can simulate bronchospasm: These include obstruction of the tracheal tube from kinking, secretions, or an overinflated balloon; bronchial intubation; active expiratory efforts (straining); pulmonary edema or embolism; and pneumothorax.

5. Chronic obstructive pulmonary disease (COPD) is currently defined as a disease state characterized by airflow limitation that is not fully reversible. The chronic airflow limitation of this disease is due to a mixture of small and large airway disease (chronic bronchitis/bronchiolitis) and parenchymal destruction (emphysema), with the representation of these two components varying from patient to patient.

6. Cessation of smoking is the long-term intervention that has been shown to reduce the rate of decline in lung function.

7. Preoperative interventions in patients with COPD aimed at correcting hypoxemia, relieving bronchospasm, mobilizing and reducing secretions, and treating infections may decrease the incidence of postoperative pulmonary complications. Patients at greatest risk of complications are those with preoperative pulmonary function measurements less than 50% of predicted.

8. Restrictive pulmonary diseases are characterized by decreased lung compliance. Lung volumes are typically reduced, with preservation of normal expiratory flow rates. Thus, both forced expiratory volume in the first second of exhalation (FEV_1) and forced vital capacity (FVC) are reduced, but the FEV_1/FVC ratio is normal.

9. Intraoperative pulmonary embolism usually presents as sudden cardiovascular collapse, hypoxemia, or bronchospasm. A decrease in end-tidal CO_2 concentration is also suggestive of pulmonary embolism but is not specific.

The increased risks posed by preexisting pulmonary disease during anesthesia and in the postoperative period are well known: Greater degrees of preoperative pulmonary impairment are associated with increased intraoperative alterations in respiratory function and higher rates of postoperative pulmonary complications. Failure to recognize patients who are at increased risk may result in patients not receiving optimal perioperative care. This chapter examines pulmonary risk and reviews the anesthetic approach for patients with the more common types of respiratory disease.

PULMONARY RISK FACTORS

Certain risk factors (Table 24–1) may predispose patients to postoperative pulmonary complications. Atelectasis, pneumonia, pulmonary embolism, and respiratory failure are common following surgery, but the incidence varies widely, depending on the patient population studied and the surgical procedures performed. In the abdominal surgery population, the incidence of postoperative pulmonary complications ranges from 2% to 6%. The two strongest predictors of complications are the operative site and a history of dyspnea, the latter of which correlates with the degree of preexisting pulmonary disease.

The association between smoking and respiratory disease is well established; abnormalities in maximal midexpiratory flow (MMEF) rates are often demonstrable well before symptoms of COPD appear. Most smokers will not have pulmonary function tests (PFTs) performed preoperatively; therefore, it is best to assume that these patients have some degree of pulmonary compromise. In otherwise normal individuals, advanced age is associated with an increased prevalence of pulmonary disease and an increased closing capacity. Obesity *per se* does not increase the likelihood of postoperative pulmonary complications. However, obstructive sleep apnea does contribute to adverse perioperative outcomes.

Thoracic and upper abdominal surgical procedures can have marked effects on pulmonary function. Operations near the diaphragm often produce diaphragmatic dysfunction and a restrictive ventilatory defect (see later discussion). Upper abdominal procedures significantly (>30%) decrease functional residual capacity (FRC). This effect is maximal on the first postoperative day and usually persists for 7 to 10 days. Rapid shallow breathing with an ineffective cough caused by pain (splinting), a decrease in the number of sigh breaths, and impaired mucociliary

TABLE 24–1 Risk factors for postoperative pulmonary complications.

Patient-Related Factors[1]	Procedure-Related Factors[1]
Supported by good evidence	
Advanced age	Aortic aneurysm repair
ASA[2] class ≥2	Thoracic surgery
Congestive heart failure	Abdominal surgery
Functional dependency	Upper abdominal surgery
Chronic obstructive pulmonary disease	Neurosurgery
	Prolonged surgery
	Head and neck surgery
	Emergency surgery
	Vascular surgery
	Use of general anesthesia
Supported by fair evidence	
Weight loss	Perioperative transfusion
Impaired sensorium	
Cigarette use	
Alcohol use	
Abnormal chest examination	
Good evidence *against* being a risk factor	
Well-controlled asthma	Hip surgery
Obesity	Genitourinary/gynecologic surgery
Insufficient data	
Obstructive sleep apnea[3]	Esophageal surgery
Poor exercise capacity	

[1]Within each evidence category, risk factors are listed according to strength of evidence, with the first factor listed having the strongest evidence.

[2]ASA, American Society of Anesthesiologists.

[3]Subsequent evidence indicates that this is a probable risk factor.

Data from Smetana GW, Lawrence VA, Cornell JE, et al. Preoperative pulmonary risk stratification for noncardiothoracic surgery: Systematic review for the American College of Physicians. *Ann Intern Med.* 2006 Apr 18;144(8):581-595.

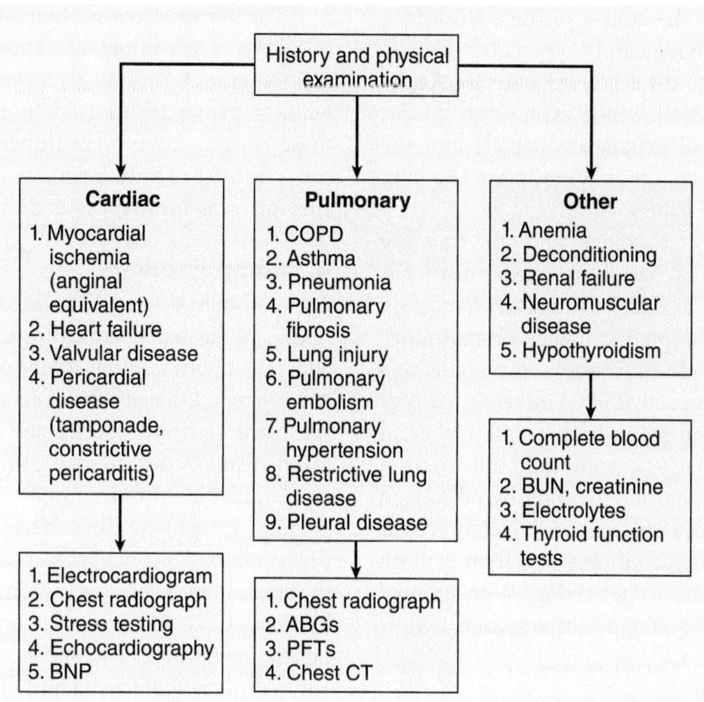

FIGURE 24–1 Evaluation of dyspnea. ABGs, arterial blood gases; BNP, brain natriuretic peptide; BUN, blood urea nitrogen; COPD, chronic obstructive pulmonary disease; CT, computed tomography; PFTs, pulmonary function tests. (Reproduced with permission from Sweitzer BJ, Smetana GW. Identification and evaluation of the patient with lung disease, *Anesthesiol Clin.* 2009 Dec;27(4):673-686.)

clearance leads to atelectasis and loss of lung volume. Subsequent ventilation–perfusion mismatch (shunt) produces hypoxemia. Residual anesthetic effects, recumbent position, sedation from opioids, abdominal distention, and restrictive dressings are also contributory. Complete relief of pain with regional anesthesia can decrease, but usually does not completely reverse, these abnormalities. Persistent atelectasis and retention of secretions promote the development of postoperative pneumonia.

Although many adverse effects of general anesthesia on pulmonary function have been described, the superiority of (unspecified) regional over general anesthesia in patients with pulmonary impairment is not firmly established. Nonetheless, enhanced recovery protocols routinely incorporate regional techniques where possible to provide multimodal, opioid-sparing postoperative analgesia.

When patients with a history of dyspnea present without the benefit of a previous workup, the differential diagnosis can be quite broad and may include both primary pulmonary and cardiac pathologies. Diagnostic approaches to evaluating such patients are summarized in Figure 24–1.

Obstructive Pulmonary Disease

Obstructive and restrictive diseases are the two most common abnormal patterns as determined by PFTs, and the former are by far more common. Obstructive diseases include asthma, emphysema, chronic bronchitis, cystic fibrosis, bronchiectasis, and bronchiolitis. The primary characteristic of these disorders is resistance to airflow. An MMEF of less than 70% (forced expiratory flow [$FEF_{25-75\%}$]) is often the only abnormality early in the course of these disorders. Values for $FEF_{25-75\%}$ in men and women are normally greater than 2.0 L/s and 1.6 L/s, respectively. As the disease progresses, both forced expiratory volume in the first second of exhalation (FEV_1) and the FEV_1/FVC (forced vital capacity) ratio are less than 70% of the predicted values.

Elevated airway resistance and air trapping increase the work of breathing; respiratory gas exchange is impaired because of ventilation/perfusion ($\dot{V}/\dot{Q}$) imbalance. The predominance of expiratory airflow resistance results in air trapping; residual volume and total lung capacity (TLC) increase. Wheezing is a common finding and represents turbulent airflow. It is often absent with mild obstruction that may be manifested initially only by prolonged exhalation. Progressive obstruction typically results first in expiratory wheezing only and then in both inspiratory and expiratory wheezing. With marked obstruction, wheezing may be absent when airflow has nearly ceased.

ASTHMA

Preoperative Considerations

Asthma is a common disorder, affecting 5% to 7% of the population. Its primary characteristic is airway (bronchiolar) inflammation and hyperreactivity in response to a variety of stimuli. Clinically, asthma is manifested by episodic attacks of dyspnea, cough, and wheezing. Airway obstruction, which is generally reversible, is the result of bronchial smooth muscle constriction, edema, and increased secretions. Classically, the obstruction is precipitated by a variety of airborne substances, including pollens, animal dander, dusts, pollutants, and various chemicals. Some patients also develop bronchospasm following ingestion of aspirin, nonsteroidal anti-inflammatory agents, sulfites, or other compounds. Exercise, cold air, emotional excitement, and viral infections may also precipitate bronchospasm. Some patients have exercised-induced exacerbations of asthma. Asthma is classified as acute or chronic. Chronic asthma is further classified as intermittent (mild) and mild, moderate, and severe persistent disease.

The terms *extrinsic* (allergic) asthma (attacks related to environmental exposures) and *intrinsic* (idiosyncratic) asthma (attacks usually occurring without provocation) were used in the past, but these classifications were imperfect; many patients show features of both forms. Moreover, overlap with chronic bronchitis (see later discussion) is common.

A. Pathophysiology

The pathophysiology of asthma involves the local release of various chemical mediators in the airway and, possibly, overactivity of the parasympathetic nervous system. Inhaled substances can initiate bronchospasm through both specific and nonspecific immune mechanisms by degranulating bronchial mast cells. In classic allergic asthma, antigen binding to immunoglobulin E (IgE) on the surface of mast cells causes degranulation. Bronchoconstriction is the result of the subsequent release of histamine; bradykinin; leukotrienes C, D, and E; platelet-activating factor; prostaglandins (PG) E_2, $F_2\alpha$, and D_2; and neutrophil and eosinophil chemotactic factors. The parasympathetic nervous system plays a major role in maintaining normal bronchial tone; diurnal variation in tone is a normal phenomenon, with peak airway resistance occurring early in the morning (at about 6:00 AM). **Vagal afferents in the bronchi are sensitive to histamine and multiple noxious stimuli, including cold air, inhaled irritants, and instrumentation (eg, tracheal intubation)**. Reflex vagal activation results in bronchoconstriction, which is mediated by an increase in intracellular cyclic guanosine monophosphate (cGMP).

During an asthma attack, bronchoconstriction, mucosal edema, and secretions increase resistance to gas flow at all levels of the lower airways. As an attack resolves, airway resistance normalizes first in the larger airways (mainstem, lobar, segmental, and subsegmental bronchi) and then in more peripheral airways. Consequently, expiratory flow rates are initially decreased throughout an entire forced exhalation, but during resolution of the attack, the expiratory flow rate is reduced only at low lung volumes. TLC, residual volume (RV), and FRC are all increased. In acutely ill patients, RV and FRC are often increased by more than 400% and 100%, respectively. Prolonged or severe attacks markedly increase the work of breathing and can fatigue respiratory muscles. The number of alveolar units with low ($\dot{V}/\dot{Q}$) ratios increases, resulting in hypoxemia. Tachypnea is likely and typically produces hypocapnia. 1 A normal or high $PaCO_2$ indicates that the patient can no longer maintain the work of breathing and is often a sign of impending respiratory failure. A pulsus paradoxus and electrocardiographic signs of right ventricular strain (ST-segment changes, right axis deviation, and right bundle-branch block) are also indicative of severe airway obstruction.

B. Treatment

Drugs used to treat asthma include β-adrenergic agonists, methylxanthines, glucocorticoids, anticholinergics, leukotriene modifiers, and mast-cell–stabilizing agents. Although devoid of any bronchodilating properties, cromolyn sodium and nedocromil are effective in preventing bronchospasm by blocking the degranulation of mast cells.

Sympathomimetic agents (eg, albuterol) are the most commonly used for acute exacerbations. They produce bronchodilation via β_2-agonist activity. Activation of β_2-adrenergic receptors on bronchiolar smooth muscle stimulates the activity of adenylate cyclase, which results in the formation of intracellular cyclic adenosine monophosphate (cAMP). These agents are usually administered via a metered-dose inhaler or by aerosol. The use of more selective β_2-agonists, such as terbutaline or albuterol, may decrease the incidence of undesirable β_1 cardiac effects, but they are often less selective in high doses.

Traditionally, methylxanthines are thought to produce bronchodilation by inhibiting phosphodiesterase, the enzyme responsible for the breakdown of cAMP. Their pulmonary effects seem much more complex and include catecholamine release, blockade of histamine release, and diaphragmatic stimulation. Unfortunately, theophylline has a narrow therapeutic range with blood levels between 10 and 20 mcg/mL. Aminophylline is the only available intravenous theophylline preparation. Methylxanthines are less frequently employed today than in the past.

Glucocorticoids are used for both acute treatment and maintenance therapy of patients with asthma because of their anti-inflammatory effects. Beclomethasone, triamcinolone, fluticasone, and budesonide are synthetic steroids commonly used in metered-dose inhalers for maintenance therapy. Although they are associated with a low incidence of undesirable systemic effects, inhaled administration does not necessarily prevent adrenal suppression. Intravenous hydrocortisone or methylprednisolone is used acutely for severe attacks, followed by tapering doses of oral prednisone. Glucocorticoids usually require several hours to become effective. The response (or lack of response) to glucocorticoids has a multifactorial genetic basis, and there are many patients with asthma who are "steroid resistant."

Anticholinergic agents produce bronchodilation through their antimuscarinic action and may block reflex bronchoconstriction. Ipratropium, a congener of atropine that can be given by a metered-dose inhaler or aerosol, is a moderately effective bronchodilator without appreciable systemic anticholinergic effects.

Intravenous magnesium sulfate has been employed to treat acute asthma because of its ability to enhance bronchodilation in combination with other agents. Inhaled magnesium sulfate has less evidence for efficacy.

Anesthetic Considerations

A. Preoperative Management

When evaluating patients with asthma, one should determine the severity and recent course of the disease, as well as whether the patient is receiving optimal medical management. Patients with poorly controlled asthma or wheezing at the time of anesthesia induction have a greater risk of perioperative complications. Conversely, well-controlled asthma has not been shown to be a risk factor for intraoperative or postoperative complications. The history and physical examination provide important information. The patient should have no or minimal dyspnea, wheezing, or cough. Complete resolution of recent exacerbations should be confirmed by chest auscultation. Patients with frequent or chronic bronchospasm should be placed on an optimal bronchodilating regimen. A chest radiograph identifies air trapping; hyperinflation results in a flattened diaphragm, a small-appearing heart, and hyperlucent lung fields. PFTs—particularly expiratory airflow measurements such as FEV_1, FEV_1/FVC, $FEF_{25-75\%}$, and peak expiratory flow rate—help in assessing the severity of airway obstruction and reversibility after bronchodilator treatment. Comparisons with previous measurements are invaluable.

2 Asthmatic patients with active bronchospasm presenting for emergency surgery should be treated aggressively. Supplemental oxygen, aerosolized β_2-agonists, and intravenous glucocorticoids can dramatically improve lung function in a few hours. Arterial blood gases may be useful in evaluating the severity and adequacy of treatment. Hypoxemia and hypercapnia are typical of severe disease; even slight hypercapnia is indicative of severe air trapping and may be a sign of impending respiratory failure.

Anticholinergic agents are not customarily given unless very copious secretions are present or if ketamine is to be used for induction of anesthesia. In typical intramuscular doses, anticholinergics are not effective in preventing reflex bronchospasm following intubation. The use of an H_2-blocking agent (such as cimetidine, ranitidine, or famotidine) is theoretically detrimental because H_2-receptor activation normally produces bronchodilation; in the event of histamine release, unopposed H_1 activation with H_2 blockade may accentuate bronchoconstriction.

Bronchodilators should be continued up to the time of surgery. Patients who receive chronic glucocorticoid therapy with more than 5 mg/d of prednisone (or its equivalent) should receive glucocorticoid supplementation based on the preoperative dosage regimen, the severity of the illness, and the degree of physiologic trespass of the surgical procedure. Supplemental doses should be tapered to baseline within 1 to 2 days.

B. Intraoperative Management

The most critical time for asthmatic patients undergoing anesthesia is during instrumentation of the airway. General anesthesia with noninvasive ventilation or regional anesthesia will circumvent this problem, but neither eliminates the possibility of bronchospasm. In fact, some clinicians believe that high spinal or epidural anesthesia may aggravate bronchoconstriction by blocking sympathetic tone to the lower airways (T1–T4) and allowing unopposed parasympathetic activity. Pain, emotional stress, or stimulation during light general anesthesia can precipitate bronchospasm. Drugs often associated with histamine release (eg, atracurium, morphine, meperidine) should be administered very slowly when used but are best avoided entirely.

The choice of induction agent is less important if adequate depth of anesthesia is achieved before intubation or surgical stimulation. Propofol, ketamine, and etomidate are suitable induction agents; propofol and ketamine may also produce bronchodilation. Ketamine is a good choice for patients with asthma who are also hemodynamically unstable. Sevoflurane usually provides the smoothest inhalation induction with bronchodilation in asthmatics. Isoflurane and desflurane more commonly produce cough, laryngospasm, and bronchospasm during inhalation induction, and we do not recommend them for this indication.

Reflex bronchospasm can be blunted before intubation by an additional dose of the induction agent, ventilating the patient with a 2 to 3 minimum alveolar concentration (MAC) of a volatile agent for 5 min, or administering intravenous or intratracheal lidocaine (1–2 mg/kg), or both. Note that intratracheal lidocaine itself can initiate bronchospasm if an inadequate dose of induction agent has been used. Administration of an anticholinergic agent may block reflex bronchospasm, but it may also cause excessive tachycardia. Although succinylcholine may rarely produce marked histamine release, it is generally safe in asthmatic patients. In the absence of capnography, confirmation of correct tracheal placement by chest auscultation can be difficult in the presence of marked bronchospasm.

Volatile anesthetics are often used for maintenance of anesthesia to take advantage of the potent bronchodilating properties shared by all of these agents. Ventilation should incorporate warmed humidified gases whenever possible. Airflow obstruction during expiration is apparent on capnography as a delayed rise of the end-tidal CO_2 value (Figure 24–2); the severity of obstruction is generally inversely related to the rate of rise in end-tidal CO_2. Severe bronchospasm is manifested by rising peak inspiratory pressures and incomplete exhalation. Tidal volumes of 6 mL/kg, with prolongation of

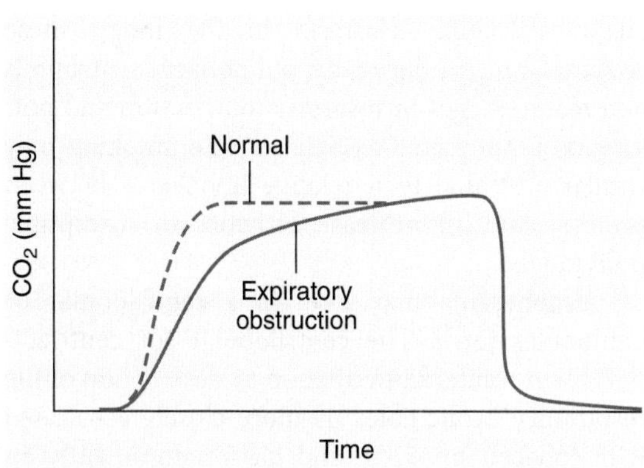

FIGURE 24–2 Capnograph of a patient with expiratory airway obstruction.

the expiratory time, may allow a more uniform distribution of gas flow to both lungs and may help avoid air trapping. The $PaCO_2$ may increase, which is acceptable if there is no contraindication from a cardiovascular or neurologic perspective.

3 Intraoperative bronchospasm is usually manifested as wheezing, increasing peak airway pressures (plateau pressure may remain unchanged), decreasing exhaled tidal volumes, or a slowly rising
4 waveform on the capnograph. Other causes can simulate bronchospasm: These include obstruction of the tracheal tube from kinking, secretions, or an overinflated balloon; bronchial intubation; active expiratory efforts (straining); pulmonary edema or embolism; and pneumothorax. Bronchospasm should be treated by increasing the concentration of the volatile agent and administering an aerosolized bronchodilator. Infusion of low-dose epinephrine may be needed if bronchospasm is refractory to other interventions.

Intravenous hydrocortisone can be given, particularly in patients known to respond to glucocorticoids. At the completion of the surgery, the patient should ideally be free of wheezing. Reversal of nondepolarizing neuromuscular blocking agents with anticholinesterase agents generally does not precipitate bronchoconstriction if preceded by the appropriate dose of an anticholinergic agent. Sugammadex avoids the issue of increasing acetylcholine concentration; however, cases of allergic reaction to sugammadex have been reported. Deep extubation (before the return of airway reflexes) reduces the risk of bronchospasm on emergence. Lidocaine as a bolus (1.5–2 mg/kg) may help to obtund airway reflexes upon emergence.

CHRONIC OBSTRUCTIVE PULMONARY DISEASE (COPD)

Preoperative Considerations

COPD is the most common pulmonary disorder encountered in adult anesthetic practice, and its prevalence increases with age. The disorder is strongly associated with cigarette smoking and has a male
5 predominance. COPD is currently defined as a disease state characterized by airflow limitation that is not fully reversible. The chronic airflow limitation of this disease is due to a mixture of small and large airway disease (chronic bronchitis/bronchiolitis) and parenchymal destruction (emphysema), with the presence of these two components varying from patient to patient.

Most patients with COPD are asymptomatic or only mildly symptomatic but demonstrate expiratory airflow obstruction when assessed with PFTs. In many patients, the obstruction has an element of reversibility, presumably from bronchospasm (as shown by improvement in response to administration of a bronchodilator). With advancing disease, maldistribution of both ventilation and pulmonary blood flow results in areas of low ($\dot{V}/\dot{Q}$) ratios (intrapulmonary shunt), as well as areas of high ($\dot{V}/\dot{Q}$) ratios (dead space).

A. Chronic Bronchitis

The clinical diagnosis of chronic bronchitis is defined as the presence of a productive cough on most days in 3 consecutive months for at least 2 consecutive years. In addition to cigarette smoking, exposure to air pollutants, occupational exposure to dusts, recurrent pulmonary infections, and familial factors may be responsible. Secretions from hypertrophied bronchial mucous glands and mucosal edema from inflammation of the airways produce airflow obstruction. Recurrent pulmonary infections (viral and bacterial) are common and often associated with bronchospasm. RV is increased, but

TABLE 24–2 Signs and symptoms of chronic obstructive pulmonary disease.

Feature	Chronic Bronchitis	Emphysema
Cough	Frequent	With exertion
Sputum	Copious	Scant
Hematocrit	Elevated	Normal
$PaCO_2$ (mm Hg)	Often elevated (>40)	Usually normal or <40
Chest radiograph	Increased lung markings	Hyperinflation
Elastic recoil	Normal	Decreased
Airway resistance	Increased	Normal to slightly increased
Cor pulmonale	Early	Late

TLC is often normal. Intrapulmonary shunting and hypoxemia are common.

In patients with COPD, chronic hypoxemia leads to erythrocytosis, pulmonary hypertension, and eventually right ventricular failure (cor pulmonale); this combination of findings is often referred to as the "blue bloater" syndrome, but less than 5% of patients with COPD fit this description (Table 24–2). In the course of disease progression, patients gradually develop chronic CO_2 retention; the normal ventilatory drive becomes less sensitive to arterial CO_2 tension and may be depressed by oxygen administration (see below).

B. Emphysema

Emphysema is a pathological disorder characterized by irreversible enlargement of the airways distal to terminal bronchioles and destruction of alveolar septa. The diagnosis can be reliably made with computed tomography (CT) of the chest. Mild apical emphysematous changes are a normal, clinically insignificant consequence of aging. Significant emphysema is more frequently related to cigarette smoking. Less commonly, emphysema occurs at an early age and is associated with a homozygous deficiency of α_1-antitrypsin. This is a protease inhibitor that prevents excessive activity of proteolytic enzymes (mainly elastase) in the lungs; these enzymes are produced by pulmonary neutrophils and macrophages in response to infection and pollutants. Emphysema associated with smoking may similarly be due to a relative imbalance between protease and antiprotease activities in susceptible individuals.

Emphysema may exist in a centrilobular or panlobular form. The centrilobular (or centriacinar) form results from dilation or destruction of the respiratory bronchioles, is more closely associated with tobacco smoking, and has predominantly an upper lobe distribution. The panlobular (or panacinar) form results in a more even dilation and destruction of the entire acinus, is associated with α_1-antitrypsin deficiency, and has a lower lobe distribution predominantly.

Loss of the elastic recoil that normally supports small airways by radial traction allows premature collapse during exhalation, leading to expiratory flow limitation with air trapping and hyperinflation (see Table 24–2). Patients characteristically have increases in RV, FRC, TLC, and the RV/TLC ratio.

Disruption of the alveolar–capillary structure and loss of the acinar structure lead to decreased diffusion lung capacity, ($\dot{V}/\dot{Q}$) mismatch, and impairment of gas exchange. Also, normal parenchyma may become compressed by the hyperinflated portions of the lung, resulting in a further increase in the ($\dot{V}/\dot{Q}$) mismatch. Due to the higher diffusibility of CO_2, its elimination is well preserved until ($\dot{V}/\dot{Q}$) abnormalities become severe. Chronic CO_2 retention occurs slowly and generally results in a compensated respiratory acidosis on blood gas analysis. Arterial oxygen tension is usually normal or slightly reduced. Acute CO_2 retention is a sign of impending respiratory failure.

Destruction of pulmonary capillaries in the alveolar septa leads to mild to moderate pulmonary hypertension. When dyspneic, patients with emphysema often purse their lips to delay the closure of the small airways, which accounts for the term "pink puffers" that is often used. However, as mentioned above, most patients diagnosed with COPD have a combination of bronchitis and emphysema and cannot be sorted into "blue bloaters" versus "pink puffers."

C. Treatment

6 Treatment for COPD is primarily supportive. Cessation of smoking is the long-term intervention that will reduce the rate of decline in lung function. Various guidelines have been suggested to aid in the primary medical management of patients with COPD. In general, spirometry is employed to assess the severity of airflow reduction characteristic of obstruction and to determine whether there is a response to bronchodilators. For bronchodilator-responsive patients, short-acting bronchodilators are recommended for acute exacerbations when FEV_1 is greater than 80% of predicted; long-acting bronchodilators and inhaled corticosteroids are suggested as FEV_1 and patient symptoms worsen. Inhaled β_2-adrenergic agonists, glucocorticoids, and ipratropium are routinely employed. Hypoxemia is treated with supplemental oxygen. Patients with chronic hypoxemia (PaO_2 <55 mm Hg) and pulmonary hypertension require low-flow oxygen therapy (1–2 L/min). CO_2 retention may be exacerbated in patients with reduced hypoxic ventilatory drive. Consequently, oxygen therapy is targeted to a hemoglobin oxygen saturation of 90%.

Pulmonary rehabilitation may improve the functional status of the patient by improving physical symptoms and exercise capacity.

Anesthetic Considerations

A. Preoperative Management

Patients with COPD should be optimized prior to elective surgical procedures in the same way as patients with asthma (see earlier discussion). They should be questioned about recent changes in dyspnea, sputum, and wheezing. Patients with an FEV_1 less than 50% of predicted (1.2–1.5 L) usually have dyspnea on exertion, whereas those with an FEV_1 less than 25% (<1 L in men) typically have dyspnea with minimal activity. The latter finding, in patients with predominantly chronic bronchitis, is also often associated with CO_2 retention and pulmonary hypertension. PFTs, chest radiographs, and arterial blood gas measurements, if available, should be reviewed carefully. The presence of bullous changes on the radiograph should be noted. Many patients have concomitant cardiac disease and should also receive a careful cardiovascular evaluation.

7 In contrast to asthma, only limited improvement in respiratory function may be seen after a short period of intensive preoperative preparation. Nonetheless, preoperative interventions in patients with COPD aimed at correcting hypoxemia, relieving bronchospasm, mobilizing and reducing secretions, and treating infections may decrease the incidence of postoperative pulmonary complications. Patients at greatest risk of complications are those with preoperative pulmonary function measurements less than 50% of predicted. The possibility that postoperative ventilation and intensive care unit admission may be necessary for high-risk patients should be discussed with both the patient and the surgeon.

Smoking should be discontinued for at least 6 to 8 weeks before the operation to decrease secretions and reduce pulmonary complications. Cigarette smoking increases mucus production and decreases clearance. Both gaseous and particulate phases of cigarette smoke can deplete glutathione and vitamin C and may promote oxidative injury to tissues. Cessation of smoking for as little as 24 h has theoretical beneficial effects on the oxygen-carrying capacity of hemoglobin; acute inhalation of cigarette smoke releases carbon monoxide, which increases carboxyhemoglobin levels, as well as nitric oxide, and nitrogen dioxide, which can lead to the formation of methemoglobin.

Long-acting bronchodilators and mucolytics should be continued, including on the day of surgery. COPD exacerbations should be treated aggressively.

Preoperative chest physiotherapy and lung expansion interventions with incentive spirometry, deep breathing exercises, cough, chest percussion, and postural drainage may be beneficial in decreasing postoperative pulmonary complications.

B. Intraoperative Management

Although regional anesthesia is often considered preferable to general anesthesia, high spinal or epidural anesthesia can decrease lung volumes, restrict the use of accessory respiratory muscles, and produce an ineffective cough, leading to dyspnea and retention of secretions. Loss of proprioception from the chest and positions such as lithotomy or lateral decubitus may accentuate dyspnea in awake patients. Concerns about hemidiaphragmatic paralysis may make interscalene blocks a less attractive option in the lung disease patient.

Preoxygenation prior to induction of general anesthesia prevents the rapid oxygen desaturation often seen in these patients. The selection of anesthetic agents and general intraoperative management must be tailored to the specific needs and goals of every patient. Unfortunately, the use of bronchodilating anesthetics improves only the reversible component of airflow obstruction; significant expiratory obstruction may still present, even under deep anesthesia. Expiratory airflow limitation, especially under positive pressure ventilation, may lead to air trapping, dynamic hyperinflation, and elevated intrinsic positive end-expiratory pressure (iPEEP). Dynamic hyperinflation may result in lung injury, hemodynamic instability, hypercapnia, and acidosis. Interventions to mitigate air trapping include: (1) allowing more time to exhale by decreasing both the respiratory rate and inspiratory/expiratory (I:E) ratio; (2) permissive hypercapnia; (3) applying low levels of extrinsic PEEP; and (4) aggressively treating bronchospasm.

Intraoperative causes of hypotension in these patients include (in addition to the "usual suspects") pneumothorax and right heart failure due to hypercapnia and acidosis. A pneumothorax may manifest as hypoxemia, increased peak airway pressures, decreasing tidal volumes, and abrupt cardiovascular collapse unresponsive to fluid and vasopressor administration.

Nitrous oxide should be avoided in patients with either bullae or pulmonary hypertension. Inhibition of hypoxic pulmonary vasoconstriction by inhalation anesthetics is usually not clinically apparent at usual doses. However, due to increased dead space, patients with severe COPD have unpredictable uptake and distribution of inhalational agents, and the end-tidal volatile anesthetic concentration is less reliable.

Although pulse oximetry accurately detects significant arterial desaturation, direct measurement of arterial oxygen tensions may be necessary to detect more subtle changes in intrapulmonary shunting. Moreover, arterial CO_2 measurements can guide ventilation because increased dead space widens the normal arterial-to-end-tidal CO_2 gradient. Moderate hypercapnia with a $PaCO_2$ of up to 70 mm Hg may be well tolerated in the short term, assuming a reasonable cardiovascular reserve. Hemodynamic support with inotropic agents may be required in more compromised patients. Hemodynamic monitoring should be dictated by any underlying cardiac dysfunction, as well as the extent of the surgery and the established enhanced recovery protocols in your unit. Successful extubation at the end of the procedure depends on multiple factors: adequate pain control, reversal of neuromuscular blockade, absence of significant bronchospasm and secretions, absence of significant hypercapnia and acidosis, and absence of respiratory depression due to residual anesthetic agents. Patients with an FEV_1 below 50% may require a period of postoperative ventilation, particularly following upper abdominal and thoracic operations.

Restrictive Pulmonary Disease

8 Restrictive pulmonary diseases are characterized by decreased lung compliance. Lung volumes are typically reduced, with preservation of normal expiratory flow rates. Thus, both FEV_1 and FVC are reduced, but the FEV_1/FVC ratio is normal.

Restrictive pulmonary diseases include many acute and chronic intrinsic pulmonary disorders, as well as extrinsic (extrapulmonary) disorders involving the pleura, chest wall, diaphragm, or neuromuscular function. Reduced lung compliance increases the work of breathing, resulting in a characteristic rapid, but shallow, breathing pattern. Respiratory gas exchange is usually maintained until the disease process is advanced.

ACUTE INTRINSIC PULMONARY DISORDERS

Acute intrinsic pulmonary disorders include pulmonary edema (including the acute respiratory distress syndrome [ARDS]), infectious pneumonia, and aspiration pneumonitis.

Preoperative Considerations

Reduced lung compliance in these disorders is primarily due to an increase in extravascular lung water, resulting from an increase in either pulmonary capillary pressure or pulmonary capillary permeability. Increased pressure occurs with left ventricular failure, whereas fluid overload and increased permeability are present with ARDS. Localized or generalized increases in permeability also occur following aspiration or infectious pneumonitis.

Anesthetic Considerations

A. Preoperative Management

Patients with acute pulmonary disease should not undergo elective surgery. In preparation for emergency procedures, oxygenation and ventilation should be optimized to the greatest extent possible. Fluid overload should be treated with diuretics; heart failure may also require treatment. Large pleural effusions usually require drainage before anesthesia. Similarly, massive abdominal distention should be relieved by nasogastric suction or drainage of ascites. Persistent hypoxemia may require mechanical ventilation.

B. Intraoperative Management

Selection of anesthetic agents should be tailored to each patient. Surgical patients with acute pulmonary disorders, such as ARDS, cardiogenic pulmonary edema, or pneumonia, are critically ill; anesthetic management should be a continuation of their preoperative intensive care. Increased inspired oxygen concentrations and PEEP may be required. The decreased lung compliance results in high peak inspiratory pressures during positive-pressure ventilation and increases the risk of barotrauma and volutrauma. Tidal volumes for these patients should be reduced to 4 to 6 mL/kg, with a compensatory increase in the ventilatory rate (14–18 breaths/min), even if the result is an increase in end-tidal CO_2. Airway pressure should generally not exceed 30 cm H_2O. Right ventricular function may be impaired due to increases in pulmonary vascular resistance secondary to permissive hypercapnia.

CHRONIC INTRINSIC PULMONARY DISORDERS

Chronic intrinsic pulmonary disorders are also often referred to as interstitial lung diseases. Regardless of etiology, the disease process is generally characterized by an insidious onset, chronic inflammation of alveolar walls and perialveolar tissue, and progressive pulmonary fibrosis. The latter can eventually interfere with gas exchange and ventilatory function. The inflammatory process may be primarily confined to the lungs or may be part of a generalized multiorgan process. Causes include hypersensitivity pneumonitis from occupational and environmental pollutants, drug toxicity (bleomycin and nitrofurantoin), radiation pneumonitis, idiopathic pulmonary fibrosis, autoimmune diseases, and sarcoidosis. Chronic pulmonary aspiration, oxygen toxicity, and severe ARDS can also produce chronic fibrosis.

Preoperative Considerations

Patients typically present with dyspnea on exertion and sometimes a nonproductive cough. Symptoms of cor pulmonale are present only with advanced disease. Physical examination may reveal fine (dry) crackles over the lung bases and, in late stages, evidence of right ventricular failure. The chest radiograph progresses from a "ground-glass" appearance to prominent reticulonodular markings and, finally, to a "honeycomb" appearance. Arterial blood gases usually show mild hypoxemia with normocarbia. PFTs are typical of a restrictive ventilatory defect (see above), and carbon monoxide diffusing capacity is reduced.

Treatment is directed at the disease process and preventing further exposure to the causative agent (if known). If the patient has chronic hypoxemia, oxygen therapy may be started to prevent, or attenuate, right ventricular failure.

Anesthetic Considerations

A. Preoperative Management

Preoperative evaluation should focus on the underlying disease process and the degree of pulmonary impairment. A history of dyspnea should be evaluated further with PFTs and arterial blood gas analysis. A vital capacity of less than 15 mL/kg is indicative of severe dysfunction (normal is >70 mL/kg). A chest radiograph is helpful in assessing disease severity.

B. Intraoperative Management

The management of these patients is complicated by their predisposition to hypoxemia and their need for controlled ventilation to ensure optimum gas exchange. The reduction in FRC (and oxygen stores) predisposes these patients to rapid hypoxemia following induction of anesthesia. Because these patients may be more susceptible to oxygen-induced toxicity, particularly patients who have received bleomycin, the inspired fractional concentration of oxygen should be kept to the minimum concentration compatible with acceptable oxygenation (Spo_2 of >90%). Protective ventilation strategies employed in ventilated patients in the intensive care unit should be continued through to the operating room. Nitric oxide may be used to reduce pulmonary vascular resistance and reduce the work of the right ventricle.

Extracorporeal membrane oxygenation (ECMO) is increasingly used in the management of acute respiratory failure. Following anticoagulation, blood is drained via venous cannulae and delivered to a membrane oxygenator. Oxygenated blood can then either be returned to the venous system, if cardiac function is preserved, or pumped into the arterial circulation, bypassing the heart and lungs. Consequently, ECMO can provide transient support for both cardiac and pulmonary failure.

EXTRINSIC RESTRICTIVE PULMONARY DISORDERS

Extrinsic restrictive pulmonary disorders alter gas exchange by interfering with normal lung expansion. They include pleural effusions, pneumothorax, mediastinal masses, kyphoscoliosis, pectus excavatum, neuromuscular disorders, and increased intraabdominal pressure from ascites, pregnancy, or bleeding. Marked obesity also produces a restrictive ventilatory defect. Anesthetic considerations are similar to those discussed for intrinsic restrictive disorders.

Pulmonary Embolism

Preoperative Considerations

Pulmonary embolism results from the entry of blood clots, fat, tumor cells, air, amniotic fluid, or foreign material into the venous system. Clots from the lower extremity or pelvic veins or, less commonly, the right side of the heart are usually responsible. Venous stasis or hypercoagulability is often contributory (Table 24–3). Pulmonary embolism can also occur intraoperatively.

A. Pathophysiology

Embolic occlusions in the pulmonary circulation increase dead space, and if minute ventilation does not change, this increase in dead space should theoretically increase $PaCO_2$. However, in practice, hypoxemia is more often seen. Pulmonary emboli acutely increase pulmonary vascular resistance by reducing the cross sectional area of the pulmonary vasculature, causing reflex and humoral vasoconstriction. Localized or generalized reflex bronchoconstriction further increases areas with low ($\dot{V}/\dot{Q}$) ratios. The net effect is an increase in ($\dot{V}/\dot{Q}$) mismatch and hypoxemia. The affected area loses its surfactant within hours and may become atelectatic within 24 to 48 h. Pulmonary infarction occurs if the embolus involves a large vessel and collateral blood

TABLE 24–3 Factors associated with deep venous thrombosis and pulmonary embolism.

Prolonged bed rest
Postpartum state
Fracture of the lower extremities
Surgery on the lower extremities
Carcinoma
Heart failure
Obesity
Surgery lasting more than 30 min
Hypercoagulability
Antithrombin III deficiency
Protein C deficiency
Protein S deficiency
Factor V Leiden mutation

flow from the bronchial circulation is insufficient for that part of the lung (incidence <10%). In previously healthy persons, occlusion of more than 50% of the pulmonary circulation (massive pulmonary embolism) is necessary before sustained pulmonary hypertension is seen. Patients with preexisting cardiac or pulmonary disease can develop acute pulmonary hypertension with occlusions of lesser magnitude. A sustained increase in right ventricular afterload can precipitate acute right ventricular failure and hemodynamic collapse. If the patient survives acute pulmonary thromboembolism, the thrombus usually begins to resolve within 1 to 2 weeks. Incomplete resolution of pulmonary emboli can produce chronic thromboembolic pulmonary hypertension.

B. Diagnosis

Clinical manifestations of pulmonary embolism include sudden tachypnea, dyspnea, chest pain, or hemoptysis. The latter generally implies lung infarction. Symptoms are often absent or mild and nonspecific unless massive embolism has occurred. Wheezing may be present on auscultation. Arterial blood gas analysis typically shows mild hypoxemia with respiratory alkalosis (the latter due to an increase in ventilation). The chest radiograph is commonly normal, especially in the acute phase, but may show an area of oligemia (radiolucency), a wedge-shaped density with an infarct, atelectasis with an elevated diaphragm, or an asymmetrically enlarged proximal pulmonary artery with acute pulmonary hypertension. Cardiac signs include tachycardia and wide fixed splitting of the S_2 heart sound; hypotension with elevated central venous pressure is usually indicative of right ventricular failure. The electrocardiogram frequently shows tachycardia and may show signs of acute cor pulmonale, such as new right axis deviation, right bundle-branch block, and tall peaked T waves. Ultrasound studies of the lower extremities may be helpful in demonstrating deep venous thrombosis (DVT). The diagnosis of embolism is more difficult to make intraoperatively (see below).

Emergency CT angiography is performed when pulmonary embolism is suspected. Echocardiography can also be used to assist in the diagnosis under emergent conditions in unstable patients perioperatively. Right ventricular overload is seen following significant pulmonary embolism. Sometimes a clot can be seen in the right heart and pulmonary artery, confirming the diagnosis. At other times, only the signs of right ventricular overload are seen (eg, tricuspid regurgitation, right ventricular dilation). The left ventricle may be relatively under-loaded secondary to the inadequate delivery of blood across the pulmonary circulation as a consequence of the embolus.

C. Treatment and Prevention

The best treatment for perioperative pulmonary embolism is prevention. Various regimens for DVT prophylaxis are employed, including heparin (unfractionated heparin 5000 units subcutaneously every 12 h begun preoperatively or immediately postoperatively in high-risk patients), enoxaparin, fondaparinux, and, most importantly, early ambulation after surgery. Patients at risk for thrombus formation are treated with warfarin. Newer anticoagulants such as factor Xa inhibitors (eg, rivaroxaban, apixaban) and the direct thrombin inhibitor dabigatran will likely assume a greater role in DVT prophylaxis. The use of intermittent pneumatic compression of the legs may decrease the incidence of venous thrombosis in the legs but not in the pelvis or the heart.

After a pulmonary embolism, parenteral anticoagulation prevents the formation of new blood clots or the extension of existing clots. Low-molecular-weight heparin (LMWH) or fondaparinux are now preferred over intravenous unfractionated heparin for initial anticoagulation following a pulmonary embolism for most patients. All patients should start warfarin therapy concurrent with starting parenteral therapy, and the two should overlap for a minimum of 5 days. The international normalized ratio should also be within the therapeutic range (>2.0) for at least 24 h before discontinuation of parenteral DVT prophylaxis. Warfarin should be continued for 3 to 12 months. Thrombolytic therapy is indicated in patients with massive pulmonary embolism and hypotension. Recent surgery and active bleeding are contraindications to anticoagulation and thrombolytic therapy. In these cases, an inferior vena cava filter may be placed to prevent recurrent pulmonary emboli. Pulmonary embolectomy may be lifesaving for hemodynamically unstable patients with massive embolism in whom thrombolytic therapy is contraindicated or ineffective.

Anesthetic Considerations

A. Preoperative Management

Patients with acute pulmonary embolism may present in the operating room or interventional radiology suite for placement of an inferior vena cava filter or for a thrombolytic procedure, or, rarely, they may be taken to the operating room for a pulmonary embolectomy. In some instances, the patient will have a history of pulmonary embolism and present for unrelated surgery; in this group of patients, the risk of interrupting anticoagulant therapy perioperatively is unknown. If the acute episode occurred more than 1 year earlier, the risk associated with temporarily stopping anticoagulant therapy is probably small. Moreover, except in the case of chronic recurrent pulmonary emboli, pulmonary function has usually returned to normal. The emphasis in the perioperative management of these patients should be on preventing new episodes of embolism (see earlier discussion).

B. Intraoperative Management

Vena cava filters are usually placed percutaneously under local anesthesia with sedation.

Patients presenting for emergency pulmonary embolectomy are critically ill. They are usually already intubated but tolerate positive-pressure ventilation poorly. Inotropic support is usually necessary until they are placed on cardiopulmonary bypass to facilitate clot removal. Inotropic support may be required to separate from cardiopulmonary bypass.

C. Intraoperative Pulmonary Embolism

Significant pulmonary embolism is rare during anesthesia. Diagnosis requires a high index of suspicion. Air emboli are common but are often overlooked unless a large amount of air is entrained. Fat embolism, as well as embolism of microthrombi and bone debris, can occur during orthopedic procedures; amniotic fluid embolism is a rare, unpredictable, and often fatal complication of late pregnancy and obstetrical delivery. Thromboembolism may occur intraoperatively during prolonged procedures. The clot may have been present prior to surgery or may form intraoperatively; surgical manipulations or a change in the patient's position may then dislodge the venous thrombus. Manipulation of tumors with intravascular extension (eg, renal cell carcinoma invading the vena cava) can similarly produce pulmonary embolism.

9 Intraoperative pulmonary embolism usually presents as sudden cardiovascular collapse, hypoxemia, or bronchospasm. A decrease in end-tidal CO_2 concentration is also suggestive of pulmonary embolism but is not specific. Invasive monitoring may reveal elevated central venous pressure. Depending on the type and location of an embolism, a transesophageal echocardiogram may be helpful; this may not reveal the embolus but will often demonstrate right heart distention and dysfunction. **If air is identified in the right atrium, or if it is suspected, emergency central vein cannulation and aspiration of the air may be lifesaving.** For all other emboli, treatment is supportive, with intravenous fluids and inotropes. Placement of a vena cava filter may be considered postoperatively.

Anesthesia and the Patient with Pulmonary Hypertension

Pulmonary hypertension may occur secondary to left ventricular failure, mitral stenosis, chronic thromboembolism, and pulmonary disease. Right ventricular dilation and hypertrophy develop, leading to tricuspid regurgitation and flattening of the intraventricular septum. Left ventricular filling becomes impaired as a consequence of the change in right ventricular geometry. Patients may be treated with inhaled nitric oxide, prostacyclin, and milrinone perioperatively to lower pulmonary pressures and improve ventricular function.

Anesthesia and SARS-CoV-2 (COVID-19)

At the time of this writing, COVID-19 continues to be a major public health emergency. The pandemic has produced morbidity and mortality worldwide. Anesthesia staff are heavily engaged in combating the pandemic in both intensive care units and operating rooms. Asymptomatic patients with COVID-19 are commonly identified during preoperative testing for surgery unrelated to COVID-19. Patients may present for emergency (eg, trauma) surgery and subsequently be found to have COVID-19. Consequently, anesthesia staff must be prepared for COVID-19 both in the operating room and the intensive care unit.

The SARS-CoV-2 virus uses its spike protein to enter cells via the angiotensin-converting enzyme 2 receptor. The symptoms of infection are variable in both presentation and severity and affect numerous organ systems. Although some patients have no or minimal symptoms and most patients recover uneventfully, others will develop bilateral pulmonary disease and impaired oxygenation that may progress to respiratory failure, shock, and death. Additionally, COVID-19 has been linked to a profound inflammatory response (cytokine storm) and a hypercoagulable state. These conditions may contribute to the wide variety of systemic effects seen in critically ill patients with COVID-19. Therapy is largely supportive, including high-flow oxygen, prone positioning, dexamethasone, and anticoagulation. Lung-protective ventilation with tidal volumes less than 6 mL/kg is suggested for ventilated patients.

Management of the patient with COVID-19 starts with educating the staff about appropriate patient isolation practices. Proper donning and doffing of personal protective equipment (PPE) requires both patience and practice. Most hospitals have established specialized negative pressure rooms (unlike the typical positive pressure rooms) to ensure that patients with COVID-19 who are undergoing surgery will not contaminate the operating room suite.

Potential outpatient treatments for COVID-19 remain investigational at this time. Several vaccines have received emergency approval from regulators. However, the long-term effectiveness of current vaccines is unknown given the rapid development of genetic variants of SARS-CoV-2. As treatments are evolving rapidly, readers are encouraged to update themselves with the latest reviews in the various specialty journals.

CASE DISCUSSION

Laparoscopic Surgery

A 45-year-old woman is scheduled for a laparoscopic cholecystectomy. Known medical problems include morbid obesity and a history of smoking.

What are the advantages of laparoscopic cholecystectomy compared with open cholecystectomy?

Laparoscopic techniques are associated with much smaller incisions than with traditional open techniques. These benefits include decreased postoperative pain, less postoperative pulmonary impairment, reduced duration of postoperative ileus, shorter hospital length of stay, earlier ambulation, and smaller surgical scars. Thus, laparoscopic surgery provides substantial medical and economic advantages.

How does laparoscopic surgery affect intraoperative pulmonary function?

The hallmark of laparoscopy is the creation of a pneumoperitoneum with pressurized CO_2. The resulting increase in intraabdominal pressure displaces the diaphragm cephalad, causing a decrease in lung compliance and an increase in peak inspiratory pressure. **Atelectasis, diminished FRC, ventilation/perfusion mismatch, and pulmonary shunting contribute to a decrease in arterial oxygenation.** These changes might be exaggerated in this obese patient with a long history of tobacco use.

The high solubility of CO_2 results in its absorption by the vasculature of the peritoneum. This, combined with smaller tidal volumes because of poor lung compliance, leads to increased arterial CO_2 levels and decreased arterial pH.

Why does patient position affect oxygenation?

A head-down (Trendelenburg) position causes a cephalad shift in the abdominal viscera and the diaphragm. FRC, total lung volume, and pulmonary compliance will be decreased. Although these changes are usually well tolerated by healthy patients, this patient's obesity and presumed preexisting lung disease increase the likelihood of hypoxemia. A head-down position also tends to shift the trachea upward, so a tracheal tube anchored at the mouth may migrate into the right mainstem bronchus. This tracheobronchial shift may be exacerbated during insufflation of the abdomen.

After insufflation, the patient's position is usually changed to a steep head-up position (reverse Trendelenburg) to facilitate surgical dissection. The respiratory effects of the head-up position are the opposite of the head-down position.

Does laparoscopic surgery affect cardiac function?

Moderate insufflation pressures usually leave heart rate, central venous pressure, and cardiac output unchanged or slightly elevated. This seems to result from increased effective cardiac filling because blood tends to be forced out of the abdomen and into the chest. **Higher insufflation pressures (>25 cm H_2O or 18 mm Hg), however, tend to collapse the major abdominal veins (particularly the inferior vena cava), which impedes venous return and leads to a drop in preload and cardiac output in some patients. Higher insufflation pressures may also produce an intraabdominal compartment syndrome, adversely impacting kidney perfusion and resulting in acute impairment of kidney function.**

Hypercarbia will stimulate the sympathetic nervous system and increase blood pressure, heart rate, and the risk of arrhythmias. Attempting to compensate by increasing the tidal volume or respiratory rate will increase the mean intrathoracic pressure, further hindering venous return and increasing mean pulmonary artery pressures. These effects can prove particularly challenging in patients with restrictive lung disease, impaired cardiac function, or intravascular volume depletion.

Although the Trendelenburg position increases preload, mean arterial pressure and cardiac output usually either remain unchanged or decrease. These seemingly paradoxical responses may be explained by carotid and aortic baroreceptor-mediated reflexes. The reverse Trendelenburg position decreases preload, cardiac output, and mean arterial pressure.

Describe the advantages and disadvantages of alternative anesthetic techniques for this patient.

Anesthetic approaches to laparoscopic surgery include infiltration of local anesthetic with an intravenous sedative, epidural or spinal anesthesia, or (much more commonly) general anesthesia. Epidural or spinal anesthesia represents a rarely chosen alternatives for laparoscopic surgery because of dyspnea and discomfort caused by the pneumoperitoneum. A high level is required for complete muscle relaxation and to prevent diaphragmatic irritation caused by gas insufflation and surgical manipulations. An obese patient with lung disease may not be able to increase spontaneous ventilation to maintain normocarbia in the face of a T2 level regional block during insufflation and a 20° Trendelenburg position. Another disadvantage of neuraxial techniques is the occasional occurrence of referred shoulder pain from diaphragmatic irritation.

Does a general anesthetic technique require tracheal intubation?

Tracheal intubation with positive-pressure ventilation is usually favored for many reasons: the risk of regurgitation from increased intraabdominal pressure during insufflation; the necessity for controlled ventilation to prevent hypercapnia; the relatively high peak inspiratory pressures required because of the pneumoperitoneum; the need for neuromuscular blockade during surgery to allow lower insufflation pressures, provide better visualization, and prevent unexpected patient movement; and the placement of a nasogastric tube and gastric decompression to minimize the risk of visceral perforation during trocar introduction and optimize visualization. The obese patient presented here would benefit from intubation to decrease the likelihood of hypoxemia, hypercarbia, and aspiration. In lower-risk patients, second-generation supraglottic airway devices are increasingly employed for a variety of surgical procedures, including those performed laparoscopically.

What special monitoring should be considered for this patient?

Monitoring end-tidal CO_2 normally provides an adequate guide for determining the minute ventilation required to maintain normocarbia. This assumes a constant gradient between arterial CO_2 and end-tidal CO_2, which is generally valid in healthy patients undergoing laparoscopy. This assumption would not apply if alveolar dead space changes during surgery. For example, any significant reduction in lung perfusion increases alveolar dead space and therefore increases the gradient between arterial and end-tidal CO_2. This may occur during laparoscopy if cardiac output drops because of high inflation pressures, the reverse Trendelenburg position, or gas embolism. Furthermore, abdominal distention lowers pulmonary compliance. Large tidal volumes are usually avoided because they are associated with high peak inspiratory pressures and can cause considerable movement of the surgical field.

What are some possible complications of laparoscopic surgery?

Surgical complications include hemorrhage if a major abdominal vessel is lacerated or peritonitis if a viscus is perforated during trocar introduction. Significant intraoperative hemorrhage may go unrecognized because of the limitations of laparoscopic visualization. Fulguration has been associated with bowel burns and bowel gas explosions. The use of pressurized gas introduces the possibility of extravasation of CO_2 along tissue planes, resulting in subcutaneous emphysema, pneumomediastinum, or pneumothorax. Nitrous oxide should be discontinued and insufflating pressures decreased as much as possible if gas extravasation is suspected. These patients may benefit from the continuation of mechanical ventilation into the immediate postoperative period.

Venous CO_2 embolism resulting from unintentional insufflation of gas into an open vein may lead to hypoxemia, pulmonary hypertension, pulmonary edema, and cardiovascular collapse. Unlike air embolism, end-tidal CO_2 may transiently increase during CO_2 gas embolism. Treatment includes the immediate release of the pneumoperitoneum, discontinuation of nitrous oxide, insertion of a central venous catheter for gas aspiration, and placement of the patient in a head-down left lateral decubitus position.

Vagal stimulation during trocar insertion, peritoneal insufflation, or manipulation of viscera can result in bradycardia and possible sinus arrest. Although this usually resolves spontaneously, elimination of the stimulus (eg, deflation of the peritoneum) and administration of atropine sulfate may be needed. Intraoperative hypotension may be more common during laparoscopic compared with open procedures secondary to impaired venous return as a consequence of increased abdominal pressure related to CO_2 insufflation. Support of the blood pressure may be necessary to maintain a suitable mean arterial pressure (≥65 mm Hg).

Even though laparoscopic procedures are associated with less muscle trauma and incisional pain than open surgery, pulmonary dysfunction can persist for at least 24 h postoperatively. For example, FEV_1, FVC, and forced expiratory flow are reduced by approximately 25% following laparoscopic cholecystectomy, compared with a 50% reduction following open cholecystectomy.

GUIDELINES

Guyatt G, Akl E, Crowther M, et al. Antithrombotic therapy and prevention of thrombosis: 9th ed: American College of Chest Physicians evidence-based clinical practice guidelines. *Chest.* 2012;141(suppl):7s.

Qaseem A, Snow V, Fitterman N, et al. Risk assessment for and strategies to reduce perioperative pulmonary complication for patients undergoing noncardiothoracic surgery: a guideline from the American College of Physicians. *Ann Intern Med.* 2006;144:576.

See www.guidelines.gov for additional guidelines from multiple organizations on deep vein thrombosis prophylaxis and pulmonary embolism.

SUGGESTED READINGS

Canet J, Gallart L, Gomar C, et al. Prediction of postoperative pulmonary complications in a population-based surgical cohort. *Anesthesiology*. 2010;113:1338.

Chen X, Liu Y, Gong Y, et al; Chinese Society of Anesthesiology, Chinese Association of Anesthesiologists. Perioperative management of patients infected with the novel coronavirus: recommendation from the joint task force of the Chinese Society of Anesthesiology and the Chinese Association of Anesthesiologists. *Anesthesiology.* 2020;132:1307.

Cox J, Jablons D. Operative and perioperative pulmonary emboli. *Thorac Surg Clin*. 2015;15:289.

Duong TN, Zeki AA, Louie S. Medical management of hospitalized patients with asthma or chronic obstructive pulmonary disease. *Hosp Med Clin*. 2017;6:437.

Gallart L, Canet J. Post-operative pulmonary complications: understanding definitions and risk assessment. *Best Pract Res Clin Anaesthesiol.* 2015;29:315.

Gordon RJ, Lombard FW. Perioperative venous thromboembolism: a review. *Anesth Analg.* 2017;125:403.

Hedenstierna G, Edmark L. Effects of anesthesia on the respiratory system. *Best Pract Res Clin Anaesthesiol.* 2015;29:273.

Henzler T, Schoenberg S, Schoepf U, Fink C. Diagnosing acute pulmonary embolism: systematic review of evidence base and cost-effectiveness of imaging tests. *J Thorac Imaging*. 2012;27:304.

Hopkinson NS, Molyneux A, Pink J, Harrisingh MC; Guideline Committee (GC). Chronic obstructive pulmonary disease: diagnosis and management: summary of updated NICE guidance. *BMJ.* 2019;366:l4486.

Lakshminarasimhachar A, Smetana G. Preoperative evaluation: estimation of pulmonary risk. *Anesthesiol Clin*. 2016;34:71.

Lee H, Kim J, Tagmazyan K. Treatment of stable chronic obstructive pulmonary disease: the GOLD guidelines. *Am Fam Physician*. 2013;88:655.

Numata T, Nakayama K, Fujii S, et al. Risk factors of postoperative pulmonary complications in patients with asthma and COPD. *BMC Pulm Med.* 2018;18:4.

Phua J, Weng L, Ling L, et al; Asian Critical Care Clinical Trials Group. Intensive care management of coronavirus disease 2019 (COVID-19): challenges and recommendations. *Lancet Respir Med.* 2020;8:506.

Radosevich M, Brown D. Anesthetic management of the adult patient with concomitant cardiac and pulmonary disease. *Anesthesiol Clin*. 2016;34:633.

Ranka S, Mohananey D, Agarwal N, et al. Chronic thromboembolic pulmonary hypertension-management strategies and outcomes. *J Cardiothorac Vasc Anesth*. 2020;34:2513.

Regli A, von Ungern-Sternberg B. Anesthesia and ventilation strategies in children with asthma: part 1—preoperative assessment. *Curr Opin Anesthesiol.* 2014;27:288.

Regli A, von Ungern-Sternberg B. Anesthesia and ventilation strategies in children with asthma: part II—intraoperative management. *Curr Opin Anesthesiol*. 2014;27:295.

Salmasi V, Maheshwari K, Yang D, et al. Relationship between intraoperative hypotension, defined by either reduction from baseline or absolute thresholds, and acute kidney and myocardial injury after non-cardiac surgery. *Anesthesiology*. 2017;126:47.

Smetana G. Postoperative pulmonary complications: an update on risk assessment and reduction. *Cleveland Clin J Med*. 2009;76(suppl 4):S60.

Sweitzer B, Smetana G. Identification and evaluation of the patient with lung disease. *Anesthesiol Clin.* 2009;27:673.

Vogelmeier CF, Criner GJ, Martinez FJ, et al. Global strategy for the diagnosis, management, and prevention of chronic obstructive lung disease 2017 report: GOLD executive summary. *Eur Respir J.* 2017;49:1700214.

CHAPTER

25

Anesthesia for Thoracic Surgery

KEY CONCEPTS

1. During one-lung ventilation, the mixing of unoxygenated blood from the collapsed upper lung with oxygenated blood from the still-ventilated dependent lung widens the alveolar-to-arterial (A-a) O_2 gradient and often results in hypoxemia.
2. There are certain clinical situations in which the use of a right-sided double-lumen tube is recommended: (1) distorted anatomy of the left main bronchus by an intrabronchial or extrabronchial mass; (2) compression of the left main bronchus due to a descending thoracic aortic aneurysm; (3) left-sided pneumonectomy; (4) left-sided single lung transplantation; and (5) left-sided sleeve resection.
3. If epidural or intrathecal opioids are to be used for postoperative pain control, intravenous opioids should be limited during surgery to prevent excessive postoperative respiratory depression.
4. Postoperative hemorrhage complicates about 3% of thoracotomies and may be associated with up to 20% mortality. Signs of hemorrhage include increased chest tube drainage (>200 mL/h), hypotension, tachycardia, and a falling hematocrit level.
5. Bronchopleural fistula presents as a sudden large air leak from the chest tube that may be associated with an increasing pneumothorax and partial lung collapse.
6. Acute herniation of the heart into the operative hemithorax can occur through the pericardial defect that is left following a radical pneumonectomy.
7. Nitrous oxide is contraindicated in patients with cysts or bullae because it can expand the air space and cause rupture. The latter may be signaled by sudden hypotension, bronchospasm, or an abrupt rise in peak inflation pressure and requires immediate placement of a chest tube.
8. Following transplantation, peak inspiratory pressures should be maintained at the minimum pressure compatible with good lung expansion, and the inspired oxygen concentration should be maintained as close to room air as allowed by a PaO_2 greater than 60 mm Hg.
9. Regardless of the procedure, a common anesthetic concern for patients with esophageal disease is the risk of pulmonary aspiration.

Common indications for thoracic surgery include malignancies (mainly of the lungs and esophagus), chest trauma, esophageal disease, and mediastinal tumors. Diagnostic procedures such as bronchoscopy, mediastinoscopy, and open-lung biopsies are also common. Improved techniques for providing lung separation have permitted an increasing fraction of surgical procedures to be performed thoracoscopically. Nonintubated video-assisted thoracic surgery is also being performed more often.

Physiological Considerations During Thoracic Anesthesia

Thoracic surgery presents a unique set of physiological problems for the anesthesiologist. These include physiological derangements caused by placing the patient in the lateral decubitus position, opening the chest **(open pneumothorax)**, and the need for one-lung ventilation.

THE LATERAL DECUBITUS POSITION

The lateral decubitus position provides optimal access for most operations on the lungs, pleura, esophagus, great vessels, other mediastinal structures, and vertebrae; however, this position may significantly alter the normal pulmonary ventilation/perfusion relationships. These derangements are further accentuated by anesthetics, mechanical ventilation, neuromuscular blockade, opening the chest, and surgical retraction. Although perfusion continues to favor the dependent lung (under anesthesia in the supine position, the dependent part of the lung is toward the back, rather than toward the feet, as would be true in an awake, standing patient), ventilation progressively favors the less perfused, superior part of the lung. The resulting ventilation/perfusion mismatch increases the risk of hypoxemia.

The Awake State

When a supine patient assumes the lateral decubitus position, ventilation/perfusion matching is preserved during spontaneous ventilation. The dependent (lower) lung receives more perfusion than does the upper lung because of gravitational influences on blood flow distribution in the pulmonary circulation. The dependent lung also receives more ventilation because (1) contraction of the dependent hemidiaphragm is more efficient compared with the nondependent (upper) hemidiaphragm and (2) the dependent lung is on a more favorable part of the compliance curve (Figure 25–1). However, spontaneous ventilation in this position is the exception, not the rule.

Induction of Anesthesia

The decrease in functional residual capacity (FRC) with induction of general anesthesia moves the upper lung to a more favorable part of the compliance curve, but it moves the lower lung to a less favorable position (Figure 25–2). As a result, the upper lung is ventilated more than the dependent lower lung; ventilation/perfusion mismatching occurs because the dependent lung continues to have greater perfusion.

Positive-Pressure Ventilation

Controlled positive-pressure ventilation favors the upper lung in the lateral position because it is more compliant than the lower lung. Neuromuscular blockade enhances this effect by allowing the abdominal contents to rise up further against the dependent hemidiaphragm and impede ventilation of the lower lung. Using a rigid "bean bag" to maintain the patient in the lateral decubitus position further restricts movement of the dependent hemithorax. Finally, opening the nondependent side of the chest further accentuates differences in compliance between the two sides because the upper lung is now less restricted in movement. All of these effects worsen ventilation/perfusion mismatching and predispose the patient to hypoxemia.

THE OPEN PNEUMOTHORAX

The lungs are normally kept expanded by negative pleural pressure—the net result of the tendency of the lung to collapse and the chest wall to expand. When one side of the chest is opened, the negative pleural pressure is lost, and the elastic recoil of the lung on that side tends to collapse it. Spontaneous ventilation with an open pneumothorax in the lateral position results in paradoxical respirations and mediastinal shift. These two phenomena could cause progressive hypoxemia and hypercapnia, but their effects are overcome by the use of positive-pressure ventilation. Open pneumothorax is used

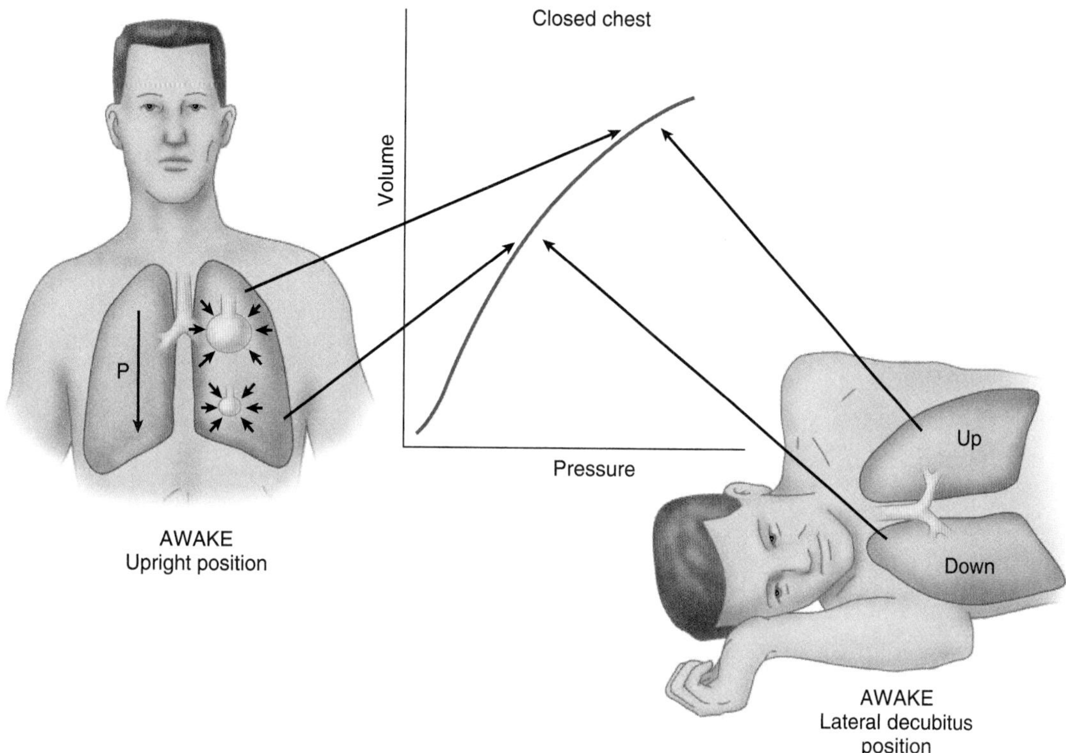

FIGURE 25–1 The effect of the lateral decubitus position on lung compliance.

to produce lung collapse during nonintubated thoracic surgery.

Mediastinal Shift

During spontaneous ventilation in the lateral position, inspiration causes pleural pressure to become more negative on the dependent side but not on the side of the open pneumothorax. This results in a downward shift of the mediastinum during inspiration and an upward shift during expiration (Figure 25–3). The major effect of the mediastinal shift is to decrease the contribution of the dependent lung to the tidal volume.

Paradoxical Respiration

Spontaneous ventilation in a patient with an open pneumothorax also results in to-and-fro gas flow between the dependent and nondependent lung (paradoxical respiration [*pendeluft*]). During inspiration, the pneumothorax increases, and gas flows from the upper lung across the carina to the dependent lung. During expiration, the gas flow reverses and moves from the dependent to the upper lung (Figure 25–4).

ONE-LUNG VENTILATION

Intentional collapse of the lung on the operative side facilitates most thoracic procedures, but it complicates anesthetic management. Because the collapsed lung continues to be perfused and is deliberately no longer ventilated, the patient develops a large right-to-left intrapulmonary shunt (20–30%). During one-lung ventilation, the mixing of unoxygenated blood from the collapsed upper lung with oxygenated blood from the still-ventilated dependent lung widens the alveolar-to-arterial (A-a) O_2 gradient and often results in hypoxemia. Fortunately, blood flow to the nonventilated lung is decreased by hypoxic pulmonary vasoconstriction (HPV). The

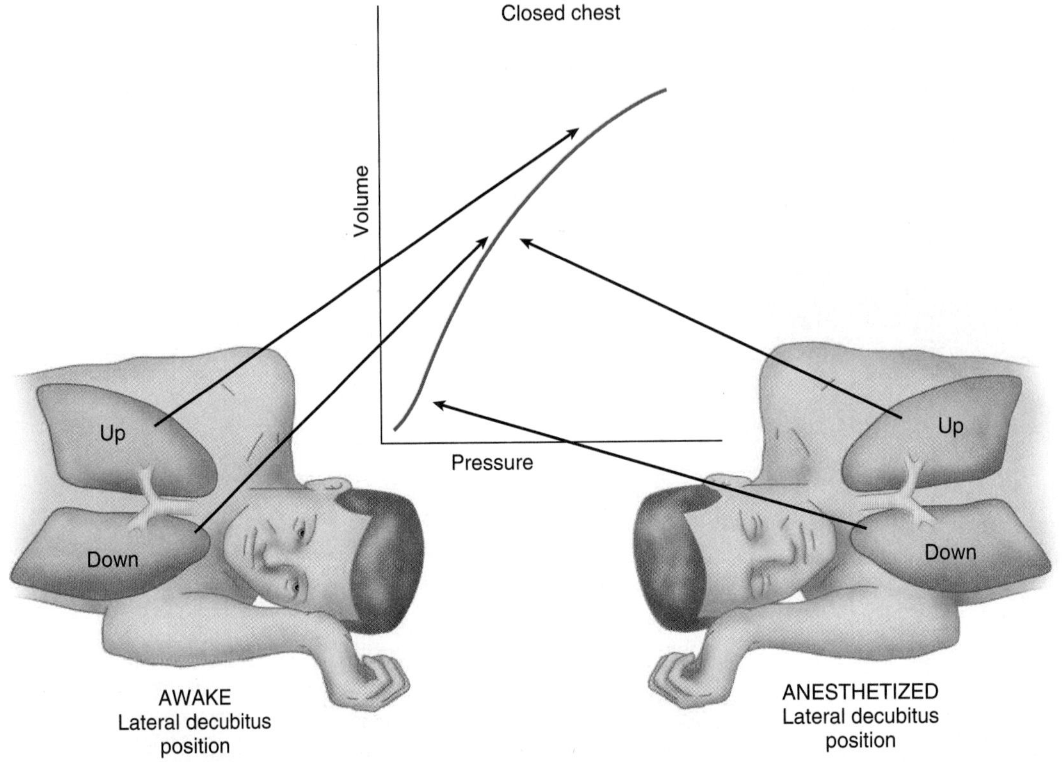

FIGURE 25–2 The effect of anesthesia on lung compliance in the lateral decubitus position. The upper lung assumes a more favorable position, and the lower lung becomes less compliant.

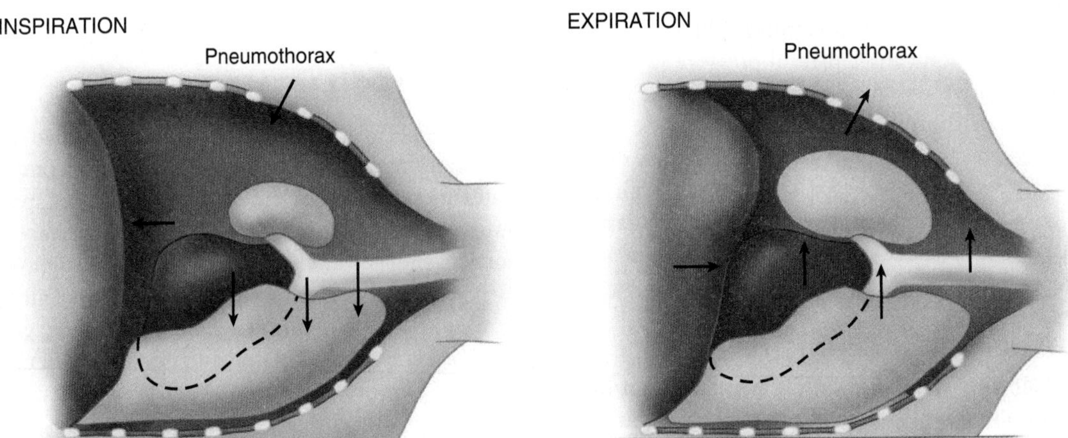

FIGURE 25–3 Mediastinal shift in a spontaneously breathing patient in the lateral decubitus position. (Reproduced with permission from Tarhan S, Moffitt EA. Principles of thoracic anesthesia. *Surg Clin North Am.* 1973 Aug;53(4):813-826.)

INSPIRATION

Pneumothorax

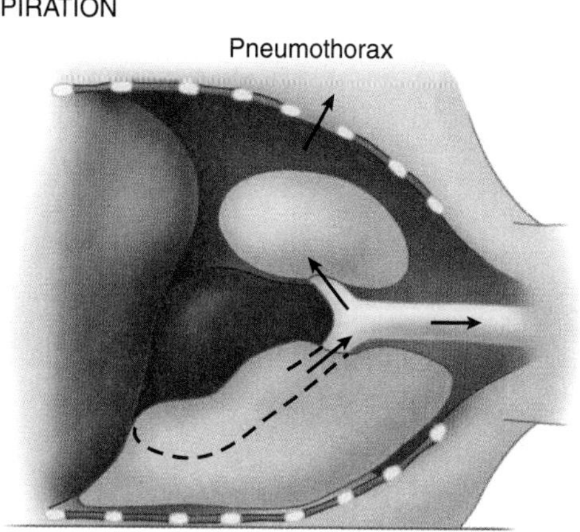

FIGURE 25–4 Paradoxical respiration in spontaneously breathing patients on their side. (Reproduced with permission from Tarhan S, Moffitt EA. Principles of thoracic anesthesia. *Surg Clin North Am.* 1973 Aug;53(4):813-826.)

surgeon can also clamp the pulmonary arterial supply to the collapsed lung when all else fails.

Factors known to inhibit HPV (thereby increasing venous admixture) and thus worsen the right-to-left shunting include pulmonary hypertension; hypocapnia alkalosis; increased cardiac output and increased mixed venous PO_2; hypothermia; vasodilators such as nitroglycerin, nitroprusside, and nitric oxide; phosphodiesterase inhibitors (milrinone, enoximone, inamrinone), β-adrenergic agonists; calcium channel blockers; and inhalation anesthetics.

Factors that decrease blood flow to the ventilated lung can be equally detrimental; they counteract the effect of HPV by indirectly increasing blood flow to the collapsed lung. Such factors include (1) high mean airway pressures in the ventilated lung due to high positive end-expiratory pressure (PEEP), hyperventilation, or high peak inspiratory pressures; (2) a low FiO_2, which produces hypoxic pulmonary vasoconstriction in the ventilated lung; (3) vasoconstrictors that may have a greater effect on normoxic vessels than hypoxic ones; and (4) intrinsic PEEP that develops due to inadequate expiratory times.

Elimination of CO_2 is usually unchanged by one-lung ventilation, provided that minute ventilation is unchanged; arterial CO_2 tension is usually not appreciably altered. One-lung ventilation can result in injury to both ventilated and nonventilated lungs. The dependent, ventilated lung is subject to hyperperfusion as well as the potential for ventilator-induced trauma secondary to large tidal volumes. The nonventilated, nondependent lung is exposed to both surgical trauma and ischemia–reperfusion injuries. We recommend the use of tidal volumes of no more than 4 to 5 mL/kg of predicted body weight during one-lung ventilation, rather than earlier recommendations to use the same tidal volume as during two-lung ventilation. Lung-protective ventilation necessitates both a reduced tidal volume delivered to the ventilated lung as well as sufficient positive end-expiratory pressure to prevent atelectasis. Failure to provide lung-protective ventilation during one-lung ventilation can lead to iatrogenic lung injury.

Techniques for One-Lung Ventilation

One-lung ventilation can also be utilized to isolate a lung or to facilitate ventilatory management under certain conditions (Table 25–1). Four techniques can be employed: (1) placement of a double-lumen bronchial tube; (2) use of a single-lumen tracheal tube in conjunction with a bronchial blocker; (3) insertion of a conventional endotracheal tube into a mainstem bronchus; or (4) the use of so-called tubeless techniques for video-assisted thoracic procedures. Double-lumen tubes are most often used.

TABLE 25–1 Indications for one-lung ventilation.

Patient-related
Confine infection to one lung
Confine bleeding to one lung
Separate ventilation to each lung
Bronchopleural fistula
Tracheobronchial disruption
Large lung cyst or bulla
Severe hypoxemia due to unilateral lung disease
Procedure-related
Repair of thoracic aortic aneurysm
Lung resection
Pneumonectomy
Lobectomy
Segmental resection
Thoracoscopy
Esophageal surgery
Single-lung transplantation
Anterior approach to the thoracic spine
Bronchoalveolar lavage

DOUBLE-LUMEN BRONCHIAL TUBES

The principal advantages of double-lumen tubes are relative ease of placement, the ability to ventilate one or both lungs, and the ability to suction either lung.

All double-lumen tubes share the following characteristics:

- A longer endobronchial lumen that enters either the right or left main bronchus and another shorter endotracheal lumen that terminates in the lower trachea
- A preformed curve that, when properly "aimed," allows preferential entry into a bronchus
- An endobronchial cuff
- An endotracheal cuff

Ventilation can be delivered to only one lung by clamping the tube delivering gas to either the bronchial or tracheal lumen with both cuffs inflated; disconnecting the appropriate connection distal to the clamp site allows the ipsilateral lung to collapse. Because of differences in bronchial anatomy between the two sides, tubes are designed specifically for either the right or left bronchus. A right-sided double-lumen tube incorporates a modified cuff and a proximal portal on the endobronchial side for ventilation of the right upper lobe. The most commonly used double-lumen tubes are available in several sizes: 35F, 37F, 39F, and 41F.

Anatomic Considerations

On average, the adult trachea is 11 to 13 cm long. It begins at the level of the cricoid cartilage (C6) and bifurcates at the level of the carina behind the sternomanubrial joint (T5). Major differences between the right and left main bronchi are as follows: (1) the larger diameter right bronchus diverges away from the trachea at a less acute angle in relation to the trachea, whereas the left bronchus diverges at a more horizontal angle (Figure 25–5); (2) the right bronchus has upper, middle, and lower lobe branches, whereas the left bronchus divides into only upper and lower lobe branches; and (3) the orifice of the right upper lobe bronchus is typically about 1 to 2.5 cm from the carina, whereas the bifurcation of the left main bronchus is typically about 5 cm distal to the carina. There is considerable anatomic variation: for example, the right upper lobe bronchus will occasionally arise from the trachea itself.

As previously noted, right-sided double-lumen tubes must have a portal through the endobronchial cuff for ventilating the right upper lobe (Figure 25–6). Anatomic variations among individuals in the distance between the carina and the right upper lobe orifice will occasionally result in difficulty ventilating that lobe with right-sided tubes. Either a left-sided or right-sided double-lumen tube can be used in most surgical procedures, irrespective of the operative side; for simplicity, many practitioners prefer to use left-sided tubes for nearly every case.

2 There are certain clinical situations in which the use of a right-sided double-lumen tube is recommended: (1) distorted anatomy of the left main bronchus by an intrabronchial or extrabronchial mass; (2) compression of the left main bronchus due to a descending thoracic aortic aneurysm; (3) left-sided pneumonectomy; (4) left-sided single lung transplantation; and (5) left-sided sleeve resection.

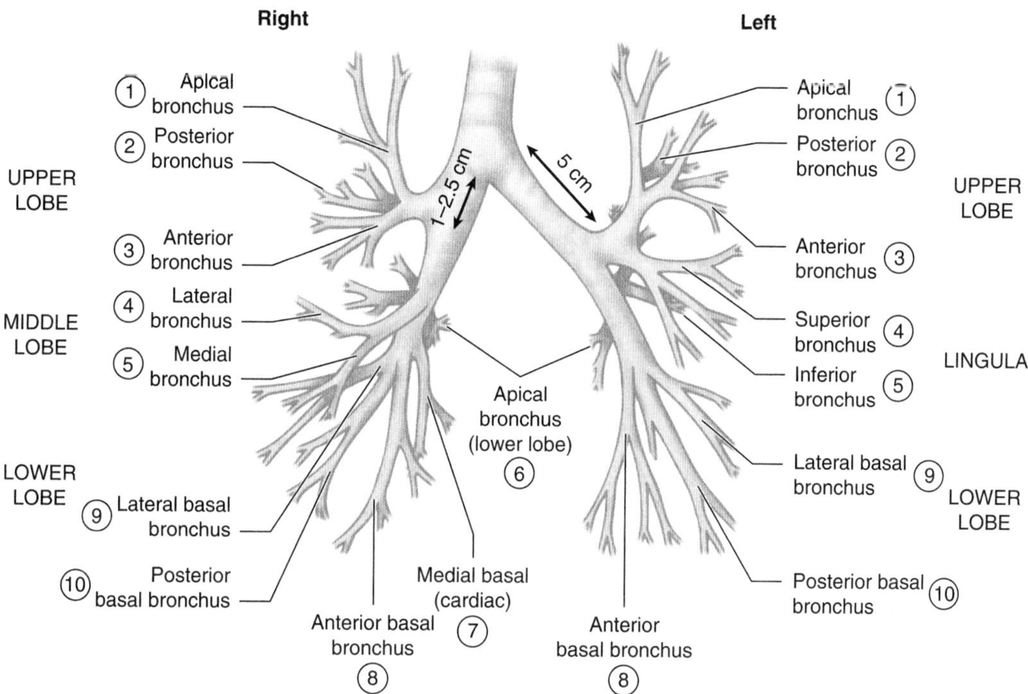

FIGURE 25–5 Anatomy of the tracheobronchial tree. Note bronchopulmonary segments (1–10) as numbered. (Adapted with permission from Gothard JWW, Branthwaite MA. *Anesthesia for Thoracic Surgery.* Oxford, UK: Blackwell; 1982.)

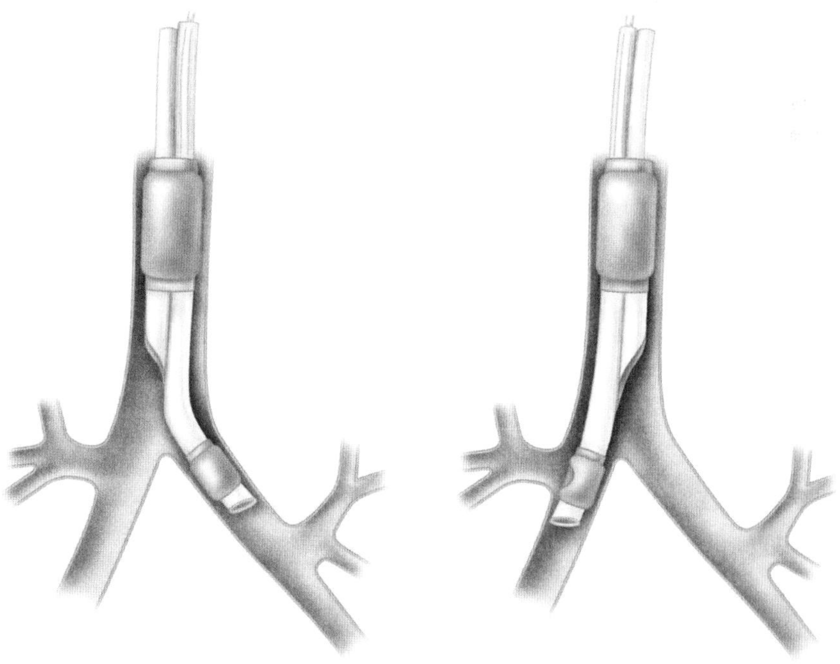

FIGURE 25–6 Correct position of a left- and right-sided double-lumen tube.

Finally, despite theoretical concerns about right upper lobe atelectasis and potentially difficult placement, studies have failed to detect differences in the clinical performance of right- and left-sided double-lumen tubes.

Placement of Double-Lumen Tubes

Laryngoscopy with a curved (MacIntosh) blade usually provides better intubating conditions than does a straight blade because the curved blade typically provides more room for manipulation of the large double-lumen tube. Video laryngoscopy can also be employed to facilitate tube placement. The double-lumen tube is passed with the distal curvature concave anteriorly and is rotated 90° (toward the side of the bronchus to be intubated) after the tip passes the vocal cords and enters the larynx (Figure 25–7). At this point, the operator has two options: the tube can be advanced until resistance is felt (the average depth of insertion is about 29 cm [at the teeth]), or alternatively, the fiberoptic bronchoscope can be inserted through the endobronchial limb and advanced into the desired bronchus. The double-lumen tube can be advanced over the bronchoscope into the desired bronchus. Correct tube placement should be established using a preset protocol (Figure 25–8 and Table 25–2) and confirmed by flexible fiberoptic

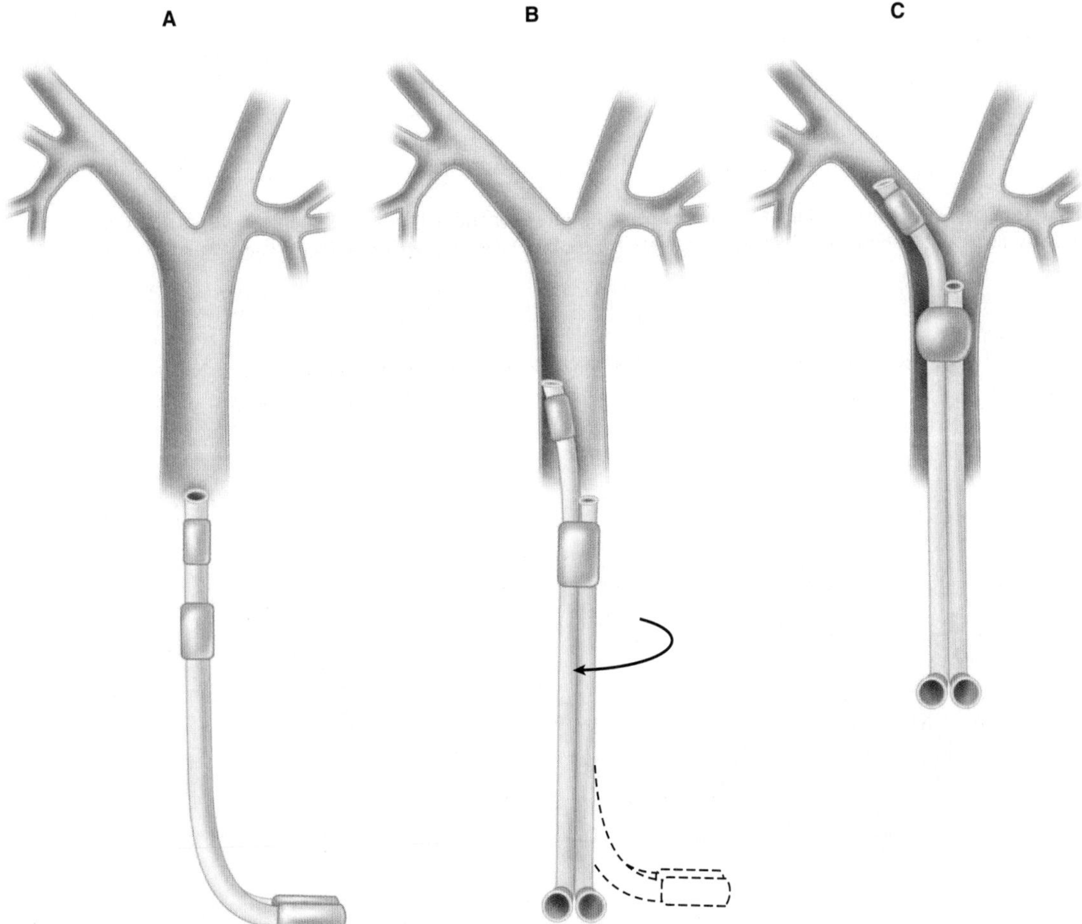

FIGURE 25–7 Placement of a left-sided double-lumen tube. Note that the tube is turned 90° as soon as it enters the larynx. **A**: Initial position. **B**: Rotated 90°. **C**: Final position.

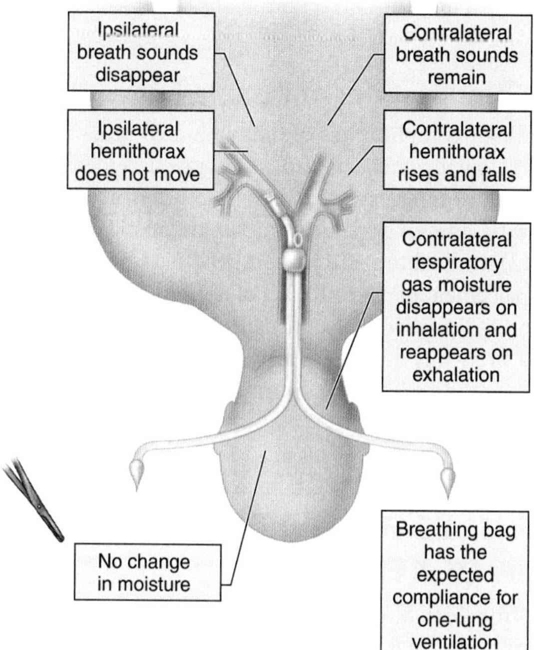

FIGURE 25–8 Results of unilateral clamping of the bronchial lumen tube when the double-lumen tube is in the correct position.

TABLE 25–2 Protocol for checking placement of a left-sided double-lumen tube.

1. Inflate the tracheal cuff (5–10 mL of air).
2. Check for bilateral breath sounds. Unilateral breath sounds indicate that the tube is too far down (tracheal opening is bronchial).
3. Inflate the bronchial cuff (1–2 mL).
4. Clamp the tracheal lumen.
5. Check for unilateral left-sided breath sounds.
   a. The persistence of right-sided breath sounds indicates that the bronchial opening is still in the trachea (the tube should be advanced).
   b. Unilateral right-sided breath sounds indicate incorrect entry of the tube in the right bronchus.
   c. The absence of breath sounds over the entire right lung and the left upper lobe indicates that the tube is too far down the left bronchus.
6. Unclamp the tracheal lumen, and clamp the bronchial lumen.
7. Check for unilateral right-sided breath sounds. The absence or diminution of breath sounds indicates that the tube is not far enough down and that the bronchial cuff is occluding the distal trachea.

bronchoscopy. When problems are encountered in intubating the patient with the double-lumen tube, placement of a single-lumen endotracheal tube should be attempted; once positioned in the trachea, the latter can be exchanged for the double-lumen tube by using a specially designed catheter guide ("tube exchanger"). We have found that double-lumen tubes placed in this way will often, as expected, find their way into the right mainstem bronchus.

Most double-lumen tubes easily accommodate bronchoscopes with a 3.6- to 4.2-mm outer diameter. When the bronchoscope is introduced into the tracheal lumen and advanced through the tracheal orifice, the carina should be visible (Figure 25–9), and the bronchial limb of the tube should be seen entering the respective bronchus; additionally, the top of the bronchial cuff (usually colored blue) should be visible but should not extend above the carina. If the bronchial cuff of a left-sided double-lumen tube is not visible, the bronchial limb may have been inserted sufficiently far to allow the bronchial cuff to obstruct the orifice of the left upper or lower lobe; the tube should be withdrawn until the cuff can be identified distal to the carina. The optimal position of a right-sided double-lumen tube is confirmed by placing the fiberoptic scope through the endobronchial lumen, which should show alignment of the endobronchial side portal with the opening of the right upper lobe bronchus. The bronchial cuff should be inflated only

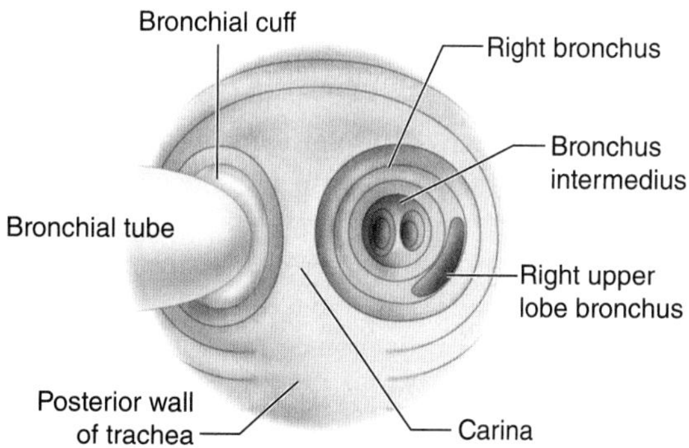

FIGURE 25–9 The view of the carina looking down the tracheal lumen of a properly positioned left double-lumen bronchial tube.

to the point at which the audible leak from the open tracheal lumen disappears while ventilating only through the bronchial lumen.

Tube position should be reconfirmed after the patient is positioned for surgery because the tube may move relative to the carina as the patient is turned into the lateral decubitus position. Malpositioning of a double-lumen tube within the tracheobronchial tree may lead to failure of the operative lung to collapse, apparent poor lung compliance, and low exhaled tidal volume. Problems with left-sided double-lumen tubes are usually related to one of three possibilities: (1) the tube tip is too distal; (2) the tube tip is too proximal; or (3) the tube is in the right bronchus (the wrong side). If the tube tip is located too distally, the bronchial cuff can obstruct the left upper or the left lower lobe orifice, and the bronchial lumen can be inserted into the orifice of the left lower or left upper lobe bronchus, respectively. When the tube is not advanced distally enough, the inflated bronchial cuff may be above the carina and also occlude the tracheal lumen. In both instances, deflation of the bronchial cuff improves ventilation to the lung and helps identify the problem. In some patients, the bronchial lumen may be within the left upper or left lower lobe bronchus but with the tracheal opening remaining above the carina; this situation is suggested by the collapse of only one of the left lobes when the bronchial lumen is clamped. In the same situation, if the surgical procedure is in the right thorax, clamping of the tracheal lumen will lead to ventilation of only the left upper or left lower lobe; hypoxia usually develops rapidly.

Right-sided double-lumen tubes can be accidentally inserted into the left mainstem bronchus, inserted too distally or too proximally, or have misalignment of the endobronchial side portal with the opening of the right upper lobe bronchus. If the tube enters the wrong bronchus, the fiberoptic bronchoscope can be used to redirect it into the correct side: (1) the bronchoscope is passed through the bronchial lumen to the tip of the tube; (2) under direct vision, the tube and the bronchoscope are withdrawn together into the trachea just above the carina; (3) the bronchoscope alone is then advanced into the correct bronchus; and (4) the double-lumen tube is gently advanced over the bronchoscope, which functions as a stylet to guide the bronchial lumen into the correct bronchus.

Complications of Double-Lumen Tubes

Major complications of double-lumen tubes include (1) hypoxemia due to tube malplacement, tube occlusion, or excessive degrees of venous admixture with one-lung ventilation; (2) traumatic laryngitis; (3) tracheobronchial rupture resulting from traumatic placement or overinflation of the endobronchial cuff; and (4) inadvertent suturing or stapling of the tube to a bronchus during surgery (detected as the inability to withdraw the tube during attempted extubation).

SINGLE-LUMEN TRACHEAL TUBES WITH A BRONCHIAL BLOCKER

Bronchial blockers are inflatable devices that are passed alongside or through a single-lumen tracheal tube to selectively occlude a bronchial orifice. The bronchial blocker must be advanced, positioned, and inflated under direct visualization via a flexible bronchoscope.

The major advantage of a single-lumen tube with a bronchial blocker is that, unlike a double-lumen tube, it need not be replaced with a conventional tracheal tube if the patient will remain intubated postoperatively (see later discussion). Its major disadvantage is that the "blocked" lung collapses slowly (and sometimes incompletely) because of the small size of the channel within the blocker catheter.

There are several types of bronchial blockers. They come in different sizes (7F and 9F) and have a 1.4-mm diameter inner lumen. Bronchial blockers have a high-volume low-pressure cuff with either an elliptical or spherical shape. The spherical shape of the cuff facilitates adequate blockade of the right mainstem bronchus. The spherical or the elliptical cuff can be used for the left mainstem bronchus. The inner lumen contains a nylon wire, which exits the distal end as a wire loop. The placement of the bronchial blocker involves inserting the endobronchial blocker through the endotracheal tube and using the fiberoptic bronchoscope and the distal loop of the guidewire to direct the blocker into a mainstem bronchus. The fiberoptic bronchoscope must be advanced beyond the bronchus opening so that the blocker enters the bronchus while it is being advanced. When the deflated cuff is beyond the entrance of the bronchus, the fiberoptic bronchoscope is withdrawn, and the blocker is secured in position. The cuff is fully inflated under fiberoptic visualization with 4 to 8 mL of air to obtain bronchial blockade. The placement must be reconfirmed when the patient is placed in the lateral position. We find bronchial blockers to be good choices for lung separation in intubated critically ill patients who require one-lung ventilation, patients who are difficult to intubate using direct laryngoscopy, patients with prior tracheostomies, and patients who may require postoperative mechanical ventilation. However, bronchial blockers are more prone to dislodgement compared with double-lumen endotracheal tubes, and their small central lumens do not allow efficient suctioning of secretions or rapid collapse of the lung.

In smaller children, an inflatable Fogarty embolectomy catheter can be used as a bronchial blocker in conjunction with a conventional tracheal tube (with the embolectomy catheter placed either inside or alongside the tracheal tube); a guidewire in the catheter can be used to facilitate placement. This technique is occasionally used to collapse one lung when other techniques do not work. As the embolectomy catheter does not have a communicating channel in the center, it also does not allow suctioning or ventilation of the isolated lung, and the catheter can be easily dislodged. Nonetheless, such bronchial blockers may be useful for one-lung anesthesia in pediatric patients and for tamponading bronchial bleeding in adult patients (see later discussion).

TUBELESS VIDEO-ASSISTED THORACIC SURGERY (NIVATS)

Thoracoscopic surgeries are increasingly being undertaken using "tubeless" anesthetic techniques. With patients anesthetized through the use of paravertebral blocks or thoracic epidural anesthesia, a spontaneous pneumothorax leading to lung collapse is created by the introduction of the thoracoscope. Sedation with propofol or dexmedetomidine is also routinely employed. Close patient monitoring is essential, and some patients will not tolerate the procedure. However, studies have shown that NIVATS may reduce surgical morbidity and hospital length of stay.

Anesthesia for Lung Resection

PREOPERATIVE CONSIDERATIONS

Lung resections are usually carried out for the diagnosis and treatment of pulmonary tumors and, less commonly, for traumatic lung injury, bullae, complications of necrotizing pulmonary infections, or bronchiectasis.

1. Tumors

Pulmonary tumors can be either benign or malignant, and, with the widespread use of bronchoscopic sampling (often guided by endobronchial ultrasound), diagnosis is usually available prior to surgery. Hamartomas account for 90% of benign tumors; they are usually peripheral pulmonary lesions and represent disorganized normal pulmonary tissue. Bronchial adenomas are usually central pulmonary lesions that are typically benign, but occasionally they may be locally invasive and rarely metastasize. These tumors include pulmonary carcinoids, cylindromas, and mucoepidermoid adenomas. They often obstruct the bronchial lumen and cause recurrent pneumonia distal to the obstruction in the same area. Primary pulmonary carcinoids may secrete multiple hormones, including adrenocorticotropic hormone (ACTH) and arginine vasopressin; however, manifestations of the carcinoid syndrome are uncommon and are more likely with metastatic disease.

Malignant pulmonary tumors are divided into bronchogenic versus metastatic. Bronchogenic cancers include small ("oat") cell and non–small cell carcinomas. The latter group includes squamous cell (epidermoid) tumors, adenocarcinomas, and large cell (anaplastic) carcinomas. Epidermoid and small cell carcinomas usually present as central masses with bronchial lesions; adenocarcinoma and large cell carcinomas are more typically peripheral lesions that often involve the pleura. Metastatic tumors may arise from almost any source, but commonly they are from cancers of the kidney, breast, ovary, testis, colon, rectum, head and neck, and uterus. Metastases may be present in lung tissue, lymph nodes, or both.

Clinical Manifestations

Symptoms may include cough, hemoptysis, wheezing, weight loss, productive sputum, dyspnea, or fever. Pleuritic chest pain or pleural effusion suggests pleural extension. Involvement of mediastinal structures is suggested by hoarseness that results from compression of the recurrent laryngeal nerve, Horner syndrome caused by involvement of the sympathetic chain, an elevated hemidiaphragm caused by compression of the phrenic nerve, dysphagia caused by compression of the esophagus, or superior vena cava syndrome caused by compression or invasion of the superior vena cava. Pericardial effusion or cardiomegaly suggests cardiac involvement. Extension of apical (superior sulcus) tumors can result in either shoulder or arm pain, or both, because of involvement of the C7–T2 roots of the brachial plexus (*Pancoast syndrome*). Distant metastases most commonly involve the brain, bone, liver, and adrenal glands.

Lung carcinomas—particularly small cell—can produce remote effects that are not related to malignant spread (*paraneoplastic syndromes*). Mechanisms include ectopic hormone production and immunological cross-reactivity between the tumor and normal tissues. Cushing syndrome, hyponatremia (syndrome of inappropriate antidiuretic hormone secretion [SIADH]), and hypercalcemia may be encountered, resulting from the ectopic secretion of ACTH, arginine vasopressin, and parathyroid hormone, respectively. Lambert–Eaton (myasthenic) syndrome is characterized by a proximal myopathy in which muscle strength increases with repeated effort (in contrast to myasthenia gravis). Other paraneoplastic syndromes include peripheral neuropathy and migratory thrombophlebitis.

Treatment

Surgery is the treatment of choice to reduce the tumor burden in nonmetastatic lung cancer. Various perioperative chemotherapy and radiation treatments are likewise employed, but there is wide variation among tissue types in their sensitivity to chemotherapy and radiation.

Resectability & Operability

Resectability is determined by the anatomic stage of the tumor, whereas operability is dependent on the interaction between the extent of the procedure required for cure and the physiological status of the patient. Anatomic staging is accomplished using chest radiography, computed tomography (CT) or magnetic resonance (MR) imaging, bronchoscopy, and (less commonly) mediastinoscopy. The extent of the surgery should maximize the chance for a cure while preserving adequate residual pulmonary function postoperatively. Lobectomy via a posterior thoracotomy, through the fifth or sixth intercostal space, or (more commonly) using video-assisted thoracoscopic surgery (VATS), is the procedure of choice for most lesions. Segmental or wedge resections may be performed for initial diagnosis or for definitive treatment of small peripheral lesions. Pneumonectomy is necessary for curative treatment of lesions involving the left or right main bronchus or when the tumor extends toward the hilum. A *sleeve resection* may be employed for patients with proximal lesions and limited pulmonary reserve as an alternative to pneumonectomy; in such instances, the involved lobar bronchus, together with part of the right or left main bronchus, is resected, and the distal bronchus is reanastomosed to the proximal bronchus or the trachea. Sleeve pneumonectomy may be considered for tumors involving the trachea.

The incidence of pulmonary complications after thoracotomy and lung resection is about 30% and is related not only to the amount of lung tissue resected but also to the disruption of chest wall mechanics because of the thoracotomy. Postoperative pulmonary dysfunction seems to be less after VATS than "open" thoracotomy. The mortality rate for pneumonectomy is generally more than twice that for a lobectomy. Mortality is greater for right-sided than left-sided pneumonectomy, possibly because of greater loss of lung tissue.

Evaluation for Lung Resection

A comprehensive preoperative assessment is necessary to assess and modify perioperative risk; minimize perioperative complications, hospital length of stay, and hospital readmission risk; and optimize outcomes. Preoperative assessment of respiratory function may include determinations of respiratory mechanics, gas exchange, and cardiorespiratory interaction. Preoperative spirometry and diffusion capacity can be used to predict postoperative values. For example:

Postoperative FEV_1 = preoperative $FEV_1 \times$ (1 − the percentage of functional lung tissue removed divided by 100).

Removal of extensively diseased lung (nonventilated but perfused) does not necessarily adversely affect pulmonary function and may actually improve oxygenation. Mortality and morbidity are significantly increased if postoperative FEV_1 is less than 30% to 40% of normative FEV_1. Gas exchange will sometimes be characterized by diffusion lung capacity for carbon monoxide (DLCO). DLCO correlates with the total functioning surface area of the alveolar–capillary interface. Predictive postoperative DLCO can be calculated in the same fashion as postoperative FEV_1. If both the predicted DLCO and FEV_1 are greater than 60%, the patient is generally at lower risk for lung resection. Cardiopulmonary exercise testing is warranted when either of the tests is less than 30%. Ventilation/perfusion $\dot{V}/\dot{Q}$ scintigraphy provides the relative contribution of each lobe to overall pulmonary function and may further refine the assessment of predicted postoperative lung function in patients when pneumonectomy is the indicated surgical procedure and there is concern about whether a single lung will be adequate to support life.

Patients considered at greater risk of perioperative complications (predicted FEV_1 or DLCO between 60% and 30%) based on standard spirometry testing and calculation of postoperative function should undergo exercise testing for evaluation of cardiopulmonary interaction. Stair climbing is the easiest way to assess exercise capacity and cardiopulmonary reserve. Patients capable of climbing two or three flights of stairs have decreased mortality and morbidity. Conversely, the ability to climb less than two flights of stairs is associated with increased perioperative risk. The gold standard for evaluating cardiopulmonary interaction is by cardiopulmonary exercise testing (CPET) and measurement of maximal minute oxygen consumption. $\dot{V}O_2$ greater than 20 mL/kg is not associated with a significant increase in perioperative mortality or morbidity, whereas minute consumption of less than 10 mL/kg is associated with an increased perioperative risk.

A combination of tests to evaluate the patient for thoracotomy and major pulmonary resection is recommended by the American College of Chest Physicians (Figure 25–10).

2. Infection

Pulmonary infections may present as a solitary nodule or cavitary lesion (necrotizing pneumonitis). VATS may be carried out to exclude malignancy and diagnose the infectious agent. Lung resection is also indicated for cavitary lesions that are refractory to antibiotic treatment, are associated with refractory empyema, or result in massive hemoptysis. Responsible organisms include both bacteria and fungi.

3. Bronchiectasis

Bronchiectasis is a permanent dilation of bronchi. It is usually the end result of severe or recurrent inflammation and obstruction of bronchi. Causes include cigarette smoking; a variety of viruses, bacteria, nontuberculous mycobacteria, and fungi; as well as inhalation of toxic gases, aspiration of gastric acid, and defective mucociliary clearance (cystic fibrosis and disorders of ciliary dysfunction). Bronchial muscle and elastic tissue are typically replaced by very vascular fibrous tissue. The latter predisposes to bouts of hemoptysis. Pulmonary resection is usually indicated for massive hemoptysis when conservative measures have failed and the disease is localized. Patients with diffuse bronchiectasis have a chronic obstructive ventilatory defect.

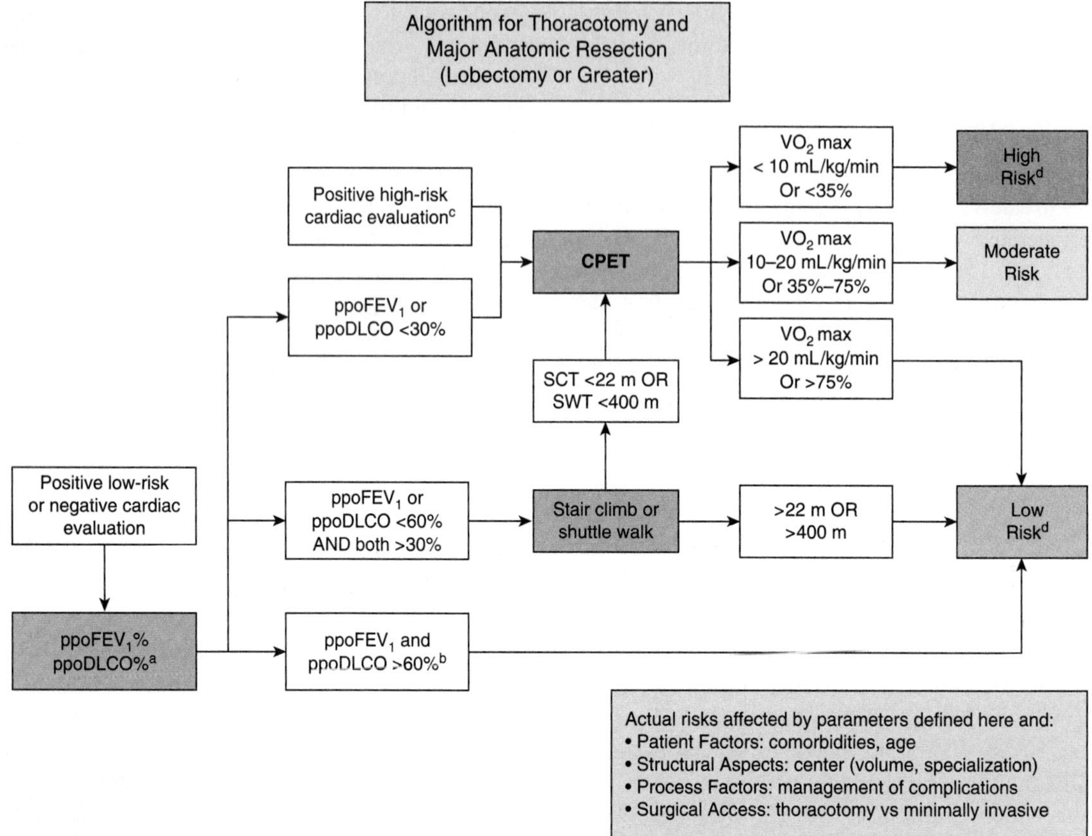

FIGURE 25–10 Physiological evaluation resection algorithm. (a) For pneumonectomy candidates, we suggest using Q scan to calculate predicted postoperative (PPO) FEV_1 or DLCO values (PPO values = preoperative values × [1 – fraction of total perfusion for the resected lung]), where the preoperative values are taken as the best-measured postbronchodilator values. For lobectomy patients, segmental counting is indicated to calculate PPO FEV_1 or DLCO values (PPO values = preoperative values × [1 – *y*/*z*]), where the preoperative values are taken as the best-measured postbronchodilator value and the number of functional or unobstructed lung segments to be removed is *y* and the total number of functional segments is *z*. (b) $ppoFEV_1$ or ppoDLCO cutoff values of 60% predicted values have been chosen based on indirect evidence and expert consensus opinion. (c) For patients with a positive high-risk cardiac evaluation deemed to be stable to proceed to surgery, we suggest performing both pulmonary function tests and cardiopulmonary exercise testing (CPET) for a more precise definition of risk. (d) Definition of risk is as follows: *Low risk*: The expected risk of mortality is below 1%. Major anatomic resections can be safely performed in this group. *Moderate risk*: Morbidity and mortality rates may vary according to the values of split lung functions, exercise tolerance, and extent of resection. The risks and benefits of the operation should be thoroughly discussed with the patient. *High risk*: The risk of mortality after standard major anatomic resections may be higher than 10%. Considerable risk of severe cardiopulmonary morbidity and residual functional loss is expected. Patients should be counseled about alternative surgical (minor resections or minimally invasive surgery) or nonsurgical options. m, meters; ppoDLCO, predicted postoperative diffusion capacity for carbon monoxide; ppoDLCO%, percent predicted postoperative diffusion capacity for carbon monoxide; $ppoFEV_1$, predicted postoperative FEV_1; ppoFEV1%, percent predicted postoperative FEV_1; SCT, stair climb test; SWT, shuttle walk test; VO_{2max}, maximal oxygen consumption. (Reproduced with permission from Brunelli A, Kim A, Berger K, et al. Physiologic evaluation of the patient with lung cancer being considered for resectional surgery: Diagnosis and management of lung cancer, 3rd ed: American College of Chest Physicians evidence-based clinical practice guidelines. *Chest.* 2013 May;143(5 Suppl):e166S-e190S.)

ANESTHETIC CONSIDERATIONS

1. Preoperative Management

Most patients undergoing pulmonary resections have underlying lung disease. It should be emphasized that smoking is a risk factor for both chronic obstructive pulmonary disease and coronary artery disease; both disorders commonly coexist in patients presenting for thoracotomy. Echocardiography is useful for assessing baseline cardiac function and may suggest evidence of cor pulmonale (right ventricular enlargement or hypertrophy) in patients with poor exercise tolerance. Investigation for coronary artery disease is indicated by the same signs and symptoms in surgical patients as in those not requiring surgery.

Patients with tumors should be queried regarding signs and symptoms of local extension of the tumor and paraneoplastic syndromes (see above). Preoperative chest radiographs and CT or MR images should be reviewed. Tracheal or bronchial deviation can make tracheal intubation and proper positioning of bronchial tubes much more difficult. Moreover, airway compression can lead to difficulty in ventilating the patient following induction of anesthesia. Pulmonary consolidation, atelectasis, and large pleural effusions predispose to hypoxemia. The location of any bullous cysts or abscesses should be noted.

Patients undergoing thoracic procedures are at increased risk of postoperative pulmonary and cardiac complications. Perioperative arrhythmias, particularly supraventricular tachycardias, are common and thought to result from surgical manipulations or distention of the right atrium following reduction of the pulmonary vascular bed. The incidence of arrhythmias increases with age and the amount of pulmonary resection.

2. Intraoperative Management

Preparation

As is true for patients requiring cardiac surgery, optimal preparation of the thoracic surgery patient may reduce the likelihood of catastrophic problems. Limited pulmonary reserve, anatomic abnormalities, or compromise of the airways, as well as the need for one-lung ventilation, predispose these patients to the rapid onset of hypoxemia. In addition to items for basic airway management, specialized and properly functioning equipment—such as multiple sizes of single- and double-lumen tubes, a flexible fiberoptic bronchoscope, a small-diameter "tube exchanger" of adequate length to accommodate a double-lumen tube, a continuous positive airway pressure (CPAP) delivery system, and an anesthesia circuit adapter for administering bronchodilators—should be immediately available.

Patients undergoing open-lung resections (segmentectomy, lobectomy, and pneumonectomy) often receive postoperative thoracic epidural analgesia unless there is a contraindication. However, patients are increasingly being treated with antiplatelet and anticoagulant medications, which may preclude epidural catheter placement. Opioid-sparing, multimodal analgesia regimens, including paravertebral blocks, local injection of aqueous or liposomal bupivacaine, and wound infusion catheters, are increasingly a part of enhanced recovery programs for thoracic surgery patients.

Venous Access

Adequate venous access (we prefer at least one 14- or 16-gauge intravenous line) is mandatory for all open thoracic surgical procedures. A blood warmer and a rapid infusion device are also desirable when extensive blood loss is anticipated.

Monitoring

Direct monitoring of arterial pressure is indicated for resections of large tumors (particularly those with mediastinal or chest wall extension) and for any procedure performed in a patient with limited pulmonary reserve or significant cardiovascular disease. Central venous access with monitoring of central venous pressure (CVP) is commonly used for pneumonectomies and resections of large tumors; however, less invasive measures of cardiac output through the use of thoracic bioimpedance, pulse contour analysis, or transpulmonary thermodilution provide better estimates of cardiac function and volume responsiveness (see Chapter 5). We suggest that if a subclavian line is placed, it should be placed on the side of the thoracotomy to avoid pneumothorax on the side that will be ventilated intraoperatively. Pulmonary artery catheters are very rarely used. In patients with significant coronary artery disease or pulmonary hypertension, intraoperative diagnosis of hypovolemia or reduced right or left ventricular performance can be easily accomplished with transesophageal echocardiography.

Induction of Anesthesia

The selection of an induction agent and its dose should be based on the patient's preoperative status. All patients should receive adequate preoxygenation before induction. An adequate depth of anesthesia will help prevent reflex bronchospasm and exaggerated cardiovascular pressor responses to laryngoscopy. This may be accomplished by incremental doses of the induction agent, an opioid, or deepening the anesthesia with a volatile inhalation agent (the latter is particularly useful in patients with reactive airways). Moreover, volatile anesthetic agents may protect the lung from injury during one-lung ventilation.

Tracheal intubation with a single-lumen endotracheal tube (or with a laryngeal mask airway [LMA]) may be necessary if the surgeon performs diagnostic bronchoscopy (see below) prior to surgery. After the bronchoscopy has been completed, the single-lumen tracheal tube (or LMA) can be replaced with a double-lumen endobronchial tube (see above). Controlled positive-pressure ventilation helps prevent atelectasis, paradoxical breathing, and mediastinal shift; it also allows control of the operative field to facilitate the surgery. LMA placement may be indicated in NIVATS procedures if deeper levels of sedation or anesthesia are required.

Positioning

Most lung resections are performed with the patient in the lateral decubitus position. Proper positioning avoids injuries and facilitates surgical exposure. The lower arm is flexed, and the upper arm is extended in front of the head, pulling the scapula away from the operative field (Figure 25–11). Pillows are placed between the arms and between the legs, and an axillary (chest) roll is usually positioned just beneath the dependent axilla to reduce pressure on the inferior shoulder (it is assumed, but not proven, that the axillary roll helps protect the brachial plexus); care is taken to avoid pressure on the eyes and the dependent ear.

Maintenance of Anesthesia

All current anesthetic techniques have been successfully used for thoracic surgery, but the ideal techniques must provide the ability to administer high concentrations of inspired oxygen, and all must permit rapid adjustments in anesthetic depth. Potent halogenated agents (isoflurane, sevoflurane, or desflurane) are often used in North American practice. Advantages of the halogenated agents versus total intravenous techniques include potent, dose-related bronchodilation and consistent depression of airway reflexes. Halogenated agents generally have minimal effects on HPV in doses less than 1 minimum alveolar concentration (MAC). Advantages of opioids include (1) generally minimal hemodynamic effects; (2) depression of airway reflexes; and (3) residual

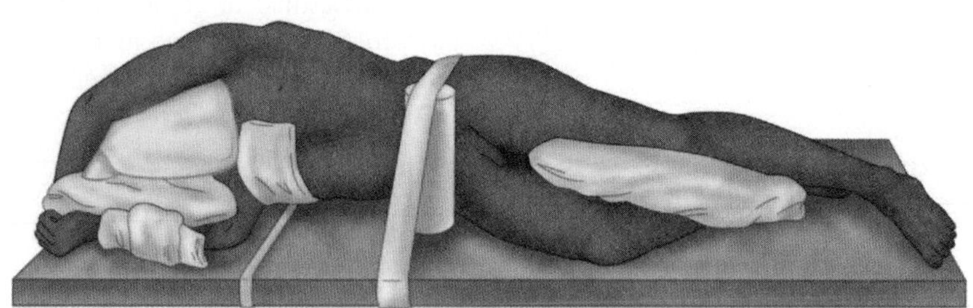

FIGURE 25–11 Proper positioning for a lateral thoracotomy. (Reproduced with permission from Gothard JWW, Branthwaite MA. *Anesthesia for Thoracic Surgery*. Oxford, UK: Blackwell; 1982.)

3 postoperative analgesia. If epidural or intrathecal opioids are to be used for postoperative analgesia, intravenous opioids should be minimized during surgery to prevent excessive postoperative respiratory depression. Maintenance of neuromuscular blockade with a nondepolarizing neuromuscular blocker (NMB) during surgery facilitates rib spreading as well as anesthetic management. Excessive fluid administration in patients undergoing thoracic surgery has been associated with acute lung injury in the postoperative period. Excessive fluid administration in the lateral decubitus position may promote a "lower lung syndrome" (ie, gravity-dependent transudation of fluid into the dependent lung). The latter increases intrapulmonary shunting and promotes hypoxemia, particularly during one-lung ventilation. Increasingly, goal-directed fluid delivery is advocated during thoracic surgery so that patients do not have too much or too little fluid resuscitation. The collapsed lung may be prone to acute lung injury due to surgical retraction during the procedure and possible ischemia–reperfusion injury. During lung resections, the bronchus (or remaining lung tissue) is usually divided with an automated stapling device. The bronchial stump is then tested for an air leak under water by transiently sustaining 30 cm of positive pressure to the airway. Prior to completion of chest closure, all remaining lung segments should be fully expanded manually under direct vision. Controlled mechanical ventilation is then resumed and continued until thoracostomy tubes are connected to suction.

Management of One-Lung Ventilation

Although still an intraoperative problem, hypoxemia has become less frequent because of better lung isolation methods, ventilation techniques, and the use of anesthetic agents with less detrimental effects on hypoxic pulmonary vasoconstriction. Attention has currently shifted toward avoidance of acute lung injury (ALI). Fortunately, ALI occurs infrequently, with an incidence of 2.5% of all lung resections combined and an incidence of 7.9% after pneumonectomy. However, when it occurs, ALI is associated with a risk of mortality or major morbidity of about 40%.

Based on current data, it seems that protective lung ventilation strategies may minimize the risk of ALI *after* lung resection. This ventilatory strategy includes the use of lower tidal volumes (<6 mL/kg), lower FiO_2 (50–80%) and lower ventilatory pressures (plateau pressure <25 cm H_2O; peak airway pressure <35 cm H_2O) through the use of pressure-controlled ventilation. Permissive hypercapnia is reasonable for those rare patients with elevated CO_2 tensions despite adequate oxygen saturation and a reasonable minute ventilation. The use of tidal volumes less than 3 mL/kg per lung may lead to lung derecruitment, atelectasis, and hypoxemia. Lung derecruitment may be avoided by the application of PEEP and recruitment maneuvers. Although the management of one-lung ventilation has long included the use of 100% oxygen, evidence for oxygen toxicity has accumulated both experimentally and clinically. Although there is no unequivocal evidence that one mode of ventilation may be more beneficial than the other, pressure-controlled ventilation may diminish the risk of barotrauma by limiting peak and plateau airway pressures, and the flow pattern results in a more homogenous distribution of the tidal volume and reduced dead space ventilation.

At the end of the procedure, the operative lung is inflated gradually to a peak inspiratory pressure of less than 30 cm H_2O to prevent disruption of the staple line. During reinflation of the operative lung, it may be helpful to clamp the lumen serving the dependent lung to limit overdistention.

Periodic arterial blood gas analysis is helpful to ensure adequate ventilation. End-tidal CO_2 measurement is useful as a trend monitor but may not be accurate due to increased dead-space and an unpredictable gradient between the arterial and end-tidal CO_2 partial pressure.

Management of Hypoxia

Hypoxemia during one-lung anesthesia requires one or more of the following interventions:

1. Adequate position of the endobronchial tube (or bronchial blocker) must be confirmed because its position relative to the carina can change as a result of surgical manipulations or traction; repeat fiberoptic bronchoscopy through the tracheal lumen can quickly detect this problem. Both lumens of the tube should

also be suctioned to exclude excessive secretions or obstruction as a factor.

2. Increase FiO_2 to 1.0.
3. Recruitment maneuvers on the dependent, ventilated lung may eliminate atelectasis and improve shunt.
4. Ensure that there is sufficient (but not excessive) PEEP to the dependent, nonoperative lung to eliminate atelectasis.
5. CPAP or blow-by oxygen to the operative lung will decrease shunting and improve oxygenation. However, uncontrolled inflation of the operative lung during VATS will make identification and visualization of the lung structures difficult for the surgeon; therefore, such maneuvers should be applied carefully and cautiously.
6. Two-lung ventilation should be instituted for severe hypoxemia. If possible, a pulmonary artery clamp can also be placed during pneumonectomy to eliminate shunt.
7. In patients with chronic obstructive lung disease, one should always be suspicious of pneumothorax on the dependent, ventilated side as a cause of severe hypoxemia. This complication requires immediate detection and treatment by aborting the surgical procedure, reexpanding the operative lung, and immediately inserting a chest tube in the contralateral chest.

Alternatives to One-Lung Ventilation

Ventilation can be stopped for short periods if 100% oxygen is insufflated at a rate greater than oxygen consumption **(apneic oxygenation) into an unobstructed tracheal tube**. Adequate oxygenation can often be maintained for prolonged periods, but progressive respiratory acidosis limits the use of this technique to 10 to 20 min in most patients. Arterial PCO_2 rises 6 mm Hg in the first minute, followed by a rise of 3 to 4 mm Hg during each subsequent minute.

High-frequency positive-pressure ventilation and high-frequency jet ventilation have been used during thoracic procedures as alternatives to one-lung ventilation. A standard tracheal tube may be used with either technique. Small tidal volumes (<2 mL/kg) allow decreased lung excursion, which may facilitate the surgery but still allow ventilation of both lungs. Unfortunately, mediastinal "bounce"—a to-and-fro movement—often interferes with the surgery.

3. Postoperative Management

General Care

Most patients are extubated shortly after surgery to decrease the risk of pulmonary barotrauma (particularly "blowout" [rupture] of the bronchial suture line). All patients (and especially those with marginal pulmonary reserve) should remain intubated until standard extubation criteria are met. When postoperative mechanical ventilation is required, double-lumen tubes should be replaced with a regular single-lumen tube at the end of surgery. We routinely use a catheter guide ("tube exchanger") for this purpose and always use this technique when the original laryngoscopy was difficult.

Patients are observed in the postanesthesia care unit and, in most instances, at least overnight in a monitored or intensive care unit. Atelectasis and shallow breathing ("splinting") from incisional pain commonly lead to hypoxemia and respiratory acidosis. Gravity-dependent transudation of fluid into the intraoperative dependent lung may also be contributory. Reexpansion edema of the collapsed nondependent lung can also occur.

4 Postoperative hemorrhage complicates about 3% of thoracotomies and may be associated with up to 20% mortality. Signs of hemorrhage include increased chest tube drainage (>200 mL/h), hypotension, tachycardia, and a falling hematocrit. Postoperative supraventricular tachyarrhythmias are common and usually require immediate treatment. Routine postoperative care should include semi-upright (>30°) positioning, sufficient supplemental oxygen to maintain satisfactory saturation, incentive spirometry, electrocardiographic and hemodynamic monitoring, a postoperative chest radiograph (to confirm the proper position of all thoracostomy tube drains and central lines and to

confirm the expansion of both lung fields), and adequate analgesia.

Postoperative Analgesia

The importance of adequate pain management in the thoracic surgical patient cannot be overstated. Inadequate pain control in these high-risk patients will result in splinting, poor respiratory effort, and the inability to cough and clear secretions, with an end result of airway closure, atelectasis, shunting, and hypoxemia. Irrespective of the modality used, there must be a comprehensive plan for pain management.

A balance between comfort and respiratory depression in patients with marginal lung function is difficult to achieve with parenteral opioids alone. Patients who have undergone thoracotomy clearly benefit from the use of other techniques (described later) that may reduce the need for parenteral opioids. If parenteral opioids are used alone, they are best administered via a patient-controlled analgesia device.

In the absence of an epidural catheter, intercostal, paravertebral, or erector spinae nerve blocks with long-acting local anesthetics may facilitate extubation and contribute to postoperative analgesia, but they have a limited duration of action, so additional means of pain management must be employed. Alternatives to regional techniques include infusion of local anesthetic through a catheter placed in the surgical wound during closure or injection of liposomal bupivacaine into the wound, either of which will markedly reduce the requirement for parenteral opioids and improve the overall quality of analgesia relative to parenteral opioids alone. The actual duration of action of liposomal bupivacaine relative to aqueous bupivacaine is controversial.

Epidural analgesia provides excellent, continuous pain relief and avoids side effects associated with systemic opioids. On the other hand, epidural techniques require around-the-clock attention from the acute pain team for the duration of the infusion and subject the patient to the long list of epidural-related side effects and complications. Most practitioners use a combination of opioid (fentanyl, morphine, hydromorphone) and local anesthetic (bupivacaine or ropivacaine), with the epidural catheter placed at a thoracic level. Gabapentin and low-dose ketamine and lidocaine intravenous infusions have all been employed as a part of multimodal analgesia regimens following thoracotomy. Oral or intravenous acetaminophen, nonsteroidal anti-inflammatory agents, or both are likewise routinely used in combination with other modalities for postoperative analgesia to reduce or eliminate opioids.

Postoperative Complications

Postoperative complications following thoracotomy are relatively common, but fortunately, most are minor and resolve uneventfully. Blood clots and thick secretions may obstruct the airways and result in atelectasis; suctioning may be necessary. Therapeutic bronchoscopy should be considered for persistent atelectasis, particularly when associated with thick secretions. Air leaks from the operative hemithorax are common following segmental and lobar resections. Most air leaks stop after a few days.
5 Bronchopleural fistula presents as a sudden large air leak from the chest tube that may be associated with an increasing pneumothorax and partial lung collapse. When it occurs within the first 24 to 72 h, it is usually the result of inadequate surgical closure of the bronchial stump. Delayed presentation is usually due to necrosis of the suture line associated with inadequate blood flow or infection.

Some complications are rare but deserve special consideration because they can be life-threatening and require immediate exploratory thoracotomy. Postoperative bleeding is reviewed above. Torsion of a lobe or segment can occur as the remaining lung on the operative side expands to occupy the hemithorax. The torsion usually occludes the pulmonary vein to that part of the lung, causing venous outflow obstruction. Hemoptysis and infarction can rapidly follow. The diagnosis is suggested by an enlarging homogeneous density on the chest radiograph and a
6 closed lobar orifice on bronchoscopy. Acute herniation of the heart into the operative hemithorax can occur through the pericardial defect that may remain following a pneumonectomy. A large pressure differential between the two hemithoraces is thought to trigger this catastrophic event. Cardiac herniation into the right hemithorax results in sudden severe hypotension with an elevated CVP

because of torsion of the central veins. Cardiac herniation into the left hemithorax following left pneumonectomy results in sudden compression of the myocardium, resulting in hypotension, ischemia, and infarction. A chest radiograph shows a shift of the cardiac shadow into the operative hemithorax.

Extensive mediastinal dissections can injure the phrenic, vagus, and left recurrent laryngeal nerves. Postoperative phrenic nerve palsy presents as elevation of the ipsilateral hemidiaphragm together with difficulty in weaning the patient from the ventilator. Large chest wall resections may include part of the diaphragm, causing a similar problem, in addition to a flail chest. If an epidural catheter has been placed, any loss of motor function or unexplained back pain should immediately trigger imaging to rule out epidural hematoma.

SPECIAL CONSIDERATIONS FOR PATIENTS UNDERGOING LUNG RESECTION

Massive Pulmonary Hemorrhage

Massive hemoptysis is usually defined as more than 500 to 600 mL of blood loss from the tracheobronchial tree within 24 h. The etiology is usually tuberculosis, bronchiectasis, a neoplasm, a complication of transbronchial or transthoracic biopsies, or (more commonly in the past) pulmonary artery rupture from overinflation of a pulmonary artery catheter balloon. Emergency surgical management with lung resection is reserved for potentially lethal massive hemoptysis. In most cases, surgery is carried out on an urgent rather than on a true emergency basis whenever possible; even then, operative mortality may exceed 20% (compared with >50% for medical management). Embolization of involved bronchial arteries may be attempted. The most common cause of death is asphyxia secondary to blood or clot in the airway. Patients may be brought to the operating room for rigid bronchoscopy when localization is not possible with fiberoptic flexible bronchoscopy. A bronchial blocker or Fogarty catheter (see earlier discussion) may be placed to tamponade the bleeding, or laser coagulation may be attempted.

Multiple large-bore intravenous catheters should be placed. Sedating drugs should not be given to awake, nonintubated, spontaneously ventilating patients because they are usually already hypoxic; 100% oxygen should be given continuously. If the patient is already intubated and has bronchial blockers in place, sedation is helpful to prevent coughing. The bronchial blocker should be left in position until the lung is resected. When the patient is not intubated, a rapid sequence induction is used. Patients usually swallow a large amount of blood and must be considered to have a full stomach. A double-lumen bronchial tube is ideal for protecting the normal lung from blood and for suctioning each lung separately. If any difficulty is encountered in placing the double-lumen tube, or if its relatively small lumens occlude easily, a large (8-mm inner diameter or larger) single-lumen tube may be used with a bronchial blocker to provide lung isolation.

Pulmonary Cyst & Bulla

Pulmonary cysts or bullae may be congenital or acquired as a result of emphysema. Large bullae can impair ventilation by compressing the surrounding lung. These air cavities often behave as if they have a one-way valve, predisposing them to enlarge progressively. Lung resection may be undertaken for progressive dyspnea or recurrent pneumothorax. The greatest risk of anesthesia is rupture of the air cavity during positive-pressure ventilation, resulting in tension pneumothorax; the latter may occur on either side prior to thoracotomy or on the nonoperative side during the lung resection. Induction of anesthesia with maintenance of spontaneous ventilation is desirable until the side with the cyst or bullae is isolated with a double-lumen tube or a chest tube is placed; most patients have a large increase in dead space, so assisted ventilation is necessary
7 to avoid excessive hypercarbia. Nitrous oxide is contraindicated in patients with cysts or bullae because it can expand the air space and cause rupture. The latter may be signaled by sudden hypotension, bronchospasm, or an abrupt rise in peak inflation pressure and requires immediate placement of a chest tube.

Lung Abscess

Lung abscesses result from primary pulmonary infections, obstructing pulmonary neoplasms (see earlier discussion), or, rarely, hematogenous spread of systemic infections. The two lungs should be isolated to prevent contamination of the healthy lung. A rapid-sequence intravenous induction with tracheal intubation with a double-lumen tube is generally recommended, with the affected lung in a dependent position. As soon as the double-lumen tube is placed, both bronchial and tracheal cuffs should be inflated. The bronchial cuff should make a tight seal before the patient is turned into the lateral decubitus position, with the diseased lung in a nondependent position. The diseased lung should be frequently suctioned during the procedure to decrease the likelihood of contaminating the healthy lung.

Bronchopleural Fistula

Bronchopleural fistulas occur following lung resection (usually pneumonectomy), rupture of a pulmonary abscess into a pleural cavity, pulmonary barotrauma, or spontaneous rupture of bullae. The majority of patients are treated (and cured) conservatively; patients come to surgery when chest tube drainage has failed. **Anesthetic management may be complicated by the inability to effectively ventilate the patient with positive pressure because of a large air leak, the potential for a tension pneumothorax, and the risk of contaminating the other lung if an empyema is present.** The empyema is usually drained prior to closure of the fistula.

A correctly placed double-lumen tube greatly simplifies anesthetic management by isolating the fistula and allowing one-lung ventilation to the normal lung. The patient should be extubated as soon as possible after the repair.

Anesthesia for Tracheal Resection

Preoperative Considerations

Tracheal resection is most commonly performed for tracheal stenosis, tumors, or, less commonly, congenital abnormalities. Tracheal stenosis can result from penetrating or blunt trauma, as well as tracheal intubation and tracheostomy. Squamous cell and adenoid cystic carcinomas account for the majority of tumors. Progressive compromise of the tracheal lumen produces dyspnea. Wheezing or stridor may be evident only with exertion. The dyspnea may be worse when the patient is lying down, with progressive airway obstruction. Hemoptysis can also complicate tracheal tumors. CT or MR imaging is valuable in localizing the lesion. **Measurement of flow–volume loops confirms the location of the obstruction and aids the clinician in evaluating the severity of the lesion (Figure 25–12).**

Anesthetic Considerations

Little premedication is given, as most patients presenting for tracheal resection have moderate to severe airway obstruction. Use of an anticholinergic agent to dry secretions is controversial because of the theoretical risk of inspissation. Monitoring should include direct arterial pressure measurements.

An inhalation induction (in 100% oxygen) is carried out in patients with severe obstruction. Sevoflurane is preferred because it is the potent anesthetic that is least irritating to the airway. Spontaneous ventilation is maintained throughout induction. NMBs are generally avoided because of the potential for complete airway obstruction following neuromuscular blockade. Laryngoscopy is performed only when the patient is judged to be under deep anesthesia. Intravenous lidocaine (1–2 mg/kg) can deepen the anesthesia without depressing respirations. The surgeon may then perform rigid bronchoscopy to evaluate and possibly dilate the lesion. Following bronchoscopy, the patient is intubated with a tracheal tube small enough to be passed distal to the obstruction whenever possible. Total intravenous anesthesia (TIVA) facilitates maintenance of anesthesia by ensuring anesthetic delivery during periods where ventilation may be impaired during surgery. Moreover, TIVA avoids leakage of anesthetic gases into the surgical field.

A collar incision is utilized for high tracheal lesions. The surgeon divides the trachea in the neck and advances a sterile armored tube into the distal trachea, passing off a sterile connecting breathing circuit to the anesthesiologist for ventilation during the

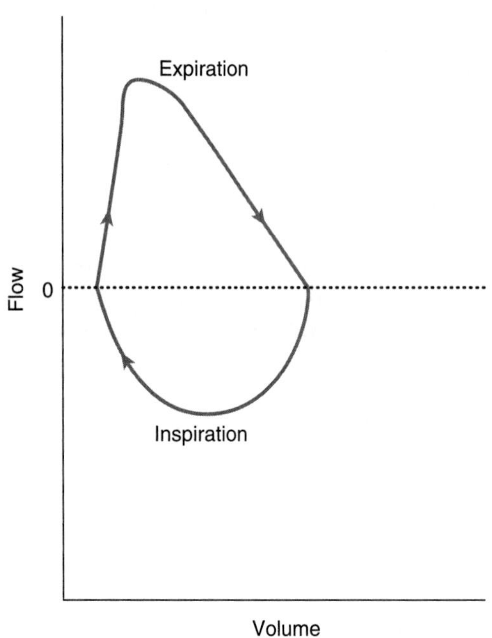

A: NORMAL

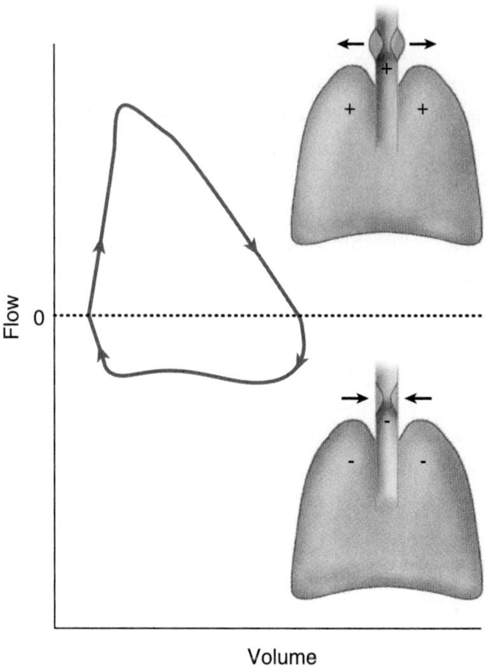

B: VARIABLE EXTRATHORACIC OBSTRUCTION

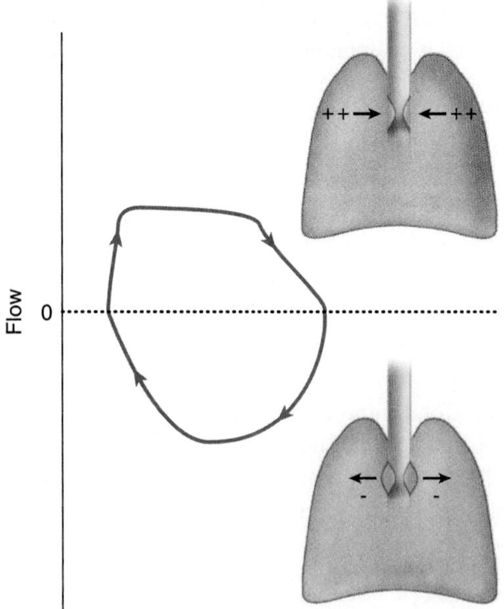

C: VARIABLE INTRATHORACIC OBSTRUCTION

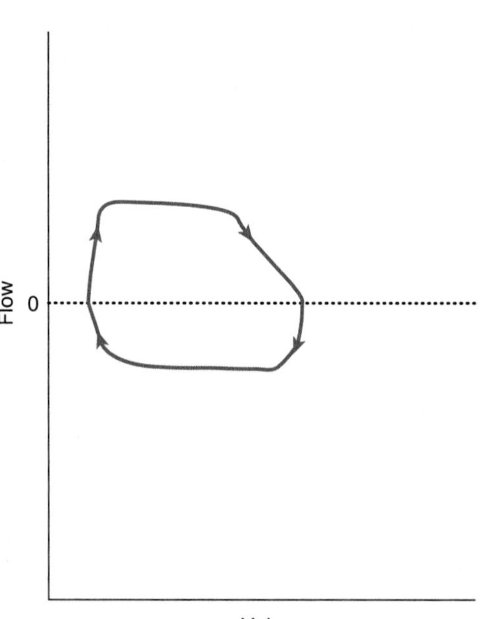

D: FIXED LARGE AIRWAY OBSTRUCTION

FIGURE 25–12 **A–D**: Flow–volume loops.

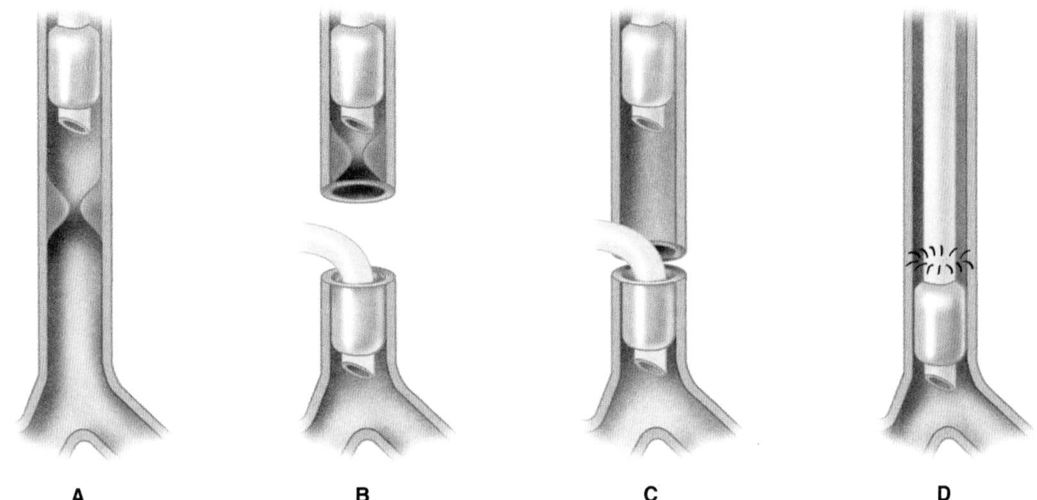

FIGURE 25–13 **A–D**: Airway management of a high tracheal lesion.

resection. Following the resection and completion of the posterior part of the reanastomosis, the armored tube is removed, and the original endotracheal tube is advanced distally, past the anastomosis (Figure 25–13). Alternatively, high-frequency jet ventilation may be employed during the anastomosis by passing the jet cannula past the obstruction and into the distal trachea (Figure 25–14). Return of spontaneous ventilation and early extubation at the end of the procedure are desirable. Patients should be positioned with the neck flexed immediately after the operation to minimize tension on the suture line (Figure 25–15).

Surgical management of low tracheal lesions requires a median sternotomy or right posterior thoracotomy. Anesthetic management may include more complicated techniques, such as high-frequency ventilation or even cardiopulmonary bypass (CPB) in complex congenital cases.

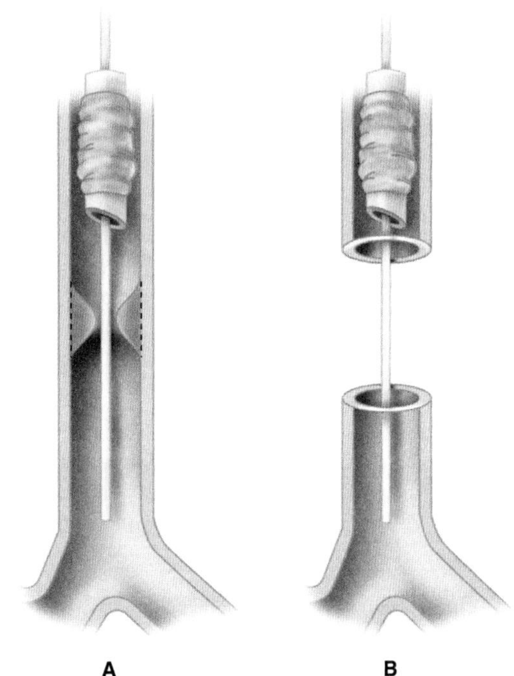

FIGURE 25–14 Tracheal resection using high-frequency jet ventilation. **A:** The catheter is advanced past the obstruction, and the cuff is deflated when jet ventilation is initiated. **B:** The catheter is advanced distally by the surgeon. Jet ventilation can be continued without interruption during resection and reanastomosis.

Anesthesia for Video-Assisted Thoracoscopic Surgery (VATS)

VATS is now used for most lung resections. Most procedures are performed through several small incisions in the chest wall, with the patient in the lateral decubitus position. Anesthetic management is similar to that for open procedures, except that one-lung

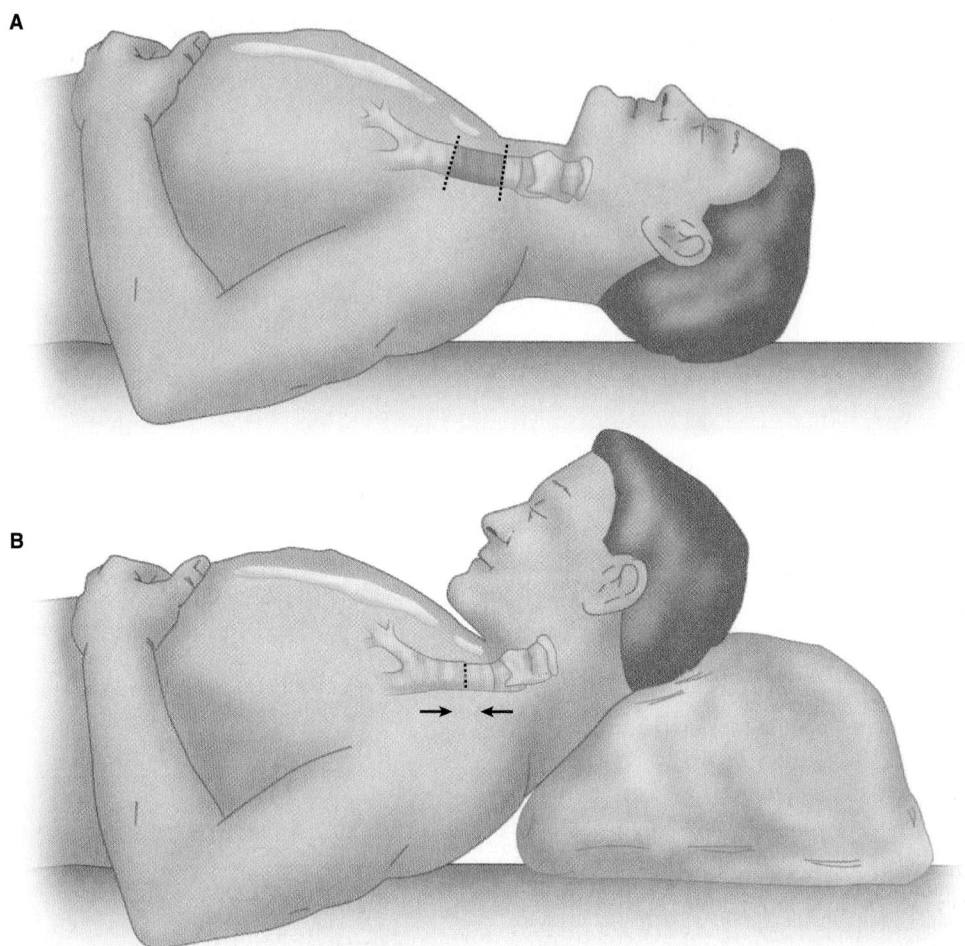

FIGURE 25–15 Position of the patient before (**A**) and after (**B**) tracheal resection and reanastomosis with the patient's neck flexed for the first 24 to 48 h.

ventilation is required (as opposed to being desirable) for nearly all procedures. As previously mentioned, "tubeless" VATS are increasingly performed.

Anesthesia for Diagnostic Thoracic Procedures

Bronchoscopy

Rigid bronchoscopy for removal of foreign bodies or tracheal dilation is usually performed under general anesthesia. These procedures are complicated by the need to share the airway with the surgeon or pulmonologist; fortunately, these procedures are often brief. After a standard intravenous induction, anesthesia is often maintained with total intravenous anesthesia and a short- or intermediate-acting NMB. One of three techniques can then be used during rigid bronchoscopy: (1) apneic oxygenation using a small catheter positioned alongside the bronchoscope to insufflate oxygen (see above); (2) conventional ventilation through the side arm of a ventilating bronchoscope (when the proximal window of this instrument is opened for suctioning or biopsies, ventilation must be interrupted); or (3) jet ventilation through an injector-type bronchoscope.

Fiberoptic bronchoscopies for placement of endobronchial stents, biopsies guided by endobronchial ultrasound, or laser treatment of airway lesions are performed with general anesthesia and either an endotracheal tube or LMA. Either an inhalation or TIVA technique can be used.

Mediastinoscopy

Mediastinoscopy, much more commonly employed in the past than at present, provides access to the mediastinal lymph nodes and is used to establish either the diagnosis or the resectability of intrathoracic malignancies (see above). Preoperative CT or MR imaging is useful for evaluating tracheal distortion or compression.

Mediastinoscopy is performed under general tracheal anesthesia with neuromuscular paralysis. Venous access with a large-bore (14- to 16-gauge) intravenous catheter is mandatory because of the risk of bleeding and the difficulty in controlling bleeding when it occurs. Because the innominate artery may be compressed during the procedure, blood pressure should be measured in the left arm.

Complications associated with mediastinoscopy include (1) vagally mediated reflex bradycardia from compression of the trachea or the great vessels; (2) excessive hemorrhage; (3) cerebral ischemia from compression of the innominate artery (detected with a right radial arterial line or pulse oximeter on the right hand); (4) pneumothorax (usually presents postoperatively); (5) air embolism (because of a 30° head elevation, the risk is greatest during spontaneous ventilation); (6) recurrent laryngeal nerve damage; and (7) phrenic nerve injury.

Bronchoalveolar Lavage

Bronchoalveolar lavage may be employed for patients with pulmonary alveolar proteinosis. These patients produce excessive quantities of surfactant and fail to clear it. They present with dyspnea and bilateral consolidation on the chest radiograph. In such patients, bronchoalveolar lavage may be indicated for severe hypoxemia or worsening dyspnea. Often, one lung is lavaged, allowing the patient to recover for a few days before the other lung is lavaged; the "sicker" lung is therefore lavaged first.

Unilateral bronchoalveolar lavage is performed under general anesthesia with a double-lumen bronchial tube. The cuffs on the tube should be properly positioned and should make a watertight seal to prevent spillage of fluid into the other side. The procedure is normally done in the supine position; although lavage with the lung in a dependent position helps to minimize contamination of the other lung, this position can cause severe ventilation/perfusion mismatch. Warm normal saline is infused into the lung to be treated and is drained by gravity. At the end of the procedure, both lungs are well suctioned, and the double-lumen tracheal tube is replaced with a single-lumen tracheal tube.

Anesthesia for Lung Transplantation

PREOPERATIVE CONSIDERATIONS

Lung transplantation is indicated for end-stage pulmonary parenchymal disease or pulmonary hypertension. Candidates are functionally incapacitated by dyspnea and have a poor prognosis. Criteria vary according to the primary disease process. Common etiologies are listed in Table 25–3. Lung transplantation (as is true for all solid organ transplants) is limited by the availability of suitable organs, not by the availability of recipients. Patients typically have dyspnea at rest or with minimal activity and resting hypoxemia (PaO_2 <50 mm Hg) with increasing oxygen requirements. Progressive CO_2 retention is also

TABLE 25–3 Indications for isolated lung transplantation.

Cystic fibrosis
Bronchiectasis
Obstructive
Chronic obstructive pulmonary disease
α_1-Antitrypsin deficiency
Pulmonary lymphangiomatosis
Restrictive
Idiopathic pulmonary fibrosis
Primary pulmonary hypertension

very common. Patients may be ventilator dependent or may be supported by extracorporeal membrane oxygenation (ECMO).

ANESTHETIC CONSIDERATIONS

1. Preoperative Management

Effective coordination between the organ-retrieval team and the transplant team minimizes graft ischemia time and avoids unnecessary prolongation of pretransplant anesthesia time. These procedures are performed on an emergency basis; therefore, patients may have little time to fast for surgery. Oral cyclosporine also may be given preoperatively. Administration of a clear antacid, an H_2 blocker, or metoclopramide should be considered. Any premedication is usually administered only in the operating room when the patient is directly attended to and monitored. Immunosuppressants and antibiotics are also administered after induction and before surgical incision.

2. Intraoperative Management

Monitoring

Strict asepsis should be observed for invasive monitoring procedures. Central venous access might be accomplished only after induction of anesthesia because patients may not be able to lie flat while awake. Patients with a patent foramen ovale are at risk of paradoxical embolism because of potentially high right atrial pressures. Transesophageal echocardiography is used to assess right ventricular function, the integrity of the intraatrial septum, and pulmonary vein flow following anastomosis.

Induction & Maintenance of Anesthesia

Induction with ketamine, etomidate, an opioid, or a combination of these agents is employed, avoiding precipitous drops in blood pressure. An NMB is used to facilitate laryngoscopy. Permissive hypercapnia and protective lung ventilation strategies are utilized. Inspired oxygen concentration is adjusted to maintain SaO_2 above 92%. Tidal volumes are maintained below 6 mL/kg using pressure-controlled ventilation. Inhalational agents are administered as tolerated for anesthesia and to provide a possible lung-protective effect.

Hypercarbia and acidosis may lead to pulmonary vasoconstriction and acute right heart failure, and hemodynamic support with inotropes may be required for these patients.

Single-Lung Transplantation

The option to employ cardiopulmonary bypass (CPB) (see Chapter 22) or extracorporeal membrane oxygenation (ECMO) during transplantation of one lung is based on the patient's response to collapsing the lung to be replaced and clamping its pulmonary artery as well as institutional practices. Persistent arterial hypoxemia (SpO_2 <88%) or right heart failure may require the institution of CPB. Drugs such as milrinone may be used for inotropic support, and inhaled nitric oxide can be delivered to dilate the pulmonary vasculature. After the recipient lung is removed, the pulmonary artery, left atrial cuff (with the pulmonary veins), and bronchus of the donor lung are anastomosed. Flexible bronchoscopy is used to examine the bronchial suture line after its completion. ECMO is increasingly preferred to provide support when needed compared with cardiopulmonary bypass.

Heart–Lung Transplantation

Heart–lung transplantation is performed through median sternotomy with CPB.

Posttransplantation Management

After anastomosis of the donor organ or organs,
8 ventilation to both lungs is resumed. Following transplantation, peak inspiratory pressures should be maintained at the minimum pressure compatible with good lung expansion, and the inspired oxygen concentration should be maintained as close to room air as allowed by a PaO_2 greater than 60 mm Hg. If transplantation has been performed on CPB, the patient is separated from CPB. Pulmonary vasodilators, inhaled nitric oxide, and inotropes (see earlier discussion) may be necessary. Transesophageal echocardiography is helpful

in identifying right or left ventricular dysfunction, as well as in evaluating blood flow in the pulmonary vessels after transplantation.

Transplantation disrupts the neural innervation, lymphatic drainage, and bronchial circulation of the transplanted lung. The respiratory pattern is unaffected, but the cough reflex is abolished below the carina. Bronchial hyperreactivity is observed in some patients. Hypoxic pulmonary vasoconstriction remains normal. Loss of lymphatic drainage increases extravascular lung water and predisposes the transplanted lung to pulmonary edema. Consequently, fluid overload should be avoided. Loss of the bronchial circulation predisposes to ischemic breakdown of the bronchial suture line.

3. Postoperative Management

Patients are extubated after surgery as soon as is feasible. A thoracic epidural catheter may be employed for postoperative analgesia when coagulation studies are normal. The postoperative course may be complicated by acute rejection, infections, and renal and hepatic dysfunction. Deteriorating lung function may result from rejection or reperfusion injury. Occasionally, temporary ECMO may be necessary. Frequent bronchoscopy with transbronchial biopsies and lavage are necessary to differentiate between rejection and infection. Nosocomial gram-negative bacteria, cytomegalovirus, *Candida*, *Aspergillus*, and *Pneumocystis jiroveci* are common pathogens. Other postoperative surgical complications include damage to the phrenic, vagus, and left recurrent laryngeal nerves.

Anesthesia for Esophageal Surgery

PREOPERATIVE CONSIDERATIONS

Common indications for esophageal surgery include tumors, gastroesophageal reflux, and motility disorders (achalasia). Surgical procedures include simple endoscopy, esophageal dilation, cervical esophagomyotomy, open or thoracoscopic distal esophagomyotomy, insertion or removal of esophageal stents, and open or minimally invasive esophagectomy. Squamous cell carcinomas account for the majority of esophageal tumors; adenocarcinomas are less common, whereas benign tumors (leiomyomas) are rare. Most tumors occur in the distal esophagus. Operative treatment may be palliative or curative. Esophageal surgery can be either transhiatal (with incisions in the neck and abdomen), transthoracic, or minimally invasive with a combination of thoracoscopy and laparoscopy. After esophageal resection, the stomach is pulled up into the thorax, or the esophagus is functionally replaced with part of the colon (*colonic interposition*).

Gastroesophageal reflux is treated surgically when the esophagitis is refractory to medical management or results in complications such as stricture, recurrent pulmonary aspiration, or a Barrett esophagus (columnar epithelium). A variety of antireflux operations may be performed (Nissen, Belsey, Hill, or Collis–Nissen) via thoracic or abdominal approaches, often laparoscopically.

Achalasia and systemic sclerosis (scleroderma) account for most surgical procedures performed for motility disorders. The former usually occurs as an isolated finding, whereas the latter is part of a generalized collagen–vascular disorder. Cricopharyngeal muscle dysfunction can be associated with a variety of neurogenic or myogenic disorders and often results in a Zenker diverticulum.

ANESTHETIC CONSIDERATIONS

9 Regardless of the procedure, a common anesthetic concern in patients with esophageal disease is the risk of pulmonary aspiration. This may result from obstruction, altered motility, or abnormal sphincter function. In fact, most patients typically report dysphagia, heartburn, regurgitation, coughing, or wheezing when lying flat. Dyspnea on exertion may also be prominent when chronic aspiration results in pulmonary fibrosis. Patients with malignancies may present with anemia and weight loss. Patients with esophageal cancer usually have a history of cigarette smoking and alcohol consumption, so patients

should be evaluated for coexisting chronic obstructive pulmonary disease, coronary artery disease, and liver dysfunction. Patients with systemic sclerosis (scleroderma) should be evaluated for involvement of other organs, particularly the kidneys, heart, and lungs; Raynaud phenomenon is also common.

In patients with reflux, consideration should be given to administering one or more of the following preoperatively: metoclopramide, an H_2-receptor blocker, sodium citrate, or a proton-pump inhibitor. In such patients, a rapid-sequence induction should be used. A double-lumen tube is used for procedures involving thoracoscopy or thoracotomy. The anesthesiologist may be asked to pass a large-diameter bougie into the esophagus as part of the surgical procedure; great caution must be exercised to help avoid pharyngeal or esophageal injury.

Transhiatal (blunt) and thoracic esophagectomies deserve special consideration. The former requires an upper abdominal incision and a left cervical incision, whereas the latter requires posterolateral thoracotomy, an abdominal incision, and, finally, a left cervical incision. Parts of the procedure may be performed using laparoscopy or VATS. Direct monitoring of arterial pressure is indicated. During the transhiatal approach to esophagectomy, substernal and diaphragmatic retractors can interfere with cardiac function. Moreover, as the esophagus is freed up blindly from the posterior mediastinum by blunt dissection, the surgeon's hand transiently interferes with cardiac filling and produces profound hypotension. The dissection can also induce marked vagal stimulation.

Colonic interposition involves forming a pedicle graft of the colon and passing it through the posterior mediastinum up to the neck to take the place of the esophagus. This procedure is lengthy, and maintenance of an adequate blood pressure, cardiac output, and hemoglobin concentration is necessary to ensure graft viability. Graft ischemia may be heralded by a progressive metabolic acidosis. Both too much and too little fluid administration can negatively impact the outcome. Goal-directed fluid therapy using hemodynamic measures (eg, stroke volume variation) may be helpful in perioperative fluid management of the esophagectomy patient.

Lung protective ventilation and multimodal perioperative analgesia should be used postoperatively.

CASE DISCUSSION

Mediastinal Adenopathy

A 9-year-old boy with mediastinal lymphadenopathy seen on a chest radiograph presents for biopsy of a cervical lymph node.

What is the most important preoperative consideration?

Is there any evidence of airway compromise? Tracheal compression may produce dyspnea (proximal obstruction) or a nonproductive cough (distal obstruction).

Asymptomatic compression is also common and may be evident only as tracheal deviation on physical or radiographic examinations. A CT scan of the chest provides invaluable information about the presence, location, and severity of airway compression. Flow–volume loops will also detect subtle airway obstruction and provide important information regarding the location and functional importance of the obstruction (see earlier discussion).

Does the absence of any preoperative dyspnea make severe intraoperative respiratory compromise less likely?

No. Severe airway obstruction can occur following induction of anesthesia in these patients, even in the absence of any preoperative symptoms. This mandates that the chest radiograph and CT scan be reviewed for evidence of asymptomatic airway obstruction. The point of obstruction is typically distal to the tip of the tracheal tube. Moreover, loss of spontaneous ventilation can precipitate complete airway obstruction.

What is superior vena cava syndrome?

Superior vena cava syndrome is the result of progressive enlargement of a mediastinal mass and compression of mediastinal structures, particularly the vena cava. Lymphomas are most commonly responsible, but primary pulmonary or mediastinal neoplasms can also produce the syndrome. Superior vena cava syndrome is often associated with severe airway obstruction and cardiovascular collapse on induction of general anesthesia. Caval compression produces venous engorgement and edema of the head, neck, and arms. Direct mechanical compression, as well as mucosal edema, severely compromise airflow in the trachea. Most patients favor an upright posture, as recumbency worsens the airway obstruction. Cardiac output may be severely depressed due to impeded venous return from the upper body, direct mechanical compression of the heart, and (with malignancies) pericardial invasion. An echocardiogram is useful in evaluating cardiac function and detecting pericardial fluid.

What is the anesthetic of choice for a patient with superior vena cava syndrome?

The absence of signs or symptoms of airway compression or superior vena cava syndrome does not preclude potentially life-threatening complications following induction of general anesthesia. Therefore, a biopsy of a peripheral node (usually cervical or scalene) under local anesthesia is safest whenever possible. Although establishing a diagnosis is of prime importance, the presence of significant airway compromise or superior vena cava syndrome may dictate empiric treatment with corticosteroids prior to tissue diagnosis at surgery (cancer is the most common cause); preoperative radiation therapy or chemotherapy may also be considered. The patient can usually safely undergo surgery with general anesthesia once airway compromise and other manifestations of the superior vena cava syndrome are alleviated.

General anesthesia may be indicated for establishing a diagnosis in young or uncooperative patients who have no evidence of airway compromise or the superior vena cava syndrome and, rarely, for patients unresponsive to steroids, radiation, or chemotherapy.

How does the presence of airway obstruction and superior vena cava syndrome influence the management of general anesthesia?

1. *Premedication*: If any drug is given, it should be only an anticholinergic. The patient should be transported to the operating room in a semi-upright position with supplemental oxygen.
2. *Monitoring*: In addition to standard monitors, an arterial line is helpful, but in young patients, it should be placed after induction. At least one large-bore intravenous catheter should be placed in a lower extremity as venous drainage from the upper body may be unreliable.
3. *Airway management*: Difficulties with ventilation and intubation should be anticipated. Following preoxygenation, awake intubation with an armored tracheal tube may be safest in a cooperative patient. The use of a flexible bronchoscope is advantageous in the presence of airway distortion and will define the site and degree of obstruction. Coughing or straining, however, may precipitate complete airway obstruction because the resultant positive pleural pressure increases intrathoracic tracheal compression. Passing the armored tube beyond the area of compression may obviate this problem. Uncooperative patients require a sevoflurane inhalation induction.
4. *Induction*: The goal should be a smooth induction maintaining spontaneous ventilation and hemodynamic stability. The ability to ventilate the patient with a good airway should be established prior to the use of an NMB. With 100% oxygen, one of three induction techniques can be used: (1) intravenous ketamine (because it results in greater hemodynamic stability in patients with reduced cardiac output); (2) inhalational induction with a volatile agent (usually sevoflurane); or (3) small incremental doses of propofol or etomidate.

   Positive-pressure ventilation can precipitate severe hypotension, and volume loading prior to induction may partly offset impaired ventricular filling secondary to caval obstruction.
5. *Maintenance of anesthesia*: The technique selected should be tailored to the patient's hemodynamic status. Following intubation, neuromuscular blockade prevents coughing or straining.
6. *Extubation*: At the end of the procedure, patients should be left intubated until the airway obstruction has resolved, as determined by flexible bronchoscopy or the presence of an air leak around the tracheal tube when the tracheal cuff is deflated.

SUGGESTED READINGS

Alam N. Lung resection in patients with marginal pulmonary function. *Thorac Surg Clin*. 2014;24:361.

Boisen ML, Rolleri N, Gorgy A, Kolarczyk L, Rao VK, Gelzinis TA. The year in thoracic anesthesia: selected highlights from 2018. *J Cardiothorac Vasc Anesth*. 2019;33:2909.

Brunelli A, Kim A, Berger K, Addrizzo-Harris D. Physiologic evaluation of the patient with lung cancer being considered for resection surgery. *Chest*. 2013;143(suppl):e166S.

Carney A, Dickinson M. Anesthesia for esophagectomy. *Anesthesiol Clin*. 2015;33:143.

Clayton-Smith A, Alston R, Adams G, et al. A comparison of the efficacy and adverse effects of double-lumen endobronchial tubes and bronchial blockers in thoracic surgery: a systematic review and meta-analysis of randomized controlled trials. *J Cardiothorac Vasc Anesth*. 2015;29:955.

Della Rocca G, Coccia C. Acute lung injury in thoracic surgery. *Curr Opin Anesthesiol*. 2013;26:40.

Della Rocca G, Vetrugno L, Coccia C, et al. Preoperative evaluation of patients undergoing lung resection surgery: defining the role of the anesthesiologist on a multidisciplinary team. *J Cardiothorac Vasc Anesth*. 2016;30:530.

Doan L, Augustus J, Androphy R, et al. Mitigating the impact of acute and chronic post-thoracotomy pain. *J Cardiothorac Vasc Anesth*. 2014;28:1048.

Falzon D, Alston RP, Coley E, Montgomery K. Lung isolation for thoracic surgery: from inception to evidence-based. *J Cardiothorac Vasc Anesth*. 2017;31:678.

Gemmill EH, Humes DJ, Catton JA. Systematic review of enhanced recovery after gastro-oesophageal cancer surgery. *Ann R Coll Surg Engl*. 2015;97:173.

Geube M, Anandamurthy B, Yared JP. Perioperative management of the lung graft following lung transplantation. *Crit Care Clin*. 2019;35:27.

Gimenez-Mila M, Klein A, Martinez G. Design and implementation of an enhanced recovery program in thoracic surgery. *J Thorac Dis*. 2016;8(suppl 1):S37.

Gothard J. Anesthetic considerations for patients with anterior mediastinal masses. *Anesthesiol Clin*. 2008;26:305.

Guldner A, Pelosi P, Abreu M. Nonventilatory strategies to prevent post-operative pulmonary complications. *Curr Opin Anesthesiol*. 2013;26:141.

Hoechter D, von Dossow V. Lung transplantation: from the procedure to managing patients with lung transplantation. *Curr Opin Anesthesiol*. 2016;29:8.

Lohser J, Slinger P. Lung injury after one-lung ventilation: a review of the pathophysiologic mechanisms affecting the ventilated and collapsed lung. *Anesth Analg*. 2015;121:302.

Mathisen D. Distal tracheal resection and reconstruction: state of the art and lessons learned. *Thorac Surg Clin*. 2018;28:199.

Marseu K, Slinger P. Perioperative pulmonary dysfunction and protection. *Anaesthesia*. 2016;71(suppl 1):46.

Módolo NS, Módolo MP, Marton MA, et al. Intravenous versus inhalation anaesthesia for one-lung ventilation. *Cochrane Database Syst Rev*. 2013;(7):CD006313.

Moreno Garijo J, Cypel M, McRae K, et al. The evolving role of extracorporeal membrane oxygenation in lung transplantation: implications for anesthetic management. *J Cardiothorac Vasc Anesth*. 2019;33:1995.

Nacarro-Martincz J, Galiana-Ivars M, Rivera-Cogollos J, et al. Management of intraoperative crisis during nonintubated thoracic surgery. *Thorac Surg Clin*. 2020;30:101.

Neto A, Schultz M, Gama de Abreu M. Intraoperative ventilation strategies to prevent postoperative pulmonary complications: systematic review, meta-analysis, and trial sequential analysis. *Best Pract Res Clin Anesthesiol*. 2015;29:331.

Rodriguez-Aldrete D, Candiotti K, Janakiraman R, et al. Trends and new evidence in the management of acute and chronic post-thoracotomy pain—an overview of the literature from 2005–2015. *J Cardiothorac Vasc Anesth*. 2016;30:762.

Salati M, Brunelli A. Risk stratification in lung resection. *Curr Surg Rep*. 2016;4:37.

Sellers D, Cassar-Demajo W, Keshavjee S, Slinger P. The evolution of lung transplantation. *J Cardiothorac Vasc Anesth*. 2017;33:1071.

Slinger P, Blank RS, Campos J, Lohsertic J, McRae K, eds. *Principles and Practice of Anesthesia for Thoracic Surgery*. 2nd ed. Springer; 2019.

Tarry D, Powell M. Hypoxic pulmonary vasoconstriction. *BJA Education*. 2017;17:208.

CHAPTER

26

Neurophysiology & Anesthesia

KEY CONCEPTS

1. Cerebral perfusion pressure is the difference between mean arterial pressure and intracranial pressure (or central venous pressure, whichever is greater).
2. The cerebral autoregulation curve is shifted to the right in patients with chronic arterial hypertension.
3. The most important extrinsic influences on cerebral blood flow (CBF) are respiratory gas tensions—particularly $PaCO_2$. CBF is directly proportionate to $PaCO_2$ between tensions of 20 and 80 mg Hg. Blood flow changes approximately 1 to 2 mL/100 g/min per mm Hg change in $PaCO_2$.
4. CBF changes 5% to 7% per 1°C change in temperature. Hypothermia decreases both cerebral metabolic rate and CBF, whereas pyrexia has the reverse effect.
5. The movement of a given substance across the blood–brain barrier is governed simultaneously by its size, charge, lipid solubility, and degree of protein binding in blood.
6. The blood–brain barrier may be disrupted by severe hypertension, tumors, trauma, strokes, infection, marked hypercapnia, hypoxia, and sustained seizure activity.
7. The cranial vault is a rigid structure with a fixed total volume, consisting of brain (80%), blood (12%), and cerebrospinal fluid (8%). Any increase in one component must be offset by an equivalent decrease in another to prevent a rise in intracranial pressure.
8. With the exception of ketamine, all intravenous agents either have little effect on or reduce cerebral metabolic rate and CBF.
9. With normal autoregulation and an intact blood–brain barrier, vasopressors increase CBF only when mean arterial blood pressure is below 50 to 60 mm Hg or above 150 to 160 mm Hg.
10. The brain is very vulnerable to ischemic injury because of its relatively high oxygen consumption and near-total dependence on aerobic glucose metabolism.
11. Hypothermia is the most effective method for protecting the brain during focal and global ischemia.

Anesthetic agents may have profound effects on cerebral metabolism, blood flow, cerebrospinal fluid (CSF) dynamics, and cerebral blood volume and pressure. In some instances, these alterations are deleterious, whereas in others they may be beneficial. This chapter reviews important neurophysiological concepts and discusses the cerebral effects of commonly used anesthetics.

Cerebral Physiology

CEREBRAL METABOLISM

The brain normally consumes 20% of total body oxygen. Most cerebral oxygen consumption (60%) is used to generate adenosine triphosphate (ATP) to support neuronal electrical activity (Figure 26–1). The cerebral metabolic rate (CMR) is usually expressed in terms of oxygen consumption ($CMRO_2$) and averages 3 to 3.8 mL/100 g/min (50 mL/min) in adults. $CMRO_2$ is greatest in the gray matter of the cerebral cortex and generally parallels cortical electrical activity. Because of the rapid oxygen consumption and the absence of significant oxygen reserves, interruption of cerebral perfusion usually results in unconsciousness within 10 s. If blood flow is not reestablished within 3 to 8 min under most conditions, ATP stores are depleted, and irreversible cellular injury occurs. The more rostral, "higher" brain regions (cortex, hippocampus) are more sensitive to hypoxic injury than the brainstem.

Neuronal cells normally utilize glucose as their primary energy source. Brain glucose consumption is approximately 5 mg/100 g/min, of which more than 90% is metabolized aerobically. $CMRO_2$ therefore normally parallels glucose consumption. This relationship is not maintained during starvation, when ketone bodies (acetoacetate and β-hydroxybutyrate) also become major energy substrates. Although the brain can also take up and metabolize lactate, cerebral function is normally dependent on a continuous supply of glucose. Acute sustained hypoglycemia is injurious to the brain. Paradoxically, hyperglycemia can exacerbate global and focal hypoxic brain injury by accelerating cerebral acidosis and cellular injury. Adequate control of perioperative blood glucose concentration is advocated in part to prevent adverse effects of hyperglycemia during ischemia; however, overzealous blood glucose control can likewise produce injury through iatrogenic hypoglycemia.

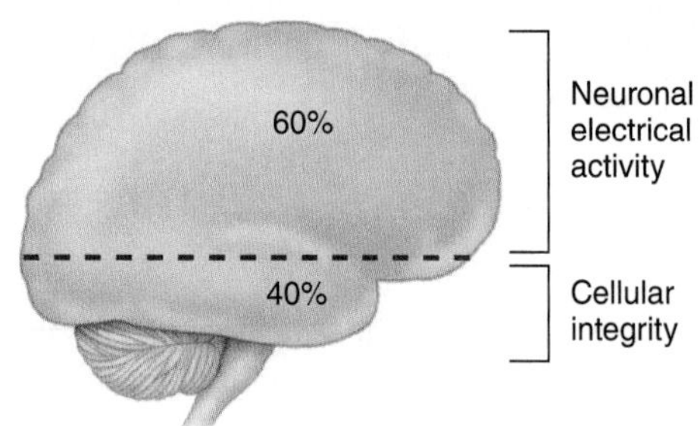

FIGURE 26–1 Normal brain oxygen requirements.

CEREBRAL BLOOD FLOW

Cerebral blood flow (CBF) varies with metabolic activity. There are a variety of methods available to directly measure CBF, including positron emission tomography, xenon washout, and computed tomography perfusion scans. Except in research environments, these methods do not lend themselves to bedside monitoring of CBF. Regional CBF parallels metabolic activity and can vary from 10 to 300 mL/100 g/min. For example, motor activity of a limb is associated with a rapid increase in regional CBF of the corresponding motor cortex. Similarly, visual activity is associated with an increase in regional CBF of the corresponding occipital visual cortex.

Although overall CBF averages 50 mL/100 g/min at a $PaCO_2$ of 40 mm Hg, flow in gray matter is roughly 80 mL/100 g/min, whereas that in white matter is 20 mL/100 g/min. Total CBF in adults averages 750 mL/min (15–20% of cardiac output). Flow rates below 20 to 25 mL/100 g/min are usually associated with cerebral impairment, as evidenced by slowing on the electroencephalogram (EEG). CBF rates below 20 mL/100 g/min typically produce a flat (isoelectric) EEG, whereas rates below 10 mL/100 g/min are usually associated with irreversible brain damage.

Indirect measures are often used to estimate the adequacy of CBF and brain tissue oxygen delivery in clinical settings. These methods include:

- The velocity of CBF can be measured using transcranial Doppler (TCD); see Chapter 5 for a discussion of the Doppler effect. An ultrasound probe (2 MHz, pulse wave Doppler) is placed in the temporal area above the zygomatic arch, which allows insonation of the middle cerebral artery. Normal velocity in the middle cerebral artery is approximately

55 cm/s. Velocities greater than 120 cm/s can indicate cerebral artery vasospasm following subarachnoid hemorrhage or hyperemic blood flow. Comparison between the velocities in the extracranial internal carotid artery and the middle cerebral artery (the Lindegaard ratio) can distinguish between these conditions. Middle cerebral artery velocity three times that of the velocity measured in the extracranial internal carotid artery more likely reflects cerebral artery vasospasm.

- Near-infrared spectroscopy is discussed in Chapter 6. Decreased saturation is associated with impaired cerebral oxygen delivery, though near-infrared spectroscopy primarily reflects cerebral venous oxygen saturation.
- Brain tissue oximetry measures the oxygen tension in brain tissue through the placement of a bolt with a Clark electrode oxygen sensor. Brain tissue CO_2 tension can also be measured using a similarly placed infrared sensor. Normal brain tissue oxygen tension varies from 20 to 50 mm Hg. Brain tissue oxygen tensions less than 20 mm Hg warrant interventions, and values less than 10 mm Hg are indicative of brain ischemia.

Cerebral blood flow is affected by numerous physiologic influences, including cerebral autoregulation, neurovascular coupling, and cerebrovascular responses to carbon dioxide and oxygen tension. Cerebral autoregulation adjusts cerebral blood flow in response to changes in mean arterial pressure (MAP). Neurovascular coupling adjusts cerebral blood flow to respond to the demands of neuronal activity. Figure 26–2 presents a summary of the integrated regulatory processes that affect cerebral perfusion.

REGULATION OF CEREBRAL BLOOD FLOW

1. Cerebral Perfusion Pressure

Cerebral perfusion pressure (CPP) is the difference between MAP and intracranial pressure (ICP) (or central venous pressure [CVP], if it is greater than ICP). MAP – ICP (or CVP) = CPP. CPP is normally 80 to 100 mm Hg. Moreover, because ICP is normally less than 10 mm Hg, CPP is primarily dependent on MAP.

Moderate to severe increases in ICP (>30 mm Hg) can compromise CPP and CBF, even in the presence of a normal MAP. Patients with CPP values less than 50 mm Hg often show slowing on the EEG, whereas those with a CPP between 25 and 40 mm Hg typically have a flat EEG. Sustained perfusion pressures less than 25 mm Hg may result in irreversible brain damage.

2. Autoregulation

Much like the heart and kidneys, the brain normally tolerates a wide range of blood pressure with little change in blood flow. The cerebral vasculature rapidly (10–60 s) adapts to changes in CPP. Decreases in CPP result in cerebral vasodilation, whereas elevations induce vasoconstriction. In normal individuals, CBF remains nearly constant between MAPs of about 60 and 160 mm Hg (Figure 26–3), though the lower limit of this autoregulation may be increased in some patients. Outside these limits, blood flow becomes pressure dependent. Pressures above 150 to 160 mm Hg can disrupt the blood–brain barrier (see below) and may result in cerebral edema and hemorrhage. Figure 26–3 is an idealized representation of the autoregulation of cerebral blood flow. There is much variation among patients in autoregulatory limits: some individuals have limited autoregulatory capacity and reduced cerebral blood flow at reduced mean arterial pressures that are well tolerated by others.

The cerebral autoregulation curve (see Figure 26–3) is shifted to the right in patients with chronic arterial hypertension. Both upper and lower limits are shifted. Flow becomes more pressure dependent at low "normal" arterial pressures in return for cerebral protection at higher arterial pressures. Studies suggest that long-term antihypertensive therapy can restore cerebral autoregulation limits toward normal. Myogenic, neurogenic, and metabolic mechanisms may contribute to cerebral autoregulation.

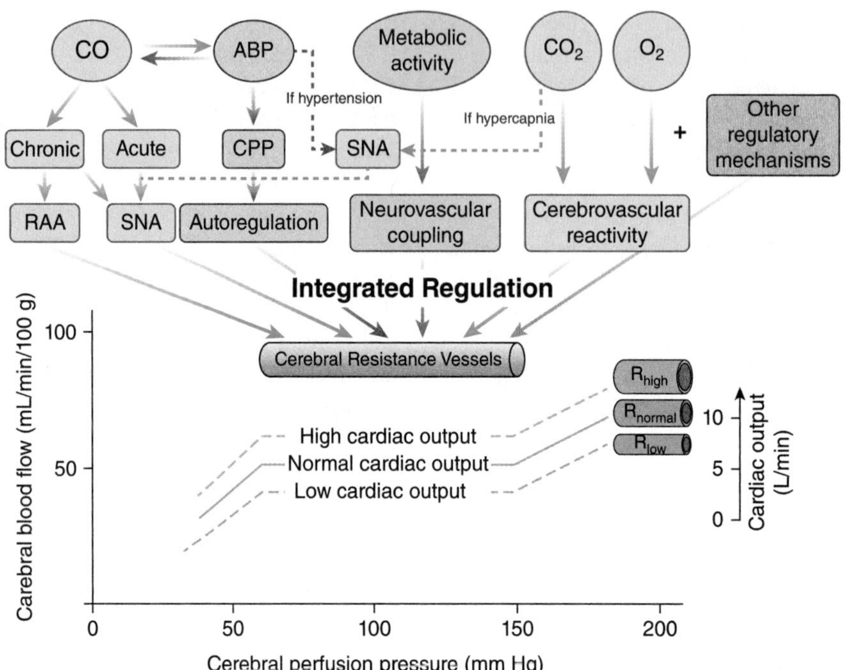

FIGURE 26–2 The conceptual framework of the integrated regulation of brain perfusion. The cerebrovascular resistance determined by the caliber of the cerebral resistance vessels is regulated by various physiologic processes: (1) cardiac output (CO) likely via sympathetic nervous activity (SNA) and the renin–angiotensin–aldosterone (RAA) system, depending on the chronicity of the change in CO, (2) arterial blood pressure (ABP) and cerebral perfusion pressure (CPP) via cerebral autoregulation, (3) cerebral metabolic activity via neurovascular coupling, and (4) arterial blood carbon dioxide (CO_2) and oxygen (O_2) via cerebrovascular reactivity. The SNA regulates cerebral blood flow and may play a prominent role during acute hypertension and hypercapnia as a protective mechanism preventing cerebral overperfusion (*dashed line*). These various regulatory mechanisms, together with other CBF-regulatory mechanisms that are not specified here, such as anesthetic effects, integrate at the level of the cerebral resistance vessels and generate only one consequence, which is the extent of the cerebrovascular resistance and, therefore, jointly regulate brain perfusion. The plateau of the autoregulation curve shifts downward when the CO is reduced and upward when augmented. The position of the plateau is determined by the caliber (R) of the cerebral resistance vessels at high (R_{high}), normal (R_{norm}), and low (R_{low}) CO. The scale of CO on the right side is smaller than that of CBF on the left side to reflect the lesser extent of change in CBF induced by an alteration of CO. (Reproduced with permission from Meng L, Hou W, Chui J, et al: Cardiac Output and Cerebral Blood Flow: The Integrated Regulation of Brain Perfusion in Adult Humans, *Anesthesiology.* 2015 Nov;123(5):1198-1208.)

3. Extrinsic Mechanisms

Respiratory Gas Tensions

3 The most important extrinsic influences on CBF are respiratory gas tensions—particularly $PaCO_2$. CBF is directly proportionate to $PaCO_2$ between tensions of 20 and 80 mm Hg (Figure 26–4). Blood flow changes approximately 1 to 2 mL/100 g/min per millimeter of mercury change in $PaCO_2$. This effect is almost immediate and is thought to be secondary to changes in the pH of CSF and cerebral tissue. Because ions do not readily cross the blood–brain barrier (see below), but CO_2 does, acute changes in $PaCO_2$ but not HCO_3^- affect CBF. Thus, acute metabolic acidosis has little effect on CBF because hydrogen ions (H^+) cannot readily cross the blood–brain barrier. After 24 to 48 h, CSF HCO_3^- ion concentration adjusts to compensate for the change in $PaCO_2$, so the effects of hypocapnia and hypercapnia are diminished. Marked hyperventilation ($PaCO_2$ <20 mm Hg) shifts the oxygen–hemoglobin dissociation curve to the left and, with changes in CBF, may result in EEG changes suggestive of cerebral impairment, even in normal individuals.

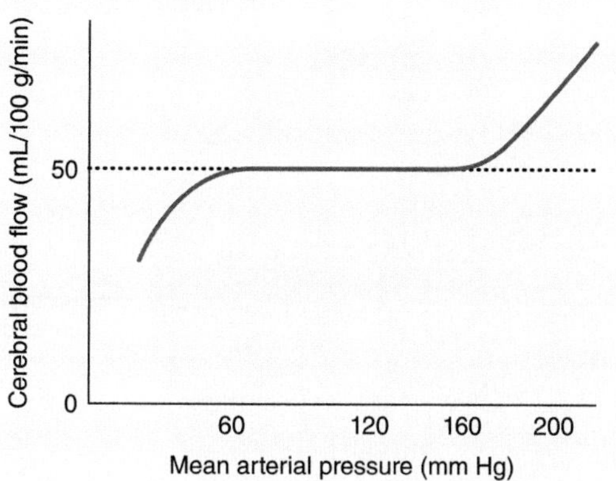

FIGURE 26–3 Normal cerebral autoregulation curve.

Only marked changes in PaO_2 alter CBF. Whereas hyperoxia may be associated with only minimal decreases (−10%) in CBF, severe hypoxemia (PaO_2 <50 mm Hg) greatly increases CBF (see Figure 26–4).

Temperature

4 CBF changes 5% to 7% per 1°C change in temperature. Hypothermia decreases both CMR and CBF, whereas hyperthermia has the reverse effect. Between 17°C and 37°C, the Q10 for humans is approximately 2—that is, for every 10° increase in temperature, the CMR doubles. Conversely, the CMR decreases by 50% if the temperature of the brain falls by 10°C (eg, from 37°C to 27°C) and another 50% if the temperature decreases from 27°C

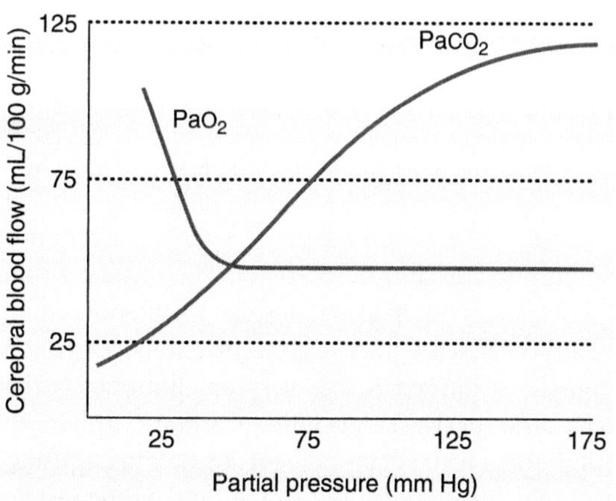

FIGURE 26–4 The relationship between cerebral blood flow and arterial respiratory gas tensions.

to 17°C. At 20°C, the EEG is isoelectric, but further decreases in temperature continue to reduce CMR throughout the brain. Hyperthermia (above 42°C) may result in neuronal cell injury.

Viscosity

The most important determinant of blood viscosity is hematocrit. A decrease in hematocrit decreases viscosity and can improve CBF; unfortunately, a reduction in hematocrit also decreases oxygen-carrying capacity and thus can potentially impair oxygen delivery. Elevated hematocrit, as is seen with marked polycythemia, increases blood viscosity and can reduce CBF. Some studies suggest that optimal cerebral oxygen delivery may occur at hematocrits of approximately 30%.

Autonomic Influences

Intracranial vessels are innervated by the sympathetic (vasoconstrictive) and parasympathetic (vasodilatory) systems. Intense sympathetic stimulation induces vasoconstriction in these vessels, which can limit CBF. Autonomic innervation may also play an important role in cerebral vasospasm following brain injury and stroke.

BLOOD–BRAIN BARRIER

Cerebral blood vessels are unique in that the junctions between vascular endothelial cells are nearly fused. The paucity of pores is responsible for what is termed the blood–brain barrier. This lipid barrier allows the passage of lipid-soluble substances, but it restricts the movement of those that are ionized or have large molecular weights. Thus, the movement of a given substance across the blood–brain barrier is governed simultaneously by its size, charge, lipid solubility, and degree of protein binding in blood. Carbon dioxide, oxygen, and lipid-soluble molecules (such as most anesthetics) freely enter the brain, whereas most ions, proteins, and large substances (such as mannitol) penetrate poorly.

Water moves freely across the blood–brain barrier as a consequence of bulk flow, whereas movement of even small ions is impeded (the equilibration half-life of Na^+ is 2–4 h). As a result, rapid changes in plasma electrolyte concentrations (and, secondarily, osmolality) produce a transient osmotic gradient between plasma and the brain. Acute hypertonicity of plasma results in net movement of water out of the brain, whereas acute hypotonicity causes a net movement of water into the brain. These effects are short-lived as equilibration eventually occurs, but when marked, they can cause rapid fluid shifts in the brain. Mannitol, an osmotically active substance that does not normally cross the blood–brain barrier, causes a sustained decrease in brain water content and is often used to acutely decrease brain volume.

6 The blood–brain barrier may be disrupted by severe hypertension, tumors, trauma, strokes, infection, marked hypercapnia, hypoxia, and sustained seizure activity. Under these conditions, fluid movement across the blood–brain barrier becomes dependent on hydrostatic pressure rather than osmotic gradients.

CEREBROSPINAL FLUID

CSF is found in the cerebral ventricles and cisterns and in the subarachnoid space surrounding the brain and spinal cord. CSF cushions the central nervous system (CNS) against trauma and helps clear waste products.

Classical (but currently controversial) teaching is that most of the CSF is formed by the choroid plexuses of the lateral ventricles. Smaller amounts are formed directly by the ventricles' ependymal cell linings, and yet smaller quantities are formed from fluid leaking into the perivascular spaces surrounding cerebral vessels (blood–brain barrier leakage). In adults, normal total CSF production is about 21 mL/h (500 mL/d), yet total CSF volume is only about 150 mL. Classical teaching (also currently controversial) is that CSF flows from the lateral ventricles through the intraventricular foramina (of Monro) into the third ventricle, through the cerebral aqueduct (of Sylvius) into the fourth ventricle, and through the median aperture of the fourth ventricle (foramen of Magendie) and the lateral apertures of the fourth ventricle (foramina of Luschka) into the cerebello-medullary cistern (cisterna magna) (Figure 26–5). From the cerebello-medullary cistern, CSF enters the subarachnoid space, circulating around the brain and spinal cord before being absorbed in arachnoid granulations over the cerebral hemispheres. Whether there is actual unidirectional "circulation" of the CSF is currently in dispute.

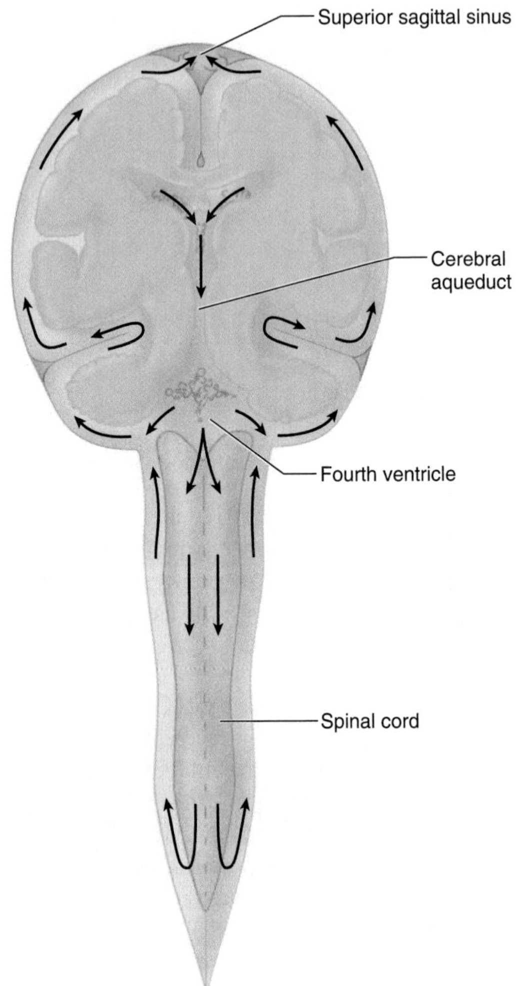

FIGURE 26–5 The flow of cerebrospinal fluid in the central nervous system, per classic dogma. As noted in the text, unidirectional flow of CSF is now questioned by investigators. (Reproduced with permission from Waxman SG. *Correlative Neuroanatomy*, 24th ed. New York, NY: McGraw Hill; 2000.)

CSF formation involves the active secretion of sodium in the choroid plexuses. The resulting fluid is isotonic with plasma despite lower potassium, bicarbonate, and glucose concentrations. Its protein content is limited to the very small amounts that leak into perivascular fluid. Carbonic anhydrase inhibitors (acetazolamide), corticosteroids, spironolactone, furosemide, isoflurane, and vasoconstrictors decrease CSF production.

Absorption of CSF involves the translocation of fluid from the arachnoid granulations into the cerebral venous sinuses. Smaller amounts are absorbed at nerve root sleeves and by meningeal lymphatics. Because the brain and spinal cord lack lymphatics, absorption of CSF is also the principal means by which perivascular and interstitial protein is returned to the blood.

INTRACRANIAL PRESSURE

7 The cranial vault is a rigid structure with a fixed total volume, containing brain (80%), blood (12%), and CSF (8%). Any increase in one component must be offset by an equivalent decrease in another to prevent a rise in ICP. By convention, ICP means supratentorial CSF pressure measured in the lateral ventricles or over the cerebral cortex and is normally 10 mm Hg or less. Minor variations may occur, depending on the site measured, but in the lateral recumbent position, lumbar CSF pressure normally approximates supratentorial pressure.

Intracranial elastance is determined by measuring the change in ICP in response to a change in intracranial volume. Normally, small increases in the volume of one component are initially well compensated (Figure 26–6). A point is eventually reached, however, at which further increases produce precipitous rises in ICP. Major compensatory mechanisms include (1) an initial displacement of CSF from the cranial to the spinal compartment, (2) an increase in CSF absorption, (3) a decrease in CSF production,

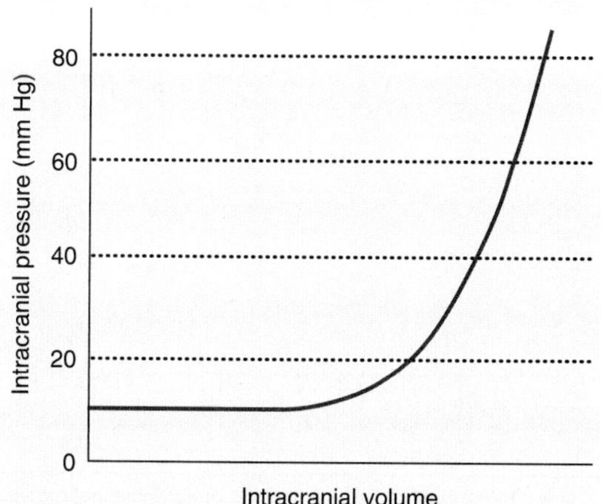

FIGURE 26–6 Normal intracranial elastance.

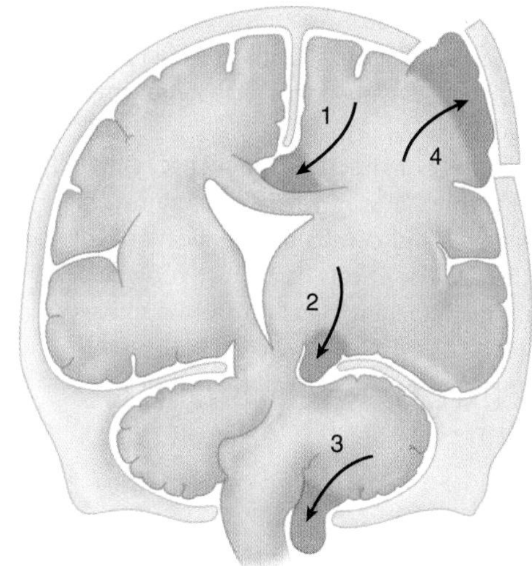

FIGURE 26–7 Potential sites of brain herniation. (Reproduced with permission from Fishman RA. Brain edema. *N Engl J Med.* 1975 Oct 2;293(14):706-711.)

and (4) a decrease in total cerebral blood volume (primarily venous).

The concept of total intracranial compliance is useful clinically, even though compliance probably varies in the different compartments of the brain and is affected by arterial blood pressure and $PaCO_2$. Blood pressure effects upon cerebral blood volume are dependent on the autoregulation of CBF.

Sustained elevations in ICP (when isolated to the intracranial space) can lead to catastrophic herniation of the brain. Herniation may occur at one of four sites (Figure 26–7): (1) the cingulate gyrus under the falx cerebri, (2) the uncinate gyrus through the tentorium cerebelli, (3) the cerebellar tonsils through the foramen magnum, or (4) any area beneath a defect in the skull (transcalvarial).

Effect of Anesthetic Agents on Cerebral Physiology

Overall, most general anesthetics have a favorable effect on brain energy consumption by reducing electrical activity. The effects of the specific agents are complicated by concomitant administration of other drugs, surgical stimulation, intracranial compliance, blood pressure, and CO_2 tension. For example, hypocapnia blunts the increases in CBF and ICP that usually occur with ketamine and volatile agents.

This section describes the changes generally associated with each drug when given alone. Table 26–1 summarizes and compares the effects of the various anesthetics. The effects of vasoactive agents and neuromuscular blocking agents are also discussed.

EFFECT OF INHALATION AGENTS

1. Volatile Anesthetics

Cerebral Metabolic Rate

Halothane, desflurane, sevoflurane, and isoflurane produce concentration-dependent decreases in CMR. Isoflurane produces the greatest maximal depression (up to 50% reduction), whereas halothane has the least effect (<25% reduction). The effects of desflurane and sevoflurane are nearly the same as those of isoflurane. No further reduction in CMR is produced by doses of anesthetics or other drugs greater than the doses that render the EEG isoelectric.

Cerebral Blood Flow & Volume

At normocarbia, volatile anesthetics dilate cerebral vessels and impair autoregulation in a concentration-dependent manner (Figure 26–8). Halothane has the greatest effect on CBF; at concentrations greater than 1%, it nearly abolishes cerebral autoregulation. Moreover, the increase in blood flow is generalized throughout all parts of the brain. At an equivalent minimum alveolar concentration (MAC) and blood pressure, halothane increases CBF up to 200%, compared with 20% for isoflurane or desflurane. Sevoflurane produces the least cerebral vasodilation. The effect of volatile agents on CBF also seems to be time dependent because, with continued administration (2–5 h), blood flow begins to return to normal.

The response of the cerebral vasculature to CO_2 is generally retained with all volatile agents. Hyperventilation (hypocapnia) can therefore abolish or blunt the initial effects of these agents on

TABLE 26–1 Comparative effects of anesthetic agents on cerebral physiology.[1]

Agent	CMR	CBF	CSF Production	CSF Absorption	CBV	ICP
Halothane	↓↓	↑↑↑	↓	↓	↑↑	↑↑
Isoflurane	↓↓↓	↑	±	↑	↑↑	↑
Desflurane	↓↓↓	↑	↑	↓	↑	↑
Sevoflurane	↓↓↓	↑	?	?	↑	↑
Nitrous oxide	↑	↑	±	±	±	↑
Barbiturates	↓↓↓↓	↓↓↓	±	↑	↓↓	↓↓↓
Etomidate	↓↓↓	↓↓	±	↑	↓↓	↓↓
Propofol	↓↓↓	↓↓↓↓	?	?	↓↓	↓↓
Benzodiazepines	↓↓	↓	±	↑	↓	↓
Ketamine	±	↑↑	±	↓	↑↑	↑↑
Opioids	±	±	±	↑	±	±
Lidocaine	↓↓	↓↓	?	?	↓↓	↓↓

[1]↑, increase; ↓, decrease; ±, little or no change; ?, unknown; CBF, cerebral blood flow; CBV, cerebral blood volume; CMR, cerebral metabolic rate; CSF, cerebrospinal fluid; ICP, intracranial pressure.

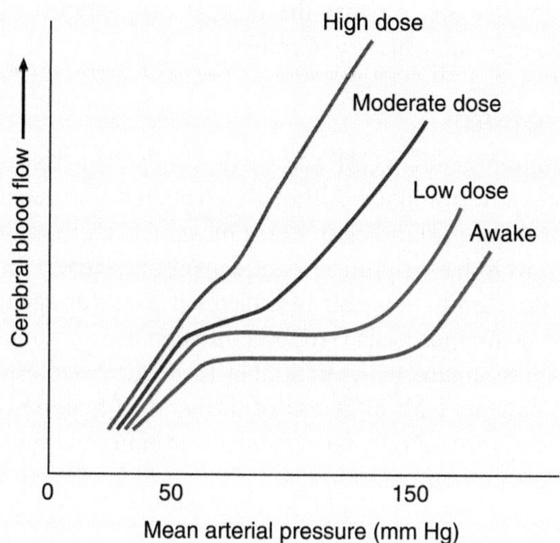

FIGURE 26–8 Dose-dependent depression of cerebral autoregulation by the volatile anesthetics.

CBF. With halothane, the timing of the hyperventilation is important. Only if hyperventilation is initiated prior to the administration of halothane will halothane-induced increases in CBF be prevented. In contrast, simultaneous hyperventilation with administration of the other agents can prevent increases in CBF and ICP.

Increases in cerebral blood volume (10–12%) generally parallel increases in CBF, but the relationship is not necessarily linear. Expansion of cerebral blood volume can markedly elevate ICP in patients with reduced intracranial compliance. Hypocapnia can blunt the increase in cerebral blood volume associated with volatile anesthetic administration.

Altered Coupling of Cerebral Metabolic Rate & Blood Flow

As is apparent from the preceding discussion, volatile agents alter, but do not uncouple, the normal relationship of CBF and CMR. The combination of a decrease in neuronal metabolic demand with an increase in CBF (metabolic supply) has been termed *luxury perfusion*. In contrast to this potentially beneficial effect during global ischemia, a detrimental **circulatory steal phenomenon** is possible with volatile anesthetics in the setting of focal ischemia. Volatile agents can increase blood flow in normal areas of the brain but not in ischemic areas, where arterioles are already maximally vasodilated. The end result may be a redistribution ("steal") of blood flow away from ischemic to normal areas.

Cerebrospinal Fluid Dynamics

Volatile anesthetics affect both formation and absorption of CSF. Halothane impedes absorption of CSF, but it only minimally retards formation. Isoflurane, on the other hand, facilitates absorption and is therefore an agent with favorable effects on CSF dynamics.

Intracranial Pressure

The net effect of volatile anesthetics on ICP is the result of immediate changes in cerebral blood volume, delayed alterations on CSF dynamics, and arterial CO_2 tension.

2. Nitrous Oxide

The effects of nitrous oxide are influenced by other agents or changes in CO_2 tension. Thus, when combined with intravenous agents, nitrous oxide has minimal effects on CBF, CMR, and ICP. Adding this agent to a volatile anesthetic, however, can in theory further increase CBF. When given alone, nitrous oxide causes cerebral vasodilation and can potentially increase ICP.

EFFECT OF INTRAVENOUS AGENTS

1. Induction Agents

8 With the exception of ketamine, all intravenous agents either have little effect on or reduce CMR and CBF. Moreover, with some exceptions, changes in blood flow generally parallel those in metabolic rate. Cerebral autoregulation and CO_2 responsiveness are preserved with all agents.

Barbiturates

Barbiturates have four major actions on the CNS: (1) hypnosis, (2) depression of CMR, (3) reduction of

CBF due to increased cerebral vascular resistance, and (4) anticonvulsant activity. Barbiturates produce dose-dependent decreases in CMR and CBF until the EEG becomes isoelectric. At that point, maximum CMR reductions of nearly 50% are observed; additional barbiturate dosing does not further reduce CMR. Unlike isoflurane, barbiturates reduce metabolic rate uniformly throughout the brain. CMR is depressed slightly more than CBF, such that metabolic supply exceeds metabolic demand (as long as CPP is maintained). Because barbiturate-induced cerebral vasoconstriction occurs only in normal areas, these agents tend to redistribute blood flow from normal to ischemic areas in the brain. The cerebral vasculature in ischemic areas remains maximally dilated because of ischemic vasomotor paralysis.

Barbiturates also seem to facilitate absorption of CSF. The resultant reduction in CSF volume, combined with decreases in CBF and cerebral blood volume, makes barbiturates highly effective in lowering ICP. Their anticonvulsant properties are also advantageous in neurosurgical patients who are at increased risk of seizures.

Opioids

Opioids generally have minimal effects on CBF, CMR, and ICP, unless $PaCO_2$ rises secondary to respiratory depression. Increases in ICP have been reported in some patients with intracranial tumors following the administration of opioids. The mechanism seems to be a precipitous drop in blood pressure; reflex cerebral vasodilation likely increases intracranial blood volume and potentially ICP. Significant decreases in blood pressure can adversely affect CPP, regardless of the opioid selected.

Etomidate

Etomidate decreases the CMR, CBF, and ICP in much the same way as barbiturates. Its effect on CMR is nonuniform, affecting the cortex more than the brainstem. Etomidate also decreases production and enhances absorption of CSF. Induction with etomidate is associated with a frequent incidence of myoclonic movements but no seizure activity on the EEG in normal individuals. Reports of seizure activity following etomidate suggest that the drug is best avoided in patients with a history of epilepsy.

Propofol

Propofol reduces CBF and CMR, similar to barbiturates and etomidate. Although it has been associated with dystonic and choreiform movements, propofol seems to have significant anticonvulsant activity. Its short elimination half-life makes it a useful agent for neuroanesthesia. Propofol infusion is commonly used for maintenance of total intravenous anesthesia in patients with or at risk of intracranial hypertension. Propofol is by far the most common induction agent for neuroanesthesia.

Benzodiazepines

Benzodiazepines lower CBF and CMR, but to a lesser extent than barbiturates, etomidate, or propofol. Benzodiazepines also have useful anticonvulsant properties. Midazolam is the benzodiazepine of choice in neuroanesthesia because of its short half-life. Midazolam used as an induction agent may cause decreases in blood pressure and CPP and may result in prolonged emergence.

Ketamine

Ketamine is the only intravenous anesthetic that dilates the cerebral vasculature and increases CBF (50–60%). Selective activation of certain areas (limbic and reticular) is partially offset by depression of other areas (somatosensory and auditory) such that total CMR does not change. Seizure activity in thalamic and limbic areas is also described. Ketamine may also impede the absorption of CSF without affecting formation. Increases in CBF, cerebral blood volume, and CSF volume can potentially increase ICP markedly in patients with decreased intracranial compliance. However, ketamine administration does not increase ICP in neurologically impaired patients under controlled ventilation with concomitant administration of propofol or a benzodiazepine. Additionally, ketamine may offer neuroprotective effects, according to some investigations. Ketamine's blockade of the *N*-methyl-D-aspartate (NMDA) receptor during periods of increased glutamate concentrations, as occurs during brain injury, may be

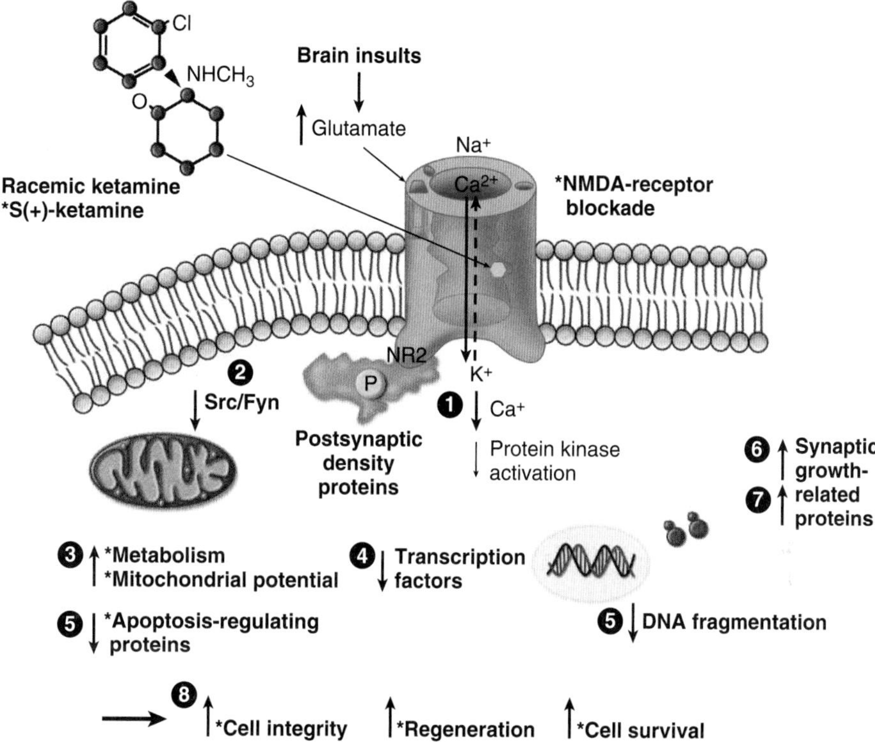

FIGURE 26–9 Pharmacological effects reported for racemic and S(+)-ketamine, which are presumed to be relevant for neuroprotection. After the onset of brain injury, blockade of excessive stimulation of *N*-methyl-D-aspartate (NMDA) receptors by ketamine reduces calcium influx through the receptor channel (1). This attenuates supraphysiological increases in the assembly and interaction of NMDA receptor subunits, postsynaptic density proteins, and other intracellular signaling systems such as protein kinases (2). Thus, several kinase transduction cascades become less activated. This improves the preservation of metabolism and maintenance of the mitochondrial transmembrane potential (3). This, in turn, reduces pathological activation of transcription factors (4). Proteins involved in apoptosis are less activated, which is associated with less DNA fragmentation (5). Better preservation of synaptic proteins occurs, and the expression of growth proteins indicating regeneration in adult neurons is enhanced (6, 7). The prevention of pathological amplification of NMDA receptor signaling finally results in increased cellular survival, preserved cellular and synaptic integrity, and regenerative efforts (8). *Superiority of effects induced by S(+)-ketamine, only. (Reproduced with permission from Himmelseher S, Durieux ME. Revising a dogma: ketamine for patients with neurological injury? *Anesth Analg.* 2005 Aug;101(2):524-534.)

protective against neuronal cell death (Figure 26–9). In spite of theoretical concerns regarding ketamine's ability to increase ICP in patients with traumatic injury, it has been used in brain-injured patients without deleterious effects upon ICP.

2. Anesthetic Adjuncts

Intravenous lidocaine decreases CMR, CBF, and ICP, but to a lesser degree than other agents. Its principal advantage is that it decreases CBF (by increasing cerebral vascular resistance) without causing other significant hemodynamic effects. Lidocaine may also have neuroprotective effects. Lidocaine infusions are used in some centers as a supplement to general anesthesia to reduce the requirement for opioids.

Droperidol has little or no effect on CMR and minimally reduces CBF. Droperidol and opioids were once mainstays of neuroanesthesia. Droperidol's prolongation of the QT interval and risk of fatal arrhythmia have retarded its use.

Dexmedetomidine reduces both CBF and CMR.

Reversal of opioids or benzodiazepines with naloxone or flumazenil, respectively, can reverse any beneficial reductions in CBF and CMR. Reversal of opioids or benzodiazepines in chronic users can lead to substance withdrawal.

3. Vasopressors

9 With normal autoregulation and an intact blood–brain barrier, vasopressors increase CBF only when mean arterial blood pressure is below 50 to 60 mm Hg or above 150 to 160 mm Hg. In the absence of autoregulation, vasopressors increase CBF by their effect on CPP. Changes in CMR generally parallel those in blood flow. β-Adrenergic agents seem to have a greater effect on the brain when the blood–brain barrier is disrupted; central β_1-receptor stimulation increases CMR and blood flow. β-Adrenergic blockers generally have no direct effect on CMR or CBF. Excessive elevations in blood pressure with any agent can disrupt the blood–brain barrier. Reductions in cardiac output reduce CBF.

4. Vasodilators

In the absence of hypotension, most vasodilators induce cerebral vasodilation and increase CBF in a dose-related fashion. When these agents decrease blood pressure, CBF is usually maintained and may even increase. The resultant increase in cerebral blood volume can elevate ICP in patients with decreased intracranial compliance.

5. Neuromuscular Blocking Agents

Neuromuscular blockers (NMBs) lack direct action on the brain but can have important secondary effects. Hypertension and histamine-mediated cerebral vasodilation increase ICP, whereas systemic hypotension (from histamine release or ganglionic blockade) lowers CPP. Succinylcholine can increase ICP to a generally minimal and clinically unimportant extent. Moreover, a small (defasciculating) dose of a nondepolarizing NMB seems to blunt the increase, though this practice seems unnecessary. In most instances, increases in ICP following administration of an NMB are the result of a hypertensive response due to light anesthesia during laryngoscopy and tracheal intubation. Acute elevations in ICP will also be seen if hypercapnia or hypoxemia results from prolonged apnea.

Physiology of Brain Protection

PATHOPHYSIOLOGY OF CEREBRAL ISCHEMIA

10 The brain is very vulnerable to ischemic injury because of its relatively high oxygen consumption and near-total dependence on aerobic glucose metabolism (see earlier discussion). Interruption of cerebral perfusion, metabolic substrate (glucose), or severe hypoxemia rapidly results in functional impairment; reduced perfusion also impairs clearance of potentially toxic metabolites. If normal oxygen tension, blood flow, and glucose supply are not quickly reestablished, under most conditions ATP stores are depleted, and irreversible neuronal injury begins. When CBF decreases below 10 mL/100 g/min, cell function is deranged, and ion pumps fail to maintain cellular vitality. The ratio of lactate to pyruvate is increased secondary to anaerobic metabolism. During ischemia, intracellular K^+ decreases, and intracellular Na^+ increases. More importantly, intracellular Ca^{2+} increases because of the failure of ATP-dependent pumps to either extrude the ion extracellularly or into intracellular cisterns, increased intracellular Na^+ concentration, and release of the excitatory neurotransmitter glutamate. Glutamate acts at the NMDA receptor, further enhancing Ca^{2+} entry into the cell, hence the potential benefit of NMDA blockers for neuroprotection.

Sustained increases in intracellular Ca^{2+} activate lipases and proteases, which initiate and propagate structural damage to neurons. Increases in free fatty acid concentration and cyclooxygenase and lipoxygenase activities result in the formation of prostaglandins and leukotrienes, some of which are potent mediators of cellular injury. Accumulation of toxic metabolites impairs cellular function and interferes with repair mechanisms. Lastly, reperfusion of ischemic tissues can cause additional tissue damage due to the formation of oxygen-derived free radicals. Likewise, inflammation and edema can promote further neuronal damage, leading to cellular apoptosis.

STRATEGIES FOR BRAIN PROTECTION

Ischemic brain injury is usually classified as focal (incomplete) or global (complete). Global ischemia may result from total circulatory arrest as well as global hypoxia. Cessation of perfusion may be caused by cardiac arrest or deliberate circulatory arrest, whereas global hypoxia may be caused by severe respiratory failure, drowning, and asphyxia (including anesthetic mishaps). Focal ischemia includes embolic, hemorrhagic, and atherosclerotic strokes, as well as blunt, penetrating, and surgical trauma.

In some instances, interventions aimed at restoring perfusion and oxygenation are possible; these include reestablishing effective circulation, normalizing arterial oxygenation and oxygen-carrying capacity, or reopening and stenting an occluded vessel. With focal ischemia, the brain tissue surrounding a severely damaged area may suffer marked functional impairment but still remain viable. Such areas are thought to have very marginal perfusion (<15 mL/100 g/min), but if further injury can be limited and normal flow is rapidly restored, these areas (the "ischemic penumbra") may recover completely. When these interventions are not applicable or available, the emphasis must be on limiting the extent of brain injury.

From a practical point of view, efforts aimed at preventing or limiting neuronal tissue damage are often similar whether the ischemia is focal or global. Clinical goals are usually to optimize CPP, decrease metabolic requirements (basal and electrical), and possibly block mediators of cellular injury. Clearly, the most effective strategy is prevention because once injury has occurred, measures aimed at cerebral protection become less effective.

Hypothermia

11 Hypothermia is a suggested method for protecting the brain during focal and global ischemia. Indeed, profound hypothermia is often used for up to 1 h of total circulatory arrest. Unlike anesthetic agents, hypothermia decreases both basal and electrical metabolic requirements throughout the brain; metabolic requirements continue to decrease even after complete electrical silence. Additionally, hypothermia reduces free radicals and other mediators of ischemic injury.

Anesthetic Agents

Barbiturates, etomidate, propofol, isoflurane, desflurane, and sevoflurane can produce burst suppression, and all but desflurane and sevoflurane can produce complete electrical silence of the brain and eliminate the metabolic cost of electrical activity. Unfortunately, these agents have no effect on basal energy requirements. Furthermore, with the exception of barbiturates, their effects are nonuniform, affecting different parts of the brain to variable extents.

Ketamine may also have a protective effect because of its ability to block the actions of glutamate at the NMDA receptor. Xenon is also suggested as a neuroprotective agent. Dexmedetomidine has been reported as a possible protective agent for children at risk for general anesthetic-induced neurotoxicity.

Studies highlighting the potential neurotoxicity of anesthetics (especially in infants) also question the role of volatile anesthetics in neuroprotection.

Specific Adjuncts

Nimodipine is used to treat vasospasm associated with subarachnoid hemorrhage.

General Measures

General patient management techniques are the neuroanesthesia interventions most likely to improve patient outcomes.

Maintenance of a satisfactory CPP is critical. Hypotension, increases in venous pressure, and increases in ICP should be avoided. Oxygen-carrying capacity should be maintained and normal arterial oxygen tension preserved. Hyperglycemia amplifies neurological injury following either focal or global ischemia, so blood glucose should be maintained at less than 180 mg/dL. Normocarbia should be maintained as both hypercarbia and hypocarbia have no beneficial effect on cerebral ischemia; hypocarbia-induced cerebral vasoconstriction may aggravate the ischemia, whereas hypercarbia may induce a steal phenomenon with focal ischemia or worsen intracellular acidosis.

TABLE 26–2 Electroencephalographic changes during anesthesia.

Activation	Depression
Inhalational agents (subanesthetic)	Inhalation agents (1–2 MAC)
Barbiturates (small doses)	Barbiturates
Benzodiazepines (small doses)	Opioids
Etomidate (small doses)	Propofol
Nitrous oxide	Etomidate
Ketamine	Hypocapnia
Mild hypercapnia	Marked hypercapnia
Sensory stimulation	Hypothermia
Hypoxia (early)	Hypoxia (late) ischemia

EFFECT OF ANESTHESIA ON ELECTROPHYSIOLOGICAL MONITORING

Electrophysiological monitors are used to assess the functional integrity of the CNS. The most commonly used monitor during neurosurgical procedures is evoked potentials. EEG is less commonly used. Proper application of these monitoring modalities is critically dependent on recognizing anesthetic-induced changes. Both monitoring modalities are described in Chapter 6.

The effects of anesthetic agents on an EEG are summarized in Table 26–2.

ELECTROENCEPHALOGRAPHY

EEG monitoring is useful for assessing the adequacy of cerebral perfusion during carotid endarterectomy (CEA), as well as anesthetic depth (most often with processed EEG). EEG changes can be simplistically described as either activation or depression. EEG activation (a shift to predominantly high-frequency and low-voltage activity) is seen with light anesthesia and surgical stimulation, whereas EEG depression (a shift to predominantly low-frequency and high-voltage activity) occurs with deep anesthesia or cerebral compromise. **Most anesthetics produce activation (at subanesthetic doses) followed by dose-dependent depression of the EEG.**

Inhalation Anesthetics

Isoflurane, desflurane, and sevoflurane produce a burst suppression pattern at high doses (>1.2–1.5 MAC). Nitrous oxide is unusual in that it increases both frequency and amplitude (high-amplitude activation).

Intravenous Agents

Benzodiazepines can produce both activation and depression of the EEG. Barbiturates, etomidate, and propofol produce a similar pattern and are the only commonly used intravenous agents capable of producing burst suppression and electrical silence at high doses. Opioids characteristically produce only dose-dependent depression of the EEG. Lastly, ketamine produces an unusual activation consisting of rhythmic high-amplitude theta activity followed by very high-amplitude gamma and low-amplitude beta activities.

EVOKED POTENTIALS

Somatosensory evoked potentials test the integrity of the spinal dorsal columns and the sensory cortex and may be useful during resection of spinal tumors, instrumentation of the spine, and carotid artery and aortic surgery. The adequacy of perfusion of the spinal cord during aortic surgery is better assessed with motor evoked potentials (which assess the anterior part of the spinal cord). Brainstem auditory evoked potentials test the integrity of the eighth cranial nerve and the auditory pathways above the pons and are used for surgery in the posterior fossa. Visual evoked potentials may be used to monitor the optic nerve and occipital cortex during resections of large pituitary tumors.

Interpretation of evoked potentials is more complicated than that of the EEG. Evoked potentials have poststimulus latencies that are described as short, intermediate, and long. Short-latency evoked potentials arise from the nerve stimulated or the brainstem. Intermediate- and long-latency evoked potentials are primarily of cortical origin. In general, short-latency potentials are least affected by anesthetic agents, whereas long-latency potentials are affected by even subanesthetic levels of most agents. Visual evoked potentials are most affected by anesthetics, whereas brainstem auditory evoked potentials are least affected.

Intravenous agents in clinical doses generally have less marked effects on evoked potentials than do volatile agents, but in high doses, they can also decrease amplitude and increase latencies (see Chapter 6). Ketamine generally increases the amplitude of short-latency signals. Frequent adjustments of inhaled anesthetic concentrations make interpretation of evoked potentials nearly impossible. We prefer to use reduced concentrations (≤0.5 MAC) of volatile anesthetic when caring for patients undergoing evoked potential monitoring, and we avoid changing the inhaled concentration.

CASE DISCUSSION

Postoperative Hemiplegia

A 62-year-old man has undergone a right carotid endarterectomy (CEA). Immediately following surgery in the recovery room, he is noted to be weak on the contralateral side.

How is a patient undergoing CEA evaluated preoperatively?

Since atherosclerosis is a systemic disease, patients with carotid stenosis are at a greatly increased risk of coexisting coronary artery and peripheral arterial disease. It would be unusual for a patient to have carotid stenosis who did not have evidence of atherosclerosis elsewhere. Patients undergoing CEA, therefore, require a preoperative cardiac evaluation, according to American College of Cardiology/American Heart Association guidelines.

With respect to patient risk factors, these guidelines provide algorithms for how patients should be evaluated and managed intraoperatively. As part of this patient's preoperative evaluation, a thorough neurological examination should have been performed, with special attention paid to motor function. This patient may well have been weak on the left side prior to surgery, in which case the hemiparesis might be due to a preexisting condition. If this is a new finding, it requires aggressive management.

Is general or regional anesthesia the optimal anesthetic technique for managing patients undergoing CEA?

Most patients undergoing CEAs in the United States have received general anesthesia because many surgeons felt more comfortable if the airway was controlled, and the patient was completely anesthetized should evidence of cerebral ischemia develop.

In some centers, regional anesthesia has been advocated as providing an adequate surgical field, a comfortable and relaxed patient (if done with monitored anesthesia care), stable hemodynamics, and ideal monitoring of cerebral function during cross-clamping because an awake patient provides the best evidence of adequate cerebral perfusion. The patient can indicate or be observed for evidence of aphasia, facial droop, or hemiparesis. Regional anesthesia is usually performed with superficial cervical plexus blockade.

How should cerebral function be monitored intraoperatively in this patient?

When the carotid is cross-clamped, the ability to identify inadequate cerebral circulation in the ipsilateral hemisphere is critical as there is a window of opportunity for immediate intervention and correction of any deficit.

Global and focal neurological status can continuously be assessed in awake patients if they are minimally sedated when undergoing regional anesthesia. In such a situation, practical assessment consists of frequent (every 2–5 min) examination of strength using the contralateral handgrip and maintenance of constant verbal contact ("cocktail conversation") with the patient to assess level of consciousness.

In patients undergoing general anesthesia, indirect cerebral monitoring techniques have been used to assess the adequacy of the cerebral circulation. These techniques include stump bleeding, stump pressure, jugular venous oxygen saturation, EEG, and transcranial Doppler (TCD). Back bleeding of the distal carotid artery following cross-clamping and incision of the artery suggests reasonable collateral circulation above the clamp, though this is very subjective and nonquantitative.

To better qualify and quantify the adequacy of collateral perfusion (see Figure 26–10), stump pressure measurements can be used. Some surgeons believe that a shunt should be used in all patients with a previous cerebrovascular accident, independent of stump pressure, and for any patient whose stump pressure is less than 25 mm Hg. However, this is controversial, as many neurosurgeons and vascular surgeons use 50 mm Hg as a cutoff. The reliability of stump pressure to predict the need for selective shunting has also been questioned. Some surgeons routinely shunt all patients, some shunt no patients, and others use selective shunting. Outcome data have not identified the best surgical approach.

The EEG is sometimes used for monitoring patients undergoing CEA under general anesthesia. In such a circumstance, inhalation or intravenous anesthesia can influence the EEG, but gross changes associated with carotid clamping can be detected easily. Analyzing subtleties of the EEG is labor and technology intensive and rarely needed. Evoked potentials have also been employed during CEA. Should neurophysiological studies identify cerebral ischemia, the surgeon can place a vascular shunt during the surgical repair to provide for ipsilateral cerebral perfusion.

Cerebral saturation monitors are sometimes employed to detect inadequate cerebral perfusion during carotid artery cross-clamping. Reductions of 10% to 20% from baseline suggest that a shunt should be placed.

How should hemodynamics be controlled intraoperatively?

During carotid clamping and immediately afterward in the recovery room, patients are often hemodynamically labile. **Bradycardia can develop during surgical manipulation of the carotid sinus because of the direct stimulation of the vagus nerve.** Tachycardia may develop as a result of stress or pain or as a direct result of manipulation of the carotid sinus with the release of catecholamines into the circulation.

Hypotension is also observed because of the direct vasodilating and negative ionotropic effects of anesthetic agents. Hypotension following carotid unclamping is common, particularly in patients with more severe carotid stenosis. This could be due to a cerebral protective process. Cerebral autoregulation protects the brain from reperfusion by reducing production of renin, vasopressin, and norepinephrine, which results in hypotension. Hypertension is also a frequent finding in patients undergoing CEA. Many patients have hypertension as a comorbid condition, which is often further exacerbated by the surgical stress and manipulation of the carotid body, which causes release of catecholamines and sympathetic stimulation.

Invasive arterial pressure monitoring and suitable venous access to infuse vasoactive medications are necessary during carotid surgery.

What is the most likely etiology of this patient's findings?

This patient most likely has had a cerebrovascular accident due to an arterio-to-arterial embolus; more than 95% of such patients will fit into this category. Weakness can also develop as a result of a hyperperfusion syndrome, which occurs in patients with severe carotid stenosis who have now reestablished flow to the affected cerebral hemisphere. Such patients usually have a greater than 95% carotid stenosis with a less than 1-mm channel in the affected carotid artery. Typically, the syndrome does not develop in the postoperative anesthesia care unit (PACU), but several hours afterward when the patient begins reporting a headache and, in severe cases, develops hemiparesis.

Because a cerebrovascular accident is most likely, when the anesthesiologist is called to see such a patient in the PACU, a thorough neurological examination quantifying any cranial nerve involvement and the degree of weakness on the

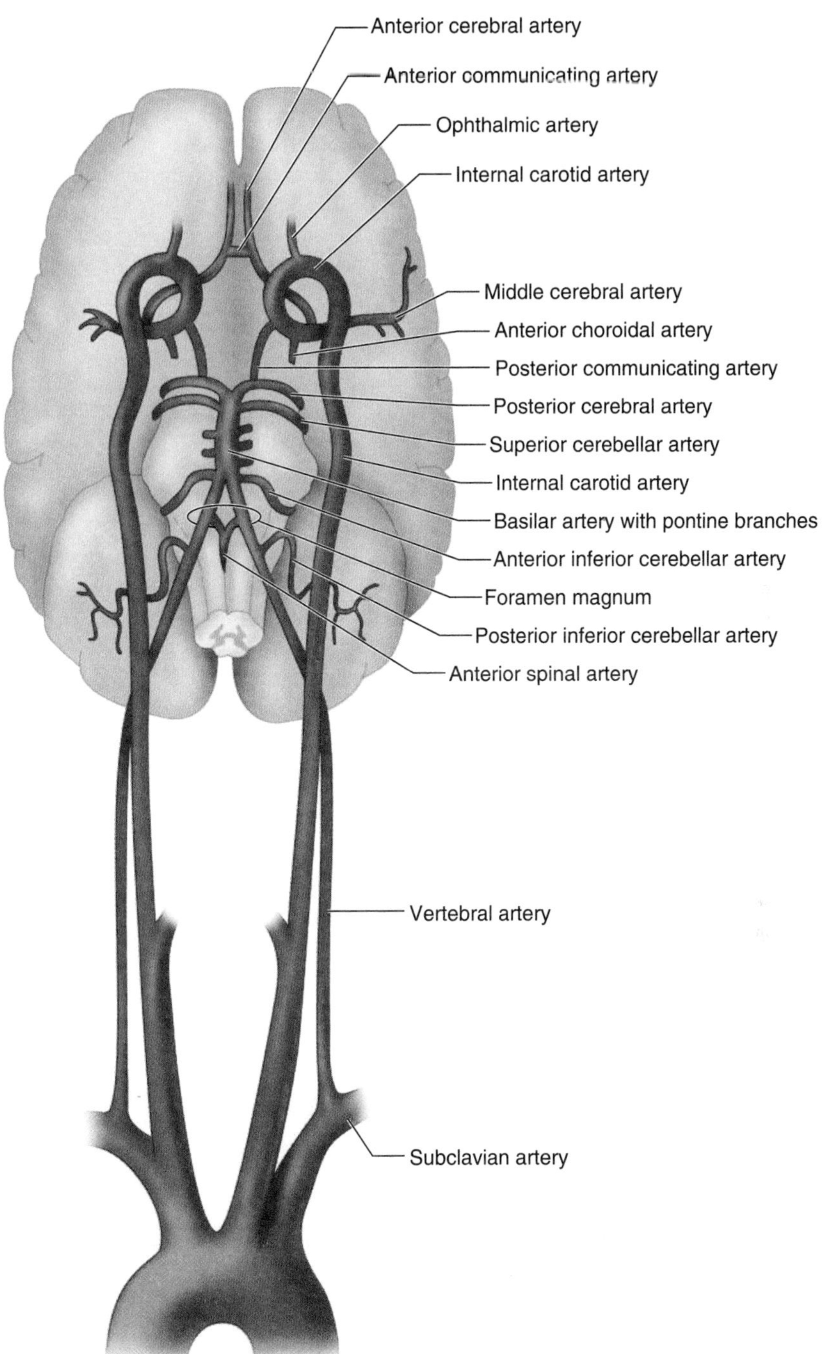

FIGURE 26–10 The cerebral circulation.

contralateral side must be immediately performed. Any hemodynamic changes need to be treated immediately, with assurance of adequate hemoglobin and oxygenation levels. The surgeon needs to be notified at once, and ultrasonic evaluation of the carotid artery is frequently required to determine whether there might be problems with the intimal suture line. It may be necessary to return to the operating room to explore the carotid artery.

SUGGESTED READINGS

Bucher J, Koyman A. Intubation of the neurologically injured patient. *J Emerg Med.* 2015;49:920.

Dagal A, Lam A. Cerebral blood flow and the injured brain: how should we monitor and manipulate it? *Curr Opin Anesthesiol.* 2011;24:131.

Drummond JC. Blood pressure and the brain: how low can you go? *Anesth Analg.* 2019;128:759.

Drummond JC, Sturaitis MK. Brain tissue oxygenation during dexmedetomidine administration in surgical patients with neurovascular injuries. *J Neurosurg Anesthesiol.* 2010;22:336.

Flexman A, Meng L, Gelb A. Outcomes in neuroanesthesia: what matters most? *Can J Anesth.* 2016;63:205.

Himmelseher S, Durieux M. Revising a dogma: ketamine for patients with neurological injury. *Anesth Analg.* 2005;101:524.

Marchesini V, Disma N. Anaesthetic neuroprotection in children: does it exist or is it all just bad? *Curr Opin Anaesthesiol.* 2019;32:363.

Meng L, Hou W, Chui J, Han R, Gelb AW. Cardiac output and cerebral blood flow: the integrated regulation of brain perfusion in adult humans. *Anesthesiology.* 2015;123:1198.

Moerman A, De Hert S. Why and how to assess cerebral autoregulation? *Best Pract Res Clin Anaesthesiol.* 2019;33:211.

Newcombe VFJ, Chow A. The features of the typical traumatic brain injury patient in the ICU are changing: what will this mean for the intensivist? *Curr Opin Crit Care.* 2021;27:80.

Orešković D, Radoš M, Klarica M. Role of choroid plexus in cerebrospinal fluid hydrodynamics. *Neuroscience.* 2017;354:69.

Picetti E, Rossi S, Abu-Zidan FM, et al. WSES consensus conference guidelines: monitoring and management of severe adult traumatic brain injury patients with polytrauma in the first 24 hours. *World J Emerg Surg.* 2019;14:53.

Quillinan N, Herson P, Traystam R. Neuropathophysiology of brain injury. *Anesthesiol Clin.* 2016;34:453.

Rao S, Avitsian R. Anesthesia for neurosurgical emergencies. *Anesthesiol Clin.* 2020;38:67.

Todd M. Outcomes after neuroanesthesia and neurosurgery: what makes a difference? *Anesthesiol Clin.* 2012;30:399.

C H A P T E R 27

Anesthesia for Neurosurgery

KEY CONCEPTS

1. Regardless of the cause, intracranial masses present symptoms and signs according to growth rate, location, and intracranial pressure. Slowly growing masses are frequently asymptomatic for long periods (despite relatively large size), whereas rapidly growing ones may present when the mass remains relatively small.
2. Computed tomography and magnetic resonance imaging scans should be reviewed for evidence of brain edema, midline shift greater than 0.5 cm, or ventricular displacement or compression.
3. Operations in the posterior fossa can injure vital circulatory and respiratory brainstem centers, as well as cranial nerves or their nuclei.
4. Venous air embolism can occur when the pressure within an open vein is subatmospheric. These conditions may exist in any position and during any procedure whenever the wound is above the level of the heart.
5. Optimal recovery of air following venous air embolism is provided by a multiorificed catheter positioned in advance at the junction between the right atrium and the superior vena cava. Confirmation of correct catheter positioning can be accomplished by intravascular electrocardiography, radiography, or transesophageal echocardiography.
6. In a patient with head trauma, correction of hypotension and control of any bleeding take precedence over radiographic studies and definitive neurosurgical treatment because systolic arterial blood pressures of less than 80 mm Hg predict a poor outcome.
7. Sudden, massive blood loss from injury to adjacent great vessels can occur intraoperatively with thoracic or lumbar spine procedures.

Anesthetic techniques must be modified in the presence of intracranial hypertension and marginal cerebral perfusion. In addition, many neurosurgical procedures require patient positions (eg, sitting, prone) that further complicate management. This chapter applies the principles developed in Chapter 26 to the anesthetic care of neurosurgical patients.

Intracranial Hypertension

Intracranial hypertension is defined as a sustained increase in intracranial pressure (ICP) above 15 mm Hg. Intracranial hypertension may result from an expanding tissue or fluid mass, a depressed skull fracture if it compresses a venous sinus, inadequate absorption of cerebrospinal fluid

(CSF), excessive cerebral blood volume (CBV), or systemic disturbances promoting brain edema (see next section). Multiple factors may be present. For example, tumors in the posterior fossa usually are associated with some degree of brain edema and mass effect, but they also may obstruct CSF outflow by compressing the fourth ventricle (obstructive hydrocephalus).

Although many patients with increased ICP are initially asymptomatic, over time, they typically develop characteristic symptoms and signs, including headache, nausea, vomiting, papilledema, focal neurological deficits, and altered consciousness. When ICP exceeds 30 mm Hg, cerebral blood flow (CBF) progressively decreases, and a vicious circle is established: ischemia causes brain edema, which in turn increases ICP, resulting in more ischemia. If left unchecked, this cycle continues until the patient dies of progressive neurological damage or catastrophic herniation. **Periodic increases in arterial blood pressure with reflex slowing of the heart rate (Cushing response) can be correlated with abrupt increases in ICP (plateau waves) lasting 1 to 15 min.** This phenomenon is the result of autoregulatory mechanisms periodically decreasing cerebral vascular resistance and increasing arterial blood pressure in response to cerebral ischemia. Eventually, severe ischemia and acidosis completely abolish autoregulation (vasomotor paralysis).

CEREBRAL EDEMA

An increase in brain water content can be produced by several mechanisms. Disruption of the blood–brain barrier (*vasogenic edema*) is most common and allows the entry of plasma-like fluid into the brain. Increases in blood pressure enhance the formation of this type of edema. Common causes of vasogenic edema include mechanical trauma, high altitudes, inflammatory lesions, brain tumors, hypertension, and infarction. Cerebral edema following metabolic insults (cytotoxic edema), such as hypoxemia or ischemia, results from failure of brain cells to actively extrude sodium, causing progressive cellular swelling. Interstitial cerebral edema can result from obstructive hydrocephalus and entry of CSF into brain interstitium. Cerebral edema can also be the result of intracellular movement of water secondary to acute decreases in serum osmolality (water intoxication).

TREATMENT

Treatment of intracranial hypertension, cerebral edema, or both is ideally directed at the underlying cause. Metabolic disturbances are corrected, and operative intervention is undertaken whenever appropriate. Vasogenic edema—particularly that associated with tumors—often responds to corticosteroids (dexamethasone). Vasogenic edema from trauma typically does not respond to corticosteroids. Blood glucose should be monitored frequently and possibly controlled with insulin infusions when steroids are used. Osmotic agents are usually effective in temporarily decreasing brain edema and ICP until more definitive measures can be undertaken. Diuresis lowers ICP chiefly by removing intracellular water from normal brain tissue. Moderate hyperventilation ($PaCO_2$ of 30–33 mm Hg) reduces CBF, CBV, and ICP acutely but may produce cerebral ischemia from cerebral vasoconstriction. Hyperventilation is currently employed as an acute measure in patients at immediate risk of herniation while other interventions are initiated.

Mannitol, in doses of 0.25 to 1 g/kg, is particularly effective in rapidly decreasing intracranial fluid volume and ICP. Its efficacy is primarily related to its effect on serum osmolality. A serum osmolality of 300 to 315 mOsm/L is generally considered desirable. Mannitol can transiently decrease blood pressure by virtue of its weak vasodilating properties, but its principal disadvantage is a transient increase in intravascular volume, which can precipitate pulmonary edema in patients with borderline cardiac or kidney function. Mannitol should generally not be used in patients with intracranial aneurysms, arteriovenous malformations (AVMs), or intracranial hemorrhage until the cranium is opened. Osmotic diuresis in such instances can expand a hematoma as the volume of the normal brain tissue around it decreases. Rapid osmotic diuresis in older adult patients can also occasionally cause a subdural hematoma due to rupture of fragile bridging veins entering the sagittal sinus.

Rebound cerebral edema may follow the use of osmotic agents.

Hypertonic saline (3% NaCl) is sometimes used to reduce cerebral edema and ICP. Hypertonic saline should be administered with care to avoid central pontine myelinolysis or osmotic demyelination syndrome in hyponatremic patients (see Chapter 49). Serum sodium concentration and osmolality should be frequently monitored. In patients with traumatic brain injury, interventions in addition to mannitol to lower intracranial pressure include head elevation, CSF drainage via ventriculostomy, and metabolic suppression with barbiturates. Decompressive craniectomy has been shown to decrease mortality in patients with sustained increases in ICP (> 25 mm Hg) following traumatic brain injury.

Anesthesia & Craniotomy for Patients with Mass Lesions

Intracranial masses may be congenital, neoplastic (benign or malignant), infectious (abscess or cyst), or vascular (hematoma or arteriovenous malformation). Primary tumors usually arise from glial cells (astrocytoma, oligodendroglioma, or glioblastoma), ependymal cells (ependymoma), or supporting tissues (meningioma, schwannoma, or choroidal papilloma). Childhood tumors include medulloblastoma, neuroblastoma, and astrocytoma.

1 Regardless of the cause, intracranial masses present symptoms and signs according to growth rate, location, and ICP. Slowly growing masses are frequently asymptomatic for long periods (despite relatively large size), whereas rapidly growing ones may present when the mass remains relatively small. Common presentations include headache, seizures, a general decline in cognitive or specific neurological functions, and focal neurological deficits. Symptoms typical of supratentorial masses include seizures, hemiplegia, or aphasia, whereas symptoms typical of infratentorial masses may include cerebellar dysfunction (ataxia, nystagmus, and dysarthria) or brainstem compression (cranial nerve palsies, altered consciousness, or abnormal respiration).

PREOPERATIVE MANAGEMENT

The preoperative evaluation for patients undergoing craniotomy should attempt to establish the presence
2 or absence of intracranial hypertension. Computed tomography (CT) and magnetic resonance imaging (MRI) scans should be reviewed for evidence of brain edema, midline shift greater than 0.5 cm, or ventricular displacement or compression. Imaging studies typically will be performed before the patient receives dexamethasone, so the mass effect may be less acute when patients who have already received dexamethasone present in the operating room. The neurological examination should document mental status and any sensory or motor deficits. Medications should be reviewed with special reference to corticosteroid, diuretic, and anticonvulsant therapy. Laboratory evaluation should rule out corticosteroid-induced hyperglycemia, electrolyte disturbances due to diuretics, or abnormal secretion of antidiuretic hormone. Anticonvulsant blood concentrations may be measured, particularly when seizures are not well controlled.

Premedication

Sedative or opioid premedication is best avoided, particularly when intracranial hypertension is suspected. Hypercapnia secondary to respiratory depression increases ICP. Corticosteroids and anticonvulsant therapy should be continued until the time of surgery.

INTRAOPERATIVE MANAGEMENT

Monitoring

In addition to standard monitors, direct intraarterial pressure monitoring and bladder catheterization are used for most patients undergoing craniotomy. Rapid changes in blood pressure during anesthetic procedures, positioning, and surgical manipulation are best managed with guidance from continuous invasive monitoring of blood pressure. Moreover, arterial blood gas analyses are necessary to closely regulate $PaCO_2$. We zero the arterial pressure transducer at the level of the head (external auditory meatus, which approximates the level of the circle of Willis)—instead of the right atrium—to facilitate calculation of cerebral perfusion pressure (CPP), and we document this practice in the anesthetic record. End-tidal CO_2 measurements alone cannot be relied upon for precise regulation of ventilation; the arterial to end-tidal CO_2 gradient must be determined. Central venous access and pressure monitoring may be considered for patients requiring vasoactive drugs. A bladder catheter is necessary because of the use of diuretics, the long duration of most neurosurgical procedures, and the utility of bladder catheterization in guiding fluid therapy and measuring core body temperature. Neuromuscular function should be monitored on the unaffected side in patients with hemiparesis because the twitch response is often abnormally resistant on the affected side. Monitoring visual evoked potentials may be useful in preventing optic nerve damage during resections of large pituitary tumors. Additional monitors for surgery in the posterior fossa are described later in this discussion.

Management of patients with intracranial hypertension may be guided by monitoring ICP perioperatively. Various ventricular, intraparenchymal, and subdural devices can be placed by neurosurgeons to provide measurements of ICP. The transducer should be zeroed to the same reference level as the arterial pressure transducer (usually the external auditory meatus, as previously noted). A ventriculostomy catheter provides the added advantage of allowing the removal of CSF to decrease ICP.

Induction

Induction of anesthesia and endotracheal intubation are critical periods for patients with compromised intracranial pressure to volume relationships, particularly if there is an elevated ICP. Intracranial elastance can be improved by osmotic diuresis or by removal of small volumes of CSF via a ventriculostomy drain. The goal of any technique should be to induce anesthesia and intubate the trachea without increasing ICP or compromising CBF. Arterial hypertension during induction increases CBV and promotes cerebral edema. Sustained hypertension can lead to marked increases in ICP, decreasing CPP and risking herniation. Excessive decreases in arterial blood pressure can be equally detrimental by compromising CPP.

The most common induction technique employs propofol or etomidate. All patients receive controlled ventilation once the induction agent has been injected. A neuromuscular blocker (NMB) is given to facilitate ventilation and prevent straining or coughing, both of which can abruptly increase ICP. An intravenous opioid given with propofol blunts the sympathetic response, particularly in young patients. Esmolol (0.5–1.0 mcg/kg) is effective in preventing tachycardia associated with intubation in lightly anesthetized patients.

The actual induction technique can be varied according to individual patient responses and coexisting diseases. Succinylcholine may theoretically increase ICP, particularly if intubation is attempted before deep anesthesia is established. Succinylcholine, however, remains the agent of choice for rapid sequence induction or when there are concerns about a potentially difficult airway as hypoxemia and hypercarbia are much more detrimental than any effect of succinylcholine to the patient with intracranial hypertension.

Hypertension during induction can be treated with β_1-blockers or by deepening the anesthetic with additional propofol. Modest concentrations of volatile agents (eg, sevoflurane) may also be used. Sevoflurane best preserves autoregulation of CBF and produces limited vasodilation; it may be the preferred volatile agent in patients with elevated ICP. Because of their potentially deleterious effect on CBV and ICP, vasodilators (eg, nicardipine, nitroprusside, nitroglycerin, hydralazine) are avoided until the dura is opened. Hypotension is generally treated with incremental doses of vasopressors (eg, phenylephrine).

Positioning

Frontal, temporal, and parietooccipital craniotomies are performed in the supine position. The head is elevated 15° to 30° to facilitate venous and CSF drainage. The head may also be turned to the side to facilitate exposure. Before and after positioning, the position of the endotracheal tube should be verified with auscultation, and all breathing circuit connections checked. The risk of unrecognized disconnections is increased because the patient's airway cannot be easily assessed after surgical draping; moreover, the operating table is usually turned 90° or 180° away from the anesthesia provider.

Maintenance of Anesthesia

Anesthesia can be maintained with inhalation anesthesia, total intravenous anesthesia techniques (TIVA), or a combination of an opioid and intravenous hypnotic (most often propofol) with a low-dose inhalation agent. Even though periods of stimulation are few, neuromuscular blockade is recommended—unless neurophysiological monitoring contradicts its use—to prevent straining, bucking, or other movement. Increased anesthetic requirements can be expected during the most stimulating periods: laryngoscopy–intubation, skin incision, dural opening, periosteal manipulations, including Mayfield pin placement and closure. TIVA with remifentanil and propofol facilitates rapid emergence and immediate neurological assessment. Likewise, the α_2-agonist dexmedetomidine can be employed during both asleep and awake craniotomies to similar effect. Normocarbia should be maintained intraoperatively. Lower $PaCO_2$ tensions provide little benefit and may be associated with cerebral ischemia and impaired oxygen dissociation from hemoglobin. Ventilatory patterns resulting in high mean airway pressures (a low rate with large tidal volumes) should be avoided because of a potentially adverse effect on ICP by increasing central venous pressure and the potential for lung injury. Lung protective ventilation (tidal volume ≤6 mL/kg) is recommended. Hypoxic patients may require positive end-expiratory pressure (PEEP) and increased mean airway pressure; in such patients, the effect of PEEP on ICP is variable.

Intravenous fluid replacement should be limited to glucose-free isotonic crystalloid. Hyperglycemia is common in neurosurgical patients and has been implicated in amplifying ischemic brain injury. Hyperglycemia should be corrected preoperatively. Neurosurgical procedures are often associated with substantial occult blood loss (underneath surgical drapes or on the floor). Hypotension and hypertension should both be expeditiously corrected. Euvolemia should be maintained, which is often tricky in the setting of osmotic diuresis.

Emergence

Most patients undergoing elective craniotomy can be extubated at the end of the procedure. Patients who will remain intubated should be sedated to prevent agitation. Extubation in the operating room requires special handling during emergence. Straining or "bucking" on the endotracheal tube may precipitate intracranial hemorrhage or worsen cerebral edema. As the skin is being closed, the patient may resume breathing spontaneously. Should the patient's head be secured in a Mayfield pin apparatus, care must be taken to avoid any patient motions (eg, bucking on the tube), which could promote neck or cranial injuries. After the head dressing is applied and full access to the patient is regained (the table is turned back to its original position as at induction), any anesthetic agents are discontinued, and the neuromuscular blockade is reversed. Rapid awakening facilitates immediate neurological assessment and is generally expected. Delayed awakening may be seen following an opioid or sedative overdose, when the end-tidal concentration of the volatile agent remains greater than 0.2 minimum alveolar concentration (MAC) or when there is a metabolic derangement or a perioperative neurological injury. Patients may need to be transported directly from the operating room for imaging when they do not respond as predicted, and immediate reexploration may be required. Most patients are taken to the intensive care unit postoperatively for close monitoring.

Anesthesia for Surgery in the Posterior Fossa

Craniotomy for a mass in the posterior fossa presents a unique set of potential problems: obstructive hydrocephalus, possible injury to vital brainstem centers, pneumocephalus, and when these procedures are performed with the patient in the sitting position, an increased risk of postural hypotension and **venous air embolism**.

Obstructive Hydrocephalus

Infratentorial masses can obstruct CSF flow through the fourth ventricle or the cerebral aqueduct of Sylvius. Small but critically located lesions can markedly increase ICP. In such cases, a ventriculostomy is often performed under local anesthesia to decrease ICP prior to induction of general anesthesia.

Brainstem Injury

3 Operations in the posterior fossa can injure vital circulatory and respiratory brainstem centers, as well as cranial nerves or their nuclei. Such injuries may occur as a result of direct surgical trauma or ischemia from retraction or other interruptions of the blood supply. Damage to respiratory centers is said to nearly always produce circulatory changes; therefore, abrupt changes in blood pressure, heart rate, or cardiac rhythm should alert the anesthesia provider to the possibility of such an injury. Such changes should be communicated to the surgeon. Isolated damage to respiratory centers may rarely occur without premonitory circulatory signs during operations on the floor of the fourth ventricle. At completion of the surgery, brainstem injuries may present as an abnormal respiratory pattern or an inability to maintain a patent airway following extubation. Monitoring brainstem auditory evoked potentials may be useful in preventing eighth nerve damage during resections of acoustic neuromas. Electromyography is also used to avoid injury to the facial nerve but requires incomplete neuromuscular blockade intraoperatively.

Positioning

Although most explorations of the posterior fossa can be performed with the patient in either a modified lateral or prone position, the sitting position may be preferred by some surgeons.

The patient is actually semirecumbent in the standard sitting position (Figure 27–1); the back is elevated to 60°, and the legs are elevated with the knees flexed. The head is fixed in a three-point holder with the neck flexed; the arms remain at the sides with the hands resting on the lap.

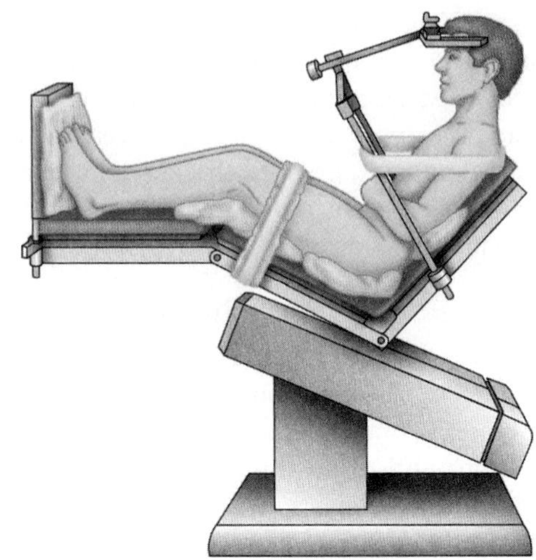

FIGURE 27–1 The sitting position for craniotomy.

Careful positioning and padding help avoid injuries. Pressure points, such as the elbows, ischial spines, heels, and forehead, must be protected. Excessive neck flexion has been associated with swelling of the upper airway (due to venous obstruction) and, rarely, quadriplegia (due to compression of the cervical spinal cord). Preexisting cervical spinal stenosis probably predisposes patients to the latter injury.

Pneumocephalus

The sitting position increases the likelihood of pneumocephalus. In this position, air readily enters the subarachnoid space as CSF is lost during surgery. In patients with cerebral atrophy, drainage of CSF is marked; air can replace CSF on the surface of the brain and in the lateral ventricles. Expansion of a pneumocephalus following dural closure can compress the brain. Postoperative pneumocephalus can cause delayed awakening and continued impairment of neurological function. Because of these and other concerns, nitrous oxide is rarely used for sitting craniotomies (see further discussion that follows).

Venous Air Embolism

4 Venous air embolism can occur when the pressure within an open vein is subatmospheric. These conditions may exist in any position and during any procedure whenever the wound is above the level of the heart. The incidence of venous air embolism is greater during sitting craniotomies (20–40%) than in craniotomies in any other position. Entry into large cerebral venous sinuses increases the risk.

The physiological consequences of venous air embolism depend on the volume and the rate of air entry and whether the patient has a right-to-left intracardiac shunt (eg, patent foramen ovale [10–25% incidence]). The latter is important because it can facilitate the passage of air into the arterial circulation (**paradoxical air embolism**). Modest quantities of air bubbles entering the venous system ordinarily lodge in the pulmonary circulation, where they are eventually absorbed. Small quantities of embolized air are well tolerated by most patients. When the amount entrained exceeds the rate of pulmonary clearance, pulmonary artery pressure rises progressively. Eventually, cardiac output decreases in response to increases in right ventricular afterload. Preexisting cardiac or pulmonary disease enhances the adverse effects of venous air embolism; relatively small amounts of air may produce marked hemodynamic changes. Nitrous oxide can markedly accentuate the effects of even small amounts of entrained air by diffusing into air bubbles and increasing their volume. The lethal volume of venous air in experimental animals receiving nitrous oxide anesthesia is reduced to one-third to one-half that of control animals not receiving nitrous oxide.

In the absence of echocardiography, definitive signs of venous air embolism are often not apparent until large volumes of air have been entrained. A decrease in end-tidal CO_2 or arterial oxygen saturation may be noticed prior to hemodynamic changes. Arterial blood gas values may show only slight increases in $PaCO_2$ as a result of increased dead space ventilation (areas with normal ventilation but decreased perfusion). Conversely, major hemodynamic manifestations, such as sudden hypotension, can occur well before hypoxemia is noted. Moreover, large amounts of intracardiac air impair tricuspid and pulmonic valve function and can produce sudden circulatory arrest by obstructing right ventricular outflow.

Paradoxical air embolism can result in a stroke or coronary occlusion, which may be apparent only postoperatively. Paradoxical air emboli are more likely to occur in patients with right-to-left intracardiac shunts, particularly when the normal transatrial (left > right) pressure gradient is consistently reversed.

A. Central Venous Catheterization

A properly positioned central venous catheter can be used to aspirate entrained air, but there is only limited evidence that this influences outcomes after venous air embolism. Some clinicians have considered right atrial catheterization mandatory for sitting craniotomies, but this is a minority viewpoint.

5 Optimal recovery of air following venous air embolism is provided by a multiorificed catheter positioned at the junction between the right atrium and the superior vena cava. Confirmation of correct catheter positioning can be accomplished by intravascular electrocardiography, radiography, or transesophageal echocardiography (TEE), with the latter being the simplest and easiest method. Intravascular electrocardiography is accomplished by using the saline-filled catheter as a "V" lead. Correct positioning near the cavoatrial junction is indicated by the appearance of a maximally biphasic P wave. If the catheter is advanced farther into the heart, the P wave changes from a biphasic to an undirectional deflection. A right ventricular or pulmonary artery waveform may also be observed when the catheter is connected to a pressure transducer and advanced too far, but pressure waveforms do not identify the cavoatrial junction.

B. Monitoring for Venous Air Embolism

The most sensitive detectors available should be used. Detecting even small amounts of venous air emboli is important because it prompts surgical control of the entry site before additional air is entrained. Currently, the devices capable of detecting the smallest volumes of air are TEE and precordial Doppler sonography. These monitors can detect air bubbles as small as 0.25 mL. TEE has the added benefit of detecting the volume of the bubbles and any transatrial passage through a patent foramen ovale, as well as evaluating any effect venous air embolism may have on cardiac function. Doppler methods employ a probe over the right atrium (usually to the right of the sternum and between the third and sixth ribs). Interruption of the regular swishing of the Doppler signal by sporadic roaring sounds indicates venous air embolism. Changes in end-tidal respiratory gas concentrations are less sensitive but are important monitors that can also detect venous air embolism before overt clinical signs are present. Venous air embolism causes a sudden decrease in end-tidal CO_2 tension in proportion to the increase in pulmonary dead space; however, decreases can also be seen with hemodynamic changes unrelated to venous air embolism, such as decreased cardiac output. A reappearance (or increase) of nitrogen in expired gases may also be seen with venous air embolism. Changes in blood pressure and heart sounds ("mill wheel" murmur) are late manifestations of venous air embolism.

C. Treatment of Venous Air Embolism

1. The surgeon should be immediately notified so that they can flood the surgical field with saline or pack it with wet gauzes and apply bone wax to the skull edges until the entry site is identified and occluded.
2. Nitrous oxide (if used) should be discontinued, and the patient should be ventilated with 100% oxygen.
3. If a central venous catheter is present, it should be aspirated in an attempt to retrieve the entrained air.
4. Intravascular volume infusion should be given to increase central venous pressure.
5. Vasopressors should be given to treat hypotension.
6. Bilateral jugular vein compression, by increasing intracranial venous pressure, may slow air entrainment and cause back bleeding, which might help the surgeon identify the entry point of the embolus.
7. Some clinicians advocate PEEP to increase cerebral venous pressure; however, reversal of the normal transatrial pressure gradient may promote paradoxical embolism in a patient with incomplete closure of the foramen ovale.
8. If the previously listed measures fail, the patient should be placed in a head-down position, and the wound should be closed quickly.
9. Persistent circulatory arrest necessitates the supine position and institution of resuscitation efforts using advanced cardiac life support algorithms.

Anesthesia for Stereotactic Surgery

Stereotaxis can be employed in treating involuntary movement disorders, intractable pain, and epilepsy and can also be used when diagnosing and treating tumors that are located deep within the brain.

These procedures are often performed under local anesthesia to allow evaluation of the patient. Propofol or dexmedetomidine infusions are often used for sedation and amnesia. Sedation should be omitted, however, if the patient already has increased ICP. The ability to rapidly provide controlled ventilation and general anesthesia for emergency craniotomy is mandatory but is complicated by the platform and localizing frame that is attached to the patient's head for the procedure. Although mask ventilation or ventilation through a laryngeal mask airway (LMA) or orotracheal intubation might be readily accomplished in an emergency, awake intubation with a fiberoptic bronchoscope or videolaryngoscope prior to positioning and surgery may be the safest approach when intubation is necessary for a patient whose head is already in a stereotactic head frame.

Functional neurosurgery is increasingly performed for the removal of lesions adjacent to speech and other vital brain centers. Sometimes patients are managed with an asleep–awake–asleep technique, with or without instrumentation of the airway. Such operations require the patient to be awake to participate in cortical mapping to identify key speech centers, such as the Broca area. Patients sleep during the painful periods of surgery (ie, during opening and closure). LMAs are often employed to assist airway management during the asleep portions of these surgeries. Local anesthetic infiltration of the scalp facilitates awake craniotomy.

Patients undergo deep brain stimulator insertion for control of movement and other disorders. A stimulator electrode is placed via a burr hole using radiological guidance to establish coordinates for electrode placement. A microelectrode recording (MER) is obtained to determine the correct placement of the stimulator in brain structures. The effect of stimulation upon the patient is noted. Sedative medications can adversely affect MER potentials, complicating the location of the correct depth of stimulator placement. Dexmedetomidine has been used to provide sedation to these patients; however, during MER and stimulation testing, sedative infusions should be discontinued to facilitate patient participation in determining correct electrode placement (Table 27–1).

Anesthesia for Head Trauma

Head injuries are a contributory factor in up to 50% of deaths due to trauma. Most patients with head trauma are young, and many (10–40%) have associated intraabdominal or intrathoracic injuries, long bone fractures, or spinal injuries. The outcome from a head injury is dependent not only on the extent of the neuronal damage at the time of injury but also on the occurrence of any secondary insults or sequelae from other injuries or complications (see Chapter 39). These secondary insults include (1) systemic factors such as hypoxemia, hypercapnia, or hypotension; (2) the formation and expansion of an epidural, subdural, or intracerebral hematoma; and (3) sustained intracranial hypertension. Head-injured patients may have a wide variety of other injuries, may arrive at the hospital in an intoxicated state, and are subject to the usual range of complications

TABLE 27–1 Advantages and disadvantages of drugs used for conscious sedation.

Agents	Advantages	Disadvantages
GABA receptor agonists	Anxiolysis	Large dose abolishes MER
Benzodiazepines		Alters the threshold for stimulation
		Induces dyskinesia
Propofol	Widely used	Abolishes tremors
	Short acting	Attenuation of MER
	Predictable emergence profile	Unpredictable dosing in patients with Parkinson disease
		Induces dyskinesia
		Tendency to cause sneezing
Opioids		
Fentanyl	? Minimal effect on MER	Rigidity
Remifentanil	Short acting	Suppression of tremors
α_2-Agonist		
Dexmedetomidine	Non–GABA-mediated action	High doses can abolish MER
	Less effect on MER	Hypotension, bradycardia
	Anxiolysis and analgesic effects	
	Sedation: easily arousable	
	Does not ameliorate clinical signs of parkinsonism	
	Maintains hemodynamic stability	
	Preserves respiration	

GABA, γ-aminobutyric acid; MER, microelectrode recording.

Reproduced with permission from Venkatraghavan L, Luciano M, Manninen P. Anesthetic management of patients undergoing deep brain stimulator insertion. *Anesth Analg.* 2010 Apr 1;110(4):1138-1145.

TABLE 27–2 Glasgow coma scale.

Category	Score
Eye opening	
Spontaneous	4
To speech	3
To pain	2
Nil	1
Best motor response	
To verbal command	
Obeys	6
To pain	
Localizes	5
Withdraws	4
Decorticate flexion	3
Extensor response	2
Nil	1
Best verbal response	
Oriented	5
Confused conversation	4
Inappropriate words	3
Incomprehensible sounds	2
Nil	1

encountered in critical care (sepsis, acute respiratory distress syndrome [ARDS], etc). Surgical and anesthetic management of these patients is directed at the immediate treatment of primary injuries and avoiding these secondary insults. The **Glasgow Coma Scale (GCS) score** (Table 27–2) generally correlates well with the severity of injury and outcome. A GCS score of 8 or less on admission is associated with approximately 35% mortality. Evidence of greater than a 5-mm midline shift (on imaging) and ventricular compression on imaging are associated with substantially worse outcomes.

Specific lesions include skull fractures, subdural and epidural hematomas, brain contusions (including intracerebral hemorrhages), penetrating head injuries, and traumatic vascular occlusions and dissections. The presence of a skull fracture greatly increases the likelihood of an intracranial lesion. Linear skull fractures are commonly associated with subdural or epidural hematomas. Basilar skull fractures may be associated with CSF rhinorrhea, pneumocephalus, cranial nerve palsies, or even a cavernous sinus–carotid artery fistula. Depressed skull fractures often present with an underlying brain contusion. Contusions may be limited to the surface of the brain or may involve hemorrhage in deeper hemispheric structures or the brainstem. Rapid deceleration injuries often produce both coup (frontal) and contrecoup (occipital) lesions. Epidural and subdural hematomas can occur as isolated lesions, as well as in association with cerebral contusions (more commonly with subdural than epidural lesions).

Operative treatment is usually elected for depressed skull fractures; evacuation of epidural, subdural, and some intracerebral hematomas; and debridement of penetrating injuries. Decompressive craniectomy is used to provide room for cerebral swelling. The cranium is subsequently reconstructed following the resolution of cerebral edema.

ICP monitoring is usually indicated in patients with lesions associated with intracranial hypertension: large contusions, mass lesions, intracerebral hemorrhage, or evidence of edema on imaging studies. ICP monitoring should also be considered in patients with signs of intracranial hypertension who are undergoing nonneurological procedures. Acute intracranial hypertension should be treated with hyperventilation, osmolar therapy, and barbiturates with the goal of avoiding herniation. Hyperventilation is associated with cerebral vasoconstriction, and if used, it should be employed in efforts to prevent imminent cerebral herniation. Immediate neurosurgical intervention is mandated. Multiple studies have found that sustained increases in ICP of greater than 60 mm Hg result in severe disability or death. Randomized trials have failed to detect the efficacy of early use of large doses of glucocorticoids in patients with head trauma. Hypothermia has likewise failed to improve survival following traumatic brain injury.

PREOPERATIVE MANAGEMENT

Anesthetic care of patients with severe head trauma begins in the emergency department. Measures to ensure patency of the airway, adequacy of ventilation and oxygenation, stabilization of the cervical spine, and correction of systemic hypotension should proceed simultaneously with neurological and trauma surgical evaluation. Airway obstruction and hypoventilation are common. Up to 70% of such patients have hypoxemia, which may be complicated by pulmonary contusion, fat emboli, or neurogenic pulmonary edema. The latter is attributed to marked systemic and pulmonary hypertension secondary to intense sympathetic nervous system activity. Supplemental oxygen should be given to all patients while the airway and ventilation are evaluated. Many patients will have drug or alcohol intoxication. All patients must be assumed to have a cervical spine injury (up to 10% incidence) until it has been ruled out radiographically. Patients with hypoventilation, an absent gag reflex, or a persistent score below 8 on the GCS (see Table 27–2) require tracheal intubation. All other patients should be carefully observed for deterioration.

Intubation

All patients should be regarded as having a full stomach and should have appropriate precautions during ventilation and tracheal intubation. Nevertheless, the effectiveness of the Sellick maneuver in preventing aspiration is questionable. In-line stabilization should be used during airway manipulation to maintain the head in a neutral position unless radiographs confirm that there is no cervical spine injury. Following preoxygenation, the adverse effects of intubation on ICP are blunted by prior administration of propofol, 1.5 to 3.0 mg/kg, and a rapid-onset NMB. Succinylcholine may produce mild and transient increases in ICP in patients with closed head injury; however, the necessity for expeditious airway management trumps theoretical concerns. Rocuronium is often used to facilitate intubation. The presence of a hard collar for cervical spine stabilization will increase the difficulty of intubation. Video laryngoscopy performed with in-line stabilization generally permits the maintenance of a neutral position during intubation. An intubating bougie should be available. If a difficult intubation is encountered with video laryngoscopy, fiberoptic or other techniques (eg, intubating LMA) can be attempted. If airway attempts are unsuccessful, a surgical airway should be obtained. Blind nasal intubation or blind passage of a nasogastric tube should be avoided in the presence of a basilar skull fracture because of the possibility of passing tubes directly through the fracture into the brain. The diagnosis of basilar skull fracture is suggested by CSF rhinorrhea or otorrhea, hemotympanum, or ecchymosis into periorbital tissues (raccoon sign) or behind the ear (Battle sign).

Hypotension

Hypotension in the setting of head trauma is nearly always related to other associated injuries (often intraabdominal). Profuse bleeding from scalp lacerations may cause hypovolemic hypotension in children. Hypotension may be seen with spinal cord injuries because of the sympathectomy associated with spinal shock. In a patient with head trauma, correction of hypotension and control of any bleeding take precedence over radiographic studies and definitive neurosurgical treatment because systolic arterial blood pressures of less than 80 mm Hg predict a poor outcome. Glucose-containing or hypotonic solutions should not be used (see earlier discussion). Otherwise, crystalloids and blood products can be administered as necessary. Massive blood loss in a patient with multiple injuries should result in the activation of a massive transfusion protocol to provide a steady supply of platelets, fresh frozen plasma, and packed red blood cells. Invasive monitoring of arterial pressure, central venous pressure, and ICP are valuable but should not delay diagnosis and treatment. Arrhythmias and electrocardiographic abnormalities in the T wave, U wave, ST segment, and QT interval are common following head injuries but are not necessarily associated with cardiac injury; they likely represent altered autonomic function.

Diagnostic Studies

The choice between operative and medical management of head trauma is based on radiographic and clinical findings. Patients should be stabilized prior to any CT or other imaging studies. Critically ill patients must be closely monitored during such studies. Restless or uncooperative patients may require general anesthesia for imaging. Sedation in such cases without control of the airway should be avoided because of the risk of further increases in ICP from hypercapnia or hypoxemia and because of the risk of aspiration.

INTRAOPERATIVE MANAGEMENT

Anesthetic management is generally similar to that for other mass lesions associated with intracranial hypertension. Invasive monitoring should be established, if not already present, but should not delay surgical decompression in a rapidly deteriorating patient.

Anesthetic techniques are designed to preserve cerebral perfusion and mitigate increases in ICP. Hypotension may occur after induction of anesthesia as a result of the combined effects of vasodilation and hypovolemia and should be treated with an α-adrenergic agonist and volume infusion if necessary. Hypertension is common with surgical stimulation, but it may also occur in response to acute elevations in ICP. Hypertension associated with elevated ICP and bradycardia is termed the *Cushing reflex*.

Hypertension can be treated with additional doses of the induction agent, with increased concentrations of an inhalation anesthetic (provided there is no hypercarbia) or with antihypertensives. Esmolol is usually effective in controlling hypertension associated with tachycardia. CPP should be maintained between 70 and 110 mm Hg. Vasodilators should be avoided until the dura is opened. Excessive hyperventilation ($PaCO_2$ <35 mm Hg) should be avoided in trauma patients (unless the patient manifests signs of impending herniation) to prevent excessive decreases in oxygen delivery.

Disseminated intravascular coagulation occasionally may be seen with severe head injuries. Such injuries cause the release of large amounts of brain thromboplastin and may also be associated with ARDS. Pulmonary aspiration and neurogenic pulmonary edema may also be responsible for deteriorating lung function. When PEEP is used, ICP monitoring can be useful to confirm an adequate CPP. Diabetes insipidus, characterized by inappropriately dilute polyuria, is frequently seen following brain trauma, especially with injuries to the pituitary. Other likely causes of polyuria should be excluded and the diagnosis confirmed by measurement of urine and serum osmolality (see Chapter 49). Gastrointestinal bleeding from stress ulceration is common in patients not receiving prophylaxis.

The decision whether to extubate the trachea at the conclusion of the surgical procedure depends on the severity of the injury, the presence of concomitant abdominal or thoracic injuries, preexisting illnesses, and the preoperative level of consciousness. Young patients who were conscious preoperatively may be extubated following the removal of a localized lesion, whereas patients with diffuse brain injury should remain intubated. Moreover, persistent intracranial hypertension requires continued paralysis, sedation, CSF drainage, and elevated head position.

Anesthesia for Intracranial Aneurysms & Arteriovenous Malformations

Saccular aneurysms and AVMs are common causes of nontraumatic intracranial hemorrhages. Surgical or interventional neuroradiological treatment may be undertaken either electively to prevent hemorrhage or as an emergency to prevent further complications once hemorrhage has taken place. Other nontraumatic hemorrhages (from hypertension, sickle cell disease, or vasculitis) are usually treated medically.

CEREBRAL ANEURYSMS

Preoperative Considerations

Cerebral aneurysms typically occur at the bifurcation of the arteries at the base of the brain; most are located in the anterior circle of Willis. Approximately 10% to 30% of patients have more than one aneurysm. The general incidence of saccular aneurysms in some estimates is reported to be 5%, but only a minority of those with aneurysms will have complications. Rupture of a saccular aneurysm is the most common cause of subarachnoid hemorrhage (SAH). The acute mortality following rupture is approximately 10%. Of those who survive the initial hemorrhage, about 25% die within 3 months from delayed complications. Moreover, up to 50% of survivors are left with neurological deficits. As a result, the emphasis in management is on the prevention of rupture. Unfortunately, most patients present only after rupture has already occurred.

Unruptured Aneurysms

Patients may present with prodromal symptoms and signs suggesting progressive enlargement. The most common symptom is headache, and the most common physical sign is a third-nerve palsy. Other manifestations could include brainstem dysfunction, visual field defects, trigeminal nerve dysfunction, cavernous sinus syndrome, seizures, and hypothalamic–pituitary dysfunction. The most commonly used techniques to diagnose an aneurysm are MRI, angiography, and helical CT angiography. Following diagnosis, patients are brought to the operating room, or more likely the "hybrid" suite, for coiling or clipping of the aneurysm. Most patients are in the 40- to 60-year-old age group and in otherwise good health.

Ruptured Aneurysms

Ruptured aneurysms usually present acutely as SAH. Patients typically report a sudden severe headache without focal neurological deficits but often associated with nausea and vomiting. Transient loss of consciousness may occur and may result from a sudden rise in ICP and precipitous drop in CPP. If ICP does not decrease rapidly after the initial sudden increase, death usually follows. Large blood clots can cause focal neurological signs in some patients. Minor bleeding may cause only a mild headache, vomiting, and nuchal rigidity. The severity of SAH is graded according to the Hunt and Hess scale (Table 27–3), as well as the World Federation of Neurological Surgeons grading scale of SAH (Table 27–4). The Fisher grading scale, which uses CT to assess the amount of blood detected, gives the best indication of the likelihood of the development of cerebral vasospasm and patient outcome (Table 27–5).

Delayed complications include delayed cerebral ischemia (DCI), rerupture, and hydrocephalus. DCI occurs in 30% of patients (usually after 4–14 days) and is a major cause of morbidity and mortality. Previously, cerebral arterial vasospasm was considered the primary cause of DCI following SAH. Although cerebral artery vasospasm does occur, it often does not correlate with areas of cerebral infarction. Consequently,

TABLE 27–3 Hunt and Hess grading scale for SAH.

Grade	Clinical Description
I	Asymptomatic or minimal headache and slight nuchal rigidity
II	Moderate to severe headache, nuchal rigidity, and no neurological deficit other than cranial nerve palsy
III	Drowsiness, confusion, or mild focal deficit
IV	Stupor, moderate to severe hemiparesis, and possibly early decerebrate rigidity and vegetative disturbances
V	Deep coma, decerebrate rigidity, and moribund appearance

Reproduced with permission from Priebe H-J. Aneurysmal subarachnoid haemorrhage and the anaesthetist. *Br J Anaesth.* 2007 July;99(1):102-118.

TABLE 27–4 World Federation of Neurological Surgeons grading scale for aneurismal SAH.

Grade	GCS Score[1]	Motor Deficit[2]
I	15	Absent
II	13 or 14	Absent
III	13 or 14	Present
IV	7-12	Present or absent
V	3-6	Present or absent

[1]GCS, Glasgow Coma Scale.

[2]Excludes cranial neuropathies, but includes dysphasia.

Reproduced with permission from Priebe H-J. Aneurysmal subarachnoid haemorrhage and the anaesthetist. *Br J Anaesth.* 2007 July;99(1):102-118

TABLE 27–5 Fisher grading scale of cranial computerized tomography (CCT).

Grade	Findings on CCT
1	No subarachnoid blood detected
2	Diffuse or vertical layers ≤1 mm
3	Localized clot and/or vertical layer >1 mm
4	Intracerebral or intraventricular clot with diffuse or no subarachnoid hemorrhage

Reproduced with permission from Priebe H-J. Aneurysmal subarachnoid haemorrhage and the anaesthetist. *Br J Anaesth.* 2007 July;99(1):102-118.

other mechanisms are considered as also contributing to DCI. These include cortical spreading depolarizations (CSDs) and microthrombosis. CSDs are waves of neuronal depolarizations of grey matter followed by a wave of inhibition. CSDs can both increase and decrease cerebral blood flow. Cerebral ischemia results secondary to inadequate perfusion following CSDs in injured brains. *N*-methyl-D-aspartate (NMDA) receptor antagonists such as ketamine may modulate CSDs. SAH is also thought to contribute to platelet activation and formation of microthrombi, which likewise produce cerebral ischemia. Manifestations of DCI are due to cerebral ischemia and infarction and depend on the severity and distribution of the involved vessels. The Ca^{2+} channel antagonist nimodipine is used following SAH to mitigate the effects of DCI. Both transcranial Doppler and brain tissue oxygen monitoring can be used to guide vasospasm therapy. Increased velocity of flow greater than 200 cm/s is indicative of severe spasm. The Lindegaard ratio compares the blood velocity of the cervical carotid artery with that of the middle cerebral artery. A ratio greater than 3 is likewise indicative of severe spasm. Brain tissue oxygen tension less than 20 mm Hg is also worrisome. **In patients with symptomatic vasospasm with an inadequate response to nimodipine, intravascular volume expansion and induced hypertension ("triple H" therapy: hypervolemia, hemodilution, and hypertension) are added as part of the therapeutic regimen.** Recent reviews have questioned the role of hypervolemia, recommending maintenance of euvolemia while acknowledging that hypertension may be most beneficial in the management of DCI. Milrinone has been suggested to improve blood flow, but it is not a standard treatment. Refractory vasospasm may be treated with catheter-delivered vasodilators, angioplasty, or both. However, radiological improvement in the vessel diameter does not necessarily correlate with an improvement in clinical status.

PREOPERATIVE MANAGEMENT

In addition to assessing and documenting neurological findings, the preoperative evaluation should include a search for coexisting diseases, such as hypertension and renal, cardiac, or ischemic cerebrovascular disease. Electrocardiographic abnormalities are commonly seen in patients with SAH, but they do not necessarily reflect underlying heart disease. However, increases of cardiac troponin during SAH are associated with myocardial injury and may herald a poor outcome. Stress-induced cardiomyopathy may also be present. Most conscious patients with normal ICP are sedated following rupture to prevent rebleeding; such sedation should be continued until induction of anesthesia. Patients with persistent elevation in ICP should receive little or no premedication to avoid hypercapnia.

INTRAOPERATIVE MANAGEMENT

Aneurysm surgery can result in exsanguinating hemorrhage as a consequence of rupture or rebleeding. Blood should be immediately available prior to the start of these operations.

Regardless of the anesthetic technique employed, anesthetic management should focus on preventing rupture (or rebleeding) and avoiding factors that promote cerebral ischemia or vasospasm. Intraarterial pressure monitoring is useful. Sudden increases in blood pressure with tracheal intubation or surgical stimulation should be avoided. Judicious intravascular volume loading permits surgical levels of anesthesia without excessive decreases in blood pressure. Because calcium channel blockers, angiotensin receptor blockers, and angiotensin-converting enzyme inhibitors cause systemic vasodilation and reduce systemic vascular resistance, patients receiving these agents preoperatively may be particularly prone to hypotension.

The great majority of cerebral aneurysms are addressed via an endovascular approach. The anesthetic concerns of patients taken for coiling in the neurointerventional suite are similar to those of patients undergoing craniotomy. General anesthesia is often employed. Patients require heparin anticoagulation and radiological contrast. Communication with the surgeon or neurointerventionalist as to the desired activated clotting time and need for protamine reversal is essential. Moreover, anesthesia staff in the neuroradiology suite must be prepared to manipulate and monitor the blood pressure, as with an open surgical procedure.

For the less common situation in which open craniotomy is required, once the dura is opened, mannitol is often given to facilitate surgical exposure and reduce the need for surgical retraction. Rapid decreases in ICP prior to dural opening are avoided as they may promote rebleeding by removing a tamponading effect on the aneurysm.

Elective (controlled) hypotension has been used in aneurysm surgery. Decreasing mean arterial blood pressure reduces the transmural tension across the aneurysm, making rupture (or rebleeding) less likely and facilitating surgical clipping. Controlled hypotension can also decrease blood loss and improve surgical visualization in the event of bleeding. The combination of a slightly head-up position with a volatile anesthetic enhances the effects of any of the commonly used hypotensive agents. Should accidental rupture of the aneurysm occur, the surgeon may request transient hypotension to facilitate control of the bleeding. Neurophysiological monitoring may be employed during aneurysm surgery to identify potential ischemia during clip application. Rarely, hypothermic circulatory arrest is used for large basilar artery aneurysms.

Depending on their neurological condition, most patients should be extubated at the end of surgery (see earlier discussion). A rapid awakening allows neurological evaluation in the operating room prior to transfer to the intensive care unit.

ARTERIOVENOUS MALFORMATIONS

AVMs cause intracerebral hemorrhage more often than SAH. These lesions are developmental abnormalities that result in arteriovenous fistulas; they typically increase in size with time. AVMs may present at any age, but bleeding is most common between 10 and 30 years of age. Other common presentations include headache and seizures. The combination of high blood flow with low vascular resistance can rarely result in high-output cardiac failure. In most cases, an endovascular approach to occlude the vessels feeding the AVM will be attempted in the "hybrid" operating room or neurointerventional suite. This may provide definitive therapy or may render the AVM more amenable to surgical excision. Neuroradiological embolization employs various coils, glues, and balloons to obliterate the AVM. Risks include embolization into cerebral arteries feeding the normal brain, as well as systemic or pulmonary embolism.

Anesthetic management of patients undergoing resection of AVMs may be complicated by extensive blood loss. Venous access with multiple large-bore cannulas is necessary. Hyperventilation and mannitol may be used to facilitate surgical access. Hyperemia and swelling can develop following resection, possibly because of altered autoregulation in the remaining normal brain. Emergence hypertension is typically controlled with agents that do not induce increases in CBF, such as β-blockers.

Acute Ischemic Stroke

Acute ischemic strokes are treated endovascularly or with thrombolysis using tissue plasminogen activator (tPA), or both. Multiple well-performed randomized clinical trials have confirmed that immediate endovascular intervention greatly improves outcomes relative to thrombolysis alone in patients with occlusions of proximal large cerebral arteries. The mantra in neurology and neurosurgery is "time is brain." The goal is to have the patient revascularized as soon as possible. Endovascular treatment should not be delayed for placement of arterial lines, etc. These patients are at immediate risk of death and disability without treatment and certainly meet the criteria for an American Society of Anesthesiologists physical status of 5E! Several post hoc analyses of the original clinical trials have suggested an association between the use of general anesthesia (versus sedation and monitoring) and worse outcomes in patients undergoing endovascular embolectomy. Nevertheless, general anesthesia remains the preference in many centers and will be required for many patients. The goals of anesthesia for endovascular treatment of acute ischemic stroke are to maintain the blood pressure less than 180 mm Hg if tPA has been given. If tPA has not been given, relative hypertension may be preferable to maintain cerebral perfusion pending clot retrieval and stenting. Once the occluded vessel has been reopened, we recommend tight control of blood pressure, in most cases keeping it at 140/90 mm Hg or less.

Anesthesia for Surgery on the Spine

Spinal surgery is most often performed for symptomatic nerve root or cord compression secondary to trauma or degenerative disorders. Compression may occur from the protrusion of an intervertebral disk or osteophytic bone (spondylosis) into the spinal canal or an intervertebral foramen. Prolapse of an intervertebral disk often occurs at either the fourth or fifth lumbar or the fifth or sixth cervical levels in adults. Spondylosis tends to affect the lower cervical spine more than the lumbar spine and typically afflicts older patients. Operations on the spinal column can help correct deformities (eg, scoliosis), decompress the cord, and fuse the spine if disrupted by trauma or degenerative conditions. Spinal surgery may also be performed to resect a tumor or vascular malformation or to drain an abscess or hematoma.

PREOPERATIVE MANAGEMENT

Preoperative evaluation should focus on any anatomic abnormalities and limited neck movements (from disease, traction, "collars," or other devices) that might complicate airway management. Neurological deficits should be documented. Neck mobility should be assessed. Patients with unstable cervical spines can be managed with either awake fiberoptic intubation or intubation after induction with in-line stabilization.

INTRAOPERATIVE MANAGEMENT

Spinal operations involving multiple levels, fusion, and instrumentation are also complicated by the potential for large intraoperative blood loss; a red cell salvage device is often used. Excessive distraction during spinal instrumentation (Harrington rod or pedicle screw fixation) can injure the spinal cord. Transthoracic approaches to the spine require one-lung ventilation. Anterior/posterior approaches require the patient to be repositioned in the middle of surgery.

Positioning

Most spine surgical procedures are carried out in the prone position. The supine position may be used for an anterior approach to the cervical spine, making anesthetic management easier but increasing the risk of injury to the trachea, esophagus, recurrent laryngeal nerve, sympathetic chain, carotid artery, or jugular vein. A sitting (for cervical spine procedures) or lateral decubitus (for lumbar spine procedures) position may occasionally be used.

Following induction of anesthesia and tracheal intubation in the supine position, the patient is turned to the prone position. Care must be taken to maintain the neck in a neutral position. Once in the prone position, the head may be turned to the side (not exceeding the patient's normal range of motion) or (more commonly) can remain face down on a cushioned holder or secured by pins or tongs. Caution is necessary to avoid corneal abrasions or retinal ischemia from pressure on either globe or pressure injuries of the nose, ears, forehead, chin, breasts, or genitalia. The chest should rest on parallel rolls ("chest rolls" of foam, gel, or other padding) or special supports—if a frame is used—to facilitate ventilation. The arms may be tucked by the sides in a comfortable position or extended with the elbows flexed (avoiding excessive abduction at the shoulder).

Turning the patient prone is a critical maneuver, sometimes complicated by hypotension. Abdominal compression, particularly in obese patients, may impede venous return and contribute to excessive intraoperative blood loss from engorgement of epidural veins. Prone positioning with chest rolls that permits the abdomen to hang freely can mitigate this increase in venous pressure. Deliberate hypotension has been advocated in the past to reduce bleeding associated with spine surgery. However, this should only be undertaken with a full understanding that controlled hypotension may increase the risk of perioperative vision loss (POVL).

POVL occurs secondary to:

- Ischemic optic neuropathy
- Perioperative glaucoma
- Cortical hypotension and embolism

Prolonged surgery in a head-down position, major blood loss, relative hypotension, diabetes, obesity, and smoking all put patients at greater risk of POVL following spine surgery.

Airway and facial edema can likewise develop after prolonged "head-down" positioning. Reintubation, if required, will likely present more difficulty than the intubation at the start of surgery.

Specialized head positioning pillows are often used when patients are placed in the prone position, permitting the face to be checked periodically to verify that the eyes, nose, and ears are free of pressure. Even foam cushions can exert pressure over time on the chin, orbit, and maxilla. Turning the head is not easily accomplished when the head is positioned on a cushion; therefore, if prolonged procedures are planned, the head can be secured with pins keeping the face free from any pressure.

Monitoring

When major blood loss is anticipated or the patient has preexisting cardiac disease, intraarterial pressure monitors should be considered prior to
7 "positioning" or "turning." Sudden, massive blood loss from injury to the adjacent great vessels can occur intraoperatively with thoracic or lumbar spine procedures.

Instrumentation of the spine requires the ability to intraoperatively detect spinal cord injury. Intraoperative wake-up techniques employing nitrous oxide-narcotic or total intravenous anesthesia allow the testing of motor function following distraction. Once preservation of motor function is established, the patient's anesthetic can be deepened. Continuous monitoring of somatosensory evoked potentials and motor evoked potentials provides alternatives that avoid the need for intraoperative awakening. These monitoring techniques require the use of propofol, opioid, or ketamine infusions, rather than deep levels of inhalation anesthetics, and the avoidance of neuromuscular paralysis.

CASE DISCUSSION

Resection of a Pituitary Tumor

A 41-year-old woman presents to the operating room for resection of a 10-mm pituitary tumor. She reports amenorrhea and galactorrhea and had recently noticed a decrease in her visual acuity, with bitemporal hemianopsia.

What hormones does the pituitary gland normally secrete?

Functionally and anatomically, the pituitary is divided into two parts: anterior and posterior. The latter is part of the neurohypophysis, which also includes the pituitary stalk and the median eminence.

The anterior pituitary is composed of several cell types, each secreting a specific hormone. Anterior pituitary hormones include adrenocorticotropic hormone (ACTH), thyroid-stimulating hormone (TSH), growth hormone (GH), the gonadotropins (follicle-stimulating hormone [FSH] and luteinizing hormone [LH]), and prolactin (PRL). Secretion of each of these hormones is regulated by hypothalamic peptides (releasing hormones) that are transported to the adenohypophysis by a capillary portal system. The secretion of FSH, LH, ACTH, TSH, and their respective releasing hormones is also under negative feedback control by the products of their target organs. For example, an increase in circulating thyroid hormone inhibits the secretion of TSH-releasing factor and TSH.

The posterior pituitary secretes antidiuretic hormone (ADH, also called vasopressin) and oxytocin. These hormones are actually formed in supraoptic and paraventricular neurons, respectively, and are transported down axons that terminate in the posterior pituitary. Hypothalamic osmoreceptors, and, to a lesser extent, peripheral vascular stretch receptors, regulate the secretion of ADH.

What is the function of these hormones?

ACTH stimulates the adrenal cortex to secrete glucocorticoids. Unlike the production of mineralocorticoids, the production of glucocorticoids is dependent on ACTH secretion. TSH accelerates the synthesis and release of thyroid hormone (thyroxine). Normal thyroid function is dependent on the production of TSH. The gonadotropins FSH and LH are necessary for the normal production of testosterone and spermatogenesis and cyclic ovarian function. GH promotes tissue growth and increases protein synthesis as well as fatty acid mobilization. Its effects on carbohydrate metabolism are to decrease cellular glucose uptake and utilization and increase insulin secretion. PRL functions to support breast development during pregnancy. Dopamine receptor antagonists are known to increase secretion of PRL.

Through its effect on water permeability in renal collecting ducts, ADH regulates extracellular osmolarity and blood volume. Oxytocin acts on areolar myoepithelial cells as part of the milk letdown reflex during suckling and enhances uterine activity during labor.

What factors determine the surgical approach in this patient?

The pituitary gland is attached to the brain by a stalk and extends downward to lie in the sella turcica of the sphenoid bone. Anteriorly, posteriorly, and inferiorly, it is bordered by bone. Laterally, it is bordered by the cavernous sinus, which contains cranial nerves III, IV, V_1, and VI, as well as the cavernous portion of the carotid artery. Superiorly, the diaphragma sella, a thick dural reflection, usually tightly encircles the stalk and forms the roof of the sella turcica. In close proximity to the stalk lie the optic nerves and chiasm. The hypothalamus lies contiguous and superior to the stalk.

Tumors less than 10 mm in diameter are usually approached via the transsphenoidal route, whereas larger tumors and those with significant suprasellar extension are approached via a bifrontal craniotomy. With the use of prophylactic antibiotics, morbidity and mortality rates are significantly less with the transsphenoidal approach; the operation is carried out with the aid of a microscope through an incision in the gingival mucosa beneath the upper lip. The surgeon enters the nasal cavity, dissects through the nasal septum, and finally penetrates the roof of the sphenoid sinus to enter the floor of the sella turcica.

What are the major problems associated with the transsphenoidal approach?

Problems include (1) the need for mucosal injections of epinephrine-containing solution to reduce bleeding, (2) the accumulation of blood and tissue debris in the pharynx and stomach, (3) the risk of hemorrhage from accidental entry into the cavernous sinus or the internal carotid artery, (4) cranial nerve damage, and (5) pituitary hypofunction. Prophylactic administration of glucocorticoids is routinely used in most centers. Diabetes insipidus develops postoperatively in up to 40% of patients but is usually transient. Less commonly, the diabetes insipidus presents intraoperatively. The supine and slightly head-up position used for this procedure may also predispose to venous air embolism.

What type of tumor does this patient have?

Tumors in or around the sella turcica account for 10% to 15% of intracranial neoplasms. Pituitary adenomas are most common, followed by craniopharyngiomas and then parasellar meningiomas. Primary malignant pituitary and metastatic tumors are rare. Pituitary tumors that secrete hormones (functional tumors) usually present early, when they are still relatively small (<10 mm). Other tumors present late, with signs of increased ICP (headache, nausea, and vomiting) or compression of contiguous structures (visual disturbances or pituitary hypofunction). Compression of the optic chiasm classically results in bitemporal hemianopia. Compression of normal pituitary tissue produces progressive endocrine dysfunction. Failure of hormonal secretion usually progresses in the order of gonadotropins, GH, ACTH, and TSH. Diabetes insipidus can also be seen preoperatively. Rarely, hemorrhage into the pituitary results in acute panhypopituitarism (pituitary apoplexy) with signs of a rapidly expanding mass, hemodynamic instability, and hypoglycemia. This patient has the most common type of secretory adenoma, producing hyperprolactinemia.

What other types of secretory hormones are seen?

Adenomas secreting ACTH (Cushing disease) produce classic manifestations of Cushing syndrome: truncal obesity, moon facies, abdominal striae, proximal muscle weakness, hypertension, and osteoporosis. Glucose tolerance is typically impaired, but frank diabetes is less common (<20%). Hirsutism, acne, and amenorrhea are also commonly seen in women.

Adenomas that secrete GH are often large and result in either gigantism (prepubertal patients) or acromegaly (adults). Excessive growth prior to epiphyseal fusion results in massive growth of the entire skeleton. After epiphyseal closure, the abnormal growth is limited to soft tissues and acral parts: hands, feet, nose, and mandible. Patients develop osteoarthritis, which often affects the temporomandibular joint and spine. Diabetes, myopathies, and neuropathies are common. Cardiovascular complications include hypertension, premature coronary disease, and cardiomyopathy in some patients. The most serious anesthetic problem encountered in these patients is difficulty in intubating the trachea.

Are any special monitors required for transsphenoidal surgery?

Monitoring should be carried out in somewhat the same way as for craniotomies. Visual evoked potentials may be employed with large tumors that involve the optic nerves. Precordial Doppler sonography may be used for detecting venous air embolism. Venous access with large-bore catheters is desirable in the event of massive hemorrhage.

What modifications, if any, are necessary in the anesthetic technique?

The same principles discussed for craniotomies apply; however, patients rarely have evidence of increased ICP. Intravenous antibiotic prophylaxis and glucocorticoid coverage (hydrocortisone, 100 mg) are usually given prior to induction. Many clinicians avoid nitrous oxide to prevent problems with postoperative pneumocephalus (see earlier discussion). Effective neuromuscular blockade is important to prevent movement while the surgeon is using the microscope. A lumbar drain is often placed to reduce ICP, facilitate surgical exposure, and reduce the likelihood of CSF leaks after closure of the dura.

SUGGESTED READINGS

Bell R, Vo A, Vexnedaroglu E, et al. The endovascular operating room as an extension of the intensive care unit: Changing strategies in the management of neurovascular disease. *Neurosurgery*. 2006;59:S3.

Bhattacharya B, Maung AA. Anesthesia for patients with traumatic brain injuries. *Anesthesiol Clin*. 2016;34:747.

Bilotta F, Guerra C, Rosa G. Update on anesthesia for craniotomy. *Curr Opin Anesthesiol*. 2013;26:517.

Datar S, Rabinstein AA. Postinterventional critical care management of aneurysmal subarachnoid hemorrhage. *Curr Opin Crit Care*. 2017;23:87.

De Sloovere V. Anesthesia for embolization of cerebral aneurysms. *Curr Opin Anesthesiol*. 2014;27:431.

Dority J, Oldham J. Subarachnoid hemorrhage: an update. *Anesthesiol Clin*. 2016;34:577.

Flexman AM, Meng L, Gelb AW. Outcomes in neuroanesthesia: what matters most? *Can J Anaesth*. 2016;63:205.

Flexman AM, Wang T, Meng L. Neuroanesthesia and outcomes: evidence, opinions, and speculations on clinically relevant topics. *Curr Opin Anaesthesiol*. 2019;32:539.

Frost E, Booij L. Anesthesia in the patient for awake craniotomy. *Curr Opin Anaesthesiol*. 2007;20:331.

Goyal M, Yu AY, Menon BK, et al. Endovascular therapy in acute ischemic stroke: challenges and transition from trials to bedside. *Stroke*. 2016;47:548.

Hutchinson P, Kolias A, Timofeev I, et al. Trial of decompressive craniectomy for traumatic intracranial hypertension. *N Engl J Med*. 2016;375:1119.

Jinadasa S, Boone M. Controversies in the management of traumatic brain injury. *Anesthesiol Clin*. 2016;34:557.

Kulikov A, Lubnin A. Anesthesia for awake craniotomy. *Curr Opin Anaesthesiol*. 2018;31:506.

Li K, Barras CD, Chandra RV, et al. A review of the management of cerebral vasospasm after aneurysmal subarachnoid hemorrhage. *World Neurosurg*. 2019;126:513.

Marcolini E, Stretz C, DeWitt KM. Intracranial hemorrhage and intracranial hypertension. *Emerg Med Clin North Am.* 2019;37:529.

Quillinan N, Herson P, Traystam. Neuropathophysiology of brain injury. *Anesthesiol Clin.* 2016;34:453.

Rabai F, Sessions R, Seubert CN. Neurophysiological monitoring and spinal cord integrity. *Best Pract Res Clin Anaesthesiol.* 2016;30:53.

Rao S, Avitsian R. Anesthesia for neurosurgical emergencies. *Anesthesiol Clin.* 2020;38:67.

Rowland M, Hadjipavlou G, Kelly M, et al. Delayed cerebral ischaemia after subarachnoid haemorrhage: looking beyond vasospasm. *Br J Anaesth.* 2012;109:315.

Sanchez-Porras R, Santos E, Scholl E, et al. The effect of ketamine on optical and electrical characteristics of spreading depolarizations in gyrencephalic swine cortex. *Neuropharmacology.* 2014;84:52.

Sharma D, Vavilala M. Perioperative management of adult traumatic brain injury. *Anesthesiol Clin.* 2012;30:333.

Smith M. Refractory intracranial hypertension: the role of decompressive craniectomy. *Anesth Analg.* 2017;125:1999.

Stocchetti N, Zoerle T, Carbonara M. Intracranial pressure management in patients with traumatic brain injury: an update. *Curr Opin Crit Care.* 2017;23:110.

Todd MM. Outcomes after neuroanesthesia and neurosurgery: what makes a difference. *Anesthesiol Clin.* 2012;30:399.

Venkatraghavan L, Luciano M, Manninen P. Anesthetic management of patients undergoing deep brain stimulation insertion. *Anesth Analg.* 2010;110:1138.

CHAPTER 28

Anesthesia for Patients with Neurological & Psychiatric Diseases

KEY CONCEPTS

1. Induction of anesthesia in patients receiving long-term levodopa therapy may result in either marked hypotension or hypertension.
2. In patients with multiple sclerosis, increases in body temperature cause exacerbation of symptoms.
3. The major risk of anesthesia in patients with autonomic dysfunction is severe hypotension, compromising cerebral and coronary blood flow.
4. Autonomic hyperreflexia should be expected in patients with spinal cord lesions above T6 and can be precipitated by surgical manipulations.
5. The most important interaction between anesthetic agents and tricyclic antidepressants is an exaggerated response to both indirect-acting vasopressors and sympathetic stimulation.

Patients with vascular and nonvascular neurological diseases or psychiatric disorders are frequently encountered by anesthesia providers. Anesthesiologists must have a basic understanding of the major neurological and psychiatric disorders and their drug therapy. Failure to recognize potential adverse anesthetic interactions may result in avoidable perioperative morbidity.

Cerebrovascular Disease

Preoperative Considerations

Patients with diagnosed cerebrovascular disease typically have a history of transient ischemic attacks (TIAs) or stroke. Patients with TIAs undergoing surgery for other indications have an increased risk of perioperative stroke. Asymptomatic carotid bruits occur in up to 4% of patients older than age 40 years, but they do not necessarily indicate significant carotid artery obstruction. Fewer than 10% of patients with asymptomatic bruits have hemodynamically significant carotid artery lesions. An asymptomatic carotid bruit may not increase the risk of stroke following surgery, but it increases the likelihood of coexisting coronary artery disease. Moreover, the absence of a bruit does not exclude significant carotid obstruction.

The risk of perioperative stroke increases with patient age and varies with the type of surgery. Rates of stroke after general anesthesia and surgery range from 0.08% to 0.4%. Even in patients with known cerebrovascular disease, the risk is only 0.4% to 3.3%. Although the overall risk of stroke associated with surgery is low, it is greatest in those undergoing open heart procedures for valvular disease, coronary artery disease with ascending aortic atherosclerosis, diseases of the thoracic aorta, and those undergoing cerebrovascular surgery. Stroke following open heart surgery is usually attributed to embolism of air, clots, or atheromatous debris. In one study, 6% of patients experienced an adverse neurological outcome following cardiac surgery. Stroke following thoracic aortic surgery may be due to emboli or ischemia secondary to prolonged circulatory arrest or a clamp placed close to the origin of the carotid artery.

The pathophysiology of postoperative strokes following noncardiovascular surgery is less clear but may involve sustained hypotension or hypertension. Hypotension with cerebral hypoperfusion can result in so-called watershed zone infarctions or thrombosis of cerebral arteries, whereas hypertension can result in intracerebral hemorrhage (hemorrhagic stroke). Sustained hypertension can disrupt the blood–brain barrier and promote cerebral edema. Perioperative atrial fibrillation can likewise lead to atrial clot formation and cerebral embolism. The period of time during which nonemergency anesthesia and surgery should best be avoided following a stroke is not clear. Abnormalities in regional blood flow and metabolic rate usually resolve after 2 weeks, whereas alterations in CO_2 responsiveness and the blood–brain barrier may require more than 4 weeks. However, urgent surgery is performed for acute intracranial hemorrhage, symptomatic carotid disease, and cardiac sources of emboli.

Patients with TIAs have a history of transient (<24 h) impairment and, by definition, no residual neurological impairment. These attacks are thought to result from emboli of fibrin-platelet aggregates that form on plaques in extracranial vessels. Unilateral visual impairment, numbness or weakness of an extremity, or aphasia is suggestive of carotid disease, whereas bilateral visual impairment, dizziness, ataxia, dysarthria, bilateral weakness, or amnesia is suggestive of vertebral–basilar disease. Patients with TIAs have a 30% to 40% chance of developing a frank stroke within 5 years; 50% of these strokes occur within the first year. Patients with TIAs should not undergo any elective surgical procedure without an adequate medical evaluation that generally includes at least noninvasive (Doppler) flow and imaging studies. The presence of an ulcerated plaque of greater than 60% occlusion is generally an indication for endovascular intervention or, less commonly, an open carotid thromboendarterectomy.

PREOPERATIVE MANAGEMENT

Preoperative assessment requires neurological and cardiovascular evaluations. The type of stroke, the presence of neurological deficits, and the extent of residual impairment should be determined. Thromboembolic strokes usually occur in patients with generalized atherosclerosis. Most patients are older adults with comorbid conditions, such as hypertension, hyperlipidemia, and diabetes. Coexisting coronary artery disease and renal impairment are common. Following ischemic strokes or TIAs, many patients are placed on long-term anticoagulant or antiplatelet therapy, or both. Management of antiplatelet therapy and antithrombotic therapy should be reviewed by the anesthesia and surgical teams, often guided by the physician who prescribed the therapy, to determine the risks and benefits of discontinuation or maintenance of such therapy perioperatively. Other systemic diseases, such as diabetes, hypertension, coronary artery disease, heart failure, and chronic obstructive lung disease, frequently manifest in patients with cerebrovascular disease.

INTRAOPERATIVE MANAGEMENT

Management of the patient following acute embolic stroke is directed toward the embolic source. Cardiac surgery is performed to remove atrial myxomas. Systemic emboli can also be produced from endocarditic vegetations, as well as from degenerated heart valves and intracardiac thrombus.

Patients with acute strokes secondary to carotid and intracranial occlusive arterial disease present for carotid endarterectomy and endovascular procedures. When an awake procedure is undertaken, the patient serves as a monitor of the adequacy of cerebral blood flow during the application of vessel clamps or the placement of a stent. When general anesthesia is used, electroencephalography, evoked potentials, carotid stump pressure, near-infrared cerebral oximetry, or transcranial Doppler may be used to estimate the adequacy of cerebral oxygen delivery. During open carotid thromboendarterectomy, the surgeon may place a shunt to deliver blood to the brain around the cross-clamped vessel. Despite adequate cerebral

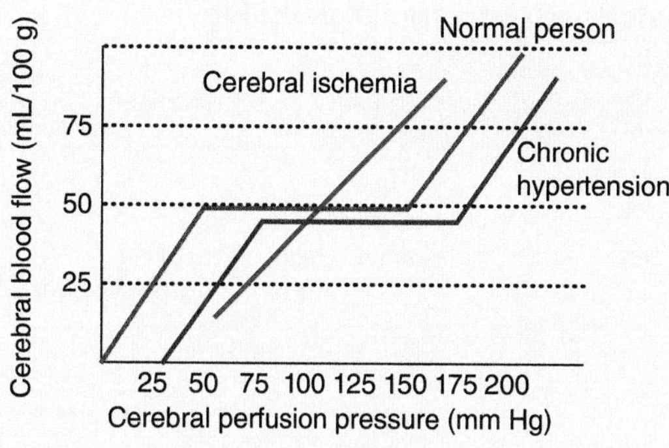

FIGURE 28–1 Cerebral autoregulation in a normal person, cerebral ischemia, and chronic hypertension. (Reproduced with permission from Shaikh S. Anesthesia considerations for the patient with acute ischemic stroke. *Semin Cardiothorac Vasc Anesth.* 2010 Mar;14(1):62-63.)

blood flow, perioperative stroke can occur during carotid surgery secondary to emboli.

The management of patients following thrombotic or hemorrhagic stroke for nonneurological surgery must be individualized. Cerebral autoregulation of blood flow may fail, leaving flow directly dependent upon cerebral perfusion pressure (Figure 28–1). The penumbra of potentially salvageable neurological tissue may therefore be very sensitive to injury from the effects of both hypotension and hypertension (Figure 28–2). We advocate tight control of blood pressure in these patients.

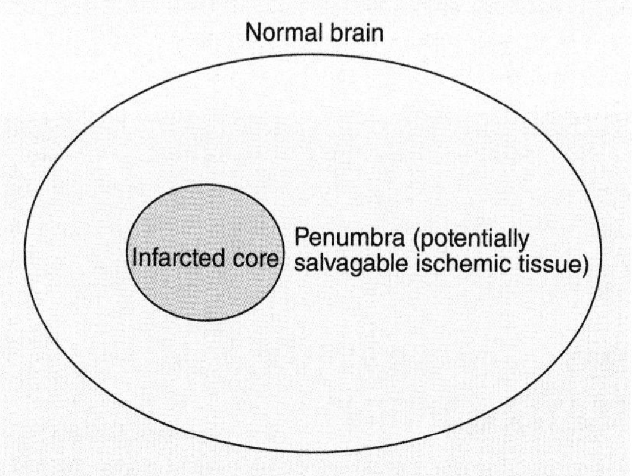

FIGURE 28–2 Penumbra. (Reproduced with permission from Shaikh S. Anesthesia considerations for the patient with acute ischemic stroke. *Semin Cardiothorac Vasc Anesth.* 2010 Mar;14(1):62-63.)

Patients taken to surgery following administration of thrombolytic therapy are at increased risk of cerebral hemorrhage, and tight blood pressure control may reduce the likelihood of cerebral bleeding.

Patients with major intracerebral hemorrhage or epidural or subdural hematomas after trauma typically undergo craniotomy and evacuation of hematoma. Invasive arterial pressure monitoring is helpful in these patients, given that cerebral autoregulation is deranged (see Figure 28–1). Hypertension is frequently treated with intravenous vasodilators and β-blockers. Subarachnoid hemorrhage is discussed in Chapter 27.

INTRACRANIAL TUMORS

Patients with intracranial mass lesions frequently present to their primary care physicians with reports of headache, visual disturbances, or seizures. Families may have noticed behavioral changes in patients with frontal lobe masses. Imaging studies confirm the presence of a mass, and initial treatment with dexamethasone is aimed at decreasing cerebral edema. Electrolytes should be reviewed perioperatively in all patients undergoing cranial surgery as both hyponatremia and hypernatremia can develop secondary to cerebral salt wasting, inappropriate antidiuretic hormone secretion, or central diabetes insipidus (Table 28–1; see also Chapter 49). Patients with altered mentation preoperatively may likewise be dehydrated. Hyperglycemia secondary to steroid use is frequently seen.

Seizure Disorders

Preoperative Considerations

Seizures represent abnormal synchronized electrical activity in the brain. They may be a manifestation of an underlying central nervous system disease, a systemic disorder, or idiopathic. Up to 2% of the population may experience a seizure in their lifetime. Epilepsy is a disorder characterized by recurrent paroxysmal seizure activity. Healthy individuals who experience an isolated nonrecurrent seizure are not considered to have epilepsy.

Seizure activity may be localized to a specific area in the brain or may be generalized. Moreover,

TABLE 28–1 Fluid and electrolyte disorders associated with intracranial pathology.

Condition	Serum Sodium Concentration	Plasma Volume	Serum Osmolality	Urine Sodium Concentration	Urine Osmolality	Treatment
SIADH	Low	Normal or increased	Low	High	High	Fluid restriction
CSWS	Low	Decreased	Normal or high	High	Normal or high	Isotonic or hypertonic saline
DI	High	Decreased	High	Normal	Low	Hypotonic saline + vasopressin

CSWS, cerebral salt wasting syndrome; DI, diabetes insipidus; SIADH, syndrome of inappropriate antidiuretic hormone secretion.

Reproduced with permission from Reddy U, Amin Y. Preoperative assessment of neurosurgical patients. *Anaesth Intensive Care Med.* 2010 Sep;11(9):357-362.

initially localized (focal) seizures can subsequently spread, becoming generalized. A simple classification scheme is presented in Table 28–2. Partial seizures (also called focal) are clinically manifested by motor, sensory, autonomic, or psychiatric symptoms, depending on the brain region affected. Focal seizures associated with impairment in consciousness are termed *complex partial* (psychomotor or temporal lobe) *seizures.* Generalized seizures characteristically produce bilaterally symmetric electrical activity without local onset. They may result in abnormal motor activity, loss of consciousness, or both. Absence (petit mal) seizures produce generalized activity resulting in isolated, transient lapses in consciousness. Other generalized seizures are usually classified according to the type of motor activity. Tonic–clonic (grand mal) seizures are most common and are characterized by a loss of consciousness followed by clonic and then tonic motor activity.

TABLE 28–2 Classification of seizures.

Partial (focal)
Simple
Complex
Secondarily generalized tonic–clonic
Generalized
Absence (petit mal)
Myoclonic
Clonic
Tonic
Tonic–clonic (grand mal)
Atonic

PREOPERATIVE MANAGEMENT

Anesthetic evaluation should focus primarily on the cause and type of seizure activity and the drugs with which the patient is being treated. Seizures in adults are most commonly due to structural brain lesions (head trauma, tumor, degeneration, or stroke) or metabolic abnormalities (uremia, hepatic failure, hypoglycemia, hypocalcemia, drug toxicity, or drug/alcohol withdrawal). Idiopathic seizures occur more often in children than in adults. Grand mal seizures are serious complicating factors in surgical patients and should be treated promptly to prevent musculoskeletal injury, hypoventilation, hypoxemia, and aspiration of gastrointestinal contents. If a seizure occurs, maintaining an open airway and adequate oxygenation are the first priorities. Propofol (50–100 mg) or a benzodiazepine such as diazepam (5–10 mg) or midazolam (1–5 mg) can be given intravenously to terminate the seizure.

Most patients with seizure disorders receive antiepileptic drugs (AEDs) preoperatively (Table 28–3). AEDs should be continued throughout the perioperative period to maintain therapeutic levels.

INTRAOPERATIVE MANAGEMENT

Hepatic microsomal enzyme induction should be expected from chronic antiseizure therapy. Enzyme induction may increase the dose requirement and frequency of intravenous anesthetics and

TABLE 28–3 AEDs: their mechanism of action, efficacy, and possible adverse affects.

AED	Mechanism of Action	Efficacy	Adverse Effects
Carbamazepine	Reduction of inward voltage-gated Na^+ currents	Focal seizures, mood stabilizer	Hypersensitivity reactions, cardiac conduction abnormalities, hyponatremia, reduced bone marrow function
Clobazam	Potentiates GABAergic neurotransmission by binding to benzodiazepine site of the $GABA_A$ receptor	Adjunctive therapy of Lennox Gastaut syndrome in patients over 2 years. Under investigation for use in focal or generalized seizures. Used in nonconvulsive status epilepticus.	Drowsiness, dizziness, depression, and aggressiveness. Sudden discontinuation can cause withdrawal seizures
Clonazepam	Potentiates GABAnergic neurotransmission by binding to benzodiazepine site of the $GABA_A$ receptor	Second-line for adjunctive treatment for focal and generalized (particularly absence and myoclonic) seizures, early status epilepticus, and Lennox–Gastaut syndrome	Sedation and cognitive impairment. Tolerance and withdrawal symptoms may develop on sudden discontinuation.
Lacosamide	Enhances slow inactivation component of voltage-gated sodium channels	Adjunctive treatment for focal seizures in patients >16 years	Dizziness, fatigue, nausea and ataxia, prolonged PR interval
Lamotrigine	Reduction of inward voltage-gated Na^+ and Ca^{2+} currents	Efficacious against focal and most generalized seizure types, devoid of enzyme-inducing properties, effective in bipolar depression	Rash and other hypersensitivity reactions
Levetiracetam	Thought to reduce inward voltage-gated Ca^{2+} currents	Efficacious against focal, myoclonic, and primarily generalized tonic–clonic seizures; virtually devoid of drug interactions; relatively well tolerated	Irritability, mood changes
Phenobarbital	Increased mean Cl^- channel opening duration	Efficacious against focal and most generalized seizures, extensive experience	Cognitive and behavioral adverse effects
Phenytoin	Reduction of inward voltage-gated Na^+ currents	Efficacious against focal seizures, extensive experience	Rash and other hypersensitivity reactions; connective tissue and cosmetic adverse effects
Topiramate	Multiple sites of action including Na^+ channels, Ca^{2+} channels, and GABA receptors	Efficacious against focal and most generalized seizure types; effective for migraine prophylaxis	Metabolic acidosis, cognitive effects, weight loss, paresthesia, nephrolithiasis, glaucoma
Valproic acid	Multiple sites of action including increased GABA levels by inhibiting reuptake and breakdown, Na^+ channel blocker	Unsurpassed efficacy against most generalized seizure types; also effective against focal seizures; effective for migraine prophylaxis; mood stabilizer	Hepatotoxicity, hyperammonemic encephalopathy, pancreatitis, platelet dysfunction, thrombocytopenia, greater teratogenic potential than for other antiepileptic drugs, postnatal cognitive effects after fetal exposure

Reproduced with permission from Bloor M, Nandi R, Thomas M. Antiepileptic drugs and anesthesia, *Paediatr Anaesth*. 2017 Mar;27(3):248-250.

nondepolarizing neuromuscular blockers (NMBs) and may increase the risk for hepatotoxicity from halothane. The epileptogenic potential of metabolites of atracurium and meperidine (laudanosine and normeperidine, respectively) is largely of theoretical interest.

Degenerative & Demyelinating Diseases

PARKINSON DISEASE

Preoperative Considerations

Parkinson disease (PD) is a common movement disorder that typically afflicts individuals aged 50 to 70 years; it has a prevalence of 3% in North America. This neurodegenerative disease is characterized by bradykinesia, rigidity, postural instability, and a resting (pill-rolling) tremor. Additional frequently occurring findings include facial masking, hypophonia, dysphagia, and gait disturbances. Increasing problems with freezing, rigidity, and tremor eventually result in physical incapacitation. Early in the course of the disease, intellectual function is usually preserved, but the disease may progress to Lewy body dementia. PD is caused by a progressive loss of dopamine in the nigrostriatal pathway. Concurrent with the loss of dopamine, the activity of the γ-aminobutyric acid (GABA) nuclei in the basal ganglia increases, leading to an inhibition of thalamic and brainstem nuclei. Thalamic inhibition, in turn, suppresses the motor system in the cortex, resulting in the characteristic signs and symptoms.

Medical treatment is directed at controlling the symptoms. A variety of drugs may be used for mild disease, including levodopa, dopamine receptor agonists, monoamine oxidase (MAO) B inhibitors, anticholinergic agents, amantadine, and catechol-O-methyltransferase (COMT) inhibitors.

Moderate to severe disease is typically treated pharmacologically with dopaminergic agents, either levodopa (a precursor of dopamine) or a dopamine-receptor agonist. COMT inhibitors are also used to prevent the decarboxylation of levodopa. Levodopa side effects include nausea, vomiting, dyskinesias, sudden sleepiness, cardiac irritability, and orthostatic hypotension. Dopamine receptor agonists include both ergot derivatives (bromocriptine and cabergoline) and nonergot derivatives (pramipexole and ropinirole). The nonergot derivatives have been shown to be beneficial when used as monotherapy in early PD; all dopamine receptor agonists are effective when given as combination therapy with levodopa in the treatment of moderate to severe PD. Side effects are similar to those found with the use of levodopa alone and include headache, confusion, and hallucinations. Pulmonary, cardiac, and retroperitoneal fibrosis; pleural effusion and thickening; Raynaud syndrome; and erythromelalgia are more common side effects with the use of ergot derivatives than with nonergot derivatives.

The surgical treatment of PD formerly included ablative procedures (thalamotomy and pallidotomy), but implantation of electrodes for deep brain stimulation is currently the most common approach. Stimulation of the subthalamic nucleus improves all of the primary symptoms of PD and results in a greater decrease in the amount of medication required for symptom relief when compared with stimulation of the globus pallidus pars internus. However, globus pallidus pars internus stimulation may produce greater improvement in dyskinesia as compared with stimulation of the subthalamic nucleus.

Anesthetic Considerations

Medications for PD should be continued perioperatively, including the morning of surgery, because of the short half-life of levodopa. Abrupt withdrawal of levodopa can cause worsening muscle rigidity and may interfere with ventilation. Phenothiazines, butyrophenones (droperidol), and metoclopramide can exacerbate symptoms as a consequence of their antidopaminergic activity and should be avoided. Anticholinergics (atropine) or antihistamines (diphenhydramine) may be used for acute exacerbation of symptoms. Diphenhydramine may be used for intraoperative sedation in patients with tremor. Induction

1 of anesthesia in patients receiving long-term levodopa therapy may result in either marked hypotension or hypertension. Relative hypovolemia, catecholamine depletion, autonomic instability, and sensitization to catecholamines are probably

contributory. Hypotension should be treated with small doses of a direct-acting vasopressor, such as phenylephrine, rather than ephedrine. The response to NMBs is generally normal. As mentioned previously, patients who fail medical treatment are candidates for surgical intervention—for example, implantation of a deep brain stimulator. Because general anesthesia alters the threshold for stimulation, it can make the correct placement of the electrodes difficult or impossible. Awake craniotomy has been the norm for epilepsy surgery and is commonly used for deep brain stimulation procedures. Two techniques are advocated: (1) a true awake craniotomy with heavy sedation (we recommend dexmedetomidine), and (2) an approach in which the patient receives a general anesthetic, usually a total intravenous anesthetic with propofol and remifentanil and a laryngeal mask airway for control of the airway. Following appropriate surgical exposure, the intravenous infusions are discontinued, and the laryngeal mask airway is removed. The patient can be reanesthetized once the implantation of leads is complete.

ALZHEIMER DISEASE & OTHER COMMON DEMENTIAS

Preoperative Considerations

Neurodegenerative diseases often lead to dementia. The incidence of dementia varies by population but seems to double every decade of life, starting at age 60. Alzheimer disease (AD) is the most common neurodegenerative disease, causing more than half of all cases of dementia; dementia with Lewy bodies (often associated with PD) and vascular dementia comprise most of the rest. Slow, progressive impairment of memory, judgment, and decision making, as well as emotional lability, are hallmarks of AD. Late in the course of the disease, severe extrapyramidal signs, apraxias, and aphasia are often present. Patients with AD usually show marked cortical atrophy with ventricular enlargement; the pathological hallmarks of AD seen at necropsy include neurofibrillary tangles that contain phosphorylated microtubular tau proteins, neuritic plaques, and excessive brain concentrations of amyloid β-peptides.

Anesthetic Considerations

Anesthetic management of patients with moderate to severe dementia is often complicated by disorientation and uncooperativeness. New onset of temporary cognitive impairment is frequent in older adult patients and often persists for 1 to 3 days following surgery. Such patients require repeated reassurance and explanation. Legally incompetent patients cannot provide informed consent for anesthesia or surgery. We avoid premedication if possible. Centrally acting anticholinergics, such as atropine and scopolamine, may contribute to postoperative confusion. Glycopyrrolate, which does not cross the blood–brain barrier, is the preferred agent when an anticholinergic is required (other than for resuscitation). Patients having dementia with Lewy bodies often have PD, and thus the anesthetic issues with PD that were addressed earlier in the chapter would apply.

Animal studies have shown that conventional general anesthetic agents are associated with neuronal injury and cell death. The outcome implications of general anesthesia in both older adults and small children are currently the subject of much investigation and debate. Apoptotic neurodegeneration has been linked to the use of GABA receptor modulators and *N*-methyl-D-aspartic acid receptor antagonists, mechanisms by which common general anesthetics produce their effects. Moreover, increased β-amyloid production is associated with anesthetic exposure; tau protein phosphorylation increases after general anesthesia; and hypothermia transiently increases tau protein phosphorylation. Despite concerns about anesthetic exposure in patients with or at risk for AD, current studies do not support avoiding needed surgery in this group.

MULTIPLE SCLEROSIS

Preoperative Considerations

Multiple sclerosis (MS) is characterized by demyelination at multiple sites in the brain and spinal cord; chronic inflammation eventually produces scarring (gliosis). MS primarily affects patients between 20 and 40 years of age, with a 2:1 female predominance, and typically follows an unpredictable course of attacks and remissions. With time,

remissions become less complete, and the disease progresses to incapacitation; almost 50% of patients will require help with walking within 15 years of diagnosis. Clinical manifestations depend on the sites affected but frequently include sensory disturbances (paresthesia), visual problems (optic neuritis and diplopia), and motor weakness. Symptoms develop over the course of days and remit over weeks to months. Early diagnosis of exacerbations can often be confirmed by analysis of cerebrospinal fluid and magnetic resonance imaging. Remyelination is limited and often fails to occur. Moreover, axonal loss can develop. Changes in neurological function seem to be related to changes in axonal conduction. Conduction can occur across demyelinated axons but seems to be affected by multiple
2 factors, particularly temperature. In patients with MS, increases in body temperature cause exacerbation of symptoms.

The treatments of MS focus separately on symptoms and attempts to arrest the disease process. Diazepam, dantrolene, or baclofen, and, in refractory cases, an intrathecal delivery system for baclofen are used to control spasticity; bethanechol is useful for urinary retention. Painful dysesthesia may respond to carbamazepine, phenytoin, or antidepressants. Glucocorticoids may decrease the severity and duration of acute attacks. Corticosteroid-resistant relapses may respond to five to seven courses of plasma exchange offered on alternate days. Interferon has also been used to treat MS. Immunomodulation with a variety of drugs has been used in an attempt to halt disease progression. The systemic effects of these therapies on coagulation, immunological, hepatic, and cardiac function should be reviewed preoperatively.

Anesthetic Considerations

The effect of stress, anesthesia, and surgery on the course of MS is controversial. Overall, the effect of anesthesia is unpredictable. Elective surgery should be avoided during relapse, regardless of the anesthetic technique employed. The preoperative consent record should document counseling of the patient to the effect that the stress of surgery and anesthesia might worsen symptoms. Spinal anesthesia has been associated with exacerbation of the disease; however, the entire surgery/delivery/anesthetic process may likewise lead to exacerbations. Peripheral nerve blocks are less of a concern because MS is a disease of the central nervous system; however, patients may have preexisting peripheral neuropathies. Epidural and other regional techniques seem to have no adverse effect on the course of the disease. No specific interactions with general anesthetics are recognized. Patients with advanced disease may have a labile cardiovascular system due to autonomic dysfunction. In the setting of paresis or paralysis, succinylcholine should be avoided because of possible hyperkalemia. Increases in body temperature should be avoided. Irrespective of the anesthetic technique, patients may experience a worsening of symptoms perioperatively and should be counseled accordingly.

AMYOTROPHIC LATERAL SCLEROSIS

Amyotrophic lateral sclerosis (ALS) is the most prevalent motor neuron neurodegenerative disease. The cause of ALS is unknown, though small numbers of patients with the familial form of the disease have a defect in the superoxide dismutase-1 gene. ALS is a rapidly progressive disorder of both upper and lower motor neurons. Patients often present in the fifth or sixth decade of life with muscular weakness, atrophy, fasciculation, and spasticity. The disease may initially be asymmetric but over the course of 2 to 3 years becomes generalized, involving all skeletal and bulbar muscles. Progressive respiratory muscle weakness makes the patient susceptible to aspiration and eventually leads to death from pneumonia or ventilatory failure. Although the heart is unaffected, autonomic dysfunction can be seen. The primary emphasis in perioperative management is on judicious respiratory care. As with other patients with lower motor neuron disease, succinylcholine is contraindicated because of the risk of hyperkalemia. Adequacy of ventilation should be carefully assessed both intraoperatively and postoperatively; an awake extubation is desirable. Difficulty in weaning patients from mechanical ventilation postoperatively may be anticipated in patients with advanced disease.

GUILLAIN–BARRÉ SYNDROME

Guillain–Barré syndrome (GBS), a relatively common disorder affecting 1 to 4 individuals per 100,000 population, is characterized by a sudden onset of ascending motor paralysis, areflexia, and variable paresthesias. Subtypes of GBS include acute inflammatory demyelinating polyneuropathy (about 75% of cases), acute motor axonal neuropathy (with antibodies against gangliosides), and acute motor sensory axonal neuropathy. Bulbar involvement, including respiratory muscle paralysis, is common. Pathologically, the disease is the result of an immunological reaction against the myelin sheath of peripheral nerves, particularly lower motor neurons. In most instances, the syndrome seems to follow an infection; the disorder can also present as a paraneoplastic syndrome associated with Hodgkin disease or as a complication of human immunodeficiency virus infection. Some patients respond to plasmapheresis. The prognosis is relatively good, with most patients recovering completely; however, approximately 10% of patients die of complications, and another 10% are left with long-term neurological sequelae.

Anesthetic management is complicated by lability of the autonomic nervous system in addition to concerns about respiratory insufficiency. Exaggerated hypotensive and hypertensive responses during anesthesia may be seen. As with other lower motor neuron disorders, succinylcholine should not be used because of the risk of hyperkalemia. The use of regional anesthesia in these patients remains controversial as it might worsen symptoms. As with all decisions, the risks and benefits of regional versus general anesthesia must be weighed on an individual basis. As damaged nerves are more susceptible to a second injury (the "double crush" effect), the performance of regional techniques in patients with preexistent neurological dysfunction should be carefully considered.

AUTONOMIC DYSFUNCTIONS

Preoperative Considerations

Autonomic dysfunction, or dysautonomia, may be due to generalized or segmental disorders of the central or peripheral nervous system. Symptoms can be generalized, segmental, or focal. These disorders may be congenital, familial, or acquired. Common manifestations include impotence; bladder and gastrointestinal dysfunction; abnormal regulation of body fluids; decreased sweating, lacrimation, and salivation; and orthostatic hypotension. The latter can be the most serious manifestation of the disorder.

Acquired autonomic dysfunction can be isolated (pure autonomic failure), part of a more generalized degenerative process (Shy–Drager syndrome, PD, olivopontocerebellar atrophy), part of a segmental neurological process (MS, syringomyelia, reflex sympathetic dystrophy, or spinal cord injury), or a manifestation of disorders affecting peripheral nerves (GBS, diabetes, chronic alcoholism, amyloidosis, or porphyria).

There are at least three forms of hereditary sensory and autonomic neuropathies, each with its own underlying genetic mutation(s). Autonomic dysfunction is prominent and is associated with generalized diminished sensation and emotional lability. Moreover, patients are predisposed to dysautonomic crises triggered by stress and characterized by marked hypertension, tachycardia, abdominal pain, diaphoresis, vomiting, and the risk of dehydration.

Anesthetic Considerations

3 The major risk of anesthesia in patients with autonomic dysfunction is severe hypotension, compromising cerebral and coronary blood flow. Marked hypertension can be equally deleterious. Most patients are chronically hypovolemic, and if volume deficits are not corrected, the vasodilatory effects of spinal and epidural anesthesia are poorly tolerated. The vasodilatory and cardiac depressant effects of most general anesthetic agents combined with positive airway pressure can be equally problematic. Continuous intraarterial blood pressure monitoring is useful. Hypotension should be treated with fluids and direct-acting vasopressors (in preference to indirect-acting agents). The dose–response relationship for vasopressors may be abnormal due to denervation. Blood loss also is usually poorly tolerated. Body temperature should be monitored closely. Patients with anhidrosis are particularly susceptible to hyperpyrexia.

SYRINGOMYELIA

Syringomyelia results in progressive cavitation of the spinal cord. In many cases, obstruction of cerebrospinal fluid outflow from the fourth ventricle seems to be contributory. Many patients have craniovertebral abnormalities, particularly the Arnold–Chiari malformation. Increased pressure in the central canal of the spinal cord produces enlargement or diverticulation to the point of cavitation. Syringomyelia typically affects the cervical spine, producing sensory and motor deficits in the upper extremities and, frequently, thoracic scoliosis. Extension upward into the medulla (syringobulbia) leads to cranial nerve deficits. Syringoperitoneal shunting and other decompressive procedures have variable success in arresting the disease.

Anesthetic evaluation should focus on defining existing neurological deficits and any pulmonary impairment due to scoliosis. Autonomic instability should be expected in patients with extensive lesions. Succinylcholine should be avoided when muscle wasting is present because of the risk of hyperkalemia. As always, adequate ventilation and full reversal of nondepolarizing NMBs should be achieved prior to extubation. Spinal puncture is contraindicated with intracranial hypertension because of the risk of brain herniation. Epidural anesthetics have been used successfully for labor analgesia in patients with Arnold–Chiari malformations, with and without syringomyelia. Risks of cerebral herniation, worsening nerve injury, and infection must be weighed against potential benefits.

Spinal Cord Injury

Preoperative Considerations

Spinal cord injuries are most often traumatic and may arise from partial or complete transection. Most injuries are due to fracture and dislocation of the vertebral column. The mechanism is usually either compression and flexion at the thoracic spine or extension at the cervical spine. Clinical manifestations depend on the level of the injury. Injuries above C3–5 (diaphragmatic innervation) require patients to receive ventilatory support to stay alive. Transections above T1 result in quadriplegia, whereas those at T2 or below result in paraplegia. The most common sites of injury are C5–6 and T12–L1. Acute spinal cord transection produces loss of sensation, flaccid paralysis, and loss of spinal reflexes below the level of injury. These findings characterize a period of spinal shock that typically lasts 1 to 3 weeks.

Over the course of the next few weeks, spinal reflexes gradually return, together with muscle spasms and signs of sympathetic overactivity. Injury in the low thoracic or lumbar spine may result in cauda equina (conus medullaris) syndrome. The latter usually consists of incomplete injury to nerve roots rather than the spinal cord.

Overactivity of the sympathetic nervous system is common with transections at T5 or above but is unusual with injuries below T10. Interruption of normal descending inhibitory impulses in the cord results in autonomic hyperreflexia. Cutaneous or visceral stimulation below the level of injury can induce intense autonomic reflexes: sympathetic discharge produces hypertension and vasoconstriction below the transection and baroreceptor-mediated reflex bradycardia and vasodilation above the transection. Cardiac arrhythmias are common.

Emergency surgical management is undertaken whenever there is reversible compression of the spinal cord due to dislocation of a vertebral body or bony fragment. Operative treatment is also indicated for spinal instability to prevent further injury.

Anesthetic Considerations

A. Acute Transection

Anesthetic management depends on the age of the injury. In the early care of acute injuries, the emphasis should be on preventing further spinal cord damage during patient movement, airway manipulation, and positioning. Airway management of the patient with an unstable cervical spine is discussed in Chapter 19. Patients with high transections often have impaired airway reflexes and are further predisposed to hypoxemia because of a decrease in functional residual capacity and atelectasis. Spinal shock can lead to hypotension and bradycardia prior to any anesthetic administration.

Direct arterial pressure monitoring is helpful. An intravenous fluid bolus and the use of ketamine for anesthesia may help prevent further decreases in blood pressure; vasopressors may also be required. Succinylcholine can be used safely in the first 24 h but should not be used thereafter because of the risk of hyperkalemia. The latter can occur within the first week following injury and is due to excessive release of potassium secondary to the proliferation of acetylcholine receptors beyond the neuromuscular synaptic cleft.

B. Chronic Transection

Anesthetic management of patients with nonacute transections is complicated by the possibility of autonomic hyperreflexia and the risk of hyperkalemia.
4 Autonomic hyperreflexia should be expected in patients with spinal cord lesions above T6 and can be precipitated by surgical manipulations. **Regional anesthesia and deep general anesthesia are effective in preventing hyperreflexia.** Many clinicians, however, are reluctant to administer spinal and epidural anesthesia in these patients because of the difficulties encountered in determining anesthetic level, exaggerated hypotension, and technical problems resulting from deformities. Severe hypertension can result in pulmonary edema, myocardial ischemia, or cerebral hemorrhage and should be treated promptly. Vasodilators should be readily available. Nondepolarizing muscle relaxants may be used. Body temperature should be monitored carefully, particularly in patients with transections above T1, because chronic vasodilation and loss of normal reflex cutaneous vasoconstriction predispose to hypothermia. Many patients with a long-standing spinal cord injury have a long history of undergoing surgery without hyperreflexia. These patients can often be managed with monitoring and sedation.

Encephalitis

Various forms of encephalitis can present secondary to infectious or autoimmune mechanisms. Patients with encephalitis are managed with the normal care given any patient with potentially increased intracranial pressure at risk of cerebral hypoperfusion.

Psychiatric Disorders

DEPRESSION

Depression is a very common mood disorder characterized by sadness and pessimism. Its cause is multifactorial, but pharmacological treatment is based on the presumption that its manifestations are due to a brain deficiency of dopamine, norepinephrine, and serotonin or altered receptor activities. Current pharmacological therapy utilizes drugs that increase brain levels of these neurotransmitters: tricyclic antidepressants, selective serotonin reuptake inhibitors (SSRIs), MAO inhibitors, and atypical antidepressants. The mechanisms of action of these drugs result in some potentially serious anesthetic interactions. An imbalance between glutamatergic and GABAergic activity in the brain leading to structural changes may also contribute to the development of depression. Up to 50% of patients with major depression hypersecrete cortisol and have abnormal circadian secretion. Electroconvulsive therapy (ECT) is increasingly used for refractory cases and may be continued prophylactically after the patient's mood recovers. The use of general anesthesia for ECT is largely responsible for its safety and widespread acceptance. Ketamine has also demonstrated efficacy in the treatment of depression.

Selective Serotonin Reuptake Inhibitors

SSRIs include fluoxetine, sertraline, and paroxetine, which some clinicians consider first-line agents of choice for depression. A surprisingly large fraction of patients undergoing elective surgery receives one of these agents. These agents have little or no anticholinergic activity and do not generally affect cardiac conduction. Their principal side effects are headache, agitation, and insomnia. Other agents include the norepinephrine–dopamine reuptake inhibitors and the serotonin–norepinephrine reuptake inhibitors.

Tricyclic Antidepressants

Tricyclic antidepressants are used for the treatment of depression and chronic pain syndromes. All tricyclic antidepressants work at nerve synapses by blocking neuronal reuptake of catecholamines, serotonin, or both. Desipramine and nortriptyline are used because they are less sedating and tend to have fewer side effects. Other agents are generally more sedating and include amitriptyline, imipramine, protriptyline, amoxapine, doxepin, and trimipramine. Clomipramine is used in the treatment of obsessive–compulsive disorders. Most tricyclic antidepressants also have significant anticholinergic (antimuscarinic) actions: dry mouth, blurred vision, prolonged gastric emptying, and urinary retention. Quinidine-like cardiac effects include tachycardia, T-wave flattening or inversion, and prolongation of the PR, QRS, and QT intervals. Amitriptyline has the most marked anticholinergic effects, whereas doxepin has the fewest cardiac effects.

Herbal Approaches

St. John's wort is being used with increased frequency as an over-the-counter therapy for depression. Because it induces hepatic enzymes, blood levels of other drugs may decrease, sometimes with serious complications. The use of all over-the-counter medications must be reviewed during the preoperative evaluation.

Perioperative Management

Antidepressant drugs are generally continued perioperatively. Increased anesthetic requirements, presumably from enhanced brain catecholamine activity, have been reported with these agents. Potentiation of centrally acting anticholinergic agents (atropine and scopolamine) may increase the likelihood of postoperative sedation, confusion, delirium, blurred vision, and urinary retention.
5 The most important interaction between anesthetic agents and tricyclic antidepressants is an exaggerated response to both indirect-acting vasopressors and sympathetic stimulation. Chronic therapy with tricyclic antidepressants is reported to deplete cardiac catecholamines, theoretically potentiating the cardiac depressant effects of anesthetics. If hypotension occurs, small doses of a direct-acting vasopressor should be used instead of an indirect-acting agent. Amitriptyline's anticholinergic action may occasionally contribute to postoperative delirium.

Monoamine Oxidase Inhibitors

MAO inhibitors were the first medications shown to be effective for depression. They are no longer considered first- or second-line agents because of their side effects. MAO inhibitors block the oxidative deamination of naturally occurring amines. At least two MAO isoenzymes (types A and B) with differential substrate selectivities have been identified. MAO-A is selective for serotonin, dopamine, and norepinephrine, whereas MAO-B is selective for dopamine and phenylethylamine. Nonselective MAO inhibitors include phenelzine, isocarboxazid, and tranylcypromine. Selective MAO-B inhibitors are useful in the treatment of PD. Additionally, unlike older nonreversible MAO inhibitors, reversible MAO-A inhibitors have been developed. Side effects include orthostatic hypotension, agitation, tremor, seizures, muscle spasms, urinary retention, paresthesia, and jaundice. The most serious sequela is a hypertensive crisis that occurs following ingestion of tyramine-containing foods (cheeses and red wines) because tyramine is used to generate norepinephrine.

Phenelzine can decrease plasma cholinesterase activity and prolong the duration of succinylcholine. Opioids should generally be used with caution in patients receiving MAO inhibitors as rare but serious reactions to opioids have been reported. Most serious reactions are associated with meperidine, resulting in hyperthermia, seizures, and coma; therefore, meperidine should not be administered to patients receiving MAO inhibitors. As with tricyclic antidepressants, exaggerated responses to vasopressors and sympathetic stimulation should be expected. If a vasopressor is necessary, a direct-acting agent in small doses should be employed. MAO inhibitors are used infrequently today.

Patients taking St. John's wort are at increased risk of serotonin syndrome, as are those taking drugs with similar effects (eg, MAO inhibitors, meperidine). Serotonin syndrome manifestations include agitation, hypertension, hyperthermia, tremor, acidosis, and autonomic instability. Treatment is supportive, along with the administration of a 5-HT antagonist (eg, cyproheptadine).

BIPOLAR DISEASE

Mania is a mood disorder characterized by elation, hyperactivity, and flight of ideas. Manic episodes may alternate with depression in patients with a bipolar (formerly manic–depressive) disorder. Mania is thought to be related to excessive norepinephrine activity in the brain. The most common agents used for maintenance therapy for this condition are lithium, valproate, quetiapine, and lamotrigine. Aripiprazole, olanzapine, and risperidone are used if the first group fails.

The mechanism of action of lithium is poorly understood. It has a narrow therapeutic range, with a desirable blood concentration between 0.8 and 1.0 mEq/L. Side effects include reversible T-wave changes, mild leukocytosis, and, on rare occasions, hypothyroidism or a vasopressin-resistant diabetes insipidus-like syndrome. Toxic blood concentrations produce confusion, sedation, muscle weakness, tremor, and slurred speech. Still higher concentrations result in widening of the QRS complex, atrioventricular block, hypotension, and seizures.

Although lithium is reported to decrease minimum alveolar concentration and prolong the duration of some NMBs, in actual practice, these effects seem to be minor. Blood levels should be checked perioperatively. Sodium depletion (secondary to loop or thiazide diuretics) decreases renal excretion of lithium and can lead to lithium toxicity. Fluid restriction and overdiuresis should be avoided. Lithium dilution cardiac output measurements are contraindicated in patients on lithium therapy.

SCHIZOPHRENIA

Patients with schizophrenia display delusions, hallucinations, disorganized or withdrawn behavior, disorganized speech, and severe emotional withdrawal. The diagnoses of schizoaffective disorder, bipolar disorder, and severe depression will need to be excluded. Schizophrenia is thought to result from an excess of dopaminergic activity in the brain.

The most commonly used antipsychotics include phenothiazines, thioxanthenes, phenylbutylpiperidines, dihydroindolones, dibenzapines, benzisoxazoles, and butyrophenones. There are numerous trade names for these drugs. First-generation antipsychotic medications had strong dopamine antagonistic effects, leading to extrapyramidal side effects (eg, muscle rigidity and progression to tardive dyskinesia). Second-generation agents have less dopamine antagonism and reduced extrapyramidal effects. The antipsychotic effect of these agents seems to be due to dopamine antagonist activity. Most cause weight gain and sedation and are mildly anxiolytic. Mild α-adrenergic blockade and anticholinergic activity are also observed. Side effects include orthostatic hypotension, acute dystonic reactions, and parkinsonism-like manifestations. Risperidone and clozapine have little extrapyramidal activity, but the latter is associated with a significant incidence of granulocytopenia. T-wave flattening, ST-segment depression, and prolongation of the PR and QT intervals may be seen, increasing the risk of torsades des pointes.

Continuing antipsychotic medication perioperatively is desirable. Reduced anesthetic requirements may be observed in some patients, and some patients may experience perioperative hypotension.

NEUROLEPTIC MALIGNANT SYNDROME

Neuroleptic malignant syndrome is a rare and life-threatening complication of antipsychotic therapy that may occur hours or weeks after drug administration. It has also accompanied abrupt withdrawal of medication for PD. Meperidine and metoclopramide can also precipitate the disorder. The mechanism is related to dopamine blockade in the basal ganglia and hypothalamus and impairment of thermoregulation. In its most severe form, the presentation is similar to that of malignant hyperthermia. Muscle rigidity, hyperthermia, rhabdomyolysis, autonomic instability, and altered consciousness are seen. Creatine kinase levels are often high. The mortality rate approaches 20% to 30%, with deaths occurring primarily as a result of kidney failure or arrhythmias. Treatment begins with stopping the offending agent and initiating supportive care. Dantrolene and bromocriptine have been used. Differential diagnoses include serotonin syndrome, malignant hyperthermia, malignant catatonia, and some other acute intoxications (eg, cocaine).

SUBSTANCE ABUSE

Behavioral disorders from abuse of psychotropic (mind-altering) substances may involve a socially acceptable drug (alcohol), a medically prescribed drug (eg, an opioid or diazepam), or an illegal substance (eg, cocaine, heroin, methamphetamine) etc. With chronic abuse, patients develop tolerance to the drug and varying degrees of psychological and physical dependence. Physical dependence is most often seen with opioids, barbiturates, alcohol, and benzodiazepines. Life-threatening complications primarily due to sympathetic overactivity can develop during abstention.

Knowledge of a patient's substance abuse preoperatively may prevent adverse drug interactions, predict tolerance to anesthetic agents, and facilitate the recognition of drug withdrawal. The history of substance abuse may be volunteered by the patient (usually only on direct questioning) or deliberately hidden.

Anesthetic requirements for substance abusers vary, depending on whether the drug exposure is acute or chronic (Table 28–4). Elective procedures should be postponed for acutely intoxicated patients and those with signs of withdrawal. When surgery is deemed necessary in patients with physical dependence, perioperative doses of the abused substance should be provided, or specific agents should be given to prevent withdrawal. In the case of opioid dependence, any opioid can be used, whereas for alcohol, a benzodiazepine is usually substituted due to the reluctance of hospital pharmacies to dispense alcohol-containing beverages to patients. Alcoholic patients should receive B vitamin/folate supplementation to prevent Korsakoff syndrome. Tolerance to most anesthetic agents is often seen but is not predictable. For general anesthesia, a technique primarily relying on a volatile inhalation agent may be preferable so that anesthetic depth can be readily adjusted according to individual need. Awareness monitoring should be likewise considered. Opioids with mixed agonist–antagonist activity can precipitate acute withdrawal. Nevertheless, buprenorphine is often used to manage substance disorders. Clonidine is a useful adjuvant in the treatment of postoperative withdrawal syndromes.

TABLE 28–4 Effect of acute and chronic substance abuse on anesthetic requirements.[1]

Substance	Acute	Chronic
Opioids	↓	↑
Barbiturates	↓	↑
Alcohol	↓	↑
Marijuana	↓	0
Benzodiazepines	↓	↑
Amphetamines	↑[2]	↓
Cocaine	↑[2]	0
Phencyclidine	↓	?

[1]↓, decreases; ↑, increases; 0, no effect; ?, unknown.
[2]Associated with marked sympathetic stimulation.

Trauma patients routinely present acutely intoxicated for emergency surgery. Patients may have consumed more than one intoxicating agent. Acute cocaine intoxication may produce hypertension secondary to the increase in central neurotransmitters, such as norepinephrine and dopamine. Hypertension and arrhythmias can occur perioperatively. Chronic abusers deplete their sympathomimetic neurotransmitters, potentially developing hypotension. Amphetamine abusers have similar anesthetic concerns as amphetamines also affect the sympathetic nervous system.

Patients on chronic, prescribed opioid therapy or those taking medications illicitly have substantially increased postoperative opioid requirements. We strongly advocate for multimodal approaches to pain control perioperatively. Whenever possible, patients should remain on their maintenance methadone or buprenorphine.

Consultation with pain management and addiction specialists is often indicated.

CASE DISCUSSION

Anesthesia for Electroconvulsive Therapy

A 64-year-old man with depression refractory to drug therapy is scheduled for electroconvulsive therapy (ECT).

How is ECT administered?

The electroconvulsive shock is applied to one or both cerebral hemispheres to induce a seizure. Variables include stimulus pattern, amplitude, and duration. The goal is to produce a therapeutic generalized seizure 30 to 60 s in duration. Electrical stimuli are usually administered until a therapeutic seizure is induced. A good therapeutic effect is generally not achieved until a total of 400 to 700 seizure seconds have been induced. Because only one treatment is given per day, patients are usually scheduled for a series of treatments, generally two or three a week. Progressive memory loss often occurs with an increasing number of treatments, particularly when electrodes are applied bilaterally.

Why is anesthesia necessary?

When the efficacy of ECT was discovered, enthusiasm was tempered in the medical community because drugs were not used to control the violent seizures caused by the procedure, thus engendering a relatively high incidence of musculoskeletal injuries. Moreover, when an NMB was used alone, patients sometimes recalled being paralyzed and awake just prior to the shock. The routine use of general anesthesia to ensure amnesia and neuromuscular blockade to prevent injuries has renewed interest in ECT. The current mortality rate for ECT is estimated to be one death per 10,000 treatments.

What are the physiological effects of ECT-induced seizures?

Seizure activity is characteristically associated with an initial parasympathetic discharge followed by a more sustained sympathetic discharge. The initial phase is characterized by bradycardia and increased secretions. Marked bradycardia (<30 beats/min), including transient asystole, is occasionally seen. The hypertension and tachycardia that follow are typically sustained for several minutes. Transient autonomic imbalance can produce arrhythmias and T-wave abnormalities on the electrocardiogram. Cerebral blood flow and ICP, intragastric pressure, and intraocular pressure all transiently increase.

Are there any contraindications to ECT?

Contraindications are a recent myocardial infarction (usually <3 months), a recent stroke (usually <1 month), an intracranial mass or aneurysm, or increased ICP from any cause. More relative contraindications include angina, poorly controlled heart failure, significant pulmonary disease, bone fractures, severe osteoporosis, pregnancy, glaucoma, and retinal detachment.

What are the important considerations in selecting anesthetic agents?

Amnesia is required only for the brief period (1–5 min) from when the NMB is given to when a therapeutic seizure has been successfully induced. The seizure itself usually results in a brief period of anterograde amnesia, somnolence, and often confusion. Consequently, only a short-acting induction agent is necessary. Moreover, because most induction agents (barbiturates, etomidate, benzodiazepines, and propofol) have anticonvulsant properties, small doses must be used. The seizure threshold is increased and the **seizure duration** is decreased by all of these agents.

Following adequate preoxygenation, methohexital (0.5–1 mg/kg) is most commonly employed. Propofol (1–1.5 mg/kg) may be used, but higher doses reduce seizure duration. Benzodiazepines raise the seizure threshold and decrease duration. Ketamine increases seizure duration but is generally not used because it also increases the incidence of delayed awakening, nausea, and ataxia and is also associated with hallucinations during emergence. The use of etomidate also prolongs recovery. In very small doses, methohexital may actually enhance seizure activity. Increases in seizure threshold are often observed with each subsequent ECT.

Neuromuscular blockade is required from the time of electrical stimulation until the end of the seizure. Succinylcholine (0.25–0.5 mg/kg) is most often selected. Controlled mask ventilation, using a self-inflating bag device or an anesthesia circle system, is required until spontaneous respirations resume.

Can seizure duration be increased without increasing the electrical stimulus?

Hyperventilation can increase seizure duration and is routinely employed in some centers. Intravenous caffeine (125–250 mg), given slowly, has also been reported to increase seizure duration.

What monitors should be used during ECT?

Monitoring should be similar to what is appropriate with the use of any other general anesthetic. Seizure activity is sometimes monitored by an unprocessed electroencephalogram. It can also be monitored in an isolated limb: a tourniquet is inflated around one arm prior to injection of succinylcholine, preventing entry of the NMB and allowing observation of convulsive motor activity in that arm.

How can the adverse hemodynamic effects of the seizure be controlled in patients with limited cardiovascular reserve?

Exaggerated parasympathetic effects should be treated with atropine. In fact, premedication with glycopyrrolate is desirable both to prevent the profuse secretions associated with seizures and to attenuate bradycardia. Nitroglycerin, nifedipine, and α- and β-adrenergic blockers have all been employed successfully to control sympathetic manifestations. High doses of β-adrenergic blockers (esmolol, 200 mg), however, are reported to decrease seizure duration.

What if the patient has a pacemaker?

Patients with pacemakers may safely undergo electroconvulsive treatments, but a magnet should be readily available to convert the pacemaker to a fixed mode, if necessary.

SUGGESTED READINGS

Armstrong MJ, Okun MS. Diagnosis and treatment of Parkinson disease: a review. *JAMA*. 2020;323:548.

Bao FP, Zhang HG, Zhu SM. Anesthetic considerations for patients with acute cervical spinal cord injury. *Neural Regen Res*. 2017;12:499.

Bloor M, Nandi R, Thomas M. Antiepileptic drugs and anesthesia. *Paediatr Anaesth*. 2017;27:248.

Bornemann-Cimenti H, Sivro N, Toft F, et al. Neuraxial anesthesia in patients with multiple sclerosis—a systematic review. *Rev Bras Anesthesiol*. 2017;67:404.

Bryson EO, Aloysi AS, Farber KG, Kellner CH. Individualized anesthetic management for patients undergoing electroconvulsive therapy: a review of current practice. *Anesth Analg*. 2017;124:1943.

Crespo V, James ML. Neuromuscular disease in the neurointensive care unit. *Anesthesiol Clin*. 2016;34:60.

Elahi FM, Miller BL. A clinicopathological approach to the diagnosis of dementia. *Nat Rev Neurol*. 2017;13:457.

Evered L, Scott DA, Silbert B. Cognitive decline associated with anesthesia and surgery in the elderly: does this contribute to dementia prevalence? *Curr Opin Psychiatry*. 2017;30:220.

Fodale V, Tripodi VF, Penna O, et al. An update on anesthetics and impact on the brain. *Expert Opin Drug Saf*. 2017;18:1.

Hebl J, Horlocker T, Kopp S, et al. Neuraxial blockade in patients with preexisting spinal stenosis, lumbar disk disease, or prior spine surgery: efficacy and neurologic complications. *Anesth Analg*. 2010;111:1511.

Horlocker TT. Complications of regional anesthesia and acute pain management. *Anesthesiol Clin*. 2011;29:257.

Hudson KA, Greene JG. Perioperative consultation for patients with preexisting neurologic disorders. *Semin Neurol*. 2015;35:690.

Indja B, Seco M, Seamark R, et al. Neurocognitive and psychiatric issues post cardiac surgery. *Heart Lung Circ*. 2017;26:779.

Kumar R, Taylor C. Cervical spine disease and anaesthesia. *Neurosurg Anaesth*. 2011;12:225.

Rajan S, Kaas B, Moukheiber E. Movement disorders emergencies. *Semin Neurol*. 2019;39:125.

Reide P, Yentis S. Anaesthesia for the obstetric patient with nonobstetric systemic disease. *Best Pract Res Clin Obstet Gynaecol*. 2010;24:313.

Roberts DP, Lewis SJG. Considerations for general anaesthesia in Parkinson's disease. *J Clin Neurosci*. 2018;48:34.

Sial OK, Parise EM, Parise LF, Gnecco T, Bolaños-Guzmán CA. Ketamine: the final frontier or another depressing end? *Behav Brain Res*. 2020;383:112508.

Veenith T, Burnstein RM. Management of patients with neurological and psychiatric disorders. *Surgery*. 2010;28:441.

CHAPTER

29 Anesthesia for Patients with Neuromuscular Disease

KEY CONCEPTS

1. Weakness associated with myasthenia gravis is due to autoimmune destruction or inactivation of postsynaptic acetylcholine receptors at the neuromuscular junction, leading to reduced numbers of receptors and degradation of their function and to complement-mediated damage to the postsynaptic membrane.
2. Patients who have myasthenia gravis with respiratory muscle or bulbar involvement are at increased risk for pulmonary aspiration and pneumonia.
3. Many patients with myasthenia gravis are exquisitely sensitive to nondepolarizing neuromuscular blockers (NMBs).
4. Patients who have myasthenia gravis are at risk for postoperative respiratory failure. Disease duration of more than 6 years, concomitant pulmonary disease, a peak inspiratory pressure of less than −25 cm H_2O (eg, −20 cm H_2O), a vital capacity less than 4 mL/kg, and a pyridostigmine dose greater than 750 mg/d are predictive of the need for postoperative ventilation following thymectomy.
5. Patients with Lambert–Eaton myasthenic syndrome and other paraneoplastic neuromuscular syndromes are very sensitive to both depolarizing and nondepolarizing NMBs.
6. Respiratory muscle degeneration in patients with muscular dystrophy interferes with an effective cough mechanism and leads to retention of secretions and frequent pulmonary infections.
7. Degeneration of cardiac muscle in patients with muscular dystrophy is common but results in dilated or hypertrophic cardiomyopathy in only 10% of patients.
8. Succinylcholine should be avoided in patients with Duchenne or Becker muscular dystrophies because of unpredictable response and the risk of inducing severe hyperkalemia or triggering malignant hyperthermia.
9. Anesthetic management in patients with periodic paralysis is directed toward preventing attacks. Perioperative management must include frequent determinations of plasma potassium concentration and correction of abnormal values, with careful electrocardiographic monitoring to detect arrhythmias.
10. In patients with periodic paralysis, the response to NMBs is unpredictable, and neuromuscular function should be carefully monitored during their use. Increased sensitivity to nondepolarizing NMBs is likely to be encountered in patients with hypokalemic periodic paralysis.

Neuromuscular diseases adversely affect muscle function either primarily or via nerve or neuromuscular junction abnormalities. They include myasthenia gravis; Lambert–Eaton syndrome; amyotrophic lateral sclerosis (ALS, or Lou Gehrig disease); infectious motor neuronopathies including acute flaccid paralysis, tetanus, and botulism; Guillain-Barré syndrome, Becker, Duchenne, facioscapulohumeral, and myotonic muscular dystrophies; Charcot–Marie–Tooth disease; polymyositis; and a large number of other pathological conditions. Although relatively uncommon, patients with these diseases will present to the operating room and to non–operating room procedure areas for diagnostic studies, treatment of complications, or procedural management of related or unrelated disorders, and they may also be evaluated and managed by anesthesia providers in the emergency department, intensive care unit, and on hospital wards in response to a rapidly progressive and life-threatening decline in respiratory status. Overall debility, with diminished respiratory muscle strength and increased sensitivity to neuromuscular blockers (NMBs), predisposes these patients to postoperative ventilatory failure, pulmonary aspiration, and pneumonia and may slow their postprocedure recovery because of difficulty with ambulation and increased risk of falling. Cardiac involvement may include cardiomyopathy or dysrhythmias. A basic understanding of the major disorders and their potential interaction with anesthetic agents is necessary to minimize the risk of perioperative morbidity and mortality. In addition, inherited or acquired neuromuscular pathology must be considered in the differential diagnosis of any patient with unexplained acute respiratory failure (Table 29–1).

TABLE 29–1 Differential diagnosis of acute neuromuscular respiratory failure.

Guillain–Barré syndrome
Myasthenia gravis
West Nile myelopathy
Organophosphate or sarin poisoning
Paraneoplastic neuropathy
Motor neuron disease
Endocrine myopathies
Hypophosphatemia
Hypokalemia or hyperkalemia
Hypermagnesemia
Mitochondrial myopathies
Acid maltase deficiencies
Tick paralysis
Botulism
Fish poisoning (tetrodotoxin and ciguatera)
Snake bite
Vasculitis
Acute porphyria

Adapted with permission from Wijdicks EFM, Kramer AH: Handbook of Clinical Neurology, Vol 140 (3rd series) *Critical Care Neurology,* Part I. Philadelphia, PA: Elsevier; 2017.

MYASTHENIA GRAVIS

Myasthenia gravis is an autoimmune disorder characterized by weakness and easy fatigability of skeletal muscle. It is classified according to disease distribution and severity (Table 29–2). The prevalence is estimated at 50 to 200 per million population. The incidence is greatest in women during their third decade; men exhibit two peaks, one in the third decade and another in the sixth decade.

1 Weakness from myasthenia gravis is due to autoimmune destruction or inactivation of postsynaptic acetylcholine receptors at the neuromuscular junction, leading to reduced numbers of receptors and degradation of their function and to complement-mediated damage to the postsynaptic end-plate. IgG antibodies against the nicotinic acetylcholine receptor in neuromuscular junctions are found in 85% to 90% of patients with generalized myasthenia gravis and up to 50% to 70% of patients with ocular myasthenia. Among patients with myasthenia gravis, 10% to 15% percent develop thymoma, whereas approximately 70% exhibit histologic evidence of thymic lymphoid follicular hyperplasia. Other autoimmune-related disorders (hypothyroidism, hyperthyroidism, rheumatoid arthritis, systemic lupus erythematosus) are also present in up to 10% of patients. In addition, acute seronegative myasthenia gravis has been associated with infusion of immune checkpoint inhibitor cancer chemotherapeutic agents, including nivolumab, pembrolizumab, and ipilimumab. The differential diagnosis

TABLE 29–2 Myasthenia Gravis Foundation of America clinical classification of myasthenia gravis.

Class	Definition
I	Any ocular muscle weakness May have weakness of eye closure All other muscle strength is normal
II	Mild weakness affecting other than ocular muscles May also have ocular muscle weakness of any severity
IIa	Predominantly affecting limb, axial muscles, or both May also have lesser involvement of oropharyngeal muscles
IIb	Predominantly affecting oropharyngeal, respiratory muscles, or both May also have lesser or equal involvement of limb, axial muscles, or both
III	Moderate weakness affecting other than ocular muscles May also have ocular muscle weakness of any severity
IIIa	Predominantly affecting limb, axial muscles, or both May also have lesser involvement of oropharyngeal muscles
IIIb	Predominantly affecting oropharyngeal, respiratory muscles, or both May also have lesser or equal involvement of limb, axial muscles, or both
IV	Severe weakness affecting other than ocular muscles May also have ocular muscle weakness of any severity
IVa	Predominantly affecting limb or axial muscles, or both May also have lesser involvement of oropharyngeal muscles
IVb	Predominantly affecting oropharyngeal, respiratory muscles, or both May also have lesser or equal involvement of limb, axial muscles, or both
V	Defined by intubation, with or without mechanical ventilation, except when employed during routine postoperative management. The use of a feeding tube without intubation places the patient in class IVb

Reproduced with permission from Jaretzki III A, Barohn RJ. Myasthenia gravis: Recommendations for clinical research standards. *Neurology.* 2000 July 12;55(1):16-23.

of myasthenia gravis includes a number of other clinical conditions that may mimic its signs and symptoms (Table 29–3). *Myasthenia gravis crisis* is an exacerbation requiring mechanical ventilation and should be included in the differential diagnosis of any patient with acute respiratory failure of unclear etiology.

The course of myasthenia gravis is marked by exacerbations and remissions, which may be partial or complete. The weakness can be asymmetric, confined to one group of muscles, or generalized. Ocular muscles are most commonly affected, resulting in fluctuating ptosis and diplopia. With bulbar involvement, laryngeal and pharyngeal muscle weakness can result in dysarthria, difficulty in chewing and swallowing, problems clearing secretions, or pulmonary aspiration. Severe disease is usually also associated with proximal muscle weakness (primarily

TABLE 29–3 Differential diagnosis of myasthenia gravis.

Other neuromuscular disorders
Congenital myasthenic syndromes
Botulism
Lambert–Eaton syndrome
Cranial nerve palsies
Diabetes
Intracranial aneurism
Trauma (eg, orbital factures)
Congenital (eg, Dwayne syndrome)
Infections (eg, basilar meningitis)
Inflammation (eg, cavernous sinus syndromes)
Neoplasm (eg, basilar meningioma)
Horner syndrome
Muscle disease
Myotonic muscular dystrophy
Oculopharyngeal muscular dystrophy
Mitochondrial myopathies (eg, chronic progressive external ophthalmoplegia)
Central nervous system pathology
Stroke
Demyelinating disease
Other
Motor neuron disease
Metabolic disease (eg, thyroid disease)

Reproduced with permission from Mahadeva B, Phillips II L, Juel VC. Autoimmune disorders of neuromuscular transmission. *Semin Neurol.* 2008 Apr;28(2):212-217.

in the neck and shoulders) and involvement of respiratory muscles. As with other neuromuscular diseases, active management of potential respiratory complications is a critical element of disease therapy (Table 29–4). Muscle strength characteristically improves with rest but deteriorates rapidly with exertion. Infection, stress, surgery, and pregnancy have unpredictable effects on the disease but often lead to exacerbations. A number of medications may exacerbate the signs and symptoms of myasthenia gravis (Table 29–5).

TABLE 29–4 Management of respiratory complications of neuromuscular disease.

Physiological Compromise	Respiratory Complication	Treatment
Low upper airway muscle tone	Upper airway obstruction Obstructive sleep apnea	Consideration of tonsillectomy or adenoidectomy, or both Noninvasive ventilation
Abnormal chest wall compliance	Lung restriction Atelectasis Scoliosis	Lung volume recruitment Scoliosis surgery
Weak inspiratory muscles	Lung restriction Atelectasis Ineffective airway clearance	Respiratory muscle training Lung volume recruitment Airway clearance therapies
Dysphagia	Pulmonary aspiration Recurrent respiratory infections Bronchiectasis and fibrosis Impaired oxygenation	Feeding therapy Enteric tube feeding Airway clearance therapies
Respiratory insufficiency	Acute or chronic respiratory failure	Noninvasive ventilation Tracheostomy tube placement and invasive ventilation

Reproduced with permission from Buu MC: Respiratory complications, management and treatments for neuromuscular disease in children. *Curr Opin Pediatr.* 2017 Jun;29(3):326-333.

TABLE 29–5 Drugs that may potentiate weakness in myasthenia gravis.

Cardiovascular agents
β-Blockers
Lidocaine
Procainamide
Quinidine
Verapamil
Antibiotics
Ampicillin
Azithromycin
Ciprofloxacin
Clarithromycin
Erythromycin
Gentamycin
Neomycin
Streptomycin
Sulfonamides
Tetracycline
Tobramycin
Central nervous system drugs
Chlorpromazine
Lithium
Phenytoin
Trihexyphenidyl
Immunomodulators
Corticosteroids
Interferon-α
Rheumatological agents
Chloroquine
D-Penicillamine
Miscellaneous
Iodinated radiocontrast agents
Magnesium
Nondepolarizing neuromuscular blockers

Data from Mahadeva B, Phillips II L, Juel VC: Autoimmune disorders of neuromuscular transmission. *Semin Neurol.* 2008;28:212; and Matney S, Huff D. Diagnosis and treatment of myasthenia gravis. *Consult Pharm.* 2007;22:239.

Anticholinesterase drugs are used to treat the muscle weakness of this disorder. These drugs increase the amount of acetylcholine at the neuromuscular junction through inhibition of end-plate acetylcholinesterase. Pyridostigmine is prescribed most often; when given orally, it has an effective duration of 2 to 4 h. Excessive administration of an anticholinesterase may precipitate *cholinergic crisis*, which is characterized by increased weakness and excessive muscarinic effects, including salivation, diarrhea, miosis, and bradycardia. An *edrophonium (Tensilon) test* may help differentiate a cholinergic from a myasthenic crisis. Increased weakness after administration of up to 10 mg of intravenous edrophonium indicates cholinergic crisis, whereas increasing strength implies myasthenic crisis. If this test is equivocal or the patient clearly has manifestations of cholinergic hyperactivity, all cholinesterase drugs should be discontinued and the patient should be monitored in an intensive care unit or close-observation area. Anticholinesterase drugs are often the only agents used to treat patients with mild disease. Moderate to severe disease is treated with a combination of an anticholinesterase drug and immunomodulating therapy. Corticosteroids are usually tried first, followed by other agents (Table 29–6). Plasmapheresis is reserved for patients with dysphagia or respiratory failure, or to normalize muscle strength preoperatively in patients undergoing a surgical procedure, including thymectomy. Up to 85% of myasthenia gravis patients younger than 55 years of age show clinical improvement following thymectomy even in the absence of a tumor, but improvement may be delayed up to several years.

TABLE 29–6 Drugs used most frequently for the treatment of myasthenia gravis.

Drug	Mode of Action	Side Effects	Risks and Contraindications
Pyridostigmine	Symptomatic; acetylcholinesterase inhibition	Cholinergic autonomic effects	Cholinergic crisis
Prednisone or prednisolone	Immunomodulation	Widespread dose-dependent glucocorticoid effects	Gastrointestinal bleeding, Cushingoid appearance
Azathioprine	Suppression of B and T cells	Nausea, vomiting, tiredness, infections, night sweats	Leukopenia, liver toxicity
Mycophenolate mofetil	Suppression of B and T cells	Nausea, vomiting, diarrhea, joint pain, infections, tiredness	Leukopenia, progressive multifocal leukoencephalopathy; contraindicated during pregnancy
Rituximab	Suppression of B cells	Nausea, infections, infusion-related problems	Progressive multifocal leukoencephalopathy
Methotrexate	Inhibition of folate metabolism	Nausea, infections, lung disease	Leukopenia, liver toxicity; contraindicated during pregnancy
Cyclosporine	Suppression of T cells and natural killer cells	Nausea, hypertension, infections, hypertrichosis	Kidney toxicity
Tacrolimus	Suppression of T cells and natural killer cells	Nausea, infections, lung disease, hypertension, neuropsychiatric problems	Liver and kidney toxicity
Cyclophosphamide	Suppression of B and T cells	Nausea, vomiting, alopecia, discoloration of nails and skin, infections	Leukopenia
Intravenous immune globulin	Suppression of B and T cells, neutralization of autoantibodies	Nausea, headache, fever, hypotension or hypertension, local skin reactions	IgA deficiency, allergic reactions

Adapted with permission from Gillhus, NE. Myesthenia gravis. *N Engl J Med.* 2016 Dec 29;375(26):2570-2581.

Anesthetic Considerations

Patients with myasthenia gravis may present for thymectomy or for unrelated surgical or obstetric procedures. Medical management of their condition should be optimized prior to the intended procedure. Myasthenic patients with respiratory and oropharyngeal weakness should be treated preoperatively with intravenous immunoglobulin or plasmapheresis. If strength normalizes, the incidence of postoperative respiratory complications should be similar to that of a nonmyasthenic patient undergoing a similar surgical procedure. Patients scheduled for thymectomy may have deteriorating muscle strength, whereas those undergoing other elective procedures may be well controlled or in remission. Adjustments in anticholinesterase medication, immunosuppressants, or steroid therapy in the perioperative period may be necessary. Patients with advanced, generalized disease may deteriorate significantly when anticholinesterase agents are withheld. These medications should be restarted immediately when the patient resumes oral intake postoperatively. When necessary, cholinesterase inhibitors can also be given parenterally at 1/30th the oral dose. Potential problems associated with the management of anticholinesterase therapy in the postoperative period include altered patient requirements, increased vagal reflexes, and the possibility of disrupting bowel anastomoses secondary to hyperperistalsis. Moreover, because these agents also inhibit plasma cholinesterase, they could *theoretically* prolong the duration of ester-type local anesthetics and succinylcholine.

Preoperative evaluation should focus on the recent course of the disease, the muscle groups affected, drug therapy, and coexisting illnesses.

2 Patients who have myasthenia gravis with respiratory muscle or bulbar involvement are at increased risk for pulmonary aspiration and pneumonia. Premedication with an H_2 blocker or proton pump inhibitor and increased emphasis on pulmonary hygiene may decrease this risk. Because patients with myasthenia gravis are often very sensitive to the respiratory depressant effect of opioids and benzodiazepines, premedication with these drugs should be done with caution, if at all.

With the exception of NMBs, standard anesthetic agents may be used in patients with myasthenia gravis. Marked respiratory depression, however, may be encountered following even moderate doses of propofol or opioids. When general anesthesia is required, a volatile agent-based anesthetic is frequently employed. Deep anesthesia with a volatile agent alone in patients with myasthenia (and patients with other neuromuscular diseases, as well) may provide sufficient relaxation for tracheal intubation and most surgical procedures, and many clinicians routinely avoid NMBs entirely. The response to succinylcholine is said to be unpredictable, and patients may manifest a relative resistance or a moderately prolonged effect (see Chapter 11). The dose of succinylcholine may be increased to 2 mg/kg to overcome any resistance, expecting that the duration of paralysis could be increased by 5 to 10 min.

3 Many patients with myasthenia gravis are exquisitely sensitive to nondepolarizing NMBs. Even a defasciculating dose in some patients may result in nearly complete paralysis. If NMBs are necessary, small doses of a relatively short-acting nondepolarizing agent are preferred. We have not found nondepolarizing NMBs to be necessary during thymectomy with volatile anesthesia. Neuromuscular blockade should be monitored very closely with a nerve stimulator, and ventilatory function should be evaluated carefully prior to extubation.

4 Patients who have myasthenia gravis are at risk for postoperative respiratory failure. Disease duration of more than 6 years, concomitant pulmonary disease, peak inspiratory pressure of less than −25 cm H_2O (eg, −20 cm H_2O), vital capacity less than 4 mL/kg, and pyridostigmine dose greater than 750 mg/d are predictive of the need for postoperative ventilation following thymectomy.

Women with myasthenia can experience increased weakness in the last trimester of pregnancy and in the early postpartum period. Epidural anesthesia is generally preferable for these patients because it avoids potential problems with respiratory depression and NMBs related to general anesthesia. Excessively high levels of motor blockade, however, can also result in hypoventilation. Infants of myasthenic mothers may show transient myasthenia for

1 to 3 weeks following birth, induced by transplacental transfer of acetylcholine receptor antibodies, which may necessitate intubation and mechanical ventilation.

PARANEOPLASTIC NEUROMUSCULAR SYNDROMES

Paraneoplastic syndromes are immune-mediated diseases associated with an underlying cancer in which organ or tissue dysfunction or damage occurs distant from the primary or metastatic tumor. Myasthenia gravis may be considered a paraneoplastic syndrome because it is an autoimmune disorder associated with thymic hyperplasia, including thymoma. Other neurological or neuromuscular paraneoplastic syndromes include Lambert–Eaton myasthenic syndrome, limbic encephalitis, neuromyotonia, stiff person syndrome, myotonic dystrophy, and polymyositis.

Lambert–Eaton Myasthenic Syndrome

Lambert–Eaton myasthenic syndrome (LEMS) is a paraneoplastic syndrome characterized by proximal muscle weakness that typically begins in the lower extremities but may spread to involve upper limb, bulbar, and respiratory muscles. Dry mouth, male impotence, and other manifestations of autonomic dysfunction are also common. LEMS is usually associated with small cell carcinoma of the lung but may also be seen with other malignancies or as an idiopathic autoimmune disease. The disorder results from a presynaptic defect of neuromuscular transmission in which antibodies to voltage-gated calcium channels on the nerve terminal markedly reduce the quantal release of acetylcholine at the motor end-plate. Small cell lung carcinoma cells express identical voltage-gated calcium channels, serving as a trigger for the autoimmune response in patients with paraneoplastic LEMS.

In contrast to myasthenia gravis, muscle weakness associated with LEMS improves with repeated effort and is improved less dramatically by anticholinesterase drugs. Guanidine hydrochloride and 3,4-diaminopyridine (3,4-DAP), which increase the presynaptic release of acetylcholine, often produce significant improvement in LEMS. Corticosteroid or other immunosuppressive medications, or plasmapheresis, may also be of benefit.

Limbic Encephalitis

Limbic encephalitis is a degenerative central nervous system disorder characterized by personality changes, hallucinations, seizures, autonomic dysfunction, varying degrees of dementia, and asymmetric loss of sensation in the extremities. It may involve the brain, brainstem, cerebellum, and spinal cord. In approximately 60% of cases, limbic encephalitis is paraneoplastic. There is a strong association with small cell lung carcinoma, and neurological dysfunction often precedes the cancer diagnosis. Therapy includes treatment of the underlying cancer, if present, and administration of immunosuppressive medications.

Neuromyotonia

Neuromyotonia is a condition of peripheral nerve hyperexcitability that is frequently associated with an underlying cancer but may also be inherited or associated with diabetic, drug- or toxin-induced, or other acquired neuropathies. Its features include *myokymia* (a continuous undulating movement of muscles described as being like a "bag of worms"), stiffness, impaired muscle relaxation, painful muscle cramping, hyperhidrosis, and muscle hypertrophy. Treatment includes immunoglobulin therapy, plasma exchange, and administration of anticonvulsants.

Stiff Person Syndrome

Stiff person syndrome is a progressive disorder characterized by axial stiffness and rigidity that may subsequently involve the proximal limb muscles. In advanced cases, paraspinal rigidity may cause marked spinal deformities, and the patient may have difficulty with ambulation and a history of frequently falling. Stiff person syndrome is rare, and it is typically associated with cancer. Therapy includes treatment of the underlying cancer, if present, and administration of immunoglobulin and benzodiazepines.

Polymyositis

Polymyositis is an inflammatory myopathy of skeletal musculature, especially proximal limb muscles, characterized by weakness and easy fatigability. Patients are prone to aspiration and frequent pneumonias because of thoracic muscle weakness and dysphagia secondary to oropharyngeal muscle involvement. They may also exhibit cardiac arrhythmias due to conduction defects. Therapy includes treatment of the underlying neoplasm, if present; plasma exchange; and administration of immunoglobulin, corticosteroids, and immunomodulators such as methotrexate, cyclosporine, and tumor necrosis factor-α inhibitors.

Anesthetic Considerations for Patients with Neuromuscular Paraneoplastic Syndromes

5 Patients with LEMS and other neuromuscular paraneoplastic syndromes are very sensitive to both depolarizing and nondepolarizing NMBs. Volatile agents alone are often sufficient to provide muscle relaxation for both intubation and most surgical procedures. NMBs should be given only in small increments and with careful neuromuscular monitoring. Because these patients frequently exhibit marked debility, benzodiazepines, opioids, and other medications with sedative effects should be administered with caution, if at all.

INFECTIOUS MOTOR NEURONOPATHIES

Acute Flaccid Paralysis

Acute flaccid paralysis (AFP) is caused by viral infection of brainstem and spinal cord lower motor neurons. Poliomyelitis was formerly the most common example of AFP, but it has been eclipsed by syndromes caused by West Nile virus and several enterovirus types. AFPs begin with a common systemic viral infection prodrome that incudes nausea and vomiting, malaise, headache, and diarrhea with abdominal cramping. Initial signs commonly include fever, rash, and lymphadenopathy, which is followed by severe weakness and by aseptic meningitis that may progress to involve the entire neuraxis. Diagnosis is suspected by the initial overall clinical presentation and confirmed with cerebrospinal fluid analysis, viral isolates from oropharyngeal and stool samples, and rising serum antibody titers.

Tetanus

Tetanus is a bacterial infection characterized by painful, episodic skeletal muscle spasms and stiffness, especially of the masseter and neck muscles (hence the common name, "lockjaw"). It is also characterized by facial muscle spasms resembling a grin (*risus sardonicus*) and spastic hyperextension of the neck and back (*opisthotonus*). Tetanus is rarely seen in developed countries because of high vaccination rates, though cases may occur in substance abusers who inject drugs subcutaneously ("skin popping"). However, it remains a major health problem in developing countries, causing approximately 250,000 deaths annually worldwide. Symptoms and signs usually occur within 7 to 21 days of an injury and are due to the gram-negative, anaerobic bacterium, *Clostridium tetani*, which is commonly found worldwide in soil and animal droppings. *C. tetani* usually enters the patient via wound inoculation and produces an exotoxin, *tetanospasmin*, which travels to the spinal cord via motor neuron retrograde intraaxonal transport. This results in sustained motor neuron discharge and the characteristic diffuse stiffness and episodic spastic motor activity, often provoked by emotion and by sensory stimuli such as sound and touch.

Tetanus is diagnosed primarily by its clinical presentation, though positive wound cultures may be found in approximately 30% to 50% of patients. Autonomic dysfunction is common, and urinary catecholamine levels are often extremely high. A hyperadrenergic state may result from reduced inhibition of preganglionic sympathetic neurons. Complications of tetanus may include muscle or tendon ruptures, fractures, pneumonia, extreme hypertension and tachycardia, hyperpyrexia, rhabdomyolysis, urinary retention and kidney failure, and sustained pharyngeal or thoracic muscle spasm often leads to acute airway obstruction and respiratory failure in severe cases.

Botulism

Botulism is a rare but potentially fatal disorder of neuromuscular transmission caused by *botulinum toxin*, which is produced by the anaerobic, gram-positive bacteria *Clostridium botulinum*. Botulinum toxin inhibits the presynaptic release of acetylcholine, and the typical presentation of botulism includes the acute onset of symmetric facial weakness, ophthalmoplegia, ptosis, and bulbar weakness. This is followed by a symmetric, progressive, and descending flaccid paralysis, and the clinical scenario may rapidly progress to airway obstruction or respiratory failure. The most clinically important characteristics of botulism are due to the effects of botulinum toxin on motor neurons, though sensory and cholinergic autonomic neurons may also be involved. Dysautonomia may present with mydriasis, blurred vision, anhidrosis, and orthostatic hypotension. Approximately 200 botulism cases are reported annually in the United States. When patients are treated with antitoxin and appropriate supportive care, the mortality rate of botulism is less than 5%, though patients may need airway support and mechanical ventilation for several months. Left untreated, however, the mortality rate of botulism is 40% to 50%.

Botulism in adults is usually due to ingestion of botulinum toxin and *C. botulinum* spores in improperly preserved food (classically, inadequately prepared home-canned food) but may also be due to wound colonization by *C. botulinum* (especially with drug users' "skin popping"). Alteration of normal intestinal flora due to long-term antibiotic therapy in infants and adults may promote intestinal colonization by *C. botulinum*, and botulism in infants may also be caused by ingestion of honey, which commonly contains *C. botulinum* spores—which is why infants should never be fed honey. Very rarely, cases of botulism have resulted from misadventures with cosmetic Botox® injections. More worrisome, however, is the potential for bioterrorism involving food or aerosolization, as the median lethal dose of inhaled botulinum toxin may be as little as 2 ng/kg and only slightly greater for ingested toxin.

Anesthetic Considerations for Patients with Infectious Motor Neuronopathies

Patients with infectious motor neuronopathies are acutely at risk for aspiration and respiratory failure due to bulbar and respiratory motor involvement. Therapy is supportive, with anesthesia providers most frequently encountering these patients during routine intensive care unit care or in consultation for acute airway management, including intubation and mechanical ventilation, and in the case of tetanus, for management of muscle relaxant therapy. Patients with clinically significant disease will rarely be seen in the operating room, and then only for urgent or emergency procedures. Patients with AFP or botulism may not need muscle relaxants for intubation or for the operative procedure, and if muscle relaxants are administered, doses should be less than usual and carefully monitored. Postoperative patients must be carefully observed for airway problems and respiratory failure. Opioids and other analgesic and sedative medications must be administered with great caution.

GUILLAIN-BARRÉ SYNDROME

Guillain-Barré syndrome is an autoimmune-mediated disorder involving peripheral nerves and nerve roots characterized by the sudden onset of symmetric, ascending motor paralysis with limb numbness, pain, and paresthesia (Chapter 28). These symptoms and signs are accompanied by dysautonomia, exemplified by pronounced variations in heart rate and blood pressure. As one of the most common neuromuscular emergencies, it has an annual incidence of 1 to 2 cases per 100,000 population in the United States and results in more than 6000 hospitalizations annually. Believed to be triggered by an altered immune reaction to infection, it often presents 10 to 14 days following an acute episode of upper respiratory infection or diarrhea associated with cytomegalovirus, Epstein-Barr virus, Zika virus, varicella-zoster virus, *Mycoplasma pneumoniae*, or *Campylobacter jejuni* and has recently been reported in association with COVID-19 infection. Thirty percent of cases progress rapidly to quadriplegia, and up to 40% require intubation and mechanical ventilation. As with other acute neuromuscular disorders, acute Guillain-Barré syndrome will rarely be seen in the operating room, and anesthesia providers will usually encounter acute cases requiring airway management and mechanical ventilation in the emergency room or intensive care unit. In the operating room, NMBs, if used at all, must be carefully monitored. Perioperative use of anxiolytic and opioid medication must be administered with extreme caution and carefully monitored.

AMYOTROPHIC LATERAL SCLEROSIS

Amyotrophic lateral sclerosis (ALS; also known as Lou Gehrig disease) is a disease of progressive, painless weakness caused by motor neuron degeneration in the motor cortex of the brain and in the spinal cord (Chapter 28). It has an annual incidence of 1 to 2 cases per 100,000 population in the United States. As with other neuromuscular disorders, anesthesia providers will most commonly encounter patients with ALS in the intensive care unit or emergency room requiring airway management and mechanical ventilation. In the operating room, neuromuscular blockers, if used at all, must be carefully monitored. Perioperative anxiolytic and opioid medication must be administered with caution and carefully monitored.

MUSCULAR DYSTROPHIES

Preoperative Considerations

Muscular dystrophies are a heterogeneous group of hereditary disorders characterized by muscle fiber necrosis and regeneration, leading to muscle degeneration and progressive weakness. Anticipated anesthetic risk is increased by the patient's overall debilitated status, which may impede clearance of secretions and postoperative ambulation, as well as by increased risk of respiratory failure and pulmonary aspiration. Duchenne muscular dystrophy is the most common and most severe form of muscular dystrophy. Other muscular dystrophy variants include Becker, myotonic, facioscapulohumeral, and limb-girdle dystrophies.

Duchenne Muscular Dystrophy

An X-linked recessive disorder, Duchenne muscular dystrophy affects males almost exclusively. It has an incidence of approximately 1 to 3 cases per 10,000 live male births and most commonly presents between 3 and 5 years of age. Affected individuals produce abnormal dystrophin, a protein found on the sarcolemma of muscle fibers. Patients characteristically develop symmetric proximal muscle weakness that is manifested as a gait disturbance. Fatty infiltration typically causes enlargement (*pseudohypertrophy*) of muscles, particularly the calves. Progressive weakness and contractures eventually result in kyphoscoliosis. Many patients are confined to wheelchairs by age 12. Disease progression may be delayed by up to 2 to 3 years with glucocorticoid therapy in some patients. Intellectual impairment is common but generally nonprogressive. Plasma creatine kinase (CK) levels are 10 to 100 times normal even early in the disease and may reflect an abnormal increase in the permeability of muscle cell membranes. Female genetic carriers often also have high plasma CK levels, variable degrees of muscle weakness, and, rarely, cardiac involvement. Plasma myoglobin concentration may also be elevated. The diagnosis is confirmed by muscle biopsy.

6 Respiratory muscle degeneration in patients with muscular dystrophy interferes with an effective cough mechanism and leads to retention of secretions and frequent pulmonary infections. The combination of marked kyphoscoliosis and muscle wasting may produce a severe restrictive ventilatory defect. Pulmonary hypertension is common with
7 disease progression. Degeneration of cardiac muscle in patients with muscular dystrophy is also common but results in dilated or hypertrophic cardiomyopathy in only 10% of patients. Mitral regurgitation secondary to papillary muscle dysfunction is also found in up to 25% of patients. Electrocardiogram abnormalities include P–R interval prolongation, QRS and ST-segment abnormalities, and prominent R waves over the right precordium

with deep Q waves over the left precordium. Atrial arrhythmias are common. Death at a relatively young age is usually due to recurrent pulmonary infections, respiratory failure, or cardiomyopathy.

Becker Muscular Dystrophy

Becker muscular dystrophy is, like Duchenne, an X-linked recessive disorder, but it is less common (1:30,000 male births). Manifestations are nearly identical to those of Duchenne muscular dystrophy except that they usually present later in life (adolescence) and progress more slowly. Mental retardation is less common. Patients often reach the fourth or fifth decade, though some may survive into their 80s. Death is usually from respiratory complications. Cardiomyopathy may occur in some cases and may precede severe skeletal weakness.

Myotonic Dystrophy

Myotonic dystrophy is a multisystem disorder that is the most common cause of *myotonia*, a slowing of relaxation after muscle contraction in response to electrical or percussive stimuli. The disease is autosomal dominant, with an incidence of 1:8000, and usually becomes clinically apparent in the second to third decade of life, but it has also been reported as a paraneoplastic disorder in association with thymoma. Myotonia is the principal early manifestation; muscle weakness and atrophy become more prominent as the disease progresses. This weakness and atrophy usually affect cranial muscles (orbicularis oculi and oris, masseter, and sternocleidomastoid) and, in contrast to most myopathies, distal muscles more than proximal muscles. Plasma CK levels are normal or slightly elevated.

Multiple organ systems are involved in myotonic dystrophy, as evidenced by presenile cataracts, premature frontal baldness, hypersomnolence with sleep apnea, and endocrine dysfunction leading to pancreatic, adrenal, thyroid, and gonadal insufficiency. Respiratory involvement leads to decreased vital capacity, and chronic hypoxemia may cause cor pulmonale. Gastrointestinal hypomotility may predispose patients to pulmonary aspiration. Uterine atony can prolong labor and increase the incidence of retained placenta. Cardiac manifestations, which are often present before other clinical symptoms appear, may include cardiomyopathy, atrial arrhythmias, and varying degrees of heart block.

The myotonia is usually described by patients as a "stiffness" that may lessen with continued activity—the so-called "warm-up phenomenon". Patients often report that cold temperatures worsen stiffness. Antimyotonic treatment may include mexiletine, phenytoin, baclofen, dantrolene, or carbamazepine. A cardiac pacemaker may be placed in patients with significant conduction defects, even if they are asymptomatic.

Facioscapulohumeral Dystrophy

Facioscapulohumeral dystrophy, an autosomal dominant disorder with an incidence of approximately 1 to 3 cases per 100,000, affects both sexes, though more females than males are asymptomatic. Patients usually present in the second or third decade of life with weakness that is confined primarily to the muscles of the face and the shoulder girdle. Muscles in the lower extremities are less commonly affected, and respiratory muscles are usually spared. The disease is slowly progressive with a variable course. Plasma CK levels are usually normal or only slightly elevated. Cardiac involvement is rare, but loss of atrial electrical activity with an inability to atrially pace the heart has been reported; ventricular pacing is still possible in these patients. Longevity is minimally affected.

Limb-Girdle Dystrophy

Limb-girdle muscular dystrophy is a heterogeneous group of genetic neuromuscular diseases. Limb-girdle syndromes include severe childhood autosomal recessive muscular dystrophy and other incompletely defined autosomal recessive syndromes such as Erb (scapulohumeral type) and Leyden–Mobius (pelvifemoral type) dystrophies. Most patients present between childhood and the second or third decade of life with slowly progressive muscle weakness that may involve the shoulder girdle, the hip girdle, or both. Plasma CK levels are usually elevated. Cardiac involvement is relatively uncommon but may present as frequent arrhythmias or congestive heart failure. Respiratory complications, such as hypoventilation and recurrent respiratory infections, may occur.

Anesthetic Considerations

A. Duchenne and Becker Muscular Dystrophies

The anesthetic management of these patients is complicated not only by muscle weakness but also by cardiac and pulmonary manifestations. An association with malignant hyperthermia has been suggested but is unproven. Preoperative premedication with sedatives or opioids should be avoided because of increased aspiration risk due to respiratory muscle weakness, gastric hypomotility, or both. Intraoperative positioning may be complicated by kyphoscoliosis or by flexion contractures of the
8 extremities or neck. Succinylcholine should be avoided in patients with Duchenne or Becker muscular dystrophies because of unpredictable response and the risk of inducing severe hyperkalemia or triggering malignant hyperthermia. Inhalational anesthetics have been associated with rhabdomyolysis and hyperkalemia in patients with Duchene muscular dystrophy in cases where no succinylcholine was employed. Although some patients exhibit a normal response to nondepolarizing NMBs, others may be very sensitive. Marked respiratory and circulatory depression may be seen with volatile anesthetics in patients with advanced disease, and regional or local anesthesia may be preferable in these patients. Perioperative morbidity is usually due to respiratory complications. Patients with vital capacities less than 30% of predicted are at greatest risk and often require temporary postoperative mechanical ventilation.

B. Myotonic Dystrophy

Patients with myotonic dystrophy are at increased risk for perioperative respiratory and cardiac complications. Most perioperative problems arise in patients with severe weakness and in those cases in which the surgical team and anesthesia providers are unaware of the diagnosis. The diagnosis of myotonic dystrophy has been made in some patients in the course of investigating prolonged apnea following general anesthesia.

Patients with myotonic dystrophy are often sensitive to even small doses of opioids, sedatives, and inhalation and intravenous anesthetic agents, all of which may cause sudden and prolonged apnea. Premedication should therefore be avoided. Succinylcholine is relatively contraindicated because it may precipitate intense myotonic contraction of the diaphragm, chest wall, or laryngeal muscles, making ventilation difficult or impossible. Other drugs that act on the motor end-plate, such as neostigmine, and physostigmine, can aggravate myotonia. Regional anesthesia may be preferentially employed but does not always prevent myotonic contractions.

The response to nondepolarizing NMBs is reported to be normal; however, they do not consistently prevent or relieve myotonic contractions. As reversal of nondepolarizing NMBs can induce myotonic contractions, the use of short-acting nondepolarizing agents is recommended. Postoperative shivering may induce myotonic contractions in the recovery room, and doses of meperidine can often prevent such shivering and may preempt myotonic contractions.

Induction of anesthesia without complications has been reported with a number of agents, including inhalation agents and propofol. Neuromuscular blockade, if needed, should employ short-acting nondepolarizing NMBs. An association between myotonic dystrophy and malignant hyperthermia has been suggested but not established. Nitrous oxide and inhalation agents can be used as maintenance anesthesia. Reversal with anticholinesterases should be avoided, if possible.

The principal postoperative complications of myotonic dystrophy are prolonged hypoventilation, atelectasis, aspiration, and pneumonia. Patients undergoing upper abdominal surgery or those with severe proximal weakness are more likely to experience pulmonary complications. Close postoperative monitoring for arrhythmias should be accompanied by aggressive pulmonary hygiene with physical therapy and incentive spirometry. Aspiration prophylaxis is indicated.

C. Other Forms of Muscular Dystrophy

Patients with facioscapulohumeral and limb-girdle muscular dystrophy generally have normal responses to anesthetic agents. Nevertheless, because of the great variability and overlap among the various forms of muscular dystrophy, sedative-hypnotics, opioids, and nondepolarizing NMBs should be used cautiously, and succinylcholine should be avoided.

MYOTONIAS

Myotonia Congenita & Paramyotonia Congenita

Myotonia congenita is a disorder manifested early in life with generalized myotonia. Both autosomal dominant (Thomsen) and recessive (Becker) forms exist. The disease is confined to skeletal muscle, and weakness is minimal or absent. Many patients have very well-developed musculature because of near constant muscle contraction. Antimyotonic therapy includes phenytoin, mexiletine, quinine sulfate, or procainamide. Other medications that have been used include tocainide, dantrolene, prednisone, acetazolamide, and taurine. There is no cardiac involvement in myotonia congenita, and a normal life span is expected.

Paramyotonia congenita is a very rare autosomal dominant disorder characterized by transient stiffness (myotonia) and, occasionally, weakness after exposure to cold temperatures. The stiffness worsens with activity in contrast to true myotonia, thus the term *paramyotonia*. Serum potassium concentration may rise following an attack similar to hyperkalemic periodic paralysis (discussed next). Medications that have been used to block the cold response include mexiletine and tocainide.

Anesthetic management of patients with myotonia congenita and paramyotonia is complicated by an abnormal response to succinylcholine, intraoperative myotonic contractions, and the need to avoid hypothermia. NMBs may paradoxically cause generalized muscle spasms, including trismus, leading to difficulty with intubation and ventilation.

Infiltration of muscles in the operative field with a dilute local anesthetic may alleviate refractory myotonic contraction. Among patients with these types of myotonia, none have been reported with positive in vitro tests for malignant hyperthermia. Excised muscle in these patients does, however, display a prolonged myotonic contraction when exposed to succinylcholine. Excessive muscle contraction during anesthesia, therefore, likely represents aggravation of myotonia and not malignant hyperthermia.

PERIODIC PARALYSIS

Periodic paralysis is a group of disorders characterized by spontaneous episodes of transient muscle weakness or paralysis. Symptoms usually begin in childhood, with episodes lasting a few hours and typically sparing respiratory muscle involvement. The weakness usually lasts less than 1 h but can last several days, and frequent attacks may lead to progressive, long-term weakness in some patients. Hypothermia exacerbates the frequency and severity of episodes. Muscle strength and serum potassium concentrations are usually normal between attacks. The episodes of weakness are due to a loss of muscle fiber excitability secondary to partial depolarization of the resting potential. This partial depolarization prevents the generation of action potentials and thereby precipitates weakness.

Periodic paralysis is classified into primary genetic channelopathies and secondary acquired forms. The genetic types are due to dominantly inherited mutations in the voltage-gated sodium, calcium, or potassium ion channels. Classifications have been based on clinical differences, but these have not been shown to relate to specific ion channels. Different defects in the same channel can cause different clinical pictures, whereas mutations in different channels may have similar clinical pictures. However, the clinical classifications remain useful as guides to prognosis and therapy.

Hypokalemic periodic paralysis is typically associated with low serum potassium levels, and *hyperkalemic periodic paralysis* is associated with elevated serum potassium levels during episodes of weakness. In these defects, muscle membranes are inexcitable to both direct and indirect stimulation due to either decreased potassium conductance or increased sodium conductance, respectively. Both defects are associated with fluid and electrolyte shifts.

Thyrotoxic periodic paralysis occurs most commonly in Asian men and is characterized by episodes of marked weakness associated with increased thyroid hormones, low thyroid-stimulating hormone, and hypokalemia. Primary therapy is treatment of the underlying hyperthyroid state.

Secondary hypokalemic paralysis can also develop if there are marked losses of potassium through the kidneys or the gastrointestinal tract. The associated weakness is, at times, episodic, and potassium levels are much lower than in other variants of hypokalemic periodic paralysis. Management of the primary disease with potassium replacement and treatment of acidosis or alkalosis is important in preventing attacks.

Patients who consume large amounts of barium salts, which block potassium channels, can also develop hypokalemic periodic paralysis. This condition is treated by stopping the barium salts and administering oral potassium.

Potassium levels that exceed 7 mEq/L between episodes of weakness suggest a secondary form of hyperkalemic periodic paralysis. Treatment is targeted toward the primary disease and involves restriction of potassium.

Anesthetic Considerations

9 Anesthetic management of patients with periodic paralysis is directed toward preventing attacks. Perioperative management must include frequent determinations of plasma potassium concentration and correction of abnormal values, with careful electrocardiographic monitoring to detect arrhythmias. Because of the potential for glucose infusions and alkalosis to lower the plasma potassium concentration, glucose-containing intravenous solutions and hyperventilation should be avoided in patients with hypokalemic paralysis, including thyrotoxic periodic paralysis, and use of drugs such as insulin and epinephrine that lower serum potassium should be minimized. Tachycardia associated with thyrotoxic periodic paralysis is treated with nonselective
10 β-blockade. The response to NMBs is unpredictable, and neuromuscular function should be carefully monitored during their use. Increased sensitivity to nondepolarizing NMBs is likely to be encountered in patients with hypokalemic periodic paralysis. Succinylcholine is contraindicated in hyperkalemic paralysis and perhaps other variants as well because of the risk of hyperkalemia. Intraoperative maintenance of core temperature is important because shivering and hypothermia may trigger or exacerbate episodes of periodic paralysis.

CASE DISCUSSION

Anesthesia for Muscle Biopsy

A 16-year-old boy with progressive proximal muscle weakness is suspected of having a primary myopathy and is scheduled for biopsy of the quadriceps muscle.

What other potential abnormalities should concern the anesthesiologist?

The diagnosis of myopathy can be difficult to make, and the differential diagnosis may include any one of several hereditary, inflammatory, endocrine, metabolic, or toxic disorders. A muscle biopsy may be necessary to supplement clinical, laboratory, nerve conduction, and electromyographic findings and help establish the diagnosis. Although the cause of the myopathy in this case is not yet clear, the clinician must always consider potential problems that can be associated with primary myopathies.

Respiratory muscle involvement should always be suspected in patients with muscle weakness. Pulmonary reserve can be assessed clinically by asking about dyspnea and activity level. Pulmonary function tests are indicated if significant dyspnea on exertion is present. An increased risk of pulmonary aspiration is suggested by a history of dysphagia, regurgitation, recurrent pulmonary infections, or abdominal distention. Cardiac abnormalities may be manifested as arrhythmias, mitral valve prolapse, or cardiomyopathy. A 12-lead electrocardiogram is also helpful in excluding conduction abnormalities. A chest radiograph can evaluate inspiratory effort, the pulmonary parenchyma, and cardiac size; gastric distention secondary to smooth muscle or autonomic dysfunction may also be evident. Preoperative laboratory evaluation should have excluded a metabolic cause with measurement of serum sodium, potassium, magnesium, calcium, and phosphate concentrations. Similarly, thyroid, adrenal, and pituitary disorders should have been excluded. Plasma CK measurement may not be helpful, but very high levels (10 times normal) generally suggest a muscular dystrophy or polymyositis.

What anesthetic technique should be used?

The choice of anesthesia should be based on both patient and procedural requirements. Most muscle biopsies can be performed under local or regional anesthesia with supplemental intravenous sedation, using small doses of midazolam. Spinal or epidural anesthesia may be utilized. A femoral nerve block can provide excellent anesthesia for biopsy of the quadriceps muscle; a separate injection may be necessary for the lateral femoral cutaneous nerve to anesthetize the anterolateral thigh. General anesthesia should be reserved for uncooperative patients or for times when local or regional anesthesia is inadequate. The anesthesia provider must therefore always be prepared with a plan for general anesthesia.

What agents may be safely used for general anesthesia?

Major goals include preventing pulmonary aspiration, avoiding excessive respiratory or circulatory depression, avoiding NMBs if possible, and perhaps avoiding agents known to trigger malignant hyperthermia. A normal response to a previous general anesthetic in the patient or a family member may be reassuring but does not guarantee the same response subsequently. General anesthesia may be induced and maintained with a combination of a benzodiazepine, propofol, and a short-acting opioid with or without nitrous oxide. Patients at increased risk for aspiration should be intubated. When an NMB is necessary, a short-acting nondepolarizing agent should be used. Succinylcholine should be avoided because of the potential risk of an unusual response (myotonic contractions, prolonged duration, or phase II block), of inducing severe hyperkalemia, or of triggering malignant hyperthermia.

SUGGESTED READINGS

Al-Ghamdi F, Darras BT, Ghosh PS. Spectrum of nondystrophic skeletal muscle channelopathies in children. *Pediatr Neurol.* 2017;70:26.

Auger C, Hernando V, Galmiche H. Use of mechanical insufflation-exsufflation devices for airway clearance in subjects with neuromuscular disease. *Respir Care.* 2017;62:236.

Bandschapp O, Iaizzo PA. Pathophysiologic and anesthetic considerations for patients with myotonia congenita or periodic paralysis. *Pediatr Anesth.* 2013;23:824.

Bodkin C, Pascuzzi RM. Update in the management of myasthenia gravis and Lambert-Eaton myasthenic syndrome. *Neurol Clin.* 2021;39:133.

Boentert M, Wenninger S, Sansone VA. Respiratory involvement in neuromuscular disorders. *Curr Opin Neurol.* 2017;30:529.

Borden SB, Muldowney BL. Transversus abdominis plane block for analgesia in spinal muscular atrophy patient. *J Clin Anesth.* 2016;33:216.

Bucelli R, Harms MB. Neuromuscular emergencies. *Semin Neurol.* 2015;35:683.

Buu MC. Respiratory complications, management and treatments for neuromuscular disease in children. *Curr Opin Pediatr.* 2017;29:326.

Cassavaugh JM, Oravitz TM. Multiple anesthetics for a patient with stiff-person syndrome. *J Clin Anesth.* 2016;31:197.

Chaudhry MA, Wayangankar S. Thyrotoxic periodic paralysis: a concise review of the literature. *Curr Rheumatol Rev.* 2016;12:190.

Damian MS, Srinivasan R. Neuromuscular problems in the ICU. *Curr Opin Neurol.* 2017;30:538.

De Wel B, Claeys KG. Malignant hyperthermia: still an issue for neuromuscular diseases? *Curr Opin Neurol.* 2018;31:628.

Dharmadasa T, Henderson RD, Talman PS, et al. Motor neurone disease: progress and challenges. *Med J Aust.* 2017;206:357.

Durieux V, Coureau M, Meert AP et al. Autoimmune paraneoplastic syndromes associated to lung cancer: a systematic review of the literature. *Lung Cancer.* 2017;106:102.

Edmundson C, Bird SJ. Acute manifestations of neuromuscular disease. *Semin Neurol.* 2019;39:115.

Evoli A, Meacci E. An update on thymectomy in myasthenia gravis. *Expert Rev Neurotherapeutics.* 2019;19:823.

Farmakidis C, Pasnoor M, Dimachkie MM, et al. Treatment of myasthenia gravis. *Neurol Clin.* 2018;36:311.

Gilhus NE. Myasthenia gravis. *N Engl J Med.* 2016;375:2570.

Gonzalez NL, Puwanant A, Lu A, et al. Myasthenia triggered by immune checkpoint inhibitors: new case and literature review. *Neuromusc Disord.* 2017;27:266.

Goutman SA. Diagnosis and clinical management of amyotrophic lateral sclerosis and other motor neuron disorders. *Continuum.* 2017;23:1332.

Greene-Chandos D, Torbey M. Critical care of neuromuscular disorders. *Continuum.* 2018;24:1753.

Grisold W, Grisold A, Löscher WN. Neuromuscular complications in cancer. *J Neurolog Sci.* 2016;367:184.

Guidon AC. Lambert-Eaton myasthenic syndrome, botulism, and immune checkpoint inhibitor-related myasthenia gravis. *Continuum.* 2019;25:1785.

Guidon AC, Amato AA. COVID-19 and neuromuscular disorders. *Neurology.* 2020;94:959.

Jitpimolmard N, Matthews E, Fialho D. Treatment updates for neuromuscular channelopathies. *Curr Treatment Options Neurol.* 2020;22:34.

Jones S, Iyadurai P, Kissel JT. The limb-girdle muscular dystrophies and the dystrophinopathies. *Continuum.* 2016;22:1954.

Jungbluth H, Ochala J, Treves S, et al. Current and future approaches to the congenital myopathies. *Semin Cell Dev Biol.* 2017;64:191.

Katz JA, Murphy GS. Anesthetic consideration for neuromuscular diseases. *Curr Opin Anesthesiol.* 2017;30:435.

Kesner VG, Oh SJ, Dimachke MM, et al. Lambert-Eaton myasthenic syndrome. *Neurol Clin.* 2018;36:379.

Kim A, Choi S-J, Kang CH, et al. Risk factors for developing post-thymectomy myasthenia gravis in patients with thymoma. *Muscle Nerve.* 2021;63:531.

Liu Y, Liu P, Zhang X, et al. Assessment of the risks of a myasthenic crisis after thymectomy in patients with myasthenia gravis: a systematic review and meta-analysis of 25 studies. *J Cardiothorac Surg.* 2020;15:270.

Liu Y, Sawalha AH, Lu Q. COVID-19 and autoimmune diseases. *Curr Opin Rheumatol.* 2021;33:155.

Matsumoto N, Nishimoto R, Matsuoka Y, et al. Anesthetic management of a patient with sodium-channel myotonia: a case report. *JA Clin Rep.* 2019;5:77.

Mendonça FT, de Moura IB, Pellizarro D, et al. Anesthetic management in patient with neurofibromatosis: a case report and literature review. *Acta Anaesthesiol Belg.* 2016;67:48.

Morrison BM. Neuromuscular disease. *Semin Neurol.* 2016;36:409.

Norris SP, Likanje M-FN, Andrews JA. Amyotrophic lateral sclerosis: update on clinical management. *Curr Opin Neurol.* 2020;33:641.

Ohshita N, Oka S, Tsuji K, et al. Anesthetic management of a patient with Charcot-Marie-Tooth disease. *Anesth Prog.* 2016;63:80.

Pasnoor M, Dimachkie MM. Approach to muscle and neuromuscular junction disorders. *Continuum.* 2019;25:536.

Peragallo JH. Pediatric myasthenia gravis. *Semin Pediatr Neurol.* 2017;24:116.

Roper MH, Vandelaer JH, Gasse FL. Maternal and neonatal tetanus. *Lancet.* 2007;370:1947.

Sahni AS, Wolfe L. Respiratory care in neuromuscular diseases. *Respir Care.* 2018;63:601.

Sinskey JL, Holzman RS. Perioperative considerations in infantile neuroaxonal dystrophy. *Pediatr Anesth.* 2017;27:322.

Smith SV, Lee AG. Update on ocular myasthenia gravis. *Neurol Clin.* 2017;35:115.

Statland JM, Tawil R. Facioscapulohumeral muscular dystrophy. *Continuum.* 2016;22:1916.

Stunnenberg BC, LoRusso S, Arnold WD, et al. Guidelines on clinical presentation and management of nondystrophic myotonias. *Muscle Nerve.* 2020;62:430.

Supakornnumporn S, Katirji B. Autoimmune neuromuscular diseases induced by immunomodulating drugs. *J Clin Neuromusc Dis.* 2018;20:28.

Taioli E, Paschal PK, Liu B. Comparison of conservative treatment and thymectomy on myasthenia gravis outcome. *Ann Thorac Surg.* 2016;102:1805.

Vivekanandam V, Munot P, Hanna MG, et al. Skeletal muscle channelopathies. *Neurologic Clin.* 2020;38:481.

Wang L, Zhang Y, He M. Clinical predictors for the prognosis of myasthenia gravis. *BMC Neurol.* 2017;17:77.

Weingarten TN, Araka CN, Mogensen ME, et al. Lambert-Eaton myasthenic syndrome during anesthesia: a report of 37 patients. *J Clin Anesth.* 2014;26:648.

Wijdicks EFM. Management of acute neuromuscular disorders. In: Wijdicks EFM, Kramer AH, eds. *Handbook of Clinical Neurology* (vol 140, chap 13, 3rd series). *Critical Care Neurology, Part I.* Elsevier; 2017:229.

Wijdicks EFM, Klein CJ. Guillain-Barré syndrome. *Mayo Clin Proc.* 2017;92:467.

CHAPTER 30

Kidney Physiology & Anesthesia

KEY CONCEPTS

1. The combined blood flow through both kidneys normally accounts for 20% to 25% of total cardiac output.
2. Autoregulation of renal blood flow normally occurs between mean arterial blood pressures of 80 and 180 mm Hg and is principally due to intrinsic myogenic responses of the afferent glomerular arterioles to blood pressure changes.
3. Renal synthesis of vasodilating prostaglandins (PGD_2, PGE_2, and PGI_2) is an important protective mechanism during periods of systemic hypotension and kidney ischemia.
4. Dopamine and fenoldopam dilate afferent and efferent arterioles via D_1-receptor activation.
5. Reversible decreases in renal blood flow, glomerular filtration rate, urinary flow, and sodium excretion occur during both neuraxial and general anesthesia. Acute kidney injury is less likely to occur if adequate intravascular volume and normal blood pressure are maintained.
6. The endocrine response to surgery and anesthesia is at least partly responsible for the transient fluid retention often seen postoperatively.
7. Compound A, a breakdown product of sevoflurane, causes acute kidney injury in laboratory animals. Low fresh gas flow rates promote its accumulation in the anesthesia machine breathing circuit. No clinical study has detected significant kidney injury in humans as a consequence of sevoflurane anesthesia; nonetheless, some authorities recommend a fresh gas flow of at least 2 L/min with sevoflurane to minimize the risk of this theoretical problem.
8. Pneumoperitoneum produced during laparoscopy causes an abdominal compartment syndrome-like state. The increase in intraabdominal pressure often produces oliguria or anuria that is generally proportional to insufflation pressure. Mechanisms include vena cava and renal vein compression, kidney parenchymal compression, decreased cardiac output, and increases in plasma levels of renin, aldosterone, and antidiuretic hormone.

The kidneys play a vital and varied role in regulating the volume and composition of body fluids, eliminating toxins, and elaborating hormones, including renin, erythropoietin, and the active form of vitamin D. Factors related to operative procedures and to anesthetic management frequently have a significant impact on kidney physiology and function and may lead to perioperative fluid overload, hypovolemia, and acute kidney injury, which are major causes of perioperative morbidity, mortality, extended hospital length of stay, and increased costs.

Diuretics are often used in the perioperative period. They are commonly administered on a chronic basis to patients with hypertension or chronic heart failure and to patients with liver or kidney disease. Diuretics may be used intraoperatively during neurosurgical, cardiac, major vascular, ophthalmic, and urological procedures. Familiarity with the various types of diuretics and their mechanisms of action, side effects, and potential anesthetic interactions is essential.

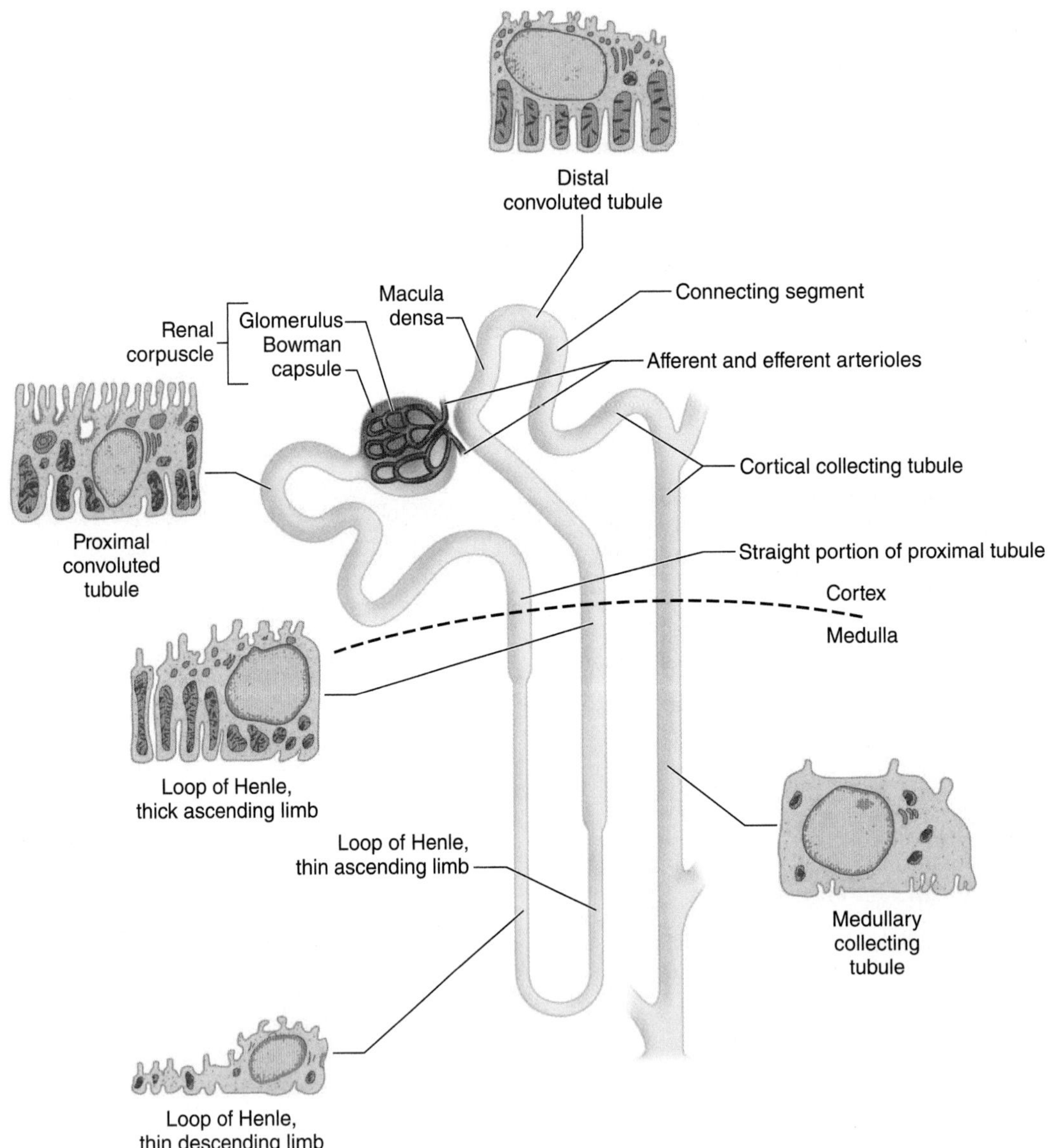

FIGURE 30–1 Major anatomical divisions of the nephron. (Reproduced with permission from Ganong WF. *Review of Medical Physiology*, 24th ed. New York, NY: McGraw Hill; 2012.)

The Nephron

Each kidney is made up of approximately 1 million functional units called *nephrons*. Anatomically, a nephron consists of a tortuous tubule with at least six specialized segments. In the *renal corpuscle*, a structure at its proximal end composed of a *glomerulus* and a *Bowman capsule*, an ultrafiltrate of blood is formed, which flows through the nephron's tubules. During this process, the ultrafiltrate's volume and composition are modified by both reabsorption and secretion of solutes, and the collected final product is eliminated as urine.

Nephrons are classified as *cortical* or *juxtamedullary*, and the renal corpuscles of all nephrons are located in the renal cortex. In addition to the renal corpuscle, the other major anatomical and functional divisions of the nephron are the *proximal convoluted tubule*, the *loop of Henle*, the *distal renal tubule*, the *collecting tubule*, and the *juxtaglomerular apparatus* (Figure 30–1 and Table 30–1).

TABLE 30–1 Functional divisions of a nephron.

Segment	Function
Renal corpuscle (glomerulus, Bowman's capsule)	Ultrafiltration of blood
Proximal tubule	Reabsorption Sodium[2] chloride Water Bicarbonate Glucose, protein, amino acids Potassium, magnesium, calcium Phosphates,[3] uric acid, urea Secretion Organic anions Organic cations Ammonia production
Loop of Henle	Reabsorption Sodium, chloride Water Potassium, calcium, magnesium Countercurrent multiplier
Distal tubule	Reabsorption Sodium[4] chloride Water Potassium Calcium[5] Bicarbonate Secretion Hydrogen ion[4] Potassium[4] Calcium
Collecting tubule	Reabsorption Sodium[4,6] chloride Water[6,7] Potassium Bicarbonate Secretion Potassium[4] Hydrogen ion[4] Ammonia production
Juxtaglomerular apparatus	Secretion of renin

[1]Partially augmented by angiotensin II.
[2]Inhibited by parathyroid hormone.
[3]At least partly aldosterone mediated.
[4]Augmented by parathyroid hormone.
[5]Inhibited by atrial natriuretic peptide.
[6]Antidiuretic hormone mediated.
Adapted with permission from Rose BD. *Clinical Physiology of Acid-Base and Electrolyte Disorders*. 3rd ed. New York, NY: McGraw Hill; 1989.

THE RENAL CORPUSCLE

Each renal corpuscle contains a glomerulus, which is composed of tufts of capillaries that jut into Bowman's capsule, providing a large surface area for blood filtration. Blood enters by a single afferent arteriole and departs by a single efferent arteriole. The glomerular endothelial cells are separated from the epithelial cells of Bowman's capsule only by their fused basement membranes. The endothelial cells are perforated with relatively large fenestrae (70–100 nm), but the epithelial cells interdigitate tightly with one another, leaving relatively small filtration slits (approximately 25 nm). The two cell types with their basement membranes provide an effective filtration barrier to cells and large-molecular-weight substances. This barrier has multiple anionic sites that give it a net negative charge, favoring the filtration of cations over anions. A third cell type, called *intraglomerular mesangial cells*, is located between the basement membrane and epithelial cells near adjacent capillaries. These contractile cells regulate glomerular blood flow and also exhibit phagocytic activity. Mesangial cells contract, reducing

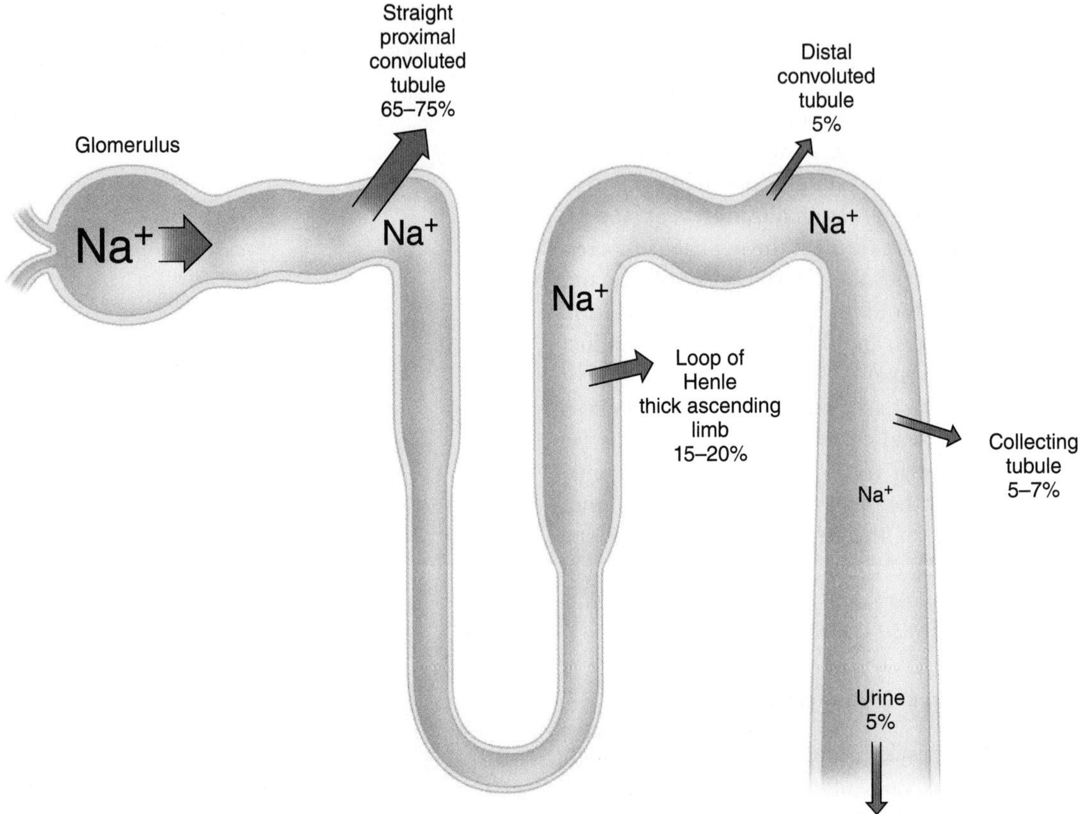

FIGURE 30–2 Sodium reabsorption in the nephron. Numbers represent the percentage of the filtered sodium reabsorbed at each site. (Reproduced with permission from Cogan MG. *Fluid and Electrolytes: Physiology and Pathophysiology.* New York, NY: Appleton & Lange; 1991.)

glomerular filtration, in response to angiotensin II, vasopressin, norepinephrine, histamine, endothelins, thromboxane A_2, leukotrienes (C_4 and D_4), prostaglandin F_2, and platelet-activating factor. They relax, thereby increasing glomerular filtration, in response to atrial natriuretic peptide (ANP), prostaglandin E_2, and dopaminergic agonists.

Glomerular filtration pressure (approximately 60 mm Hg) is normally approximately 60% of mean arterial pressure and is opposed by both plasma oncotic pressure (approximately 25 mm Hg) and renal interstitial pressure (approximately 10 mm Hg). Afferent and efferent arteriolar tone are both important in determining glomerular filtration pressure: filtration pressure is directly proportional to efferent arteriolar tone but inversely proportional to afferent tone. Approximately 20% of plasma is normally filtered into the Bowman capsule as blood passes through the glomerulus.

The Proximal Tubule

Of the ultrafiltrate formed in Bowman's capsule, 65% to 75% is normally reabsorbed isotonically (ie, proportional amounts of water and sodium) in the proximal renal tubule (Figure 30–2). To be reabsorbed, most substances must first traverse the tubular (apical) side of the cell membrane and then cross the basolateral cell membrane into the renal interstitium before entering peritubular capillaries. The major function of the proximal tubule is Na^+ reabsorption. Sodium is actively transported out of proximal tubular epithelial cells at their capillary side by

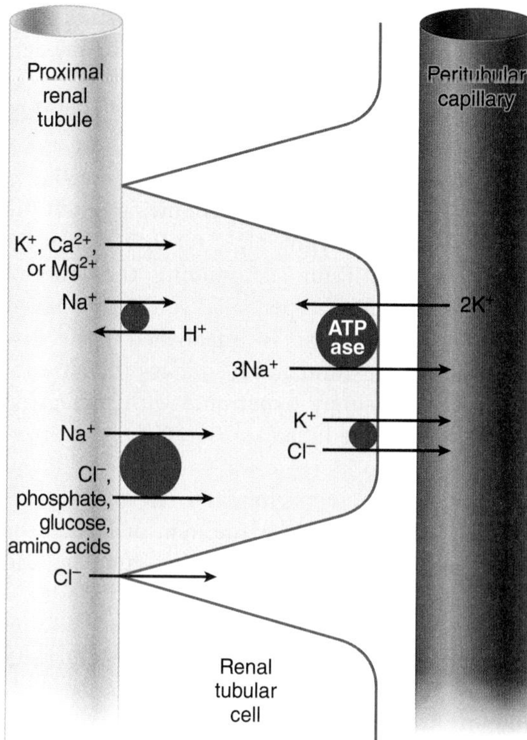

FIGURE 30–3 Reabsorption of solutes in proximal tubules. Note that Na^+–K^+-ATPase supplies the energy for reabsorption of most solutes by maintaining a low intracellular concentration of sodium.

membrane-bound Na^+–K^+-adenosine triphosphatase (Na^+–K^+-ATPase) (Figure 30–3). The resulting low intracellular concentration of Na^+ allows passive movement of Na^+ down its gradient from tubular fluid into the tubular epithelial cells. Angiotensin II and norepinephrine enhance Na^+ reabsorption in the early proximal tubule. In contrast, dopamine and fenoldopam decrease the proximal reabsorption of sodium via D_1-receptor activation.

Sodium reabsorption is coupled with the reabsorption of other solutes and the secretion of H^+ (see Figure 30–3). Specific carrier proteins use the low concentration of Na^+ inside cells to transport phosphate, glucose, and amino acids. The net loss of intracellular positive charges, the result of Na^+–K^+-ATPase activity (exchanging $3Na^+$ for $2K^+$), favors the absorption of other cations (K^+, Ca^{2+}, and Mg^{2+}). Thus, the Na^+–K^+-ATPase at the basolateral side of the renal tubular epithelial cells provides the energy for the reabsorption of most solutes. Sodium reabsorption at the luminal membrane is also coupled with countertransport (secretion) of H^+. The latter mechanism is responsible for the reabsorption of 90% of the filtered bicarbonate ions (see Figure 50–3). Unlike other solutes, chloride can traverse the tight junctions between adjacent tubular epithelial cells, and accordingly, is passively resorbed via its concentration gradient. Active chloride reabsorption may also take place as a result of a K^+–Cl^- cotransporter that extrudes both ions at the capillary side of the cell membrane (see Figure 30–3). Water moves passively out the proximal tubule along osmotic gradients. Apical membranes of epithelial cells contain specialized water channels, composed of a membrane protein called aquaporin-1, that facilitate water movement.

The proximal tubules are capable of secreting organic cations and anions. Creatinine excretion can be inhibited by other organic cations (eg, trimethoprim or pyrimethamine), leading to increases in serum creatinine concentration. Organic anions such as urates, ketoacids, penicillins, cephalosporins, diuretics, salicylates, and most radiocontrast dyes also share common secretory mechanisms and can compete with one another. Low-molecular-weight proteins, which are filtered by glomeruli, are normally reabsorbed by proximal tubular epithelial cells to be metabolized intracellularly.

The Loop of Henle

The loop of Henle consists of *descending* and *ascending* portions. They are responsible for maintaining a hypertonic medullary interstitium, and they also indirectly provide the collecting tubules with the ability to concentrate urine. The thin descending segment is a continuation of the proximal tubule and descends from the renal cortex into the renal medulla. In the medulla, the descending portion acutely turns back upon itself and rises back up toward the cortex as the ascending portion. The ascending portion consists of a functionally distinct thin ascending limb, a medullary thick ascending limb, and a cortical thick ascending limb (see Figure 30–1). *Cortical* nephrons have relatively short loops of Henle that extend only into the more superficial regions of the renal medulla and often lack a thin ascending limb. *Juxtamedullary* nephrons, which have renal corpuscles located near the renal medulla, possess loops of Henle that project deeply into the renal medulla. Cortical nephrons outnumber juxtamedullary nephrons by approximately 7:1.

Only 25% to 35% of the ultrafiltrate formed in Bowman's capsule normally reaches the loop of Henle, where 15% to 20% of the filtered sodium load is normally reabsorbed. With the notable exception of the ascending thick medullary and cortical segments, solute and water reabsorption in the loop of Henle is passive and follows concentration and osmotic gradients. In the ascending thick segment, however, Na^+ and Cl^- are reabsorbed in excess of water; Na^+ reabsorption in this part of the nephron is directly coupled to both K^+ and Cl^- reabsorption (Figure 30–4), and $[Cl^-]$ in tubular fluid appears to be the rate-limiting factor. Active Na^+ reabsorption still results from Na^+–K^+-ATPase activity on the capillary side of tubular epithelial cells.

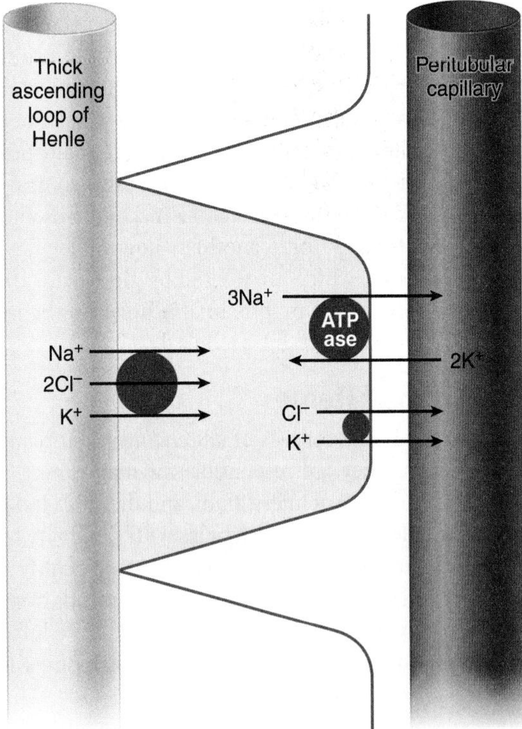

FIGURE 30–4 Sodium and chloride reabsorption in the thick ascending loop of Henle. All four sites on the luminal carrier protein must be occupied for transport to occur. The rate-limiting factor appears to be chloride concentration in tubular fluid.

Unlike the descending limb and the thin ascending limb of the loop of Henle, the thick parts of the ascending limb are impermeable to water. As a result, tubular fluid flowing out of the loop of Henle is hypotonic (100–200 mOsm/L), and the interstitium surrounding the loop of Henle is therefore hypertonic. A *countercurrent multiplier mechanism* is established such that both the tubular fluid and medullary interstitium become increasingly hypertonic with increasing depth into the medulla (Figure 30–5). Urea concentrations also increase within the medulla and contribute to the hypertonicity. The countercurrent mechanism includes the loop of Henle, the cortical and medullary collecting tubules, and adjacent capillaries (vasa recta).

The thick ascending loop of Henle is also an important site for calcium and magnesium reabsorption, and parathyroid hormone promotes calcium reabsorption at this location.

The Distal Tubule

The distal tubule receives hypotonic fluid from the loop of Henle and is normally responsible for only minor modifications of tubular fluid. In contrast to more proximal portions, the distal nephron has very tight junctions between tubular epithelial cells and is relatively impermeable to water and sodium and therefore maintains the gradients generated by the loop of Henle. Sodium reabsorption in the distal tubule normally accounts for only about 5% of the filtered sodium load. As in other parts of the nephron, the energy is derived from Na^+–K^+-ATPase activity on the capillary side, but on the luminal side, Na^+ is reabsorbed by an Na^+–Cl^- carrier. Sodium reabsorption in this segment is directly proportional to Na^+ delivery. The distal tubule is the major site of parathyroid hormone– and vitamin D–mediated calcium reabsorption.

The latter portion of the distal tubule is referred to as the *connecting segment*. Although it is involved in hormone-mediated calcium reabsorption, unlike more proximal portions, it also participates in aldosterone-mediated Na^+ reabsorption.

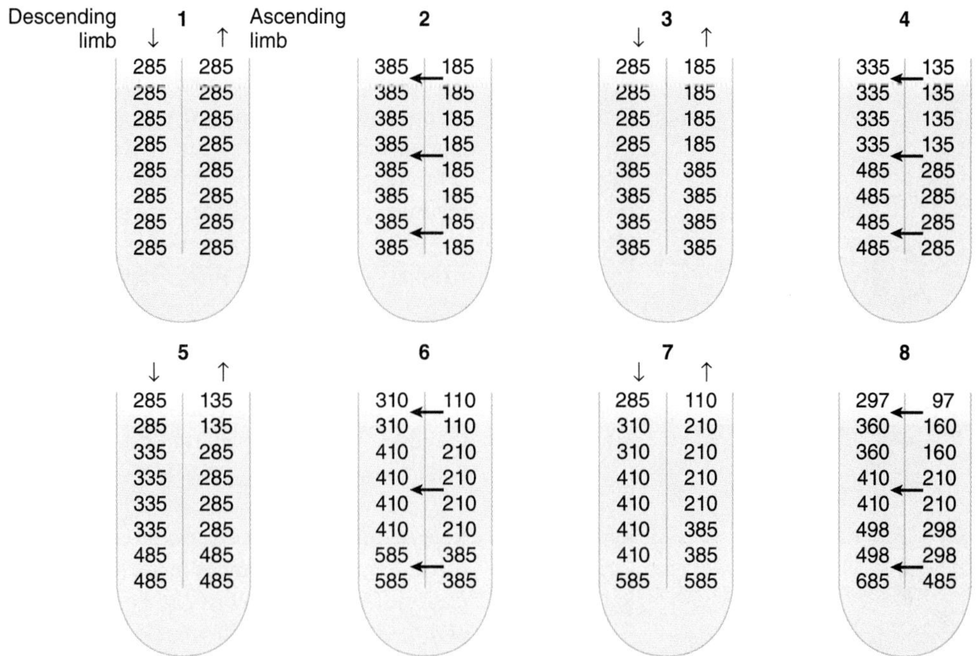

FIGURE 30–5 The countercurrent multiplier mechanism. This mechanism is dependent on differential permeability and transport characteristics between the descending and ascending limbs. The descending limb and the thin ascending limb are permeable to water, Na^+, Cl^-, and urea. The thick ascending limb is impermeable to water and urea and actively reabsorbs Na^+ and Cl^- and therefore can generate an osmotic gradient. This figure depicts from "time zero," a progressive 200-mOsm/kg gradient between the descending and ascending limbs. Note that as urine flows, the gradient remains unchanged, but the osmolality progressively increases at the bottom of the loop. (Reproduced with permission from Pitts RF. *Physiology of the Kidney and Body Fluids.* 3rd ed. Philadelphia, PA: Year Book; 1974.)

The Collecting Tubule

The collecting tubule can be divided into *cortical* and *medullary* portions, and together they normally account for the reabsorption of 5% to 7% of the filtered sodium load.

A. Cortical Collecting Tubule

This part of the nephron consists of two cell types: (1) *principal cells* that primarily secrete potassium and participate in aldosterone-stimulated Na^+ reabsorption, and (2) *intercalated cells* that are responsible for acid–base regulation. Because principal cells reabsorb Na^+ via an electrogenic pump, either Cl^- must also be reabsorbed, or K^+ must be secreted to maintain electroneutrality. Increased intracellular $[K^+]$ favors K^+ secretion. Aldosterone enhances Na^+–K^+-ATPase activity in this part of the nephron by increasing the number of open K^+ and Na^+ channels in the luminal membrane. Aldosterone also enhances the H^+-secreting ATPase on the luminal border of I cells (Figure 30–6). Intercalated cells additionally have a luminal K^+–H^+-ATPase pump, which reabsorbs K^+ and secretes H^+, and are also capable of secreting bicarbonate ion in response to large alkaline loads.

B. Medullary Collecting Tubule

The medullary collecting tubule courses down from the cortex through the hypertonic medulla before joining collecting tubules from other nephrons to form a single ureter in each kidney. This part of the collecting tubule is the principal site of action for antidiuretic hormone (ADH), also called vasopressin or arginine vasopressin (AVP). Vasopressin stimulates the expression of a water channel protein, aquaporin-2, in the cell membrane. The permeability of the luminal membrane to water is entirely dependent on the presence of vasopressin (see Chapter 49). Dehydration increases vasopressin secretion,

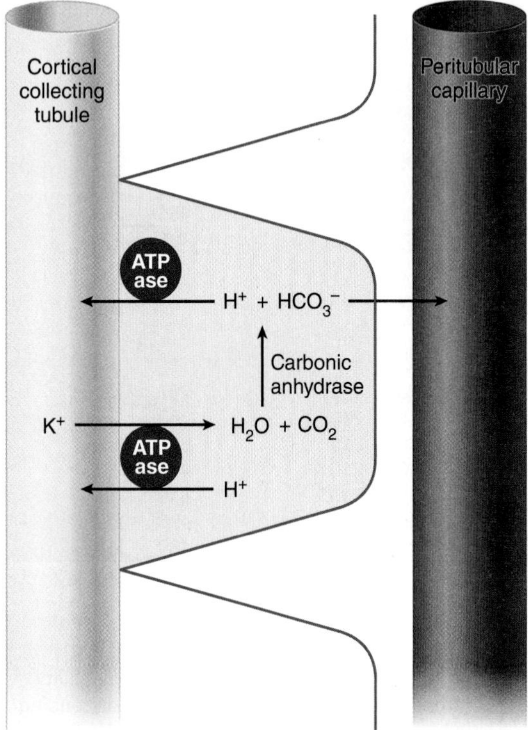

FIGURE 30–6 Secretion of hydrogen ions and reabsorption of bicarbonate and potassium in the cortical collecting tubule.

rendering the luminal membrane permeable to water. As a result, water is osmotically drawn out of the collecting tubule fluid passing through the medulla, resulting in the production of concentrated urine (up to 1400 mOsm/L). Conversely, adequate hydration suppresses vasopressin secretion, allowing fluid in the collecting tubules to pass through the medulla relatively unchanged and remain hypotonic (100–200 mOsm/L). This part of the nephron is responsible for acidifying urine; the hydrogen ions secreted are excreted in the form of titratable acids (phosphates) and ammonium ions (see Chapter 50).

C. Role of the Collecting Tubule in Maintaining a Hypertonic Medulla

Differences in permeability to urea in the cortical and medullary collecting tubules account for up to half the hypertonicity of the renal medulla. Cortical collecting tubules are freely permeable to urea, whereas medullary collecting tubules are normally impermeable. In the presence of vasopressin, the innermost part of the medullary collecting tubules becomes even more permeable to urea. Thus, when vasopressin is secreted, water moves out of the collecting tubules, and the urea becomes highly concentrated. Urea can then diffuse out deeply into the medullary interstitium, increasing its tonicity.

The Juxtaglomerular Apparatus

This small organ within each nephron consists of a specialized segment of the afferent arteriole, containing juxtaglomerular cells within its wall, and the end of the thick, ascending cortical segment of the loop of Henle, the *macula densa* (Figure 30–7). Juxtaglomerular cells synthesize the enzyme renin and are innervated by the sympathetic nervous system. Release of renin depends on β_1-adrenergic sympathetic stimulation, changes in afferent arteriolar wall pressure (see Chapter 49), and changes in chloride flow past the macula densa. Renin released into the bloodstream catalyzes the conversion of angiotensinogen, a protein synthesized by the liver, to angiotensin I. This inert decapeptide is then rapidly converted, primarily in the lungs, by angiotensin-converting enzyme (ACE) to form the octapeptide angiotensin II. Angiotensin II plays a major role in blood pressure regulation (see Chapter 15) and aldosterone secretion (see Chapter 49). Proximal renal tubular cells have ACE as well as angiotensin II receptors. Moreover, intrarenal formation of angiotensin II enhances sodium reabsorption in proximal tubules.

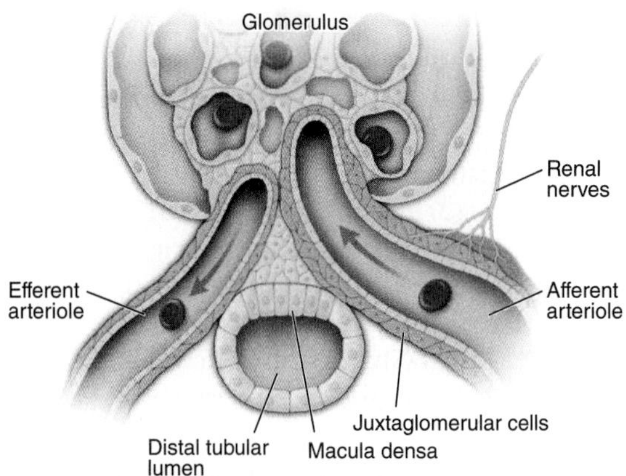

FIGURE 30–7 The juxtaglomerular apparatus.

Extrarenal production of renin and angiotensin II also takes place in the vascular endothelium, the adrenal glands, and the brain.

The Renal Circulation

Renal function is intimately related to renal blood flow (RBF). In fact, the kidneys are the only organs for which oxygen consumption is determined by blood flow; the reverse is true in other organs. The 1 combined blood flow through both kidneys normally accounts for 20% to 25% of total cardiac output. Approximately 80% of RBF normally goes to cortical nephrons, and only 10% to 15% goes to juxtamedullary nephrons. The renal cortex extracts relatively little oxygen, having an oxygen tension of approximately 50 mm Hg, because its relatively high blood flow principally serves the filtration function. In contrast, the renal medulla maintains high metabolic activity because of solute reabsorption and requires low blood flow to maintain high osmotic gradients. It has an oxygen tension of approximately 15 mm Hg and is relatively vulnerable to ischemia.

Redistribution of RBF away from cortical nephrons with short loops of Henle to larger juxtamedullary nephrons with long loops is associated with sodium retention and occurs under conditions that include sympathetic stimulation, increased levels of catecholamines and angiotensin II, and heart failure.

In most individuals, each kidney is supplied by a single renal artery arising from the aorta. The renal artery divides at the renal pelvis into *interlobar arteries*, which in turn give rise to *arcuate arteries* at the junction between the renal cortex and medulla (Figure 30–8). Arcuate arteries further divide into

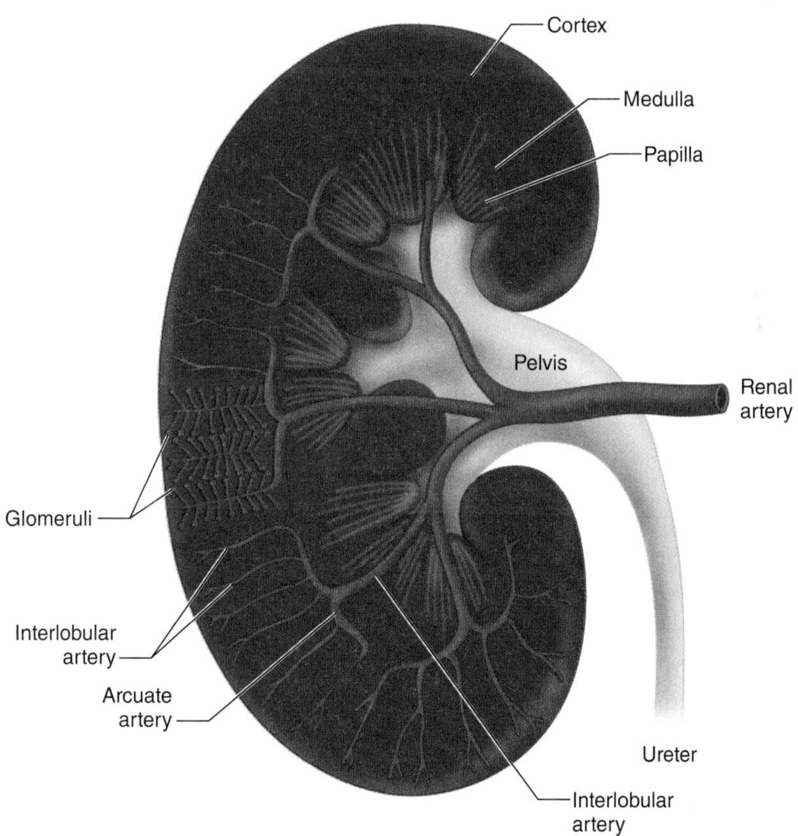

FIGURE 30–8 The renal circulation. (Reproduced with permission from Leaf A, Cotran RS. *Renal Pathophysiology*. New York, NY: Oxford University Press; 1976.)

interlobular branches that eventually supply each nephron via a single *afferent arteriole*. Blood from each glomerular capillary tuft is drained via a single *efferent arteriole* and then travels alongside adjacent renal tubules in a second *peritubular* system of capillaries. In contrast to the glomerular capillaries, which favor filtration, peritubular capillaries are primarily "reabsorptive." Venules draining this second capillary plexus return blood to the inferior vena cava via a single renal vein from each kidney.

KIDNEY BLOOD FLOW & GLOMERULAR FILTRATION

Clearance

The concept of *clearance* is frequently used in measurements of RBF and the glomerular filtration rate (GFR). The renal clearance of a substance is defined as the volume of blood that is completely cleared of that substance per unit of time (usually, per minute).

Renal Blood Flow

Renal plasma flow (RPF) is commonly measured by *p*-aminohippurate (PAH) clearance. PAH at low plasma concentrations can be assumed to be completely cleared from plasma by filtration and secretion in one passage through the kidneys. Consequently,

$$\text{RPF} = \text{Clearance of PAH} = \left(\frac{[\text{PAH}]_U}{[\text{PAH}]_P}\right) \times \text{Urine flow}$$

where $[\text{PAH}]_U$ is the urinary concentration of PAH and $[\text{PAH}]_P$ is the plasma PAH concentration.

If the hematocrit (measured as a decimal rather than as a percent) is known,

$$\text{RBF} = \frac{\text{RPF}}{(1 - \text{Hematocrit})}$$

RPF and RBF are normally about 660 and 1200 mL/min, respectively.

Glomerular Filtration Rate

The GFR, the volume of fluid filtered from the glomerular capillaries into the Bowman capsule per unit time, normally approximates 20% of RPF. Clearance of inulin, a fructose polysaccharide that is completely filtered but is neither secreted nor reabsorbed, is a good measure of GFR. Normal values for GFR are approximately 120 ± 25 mL/min in men and 95 ± 20 mL/min in women. Although less accurate than measuring inulin clearance, *creatinine clearance* is a much more practical measurement of GFR. Creatinine clearance tends to overestimate GFR because some creatinine is normally secreted by renal tubules (see Chapter 30). Creatinine is a product of phosphocreatine breakdown in muscle. Creatinine clearance is calculated as follows:

$$\text{Creatinine clearance} = \frac{([\text{Creatinine}]_U \times \text{Urinary flow rate})}{[\text{Creatinine}]_P}$$

where $[\text{creatinine}]_U$ is the creatinine concentration in urine and $[\text{creatinine}]_P$ is the creatinine concentration in plasma.

The ratio of GFR to RPF is called the *filtration fraction* (FF) and is normally 20%. GFR is dependent on the relative tones of both the afferent and efferent arterioles, as discussed earlier. Afferent and efferent arteriolar tone is responsible for maintaining a relatively constant GFR over a wide range of blood pressures. Afferent arteriolar dilation or efferent arteriolar vasoconstriction can increase the FF and maintain GFR, even when RPF decreases, for example.

Control Mechanisms

Regulation of RBF represents a complex interplay among intrinsic autoregulation, tubuloglomerular feedback, hormonal and neuronal influences on the kidney, and systemic blood pressure (Figure 30–9).

A. Intrinsic Regulation

2 Autoregulation of RBF normally occurs between mean arterial blood pressures of 80 and 180 mm Hg and is principally due to intrinsic myogenic responses of afferent glomerular arterioles to blood pressure changes. Within these limits, RBF and GFR are kept relatively constant by afferent arteriolar vasoconstriction or vasodilation. Outside the autoregulation limits, RBF becomes pressure dependent. Glomerular filtration generally ceases when mean systemic arterial pressure is less than 40 to 50 mm Hg.

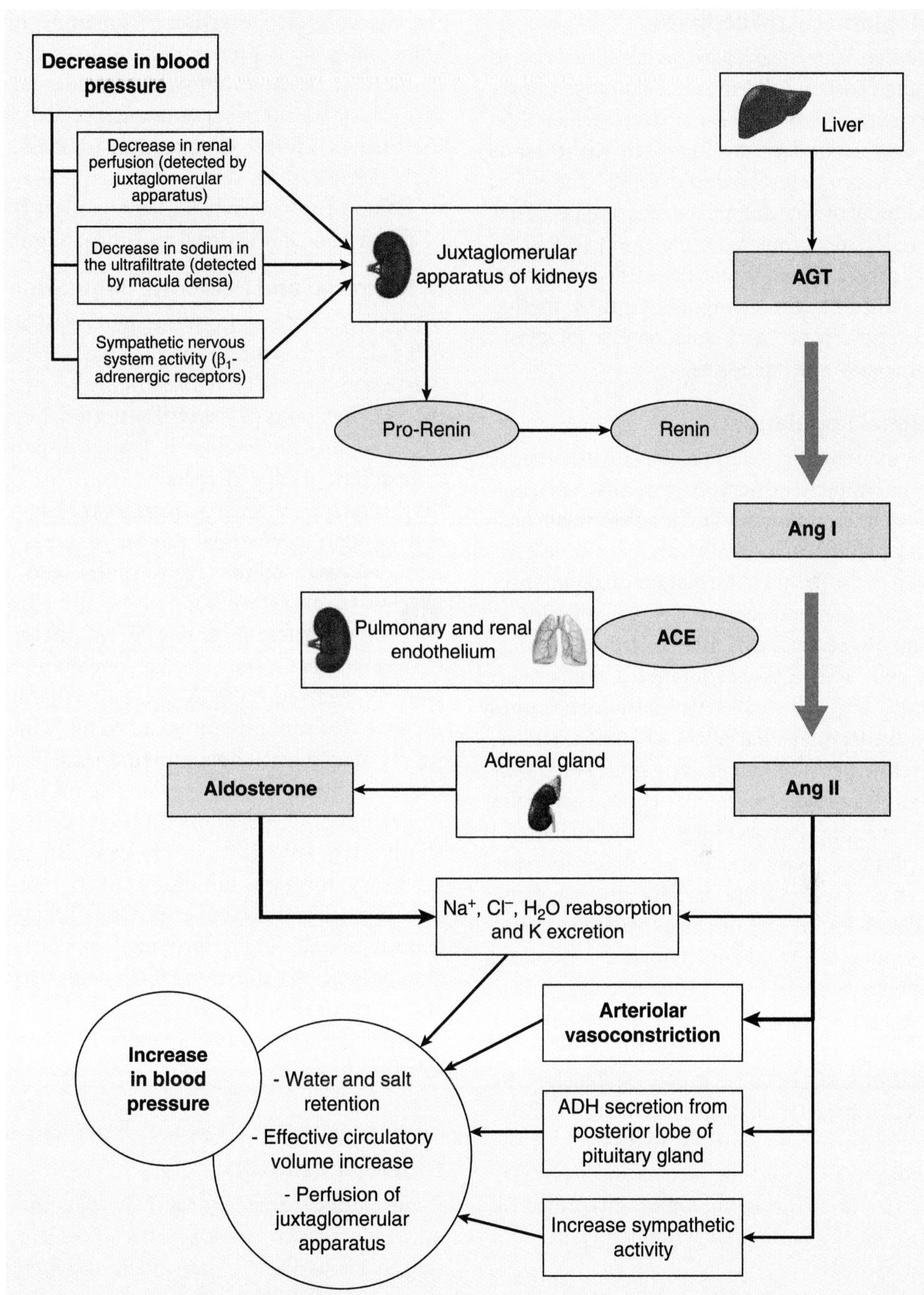

FIGURE 30–9 The role of the renin-angiotensin-aldosterone system in regulation of blood pressure and fluid balance. AGT, angiotensinogen; Ang I, angiotensin I; Ang II, angiotensin II; ACE, angiotensin-converting enzyme. (Reproduced with permission from Rastogi A, Arman F, Alipourfetrati S. New agents in treatment of hyperkalemia: An opportunity to optimize use of RAAS inhibitors for blood pressure control and organ protection in patients with chronic kidney disease. *Curr Hypertens Rep.* 2016 Jul;18(7):55.)

B. Tubuloglomerular Feedback

Tubuloglomerular feedback plays an important role in maintaining constant GFR over a wide range of perfusion pressures. Through this mechanism, increased tubular flow secondary to increased GFR tends to reflexively promote a reduced GFR; conversely, decreased tubular flow secondary to decreased GFR tends to reflexively promote an increased GFR. This regulatory process involves macula densa and mesangial cells, which react to changes in GFR by altering afferent arteriolar tone via modulation of local release of calcium, renin, and adenosine.

C. Hormonal Regulation

Decreases in afferent glomerular arteriolar pressure, increases in sympathetic nervous system activity, and decreases in distal tubule sodium load stimulate prorenin (the precursor to renin) and renin release, resulting in the subsequent formation of angiotensin II, which causes generalized arterial vasoconstriction and secondarily reduces RBF. Both afferent and efferent glomerular arterioles are constricted, but because the efferent arteriole is smaller, its resistance becomes relatively greater than that of the afferent arteriole; GFR therefore tends to be relatively preserved. Very high levels of angiotensin II constrict both arterioles and can markedly decrease GFR. Epinephrine and norepinephrine directly and preferentially increase afferent arteriolar tone but usually do not cause marked decreases in GFR because these agents also increase renin release and angiotensin II formation. Relative preservation of GFR during increased aldosterone or catecholamine secretion appears at least partly to be mediated by angiotensin-induced prostaglandin synthesis because it can be blocked by inhibitors of prostaglandin synthesis such as nonsteroidal anti-inflammatory drugs (NSAIDs). Renal
3 synthesis of vasodilating prostaglandins (PGD_2, PGE_2, and PGI_2) is an important protective mechanism during periods of systemic hypotension and kidney ischemia.

Atrial natriuretic peptide (ANP) helps regulate blood pressure and expanded extracellular fluid volume by promoting vasodilation and renal excretion of sodium and water. It is released from atrial myocytes in response to atrial distension and is a direct smooth muscle dilator that antagonizes the vasoconstrictive action of norepinephrine and angiotensin II. It preferentially dilates the afferent glomerular arteriole, constricts the efferent glomerular arteriole, and relaxes mesangial cells, effectively increasing GFR (see Chapter 49). ANP also inhibits both the release of renin and angiotensin-induced secretion of aldosterone and antagonizes the action of aldosterone in the distal and collecting tubules.

D. Neuronal and Paracrine Regulation

Sympathetic outflow from the spinal cord at the level of T4–L1 reaches the kidneys via the celiac and renal plexuses. Sympathetic nerves innervate the juxtaglomerular apparatus (β_1) as well as the renal vasculature (α_1), and this innervation is largely responsible for sympathetic-mediated reductions in RBF (see later discussion). α_1-Adrenergic receptors enhance sodium reabsorption in proximal tubules, whereas α_2 receptors decrease sodium reabsorption and promote
4 water excretion. Dopamine and fenoldopam dilate afferent and efferent arterioles via D_1-receptor activation. Unlike dopamine, fenoldopam is selective for the D_1-receptor. Although these agents are commonly administered for "renal preservation" during catecholamine infusions, there is no clinical evidence that they are effective in this role. Activation of D_2-receptors on presynaptic postganglionic sympathetic neurons can also vasodilate arterioles through inhibition of norepinephrine secretion (negative feedback). Dopamine is formed extraneuronally in the proximal tubule cells from circulating L-3,4-dihydroxyphenylalanine (L-dopa) and is released into the tubule where it can bind dopaminergic receptors to reduce proximal reabsorption of Na^+.

Effects of Anesthesia & Surgery on Kidney Function

Acute kidney injury (AKI) is a common and underappreciated perioperative problem, occurring in 1% to 5% of all hospitalized patients and in approximately 50% of all ICU patients. Recent data suggest that the prevalence of AKI in hospitalized patients with COVID-19 is approximately 30%. AKI is a major contributor to increased hospital length of stay, markedly increasing morbidity, mortality, and cost of care. Patients may develop AKI and

TABLE 30–2 Causes of acute kidney injury secondary to intrinsic kidney disease.

Vascular Effects	Renal Parenchymal Effects
Hemodynamic effects	**Glomerular diseases**
Acute kidney failure (eg, in older adult patients and those taking nonsteroidal anti-inflammatory drugs [NSAIDs])	Rapidly progressive glomerulonephritis (systemic vasculitis, Goodpasture disease, systemic lupus erythematosus, other forms of glomerulonephritis)
Contrast agent–induced (producing renal vasoconstriction and avid sodium retention)	Hemolytic uremic syndrome
	Cryoglobulinemia
Hepatorenal syndrome	**Malignant hypertension**
Cirrhosis (producing intense renal vasoconstriction and sodium retention)	Untreated primary ("essential") hypertension
	Chronic glomerulonephritis
Impaired renal perfusion and autoregulation	**Acute tubular necrosis**
Angiotensin-converting enzyme inhibitors, NSAIDs *plus*	Surgery (general, cardiac, vascular)
Atherosclerotic renal vascular disease or hypovolemia	Obstetric complications
	Sepsis
Abdominal compartment syndrome	Acute heart failure
Postoperative abdominal exploration	Burns
Tense ascites	**Rhabdomyolysis**
Atheroembolism ("cholesterol embolism")	Post crush injury
Angiography	Drug overdose
Anticoagulation	Status epilepticus
Thrombolysis	**Osmotic damage to proximal tubular cells**
Renal embolism	Sucrose-containing intravenous immunoglobulin solutions
Endocarditis	**Acute pyelonephritis**
Cardiac thrombus	Infection (eg, in patients with diabetes and partial obstruction from papillary necrosis)
Renal vein thrombosis	
Malignancy	**Myeloma**
Preexisting nephritis syndrome	Cast nephropathy
	Light-chain deposition disease
	Amyloidosis
	Sepsis
	Interstitial nephropathy
	Drug-induced (aminoglycosides, amphotericin, and many other agents)
	Acute interstitial nephritis
	Urate nephropathy
	Chemotherapy for acute leukemia or lymphoma
	Hypercalcemia
	Sarcoidosis
	Milk-alkali syndrome

Data from Armitage AJ, Tomson C. Acute renal failure, *Medicine.* 2003 June 1;31(6):43-48.

kidney failure secondary to intrinsic kidney disease (Table 30–2), and risk factors for AKI in the perioperative setting include preexisting kidney impairment, diabetes mellitus, cardiovascular disease, hypovolemia, as well as the use of potentially nephrotoxic medications by older adult patients. The risk index in Table 30–3 identifies preoperative predictors of AKI following general surgery.

Clinical studies attempting to define the effects of anesthetic agents on kidney function are complicated

TABLE 30–3 Acute kidney injury risk index for patients undergoing general surgery.[1]

Risk Factor
• Age ≥56 y
• Male sex
• Active congestive heart failure
• Ascites
• Hypertension
• Emergency surgery
• Intraperitoneal surgery
• Renal insufficiency—mild or moderate[2]
• Diabetes mellitus—oral or insulin therapy

[1]Risk Index classification is based on the number of risk factors present: class I (0–2 risk factors), class II (3 risk factors), class III (4 risk factors), class IV (5 risk factors), class V (≥6 risk factors).

[2]Preoperative serum creatinine >1.2 mg/dL.

Reproduced with permission from Kheterpal S, Tremper KK, Heung M, et al. Development and validation of an acute kidney injury risk index for patients undergoing general surgery. Results from a national data set. *Anesthesiology.* 2009 Mar;110(3):505-515.

and difficult. However, several conclusions can be stated:

1. Reversible decreases in RBF, GFR, urinary flow, and sodium excretion occur during both neuraxial and general anesthesia.
2. Such changes are usually less pronounced during neuraxial anesthesia.
3. Most of these changes are indirect and are mediated by autonomic and hormonal responses to surgery and anesthesia.
4. AKI is less likely to occur when an adequate intravascular volume and normal blood pressure are maintained.
5. There is no evidence that currently utilized vapor anesthetic agents cause AKI in humans. However, compound A, a breakdown product of sevoflurane, produces renal toxicity when sevoflurane is administered with reduced fresh gas flow rates to laboratory animals.

INDIRECT ANESTHETIC EFFECTS

Cardiovascular

Most inhalation and intravenous anesthetics produce concentration-dependent decreases in systemic blood pressure via cardiac depression and vasodilation. Depending on the level of sympathetic blockade, spinal or epidural anesthesia may cause a drop in systemic blood pressure secondary to decreased cardiac output as a result of decreased sympathetic tone. This leads to increased venous pooling of blood and decreased systemic vascular resistance, decreased heart rate and contractility, and decreased cardiac output. Decreases in blood pressure below the limits of autoregulation reduce RBF, GFR, urinary flow, and sodium excretion, and this adverse impact on kidney function can be reversed by the administration of pressor agents and intravenous fluids.

Neurological

Increased sympathetic tone commonly occurs in the perioperative period as a result of anxiety, pain, light anesthesia, and surgical stimulation. Heightened sympathetic activity increases renal vascular resistance and activates several hormonal systems, reducing RBF, GFR, and urine output.

Endocrine

Endocrine changes during sedation and general anesthesia are a component of the stress response induced by factors that may include anxiety, pain, surgical stimulation, circulatory depression, hypoxia, acidosis, and hypothermia. Increases in epinephrine and norepinephrine, renin, angiotensin II, aldosterone, ADH, adrenocorticotropic hormone, and cortisol are common. Catecholamines, ADH, and angiotensin II all reduce RBF by inducing renal arterial constriction. Aldosterone enhances sodium reabsorption in the distal tubule and collecting tubule, resulting in sodium retention and expansion of the extracellular fluid compartment. Nonosmotic release of ADH also favors water retention and may result in hyponatremia. 6 The endocrine response to surgery and anesthesia is at least partly responsible for the transient fluid retention often seen postoperatively in many patients.

DIRECT ANESTHETIC EFFECTS

The direct effects of anesthetics on renal function are minor compared with the secondary effects described earlier.

Volatile Agents

Halothane, isoflurane, sevoflurane, and desflurane 7 decrease renal vascular resistance. As previously noted, compound A, a breakdown product of sevoflurane, causes acute kidney injury in laboratory animals. Low fresh gas flow rates promote its accumulation in the anesthesia machine breathing circuit. No clinical study has detected kidney injury in humans as a consequence of sevoflurane anesthesia; nonetheless, some authorities recommend a fresh gas flow of at least 2 L/min with sevoflurane to minimize the risk of this theoretical problem, especially when anesthetizing laboratory rats!

Intravenous Agents

Opioids and propofol exhibit minor, if any, effects on the kidney when used alone. Ketamine minimally affects kidney function and may, relative to other anesthetic agents, preserve kidney function during hemorrhagic hypovolemia. Agents with α-adrenergic blocking activity may prevent catecholamine-induced redistribution of RBF. Drugs with antidopaminergic activity—such as metoclopramide, phenothiazines, and droperidol—may impair the renal response to dopamine. Inhibition of prostaglandin synthesis by NSAIDs such as ketorolac prevents renal production of vasodilatory prostaglandins in patients with high levels of angiotensin II and norepinephrine; attenuation of prostaglandin synthesis in this setting may promote AKI. ACE inhibitors block the protective effects of angiotensin II and may result in reductions in GFR during anesthesia. The effects of intravenous fluids on kidney function are reviewed in Chapter 31.

Other Drugs

Many medications, including radiocontrast agents, used in the perioperative period can adversely affect kidney function, especially in the setting of preexisting kidney disease (Table 30–4). Mechanisms of injury include vasoconstriction, direct tubular injury, drug-induced immunological and inflammatory responses, and renal microvascular or tubular obstruction. Radiocontrast agents are probably the most common cause of AKI in the acute care setting. In addition to intravenous hydration, pretreatment with *N*-acetylcysteine (600 mg orally every 12 h in four doses beginning prior to contrast administration) has been shown to decrease the risk of radiocontrast agent–induced AKI in patients with preexisting kidney disease. *N*-Acetylcysteine's protective action may be due to free radical scavenging or sulfhydryl donor–reducing properties. Fenoldopam, mannitol, loop diuretics, and low-dose dopamine infusion do not help maintain renal function or confer protection against AKI, and *N*-acetylcysteine has not been shown to be protective in the perioperative setting except for patients who receive radiocontrast dyes.

TABLE 30–4 Drugs and toxins associated with acute kidney injury.

Type of Injury	Drug or Toxin
Decreased renal perfusion	Nonsteroidal anti-inflammatory drugs (NSAIDs), angiotensin-converting enzyme inhibitors, radiocontrast agents, amphotericin B, cyclosporine, tacrolimus
Direct tubular injury	Aminoglycosides, radiocontrast agents, amphotericin B, methotrexate, cisplatin, foscarnet, pentamidine, heavy metals, myoglobin, hemoglobin, intravenous immunoglobulin, HIV protease inhibitors
Intratubular obstruction	Radiocontrast agents, methotrexate, acyclovir, sulfonamides, ethylene glycol, uric acid, cocaine, lovastatin
Immunological–Inflammatory	Penicillin, cephalosporins, allopurinol, NSAIDs, sulfonamides, diuretics, rifampin, ciprofloxacin, cimetidine, proton pump inhibitors, tetracycline, phenytoin

Reproduced with permission from Anderson RJ, Barry DW. Clinical and laboratory diagnosis of acute renal failure. *Best Pract Res Clin Anaesthesioll.* 2004 Mar;18(1):1-20.

DIRECT SURGICAL EFFECTS

In addition to the physiological changes associated with the neuroendocrine stress response to surgery, certain surgical procedures can significantly alter 8 kidney physiology. Pneumoperitoneum produced during laparoscopy creates an abdominal compartment syndrome-like state. The increase in intraabdominal pressure often produces oliguria or anuria that is proportional to insufflation pressure. Mechanisms include vena cava and renal vein compression; kidney parenchymal compression; decreased cardiac output; and increases in plasma levels of renin, aldosterone, and ADH. Abdominal compartment syndrome can also be produced by a number of comorbid problems, with similar adverse impact on kidney function via the same mechanisms (Table 30–5; see Chapters 31 and 39).

TABLE 30–5 Risk factors for intraabdominal hypertension and abdominal compartment syndrome.

Diminished abdominal well compliance
Acute respiratory failure, especially mechanical ventilation with high mean airway pressure (ie, high positive end-expiratory pressure)
Abdominal surgery with primary fascial or tight closure
Major trauma/burns
Prone positioning or head of bed >30°
High BMI, central obesity
Abdominal wall edema
Increased intraluminal visceral contents
Gastroparesis
Ileus
Colonic pseudo-obstruction
Bowel obstruction
Increased abdominal cavity contents
Hemoperitoneum/pneumoperitoneum
Ascites (from any mechanism)
Space-occupying mass (ie, malignancy)
Intraabdominal abscess or other infection
Peritoneal dialysis
Fluid resuscitation/capillary leak
Acidosis (pH <7.2)
Hypotension
Hypothermia (core temperature <33°C)
Polytransfusion (>10 units of blood in 24 h)
Coagulopathy (INR >1.5, platelets <55,000, PTT >2 times normal)
Massive fluid resuscitation (>5 L/24 h)
Pancreatitis
Oliguria
Sepsis
Damage control laparotomy

BMI, body mass index; INR, international normalized ratio; PTT, partial thromboplastin time.

Reproduced with permission from Patel DM, Connor Jr., MJ. Intra-abdominal hypertension and abdominal compartment syndrome: An underappreciated cause of acute kidney injury. *Adv Chronic Kidney Dis.* 2016 May;23(3):160-166.

Other surgical procedures that can impair kidney function and may also increase the risk of AKI include cardiopulmonary bypass (see Chapter 22), cross-clamping of the aorta (see Chapter 22), and dissection near the renal arteries (see Chapter 32). The potential effects of neurosurgical procedures on ADH physiology are discussed in Chapters 27 and 49.

Diuretics

Diuretics increase urinary output by decreasing reabsorption of Na^+ and water. Although classified according to their mechanism of action, many diuretics have more than one such mechanism; hence this classification system is imperfect. Only major mechanisms will be reviewed here.

Most diuretics exert their action on the luminal cell membrane from within the renal tubules. Because nearly all diuretics are highly protein bound, relatively little of the free drug enters the tubules by filtration. Most diuretics must therefore be secreted by the proximal tubule (usually via the organic anion pump) to exert their action. Impaired delivery into the renal tubules accounts for resistance to diuretics in patients with decreased kidney function.

OSMOTIC DIURETICS (MANNITOL)

Osmotically active diuretics are filtered at the glomerulus and undergo limited or no reabsorption in the proximal tubule. Their presence in the proximal tubule limits the passive water reabsorption that normally follows active sodium reabsorption. Although their major effect is to increase water excretion, in large doses, osmotically active diuretics also increase electrolyte excretion. The same mechanism also impairs water and solute reabsorption in the loop of Henle.

Mannitol is a six-carbon sugar that is the most commonly used osmotic diuretic. It also increases RBF in addition to its diuretic effect, which can promote washing out some of the medullary hypertonicity and thus interfere with renal concentrating ability. Mannitol activates the intrarenal synthesis of vasodilating prostaglandins and may be a free radical scavenger.

Uses

A. Prophylaxis Against Acute Kidney Injury in High-Risk Patients

Many clinicians continue to administer mannitol for kidney protection and, less frequently, to convert oliguric acute kidney failure to nonoliguric kidney failure, with the goal of lowering associated morbidity and mortality. However, there is no clinical evidence that such use of mannitol provides kidney protection, lessens the severity of AKI, or lessens the morbidity or mortality associated with AKI when compared with correction of hypovolemia and preservation of adequate kidney perfusion alone. In addition, high-dose mannitol can be nephrotoxic, especially in patients with impaired kidney function.

B. Evaluation of Acute Oliguria

Mannitol will augment urinary output in the setting of hypovolemia but will have little effect in the presence of severe glomerular or tubular injury. The optimal initial approach to evaluation (and treatment) of acute oliguria is to correct any existing hypovolemia and optimize cardiac output and kidney perfusion.

C. Acute Reduction of Intracranial Pressure & Cerebral Edema

See Chapter 27.

D. Acute Reduction of Intraocular Pressure in the Perioperative Period

See Chapter 36.

Intravenous Dosage

The intravenous dose for mannitol is 0.25 to 1 g/kg of ideal body weight.

Side Effects

Mannitol solutions are hypertonic and acutely raise plasma and extracellular osmolality. A rapid intracellular-to-extracellular shift of water can transiently increase intravascular volume and precipitate cardiac decompensation and pulmonary edema in patients with limited cardiac reserve. Transient hyponatremia and reductions in hemoglobin concentration are also common and represent acute hemodilution resulting from rapid movement of water out of cells; a small and transient increase in plasma potassium concentration may also be observed. It is also important to note that the initial hyponatremia does not represent hypoosmolality but reflects the presence of mannitol (see Chapter 49). If fluid and electrolyte losses are not replaced following diuresis, mannitol administration can result in hypovolemia, hypokalemia, and hypernatremia. The hypernatremia occurs because water is lost in excess of sodium. As previously noted, high-dose mannitol can be nephrotoxic, especially in patients with impaired kidney function.

LOOP DIURETICS

The loop diuretics include furosemide (Lasix), bumetanide (Bumex), ethacrynic acid (Edecrin), and torsemide (Demadex). All loop diuretics inhibit Na^+ and Cl^- reabsorption in the thick ascending limb. Sodium reabsorption at that site requires that all four sites on the Na^+–K^+–$2Cl^-$ luminal carrier protein be occupied. Loop diuretics compete with Cl^- for its binding site on the carrier protein (see Figure 30–4). With a maximal effect, they can promote excretion of 15% to 20% of the filtered sodium load. Both urinary-concentrating and urinary-diluting capacities are impaired. The large amounts of Na^+ and Cl^- presented to the distal nephron overwhelm its limited reabsorptive capability. The resulting urine remains hypotonic due to rapid urinary flow rates that prevent equilibration with the hypertonic renal medulla and due to interference with the action of ADH on the collecting tubules. A marked increase in diuresis may occur when a loop diuretic is combined with a thiazide diuretic, especially metolazone (Mykrox, Zaroxolyn, Zytanix).

Loop diuretics also increase urinary calcium and magnesium excretion. Ethacrynic acid is the only loop diuretic that is not a sulfonamide derivative, and thus it may be the diuretic of choice for patients allergic to sulfonamide drugs. Torsemide may have an antihypertensive action independent of its diuretic effect.

Uses

A. Edematous States (Sodium Overload)

These disorders include heart failure, cirrhosis, nephrotic syndrome, and kidney disease. When given intravenously, loop diuretics can rapidly reverse cardiac and pulmonary manifestations of fluid overload.

B. Hypertension

Loop diuretics may be used as adjuncts to other hypotensive agents, particularly when thiazides alone are ineffective (see later discussion).

C. Evaluation of Acute Oliguria

The optimal initial approach to acute oliguria is to correct hypovolemia and optimize cardiac output and renal perfusion.

D. Conversion of Oliguric Kidney Failure to Nonoliguric Kidney Failure

As with mannitol, discussed earlier, many clinicians continue to administer loop diuretics for kidney protection and to convert oliguric acute kidney failure to nonoliguric kidney failure, despite lack of evidence that such use provides kidney protection, lessens the severity of AKI, or lessens the morbidity or mortality associated with AKI, when compared with correction of hypovolemia and preservation of adequate kidney perfusion alone.

E. Treatment of Hypercalcemia

See Chapter 49.

F. Rapid Correction of Hyponatremia

See Chapter 49.

Intravenous Dosages

The intravenous doses are furosemide, 10 to 100 mg; bumetanide, 0.5 to 1 mg; ethacrynic acid, 50 to 100 mg; and torsemide 10 to 100 mg.

Side Effects

Increased delivery of Na^+ to the distal and collecting tubules increases K^+ and H^+ secretion at those sites and thus produces hypokalemia and metabolic alkalosis. Marked Na^+ losses will also lead to hypovolemia and prerenal azotemia; secondary hyperaldosteronism often accentuates the hypokalemia and metabolic alkalosis. Urinary calcium and magnesium loss promoted by loop diuretics may result in hypocalcemia or hypomagnesemia, or both. Hypercalciuria can promote urolithiasis. Hyperuricemia may result from increased urate reabsorption and from competitive inhibition of urate secretion in the proximal tubule. Reversible and irreversible hearing loss has been reported with loop diuretics, especially furosemide and ethacrynic acid.

THIAZIDE & THIAZIDE-LIKE DIURETICS

This group of agents includes thiazides containing a benzothiadiazine molecular structure and also thiazide-like drugs with similar actions but without the benzothiadiazine structure, including chlorthalidone (Thalitone), quinethazone (Hydromox), metolazone, and indapamide (Lozol). These diuretics act at the distal tubule, including the connecting segment, and inhibition of sodium reabsorption at this site impairs diluting but not concentrating ability. They compete for the Cl^- site on the luminal Na^+–Cl^- carrier protein. When given alone, thiazide and thiazide-like diuretics increase Na^+ excretion to only 3% to 5% of the filtered load because of enhanced compensatory Na^+ reabsorption in the collecting tubules. They also possess carbonic anhydrase–inhibiting activity in the proximal tubule, which is usually masked by sodium reabsorption in the loop of Henle and which is probably responsible for the marked diuresis often seen when they are combined with loop diuretics. In contrast to their effects on sodium excretion, thiazide and thiazide-like diuretics augment Ca^{2+} reabsorption in the distal tubule. Indapamide has some vasodilating properties and is the only thiazide or thiazide-like diuretic with significant hepatic excretion.

Uses

A. Hypertension

Thiazide and thiazide-like diuretics are often selected as first-line agents in the treatment of hypertension (see Chapter 21), and they have been shown to improve long-term outcomes in this disorder.

B. Edematous Disorders (Sodium Overload)

These drugs are used to treat mild to moderate edema and congestive heart failure related to mild to moderate sodium overload.

C. Hypercalciuria

Thiazide and thiazide-like diuretics are often used to decrease calcium excretion in patients who form calcium-containing kidney stones.

D. Nephrogenic Diabetes Insipidus

The efficacy of these agents in this disorder is based upon their ability to impair diluting capacity and increase urine osmolality (see Chapter 49).

Intravenous Dosages

These agents are only given orally.

Side Effects

Although thiazide and thiazide-like diuretics deliver less sodium to the collecting tubules than loop diuretics, the increase in sodium excretion is enough to enhance K^+ secretion and frequently results in hypokalemia. Enhanced H^+ secretion can also occur, resulting in metabolic alkalosis. Impairment of renal diluting capacity may produce hyponatremia. Hyperuricemia, hyperglycemia, hypercalcemia, and hyperlipidemia may also be seen.

POTASSIUM-SPARING DIURETICS

These are weak diuretic agents and characteristically do not increase potassium excretion. Potassium-sparing diuretics inhibit Na^+ reabsorption in the collecting tubules and therefore can maximally excrete only 1% to 2% of the filtered Na^+ load. They are usually used in conjunction with more potent diuretics for their potassium-sparing effect.

1. Aldosterone Antagonists (Spironolactone & Eplerenone)

Spironolactone (Aldactone) and eplerenone (Inspra) are direct antagonists of collecting tubule aldosterone receptors. They inhibit aldosterone-mediated Na^+ reabsorption and K^+ secretion. Both agents have been shown to improve survival in patients with chronic heart failure.

Uses

These agents may be used as adjuvants in the treatment of refractory edematous states associated with secondary hyperaldosteronism (see Chapter 49). Spironolactone is particularly effective in patients with ascites related to advanced liver disease. Eplerenone is commonly used in the management of chronic heart failure, where it may improve outcomes.

Intravenous Dosage

These agents are only given orally.

Side Effects

These agents can result in hyperkalemia in patients with high potassium intake or kidney disease and in those receiving β-blockers or ACE inhibitors. Metabolic acidosis may also be seen. Eplerenone lacks spironolactone's side effects of gynecomastia and sexual dysfunction.

2. Noncompetitive Potassium-Sparing Diuretics

Triamterene (Dyrenium) and amiloride (Midamor) inhibit Na^+ reabsorption and K^+ secretion by decreasing the number of open sodium channels in the luminal membrane of collecting tubules and are not dependent upon aldosterone activity. Amiloride may also inhibit Na^+–K^+-ATPase activity in the collecting tubule.

Uses

In patients with hypertension, these agents are often combined with a thiazide or similar diuretic to minimize hypokalemia produced by the other agent. They have been added to more potent loop diuretics in congestive heart failure patients with marked potassium wasting. These agents are only given orally.

Side Effects

Amiloride and triamterene can cause hyperkalemia and metabolic acidosis similar to that seen with spironolactone (see above). Both can also cause nausea, vomiting, and diarrhea. Amiloride is generally associated with fewer side effects, but paresthesias, depression, muscle weakness, and cramping may occasionally be seen. Triamterene, on rare occasions, has resulted in renal stones and is potentially nephrotoxic, particularly when combined with nonsteroidal anti-inflammatory agents.

CARBONIC ANHYDRASE INHIBITORS

Carbonic anhydrase inhibitors such as acetazolamide (Diamox) interfere with Na^+ reabsorption and H^+ secretion in proximal tubules. They are weak diuretics because the former effect is limited by the reabsorptive capacities of more distal segments of nephrons. Nonetheless, these agents significantly interfere with H^+ secretion in the proximal tubule and impair HCO_3^- reabsorption.

Uses

A. Correction of Metabolic Alkalosis in Edematous Patients

Carbonic anhydrase inhibitors often potentiate the effects of other diuretics.

B. Alkalinization of Urine

Alkalinization enhances urinary excretion of weakly acidic compounds such as uric acid.

C. Reduction of Intraocular Pressure

Inhibition of carbonic anhydrase in the ciliary processes reduces the formation of aqueous humor and, secondarily, intraocular pressure. Carbonic anhydrase inhibitors, including oral or intravenous acetazolamide, oral methazolamide (Neptazane), and ophthalmic topical brinzolamide (Azopt) and dorzolamide (Trusopt), are often used to treat glaucoma.

Intravenous Dosage

For acetazolamide, the intravenous dose is 250 to 500 mg.

Side Effects

Carbonic anhydrase inhibitors generally produce only a mild hyperchloremic metabolic acidosis because of an apparently limited effect on the distal nephron. Large doses of acetazolamide have been reported to cause drowsiness, paresthesias, and confusion. Alkalinization of the urine can interfere with the excretion of amine drugs, such as quinidine. Acetazolamide is frequently used for prophylaxis against altitude sickness.

OTHER DRUGS WITH DIURETIC EFFECTS

These agents may increase GFR by elevating cardiac output or arterial blood pressure, thereby increasing RBF. Drugs in this category are not primarily classified as diuretics because of their other major actions. They include methylxanthines (theophylline), cardiac glycosides (digitalis), fenoldopam (Corlopam), inotropes (dopamine, dobutamine), and intravenous crystalloid and colloid infusions. Methylxanthines also appear to decrease sodium reabsorption in both the proximal and distal renal tubules.

CASE DISCUSSION

Intraoperative Oliguria

A 58-year-old woman is undergoing radical hysterectomy under general anesthesia. She was in good health prior to the diagnosis of uterine carcinoma. An indwelling urinary catheter is placed following induction of general anesthesia. Total urinary output was 60 mL for the first 2 h of surgery. After the third hour of surgery, only 5 mL of urine is noted in the drainage reservoir.

Should the anesthesia provider be concerned?

Decreases in urinary output during anesthesia are very common. Although decreases may be expected owing to the physiological effects of surgery and anesthesia, a urinary output of less than 20 mL/h in adults usually requires evaluation.

What issues should be addressed?

The following questions should be answered:

1. Is there a problem with the urinary catheter and drainage system?

2. Are hemodynamic parameters compatible with adequate kidney function?
3. Could the decrease in urinary output be directly related to surgical manipulations?

How can the urinary catheter and drainage system be evaluated intraoperatively?

Incorrect urinary catheter placement is not uncommon and should be suspected if there has been a total absence of urine flow since the time of catheter insertion. The catheter may be inadvertently placed and inflated in the urethra in men or the vagina in women. Catheter displacement, kinking, obstruction, or disconnection from the reservoir tubing can all present with features similar to this case, with complete or near-complete cessation of urinary flow. The diagnosis of such mechanical problems requires retracing and inspecting the path of urine (often under the surgical drapes) from the catheter to the collection reservoir. Obstruction of the catheter can be confirmed by an inability to irrigate the bladder with saline through the catheter.

What hemodynamic parameters should be evaluated?

Decreased urinary output during surgery is most commonly the result of hormonal and hemodynamic changes. In many instances, a decrease in intravascular volume, cardiac output, or mean arterial blood pressure is responsible. Redistribution of renal blood flow from the renal cortex to the medulla may also play a role.

Intravascular volume depletion can rapidly develop when intravenous fluid replacement does not match intraoperative blood loss and insensible fluid loss. Oliguria requires careful assessment of intravascular volume to exclude hypovolemia. An increase in urinary output following an intravenous fluid bolus is highly suggestive of hypovolemia. In contrast, oliguria in patients with a history of congestive heart failure may require inotropes, vasodilators, or diuretics. Intravascular volume status is often difficult to optimize, and goal-directed hemodynamic and fluid therapy utilizing arterial pulse contour analysis (eg, LIDCO Rapid, Vigileo FloTrak), esophageal Doppler, or transesophageal echocardiography should be considered when an accurate determination of hemodynamic and fluid volume status is critically important, particularly in patients with underlying heart, kidney, or advanced liver disease (see Chapter 5). In addition to providing a more accurate assessment of the patient's volume and hemodynamic status than that obtained with central venous pressure monitoring, these modalities avoid the risks associated with central venous access procedures and with pulmonary artery catheter placement and use.

When mean arterial blood pressure drops below the lower limit of renal autoregulation (80 mm Hg), urinary flow becomes blood pressure dependent. The latter may be particularly true in patients with chronic systemic hypertension, in whom renal autoregulation has shifted to a higher range of mean arterial blood pressure. Reductions in anesthetic depth, intravenous fluid boluses, or the administration of a vasopressor or inotrope will usually increase blood pressure and urinary output in such instances.

Otherwise normal patients may exhibit decreased urinary output in spite of normal intravascular volume, cardiac output, and mean arterial blood pressure. A small dose of a loop diuretic (eg, furosemide, 5–10 mg) usually restores urinary flow in such instances but is not necessary since such therapy does not convey protection against acute kidney injury.

How can surgical manipulations influence urinary output?

In addition to the neuroendocrine response to surgery, mechanical factors related to the surgery itself can alter urinary output. This is particularly true during pelvic surgery, when compression of the bladder by retractors, unintentional cystotomy, and ligation or severing of one or both ureters can dramatically affect urinary output. Retractor compression combined with a head-down (Trendelenburg) position commonly impedes emptying of the bladder. Excessive pressure on the bladder will often produce hematuria. Excessive insufflation pressure during laparoscopy may result in abdominal compartment syndrome, with decreased or absent urine output, as previously described.

When mechanical problems with the urinary catheter drainage system and hemodynamic factors are excluded, a surgical explanation should be sought. The surgeon should be notified so that the position of the retractors can be checked, the ureters identified, and their path retraced in the operative area. Intravenous methylene blue or indigo carmine dyes (excreted in urine) are useful in identifying the site of an unintentional cystotomy or the end of a severed ureter. Note that the appearance of dye in the urinary drainage reservoir does not exclude unilateral ligation of one ureter. Methylene blue and, to a much lesser extent, indigo carmine can transiently give falsely low pulse oximeter readings (see Chapter 6). In the case of laparoscopic surgery, the surgeon should be asked to verify and minimize insufflation pressure.

What was the outcome?

After the integrity of the urinary catheter and drainage system was checked, 1 L of Plasma-Lyte along with 500 mL of 5% albumin and 10 mg of furosemide were administered intravenously but failed to significantly increase urinary output. Indigo carmine was given intravenously, and the proximal end of a severed left ureter was subsequently identified. A urologist was called, and the ureter was reanastomosed.

SUGGESTED READINGS

Agarwal A, Dong Z, Harris R, et al. Cellular and molecular mechanisms of AKI. *J Am Soc Nephrol.* 2016;27:1288.

Busse LW, Ostermann M. Vasopressor therapy and blood pressure management in the setting of acute kidney injury. *Semin Nephrol.* 2019;39:462.

Chen Y-T, Shao S-C, Lai EC-C, et al. Mortality rate of acute kidney injury in SARS, MERS, and COVID-19 infection: a systematic review and meta-analysis. *Crit Care.* 2020;24:439.

Faubel S, Shah PB. Immediate consequences of acute kidney injury: the impact of traditional and nontraditional complications on mortality in acute kidney injury. *Adv Chron Kidney Dis.* 2016;23:179.

Golden D, Corbett J, Forni LG. Peri-operative renal dysfunction: prevention and management. *Anaesthesia.* 2016;71(suppl):51.

Goldstein SL. The renal angina index to predict acute kidney injury: are adults just large children? *Kidney Int Rep.* 2018;3:516.

Haines RW, Kirwan J, Prowle JR. Managing chloride and bicarbonate in the prevention and treatment of acute kidney injury. *Semin Nephrol.* 2019;39:473.

Hodgson LE, Selby N, Huang T-M, et al. The role of risk prediction models in prevention and management of AKI. *Semin Nephrol.* 2019;39:421.

Ichai C, Vinsonneau C, Souweine B, et al. Acute kidney injury in the perioperative period and in intensive care units (excluding renal replacement therapies). *Ann Intens Care.* 2016;6:48.

Joannidis M, Forni LG, Haase M, et al. Use of cell cycle arrest biomarkers in conjunction with classical markers of acute kidney injury. *Crit Care Med.* 2019;47:e820.

Joyce E, Kane-Gill S, Fuhrman D, et al. Drug-associated acute kidney injury: who's at risk? *Pediatr Nephrol.* 2017;32:59.

Katz NM, Kellum JA, Ronco C. Acute kidney stress and prevention of acute kidney injury. *Crit Care Med.* 2019;47:993.

Kellum J, Bellomo R, Ronco C. Does this patient have acute kidney injury? An AKI checklist. *Intens Care Med.* 2016;42:96.

Kellum JA, Fuhrman DY. The handwriting is on the wall: there will soon be a drug for AKI. *Nature Rev Nephrol.* 2019;15:65.

Kitchlu A, McArthur E, Amir E, et al. Acute kidney injury in patients receiving systemic treatment for cancer: a population-based cohort study. *J Natl Cancer Inst.* 2019;111:1.

Leatherby RJ, Theodorou C, Dhanda R. Renal physiology: blood flow, glomerular filtration and plasma clearance. *Anaesth Intens Care Med.* 2021;22:439.

Legrand M, Ince C. Intravenous fluids in AKI: a mechanistically guided approach. *Semin Nephrol.* 2016;36:53.

Murray PT. Prediction of acute kidney injury in hospitalized, non-critically ill patients. *Mayo Clin Proc.* 2020;95:435.

Nagalingam K. Acute kidney injury: the hidden killer in the ward. *J Ren Care.* 2020;46:72.

Ng JH, Hirsch JS, Hazzan A, et al. Outcomes among hospitalized patients with COVID-19 and acute kidney injury. *Am J Kidney Dis.* 2020;77:204.

Noble RA, Lucas BJ, Selby NM. Long-term outcomes in patients with acute kidney injury. *Clin J Am Soc Nephrol.* 2020;15:423.

O'Connor ME, Kirwan CJ, Pearse RM, et al. Incidence and associations of acute kidney injury after major abdominal surgery. *Intens Care Med.* 2016;42:521.

Oh D-J. A long journey for acute kidney injury biomarkers. *Renal Failure.* 2020;42:154.

O'Neal JB, Shaw AD, Billings IV FT. Acute kidney injury following cardiac surgery: current understanding and future directions. *Crit Care.* 2016;20:187.

Osborn JW, Tyshynsky R, Vulchanova L. Function of renal nerves in kidney physiology and pathophysiology. *Ann Rev Physiol.* 2021;83:429.

Pakula AM, Skinner RA. Acute kidney injury in the critically ill patient: a current review of the literature. *J Intens Care Med.* 2016;31:319.

Patel D, Connor M Jr. Intra-abdominal hypertension and abdominal compartment syndrome: an underappreciated cause of acute kidney injury. *Adv Chron Kidney Dis.* 2016;23:160.

Peerapornratana S, Manrique-Caballero CL, Gómez H, et al. Acute kidney injury from sepsis: current concepts, epidemiology, pathophysiology, prevention, and treatment. *Kidney Int.* 2019;96:1083.

Rein JL, Coca SG. "I don't get no respect": the role of chloride in acute kidney injury. *Am J Physiol Renal Physiol* 2019;316:F587.

Ronco F, Tarantini G, McCullough PA. Contrast-induced acute kidney injury in interventional cardiology: an update and key guidance for clinicians. *Rev Cardiovasc Med.* 2020;21:9.

Saffadi S, Hommos MS, Enders FT, et al. Risk factors for acute kidney injury in hospitalized non-critically ill patients: a population-based study. *Mayo Clin Proc.* 2020;95:459.

Scholz H, Boivin FJ, Schmidt-Ott KM, et al. Kidney physiology and susceptibility to acute kidney injury: implications for renoprotection. *Nature Rev Nephrol.* 2021;17:335.

See EJ, Jayasinghe K, Glassford N, et al. Long-term risk of adverse outcomes after acute kidney injury: a systematic review and meta-analysis of cohort studies using consensus definitions of exposure. *Kidney Int.* 2019;95:160.

Selby NM, Taal MW. Long-term outcomes after AKI–a major unmet clinical need. *Kidney Int.* 2019;95:21.

Semler MQ, Kellum JA. Balanced crystalloid solutions. *Am J Resp Crit Care Med.* 2019;199:952.

Silver SA, Beaubien-Souligny W, Shah PS, et al. The prevalence of acute kidney injury in patients hospitalized with COVID-19 infection: a systematic review and meta-analysis. *Kidney Med.* 2021;3:83.

Tomasev N, Glorot X, Rae JW, et al. A clinically applicable approach to continuous prediction of future acute kidney injury. *Nature.* 2019;572:116.

Wang Y, Liu K, Xie X, et al. Contrast-associated acute kidney injury: an update of risk factors, risk factor scores, and preventative measures. *Clin Imaging.* 2021;69:354.

CHAPTER 31

Anesthesia for Patients with Kidney Disease

KEY CONCEPTS

1. The utility of a single serum creatinine measurement as an indicator of glomerular filtration rate (GFR) is limited in critical illness: The rate of creatinine production, and its volume of distribution, may be abnormal in the critically ill patient, and the serum creatinine concentration often does not accurately reflect GFR in the physiological disequilibrium of acute kidney injury (AKI).
2. Creatinine clearance measurement is the most accurate method available for clinically assessing overall kidney function.
3. Accumulation of morphine (morphine-6-glucuronide) and meperidine (normeperidine) metabolites may prolong respiratory depression in patients with kidney failure, and increased levels of normeperidine may promote seizure activity.
4. Succinylcholine can be safely used in patients with kidney failure in the absence of hyperkalemia at the time of induction.
5. Extracellular fluid overload from sodium retention, in association with increased cardiac demand imposed by anemia and hypertension, makes patients with end-stage kidney disease particularly prone to congestive heart failure and pulmonary edema.
6. Delayed gastric emptying secondary to kidney disease–associated autonomic neuropathy may predispose patients to perioperative aspiration.
7. Controlled ventilation should be considered for patients with kidney failure under general anesthesia. Inadequate spontaneous or assisted ventilation with progressive hypercarbia under anesthesia can result in respiratory acidosis that may exacerbate preexisting acidemia, lead to potentially severe circulatory depression, and result in dangerously increased serum potassium concentration.
8. Correct anesthetic management of patients with renal insufficiency is as critical as management of those with frank kidney failure, especially during procedures associated with a relatively high incidence of postoperative kidney failure, such as cardiac and aortic reconstructive surgery.
9. Intravascular volume depletion, sepsis, obstructive jaundice, crush injuries, and renal toxins, such as radiocontrast agents, certain antibiotics, angiotensin-converting enzyme inhibitors, and nonsteroidal anti-inflammatory drugs, are major risk factors for acute deterioration in kidney function and kidney failure.
10. Kidney protection with adequate hydration and maintenance of renal blood flow is especially important for patients at high risk for perioperative AKI and kidney failure, such as those undergoing cardiac, major aortic reconstructive, and other surgical procedures associated with significant physiological trespass. The use of mannitol, low-dose dopamine infusion, loop diuretics, or fenoldopam for kidney protection is controversial and without proof of efficacy.

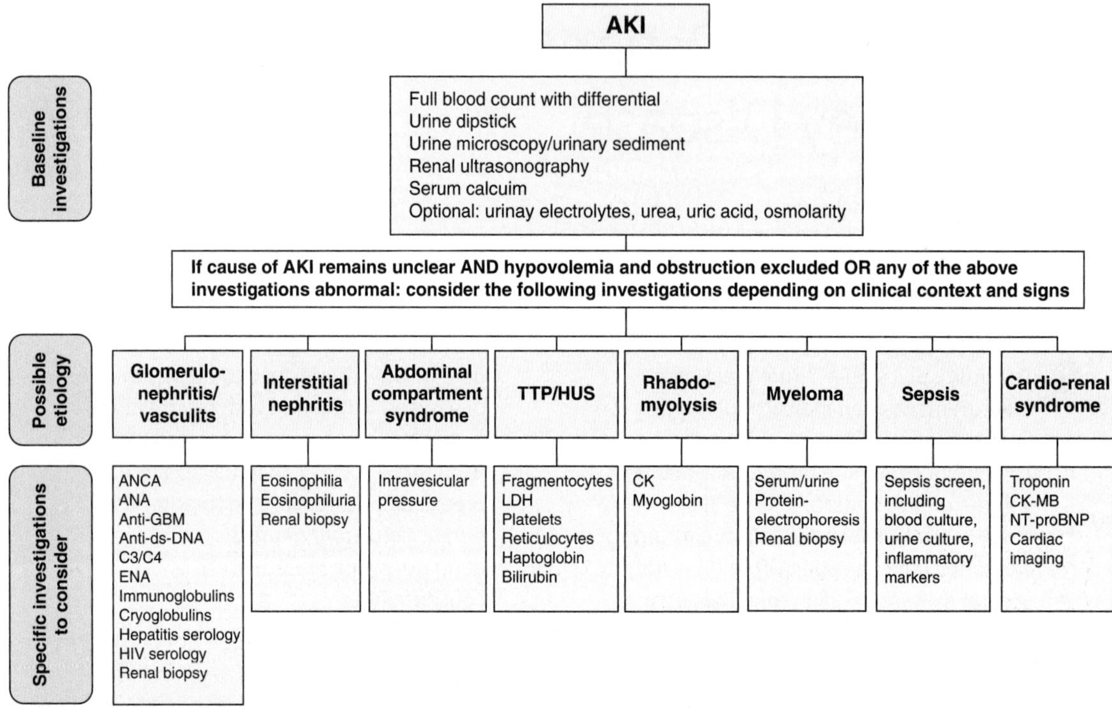

FIGURE 31–1 Differential diagnosis and evaluation of acute kidney injury (AKI). ANA, antinuclear antibody; ANCA, antineutrophil cytoplasmic antibody; Anti-ds-DNA, anti–double-stranded DNA; Anti-GMB, anti–glomerular basement membrane; C3, complement component 3; C4, complement component 4; CK, creatine kinase; CK-MB, creatine kinase MB fraction; ENA, extractable nuclear antigen; HIV, human immunodeficiency virus; HUS, hemolytic uremic syndrome; LDH, lactate dehydrogenase; NT-proBNP, *N*-terminal pro-brain natriuretic peptide; TTP, thrombotic thrombocytopenic purpura. (Reproduced with permission from Ostermann M, Joannidis M. Acute kidney injury 2016: Diagnosis and diagnostic workup. *Crit Care.* 2016 Sep 27;20(1):299.)

Acute kidney injury (AKI) is a common problem, with an incidence of up to 5% in all hospitalized patients and approximately 50% of patients in the intensive care unit. Postoperative AKI may occur in 1% to 5% or more of general surgery patients and in up to 30% of patients undergoing cardiothoracic and vascular procedures. Perioperative AKI is a markedly underappreciated problem that greatly increases perioperative morbidity, mortality, and costs. It is a systemic disorder that can include fluid and electrolyte derangements, respiratory failure, major cardiovascular events, weakened immunocompetence leading to infection and sepsis, altered mental status, hepatic dysfunction, and gastrointestinal hemorrhage. It is also a major cause of chronic kidney disease (CKD). Preoperative risk factors for perioperative AKI include preexisting kidney disease, hypertension, diabetes mellitus, liver disease, sepsis, trauma, hypovolemia, multiple myeloma, and age greater than 55 years. The risk of perioperative AKI is also increased by exposure to nephrotoxic agents such as nonsteroidal anti-inflammatory drugs (NSAIDs), radiocontrast agents, and antibiotics (see Table 30–4). The clinician must possess a thorough understanding of the risks of AKI, its differential diagnosis, and its evaluation strategy (Figure 31–1).

Evaluating Kidney Function

The underlying cause of impaired kidney function may be glomerular dysfunction, tubular dysfunction, or urinary tract obstruction. Accurate clinical assessment of kidney function is often difficult and relies heavily on clinical laboratory determinations of glomerular filtration rate (GFR), including creatinine clearance, and other evaluations (Tables 31–1 **and** 31–2). Even small

TABLE 31–1 Severity of kidney injury according to glomerular function.

	Creatinine Clearance (mL/min)
Normal	100–120
Decreased kidney reserve	60–100
Mild kidney impairment	40–60
Moderate kidney insufficiency	25–40
Kidney failure	<25
End-stage kidney disease[1]	<10

[1]This term applies to patients with chronic kidney failure.

postoperative increases in serum creatinine are associated with increased morbidity and mortality, though many factors may confound its measurement (Figure 31–2). Systems employed in defining and staging the degree of kidney dysfunction include the Acute Dialysis Quality Initiative Risk, Injury, Failure, Loss, End-Stage (RIFLE) criteria, and the Acute Kidney Injury Network (AKIN) staging system. These systems were merged into the Kidney Disease Improving Global Outcomes (KDIGO) classification (Table 31–3). Thus, the traditional diagnosis of AKI, based upon serum creatinine and urine output, has been refined into an increase of serum creatinine of 0.3 mg/dL or

TABLE 31–2 Laboratory evaluation of kidney impairment.

Diagnostic Test	Strengths	Weaknesses
Serum creatinine	Easily available Low cost	Not renal specific Late marker after renal injury Serum levels confounded by muscle mass, drugs, laboratory technique, fluid status
Blood urea nitrogen	Easily available Low cost	Not renal specific Serum levels confounded by liver disease, gastrointestinal bleed, and hypovolemia
FeNa	Easily available Low cost	Difficult to interpret in patients with chronic kidney disease Confounded by diuretic treatment
Urine microscopy	Noninvasive Low cost Can provide very valuable information if done properly, (ie, red cell casts in case of glomerulonephritis)	Operator dependent Requires training and experience
Renal histology	Can provide very valuable information about cause of AKI and degree of chronic changes	Invasive Requires competency Bleeding complications
Novel AKI biomarkers	Opportunity to diagnose AKI before creatinine rise May provide additional diagnostic and prognostic information	Costs Significant confounders
Techniques to measure real-time GFR	Opportunity to monitor GFR in real time and to diagnose AKI early	Costs Not yet available in clinical practice Requires training and experience

AKI, acute kidney injury; FeNa, fractional excretion of sodium; GFR, glomerular filtration rate.

Reproduced with permission from Ostermann M. Diagnosis of acute kidney injury: Kidney Disease Improving Global Outcomes criteria and beyond. *Curr Opin Crit.* 2014 Dec;20(6):581-587.

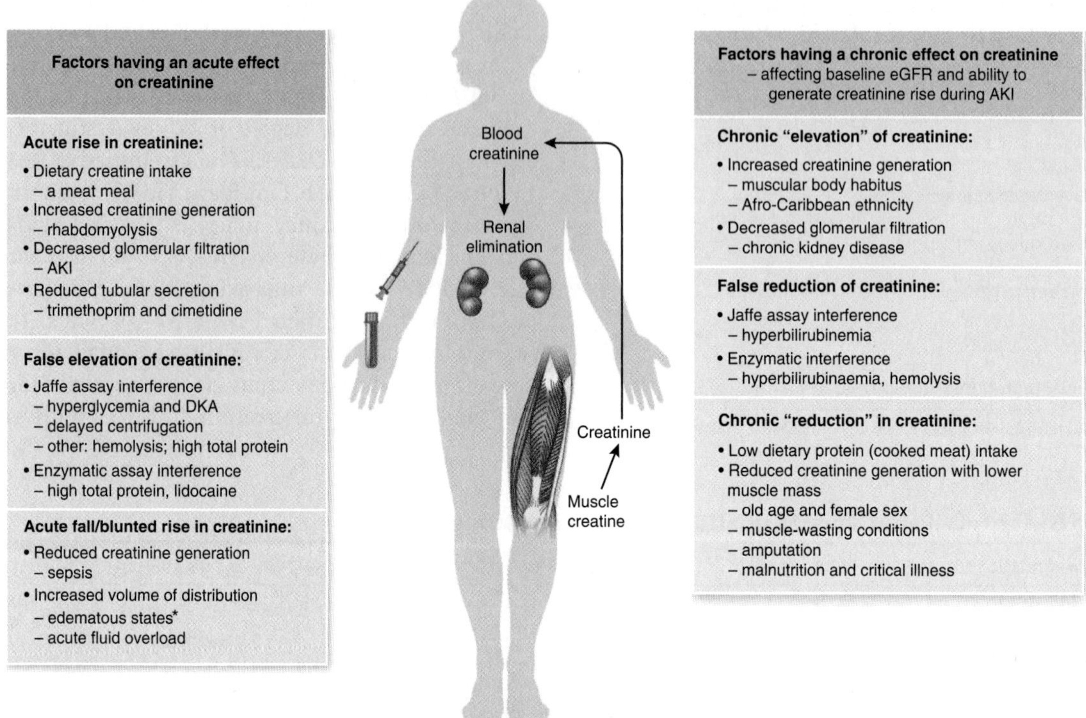

Factors having an acute effect on creatinine
Acute rise in creatinine:
• Dietary creatine intake
– a meat meal
• Increased creatinine generation
– rhabdomyolysis
• Decreased glomerular filtration
– AKI
• Reduced tubular secretion
– trimethoprim and cimetidine
False elevation of creatinine:
• Jaffe assay interference
– hyperglycemia and DKA
– delayed centrifugation
– other: hemolysis; high total protein
• Enzymatic assay interference
– high total protein, lidocaine
Acute fall/blunted rise in creatinine:
• Reduced creatinine generation
– sepsis
• Increased volume of distribution
– edematous states*
– acute fluid overload
Blood creatinine
Renal elimination
Creatinine
Muscle creatine
Factors having a chronic effect on creatinine – affecting baseline eGFR and ability to generate creatinine rise during AKI
Chronic "elevation" of creatinine:
• Increased creatinine generation
– muscular body habitus
– Afro-Caribbean ethnicity
• Decreased glomerular filtration
– chronic kidney disease
False reduction of creatinine:
• Jaffe assay interference
– hyperbilirubinemia
• Enzymatic interference
– hyperbilirubinaemia, hemolysis
Chronic "reduction" in creatinine:
• Low dietary protein (cooked meat) intake
• Reduced creatinine generation with lower muscle mass
– old age and female sex
– muscle-wasting conditions
– amputation
– malnutrition and critical illness

FIGURE 31–2 Factors affecting serum creatinine interpretation in acute kidney injury. *Edematous states: cirrhosis, nephrotic syndrome, heart failure. DKA, diabetic ketoacidosis; eGFR, estimated glomerular filtration rate. (Reproduced with permission from Thomas MD, Blaine C, Dawnay A, et al. The definition of acute kidney injury and its use in practice. *Kidney Int.* 2015 Jan;87(1):62-73.)

more within 48 h or a 1.5-fold or greater increase in baseline within 7 days. Since AKI is a systemic disorder, it is important to recall that the kidney excretory function assessed via serum creatinine and urine output ignores endocrine, metabolic, and immunological kidney functions. A great deal of research is currently evaluating plasma and urine biomarkers associated with AKI, and several are now commercially available (Figure 31–3). It is likely that biomarkers will play an increasingly prominent role in the diagnosis, staging, and prognostic assessment of AKI.

BLOOD UREA NITROGEN

The primary source of urea in the body is the liver. During protein catabolism, ammonia is produced from the deamination of amino acids. Hepatic conversion of ammonia to urea prevents the buildup of toxic ammonia levels:

$$2NH_3 + CO_2 \rightarrow H_2N - CO - NH_2 + H_2O$$

Blood urea nitrogen (BUN) is therefore directly related to protein catabolism and inversely related to glomerular filtration. As a result, BUN is not a reliable indicator of the GFR unless protein catabolism is normal and constant. Recall that 40% to 50% of the urea filtrate is normally reabsorbed passively by the renal tubules and that hypovolemia increases this fraction.

The normal BUN concentration is 10 to 20 mg/dL. Lower values may be seen with starvation or liver disease; elevations usually result from decreases in GFR or increases in protein catabolism. The latter may be due to a high catabolic state (trauma or sepsis), degradation of blood either in the gastrointestinal tract or in a large hematoma,

TABLE 31–3 RIFLE, AKIN, and KDIGO classifications for acute kidney injury.

	Serum Creatinine Criteria			Urine Output Criteria of All Classifications
	RIFLE Classification	AKIN Classification	KDIGO Classification	
Definition of AKI		Increase in serum creatinine of either ≥0.3 mg/dL (≥26.4 μmol/L) or a percentage increase of ≥50% (1.5-fold from baseline) in 48 h	Rise in serum creatinine by ≥26 μmol/L over ≤48 h, or to ≥1.5-fold from baseline that is known or presumed to have occurred in the preceding 7 days	
Stage I or RIFLE risk	Increase in serum creatinine to ≥1.5 to 2-fold from baseline, or GFR decrease by >25%	Increase in serum creatinine by ≥26 μmol/L (>0.3 mg/dL) or increase to more than or equal to 1.5-fold to 2-fold from baseline	Rise in serum creatinine by ≥26.5 μmol/L in 48 h, or rise to 1.5–1.9 times from baseline	<0.5 mL/kg/h for >6 h
Stage II or RIFLE injury	Increase in serum creatinine to >2-fold to 3-fold from baseline, or GFR decrease by >50%	Increase in serum creatinine to more than 2-fold to 3-fold from baseline	Rise in serum creatinine 2.0–2.9 times from baseline	<0.5 mL/kg/h for >12 h
Stage III or RIFLE failure	Increase in serum creatinine to >3-fold from baseline, or to ≥354 μmol/L with an acute rise of at least 44 μmol/L, or GFR decrease by >75%	Increase in serum creatinine to more than 3-fold from baseline, or to ≥354 μmol/L with an acute rise of at least 44 μmol/L, or treatment with RRT irrespective of the stage at the time of RRT	Rise in serum creatinine three times from baseline, or increase in serum creatinine to ≥353.6 μmol/L, or initiation of RRT irrespective of serum creatinine	<0.3 mL/kg/h for 24 h or more, or anuria for 12 h
RIFLE loss	Complete loss of kidney function for >4 wk	—	—	
End-stage kidney disease	End-stage kidney disease for >3 mo	—	—	

AKI, acute kidney injury; AKIN, Acute Kidney Injury Network; GFR, glomerular filtration rate; KDIGO, Kidney Disease Improving Global Outcomes; RIFLE, Risk, Injury, Failure, Loss, End-Stage; RRT, renal replacement therapy.

Reproduced with permission from Ostermann M. Diagnosis of acute kidney injury: Kidney Disease Improving Global Outcomes and beyond. *Curr Opin Crit Care.* 2014 Dec;20(6):581-587.

or a high-protein diet. BUN concentrations greater than 50 mg/dL are generally associated with impaired kidney function.

SERUM CREATININE

Creatine is a product of muscle metabolism that is nonenzymatically converted to creatinine. Daily creatinine production in most people is relatively constant and related to muscle mass, averaging 20 to 25 mg/kg in men and 15 to 20 mg/kg in women. Creatinine is then filtered (and to a minor extent secreted) but not reabsorbed in the kidneys. Serum creatinine concentration is therefore directly related to body muscle mass and inversely related to glomerular filtration (Figure 31–4). Because body muscle mass is usually relatively constant, serum creatinine measurements are generally reliable indices of GFR

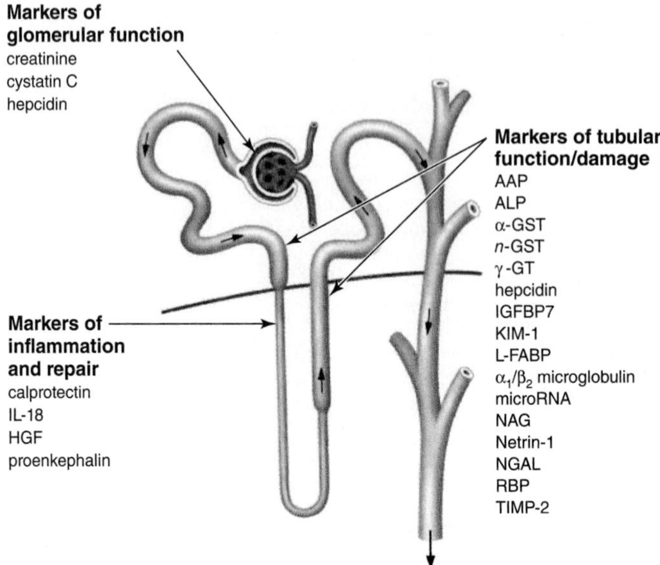

FIGURE 31–3 AKI biomarkers. α-GST, α-glutathione S-transferase; AAP, alanine aminopeptidase; ALP, alkaline phosphatase; γ-GT, γ-glutamyl transpeptidase; *n*-GST, *n*-glutathione S-transferase; HGF, hepatocyte growth factor; IGFBP-7, insulin-like growth factor binding protein 7; IL-18, interleukin-18; KIM-1, kidney injury molecule-1; L-FABP, liver fatty acid-binding protein; NAG, *N*-acetyl-β-D-glucosaminidase; NGAL, neutrophil gelatinase-associated lipocalin; RBP, retinol-binding protein; TIMP-2, tissue inhibitor metalloproteinase-2. (Reproduced with permission from Ostermann M, Joannidis M. Acute kidney injury 2016: Diagnosis and diagnostic workup. *Crit Care.* 2016 Sep 27;20(1):299.)

1 in the ambulatory patient. However, the utility of a single serum creatinine measurement as an indicator of GFR is limited in critical illness: The rate of creatinine production and its volume of distribution is frequently abnormal in the critically ill patient, and a single serum creatinine measurement often will not accurately reflect GFR in the physiological disequilibrium of AKI.

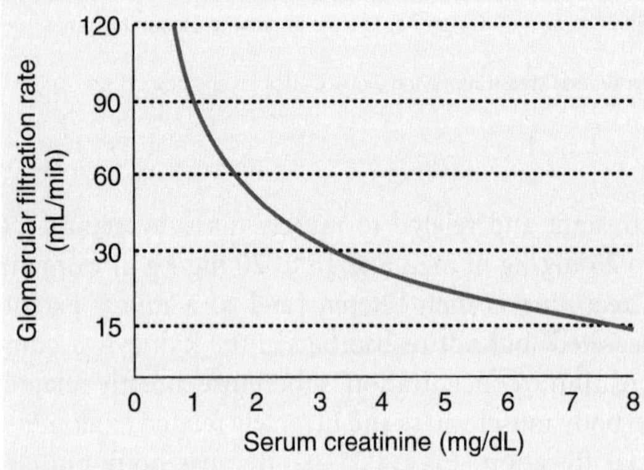

FIGURE 31–4 The relationship between the serum creatinine concentration and the glomerular filtration rate.

The normal serum creatinine concentration is 0.8 to 1.3 mg/dL in men and 0.6 to 1 mg/dL in women. Note from Figure 31–4 that each doubling of the serum creatinine represents a 50% reduction in GFR. As previously noted, many factors may affect serum creatinine measurement.

GFR declines with increasing age in most individuals (5% per decade after age 20), but because muscle mass also declines, the serum creatinine remains relatively normal; creatinine production may decrease to 10 mg/kg. Thus, in older adult patients, small increases in serum creatinine may represent large changes in GFR. Using age and lean body weight (in kilograms), GFR can be estimated by the following formula for men:

$$\text{Creatinine clearance} = \frac{[(140 - \text{Age}) \times \text{Lean body weight}]}{(72 \times \text{Plasma creatinine})}$$

For women, this equation must be multiplied by 0.85 to compensate for a smaller muscle mass.

The serum creatinine concentration requires 48 to 72 h to equilibrate at a new level following acute changes in GFR.

CREATININE CLEARANCE

2 Creatinine clearance measurement is the most accurate method available for clinically assessing GFR. Although measurements are usually performed over 24 h, 2-h creatinine clearance determinations are reasonably accurate and more convenient to perform. Mild impairment of kidney function generally results in creatinine clearances of 40 to 60 mL/min. Clearances between 25 and 40 mL/min produce moderate kidney dysfunction and nearly always cause symptoms. Creatinine clearances less than 25 mL/min are indicative of overt kidney failure.

Later-stage kidney disease leads to increased creatinine secretion in the proximal tubule. As a result, with declining kidney function the creatinine clearance progressively overestimates the true GFR. Moreover, relative preservation of GFR despite progressive kidney disease may result from compensatory hyperfiltration in the remaining nephrons and increases in glomerular filtration pressure. It is therefore important to look for other signs of deteriorating kidney function, including hypertension, proteinuria, or abnormalities in urine sediment.

BLOOD UREA NITROGEN: CREATININE RATIO

Low renal tubular flow rates enhance urea reabsorption but do not affect creatinine excretion. As a result, the ratio of serum BUN to serum creatinine increases to more than 10:1. Decreases in tubular flow can be caused by decreased kidney perfusion or obstruction of the urinary tract. *BUN:creatinine ratios greater than 15:1 are therefore seen in volume depletion and in edematous disorders associated with decreased tubular flow (eg, congestive heart failure, cirrhosis, nephrotic syndrome) as well as in obstructive uropathies.* Increases in protein catabolism can also increase this ratio.

URINALYSIS

Urinalysis continues to be routinely performed for evaluating kidney function. Although its utility and cost-effectiveness for this purpose are questionable, urinalysis can be helpful in identifying some disorders of renal tubular dysfunction as well as some nonrenal disturbances. A routine urinalysis typically includes pH; specific gravity; detection and quantification of glucose, protein, and bilirubin content; and microscopic examination of the urinary sediment. Urinary pH is helpful only when arterial pH is also known. A urinary pH greater than 7.0 in the presence of systemic acidosis is suggestive of renal tubular acidosis (see Chapter 50). Specific gravity is related to urinary osmolality; 1.010 usually corresponds to 290 mOsm/kg. A specific gravity greater than 1.018 after an overnight fast is indicative of adequate renal concentrating ability. A lower specific gravity in the presence of hyperosmolality in plasma is consistent with diabetes insipidus.

Glycosuria is the result of either a reduced tubular threshold for glucose (normally 180 mg/dL), sodium-glucose cotransporter-2 (SGLT2) inhibitor administration in patients with type 2 diabetes, or hyperglycemia. Proteinuria detected by routine urinalysis should be evaluated by means of 24-h urine collection. Urinary protein excretions greater than 150 mg/d are significant. Elevated levels of bilirubin in the urine are seen with biliary obstruction.

Microscopic analysis of the urinary sediment detects the presence of red or white blood cells, bacteria, casts, and crystals. Red cells may be indicative of bleeding due to tumor, stones, infection, coagulopathy, or trauma (commonly, urinary catheterization). White cells and bacteria are generally associated with infection. Disease processes at the level of the nephron produce tubular casts. Crystals may be indicative of abnormalities in oxalic acid, uric acid, or cystine metabolism.

Altered Kidney Function & the Effects of Anesthetic Agents

Most drugs commonly employed during anesthesia (other than volatile anesthetics) are at least partly dependent on renal excretion for elimination.

In the presence of kidney impairment, dosage modifications may be required to prevent accumulation of the drug or its active metabolites. Moreover, the systemic effects of AKI can potentiate the pharmacological actions of many of these agents. This latter observation may be the result of decreased protein binding of the drug, greater brain penetration due to some breach of the blood–brain barrier, or a synergistic effect with the toxins retained in kidney failure.

INTRAVENOUS AGENTS

Propofol & Etomidate

The pharmacokinetics of both propofol and etomidate are minimally affected by impaired kidney function. Decreased protein binding of etomidate in patients with hypoalbuminemia may enhance its pharmacological effects.

Barbiturates

Patients with kidney disease often exhibit increased sensitivity to barbiturates during induction, even though pharmacokinetic profiles appear to be unchanged. The mechanism appears to be an increase in free circulating barbiturate secondary to decreased protein binding. Acidosis may also favor a more rapid entry of these agents into the brain by increasing the nonionized fraction of the drug (see Chapter 26).

Ketamine

Ketamine pharmacokinetics are minimally altered by kidney disease. Some active hepatic metabolites are dependent on renal excretion and can potentially accumulate in kidney failure.

Benzodiazepines

Benzodiazepines undergo hepatic metabolism and conjugation prior to elimination in urine. Because they are highly protein bound, increased benzodiazepine sensitivity may be seen in patients with hypoalbuminemia. Diazepam and midazolam should be administered cautiously in the presence of kidney impairment because of the potential for the accumulation of active metabolites.

Opioids

Most opioids used in anesthetic practice (morphine, meperidine, fentanyl, sufentanil, and alfentanil) are inactivated by the liver; some of these metabolites are then excreted in urine. Remifentanil pharmacokinetics are unaffected by kidney function due to rapid ester hydrolysis in blood. With the exception of morphine and meperidine, significant accumulation of active metabolites generally does not occur
3 with these agents. Accumulation of morphine (morphine-6-glucuronide) and meperidine (normeperidine) metabolites may prolong respiratory depression in patients with kidney failure, and increased levels of normeperidine may promote seizure activity. The pharmacokinetics of the most commonly used opioid agonist–antagonists (butorphanol, nalbuphine, and buprenorphine) are unaffected by kidney failure.

Anticholinergic Agents

In doses used for premedication, atropine and glycopyrrolate can generally be used safely in patients with kidney impairment. Because up to 50% of these drugs and their active metabolites are normally excreted in urine, however, the potential for accumulation exists following repeated doses. Scopolamine is less dependent on renal excretion, but its central nervous system effects can be enhanced by decreased kidney function.

Phenothiazines, H_2 Blockers, & Related Agents

Most phenothiazines, such as promethazine, are metabolized to inactive compounds by the liver. Droperidol may be partly dependent on the kidneys for excretion. Although their pharmacokinetic profiles are not appreciably altered by kidney impairment, potentiation of the central depressant effects of phenothiazines by the systemic effects of kidney disease may occur.

All H_2-receptor blockers are dependent on kidney excretion, and their dose must be reduced for patients with kidney disease. Proton pump inhibitor dosage does not need to be reduced for patients with kidney disease. Metoclopramide is partly excreted unchanged in urine and will accumulate in kidney failure. Although up to 50% of dolasetron is excreted in urine, no dosage adjustments are recommended for any of the 5-HT_3 blockers in patients with kidney disease.

INHALATION AGENTS

Volatile Agents

Volatile anesthetic agents are ideal for patients with kidney disease because they are not dependent on the kidneys for elimination and they have minimal direct effects on kidney blood flow. Although patients with mild to moderate kidney impairment do not exhibit altered uptake or distribution, accelerated induction and emergence may be seen in severely anemic patients (hemoglobin <5 g/dL) with chronic kidney failure, possibly because of a decrease in the blood:gas partition coefficient. Some clinicians avoid sevoflurane (and avoid <2 L/min gas flows) for patients with kidney disease who undergo lengthy procedures (see Chapters 8 and 30).

Nitrous Oxide

Some clinicians omit entirely or limit the use of nitrous oxide (or air) to maintain an FiO_2 of 50% or greater in severely anemic patients with end-stage kidney disease in an attempt to increase arterial oxygen content. This may be justified in patients with hemoglobin less than 7 g/dL, in whom even a small increase in the dissolved oxygen content may represent a significant percentage of the arterial to venous oxygen difference (see Chapter 23).

MUSCLE RELAXANTS

Succinylcholine

4 Succinylcholine can be safely used in patients with kidney failure in the absence of hyperkalemia at the time of induction. It should be avoided in patients with kidney failure when the serum potassium is known to be increased or is undetermined. Although decreased plasma cholinesterase levels have been reported in uremic patients following dialysis, significant prolongation of neuromuscular blockade with succinylcholine use is rarely seen in this circumstance.

Cisatracurium & Atracurium

Cisatracurium and atracurium are degraded by plasma ester hydrolysis and nonenzymatic Hofmann elimination. These agents are often the drugs of choice for muscle relaxation in patients with kidney failure, especially in clinical situations where neuromuscular function monitoring is difficult or impossible.

Vecuronium & Rocuronium

The elimination of vecuronium is primarily hepatic, but up to 20% of the drug is eliminated in urine. The effects of large doses of vecuronium (>0.1 mg/kg) are only modestly prolonged in patients with kidney disease. Rocuronium primarily undergoes hepatic elimination, but prolongation in patients with severe kidney disease has been reported. In general, with appropriate neuromuscular monitoring, these two agents can be used with few problems in patients with severe kidney disease.

Curare (d-Tubocurarine)

Elimination of d-tubocurarine is dependent on both kidney and biliary excretion; 40% to 60% of a dose of curare is normally excreted in urine. Increasingly prolonged effects are observed following repeated doses in patients with decreased kidney function. Smaller doses and longer dosing intervals are therefore required for maintenance of optimal muscle relaxation.

Pancuronium

Pancuronium is primarily dependent on renal excretion (60–90%). Although pancuronium is metabolized by the liver into less active intermediates, its elimination half-life is still primarily dependent on renal excretion (60–80%). Neuromuscular function should be closely monitored if pancuronium is used in patients with abnormal kidney function.

Reversal Agents

Renal excretion is the principal route of elimination for edrophonium, neostigmine, and pyridostigmine. The half-lives of these agents in patients with kidney impairment are therefore prolonged at least as much as any of the above relaxants, and problems with inadequate reversal of neuromuscular blockade are usually related to other factors (see Chapter 11). Thus, "recurarization" due to inadequate duration of the reversal agent is unlikely. Sugammadex is a steroidal muscle relaxant encapsulator drug that, even after binding vecuronium or rocuronium, is rapidly and entirely eliminated (along with the neuromuscular blocker) in its unmetabolized form by the kidney (see Chapter 11). Early studies suggest that the onset of sugammadex muscle relaxant reversal may be delayed and that the sugammadex–muscle relaxant complex may persist for several days in the plasma of patients with decreased kidney function. Because of the potential patient safety implications of prolonged sugammadex–muscle relaxant complex exposure in this situation, the use of sugammadex is not recommended at this time in patients with low creatine clearance (<30 mL/min) or on renal replacement therapy (RRT).

TABLE 31–4 Management priorities in patients with acute kidney failure.

- Search for and correct prerenal and postrenal causes
- Review medications and patient-administered substances and stop any potential nephrotoxins
- Administer medications in doses appropriate for their clearance
- Optimize cardiac output and renal blood flow
- Monitor fluid intake and output; measure body weight daily
- Search for and treat acute complications (hyperkalemia, hyponatremia, acidosis, hyperphosphatemia, pulmonary edema)
- Search for and aggressively treat infections and sepsis
- Provide early nutritional support
- Provide expert supportive care (management of catheter and skin care; pressure sore and deep venous thromboembolic prophylaxis; psychological support).

Reproduced with permission from Lameire N, Van Biesen W, Vanholder R. Acute renal failure. Lancet. 2005 Jan 29-Feb 4;365(9457):417-430.

Anesthesia for Patients with Kidney Failure

PREOPERATIVE CONSIDERATIONS

Acute Kidney Failure

This syndrome is a rapid deterioration in kidney function that results in the retention of nitrogenous waste products (azotemia). These substances, many of which behave as toxins, are byproducts of protein and amino acid metabolism. Impaired kidney metabolic activity may contribute to widespread organ dysfunction (see Chapter 30).

Kidney failure can be classified as prerenal, renal, and postrenal, depending on its cause(s), and the initial therapeutic approach varies accordingly (see Figure 31–1 and Table 31–4). Prerenal kidney failure results from an acute decrease in renal perfusion; intrinsic kidney failure is usually due to underlying kidney disease, kidney ischemia, or nephrotoxins; and postrenal failure is the result of urinary collecting system obstruction or disruption. Both prerenal and postrenal forms of kidney failure are readily reversible in their initial stages, but with time both progress to intrinsic kidney failure. Most adult patients with kidney failure first develop oliguria. Nonoliguric patients with kidney failure (urinary outputs >400 mL/d) continue to form urine that is qualitatively poor; these patients tend to have greater preservation of GFR. Although glomerular filtration and tubular function are impaired in both cases, these abnormalities tend to be less severe in nonoliguric kidney failure.

The course of intrinsic acute kidney failure varies widely, but oliguria typically lasts for 2 weeks and is followed by a diuretic phase marked by a progressive increase in urinary output. This diuretic phase often results in very large urinary outputs and is usually absent in nonoliguric kidney failure. Kidney function improves over the course of several weeks but may not return to normal for up to 1 year, and subsequent chronic kidney disease is common. The course of prerenal and postrenal kidney failure is dependent upon promptness in diagnosis and correction of the causal condition. Diagnostic ultrasound, including point-of-care ultrasound, is increasingly used to rapidly and noninvasively evaluate possible obstructive uropathy.

Chronic Kidney Disease

The most common causes of chronic kidney disease (CKD) are hypertensive nephrosclerosis, diabetic nephropathy, chronic glomerulonephritis, and

TABLE 31–5 Manifestations of chronic kidney disease.

Neurological	**Metabolic**
Peripheral neuropathy	Metabolic acidosis
Autonomic neuropathy	Hyperkalemia
Muscle twitching	Hyponatremia
Encephalopathy	Hypermagnesemia
Asterixis	Hyperphosphatemia
Myoclonus	Hypocalcemia
Lethargy	Hyperuricemia
Confusion	Hypoalbuminemia
Seizures	**Hematological**
Coma	Anemia
Cardiovascular	Platelet dysfunction
Fluid overload	Leukocyte dysfunction
Congestive heart failure	**Endocrine**
Hypertension	Glucose intolerance
Pericarditis	Secondary hyperparathyroidism
Arrhythmia	Hypertriglyceridemia
Conduction blocks	**Skeletal**
Vascular calcification	Osteodystrophy
Accelerated atherosclerosis	Periarticular calcification
Pulmonary	**Skin**
Hyperventilation	Hyperpigmentation
Interstitial edema	Ecchymosis
Alveolar edema	Pruritus
Pleural effusion	
Gastrointestinal	
Anorexia	
Nausea and vomiting	
Delayed gastric emptying	
Hyperacidity	
Mucosal ulcerations	
Hemorrhage	
Adynamic ileus	

polycystic kidney disease. The uncorrected manifestations of this syndrome (Table 31–5) are usually seen only after GFR decreases below 25 mL/min. Patients with GFR less than 10 mL/min are dependent upon RRT for survival in the form of hemodialysis, hemofiltration, or peritoneal dialysis.

The generalized effects of severe CKD can usually be controlled by RRT. Most patients with end-stage kidney disease who do not undergo renal transplantation receive RRT three times per week. There are complications directly related to RRT itself (Table 31–6). Hypotension, neutropenia, hypoxemia, and disequilibrium syndrome are generally transient if they occur and resolve within hours after RRT. Factors contributing to hypotension during dialysis include the vasodilating effects of dialysate

TABLE 31–6 Complications of renal replacement therapy.

Neurological
Dialysis disequilibrium syndrome
Dementia
Cardiovascular
Intravascular volume depletion
Hypotension
Arrhythmia
Pulmonary
Hypoxemia
Gastrointestinal
Ascites
Hematological
Anemia
Transient neutropenia
Residual anticoagulation
Hypocomplementemia
Metabolic
Hypokalemia
Large protein losses
Skeletal
Osteomalacia
Arthropathy
Myopathy
Infectious
Peritonitis
Transfusion-related hepatitis

solutions, autonomic neuropathy, and rapid removal of fluid. The interaction of white cells with dialysis membranes can result in neutropenia and leukocyte-mediated pulmonary dysfunction leading to hypoxemia. *Dialysis disequilibrium syndrome* (DDS) is most frequently seen following aggressive dialysis and is characterized by transient alterations in mental status and focal neurological deficits that are secondary to cerebral edema.

Manifestations of Kidney Failure

A. Metabolic

Multiple metabolic abnormalities, including hyperkalemia, hyperphosphatemia, hypocalcemia, hypermagnesemia, hyperuricemia, and hypoalbuminemia, typically develop in patients with kidney failure. Water and sodium retention can result in worsening hyponatremia and extracellular fluid overload, respectively. Failure to excrete nonvolatile acids produces an increased anion gap metabolic acidosis (see Chapter 50). Hypernatremia and hypokalemia are uncommon complications.

Hyperkalemia is a potentially lethal consequence of kidney failure (see Chapter 49). It usually occurs in patients with creatinine clearances of less than 5 mL/min, but it can also develop rapidly in patients with higher clearances in the setting of large potassium loads (eg, trauma, hemolysis, infections, or potassium administration).

Hypermagnesemia is generally mild unless magnesium intake is increased (commonly from magnesium-containing antacids). Hypocalcemia is secondary to resistance to parathyroid hormone, decreased intestinal calcium absorption secondary to decreased kidney synthesis of 1,25-dihydroxycholecalciferol, and hyperphosphatemia-associated calcium deposition into bone. Symptoms of hypocalcemia rarely develop unless patients are also alkalotic.

Patients with kidney failure also rapidly lose tissue protein and readily develop hypoalbuminemia. Anorexia, protein restriction, and dialysis are contributory.

B. Hematologic

Anemia is nearly always present when the creatinine clearance is below 30 mL/min. Hemoglobin concentrations are generally 6 to 8 g/dL due to decreased erythropoietin production, red cell production, and red cell survival. Additional factors may include gastrointestinal blood loss, hemodilution, bone marrow suppression from recurrent infections, and blood loss for laboratory testing. Even with transfusions, it is often difficult to maintain hemoglobin concentrations greater than 9 g/dL. Erythropoietin administration may partially correct the anemia. Increased levels of 2,3-diphosphoglycerate (2,3-DPG), which facilitates the unloading of oxygen from hemoglobin (see Chapter 23), develop in response to the decrease in blood oxygen-carrying capacity. The metabolic acidosis associated with CKD also favors a rightward shift in the hemoglobin–oxygen dissociation curve. In the absence of symptomatic heart disease, most CKD patients tolerate anemia well.

Both platelet and white cell function are impaired in patients with kidney failure. Clinically, this is manifested as a prolonged bleeding time and increased susceptibility to infections, respectively. Most patients have decreased platelet factor III activity as well as decreased platelet adhesiveness and aggregation. Patients who have recently undergone hemodialysis may also have residual anticoagulant effects from heparin.

C. Cardiovascular

Cardiac output increases in kidney failure to maintain oxygen delivery due to decreased blood oxygen-carrying capacity. Sodium retention and abnormalities in the renin–angiotensin system result in systemic arterial hypertension. Left ventricular hypertrophy is a common finding in CKD. 5 Extracellular fluid overload from sodium retention, in association with increased cardiac demand imposed by anemia and hypertension, makes CKD patients prone to congestive heart failure and pulmonary edema. Increased permeability of the alveolar–capillary membrane may also be a predisposing factor for pulmonary edema associated with CKD (see later discussion). Arrhythmias, including conduction blocks, are common and may be related to metabolic abnormalities and to the deposition of calcium in the conduction system. Uremic pericarditis may develop in some patients, who may be asymptomatic, may present with chest pain, or may present with cardiac tamponade. Patients with CKD also characteristically develop accelerated peripheral vascular and coronary artery atherosclerotic disease.

Intravascular volume depletion may occur in high-output acute kidney failure if fluid replacement is inadequate. Hypovolemia may also occur secondary to excessive fluid removal during dialysis.

D. Pulmonary

Without RRT or bicarbonate therapy, CKD patients may be dependent on increased minute ventilation as compensation for metabolic acidosis (see Chapter 50). Pulmonary extravascular water is often increased in the form of interstitial edema, resulting in a widening of the alveolar to arterial oxygen gradient and predisposing to hypoxemia. Increased permeability of the alveolar–capillary membrane in some patients can result in pulmonary edema even with normal pulmonary capillary pressures.

E. Endocrine

Abnormal glucose tolerance is common in CKD, usually resulting from peripheral insulin resistance (type 2 diabetes mellitus is one of the most common causes of CKD). Secondary hyperparathyroidism in patients with chronic kidney failure can produce metabolic bone disease, predisposing them to fractures. Abnormalities in lipid metabolism frequently lead to hypertriglyceridemia and contribute to accelerated atherosclerosis. Increased circulating levels of proteins and polypeptides normally degraded by the kidneys are often present, including parathyroid hormone, insulin, glucagon, growth hormone, luteinizing hormone, and prolactin.

F. Gastrointestinal

Anorexia, nausea, vomiting, and ileus are commonly associated with uremia. Hypersecretion of gastric acid increases the incidence of peptic ulceration and gastrointestinal hemorrhage, which occurs in 10%
6 to 30% of patients. Delayed gastric emptying secondary to kidney disease–associated autonomic neuropathy may predispose patients to perioperative aspiration. Patients with CKD also have an increased incidence of hepatitis B and C, often with associated hepatic dysfunction.

G. Neurological

Asterixis, lethargy, confusion, seizures, and coma are manifestations of uremic encephalopathy, and symptoms usually correlate with the degree of azotemia. Autonomic and peripheral neuropathies are common in patients with CKD. Peripheral neuropathies are typically sensory and involve the distal lower extremities.

Preoperative Evaluation

Most perioperative patients with acute kidney failure are critically ill, and their kidney failure is frequently associated with trauma or perioperative medical or surgical complications. They are typically in a state of metabolic catabolism. Optimal perioperative management is dependent upon RRT. Hemodialysis is more effective than peritoneal dialysis and can be readily accomplished via a temporary internal jugular, subclavian, or femoral dialysis catheter.

TABLE 31–7 Indications for renal replacement therapy.

Fluid overload
Hyperkalemia
Severe acidosis
Metabolic encephalopathy
Pericarditis
Coagulopathy
Refractory gastrointestinal symptoms
Drug toxicity

Continuous renal replacement therapy (CRRT) is often used when patients are too hemodynamically unstable to tolerate intermittent hemodialysis. Indications for RRT are listed in Table 31–7.

Patients with CKD commonly present to the operating room for creation or revision of an arteriovenous dialysis fistula under local or regional anesthesia. Preoperative dialysis on the day of surgery or on the previous day is typical. However, regardless of the intended procedure or the anesthetic employed, one must be certain that the patient is in optimal medical condition; potentially reversible manifestations of uremia (see Table 31–5) should be addressed.

The history and physical examination should address both cardiac and respiratory function. Signs of fluid overload or hypovolemia should be sought. Patients are often relatively hypovolemic immediately following dialysis. A comparison of the patient's current weight with previous predialysis and postdialysis weights may be helpful. Hemodynamic data and a chest radiograph, if available, are useful in confirming clinical suspicion of volume overload. Arterial blood gas analysis is useful in evaluating oxygenation, ventilation, hemoglobin level, and acid–base status in patients with dyspnea or tachypnea. The electrocardiogram should be examined for signs of hyperkalemia or hypocalcemia (see Chapter 49) as well as ischemia, conduction block, and ventricular hypertrophy. Echocardiography can assess cardiac function, ventricular hypertrophy, wall motion abnormalities, and pericardial fluid. A pericardial friction rub may not be audible on auscultation of patients with a pericardial effusion.

TABLE 31–8 Drugs with a potential for significant accumulation in patients with renal impairment.

Muscle relaxants Pancuronium **Anticholinergics** Atropine Glycopyrrolate **Metoclopramide** **H_2-receptor antagonists** Cimetidine Ranitidine **Digitalis** **Diuretics** **Calcium channel antagonists** Diltiazem Nifedipine **β-Adrenergic blockers** Atenolol Nadolol Pindolol Propranolol **Antihypertensives** Captopril Clonidine Enalapril Hydralazine Lisinopril Nitroprusside (thiocyanate)	**Antiarrhythmics** Bretylium Disopyramide Encainide (genetically determined) Procainamide Tocainide **Bronchodilators** Terbutaline **Psychiatric** Lithium **Antibiotics** Aminoglycosides Cephalosporins Penicillins Tetracycline Vancomycin **Anticonvulsants** Carbamazepine Ethosuximide Primidone **Other** Sugammadex

Preoperative red blood cell transfusions are usually administered only for severe anemia as guided by the patient's clinical status. Bleeding time and coagulation studies (or perhaps a thromboelastogram) may be advisable, particularly if neuraxial anesthesia is being considered. Serum electrolyte, BUN, and creatinine measurements can assess the adequacy of dialysis. Glucose measurements guide the potential need for perioperative insulin therapy.

Drugs with significant renal elimination should be avoided if possible (Table 31–8). Dosage adjustments and measurements of blood levels (when available) are necessary to minimize the risk of drug toxicity.

Premedication

Alert patients who are stable can be given reduced doses of a benzodiazepine if needed. Chemoprophylaxis for patients at risk for aspiration is reviewed in Chapter 17. Preoperative medications—particularly antihypertensive agents—should be continued until the time of surgery (see Chapter 21). The management of patients with diabetes is discussed in Chapter 35.

INTRAOPERATIVE CONSIDERATIONS

Monitoring

Patients with kidney disease and failure are at increased risk for perioperative complications, and their general medical condition and the planned operative procedure dictate monitoring requirements. Because of the risk of thrombosis, blood pressure should not be measured by a cuff on an arm with an arteriovenous fistula. Continuous invasive or noninvasive blood pressure monitoring may be indicated in patients with poorly controlled hypertension.

Induction

Patients with nausea, vomiting, or gastrointestinal bleeding should undergo rapid-sequence induction and intubation. The dose of the induction agent should be reduced for debilitated or critically ill patients or for patients who have recently undergone hemodialysis and who remain relatively hypovolemic. Propofol, 1 to 2 mg/kg, or etomidate, 0.2 to 0.4 mg/kg, is often used. An opioid, β-blocker (esmolol), or lidocaine may be used to blunt the hypertensive response to airway instrumentation and intubation. Succinylcholine, 1.5 mg/kg, can be used to facilitate endotracheal intubation in the absence of hyperkalemia. Rocuronium (1 mg/kg), vecuronium (0.1 mg/kg), cisatracurium (0.15 mg/kg), or propofol–lidocaine induction without a relaxant may be considered for intubation in patients with hyperkalemia.

Anesthesia Maintenance

The ideal anesthetic maintenance technique should control hypertension with minimal deleterious effect on cardiac output because increased cardiac output is the principal compensatory mechanism for tissue oxygen delivery in anemia. Volatile anesthetics, propofol, fentanyl, sufentanil, alfentanil, and remifentanil are satisfactory maintenance agents. Meperidine should be avoided because of the accumulation of its metabolite normeperidine. Morphine may be used, but prolongation of its effects may occur.

7 Controlled ventilation should be considered for patients with kidney failure under general anesthesia. Inadequate spontaneous ventilation with progressive hypercarbia under anesthesia can result in respiratory acidosis that may exacerbate preexisting acidemia, lead to potentially severe circulatory depression, and result in dangerously increased serum potassium concentration (see Chapter 50). On the other hand, respiratory alkalosis may also be detrimental because it shifts the hemoglobin dissociation curve to the left, can exacerbate preexisting hypocalcemia, and may reduce cerebral blood flow.

Fluid Therapy

Superficial procedures involving minimal physiological trespass require the replacement of insensible fluid losses only. In situations requiring significant fluid volume for maintenance or resuscitation, isotonic crystalloids, colloids, or both may be used (see Chapter 51). Current evidence suggests balanced crystalloids such as Plasma-Lyte or lactated Ringer's solution are preferable in such circumstances to chloride-rich crystalloids such as 0.9% saline because of the deleterious effects of hyperchloremia on kidney function. However, 0.9% saline is preferable to balanced crystalloids in patients with alkalosis and hypochloremia. Lactated Ringer's solution should be avoided in hyperkalemic patients when large fluid volumes are required because it contains potassium 4 mEq/L. Glucose-free solutions should be used because of the glucose intolerance associated with uremia. Blood that is lost should be replaced with colloid or packed red blood cells as clinically indicated. An allogeneic blood transfusion may decrease the likelihood of kidney rejection following transplantation because of associated immunosuppression. Hydroxyethyl starch has been associated with an increased risk of AKI and death when administered to critically ill patients or those with preexisting impaired kidney function or when used for volume resuscitation. Its use in other circumstances is controversial at this time and the subject of many investigations. Intraoperative fluid therapy can be guided by noninvasive measurements of stroke volume and cardiac output.

Anesthesia for Patients with Mild to Moderate Kidney Impairment

PREOPERATIVE CONSIDERATIONS

The kidney normally possesses a large functional reserve. GFR, as determined by creatinine clearance, can decrease from 120 to 60 mL/min without clinical signs or symptoms of diminished kidney function. Even patients with creatinine clearances of 40 to 60 mL/min usually are asymptomatic. These patients have only mild kidney impairment but should still be thought of as having decreased kidney reserve. Preservation of remaining kidney function is paramount and best accomplished by maintaining normovolemia and normal kidney perfusion.

When creatinine clearance decreases to 25 to 40 mL/min, kidney impairment is moderate, and patients are said to have renal insufficiency. Azotemia is always present, and hypertension and anemia are
8 common. Correct anesthetic management of this group of patients is as critical as management of those with frank kidney failure, especially during procedures associated with a relatively high incidence of postoperative kidney failure, such as car-
9 diac and aortic reconstructive surgery. Intravascular volume depletion, sepsis, obstructive jaundice, crush injuries, and renal toxins such as radiocontrast agents, certain antibiotics, angiotensin-converting enzyme inhibitors, and NSAIDs (see Table 30–4) are additional major risk factors for acute deterioration in kidney function. Hypovolemia and decreased kidney perfusion are particularly important causative factors in the development of acute postoperative kidney failure. The emphasis in the management of these patients is on prevention

because the mortality rate of postoperative kidney failure may surpass 50%. The combination of diabetes and preexisting kidney disease markedly increases the perioperative risk of kidney function deterioration and kidney failure.

10 Kidney protection with adequate hydration and maintenance of renal blood flow is especially important for patients at high risk for perioperative AKI and kidney failure, such as those undergoing cardiac, major aortic reconstructive, and other surgical procedures associated with significant physiological trespass. The use of mannitol, low-dose dopamine or fenoldopam infusion, loop diuretics, or bicarbonate infusion for kidney protection is controversial and without proof of efficacy (see earlier discussion). *N*-acetylcysteine, when given prior to the administration of radiocontrast agents, reduces the risk of radiocontrast agent–induced AKI (see Chapter 30).

INTRAOPERATIVE CONSIDERATIONS

Monitoring

The American Society of Anesthesiologists' basic monitoring standards are used for procedures involving minimal fluid losses. For procedures associated with significant blood or fluid loss, close monitoring of hemodynamic performance and urinary output is important (see Chapter 51). Although maintenance of urinary output does not ensure the preservation of kidney function, urinary outputs greater than 0.5 mL/kg/h are preferable. Continuous invasive blood pressure monitoring is also important if rapid changes in blood pressure are anticipated, such as in patients with poorly controlled hypertension and in those undergoing procedures associated with abrupt changes in sympathetic stimulation or in cardiac preload or afterload.

Induction

Selection of an induction agent is not as important as ensuring an adequate intravascular volume prior to induction; induction of anesthesia in hypovolemic patients with impaired kidney function frequently results in hypotension. Unless a vasopressor is administered, such hypotension typically resolves only following intubation or surgical stimulation. Kidney perfusion, which may already be compromised by preexisting hypovolemia, may deteriorate further, first as a result of hypotension, and subsequently from sympathetically or pharmacologically mediated renal vasoconstriction. If sustained, the decrease in renal perfusion may contribute to postoperative kidney impairment or failure. Adequate preoperative hydration usually prevents this sequence of events.

Maintenance of Anesthesia

All anesthetic maintenance agents are acceptable, with the possible exception of sevoflurane administered with low gas flows over a prolonged time period (see Chapter 30). Intraoperative deterioration in kidney function may result from adverse effects of the operative procedure (hemorrhage, vascular occlusion, abdominal compartment syndrome, arterial emboli) or anesthetic (hypotension secondary to myocardial depression or vasodilation), from indirect hormonal effects (sympathoadrenal activation or antidiuretic hormone secretion), or from impeded venous return secondary to positive-pressure ventilation. Many of these effects are avoidable or reversible when adequate intravenous fluids are given to maintain a normal or slightly expanded intravascular volume. The administration of large doses of predominantly α-adrenergic vasopressors (phenylephrine and norepinephrine) may also be detrimental to the preservation of kidney function. Small, intermittent doses, or brief infusions, of vasoconstrictors may be useful in maintaining renal blood flow until other measures (eg, transfusion) are undertaken to correct hypotension.

Fluid Therapy

As reviewed earlier, appropriate fluid administration is important in managing patients with preexisting AKI or kidney failure or who are at risk for AKI. We find guidance from noninvasive monitors of stroke volume and cardiac output useful. Concern over fluid overload is justified, but acute problems are rarely encountered in such patients with normal urinary outputs if rational fluid administration guidelines and appropriate monitoring are employed (see Chapter 51). Moreover, the adverse consequences of excessive fluid overload are far easier to treat than those of AKI and kidney failure.

CASE DISCUSSION

A Patient with Uncontrolled Hypertension

A 59-year-old man with a recent onset of hypertension is scheduled for stenting of a stenotic left renal artery. His preoperative blood pressure is 180/110 mm Hg.

What is the likely cause of this patient's hypertension?

Renovascular hypertension is one of the few forms of hypertension that can be corrected with surgery or mechanical intervention. Others include coarctation of the aorta, pheochromocytoma, Cushing disease, and primary hyperaldosteronism.

Most studies suggest that renovascular hypertension accounts for 2% to 5% of all cases of hypertension. Characteristically, it manifests as a relatively sudden onset of hypertension in a person younger than 35 or older than 55 years of age. Renal artery stenosis can also be responsible for the development of accelerated or malignant hypertension in previously hypertensive persons of any age.

What is the pathophysiology of the hypertension?

Unilateral or bilateral stenosis of the renal artery decreases the perfusion pressure to the kidney(s) distal to the obstruction. Activation of the juxtaglomerular apparatus and release of renin increases circulating levels of angiotensin II and aldosterone, resulting in peripheral vascular constriction and sodium retention, respectively. The resulting systemic arterial hypertension is often severe.

In nearly two-thirds of patients, the stenosis results from an atheromatous plaque in the proximal renal artery. These patients are typically men over the age of 55 years. In the remaining one-third of patients, the stenosis is more distal and is due to malformations of the arterial wall, commonly referred to as fibromuscular hyperplasia (or dysplasia). This latter lesion most commonly presents in women younger than 35 years. Bilateral renal artery stenosis is present in 30% to 50% of patients with renovascular hypertension. Less common causes of stenosis include dissecting aneurysms, emboli, polyarteritis nodosa, radiation, trauma, extrinsic compression from retroperitoneal fibrosis or tumors, and hypoplasia of the renal arteries.

What clinical manifestations other than hypertension may be present?

Signs of secondary hyperaldosteronism can be prominent. These include sodium retention in the form of edema, metabolic alkalosis, and hypokalemia. The latter can cause muscle weakness, polyuria, and even tetany.

How is the diagnosis made?

The diagnosis is suggested by the clinical presentation previously described. A mid-abdominal bruit may also be present, but the diagnosis requires laboratory and radiographic confirmation. A definitive diagnosis is made by renal arteriography, and percutaneous balloon angioplasty with stenting may be performed at the same time. The functional significance of the restrictive lesion(s) may be evaluated by selective catheterization of both renal veins and subsequent measurement of plasma renin activity in blood from each kidney. Restenosis rates following angioplasty are estimated to be less than 15% after 1 year. Patients who are not candidates for angioplasty and stenting are referred for surgery.

Should this patient undergo intervention or surgical correction given his present blood pressure?

Optimal medical therapy is important in preparing these patients for operation. Relative to patients with well-controlled hypertension, those with poorly controlled hypertension have an increased incidence of intraoperative problems, including marked hypertension, hypotension, myocardial ischemia, and arrhythmias. Ideally, arterial blood pressure should be well controlled prior to surgery. Patients should be evaluated for preexisting kidney dysfunction, and metabolic disturbances such as hypokalemia should be corrected. Patients should also be evaluated as indicated for the presence and severity of coexisting atherosclerotic disease, according to current American College of Cardiology/American Heart Association (ACC/AHA) guidelines (see Chapter 21).

What antihypertensive agents are most useful for controlling blood pressure perioperatively in these patients?

β-Adrenergic blocking drugs are frequently utilized for blood pressure control in the perioperative period. They are particularly effective because secretion of renin is partly mediated by β_1-adrenergic receptors. Although parenteral selective β_1-blocking agents such as metoprolol and esmolol would be expected to be most effective, nonselective agents appear equally effective. Esmolol may be the intraoperative β_1-blocking agent of choice because of its short half-life and titratability. Direct vasodilators clevidipine and nicardipine are also useful in controlling intraoperative hypertension (see Chapter 15).

ACE inhibitors and angiotensin-converting enzyme receptor blockers are contraindicated in bilateral renal artery stenosis or in unilateral renal artery stenosis where there is only one functioning kidney because they can precipitate kidney failure.

What intraoperative considerations are important for the anesthesia provider?

Open surgical revascularization of a kidney is a major procedure, with the potential for major blood loss, fluid shifts, and hemodynamic changes. One of several procedures may be performed, including transaortic renal endarterectomy, aortorenal bypass (using a saphenous vein, synthetic graft, or segment of the hypogastric artery), a splenic to (left) renal artery bypass, a hepatic or gastroduodenal to (right) renal artery bypass, or excision of the stenotic segment with reanastomosis of the renal artery to the aorta. Rarely, nephrectomy may be performed. Isolated stenosis of a renal artery may be corrected with percutaneous stenting performed with local anesthesia and conscious or deep sedation.

With all "open" procedures, an extensive retroperitoneal dissection often necessitates relatively large volumes of intravenous fluid replacement. Large-bore intravenous access is mandatory because of the potential for extensive blood loss. Heparinization contributes to increased blood loss. Depending on the surgical technique, aortic cross-clamping, with its associated hemodynamic consequences, often complicates anesthetic management (see Chapter 22). Continuous intraarterial blood pressure monitoring will always be used, and central venous pressure monitoring is often helpful. Goal-directed hemodynamic and fluid therapy utilizing arterial pulse contour analysis, esophageal Doppler, or transesophageal echocardiography should be considered for patients with poor ventricular function and may be advisable in most patients to guide fluid management (see Chapter 51). The choice of anesthetic technique is generally determined by the patient's cardiovascular function.

Generous hydration and maintenance of adequate cardiac output and blood pressure are important to protect both the affected and the normal kidney against acute ischemic injury. Topical cooling of the affected kidney during the anastomosis may also be employed.

What postoperative considerations are important?

Although in most patients hypertension is ultimately cured or significantly improved, arterial blood pressure is often quite labile in the early postoperative period. Close hemodynamic monitoring should be continued well into the postoperative period. Reported operative mortality rates range from 1% to 6%, and most deaths are associated with myocardial infarction. The latter probably reflects the relatively high prevalence of coronary artery disease in older patients with renovascular hypertension.

SUGGESTED READINGS

Albert C, Haase M, Albert A, et al. Biomarker-guided risk assessment for acute kidney injury: time for clinical implementation? *Ann Laboratory Med*. 2021;41:1.

Astapenko D, Navratil P, Pouska J, et al. Clinical physiology aspects of chloremia in fluid therapy: a systematic review. *Perioper Med* (Lond). 2020;9:40.

Bie P, Evans RG. Normotension, hypertension and body fluid regulation: brain and kidney. *Acta Physiol.* 2017;219:288.

Chong MA, Wang Y, Berbenetz NM, et al. Does goal-directed haemondynamic and fluid therapy improve peri-operative outcomes? A systematic review and meta-analysis. *Eur J Anaesthesiol.* 2018;35:469.

Duncan AE, Jia Y, Soltesz E, et al. Effect of 6% hydroxyethyl starch 130/0.4 on kidney and haemostatic function in cardiac surgical patients: a randomized controlled trial. *Anaesthesia.* 2020;75:1180.

Heming N, Moine P, Coscas R, et al. Perioperative fluid management for major elective surgery. *Br J Surg.* 2020;107:e56.

Jamme M, Legrand M, Geri G. Outcome of acute kidney injury: how to make a difference? *Ann Intensive Care.* 2021;11:60.

Joannidis M, Forni LG, Haase M, et al. Use of cell cycle arrest biomarkers in conjunction with classical markers of acute kidney injury. *Crit Care Med.* 2019;47:e820.

Kabon B, Sessler DI, Kurz A, et al. Effect of intraoperative goal-directed balanced crystalloid *versus* colloid administration on major postoperative morbidity. A randomized trial. *Anesthesiology.* 2019;130:728.

Kellum JA, Shaw AD. Assessing toxicity of intravenous crystalloids in critically ill patients. *J Am Med Soc.* 2015;314;1695.

Khan S, Floris M, Pani A, et al. Sodium and volume disorders in advanced chronic kidney disease. *Adv Chron Kidney Dis.* 2016;23:240.

Legrand M, Ince C. Intravenous fluids in AKI: a mechanistically guided approach. *Sem Nephrol.* 2016;36:53.

Lobo DN, Awad S. Should chloride-rich crystalloids remain the mainstay of fluid resuscitation to prevent 'pre-renal' acute kidney injury? Con. *Kidney Int.* 2014;86:1096.

Maheshwari K, Sessler DI. Goal-directed therapy: why benefit remains uncertain. *Anesthesiology.* 2020;133:5.

Massoth C, Zarbock A, Meersch M. Risk stratification for targeted AKI prevention after surgery: biomarkers and bundled interventions. *Semin Nephrol.* 2019;39:454.

Nagore D, Candela A, Bürge M, et al. Hydroxyethyl starch and acute kidney injury in high-risk patients undergoing cardiac surgery: a prospective multicenter study. *J Clin Anesth.* 2021;73:1.

Ostermann M, Cennamo A, Meersch M, et al. A narrative review of the impact of surgery and anaesthesia on acute kidney injury *Anaesthesia.* 2020;75 Suppl 1:e121.

Raghunathan K, Nailer P, Konoske R. What is the ideal crystalloid? *Curr Opin Crit Care.* 2015;21:309.

Saadat-Gilani K, Zarbock A, Meersch M. Perioperative renoprotection: clinical implications. *Anesth Analg.* 2020;131:1667.

Soussi S, Ferry A, Chaussard M, et al. Chloride toxicity in critically ill patients: what's the evidence? *Anaesth, Crit Care Pain Med.* 2016;36:125.

Turan A, Cohen B, Adegboye J, et al. Mild acute kidney injury after noncardiac surgery is associated with long-term renal dysfunction: a retrospective cohort study. *Anesthesiology.* 2020;132:1053.

Wanner C, Amann K, Shoji T. The heart and vascular system in dialysis. *Lancet.* 2016;388:276.

Xu Y, Wang S, He L, et al. Hydroxyethyl starch 130/0.4 for volume replacement therapy in surgical patients: a systematic review and meta-analysis of randomized controlled trials. *Perioper Med* (Lond). 2021;10:16.

CHAPTER

32 Anesthesia for Genitourinary Surgery

KEY CONCEPTS

1. Next to the supine position, the lithotomy position is the most commonly used position for patients undergoing urological and gynecological procedures. Failure to properly position and pad the patient can result in pressure sores, nerve injuries, or compartment syndromes.
2. The lithotomy position is associated with major physiological alterations. Functional residual capacity decreases, predisposing patients to atelectasis and hypoxia. Elevation of the legs drains blood into the central circulation acutely, and mean blood pressure and cardiac output may increase. Conversely, rapid lowering the legs from the lithotomy or Trendelenburg position acutely decreases venous return and can result in hypotension.
3. Because of the short duration (15–20 min) and outpatient setting of most cystoscopies, general anesthesia is often chosen, commonly employing a laryngeal mask airway.
4. Both epidural and spinal blockade with a T10 sensory level provide excellent anesthesia for cystoscopy. However, when neuraxial regional anesthesia is chosen, most anesthesiologists prefer spinal to epidural anesthesia because of its more rapid onset of dense sensory blockade.
5. Manifestations of TURP (transurethral resection of the prostate) syndrome are primarily those of circulatory fluid overload, water intoxication, and, occasionally, toxicity from the solute in the irrigating fluid.
6. Absorption of TURP irrigation fluid is dependent on the duration of the resection and the pressure of the irrigation fluid.
7. When compared with general anesthesia, regional anesthesia for TURP may reduce the incidence of postoperative venous thrombosis. It is also less likely to mask symptoms and signs of TURP syndrome or bladder perforation.
8. Patients with a history of cardiac arrhythmias and those with a pacemaker or implantable cardioverter defibrillator (ICD) may be at risk for developing arrhythmias induced by shock waves during extracorporeal shock wave lithotripsy (ESWL). Shock waves can damage the internal components of pacemaker and ICD devices.
9. Patients who are undergoing retroperitoneal lymph node dissection and who have received bleomycin preoperatively are at increased risk for developing postoperative pulmonary insufficiency. These patients may be particularly at risk for oxygen toxicity and fluid overload and for developing acute respiratory distress syndrome postoperatively.

—*Continued next page*

Continued—

For patients undergoing kidney transplantation, the preoperative serum potassium concentration should be below 5.5 mEq/L, and existing coagulopathies should be corrected. Hyperkalemia has been reported after the release of the vascular clamp following completion of the arterial anastomosis, particularly in pediatric and other small patients. The release of potassium contained in the preservative solution has been implicated as the cause of this phenomenon.

Urological procedures range in impact and risk from simple outpatient cystoscopy to radical cystectomy and nephrectomy for renal cell carcinoma with vena caval thrombosis. Patients undergoing genitourinary procedures may be of any age, but many are older adults with coexisting medical illnesses, including chronic kidney disease. The impact of anesthesia on kidney function is discussed in Chapter 31. This chapter reviews the anesthetic management of common urological procedures. Lithotomy and steep head-down (Trendelenburg) positions are used in many of these procedures. Moreover, advances in preoperative patient optimization, perioperative management, and postoperative rehabilitation allow more patients with coexisting disease to be considered acceptable candidates for kidney transplantation, extensive tumor debulking operations, and reconstructive genitourinary procedures.

CYSTOSCOPY

Preoperative Considerations

Cystoscopy is a very common urological procedure, the indications for which include hematuria, recurrent urinary infections, renal calculi, and urinary obstruction. Bladder biopsies, retrograde pyelograms, transurethral resection of bladder tumors, extraction or laser lithotripsy of kidney stones, and placement or manipulation of ureteral catheters (stents) are also commonly performed through the cystoscope.

Anesthetic management varies with the age and gender of the patient and the purpose of the procedure. General anesthesia is usually necessary for children. Operative cystoscopies involving biopsies, cauterization, or manipulation of ureteral catheters require regional or general anesthesia, regardless of patient anatomy.

Intraoperative Considerations

A. Lithotomy Position

1 Next to the supine position, the lithotomy position is the most commonly used position for patients undergoing urological and gynecological procedures. Failure to properly position and pad the patient can result in pressure sores, nerve injuries, or compartment syndromes. Ideally, two people will move the patient's legs simultaneously up into or down from the lithotomy position. Straps around the ankles or special holders support the legs in lithotomy position (Figure 32–1). The leg supports should be padded wherever there is skin contact, and straps must not impede circulation. When the patient's arms are tucked by the side, one must prevent the fingers from being caught between the mid and lower sections of the operating room table when the lower section is lowered and raised. Many clinicians will completely enclose the patient's hands and fingers with protective padding when the arms are tucked by the side in order to minimize this risk. Injury to the tibial (common peroneal) nerve, resulting in loss of dorsiflexion of the foot, may result if the lateral knee rests against the strap support. If the legs are allowed to rest on medially placed strap supports, compression of the saphenous nerve can result in numbness along the medial calf. Excessive flexion of the thigh against the groin can injure the obturator and, less commonly, the femoral nerves. Extreme flexion at the thigh can also stretch the sciatic nerve. The most

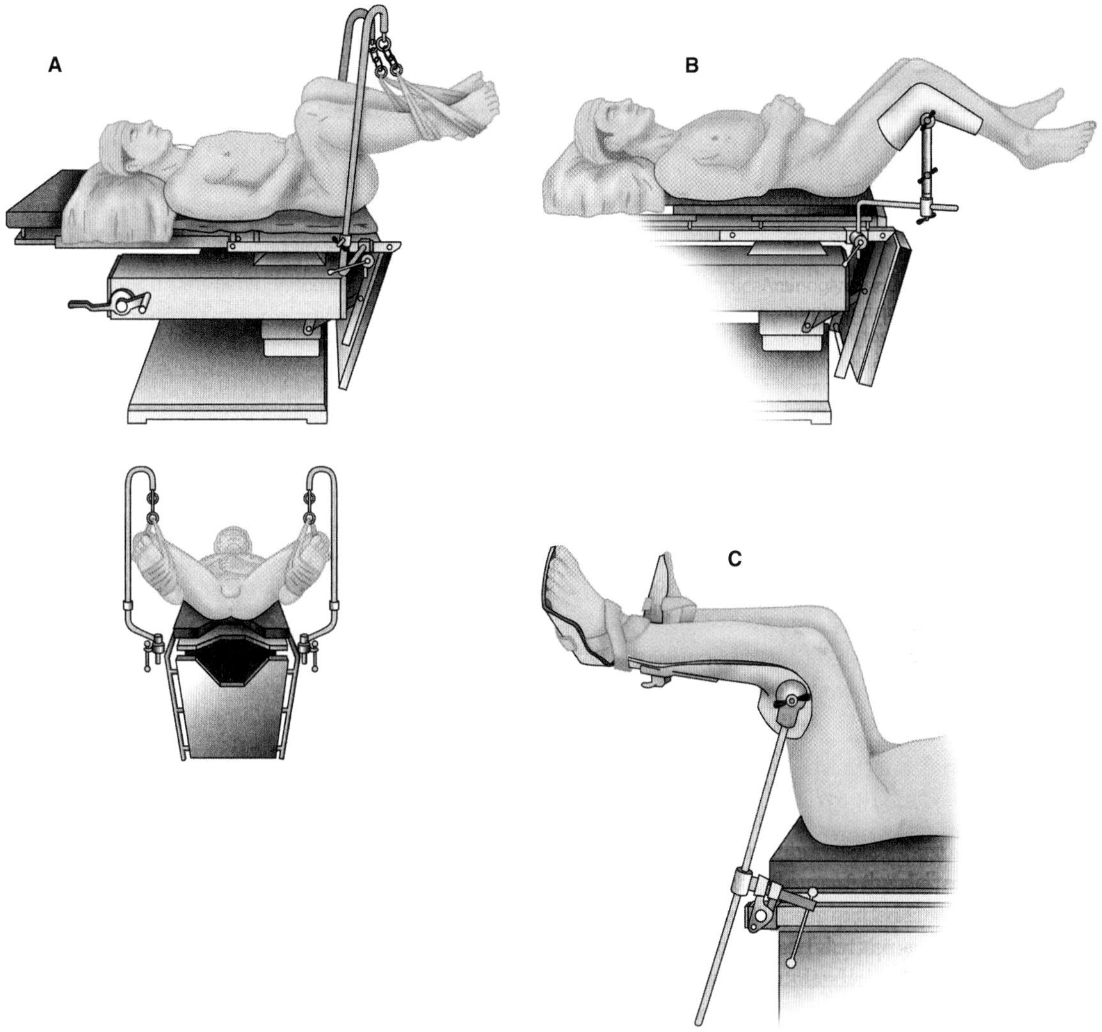

FIGURE 32–1 The lithotomy position. **A**: Strap stirrups. **B**: Bier–Hoff stirrups. **C**: Allen stirrups. (Reproduced with permission from Martin JT. *Positioning in Anesthesia*. Philadelphia, PA: WB Saunders; 1988.)

common nerve injuries directly associated with the lithotomy position involve the lumbosacral plexus. Brachial plexus injuries can occur if the upper extremities are improperly positioned (eg, hyperextension at the axilla). Unfortunately, nerve damage may be newly diagnosed postoperatively even when the extremities have been properly positioned and padded. Compartment syndrome of the lower extremities with rhabdomyolysis has been reported with prolonged time in the lithotomy position, after which lower extremity nerve damage is also more likely. It is important to document any preexisting neuropathy at the time of the pre-anesthetic history and physical examination.

2 The lithotomy position is associated with major physiological alterations. Functional residual capacity decreases, predisposing patients to atelectasis and hypoxia. This effect is amplified by

steep Trendelenburg positioning (30–45°), which is commonly utilized in combination with the lithotomy position. Elevation of the legs acutely drains blood into the central circulation, and mean blood pressure and cardiac output may increase. Conversely, rapid lowering the legs from the lithotomy or Trendelenburg position acutely decreases venous return and cardiac output and can result in hypotension. Vasodilation from either general or regional anesthesia potentiates the hypotension in this situation, and for this reason, blood pressure measurement should be taken immediately after the legs are lowered.

B. Choice of Anesthesia

1. General anesthesia—Any anesthetic technique 3 suitable for outpatients may be utilized. Because of the short duration (15–20 min) and outpatient setting of most cystoscopies, general anesthesia is often chosen, commonly employing a laryngeal mask airway. Oxygen saturation should be closely monitored when obese or older adult patients or those with marginal pulmonary reserve are placed in the lithotomy or Trendelenburg position.

4 **2. Regional anesthesia**—Both epidural and spinal anesthesia provide satisfactory conditions for cystoscopy. However, when neuraxial regional anesthesia is chosen, most anesthesiologists prefer spinal to epidural anesthesia because of its more rapid onset of dense sensory blockade. Studies fail to demonstrate that immediate elevation of the legs into lithotomy position following administration of hyperbaric spinal anesthesia either increases the dermatomal extent of anesthesia to a clinically significant degree or increases the likelihood of severe hypotension. A T10 sensory level block provides excellent anesthesia for all cystoscopic procedures.

TRANSURETHRAL RESECTION OF THE PROSTATE

Preoperative Considerations

Benign prostatic hyperplasia (BPH) frequently leads to bladder outlet obstruction in men older than 60 years. Although most patients are treated medically, some require surgical intervention. Indications for transurethral resection of the prostate (TURP) include bladder outlet obstruction due to BPH, bladder calculi, recurrent episodes of urinary retention, urinary tract infections, and hematuria. Patients with prostate cancer who are not candidates for radical prostatectomy may also benefit from TURP to relieve urinary obstruction.

TURP requires regional or general anesthesia. Despite advanced age and prevalence of significant comorbidity, perioperative mortality and medical morbidity (most frequently myocardial infarction, pulmonary edema, and kidney failure) for this procedure are both less than 1%.

The most common surgical complications of TURP are clot retention, failure to void, uncontrolled hematuria requiring surgical revision, urinary tract infection, and chronic hematuria. Other complications may include TURP syndrome, bladder perforation, sepsis, hypothermia, and disseminated intravascular coagulation (DIC). A blood type and screen (see Chapter 51) is adequate for most patients, though crossmatched blood should be available for anemic patients and for patients with a large prostate in which extensive resection is contemplated. Prostatic bleeding can be difficult to control through the cystoscope.

Intraoperative Considerations

TURP is conventionally performed by passing a monopolar electrical loop through a special cystoscope (resectoscope). With continuous irrigation and direct visualization, prostatic tissue is resected by applying a cutting current to the loop. Because of the characteristics of the prostate and the large amounts of irrigation fluid often used, TURP can be associated with serious complications (Table 32–1).

A. TURP Syndrome

Transurethral prostatic resection, now a relatively uncommon procedure, often opens the extensive network of venous sinuses in the prostate, potentially allowing systemic absorption of the irrigating fluid. The absorption of large amounts of fluid (2 L or more) results in a constellation of symptoms and signs commonly referred to as *TURP syndrome* 5 (Table 32–2). The manifestations are primarily those of circulatory fluid overload, water

TABLE 32–1 Surgical complications associated with transurethral resection of the prostate (TURP).

Most common
Clot retention
Failure to void
Uncontrolled acute hematuria
Urinary tract infection
Chronic hematuria
Less common
TURP syndrome
Bladder perforation
Hypothermia
Sepsis
Disseminated intravascular coagulation

intoxication, and, occasionally, toxicity from the solute in the irrigating fluid. The incidence of TURP syndrome is less than 1%. This syndrome presents intraoperatively or postoperatively as headache, restlessness, confusion, cyanosis, dyspnea, arrhythmias, hypotension, seizures, or a combination of these, and it can rapidly be fatal. TURP syndrome is most commonly associated with large-volume prostate resection and use of large volumes of irrigation fluid, and it has also been much less commonly reported with cystoscopy, arthroscopy, transurethral resection of bladder tumors, and transcervical resection of the endometrium.

Electrolyte solutions cannot be used for irrigation during monopolar TURP because they disperse the electrocautery current. Water provides excellent visibility because its hypotonicity lyses red blood cells, but significant water absorption can readily result in acute water intoxication. Water irrigation is generally restricted to transurethral resection of bladder tumors only. For monopolar TURP, slightly hypotonic nonelectrolyte irrigating solutions such as glycine 1.5% (230 mOsm/L) or a mixture of sorbitol 2.7% and mannitol 0.54% (195 mOsm/L) are most commonly used. Less commonly used solutions include sorbitol 3.3%, mannitol 3%, dextrose 2.5% to 4%, and urea 1%. Significant absorption of water can occur because all these fluids are hypotonic. The fluid absorption rate is also influenced by irrigation fluid pressure: High pressure (high bottle or bag height) increases the rate of fluid absorption.

TABLE 32–2 Manifestations of TURP syndrome.[1]

Hyponatremia
Hypoosmolality
Fluid overload
Congestive heart failure
Pulmonary edema
Hypotension
Hemolysis
Solute toxicity
Hyperglycinemia (glycine)
Hyperammonemia (glycine)
Hyperglycemia (sorbitol)
Intravascular volume expansion (mannitol)

[1]TURP, transurethral resection of the prostate.

6 Absorption of TURP irrigation fluid is dependent on the duration of the resection and the pressure of the irrigation fluid. Pulmonary edema can readily result from the absorption of large amounts of irrigation fluid, particularly in patients with limited cardiac reserve. The hypotonicity of these fluids also results in acute hyponatremia and hypoosmolality, which can lead to serious neurological manifestations. Symptoms of hyponatremia usually do not develop until the serum sodium concentration decreases below 120 mEq/L. Marked hypotonicity in plasma ($[Na^+]$ <100 mEq/L) may also result in acute intravascular hemolysis.

Toxicity may also arise from absorption of the solutes in these fluids. Marked *hyperglycinemia* has been reported with glycine solutions and may contribute to circulatory depression and central nervous system toxicity. Glycine has been implicated in rare instances of transient blindness following TURP. *Hyperammonemia*, presumably from the degradation of glycine, has also been documented in a few patients with marked central nervous system toxicity following TURP.

Treatment of TURP syndrome depends on early recognition and should be based on the severity of the symptoms. The absorbed water must be eliminated, and hypoxemia and hypoperfusion must be treated. Most patients can be managed with fluid restriction and intravenous furosemide. Symptomatic hyponatremia resulting in seizures or coma should be treated with hypertonic saline (see Chapter 49). Seizure activity can be terminated with small doses of midazolam (2–4 mg). Endotracheal intubation may be considered to prevent aspiration until the patient's mental status normalizes. The amount and rate of hypertonic saline solution (3% or 5%) needed to correct the hyponatremia to a safe level should be based on the patient's serum sodium concentration (see Chapter 49).

Recently, additional procedural methods for the treatment of BPH have included bipolar TURP, laser and radiofrequency ablation, photodynamic and thermal therapy, and cryotherapy, and these evolutionary changes in TURP technique have markedly reduced the incidence and severity of TURP syndrome. Low-voltage bipolar TURP allows the use of isotonic saline irrigation fluid, thus avoiding TURP syndrome with the exception of the persisting risk of fluid overload. Because this procedure simultaneously cauterizes as it resects, it decreases the risk of clot retention.

B. Hypothermia

Large volumes of irrigating fluids at room temperature can be a major source of heat loss in patients. Irrigating solutions should be warmed to body temperature prior to use to prevent hypothermia. Postoperative shivering associated with hypothermia may dislodge clots and promote postoperative bleeding.

C. Bladder Perforation

The incidence of bladder perforation during TURP is less than 1% and may result from either the resectoscope going through the bladder wall or from overdistention of the bladder with irrigation fluid. Most bladder perforations are extraperitoneal and are signaled by poor return of the irrigating fluid. Awake patients will typically report nausea, diaphoresis, and retropubic or lower abdominal pain. Large extraperitoneal and most intraperitoneal perforations are usually even more obvious, presenting as sudden unexplained hypotension or hypertension and with generalized abdominal pain in awake patients. Regardless of the anesthetic technique employed, perforation should be suspected in settings of sudden hypotension or hypertension, particularly with acute, vagal-mediated bradycardia.

D. Coagulopathy

DIC following TURP may result from the release of thromboplastins from prostate tissue during the procedure. Rarely, patients with metastatic carcinoma of the prostate develop a coagulopathy from primary fibrinolysis due to secretion of a fibrinolytic enzyme. Coagulopathy may be suspected from diffuse, uncontrollable bleeding but must be defined with laboratory tests. Primary fibrinolysis should be treated with ε-aminocaproic acid (Amicar) or tranexamic acid. Treatment of DIC in this setting may require heparin in addition to the replacement of clotting factors and platelets, and consultation with a hematologist should be considered.

E. Septicemia

The prostate is often colonized with bacteria and may harbor chronic infection. Extensive surgical resection with the opening of venous sinuses can allow the entry of organisms into the bloodstream, and thus bacteremia is commonly associated with transurethral surgery. Prophylactic antibiotic therapy (most commonly gentamicin, levofloxacin, or cefazolin) is usually administered prior to TURP.

F. Choice of Anesthesia

Either spinal or epidural anesthesia with a T10 sensory level, or general anesthesia, provides excellent anesthesia and good operating conditions for TURP. 7 When compared with general anesthesia, regional anesthesia may reduce the incidence of postoperative venous thrombosis. It is also less likely to mask symptoms and signs of TURP syndrome or bladder perforation. Clinical studies have failed to show any differences in blood loss, postoperative cognitive function, and mortality between regional and general anesthesia for TURP. Acute hyponatremia from TURP syndrome may delay or prevent emergence from general anesthesia.

G. Monitoring

Evaluation of mental status in the awake or moderately sedated patient is the best monitor for detection of early signs of TURP syndrome and bladder perforation. Blood loss is particularly difficult to assess during TURP because of the use of irrigating solutions, so it is necessary to rely on clinical signs of hypovolemia (see Chapter 51). Blood loss averages approximately 3 to 5 mL/min of resection (usually 200–300 mL total) and is rarely life-threatening. Transient, postoperative decreases in hematocrit may simply reflect hemodilution from absorption of irrigation fluid. Very few patients will require an intraoperative blood transfusion.

LITHOTRIPSY

The treatment of kidney stones has evolved from primarily open surgical procedures to less invasive or entirely noninvasive techniques. Cystoscopic procedures, including flexible ureteroscopy with stone extraction, stent placement, and intracorporeal lithotripsy (laser or electrohydraulic), along with medical expulsive therapy (MET), have become first-line therapy. Extracorporeal shock wave lithotripsy (ESWL) is used primarily for 4-mm to 2-cm intrarenal stones, and percutaneous and laparoscopic nephrolithotomy is used for larger or impacted stones. MET has become the treatment of choice among many clinicians for acute episodes of urolithiasis: for stones up to 10 mm in diameter, administration of the α-blockers tamsulosin (Flomax), doxazosin (Cardura), or terazosin (Hytrin) or the calcium channel blocker nifedipine (Procardia, Adalat) increases the likelihood of stone expulsion.

During ESWL, repetitive high-energy shocks (sound waves) are generated and focused on the stone, causing it to fragment. Water or (more commonly) a conducting gel couples the generator to the patient. The change in acoustic impedance at the tissue–stone interface creates shear and tear forces on the stone, fragmenting it sufficiently to allow its passage in small pieces down the urinary tract. Ureteral stents are often placed prior to the procedure. Contraindications to the procedure include the inability to position the patient so that lung and intestine are away from the sound wave focus, urinary obstruction below the stone, untreated infection, a bleeding diathesis, and pregnancy. The presence of a nearby aortic aneurysm or an orthopedic prosthetic device is a relative contraindication.

Electrohydraulic, electromagnetic, or piezoelectric shock wave generators may be used for ESWL. With older electrohydraulic units, the patient is placed in a heated water bath, which conducts the shock waves to the patient. Modern lithotripters generate shock waves either electromagnetically or from piezoelectric crystals. The generator is enclosed in a water-filled casing and comes in contact with the patient via a conducting gel on a plastic membrane (Figure 32–2). In the case of electromagnetic machines, the vibration of a metallic plate in front of an electromagnet produces the shock waves. With piezoelectric models, the waves are the result of changes in the external dimensions of ceramic crystals when an electric current is applied.

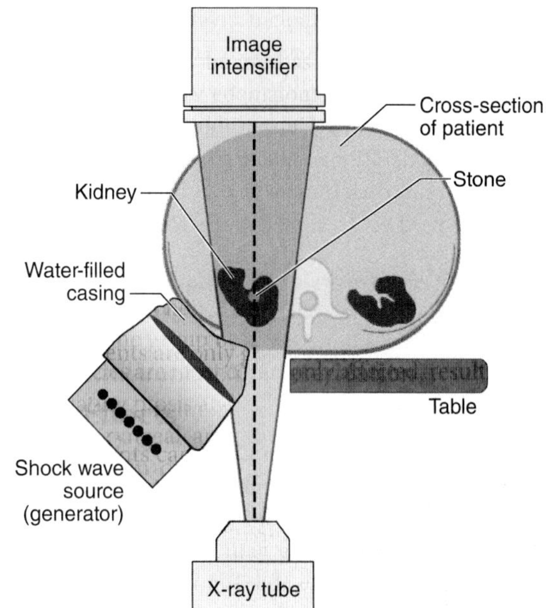

FIGURE 32–2 Schematic representation of a tubless lithotripsy unit.

Preoperative Considerations

8 Patients with a history of cardiac arrhythmias and those with a pacemaker or implantable cardioverter defibrillator (ICD) may be at greater risk for arrhythmias during ESWL. Synchronization of the shock waves with the electrocardiogram (ECG) R wave decreases the incidence of arrhythmias during ESWL. The shock waves are usually timed to occur 20 ms after the R wave to correspond with the ventricular refractory period, though studies suggest that asynchronous delivery of shocks may be safe in patients without heart disease. Shock waves can damage the internal components of implanted cardiac devices. The manufacturer should be contacted as to the best method for managing the device (eg, reprogramming or applying a magnet).

Intraoperative Considerations

Anesthetic considerations for ureteroscopy, stone manipulation, and laser lithotripsy are similar to those for cystoscopic procedures. ESWL requires special considerations, particularly when older lithotriptors requiring the patient to be immersed in water are used.

A. Effects of Immersion During ESWL

Immersion into a heated water bath (36–37°C) initially results in vasodilation that can transiently lead to hypotension. Arterial blood pressure, however, subsequently rises as venous blood is redistributed centrally due to the hydrostatic pressure of water on the legs and abdomen. Systemic vascular resistance (SVR) rises, and cardiac output may decrease. Moreover, the increase in intrathoracic blood volume reduces functional residual capacity and may predispose some patients to hypoxemia.

B. Choice of Anesthesia

Pain during lithotripsy is from the dissipation of a small amount of energy as shock waves enter the body through the skin. The pain is therefore localized to the skin and is proportionate to the shock wave intensity. Older water bath lithotripsy units require 1000 to 2400 relatively high-intensity shock waves, which most patients cannot tolerate without either regional or general anesthesia. In contrast, newer lithotripsy units that are coupled directly to the skin utilize 2000 to 3000 lower-intensity shock waves that usually require only light sedation.

C. Regional Anesthesia

Continuous epidural anesthesia is commonly employed during ESWL with older water bath lithotriptors. A T6 sensory level ensures adequate anesthesia as renal innervation is derived from T10 to L2. When using the loss of resistance technique for placement of the epidural catheter, saline should be used instead of air during epidural catheter insertion as air in the epidural space can dissipate shock waves and may promote injury to neural tissue. Foam tape should not be used to secure the epidural catheter as this type of tape has been shown to dissipate the energy of the shock waves when it is in their path. Spinal anesthesia can also be used satisfactorily but offers less control over the sensory level and an uncertain duration of surgery; for this reason, epidural anesthesia is usually preferred in this setting.

Disadvantages of regional anesthesia or sedation include the inability to control diaphragmatic movement (excessive diaphragmatic excursion can move the stone out of the wave focus and may prolong the procedure) and bradycardia (this will prolong the procedure when shock waves are coupled to the ECG). Glycopyrrolate may be administered to accelerate the ESWL procedure.

D. General Anesthesia

General endotracheal anesthesia allows control of diaphragmatic excursion during lithotripsy using older water bath lithotriptors. The procedure is complicated by the inherent risks associated with placing a supine anesthetized patient in a chair, elevating and then lowering the chair into a water bath to shoulder depth, and then reversing the sequence at the end. A light general anesthetic technique in conjunction with a muscle relaxant is preferable. The muscle relaxant ensures patient immobility and control of diaphragmatic movement.

E. Monitored Anesthesia Care

Monitored anesthesia care with intravenous midazolam and fentanyl is usually adequate for modern low-energy lithotripsy. Deeper sedation may also be used.

F. Monitoring

Standard anesthesia monitoring must be used for conscious or deep sedation or for general anesthesia. *Supraventricular arrhythmias may occur even with R wave synchronized shocks.* With immersion lithotripsy, ECG pads should be attached securely with a waterproof dressing. The temperature of the bath and the patient should be monitored to prevent hypothermia or hyperthermia.

G. Fluid Management

Intravenous fluid therapy is typically generous. Following an initial intravenous crystalloid fluid bolus, an additional 1000 to 2000 mL is often given with a small dose of furosemide to maintain brisk urinary flow and flush stone debris and blood clots. Patients with impaired cardiac reserve require more conservative fluid therapy.

NONCANCER SURGERY OF THE UPPER URETER & KIDNEY

Laparoscopic urological procedures, including partial and total nephrectomy, live donor nephrectomy, lithotomy, and pyeloplasty, are increasingly utilized because of advantages that include less perioperative pain, shorter hospital length of stay, and relatively rapid convalescence and return to function. Both transperitoneal and retroperitoneal approaches have been developed. A hand-assisted technique employs an additional larger incision that allows the surgeon to insert one hand for tactile sensation and facilitation of dissection. Anesthetic management is similar to that for any laparoscopic procedure.

Open procedures for kidney stones in the upper ureter and renal pelvis and nephrectomies for nonmalignant disease are often carried out in the "kidney rest" or lateral flexed position. With the patient in a full lateral position, the dependent leg is flexed, the other leg is extended, and padding is placed between the legs. An axillary roll is placed beneath the dependent upper chest to minimize the risk of brachial plexus injury. The operating table is then extended to achieve maximal separation between the iliac crest and the costal margin on the operative side, and the kidney rest (a bar in the groove where the table bends) is elevated to raise the nondependent iliac crest higher and improve surgical exposure.

The lateral flexed position is associated with adverse respiratory and circulatory effects. Functional residual capacity is reduced in the dependent lung but may increase in the nondependent lung. In the anesthetized patient receiving controlled ventilation, ventilation/perfusion mismatching occurs because the dependent lung receives greater blood flow than the nondependent lung, whereas the nondependent lung receives greater ventilation, predisposing the patient to atelectasis in the dependent lung and to shunt-induced hypoxemia. The arterial-to-end-tidal gradient for carbon dioxide progressively increases during general anesthesia in this position, indicating that dead space ventilation also increases in the nondependent lung. Moreover, elevation of the kidney rest can significantly decrease cardiac output in some patients by compressing the inferior vena cava. Venous pooling in the legs potentiates anesthesia-induced vasodilation.

Initial placement of at least one large-bore intravenous catheter is advised because of the potential for large blood loss and limited vascular access in the lateral flexed position. Arterial catheters are typically utilized. Endotracheal tube location may be altered during positioning; thus, proper endotracheal tube placement must again be verified following final patient positioning prior to skin preparation and surgical draping. Intraoperative pneumothorax may occur as a result of surgical entry into the pleural space.

SURGERY FOR UROLOGICAL MALIGNANCIES

Improved survival rates for patients with urological cancer following radical surgical resections have resulted in an increase in the number of procedures performed for prostatic, bladder, testicular, and kidney cancer. The desire for accelerated, less complicated recovery with smaller, less painful incisions has prompted the development of laparoscopic pelvic and abdominal operations, including radical prostatectomy, cystectomy, pelvic lymph node dissection, nephrectomy, and adrenalectomy. Robot-assisted technology is increasingly being applied to these procedures.

Many urological procedures are carried out with the patient in a hyperextended supine position to facilitate exposure of the pelvis during pelvic lymph node dissection, retropubic prostatectomy, or cystectomy (Figure 32–3). The patient is positioned supine with the iliac crest over the break in the operating table, and the table is extended such that the distance between the iliac crest and the costal margin increases maximally. Care must be taken to avoid putting excessive strain on the patient's back. The operating room table is also tilted head-down to make the operative field horizontal. In the frog-leg

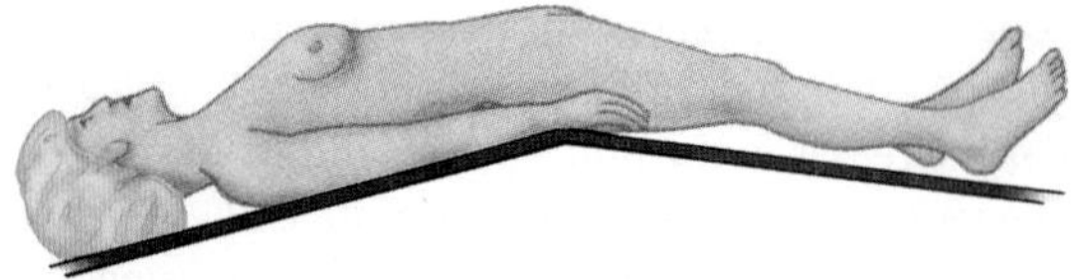

FIGURE 32–3 The hyperextended position. (Reproduced with permission from Skinner DG, Lieskovsky G. *Diagnosis and Management of Genitourinary Cancer.* Philadelphia, PA: WB Saunders; 1988.)

position, a variation of the hyperextended supine position, the knees are also flexed, and the hips are abducted and externally rotated.

1. Prostate Cancer

Preoperative Considerations

Adenocarcinoma of the prostate is the most common nonskin cancer in men and is second only to lung cancer as the most common cause of cancer deaths in men older than 55 years. Approximately one in six men will be diagnosed with prostate cancer in their lifetime. Management varies from surveillance to radical surgery. Important variables include the grade and stage of the malignancy, the patient's age, the level of prostate-specific antigen (PSA) in blood, and the presence of medical comorbidity. Transrectal ultrasound, sometimes guided by previous magnetic resonance imaging (MRI), is used to guide transrectal biopsies. Clinical staging is based on the *Gleason score* of the biopsy specimens, MRI to determine whether there is tumor migration to regional lymph nodes, and a bone scan.

Intraoperative Considerations

Patients with prostate cancer may present to the operating room for open radical retropubic prostatectomy with lymph node dissection, robot-assisted laparoscopic radical prostatectomy with pelvic lymph node dissection, salvage prostatectomy (following failure of radiation therapy), cryoablation, or bilateral orchiectomy for androgen deprivation therapy.

A. Radical Retropubic Prostatectomy

Open radical retropubic prostatectomy is usually performed through a lower midline abdominal incision. It may be curative for localized prostate cancer or occasionally used as a salvage procedure after failure of radiation. The prostate is removed en bloc with the seminal vesicles, ejaculatory ducts, and part of the bladder neck. A "nerve-sparing" technique may be used for smaller, well-defined lesions with the intention of preserving sexual function. Following prostatectomy, the remaining bladder neck is anastomosed directly to the urethra over an indwelling urinary catheter. The surgeon may ask for intravenous administration of indigo carmine for visualization of the ureters, and this dye can be associated with hypertension or hypotension.

Radical retropubic prostatectomy may be accompanied by sufficient operative blood loss to require transfusion. Most centers use direct arterial blood pressure monitoring, and central venous pressure monitoring may also be employed. Other centers routinely utilize noninvasive cardiac output monitoring (eg, LiDCOrapid or FloTrac/Vigileo). Operative blood loss varies considerably from surgeon to surgeon, with typical values less than 500 mL. Factors influencing blood loss include prostate size, duration of operation, and the skill and experience of the surgeon. Blood loss and operative morbidity and mortality are similar in patients receiving general anesthesia and those receiving regional anesthesia. Neuraxial anesthesia requires a T6 sensory level, but these patients typically do not tolerate regional anesthesia without deep sedation unless the hyperextended supine position is moderated. The combination of a prolonged Trendelenburg position together with the administration of large amounts of intravenous fluids may rarely produce edema of the upper airway. The risk of hypothermia should be minimized by utilizing a forced-air warming blanket and an intravenous fluid warmer.

Postoperative complications include hemorrhage; deep venous thrombosis (DVT) that may result in pulmonary embolus; injuries to the obturator nerve, ureter, and rectum; and urinary incontinence and impotence. Extensive surgical dissection around the pelvic veins increases the risk of intraoperative venous air embolism and postoperative thromboembolic complications. An enhanced recovery approach to perioperative care should be standard. Although epidural anesthesia may reduce the incidence of postoperative deep venous thrombosis following open prostatectomy, this beneficial technique may be limited by the routine use of DVT drug prophylaxis postoperatively, and in the era of enhanced recovery, it is used less often. Ketorolac and acetaminophen are used as analgesic adjuvants and have been reported to improve analgesia and, because of their opioid-sparing effects, decrease opioid requirements and promote the earlier return of bowel function.

B. Robot-Assisted Laparoscopic Radical Prostatectomy

Robot-assisted laparoscopic radical prostatectomy with pelvic lymph node dissection differs from most other laparoscopic procedures by the frequent use of steep (>30°) Trendelenburg position for surgical exposure. Patient positioning, the duration of the procedure, the need for abdominal distention, and the desirability of increasing minute ventilation require the use of general endotracheal anesthesia. Nitrous oxide is avoided to prevent bowel distention. Most radical prostatectomies are performed laparoscopically, and nearly all laparoscopic prostatectomies in the United States are performed with robot assistance. When compared with open retropubic prostatectomy, laparoscopic robot-assisted prostatectomy is associated with a longer procedure time but with less blood loss and fewer blood transfusions, lower postoperative pain scores and lower opioid requirements, less postoperative nausea and vomiting, and shorter hospital length of stay. The steep Trendelenburg position can lead to head and neck tissue edema and increased intraocular pressure. Complications reported to be associated with such positioning include upper airway edema and postextubation respiratory distress, postoperative visual loss involving ischemic optic neuropathy or retinal detachment, and brachial plexus injury. The surgeon should be routinely advised as to the length of time during which steep Trendelenburg positioning is maintained, and some centers have abandoned the routine use of steep Trendelenburg positioning entirely.

Most clinicians use a single large-bore intravenous catheter. The risk of hypothermia should be minimized by utilizing a forced-air warming blanket and an intravenous fluid warmer. Adequate postoperative analgesia is provided by ketorolac or acetaminophen, or both, and supplemented as needed with opioids. Postoperative epidural analgesia is not warranted because of relatively low postoperative pain scores and because patients may be discharged 24 h after surgery.

C. Bilateral Orchiectomy

Bilateral orchiectomy may be performed for androgen deprivation in cases of metastatic prostate cancer. The procedure is relatively short (20–45 min) and is performed through a single midline scrotal incision. Although bilateral orchiectomy can be performed with local or regional anesthesia, most patients and many clinicians prefer general anesthesia, usually administered via a laryngeal mask airway, or spinal anesthesia.

2. Bladder Cancer

Preoperative Considerations

Bladder cancer occurs at an average patient age of 65 years with a 3:1 male to female ratio. Transitional cell carcinoma of the bladder is second to prostate adenocarcinoma as the most common malignancy of the male genitourinary tract. The association of cigarette smoking with bladder carcinoma results in coexistent coronary artery and chronic obstructive pulmonary disease in many of these patients. There may be underlying kidney disease related to age or urinary tract obstruction. Staging includes cystoscopy and imaging. Intravesical chemotherapy is used for superficial tumors, and *transurethral resection of bladder tumors* (TURBT) is carried out via cystoscopy for low-grade, noninvasive bladder tumors. Some patients may receive preoperative radiation to shrink the tumor before radical cystectomy. Urinary diversion is usually performed immediately following cystectomy.

Intraoperative Considerations

A. Transurethral Bladder Resection

Bladder tumors may occur at various sites within the bladder, and laterally located tumors may lie in proximity to the obturator nerve. In such cases, if spinal anesthesia is administered or if general anesthesia is administered without the use of a muscle relaxant, use of the cautery resectoscope may result in stimulation of the obturator nerve and adduction of the legs. Urologists rarely derive amusement from having their ear struck by the patient's knee; thus, in contrast to TURP, TURBT procedures are more commonly performed with general anesthesia and neuromuscular blockade. TURBT, unlike TURP, is rarely associated with the absorption of significant amounts of irrigating solution.

B. Radical Cystectomy

With radical cystectomy, all anterior pelvic organs—including the bladder, prostate, and seminal vesicles—are removed in men; the bladder, uterus, cervix, ovaries, and part of the anterior vaginal vault may be removed in women. Pelvic node dissection and urinary diversion are also carried out. Radical cystectomy is associated with the greatest risk of perioperative morbidity and mortality of all major urological procedures, especially in the older adult population. However, continuous improvements in neoadjuvant chemotherapy and enhanced recovery after surgery programs have resulted in progressively lower rates of perioperative morbidity and mortality as well as higher rates of 1- and 5-year survival. When compared with open radical cystectomy, robot-assisted radical cystectomy is associated with reduced perioperative complications, less blood loss and transfusion, and shorter hospital length of stay.

The duration of radical cystectomy is typically 4 to 6 h, and blood transfusion is frequently needed. General endotracheal anesthesia with a muscle relaxant provides optimal operating conditions. Controlled hypotensive anesthesia may reduce intraoperative blood loss and transfusion requirements in open cystectomy, and some surgeons also believe it improves surgical visualization. However, maintenance of mean arterial pressure below 55 to 65 mm Hg may be associated with an increased risk of acute kidney injury and stroke. Continuous epidural anesthesia can facilitate induced hypotension, decrease general anesthetic requirements, and facilitate postoperative analgesia. Optimized intraoperative fluid administration (using noninvasive cardiac output monitoring) may decrease blood transfusion requirements, postoperative complications, and hospital length of stay. Continuous epidural infusion or transversus abdominis plane (TAP) block is frequently used for postoperative analgesia.

Most clinicians will place an arterial catheter along with two large-bore intravenous lines. Urinary output is correlated with the progress of the operation as the urinary collection path is interrupted at an early point during most of these procedures. As with all lengthy operative procedures, the risk of hypothermia is minimized by the use of a forced-air warming blanket and intravenous fluid warming.

C. Urinary Diversion

Urinary diversion (ie, implanting the ureters into a segment of bowel) is usually performed immediately following radical cystectomy. The selected bowel segment is either left *in situ*, such as in ureterosigmoidostomy, or divided with its mesenteric blood supply intact and attached to a cutaneous stoma or urethra. Moreover, the isolated bowel can either function as a conduit (eg, *ileal conduit*) or be reconstructed to form a continent reservoir (*neobladder*). Conduits may be formed from the ileum, jejunum, or colon.

Major anesthetic goals for urinary diversion procedures include keeping the patient well hydrated and maintaining a brisk urinary output once the ureters are opened. Neuraxial anesthesia often produces unopposed parasympathetic activity due to sympathetic blockade, which results in a contracted, hyperactive bowel that makes construction of a continent ileal reservoir technically difficult. Papaverine (100–150 mg as a slow intravenous infusion over 2–3 h), glycopyrrolate (1 mg), or glucagon (1 mg) may alleviate this problem.

Prolonged contact of urine with bowel mucosa due to slow urine flow may produce significant metabolic disturbances. Hyponatremia, hypochloremia, hyperkalemia, and metabolic acidosis can occur following the construction of jejunal conduits. In contrast, colonic and ileal conduits may be associated with hyperchloremic metabolic acidosis. The use of temporary ureteral stents and maintenance of high urinary flow help alleviate this problem in the early postoperative period.

3. Testicular Cancer

Preoperative Considerations

Testicular tumors are classified as either seminomas or nonseminomas. The initial treatment for all tumors is radical (inguinal) orchiectomy, and subsequent management depends on tumor histology. Retroperitoneal lymph node dissection (RPLND) plays a major role in the staging and management of patients with nonseminomatous germ cell tumors. Low-stage disease is managed with RPLND or, in some instances, by surveillance. High-stage disease is usually treated with chemotherapy followed by RPLND.

In contrast to other tissue types, seminomas are very radiosensitive tumors that are primarily treated with retroperitoneal radiotherapy. Chemotherapy is used for patients who relapse after radiation. Patients with large bulky seminomas or those with increased α-fetoprotein levels (usually associated with nonseminomas) are treated primarily with chemotherapy. Chemotherapeutic agents commonly include cisplatin, vincristine, vinblastine, cyclophosphamide, dactinomycin, bleomycin, and etoposide. RPLND is usually undertaken for patients with residual tumor after chemotherapy.

Patients undergoing RPLND for testicular cancer are typically young (15–35 years old) but are at increased risk for morbidity from the residual effects of preoperative chemotherapy and radiation therapy. In addition to bone marrow suppression, specific organ toxicity may be encountered, such as impaired kidney function following cisplatin, pulmonary fibrosis following bleomycin, and neuropathy following vincristine.

Intraoperative Considerations

A. Radical Orchiectomy

Inguinal orchiectomy can be carried out with regional or general anesthesia. Anesthetic management may be complicated by reflex bradycardia from traction on the spermatic cord.

B. Retroperitoneal Lymph Node Dissection

The retroperitoneum is usually accessed through a midline incision, but regardless of the surgical approach, all lymphatic tissue between the ureters from the renal vessels to the iliac bifurcation is removed. With the standard RPLND, all sympathetic fibers are disrupted, resulting in loss of normal ejaculation and infertility. A modified technique that may help preserve fertility limits the dissection below the inferior mesenteric artery to include lymphatic tissue only on the ipsilateral side of the testicular tumor.

9 Patients who have received bleomycin preoperatively may be particularly at risk for oxygen toxicity and fluid overload. Excessive intravenous fluid administration may promote pulmonary insufficiency or acute respiratory distress syndrome postoperatively and should be avoided. Anesthetic management should include the use of the lowest inspired concentration of oxygen compatible with oxygen saturation above 90%. Positive end-expiratory pressure (5–10 cm H_2O) may help optimize oxygenation.

Evaporative and redistributive fluid losses with open RPLND can be considerable as a result of the large incision and the extensive surgical dissection. Retraction of the inferior vena cava during surgery often results in transient arterial hypotension.

Postoperative pain associated with open RPLND incisions is severe, and continuous epidural analgesia, intrathecal morphine or hydromorphone, or TAP block should be considered. Because ligation of intercostal arteries during left-sided dissections has rarely resulted in paraplegia, it may be prudent to document normal motor function postoperatively prior to the institution of epidural analgesia. The arteria radicularis magna (artery of Adamkiewicz), which is supplied by these vessels and is responsible for most of the arterial blood to the lower half of the spinal cord, arises on the left side in most individuals. It should be noted that unilateral sympathectomy following modified RPLND usually results in the ipsilateral leg being warmer than the contralateral one. Patients who have undergone RPLND frequently report severe bladder spasm pain in the postanesthesia care unit.

4. Kidney Cancer

Preoperative Considerations

Renal cell carcinoma is the cause of approximately 3% of all adult cancers and 95% of all kidney cancers.

It has a peak incidence between the fifth and sixth decades of life, with a 2:1 male to female ratio. It is commonly discovered as an incidental finding in the course of evaluating a supposedly unrelated medical problem, such as MRI performed for evaluation of low back pain. The classic triad of hematuria, flank pain, and palpable mass occurs in only 10% of patients, and the tumor often causes symptoms only after it has grown considerably in size. Renal cell carcinoma is frequently associated with paraneoplastic syndromes, such as erythrocytosis, hypercalcemia, hypertension, and nonmetastatic hepatic dysfunction. Tumors confined to the kidney may be treated by open or laparoscopic partial or total nephrectomy or by percutaneous cryoablation or radiofrequency ablation. Palliative surgical treatment may involve more extensive tumor debulking. In approximately 5% to 10% of patients, the tumor extends into the renal vein and inferior vena cava as a thrombus (Figure 32–4) and in some cases approaches or enters the right atrium. Staging includes CT or MRI scans and an arteriogram. Preoperative arterial embolization may shrink the tumor mass and reduce operative blood loss.

Preoperative evaluation of the patient with renal carcinoma should focus on tumor staging, kidney function, the presence of coexisting systemic diseases, and anesthetic management needs dictated by the scope of anticipated surgical resection. Preexisting kidney function impairment depends upon tumor size in the affected kidney as well as coexisting systemic disorders such as hypertension, diabetes, and coronary artery disease. Smoking is a well-established risk factor for renal cell carcinoma, and these patients have a high incidence of underlying coronary artery and chronic obstructive lung disease. Although some patients present with erythrocytosis, most are anemic.

Intraoperative Considerations

A. Percutaneous Cryoablation or Radiofrequency Ablation

Relatively small kidney tumors without metastasis are commonly ablated by interventional radiologists using percutaneous cryoprobes or radiofrequency probes with ultrasonography or CT guidance. This may be performed on an outpatient or 23-h stay basis. Routine American Society of Anesthesiologists (ASA) monitors are used, and general endotracheal anesthesia with muscle relaxation is usually employed to minimize the risk of patient movement during the procedure. An indwelling urinary catheter is typically used if the procedure duration is anticipated to be more than approximately 2 to 3 h. Precautions must be taken for patients with pacemakers or ICDs who are undergoing radiofrequency ablation (see Chapter 21). The patient is typically placed in the lateral decubitus or prone position. The patient may experience significant postoperative pain of limited duration requiring intravenous analgesia.

B. Radical Nephrectomy

This operation may be carried out via an anterior subcostal, flank, or (rarely) midline incision. Hand-assisted laparoscopic technique is often utilized for partial or total nephrectomy associated with a smaller tumor mass. Many centers prefer a thoracoabdominal approach for large tumors, particularly when a tumor thrombus is present. The kidney, adrenal gland, and perinephric fat are removed en bloc with the surrounding (Gerota) fascia. General endotracheal anesthesia is used, often in combination with epidural anesthesia.

This operation has the potential for extensive blood loss because these tumors are very vascular and often very large. Two large-bore intravenous lines with an indwelling peripheral arterial catheter are typically used. Transesophageal echocardiography (TEE), esophageal Doppler, or peripheral pulse wave analysis (Lidco or Vigileo) are often used for hemodynamic monitoring. We use TEE in all patients with vena cava thrombus. Retraction of the inferior vena cava may be associated with transient arterial hypotension. Only brief periods of controlled hypotension should be used to reduce blood loss because of the potential for acute kidney injury in the contralateral kidney. Reflex vasoconstriction in the unaffected kidney can also result in acute kidney injury.

If combined general–epidural anesthesia is employed, administration of epidural local anesthetic is usually postponed until the risk of significant operative blood loss has passed. As with all lengthy operative procedures, the risk of hypothermia should be minimized by utilizing core temperature

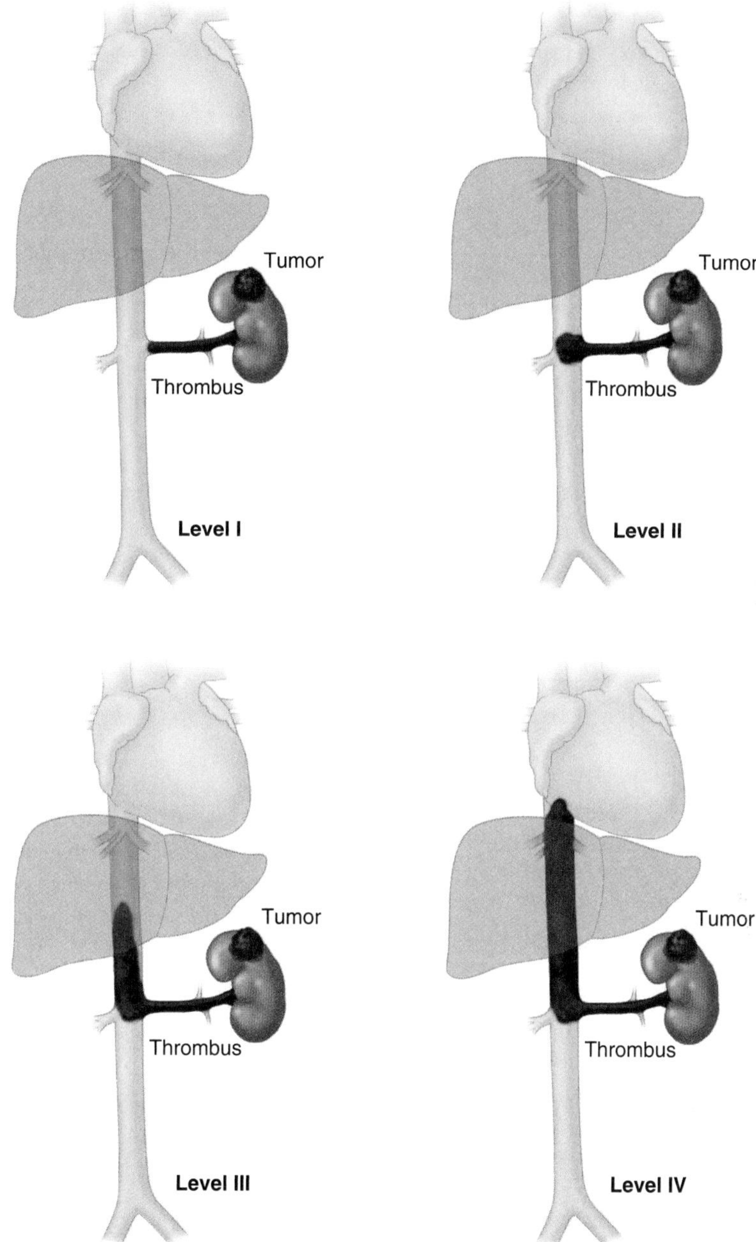

FIGURE 32-4 Mayo classification of venous thrombus invasion in renal cell carcinoma. Level I: Tumor thrombus is either at the entry of the renal vein or within the inferior vena cava (IVC) less than 2 cm from the confluence of the renal vein and the IVC. Level II: Thrombus extends within the IVC more than 2 cm above the confluence of the renal vein and IVC but still remains below the hepatic veins. Level III: Thrombus involves the intrahepatic IVC. The size of the thrombus ranges from a narrow tail that extends into the IVC to one that fills the lumen and enlarges the IVC. Level IV: Thrombus extends above the diaphragm or into the right atrium. (Reproduced with permission from Morita Y, Ayabe K, Nurok M, et al. Perioperative anesthetic management for renal cell carcinoma with venal caval thrombus extending into the right atrium: case series. *J Clin Anesth.* 2017 Feb;36:39-46.)

monitoring, a forced-air warming blanket, and intravenous fluid warming. Subcostal, flank, or midline incisions for open nephrectomy are extremely painful, and epidural analgesia is very useful in minimizing discomfort and accelerating convalescence.

C. Radical Nephrectomy with Excision of Tumor Thrombus

Anesthetic management of this operation can be challenging because of the degree of physiological trespass and potential for major blood loss. A thoracoabdominal approach allows the use of cardiopulmonary bypass when necessary.

Surgery can significantly prolong and improve quality of life, and in some patients, metastases may regress after resection of the primary tumor. A preoperative ventilation-perfusion scan may detect preexisting pulmonary embolization of the thrombus. Intraoperative TEE is helpful in determining whether the uppermost margin of the tumor thrombus extends to the diaphragm, above the diaphragm, into the right atrium, or even across the tricuspid valve. TEE is also used to confirm the absence of tumor in the vena cava, right atrium, and right ventricle after successful surgery.

The presence of a large thrombus (level II, III, or IV) complicates anesthetic management. Problems associated with massive blood transfusion should be anticipated (see Chapter 51). Central venous catheterization should be performed cautiously to prevent dislodgement and embolization of tumor thrombus extending into the right atrium. An increased central venous pressure is typical with significant caval thrombus and reflects the degree of venous obstruction. Pulmonary artery catheters risk dislodgement of right atrial tumor thrombus and provide no useful information that cannot be obtained from TEE.

Complete obstruction of the inferior vena cava markedly increases operative blood loss because of dilated venous collaterals. Patients are also at significant risk for potentially catastrophic intraoperative pulmonary embolization of the tumor. Tumor embolization may be heralded by sudden supraventricular arrhythmias, arterial desaturation, and profound systemic hypotension. TEE is critical in this situation. Cardiopulmonary bypass may be used when the tumor cannot be pulled back from the right atrium into the cava and is often kept on immediate standby for cases involving extensive tumor thrombus. Heparinization and hypothermia greatly increase surgical blood loss.

KIDNEY TRANSPLANTATION

The success of kidney transplantation, which is largely due to advances in immunosuppressive therapy, has greatly improved the quality of life for patients with end-stage kidney disease. With modern immunosuppressive regimens, cadaveric transplants have achieved almost the same 80% to 90% 3-year graft survival rate as living-related donor grafts.

Preoperative Considerations

Current organ preservation techniques allow ample time (24–48 h) for preoperative dialysis of cadaveric kidney recipients. Living-related transplants are performed electively with simultaneous donor and
10 recipient operations. The recipient's serum potassium concentration should be below 5.5 mEq/L, and existing coagulopathies should be corrected.

Intraoperative Considerations

Transplantation is carried out by placing the donor kidney retroperitoneally in the iliac fossa and anastomosing the renal vessels to the iliac vessels and the ureter to the bladder. Heparin is administered prior to temporary clamping of the iliac vessels. Intravenous mannitol administered to the transplant recipient helps establish an osmotic diuresis following reperfusion. Immunosuppression is initiated on the day of surgery with a combination of medications that may include corticosteroids, cyclosporine or tacrolimus, azathioprine or mycophenolate mofetil, antithymocyte globulin, monoclonal antibodies directed against specific subsets of T lymphocytes (OKT3), and interleukin-2 receptor antibodies (daclizumab or basiliximab). The anesthesia provider should discuss in advance with the surgery team the timing and dosage of any immunosuppressive agents that will need to be given perioperatively. Recipient nephrectomy for a failed transplant may be performed for intractable hypertension or chronic infection.

A. Choice of Anesthesia

Most kidney transplants are performed with general anesthesia, though spinal and epidural anesthesia have been utilized. All general anesthetic agents have been employed without any apparent detrimental effect on graft function. Cisatracurium may be the muscle relaxant of choice as it is not dependent upon renal excretion for elimination. With careful neuromuscular monitoring, other relaxants can be used safely.

B. Monitoring

A urinary catheter is placed preoperatively in addition to routine monitors, and brisk urine flow following the arterial anastomosis generally indicates good graft function. If the graft ischemic time was prolonged, an oliguric phase may precede the diuretic phase, in which case intravenous fluid therapy must be appropriately adjusted. Administration of furosemide or additional mannitol may be indicated in such cases. Hyperkalemia has been reported after release of the vascular clamp following completion of the arterial anastomosis, particularly in pediatric and other small patients, and release of potassium contained in the preservative solution has been implicated as the cause of this phenomenon. Donor kidney washout of the preservative solution with ice-cold lactated Ringer's solution just prior to the vascular anastomosis may help avoid this problem. Serum electrolyte concentrations (particularly potassium) should be monitored closely after completion of the anastomosis. Hyperkalemia may be suspected from peaking of the T wave on the ECG.

CASE DISCUSSION

Hypotension in the Recovery Room

A 79-year-old man with a history of an inferior myocardial infarction was admitted to the recovery room following TURP under general anesthesia. The procedure took 90 min and was reported to be uncomplicated. On admission, the patient is extubated but still unresponsive, and vital signs are stable. Twenty minutes later, he is noted to be awake but restless. He begins to shiver intensely, his blood pressure decreases to 80/35 mm Hg, and his respirations increase to 40 breaths/min. The bedside monitor shows a sinus tachycardia of 140 beats/min and an oxygen saturation of 92%.

What is the differential diagnosis?

The differential diagnosis of hypotension following TURP should always include (1) hemorrhage, (2) TURP syndrome, (3) bladder perforation, (4) myocardial infarction or ischemia, (5) septicemia, and (6) disseminated intravascular coagulation (DIC).

Other possibilities (see Chapter 56) are less likely in this setting but should always be considered, particularly when the patient fails to respond to appropriate measures (see below).

Based on the history, what is the most likely diagnosis?

A diagnosis cannot be made with reasonable certainty at this point, and the patient requires further evaluation. Nonetheless, the hypotension and shivering must be treated rapidly because of the history of coronary artery disease. The hypotension seriously compromises coronary perfusion, and the shivering markedly increases myocardial oxygen demand (see Chapter 21).

What diagnostic aids would be helpful?

Rapid examination of the patient is extremely useful in narrowing down the possibilities. Hemorrhage from the prostate should be apparent from the effluent of the continuous bladder irrigation system placed after the procedure. Relatively little blood in the urine makes it look pink or red; brisk hemorrhage is often apparent as grossly bloody drainage. Occasionally, the drainage may be scant because of clots blocking the drainage catheter; irrigation of the catheter is indicated in such cases.

Clinical signs of peripheral perfusion are invaluable. Hypovolemic patients have decreased peripheral pulses, and their extremities are usually cool and may be cyanotic. Poor perfusion is consistent with hemorrhage, bladder perforation, DIC, and severe myocardial ischemia or infarction. A full, bounding peripheral pulse with warm extremities is suggestive of, but not always present in, septicemia. Signs of fluid overload should be searched for, such as jugular venous distention, pulmonary crackles, and an S_3 gallop. Fluid overload is more consistent with TURP syndrome but may also be seen in myocardial infarction or ischemia when resulting in congestive heart failure.

The abdomen should be examined for signs of perforation. A rigid and tender or distended abdomen is very suggestive of perforation and should prompt immediate surgical evaluation. When the abdomen is soft and nontender, perforation can reasonably be excluded.

Further evaluation requires laboratory measurements, an ECG, a chest radiograph, and possibly a transthoracic echocardiogram. Blood should be immediately obtained for arterial blood gas analysis and measurements of hematocrit, hemoglobin, electrolytes, glucose, platelet count, and prothrombin and partial thromboplastin tests. If DIC is suggested by diffuse oozing, fibrinogen and fibrin split product measurements will confirm the diagnosis. A 12-lead ECG should be evaluated for evidence of ischemia or evolving myocardial infarction. A chest radiograph should be obtained to search for evidence of pulmonary congestion, aspiration, pneumothorax, or cardiomegaly. An echocardiogram helps determine end-diastolic volume and systolic function (particularly the presence or absence of regional wall motion abnormalities) and can detect valvular abnormalities; comparison with prior studies would be invaluable. Sonography of the abdomen can be used to detect extravasation.

While laboratory measurements are being performed, what therapeutic and diagnostic measures should be undertaken?

Immediate measures aimed at avoiding hypoxemia and hypoperfusion should be instituted. Supplemental oxygen should be administered, and endotracheal intubation is indicated if significant hypoventilation or respiratory distress is present. Frequent blood pressure measurements should be obtained. If signs of fluid overload are absent, a diagnostic fluid challenge with 300 to 500 mL of crystalloid or 250 mL of colloid is helpful. A favorable response, as indicated by an increase in blood pressure and a decrease in heart rate (or an increase in cardiac output as measured using a noninvasive monitor), supports a diagnosis of hypovolemia and may indicate the need for additional fluid boluses. Obvious bleeding in the setting of anemia and hypotension necessitates blood transfusion. The absence of a quick response to intravenous fluid volume challenge should prompt further evaluation. Administration of an inotrope is appropriate should ventricular dysfunction be detected by echocardiography. Direct intraarterial pressure measurement is invaluable in this setting.

If signs of fluid overload are present, intravenous furosemide in addition to an inotrope is indicated.

The patient's axillary temperature is 35.5°C. Does the absence of obvious fever exclude sepsis?

No. Anesthesia is commonly associated with altered temperature regulation. Moreover, correlation between axillary and core temperatures is unreliable (see Chapter 52). A high index of suspicion is therefore required to diagnose sepsis. Leukocytosis is common following surgery and is not a reliable indicator of sepsis in this setting.

The mechanism of shivering in patients recovering from anesthesia is poorly understood. Although shivering is common in patients who become hypothermic during surgery (and presumably functions to raise body temperature back to normal), its relation to body temperature is inconsistent. Anesthetics probably alter the normal behavior of hypothalamic thermoregulatory centers. In contrast, infectious agents, circulating toxins, or immune reactions cause the release of cytokines that stimulate the hypothalamus to synthesize prostaglandin (PG) E_2. The latter, in turn, activates neurons responsible for heat production, resulting in intense shivering.

How can the shivering be stopped?

Regardless of its cause, shivering has the undesirable effects of markedly increasing metabolic oxygen demand (100–200%) and CO_2 production. Both cardiac output and minute ventilation must therefore increase, and these effects are often poorly tolerated by patients with limited cardiac or pulmonary reserve. Although the ultimate therapeutic goal is to correct the underlying problem, additional measures are indicated in this patient. Supplemental oxygen therapy addresses hypoxemia. Meperidine in small doses (12.5–25 mg intravenously) frequently terminates shivering regardless of the cause. Shivering associated with sepsis and immune reactions can also be moderated or abolished by prostaglandin synthetase inhibitors (aspirin, acetaminophen, and nonsteroidal anti-inflammatory agents), of which only acetaminophen would likely be appropriate until hemorrhage was ruled out because it does not affect platelet function.

What was the outcome?

Examination of the patient reveals warm extremities with a good pulse, even with the low blood pressure. The abdomen is soft and nontender. The irrigation fluid from the bladder is only slightly pink. A diagnosis of probable sepsis is made. Blood cultures are obtained, and antibiotic therapy is initiated to cover gram-negative organisms and enterococci, the most common pathogens. A dopamine infusion is initiated. In settings of redistributive, vasodilatory shock, additional vasoconstrictors (eg, vasopressin) may be needed. The shivering ceases following administration of meperidine, 12.5 mg intravenously. The blood pressure increases to 110/60 mm Hg, and the heart rate slows to 90 beats/min following a 1000 mL intravenous fluid bolus and initiation of a 5-mcg/kg/min dopamine infusion. The serum sodium concentration was found to be 130 mEq/L. Four hours later, dopamine was no longer needed and was discontinued. The patient's subsequent recovery was uneventful.

SUGGESTED READINGS

Aceto P, Beretta L, Cariello C, et al. Joint consensus on anesthesia in urologic and gynecologic robotic surgery: specific issues in management from a task force of the SIAARTI, SIGO, and SIU. *Minerva Anestesiol.* 2019;85:871.

Arviso C, Mehta ST, Yunker A. Adverse events related to Trendelenburg position during laparoscopic surgery: recommendations and review of the literature. *Curr Opin Obstet Gynecol.* 2018;30:272.

Bruce A, Krishan A, Sadiq S, et al. Safety and efficacy of bipolar transurethral resection of the prostate vs monopolar transurethral resection of prostate in the treatment of moderate-large volume prostatic hyperplasia: a systematic review and meta-analysis. *J Endourol.* 2021;35:663.

Calderone CE, Tuck BC, Gray SH, et al. The role of transesophageal echocardiography in the management of renal cell carcinoma with venous tumor thrombus. *Echocardiography.* 2018;35:2047.

Calixto Fernandes MH, Schricker T, Magder S, et al. Perioperative fluid management in kidney transplantation: a black box. *Crit Care.* 2018;22:14.

Castellani D, Gasparri L, Faloia L, et al. Fluid overload syndrome: a potentially life-threatening complication of Thulium laser enucleation of the prostate. *Andrologia.* 2021;53:e13807.

Chui J, Murkin JM, Posner KL, et al. Perioperative peripheral nerve injury after general anesthesia: a qualitative systemic review. *Anesth Analg.* 2018;127:134.

Cornelius J, Mudlagk J, Afferi L, et al. Postoperative peripheral neuropathies associated with patient positioning during robot-assisted laparoscopic radical prostatectomy (RARP): a systematic review of the literature. *Prostate.* 2021;81:361.

Feng D, Liu S, Lu Y, et al. Clinical efficacy and safety of enhanced recovery after surgery for patients treated with radical cystectomy and ileal urinary diversion: a systematic review and meta-analysis of randomized controlled trials. *Transl Androl Urol.* 2020;9:1743.

Gul ZG, Katims AB, Winoker JS, et al. Robotic-assisted radical cystectomy versus open radical cystectomy: a review of what we do and don't know. *Transl Androl Urol.* 2021;10:2209.

Haberal M, Boyvat F, Akdur A, et al. Surgical complications after kidney transplantation. *Exper Clin Transpl.* 2016;6:587.

Ilic D, Evans SM, Allan CA, Jung JH, Murphy D, Frydenberg M. Laparoscopic and robotic-assisted versus open radical prostatectomy for the treatment of localised prostate cancer. *Cochrane Database Syst Rev.* 2017;(9):CD009625.

Ince ME, Ozkan G, Ors N, et al. Anesthesia management for robotic-assisted radical prostatectomy. Single center experience. *Ann Ital Chir.* 2020;91:196.

Jara RD, Guerrón AD, Portenier D. Complications of robotic surgery. *Surg Clin North Am*. 2020;100:461.

Jo YY, Kwak HJ. What is the proper ventilation strategy during laparoscopic surgery? *Korean J Anesthesiol.* 2017;70:596.

Kostibas MP, Arora V, Gorin MA, et al. Defining the role of intraoperative transesophageal echocardiography during radical nephrectomy with inferior vena cava tumor thrombectomy for renal cell carcinoma. *Urology*. 2017;107:161.

Kumar V, Vineet K, Deb A. TUR syndrome – a report. *Urol Case Rep*. 2019;26:100982.

McGowan-Smyth S, Vasdev N, Gowrie-Mohan S. Spinal anesthesia facilitates the early recognition of TUR syndrome. *Curr Urol*. 2015;9:57.

Nasrallah G, Souki FG. Perianesthetic management of laparoscopic kidney surgery. *Curr Urol Rep*. 2018;19:1.

Nik-Ahd F, Souders CP, Houman J, et al. Robotic urologic surgery: trends in Food and Drug Administration-reported adverse events over the last decade. *J Endourol*. 2019;33:649.

Practice advisory for the prevention of perioperative peripheral neuropathies 2018: an updated report by the American Society of Anesthesiologists task force on prevention of perioperative peripheral neuropathies. *Anesthesiology*. 2018;128:11.

Pridgeon S, Bishop CV, Adshead J. Lower limb compartment syndrome as a complication of robot-assisted radical prostatectomy: the UK experience. *Br J Urol Int*. 2013;112:485.

Rajan S, Babazade R, Govindarajan SR, et al. Perioperative factors associated with acute kidney injury after partial nephrectomy. *Br J Anaesthesia*. 2016;116:70.

Satkunasivam R, Tallman CT, Taylor JM, et al. Robot-assisted radical cystectomy versus open radical cystectomy: a meta-analysis of oncologic, perioperative, and complication-related outcomes. *Eur Urol Oncol*. 2019;2:443.

Souki FG, Rodriguez-Blanco YF, Reddy Polu S, et al. Survey of anesthesiologists' practices related to steep Trendelenburg positions in the USA. *BMC Anesthesiol*. 2018;18:117.

Teo JS, Lee YM, Ho HSS. An update on transurethral surgery for benign prostatic obstruction. *Asian J Urol*. 2017;4:195.

Wang Y, Wang X, Chang Y. Radical nephrectomy combined with removal of tumor thrombus from inferior vena cava under real-time monitoring with transesophageal echocardiography: a case report. *Medicine* (Baltimore). 2020;99:e19392.

Weiman A, Braga M, Carli F, et al. ESPEN guideline: clinical nutrition in surgery. *Clin Nutr*. 2017;36:623.

CHAPTER 33

Hepatic Physiology & Anesthesia

Michael Ramsay, MD, FRCA

KEY CONCEPTS

1. The hepatic artery, coming directly off the celiac trunk, supplies approximately 30% of the blood supply and 50% to 70% of the liver's oxygen requirements, and the portal vein supplies 70% of the blood supply and the remaining 50% or less of oxygen requirements.
2. All coagulation factors, with the exception of factor VIII and von Willebrand factor, are produced by the liver. Vitamin K is a necessary cofactor in the synthesis of prothrombin (factor II) and factors VII, IX, and X.
3. Many "liver function" tests, such as serum transaminase measurements, reflect hepatocellular necroinflammatory activity more than hepatic function. Liver tests that measure hepatic synthetic function include serum albumin, prothrombin time (PT) or international normalized ratio (INR), serum cholesterol, and plasma pseudocholinesterase. Serum bilirubin reflects liver excretory function.
4. Albumin values less than 2.5 g/dL are generally indicative of chronic liver disease, acute stress, or severe malnutrition. Increased losses of albumin in the urine (nephrotic syndrome) or the gastrointestinal tract (protein-losing enteropathy) can also produce hypoalbuminemia.
5. The PT, which normally ranges between 11 and 14 s, depending on the control value, measures the activity of fibrinogen, prothrombin, and factors V, VII, and X. A prolonged INR reflects a dysfunctional liver. The effect on coagulation will depend on the balance between coagulation and anticoagulation factors. If production of protein C, protein S, and antithrombin 3 are affected more than the coagulation factors, a normal or hypercoagulable state might exist. The INR was developed to monitor the effect of warfarin, which only affects clotting factors made in the liver, not hepatic-synthetized anticoagulant factors. So if a patient has an INR of 3 and is not taking warfarin, the liver clotting mechanism is dysfunctional. Such a patient could have a potential bleeding tendency, as most will have, but some will have an increased clotting potential. This is because the pro-coagulation factors may not be impeded as much as the anticoagulation factors, so additional assessment should be done in this situation before withholding venous thromboembolism (VTE) prophylaxis or administering fresh frozen plasma.
6. Operative procedures near the liver can reduce hepatic blood flow up to 60%. Although the mechanisms are not clear, they most likely involve sympathetic activation, local reflexes, and direct compression of vessels in the portal and hepatic circulations.

—Continued next page

Continued—

7. The neuroendocrine stress response to surgery and trauma is characterized by elevated circulating levels of catecholamines, glucagon, and cortisol and results in the mobilization of carbohydrate stores and proteins, causing hyperglycemia and a negative nitrogen balance (catabolism).

8. All opioids can potentially cause spasm of the sphincter of Oddi and increase biliary pressure.

9. When liver tests are abnormal postoperatively, the usual cause is underlying liver disease or the surgical procedure itself.

10. Liver cirrhosis may result in portal hypertension, bleeding varices, and major organ dysfunction.

FUNCTIONAL ANATOMY

The liver is the heaviest organ in the body, weighing approximately 1500 g in adults. It is separated by the *falciform ligament* into right and left anatomic lobes; the larger right lobe has two additional smaller lobes at its posterior–inferior surface, the caudate and quadrate lobes.

In contrast, surgeons describe the liver based on its blood supply. Thus, the right and left surgical lobes are defined by the point of bifurcation of the hepatic artery and portal vein (*porta hepatis*); the falciform ligament therefore divides the left surgical lobe into medial and lateral segments. Surgical anatomy defines a total of eight segments.

The liver is made up of 50,000 to 100,000 discrete anatomic units called *lobules*. Each lobule is composed of plates of hepatocytes arranged cylindrically around a *centrilobular vein* (Figure 33–1). Four to five portal tracts, composed of hepatic arterioles, portal venules, bile canaliculi, lymphatics, and nerves, surround each lobule.

In contrast to a lobule, an *acinus*, the functional unit of the liver, is defined by a portal tract in the middle and centrilobular veins at the periphery. Cells closest to the portal tract (zone 1) are well oxygenated; those closest to centrilobular veins (zone 3) receive the least oxygen and are therefore most susceptible to ischemic injury.

Blood from hepatic arterioles and portal venules comingle in the *sinusoidal channels*, which lie between the cellular plates and serve as capillaries. These channels are lined by endothelial cells and by macrophages known as *Kupffer cells*. The Kupffer cells remove bacterial endotoxins, viruses, proteins, and particulate matter from the blood. The *space of Disse* lies between the sinusoidal capillaries and the hepatocytes. Venous drainage from the central veins of hepatic lobules coalesces to form the hepatic veins (right, middle, and left), which empty into the inferior vena cava (Figure 33–2). The caudate lobe is usually drained by its own set of veins.

Bile canaliculi originate between hepatocytes within each plate and join to form bile ducts. An extensive system of lymphatic channels also forms within the plates and is in direct communication with the space of Disse.

The liver is supplied by T6–T11 sympathetic nerve fibers, right and left vagal nerve parasympathetic fibers, and right phrenic nerve fibers. Some autonomic fibers synapse first in the celiac plexus, whereas others reach the liver directly via splanchnic nerves and vagal branches before forming the hepatic plexus. The majority of sensory afferent fibers travel with sympathetic fibers.

Hepatic Blood Flow

Normal hepatic blood flow is 25% to 30% of the cardiac output and is provided by the hepatic artery and
1 portal vein. The hepatic artery supplies approximately 30% of the blood supply and 50% to 70% of the liver's oxygen requirements, and the portal vein supplies 70% of the blood supply and the remaining

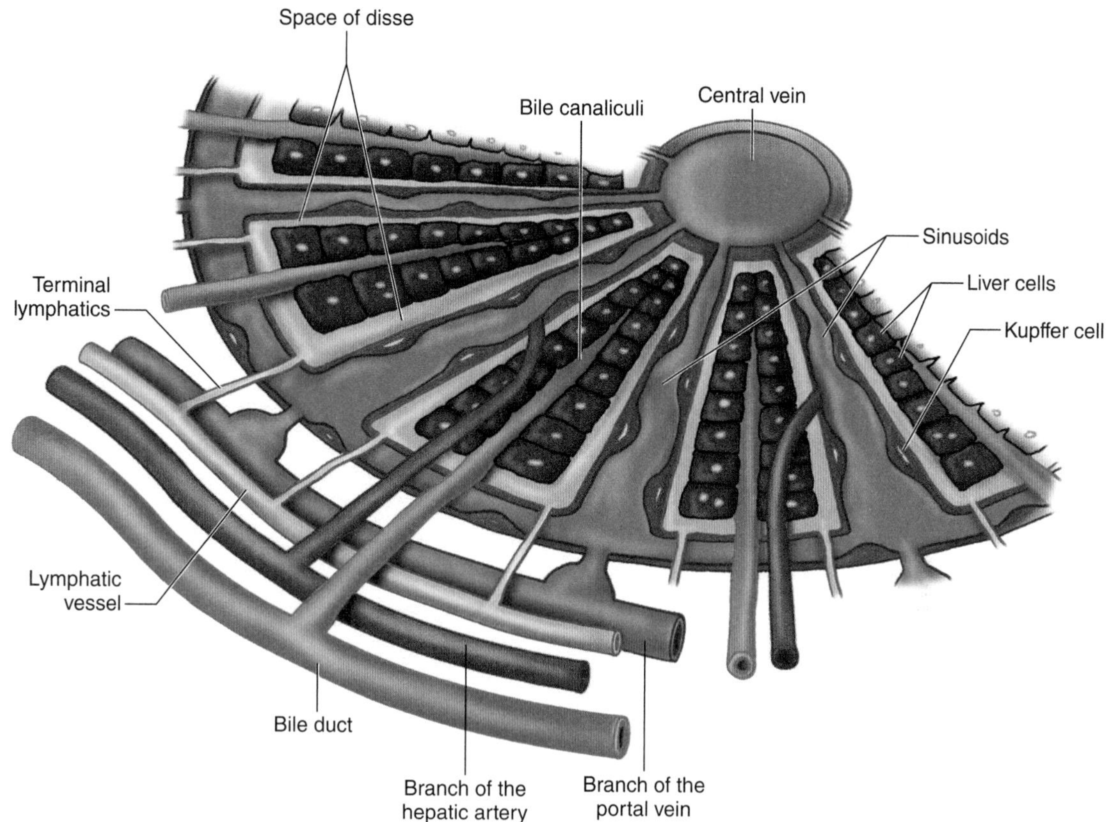

FIGURE 33–1 The hepatic lobule.

30% to 50% (see Figure 33–2) of the liver's oxygen requirements. Hepatic arterial flow is dependent on metabolic demand (autoregulation), whereas flow through the portal vein is dependent on blood flow to the gastrointestinal tract and the spleen. A reciprocal, though somewhat limited, mechanism exists, such that a decrease in either hepatic arterial or portal venous flow results in a compensatory increase in the other.

The hepatic artery has α_1-adrenergic vasoconstriction receptors as well as β_2-adrenergic, dopaminergic (D_1), and cholinergic vasodilator receptors. The portal vein has only α_1-adrenergic and dopaminergic (D_1) receptors. Sympathetic activation results in vasoconstriction of the hepatic artery and mesenteric vessels, decreasing hepatic blood flow. β-Adrenergic stimulation vasodilates the hepatic artery; β-blockers reduce blood flow and therefore decrease portal pressure. The drug vasopressin causes a reduction in splanchnic blood flow.

Reservoir Function

Portal vein pressure is normally only about 7 to 10 mm Hg, but the low resistance of the hepatic sinusoids allows relatively large blood flows through the portal vein. Small changes in hepatic venous tone and hepatic venous pressure thus can result in large changes in hepatic blood volume, allowing the liver to act as a blood reservoir (Figure 33–3). A decrease in hepatic venous pressure, as occurs during hemorrhage, shifts blood from hepatic veins and sinusoids into the central venous circulation and augments circulating blood volume. Blood loss can be reduced during liver surgery by lowering the central venous pressure, thereby reducing hepatic venous pressure and hepatic blood volume. In patients with congestive heart failure, the increase in central venous pressure is transmitted to the hepatic veins and causes congestion of the liver that can adversely affect liver function.

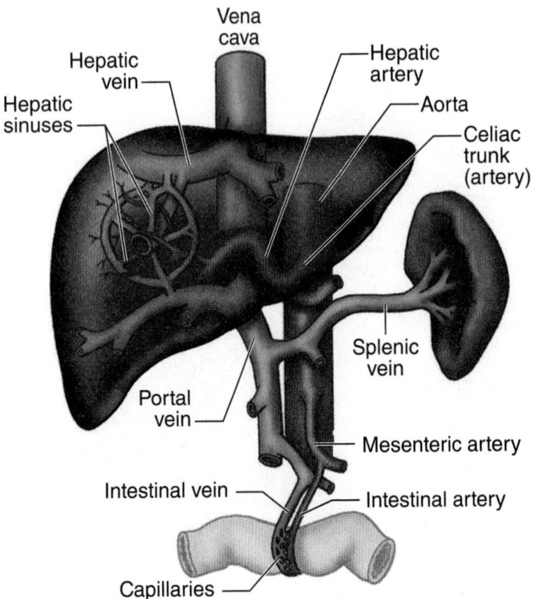

FIGURE 33–2 Hepatic blood flow. (Modified with permission from Guyton AC. *Textbook of Medical Physiology.* 7th ed. Philadelphia, PA: WB Saunders; 1986.)

Metabolic Function

The abundance of enzymatic pathways in the liver allows it to play a key role in the metabolism of carbohydrates, fats, proteins, and other substances (Figure 33–4 and Table 33–1). The final products of carbohydrate digestion are glucose, fructose, and galactose. With the exception of the large amount of fructose that is converted by the liver to lactate, the hepatic conversion of fructose and galactose into glucose makes glucose metabolism the final common pathway for most carbohydrates.

All cells utilize glucose to produce energy in the form of adenosine triphosphate (ATP), either aerobically via the citric acid cycle or anaerobically via glycolysis. The liver and adipose tissue can also utilize the phosphogluconate pathway, which provides energy and fatty acid synthesis. Normally, most of the glucose absorbed following a meal is stored as glycogen, which only the liver and muscle are able to store in significant amounts. When glycogen storage capacity is exceeded, excess glucose is converted into fat. Insulin enhances glycogen synthesis, and epinephrine and glucagon enhance glycogenolysis. Glucose consumption

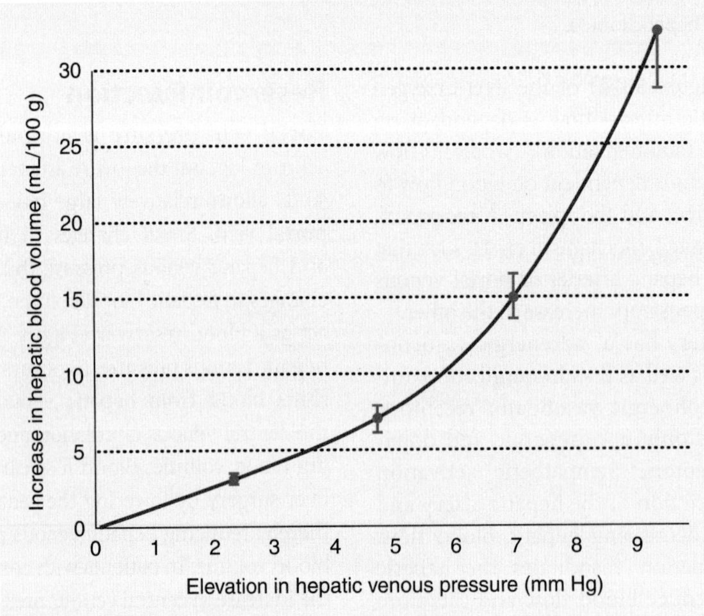

FIGURE 33–3 The role of the liver as a blood reservoir. (Modified with permission from Lautt WW, Greenway CV. Hepatic venous compliance and role of liver as a blood reservoir. *Am J Physiol.* 1976 Aug;231(2):292-295.)

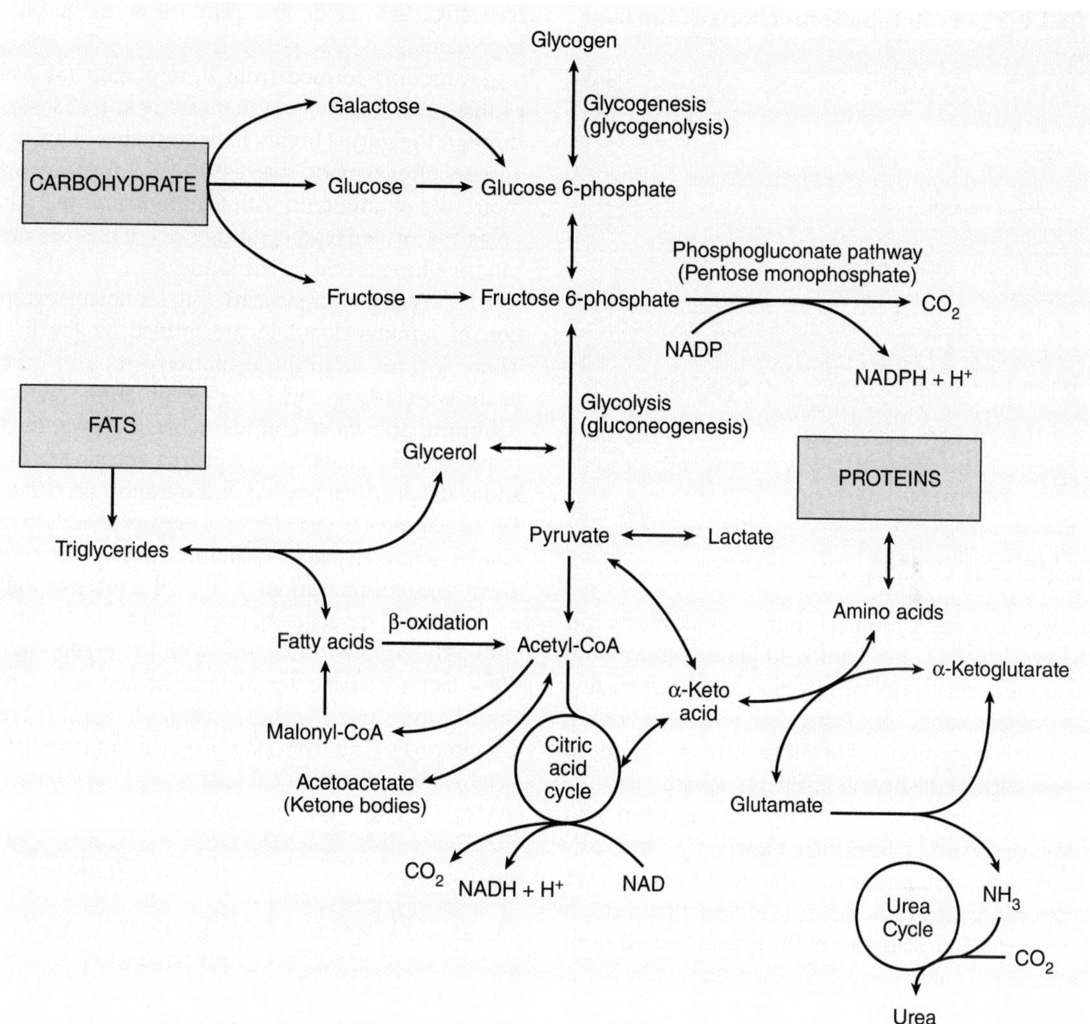

FIGURE 33–4 Important metabolic pathways in hepatocytes. Although small amounts of adenosine triphosphate (ATP) are derived directly from some intermediary reactions, the overwhelming majority of ATP produced is the result of oxidative phosphorylation of the reduced forms of nicotinamide adenine dinucleotide (NADH) and nicotinamide adenine dinucleotide phosphate (NADPH).

averages 150 g/d, and hepatic glycogen stores are normally depleted after 24 h of fasting. After this period of fasting, *gluconeogenesis*, the *de novo* synthesis of glucose, is necessary to provide an uninterrupted supply of glucose for other organs.

The liver and kidney are unique in their capacity to form glucose from lactate, pyruvate, amino acids (mainly alanine), and glycerol (derived from fat metabolism). Hepatic gluconeogenesis is vital in the maintenance of a normal blood glucose concentration. Glucocorticoids, catecholamines, glucagon, and thyroid hormone greatly enhance gluconeogenesis, whereas insulin inhibits it.

When carbohydrate stores are saturated, the liver converts the excess ingested carbohydrates and proteins into fat. The fatty acids thus formed can be used immediately for fuel or stored in adipose tissue or the liver for later consumption. Nearly all cells utilize fatty acids derived from ingested fats or synthesized from intermediary metabolites of carbohydrates and

TABLE 33–1 Metabolic functions of the liver.

Creation and secretion of bile
Nutrient metabolism
Amino acids
Monosaccharides (sugars)
Lipids (fatty acids, cholesterol, phospholipids, lipoproteins)
Vitamins
Phase I and II biotransformation
Toxins
Drugs
Hormones (steroids)
Synthesis
Albumin, α_1-antitrypsin, proteases
Clotting factors
Acute phase proteins
Plasma cholinesterase
Immune function
Kupffer cells

protein as an energy source—only red blood cells and the renal medulla are limited to glucose utilization. Neurons normally utilize only glucose, but after a few days of starvation, they can switch to ketone bodies, the breakdown products of fatty acids that have been synthesized by the liver as an energy source.

To oxidize fatty acids, they are converted into acetyl-coenzyme A (acetyl-CoA), which is then oxidized via the citric acid cycle to produce ATP. The liver is capable of high rates of fatty acid oxidation and can form acetoacetic acid (one of the ketone bodies) from excess acetyl-CoA. The acetoacetate released by hepatocytes serves as an alternative energy source for other cell types by reconversion into acetyl-CoA. Insulin inhibits hepatic ketone body production. Acetyl-CoA is also used by the liver for the production of cholesterol and phospholipids, which is necessary for the synthesis of cellular membranes throughout the body.

The liver performs a critical role in protein metabolism. The steps involved in protein metabolism include (1) deamination of amino acids, (2) formation of urea (to eliminate the ammonia produced from deamination), (3) interconversions between nonessential amino acids, and (4) formation of plasma proteins. Deamination is necessary for the conversion of excess amino acids into carbohydrates and fats. The enzymatic processes, most commonly transamination, convert amino acids into their respective keto acids and produce ammonia as a byproduct.

Ammonia formed from deamination (as well as that produced by colonic bacteria and absorbed through the gut) is highly toxic to tissues. Through a series of enzymatic steps, the liver combines two molecules of ammonia with CO_2 to form urea. The urea thus formed readily diffuses out of the liver and can then be excreted by the kidneys.

Nearly all plasma proteins, with the notable exception of immunoglobulins, are formed by the liver. These include albumin, α_1-antitrypsin, and other proteases/elastases and the coagulation factors. Albumin, the most abundant plasma protein, is responsible for maintaining a plasma oncotic pressure and is the principal binding and transport protein for fatty acids and a large number of hormones and drugs. Consequently, changes in albumin concentration can affect the concentration of the pharmacologically active, unbound fraction of many drugs.

2 All coagulation factors, with the exception of factor VIII and von Willebrand factor, are produced by the liver (Table 33–2 and Figure 33–5; see Chapter 51). The liver also produces anticoagulant

TABLE 33–2 Coagulation factors.

Factor		Approximate Half-Life (h)
I	Fibrinogen	100
II	Prothrombin	80
III	Tissue thromboplastin	—
IV	Calcium	—
V	Proaccelerin	18
VII	Proconvertin	6
VIII	Antihemophilic factor	10
IX	Christmas factor	24
X	Stuart factor	50
XI	Plasma thromboplastin antecedents	25
XII	Hageman factor	60
XIII	Fibrin-stabilizing factor	90

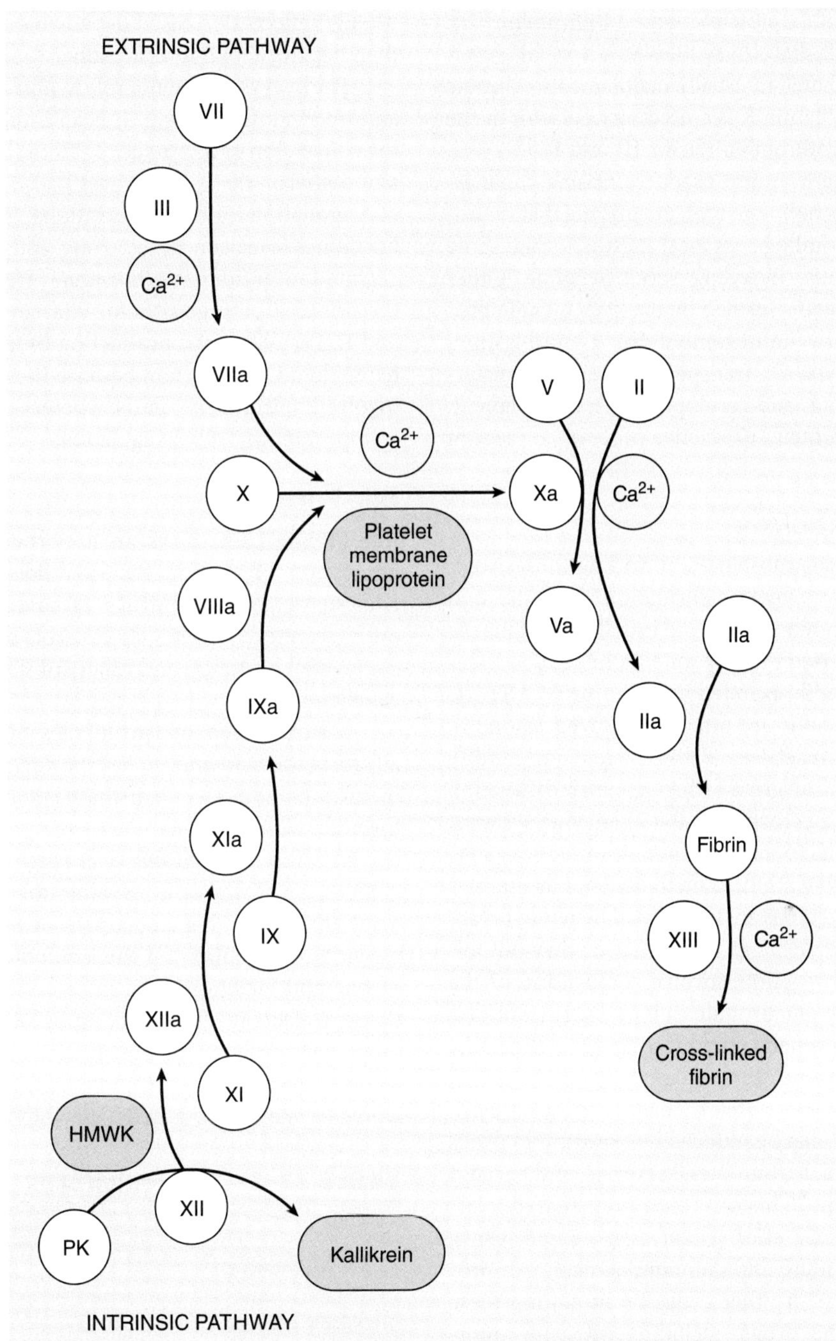

FIGURE 33–5 The intrinsic and extrinsic coagulation pathways. HMWK, high-molecular-weight kininogen.

factors (protein C, protein S, and antithrombin III). Vascular endothelial cells synthesize factor VIII, levels of which are therefore usually maintained in chronic liver disease. Vitamin K is a necessary cofactor in the synthesis of prothrombin (factor II) and factors VII, IX, and X. The liver also produces plasma cholinesterase (pseudocholinesterase), an enzyme that hydrolyzes esters, including ester local anesthetics and some muscle relaxants, including succinylcholine. Other important proteins formed by the liver include protease inhibitors (antithrombin III, α_2-antiplasmin, and α_1-antitrypsin), transport proteins (transferrin, haptoglobin, and ceruloplasmin), complement, α_1-acid glycoprotein, C-reactive protein, and serum amyloid A.

Drug Metabolism

Many exogenous substances, including most drugs, undergo hepatic biotransformation, and the end products of these reactions are usually either inactivated or converted to more water-soluble substances that can be readily excreted in bile or urine. Hepatic biotransformations are often categorized as one of two types of reactions. *Phase I reactions* modify reactive chemical groups through mixed-function oxidases or the cytochrome P-450 enzyme systems, resulting in oxidation, reduction, deamination, sulfoxidation, dealkylation, or methylation. Barbiturates and benzodiazepines are inactivated by phase I reactions. *Phase II reactions*, which may or may not follow a phase I reaction, involve conjugation of the substance with glucuronide, sulfate, taurine, or glycine. The conjugated compound can then be readily eliminated in urine or bile.

Some enzyme systems, such as those of cytochrome P-450, can be induced by exposure to drugs such as ethanol, barbiturates, ketamine, and perhaps benzodiazepines. This can result in increased tolerance to the drugs' effects. Conversely, some agents, such as cimetidine and chloramphenicol, can prolong the effects of other drugs by inhibiting these enzymes. Some drugs, including lidocaine, morphine, verapamil, labetalol, and propranolol, have very high rates of hepatic extraction from the circulation, and their metabolism is therefore highly dependent upon the rate of hepatic blood flow. As a result, a decrease in their metabolic clearance usually reflects decreased hepatic blood flow rather than hepatocellular dysfunction.

The liver plays a major role in hormone, vitamin, and mineral metabolism. It is an important site for the conversion of thyroxine (T_4) into the more active triiodothyronine (T_3). The liver is also the major site of degradation for thyroid hormone, insulin, steroid hormones (estrogen, aldosterone, and cortisol), glucagon, and antidiuretic hormone. Hepatocytes are the principal storage sites for vitamins A, B_{12}, E, D, and K. Lastly, hepatic production of transferrin and haptoglobin is important because these proteins are involved in iron hemostasis, whereas ceruloplasmin is important in copper regulation.

Bile Formation

Bile (Table 33–3) plays an important role in the absorption of fat and the excretion of bilirubin, cholesterol, and many drugs. Hepatocytes continuously secrete bile salts, cholesterol, phospholipids, conjugated bilirubin, and other substances into bile canaliculi.

Bile ducts from hepatic lobules join and eventually form the *right and left hepatic ducts*. These ducts, in turn, combine to form the *hepatic duct,* which, together with the *cystic duct* from the gallbladder, becomes the *common bile duct* (Figure 33–6). The gallbladder serves as a reservoir for bile. The bile acids formed by hepatocytes from cholesterol are essential for emulsifying the insoluble components of bile and facilitating the intestinal absorption of lipids. Defects in the formation or secretion of bile salts interfere with the absorption of fats and fat-soluble vitamins (A, D, E, and K). Because of limited stores of vitamin K, a deficiency of this fat-soluble

TABLE 33–3 Composition of bile.

97% water
<1% bile salts
Pigments
Inorganic salts
Lipids
Cholesterol
Fatty acids
Lecithin
Alkaline phosphatase

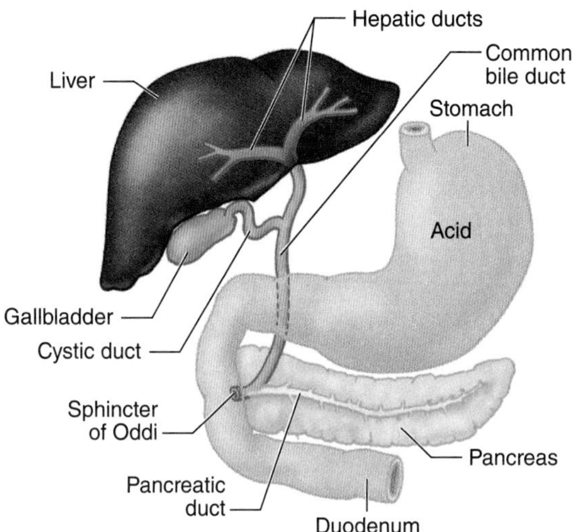

FIGURE 33–6 The biliary system. (Modified with permission from Guyton AC. *Textbook of Medical Physiology.* 7th ed. Philadelphia, PA: WB Saunders; 1986.)

vitamin can develop within a few days. *Vitamin K deficiency is manifested as a coagulopathy due to impaired formation of prothrombin and of factors VII, IX, and X.*

Bilirubin is primarily the end product of hemoglobin metabolism, and it is formed from the degradation of the heme ring in Kupffer cells. Bilirubin is then released into the blood, where it readily binds to albumin. Hepatic uptake of bilirubin from the circulation is passive, but binding to intracellular proteins traps the bilirubin inside hepatocytes. Bilirubin is conjugated by the hepatocytes, primarily with glucuronide, and actively excreted into bile canaliculi.

LIVER TESTS

The most commonly performed liver tests are neither sensitive nor specific. No one laboratory test evaluates overall hepatic function, reflecting instead one aspect of hepatic function that must be interpreted in conjunction with other tests and clinical assessment of the patient.

3 Many "liver function" tests, such as serum transaminase measurements, reflect hepatocellular integrity more than hepatic function. Liver tests that do assess hepatic synthetic function include serum albumin, prothrombin time (PT) or international normalized ratio (INR), serum cholesterol, and plasma pseudocholinesterase. Moreover, because of the liver's large functional reserve, substantial cirrhosis may be present with few or no laboratory abnormalities evident.

Liver abnormalities can often be divided into either *parenchymal* disorders or *obstructive* disorders based on laboratory tests (Table 33–4). Obstructive disorders primarily affect the biliary excretion of substances, whereas parenchymal disorders result in generalized hepatocellular dysfunction.

TABLE 33–4 Abnormalities in liver tests.[1,2]

	Parenchymal (Hepatocellular) Dysfunction	Biliary Obstruction or Cholestasis
AST (SGOT)	↑ to ↑↑↑	↑
ALT (SGPT)	↑ to ↑↑↑	↑
Albumin	0 to ↓↓↓	0
Prothrombin time	0 to ↑↑↑	0 to ↑↑[3]
Bilirubin	0 to ↑↑↑	0 to ↑↑↑
Alkaline phosphatase	↑	↑ to ↑↑↑
5′-Nucleotidase	0 to ↑	↑ to ↑↑↑
γ-Glutamyl transpeptidase	↑ to ↑↑↑	↑↑↑

[1]ALT, alanine aminotransferase; AST, aspartate aminotransferase; SGOT, serum glutamic-oxaloacetic transaminase; SGPT, serum glutamic pyruvic-transferase.

[2]↑, increases; 0, no change; ↓, decreases.

[3]Usually corrects with vitamin K.

Adapted with permission from Wilson JD, Braunwald E, Isselbacher KJ et al. *Harrison's Principles of Internal Medicine,* 12th ed. New York, NY: McGraw Hill; 1991.

Serum Bilirubin

The normal total bilirubin concentration, composed of conjugated (*direct*), water-soluble, and unconjugated (*indirect*) lipid-soluble forms, is less than 1.5 mg/dL (<25 mmol/L) and reflects the balance between bilirubin production and excretion. *Jaundice is usually clinically obvious when total bilirubin exceeds 3 mg/dL.* A predominantly conjugated hyperbilirubinemia (>50%) is associated with increased urinary urobilinogen and may reflect hepatocellular dysfunction, congenital (Dubin–Johnson or Rotor syndrome) or acquired intrahepatic cholestasis, or extrahepatic biliary obstruction. Hyperbilirubinemia that is primarily unconjugated may be seen with hemolysis or with congenital (Gilbert or Crigler–Najjar syndrome) or acquired defects in bilirubin conjugation. Unconjugated bilirubin is neurotoxic, and high levels may produce encephalopathy.

Serum Aminotransferases (Transaminases)

These enzymes are released into the circulation as a result of hepatocellular injury or death. Two aminotransferases are most commonly measured: aspartate aminotransferase (AST), also known as *serum glutamic-oxaloacetic transaminase* (SGOT), and alanine aminotransferase (ALT), also known as *serum glutamic pyruvic-transferase* (SGPT).

Serum Alkaline Phosphatase

Alkaline phosphatase is produced by the liver, bone, small bowel, kidneys, and placenta and is excreted into bile. Normal serum alkaline phosphatase activity is 25 to 85 IU/L; children and adolescents have much higher levels, reflecting active growth. Most circulating alkaline phosphatase is normally derived from bone; however, with biliary obstruction, more hepatic alkaline phosphatase is synthesized and released into the circulation.

Serum Albumin

The normal serum albumin concentration is 3.5 to 5.5 g/dL. Because its half-life is approximately 2 to 3 weeks, albumin concentration may initially be
4 normal with acute liver disease. Albumin values less than 2.5 g/dL are generally indicative of chronic liver disease, acute stress, or severe malnutrition. Increased losses of albumin in the urine (*nephrotic syndrome*) or the gastrointestinal tract (*protein-losing enteropathy*) can also produce hypoalbuminemia.

Blood Ammonia

Significant elevations of blood ammonia levels usually reflect disruption of hepatic urea synthesis. Normal whole blood ammonia levels are 47 to 65 mmol/L (80–110 mg/dL). Marked elevations usually reflect severe hepatocellular damage and may cause encephalopathy.

Prothrombin Time

5 The PT, which normally ranges between 11 and 14 s, measures the activity of fibrinogen, prothrombin, and factors V, VII, and X. The relatively short half-life of factor VII (4–6 h) makes the PT useful in evaluating the hepatic synthetic function of patients with acute or chronic liver disease. Prolongations of the PT greater than 3 to 4 s from the control are considered significant and usually correspond to an INR greater than 1.5. This INR reflects liver dysfunction but not the degree of coagulopathy. If protein C, protein S, and antithrombin 3 are more depressed than the coagulation factors, the patient may have normal clotting or even be hypercoagulable. *The INR was designed to reflect warfarin activity, not liver function.* This is of great clinical importance as a prolonged INR after liver surgery may result in venous thromboembolic prophylaxis being withheld until the INR normalizes. This may leave the patient at increased risk for a pulmonary embolus. *Because only 20% to 30% of normal factor activity is required for normal coagulation, prolongation of the PT usually reflects either severe liver disease or vitamin K deficiency.* See Table 33–5 for a list of coagulation test abnormalities. To prevent VTE, clinicians are increasingly treating patients with factor Xa inhibitors (eg, apixaban, rivaroxaban) for the prevention of thrombosis. Direct assays of anti-factor Xa activity may be employed to monitor their effects. The direct thrombin inhibitor dabigatran is also currently prescribed for prophylaxis.

Point-of-Care Viscoelastic Coagulation Monitoring

This technology provides a "real-time" assessment of the coagulation status and utilizes thromboelastography (TEG), rotation thromboelastometry (ROTEM), or Sonoclot analysis to assess global coagulation via the viscoelastic properties of whole blood (Figure 33–7). A clear picture is provided of

TABLE 33–5 Coagulation test abnormalities.[1]

	PT	PTT	TT	Fibrinogen
Advanced liver disease	↑	↑	N or ↑	N or ↓
DIC	↑	↑	↑	↓
Vitamin K deficiency	↑↑	↑	N	N
Warfarin therapy	↑↑	↑	N	N
Heparin therapy	↑	↑↑	↑	N
Hemophilia				
Factor VIII deficiency	N	↑	N	N
Factor IX deficiency	N	↑	N	N
Factor VII deficiency	↑	N	N	N
Factor XIII deficiency	N	N	N	N

[1]DIC, disseminated intravascular coagulation; N, normal; PT, prothrombin time; PTT, partial thromboplastin time; TT, thrombin time.

the global effect of balance between the procoagulant and anticoagulant systems and the profibrinolytic and antifibrinolytic systems and the resultant clot tensile strength, allowing precise management of hemostatic therapy. The rate of clot formation, the strength of the clot, and the impact of any clot lysis can be observed. The presence of disseminated intravascular coagulation can be evaluated, as can the effect of heparin or heparinoid activity. In addition, platelet function can be assessed, including the effects of platelet inhibition. Viscoelastic coagulation monitoring is particularly important when assessing the coagulation and thromboembolic risk of the patient who has a prolonged INR from liver dysfunction or the effect of warfarin and has undergone, or is about to undergo, procedural care. Coagulopathy is a balance of the procoagulant and anticoagulant factors produced by the liver, and the INR only examines the procoagulant side. A patient with an INR of 3, for example, may also have anticoagulant factors so reduced that the patient is in a hypercoagulable state and thereby actually at increased risk for venous thromboembolism. This risk can be readily evaluated by viscoelastic testing.

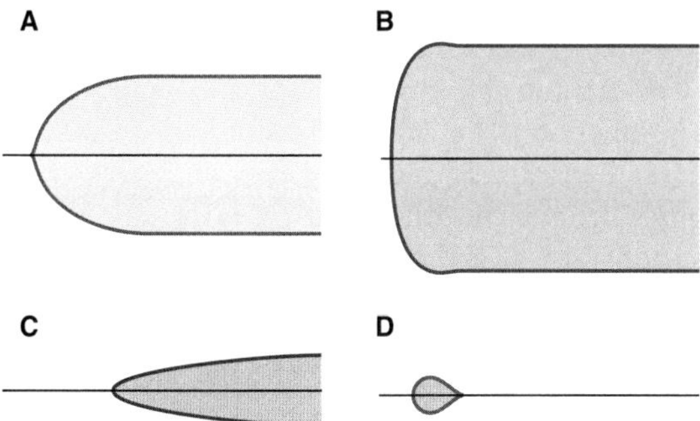

FIGURE 33–7 Examples of typical thromboelastography tracings. **A**: Normal. **B**: Hypercoagulation. **C**: Hypocoagulation (eg, thrombocytopenia). **D**: Fibrinolysis. (Reproduced with permission from Johansson PI, Stissing T, Bochsen L, et al. Thrombelastography and thromboelastometry in assessing coagulopathy in trauma. *Scand J Trauma Resusc Emerg Med.* 2009 Sep 23:17:45.)

EFFECT OF ANESTHESIA ON HEPATIC FUNCTION

Hepatic blood flow usually decreases during regional and general anesthesia, and multiple factors are responsible, including both direct and indirect effects of anesthetic agents, the type of ventilation employed, and the type of surgery being performed.

Decreases in cardiac output reduce hepatic blood flow. Controlled positive-pressure ventilation with high mean airway pressures reduces venous return and cardiac output and can compromise hepatic blood flow. The former increases hepatic venous pressure, whereas the latter can reduce blood pressure and increase sympathetic tone. Positive end-expiratory pressure (PEEP) further accentuates these effects. All these parameters may be seen in patients undergoing laparoscopic and robotic surgery, especially in the steep Trendelenburg position.

6 Operative procedures near the liver can reduce hepatic blood flow up to 60%. Although the mechanisms are not clear, they most likely involve sympathetic activation, local reflexes, and direct compression of vessels in the portal and hepatic circulations.

β-Adrenergic blockers, α_1-adrenergic agonists, H_2-receptor blockers, and vasopressin reduce hepatic blood flow. Dopamine infusions (0.5–2.5 mcg/kg/min) may increase liver blood flow.

Metabolic Functions

The effects of the various anesthetic agents on hepatic metabolism are poorly defined. An endocrine stress response secondary to fasting and
7 surgical trauma is generally observed. The neuroendocrine stress response to surgery and trauma is characterized by elevated circulating levels of catecholamines, glucagon, and cortisol and results in the mobilization of carbohydrate stores and protein, causing hyperglycemia and negative nitrogen balance (catabolism). The neuroendocrine stress response may be at least partially blunted by regional anesthesia, deep general anesthesia, or pharmacological blockade of the sympathetic system, with regional anesthesia having the most salutary effect
8 on catabolism. All opioids can potentially cause spasm of the sphincter of Oddi and increase biliary pressure. Naloxone and glucagon may relieve opioid-induced biliary spasm.

Procedures in close proximity to the liver frequently result in modest elevations in lactate dehydrogenase and transaminase concentrations regardless of the anesthetic agent or technique
9 employed. When liver function tests are abnormal postoperatively, the usual cause is underlying liver disease or the surgical procedure itself. Persistent abnormalities in liver tests may be indicative of viral hepatitis, sepsis, idiosyncratic drug reactions, or surgical complications. *Postoperative jaundice can result from a variety of factors (Table 33–6), but the most common cause is either overproduction of bilirubin because of resorption of a large hematoma or hemolysis following transfusion.* Nonetheless, all other causes should be considered. A correct diagnosis requires a careful review of preoperative liver function and of intraoperative and postoperative events, such as transfusions, sustained hypotension or hypoxemia, and drug exposure. Desflurane, sevoflurane, and isoflurane have minimal, if any, direct adverse effect upon hepatocytes.

TABLE 33–6 Causes of postoperative jaundice.

Prehepatic (increased bilirubin production)
Resorption of hematomas
Hemolytic anemia transfusion
Senescent red cell breakdown
Hemolytic reactions
Hepatic (hepatocellular dysfunction)
Preexisting liver disease
Ischemic or hypoxemic injury
Drug-induced
Gilbert syndrome
Intrahepatic cholestasis
Halothane
Posthepatic (biliary obstruction)
Postoperative cholecystitis
Postoperative pancreatitis
Retained common bile duct stone
Bile duct injury
Miscellaneous

Hepatic Cirrhosis

10 Liver cirrhosis may result in portal hypertension, bleeding varices, and major organ dysfunction. The major causes of cirrhosis are viral hepatitis B and C, excessive alcohol use, nonalcoholic steatohepatitis (NASH), and hemochromatosis. Cirrhosis is complicated by portal hypertension that may result in ascites, sometimes in massive volumes together with pleural effusions, variceal hemorrhage, splenomegaly, hepatorenal syndrome, encephalopathy, and, if the cirrhosis is viral in etiology, hepatocellular cancer. Treatment options include transjugular intrahepatic portosystemic shunt (TIPS) procedure, liver transplantation, or both. The prognosis of the patient may be indicated by the Child-Turcotte-Pugh Score or the MELD Score (see Chapter 34).

CASE DISCUSSION

Coagulopathy in a Patient with Liver Disease (also see Chapter 51)

A 52-year-old man with a long history of alcohol use disorder presents for a splenorenal shunt after three major episodes of upper gastrointestinal hemorrhage from esophageal varices. Coagulation studies reveal a PT of 17 s (control: 12 s), INR of 1.7, and a partial thromboplastin time (PTT) of 43 s (control: 29 s). The platelet count is 75,000/μL.

What factors can contribute to excessive bleeding during and following surgery?

Hemostasis following trauma or surgery is dependent on three major processes: (1) vascular spasm, (2) formation of a platelet plug (*primary hemostasis*), and (3) coagulation of blood (*secondary hemostasis*) in addition to adequate surgical control of bleeding sites. The first two occur immediately (in seconds), whereas the third is delayed (in minutes). A defect in any of these processes can lead to a bleeding diathesis and increased blood loss.

Outline the mechanisms involved in primary hemostasis.

Injury to smaller blood vessels normally causes localized spasm as a result of the release of humoral factors from platelets and local myogenic reflexes. Sympathetic-mediated vasoconstriction is also a factor in medium-sized vessels. Exposure of circulating platelets to the damaged endothelial surface causes them to undergo a series of changes that results in the formation of a platelet plug. If the break in a vessel is small, the plug itself can often completely stop bleeding. If the break is large, however, coagulation of blood is also necessary to stop the bleeding.

The formation of the platelet plug can be broken down into three stages: (1) adhesion, (2) release of platelet granules, and (3) aggregation. Following injury, circulating platelets adhere to subendothelial collagen via specific glycoprotein (GP) receptors on their membrane. This interaction is stabilized by a circulating GP called *von Willebrand factor* (vWF), which forms additional bridges between subendothelial collagen and platelets via GPIb. Collagen (as well as epinephrine and thrombin) activates platelet membrane-bound phospholipases A and C, which, in turn, results in the formation of thromboxane A_2 (TXA_2) and platelet degranulation. TXA_2 is a potent vasoconstrictor that also promotes platelet aggregation. Platelet granules contain a large number of substances, including adenosine diphosphate (ADP), factor V, vWF, fibrinogen, and fibronectin. These factors attract and activate additional platelets. ADP alters platelet membrane GPIIb/IIIa, which facilitates the binding of fibrinogen to activated platelets.

Describe the mechanisms involved in normal coagulation.

Coagulation, often referred to as *secondary hemostasis*, involves the formation of a fibrin clot, which usually binds and strengthens a platelet plug. Fibrin can be formed via one of two pathways (*extrinsic* or *intrinsic*; see Figure 33–5) that involve calcium and activation of soluble coagulation precursor proteins in blood (see Table 33–2). Regardless of which pathway is activated, the coagulation cascade ends in the conversion of *fibrinogen* to *fibrin*. The extrinsic pathway of the coagulation cascade is triggered by the release of a tissue lipoprotein, *thromboplastin*, from the membranes of injured cells and is likely the more important pathway. The intrinsic pathway can be triggered by the interaction between subendothelial collagen with circulating Hageman factor (XII), high-molecular-weight kininogen, and prekallikrein. The latter two substances are also involved in the formation of bradykinin.

Thrombin plays a central role in coagulation because it not only activates platelets it also accelerates the conversion of factors V, VIII, and XIII to their active forms. Conversion of prothrombin to thrombin is markedly accelerated by activated platelets. Thrombin then converts fibrinogen to soluble fibrin monomers that polymerize on the platelet plug. The cross-linking of fibrin polymers by factor XIII is necessary to form a strong, insoluble fibrin clot. Finally, retraction of the clot, which requires platelets, expresses fluid from the clot and helps pull the walls of the damaged blood vessel together.

What prevents coagulation of blood in normal tissues?

The coagulation process is limited to injured areas by localization of platelets to the injured area and by the maintenance of normal blood flow in uninjured areas. Normal endothelium produces *prostacyclin* (prostaglandin I_2, PGI_2), which is a potent vasodilator that also inhibits platelet activation and helps confine the primary hemostatic process to the injured area. Normal blood flow is important in clearing activated coagulation factors, which are taken up by the monocyte–macrophage scavenger system. Multiple inhibitors of coagulation are normally present in plasma, including antithrombin III, protein C, protein S, and tissue factor pathway inhibitor. Antithrombin III complexes with and inactivates circulating coagulation factors (with the notable exception of factor VII), and protein C specifically inactivates factors V and VIII. *Heparin exerts its anticoagulant activity by augmenting the activity of antithrombin III.* Protein S enhances the activity of protein C, and deficiencies of protein C and protein S lead to hypercoagulability. Tissue factor pathway inhibitor antagonizes the action of activated factor VII.

What is the role of the fibrinolytic system in normal hemostasis?

The fibrinolytic system is normally activated simultaneously with the coagulation cascade and functions to maintain the fluidity of blood during coagulation. It is also responsible for clot lysis once tissue repair begins. When a clot is formed, a large amount of the protein *plasminogen* is incorporated. Plasminogen is then activated by *tissue plasminogen activator* (tPA), which is usually released by endothelial cells in response to thrombin, and by Hageman factor (XII). The resulting formation of *plasmin* degrades fibrin and fibrinogen, as well as other coagulation factors. Urokinase (found in urine) and streptokinase (a product of bacteria) are also potent activators of plasminogen to plasmin. The action of tPA is localized because (1) it is absorbed into the fibrin clot, (2) it activates plasminogen more effectively on the clot, (3) free plasmin is rapidly neutralized by a circulating α_2-antiplasmin, and (4) circulating tPA is cleared by the liver. Plasmin degrades fibrin and fibrinogen into small fragments. These fibrin degradation products possess anticoagulant activity because they compete with fibrinogen for thrombin; they are normally cleared by the monocyte–macrophage system. The drugs ε-aminocaproic acid (EACA) and tranexamic acid inhibit the conversion of plasminogen to plasmin. Endothelium also normally secretes a plasminogen activator inhibitor (PAI-1) that antagonizes tPA.

What hemostatic defects are likely to be present in this patient?

Multifactorial coagulopathy often develops in patients with advanced liver disease. Three major causes are usually responsible: (1) vitamin K deficiency due to dietary deficiency or impaired absorption or storage, (2) impaired hepatic synthesis of coagulation factors, and (3) splenic sequestration of platelets resulting from hypersplenism. To complicate matters further, patients with cirrhosis typically have multiple potential bleeding sites (esophageal varices, gastritis, peptic ulcers, and hemorrhoids) and frequently require multiple blood transfusions. With severe liver disease, patients may also have decreased synthesis of coagulation inhibitors and may fail to clear activated coagulation factors and fibrin split products because of impaired Kupffer cell function; the resultant coagulation defect resembles and becomes indistinguishable from *disseminated intravascular coagulation* (DIC).

What is DIC?

In DIC, the coagulation cascade is activated by the release of endogenous tissue thromboplastin or thromboplastin-like substances or by direct activation of factor XII by endotoxin or foreign surfaces. Widespread deposition of fibrin in the microcirculation results in consumption of coagulation factors, secondary fibrinolysis, acute severe thrombocytopenia, and microangiopathic hemolytic anemia. Diffuse bleeding and, in some cases, thromboembolic phenomena usually follow. Treatment is generally aimed at the underlying cause. Supportive measures include transfusion of coagulation factors and platelets. Heparin therapy is controversial but may benefit patients with thromboembolic phenomena.

What is primary fibrinolysis?

This bleeding disorder is due to uncontrolled fibrinolysis. Patients may have a deficiency of α_2-antiplasmin or impaired clearance of tPA. The latter may be common in patients with severe liver disease and during the anhepatic phase of liver transplantation. The disorder may occasionally be encountered in patients with carcinoma of the prostate. Diagnosis is often difficult but is suggested by a bleeding diathesis with a low fibrinogen level but relatively normal coagulation tests and platelet count (as noted next). Treatment includes fresh frozen plasma or cryoprecipitate and possibly either EACA or tranexamic acid.

How are coagulation tests helpful in evaluating inadequate hemostasis?

The diagnosis of coagulation abnormalities can be facilitated by measurement of the activated partial thromboplastin time (aPTT), PT, thrombin time (TT), fibrin degradation products, and fibrinogen level (see Table 33–5). The aPTT measures the intrinsic pathway (factors I, II, V, VIII, IX, X, XI, and XII). The whole blood clotting time and activated clotting time (ACT) also measure the intrinsic pathway. In contrast, the PT measures the extrinsic pathway (factors I, II, V, and VII). The TT specifically measures the conversion of fibrinogen to fibrin (factors I and II). The normal plasma fibrinogen level is 200 to 400 mg/dL (5.9–11.7 μmol/L). Because heparin therapy primarily affects the intrinsic pathway, in low doses, it usually prolongs the aPTT only. In high doses, heparin also prolongs the PT. In contrast, warfarin primarily affects vitamin K–dependent factors (II, VII, IX, and X), so the PT is prolonged at usual doses, and the aPTT is prolonged only at high doses. In vivo plasmin activity can be evaluated by measuring circulating levels of peptides cleaved from fibrin and fibrinogen by plasmin, namely *fibrin degradation products* (FDPs) and D-dimers. Patients with primary fibrinolysis usually have elevated FDPs, but normal D-dimer levels.

What tests are most helpful in evaluating inadequate primary hemostasis?

The most commonly performed tests include a platelet count and a bleeding time but also include TEG, ROTEM, and Sonoclot analysis (see Figure 33–7 and Chapter 51). Patients with normally functioning platelets and platelet counts above 100,000/μL have normal primary hemostasis. The normal platelet count is 150,000 to 450,000/μL, and the bleeding time is generally not affected by the platelet count when the latter is greater than 100,000/μL. When the platelet count is 50,000/μL or greater, excessive bleeding generally occurs only with severe trauma or extensive surgery. In contrast, patients with platelet counts less than 20,000/μL often develop significant bleeding following even minor trauma. However, patients with liver cirrhosis may be thrombocytopenic but have increased levels of vWF, resulting in very active platelets that may compensate for the low count. Thrombocytopenia usually results from one of three mechanisms: (1) decreased platelet production, (2) splenic sequestration of platelets, or (3) increased platelet destruction. The third mechanism may fall under one of two categories of destruction: immune or nonimmune. Nonimmune destruction includes vasculitis or DIC.

A prolonged bleeding time with a normal platelet count implies a qualitative platelet defect. Although the bleeding time is somewhat dependent on the technique employed, values longer than 9 min are generally considered abnormal. Significant intraoperative and postoperative bleeding may be expected when the bleeding time exceeds 15 min. Specialized testing is required to diagnose specific platelet functional defects.

What are the most common causes of qualitative platelet defects?

The most common platelet defect is due to inhibition of TXA_2 production by aspirin and other nonsteroidal anti-inflammatory drugs (NSAIDs). In contrast to aspirin, which irreversibly acetylates and inactivates cyclooxygenase for the life of the platelet (up to 8 days), enzyme inhibition by other NSAIDs is reversible and generally lasts only 24 h. Increasingly patients with cardiac stents are treated with a variety of antiplatelet agents such as clopidogrel, which impair platelet function for the life of the platelet. Assays of platelet function are available to determine the degree to which platelet function is inhibited.

What is von Willebrand disease?

The most common inherited bleeding disorder (1:800–1000 patients) is *von Willebrand disease*. Patients with this disorder produce either a defective vWF or low levels of a normal vWF (normal: 5–10 mg/L). Most patients are heterozygous and have relatively mild hemostatic defects that become clinically apparent only when they are subjected to major surgery or trauma or following ingestion of NSAIDs. In addition to helping link platelets, vWF serves as a carrier for coagulation factor VIII. As a result, these patients typically have a prolonged bleeding time, decreased plasma vWF concentration, and decreased factor VIII activity. Acquired forms of von Willebrand disease may be encountered in patients with some immune disorders and those with tumors that absorb vWF onto their surface. At least three forms of the disease are recognized, ranging in severity from mild to severe.

Treatment with desmopressin (DDAVP) can raise vWF levels in some patients with mild von Willebrand disease (as well as normal individuals). The drug is usually administered at a dose of 0.3 mcg/kg intravenously 30 min prior to surgery. Patients who do not respond to DDAVP should receive cryoprecipitate or factor VIII concentrates, both of which are rich in vWF; prophylactic infusions are generally recommended before and after surgery twice a day for 2 to 4 days to help assure surgical hemostasis.

What other hereditary hemostatic defects may be encountered in anesthetic practice?

The most common inherited secondary hemostasis defect is *factor VIII deficiency (hemophilia A)*, an X-linked abnormality estimated to affect 1:10,000 males. Disease severity is generally inversely related to factor VIII activity. Most symptomatic patients experience hemarthrosis, bleeding into deep tissues, and hematuria, and they usually have less than 5% of normal factor VIII activity. Classically, patients present with a prolonged aPTT but a normal PT and bleeding time. The diagnosis is confirmed by measuring factor VIII activity in blood. Affected patients generally do not experience increased bleeding during surgery when factor VIII levels are more than 30% of normal, but most clinicians recommend increasing factor VIII levels to more than 50% of normal prior to surgery. Normal (fresh frozen) plasma, by definition, is considered to have 1 U of factor VIII activity per milliliter. In contrast, cryoprecipitate has 5 to 10 U/mL, whereas factor VIII concentrates have approximately 40 U/mL. Each unit of factor VIII transfused is estimated to raise factor VIII levels 2% per kilogram of body weight. Twice-a-day transfusions are generally recommended following surgery because of the relatively short half-life of factor VIII (8–12 h). Administration of DDAVP can raise factor VIII levels two- to threefold in some patients. EACA or tranexamic acid may also be used as adjuncts. Recombinant factor VIII is now undergoing clinical trials.

Hemophilia B (also known as *Christmas disease*) is the result of an X-linked hereditary deficiency of factor IX. It is very similar to hemophilia A but much less common (1:100,000 males). Measurement of factor IX levels establishes the diagnosis. Perioperative administration of fresh frozen plasma is generally recommended to maintain factor IX activity at more than 30% of normal. Recombinant or monoclonal purified factor IX is available.

Factor XIII deficiency is extremely rare but notable in that the aPTT, PT, TT, and bleeding times are normal. The diagnosis requires the measurement of factor XIII levels. Because only 1% of normal factor XIII activity is generally required, patients are treated by a single transfusion of fresh frozen plasma.

Do normal laboratory values exclude a hemostatic defect?

A bleeding diathesis may exist even in the absence of gross abnormalities on routine laboratory tests. Some hemostatic defects are often not detected by routine testing but require additional specialized tests. A history of excessive bleeding after dental extractions, childbirth, minor surgery, minor trauma, or even during menstruation suggests a hemostatic defect. Conversely, there may be no excess bleeding despite abnormal laboratory testing. A family history of a bleeding diathesis may suggest an inherited coagulation defect, but such history is often absent because the increased bleeding is often minor and goes unnoticed.

Hemostatic defects can often be differentiated by their clinical presentation. Bleeding in patients with primary hemostatic defects usually immediately follows minor trauma, is confined to superficial sites (skin or mucosal surfaces), and often can be controlled by local compression. Small pinpoint hemorrhages from capillaries in the dermis (petechiae) are typically present on examination. Bleeding into subcutaneous tissues (ecchymosis) from small arterioles or venules is also common in patients with platelet disorders. In contrast, bleeding that results from secondary hemostatic defects is usually delayed following injury, is typically deep (subcutaneous tissues, joints, body cavities, or muscles), and is often difficult to stop even with compression. Hemorrhages may be palpable as hematomas or may go unnoticed when located deeper (retroperitoneal). Coagulation may be impaired by systemic hypothermia or by subnormal temperature at the site of bleeding, even when coagulation test results (PT, aPTT, bleeding time) are normal and there is no history of hemostatic defects. Most laboratory tests are carried out at body temperature and may not reflect the effects of hypothermia.

SUGGESTED READINGS

Barton CA. Treatment of coagulopathy related to hepatic insufficiency. *Crit Care Med*. 2016;44:1927.

Bona R. Hypercoagulable states: what the oral surgeon needs to know. *Oral Maxillofac Surg Clin N Am*. 2016;28:491.

Cohen MJ, Christie SA. Coagulopathy of trauma. *Crit Care Clin*. 2017;333:101.

Drumheller BC, Stein DM, Moore LJ, et al. Thromboelastography and rotational thromboelastometry for the surgical intensivist: a narrative review. *J Trauma Acute Care Surg*. 2019;86:710.

Friedman LS. Martin P. *Handbook of Liver Disease*. 4th ed. Elsevier; 2018.

Goobie SM, Haas T. Perioperative bleeding management in pediatric patients. *Curr Opin Anaesthesiol*. 2016;29:352.

Hackl C, Schlitt HJ, Renner P, et al. Liver surgery in cirrhosis and portal hypertension. *World J Gastroenterol*. 2016;22:2725.

Iba T, Levi M, Levy JH. Sepsis-induced coagulopathy and disseminated intravascular coagulation. *Semin Thromb Hemost*. 2020;46:89.

Kandiah PA, Olson JC, Subramanian RM. Emerging strategies for the treatment of patients with acute hepatic failure. *Curr Opin Crit Care*. 2016;22:142.

Levi M, Sivapalaratnam S. Disseminated intravascular coagulation: an update on pathogenesis and diagnosis. *Expert Rev Hematol*. 2018;11:663.

O'Leary JG, Greenberg CS, Patton HM, et al. AGA clinical practice update: coagulation in cirrhosis. *Gastroenterology*. 2019;157:34.

Peyvandi F, Garagiola I, Biguzzi E. Advances in the treatment of bleeding disorders. *J Thromb Haemost*. 2016;14:2095.

Tapper EB, Jiang ZG, Patwardhan VR. Refining the ammonia hypothesis: a pathology-driven approach to the treatment of hepatic encephalopathy. *Mayo Clin Proc*. 2015;90:646.

Wijdicks EFM. Hepatic encephalopathy. *N Engl J Med*. 2016;375:1660.

Wikkelsø A, Wettersley J, Møller AM, et al. Thromboelastography (TEG) or rotational thromboelastometry (ROTEM) to monitor haemostatic treatment in bleeding patients: a systemic review with meta-analysis and trial sequential analysis. *Anaesthesia*. 2017;72:519.

Williams B, McNeil J, Crabbe A, et al. Practical use of thromboelastometry in the management of perioperative coagulopathy and bleeding. *Transfus Med Rev*. 2017;31:11.

CHAPTER 34

Anesthesia for Patients with Liver Disease

Michael Ramsay, MD, FRCA

KEY CONCEPTS

1. Because of increased perioperative risk, patients with acute hepatitis should have elective surgery postponed until the acute hepatitis has resolved, as indicated by the normalization of liver tests.
2. Isoflurane and sevoflurane are the volatile agents of choice for patients with significant liver disease because they preserve hepatic blood flow and oxygen delivery. Factors known to reduce hepatic blood flow, such as hypotension, excessive sympathetic activation, and high mean airway pressures during controlled ventilation, should be avoided.
3. In evaluating patients for chronic hepatitis, laboratory test results may show only a mild elevation in serum aminotransferase activity and often correlate poorly with disease severity.
4. Liver cirrhosis refers to the damaging effects to the liver of inflammation, hepatocellular injury, and the resulting fibrosis and regeneration of hepatocytes.
5. Liver cirrhosis leads to portal hypertension, varices, and widespread endothelial damage from toxins not cleared by the liver that may cause multiorgan dysfunction.
6. Massive bleeding from gastroesophageal varices is a major cause of morbidity and mortality in patients with liver disease, and, in addition to the cardiovascular effects of acute blood loss, the absorbed nitrogen load from the breakdown of blood in the gastrointestinal tract can precipitate hepatic encephalopathy.
7. Cardiovascular changes observed in cirrhotic patients are usually those of hyperdynamic circulation, though clinically significant cirrhotic cardiomyopathy is often present and not recognized. A left ventricular ejection fraction of 50% is low for a patient with cirrhosis!
8. The effects of hepatic cirrhosis on pulmonary arterioles may result in vasodilation, causing shunts and chronic hypoxemia, or conversely lead to pulmonary vasoconstriction and medial hyperplasia, causing an increase in vascular resistance and pulmonary hypertension.
9. Hepatorenal syndrome is a functional renal defect in patients with cirrhosis that usually follows gastrointestinal bleeding, aggressive diuresis, sepsis, or major surgery. It is characterized by progressive oliguria with avid sodium retention, azotemia, intractable ascites, and a very high mortality rate.
10. Factors known to precipitate hepatic encephalopathy in patients with cirrhosis include gastrointestinal bleeding, increased dietary protein intake, hypokalemic alkalosis from vomiting or diuresis, infections, worsening liver function, and drugs with central nervous system depressant activity.
11. Following the removal of large amounts of ascitic fluid, aggressive intravenous fluid replacement is often necessary to prevent profound hypotension and acute kidney injury or failure.

The prevalence of liver disease is increasing. Cirrhosis, the terminal pathology of most liver diseases, has a general population incidence as high as 5% in some autopsy series. It is a major cause of death in men in their fourth and fifth decades of life, and mortality rates are increasing. Ten percent of the patients with liver disease undergo operative procedures during the final 2 years of their lives. The liver has remarkable functional reserve, and thus overt manifestations of hepatic disease are often absent until extensive damage has occurred. When patients with little hepatic reserve come to the operating room, effects from anesthesia and the surgical procedure can precipitate hepatic decompensation and frank hepatic failure.

COAGULATION IN LIVER DISEASE

The hemostatic changes that occur with liver disease may cause hypercoagulation and thrombosis, as well as an increased risk of bleeding. The causes of excessive bleeding primarily involve thrombocytopenia, endothelial dysfunction, portal hypertension, kidney failure, and sepsis (see Chapters 31 and 51). Clot breakdown may be enhanced by an imbalance of the fibrinolytic system.

Chronic liver disease is characterized by the impaired synthesis of coagulation factors, resulting in prolongation of the prothrombin time (PT) and international normalized ratio (INR) (Table 34–1). The INR was designed to monitor the anticoagulant effect of warfarin, not the anticoagulant effect of liver dysfunction. In liver dysfunction, the anticoagulant factors (protein C, antithrombin, and tissue factor pathway inhibitor) are also reduced and may balance out any effect of a prolonged PT. This may be confirmed by assessing thrombin generation in the presence of endothelial-produced thrombomodulin. Adequate thrombin production requires an adequate number of functioning platelets. If the platelet count is greater than 40,000/μL, coagulation may well be normal in a patient with severe cirrhosis. In fact, more recently it has been shown that an increased von Willebrand factor (vWF) in liver disease may result in activated platelets allowing normal or increased coagulation despite a much lower platelet count. It is important to use point-of-care global viscoelastic coagulation testing to fully reveal the state of coagulation (see later discussion).

Cirrhotic patients will typically have hyperfibrinolysis. However, individual laboratory tests may not give a true picture of the state of fibrinolysis. Thromboelastography (TEG), rotational thromboelastometry

TABLE 34–1 Coagulation test abnormalities.[1]

	PT	PTT	TT	Fibrinogen
Advanced liver disease	↑	↑	N or ↑	N or ↓
DIC	↑	↑	↑	↓
Vitamin K deficiency	↑↑	↑	N	N
Warfarin therapy	↑↑	↑	N	N
Heparin therapy	↑	↑↑	↑	N
Hemophilia				
Factor VIII deficiency	N	↑	N	N
Factor IX deficiency	N	↑	N	N
Factor VII deficiency	↑	N	N	N
Factor XIII deficiency	N	N	N	N

[1]DIC, disseminated intravascular coagulation; N, normal; PT, prothrombin time; PTT, partial thromboplastin time; TT, thrombin time.

(ROTEM), and Sonoclot viscoelastic coagulation testing technologies are the optimal methods of demonstrating the global state of the coagulation system at a specific moment in time in any patient with liver disease (see Chapter 51). An INR of 3 with a platelet count of 40,000/uL may be associated with a hypercoagulable state in some cirrhotic patients. Therefore, venous thromboembolism prophylaxis should not be withheld or fresh frozen plasma administered until the patient's coagulopathy has been properly assessed.

Hepatitis

ACUTE HEPATITIS

Acute hepatitis is usually the result of a viral infection, drug reaction, or exposure to a hepatotoxin. The illness represents acute hepatocellular injury with a variable degree of cellular necrosis. Clinical manifestations depend on the severity of the inflammatory reaction and on the extent of necrosis. Mild inflammatory reactions may present merely as asymptomatic elevations in the serum transaminases, whereas massive hepatic necrosis presents as acute fulminant hepatic failure.

Viral Hepatitis

Viral hepatitis is most commonly due to hepatitis A, B, or C viral infection. At least two other hepatitis viruses have also been identified: hepatitis D (delta virus) and hepatitis E (enteric non-A, non-B). Hepatitis types A and E are transmitted by the fecal–oral route, whereas hepatitis types B and C are transmitted primarily percutaneously and by contact with body fluids. Hepatitis D is unique in that it may be transmitted by either route and requires the presence of the hepatitis B virus in the host to be infective. Other viruses may also cause hepatitis, including Epstein–Barr, herpes simplex, cytomegalovirus, coxsackieviruses. Elevations in hepatic enzymes are also associated with COVID-19 disease.

Patients with viral hepatitis often have a 1- to 2-week mild prodromal illness (fatigue, malaise, low-grade fever, or nausea and vomiting) that may or may not be followed by jaundice. The jaundice typically lasts 2 to 12 weeks, but complete recovery, as evidenced by serum transaminase measurements, usually takes 4 months. Serological testing is necessary to determine the causative viral agent. The clinical course tends to be more complicated and prolonged with hepatitis B and C viruses relative to other types of viral hepatitis. Cholestasis (see later discussion) may be a major manifestation. Rarely, fulminant hepatic failure (massive hepatic necrosis) can develop.

The incidence of chronic active hepatitis is 3% to 10% following infection with hepatitis B virus and at least 50% following infection with hepatitis C virus. A small percentage of patients (mainly immunosuppressed patients and those on long-term hemodialysis regimens) become asymptomatic infectious carriers following infection with hepatitis B virus, and up to 30% of these patients remain infectious with the hepatitis B surface antigen (HBsAg) persisting in their blood. Most patients with chronic hepatitis C infection seem to have very low, intermittent, or absent circulating viral particles and are therefore not highly infective. Approximately 0.5% to 1% of patients with hepatitis C infection become asymptomatic infectious carriers, and infectivity correlates with the detection of hepatitis C viral RNA in peripheral blood. Such infectious carriers pose a major health hazard to operating room personnel.

In addition to "universal precautions" for avoiding direct contact with blood and secretions (gloves, mask, protective eyewear, and not recapping needles), immunization of health care personnel is highly effective against hepatitis B infection. A vaccine for hepatitis C is not available; moreover, unlike hepatitis B infection, hepatitis C infection does not seem to confer immunity to subsequent exposure. Postexposure prophylaxis with hyperimmune globulin is effective for hepatitis B, but not hepatitis C. Effective therapies now exist for hepatitis C, but continued hepatocellular carcinoma surveillance remains important for these patients.

Drug-Induced Hepatitis

Drug-induced hepatitis (Table 34–2) can result from direct, dose-dependent toxicity of a drug or drug metabolite, an idiosyncratic drug reaction, or a combination of these two causes. The clinical course often resembles viral hepatitis, making

TABLE 34–2 Drugs and other substances associated with hepatitis.

Toxic
Alcohol
Acetaminophen
Salicylates
Tetracyclines
Trichloroethylene
Vinyl chloride
Carbon tetrachloride
Yellow phosphorus
Poisonous mushrooms (*Amanita, Galerina*)
Idiosyncratic
Volatile anesthetics (halothane)
Phenytoin
Sulfonamides
Rifampin
Indomethacin
Toxic and idiosyncratic
Methyldopa
Isoniazid
Sodium valproate
Amiodarone
Primarily cholestatic
Chlorpromazine
Cyclosporine
Oral contraceptives
Anabolic steroids
Erythromycin estolate
Methimazole

diagnosis difficult. Alcoholic hepatitis is probably the most common form of drug-induced hepatitis, but the etiology may not be obvious from the history. Chronic alcohol ingestion can also result in hepatomegaly from fatty infiltration of the liver, which reflects impaired fatty acid oxidation, increased uptake and esterification of fatty acids, and diminished lipoprotein synthesis and secretion. Acetaminophen ingestion of 25 g or more usually results in fatal fulminant hepatotoxicity. A few drugs, such as chlorpromazine and oral contraceptives, may cause cholestatic-type reactions (see later discussion). Ingestion of potent hepatotoxins, such as carbon tetrachloride and certain species of mushrooms (*Amanita, Galerina*), also may result in fatal hepatotoxicity.

1 Because of increased perioperative risk, patients with acute hepatitis should have elective surgery postponed until the illness has resolved, as indicated by the normalization of liver tests. In addition, acute alcohol toxicity greatly complicates anesthetic management, and acute alcohol withdrawal during the perioperative period may be associated with a mortality rate as high as 50%. Only emergency surgery should be considered for patients presenting with acute alcohol withdrawal. Patients with hepatitis are at risk of deterioration of hepatic function and the development of complications from hepatic failure, such as encephalopathy, coagulopathy, or hepatorenal syndrome.

Laboratory evaluation of the patient with hepatitis should include blood urea nitrogen, serum electrolytes, creatinine, glucose, transaminases, bilirubin, alkaline phosphatase, albumin, platelet count, and PT. Serum should also be checked for HBsAg whenever possible. A blood alcohol level is useful if the history or physical examination is compatible with recent ethanol intoxication. Hypokalemia and metabolic alkalosis are not uncommon and are usually due to vomiting. Concomitant hypomagnesemia may be present in patients with chronic alcohol use disorder and predisposes them to cardiac arrhythmias. The elevation in serum transaminases does not necessarily correlate with the amount of hepatic necrosis. The serum alanine aminotransferase (ALT) is generally higher than the serum aspartate aminotransferase (AST), except in alcoholic hepatitis, where the reverse occurs. Bilirubin and alkaline phosphatase are usually only moderately elevated, except with the cholestatic variant of hepatitis. The PT is the best indicator of hepatic synthetic function. Persistent prolongation of the PT (INR ≥1.5) following administration of vitamin K is indicative of severe hepatic dysfunction. Hypoglycemia is not uncommon. Hypoalbuminemia is usually not present except in protracted cases, with severe malnutrition, or when chronic liver disease is present.

If a patient with acute hepatitis must undergo an emergency operation, the preanesthetic evaluation should focus on determining the cause and the degree of hepatic impairment. Information should be obtained regarding recent drug exposures, including alcohol intake, intravenous drug use, recent transfusions, and prior anesthetics. The presence of nausea or vomiting should be noted, and, if present, dehydration and electrolyte abnormalities should be anticipated and corrected. Changes in mental status may indicate severe hepatic impairment. Inappropriate behavior or obtundation in patients with alcohol use disorder may be signs of acute intoxication, whereas tremulousness, irritability, tachycardia, and hypertension usually reflect withdrawal. Fresh frozen plasma may be necessary to correct coagulopathy. Premedication is generally not given to patients with advanced liver disease. However, benzodiazepines and thiamine are indicated in patients with, or at risk for, acute alcohol withdrawal; nevertheless, benzodiazepines must be administered cautiously as they may precipitate hepatic coma in an encephalopathic patient. This may be reversed in some patients with flumazenil.

Intraoperative Considerations

The goal of intraoperative management is to preserve existing hepatic function. Some patients with viral hepatitis may exhibit increased central nervous system sensitivity to anesthetics, whereas patients with alcohol use disorder will often display cross-tolerance to both intravenous and volatile anesthetics. These patients also require close cardiovascular monitoring because the cardiac depressant effects of alcohol are additive to those of anesthetics; moreover, alcoholic cardiomyopathy may also be present in these patients.

Inhalation anesthetics are generally preferable to intravenous agents because most of the latter are dependent on the liver for metabolism, elimination, or both. Standard induction doses of intravenous induction agents can generally be used because their action is terminated by redistribution rather than metabolism or excretion. A prolonged duration of action, however, may be encountered with large or repeated doses of intravenous agents, particularly
2 opioids. Isoflurane and sevoflurane are the volatile agents of choice for patients with significant liver disease because they preserve hepatic blood flow and oxygen delivery. Factors known to reduce hepatic blood flow, such as hypotension, excessive sympathetic activation, and high mean airway pressures during controlled ventilation, should be avoided. Regional anesthesia, including major conduction blockade, may be employed in the absence of coagulopathy, provided hypotension is avoided.

CHRONIC HEPATITIS

Chronic hepatitis is defined as persistent hepatic inflammation for longer than 6 months, as evidenced by elevated serum aminotransferases. Patients can usually be classified as having one of three distinct syndromes based on a liver biopsy: chronic persistent hepatitis, chronic lobular hepatitis, or chronic active hepatitis. Patients with chronic active hepatitis have chronic hepatic inflammation with destruction of normal cellular architecture and "piecemeal necrosis" on the biopsy. Evidence of cirrhosis is either present initially or eventually develops in 20% to 50% of patients. Although chronic active hepatitis seems to have many causes, it occurs most commonly as a sequela of hepatitis B or hepatitis C. Other causes include medications (methyldopa, isoniazid, and nitrofurantoin) and autoimmune disorders. Both immunological factors and a genetic predisposition may be responsible in most cases. Patients usually present with a history of fatigue and recurrent jaundice; extrahepatic manifestations, such as arthritis and serositis, are not uncommon. Manifestations of cirrhosis eventually predominate in
3 patients with progressive disease. In evaluating patients for chronic hepatitis, laboratory test results may show only a mild elevation in serum aminotransferase activity and often correlate poorly with disease severity. Patients without chronic hepatitis B or C infection usually have a favorable response to immunosuppressants and are treated with long-term corticosteroid therapy with or without azathioprine.

Anesthetic Management

Patients with chronic persistent or chronic lobular hepatitis should be treated similarly to those with acute hepatitis. In contrast, those with chronic active hepatitis should be assumed to already have cirrhosis and should be treated accordingly (as discussed next). Patients with autoimmune chronic active hepatitis may also present with problems related to other autoimmune manifestations (such as diabetes or thyroiditis) or to the long-term corticosteroid therapy that they have likely received.

Cirrhosis

4 Liver cirrhosis refers to the damaging effects to the liver of inflammation, hepatocellular injury, and the resulting fibrosis and regeneration of hepatocytes. Cirrhosis is a progressive disease that eventually results in hepatic failure. The most common cause of cirrhosis in the United States was chronic alcohol abuse, but that has now been overtaken by nonalcoholic steatohepatitis (NASH, fatty liver) accompanying the massive increase in morbid obesity prevalence. Other causes include chronic active hepatitis (postnecrotic cirrhosis), chronic biliary inflammation or obstruction (primary biliary cirrhosis, sclerosing cholangitis), chronic right-sided congestive heart failure (cardiac cirrhosis), autoimmune hepatitis, hemochromatosis, Wilson disease, α_1-antitrypsin deficiency, and cryptogenic cirrhosis. Regardless of the cause, hepatocyte necro-
5 sis is followed by fibrosis and nodular regeneration. Distortion of the liver's normal cellular and vascular architecture obstructs portal venous flow and leads to portal hypertension and varices. Impairment of the liver's normal synthetic and other diverse metabolic functions, along with widespread endothelial damage from toxins not cleared by the liver, may cause multiorgan dysfunction.

Clinically, signs and symptoms often do not correlate with disease severity. Manifestations are typically absent initially, but jaundice and ascites eventually develop in most patients. Other signs include spider angiomas, palmar erythema, gynecomastia, and splenomegaly. Moreover, cirrhosis is generally associated with the development of three major complications: (1) variceal hemorrhage from portal hypertension, (2) intractable fluid retention in the form of ascites and hepatorenal syndrome, and (3) hepatic encephalopathy or coma. Approximately 10% of patients with cirrhosis also develop at least one episode of spontaneous bacterial peritonitis, and some patients, especially those with a viral etiology, will eventually develop hepatocellular carcinoma. This may occur even after the virus has been eradicated by the new antiviral therapies.

A few diseases can produce hepatic fibrosis without hepatocellular necrosis or nodular regeneration, resulting in portal hypertension and its associated complications with hepatocellular function often preserved. These disorders include schistosomiasis, idiopathic portal fibrosis (Banti syndrome), and congenital hepatic fibrosis. Obstruction of the hepatic veins or inferior vena cava (Budd–Chiari syndrome) can also cause portal hypertension. The latter may be the result of venous thrombosis (hypercoagulable state), a tumor thrombus (eg, renal carcinoma), or occlusive disease of the sublobular hepatic veins.

Preoperative Considerations

The detrimental effects of anesthesia and surgery on hepatic blood flow are discussed later in this section. Patients with cirrhosis are at increased risk of deterioration of liver function because of limited functional reserve. Successful anesthetic management of these patients is dependent on recognizing the multisystem nature of cirrhosis (Table 34–3) and controlling or preventing its complications. Patients with severe disease and limited survival without liver transplantation, with urgency for transplantation quantified by high MELD (*Model for End-stage Liver Disease*, see below) scores, present with severe deconditioning, increased frailty, severe loss of muscle mass, and a markedly distended abdomen containing liters of ascites.

A. Gastrointestinal Manifestations

Portal hypertension leads to the development of extensive portosystemic venous collateral channels. Four major collateral sites are generally recognized: gastroesophageal, hemorrhoidal, periumbilical, and retroperitoneal. Portal hypertension is often apparent preoperatively, as evidenced by dilated abdominal
6 wall veins (*caput medusae*). Massive bleeding from gastroesophageal varices is a major cause of morbidity and mortality in patients with liver disease, and, in addition to the effects of acute blood loss, the absorbed nitrogen load from the breakdown of blood in the gastrointestinal tract can precipitate hepatic encephalopathy.

The treatment of variceal bleeding is primarily supportive, but it frequently involves endoscopic procedures for identification of the bleeding site(s) and therapeutic maneuvers, such as injection sclerosis of varices, electrocoagulation, or application

TABLE 34–3 Manifestations of cirrhosis.

Gastrointestinal
Portal hypertension
Ascites
Esophageal varices
Hemorrhoids
Gastrointestinal bleeding
Circulatory
Hyperdynamic state (high cardiac output)
Systemic arteriovenous shunts
Low systemic vascular resistance
Cirrhotic cardiomyopathy; pulmonary hypertension
Pulmonary
Increased intrapulmonary shunting; hepatopulmonary syndrome
Decreased functional residual capacity
Pleural effusions
Restrictive ventilatory defect
Respiratory alkalosis
Renal
Increased proximal reabsorption of sodium
Increased distal reabsorption of sodium
Impaired free water clearance
Decreased renal perfusion
Hepatorenal syndrome
Hematological
Anemia
Coagulopathy
Hypersplenism
Thrombocytopenia
Leukopenia
Infectious
Spontaneous bacterial peritonitis
Metabolic
Hyponatremia and hypernatremia
Hypokalemia and hypocalcemia
Hypomagnesemia
Hypoalbuminemia
Hypoglycemia
Neurological
Encephalopathy

of hemoclips or bands. In addition to the risks posed by a patient who is physiologically fragile and acutely hypovolemic and hypotensive, anesthesia for such endoscopic procedures frequently involves the additional challenges of an encephalopathic, uncooperative patient and a stomach full of food and blood. Endoscopic unipolar electrocautery may adversely affect implanted cardiac pacing and defibrillator devices.

Blood loss should be replaced with intravenous fluids and blood products. Nonoperative treatment includes vasopressin, somatostatin, propranolol, or balloon tamponade with a Sengstaken–Blakemore tube. Vasopressin, somatostatin, and propranolol reduce the rate of blood loss. High doses of vasopressin can result in congestive heart failure or myocardial ischemia; concomitant infusion of intravenous nitroglycerin may reduce the likelihood of these complications and bleeding. Placement of a percutaneous transjugular intrahepatic portosystemic shunt (TIPS) can reduce portal hypertension and subsequent bleeding but may increase the incidence of encephalopathy. Emergency surgery may be indicated when the bleeding fails to stop or recurs. Perioperative risk correlates with the degree of hepatic impairment, based on clinical and laboratory findings. Child's classification for evaluating hepatic reserve is shown in Table 34–4. Shunting procedures are generally performed on low-risk patients, whereas ablative surgery, esophageal transection, and gastric devascularization are reserved for high-risk patients.

B. Hematologic Manifestations

Anemia, thrombocytopenia, and, less commonly, leukopenia may be present. The cause of the anemia is usually multifactorial and includes blood loss, increased red blood cell destruction, bone marrow suppression, and nutritional deficiencies. Congestive splenomegaly secondary to portal hypertension is largely responsible for the thrombocytopenia and leukopenia. Coagulation factor deficiencies arise as a result of impaired hepatic synthesis. Enhanced fibrinolysis secondary to decreased clearance of activators of the fibrinolytic system may also contribute to the coagulopathy.

The need for preoperative blood transfusions should be balanced against the obligatory increase in nitrogen load. Protein breakdown from excessive blood transfusions can precipitate encephalopathy. Nevertheless, coagulopathy should be corrected before surgery. Clotting factors should be replaced with appropriate blood products, such as fresh frozen plasma and cryoprecipitate. Platelet transfusions

TABLE 34–4 Child's classification for evaluating hepatic reserve.

Risk Group	A	B	C
Bilirubin (mg/dL)	<2.0	2.0–3.0	>3.0
Serum albumin (g/dL)	>3.5	3.0–3.5	<3.0
Ascites	None	Controlled	Poorly controlled
Encephalopathy	Absent	Minimal	Coma
Nutrition	Excellent	Good	Poor
Mortality rate (%)	2–5	10	50

Adapted with permission from Child CG. *The Liver and Portal Hypertension*. Philadelphia, PA: WB Saunders; 1964.

should be considered immediately prior to surgery for platelet counts less than 50,000/μL. Assessment of the integrity of the coagulation system by viscoelastic technology will provide specific management information.

C. Circulatory Manifestations

End-stage liver disease and, in particular, cirrhosis of the liver may be associated with disorders of all major organ systems (see Table 34–3 and Table 34–5). Cardiovascular changes observed in cirrhotic patients 7 are usually those of a hyperdynamic circulation, though clinically significant cirrhotic cardiomyopathy is often present and not recognized (Table 34–6). There may be a reduced cardiac contractile response to stress, altered diastolic relaxation, downregulation of β-adrenergic receptors, and electrophysiological changes as a result of cirrhotic cardiomyopathy.

Echocardiographic examination of cardiac function may initially be interpreted as normal because of significant afterload reduction caused by low systemic vascular resistance. However, both systolic and diastolic dysfunction are often present. Noninvasive stress imaging is frequently used to assess coronary artery disease in patients older than age 50 years and in those with cardiac risk factors.

TABLE 34–5 Differential diagnosis of cardiopulmonary dysfunction in chronic liver disease and portal hypertension.

Primary cardiopulmonary disorders
Chronic obstructive pulmonary disease
Congestive heart failure
Asthma
Restrictive lung disease
Pneumonia
Complications of cirrhosis
Ascites
Pleural effusions
Muscle wasting
Cardiopulmonary/liver disease
Alcoholic liver disease with alcoholic cardiomyopathy
Hemochromatosis with iron overload cardiomyopathy
α_1-Antitrypsin deficiency with panacinar emphysema
Primary biliary cirrhosis with fibrosing alveolitis
Pulmonary vascular disorders
Hepatopulmonary syndrome
Portopulmonary hypertension

Hepatopulmonary Syndrome

The effects of hepatic cirrhosis on pulmonary vascular resistance (PVR) vessels may result

TABLE 34–6 Hemodynamic and pathological changes in the typical cirrhotic patient.

Increased cardiac output
Increased heart rate
Decreased systemic vascular resistance
Increased circulating volume
Coronary artery disease
Cirrhotic cardiomyopathy (often unrecognized)
Low systemic vascular resistance conceals poor left ventricular function
Reduced responsiveness to β-agonists

TABLE 34–7 Hepatopulmonary syndrome.

Clinical features
Cyanosis
Digital clubbing
Cutaneous telangiectasia
Orthodeoxia (oxygen desaturation on sitting or standing)
Platypnea (breathing more easily while lying flat)
Dyspnea
Diagnostic criteria
Presence of liver disease, usually with portal hypertension and cirrhosis
An alveolar to arterial oxygen gradient of >15 mm Hg
Pulmonary arteriovenous connections demonstrated by:
• A delayed contrast-enhanced (agitated saline) echocardiogram showing contrast in the left heart chambers 4–6 heartbeats after contrast appears in the right heart chambers
• Brain uptake >6% following technetium-99m macroaggregated albumin lung perfusion scan
Indications
Liver transplantation is the only therapy that will cure hepatopulmonary syndrome

in vasodilation, causing shunts and chronic hypoxemia, or conversely lead to pulmonary vasoconstriction and medial hyperplasia, causing an increase in vascular resistance and pulmonary hypertension. *Hepatopulmonary syndrome* (HPS; Table 34–7) is found in approximately 30% of liver transplant candidates and is characterized by a triad of decreased oxygen saturation in the presence of advanced liver disease and intrapulmonary arteriolar dilation. Intrapulmonary vascular dilation causes intrapulmonary right-to-left shunting and an increase in the alveolar-to-arterial oxygen gradient.

Pulse oximetry may be used to screen for HPS, and room air SpO_2 less than 96% in the sitting position requires investigation. There is no medical treatment for HPS, which is progressive, but it is reversed over 6 months to 2 years by liver transplantation.

Portopulmonary Hypertension

Pulmonary vascular remodeling may occur in association with chronic liver disease, involving vascular smooth muscle proliferation, vasoconstriction, intimal proliferation, and eventual fibrosis, all presenting as obstruction causing increased resistance to

TABLE 34–8 Clinical features of portopulmonary hypertension.

Increased pulmonary vascular resistance: vasoconstriction, structural vascular remodeling, and eventual fibrosis
Mean pulmonary artery pressure >25 mm Hg with normal pulmonary capillary wedge pressure
Right ventricular overload
Right heart failure
Hepatic congestion
Increased liver transplantation mortality risk, especially if mean pulmonary artery pressure is >35 mm Hg

pulmonary blood flow. These pathological changes may result in pulmonary hypertension, and if associated with portal hypertension, the condition is termed *portopulmonary hypertension* (POPH; Table 34–8).

The diagnostic criteria for POPH include a mean pulmonary artery pressure (mPAP) greater than 25 mm Hg at rest and a PVR greater than 240 dyn·s·cm^{-5}. The transpulmonary gradient of greater than 12 mm Hg (mPAP minus pulmonary arteriolar occlusion pressure [PAOP]) reflects the obstruction to flow and distinguishes the contribution of volume and resistance to the increase in mPAP.

POPH may be classified as mild (mPAP 25–35 mm Hg), moderate (mPAP >35 and <45 mm Hg), and severe (mPAP >45 mm Hg). Mild POPH is not associated with increased mortality at liver transplantation, though the immediate recovery period may be challenging if there is a significant increase in cardiac output after reperfusion of the new graft. Moderate and severe POPH are associated with significant mortality at transplantation. However, the key factor is not mPAP but rather right ventricular (RV) function.

The success of liver transplantation will depend on the right ventricle maintaining good function during and after the transplant procedure despite increases in cardiac output, volume, and PVR. If RV dysfunction or failure occurs, graft congestion with possible graft failure and possible mortality may ensue. Assessment of the right ventricle using transesophageal echocardiography (TEE) is necessary.

The role of liver transplantation in the management of POPH is not well defined. In some patients, pulmonary hypertension will reverse quickly after transplant; however, other patients may require months or years of ongoing vasodilator therapy. Yet other patients may continue to progress and eventually develop RV failure. Some patients with HPS develop pulmonary hypertension after liver transplantation, suggesting that both pathologies may occur simultaneously. Liver transplantation offers the best outcome in patients with POPH that is responsive to vasodilator therapy.

A. Respiratory Manifestations

Disturbances in pulmonary gas exchange and ventilatory mechanics are often present. Hyperventilation is common and results in primary respiratory alkalosis. As previously noted, hypoxemia is frequently present and is due to right-to-left shunting of up to 40% of cardiac output. Shunting is due to an increase in both pulmonary arteriovenous communications (absolute) and ventilation/perfusion mismatching (relative). Elevation of the diaphragm from ascites decreases lung volumes, particularly functional residual capacity, and predisposes to atelectasis. Moreover, large amounts of ascites produce a restrictive ventilatory defect that increases the work of breathing. Large pleural effusions are also frequently found.

Review of the chest radiograph and arterial blood gas measurements is useful preoperatively because atelectasis, effusions, and hypoxemia may not be evident on clinical examination. Paracentesis in patients with massive ascites and pulmonary compromise should be performed with caution because excessive fluid removal can lead to circulatory collapse.

B. Renal Manifestations and Fluid Balance

Derangements of fluid and electrolyte balance may manifest as ascites, edema, electrolyte disturbances, and *hepatorenal syndrome* (see below). Important mechanisms responsible for ascites include (1) portal hypertension, which increases hydrostatic pressure and favors transudation of fluid across the intestine into the peritoneal cavity; (2) hypoalbuminemia, which decreases plasma oncotic pressure and favors fluid transudation; (3) seepage of protein-rich lymphatic fluid from the serosal surface of the liver secondary to distortion and obstruction of lymphatic channels in the liver; and (4) avid renal sodium and water retention.

Patients with cirrhosis and ascites have decreased kidney perfusion, altered intrarenal hemodynamics, enhanced proximal and distal sodium reabsorption, and impairment of free water clearance. Hyponatremia and hypokalemia are common. The former is dilutional, whereas the latter is due to excessive urinary potassium losses from secondary hyperaldosteronism or from diuretics. The most severe expression of these abnormalities is seen with the development of hepatorenal syndrome. Patients with ascites have elevated levels of circulating catecholamines, probably due to enhanced sympathetic outflow. In addition to increased renin and angiotensin II, these patients are insensitive to circulating atrial natriuretic peptide.

9 **Hepatorenal syndrome** is a functional renal defect in patients with cirrhosis that usually follows gastrointestinal bleeding, aggressive diuresis, sepsis, or major surgery. It is characterized by increased renal vasoconstriction, which may be a response to splanchnic vasodilation, reduced glomerular filtration rate, progressive oliguria with avid sodium retention, azotemia, intractable ascites, and a very high mortality rate. Treatment is supportive and often unsuccessful unless liver transplantation is undertaken.

Judicious perioperative fluid management in patients with advanced liver disease is critical. The importance of preserving kidney function cannot be overemphasized. Overzealous preoperative diuresis should be avoided, and acute intravascular fluid deficits should be corrected with colloid infusions. Diuresis to reduce ascites and edema fluid should be accomplished over several days. Loop diuretics are administered only after measures such as bed rest, sodium restriction (<2 g NaCl/d), and spironolactone administration have been ineffective. Daily body weight measurements are useful in preventing intravascular volume depletion during diuresis; in patients with both ascites and peripheral edema, no more than 1 kg/d should be lost during diuresis, and in those with ascites alone, no more than 0.5 kg/d should be lost. Hyponatremia (serum $[Na^+]$ <130 mEq/L) also requires water restriction (<1.5 L/d), and potassium deficits should be replaced preoperatively. Medical treatment includes albumin infusions in combination with vasoconstrictors such as vasopressin, midodrine, and norepinephrine, and perhaps the vasopressin analogue, terlipressin. Prolonged kidney impairment will result in acute tubular necrosis, and if this occurs, a liver–kidney transplant may be indicated.

C. Central Nervous System Manifestations

Hepatic encephalopathy is characterized by mental status alterations with fluctuating neurological signs (asterixis, hyperreflexia, or inverted plantar reflex) and characteristic electroencephalographic changes (symmetric high-voltage, slow-wave activity). This is associated with the accumulation of neurotoxins, including ammonia and short-chain fatty acids. Some patients also have elevated intracranial pressure. Metabolic encephalopathy seems to be proportionately related to both the amount of hepatocellular damage present and the degree of shunting of portal blood away from the liver and directly into the systemic circulation. The accumulation of substances originating in the gastrointestinal tract (but normally metabolized by the liver) has been implicated.
10 Factors known to precipitate hepatic encephalopathy include gastrointestinal bleeding, increased dietary protein intake, hypokalemic alkalosis from vomiting or diuresis, infections, worsening liver function, and drugs with central nervous system depressant activity.

Hepatic encephalopathy should be aggressively treated preoperatively. Precipitating causes should be corrected. Oral lactulose (30–50 mL every 8 h) or neomycin (500 mg every 6 h) is useful in reducing intestinal ammonia absorption. Lactulose acts as an osmotic laxative and, like neomycin, likely inhibits ammonia production by intestinal bacteria. Sedatives, especially benzodiazepines, should be avoided as they may precipitate hepatic coma.

Intraoperative Considerations

Patients with postnecrotic cirrhosis due to hepatitis B or hepatitis C who are carriers of the virus may be infectious. Universal precautions are always indicated in preventing contact with blood and body fluids from all patients.

A. Drug Responses

The response to anesthetic agents is unpredictable in patients with cirrhosis. Changes in central nervous system sensitivity, volumes of distribution, protein binding, drug metabolism, and drug elimination are common. An increase in the volume of distribution for highly ionized drugs, such as neuromuscular blockers (NMBs), is due to the expanded extracellular fluid compartment; an apparent resistance may be observed, requiring larger than normal loading doses. However, smaller than normal maintenance doses of NMBs dependent on hepatic elimination (rocuronium and vecuronium) should be used. The duration of action of succinylcholine may be prolonged because of reduced levels of pseudocholinesterase, but this is rarely of clinical consequence.

B. Anesthetic Technique

The cirrhotic liver is very dependent on hepatic arterial perfusion because of reduced portal venous blood flow. Preservation of hepatic arterial blood flow and avoidance of agents with potentially adverse effects on hepatic function are critical. Regional anesthesia may be used in patients without thrombocytopenia or coagulopathy, but hypotension must be avoided. A propofol induction followed by isoflurane or sevoflurane with an oxygen–air mixture is commonly employed for general anesthesia. Opioid supplementation reduces the dose of the volatile agent required, but the half-lives of opioids are often significantly prolonged, which may cause postoperative respiratory depression. Cisatracurium may be the NMB of choice because of its nonhepatic metabolism.

Preoperative nausea, vomiting, upper gastrointestinal bleeding, and abdominal distention due to massive ascites require a well-planned anesthetic induction. Preoxygenation and rapid-sequence induction/intubation with cricoid pressure are often performed. For unstable patients and those with active bleeding, either an awake intubation or a rapid-sequence induction using ketamine or etomidate and succinylcholine or rocuronium is suggested.

C. Monitoring

Pulse oximetry should be supplemented with arterial blood gas measurements to monitor acid–base status. Patients with large right-to-left intrapulmonary shunts may not tolerate nitrous oxide and may require positive end-expiratory pressure (PEEP) to treat ventilation/perfusion inequalities and associated hypoxemia. Patients receiving vasopressin infusions should be monitored for myocardial ischemia due to coronary vasoconstriction.

Continuous intraarterial pressure monitoring is often used because hemodynamic instability frequently occurs as a result of excessive bleeding and operative manipulations. Intravascular volume status is often difficult to optimize, and goal-directed hemodynamic and fluid therapy utilizing esophageal Doppler, arterial waveform analysis, pleth variability index (PVI), or TEE should be considered. Such approaches may be helpful in preventing acute kidney injury. Urinary output must be followed closely; mannitol may be considered for persistently low urinary outputs despite adequate intravascular fluid replacement. Vasopressor support may be necessary, and norepinephrine and vasopressin infusions are frequently helpful.

D. Fluid Replacement

Most patients are sodium-restricted preoperatively, but preservation of intravascular volume and urinary output takes intraoperative priority. The use of predominantly colloid intravenous fluids (albumin) may be preferable to avoid sodium overload and to increase plasma oncotic pressure. Intravenous fluid replacement should take into account the excessive bleeding and fluid shifts that often occur in these patients during abdominal procedures. Venous engorgement from portal hypertension, varices, lysis of adhesions from previous surgery, and coagulopathy lead to excessive bleeding during surgical procedures, whereas evacuation of ascites and prolonged surgical procedures result in large fluid shifts.
11 Following the removal of large amounts of ascitic fluid, aggressive intravenous fluid replacement is often necessary to prevent profound hypotension and acute kidney injury or failure. Liberal use of crystalloid solutions may result in widespread edema because of the low serum albumin, and colloid solutions are usually preferable.

Most preoperative patients are anemic and coagulopathic, and perioperative red blood cell transfusion may lead to hypocalcemia from impaired citrate metabolism in the cirrhotic liver. Citrate, the anticoagulant in stored red blood cell preparations, binds with plasma calcium, producing hypocalcemia. Intravenous calcium may be necessary (see Chapter 51).

Hepatic Surgery

Common hepatic procedures include repair of lacerations, drainage of abscesses, and resection of primary or metastatic neoplasms, and up to 80% to 85% of the liver can be resected in many patients. In addition, liver transplantation is performed in many centers. The perioperative care of patients undergoing hepatic surgery is often challenging because of the coexisting medical problems and debilitation found in many patients with intrinsic liver disease and because of the potential for significant operative blood loss. Hepatitis and cirrhosis greatly complicate anesthetic management and increase perioperative mortality. Multiple large-bore intravenous catheters, central venous access, and blood warmers are necessary; rapid infusion devices facilitate management when massive blood transfusion is anticipated. Continuous intraarterial pressure monitoring is typically used.

Hemodynamic optimization is often complicated by the conflict between the need to maintain sufficient intravascular volume to ensure adequate hepatic perfusion and the need to keep central venous pressure low to minimize liver engorgement and surgical bleeding. Central venous pressure measurement is not an accurate monitor of volume status; we suggest goal-directed fluid therapy utilizing esophageal Doppler, arterial waveform analysis, PVI, or TEE. Care should be taken in placing an esophageal Doppler or TEE probe in a patient with esophageal variceal disease.

Hypotensive anesthesia should be avoided because of its potentially deleterious effects on liver function. Administration of antifibrinolytics, such as ε-aminocaproic acid or tranexamic acid, may reduce operative blood loss, especially if fibrinolysis can be demonstrated by viscoelastic coagulation monitoring. Hypoglycemia, coagulopathy, and sepsis may occur following large liver resections. Drainage of an abscess or cyst may be complicated by peritoneal contamination. In the case of a hydatid cyst, spillage can cause anaphylaxis due to the release of *Echinococcus* antigens.

Postoperative complications include hepatic dysfunction, sepsis, and blood loss secondary to coagulopathy or surgical bleeding. Postoperative pain from the surgical incision may hinder postoperative mobilization and convalescence, but perioperative coagulopathy may limit the use of epidural analgesia. Transversus abdominis plane (TAP) blocks may be very effective (see Chapter 46). Postoperative mechanical ventilation may be necessary for patients who have undergone extensive resections or who are markedly debilitated.

Liver Transplantation

When a center opens a liver transplantation program, a credentialed liver anesthesia director should be appointed who should be an anesthesiologist with experience and training in liver transplantation anesthesia. A dedicated team of anesthesiologists should be assembled to manage the perioperative course of all liver transplantation patients. This team should have a thorough understanding of the indications for and contraindications to liver transplantation (Tables 34–9 and 34–10), as well as the perioperative implications of associated comorbidities such as coronary artery disease, cirrhotic cardiomyopathy, portopulmonary hypertension, hepatopulmonary syndrome, hepatorenal syndrome, hepatic encephalopathy, and cerebral edema. It has been demonstrated that such an approach improves outcomes, as measured by reduced blood transfusions, the need for postoperative mechanical ventilation, and the intensive care unit length of stay.

TABLE 34–9 Indications for liver transplantation.

Pediatric	Adult
Congenital hepatic fibrosis	Primary biliary cirrhosis
Alagille disease	Primary sclerosing cholangitis
Biliary atresia	Autoimmune hepatitis
α_1-Antitrypsin deficiency	Cryptogenic cirrhosis
Byler disease	Viral hepatitis with cirrhosis
Metabolic disorders	Alcoholic cirrhosis
Wilson disease	Primary hepatocellular malignancies
Tyrosinemia	Nonalcoholic steatohepatitis
Glycogen storage diseases	Fulminant hepatitis
Crigler–Najjar disease	Hepatic vein thrombosis
Hemophilia	Familial amyloid polyneuropathy
Lysosomal storage diseases	Chronic viral hepatitis
Protoporphyria	
Familial hypercholesterolemia	
Primary hyperoxaluria	

TABLE 34–10 Contraindications to liver transplantation.

Absolute	Relative
Active sepsis	Severe obesity
Active substance or alcohol abuse	Severe pulmonary hypertension
Advanced cardiac disease	Severe cardiomyopathy
Extrahepatic malignancy	High viral load HIV
Metastatic malignancy	
Cholangiocarcinoma	

Preoperative Considerations

The *Model for End-stage Liver Disease (MELD)* score is used by the United Network for Organ Sharing (UNOS) to prioritize patients on the liver transplantation waiting list. The score is based on the patient's serum bilirubin, serum creatinine, and INR and is a predictor of survival time if the patient does not receive a liver transplant. A score of 20 predicts a 20% risk of mortality at 3 months, whereas a score of 40 predicts a 71% risk of mortality at 3 months (Figure 34–1).

$$\begin{aligned}\text{The MELD score}\\ &= 0.957 \times \log_e[\text{serum creatinine (mg/dL)}]\\ &\quad + 0.378 \times \log_e[\text{total serum bilirubin (mg/dL)}]\\ &\quad + 1.120 \times \log_e[\text{INR}]\end{aligned}$$

Multiply the resulting value by 10, and round to the nearest whole number. The minimum for all values is 1.0; the maximum value for creatinine is 4.0.

Most liver transplant candidates have high MELD scores and present with jaundice, kidney failure, and coagulopathy. They may also be emaciated and have massive ascites, and some may have encephalopathy, HPS, cirrhotic cardiomyopathy, and POPH. These patients often have an increased cardiac index and reduced systemic vascular resistance.

Significant blood loss must be anticipated, and large-bore intravenous catheters should be placed

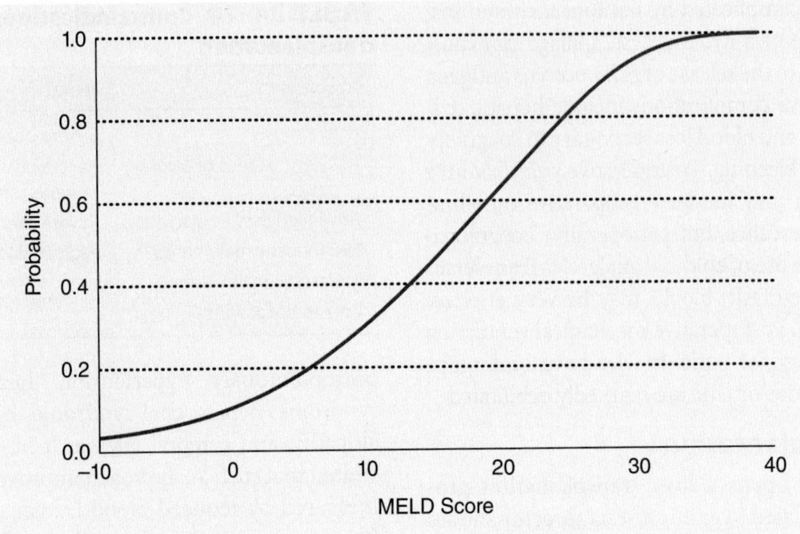

FIGURE 34–1 Relationship between Model for End-stage Liver Disease (MELD) score and 3-month mortality in patients with cirrhotic liver disease. (Reproduced with permission from Wiesner RH, McDiarmid SV, Kamath PS, et al. MELD and PELD: Application of survival models to liver allocation. *Liver Transpl.* 2001 July;7(7):567-580.)

for access. A rapid infusion pump should be available. Routine hemodynamic monitoring should include intraarterial pressure monitoring. TEE is routinely utilized in many centers. Pulmonary artery catheterization, once routine, has now been replaced by a central venous catheter and TEE at many centers, except when there is concern for POPH or cirrhotic cardiomyopathy.

The immediate availability of intraoperative continuous venovenous hemodialysis (CVVHD) may be very helpful for volume and electrolyte management in patients with marginal or no kidney function. In patients with significant electrolyte abnormalities, serum sodium and potassium can be closely managed by adjusting the CVVHD dialysate solution.

Intraoperative Management

As previously noted, hepatic disease causes endothelial dysfunction that impairs all organs of the body. The heart develops cirrhotic cardiomyopathy; the brain, encephalopathy and eventual cerebral edema; the kidneys, hepatorenal syndrome and eventual acute tubular necrosis; and the lungs, HPS or portopulmonary hypertension, or both. Therefore, each organ must be carefully managed throughout the operative procedure and postoperative period.

Maintenance of cerebral perfusion pressure (CPP) is particularly important in patients with cerebral edema, and some centers will monitor intracranial pressure. Additional cerebral protective measures include head elevation of 20°, mild hypothermia, and mild hypocarbia with vasopressor support to maintain mean arterial pressure. When the patient's head is elevated, the arterial pressure transducer should be zeroed at the level of the external auditory meatus for accurate determination of CPP.

Coagulopathy is managed with the aid of a point-of-care viscoelastic coagulation assay device (TEG, ROTEM, or Sonoclot) or frequent assessment of conventional tests of coagulation. Blood loss may be large, and transfusions are targeted to maintain the hemoglobin level greater than 7 g/dL.

Transfusions must be tempered to keep the central venous pressure (CVP) low during the liver dissection to reduce blood loss and minimize liver congestion, and during reperfusion and the remainder of the procedure to prevent graft congestion and hepatic dysfunction. Most coagulopathies will correct with the new liver if its function is good. Fibrinolysis, a low ionized calcium level, and hypothermia must be corrected, as these may promote bleeding. However, coagulation defects usually do not need to be treated preoperatively or intraoperatively unless bleeding is a problem. Intraoperative transfusion of platelets and fresh frozen plasma is associated with decreased long-term patient survival.

The liver transplantation surgical procedure is divided into three stages: *preanhepatic*, *anhepatic*, and *neohepatic* periods.

The preanhepatic (dissection) phase is highlighted by the management of hemodynamic changes related to blood loss and surgical compression of major vessels. Surgical entry into a large varix may lead to large blood loss. Hyponatremia should be carefully managed without rapid serum sodium correction because this may promote the development of osmotic demyelination syndrome (see Chapter 49). Hyperkalemia may require aggressive intervention with diuresis, transfusion of only washed packed red blood cells, or CVVHD. Citrate toxicity (hypocalcemia) may occur if blood is transfused; therefore, ionized calcium should be closely monitored, and calcium salts should be administered as necessary. A low CVP is helpful to minimize blood loss while systemic arterial pressure is maintained.

The anhepatic phase begins with vascular occlusion of the inflow to the liver and ends with reperfusion. Some centers utilize venovenous bypass to prevent congestion of the visceral organs, improve venous return, and possibly protect kidney function. If there are few varices, as may be seen in a patient with hepatocellular cancer, the total or partial occlusion of the vena cava may be associated with a significant low-flow state because of the lack of venous return to the heart. Many transplant centers administer 3000 units of intravenous heparin 3 minutes before the cava clamp is applied to prevent "low-flow state" clotting from occurring.

In the neohepatic phase, two pathophysiological events may occur on opening the portal vein and allowing reperfusion of the graft. The first is a reperfusion syndrome caused by the cold, acidotic, hyperkalemic solution that may contain emboli and vasoactive substances being flushed from the graft directly into the vena cava. This may cause hypotension, right heart dysfunction, arrhythmias, and even cardiac arrest and may be preempted to some extent by the prophylactic administration of calcium chloride and sodium bicarbonate. The second syndrome that may occur is hepatic ischemia/reperfusion injury. This may result from impaired reperfusion due to severe endothelial dysfunction and, in rare cases, may lead to primary nonfunction of the graft.

Postoperative Management

Patients who undergo liver transplantation are often severely debilitated and malnourished and have multiorgan dysfunction. They will need careful support and continuous monitoring until they have recovered. Early extubation is appropriate in patients who are comfortable, cooperative, and not bleeding. Immunosuppression must be carefully managed to minimize the risk of sepsis. A close watch of graft function must be maintained, with a low threshold for checking hepatic artery patency and flow. Postoperative bleeding, biliary leaks, and vascular thromboses may require surgical reexploration.

SPECIAL SITUATIONS

Patients with elevated intracranial pressure (ICP) and those at risk of its development should have ICP monitoring in place, if possible, to enable the appropriate management of CPP. The management of patients who are at risk of or have elevated ICP should include the following:

- ICP less than 20 mm Hg
- CPP greater than 50 mm Hg
- Mean arterial pressure greater than 60 mm Hg
- Proper bed position (elevate the head of the bed by 20–25°)
- Controlled airway and ventilation
- Controlled sedation (eg, propofol)
- Vasopressor support (eg, vasopressin, norepinephrine) when necessary
- Controlled hypothermia (32–33°C)
- Glycemic control
- Aggressive treatment of metabolic acidosis and coagulopathy
- CVVHD

Pediatric Liver Transplantation

Selected pediatric centers report 1-year survival rates of 90%. The use of reduced-size and living donor grafts has increased organ availability in this patient population.

Living Donor Transplantation

The use of living donors has increased the pool of organs available for transplantation. However, this procedure does expose healthy individuals to morbidity and mortality risks. Informed consent from the donor must be obtained with the understanding that there is often a great deal of emotional pressure on family members to donate and consent must be freely given without coercion.

In most donor anesthesia protocols, maintenance of a CVP less than 5 cm H_2O is utilized to reduce intraoperative blood loss. Adequate postoperative analgesia is required so that comfortable donor patients may be extubated at the end of the procedure. Transversus abdominus plane (TAP) block with rectus sheath block (see Chapter 46) meet this need. Complications of this surgery for the donor patient include transient hepatic dysfunction, wound infection, postoperative bleeding, portal vein thrombosis, biliary leaks, and, very rarely, death. An increased incidence of perioperative brachial plexus injury has been reported in donor patients, perhaps the result of rib cage retraction. Many centers will monitor the hepatic artery flow in the recipient postoperatively overnight with an implantable Doppler probe.

CASE DISCUSSION

Liver Transplantation

A 23-year-old woman develops fulminant hepatic failure after ingesting wild mushrooms. She is not expected to survive without a liver transplant.

What are the indications for liver transplantation?

Orthotopic liver transplantation is usually performed in patients with end-stage liver disease who begin to experience life-threatening complications, especially when such complications become unresponsive to medical or nontransplant surgery. Transplantation is also carried out in patients with fulminant hepatic failure (from viral hepatitis or a hepatotoxin) when survival with medical management alone is judged unlikely. The MELD score is used to assess the urgency for transplantation.

The most common indications for liver transplantation in children, in order of decreasing frequency, are biliary atresia, inborn errors of metabolism (usually α_1-antitrypsin deficiency, Wilson disease, tyrosinemia, and Crigler–Najjar type I syndrome), and postnecrotic cirrhosis.

The most common indications in adults are postnecrotic (nonalcoholic) cirrhosis, primary biliary cirrhosis, sclerosing cholangitis, and, less commonly, primary malignant tumors in the liver.

What factors have contributed to the recent success of liver transplantation?

One-year survival rates for liver transplantations exceed 80% to 85% in some centers. Currently, 5-year survival rates are 50% to 60%. The success of this procedure owes much to the use of cyclosporine and tacrolimus for immunosuppressant therapy. These drugs selectively suppress the activities of helper T cells (CD4 lymphocytes) by inhibiting the production of interleukin-2 (IL-2) and other cytokines. IL-2 is required for the generation and proliferation of cytotoxic T cells responsible for graft rejection and for activating B cells responsible for T cell-dependent humoral responses. Cyclosporine is usually initially combined with corticosteroids and other agents (eg, mycophenolate and azathioprine). Tacrolimus has proved effective in cyclosporine-resistant rejection and is the preferred alternative to cyclosporine as the primary immunosuppressant agent. The use of anti-OKT-3, a monoclonal antibody directed against lymphocytes, has been extremely useful in treating steroid-resistant acute rejection.

Additional factors influencing the improvement in liver transplantation outcome include a greater understanding and experience with transplantation and improved assessment and monitoring with transesophageal echocardiography.

What are the phases of the transplantation surgical procedure?

These procedures can be divided into three phases: a dissection (preanhepatic) phase, an anhepatic phase, and a neohepatic phase.

1. *Dissection (preanhepatic) phase:* Through a hockey stick incision, the liver is dissected so that it remains attached only by the inferior vena cava (IVC) and portal vein. The hepatic artery and common bile duct are ligated. Large abdominal varices may prolong the duration of and increase the blood loss associated with this phase.
2. *Anhepatic phase:* Once the donor liver graft is ready, the portal vein is clamped, followed by the IVC above and below the liver. The liver is then lifted out of the abdomen. Venovenous bypass may be employed during this phase or a "piggy-back" technique where the IVC is only partially occluded. The donor liver is then anastomosed to the supra- and infrahepatic inferior venae cava and the portal vein.
3. *Revascularization and biliary reconstruction (neohepatic or postanhepatic) phase:* Following completion of the venous anastomoses, venous clamps are removed from the cava, allowing venous blood to return to the heart. Next, the portal vein is slowly opened, allowing blood to flush out preservation fluid and other substances accumulated in the liver during its ischemic time. This reperfusion may result in hypotension, arrhythmias, or cardiac arrest—a scenario termed the *reperfusion syndrome*. The circulation to the new liver is completed by anastomosing the hepatic artery. Lastly, the common bile duct of the donor liver is then usually anastomosed to the recipient using the recipient's common bile duct or a Roux-en-Y choledochojejunostomy.

What major problems complicate anesthesia for liver transplantation?

Potential problems include multiorgan dysfunction caused by cirrhosis, massive blood loss, hemodynamic instability from clamping and unclamping the inferior vena cava and portal vein, metabolic consequences of the anhepatic phase, and air embolism and hyperkalemia.

Preoperative coagulation defects, thrombocytopenia, and previous abdominal surgery greatly increase blood loss. Extensive venous collaterals between the portal and systemic venous circulations also contribute to increased bleeding from the abdominal wall. Potential complications of massive blood transfusion include hypothermia, coagulopathies, hyperkalemia, citrate intoxication (hypocalcemia), and the potential transmission of infectious agents. Blood salvaging techniques are useful in reducing the need for donor red blood cell transfusion.

What is adequate venous access for these procedures?

Bleeding is a recurring problem during each phase of liver transplantation. Adequate venous access is paramount in anesthetic management. Several large-bore (14-gauge or larger) intravenous catheters should be placed above the diaphragm. Specialized 8.5F catheters can be placed in antecubital veins and used in conjunction with rapid infusion devices. Most centers place a large-bore central venous catheter. Efforts to minimize the risk of hypothermia should include the use of fluid warming and forced-air surface warming devices.

What monitoring techniques are most useful during surgery?

All patients require direct intraarterial pressure monitoring. A central venous catheter should be available. Goal-directed hemodynamic and fluid management utilizing arterial pulse wave analysis, esophageal Doppler, PVI, or TEE is common. Urinary output should be monitored throughout surgery via an indwelling urinary catheter.

Laboratory measurements constitute an important part of intraoperative monitoring. Serial hematocrit measurements guide red blood cell replacement. Similarly, frequent measurements of arterial blood gases, serum electrolytes, serum ionized calcium, and serum glucose are necessary to detect and appropriately treat metabolic derangements. Coagulation can be monitored by measuring PT, activated partial thromboplastin time, fibrinogen level, and platelet counts, and by point-of-care viscoelastic coagulation analysis—TEG, ROTEM, or Sonoclot analysis. These latter modalities not only assess overall clotting and platelet function but can also detect fibrinolysis.

What anesthetic technique may be used for liver transplantation?

Most patients should be considered as having a "full stomach," often because of marked abdominal distention or recent upper gastrointestinal bleeding. General anesthesia is usually induced via a rapid sequence induction. The semi-upright (back up) position during induction prevents rapid oxygen desaturation and facilitates ventilation until the abdomen is open. Hyperventilation should be avoided unless there is increased intracranial pressure. Anesthesia is generally maintained with a volatile agent (usually isoflurane or sevoflurane) and an intravenous opioid (usually fentanyl or sufentanil). The concentration of the volatile agent should be limited to less than 1 minimum alveolar concentration in patients with severe encephalopathy. Nitrous oxide is usually avoided. Many patients are routinely transferred to the intensive care unit intubated and mechanically ventilated at the end of the operative procedure, though immediate postoperative extubation may be considered if the patient is comfortable, cooperative, physiologically stable, and not bleeding.

What physiological derangements are associated with the anhepatic phase?

When the liver is removed, the large citrate load from blood products is no longer metabolized and results in hypocalcemia and secondary myocardial depression. Periodic calcium chloride administration (1 g) is necessary but should be guided by ionized calcium concentration measurements to avoid hypercalcemia. A low-flow state may exist with a severely limited venous return if the patient does not have significant varices. This may require volume to be transfused, but with the knowledge that the new liver must not be congested when venous return is restored. Thus, vasopressors may be necessary during this stage. The low-flow state, if it occurs, may be preempted by 3000 units of heparin if the coagulation is normal. Progressive acidosis is also encountered because acid metabolites from the intestines and lower body are not cleared by the absent liver. Sodium bicarbonate therapy will be necessary and should similarly be guided by arterial blood gas analysis. Excessive administration of sodium bicarbonate results in hypernatremia, hyperosmolality, and accentuation of the metabolic alkalosis that typically follows massive blood transfusions. Tromethamine should be considered when large amounts of alkali therapy are necessary. Although hypoglycemia can occur during the anhepatic phase, hyperglycemia is a more common occurrence following reperfusion.

The anhepatic phase ends when the three venous clamps are removed and the donor liver is reperfused. Pulmonary and systemic (paradoxical) air embolism can occur when the circulation is fully reestablished to the donor liver because air often enters hepatic sinusoids after harvesting. Systemic air embolism probably reflects the fact that many of these patients have extensive arteriovenous communications. Thromboembolic phenomena are also possible following reperfusion.

What problems may be anticipated during the revascularization phase?

Perfusion of the donor liver by the recipient's blood often results in transiently increased serum potassium concentration of up to 1 to 2 mEq/L and increased systemic acidosis. Reperfusion releases potassium from any remaining preservative solution still within the liver, as well as potassium released from tissues distal to venous clamps. Unclamping may also release a large acid load from ischemic tissue in the lower body (especially without venovenous bypass); preemptive administration of sodium bicarbonate is advocated by some.

When the circulation to the new liver is established, the sudden increase in blood volume, acidosis, and hyperkalemia can produce tachyarrhythmias or, more commonly, bradyarrhythmias. In addition to calcium chloride and sodium bicarbonate, inotropic support is also often required. Hyperfibrinolysis is commonly present and seems to be due to a marked increase in tissue plasminogen activator and a decrease in plasminogen activator inhibitor and α_2-antiplasmin during the anhepatic phase. Fibrinolysis can be detected by point-of-care viscoelastic coagulation analysis. ε-Aminocaproic acid or tranexamic acid, which inhibit the formation of plasmin, may be indicated in those instances but should not be used prophylactically.

What problems are encountered postoperatively?

Patients often have an uncomplicated postoperative course and, after sufficient observation in the intensive care unit, may be transferred directly to the nursing unit designed for liver transplant patients. Problems to anticipate include graft dysfunction or failure, persistent hemorrhage, fluid overload, metabolic abnormalities (particularly metabolic alkalosis and hypokalemia), respiratory failure, pleural effusions, acute kidney injury or failure, systemic infections, and surgical complications (eg, bile leaks or stricture, or thrombosis of the hepatic or portal vessels). The last two complications may become suspect during ultrasound examination and are confirmed by angiography. Neurological complications include seizures, intracranial hemorrhage, encephalopathy, osmotic demyelination syndrome from a sudden increase in serum sodium, and immunosuppressant-related neurotoxicity. Contributory factors for acute kidney injury or failure include periods of hypotension, impaired kidney perfusion when the inferior vena cava is clamped (resulting in high pressures in the renal veins), and cyclosporine or antibiotic nephropathy. Measurement of immunosuppressant levels may be helpful in avoiding toxicity.

Prophylactic antibiotics and antifungal agents are routinely given in many centers because of a high incidence of infections.

Graft function is usually monitored by the PT, serum bilirubin, aminotransferase activity, and serum lactate measurements. A specific diagnosis requires a liver biopsy.

SUGGESTED READINGS

Adelmann D, Kronish K, Ramsay MA. Anesthesia for liver transplantation. *Anesthesiol Clin* 2017;35:491.

Bezinover D, Dirkman D, Findlay J, et al. Perioperative coagulation management in liver transplant recipients. *Transplantation* 2018;102:578.

Dienstag JL, Cosimi AB. Liver transplantation—a vision realized. *N Engl J Med*. 2012;367:1483.

Goldberg DS, Fallon MB. Lung and heart disease secondary to liver disease. *Clin Gastroenterol Hepatol*. 2015;13:2118.

Groose MK, Aldred BW, Mezrich JD, et al. Risk factors for intracardiac thrombus during liver transplantation. *Liver Transplantation* 2019;25:1682.

Im GY, Lubezky N, Facciuto ME, et al. Surgery in patients with portal hypertension. A pre-operative checklist and strategies for attenuating risk. *Clin Liver Dis*. 2014;18:477.

Khemichian S, Francoz C, Durand F, Karvellas CJ, Nadim MK. Hepatorenal syndrome. *Crit Care Clin*. 2021;37:321.

Krowka MJ, Fallon MB, Kawut SM, et al. International Liver Transplant Society practice guidelines: diagnosis and management of hepatopulmonary syndrome and portopulmonary hypertension. *Transplantation*. 2016;100:1440.

Mallett S. Clinical utility of viscoelastic tests of coagulation in patients with liver disease and during liver transplantation. *Semin Thromb Hemostasis*. 2015;41:527.

Robertson AC, Eagle SS. Transesophageal echocardiography during orthotopic liver transplantation: maximizing information without the distraction. *J Cardiothorac Vasc Anesth*. 2014;28:141.

Shah N, Silva RG, Kowalski A, et al. Hepatorenal syndrome. *Disease-A-Month*. 2016;62:364.

Spring A, Saran JS, McCarthy S, McCluskey SA. Anesthesia for the patient with severe liver failure. *Anesthesiol Clin*. 2020;38:35.

Suraweera D, Sundaram V, Saab S. Evaluation and management of hepatic encephalopathy. Current status and future directions. *Gut Liver*. 2016;10:509.

Tripodi A. Liver disease and hemostatic (dys)function. *Semin Thromb Hemostasis*. 2015;41:462.

Zardi EM, Zardi DM, Chin D, et al. Cirrhotic cardiomyopathy in the pre- and post-liver transplantation phase. *J Cardiol*. 2016;67:125.

CHAPTER 35

Anesthesia for Patients with Endocrine Disease

KEY CONCEPTS

1. Diabetic autonomic neuropathy may limit the patient's ability to compensate (with tachycardia and increased peripheral resistance) for intravascular volume changes and may predispose the patient to cardiovascular instability (eg, postinduction hypotension) and even sudden cardiac death.
2. Temporomandibular joint and cervical spine mobility should be assessed preoperatively in patients with diabetes to reduce the likelihood of unanticipated difficult intubation. Difficult intubation has been reported in as many as 30% of persons with type 1 diabetes.
3. Sulfonylureas and metformin have long half-lives, and many clinicians will discontinue them 24 to 48 h before surgery. They can be started postoperatively when the patient resumes oral intake.
4. Incompletely treated hyperthyroid patients may be chronically hypovolemic and prone to an exaggerated hypotensive response to induction of anesthesia.
5. Clinically hypothyroid patients are more susceptible to the hypotensive effect of anesthetic agents because of diminished cardiac output, blunted baroreceptor reflexes, and decreased intravascular volume.
6. Patients with glucocorticoid deficiency must receive adequate steroid replacement therapy during the perioperative period.
7. In patients with pheochromocytoma, drugs or techniques that indirectly stimulate or promote the release of catecholamines (eg, ephedrine, hypoventilation, bolus doses of ketamine), potentiate the arrhythmic effects of catecholamines (halothane), or consistently release histamine (eg, large doses of atracurium or morphine sulfate) may precipitate hypertension and are best avoided.
8. Obese patients may be difficult to intubate as a result of limited mobility of the temporomandibular and atlantooccipital joints, a narrowed upper airway, and a shortened distance between the mandible and sternal fat pads.
9. The key to perioperative management of patients with carcinoid syndrome is to avoid anesthetic and surgical techniques or agents that could cause the tumor to release vasoactive substances.

The underproduction or overproduction of hormones can have life-threatening consequences. Therefore, it is not surprising that endocrinopathies affect anesthetic management. This chapter briefly reviews the normal physiology and pathophysiology of four endocrine organs: the pancreas, the thyroid, the parathyroids, and the adrenal glands. It also considers obesity and carcinoid syndrome.

The Pancreas

Physiology

Insulin, the most important anabolic hormone, has multiple metabolic effects, including facilitating glucose and potassium entry into adipose and muscle cells; increasing glycogen, protein, and fatty acid synthesis; and decreasing glycogenolysis, gluconeogenesis, ketogenesis, lipolysis, and protein catabolism. Adults normally secrete approximately 50 units of insulin each day from the β cells of the pancreas. The rate of insulin secretion is primarily determined by the plasma glucose concentration.

In general, insulin stimulates anabolism and weight gain, whereas lack of insulin is associated with catabolism, a negative nitrogen balance, and weight loss (Table 35–1).

TABLE 35–1 Effects of insulin.

Effects on liver
Anabolic
Promotes glycogenesis
Increases synthesis of triglycerides, cholesterol, and VLDL[1]
Increases protein synthesis
Promotes glycolysis
Anticatabolic
Inhibits glycogenolysis
Inhibits ketogenesis
Inhibits gluconeogenesis
Effects on muscle
Anabolic
Increases amino acid transport
Increases protein synthesis
Anticatabolic
Increases glucose transport
Enhances activity of glycogen synthetase
Inhibits activity of glycogen phosphorylase
Effects on fat
Promotes triglyceride storage
Induces lipoprotein lipase, making fatty acids available for absorption into fat cells
Increases glucose transport into fat cells, thus increasing availability of α-glycerol phosphate for triglyceride synthesis
Inhibits intracellular lipolysis

[1]VLDL, very low-density lipoprotein.

Reproduced with permission from Gardner DG, Shoback D. *Greenspan's Basic & Clinical Endocrinology,* 9th ed. New York, NY: McGraw Hill; 2011.

DIABETES MELLITUS

Clinical Manifestations

Diabetes mellitus is characterized by hyperglycemia and glycosuria arising from an absolute or relative deficiency of insulin or insulin responsiveness. The diagnosis is based on an elevated fasting plasma glucose greater than 126 mg/dL or glycated hemoglobin (HgbA1c) of 6.5% or greater. Values are sometimes reported for blood glucose, which runs 12% to 15% lower than plasma glucose. Even when testing whole blood, newer glucose meters calculate and display plasma glucose. Long-term complications of diabetes include retinopathy, kidney disease, hypertension, coronary artery disease, peripheral and cerebral vascular disease, and peripheral and autonomic neuropathies. Patients with diabetes who are also hyperglycemic have an increased susceptibility to infections.

Diabetes is classified in multiple ways (Table 35–2). Type 1 (insulin-requiring due to endogenous insulin deficiency) and type 2 (insulin-resistant) diabetes are the most common and well known.

There are three life-threatening acute complications of diabetes and its treatment—diabetic ketoacidosis (DKA), hyperosmolar nonketotic coma, and hypoglycemia—in addition to other acute medical problems (such as sepsis) in which the presence of diabetes makes treatment more difficult.

TABLE 35–2 Diagnosis and classification of diabetes mellitus.

Diagnosis (based on blood glucose level)	
Fasting	126 mg/dL (7.0 mmol/L)
Glucose tolerance test	200 mg/dL (11.1 mmol/L)
Classification	
Type 1 (juvenile)	Absolute insulin deficiency secondary to immune-mediated or idiopathic causes
Type 2	Onset in childhood or adulthood secondary to insulin resistance (relative insulin insensitivity)
Gestational	Onset of disease during pregnancy; may or may not persist postpartum

Decreased insulin activity allows the catabolism of free fatty acids into ketone bodies (acetoacetate and β-hydroxybutyrate), some of which are weak acids (see Chapter 50). Accumulation of these organic acids results in DKA, an anion-gap metabolic acidosis. DKA can easily be distinguished from lactic acidosis; lactic acidosis is identified by elevated plasma lactate (>6 mmol/L) and the absence of urine and plasma ketones. However, both DKA and starvation ketosis may occur concurrently with lactic acidosis, underscoring the need for measurement of lactate. DKA is associated with type 1 diabetes mellitus, but a rare individual with DKA may appear phenotypically to have type 2 diabetes mellitus. Alcoholic ketoacidosis can follow binge drinking in a nondiabetic patient and may include a normal or slightly elevated blood glucose level. Such patients may also have a disproportionate increase in β-hydroxybutyrate compared with acetoacetate, in contrast to those with DKA.

Infection is a common precipitating cause of DKA in otherwise well-managed patients with type 1 diabetes. DKA may be the initial presentation of type 1 diabetes. Clinical manifestations of DKA include tachypnea (respiratory compensation for the metabolic acidosis), abdominal pain, nausea and vomiting, and changes in sensorium. The treatment of DKA should include correcting the often substantial hypovolemia, hyperglycemia, and total body potassium deficit. This is typically accomplished with a continuous infusion of isotonic fluids with potassium and an insulin infusion.

The goal for decreasing blood glucose in ketoacidosis should be 100 mg/dL/h or less or 10%/h or less with an intravenous insulin infusion starting at 0.1 units/kg/h. DKA patients may be resistant to insulin, and the insulin infusion rate may need to be increased if glucose concentrations do not decrease. As glucose moves intracellularly, so does potassium. Although this can quickly lead to a critical level of hypokalemia if not corrected, overaggressive potassium replacement can lead to equally life-threatening hyperkalemia. Potassium and blood glucose should be monitored frequently during treatment of DKA.

Several liters of 0.9% saline (1–2 L the first hour, followed by 200–500 mL/h) may be required to correct dehydration in adult patients. When plasma glucose decreases to 250 mg/dL, an infusion of D_5W should be added to the insulin infusion to decrease the possibility of hypoglycemia and to provide a continuous source of glucose (with the infused insulin) for eventual normalization of intracellular metabolism. Bicarbonate is rarely needed to correct severe acidosis (pH <7.1) as the acidosis will correct with volume expansion and with normalization of the plasma glucose concentration.

Ketoacidosis is not a feature of **hyperosmolar nonketotic coma,** possibly because enough insulin is available to prevent ketone body formation. Instead, a hyperglycemia-induced diuresis leads to dehydration and hyperosmolality and may ultimately lead to kidney failure, lactic acidosis, and disseminated intravascular coagulation. Hyperosmolality (frequently exceeding 360 mOsm/L) dehydrates neurons, causing altered mental status and seizures. Severe hyperglycemia causes factitious hyponatremia: each 100 mg/dL increase in plasma glucose lowers plasma sodium concentration by 1.6 mEq/L. Treatment includes fluid resuscitation with normal saline, small doses of insulin, and potassium supplementation.

Hypoglycemia in a patient with diabetes is the result of an absolute or relative excess of insulin relative to carbohydrate intake and exercise. Furthermore, patients with diabetes are incompletely able to counter hypoglycemia despite secreting glucagon or epinephrine (*counterregulatory failure*). The brain depends on glucose as an energy source, and it is the organ most susceptible to injury from hypoglycemia. If hypoglycemia is not treated, mental status changes can progress from anxiety, lightheadedness, headache, or confusion to convulsions and coma. The counterregulatory release of epinephrine produces the systemic manifestations of hypoglycemia: diaphoresis, tachycardia, and nervousness. Most of the signs and all of the symptoms of hypoglycemia will be masked by general anesthesia. Although the lower boundary of normal plasma glucose levels is ill-defined, medically important hypoglycemia is present when plasma glucose is less than 50 mg/dL. The treatment of hypoglycemia in anesthetized or critically ill patients consists of intravenous administration of 50% glucose (each milliliter of 50% glucose will raise the blood glucose of a 70-kg patient by approximately 2 mg/dL). Awake patients can be treated orally with tablets or fluids containing glucose or sucrose.

Anesthetic Considerations

A. Preoperative

Abnormally elevated hemoglobin A_{1c} concentrations identify patients with poor long-term control of blood glucose. These patients are more likely to have hyperglycemia on the day of surgery and have an increased risk of complications, adverse outcomes, and increased costs. The perioperative morbidity of patients with diabetes is related to their preexisting end-organ damage. Unfortunately, many surgical patients with type 2 diabetes mellitus may be unaware of their condition.

A preoperative chest radiograph is not routinely indicated in patients with diabetes. These patients have an increased incidence of ST-segment and T-wave-segment abnormalities on preoperative electrocardiograms (ECGs). Myocardial ischemia or old infarction may be evident on an ECG despite a negative history. Patients with diabetes and hypertension have a 50% likelihood of coexisting **diabetic autonomic neuropathy** (Table 35–3). Reflex dysfunction of the autonomic nervous system may be increased by old age, diabetes
1 of longer than 10 years' duration, coronary artery disease, or β-adrenergic blockade. Diabetic autonomic neuropathy may limit the patient's ability to compensate (with tachycardia and increased peripheral resistance) for intravascular volume changes and may predispose the patient to cardiovascular instability (eg, postinduction hypotension) and even sudden cardiac death. Autonomic dysfunction contributes to delayed gastric emptying (diabetic gastroparesis). Premedication with a nonparticulate antacid and metoclopramide is often used in obese patients with diabetes who have signs of cardiac autonomic dysfunction. However, autonomic dysfunction of the gastrointestinal tract may be present without signs of cardiac involvement. Diabetic neuropathy may also lead to silent (painless) myocardial ischemia.

TABLE 35–3 Clinical signs of diabetic autonomic neuropathy.

Hypertension
Painless myocardial ischemia
Orthostatic hypotension
Lack of heart rate variability[1]
Reduced heart rate response to atropine and propranolol
Resting tachycardia
Early satiety
Neurogenic bladder
Lack of sweating
Impotence

[1]Normal heart rate variability during voluntary deep breathing (6 breaths/min) should be >10 beats/min.

Diabetic kidney dysfunction is manifested first by proteinuria and later by elevated serum creatinine. By these criteria, most patients with type 1 diabetes have evidence of kidney disease by 30 years of age. Chronic hyperglycemia leads to glycosylation of tissue proteins
2 and reduced mobility of joints. Temporomandibular joint and cervical spine mobility should be assessed preoperatively in patients with diabetes to reduce the likelihood of unanticipated difficult intubations.

B. Intraoperative

The goal of intraoperative blood glucose management is to avoid hypoglycemia while maintaining blood glucose at 180 mg/dL or less. True "tight" control (blood glucose <150 mg/dL) during surgery or critical illness has been associated with a worse outcome than "looser" control in both critically ill adults and children. Excessively "loose" blood glucose that is greater than 180 mg/dL also carries risk. The range over which blood glucose should be maintained in critical illness has been the subject of several much-discussed clinical trials. Hyperglycemia has been associated with hyperosmolarity, infection, poor wound healing, and increased mortality. Severe hyperglycemia may worsen neurological outcome following an episode of cerebral ischemia and may compromise outcome after cardiac surgery or an acute myocardial infarction. Maintaining blood glucose control (<180 mg/dL) in patients undergoing cardiopulmonary bypass decreases infectious complications.

Perioperative glucose management has been used as a measurement of "quality" anesthetic care. Consequently, one should ensure that one's glucose management protocols align with institutional and national expectations. Control of blood glucose in patients with diabetes who are pregnant improves fetal outcomes. Nonetheless, as noted earlier, the brain's dependence on glucose as an energy supply makes it essential that hypoglycemia be avoided. Because of an increased incidence of and increased risk from infections, strict attention to aseptic technique and meticulous wound care are especially important in patients with diabetes.

There are several common perioperative management regimens for insulin-dependent patients. In the most time-honored approach (which we do *not* recommend because it is not terribly effective), the patient receives half of the usual morning intermediate-acting insulin dose (Table 35–4). Insulin is administered *after* intravenous access has been established and the morning blood glucose level is checked to decrease the risk of hypoglycemia. For example, a patient who normally takes 30 units of NPH (neutral protamine Hagedorn; intermediate-acting) insulin and 10 units of regular or Lispro (short-acting) insulin or insulin analogue each morning and whose blood glucose is at least 150 mg/dL would receive 15 units (half the normal 30-unit morning dose) of NPH subcutaneously before surgery along with an infusion of 5% dextrose solution (1.5 mL/kg/h). Absorption of subcutaneous or intramuscular insulin depends on tissue blood flow, however, and can be unpredictable during surgery. Intraoperative hyperglycemia (>180 mg/dL) may be treated with boluses of intravenous regular insulin. One unit of regular insulin given to an adult usually lowers plasma glucose by 25 to 30 mg/dL.

A better method, appropriate for all but short procedures, is to withhold insulin prior to the operation and to administer regular insulin as a continuous infusion. The advantage of this technique is more precise control of insulin delivery than can be achieved with a subcutaneous or intramuscular injection of NPH insulin, particularly in conditions associated with poor skin and muscle perfusion. Regular insulin can be added to normal saline in a concentration of 1 unit/mL and the infusion begun at 0.1 unit/kg/h or less. As blood glucose fluctuates, the insulin infusion can be adjusted as required. A dedicated intravenous line for the dextrose and insulin infusions prevents unintended rate changes caused by other intraoperative fluids and drugs. Supplemental dextrose can be administered if the patient becomes hypoglycemic (<100 mg/dL). It must be stressed that these doses are approximations and do not apply to patients in catabolic states (eg, sepsis, hyperthermia).

The dose required may be approximated by the following formula:

$$\text{Unit per hour} = \frac{\text{Plasma glucose (mg/dL)}}{150}$$

A reasonable target for the intraoperative maintenance of blood glucose is less than 180 mg/dL and greater than 85 mg/dL.

When administering an intravenous insulin infusion to surgical patients, adding some (eg, 20 mEq) KCl to each liter of maintenance fluid may be useful as insulin causes an intracellular potassium shift. Because individual insulin needs can vary dramatically, any formula should be considered only a crude guideline. Periodic glucose measurements are required.

If the patient is taking an oral hypoglycemic agent preoperatively rather than insulin, the drug can

3 be continued until the day of surgery. However, sulfonylureas and metformin have long half-lives, and many clinicians will discontinue them 24 to 48 h before surgery. They can be started postoperatively when the patient resumes oral intake. Metformin is restarted if renal and hepatic function remain adequate. The effects of oral hypoglycemic drugs with a short duration of action can be prolonged in the

TABLE 35–4 Two common techniques for perioperative insulin management in diabetes mellitus.

	Bolus Administration	Continuous Infusion
Preoperative	D_5W (1.5 mL/kg/h) NPH[1] insulin (half usual AM dose)	D_5W (1 mL/kg/h) Regular insulin: $\text{Units/h} = \frac{\text{Plasma glucose}}{150}$
Intraoperative	Regular insulin (as per sliding scale)	Same as preoperative
Postoperative	Same as intraoperative	Same as preoperative

[1]NPH, neutral protamine Hagedorn.

presence of kidney failure. In addition, patients with type 2 diabetes taking a sodium-glucose cotransporter 2 (SGLT2) inhibitor hypoglycemic medication (canagliflozin, dapagliflozin, empagliflozin, ertugliflozin) are at higher risk of diabetic ketoacidosis, including euglycemic diabetic ketoacidosis, provoked by fluid and hormonal changes related to surgery, so these medications should be stopped in advance of any planned operation. Canagliflozin, dapagliflozin, and empagliflozin should be stopped at least 3 days in advance of scheduled surgery, and ertugliflozin should be stopped at least 4 days before scheduled surgery. Adequate glucose control should be maintained by other means from the time these medications are discontinued until the postoperative period when the patient has resumed normal oral intake and the patient's SGLT2 medication can be resumed.

Many patients maintained on oral antidiabetic agents will require insulin treatment during the intraoperative and postoperative periods. The stress of surgery causes elevations in counterregulatory hormones and inflammatory mediators such as tumor necrosis factor and interleukins. The result is stress hyperglycemia, increasing insulin requirements. In general, patients with type 2 diabetes tolerate minor, brief surgical procedures without requiring exogenous insulin. Conversely, many ostensibly "nondiabetic" patients show pronounced hyperglycemia during critical illness and require a period of insulin therapy.

The key to any diabetic management regimen is to monitor glucose levels frequently. Patients receiving insulin infusions intraoperatively may need to have their glucose measured hourly. Those with type 2 diabetes vary in their ability to produce and respond to insulin. Likewise, insulin requirements vary with the extensiveness of the surgical procedure. Bedside glucose meters are capable of determining the glucose concentration in a drop of blood within a minute. These devices measure the color conversion of a glucose oxidase–impregnated strip. Their accuracy depends, to a large extent, on adherence to the device's specific testing protocol but in no way reproduces the accuracy of standard laboratory testing, particularly at the extremes of glucose concentrations. Monitoring urine glucose is of value only for detecting glycosuria.

Patients who take NPH or other protamine-containing insulin preparations have an increased risk of adverse reactions to protamine sulfate, including anaphylactoid reactions and death. Unfortunately, operations that require the use of heparin and subsequent reversal with protamine (eg, cardiac and vascular surgery) are more common in patients with diabetes. Based on immunological principles and our clinical experience, we do not advocate administering protamine test doses prior to the full reversal dose.

Patients who use subcutaneous insulin infusion pumps to manage type 1 diabetes can program the pump to deliver "basal" amounts of regular insulin (or insulin glargine) when fasting. By definition, the basal rate is the amount of insulin required during fasting. Patients can safely undergo short outpatient surgery with the pump on the basal setting. If more extensive inpatient procedures are required, these patients will normally suspend their pumps and be managed with intravenous insulin infusions and periodic blood glucose measurements, as described earlier.

C. Postoperative

Close monitoring of blood glucose must continue postoperatively. There is considerable patient-to-patient variation in onset and duration of action of insulin preparations (Table 35–5). For example,

TABLE 35–5 Summary of bioavailability characteristics of the insulins.[1]

	Insulin Type	Onset	Peak Action	Duration
Short-acting	Lispro	10–20 min	30–90 min	4–6 h
	Regular	15–30 min	1–3 h	5–7 h
	Semilente, Semitard	30–60 min	4–6 h	12–16 h
Intermediate-acting	Lente, Lentard, NPH[2]	2–4 h	8–10 h	18–24 h
Long-acting	Ultralente, Glargine, Insulatard	4–5 h	8–14 h	25–36 h

[1]There is considerable patient-to-patient variation. Not all formulations are available in every country.

[2]NPH, neutral protamine Hagedorn.

the onset of action of subcutaneous regular insulin is less than 1 h, but in rare patients, its duration of action may continue for 6 h. NPH insulin typically has an onset of action within 2 h, but its action can endure longer than 24 h.

The Thyroid

Physiology

Dietary iodine is absorbed by the gastrointestinal tract, converted to iodide ion, and actively transported into the thyroid gland. Once in the gland, iodine is combined with the amino acid tyrosine. The end result is triiodothyronine (T_3) and thyroxine (T_4), which are bound to proteins and stored within the thyroid. Although the gland releases more T_4 than T_3, the latter is more potent and less protein bound. Of all circulating T_3, most is formed peripherally from partial deiodination of T_4. An elaborate feedback mechanism controls thyroid hormone synthesis and involves the hypothalamus (thyrotropin-releasing hormone [TRH]), the anterior pituitary (thyroid-stimulating hormone [TSH]), autoregulation, and the adequacy of iodine intake.

Thyroid hormone (T_3) increases carbohydrate and fat metabolism and is an important factor in determining growth and metabolic rate. An increase in metabolic rate is accompanied by an increase in oxygen consumption and CO_2 production. Heart rate and contractility are also increased.

HYPERTHYROIDISM

Clinical Manifestations

Excess thyroid hormone levels can be caused by Graves disease, toxic multinodular goiter, TSH-secreting pituitary tumors, "toxic" or "hot" thyroid adenomas, or overdosage (accidental or intentional) of thyroid hormone. Clinical manifestations of excess thyroid hormone concentrations include weight loss, heat intolerance, muscle weakness, diarrhea, hyperactive reflexes, cardiac arrhythmias, and nervousness. A fine tremor, exophthalmos, or goiter may be noted, particularly when the cause is Graves disease. New-onset atrial fibrillation is a classic presentation of hyperthyroidism, but cardiac signs may also include sinus tachycardia and congestive heart failure. The diagnosis of hyperthyroidism is confirmed by abnormal thyroid function tests, which may include an elevation in serum T_4 and serum T_3 and a reduced TSH level.

Medical treatment of hyperthyroidism relies on drugs that inhibit thyroid hormone synthesis (eg, propylthiouracil, methimazole), prevent hormone release (eg, potassium or sodium iodide), or mask the signs of adrenergic overactivity (eg, propranolol). In addition, although β-adrenergic antagonists do not affect thyroid gland function, they do decrease the peripheral conversion of T_4 to T_3. Radioactive iodine destroys thyroid cell function and may result in hypothyroidism. Radioactive iodine is not recommended for pregnant patients. Subtotal thyroidectomy is rarely used as an alternative to medical therapy but is typically reserved for patients with large toxic multinodular goiters or solitary toxic adenomas. Graves disease is usually treated with antithyroid drugs or radioactive iodine.

Anesthetic Considerations

A. Preoperative

All elective surgical procedures, including subtotal thyroidectomy, should be postponed until the patient is rendered clinically and chemically euthyroid with medical treatment. The patient should have normal T_3 and T_4 concentrations and should not have resting tachycardia. Antithyroid medications and β-adrenergic antagonists are continued through the morning of surgery. Administration of propylthiouracil and methimazole is particularly important because of their short half-lives.

Patients with larger goiters or thyroid masses will often have preoperative imaging studies to rule out extension into the mediastinum. Such extension might mandate sternotomy for complete resection.

B. Intraoperative

Cardiovascular function and body temperature should be closely monitored in patients with a history of hyperthyroidism. When emergency surgery must proceed despite clinical hyperthyroidism, the hyperdynamic circulation can be controlled intraoperatively with an esmolol infusion. The exophthalmos of

Graves disease increases the risk of corneal abrasion or ulceration.

Ketamine, indirect-acting adrenergic agonists (ephedrine), and other drugs that stimulate the sympathetic nervous system are best avoided in patients with current or recently corrected hyperthyroidism because

4 of the possibility of exaggerated elevations in blood pressure and heart rate. Incompletely treated hyperthyroid patients may be hypovolemic and prone to hypotension with the induction of anesthesia. On the other hand, inadequate anesthetic depth during laryngoscopy or surgical incision in such patients may lead to tachycardia, hypertension, or ventricular arrhythmias.

Thyrotoxicosis is associated with myopathies and myasthenia gravis; therefore, neuromuscular blocking agents (NMBs) should be administered cautiously. Hyperthyroidism does not increase the minimum alveolar concentration (MAC) of inhaled anesthetics.

C. Postoperative

The most serious threat to a hyperthyroid patient undergoing surgery is **thyroid storm**, characterized by hyperpyrexia, tachycardia, altered consciousness (eg, agitation, delirium, coma), and hypotension. Thyroid storm is a medical emergency that requires aggressive management and monitoring (see Case Discussion, Chapter 56). The onset is usually 6 to 24 h after surgery, but it can occur intraoperatively, mimicking malignant hyperthermia. Unlike malignant hyperthermia, thyroid storm is not associated with muscle rigidity, elevated creatine kinase, or marked metabolic (lactic) and respiratory acidosis. Treatment includes hydration and cooling, an intravenous β-blocker (typically an esmolol infusion with a target heart rate <100/min), propylthiouracil (250–500 mg every 6 h orally or by nasogastric tube) followed by sodium iodide (1 g intravenously over 12 h) and correction of any precipitating cause (eg, infection). Hydrocortisone (100–200 mg every 8 h) or the equivalent is given to counteract any coexisting adrenal gland suppression.

Thyroidectomy is associated with several potential surgical complications. Recurrent laryngeal nerve palsy produces hoarseness (unilateral) or aphonia and stridor (bilateral). Vocal cord function can be evaluated by laryngoscopy immediately following "deep extubation"; however, this is rarely necessary. Immobility of one or both cords may require reintubation and exploration of the wound. Wound hematomas may compress the trachea, obstructing the airway, particularly in patients with tracheomalacia. The hematoma may distort the airway anatomy, making intubation difficult. Immediate treatment includes opening the neck wound, evacuating the clot, and reassessing the need for reintubation. In the immediate postoperative setting, anesthesia personnel must be prepared to open the surgical wound to relieve airway compression if the surgeon is unavailable.

Hypoparathyroidism from unintentional removal of all four parathyroid glands will cause acute hypocalcemia within 12 to 72 h (see the section on Clinical Manifestations under Hypoparathyroidism). Pneumothorax is a rare complication of neck exploration.

HYPOTHYROIDISM

Clinical Manifestations

Hypothyroidism can be caused by autoimmune disease (eg, Hashimoto thyroiditis), thyroidectomy, radioactive iodine, antithyroid medications, iodine deficiency, or failure of the hypothalamic–pituitary axis (secondary hypothyroidism). Hypothyroidism during neonatal development results in cretinism, a condition marked by physical and mental retardation. Clinical manifestations of hypothyroidism in the adult are usually subtle and include infertility, weight gain, cold intolerance, muscle fatigue, lethargy, constipation, hypoactive reflexes, dull facial expression, and depression. In advanced cases, heart rate, myocardial contractility, stroke volume, and cardiac output are all decreased, and extremities are cool and mottled because of peripheral vasoconstriction. Pleural, abdominal, and pericardial effusions are common. Hypothyroidism is typically diagnosed by an elevated TSH concentration, often with a reduced free (or total) T_3 level. Primary hypothyroidism, the more common condition, is differentiated from secondary disease by an elevation in TSH in the former. The treatment of hypothyroidism consists of oral replacement therapy with a thyroid hormone preparation, which takes several days to produce a physiological effect and several weeks to evoke clear-cut clinical improvement. Normal concentrations of TSH despite reduced T_3 concentrations (termed "euthyroid sick" syndrome or nonthyroidal illness syndrome) are often seen after major operations and with a long list of chronic and critical illnesses.

Myxedema coma results from extreme hypothyroidism and is characterized by coma, hypoventilation, hypothermia, hyponatremia (from inappropriate antidiuretic hormone secretion), and congestive heart failure. It is more common in older adult patients and may be precipitated by infection, surgery, or trauma. Myxedema coma is a life-threatening disease that can be treated with intravenous T_3. T_4 should not be used in this circumstance to avoid the need for peripheral conversion to T_3. The ECG should be monitored during therapy to detect myocardial ischemia or arrhythmias. Steroid replacement (eg, hydrocortisone, 100 mg intravenously every 8 h) is routinely given due to frequent coexisting adrenal gland suppression. Some patients may require ventilatory support and external warming.

Anesthetic Considerations

A. Preoperative

Patients with severe uncorrected hypothyroidism or myxedema coma must not undergo elective surgery. Such patients should be treated with T_3 intravenously prior to urgent or emergency surgery. Although the euthyroid state is ideal, mild to moderate hypothyroidism is not an absolute contraindication to necessary surgery, for example, urgent coronary bypass surgery.

Symptomatic hypothyroid patients should receive minimal preoperative sedation because they are prone to drug-induced respiratory depression. In addition, they may fail to respond to hypoxia with increased minute ventilation. Patients who have been rendered euthyroid may receive their usual dose of thyroid medication on the morning of surgery; however, most commonly used preparations have long half-lives (the half-life of T_4 is about 8 days), and omission of a single daily dose has no medical importance.

B. Intraoperative

5 Clinically hypothyroid patients are more susceptible to the hypotensive effect of anesthetic agents because of diminished cardiac output, blunted baroreceptor reflexes, and decreased intravascular volume. In this circumstance, ketamine or etomidate can be recommended for induction of anesthesia. The possibility of coexistent primary adrenal insufficiency should be considered in cases of refractory hypotension. **Other potential coexisting conditions include hypoglycemia, anemia, hyponatremia, difficulty during intubation because of a large tongue, and hypothermia from a low basal metabolic rate.**

C. Postoperative

Recovery from general anesthesia may be delayed in hypothyroid patients by hypothermia, respiratory depression, or slowed drug biotransformation. Because hypothyroidism increases vulnerability to respiratory depression, a multimodal approach to postoperative pain management, rather than strict reliance on opioids, is appropriate.

The Parathyroid –Vitamin D–Bone–Kidney Axis

Physiology

Parathyroid hormone (PTH) is the principal regulator of calcium homeostasis. It increases serum calcium concentrations directly by promoting resorption of bone and teeth, limiting renal excretion of calcium, and indirectly by stimulating vitamin D synthesis in the kidney to enhance gastrointestinal calcium absorption. PTH decreases serum phosphate by increasing renal excretion. The hormone fibroblast growth factor 23 (FGF23) arises from bone and acts on the kidney to induce phosphaturia and reduce the production of vitamin D_3. FGF23 actions require that α-klotho activate the FGF receptor.

The effects of PTH on calcium serum levels are countered in lower animals by calcitonin, a hormone excreted by parafollicular C cells in the thyroid. Although calcitonin is effective given as a pharmaceutical in humans, its role in normal human physiology appears negligible (Table 35–6). Of total body calcium, 99% is in the skeleton. Of the calcium in the blood, 40% is bound to proteins, and 60% is ionized or complexed to organic ions. Unbound ionized calcium is physiologically the most important fraction.

TABLE 35–6 Actions of major calcium-regulating hormones.

	Bone	Kidney	Intestines
Parathyroid hormone (PTH)	Increases resorption of calcium and phosphate	Increases reabsorption of calcium; decreases reabsorption of phosphate; increases conversion of 25-OHD_3 to 1,25$(OH)_2$ D_3;[1] decreases reabsorption of bicarbonate	No direct effects; increases renal production of vitamin D
Calcitonin	Inhibits osteoclastic resorption	Decreases reabsorption of calcium and phosphate	Inhibits reabsorption of phosphate; increases renal excretion of sodium and calcium
Vitamin D	Maintains Ca^{2+} homeostasis	Decreases reabsorption of calcium (probably less important than PTH)	Increases absorption of calcium

[1]25-OHD_3, 25-hydroxyvitamin D_3; 1,25$(OH)_2D_3$, 1,25-dihydroxyvitamin D_3.

The remaining major player in this system, vitamin D, is a steroid hormone that can be absorbed via the gastrointestinal tract from food or synthesized from cholesterol derivatives. Conversion of 7-dehydrocalciferol to vitamin D_3 is facilitated by exposure to ultraviolet light. Hydroxylation in the liver and kidneys yields 1,25$(OH)_2D_3$ (1,25-dihydroxyvitamin D_3), the active molecule that binds vitamin D receptors (VDRs) and produces its physiological actions. VDRs are located in the nucleus where, after binding vitamin D, they regulate the expression of specific genes. 1,25$(OH)_2D_3$ promotes normal growth and remodeling of bone, in addition to helping to regulate calcium and phosphate concentrations. Vitamin D also plays a physiologic role in the regulation of the immune system, though its precise function and the impact of vitamin D supplementation on immunocompetence are not well understood at this time.

HYPERPARATHYROIDISM

Clinical Manifestations

Causes of primary hyperparathyroidism include parathyroid adenomas, hyperplasia of the parathyroid gland, and certain carcinomas. Secondary hyperparathyroidism is an adaptive response to hypocalcemia produced by conditions such as end-stage kidney disease or intestinal malabsorption syndromes. Ectopic hyperparathyroidism is due to the production of PTH by rare tumors outside the parathyroid gland. Overall, the most common cause of hypercalcemia in hospitalized patients is malignancy. Parathyroid hormone–related peptide may cause significant hypercalcemia when secreted by a tumor (eg, carcinoma of the lung or liver). Bone invasion with accompanying osteolytic hypercalcemia may complicate multiple myeloma, lymphoma, or leukemia. Nearly all clinical manifestations of hyperparathyroidism are due to hypercalcemia (Table 35–7). Rarer causes of hypercalcemia include bone metastases of solid organ tumors, vitamin D intoxication, milk-alkali syndrome, lithium therapy, sarcoidosis, and prolonged immobilization. The treatment of hyperparathyroidism depends on the cause, but surgical removal of all four glands is often required in the setting of parathyroid hyperplasia. When there is a single adenoma, its removal cures many patients with sporadic primary hyperparathyroidism.

Anesthetic Considerations

In patients with hypercalcemia due to hyperparathyroidism, hydration with normal saline and diuresis facilitated by furosemide will usually decrease serum calcium to acceptable values (<14 mg/dL, 7 mEq/L, or 3.5 mmol/L). More aggressive therapy with the intravenous bisphosphonates pamidronate (Aredia) or etidronate (Didronel) may be necessary for patients with hypercalcemia of malignancy. Plicamycin (Mithramycin), glucocorticoids, calcitonin, or dialysis may be necessary when intravenous bisphosphonates are not sufficient or are contraindicated. Hypoventilation should be avoided as acidosis increases ionized calcium. Elevated calcium

TABLE 35–7 Effects of hyperparathyroidism.

Cardiovascular
Hypertension
Ventricular arrhythmias
ECG[1] changes (shortened QT interval,[2] widened T wave)
Renal
Polyuria
Impaired renal concentrating ability
Kidney stones
Hyperchloremic metabolic acidosis
Dehydration
Polydipsia
Kidney failure
Gastrointestinal
Constipation
Nausea and vomiting
Anorexia
Pancreatitis
Peptic ulcer disease
Musculoskeletal
Muscle weakness
Osteoporosis
Neurological
Mental status change (eg, delirium, psychosis, coma)

[1]ECG, electrocardiogram.

[2]The QT interval may be prolonged at serum calcium concentrations >16 mg/dL.

levels can cause cardiac arrhythmias. The response to NMBs may be altered in patients with preexisting muscle weakness caused by the effects of calcium at the neuromuscular junction. Osteoporosis worsened by hyperparathyroidism predisposes patients to vertebral and long bone fractures during anesthetic procedures, positioning, and transport. The notable postoperative complications of parathyroidectomy are similar to those of subtotal thyroidectomy.

HYPOPARATHYROIDISM

Clinical Manifestations

Hypoparathyroidism is usually due to deficiency of PTH following parathyroidectomy. Clinical manifestations of hypoparathyroidism are a result of hypocalcemia (Table 35–8), which can also be caused by kidney failure, hypomagnesemia, vitamin D deficiency, and acute pancreatitis (see Chapter 49). Hypoalbuminemia decreases total serum calcium (a 1-g/dL drop in serum albumin causes a 0.8-mg/dL decrease in total serum calcium), but ionized calcium, the active entity, is unaltered. The archetypical presentation of hypocalcemia is tetany, classically diagnosed by the Chvostek sign (painful twitching of the facial musculature following tapping over the facial nerve) or the Trousseau sign (carpal spasm following inflation of an arm tourniquet above systolic blood pressure for 3 min). Treatment of symptomatic hypocalcemia consists of intravenous administration of calcium salts.

TABLE 35–8 Effects of hypoparathyroidism.

Cardiovascular
ECG[1] changes (prolonged QT interval)
Hypotension
Congestive heart failure
Neurological
Neuromuscular irritability (eg, laryngospasm, inspiratory stridor, tetany, seizures)
Perioral paresthesia
Mental status changes (eg, dementia, depression, psychosis)

[1]ECG, electrocardiogram.

Mild hypocalcemia is common following cardiopulmonary bypass or infusion of albumin solutions. In many adult patients, this need not be treated because the response of the PTH–vitamin D axis will usually be sufficient to restore ionized calcium to normal values and mild hypocalcemia will usually have no hemodynamic consequences.

Anesthetic Considerations

Serum calcium must be normalized in any patient who presents with cardiac manifestations of severe hypocalcemia. Alkalosis from hyperventilation or sodium bicarbonate therapy will further decrease ionized calcium. Although citrate-containing blood products usually do not lower serum calcium significantly, they should be administered cautiously in patients with preexisting hypocalcemia. Other considerations include avoiding the bolus administration of albumin solutions (which bind and reduce ionized calcium concentrations) and being mindful of the possibility of hypocalcemia-induced coagulopathy.

VITAMIN D DEFICIENCY

A diet deficient in vitamin D combined with a lack of sun (ultraviolet light) exposure will lead to rickets in children and osteomalacia in adults. Decreased concentrations of vitamin D, more common in older adults, those who live in far northern latitudes, and those too frail or ill to spend time outdoors, have been associated with a great many conditions and diseases. Causal linkages have been hard to identify. Despite the great number of articles that have been written on this topic, we lack proper evidence regarding the vitamin D concentrations below which vitamin D replacement is mandatory, how best to replace vitamin D in those who require replacement, and indeed whether vitamin D replacement improves outcomes in those conditions in which reduced vitamin D concentrations have been associated with worse outcomes. The data are even murkier regarding vitamin D replacement in patients undergoing surgery.

The Adrenal Gland

Physiology

The adrenal gland is divided into the cortex and medulla. The adrenal cortex secretes androgens, mineralocorticoids (eg, aldosterone), and glucocorticoids (eg, cortisol). The adrenal medulla secretes catecholamines (primarily epinephrine but also small amounts of norepinephrine and dopamine). The adrenal androgens have almost no relevance for anesthetic management and will not be considered further.

Aldosterone is primarily involved with fluid and electrolyte balance. Aldosterone secretion causes sodium ions and water to be reabsorbed in the distal renal tubule and collecting duct and potassium and hydrogen ions to be secreted. The net effect is an expansion in extracellular fluid volume caused by fluid retention, a decrease in plasma potassium, and metabolic alkalosis. Aldosterone secretion is stimulated by the renin–angiotensin system (specifically, angiotensin III, a product of angiotensin II, pituitary adrenocorticotropic hormone (ACTH), metabolic acidosis, and hyperkalemia. Hypovolemia, hypotension, congestive heart failure, and the neuroendocrine stress response to surgery result in an elevation of aldosterone concentrations. Blockade of the renin–angiotensin–aldosterone system with angiotensin-converting enzyme inhibitors or angiotensin receptor blockers, or both, is a cornerstone of therapy (and increases survival) in hypertension and chronic heart failure. Aldosterone receptor blockers (spironolactone or eplerenone) added to standard therapy prolong survival in patients with chronic heart failure.

Glucocorticoids are essential for life and have multiple physiological effects, including enhanced gluconeogenesis and inhibition of peripheral glucose utilization. These actions tend to raise blood glucose and worsen diabetic control. Glucocorticoids are required for vascular and bronchial smooth muscle to respond to catecholamines. Because glucocorticoids are structurally related to aldosterone, most tend to promote sodium retention and potassium excretion (a mineralocorticoid effect). ACTH released by the anterior pituitary is the principal regulator of glucocorticoid secretion. Basal secretion of ACTH and glucocorticoids exhibits a diurnal rhythm. Stressful conditions promote the secretion of ACTH and cortisol while circulating glucocorticoids inhibit ACTH and cortisol secretion. Under nonstressed conditions, endogenous production of cortisol, the most important endogenous glucocorticoid, averages 20 mg/d.

The structure, biosynthesis, physiological effects, and metabolism of catecholamines are discussed in Chapter 14. Epinephrine constitutes 80% of adrenal catecholamine output in humans. Catecholamine release is regulated mainly by sympathetic cholinergic preganglionic fibers that innervate the adrenal medulla. Stimuli include exercise, hemorrhage, surgery, hypotension, hypothermia, hypoglycemia, hypercapnia, hypoxemia, pain, and fear.

MINERALOCORTICOID EXCESS

Clinical Manifestations

Hypersecretion of aldosterone by the adrenal cortex (primary aldosteronism) can be due to a unilateral adenoma (aldosteronoma or Conn syndrome), bilateral hyperplasia, or in very rare cases, carcinoma of the adrenal gland. Some disease states stimulate aldosterone secretion by affecting the renin–angiotensin system. For example, congestive heart failure, hepatic cirrhosis with ascites, nephrotic syndrome, and some forms of hypertension (eg, renal artery stenosis) can cause secondary hyperaldosteronism. Although both primary and secondary hyperaldosteronism are characterized by increased levels of aldosterone, only the latter is associated with increased renin activity. The usual clinical manifestations of mineralocorticoid excess include hypokalemia and hypertension, and an increased ratio of aldosterone–plasma renin activity has been noted in laboratory studies.

Anesthetic Considerations

Fluid and electrolyte disturbances can be corrected preoperatively using spironolactone. This aldosterone antagonist is a potassium-sparing diuretic with antihypertensive properties. Intravascular volume can be assessed preoperatively by testing for orthostatic hypotension.

MINERALOCORTICOID DEFICIENCY

Clinical Manifestations & Anesthetic Considerations

Atrophy or destruction of both adrenal glands results in a combined deficiency of mineralocorticoids and glucocorticoids (see the section on Glucocorticoid Deficiency). Isolated deficiency of mineralocorticoid activity almost never occurs.

GLUCOCORTICOID EXCESS

Clinical Manifestations

Glucocorticoid excess may be due to exogenous administration of steroid hormones, intrinsic hyperfunction of the adrenal cortex (eg, adrenocortical adenoma), ACTH production by a nonpituitary tumor (ectopic ACTH syndrome), or hypersecretion by a pituitary adenoma (Cushing disease). Regardless of the cause, an excess of corticosteroids produces Cushing syndrome, characterized by muscle wasting and weakness, osteoporosis, central obesity, abdominal striae, glucose intolerance, menstrual irregularity, hypertension, and mental status changes.

Anesthetic Considerations

Patients with Cushing syndrome may be volume overloaded and have hypokalemic metabolic alkalosis resulting from the mineralocorticoid activity of glucocorticoids. These abnormalities should be corrected preoperatively in the manner previously described. Patients with osteoporosis are at risk for fracture during positioning. If the cause of Cushing syndrome is exogenous glucocorticoids, the patient's adrenal glands may not be able to respond to perioperative stresses, and supplemental steroids are indicated (see the section on Glucocorticoid Deficiency). Likewise, patients undergoing adrenalectomy require intraoperative glucocorticoid replacement (in adults, intravenous hydrocortisone succinate, 100 mg every 8 h has been the traditional stress dose). Although many adrenal tumors are removed uneventfully during laparoscopic surgery, complications of adrenalectomy may include major blood loss and unintentional pneumothorax.

GLUCOCORTICOID DEFICIENCY

Clinical Manifestations

Primary adrenal insufficiency (Addison disease), caused by the destruction of the adrenal gland, results in a combined mineralocorticoid and glucocorticoid deficiency. Clinical manifestations are due to aldosterone deficiency (hyponatremia, hypovolemia, hypotension, hyperkalemia, and metabolic acidosis) and cortisol deficiency (weakness, fatigue, hypoglycemia, hypotension, and weight loss).

Secondary adrenal insufficiency is a result of inadequate ACTH secretion by the pituitary. The most common cause of secondary adrenal insufficiency is prior administration of exogenous glucocorticoids. Because mineralocorticoid secretion is usually adequate in secondary adrenal insufficiency, fluid and electrolyte disturbances are not present. Acute adrenal insufficiency (Addisonian crisis), however, can be triggered in steroid-dependent patients who do not receive appropriate glucocorticoid doses during periods of stress (eg, infection, trauma, surgery) and in patients who receive infusions of etomidate. The clinical features of this medical emergency include fever, abdominal pain, orthostatic hypotension, and hypovolemia that may progress to circulatory shock unresponsive to resuscitation.

Anesthetic Considerations

6 Patients with glucocorticoid deficiency must receive adequate steroid replacement therapy during the perioperative period. Patients who have received potentially suppressive doses of steroids (eg, the daily equivalent of 5 mg of prednisone) by any route of administration (topical, inhalational, or oral) for a period of more than 2 weeks any time in the previous 12 months may be unable to respond appropriately to surgical stress and should receive perioperative glucocorticoid supplementation.

What represents adequate steroid coverage is controversial, and there are those who advocate variable dosing based on the extent of the surgery. Although adults normally secrete 20 mg of cortisol daily, this may increase to more than 300 mg under conditions of maximal stress. Thus, a traditional recommendation was to administer 100 mg of hydrocortisone every 8 h beginning on the morning of surgery. An alternative low-dose regimen (25 mg of hydrocortisone at the time of induction followed by an infusion of 100 mg during the subsequent 24 h) maintains plasma cortisol levels equal to or higher than those reported in healthy patients undergoing similar elective surgery. This second regimen might be particularly appropriate for patients with diabetes, in whom glucocorticoid administration often interferes with the control of blood glucose.

CATECHOLAMINE EXCESS

Clinical Manifestations

Paragangliomas and pheochromocytomas are tumors that consist of cells originating from the embryonic neural crest. Pheochromocytomas arise in the adrenal gland; paragangliomas can be thought of as extraadrenal pheochromocytomas. These tumors account for 0.1% of all cases of hypertension, and hypertension arises from excessive secretion of catecholamines by the tumors. Although the tumors are usually localized in a single adrenal gland, 10% to 15% are bilateral or extraadrenal. Approximately 10% of tumors are malignant. The cardinal manifestations of pheochromocytoma are paroxysmal hypertension, headache, sweating, and palpitations. Unexpected intraoperative hypertension and tachycardia during manipulation of abdominal structures may occasionally be the first indications of an undiagnosed pheochromocytoma. The pathophysiology, diagnosis, and treatment of these tumors require an understanding of catecholamine metabolism and of the pharmacology of adrenergic agonists and antagonists. The Case Discussion in Chapter 14 examines these aspects of pheochromocytoma management.

Anesthetic Considerations

Preoperative assessment should focus on the adequacy of α-adrenergic blockade and volume replacement. Specifically, resting arterial blood pressure, orthostatic blood pressure and heart rate, ventricular ectopy, and electrocardiographic evidence of ischemia should be evaluated.

A decrease in plasma volume and red cell mass contributes to the severe chronic hypovolemia seen in these patients. The hematocrit may be normal or elevated, depending on the relative contribution of hypovolemia and anemia. Preoperative α-adrenergic blockade with phenoxybenzamine (a noncompetitive inhibitor) helps correct the volume deficit, in addition to correcting hypertension. β Blockade should be initiated only after α blockade has been well established if there is a need to control heart rate. β Blockade initiated in the absence of α blockade may initiate disastrous hypertension in patients with pheochromocytoma. A decline in hematocrit should accompany the expansion of circulatory volume, potentially unmasking underlying anemia.

Potentially life-threatening fluctuations in blood pressure—particularly during induction and manipulation of the tumor—indicate the need for invasive arterial pressure monitoring. Patients with evidence of cardiac disease (or in whom cardiac disease is suspected) may benefit from having a central line (a convenient route of access for administering vasoactive drugs, should they be required) and from intraoperative transesophageal echocardiography.

Intubation should not be attempted until a deep level of general anesthesia (possibly also including local anesthesia of the trachea) has been established. Intraoperative hypertension can be treated with phentolamine, nitroprusside, nicardipine, or clevidipine. Phentolamine specifically blocks α-adrenergic receptors and blocks the effects of excessive circulating catecholamines. Nitroprusside has a rapid onset of action and a short duration of action and can be effective in cases where calcium channel blockers are ineffective. Nicardipine and clevidipine are being used more frequently preoper-
7 atively and intraoperatively. Drugs or techniques that indirectly stimulate or promote the release of catecholamines (eg, ephedrine, hypoventilation, large bolus doses of ketamine), potentiate the arrhythmic effects of catecholamines (halothane), or consistently release histamine (eg, large doses of atracurium or morphine sulfate) are best avoided.

After ligation of the tumor's venous supply, the primary problem frequently becomes *hypotension* from the combination of hypovolemia, persisting adrenergic blockade, and tolerance to the increased concentrations of endogenous catecholamines that have been abruptly withdrawn. Assessment of intravascular volume can be guided by echocardiography or other noninvasive measures of cardiac output and stroke volume. Infusions of adrenergic agonists, such as phenylephrine or norepinephrine, often prove necessary. Postoperative *hypertension* is rare and may indicate the presence of unresected occult tumors.

OBESITY

Overweight and obesity are classified using the body mass index (BMI). Overweight is defined as a BMI of 24 kg/m^2 or higher, obesity as a BMI of 30 or higher, and extreme obesity (formerly termed "morbid obesity") as a BMI of more than 40. BMI is calculated by dividing the weight (in kilograms) by the height (in meters) squared. A great many BMI calculators are available online or as apps for smartphones. Health risks increase with the degree of obesity and increased abdominal distribution of weight. Obesity has only recently been included as a factor in determining a patient's American Society of Anesthesiologists (ASA) score. Men with a waist measurement of 40 in. or more and women with a waist measurement of 35 in. or more are at increased health risk. For a patient 1.8 m tall and weighing 70 kg, the BMI would be as shown in the following formula:

$$\text{BMI} = \frac{\text{Weight (kg)}}{(\text{Height [m]})^2} = \frac{70\text{ kg}}{1.8^2} = \frac{70}{3.24}$$
$$= 21.6\text{ kg/m}^2$$

Clinical Manifestations

Obesity is associated with many diseases, including type 2 diabetes mellitus, hypertension, coronary artery disease, obstructive sleep apnea, degenerative joint disease (osteoarthritis), and cholelithiasis. Even in the absence of obvious coexisting disease, however, extreme obesity has profound physiological consequences. Oxygen demand, CO_2 production, and alveolar ventilation are elevated because metabolic rate is proportional to body weight. Excessive adipose tissue over the thorax decreases chest wall compliance even though lung compliance may remain normal. Increased abdominal mass forces the diaphragm cephalad, yielding lung volumes suggestive of restrictive lung disease. Reductions in lung volumes are accentuated by the supine and Trendelenburg positions. In particular, functional residual capacity may fall below closing capacity. If this occurs, some alveoli will close during normal tidal volume ventilation, causing a ventilation/perfusion mismatch.

Whereas obese patients are often hypoxemic, only a few are hypercapnic, which, when present, should be a warning of impending complications. Obstructive sleep apnea (OSA) is a complication of extreme obesity characterized by hypercapnia, cyanosis-induced polycythemia, right-sided heart failure, and somnolence. These patients appear to have blunted respiratory drive and often suffer from loud snoring and upper-airway obstruction during sleep. OSA patients often report dry mouths and daytime somnolence; bed partners frequently describe apneic pauses. OSA has also been associated with perioperative complications, including hypertension, hypoxia, arrhythmias, myocardial infarction, pulmonary edema, stroke, and death. The potential for difficult mask ventilation and difficult intubation, followed by upper airway obstruction during recovery, should be anticipated.

Patients with OSA are vulnerable during the postoperative period, particularly when sedatives or opioids have been given. Patients positioned supine are unusually susceptible to upper airway obstruction. For patients with known or suspected OSA, postoperative continuous positive airway pressure (CPAP) should be considered until the patient can protect the airway and maintain spontaneous ventilation without obstruction. Both the ASA and the Society of Ambulatory Anesthesia offer guidelines on perioperative management of the patient with OSA (see Chapter 44).

The heart of a patient with OSA has an increased workload as cardiac output and blood volume increase to perfuse additional fat stores. Arterial hypertension leads to left ventricular hypertrophy. Elevations in pulmonary blood flow and pulmonary artery vasoconstriction from persistent hypoxia can lead to pulmonary hypertension and cor pulmonale.

Obese patients have an increased risk of hiatal hernia, gastroesophageal reflux disease, delayed gastric emptying, hyperacidic gastric fluid, and gastric cancer. Fatty infiltration of the liver also occurs and may be associated with abnormal liver tests, but the extent of infiltration does not correlate well with the degree of liver test abnormality. Nonalcoholic fatty liver disease is now the most common cause of liver cirrhosis in the United States.

Anesthetic Considerations

A. Preoperative

For the reasons outlined above, obese patients are at an increased risk for developing aspiration pneumonia. Pretreatment with a nonparticulate antacid, H_2 antagonists, and metoclopramide should be considered. Premedication with respiratory depressant drugs must be avoided in patients with OSA.

Preoperative testing may include such items as chest radiograph, ECG, and arterial blood gas analysis, all with the goal of assessing cardiopulmonary reserve. Physical signs of cardiac failure may be difficult to identify. Blood pressures must be taken with a cuff of the appropriate size. Intravenous and intraarterial access may present technical difficulties. Obscured landmarks, difficult positioning, and extensive layers of adipose tissue may make regional anesthesia difficult
8 with standard equipment and techniques. Obese patients may be difficult to intubate as a result of limited mobility of the temporomandibular and atlantooccipital joints, a narrowed upper airway, and a shortened distance between the mandible and sternal fat pads.

B. Intraoperative

To avoid aspiration and hypoventilation, morbidly obese patients are often intubated for all but short general anesthetics. If intubation appears potentially difficult, we use either video laryngoscopy or fiberoptic bronchoscopy. Positioning the patient on an intubating ramp is very helpful. Auscultation of breath sounds may prove difficult. Even with controlled ventilation, these patients may require increased inspired oxygen concentrations to prevent hypoxia, particularly in the lithotomy, Trendelenburg, or prone positions. Subdiaphragmatic abdominal laparotomy packs can cause further deterioration of pulmonary function and a reduction of arterial blood pressure by compressing the inferior vena cava. Volatile anesthetics may be metabolized more extensively in obese patients. Increased metabolism may explain the increased incidence of halothane hepatitis observed in obese patients. Obese patients may have a prolonged induction and emergence from inhaled anesthetics.

Theoretically, greater fat stores would increase the volume of distribution for lipid-soluble drugs (eg, benzodiazepines, opioids) relative to a lean person of the same bodyweight. However, the volume of distribution of, for example, fentanyl or sufentanil is so large that obesity has minimal influence. Water-soluble drugs (eg, NMBs) have small volumes of distribution, which are minimally increased by body fat. Therefore, the dosing of water-soluble drugs should be based on ideal body weight to avoid overdosage.

Although dosage requirements for epidural and spinal anesthesia are difficult to predict, obese patients typically require 20% to 25% less local anesthetic per blocked segment because of epidural fat and distended epidural veins reducing the CSF volume. Continuous epidural anesthesia has the usual advantages of providing pain relief and potentially decreasing respiratory complications in the postoperative period. Regional nerve blocks, particularly when combined with multimodal pain control, have the additional advantages of not interfering with the standard deep vein thrombosis prophylaxis, rarely producing hypotension, and reducing the need for opioids (see Chapter 48).

C. Postoperative

Respiratory failure is the major postoperative problem of morbidly obese patients. The risk of postoperative hypoxemia is increased in these patients, especially when there is preoperative hypoxemia, and in patients undergoing surgery involving the thorax or upper abdomen. An obese patient should remain intubated until there is no doubt that an adequate airway and tidal volume will be maintained, NMBs are completely reversed, and the patient is awake. This does *not* mean that all obese patients need to be ventilated overnight in an intensive care unit. If the patient is extubated in the operating room, supplemental oxygen should be provided during transportation to the postanesthesia care unit. A 45° modified sitting position will improve ventilation and oxygenation. The risk of hypoxemia extends for several days into the postoperative period, and providing supplemental oxygen or CPAP, or both, should be routinely considered. Other common postoperative complications in obese patients include pneumonia, wound infection, deep venous thrombosis, and pulmonary embolism. Morbidly obese and OSA patients may be candidates for outpatient surgery provided they are adequately monitored and assessed postoperatively before discharge to home and provided the surgical procedure will not require large doses of opioids for postoperative pain control. It is hard to conceive of a better indication for multimodal analgesia.

Carcinoid Syndrome

Carcinoid syndrome results from the secretion of vasoactive substances (eg, serotonin, kallikrein, histamine) from neuroendocrine tumors (carcinoid tumors). Most of these tumors are located in the gastrointestinal tract, so their metabolic products are released into the portal circulation and largely metabolized by the liver before they can cause systemic effects. However, the products of nonintestinal tumors (eg, pulmonary, ovarian) or hepatic metastases bypass the portal circulation and can cause a variety of clinical manifestations. Many patients undergo surgery for resection of carcinoid tumors; most such patients will never experience carcinoid syndrome.

Clinical Manifestations

The most common manifestations of carcinoid syndrome are cutaneous flushing, bronchospasm, profuse diarrhea, dramatic swings in arterial blood pressure (usually hypotension), and supraventricular arrhythmias (Table 35–9). **Carcinoid syndrome is associated with right-sided heart disease caused by valvular and myocardial plaque formation and, in some cases, implantation of tumors on the tricuspid and pulmonary valves.** The diagnosis of carcinoid syndrome is confirmed by detection of serotonin metabolites in the urine (5-hydroxyindoleacetic acid) or plasma or suggested by elevated plasma levels of chromogranin A. Treatment varies depending on tumor location but may include surgical resection, symptomatic relief, or specific serotonin and histamine antagonists. Somatostatin, an inhibitory peptide, reduces the release of vasoactive tumor products.

Anesthetic Considerations

The key to perioperative management of patients with carcinoid syndrome is to avoid

TABLE 35–9 Principal mediators of carcinoid syndrome and their clinical manifestations.

Mediator	Clinical Manifestations
Serotonin	Vasoconstriction (coronary artery spasm, hypertension), increased intestinal tone, water and electrolyte imbalance (diarrhea), tryptophan deficiency (hypoproteinemia, pellagra)
Kallikrein	Vasodilation (hypotension, flushing), bronchoconstriction
Histamine	Vasodilation (hypotension, flushing), arrhythmias, bronchoconstriction

techniques or agents that could cause the tumor to release vasoactive substances. Regional anesthesia may limit the perioperative release of stress hormones. Large bolus doses of histamine-releasing drugs (eg, morphine and atracurium) should be avoided. Surgical manipulation of the tumor can cause a massive release of hormones. Monitoring likely will include an arterial line. We recommend transesophageal echocardiography if there are concerns about intrinsic heart disease caused by carcinoid syndrome. Alterations in carbohydrate metabolism may lead to hypoglycemia or hyperglycemia. Consultation with an endocrinologist may help clarify the role of antihistamine, antiserotonin drugs (eg, methysergide), octreotide (a long-acting somatostatin analogue), or antikallikrein drugs (eg, corticosteroids) in specific patients.

CASE DISCUSSION

Multiple Endocrine Neoplasia

An isolated thyroid nodule is discovered during physical examination of a 36-year-old woman who reports diarrhea and headaches. Workup of the tumor reveals hypercalcemia and an elevated calcitonin level, which leads to the diagnosis of medullary cancer of the thyroid and primary hyperparathyroidism. During induction of general anesthesia for total thyroidectomy, the patient's blood pressure rises to 240/140 mm Hg, and her heart rate approaches 140 beats/min, with frequent premature ventricular contractions. The operation is canceled, an arterial line is inserted, and the patient is treated with intravenous esmolol and nicardipine.

What could be the cause of this patient's hypertensive crisis during induction of general anesthesia?

Multiple endocrine neoplasia (MEN) is characterized by tumors in several endocrine organs. MEN type 1 consists of pancreatic (gastrinomas, insulinomas), pituitary, and parathyroid tumors. MEN type 2 consists of medullary thyroid carcinoma, pheochromocytoma, and hyperparathyroidism (type 2a) or multiple mucosal neuromas (type 2b or type 3). The hypertensive episode in this case may be due to a previously undiagnosed pheochromocytoma or paraganglioma. The pheochromocytoma in MEN may consist of multiple small tumors. These patients are typically young adults with strong family histories of MEN. If multiple surgeries are planned, pheochromocytoma resection will usually be scheduled first.

What is calcitonin, and why is it associated with medullary cancer?

Calcitonin is a polypeptide manufactured by the parafollicular cells (C cells) in the thyroid gland. It is secreted in response to increases in plasma ionic calcium and tends to lower calcium levels by affecting kidney and bone function. Therefore, it acts as an antagonist of parathyroid hormone (see Table 35–6).

Why is this patient hypercalcemic if calcitonin lowers serum calcium?

An excess or deficiency of calcitonin has minor effects in humans compared with the effects of parathyroid disorders. This patient's hypercalcemia is most likely due to coexisting primary hyperparathyroidism (MEN type 2a).

Are headache and diarrhea consistent with the diagnosis of MEN?

The history of headaches suggests the possibility of pheochromocytoma or paraganglioma, whereas diarrhea may be due to calcitonin or one of the other peptides often produced by medullary thyroid carcinoma (eg, ACTH, somatostatin, β-endorphin).

What follow-up is required for this patient?

Because of the life-threatening hemodynamic changes associated with pheochromocytoma, this entity must be medically controlled before any surgery can be considered (see Case Discussion, Chapter 14). Because MEN syndromes are hereditary, family members should be screened for early signs of pheochromocytoma, thyroid cancer, and hyperparathyroidism.

GUIDELINES

Practice guidelines for the perioperative management of patients with obstructive sleep apnea: an updated report by the American Society of Anesthesiologists task force on perioperative management of patients with obstructive sleep apnea. *Anesthesiology*. 2014;120:268.

Society for Ambulatory Anesthesia consensus statement on selection of patients with obstructive sleep apnea undergoing ambulatory surgery. http://www.sambahq.org/main/clinical-practice-guidelines/

SUGGESTED READINGS

Agus MS, Wypij D, Hirshberg EL, et al; HALF-PINT Study Investigators and the PALISI Network. Tight glycemic control in critically ill children. *N Engl J Med*. 2017;376:729.

Arlt W, Allolio B. Adrenal insufficiency. *Lancet*. 2003;361:1881.

Arterburn DE, Telem DA, Kushner RF, Courcoulas AP. Benefits and risks of bariatric surgery in adults: a review. *JAMA*. 2020;324:879.

Azim S, Kashyap SR. Bariatric surgery: pathophysiology and outcomes. *Endocrinol Metab Clin North Am*. 2016;45:905.

Blau JE, Collins MT. The PTH-vitamin D-FGF23 axis. *Rev Endocr Metab Disord*. 2015;16:165.

El-Menyar A, Mekkodathil A, Al-Thani H. Traumatic injuries in patients with diabetes mellitus. *J Emerg Trauma Shock*. 2016;9:64.

Fang F, Ding L, He Q, Liu M. Preoperative management of pheochromocytoma and paraganglioma. *Front Endocrinol* (Lausanne). 2020;11:586795.

Gunst J, De Bruyn A, Van den Berghe G. Glucose control in the ICU. *Curr Opin Anaesthesiol*. 2019;32:156.

Jones GC, Macklin JP, Alexander WD. Contraindications to the use of metformin. Evidence suggests that it is time to amend the list. *BMJ*. 2003;326:4.

Khan AA, Hanley DA, Rizzoli R, et al. Primary hyperparathyroidism: review and recommendations on evaluation, diagnosis, and management. A Canadian and international consensus. *Osteoporos Int*. 2017;28:1.

Kiernan CM, Solórzano CC. Pheochromocytoma and paraganglioma: diagnosis, genetics, and treatment. *Surg Oncol Clin N Am*. 2016;25:119.

King DR, Velmahos GC. Difficulties in managing the surgical patient who is morbidly obese. *Crit Care Med*. 2010;38:S478.

Kohl BA, Schwartz S. How to manage perioperative endocrine insufficiency. *Anesthesiol Clin*. 2010;28:139.

Moon TS, Joshi GP. Are morbidly obese patients suitable for ambulatory surgery? *Curr Opin Anaesthesiol*. 2016;29:141.

NICE-SUGAR Study Investigators, Finfer S, Chittock DR, et al. Intensive versus conventional glucose control in critically ill patients. *N Engl J Med*. 2009;360:1283.

Shifrin AL. Brief overview of calcium, vitamin d, parathyroid hormone metabolism, and calcium-sensing receptor function. In: Shifrin AL, ed. *Advances in Treatment and Management in Surgical Endocrinology*. Elsevier; 2020;63-70.

Van den Berghe G, Schetz M, Vlasselaers D, et al. Clinical review: intensive insulin therapy in critically ill patients: NICE-SUGAR or Leuven blood glucose target? *J Clin Endocrinol Metab*. 2009;94:3163.

Zaghiyan KN, Murrell Z, Melmed GY, Fleshner PR. High-dose perioperative corticosteroids in steroid-treated patients undergoing major colorectal surgery: necessary or overkill? *Am J Surg*. 2012;204:481.

Zaloga GP, Butterworth JF 4th. Hypovitaminosis D in hospitalized patients: a marker of frailty or a disease requiring treatment? *Anesth Analg*. 2014;119:613.

CHAPTER

36

Anesthesia for Ophthalmic Surgery

KEY CONCEPTS

1. Any factor that increases intraocular pressure in the setting of an open globe may cause drainage of aqueous or extrusion of vitreous through the wound, serious complications that can permanently damage vision.
2. Succinylcholine increases intraocular pressure by 5 to 10 mm Hg for 5 to 10 min after administration, principally through prolonged contracture of the extraocular muscles. However, in studies of hundreds of patients with open eye injuries, no patient experienced extrusion of ocular contents after administration of succinylcholine. Thus, succinylcholine is *not* contraindicated in cases of open eye injuries.
3. Traction on extraocular muscles, pressure on the eyeball, administration of a retrobulbar block, and trauma to the eye can elicit a wide variety of cardiac arrhythmias ranging from bradycardia and ventricular ectopy to sinus arrest or ventricular fibrillation.
4. Complications involving the intraocular expansion of gas bubbles injected by the ophthalmologist can be avoided by discontinuing nitrous oxide at least 15 min prior to the injection of air or sulfur hexafluoride or by avoiding the use of nitrous oxide entirely.
5. Medications applied topically to mucosa are absorbed systemically at a rate intermediate between absorption following intravenous and subcutaneous injection.
6. Echothiophate is an irreversible cholinesterase inhibitor now rarely used in the treatment of glaucoma. Topical application leads to systemic absorption and inhibition of plasma cholinesterase activity. Because succinylcholine is metabolized by this enzyme, echothiophate will prolong its duration of action.
7. The key to inducing anesthesia in a patient with an open eye injury is controlling intraocular pressure with a smooth induction. Coughing and gagging during intubation are avoided by first achieving a deep level of anesthesia and profound paralysis.
8. The postretrobulbar block apnea syndrome is probably due to the injection of local anesthetic into the optic nerve sheath, with spread into the cerebrospinal fluid.
9. Regardless of the anesthetic technique, American Society of Anesthesiologists standards for basic monitoring must be employed, and equipment and drugs necessary for airway management and resuscitation must be immediately available.

Ophthalmic surgery poses unique problems, including regulation of intraocular pressure, control of intraocular gas expansion, prevention of the oculocardiac reflex and management of its consequences, and management of systemic effects of ophthalmic drugs. Mastery of general and sedation anesthesia techniques for ophthalmic surgery and a thorough understanding of potentially complicating issues—including the comorbidities of an increasing geriatric patient population—are necessary for optimal perioperative outcomes. In addition, most ophthalmic procedures are performed under topical or regional anesthesia. The anesthesia practitioner must be familiar with their potential complications, including those of the accompanying sedation, even if not personally administering the topical anesthetic or the block.

TABLE 36–1 The effect of cardiac and respiratory variables on intraocular pressure (IOP).[1]

Variable	Effect on IOP
Central venous pressure	
Increase	↑↑↑
Decrease	↓↓↓
Arterial blood pressure	
Increase	↑
Decrease	↓
$PaCO_2$	
Increase (hypoventilation)	↑↑
Decrease (hyperventilation)	↓↓
PaO_2	
Increase	0
Decrease	↑

[1]↓, decrease (mild, moderate, marked); ↑, increase (mild, moderate, marked); 0, no effect.

INTRAOCULAR PRESSURE DYNAMICS

Physiology of Intraocular Pressure

The eye can be considered a hollow sphere with a rigid wall. If the contents of the sphere increase, the normal intraocular pressure of 12 to 20 mm Hg will rise. For example, glaucoma is caused by an obstruction to aqueous humor outflow. Similarly, intraocular pressure will rise if the volume of blood within the globe is increased. A rise in venous pressure will increase intraocular pressure by decreasing aqueous drainage and increasing choroidal blood volume. Any event that alters arterial or central venous blood pressure or ventilation (eg, laryngoscopy, intubation, airway obstruction, coughing, Trendelenburg position) can adversely affect intraocular pressure (Table 36–1).

Compressing the globe without a proportional change in the volume of its contents will increase intraocular pressure. Pressure on the eye from a malpositioned mask, improper prone positioning, or retrobulbar hemorrhage can lead to a marked increase in intraocular pressure, possible eye pain, and temporary or permanent visual changes.

Intraocular pressure helps maintain the shape and the optical properties of the eye. Temporary variations in pressure are normally well tolerated. For example, blinking raises intraocular pressure by 5 mm Hg, and squinting (forced contraction of the orbicularis oculi muscles) may transiently increase intraocular pressure greater than 50 mm Hg. However, even brief episodes of increased intraocular pressure in patients with underlying low ophthalmic artery pressure (eg, from systemic hypotension or arteriosclerotic involvement of the retinal artery) may cause retinal ischemia.

When the globe is opened by surgical incision (Table 36–2) or traumatic perforation, intraocular pressure approaches atmospheric pressure. Any factor

1 that increases intraocular pressure in the setting of an open globe may cause drainage of aqueous or extrusion of vitreous through the wound, serious complications that can permanently damage vision.

TABLE 36–2 Open-eye surgical procedures.

Cataract extraction
Corneal laceration repair
Corneal transplant (penetrating keratoplasty)
Peripheral iridectomy
Removal of foreign body
Ruptured globe repair
Secondary intraocular lens implantation
Trabeculectomy (and other filtering procedures)
Vitrectomy (anterior and posterior)
Wound leak repair

Effect of Anesthetic Drugs on Intraocular Pressure

Most anesthetic drugs either reduce intraocular pressure or have no effect (Table 36–3). Intraocular pressure decreases with inhalational anesthetics in proportion to anesthetic depth. There are multiple causes for this. Decreased blood pressure reduces choroidal volume, relaxation of the extraocular muscles lowers wall tension, and pupillary constriction facilitates aqueous outflow. Intravenous anesthetics also decrease intraocular pressure, with the exception of ketamine, which usually raises arterial blood pressure and does not relax extraocular muscles.

Topically administered anticholinergic drugs result in pupillary dilation (mydriasis), which may precipitate or worsen angle-closure glaucoma. However, systemically administered atropine or glycopyrrolate for premedication is not associated with intraocular hypertension, even in patients with glaucoma.

2 Succinylcholine increases intraocular pressure by 5 to 10 mm Hg for 5 to 10 min after administration, principally through prolonged contracture of the extraocular muscles. However, in studies of hundreds of patients with open eye injuries, no patient experienced extrusion of ocular contents after administration of succinylcholine. Thus, succinylcholine is *not* contraindicated in cases of open eye injuries. Nevertheless, dogma often trumps data, and ophthalmic surgeons may request that it not be administered in certain circumstances. Unlike other skeletal muscles, extraocular muscles contain myocytes with multiple neuromuscular junctions, and depolarization of these cells by succinylcholine causes prolonged contracture. The resulting increase in intraocular pressure may have several effects: it will cause spurious measurements of intraocular pressure during examinations under anesthesia in glaucoma patients, potentially leading to unnecessary surgery, and prolonged contracture of the extraocular muscles may result in an abnormal forced duction test, a maneuver utilized in strabismus surgery to evaluate the cause of extraocular muscle imbalance and to determine the type of surgical correction. Nondepolarizing neuromuscular blockers (NMBs) do not increase intraocular pressure, and we advocate that succinylcholine be reserved for rapid-sequence induction.

TABLE 36–3 The effect of anesthetic agents on intraocular pressure (IOP).[1]

Drug	Effect on IOP
Inhaled anesthetics	
Volatile agents	↓↓
Nitrous oxide	↓
Intravenous anesthetics	
Propofol	↓↓
Benzodiazepines	↓↓
Ketamine	?
Opioids	↓
Muscle relaxants	
Succinylcholine	↑↑
Nondepolarizers	0/↓

[1]↓, decrease (mild, moderate); ↑, increase (mild, moderate); 0/↓, no change or mild decrease; ?, conflicting reports.

THE OCULOCARDIAC REFLEX

3 Traction on extraocular muscles, pressure on the eyeball, administration of a retrobulbar block, and trauma to the eye can elicit a wide variety of cardiac arrhythmias ranging from bradycardia and ventricular ectopy to sinus arrest or ventricular fibrillation. This *oculocardiac reflex* consists of a trigeminal (V_1) afferent and a vagal efferent pathway and is most commonly encountered in children undergoing strabismus surgery, though it can be evoked in all age groups and during a variety of ocular procedures. In awake patients, the oculocardiac reflex may be accompanied by nausea.

Routine prophylaxis for the oculocardiac reflex is controversial, especially in adults. Anticholinergic medication may prevent the oculocardiac reflex. Intravenous atropine or glycopyrrolate given immediately before traction on extraocular muscles is more effective than intramuscular premedication administered preoperatively. However, anticholinergic medication should be administered with caution to any patient who has or may have coronary artery disease because of the potential for an increase in heart rate sufficient to induce myocardial ischemia. Ventricular tachycardia and ventricular fibrillation following the administration of anticholinergic medication have also been reported. Retrobulbar blockade or deep inhalational anesthesia may also preempt the oculocardiac reflex, though administration of a retrobulbar block may itself initiate the oculocardiac reflex.

Management of the oculocardiac reflex includes (1) immediate notification of the surgeon and cessation of surgical stimulation until heart rate recovers; (2) confirmation of adequate ventilation, oxygenation, and depth of anesthesia; (3) administration of intravenous atropine (10 mcg/kg) if bradycardia persists; and (4) in recalcitrant episodes, infiltration of the rectus muscles with local anesthetic.

INTRAOCULAR GAS EXPANSION

A gas bubble may be injected by the ophthalmologist into the posterior chamber during vitreous surgery. Intravitreal air injection will tend to flatten a detached retina and facilitate anatomically correct healing. Nitrous oxide administration is contraindicated in this circumstance: The bubble will increase in size if nitrous oxide is administered because nitrous oxide is 35 times more soluble than nitrogen in blood (see Chapter 8). Thus, it tends to diffuse into an air bubble more rapidly than nitrogen (the major component of air) is absorbed by the bloodstream. If the bubble expands after the globe is closed, intraocular pressure will rise.

Sulfur hexafluoride is an inert gas that is less soluble in blood than is nitrogen—and much less soluble than nitrous oxide. Its longer duration of action (up to 10 days) compared with an air bubble can provide a therapeutic advantage. The bubble size doubles within 24 h after injection because nitrogen from inhaled air enters the bubble more rapidly than the sulfur hexafluoride diffuses into the bloodstream. Even so, unless high volumes of pure sulfur hexafluoride are injected, the slow bubble expansion does not typically increase intraocular pressure. If the patient is breathing nitrous oxide, however, the bubble will rapidly increase in size and may lead to intraocular hypertension. A 70% inspired nitrous oxide concentration will almost triple the size of a 1-mL bubble and may double the pressure in a closed eye within 30 min. Subsequent discontinuation of nitrous oxide will lead to reabsorption of the bubble, which has become a mixture of nitrous oxide and sulfur hexafluoride. The consequent fall in intraocular pressure could precipitate another retinal detachment.

Complications involving the intraocular expan-
4 sion of gas bubbles can be avoided by discontinuing nitrous oxide at least 15 min before the injection of air or sulfur hexafluoride or by avoiding the use of nitrous oxide entirely. Nitrous oxide should be avoided until the bubble is absorbed (5 days after air and 10 days after sulfur hexafluoride injection). We believe avoiding nitrous oxide entirely is the simplest approach in these patients.

SYSTEMIC EFFECTS OF OPHTHALMIC DRUGS

Topically applied eye drops are systemically absorbed by vessels in the conjunctival sac and the nasolacrimal duct mucosa (see Case Discussion, Chapter 13). One drop (typically, approximately 1/20 mL) of 10% phenylephrine contains approximately 5 mg of this drug. Compare this dose with the intravenous dose of phenylephrine (0.05–0.1 mg) used to treat an adult patient with acute hypotension. Medications
5 applied topically to mucosa are absorbed systemically at a rate intermediate between absorption following intravenous and subcutaneous injection. The two patient populations most likely to require eye surgery, pediatric and geriatric, are at particular risk of the toxic effects of topically applied medications and should receive at most a 2.5% phenylephrine solution (Table 36–4).

Echothiophate (phospholine iodide) is an irre-
6 versible cholinesterase inhibitor now rarely used in the treatment of glaucoma. Topical application leads to systemic absorption and inhibition of plasma cholinesterase activity. *Because succinylcholine is metabolized by this enzyme, echothiophate will prolong its duration of action.* Paralysis usually will not exceed 20 to 30 min, and postoperative apnea is unlikely. The inhibition of cholinesterase activity lasts for 3 to 7 weeks after the discontinuation of echothiophate drops. Muscarinic side effects of echothiophate, such as bradycardia during induction, can be prevented with intravenous anticholinergic drugs (eg, atropine or glycopyrrolate).

TABLE 36–4 Systemic effects of ophthalmic medications.

Drug	Mechanism of Action	Potential Adverse Effect
Acetylcholine	Cholinergic agonist (miosis)	Bronchospasm, bradycardia, hypotension
Acetazolamide	Carbonic anhydrase inhibitor (decreases IOP[1])	Diuresis, hypokalemic metabolic acidosis
Atropine	Anticholinergic (mydriasis)	Central anticholinergic syndrome[2]
Cyclopentolate	Anticholinergic (mydriasis)	Disorientation, psychosis, convulsions
Echothiophate	Cholinesterase inhibitor (miosis, decreases IOP)	Prolongation of succinylcholine and mivacurium paralysis, bronchospasm
Epinephrine	Sympathetic agonist (mydriasis, decreases IOP)	Hypertension, bradycardia, tachycardia, headache
Phenylephrine	α-Adrenergic agonist (mydriasis, vasoconstriction)	Hypertension, tachycardia, dysrhythmias
Scopolamine	Anticholinergic (mydriasis, vasoconstriction)	Central anticholinergic syndrome[2]
Timolol	β-Adrenergic blocking agent (decreases IOP)	Bradycardia, asthma, congestive heart failure

[1]IOP, intraocular pressure.

[2]See Case Discussion, Chapter 13.

Epinephrine eye drops can cause hypertension, tachycardia, and ventricular arrhythmias; the arrhythmogenic effects are potentiated by halothane. Direct instillation of epinephrine into the anterior chamber of the eye has not been associated with cardiovascular toxicity.

Timolol, a nonselective β-adrenergic antagonist, reduces intraocular pressure by decreasing the production of aqueous humor. Topically applied timolol eye drops, commonly used to treat glaucoma, will often result in a reduced heart rate. In rare cases, timolol has been associated with atropine-resistant bradycardia, hypotension, and bronchospasm during general anesthesia.

General Anesthesia for Ophthalmic Surgery

The choice between general and local anesthesia should be made jointly by the patient, anesthesiologist, and surgeon. Patients may refuse to consider local anesthesia due to fear of being awake during the operation, fear of the eye block procedure, or unpleasant recall of a previous eye block or local eye procedure. General anesthesia is indicated in children and uncooperative patients as even small head movements can prove disastrous during microsurgery.

PREMEDICATION

Patients undergoing eye surgery may be apprehensive; however, premedication must be administered with caution and only after careful consideration of the patient's medical status. Patients are often older adults with systemic illnesses such as hypertension, diabetes mellitus, and coronary artery disease, and pediatric patients may have associated congenital disorders.

INDUCTION

The choice of induction technique for eye surgery usually depends more on the patient's coexisting medical problems than on the patient's eye disease or the specific operation contemplated. One exception is the patient with a ruptured globe. The key to

7 inducing anesthesia in a patient with an open eye injury is controlling intraocular pressure with a smooth induction. Specifically, coughing during intubation must be avoided by first achieving a deep level of anesthesia and profound paralysis.

The intraocular pressure response to laryngoscopy and endotracheal intubation can be moderated by prior administration of intravenous lidocaine (1.5 mg/kg), an opioid (eg, remifentanil 0.5–1 mcg/kg or alfentanil 20 mcg/kg), or esmolol (0.5–1.5 mg/kg). A nondepolarizing muscle relaxant or succinylcholine may be used. Many patients with open globe injuries have full stomachs and require a rapid-sequence induction technique to avoid aspiration (see the later Case Discussion). Despite theoretical concerns, succinylcholine does not increase the likelihood of vitreous loss with open eye injuries.

MONITORING & MAINTENANCE

Eye surgery often necessitates positioning the anesthesia provider away from the patient's airway, making close monitoring of pulse oximetry and the capnograph especially important. Endotracheal tube kinking, breathing circuit disconnection, and unintentional extubation may be more likely because of the surgeon working near the airway. The risk of endotracheal tube kinking and obstruction can be minimized by using a preformed oral RAE (Ring-Adair-Elwyn) endotracheal tube (Figure 36–1). The possibility of arrhythmias caused by the oculocardiac reflex increases the importance of closely monitoring the electrocardiogram.

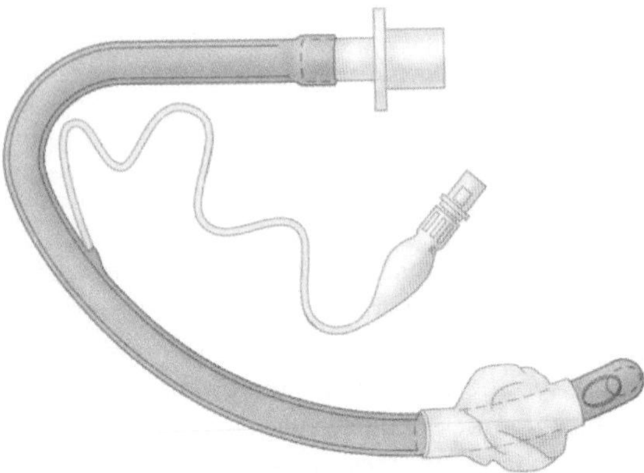

FIGURE 36–1 An oral RAE (Ring-Adair-Elwyn) endotracheal tube has a preformed right-angle bend at the level of the teeth so that it exits the mouth away from the surgical field during ophthalmic or nasal surgery.

In contrast to most other types of pediatric surgery, infant body temperature may rise during ophthalmic surgery because of head-to-toe draping and minimal body surface exposure. End-tidal CO_2 analysis helps differentiate this iatrogenic hyperthermia from malignant hyperthermia.

The pain and stress evoked by eye surgery are considerably less than during a major surgical procedure. "Lighter" anesthesia might be attractive if the consequences of patient movement were not so potentially catastrophic. The lack of cardiovascular stimulation inherent in most eye procedures combined with the need for adequate anesthetic depth can result in hypotension in older adults. This problem is usually addressed by ensuring adequate intravenous hydration and adequate depth of anesthesia and administrating intravenous vasoconstrictors to maintain blood pressure. Administration of nondepolarizing muscle relaxants to avoid patient movement is often used in such circumstances to allow a reduced depth of general anesthesia, but it mandates strict attention to the extent of neuromuscular blockade.

Emesis caused by vagal stimulation is a common postoperative problem following eye surgery, particularly with strabismus repair. The Valsalva effect and the increase in central venous pressure that accompany vomiting can be detrimental to the surgical result. Prophylactic administration of drugs that prevent postoperative nausea and vomiting is strongly recommended.

EXTUBATION & EMERGENCE

A smooth emergence from general anesthesia is important to minimize the risk of postoperative wound dehiscence. Coughing or gagging due to the endotracheal tube can be minimized by extubating the patient at a moderately deep level of anesthesia. As the time of extubation approaches, intravenous lidocaine (1.5 mg/kg) may be given to blunt cough reflexes temporarily. Extubation proceeds 1 to 2 min after the lidocaine administration and during spontaneous ventilation with 100% oxygen. Proper airway maintenance is crucial until the patient's cough and swallowing reflexes return.

Severe discomfort is unusual following eye surgery. Scleral buckling procedures, enucleation, and ruptured globe repair are the most painful operations. Modest incremental doses of intravenous opioid usually provide sufficient analgesia. The surgeon should be alerted if severe pain is noted following emergence from general anesthesia as it may signal intraocular hypertension, corneal abrasion, or other surgical complications.

Regional Anesthesia for Ophthalmic Surgery

Options for local anesthesia for eye surgery include topical application of local anesthetic or placement of a *retrobulbar*, *peribulbar*, or *sub-Tenon (episcleral) block*. Each of these techniques is commonly combined with intravenous sedation. Local anesthesia is preferred to general anesthesia for eye surgery because local anesthesia involves less physiological trespass and is less likely to be associated with postoperative nausea and vomiting. However, eye block procedures have potential complications and may not provide adequate ophthalmic akinesia or analgesia. Some patients may be unable to lie perfectly still for the duration of the surgery. For these reasons, the appropriate equipment and qualified personnel required to treat the complications of local anesthesia and induce general anesthesia must be readily available.

RETROBULBAR BLOCKADE

In this technique, local anesthetic is injected behind the eye into the cone formed by the extraocular muscles (Figure 36–2), and a facial nerve block is utilized to prevent blinking (Figure 36–3). A blunt-tipped 25-gauge needle penetrates the lower lid at the

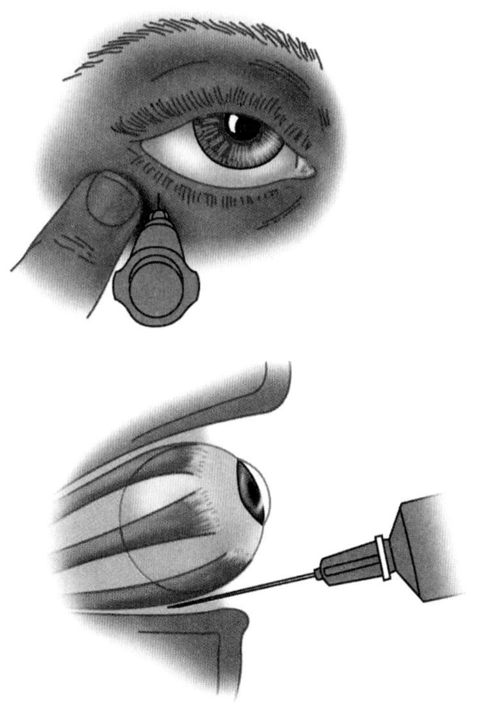

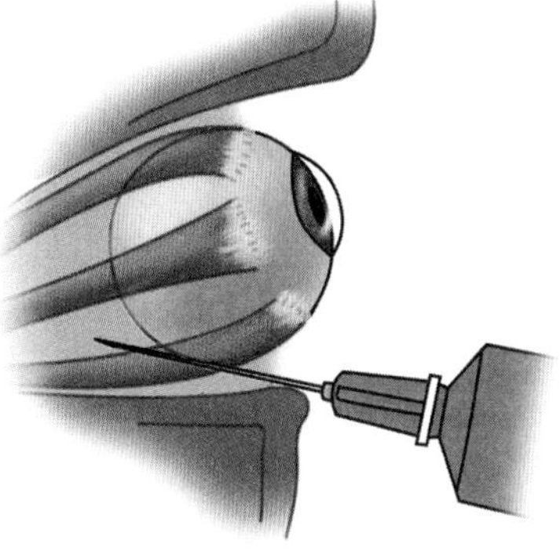

FIGURE 36–2 **A**: During the administration of a retrobulbar block, the patient looks supranasally as a needle is advanced 1.5 cm along the inferotemporal wall of the orbit. **B**: The needle is then redirected upward and nasally toward the apex of the orbit and advanced until its tip penetrates the muscle cone.

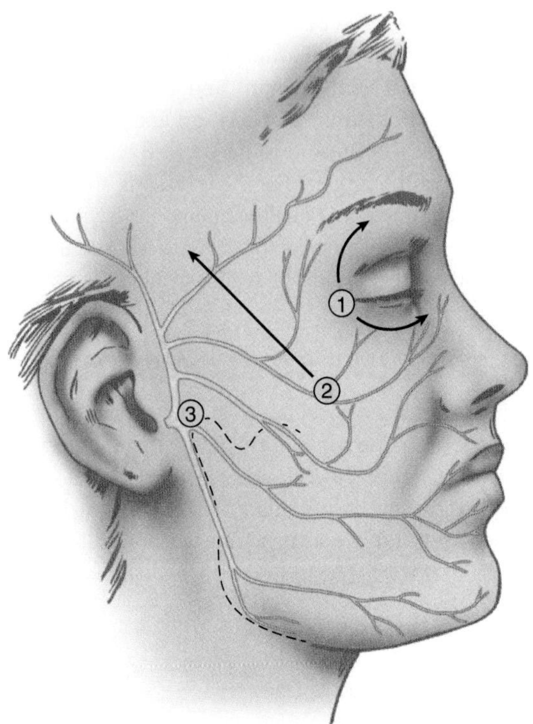

FIGURE 36–3 Facial nerve block techniques: van Lint (1), Atkinson (2), and O'Brien (3).

junction of the middle and lateral one-third of the orbit (usually 0.5 cm medial to the lateral canthus). Awake patients are instructed to stare supranasally as the needle is advanced toward the apex of the muscle cone. Commonly, patients undergoing such eye blocks will receive a brief period of deep sedation or general anesthesia during the block (using such agents as etomidate or propofol). After aspiration of the syringe to preclude intravascular injection, 2 to 5 mL of local anesthetic is injected, and the needle is removed. Choice of local anesthetic varies, but lidocaine 2% or bupivacaine (or ropivacaine) 0.75% are common. The addition of epinephrine may reduce bleeding and prolong the anesthesia. A successful retrobulbar block is accompanied by anesthesia, akinesia, and abolishment of the *oculocephalic reflex* (ie, the blocked eye does not move during head turning).

Complications of retrobulbar injection of local anesthetics include retrobulbar hemorrhage, perforation of the globe, optic nerve injury, intravascular injection with resultant convulsions, oculocardiac reflex, trigeminal nerve block, respiratory arrest, and, rarely, acute neurogenic pulmonary edema. Forceful injection of local anesthetic into the ophthalmic artery causes retrograde flow toward the brain and may result in an instantaneous seizure. 8 The *postretrobulbar block apnea syndrome* is probably due to injection of local anesthetic into the optic nerve sheath, with spread into the cerebrospinal fluid. In this situation, the central nervous system is exposed to high concentrations of local anesthetic, leading to mental status changes that may include unconsciousness. Apnea occurs within 20 min and resolves within an hour. Treatment is supportive, with positive-pressure ventilation to prevent hypoxia, bradycardia, and cardiac arrest. Adequacy of ventilation must be constantly monitored in patients who have received retrobulbar anesthesia.

The adjuvant *hyaluronidase* is frequently added to local anesthetic solutions used in eye blocks to enhance the spread and density of the block. Patients may rarely experience an allergic reaction to hyaluronidase. Retrobulbar hemorrhage, cellulitis, occult injury, and contact allergy to topical eye drops must be ruled out in the differential diagnosis. Retrobulbar injection is usually not performed in patients with bleeding disorders or receiving anticoagulation therapy because of the risk of retrobulbar hemorrhage, extreme myopia because the elongated globe increases the risk of perforation, or an open eye injury because the pressure from injecting fluid behind the eye may cause extrusion of intraocular contents through the wound.

PERIBULBAR BLOCKADE

In contrast to retrobulbar blockade, with the peribulbar blockade technique, the needle does not penetrate the cone formed by the extraocular muscles. Advantages of the peribulbar technique include less risk of penetration of the globe, optic nerve, and artery and less pain on injection. Disadvantages include a slower onset and an increased likelihood of ecchymosis. Both techniques will have equal success at producing akinesia of the eye.

The peribulbar block is performed with the patient supine and looking directly ahead (or possibly

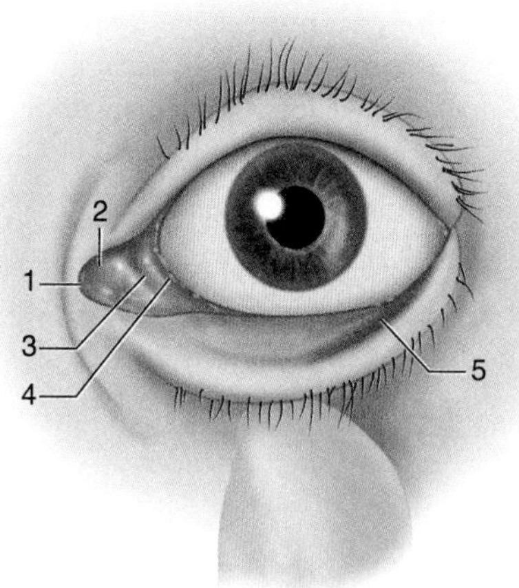

FIGURE 36–4 Anatomic landmarks for the introduction of a needle or catheter in most frequently employed eye blocks: (1) medial canthus peribulbar anesthesia, (2) lacrimal caruncle, (3) semilunaris fold of the conjunctiva, (4) medial canthus episcleral anesthesia, and (5) inferior and temporal peribulbar anesthesia.

under a brief period of deep sedation). After topical anesthesia of the conjunctiva, one or two transconjunctival injections are administered (Figure 36–4). As the eyelid is retracted, an inferotemporal injection is given halfway between the lateral canthus and the lateral limbus. The needle is advanced under the globe, parallel to the orbital floor; when it passes the equator of the eye, it is directed slightly medial (20°) and cephalad (10°), and 5 mL of local anesthetic is injected. To ensure akinesia, the anesthesia provider may give a second 5-mL injection through the conjunctiva on the nasal side, medial to the caruncle, and directed straight back parallel to the medial orbital wall, pointing slightly cephalad (20°).

Sub-Tenon (Episcleral) Block

Tenon's fascia surrounds the globe and extraocular muscles. Local anesthetic injected beneath it into the episcleral space spreads circularly around the sclera and to the extraocular muscle sheaths (see Figure 36–4). A special blunt curved cannula is used for a sub-Tenon block. After topical anesthesia, the conjunctiva is lifted along with Tenon's fascia in the inferonasal quadrant with forceps. A small nick is then made with blunt-tipped scissors, which are then slid underneath to create a path in Tenon's fascia that follows the contour of the globe and extends past the equator. While the eye is still fixed with forceps, the cannula is inserted, and 3 to 4 mL of local anesthetic is injected. Complications with sub-Tenon blocks are significantly less than with retrobulbar and peribulbar techniques. Globe perforation, hemorrhage, cellulitis, permanent visual loss, and local anesthetic spread into cerebrospinal fluid have been reported.

FACIAL NERVE BLOCK

A facial nerve block prevents squinting of the eyelids during surgery and allows placement of a lid speculum. There are several techniques of facial nerve block: *van Lint, Atkinson*, and *O'Brien* (see Figure 36–3). The major complication of these blocks is subcutaneous hemorrhage. The *Nadbath technique* blocks the facial nerve as it exits the stylomastoid foramen under the external auditory canal, in close proximity to the vagus and glossopharyngeal nerves. This block is not recommended because it has been associated with vocal cord paralysis, laryngospasm, dysphagia, and respiratory distress.

TOPICAL ANESTHESIA OF THE EYE

Increasingly, the trend has been to use simple topical local anesthetic techniques for anterior chamber (eg, cataract) and glaucoma operations rather than local anesthetic injections. A typical regimen for topical local anesthesia involves the application of 0.5% proparacaine (also known as *proxymetacaine*) local anesthetic drops, repeated at 5-min intervals for five applications, followed by the topical application of a local anesthetic gel (lidocaine plus 2% methyl-cellulose) with a cotton swab to the inferior and superior conjunctival sacs. Ophthalmic 0.5% tetracaine may also be utilized. Topical anesthesia is not appropriate for posterior chamber surgery (eg, retinal detachment repair with a buckle), and it works best for faster surgeons using a gentle surgical technique that does not require akinesia of the eye.

INTRAVENOUS SEDATION

Many techniques of intravenous sedation are available for eye surgery, and the particular drug used is less important than the dose. Deep sedation, though sometimes used during placement of ophthalmic nerve blocks, is almost never used intraoperatively because of the risks of apnea, aspiration, and unintentional patient movement during surgery. An intraoperative light sedation regimen that includes small doses of midazolam, with or without fentanyl or sufentanil, is recommended. Doses vary considerably among patients but should be administered in small increments.

Patients may find the administration of eye blocks frightening and uncomfortable, and many anesthesia providers will administer small, incremental doses of propofol to produce a brief state of unconsciousness during the regional block. Some will substitute a bolus of opioid (remifentanil 0.1–0.5 mcg/kg or alfentanil 375–500 mcg) to produce a brief period of intense analgesia during the eye block procedure.

Administration of an antiemetic should be considered if an opioid is used. Regardless of the 9 anesthetic technique, American Society of Anesthesiologists standards for basic monitoring must be employed, and equipment and drugs necessary for airway management and resuscitation must be immediately available.

CASE DISCUSSION

An Approach to a Patient with an Open Eye & a Full Stomach

A 12-year-old boy is brought to the emergency department after being shot in the eye with a pellet gun. A brief examination by the ophthalmologist reveals intraocular contents leaking from the wound. The boy is scheduled for emergency repair of the ruptured globe.

What should be emphasized in the preoperative evaluation of this patient?

Aside from taking a medical history and performing a physical examination, the time of last oral intake before or after the injury should be established. The patient must be considered to have a full stomach if the injury occurred within 8 h after the last meal, even if the patient did not eat for several hours after the injury: Gastric emptying is delayed by pain and anxiety that follows trauma.

What is the significance of a full stomach in a patient with an open globe injury?

Managing patients who have sustained penetrating eye injuries provides a challenge because of the need to deal with at least two conflicting objectives: (1) preventing further damage to the eye by avoiding increases in intraocular pressure and (2) preventing pulmonary aspiration in a patient with a full stomach. However, many of the common strategies used to achieve these objectives are in conflict with one another (Tables 36–5 and 36–6). For example, although regional anesthesia (eg, retrobulbar block) minimizes the risk of aspiration pneumonia, it is relatively contraindicated in patients with penetrating eye injuries because injecting local anesthetic behind the globe increases intraocular pressure and may lead to the expulsion of intraocular contents. Therefore, these patients require general anesthesia—despite the increased risk of aspiration pneumonia.

TABLE 36–5 Strategies to prevent increases in intraocular pressure (IOP).

Avoid direct pressure on the globe
Patch eye with Fox shield
No retrobulbar or peribulbar injections
Careful face mask technique
Avoid increases in central venous pressure
Prevent coughing during induction and intubation
Ensure a deep level of anesthesia and relaxation prior to laryngoscopy[1]
Avoid head-down positions
Extubate under deep anesthesia[1]
Avoid pharmacological agents that increase IOP

[1]These strategies are not recommended in patients with full stomachs.

TABLE 36–6 Strategies to prevent aspiration pneumonia.

Regional anesthesia with minimal sedation[1]
Premedication
Metoclopramide
Histamine H_2-receptor antagonists
Nonparticulate antacids
Evacuation of gastric contents
Nasogastric tube[1]
Rapid-sequence induction
Cricoid pressure
Rapid induction with rapid onset of paralysis
Avoidance of positive-pressure ventilation via mask
Intubation as soon as possible
Extubation awake

[1]Not recommended for patients with penetrating eye injuries.

What preoperative preparation should be considered in this patient?

One clearly will want to minimize the risk of aspiration pneumonia by decreasing gastric volume and acidity (see Case Discussion, Chapter 17). The risk of aspiration in patients with eye injuries is reduced by proper selection of drugs and anesthetic techniques. Evacuation of gastric contents with a nasogastric tube in an awake or sedated patient may lead to coughing, retching, and other responses that can dramatically increase intraocular pressure.

Metoclopramide increases lower esophageal sphincter tone, speeds gastric emptying, lowers gastric fluid volume, and exerts an antiemetic effect. It should be given intravenously (10 mg) as soon as possible and repeated every 2 to 4 h until surgery.

Ranitidine (50 mg intravenously), cimetidine (300 mg intravenously), and famotidine (20 mg intravenously) are H_2-receptor antagonists that inhibit gastric acid secretion. Because they have no effect on the pH of gastric secretions present in the stomach prior to their administration, they have limited value in patients presenting for emergency surgery.

Unlike H_2-receptor antagonists, antacids have an immediate effect. Unfortunately, they increase intragastric volume. Nonparticulate antacids (preparations of sodium citrate, potassium citrate, and citric acid) lose effectiveness within 30 to 60 min and should be given immediately prior to induction (15–30 mL orally).

Which induction agents are recommended in patients with penetrating eye injuries?

The ideal induction agent for patients with full stomachs would provide a rapid onset of action to minimize the risk of regurgitation. Propofol and etomidate have essentially equally rapid onsets of action and lower intraocular pressure. Although investigations of the effects of ketamine on intraocular pressure have provided conflicting results, ketamine is not recommended in penetrating eye injuries because of the increased risk of blepharospasm and nystagmus.

Although etomidate may prove valuable in some patients with cardiac disease, it is associated with an incidence of myoclonus ranging from 10% to 60%. An episode of severe myoclonus may have contributed to complete retinal detachment and vitreous prolapse in a report of one patient with an open globe injury and limited cardiovascular reserve.

Propofol has a rapid onset of action and decreases intraocular pressure; however, it does not entirely prevent the hypertensive response to laryngoscopy and intubation or the increase in intraocular pressure that accompanies laryngoscopy and intubation. Prior administration of fentanyl (1–3 mcg/kg), remifentanil (0.5–1 mcg/kg), alfentanil (20 mcg/kg), esmolol (0.5–1.5 mg/kg), or lidocaine (1.5 mg/kg) attenuates this response with varying degrees of success.

How does the choice of muscle relaxant differ between these patients and other patients at risk of aspiration?

Succinylcholine moderately increases intraocular pressure, but that is a small price to pay for a rapid onset of profound muscle relaxation that decreases the risk of aspiration or of a Valsalva response during intubation. Advocates of succinylcholine point to the lack of evidence documenting further eye injury when succinylcholine has been used with open eye injuries.

Nondepolarizing muscle relaxants do not increase intraocular pressure, but the onset of deep muscle relaxation is slower than with succinylcholine. Regardless of the muscle relaxant chosen, intubation should not be attempted until a level of paralysis is achieved that will reliably prevent coughing on the endotracheal tube.

How do induction strategies vary in pediatric patients without intravenous access?

A hysterical child with a penetrating eye injury and a full stomach provides an anesthetic challenge for which there is no perfect solution. Once again, the dilemma is due to the need to avoid increases in intraocular pressure yet minimize the risk of aspiration. Screaming and crying can lead to marked increases in intraocular pressure. Attempting to sedate children with rectal suppositories or intramuscular injections often heightens their state of agitation and may worsen the eye injury. Similarly, although preoperative sedation may increase the risk of aspiration by obtunding airway reflexes, it is often necessary to establish an intravenous line for a rapid-sequence induction. Although difficult to achieve, an ideal strategy would be to administer enough sedation painlessly to allow the placement of an intravenous line yet maintain a level of consciousness adequate to protect airway reflexes. However, the most prudent strategy is to do everything reasonable to avoid aspiration—even at the cost of further eye damage.

Are there special considerations during extubation and emergence?

Patients at risk of aspiration during induction are also at risk during extubation and emergence. Therefore, extubation must be delayed until the patient is awake and has intact airway reflexes (eg, spontaneous swallowing and coughing on the endotracheal tube). Deep extubation increases the risk of vomiting and aspiration. Intraoperative administration of antiemetic medication and nasogastric or orogastric tube suctioning may decrease the incidence of emesis during emergence, but they do not guarantee an empty stomach.

SUGGESTED READINGS

Alhassan MB, Kyari F, Ejere HO. Peribulbar versus retrobulbar anaesthesia for cataract surgery. *Cochrane Database Syst Rev*. 2015;(7):CD004083.

Ascaso F, Peligero J, Longas J, et al. Regional anesthesia of the eye, orbit, and periocular skin. *Clin Dermatol.* 2015;33:227.

Bryant J, Busbee B, Reichel E. Overview of ocular anesthesia: past and present. *Curr Opin Ophthalmol.* 2011;22:180.

Chua MJ, Lersch F, Chua AWY, Kumar CM, Eke T. Sub-Tenon's anaesthesia for modern eye surgery-clinicians' perspective, 30 years after re-introduction. *Eye* (Lond). 2021;35:1295.

Connor MA, Menke AM, Vrcek I, Shore JW. Operating room fires in periocular surgery. *Int Ophthalmol.* 2018;38:1085.

Gayer S, Palte HD. Ultrasound-guided ophthalmic regional anesthesia. *Curr Opin Anesthesiol.* 2016;29:655.

Kelly DJ, Farrell SM. Physiology and role of intraocular pressure in contemporary anesthesia. *Anesth Analg.* 2018;126:1551.

Kong K, Khan J. Ophthalmic patients on antithrombotic drugs: a review and guide to perioperative management. *Br J Ophthalmol.* 2015;99:1025.

Lee R, Thompson J, Eke T. Severe adverse events associated with local anesthesia in cataract surgery: 1 year national survey of practice and complications in the UK. *Br J Ophthalmol.* 2016;100:772.

Lesin M, Domazet Bugarin J, Puljak L. Factors associated with postoperative pain and analgesic consumption in ophthalmic surgery: a systematic review. *Surv Ophthalmol.* 2015;60:196.

Lesin M, Duplancic Sundov Z, Jukic M, et al. Postoperative pain in complex ophthalmic surgical procedures: comparing practice with guidelines. *Pain Med.* 2014;15:1036.

Lewis H, James I. Update on anaesthesia for paediatric ophthalmic surgery. *BJA Educ.* 2021;21(1):32.

Malafa M, Coleman J, Bowman RW, et al. Perioperative corneal abrasion: updated guidelines for prevention and management. *Plast Reconstr Surg.* 2016;137:790e.

Morris R, Sapp M, Oltmanns M, et al. Presumed air by vitrectomy embolisation (PAVE) a potentially fatal syndrome. *Br J Ophthalmol.* 2014;98:765.

Nasiri N, Sharifi H, Bazrafshan A, Noori A, Karamouzian M, Sharifi A. Ocular manifestations of COVID-19: a systematic review and meta-analysis. *J Ophthalmic Vis Res.* 2021;16:103.

Palte H. Ophthalmic regional blocks: management, challenges, and solutions. *Local Reg Anesth.* 2015;8:57.

Porela-Tiihonen S, Kaarniranta K, Kokki H. Postoperative pain after cataract surgery. *J Cataract Refract Surg.* 2013;39:789.

Riad W, Akbar F. Ophthalmic regional blockade complication rate: a single center audit of 33,363 ophthalmic operations. *J Clin Anesth.* 2012;24:193.

Singh RB, Khera T, Ly V, et al. Ocular complications of perioperative anesthesia: a review. *Graefes Arch Clin Exp Ophthalmol.* 2021;259:2069.

Spiteri N, Sidaras G, Czanner G, et al. Assessing the quality of ophthalmic anesthesia. *J Clin Anesth.* 2015;27:285.

Anesthesia for Otolaryngology–Head & Neck Surgery

CHAPTER 37

KEY CONCEPTS

1 The anesthetic goals for laryngeal endoscopy include an immobile surgical field and adequate masseter muscle relaxation for the introduction of the suspension laryngoscope (typically profound muscle paralysis will be sought), adequate oxygenation and ventilation, and cardiovascular stability despite periods of rapidly varying procedural stimulation.

2 During jet ventilation, chest wall motion must be monitored and sufficient exhalation time allowed to avoid air trapping and barotrauma.

3 The greatest concern of laser airway surgery is an airway fire. This risk can be moderated by minimizing the fraction of inspired oxygen (FiO_2 <30% if tolerated by the patient) and can be eliminated when there is no combustible material (eg, flammable endotracheal tube, catheter, or dry cotton pledget) in the airway.

4 Techniques to minimize intraoperative blood loss include topical vasoconstriction with cocaine or an epinephrine-containing local anesthetic for vasoconstriction, maintaining a slightly head-up position, and providing a mild degree of controlled hypotension.

5 If there is serious preoperative concern regarding potential airway problems, intravenous induction may be avoided in favor of awake direct or fiberoptic laryngoscopy (cooperative patient) or direct or fiberoptic intubation following an inhalational induction, maintaining spontaneous ventilation (uncooperative patient). In any case, the appropriate equipment and qualified personnel required for emergency tracheostomy must be immediately available.

6 The surgeon may request the omission of neuromuscular blockade during neck dissection, thyroidectomy, or parotidectomy to allow nerve identification (eg, spinal accessory, facial nerves) by direct nerve stimulation and thereby facilitate their preservation.

7 Manipulation of the carotid sinus and stellate ganglion during radical neck dissection has been associated with wide swings in blood pressure, bradycardia, arrhythmias, sinus arrest, and prolonged QT intervals. Infiltration of the carotid sheath with local anesthetic will usually moderate these problems. Bilateral neck dissection may result in postoperative hypertension and loss of hypoxic drive due to denervation of the carotid sinuses and bodies.

8 Patients undergoing maxillofacial reconstruction or orthognathic surgical procedures often pose airway challenges. If there are any anticipated signs of problems with mask ventilation or tracheal intubation, the airway should be secured prior to induction of general anesthesia.

—Continued next page

Continued—

 9 If there is a risk of postoperative edema involving structures that could obstruct the airway (eg, tongue, pharynx), the patient should be closely observed and perhaps kept intubated.

10 Nitrous oxide is either entirely avoided during tympanoplasty or discontinued prior to graft placement.

Cooperation and communication between surgeon and anesthesia provider are critical for all surgery within or near the airway. Establishing, maintaining, and protecting the airway in the face of abnormal anatomy during a procedural intervention are demanding tasks. An understanding of airway anatomy (see Chapter 19) and an appreciation of common otorhinolaryngologic and maxillofacial procedures are invaluable in handling these anesthetic challenges successfully.

ENDOSCOPY

Endoscopy includes diagnostic and operative laryngoscopy and microlaryngoscopy (laryngoscopy aided by an operating microscope), esophagoscopy, and bronchoscopy (discussed in Chapter 25). Endoscopic procedures may be accompanied by laser surgery.

Preoperative Considerations

Patients presenting for upper airway endoscopic procedures are frequently being evaluated for voice disorders (often presenting as hoarseness), stridor, or hemoptysis. Possible diagnoses include foreign body aspiration, trauma to the aerodigestive tract, papillomas, tracheal stenosis, tumors, or vocal cord dysfunction. Thus, a preoperative medical history and physical examination, with particular attention to potential airway problems, must precede any decisions regarding the anesthetic plan. In some patients, flow–volume loop (see Chapter 6), radiographic, computed tomography, ultrasound, or magnetic resonance imaging studies may be available for review or need to be requested. Many patients will have undergone preoperative indirect laryngoscopy or fiberoptic nasopharyngoscopy, and the information gained from these procedures is often of critical importance.

Important initial questions that must be answered are whether positive-pressure ventilation via face or laryngeal mask is feasible and whether the patient can be intubated using conventional direct or video laryngoscopy. If the answer to either question is "no" or "unlikely," the patient's airway should be secured prior to induction using an alternative technique such as awake fiberoptic bronchoscope or tracheostomy under local anesthesia (see Case Discussion, Chapter 19). However, even the initial securing of an airway with tracheostomy does not prevent intraoperative airway obstruction due to surgical manipulation, a foreign body, or hemorrhage.

Sedative premedication should be avoided in a patient with threatening upper airway obstruction. Glycopyrrolate (0.2–0.3 mg) works more effectively and persistently when given intramuscularly rather than intravenously 1 h before surgery and may prove helpful by minimizing secretions, thereby facilitating airway visualization.

Intraoperative Management

1 The anesthetic goals for laryngeal endoscopy include an immobile surgical field and adequate masseter muscle relaxation for the introduction of the suspension laryngoscope (typically profound muscle paralysis will be sought), adequate oxygenation and ventilation, and cardiovascular stability despite rapidly varying levels of procedural stimulation.

A. Muscle Relaxation

Intraoperative muscle relaxation can be achieved by intermittent boluses or infusion of intermediate-duration nondepolarizing neuromuscular blocking agents (NMBs) (eg, rocuronium, vecuronium, cisatracurium) or with a succinylcholine infusion. Rapid recovery is important as endoscopy is often an outpatient procedure. Given that profound muscle relaxation is often needed until the very end of the operative procedure, endoscopy remains one of the few remaining indications for succinylcholine infusions; however, the use of sugammadex (Bridion) to reverse profound degrees of rocuronium or vecuronium neuromuscular blockade has rendered succinylcholine infusion largely obsolete.

B. Oxygenation & Ventilation

Several methods have successfully been used to provide oxygenation and ventilation during endoscopy while simultaneously minimizing interference with the operative procedure. Most commonly, the patient is intubated with a small-diameter endotracheal tube through which conventional positive-pressure ventilation is administered. Standard endotracheal tubes of smaller diameters, however, are designed for pediatric patients and therefore are too short for the adult trachea and have a low-volume cuff that will exert increased pressure against the tracheal mucosa. A 4.0-, 5.0-, or 6.0-mm specialized microlaryngeal endotracheal tube (Mallinckrodt MLT) is the same length as an adult tube, has a disproportionately large high-volume low-pressure cuff, and is stiffer and less prone to compression than a conventional endotracheal tube of the same diameter. The advantages of intubation in endoscopy include protection against aspiration and the ability to administer inhalational anesthetics and continuously monitor end-tidal CO_2.

In some procedures, such as those involving the posterior commissure or vocal cords, intubation with an endotracheal tube may interfere with the surgeon's visualization or performance of the procedure. A simple alternative is insufflation of high flows of oxygen through a small catheter placed in the trachea. Although oxygenation may be maintained in patients with good lung function, ventilation will be inadequate for longer procedures unless the patient is allowed to breathe spontaneously.

Another option is the *intermittent apnea technique*, in which positive-pressure ventilation with oxygen by face mask or endotracheal tube is alternated with periods of apnea, during which the surgical procedure is performed. The duration of apnea, usually 2 to 3 min, is determined by how well the patient maintains oxygen saturation, as measured by pulse oximetry. Risks of this technique include hypoventilation with hypercarbia, failure to reestablish the airway, and pulmonary aspiration.

Another attractive alternative approach involves *manual jet ventilation* via a laryngoscope side port. During inspiration (1–2 s), a high-pressure (30–50 psi) jet of oxygen is directed through the glottic opening and entrains a mixture of oxygen and room air into the lungs (Venturi effect). Expiration (4–6 s duration) is passive. 2 Chest wall motion must be monitored and sufficient exhalation time allowed to avoid air trapping and barotrauma. This technique requires total intravenous anesthesia. A variation of this technique is *high-frequency jet ventilation*, which utilizes a small cannula or tube in the trachea, through which gas is injected 80 to 300 times per minute (see Chapter 58). Capnography will not provide an accurate estimate of end-tidal CO_2 during jet ventilation because of the constant and sizable dilution of alveolar gases.

C. Cardiovascular Stability

Blood pressure and heart rate often fluctuate markedly during endoscopic procedures for two reasons. First, some of the patients undergoing these procedures are older adults with a long history of heavy tobacco and alcohol use that predisposes them to cardiovascular disease. In addition, the endoscopic procedure is, in essence, a series of physiologically stressful laryngoscopies and interventions, separated by varying periods of minimal surgical stimulation. Attempting to maintain a constant level of anesthesia invariably results in alternating intervals of hypertension and hypotension. Providing a modest baseline level of anesthesia allows supplementation with short-acting anesthetics (eg, propofol, remifentanil) or sympathetic antagonists (eg, esmolol), or both, as needed during periods of intense stimulation. Less commonly, some anesthesia providers utilize a regional nerve block of the glossopharyngeal nerve and superior laryngeal nerve to help minimize intraoperative swings in blood pressure (see Case Discussion, Chapter 19).

Laser Precautions

Laser light differs from ordinary light in three ways: It is monochromatic (possesses one wavelength), coherent (oscillates in the same phase), and collimated (exists as a narrow parallel beam). These characteristics offer the surgeon excellent precision and hemostasis with minimal postoperative edema or pain. Unfortunately, lasers introduce several major hazards into the operating room environment.

The uses and side effects of a laser vary with its wavelength, which is determined by the medium in which the laser beam is generated. For example, a CO_2 laser produces a long wavelength (10,600 nm), whereas yttrium–aluminum–garnet (YAG) lasers produce a shorter wavelength (1064 or 1320 nm). As the wavelength increases, absorption by water increases, and tissue penetration decreases. Thus, the effects of the CO_2 laser are much more localized and superficial than are those of the YAG laser.

General laser precautions include suction evacuation of toxic fumes (laser plume) from tissue vaporization because they have the potential to transmit microbial diseases. When a significant laser plume is generated, individually fitted respiratory filter masks compliant with U.S. Occupational Safety and Health Administration (OSHA) standards should be worn by all operating room personnel. In addition, during laser procedures, all operating room personnel should wear laser eye protection appropriate for the type of laser used, and the patient's eyes should be taped shut. Operating room windows should be covered, and appropriately placed signage should be used to alert those entering the room that a laser device is in use.

3 The greatest risk of laser airway surgery is an airway fire. This risk can be moderated by minimizing the fraction of inspired oxygen (FiO_2 <30% if tolerated by the patient) and can be eliminated when there is no combustible material (eg, flammable endotracheal tube, catheter, or dry cotton pledget) in the airway. If an endotracheal tube is used, it must be relatively resistant to laser ignition (Table 37–1). Such specialized endotracheal tubes not only resist laser beam strikes but also possess double cuffs that should be inflated with saline instead of air to better absorb thermal energy and reduce the risk of ignition. If the proximal cuff is struck by the laser and the saline escapes, the distal cuff will continue to seal the airway. Alternatively, endotracheal tubes can be wrapped with a variety of metallic tapes; however, this is a suboptimal practice and should be avoided whenever the use of a specialized, commercially available, flexible, stainless steel, laser-resistant endotracheal tube is possible (Table 37–2).

Although specialized, laser-resistant endotracheal tubes may be used, it must be emphasized that *no endotracheal tube or currently available endotracheal tube protection device is reliably laser-proof. Therefore, whenever laser airway surgery is being*

TABLE 37–1 Advantages and disadvantages of various endotracheal tubes for laser airway surgery.

Type of Tube	Advantages	Disadvantages
Polyvinyl chloride	Inexpensive, nonreflective	Low melting point, highly combustible[1]
Red rubber	Puncture-resistant, maintains structure, nonreflective	Highly combustible[1]
Silicone rubber	Nonreflective	Combustible,[1] turns to toxic ash
Metal	Combustion-resistant,[1] kink-resistant	Thick-walled flammable cuff, transfers heat, reflects laser, cumbersome

[1]Combustibility depends on fraction of inspired oxygen and laser energy.

TABLE 37–2 Disadvantages of wrapping a tracheal tube with metallic tape.

No cuff protection
Adds thickness to tube
Not a device approved by the US Food and Drug Administration
Protection varies with type of metal foil
Adhesive backing may ignite
May reflect laser onto nontargeted tissue
Rough edges may damage mucosal surfaces

performed with an endotracheal tube in place, the following precautions should be observed:

- Inspired oxygen concentration should be as low as possible by utilizing air in the inspired gas mixture (many patients tolerate an FiO_2 of 21%).
- Nitrous oxide supports combustion and must not be used.
- The endotracheal tube cuffs should be filled with saline. Some practitioners add methylene blue to the saline to make cuff rupture more obvious. A well-sealed, cuffed endotracheal tube will minimize the oxygen concentration in the pharynx.
- Laser intensity and duration should be limited as much as possible.
- Saline-saturated pledgets, though potentially flammable, should be placed in the airway to limit the risk of endotracheal tube ignition and damage to adjacent tissue.
- A source of water (eg, water-filled 60-mL syringe and basin) should be immediately available in case of fire.

These precautions limit but do not eliminate the risk of an airway fire; anesthesia providers must proactively address the hazard of fire whenever laser or electrocautery is utilized near the airway (Table 37–3).

If an airway fire should occur, all air/oxygen should immediately be turned off at the anesthesia gas machine, and burning combustible material (eg, an endotracheal tube) must be removed from the airway. The fire can be extinguished with saline, and the patient's airway must be examined to be certain that all foreign body fragments have been removed.

TABLE 37–3 Airway fire protocol.

1. Stop ventilation and remove tracheal tube.
2. Turn off oxygen and disconnect circuit from machine.
3. Submerge tube in water.
4. Ventilate with face mask and reintubate.
5. Assess airway damage with bronchoscopy, serial chest x-rays, and arterial blood gases.
6. Consider bronchial lavage and steroids.

NASAL & SINUS SURGERY

Common nasal and sinus surgeries include polypectomy, endoscopic sinus surgery, maxillary sinusotomy (Caldwell–Luc procedure), rhinoplasty, and septoplasty.

Preoperative Considerations

Patients undergoing nasal or sinus surgery may have a considerable degree of preoperative nasal obstruction caused by polyps, a deviated septum, or mucosal congestion from infection. This may make face mask ventilation difficult, particularly if combined with other causes of difficult ventilation (eg, obesity, maxillofacial deformities).

Nasal polyps are often associated with allergic disorders, such as asthma. Patients who also have a history of allergic reactions to aspirin should not be given any nonsteroidal anti-inflammatory drugs (including ketorolac) for postoperative analgesia. Nasal polyps are a common feature of cystic fibrosis.

Because of the rich vascular supply of the nasal mucosa, the preoperative interview should concentrate on questions concerning medication use (eg, aspirin, clopidogrel) and any history of bleeding problems.

Intraoperative Management

Many nasal procedures can be satisfactorily performed under local anesthesia with sedation. The anterior ethmoidal nerve and sphenopalatine nerves (see Figure 19–3) provide sensory innervation to the nasal septum and lateral walls. Both can be blocked by packing the nose with gauze or cotton-tipped applicators soaked with local anesthetic. The topical anesthetic should be allowed to remain in place at least 10 min before instrumentation is attempted. Supplementation with submucosal injections of local anesthetic is often required. Use of an epinephrine-containing or cocaine solution will shrink the nasal mucosa and potentially decrease intraoperative blood loss. Intranasal cocaine (maximum dose, 3 mg/kg), though providing both excellent anesthesia and vasoconstriction of the nasal mucosa, is rapidly absorbed, reaching peak systemic blood levels in 30 min, and may be associated with cardiovascular side effects (see Chapter 16).

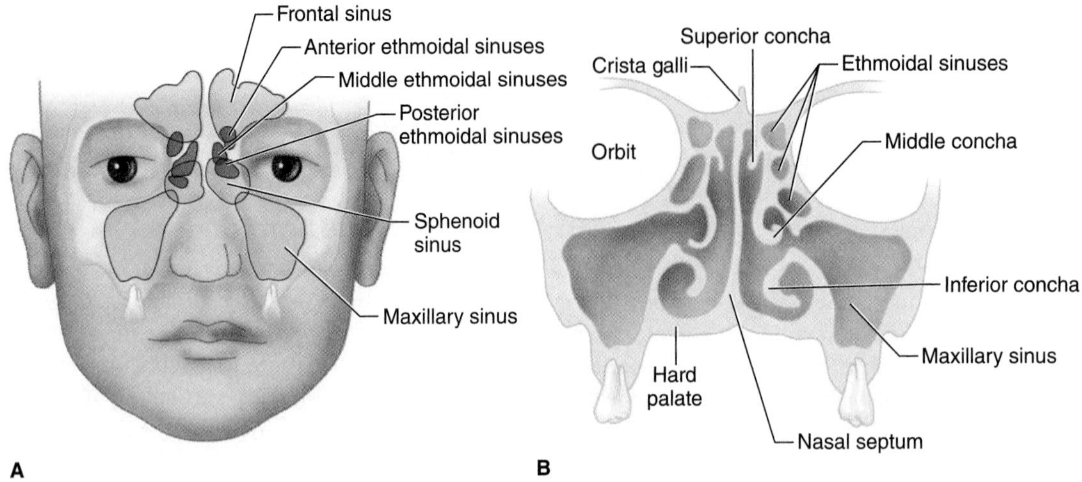

FIGURE 37–1 Orbital fracture is a risk of endoscopic sinus surgery because of the proximity of the sinuses to the orbit (**A**, frontal view; **B**, coronal section). (Modified with permission from Snell RS, Katz J. *Clinical Anatomy for Anesthesiologists.* New York, NY: Appleton & Lange; 1988.)

General anesthesia is often preferred for nasal surgery because of the discomfort and incomplete block that may accompany topical anesthesia. Special considerations during and shortly following induction include using an oral airway during face mask ventilation to mitigate the effects of nasal obstruction, intubating with a reinforced or preformed Mallinckrodt oral RAE (Ring–Adair–Elwyn) endotracheal tube (see Figure 36–1), and tucking the patient's padded arms, with protection of the fingers, to the side. Because of the proximity of the surgical field, it is important to tape the patient's eyes closed to avoid corneal abrasion. One exception to this occurs during dissection in endoscopic sinus surgery, when the surgeon may wish to periodically check for eye movement because of the close proximity of the sinuses and orbit (Figure 37–1); nonetheless, the eyes should remain protected until the surgeon is ready to observe them. NMBs are often utilized because of potential neurological or ophthalmic injury that may occur if the patient moves during sinus instrumentation.

4 Techniques to minimize intraoperative blood loss include topical vasoconstriction with cocaine or an epinephrine-containing local anesthetic, maintaining a slightly head-up position and providing a mild degree of controlled hypotension. A posterior pharyngeal pack is often placed to limit the risk of aspiration of blood. Despite these precautions, the anesthesia provider must be prepared for major blood loss, especially during resection of vascular tumors (eg, juvenile nasopharyngeal angiofibroma).

Coughing or straining during emergence from anesthesia and extubation should be avoided as these events will increase venous pressure and increase postoperative bleeding. However, relatively deep extubation strategies that are commonly and appropriately utilized to accomplish this goal may increase the risk of aspiration.

HEAD & NECK CANCER SURGERY

Surgery for cancer of the head and neck includes laryngectomy, glossectomy, pharyngectomy, parotidectomy, hemimandibulectomy, and radical neck dissection. An endoscopic examination following induction of anesthesia often precedes these surgical procedures. Timing of a tracheostomy, if planned, depends upon the patient's preoperative airway compromise. Some procedures may include extensive reconstructive surgery, such as the transplantation of a free microvascular muscle flap, with long surgical time duration.

Preoperative Considerations

The typical patient presenting for head and neck cancer surgery is older and often has had many years of heavy tobacco and alcohol use. Those patients without a history of extensive tobacco and alcohol use will usually have been infected with human papillomavirus. Common coexisting medical conditions include chronic obstructive pulmonary disease, coronary artery disease, hypertension, diabetes, alcoholism, and malnutrition. These patients will benefit from an enhanced recovery after surgery program that includes preoperative nutritional repletion over the course of several days and hydration with a carbohydrate–protein drink during the 24 h period prior to surgery.

Airway management may be complicated by abnormal airway anatomy, possibly including an obstructing lesion, or by preoperative radiation therapy that has fibrosed and distorted the patient's airway
5 structures. If there is concern regarding potential airway problems, intravenous induction may be avoided in favor of awake direct or fiberoptic laryngoscopy (cooperative patient) or direct or fiberoptic intubation following an inhalational induction, maintaining spontaneous ventilation (uncooperative patient). Elective tracheostomy under local anesthesia prior to induction of general anesthesia is often a prudent option, all the more so since many head and neck cancer surgeries will conclude with a temporary or permanent tracheostomy, anyway. In any case, the appropriate equipment and qualified personnel required for emergency tracheostomy must be *immediately* available during anesthetic induction for head and neck cancer operations where a difficult airway is known or suspected and the induction is not preceded by tracheostomy.

Intraoperative Management

A. Monitoring

Because many of these procedures are lengthy and associated with substantial blood loss and because of the prevalence of coexisting cardiopulmonary disease, arterial cannulation may be utilized for blood pressure monitoring and for obtaining blood periodically for laboratory analyses. If central venous access is deemed necessary, the surgeon should be consulted to ascertain that planned internal jugular or subclavian venous access will not interfere with the intended surgical procedures; antecubital or femoral veins are reasonable alternatives. Arterial lines and intravenous cannulas should not be placed in the operative arm if a radial forearm flap is planned. A minimum of two large-bore intravenous lines and a urinary catheter (preferably with temperature-monitoring capability) should be placed. As the arms are typically secured next to the patient's sides for these procedures, the continued functionality of upper extremity arterial and intravenous lines should be verified prior to placement of the sterile surgical drapes. A forced-air warming blanket should be used to help maintain normal body temperature. Intraoperative hypothermia and consequent vasoconstriction can be detrimental to the perfusion of a microvascular free flap.

Intraoperative nerve monitoring is increasingly utilized by surgeons in anterior neck operations to help preserve the superior laryngeal, recurrent laryngeal, and vagus nerves (Figure 37–2), and the anesthesia provider may be asked to place a specialized nerve integrity monitor endotracheal tube (Medtronic Xomed NIM endotracheal tube) to facilitate this process (Figure 37–3).

B. Tracheostomy

Head and neck cancer surgery often includes tracheostomy. Immediately prior to surgical entry into the trachea, the endotracheal tube and hypopharynx should be thoroughly suctioned to limit the risk of aspiration of blood and secretions. If electrocautery is used during the surgical dissection, the FiO_2 should be lowered to 30% or less, if possible, to minimize the risk of fire as the trachea is entered. In any case, the easiest way to minimize airway fire risk in this circumstance is for the surgeon *not* to use electrocautery to enter the trachea. After dissection down to the trachea, the endotracheal tube cuff is deflated to avoid perforation by the scalpel. When the tracheal wall is transected, the endotracheal tube is withdrawn so that its tip is immediately cephalad to the incision. Ventilation during this period is difficult because of the large leak through the tracheal incision. A sterile, cuffed tracheostomy tube is placed in the trachea, the cuff is inflated, and the tube is connected to a sterile breathing circuit extension. As soon as the correct position is confirmed by capnography and bilateral chest auscultation, the original endotracheal

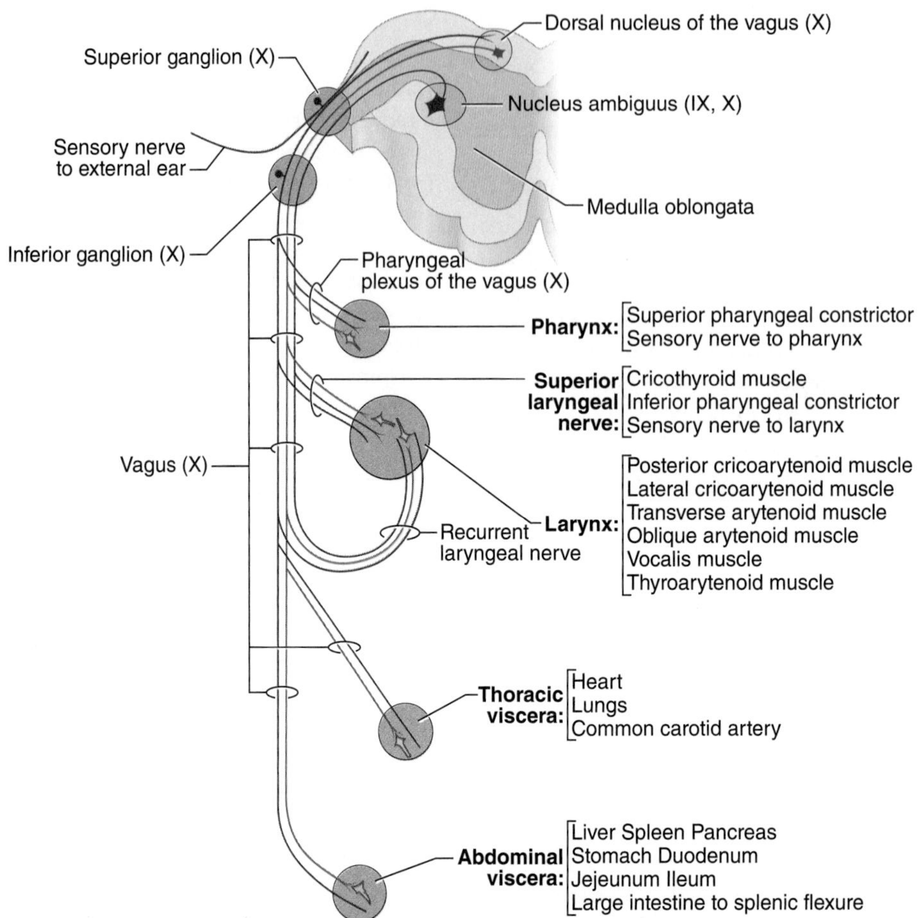

FIGURE 37–2 The **vagus nerve** (cranial nerve X) originates in the medulla oblongata and then ramifies in the superior and inferior vagal ganglia in the neck. Its first major branch is the pharyngeal plexus of the vagus. The **superior laryngeal nerve** divides into the external and internal laryngeal nerves. The *internal branch* supplies sensory innervation of the laryngeal mucosa above the vocal cords, and the *external branch* innervates the inferior pharyngeal constrictor muscles and the cricothyroid muscle of the larynx. Cricothyroid muscle contraction increases the voice pitch by lengthening, tensing, and adducting the vocal folds. The superior laryngeal nerve is at risk of damage during operations of the anterior neck, especially thyroid surgery, and injury to this nerve may result in hoarseness and loss of vocal volume. The next branch of the vagus is the **recurrent laryngeal nerve**, which innervates all of the muscles of the larynx except the cricothyroid, and is responsible for phonation and glottic opening. The recurrent laryngeal nerve runs immediately behind the thyroid gland and thus is the nerve at greatest risk for injury during thyroid surgery. Unilateral recurrent laryngeal nerve damage may result in vocal changes or hoarseness, and bilateral nerve damage may result in aphonia and respiratory distress. Inferior to this nerve, the vagus nerve provides autonomic motor and sensory nerve fibers to the thoracic and abdominal viscera. (Reproduced with permission from Dillon FX. Electromyographic (EMG) neuromonitoring in otolaryngology-head and neck surgery. *Anesthesiol Clin.* 2010 Sep;28(3):423-442.)

tube may be entirely removed. An increase in peak inspiratory pressure immediately after tracheostomy usually indicates a malpositioned endotracheal tube, bronchospasm, debris or secretions in the trachea, or, rarely, pneumothorax.

C. Maintenance of Anesthesia

6 The surgeon may request the omission of NMBs during neck dissection, thyroidectomy, or parotidectomy to allow nerve identification (eg, spinal accessory, facial nerves) by direct nerve

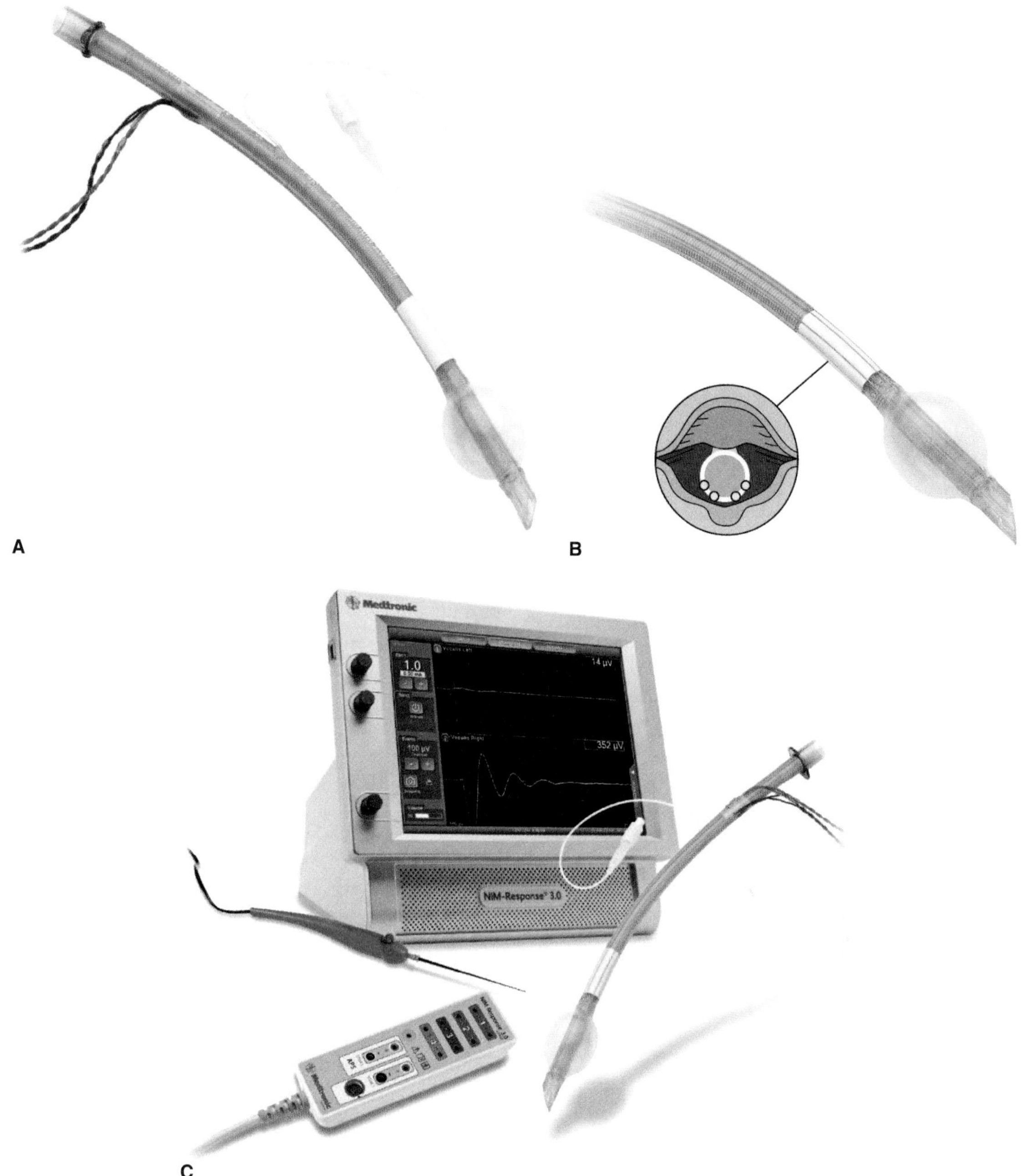

FIGURE 37–3 **A**: The Medtronic Xomed NIM electromyographic (EMG) nerve integrity monitoring endotracheal tube. Succinylcholine (or no relaxant at all) should be used for intubation, and the endotracheal tube should be secured in the midline. If lubricant is used, it must not contain local anesthetics. **B**: A slightly larger endotracheal tube size should be used to facilitate mucosal contact with the electrodes, and the electrode band of the NIM tube must be positioned at the level of the vocal cords. **C**: Nerve integrity is continuously monitored via EMG activity (Medtronic Xomed NIM-Response 3.0 Nerve Integrity Monitor). Nondepolarizing muscle relaxants are contraindicated because they prevent EMG monitoring. (Reproduced with permission from Medtronic Xomed.)

stimulation and thereby facilitate their preservation. If a nerve integrity monitor endotracheal tube is utilized, succinylcholine (or propofol with no relaxant) may be used to facilitate intubation. Moderate controlled hypotension may be helpful in limiting blood loss; however, cerebral perfusion may be compromised with moderate hypotension when a tumor invades the carotid artery or jugular vein (the latter may increase cerebral venous pressure). If the head-up tilt is utilized, it is important that the arterial blood pressure transducer be zeroed at the level of the brain (external auditory meatus) to determine cerebral perfusion pressure most accurately. In addition, head-up tilt increases the risk of venous air embolism.

Following reanastomosis of a microvascular free flap, blood pressure should be maintained at the patient's baseline level. The use of vasoconstrictive agents (eg, phenylephrine) should be minimized because of the potential decrease in flap perfusion due to vasoconstriction. Similarly, the use of vasodilators (eg, sodium nitroprusside or hydralazine) should be avoided to minimize any decrease in graft perfusion pressure.

D. Transfusion

Transfusion decisions must balance the patient's immediate surgical risks with the possibility of an increased cancer recurrence rate resulting from transfusion-induced immune suppression. Rheological factors make a moderately low hematocrit (eg, 27–30%) desirable when microvascular free flaps are performed. Excessive diuresis should be avoided during microvascular free-flap surgery to optimize graft perfusion in the postoperative period.

E. Cardiovascular Instability

7 Manipulation of the carotid sinus and stellate ganglion during radical neck dissection has been associated with wide swings in blood pressure, bradycardia, arrhythmias, sinus arrest, and prolonged QT intervals. Infiltration of the carotid sheath with local anesthetic will usually moderate these problems. Bilateral neck dissection may result in postoperative hypertension and loss of hypoxic drive due to denervation of the carotid sinuses and carotid bodies.

Postoperative Management

The principal postoperative complications associated with head and neck cancer surgery include hypocalcemia secondary to acute hypoparathyroidism, threats to airway integrity secondary to hemorrhage, hematoma formation, and bilateral vocal cord palsy with stridor resulting from bilateral recurrent laryngeal nerve injury (see Chapter 35). Postoperative hypoparathyroidism is a common condition, resulting from injury to the parathyroid glands or their blood supply during thyroidectomy or neck dissection or from unintentional or intentional removal of all four parathyroid glands. It may be either symptomatic or asymptomatic, and it occurs transiently in up to 49% of thyroidectomy patients and is permanent in up to 33% of thyroidectomy patients. Symptoms and signs depend upon the rate of onset and severity of hypocalcemia. Clinical signs of acute, severe hypocalcemia include laryngospasm, bronchospasm, QT prolongation-related arrhythmias, and congestive heart failure. Neurological symptoms and signs range from circumoral paresthesia, distal extremity numbness, and carpopedal spasm to confusion, delirium, and seizure activity. Symptomatic hypocalcemia is a medical emergency and should be treated with intravenous calcium salts, whereas asymptomatic hypocalcemia may be treated with oral calcium preparations (see Chapter 49).

MAXILLOFACIAL RECONSTRUCTION & ORTHOGNATHIC SURGERY

Maxillofacial reconstruction is often required to correct the effects of trauma (eg, fractures of the mandible or maxilla) or developmental malformations or for radical cancer surgeries (eg, maxillectomy or mandibulectomy). Orthognathic procedures (eg, Le Fort osteotomies, mandibular osteotomies) for skeletal malocclusion share many of the same surgical and anesthetic techniques.

Preoperative Considerations

8 Patients undergoing maxillofacial reconstruction or orthognathic surgical procedures often pose airway challenges. Particular attention should be focused on jaw opening, mask

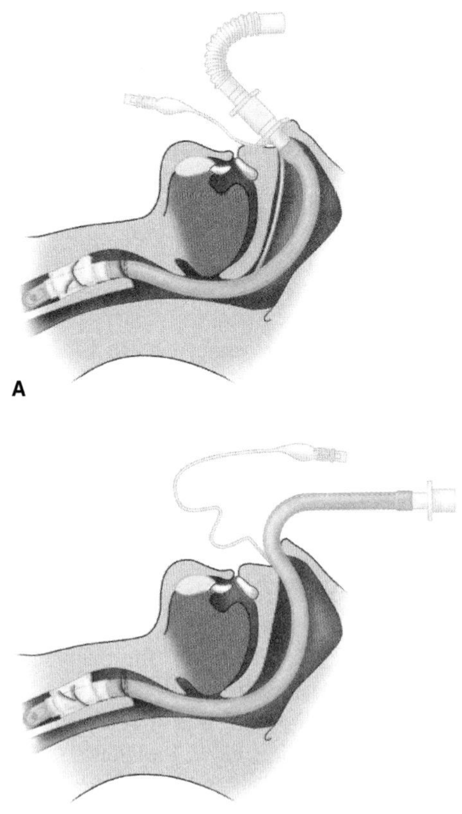

FIGURE 37–4 **A**: A regular straight endotracheal tube can be cut at the level of the nares and a flexible connector attached. **B**: Alternatively, a nasal RAE endotracheal tube has a preformed right-angle bend at the level of the nose so that the tube is directed over the forehead.

fit, neck mobility, micrognathia, retrognathia, maxillary protrusion (overbite), macroglossia, dental pathology, nasal patency, and the existence of any intraoral lesions or debris. If there are any anticipated signs of problems with mask ventilation or endotracheal intubation, the airway should be secured prior to induction of general anesthesia. This may involve fiberoptic nasal intubation, fiberoptic oral intubation, or tracheostomy with local anesthesia facilitated with cautious sedation. Nasal intubation with a straight tube with a flexible angle connector (Figure 37–4A) or a preformed nasal RAE (Figure 37–4B) tube is usually preferred in dental and oral surgery. The endotracheal tube can then be directed cephalad over the patient's forehead. With any nasal intubation, care should be taken to prevent the endotracheal tube from putting pressure on the tissues of the nasal opening, as this situation may result in local tissue pressure necrosis in the setting of a lengthy surgical procedure. Nasal intubation should be considered with caution in Le Fort II and III fractures because of the possibility of a coexisting basilar skull fracture (Figure 37–5).

Intraoperative Management

Maxillofacial reconstructive and orthognathic surgeries can be lengthy and involve substantial blood loss. An oropharyngeal ("throat") pack is often placed to minimize the amount of blood and other debris reaching the larynx and trachea, and one must remember to remove the pack at the end of surgery before the jaws are wired shut! Strategies to

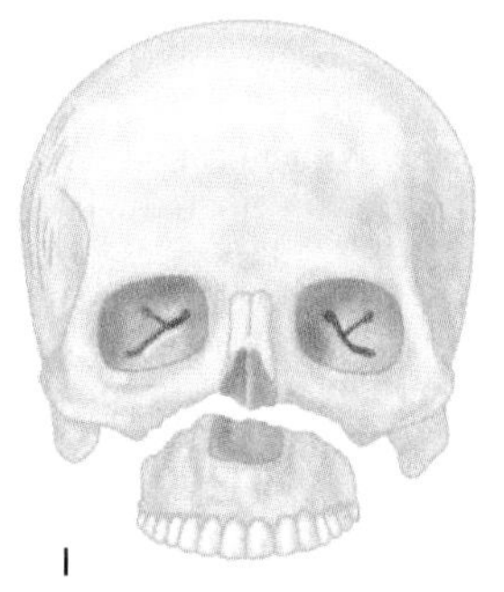

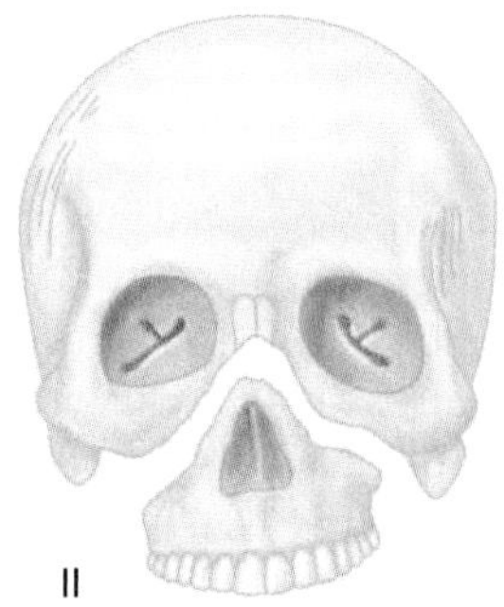

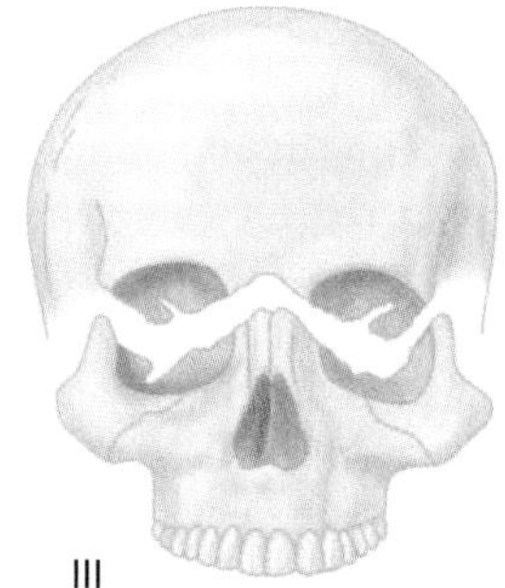

FIGURE 37–5 Diagrammatic representation of Le Fort I, II, and III fractures. Le Fort II and III fractures may coexist with a basilar skull fracture, a contraindication to nasal intubation.

minimize bleeding include a slight head-up position, controlled hypotension, and local infiltration with epinephrine solutions. Because the patient's arms are typically tucked at the side, two intravenous lines may be established prior to surgery. An arterial line is typically placed. As previously noted, if head-up tilt is utilized, it is important that the arterial blood pressure transducer be zeroed at the level of the brain (external auditory meatus) to determine cerebral perfusion pressure most accurately. In addition, the anesthesia provider must be alert to the increased risk of venous air embolism in the setting of head-up tilt.

Because of the proximity of the airway to the surgical field, positioning of surgical team personnel, and positioning of the patient's head often 90° or 180° away from the anesthesia provider, there is an increased risk of critical intraoperative airway problems, such as endotracheal tube kinking, disconnection, or perforation by a surgical instrument. Monitoring of end-tidal CO_2, peak inspiratory pressures, and breath sounds via an esophageal stethoscope assume greater importance in such cases. If the operative procedure is near the airway, the use of electrocautery or laser increases the risk of fire. At the end of surgery, the oropha-
9 ryngeal pack must be removed and the pharynx suctioned. If there is a risk of postoperative tissue edema involving structures that could potentially obstruct the airway (eg, tongue, pharynx), the patient should be closely observed and perhaps kept sedated and intubated for several hours postoperatively or overnight. In such uncertain situations, extubation may be performed over an endotracheal tube exchanger (eg, Cook Airway Exchange Catheter with Rapi-Fit Adapter, Cook Medical), which can facilitate reintubation and provide oxygenation in the setting of immediate postextubation respiratory obstruction. In addition, the operating team must be prepared for emergency tracheotomy or cricothyrotomy. Otherwise, extubation can be attempted once the patient is fully awake and there are no signs of continued bleeding. Patients with intermaxillary fixation (eg, maxillomandibular wiring) *must* have suction and appropriate wire cutting tools continuously at the bedside in case of vomiting or other airway emergencies. Extubating a patient whose jaws are wired shut and whose oropharyngeal pack has not been removed can lead to life-threatening airway obstruction. "Has the throat pack been removed?" should be asked before intermaxillary fixation is initiated and again before removing the endotracheal tube.

EAR SURGERY

Frequently performed ear surgeries include stapedectomy or stapedotomy, tympanoplasty, and mastoidectomy. Myringotomy with insertion of tympanostomy tubes is the most common pediatric surgical procedure and is discussed in Chapter 42.

Intraoperative Management

A. Nitrous Oxide

Nitrous oxide is not often used in anesthesia for ear surgery. Because nitrous oxide is more soluble than nitrogen in blood, it diffuses into air-containing cavities more rapidly than nitrogen (the major component of air) can be absorbed by the bloodstream (see Chapter 8). Normally, changes in middle ear pressures caused by nitrous oxide are well tolerated as a result of passive venting through the eustachian tube. However, patients with a history of chronic ear problems such as otitis media or sinusitis often have obstructed eustachian tubes and may, on rare occasions, experience hearing loss or tympanic membrane rupture from the administration of nitrous oxide anesthesia.

During tympanoplasty, the middle ear is open to the atmosphere, and there is no pressure buildup. However, once the surgeon has placed a tympanic membrane graft, the middle ear becomes a closed space, and if nitrous oxide is allowed to diffuse into any gas remaining in this space, middle ear pressure will rise, and the graft may be displaced. Conversely, discontinuing nitrous oxide after graft placement will create a negative middle ear pressure that could also cause graft dislodgment. Therefore,
10 nitrous oxide is either entirely avoided during tympanoplasty (which is our preference) or discontinued prior to graft placement. Obviously, the exact amount of time required to wash out the nitrous oxide depends on many factors, including alveolar ventilation and fresh gas flows (see Chapter 8), but 15 to 30 min is usually recommended.

B. Hemostasis

As with any form of microsurgery, even tiny amounts of blood can obscure the operating field. Techniques to minimize blood loss during ear surgery include mild (15°) head elevation, infiltration or topical application of epinephrine (1:50,000–1:200,000), and moderate controlled hypotension. Because coughing on the endotracheal tube during emergence (particularly during neck movement associated with head bandaging) will increase venous pressure and may cause bleeding and increased middle ear pressure, deep extubation is often utilized.

C. Facial Nerve Identification

Preservation of the facial nerve is an important consideration during some ear procedures, such as resection of a glomus tumor or acoustic neuroma. During such cases, intraoperative paralysis with NMBs will make identification of the facial nerve by direct nerve stimulation impossible. Thus, intraoperative paralysis should not be employed without discussion with the surgical team.

D. Postoperative Vertigo, Nausea, & Vomiting

Because the inner ear is intimately involved with the sense of balance, ear surgery may cause postoperative dizziness (vertigo) and postoperative nausea and vomiting (PONV). Induction and maintenance with propofol have been shown to decrease PONV in patients undergoing middle ear surgery. Prophylaxis with decadron prior to induction and a 5-HT_3 blocker prior to emergence should be considered. Patients undergoing ear surgery should be carefully assessed for vertigo postoperatively, and their ambulation should be closely monitored to minimize the risk of falling.

Oral Surgical Procedures

Most minor oral surgical procedures are performed in a clinic or office setting utilizing local anesthesia, augmented with varying degrees of sedation. If intravenous sedation is employed, or if the procedure is complex, a qualified anesthesia provider should be present. A qualified anesthesia provider *must* be present to administer deep sedation or general anesthesia if either is utilized. Typically, a bite block and an oropharyngeal throat pack protect the airway. For light to moderate levels of sedation, the oropharyngeal pack prevents irrigating fluids and dental debris from entering the airway. Deep sedation and general anesthesia require an increased level of airway management by a qualified anesthesia provider. Regardless of whether deep sedation or general anesthesia is inadvertent or intended, appropriate equipment, supplies, and medications *must* be immediately available to help ensure that any anticipated or unexpected anesthesia-related problem occurring in an office or clinic environment can be safely addressed with the same standard of care that is required in the hospital or ambulatory surgery center setting.

Minor oral surgical procedures, such as dental extractions, typically last no longer than 1 h. A nerve block or local anesthetic infiltration is typically utilized. In adults, most oral surgeons use 2% lidocaine with 1:100,000 epinephrine or 0.5% bupivacaine with 1:200,000 epinephrine in quantities no greater than 12 mL and 8 mL, respectively. Articaine is commonly used in Europe. The anesthesia provider must be informed by the surgeon of the local anesthetic used and its concentration and volume injected so that the allowed dosage based on patient weight is not exceeded. Pediatric patients are particularly at risk of local anesthesia toxicity due to excess local anesthetic dose administration or accidental intravascular injection.

Intravenous sedation during oral surgical procedures greatly increases the patient's comfort and facilitates surgery. Small doses of fentanyl and midazolam are usually adequate for adults prior to injection of the local anesthetic. The sedation can be further augmented by additional small dosages of fentanyl, midazolam, or a propofol infusion. Incremental doses of propofol, 20 to 30 mg for adults, are often used if the surgeon requires a brief episode of deep sedation or general anesthesia.

These techniques require a high level of cooperation and participation by both the surgeon and anesthesia provider. If there is the possibility of increased risk due to preexisting medical conditions, less than ideal airway, or extent of contemplated surgical procedure, it is safer to perform the procedure in a hospital or ambulatory surgery center setting with general endotracheal anesthesia.

CASE DISCUSSION

Bleeding Following Sinus Surgery

A 50-year-old man has a paroxysm of coughing in the postanesthesia care unit while awakening following uneventful endoscopic sinus surgery. Immediately afterward, his respirations seem labored with a loud inspiratory stridor.

What is the differential diagnosis of inspiratory stridor?

The acute onset of inspiratory stridor in a postoperative patient may be due to laryngospasm, laryngeal edema, foreign body aspiration, or vocal cord dysfunction. Laryngospasm, an involuntary spasm of the laryngeal musculature, may be triggered by blood or secretions stimulating the superior laryngeal nerve (see Chapter 19). Laryngeal edema may be caused by an allergic drug reaction, hereditary or iatrogenic angioedema, or a traumatic intubation. Vocal cord dysfunction could be due to residual muscle relaxant effect, hypocalcemic alkalotic tetany, intubation trauma, or paradoxical vocal cord motion.

Another paroxysm of coughing is accompanied by hemoptysis. What is your immediate management?

Bleeding after nose or throat surgery can be very serious. Patients who are not fully awake may continue to gag and cough on the secretions, increasing venous pressure and worsening the bleeding. Furthermore, they may aspirate blood and other secretions. Fortunately, because of its physiological pH, aspiration of blood is not as serious as aspiration of acidic gastric contents. Nonetheless, the airway should be immediately secured in the obtunded patient. This may be accomplished with an awake intubation or a rapid-sequence induction.

If the patient is awake and alert enough to cough and swallow and does not seem to be aspirating blood, the first priority should be to decrease the bleeding as quickly as possible. Immediate measures that should be considered include raising the head of the bed to decrease venous and arterial pressures at the site of bleeding and aggressively treating any degree of systolic hypertension with intravenous antihypertensive agents. Sedation should be avoided so that airway reflexes are not compromised. The surgeon should be notified, and the operating room should be alerted as to the possibility of reoperation.

Despite these measures, the bleeding continues, and surgical intervention seems to be necessary. Describe your strategy for induction of anesthesia in this patient.

Before induction of general anesthesia in a bleeding patient, hypovolemia should be corrected. The degree of hypovolemia may be difficult to assess because much of the blood may be swallowed, but it can be estimated by changes in vital signs, postural hypotension, and hematocrit. Cross-matched blood should be readily available, and a second large-bore intravenous line should be secured. From an anesthetic standpoint, this is an entirely different patient than the one who presented for surgery initially: the patient now has a full stomach, is hypovolemic, and may be more difficult to intubate.

The preferred technique in this patient is a rapid-sequence induction. Induction drug choice (eg, ketamine, etomidate) and dosage should anticipate the possibility of hypotension from persistent hypovolemia. Qualified personnel and appropriate equipment for an emergency tracheostomy should be immediately available. An orogastric tube should be passed to decompress the stomach following induction and intubation.

Which arteries supply blood to the nose?

The arterial supply of the nose is provided by the internal maxillary artery and the anterior ethmoid artery. These may have to be ligated in uncontrollable epistaxis.

Describe extubation.

Because this patient is still at risk for aspiration, extubation should not be attempted until the patient has fully awakened and regained airway reflexes. Although it is desirable to limit coughing and "bucking" on the endotracheal tube during emergence, this may be difficult to achieve in the awakening patient. Intravenous lidocaine or dexmedetomidine may be helpful in this situation.

SUGGESTED READINGS

Acharya K. Rigid bronchoscopy in airway foreign bodies: value of the clinical and radiological signs. *Int Arch Otorhinolaryngol*. 2016;20:196.

Ahmen-Nusrath A. Anaesthesia for head and neck cancer surgery. *BJA Education*. 2017;17:383.

Akulian JA, Yarmus L, Feller-Kopman D. The role of cricothyrotomy, tracheostomy, and percutaneous tracheostomy in airway management. *Anesthesiol Clin*. 2015;33:357.

Baker P. Assessment before airway management. *Anesthesiol Clin*. 2015;33:257.

Bradley J, Lee GS, Peyton J. Anesthesia for shared airway surgery in children. *Paediatr Anaesth*. 2020;30:288.

Carlton DA, Govindaraj S. Anesthesia for functional endoscopic sinus surgery. *Curr Opin Otolaryngol Head Neck Surg*. 2017;25:24.

Charters P, Ahmad I, Patel A, et al. Anaesthesia for head and neck surgery: United Kingdom National Multidisciplinary Guidelines. *J Laryngol Otol*. 2016;130(suppl S2):S23.

Ehsan Z, Mahmoud M, Shott SR, Amin RS, Ishman SL. The effects of anesthesia and opioids on the upper airway: a systematic review. *Laryngoscope*. 2016;126:270.

Fang CH, Friedman R, White PE et al. Emergent awake tracheostomy–the five-year experience at an urban tertiary care center. *Laryngoscope*. 2015;125:2476.

Gerasimov M, Lee B, Bittner EA. Postoperative anterior neck hematoma (ANH): timely intervention is vital. *APSF Newsletter*. 2021;36:44.

Giovannitti JA Jr. Anesthesia for off-floor dental and oral surgery. *Curr Opin Anesthesiol*. 2016;29:519.

Groom P, Schofield L, Hettiarachchi, et al. Performance of emergency surgical front of neck airway access by head and neck surgeons, general surgeons, or anaesthetists: an *in situ* simulation study. *Br J Anaesth*. 2019;125:696.

Hassanein AG, Abdel Mabood AMA. Can submandibular tracheal intubation be an alternative to tracheotomy during surgery for major maxillofacial fractures? *J Oral Maxillofac Surg*. 2017;75:508e1.

Hemantkumar I. Anesthesia for laser surgery of the airway. *Int J Otorhinolaryngol Clin*. 2017;9:1.

Hsu J, Tan M. Anesthesia considerations in laryngeal surgery. *Int Anesthesiol Clin*. 2017;55:11.

Huh H, Park SJ, Lim HH, et al. Optimal anesthetic regimen for ambulatory laser microlaryngeal surgery. *Laryngoscope*. 2017;127:1135.

Johnson AP, Boscoe E, Cabrera-Muffly C. Local blocks and regional anesthesia in the head and neck. *Otolaryngol Clin North Am*. 2020;53:739.

Kakava K, Tournis S, Papadakis G, et al. Postsurgical hypoparathyroidism: a systemic review. *In Vivo*. 2016;30:171.

Kartush JM, Rice KS, Minahan RE, et al. Best practices in facial nerve monitoring. *Laryngoscope*. 2021;131:S1.

Lin S, McKenna SJ, Yao CF, Chen YR, Chen C. Effects of hypotensive anesthesia on reducing intraoperative blood loss, duration of operation, and quality of surgical field during orthognathic surgery: a systematic review and meta-analysis of randomized controlled trials. *J Oral Maxillofac Surg*. 2017;75:73.

Mitchell RM, Parikh SR. Hemostasis in tonsillectomy. *Otolaryngol Clin N Am*. 2016;49:615.

Morrison DR, Moore LS, Walsh EM. Perioperative pain management following otologic surgery. *Otolaryngol Clin North Am*. 2020;53:803.

Muse IO, Straker T. A comprehensive review of regional anesthesia for head and neck surgery. *J Head Neck Anesth*. 2021;5:e33.

Nirgude A, Hemantkumar I. Anesthetic considerations in micro laryngoscopy and direct laryngoscopy. *Int J Otorhinolaryngol Clin*. 2017;9:10.

O'Dell K. Predictors of difficult intubation and the otolaryngology perioperative consult. *Anesthesiol Clin*. 2015;33:279.

Parry Z, Macnab R. Thyroid disease and thyroid surgery. *Endocrinology*. 2017;18:488.

Pearson KL, McGuire BE. Anaesthesia for laryngo-tracheal surgery, including tubeless field techniques. *BJA Education*. 2017;17:242.

Regli A, Becke K, von Ungern-Sternberg BS. An update on the perioperative management of children with upper respiratory tract infections. *Curr Opin Anesthesiol*. 2017;30:362.

Rosero EB, Corbett J, Mau T, et al. Intraoperative airway management considerations for adult patients presenting with tracheostomy: a narrative review. *Anesth Analg*. 2021;132:1003.

Shemesh S, Tamir S, Goldfarb A, et al. To proceed or not to proceed: ENT surgery in paediatric patients with acute upper respiratory tract infection. *J Laryngol Otol*. 2016;130:800.

Spataro E, Durakovic N, Kallogjeri D, et al. Complications and 30-day hospital readmission rates of patients undergoing tracheostomy: a prospective analysis. *Laryngoscope*. 2017;127:2746.

Stephens M, Montgomery J, Stirling Urquhart S. Management of elective laryngectomy. *BJA Education*. 2017;17:306.

Tewari A, Samy RN, Castle J, et al. Intraoperative neurophysiological monitoring of the laryngeal nerves during anterior neck surgery: a review. *Ann Otol Rhinol Laryngol*. 2017;126:672.

Waberski AT, Espinel AG, Reddy SK. Anesthesia safety in otolaryngology. *Otolaryngol Clin North Am*. 2019;52:63.

Worrall DM, Tanella A, DeMaria S Jr, et al. Anesthesia and enhanced recovery after head and neck surgery. *Otolaryngol Clin North Am*. 2019;52:1095.

CHAPTER 38

Anesthesia for Orthopedic Surgery

Edward R. Mariano, MD, MAS, FASA, and Jody C. Leng, MD, MS

KEY CONCEPTS

1. Clinical manifestations of bone cement implantation syndrome include hypoxia (increased pulmonary shunt), hypotension, arrhythmias (including heart block and sinus arrest), pulmonary hypertension (increased pulmonary vascular resistance), and decreased cardiac output.

2. The use of a pneumatic tourniquet on an extremity creates a bloodless field that may facilitate surgery. However, tourniquets can produce potential problems of their own, including hemodynamic changes, pain, metabolic alterations, arterial thromboembolism, and pulmonary embolism.

3. Fat embolism syndrome classically presents within 72 h following long-bone or pelvic fracture, with the triad of dyspnea, confusion, and petechiae.

4. Deep vein thrombosis and pulmonary embolism can cause morbidity and mortality during and following orthopedic operations, particularly those procedures involving the pelvis and lower extremities.

5. Neuraxial anesthesia alone or combined with general anesthesia may reduce thromboembolic complications by several mechanisms, including sympathectomy-induced increases in lower extremity venous blood flow, systemic anti-inflammatory effects of local anesthetics, decreased platelet reactivity, attenuated postoperative increase in factor VIII and von Willebrand factor, attenuated postoperative decrease in antithrombin III, and alterations in stress hormone release.

6. Preoperatively, neuraxial techniques may be performed after waiting at least 12 h after a prophylactic low-molecular-weight heparin (LMWH) dose. Postoperatively, neuraxial catheters may be maintained in patients who receive once-daily prophylactic dosing, and catheters should be removed at least 12 h after the previous dose. Following catheter removal, the next dose may be given after a 4 h delay. For postoperative patients who receive twice-daily prophylactic dosing, neuraxial catheters should not be left in situ and should be removed 4 or more hours before the first dose of LMWH. For therapeutic dosing of LMWH, a longer wait time of 24 h after the previous dose is recommended prior to any neuraxial technique.

7. Flexion and extension lateral radiographs of the cervical spine should be obtained preoperatively in patients with rheumatoid arthritis severe enough to require steroids, immune therapy, or methotrexate. If atlantoaxial instability is present, intubation should be performed with in-line stabilization utilizing video or fiberoptic laryngoscopy.

8. Effective communication between the anesthesia practitioner and surgeon is essential during bilateral hip arthroplasty.

—Continued next page

Continued—

If major hemodynamic instability occurs during the first hip replacement procedure, the second arthroplasty should be postponed.

9 Adjuvants such as opioids, clonidine, ketorolac, and neostigmine, when added to local anesthetic solutions for intraarticular injection, have been used in various combinations to extend analgesic duration following knee arthroscopy.

10 Effective postoperative multimodal analgesia facilitates early physical rehabilitation to maximize postoperative range of motion and prevent joint adhesions following knee replacement.

11 Interscalene brachial plexus block with or without a perineural catheter is ideally suited for shoulder procedures. Even when general anesthesia is employed, a peripheral nerve or brachial plexus block can supplement intraoperative anesthesia and provide effective postoperative analgesia.

Orthopedic surgery provides many anesthetic challenges. Patients may present as neonates with congenital limb deformities, as teenagers with sports-related injuries, as adults for procedures ranging from excision of a minor soft-tissue mass to joint replacement, or at any age with bone cancer or traumatic fracture, and comorbidities vary widely. This chapter focuses on perioperative care issues specific to patients undergoing common orthopedic surgical procedures. For example, patients with long bone fractures are predisposed to fat embolism syndrome. Patients are at increased risk for venous thromboembolism following pelvic, hip, and other lower extremity operations. The use of bone cement during arthroplasties can cause hemodynamic instability. Limb tourniquets limit blood loss but introduce additional risks. Perioperative care of patients undergoing cervical, thoracic, and lumbar spine procedures is reviewed in Chapter 27.

Neuraxial and other regional anesthetic techniques play an important role in decreasing the incidence of perioperative thromboembolic and other complications, providing postoperative analgesia, and facilitating early rehabilitation and hospital discharge. Advances in surgical techniques, such as minimally invasive approaches to knee and hip replacement, are necessitating modifications in anesthetic and perioperative management to facilitate overnight or even same-day discharge of patients who formerly required days of hospitalization. It is impossible to cover the anesthetic implications of all orthopedic operations in one chapter; hence, the focus here is on typical perioperative management considerations and strategies for the anesthetic care of patients undergoing select orthopedic surgical procedures.

PERIOPERATIVE MANAGEMENT CONSIDERATIONS IN ORTHOPEDIC SURGERY

Bone Cement

Bone cement, *polymethylmethacrylate*, is frequently required for joint arthroplasties. The cement interdigitates within the interstices of cancellous bone and strongly binds the prosthetic implant to the patient's bone. Mixing polymerized methylmethacrylate powder with liquid methylmethacrylate monomer causes polymerization and cross-linking of the polymer chains. This exothermic reaction leads to hardening of the cement and expansion against the prosthetic components. The resultant intramedullary hypertension (>500 mm Hg) can cause embolization of fat, bone marrow, cement, and air into venous channels. Systemic absorption of residual methyl methacrylate monomer can produce vasodilation and a decrease in systemic vascular resistance. The release of tissue thromboplastin may trigger platelet aggregation, embolic microthrombus formation, and cardiovascular instability as a result of the circulation of vasoactive substances. Nevertheless, most patients experience no adverse response to the application of bone cement.

1 **The clinical manifestations of *bone cement implantation syndrome* include hypoxia (increased pulmonary shunt), hypotension, arrhythmias (including heart block and sinus arrest), pulmonary hypertension (increased pulmonary vascular resistance), and decreased cardiac output.** Emboli frequently occur during the insertion of a femoral prosthesis for hip arthroplasty. Treatment strategies for this complication include increasing inspired oxygen concentration prior to cementing, monitoring to maintain euvolemia and adequate blood pressure, creating a vent hole in the distal femur to relieve intramedullary pressure, performing high-pressure lavage of the femoral shaft to remove potentially microembolic debris, or using a femoral component that does not require cement.

Another source of concern related to the use of cement is the potential for gradual aseptic loosening of the prosthesis over time. Cementless implants are designed with a porous coat that allows natural bone to grow into them. Cementless prostheses offer the potential for shorter surgical procedure duration and avoidance of cement-related complications. However, these implants are most appropriate for younger, active patients with good bone quality because active bone formation is required, and aseptic loosening is still a possible complication. Cemented prostheses are preferred for older (>80 years) and less active patients who often have osteoporosis or thin cortical bone. Practices continue to evolve regarding the selection of cemented versus cementless implants, depending on the joint affected, patient, the surgical technique, and the emergence of newer implants.

Pneumatic Tourniquets

2 **Use of a pneumatic tourniquet on an extremity creates a bloodless field that may facilitate surgery. However, tourniquets can produce potential problems of their own, including hemodynamic changes, pain, metabolic alterations, arterial thromboembolism, and pulmonary embolism.** Inflation pressure is usually set approximately 100 mm Hg higher than the patient's baseline systolic blood pressure. Prolonged inflation (>2 h) can lead to muscle ischemia and may produce rhabdomyolysis or contribute to perioperative neuropathy. Tourniquet inflation has also been associated with increases in body temperature in pediatric patients undergoing lower extremity surgery.

Exsanguination of a lower extremity and tourniquet inflation cause a rapid shift of blood volume into the central circulation. Bilateral lower extremity exsanguination, though rarely performed, can cause an increase in central venous pressure and arterial blood pressure that may not be well tolerated in patients with noncompliant ventricles and diastolic dysfunction.

Awake patients predictably experience tourniquet pain with inflation pressures of 100 mm Hg above systolic blood pressure for more than a few minutes. *During a regional anesthetic, tourniquet pain may gradually become so severe in some patients over time that they may require substantial supplemental intravenous analgesia, if not general anesthesia, despite the fact that the block is adequate to "cover" the surgical incision. Even during general anesthesia, the noxious stimulus of tourniquet compression often manifests as a gradually increasing mean arterial blood pressure beginning approximately 1 h after cuff inflation.* Signs of progressive sympathetic activation include marked hypertension, tachycardia, and diaphoresis. The likelihood of tourniquet pain and its accompanying hypertension is influenced by many factors, including the duration of cuff inflation, the anesthetic technique (regional anesthesia versus general anesthesia), the extent of dermatomal spread or peripheral nerve coverage of the regional anesthetic block, the choice of local anesthetic and dose ("density" of block), and supplementation with adjuvants either intravenously or in combination with local anesthetic solutions when applicable.

Cuff deflation invariably and immediately relieves tourniquet pain and associated hypertension. In fact, cuff deflation may be accompanied by a precipitous decrease in central venous and arterial blood pressure. Heart rate usually increases, and core temperature decreases. Washout of accumulated metabolic wastes from the ischemic extremity increases carbon dioxide partial pressure in arterial blood ($PaCO_2$), end-tidal carbon dioxide ($ETCO_2$), and serum lactate and potassium levels. These metabolic alterations can cause an increase in minute ventilation in the spontaneously breathing patient and, rarely, arrhythmias. Tourniquet-induced circulatory stasis of a lower extremity may lead to the development of deep venous thrombosis. Transesophageal echocardiography can detect subclinical pulmonary embolism (miliary emboli in the right atrium and ventricle) following tourniquet deflation, even in minor orthopedic surgical cases. Rare episodes of massive pulmonary embolism during total knee arthroplasty have been reported in association with tourniquet inflation and deflation. Tourniquets have been safely used in patients with sickle cell disease, though particular attention should be paid to maintaining oxygenation, normocarbia or hypocarbia, hydration, and normothermia.

Fat Embolism Syndrome

Some degree of fat embolism probably occurs with all long-bone fractures. *Fat embolism syndrome* is less frequent but potentially fatal (10–20% mortality). 3 **It classically presents within 72 h following long-bone or pelvic fracture, with the triad of dyspnea, confusion, and petechiae.** This syndrome can also be seen following cardiopulmonary resuscitation, parenteral feeding with lipid infusion, and liposuction. One theory of its pathogenesis proposes that fat globules are released by the disruption of fat cells in the fractured bone and enter the circulation through tears in medullary vessels. An alternative theory suggests that fat globules are chylomicrons resulting from the aggregation of circulating free fatty acids caused by changes in fatty acid metabolism. Regardless of their source, the increased free fatty acid levels can have a toxic effect on the capillary–alveolar membrane, leading to the release of vasoactive amines and prostaglandins and the development of acute respiratory distress syndrome (ARDS; see Chapter 57). Neurological manifestations (eg, agitation, confusion, stupor, or coma) are the probable result of capillary damage in the cerebral circulation and cerebral edema. These signs may be exacerbated by hypoxia.

The diagnosis of fat embolism syndrome is suggested by petechiae on the chest, upper extremities, axillae, and conjunctiva. Fat globules occasionally may be observed in the retina (with ophthalmoscopy), urine, or sputum. Coagulation abnormalities such as thrombocytopenia or prolonged clotting times are occasionally present. Serum lipase activity may be elevated but does not predict disease severity. Pulmonary involvement typically progresses from mild hypoxia and a normal chest radiograph to severe hypoxia or respiratory failure with radiographic findings of diffuse pulmonary opacities. Most of the classic signs and symptoms of fat embolism syndrome occur 1 to 3 days after the precipitating event. During general anesthesia, signs may include a decline in $ETCO_2$ and arterial oxygen saturation and a rise in pulmonary artery pressures. Electrocardiography may show ischemic ST-segment changes and a pattern of right-sided heart strain.

Management of fat embolism syndrome involves careful planning that anticipates the possible problem and immediate cardiopulmonary support should the problem occur. Early stabilization of the fracture decreases the likelihood of fat embolism syndrome and, in particular, the risk of pulmonary complications. Supportive treatment consists of oxygen therapy with continuous positive airway pressure ventilation to prevent hypoxia and specific ventilator strategies in the event of ARDS. Systemic hypotension will require appropriate pressor support, and selective pulmonary vasodilators may aid the management of pulmonary hypertension. The use of corticosteroid therapy in preventing or treating fat embolism syndrome is controversial.

Deep Venous Thrombosis & Thromboembolism

4 **Deep vein thrombosis (DVT) and pulmonary embolism (PE) can cause morbidity and mortality following orthopedic operations, particularly those involving the pelvis and lower extremities. Risk factors include obesity, age greater than 60 years, procedures lasting more than 30 min, use of a tourniquet, lower extremity fracture, and immobilization for more than 4 days. Orthopedic patients at greatest risk include those undergoing hip surgery or knee replacement or major operations for lower extremity trauma. Such patients will experience DVT rates of 40% to 80% without prophylaxis.** The incidence

of clinically important PE following hip surgery in some studies is reported to be as high as 20%, whereas that of fatal PE may be 1% to 3%. Underlying pathophysiological mechanisms include venous stasis with a hypercoagulable state due to local and systemic inflammatory responses to surgery.

Pharmacological prophylaxis and the routine use of mechanical devices such as intermittent pneumatic compression (IPC) have been shown to decrease the incidence of DVT and PE. Although mechanical thromboprophylaxis should be considered for every patient, the use of pharmacological anticoagulants must be balanced against the risk of bleeding. For patients at increased risk for DVT but having "normal" bleeding risk, low-dose subcutaneous unfractionated heparin (LUFH), warfarin, or low-molecular-weight heparin (LMWH) may be employed in addition to mechanical prophylaxis. Patients at significantly increased risk of bleeding may be managed with mechanical prophylaxis alone until bleeding risk decreases. In general, anticoagulants are started on the day of surgery in patients without indwelling epidural catheters. Newer direct oral anticoagulants that inhibit factor Xa or thrombin have a fast onset of action, are renally excreted, and deserve special consideration in the context of regional anesthesia.

5 **Neuraxial anesthesia alone or combined with general anesthesia may reduce thromboembolic complications by several mechanisms, including sympathectomy-induced increases in lower extremity venous blood flow, systemic anti-inflammatory effects of local anesthetics, decreased platelet reactivity, attenuated postoperative increases in factor VIII and von Willebrand factor, attenuated postoperative decreases in antithrombin III, and alterations in stress hormone release.**

According to the Fourth Edition of the American Society of Regional Anesthesia and Pain Medicine Evidence-Based Guidelines on regional anesthesia and anticoagulation, neuraxial anesthesia is not recommended in patients currently receiving antiplatelet agents, thrombolytics, fondaparinux, direct thrombin inhibitors, or therapeutic regimens of LMWH because of the unacceptable risk for spinal or epidural hematoma. In patients receiving LUFH for thromboprophylaxis in dosing regimens of 5000 units two or three times daily, neuraxial block (or removal of a neuraxial catheter) may be performed 4 to 6 h after the previous dose; subsequent dosing may resume 1 h after catheter removal.

6 **For patients receiving prophylactic LMWH, the guidelines vary based on regimen and perioperative phase. Preoperatively, neuraxial techniques may be performed after waiting at least 12 hours after a prophylactic dose. Postoperatively, neuraxial catheters may be maintained in patients who receive once-daily prophylactic dosing, and catheters should be removed at least 12 h after the previous dose. Following catheter removal, the next dose may be given after a 4-h delay. For postoperative patients who receive twice-daily prophylactic dosing, neuraxial catheters should not be left in situ and should be removed 4 or more hours before the first dose of LMWH. For therapeutic dosing of LMWH, a longer wait time of 24 h after the previous dose is recommended prior to any neuraxial technique. Patients on warfarin therapy should not receive a neuraxial block unless the international normalized ratio (INR) is normal, and catheters should be removed when the INR is 1.5 or lower.** The Fourth Edition of these guidelines also suggests that these recommendations be applied to deep peripheral nerve and deep plexus blocks and catheters (see Suggested Reading). Revisions to these guidelines occur regularly. *We strongly recommend that anesthesia practitioners download and use the ASRA Coags mobile application ("app") from the American Society of Regional Anesthesia and Pain Medicine as a bedside decision support tool.*

Hip Surgery

Common hip procedures performed in adults include repair of hip fracture, total hip arthroplasty (THA), and closed reduction of hip dislocation.

FRACTURE OF THE PROXIMAL FEMUR

Preoperative Considerations

Most patients presenting with femoral neck fractures are frail older adults. An occasional young patient will have sustained major trauma to the femur or pelvis.

Studies have reported mortality rates following hip fracture of up to 10% during the initial hospitalization and over 20% within 1 year. Many of these patients have concomitant diseases such as coronary artery disease, cerebrovascular disease, chronic obstructive pulmonary disease, or diabetes.

Patients presenting with femur fractures are frequently hypovolemic from occult blood loss and inadequate oral intake. In general, intracapsular (subcapital, transcervical) fractures are associated with less occult blood loss than extracapsular (base of the femoral neck, intertrochanteric, subtrochanteric) fractures (Figure 38–1). *A normal or borderline-low preoperative hematocrit may be deceiving when hemoconcentration masks occult blood loss.*

Another characteristic of hip fracture patients is the frequent presence of preoperative hypoxia that may, at least in part, be due to fat embolism; other factors can include bibasilar atelectasis from immobility, pulmonary congestion (and effusion) from congestive heart failure, consolidation due to infection, or a preexisting pulmonary condition such as chronic obstructive pulmonary disease.

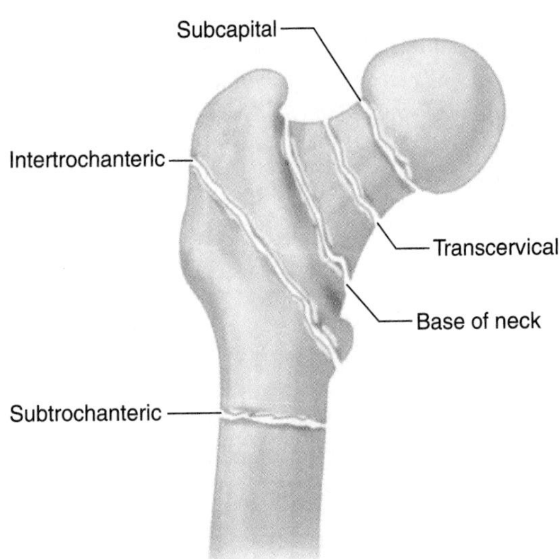

FIGURE 38–1 Blood loss from hip fracture depends on the location of the fracture (subtrochanteric, intertrochanteric > base of femoral neck > transcervical, subcapital) because the capsule restricts blood loss by acting like a tourniquet.

Intraoperative Management

The choice between regional (spinal or epidural) and general anesthesia has been extensively evaluated for hip fracture surgery. A meta-analysis of 15 randomized clinical trials showed a decrease in postoperative DVT and 1-month mortality with regional anesthesia, but these advantages do not persist beyond 3 months. A large database study involving over 50,000 patients treated for hip fracture in New York State also did not show a difference in 30-day mortality based on anesthetic technique but did show a slightly shorter length of stay for patients who received regional anesthesia. A large prospective multi-center study did not show a difference between spinal and general anesthesia in terms of 60-day mortality or incidence of delirium.

A regional anesthetic technique, with or without concomitant general anesthesia, can provide the additional advantage of postoperative pain control. If a spinal anesthetic is planned, hypobaric or isobaric local anesthetics facilitate positioning since the patient can remain in the same position for both block placement and surgery. Intrathecal opioids such as morphine can extend postoperative analgesia but require close postoperative monitoring for delayed respiratory depression. A continuous peripheral nerve block technique such as a fascia iliaca catheter offers selective long-acting analgesia without the risk of these respiratory side effects.

Consideration should also be given to the type of reduction and fixation to be used. This is dependent on the fracture site, degree of displacement, preoperative functional status of the patient, and surgeon preference. Undisplaced fractures of the proximal femur may be treated with percutaneous pinning or cannulated screw fixation with the patient in the supine position. A hip compression screw and side plate are most often employed for intertrochanteric fractures. Displaced intracapsular fractures may require internal fixation, hemiarthroplasty, or THA (Figure 38–2). Surgical treatment of extracapsular hip fractures is accomplished with either an extramedullary implant (eg, sliding screw and plate) or an intramedullary nail.

Hemiarthroplasty and THA are longer, more invasive operations than most other orthopedic procedures. They are usually performed with patients

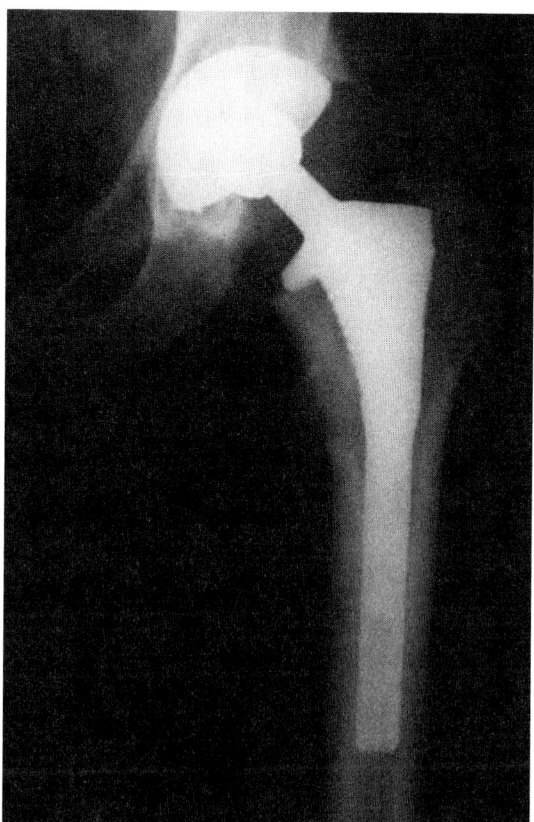

FIGURE 38–2 Uncemented total hip arthroplasty.

in the lateral decubitus position, are associated with greater blood loss, and potentially result in greater hemodynamic changes, particularly if cement is used. Venous access should be sufficient to permit rapid transfusion.

TOTAL HIP ARTHROPLASTY

Preoperative Considerations

Most patients undergoing THA have osteoarthritis (degenerative joint disease), hip fracture, avascular necrosis, or autoimmune conditions such as rheumatoid arthritis (RA). Osteoarthritis is a degenerative disease affecting the articular surface of joints (commonly the hips and knees). The etiology of osteoarthritis appears to involve repetitive joint trauma. Because osteoarthritis may also involve the spine, neck manipulation during tracheal intubation should be minimized to avoid nerve root compression or disc protrusion.

TABLE 38–1 Systemic manifestations of rheumatoid arthritis.

Organ System	Abnormalities
Cardiovascular	Pericardial thickening and effusion, myocarditis, coronary arteritis, conduction defects, vasculitis, cardiac valve fibrosis (aortic regurgitation)
Pulmonary	Pleural effusion, pulmonary nodules, interstitial pulmonary fibrosis
Hematopoietic	Anemia, eosinophilia, platelet dysfunction (from aspirin therapy), thrombocytopenia
Endocrine	Adrenal insufficiency (from glucocorticoid therapy), impaired immune system
Dermatological	Thin and atrophic skin from the disease and immunosuppressive drugs

RA is characterized by immune-mediated joint destruction with chronic and progressive inflammation of synovial membranes, as opposed to the articular wear-and-tear of osteoarthritis. RA is a systemic disease affecting multiple organ systems (Table 38–1). RA often affects the small joints of the hands, wrists, and feet, causing severe deformity.

Extreme cases of RA involve almost all synovial membranes, including those in the cervical spine and temporomandibular joint. *Atlantoaxial subluxation*, which can be diagnosed radiologically, may lead to protrusion of the odontoid process into the foramen magnum during intubation, compromising vertebral blood flow and compressing the spinal cord or brainstem (Figure 38–3). 7 Flexion and extension lateral radiographs of the cervical spine should be obtained preoperatively in patients with RA severe enough to require steroids or other immunosuppressive therapy, including methotrexate. If atlantoaxial instability is present, intubation should be performed with in-line stabilization utilizing video or fiberoptic laryngoscopy. Involvement of the temporomandibular joint can limit jaw mobility and range of motion to such a degree that conventional orotracheal intubation may be impossible. Hoarseness or inspiratory stridor may signal a narrowing of the glottic opening caused by cricoarytenoid arthritis.

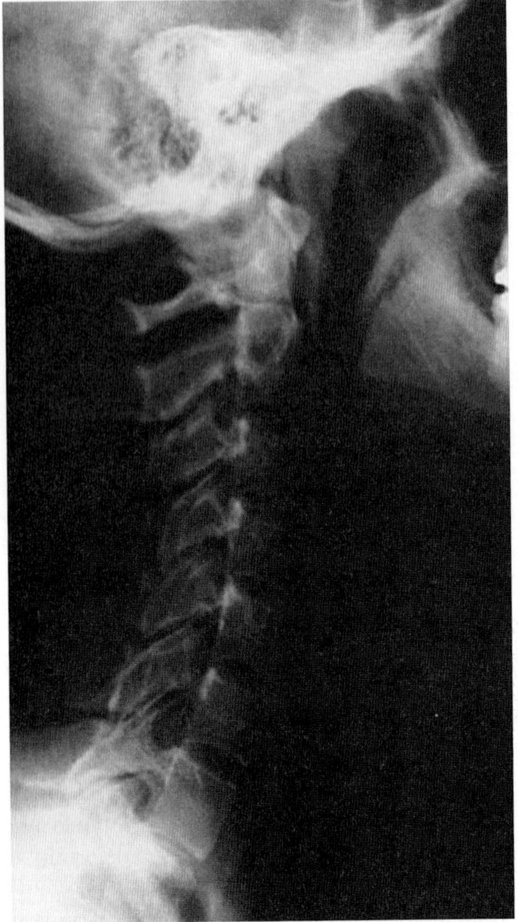

A

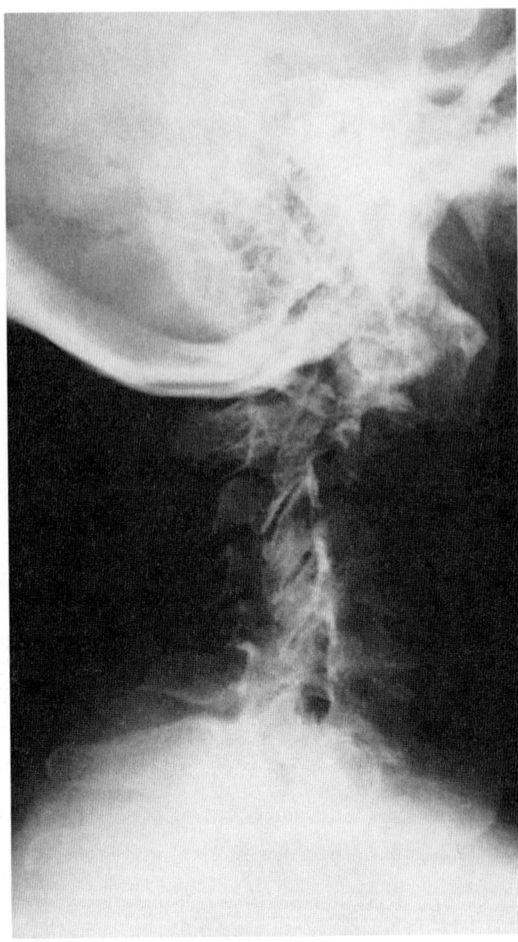

B

FIGURE 38–3 Because instability of the cervical spine may be asymptomatic, lateral radiographs are mandatory in patients with severe rheumatoid arthritis. **A**: Radiograph of a normal lateral cervical spine. **B**: Lateral cervical spine of a patient with rheumatoid arthritis; note the severe C1–C2 instability.

This condition may lead to postextubation airway obstruction even when a smaller diameter tracheal tube has been used.

Patients with RA or osteoarthritis commonly receive nonsteroidal anti-inflammatory drugs (NSAIDs) for pain management. These drugs can have serious side effects such as gastrointestinal bleeding, kidney toxicity, and platelet dysfunction.

Intraoperative Management

THA involves several surgical steps, including positioning of the patient (usually in the lateral decubitus position), dislocation and removal of the femoral head, reaming of the acetabulum and insertion of a prosthetic acetabular cup (with or without cement), and reaming of the femur and insertion of a femoral component (femoral head and stem) into the femoral shaft with or without cement. THA is associated with three potentially life-threatening complications: bone cement implantation syndrome, intra- and postoperative hemorrhage, and venous thromboembolism. Thus, invasive arterial monitoring may be justified for select patients undergoing these procedures. General anesthesia, neuraxial anesthesia, or a combination of techniques can provide suitable operating conditions. The use of neuraxial anesthesia with or without general anesthesia for THA has been recommended by an international consensus statement based on data supporting decreased mortality and decreased incidence of postoperative complications such as all-cause infections, acute kidney injury or failure, and thromboembolism. Neuraxial administration of opioids such as morphine or hydromorphone in the perioperative period extends the duration of postoperative analgesia. Clinical practice guidelines now recommend the routine administration of tranexamic acid prior to incision to reduce blood loss. Both intravenous and topical routes of administration are supported by available evidence; however, and a multiple-dose regimen has not been consistently shown to influence the amount of blood loss or need for blood transfusion compared with a single dose.

A. Hip Resurfacing Arthroplasty

The increasing number of younger patients presenting for hip arthroplasty and of other patients who require revision of standard (metal-on-polyethylene) THA implants has led to the redevelopment of hip resurfacing arthroplasty techniques. Compared with traditional hip arthroplasty implants, hip resurfacing maintains patients' native bone to a greater degree. Metal-on-metal hybrid implants are usually employed. Surgical approaches can be anterior or posterior, with the posterior approach most commonly used due to better visualization. Since the femoral head remains intact, its dislocation and repositioning during surgery may theoretically compromise its own blood supply. With the posterior approach, patients are placed in the lateral decubitus position similar to traditional hip arthroplasty.

Outcomes data related to hip resurfacing versus traditional THA are controversial. Prospective studies have not shown a difference in gait or postural balance at 3 months postoperatively. One meta-analysis favored resurfacing in terms of functional outcome and blood loss despite comparable results for postoperative pain scores and patient satisfaction. Of particular concern is the finding that patients who undergo resurfacing are nearly twice as likely to require revision surgery as those receiving traditional hip arthroplasty. There is a greater incidence of aseptic component loosening (possibly from metal hypersensitivity) and femoral neck fracture, particularly in women. Finally, the presence of metal debris in the joint space (from metal-on-metal contact wear) has led to a marked narrowing of indications for the prostheses and the procedure. Monitoring of serum cobalt and chromium levels has been suggested for these patients. Adverse local tissue reactions, including abnormal fluid collections and pseudotumors, may also occur as a result of metal debris and are best detected early to avoid permanent damage to muscle, bone, and soft tissues.

B. Bilateral Arthroplasty

Bilateral hip arthroplasty can be safely performed in fit patients as a combined procedure, assuming the absence of significant pulmonary embolization after insertion of the first femoral component. Monitoring may include echocardiography.

8 **Effective communication between the anesthesia practitioner and surgeon is essential. If major hemodynamic instability occurs during the first hip replacement procedure, the second arthroplasty should be postponed.**

C. Revision Arthroplasty

Revision of a prior hip arthroplasty is often associated with much greater blood loss than in the initial procedure. Blood loss depends on many factors, including the experience and skill of the surgeon. Evidence suggests that blood loss may be decreased during hip surgery if a neuraxial anesthetic is used (eg, spinal or epidural anesthesia) compared with general anesthesia, even at similar mean arterial blood pressures. The mechanism is unclear. Given the potential for perioperative blood transfusion, preoperative autologous blood donation and intraoperative blood salvage may be considered. Preoperative administration of vitamins B_{12} and K and iron can treat mild forms of chronic anemia. Alternatively, an intravenous iron infusion can be used. Finally, and most expensively, recombinant human erythropoietin in the form of weekly subcutaneous injections before surgery may also decrease the need for perioperative allogeneic blood transfusion. Erythropoietin increases red blood cell production by stimulating the division and differentiation of erythroid progenitors in the bone marrow. Maintaining normal body temperature during hip replacement surgery also reduces blood loss.

D. Minimally Invasive Arthroplasty

Computer-assisted surgery (CAS) has been proposed to improve surgical outcomes and promote early rehabilitation through minimally invasive techniques employing cementless implants, though this approach has not been widely adopted. Computer software can accurately reconstruct three-dimensional images of bone and soft tissue based on radiographs, fluoroscopy, computed tomography, or magnetic resonance imaging data. The computer matches preoperative images or planning information to the position of the patient on the operating room table. Tracking devices are attached to target bones (Figure 38–4) and instruments used during surgery, and the navigation system utilizes optical cameras and infrared light-emitting diodes to sense their positions. CAS thus allows accurate placement of implants through smaller incisions, and the resulting reduction in tissue and muscle damage may lead to less pain and earlier rehabilitation. The lateral approach utilizes a single incision with the patient in the lateral decubitus position (see Figure 38–4), while the anterior approach utilizes two small incisions (one for the acetabular component and another for the femoral component) with the patient supine. The evidence to date does not demonstrate outcome advantages for CAS.

E. Hip Arthroscopy

In recent years, hip arthroscopy has increased in popularity as a minimally invasive alternative to open arthrotomy for a variety of surgical indications such as femoroacetabular impingement (FAI), acetabular labral tears, loose bodies, and osteoarthritis. At present, there is some evidence in the published literature to support hip arthroscopy for FAI, but evidence is lacking for other indications.

CLOSED REDUCTION OF HIP DISLOCATION

There is a 3% incidence of hip dislocation following primary hip arthroplasty and a 20% incidence following total hip revision arthroplasty. *Because less force is required to dislocate a prosthetic hip, patients with hip implants require special precautions during positioning for subsequent surgical procedures.* Extremes of hip flexion, internal rotation, and adduction increase the risk of dislocation. Hip dislocations may be corrected with closed reduction facilitated by the use of a brief intravenous general anesthetic, often performed in a monitored setting outside of the operating room (eg, emergency department). Temporary muscle relaxation can be provided by succinylcholine, if necessary, to facilitate the reduction when the hip musculature is severely contracted. Deep sedation or general anesthesia must be provided by appropriately qualified and credentialed practitioners using ASA basic monitoring with appropriate airway management equipment

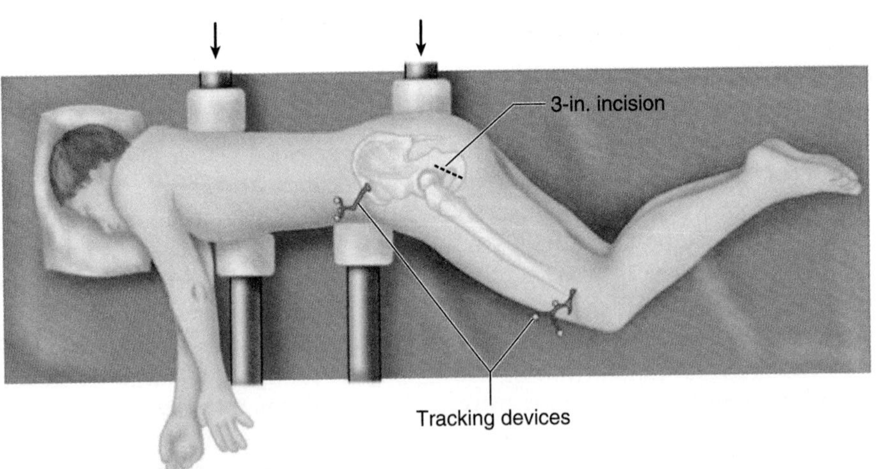

FIGURE 38–4 Minimally invasive total hip arthroplasty: lateral approach. Note the small 3-in. incision and tracking devices for the CAS navigation system.

and supplies immediately available. Successful reduction should be confirmed radiographically.

Knee Surgery

The most frequently performed knee surgeries are arthroscopy and total or partial arthroplasty.

KNEE ARTHROSCOPY

Preoperative Considerations

Arthroscopy has revolutionized surgery of many joints, including the hip, knee, shoulder, ankle, elbow, and wrist. Joint arthroscopies are usually performed as outpatient procedures. Although the typical patient undergoing knee arthroscopy is often thought of as being a healthy young athlete, knee arthroscopies may also be performed in older adult patients with multiple medical problems.

Intraoperative Management

A bloodless field facilitates arthroscopic surgery. Knee surgery lends itself to the use of a pneumatic tourniquet, though its use is optional. The surgery is performed as an outpatient procedure. Alternative anesthetic techniques include general anesthesia, neuraxial anesthesia, peripheral nerve blocks, periarticular injections, or intraarticular injections employing local anesthetic solutions with or without adjuvants combined with intravenous sedation analgesia.

For patients undergoing knee arthroscopy, neuraxial anesthetic techniques include epidural and spinal anesthesia. However, for ambulatory surgery, time to discharge following neuraxial anesthesia may be prolonged compared with general anesthesia.

Postoperative Pain Management

Successful outpatient recovery depends on early ambulation, adequate analgesia, and minimal sedation and nausea and vomiting. Techniques that avoid large doses of systemic opioids have obvious appeal. Intraarticular bupivacaine or ropivacaine usually provides satisfactory analgesia for several

9 hours postoperatively. **Adjuvants such as opioids, clonidine, ketorolac, epinephrine, and neostigmine added to local anesthetic solutions for intraarticular injection have been used in various combinations to extend the analgesic duration. Other multimodal pain management strategies include systemic NSAIDs, acetaminophen, and single or continuous peripheral nerve blocks, particularly for arthroscopic ligament reconstruction.**

TOTAL KNEE ARTHROPLASTY

Preoperative Considerations

Patients presenting for total knee arthroplasty (TKA) (Figure 38–5) have similar comorbidities to those undergoing THA.

Intraoperative Management

During TKA, patients remain in a supine position, and intraoperative blood loss is limited by the use of a tourniquet. A neuraxial anesthetic technique is recommended as it is associated with lower rates of all-cause infections, acute kidney injury and failure, pulmonary and thromboembolic complications, and falls when compared with general anesthesia. Bone cement implantation syndrome following the insertion of a femoral prosthesis is possible but is less likely than during THA. Release of emboli into the systemic circulation following tourniquet release may contribute to systemic hypotension. Tranexamic acid administration prior to incision is recommended to reduce surgical bleeding, similar to THA.

10 **Pain is typically more severe and longer-lasting after TKA than after THA. Effective postoperative multimodal analgesia facilitates early physical rehabilitation to maximize postoperative range of motion and prevent joint adhesions following knee replacement.** It is important to balance pain control with the need for an alert and cooperative patient during physical therapy. Epidural analgesia may be useful after bilateral TKA, depending on the choice of prophylactic anticoagulation in these high-risk cases. *For unilateral knee replacement, perineural catheters provide equivalent analgesia to epidural catheters while perineural catheters produce fewer side effects (eg, pruritus, nausea and vomiting, urinary retention, or orthostatic lightheadedness) and are more likely to permit earlier ambulation.* Preoperative regional analgesia performance in a

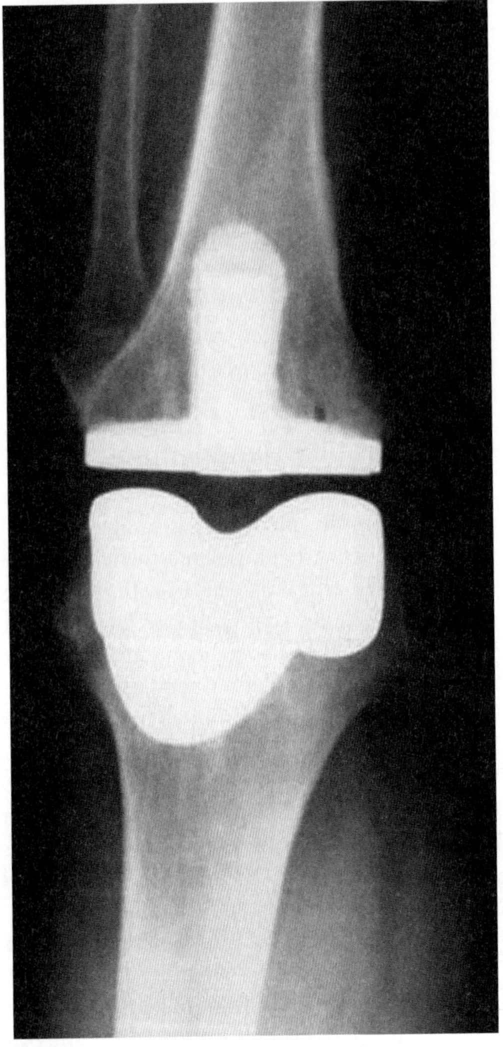

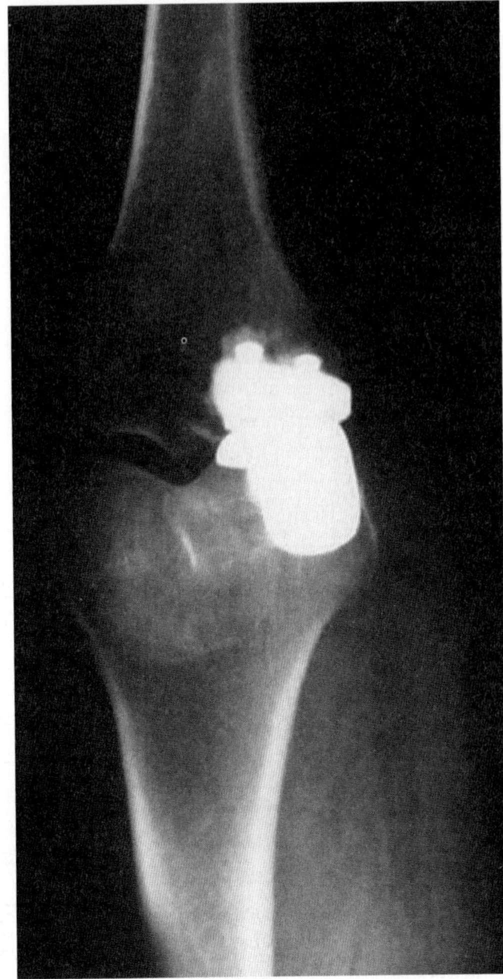

FIGURE 38–5 Total (**A**) and partial (**B**) knee replacement.

"block room" or induction room can minimize operating room delays (Figure 38–6).

Unicompartmental or partial knee replacement and minimally invasive knee arthroplasty with muscle-sparing approaches have been described. With proper patient selection, these techniques may reduce quadriceps muscle damage, facilitating earlier achievement of range-of-motion and ambulation goals, and may allow for short-stay admission or even same-day discharge in select situations. Anesthetic management and postoperative analgesia should facilitate an accelerated, enhanced recovery program. Single or continuous peripheral nerve blocks, alone or in combination, can provide target-specific pain control and facilitate early rehabilitation. Continuous peripheral nerve block catheters with subsequent perineural local anesthetic infusions have been shown to decrease time to meet discharge criteria for TKA. The management of perineural catheters takes a hands-on

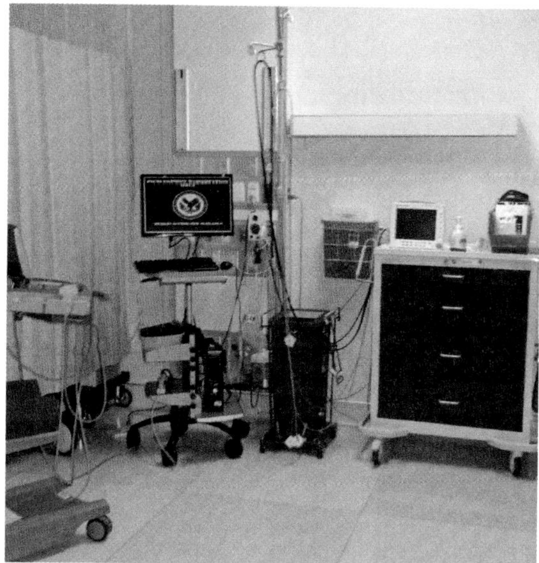

FIGURE 38–6 A "block room" can be located in a preoperative holding area, induction room, or postanesthesia care unit and should offer standard monitoring (as outlined by the American Society of Anesthesiologists) and ample storage for regional anesthesia supplies and equipment.

team approach with 24/7/365 coverage. *Among the postoperative complications of lower extremity arthroplasty procedures, patient falls are of greatest concern, and comprehensive fall prevention programs need to be in place wherever these surgeries are performed, whether or not patients receive regional anesthesia.* Administration of intrathecal opioids for postoperative pain management is also widely used with enhanced recovery programs. Finally, postoperative analgesia in the form of periarticular local anesthetic infiltration by surgeons, with or without adjuvants, is commonly practiced and supported by evidence.

Surgery on the Upper Extremity

Procedures on the upper extremities include those for disorders of the shoulder (eg, subacromial impingement or rotator cuff tears), traumatic fractures, nerve entrapment syndromes (eg, carpal tunnel syndrome), and autoimmune or degenerative joint diseases.

SHOULDER SURGERY

Shoulder operations may be open or arthroscopic. These procedures are performed either in a sitting ("beach chair") or, less commonly, the lateral decubitus position. *The beach chair position may be associated with decreases in cerebral perfusion. Blindness, stroke, and even brain death have been described, emphasizing the need to accurately measure blood pressure at the level of the brain.* When using noninvasive blood pressure monitoring, the cuff should be applied on the upper arm because systolic blood pressure readings from the calf can be 40 mm Hg higher than brachial readings on the same patient. If the surgeon requests controlled hypotension, intraarterial blood pressure monitoring must be used, and the transducer should be positioned at the level of the brainstem (external meatus of the ear). 11 **Interscalene brachial plexus block with or without a perineural catheter is ideally suited for shoulder procedures.** More distal blocks such as the superior trunk or supraclavicular block and the "shoulder block" (eg, suprascapular and axillary nerve blocks) represent alternatives. Even when general anesthesia is employed, a peripheral nerve or brachial plexus block can supplement anesthesia by providing muscle relaxation and effective intraoperative and postoperative analgesia.

Preoperative insertion of an indwelling perineural catheter with the subsequent infusion of a dilute local anesthetic infusion solution allows postoperative analgesia for 48 to 72 h with most fixed-reservoir disposable pumps following arthroscopic or open shoulder operations (see Chapter 46). Alternatively, the surgeon may insert a subacromial catheter to provide continuous infusion of local anesthetic for postoperative analgesia. Direct placement of intraarticular catheters into the glenohumeral joint with the infusion of bupivacaine has been associated with glenohumeral chondrolysis in human and animal studies and is not recommended. Multimodal analgesia, including systemic NSAIDs, acetaminophen (if no contraindications), and local anesthetic infusions in the perioperative period can help reduce postoperative opioid requirements.

DISTAL UPPER EXTREMITY SURGERY

Distal upper extremity surgical procedures generally take place on an outpatient basis. Minor soft tissue operations of the hand of short duration (eg, carpal tunnel release) may be performed with local infiltration or with intravenous regional anesthesia (IVRA, or Bier block). The limiting factor with IVRA is tourniquet tolerance.

For operations lasting more than 1 h or for more invasive procedures involving bones or joints, a brachial plexus block is the preferred regional anesthetic technique. Multiple approaches can be used to anesthetize the brachial plexus for distal upper extremity surgery (see Chapter 46). Selection of brachial plexus block technique should take into account the planned surgical site and location of the pneumatic tourniquet, if applicable. Continuous peripheral nerve blocks may be appropriate for inpatient and outpatient procedures to extend the duration of analgesia further into the postoperative period, facilitate physical therapy, or both. Brachial plexus blocks do not routinely anesthetize the intercostobrachial nerve distribution hence, subcutaneous infiltration of local anesthetic may be required for procedures involving the medial upper arm.

Anesthetic considerations for distal upper extremity surgery should include patient positioning and the use of a pneumatic tourniquet. Most procedures can be performed with the patient supine; the operative arm abducted 90° and resting on a hand table; and the operating room table rotated 90° to position the operative arm in the center of the room. Exceptions to this rule often involve surgery around the elbow, and certain operations may require the patient to be in lateral decubitus or even prone position. Because patients are often scheduled for same-day discharge, perioperative management should focus on ensuring rapid recovery and effective pain control without severe pain or nausea (see Chapter 44).

CASE DISCUSSION

Managing Blood Loss in Jehovah's Witnesses

A 58-year-old male patient who is a Jehovah's Witness presents for hemipelvectomy to resect a malignant bone tumor (osteogenic sarcoma). The patient has received chemotherapy over the past 2 months with multiple drugs, including doxorubicin. He has no other medical problems, and the preoperative hematocrit is 47%.

How does the care of patients who are Jehovah's Witnesses particularly challenge the anesthesia team?

Jehovah's Witnesses, a fellowship of more than 1 million Americans, object to the administration of blood for any indication. This objection stems from their interpretation of the Bible ("to keep abstaining from . . . blood," Acts 15:28,29) and not for medical reasons (eg, the fear of hepatitis). Physicians and nurses should honor the principle of autonomy: Patients have final authority over what is done to them. Witnesses typically sign a waiver releasing medical practitioners from liability for any consequences of blood refusal.

Which intravenous fluids will Witnesses accept?

Witnesses abstain from blood and blood products (eg, packed red blood cells, fresh frozen plasma, platelets) but not from non–blood-containing solutions. They accept crystalloids, hetastarch, and dextran replacement solutions. Witnesses often view albumin, erythropoietin (because of the use of albumin), immune globulins, and hemophiliac preparations as a gray area that requires a personal decision by the believer.

Do they allow the use of autologous blood?

According to their religion, any blood that is removed from the body should be discarded ("You should pour it out upon the ground as water," Deuteronomy 12:24) and not stored. Thus, the usual practice of autologous preoperative collection and storage would not be allowed. Techniques of acute normovolemic hemodilution and intraoperative blood salvage have been accepted by some Witnesses, however, as long as their blood maintains continuity with their circulatory systems at all times. For example, up to 4 units of blood could be drawn from the patient immediately before surgery and kept in anticoagulant-containing bags that maintain a constant link to the patient's body. The blood could be replaced by an acceptable colloid or crystalloid solution then reinfused as needed during surgery.

How would the inability to transfuse blood affect intraoperative monitoring decisions?

Hemipelvectomy involves radical resection that can lead to massive blood loss. This is particularly true for large tumors removed using the more invasive internal approach. Intraarterial and central venous catheter placement would be indicated in patients undergoing this procedure. Techniques that minimize intraoperative blood loss (eg, controlled hypotension, aprotinin) should be considered. In a Jehovah's Witness patient, the management of life-threatening anemia (Hb <5 g/dL) may be improved by optimizing cardiac output, oxygen delivery, and oxygen consumption.

What physiological effects result from severe anemia?

Assuming the maintenance of normovolemia and the absence of preexisting major end-organ dysfunction, most patients tolerate severe anemia surprisingly well. Decreased blood viscosity and vasodilation lower systemic vascular resistance and increase blood flow. Augmentation of stroke volume increases cardiac output, allowing arterial blood pressure and heart rate to remain relatively unchanged. Coronary and cerebral blood flows increase in the absence of coronary artery disease and carotid artery stenosis. A decrease in venous oxygen saturation reflects an increase in tissue oxygen extraction. Oozing from surgical wounds as a result of dilutional coagulopathy may accompany extreme degrees of anemia.

What are some of the anesthetic implications of preoperative doxorubicin therapy?

This anthracycline chemotherapeutic agent has well-recognized cardiac side effects, ranging from transient arrhythmias and electrocardiographic changes (eg, ST-segment and T-wave abnormalities) to irreversible cardiomyopathy and congestive heart failure. The risk of cardiomyopathy appears to increase with a cumulative dose greater than 550 mg/m^2, prior radiotherapy, and concurrent cyclophosphamide treatment. Mild degrees of cardiomyopathy can be detected preoperatively with endomyocardial biopsy, echocardiography, or exercise radionuclide angiography. The other important toxicity of doxorubicin is myelosuppression manifesting as thrombocytopenia, leukopenia, and anemia.

Are there any special considerations regarding postoperative pain management in the Jehovah's Witness patient?

Witnesses generally refrain from any mind-altering drugs or medications, though opioids prescribed by a physician for severe pain are accepted by some believers. Insertion of an epidural catheter can provide acceptable analgesia with local anesthetics, with or without opioids.

GUIDELINES

Fillingham YA, Ramkumar DB, Jevsevar DS, et al. Tranexamic acid in total joint arthroplasty: the endorsed clinical practice guides of the American Association of Hip and Knee Surgeons, American Society of Regional Anesthesia and Pain Medicine, American Academy of Orthopaedic Surgeons, Hip Society, and Knee Society. *Reg Anesth Pain Med.* 2019;44:7

Horlocker TT, Vandermeuelen E, Kopp SL, Gogarten W, Leffert LR, Benzon HT. Regional anesthesia in the patient receiving antithrombotic or thrombolytic therapy: American Society of Regional Anesthesia and Pain Medicine evidence-based guidelines (fourth edition). *Reg Anesth Pain Med.* 2018;43:263.

Memtsoudis SG, Cozowicz C, Bekeris J, et al. Anaesthetic care of patients undergoing primary hip and knee arthroplasty: consensus recommendations from the International Consensus on Anaesthesia-Related Outcomes after Surgery group (ICAROS) based on a systematic review and meta-analysis. *Br J Anaesth.* 2019;123:269.

SUGGESTED READINGS

Albrecht E, Mermoud J, Fournier N, Kern C, et al. A systematic review of ultrasound-guided methods for brachial plexus blockade. *Anaesthesia*. 2016;71:213.

Amundson AW, Johnson RL, Abdel MP, et al. A three-arm randomized clinical trial comparing continuous femoral plus single-injection sciatic peripheral nerve blocks versus periarticular injection with ropivacaine or liposomal bupivacaine for patients undergoing total knee arthroplasty. *Anesthesiology*. 2017;126:1139.

Andersen LØ, Kehlet H. Analgesic efficacy of local infiltration analgesia in hip and knee arthroplasty: a systematic review. *Br J Anaesth*. 2014;113:360.

Aprato A, Risitano S, Sabatini L, et al. Cementless total knee arthroplasty. *Ann Transl Med*. 2016;4:129.

Bin Abd Razak HR, Yung WY. Postoperative delirium in patients undergoing total joint arthroplasty: a systematic review. *J Arthroplasty*. 2015;30:1414.

Donaldson AJ, Thomson HE, Harper NJ, et al. Bone cement implantation syndrome. *Br J Anaesth*. 2009;102:12.

Elkassabany NM, Mariano ER. Aiming to refine the interscalene block: another bullseye or missing the mark? *Anesthesiology*. 2019;131:1207.

Guay J, Parker MJ, Gajendragadkar PR, Kopp S. Anaesthesia for hip fracture surgery in adults. *Cochrane Database Syst Rev*. 2016;(2):CD000521.

Gulihar A, Robati S, Twaij H, et al. Articular cartilage and local anaesthetic: a systematic review of the current literature. *J Orthop*. 2015;12(suppl 2):S200.

Højer Karlsen AP, Geisler A, Petersen PL, et al. Postoperative pain treatment after total hip arthroplasty: a systematic review. *Pain*. 2015;156:8.

Jones EL, Wainwright TW, Foster JD, et al. A systematic review of patient-reported outcomes and patient experience in enhanced recovery after orthopaedic surgery. *Ann R Coll Surg Engl*. 2014;96:89.

Kandarian BS, Elkassabany NM, Tamboli M, et al. Updates on multimodal analgesia and regional anesthesia for total knee arthroplasty patients. *Best Pract Res Clin Anaesthesiol*. 2019;33:111.

Mariano ER, Schatman ME. A common-sense patient-centered approach to multimodal analgesia within surgical enhanced recovery protocols. *J Pain Res*. 2019;12:3461.

Neuman M, Rosenbaum P, Ludwig, et al. Anesthesia technique, mortality, and length of stay after hip fracture surgery. *JAMA*. 2014;311:2508.

Neuman M, Feng R, Carson JL, et al. Spinal anesthesia or general anesthesia for hip surgery in older adults. N Engl J Med. 2021;385:2025.

Sershon R, Balkissoon R, Della Valle C. Current indications for hip resurfacing arthroplasty in 2016. *Curr Rev Musculoskeletal Med*. 2016;9:84.

Tria AJ, Scuderi GR. Minimally invasive knee arthroplasty: an overview. *World J Orthop*. 2015;6:804.

Van der List J, Chawla H, Joskowicz L, et al. Current state of computer navigation and robotics in unicompartmental and total knee arthroplasty: a systematic review with meta-analysis. *Knee Surg Sports Traumatol Arthros*. 2016;24:3482.

Webb C, Mariano E. Best multimodal analgesic protocol for total knee arthroplasty. *Pain Manag*. 2015;5:185.

CHAPTER 39

Anesthesia for Trauma & Emergency Surgery

KEY CONCEPTS

1. All acute trauma patients should be presumed to have a full stomach and thereby be at increased risk of pulmonary aspiration.
2. Cervical spine injury is presumed in any trauma patient presenting with neck pain or any suggestion of neurologic injury, as well as those with loss of consciousness, significant head injury, or intoxication.
3. In the patient with blunt or penetrating injury, providers should maintain a high level of suspicion for pulmonary injury that could evolve into a tension pneumothorax when mechanical ventilation is initiated. No trauma patient should die without having potential tension pneumothorax relieved.
4. In up to 25% of trauma patients, trauma-induced coagulopathy (TIC) is present shortly after injury and before any resuscitative efforts have been initiated.
5. Balanced administration of red blood cells, fresh frozen plasma, and platelet units (1:1:1) is termed *damage control resuscitation* (DCR). Administering blood products in equal ratios early in resuscitation has become an accepted approach for preventing or correcting TIC.
6. *Transfusion-associated circulatory overload* (TACO) is the greatest risk to trauma patients from DCR. The incidence of *transfusion-related acute lung injury* (TRALI) has decreased markedly with restriction of plasma and platelet donation to donors who are male, or who are female and who have either never been pregnant or who have been tested and found to be anti-HLA negative.
7. *Damage control surgery* is a surgical intervention intended to stop hemorrhage and limit gastrointestinal contamination of the abdominal compartment in severely injured and bleeding patients. An emergency exploratory laparotomy is performed in a start–stop fashion, attempting to discover and control bleeding injuries while affording the anesthesia team opportunities for resuscitation and preventing prolonged hypotension and hypothermia between surgical interventions.
8. Any trauma patient with an altered level of consciousness must be considered to have a traumatic brain injury (TBI) until proven otherwise. The presence or suspicion of TBI mandates attention to maintaining cerebral perfusion pressure and oxygenation during all aspects of care. The most reliable clinical assessment tool in determining the significance of TBI in a nonsedated, nonparalyzed patient is the Glasgow Coma Scale. Acute subdural hematoma is the most common brain injury prompting emergency neurosurgical intervention and is associated with the highest mortality.
9. Systemic hypotension (systolic blood pressures <90 mm Hg), hypoxia (PaO_2 <60 mm Hg), hypercapnia ($PaCO_2$ >50 mm Hg),

— *Continued next page*

Continued—

and hyperthermia (temperature >38.0°C) have a negative impact on morbidity and mortality following head injuries, likely because of their contributions to increasing cerebral edema and intracranial pressure (ICP).

10 Current Brain Trauma Foundation guidelines recommend maintaining cerebral perfusion pressure between 50 and 70 mm Hg and ICP at less than 20 mm Hg for patients with severe head injury.

11 Maintaining supranormal mean arterial blood pressure to help ensure adequate spinal cord perfusion in areas of otherwise reduced blood flow due to cord compression or vascular compromise is likely to be of more benefit than steroid administration.

12 Major burns (a second- or third-degree burn involving ≥20% of total body surface area [TBSA]) induce a unique hemodynamic response. Cardiac output declines abruptly by up to 50% within 30 min of injury due to massive vasoconstriction, inducing a state of normovolemic hypoperfusion (*burn shock*).

13 In contrast to blunt and penetrating trauma, where crystalloid fluids are discouraged, burn fluid resuscitation emphasizes the use of balanced crystalloid fluids in preference to albumin, hydroxyethyl starch, normal or hypertonic saline, or blood.

14 The differential diagnosis for altered mental status following burn injury, smoke inhalation, or both includes carbon monoxide and cyanide poisoning.

15 Beyond 48 h following a major burn injury, succinylcholine administration can produce lethal hyperkalemia.

16 Older adults represent the fastest-growing trauma population. A progressive decrease in trauma survivability is first seen beginning around age 50. Significant underlying medical conditions contribute to increased trauma-related morbidity and mortality after even modest injuries.

17 In situations of mass casualty incidents, point-of-care (POC) ultrasound technology provides timely, critical information related to triaging patients for surgical and nonsurgical therapies using the CAVEAT (chest, abdomen, vena cava, and extremities) assessment.

Trauma is a leading cause of morbidity and mortality in all age groups and a leading cause of death in both young people (under 20 years old) and older adults (over 70 years old). All aspects of trauma care, from that provided at the scene, through transport, resuscitation, surgery, intensive care, and rehabilitation, must be coordinated if trauma patients are to have the greatest opportunity for a full recovery. The Advanced Trauma Life Support (ATLS) program developed by the American College of Surgeons Committee on Trauma has provided training and recommendations for consistent approaches to trauma resuscitation. The development of criteria for Level 1 Trauma Centers has also improved care by directing severely injured patients to facilities with appropriate resources. Although trauma anesthesia is sometimes thought of as a unique topic, many of the principles for managing trauma patients are relevant to any unstable or hemorrhaging patient. Thus, many issues commonly encountered in typical anesthesia practices are addressed in this chapter.

PRIMARY SURVEY

Airway

Emergency Medical Technician-Paramedics (EMT-P), Critical Care flight nurses, and Emergency Medicine physicians have airway management training for the prehospital and hospital settings. As a result, in North America, the anesthesia provider's role in providing initial trauma airway interventions has declined. As a consequence, when called upon for assistance in airway management in the emergency department, anesthesia providers must expect a challenging airway since routine airway management techniques have likely proved unsuccessful.

There are three important aspects of airway management in the initial evaluation of a trauma patient: (1) the need for basic life support intervention; (2) the presumed presence of a cervical spinal cord injury until proven otherwise; and (3) the potential for failed endotracheal intubation. By improving oxygenation and reducing hypercarbia in the unresponsive trauma patient, effective basic life support may improve a patient's level of consciousness sufficiently to remove the need for intubation. In those with persistent unresponsiveness, effective basic life support improves preoxygenation and reduces the risk for hypoxia during
1 airway interventions. All acute trauma patients should be presumed to have a full stomach and be at increased risk for pulmonary aspiration.

2 Cervical spine injury is presumed in any trauma patient presenting with neck pain or any suggestion of neurologic injury as well as those with loss of consciousness, significant head injury, or intoxication. Cervical collar ("C-collar") application before transport protects the cervical spinal cord by limiting cervical extension, and first-responders should utilize well-designed "hard" collars (eg, Aspen, Miami-J, Philadelphia) for cervical spine stabilization. *Traditional "soft" cervical collars provide essentially no useful cervical spine stabilization.* Hard collar cervical spine stabilization negatively impacts positioning for direct laryngoscopy and tracheal intubation, and alternative airway management devices (eg, video laryngoscope, fiberoptic bronchoscope) must be immediately available. If tracheal intubation is required, the front part of the C-collar can be removed as long as the head and neck remain in a neutral position while a designated assistant maintains manual in-line stabilization. This is usually performed with the assistant standing by the torso or kneeling at the head of the bed, holding the patient's head at the level of the ears and allowing the patient's mouth to open during laryngoscopy.

Alternative supraglottic devices for airway management (eg, King supralaryngeal device) may be used if direct laryngoscopy has failed in any environment (prehospital to intensive care unit). These devices, blindly placed into the airway, isolate the glottis opening between a large inflatable cuff positioned at the base of the tongue and the distal cuff that most likely rests in the proximal esophagus (Figure 39–1). The prolonged presence of supraglottic devices in the airway has been associated with tongue engorgement resulting from the large, proximal cuff obstructing venous outflow from the tongue, and in some cases, tongue engorgement has been sufficiently severe to warrant tracheostomy prior to its removal.

Limited evidence exists that prehospital airway management in trauma patients improves outcomes. However, failed endotracheal intubation in the prehospital environment certainly exposes patients to significant morbidity. Failed intubation attempts often result in systemic hypoxemia, and repeated hypoxemic events after even modest neurological injury further exacerbate the initial neurological insult (the *second hit* phenomenon).

Airway management in trauma patients is uneventful in most circumstances. Cricothyroidotomies and tracheostomies are rarely required for securing trauma airways. However, when trauma significantly alters or distorts the facial or upper airway anatomy to the point of preventing effective mask ventilation, or when hemorrhage into the airway precludes the patient from lying supine, elective cricothyroidotomy or tracheostomy should be considered before administering sedation or neuromuscular blockers in preparation for attempting oral intubation.

Breathing

Pulmonary injury may not be immediately apparent
3 upon the trauma patient's arrival to the hospital. In the patient with blunt or penetrating injury, providers should maintain a high level of suspicion for pulmonary injury that could evolve into a tension pneumothorax when mechanical ventilation is initiated. Peak inspiratory pressure and tidal volumes should be monitored throughout the initial resuscitation. Abrupt cardiovascular collapse shortly

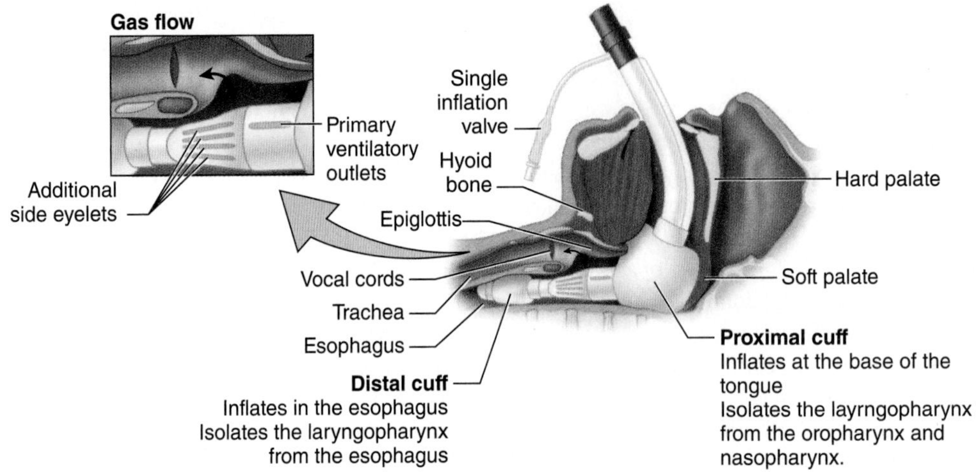

FIGURE 39–1 The King LT supralaryngeal device. The glottic opening lies between the large cuff positioned at the base of the tongue and the smaller balloon positioned in the proximal esophagus. The airway is not secured but rather isolated between the oropharynx and the proximal esophagus. (Reproduced with permission from King Systems Corporation, KLTD/KLTSD Disposable Supralaryngeal Airways Inservice Program, August 23, 2006.)

after instituting mechanical ventilation may signal the presence of a pneumothorax. Any trauma-related cardiovascular collapse is managed by disconnecting the patient from mechanical ventilation and performing bilateral needle thoracostomies. This intervention is accomplished by inserting a 14-gauge intravenous catheter into the second intercostal space in the midclavicular line, followed by a larger, more effective thoracostomy tube placed in the midaxillary line. *No trauma patient should die without having potential tension pneumothorax relieved.*

Circulation

Signs of a pulse and blood pressure are sought during the primary trauma patient survey. Unless the trauma patient arrives at the hospital other than by ambulance, the resuscitation team will likely have received information about the patient's vital signs from the prehospital first responders. The absence of a pulse following trauma is associated with minimal chances of survival. An emergency POC ultrasound evaluation of the chest and abdomen is indicated for any patient arriving in cardiac arrest after trauma, as are bilateral needle thoracostomies. The ultrasound evaluation will search for an empty heart or massive blood collection in the chest or abdomen.

The American College of Surgeons Committee on Trauma no longer endorses the use of emergency thoracotomy in treating patients without blood pressure or palpable pulse following *blunt* trauma, given the lack of evidence supporting survival following this intervention. In victims of penetrating trauma without a palpable pulse or blood pressure but with organized cardiac rhythm, a resuscitative thoracotomy may offer some survivability, but mortality remains exceedingly high.

Tourniquet use remains underutilized for compressible hemorrhage. Any extremity with significant vascular injury should have a tourniquet applied at the earliest possible moment ("stop the bleed"). The fear of tourniquet-induced limb ischemia often distracts first responders from making prompt, effective interventions in controlling hemorrhage with a tourniquet. *Hemorrhage, not limb ischemia or loss of limb function, is the most pressing threat to life, and it should be controlled by any effective measure at the earliest possible opportunity.*

Neurological Function

Once the presence of circulation is confirmed, a brief neurological examination is conducted. Level of consciousness (typically using the Glasgow Coma Scale), pupillary size and reaction, lateralizing signs suggesting intracranial or extracranial injuries, and indications of potential spinal cord injury are quickly evaluated. As noted earlier, hypercarbia often causes depressed neurological responsiveness following trauma, and it is effectively corrected with basic life support airway interventions. Additional causes of depressed neurological function (eg, alcohol/drug intoxication, effects of illicit or prescribed medications, hypoglycemia, hypoperfusion, brain or spinal cord injury) must also be considered. Mechanisms of injury must be reviewed as well as exclusion of other factors in determining the risk for central nervous system trauma. Persistently depressed levels of consciousness should be considered a result of central nervous system injury until disproved by emergency diagnostic studies (eg, computed tomography scan).

Injury Assessment

The patient must be fully exposed and examined to adequately assess the extent of injury. This physical exposure increases the risk of hypothermia, which is associated with increased bleeding in the trauma patient. The resuscitation bay and operating room must be maintained near body temperature (uncomfortably warm), all intravenous fluids and blood products (except platelets) should be warmed during administration, and under-body forced-air patient warmers should be utilized. Although these interventions are important in addressing hypothermia, meticulous trauma team efficiency in identifying life-threatening injuries is critical for patient survival. In most urban trauma centers, the initial major trauma evaluation is completed within 20 min of patient arrival.

The FAST Examination

The FAST *(Focused Assessment with Sonography for Trauma)* examination utilizes ultrasonography at the trauma victim's bedside, performed by surgeons or emergency medicine physicians, for detecting the presence or absence of free fluid in the perihepatic and perisplenic spaces, pericardium, and pelvis. **Patients with free fluid in these areas, as well as two of the following—penetrating injury, systolic blood pressures less than 90 mm Hg, or heart rate over 120 beats per minute—are likely to have high mortality and trauma-induced coagulopathy and require a massive transfusion.** These critical findings have been validated in numerous trauma studies and warrant immediate surgical intervention for hemorrhage control.

RESUSCITATION

Hemorrhage

Certain trauma terminology must be understood and utilized by the trauma care team to effectively communicate during trauma resuscitation or procedures in which blood loss is occurring. *Hemorrhage classifications I through IV, damage control resuscitation,* and *damage control surgery* are terms that quickly convey critical information, using a common understanding of the various interventions that may be required for resuscitating a trauma or surgical patient experiencing life-threatening bleeding. The American College of Surgeons identifies four classes of hemorrhage:

- **Class I hemorrhage** is the volume of blood that can be lost without hemodynamic consequence. With this volume of blood loss, the heart rate does not change, and the blood pressure does not decrease. In most circumstances, this amount of blood represents less than 15% of circulating blood volume. The typical adult has a blood volume equivalent of 70 mL/kg. For an 80-kg patient, the circulating blood volume is roughly 5.6 L. Children are considered to have an 80-mL/kg blood volume, and infants, 90 mL/kg. Intravenous resuscitation is not required if bleeding is promptly controlled, as in minor elective surgical procedures.
- **Class II hemorrhage** is the volume of blood that, when lost, prompts sympathetic responses to maintain perfusion and represents the loss of 15% to 30% of circulating blood volume. The diastolic blood pressure will increase due to vasoconstriction, and the heart rate will increase to maintain cardiac output. Intravenous fluid replacement is indicated for blood loss of this volume. Transfusions may be required if the bleeding continues, suggesting a progression to class III hemorrhage.

- **Class III hemorrhage** represents a loss of 30% to 40% of circulating blood volume, which consistently results in decreased blood pressure. Compensatory mechanisms of vasoconstriction and tachycardia are not sufficient for maintaining tissue perfusion to meet metabolic demand, and arterial blood gas analysis will reveal metabolic acidosis. Blood transfusion is necessary to restore adequate tissue perfusion and oxygenation. The other trauma team members must be notified when this pattern of fluid dependence develops, and discussion must be initiated regarding the possible need for *damage control* intervention (discussed later) for hemorrhage control.
- Life-threatening **class IV hemorrhage** represents more than 40% of circulating blood volume loss. The patient will be unresponsive and profoundly hypotensive, and rapid control of bleeding and aggressive blood-based resuscitation (*damage control resuscitation*) are required to prevent death. Patients experiencing this degree of hemorrhage will have some element of *trauma-induced coagulopathy* (TIC), require massive blood transfusion (more than 10 units of red blood cells in a 24-h period), and are at greatly increased risk for death. *The response to hemorrhage of this consequence must be damage control resuscitation and damage control surgery* (see later discussion).

Trauma-Induced Coagulopathy

Coagulation abnormalities are common following major trauma, and trauma-induced coagulopathy (TIC) coagulopathy is an independent risk factor
4 **for death.** TIC is present shortly after injury and before any resuscitative efforts have been initiated in up to 25% of major trauma patients. This means that the coagulopathy cannot be attributed to the dilutional effects of resuscitative fluids. Global tissue hypoperfusion appears to play a key role in the development of TIC. In one report, TIC was only related to the presence of severe metabolic acidosis (base deficits >6 mEq/L) and appeared to have a dose-dependent relationship with the degree of tissue hypoperfusion; 2% of patients with base deficits less than 6 mEq/L developed coagulopathy compared with 20% of patients with base deficits greater than 6 mEq/L. Although injury severity scores were likely higher in the coagulopathic patients, only the presence of metabolic acidosis correlated to developing TIC.

During hypoperfusion, the endothelium releases thrombomodulin and activated protein C, which, at the microcirculation level, prevents thrombosis. Thrombomodulin binds thrombin, thereby preventing thrombin from cleaving fibrinogen to fibrin. The thrombomodulin–thrombin complex activates protein C, which then inhibits the extrinsic coagulation pathway through effects on cofactors V and VIII (Figure 39–2). Activated protein C also inhibits plasminogen activator inhibitor-1 proteins, which increases tissue plasminogen activator, resulting in hyperfibrinolysis (Figure 39–3). One prospective clinical study found the following effects of hypoperfusion on coagulation parameters: (1) progressive coagulopathy as base deficit increases; (2) increasing plasma thrombomodulin and falling protein C (indicating activation of the protein levels with increasing base deficit), supporting the argument that the anticoagulant effects of these proteins in the presence of hypoperfusion are related to the prolongation of prothrombin and partial thromboplastin times; and (3) early-onset TIC and increased mortality.

TIC is not solely related to impaired clot formation. As previously noted, fibrinolysis is an equally important component as a result of plasmin activity on an existing clot. Tranexamic acid administration is associated with decreased bleeding during cardiac and orthopedic surgeries, presumably because of its antifibrinolytic properties. A randomized control study involving 20,000 trauma patients with or at risk of significant bleeding found a significantly reduced risk for death from hemorrhage when tranexamic acid therapy (loading dose, 1 g over 10 min, followed by an infusion of 1 g over 8 h) was initiated within the first 3 h following major trauma (the CRASH-II study). Figure 39–4 demonstrates the benefit of initiating this therapy in relation to the time of injury. Although this study resulted in the widespread use of tranexamic acid in major trauma, its shortcomings (eg, a very small number of its 20,000 patients required transfusion or were transfused) have more recently resulted in reconsideration of tranexamic acid administration in trauma care.

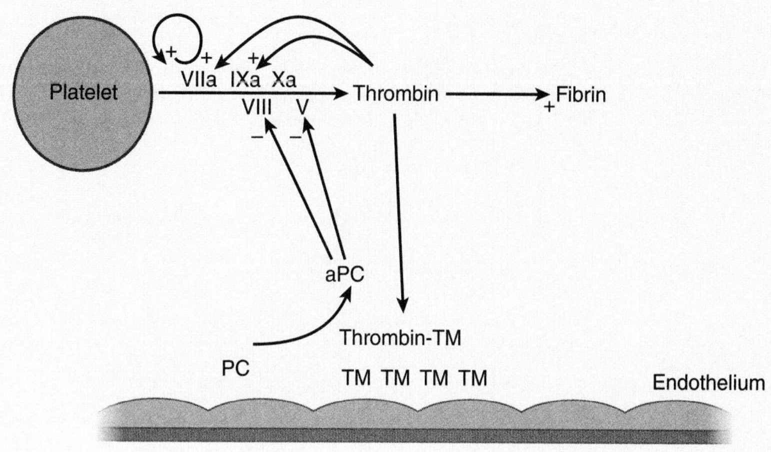
Thrombin is generated primarily via the "extrinsic" pathway with multiple feed-forward loops. When thrombomodulin (TM) is presented by the endothelium, it complexes thrombin, which is no longer available to cleave fibrinogen. This anticoagulent thrombin activates protein C (PC), which reduces further thrombin generation through inhibition of cofactors V and VIII.
Platelet
VIIa IXa Xa
VIII V
Thrombin
Fibrin
aPC
Thrombin-TM
PC
TM TM TM TM
Endothelium

FIGURE 39–2 Mechanism of trauma-induced coagulopathy. During periods of tissue hypoperfusion, thrombomodulin (TM) released by the endothelium complexes with thrombin. The thrombin–TM complexes prevent cleavage of fibrinogen to fibrin and also activate protein C (PC), reducing further thrombin generation through cofactors V and VIII. (Reproduced with permission from Brohi K, Cohen MJ, Davenport RA. Acute coagulopathy of trauma: mechanism, identification and effect. *Curr Opin Crit Care.* 2007 Dec;13(6):680-685.)

Hemostatic Resuscitation

Early coagulopathy of trauma is associated with increased mortality. Military experience treating combat-wounded soldiers and civilians has provided great insight into trauma resuscitation and TIC. Battlefield resuscitation protocols have utilized whole blood for decades. Whole blood resuscitation is instituted in circumstances where casualty load

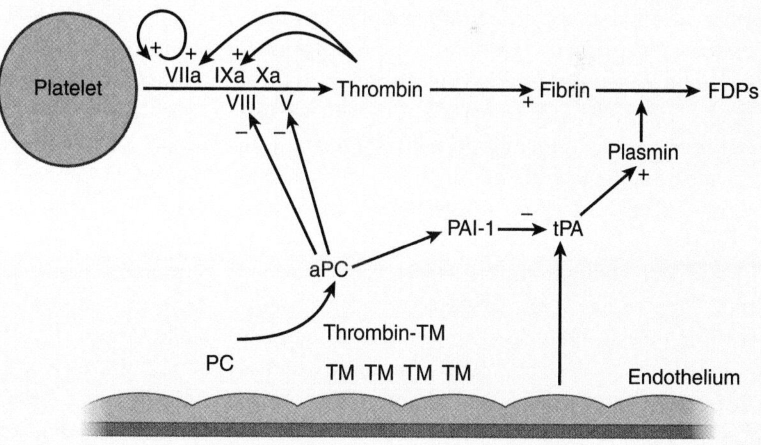
Tissue plasminogen activator (tPA) is released from the endothelium by injury and hypoperfusion and cleaves plasminogen to initiate fibrinolysis. Activated protein C (aPC) consumes plasminogen activator inhibitor-1 (PAI-1) when present in excess, and reduced PAI-1 leads to increased tPA activity and hyperfibrinolysis.
Platelet
VIIa IXa Xa
VIII V
Thrombin
Fibrin
FDPs
Plasmin
PAI-1
tPA
aPC
Thrombin-TM
PC
TM TM TM TM
Endothelium

FIGURE 39–3 Mechanism of hyperfibrinolysis in tissue hypoperfusion. Tissue plasminogen activator (tPA) released from the endothelium during hypoperfusion states cleaves plasminogen to initiate fibrinolysis. Activated protein C (aPC) consumes plasminogen activator inhibitor-1 (PAI-1) when present in excess, and reduced PAI-1 leads to increased tPA activity and hyperfibrinolysis. FDPs, fibrin degradation products; PC, protein C; TM, thrombomodulin. (Reproduced with permission from Brohi K, Cohen MJ, Davenport RA. Acute coagulopathy of trauma: Mechanism, identification and effect. *Curr Opin Crit Care.* 2007 Dec;13(6):680-685.)

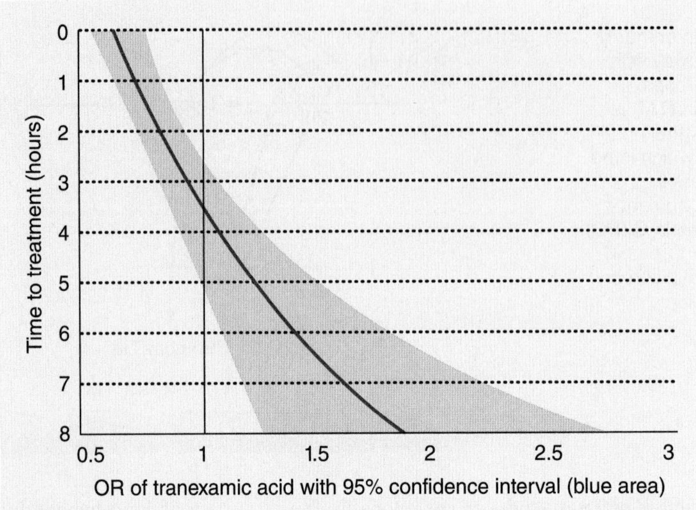

FIGURE 39–4 Influence of tranexamic acid in preventing death from bleeding. Outcomes ratios (OR) of tranexamic acid with 95% confidence interval (*blue area*) on the *x*-axis and time (h) to treatment on the *y*-axis demonstrate improved survival if tranexamic acid therapy is initiated within 3 h of injury. The area of the curve to the left of OR 1.0 demonstrates the benefits of therapy, while that to the right demonstrates harm from intervention. (Reproduced with permission from Roberts I, Shakur H, Afolabi A, et al. The importance of early treatment with tranexamic acid in bleeding trauma patients: An exploratory analysis of the CRASH-2 randomised controlled trial. *Lancet*. 2011 Mar 26;377(9771):1096-1101.)

exceeds available blood resources, usually in remote or forward bases near combat. The process requires about an hour to collect, process, and then deliver blood between soldiers. The blood is warm, and clotting factors and platelets are at optimum temperature and pH. The use of whole blood transfusions in these settings is lifesaving. However, in most circumstances, the U.S. Department of Defense utilizes more conventional blood banking techniques and utilization of blood products in combat theaters, making the need for whole blood transfusions infrequent.

Military conflicts in the 2000s have provided ample opportunities for developing updated transfusion protocols. Retrospective analysis of severely wounded service members found improved survival when fresh frozen plasma was administered early in

5 trauma resuscitations. In an attempt to recreate whole blood, balanced administration of red blood cells, fresh frozen plasma, and platelet units (1:1:1) became the standard trauma transfusion protocol in military settings and was promptly adopted thereafter by major civilian trauma centers, which also noted improved patient survival. This approach to transfusion is termed *damage control resuscitation* (DCR).

Administering blood products in equal ratios early in resuscitation has become an accepted approach for preventing or correcting TIC. Although this combination of blood products attempts replication of whole blood, the resultant fluid is pancytopenic, with only a fraction of whole blood's hematocrit and coagulation factor concentration. Red blood cells will improve oxygen delivery to hypoperfused, ischemic tissues. Fresh frozen plasma provides clotting factors V and VIII along with fibrinogen, which improves clotting, possibly due to overwhelming of the thrombin–thrombomodulin complex. Platelets and cryoprecipitate, although included in the 1:1:1 DCR protocol, are probably not necessary in the initial phase of resuscitation, given the normal platelet and fibrinogen levels noted in early coagulopathy. The use of crystalloid fluids in early trauma resuscitation has markedly decreased with the increased emphasis upon early blood product administration.

Most trauma centers have early-release type O-negative blood available for immediate transfusion to patients with severe hemorrhage. Depending on the urgency of transfusion need, blood product administration typically progresses from O-negative to type-specific and then to cross-matched units as the acute need decreases. Patients administered uncrossmatched, O-negative blood are those at greater risk of requiring massive transfusion. As the amount of uncrossmatched blood administered increases beyond eight units, resuscitation should persist using O-negative blood without attempting to switch to the patient's native blood type. Reverting to the patient's native blood type in this situation risks transfusion reactions that will further complicate resuscitation and survival.

Most clinical studies evaluating DCR have been retrospective. However, a prospective, randomized, multi-institutional massive transfusion study from 10 U.S. level 1 trauma centers (the PROMTT study) was conducted and published in 2013, confirming that the greater the injury and concomitant hemorrhagic shock, the greater the likelihood of TIC requiring massive transfusion and the greater the risk of death. The contribution of activated protein C to TIC and the benefits of blood-based, rather than crystalloid-based, resuscitation for hemorrhagic shock were also demonstrated.

Point-of-care functional clotting studies are extremely useful for guiding specific blood product use. Thromboelastography (TEG) and rotational elastometry (ROTEM) identify the specific deficiencies, freeing the practitioner from reliance solely on the 1:1:1 transfusion ratio DCR approach. Both TEG and ROTEM assess the rate of clot formation and clot stability, reflecting the interactions between the coagulation cascades, platelets, and the fibrinolytic system. Figure 39–5 demonstrates the pattern seen with TEG. Use of this technology in trauma resuscitations reduces blood product use (therefore, less exposure to potential infection and less expense) and identifies fibrinolysis.

Potential hazards may result from the aggressive administration of blood products during the resuscitation phase. Although blood-borne diseases such as acquired immunodeficiency syndrome, hepatitis B, and hepatitis C are usually cited as significant transfusion-related risks, modern blood bank

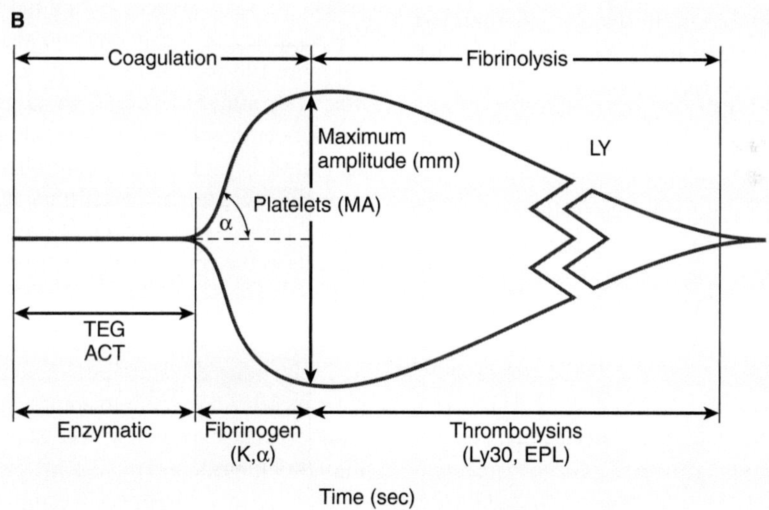

FIGURE 39–5 Thromboelastograph (TEG). The graph begins as a straight line until clot formation begins (the enzymatic stage of clotting). As a clot forms, increasing resistance develops on the strain gauge, creating a splaying of the graph. The pattern of the graph suggests the status of fibrinogen stores (α angle) and platelet function (maximum amplitude, MA). Eventually, fibrinolysis will occur, as demonstrated by decreasing MA. Deficiencies of various clotting components will affect each phase of the TEG, whereas increased fibrinolysis will be demonstrated by an earlier decline in the maximum amplitude. ACT, activated clotting time; EPL, Ly30, K, R, values related to the rate of clot breakdown. (Reproduced with permission from Kashuk JL, Moore EE, Sawyer M, et al. Postinjury coagulopathy management: Goal directed resuscitation via POC thrombelastography. *Ann Surg*. 2010 Apr;251(4):604-614.)

donor screening has decreased the incidence of such
6 infections by as much as 10,000-fold. The incidence of *transfusion-related acute lung injury* (TRALI), until recently the leading cause of transfusion-related death, has also markedly declined. With the recognition that the presence of HLA antibodies in donor plasma is the principal TRALI risk factor, most blood banks now accept plasma and platelet donations only from males or from females who have either never been pregnant or who have been tested and found to be anti-HLA negative. The greatest transfusion risk patients now face during trauma resuscitation is *transfusion-associated circulatory overload* (TACO), which occurs when blood products are administered at a rate greater than the patient's cardiac output. This is most likely to occur when the provider administering blood products has not recognized that the source of bleeding has been successfully controlled. Communication in this situation is critical between those team members resuscitating the patient with blood products and those attempting to control the hemorrhage.

Massive Transfusion Protocols

Delay in obtaining blood products other than red blood cells is a potential problem for both military and civilian trauma resuscitations. Clinical evidence supports the need for and benefit of established *massive transfusion protocols* (MTPs), allowing the blood bank to assemble blood products in prescribed ratios in supporting blood-based trauma resuscitations. With MTPs in place, hemostatic resuscitation can continue until the demand for blood products stops. *An MTP-driven, blood-based resuscitation, rather than a crystalloid-based resuscitation, improves survival from trauma, reduces total blood product utilization in the first 24 h following injury, reduces acute infectious complications (severe sepsis, septic shock, and ventilator-associated pneumonia), and decreases postresuscitation organ dysfunction (an 80% decrease in odds of developing multisystem organ failure).*

MTPs benefit both the patient (improved survival and fewer complications) and the institution (more efficient and effective processes for utilizing scarce blood bank resources). Most hospitals performing complex surgeries, transplants, or trauma resuscitations now have MTPs in place, though one must recognize that the transfusion needs of transplant, cancer, and cardiac patients may differ from those of trauma patients. Establishing which personnel are empowered to initiate MTP use during trauma resuscitation is of great importance, given the expense and implications for the blood bank in terms of blood product inventory, personnel training and availability, and disruption of routine blood bank duties. Annual reviews of MTPs are necessary for ensuring that the most current knowledge, technology, and medications are employed to optimize blood product utilization.

DEFINITIVE TRAUMA INTERVENTIONS

The initial history and physical examination, emergency procedures, and evaluations used to determine the extent of injury and the need for resuscitation and surgical intervention all occur outside the operating room and often before an anesthesia provider has been alerted. However, critical initial issues impacting anesthetic management of trauma patients include the adequacy of the airway and vascular access, the ability of the patient to tolerate anesthesia, prevention of hypothermia, access to adequate blood bank supplies, and avoidance of crystalloids and vasopressors until hemorrhage is controlled. Therefore, we strongly recommend anesthesiologist participation in the early assessment of severely injured trauma patients in the emergency department.

Anesthetic Induction & Maintenance

Severely injured, conscious, and oriented trauma patients arriving for emergency surgery should have an abbreviated interview and examination, including an emphasis on consent for blood transfusions and advice that intraoperative awareness may occur during emergency surgery. As always, such discussions should be documented in the patient's record.

The operating room should be as warm as practical. Intravenous fluid warmers and rapid infusion devices should be ready for use. As previously noted, all patients arriving for trauma surgery should be presumed to have full stomachs with increased risk for aspiration of gastric contents, and the presence of a C-collar for cervical spine stabilization may increase intubation difficulty. Alternative airway devices (eg, fiberoptic bronchoscope, videolaryngoscope) and adequate suction equipment must be immediately available and ready for use.

Intravenous access is usually established in the prehospital setting or emergency department. If the existing peripheral intravenous lines are sufficient to permit infusing blood under pressure (eg, from a rapid infusion device), a central line may not be necessary. However, patients may arrive in the operating room so profoundly hypotensive and hypovolemic that peripheral intravenous line placement may be impossible. In these circumstances, a subclavian catheter or intraosseous device should be inserted and blood-based resuscitation initiated. The subclavian vein is often preferred for central venous access in profoundly hypotensive patients due to its position between the clavicle and first rib, which tends to stent the subclavian vein open even in profound hypovolemia. An intraosseous device placed with the use of a small bone drill in the proximal tibia or humerus provides direct access to venous complexes through the bone marrow. The use of interosseous access requires that the bone proximal and distal to the insertion site be intact; otherwise, extravasation of infused fluids will occur as a result of the fluid taking the path of least resistance (the fracture site). Intraosseous infusions require pressure, not gravity, for infusions to overcome the resistance to flow originating in the bone marrow. Finally, the ubiquitous availability of point-of-care ultrasound devices in anesthesia practice may allow the safe placement of large-bore or central venous catheters in jugular veins using ultrasound guidance, even in the presence of profound hypovolemia.

Major blood loss and hemodynamic instability create a dangerous situation for the conscious trauma patient and a challenging decision for the anesthesia provider planning the induction of general anesthesia. Trauma patients with severe injuries may experience profound hypotension following even modest doses (0.25–0.5 mg/kg intravenously) of propofol. Etomidate preserves sympathetic tone, which makes it a modestly safer choice than propofol. Ketamine is also a reasonable choice, particularly if given in 10-mg intravenous boluses until the patient becomes unresponsive. Scopolamine, 0.4 mg intravenously, should be considered as an amnestic agent for the profoundly hemodynamically unstable but conscious patient at great risk for hemodynamic collapse on induction of anesthesia for emergency surgery. What is most important is not the particular intravenous anesthetic induction agent chosen but the recognition that *the hemodynamically unstable trauma patient will tolerate significantly less medication for induction and maintenance of anesthesia than in normal circumstances.*

Fluid management in major trauma resuscitations emphasizes blood products rather than crystalloid fluids, as previously noted. An MTP should be requested and followed, with the blood immediately available upon the arrival of the patient to the operating room. All fluids should be warmed, except for platelets. Ionized calcium quickly declines and must be replaced when blood products are rapidly infused. Vasopressors should be avoided, if possible, until the source of bleeding is controlled. Studies suggest that increasing the blood pressure with vasopressors during hemorrhage disrupts fresh clots, resulting in more bleeding.

An arterial line is helpful but not mandatory in the initial resuscitation of the trauma victim. Cannulating an artery in the presence of profound hypotension may prove difficult even with the assistance of ultrasonography. Attempts at placing invasive monitors can continue as the patient is prepared for incision, including gowning and gloving the person attempting arterial line placement on the surgical side of the drape, if necessary. The surgical incision must not be delayed even though arterial line placement may be challenging. Surgical control of bleeding and DCR are the top priorities in trauma resuscitation, not arterial line placement. Patients in this degree of hemodynamic compromise can be presumed to have TIC and need massive transfusion. Attempts for arterial line placement can resume and are more likely to be successful as blood pressure improves from operative hemostasis and resuscitative transfusion.

Damage Control Surgery

If a trauma patient requires emergency laparotomy for intraabdominal hemorrhage, the trauma surgeon will perform an abbreviated procedure termed *damage control surgery* (DCS). This surgical intervention is intended to stop hemorrhage and limit gastrointestinal contamination of the abdominal compartment. After making a midline incision, the surgeon quickly searches for sources of bleeding through a quadrant-by-quadrant examination. Definitive repair of complex injuries is not part of DCS. Identification and control of injured blood vessels and solid organs, as well as inspection of injuries in areas relatively inaccessible to midline approaches but potentially addressed by interventional radiology techniques (eg, deep liver lacerations, retroperitoneal hemorrhage), occurs during DCS. Hollow viscus injuries are addressed with resection, stapling, or both. Leaving the intestines disconnected until the patient is more stable reduces intraabdominal contamination and operating time.

Communication among the trauma team is essential during DCS. The surgeon must know if the patient is becoming unstable, hypothermic, or coagulopathic. The anesthesia team must speak up when there is a need to pause the surgical procedure to allow resuscitation. Pausing surgery results in the surgeon compressing or packing an area of bleeding during times of profound hypotension until transfusion restores acceptable systolic blood pressure (80–90 mm Hg). If this interruption of surgery is unsuccessful in improving blood pressure, the surgeon can directly compress the aorta. This intervention provides the surgeon direct feedback as to the effectiveness of transfusion—a soft aorta suggests profound hypovolemia, whereas the return of a firm, pulsatile aorta suggests a more acceptable circulating blood volume. A brief episode of bradycardia/asystole may accompany direct aortic compression. When transfusions are ineffective in maintaining perfusion, the operation should be interrupted and the bleeding areas packed, and a decision should be made between the surgeon and anesthesia team as to whether the patient can be transferred to the interventional radiology suite to treat bleeding from surgically inaccessible sites or to the intensive care unit where rewarming, correction of coagulopathy, and hemodynamic stabilization may occur.

A key component of DCS is planned reoperation once the patient is more stable. Bowel continuity can be restored, or a colostomy can be performed at a later time. The abdominal fascia is often not definitively closed after DCS. The wound may be covered with an occlusive dressing over a wound vacuum sponge. Bowel edema in the setting of closed abdominal fascia following massive transfusion risks abdominal compartment syndrome, respiratory compromise, and multisystem organ failure.

The interventional radiology suite is an increasingly important part of the DCS sequence. Vascular catheter-based interventional radiology techniques can reach essentially any bleeding vessel and deposit coils or foam that may control hemorrhage, most notably in liver, kidney, and retroperitoneal injuries. Hemorrhage from pelvic ring fractures or major thoracic or abdominal vascular injuries are also potentially controlled by such interventions. In addition, patients are often taken to interventional radiology following DCS to assess blood flow and hemostasis in organs either injured by the initial trauma or potentially compromised as part of the DCS.

TRAUMATIC BRAIN INJURY

8 **Any trauma patient with an altered level of consciousness must be considered to have a traumatic brain injury (TBI) until proven otherwise** (see Chapter 27). The presence or suspicion of TBI mandates attention to maintaining cerebral perfusion pressure and oxygenation during all aspects of care. The most reliable clinical assessment tool in determining the significance of TBI in a nonsedated, nonparalyzed patient is the Glasgow Coma Scale (GCS; see Table 27–2). A declining motor score is suggestive of progressing neurological deterioration, prompting urgent neurological evaluation and possible surgical intervention. Although trauma patients frequently have head injuries, few head injuries require emergency neurosurgical intervention. TBIs are categorized as either *primary* or *secondary*. Primary brain injuries are directly related to trauma. Four categories of primary brain injury are seen: (1) subdural hematoma; (2) epidural hematoma; (3) intraparenchymal hemorrhage; and (4) nonfocal,

diffuse neuronal injury disrupting axons of the central nervous system. These injuries potentially elevate intracranial pressure (ICP), compromising cerebral blood flow. Death occurring soon after head trauma is usually the result of primary brain injury.

Acute subdural hematoma is the most common brain injury prompting emergency neurosurgical intervention and is associated with the highest mortality. Small bridging veins between the skull and brain are disrupted in deceleration or blunt force injuries, resulting in blood accumulation and compression of brain tissue. The accumulation of blood raises ICP and compromises cerebral blood flow. Morbidity and mortality are related to the size of the hematoma and the magnitude of the midline shift of intracranial contents. Midline shifts of intracranial contents may exceed the size of the hematoma, suggesting a significant contribution of cerebral edema or underlying intracerebral hemorrhage.

Epidural hematoma occurs when the middle cerebral artery or other cranial vessels are disrupted, often in association with skull fracture. This injury accounts for less than 10% of neurosurgical trauma emergencies and has a better prognosis than acute subdural hematoma. The patient with an epidural hematoma may initially be conscious, followed by progressive unresponsiveness and coma. Emergency surgical decompression is indicated when supratentorial lesions occupy more than 30 mL volume and infratentorial lesions occupy more than 10 mL volume (brainstem compression may occur at much lower hematoma volumes). A small epidural hematoma may not require immediate evacuation if the patient is neurologically intact, close observation and repeated neurological examinations are possible, and neurosurgical resources are immediately available should emergency decompression become necessary.

Intraparenchymal injuries are caused by rapid deceleration of the brain within the skull, usually involving the tips of the frontal and temporal lobes, and represent nearly 20% of neurosurgical emergencies following trauma. Such injuries tend to be associated with edema, necrosis, and infarcts in areas surrounding the damaged tissue. Intraparenchymal injury may underlie a subdural hematoma. There is no consensus regarding the surgical interventions that should be performed for intraparenchymal hemorrhage, but surgical decompression may be necessary to reduce sustained, dangerously elevated ICP.

Diffuse neuronal injury results from rapid deceleration or movement of brain tissue of sufficient force to disrupt neurons and axons and is more common in children than in adults. The extent of injury may not be obvious in the period immediately following injury but will become apparent with serial magnetic resonance imaging. The greater the extent of the diffuse neuronal injury following trauma, the higher the mortality and disability severity. Surgical intervention is not indicated for these injuries unless a decompressive craniectomy is required for relief of refractory elevated ICP.

Secondary brain injuries are considered poten-
9 tially preventable injuries. Systemic hypoten-
sion (systolic blood pressures <90 mm Hg), hypoxia (PaO_2 <60 mm Hg), hypercapnia ($PaCO_2$ >50 mm Hg), and hyperthermia (temperature >38.0°C) have a negative impact on morbidity and mortality following head injuries, likely because of their contributions to increasing cerebral edema and ICP. *Hypotension and hypoxemia are recognized as major contributors to poor neurological recovery from severe TBI. Hypoxemia is the single most important parameter correlating with poor neurological outcome following head trauma and should be corrected at the earliest possible opportunity.* Hypotension (mean arterial blood pressure <60 mm Hg) should also be treated aggressively with fluids, vasopressors, or both in the presence of isolated head injury.

Management of severe head trauma in the presence of other severe injuries and hemorrhage creates a difficult resuscitation dilemma. Emergency neurosurgery and damage control laparotomy are nearly impossible to perform simultaneously, and in most circumstances, control of life-threatening hemorrhage takes precedence over neurosurgical intervention. Attempts to increase cerebral perfusion pressure in the presence of life-threatening hemorrhage will exacerbate bleeding. Once non-neurosurgical hemorrhage is controlled, attention can be directed toward the neurosurgical emergency, specifically toward restoring cerebral perfusion pressure. Prolonged periods of cerebral hypoperfusion in this situation are associated with negative neurological outcomes.

Management Considerations for Acute Traumatic Brain Injury

In the absence of an intracranial clot requiring surgical evacuation, medical interventions are the primary means of treating elevated ICP following head trauma. Normal cerebral perfusion pressure (CPP), the difference between mean arterial pressure (MAP) and ICP, is approximately 80 to 100 mm Hg (MAP − ICP = CPP; see Chapter 26). ICP monitoring is not required for conscious and alert patients. In addition, patients who are intentionally anticoagulated or who have bleeding diathesis in response to trauma should not have ICP monitoring. However, an ICP monitor should be placed when serial neurological examinations and additional clinical assessments reveal impairment or when there is an increased risk for elevated ICP (Table 39–1). Interventions for reducing ICP are indicated when readings are higher than 20 to 25 mm Hg, though multiple studies have evaluated interventions aimed at improving CPP and managing ICP without finding obvious outcome benefits for any particular treatment scheme. 10 **Current Brain Trauma Foundation guidelines recommend maintaining CPP between 50 and 70 mm Hg and ICP at less than 20 mm Hg for patients with severe head injury.**

Cerebral blood flow (CBF) is directly related to arterial carbon dioxide concentration. Cerebral vasoconstriction occurs as arterial carbon dioxide levels decrease, reducing CBF and ICP. Conversely, cerebral vasodilation occurs as arterial carbon dioxide levels rise, increasing CBF and ICP. Changes in arterial carbon dioxide levels exert a prompt CBF and ICP response, making hyperventilation an effective therapeutic intervention in cases of elevated ICP associated with TBI. *However, hyperventilation in the presence of systemic hypotension, particularly in the hemodynamically unstable, hemorrhaging trauma patient, increases the risk of neurological ischemia and should be avoided until normotension is restored.*

Osmotic diuretic therapy is another commonly used and widely accepted intervention for reducing elevated ICP. Intravenous mannitol doses of 0.25 to 1.0 g/kg body weight are effective in drawing extravascular fluid from brain tissue into the vascular system, decreasing brain edema and ICP. Because this intervention also induces brisk diuresis, plasma osmolality and serum electrolytes must be monitored.

Barbiturate coma has been used to reduce cerebral metabolic rate, cerebral blood flow, cerebral oxygen demand, and intracranial hypertension until cerebral perfusion improves. Hypotension is commonly associated with this therapy, which limits its use in hemodynamically unstable patients. Vasopressors may be used to maintain CPP between 50 and 70 mm Hg in such cases. The dose of pentobarbital (preferable to thiopental) is based upon electroencephalographic (EEG) evidence of burst suppression, the EEG threshold for maximally reduced cerebral metabolic rate for oxygen and glucose.

Crystalloid is preferable for fluid therapy in the presence of isolated TBI. Although the use of colloid might seem advantageous in preventing brain edema, in a recent study, albumin-based resuscitation following TBI nearly doubled mortality. TBI is often associated with blood–brain barrier disruption, and albumin administration in this situation

TABLE 39–1 Indications for intracranial ICP monitoring.

Severe head injury (defined as GCS score ≤8 after cardiopulmonary resuscitation) *plus*
(a) Abnormal admitting head CT scan *or*
(b) Normal CT scan plus ≥2 of: age >40 y, systolic blood pressure >90 mm Hg, decerebrate or decorticate position
Sedated patients; patient in induced coma after severe TBI
Multisystem injury with altered level of consciousness
Patient receiving treatment that increases risk of increased ICP (eg, high-volume intravenous fluids)
Postoperatively after removal or intracranial mass
Abnormal values in noninvasive ICP monitoring, increased dynamics of simulated values, or abnormal shapes in transcranial Doppler blood flow velocity waveform (increased pulsatility) with exclusion of arterial hypotension and hypocapnia

CT, computed tomography; GCS, Glasgow Coma Scale; ICP, intracranial pressure; TBI, traumatic brain injury.

Reproduced with permission from Li LM, Timofeev I, Czosnyka M, et al. Review article: The surgical approach to the management of increased intracranial pressure after traumatic brain injury. *Anesth Analg.* 2010 Sep;111(3):736-748.

may result in greater brain tissue edema and higher ICP, contributing to higher morbidity and mortality.

SPINAL CORD INJURY

The normal spine structure comprises three columns: anterior, middle, and posterior. The *anterior column* includes the anterior two-thirds of the vertebral body and the anterior longitudinal ligament. The *middle column* includes the posterior third of the vertebral body, the posterior longitudinal ligament, and the posterior component of the annulus fibrosus. The *posterior column* includes the laminae and facets, the spinous processes, and the interspinous ligaments. Spine instability results when two or all three of the columns are disrupted.

The trauma patient with a relevant mechanism of injury (typically blunt force involving acceleration–deceleration) must be approached with a high degree of suspicion for spinal cord injury unless it has been ruled out with imaging studies. *A lateral radiograph of the cervical spine demonstrating the entire cervical spine to the top of the T1 vertebrae will detect 85% to 90% of significant cervical spine abnormalities.* Cervical spine radiographs must be examined for structure and alignment of vertebral bodies, narrowing or widening of interspinous spaces and the central canal, alignment along the anterior and posterior ligament lines, and appearance of the spinolaminar line and posterior spinous processes of C2 through C7. The presence of one spinal fracture is associated with a 10% to 15% incidence of a second spinal fracture.

Thoracolumbar injuries most commonly involve the T11 through L3 vertebrae as a result of flexion forces. The presence of one thoracolumbar spinal injury is associated with a 40% chance of a second fracture caudal to the first, likely due to the force required to fracture the lower spine. Bilateral calcaneus fractures also warrant a thorough thoracolumbar spine evaluation due to the increased likelihood of associated spinal fracture associated with this injury pattern.

Cervical spine injuries occurring above C2 are associated with apnea and death. (C3–C5 roots form the phrenic nerve). *High spinal injuries are often accompanied by neurogenic shock due to the loss of sympathetic tone.* Neurogenic shock may masquerade as hemorrhagic shock in the presence of major trauma because the cause of the hypotension may be presumed hemorrhagic rather than neurological in origin. The presence of profound bradycardia 24 to 48 h after a high thoracic spinal cord lesion likely represents compromise of the cardioaccelerator function found in the T1–T4 region.

The principal therapeutic objectives following spinal cord injury are to prevent exacerbation of primary structural disruption and minimize the risk of extending neurological injury from hypotension-related hypoperfusion of ischemic areas of the spinal cord. In patients with complete spinal cord transection, very few interventions will influence recovery. Patients with incomplete spinal cord lesions require careful management of hemodynamic parameters (eg, avoiding hypotension) and surgical stabilization of the spine to prevent extension of existing injury and exacerbation of existing neurological deficits.

Surgical decompression and stabilization of spinal fractures are indicated when a vertebral body loses more than 50% of its normal height or the spinal canal is narrowed by more than 30% of its normal diameter. Methylprednisolone is often administered for spinal cord injury in this situation because the anti-inflammatory properties of this steroid potentially reduce spinal cord edema within the tight confines of a compromised spinal canal. Despite outcome studies from animal models of traumatic spinal cord injury demonstrating benefit from early surgical intervention, steroid therapy, or both, human studies have failed to demonstrate consistent benefit from either intervention. The presence of a decompressible lesion in the area of an incomplete spinal cord transection is not an indication for early operative intervention unless other, more life-threatening conditions are present.

11 Maintaining supranormal mean arterial blood pressure to help ensure adequate spinal cord perfusion in areas of otherwise reduced blood flow due to cord compression or vascular compromise is likely to be of more benefit than steroid administration. Hypotension must be avoided during induction of anesthesia, throughout operative decompression and stabilization of the spine injury, and in the postoperative phase.

Older adults are at greater risk for spinal cord injury because of decreased mobility and flexibility, greater incidence of spondylosis and osteophytes, and decreased space within the spinal canal to accommodate spinal cord edema following trauma. The incidence of spinal injury from falls in older adults is rapidly approaching that of spinal cord injury from motor vehicle accidents in younger patients. Mortality following spinal cord injury in older adults, particularly those over the age of 75 years, is greater than that in younger patients with a similar injury.

The unique injury pattern of penetrating spinal cord injury warrants separate consideration. Unlike blunt spinal trauma, penetrating trauma of the spinal cord due to bullets and shrapnel is unlikely to cause an unstable spine. As a result, C-collar or long-board immobilization may not be indicated in an isolated penetrating spinal cord injury. The C-collar placement in the presence of a cervical spine penetrating injury may actually hinder observation of soft tissue swelling, tracheal deviation, or other anatomic indications of imminent airway compromise. Unlike blunt trauma, penetrating injuries of the spinal cord induce damage at the moment of injury without risk of subsequent exacerbation of the injury. Like other spinal cord injuries, however, maintenance of spinal cord perfusion using supranormal mean arterial pressure is indicated until spinal cord function can be more thoroughly evaluated.

BURNS

Burns represent a unique but common traumatic injury that is second only to motor vehicle accidents as the leading source of accidental death. The extent of burn injury is determined by the temperature and duration of heat contact. Children, because of their increased body surface area to body mass ratio, and older adults, whose thinner skin allows deeper burns from similar thermal insult, are both at greater risk for major burn injury. The pathophysiological and hemodynamic responses to burn injuries are unique and warrant specialized care that can be optimally provided at burn treatment centers, especially when second- or third-degree burns involve more than 20% of a patient's total body surface area (TBSA). A basic understanding of burn pathophysiology and resuscitation requirements, especially early initiation of therapies such as oxygen administration and aggressive fluid resuscitation, will improve patient survival.

Burns are classified as first, second, or third degree. *First-degree* burns are injuries that do not penetrate the epidermis (eg, sunburns and superficial thermal injuries). Fluid replacement for these burns is not indicated, and the area of first-degree burns should not be included in calculating fluid replacement when more extensive or significant burns are also present. *Second-degree* burns are partial-thickness injuries (superficial or deep) that penetrate the epidermis, extend into the dermis for some depth, and are associated with blistering. Fluid replacement therapy is indicated for patients with second-degree burns when more than 20% of the TBSA is involved. Skin grafting also may be necessary in some cases of second-degree burns, depending upon wound size and location. *Third-degree* burns are those in which the thermal injury penetrates the full thickness of the dermis. Nerves, blood vessels, lymphatic channels, and other deep structures may have been destroyed, creating a severe but insensate wound, though healthy tissue surrounding the third-degree burn will be very painful. Debridement and skin grafting are almost always required for recovery from third-degree burns.

12 Major burns (a second- or third-degree burn involving ≥20% of TBSA) induce a unique hemodynamic response. Cardiac output declines by up to 50% within 30 min of the injury in response to burn-induced massive vasoconstriction, inducing a state of normovolemic hypoperfusion (*burn shock*). This intense hemodynamic response may be poorly tolerated by patients with major underlying medical conditions, and survival depends on the restoration of circulating volume and the infusion of crystalloid fluids according to recommended protocols (see below). If adequate intravenous fluid therapy is provided, cardiac function returns to normal within 48 h of injury and then typically progresses to a hyperdynamic physiology as the metabolic challenge of healing begins. Plasma volume and urine output are initially reduced after major burn injuries.

13 In contrast to fluid management of blunt and penetrating trauma, burn fluid resuscitation emphasizes the use of balanced crystalloid fluids (see Chapter 51) in preference to albumin, hydroxyethyl starch, normal or hypertonic saline, or blood.

Following burn injuries, acute kidney failure is more common when hypertonic saline is used during initial fluid resuscitation, death is more likely when blood is administered, and outcomes are unchanged when albumin (rather than crystalloid) is used in resuscitation.

Fluid resuscitation is continuous over the first 24 h following burn injury. Two formulas are commonly used in guiding burn injury fluid resuscitation: the *Parkland* and the *modified Brooke*. Both require an understanding of the *Rule of Nines* (Figure 39–6) to calculate resuscitation

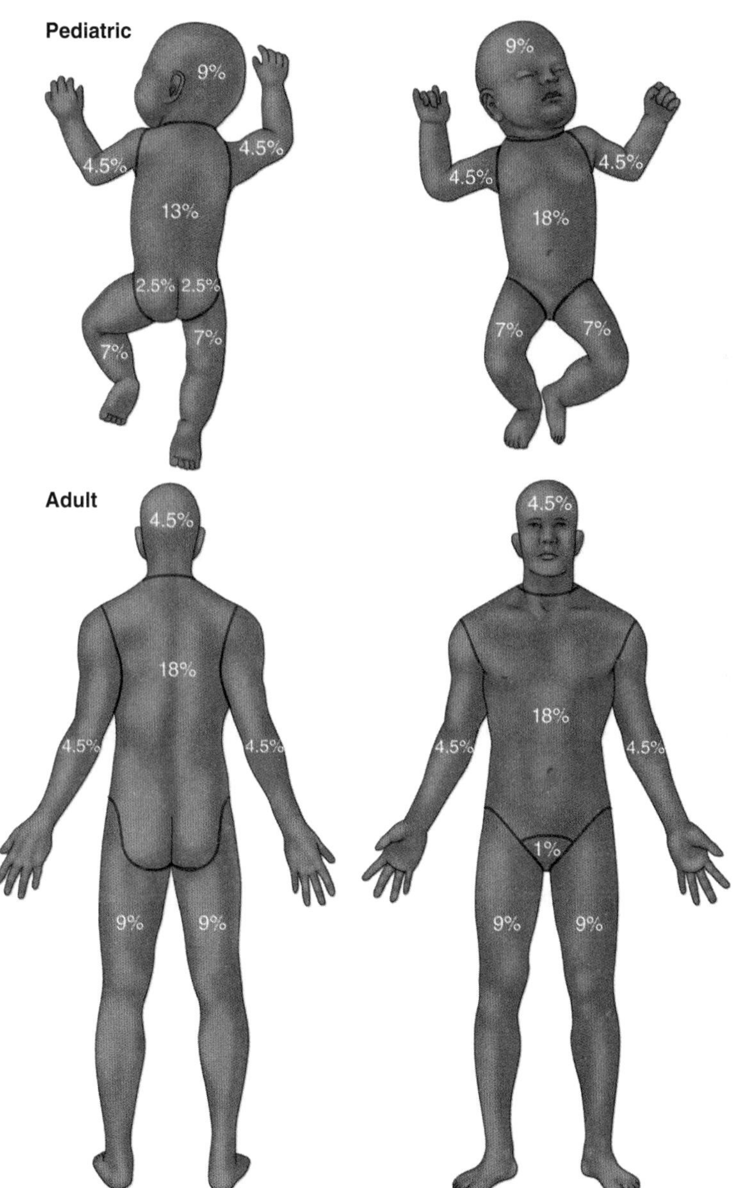

FIGURE 39–6 The Rule of Nines, utilized to estimate burned surface area as a percentage of total body surface area (TBSA). (Reproduced with permission from American College of Surgeons. *ATLS: Advanced Trauma Life Support for Doctors (Student Course Manual)*. 9th ed. Chicago, IL: ACS; 2012.)

fluid volumes. The adult Parkland protocol recommends 4 mL/kg/% burned TBSA to be given in the first 24 h, with half the volume given in the first 8 h and the remaining volume over the following 16 h. The adult modified Brooke protocol recommends 2 mL/kg/% burned TBSA, with half the calculated volume beginning in the first 8 h and the remainder over the following 16 h. Both formulas use urine output as a reliable indicator of fluid resuscitation adequacy, targeting adult urine production of 0.5 to 1.0 mL/kg/h as indicators of adequate circulating volume. If adult urine output exceeds 1.0 mL/kg/h, the infusions are slowed. In both protocols, an amount equal to half the volume administered in the first 24 h is infused in the second 24-h period following injury. The goal of maintaining adult urine output at 0.5 to 1.0 mL/kg/h continues throughout the initial phase of resuscitation.

When pediatric burn patients are encountered, the fluid resuscitation protocols are the same as for adults. Children weighing less than 30 kg should receive 5% dextrose in their intravenous fluids, and the target urine output is 1.0 mL/kg/h. The target urine output for infants younger than 1 year of age is 1 to 2 mL/kg/h.

Burn Management Considerations

A. Fluid Creep

The Parkland and modified Brooke protocols both use urine output as an indicator for adequate fluid resuscitation. However, circumstances may arise in which the volume of fluid administered exceeds the original volume goal. For example, initial fluid resuscitation volumes may be miscalculated if first-degree burns are mistakenly incorporated into the TBSA value. Prolonged use of sedation may result in hypotension, prompting the administration of additional fluids rather than vasoconstrictors. The phenomenon of *fluid creep* occurs when intravenous fluid therapy volumes are increased beyond intended calculations in response to hemodynamic changes related to issues other than circulating volumes. Fluid creep is associated with abdominal compartment syndrome and pulmonary complications, often leading to resuscitation-related morbidity.

B. Abdominal Compartment Syndrome

Abdominal compartment syndrome (ACS) is a risk for pediatric and adult patients with circumferential abdominal burns and for patients receiving intravenous fluid volumes greater than 6 mL/kg/% burned TBSA. Intraabdominal pressure can be determined by measuring intraluminal bladder pressure using a Foley catheter connected to a pressure transducer. The transducer is connected to a three-way stopcock at the point where the Foley catheter connects to the drainage tube. After the transducer is zeroed at the pelvic brim, 20 mL of fluid is instilled into the bladder. Intraabdominal pressure readings are taken 60 s after infusing fluid into the bladder, which allows the bladder to relax. Intraabdominal pressures exceeding 20 mm Hg warrant abdominal cavity decompression. However, an abdominal surgical procedure places the burn patient at increased risk for intraabdominal *Pseudomonas* infection, particularly if the laparotomy incision is near burned tissue. Early and frequent assessment of intraabdominal pressure and consideration of potential etiologies of hypotension in the burn patient other than hypovolemia are important preventative measures for ACS.

C. Pulmonary Complications

Excessive fluid resuscitation volumes are associated with an increased incidence of pneumonia. Patients with severe burns frequently have a related pulmonary injury. Decreased tracheal ciliary activity, the presence of resuscitation-induced pulmonary edema, reduced immunocompetence, and tracheal intubation predispose burn patients to pneumonia. ACS can have an adverse impact on pulmonary function. Intravenous fluid administration volumes must be monitored closely and documented to be consistent with American Burn Association recommendations (ie, the Parkland or modified Brooke protocol). Fluid administration that exceeds recommendations warrants a careful review of the rationale.

D. Carbon Monoxide and Cyanide Poisoning

14 The differential diagnosis for altered mental status following burn injury and smoke inhalation includes carbon monoxide and cyanide

poisoning (see Chapter 57). Endotracheal intubation and mechanical ventilation with high inspired oxygen concentration are indicated in this situation. Carbon monoxide binds hemoglobin with an affinity approximately 250 times that of oxygen. The resultant carboxyhemoglobin (HbCO) leaves less hemoglobin available for binding oxygen and shifts the O_2–Hb dissociation curve to the left, both causing impaired delivery of oxygen to tissues. *Pulse oximetry provides a falsely elevated indication of oxygen saturation in the setting of carbon monoxide exposure because of its inability to distinguish oxygenated hemoglobin* (HbO_2) *from* HbCO. Arterial or venous blood gas analysis can directly measure HbCO. Clinically important carbon monoxide poisoning is seen when HbCO levels exceed 10% (those who regularly smoke tobacco have HbCO levels of up to 10%). If HbCO exceeds 20%, intubation and mechanical ventilation are indicated to improve local tissue oxygenation and accelerate carbon monoxide elimination. Death from carbon monoxide occurs when HbCO levels exceed 60%. Hyperbaric oxygen therapy is indicated for carbon monoxide poisonings from any etiology. Multiple hyperbaric oxygen sessions are required to reduce the long-term consequences of carbon monoxide poisoning.

Anesthetic Considerations for Burn Therapy

A primary characteristic of all burn patients is an inability to regulate temperature. The resuscitation environment must be maintained near body temperature through the use of radiant warming, forced-air warming devices, and fluid warming devices. All burn care environments must be maintained near 40°C.

Assessment of the burn patient begins with an inspection of the airway. Although the face may be burned (singed facial hair, nasal vibrissae), facial burns are not an indication for tracheal intubation. The need for urgent airway management, mechanical ventilation, and oxygen therapy is indicated by hoarse voice, dyspnea, tachypnea, or altered level of consciousness. Arterial blood gas determination should be obtained early in the treatment process for assessment of the HbCO level. Mechanical ventilation should be adjusted to achieve adequate oxygen saturation (based upon measured oxygen levels rather than pulse oximetry) at the lowest tidal volumes.

Tracheal intubation in the early period following burn injury (up to the first 48 h) can be facilitated with succinylcholine for muscle relaxation. In patients with major burns exceeding 20% of TBSA, injury and disruption of neuromuscular end-plates occurs, followed by upregulation of acetylcholine receptors. 15 **Beyond 48 h following a major burn injury, succinylcholine administration can produce lethal hyperkalemia.** This risk for succinylcholine-induced hyperkalemia persists for up to 2 years following burn injury.

Analgesia for burn patients is challenging. Concerns regarding opioid tolerance and psychosocial complications of burn therapy are commonplace. Multimodal approaches are advantageous. Regional analgesia may provide benefit, though in the early postburn period, this technique may mask the symptoms of compartment syndrome or other clinically important signs and symptoms related to the primary burn injury.

EMERGING TRENDS IN TRAUMA CARE

Older Adults

16 **Older adults represent the fastest-growing population seen in trauma centers across the world. They are at greater risk for serious complications and death after even modest trauma.** Preexisting conditions that negatively impact physiological reserve and ability to recover from trauma contribute more to the greater complication and death rate after trauma than age itself. Although "geriatric" is not a specific age, with respect to "geriatric" trauma outcomes, several studies have observed worsening outcomes after trauma beginning between the ages of 45 and 55 years, suggesting decreased physiological reserve following trauma may start at ages far earlier than previously appreciated. With advancing age, several studies found the risk for death after trauma doubled for trauma victims older than 65 years when injury severity was case-matched to those younger than 65 years.

Preventing falls in the older adult population is an emerging public health issue. Falling from standing height is responsible for 90% of injuries in patients over the age of 65 years. Fall-related intracranial hemorrhage, skeletal fractures, and major thoracic or intraabdominal vascular injuries increase morbidity and mortality in this patient population. Patients taking oral anticoagulants have lower GCS scores and higher morbidity than older adult patients experiencing similar injuries who do not use oral anticoagulants. The use of oral anticoagulants in this patient population is an independent predictor of 30-day mortality after falling.

Mass Casualty Incidents

Preparing for *mass casualty incidents* has become a common exercise for trauma centers, and such preparations must include the anesthesiology service. Although no specific number of casualties identifies an incident as a mass casualty incident, there are characteristics that warrant some explanation and understanding; nearly all relate to a facility's usual emergency patient capacity.

Multiple injury incidents are those circumstances where more than one patient arrives at the same facility from a traumatic event. In a small hospital, this may overwhelm available resources. However, for most suburban and urban trauma facilities, such an incident may simply redirect available resources away from noncritical patients for a limited amount of time, and the overall function of the facility may not be significantly impacted.

Mass casualty incidents are events where the number of patients arriving from the traumatic event overwhelms available hospital resources, prompting diversion of noncritical patients to other facilities and interrupting normal hospital functions, including elective surgery. Patient triage is required to ensure limited resources are
17 preserved for the highest-acuity patients. **Point-of-care ultrasound imaging has become a key triage tool in these situations, where CAVEAT (*chest, abdomen, vena cava, and extremities*) examinations rapidly determine the viability of critically injured patients.**

Although mass casualty incidents are dreaded events, a few predictable patterns have been well established and warrant mentioning. First, in most mass casualty events, be it bus accidents, train crashes, civilian bombings in outdoor settings, or terrorist attacks occurring where victims are not trapped in buildings, 10% of the victims die at the scene, another 10% will be critically wounded and in need of emergency surgery, 20% will require urgent surgery within 8 h, and 30% will require nonemergency interventions. The key is identifying the nature and likely number of victims involved. Second, victims of mass casualty events often arrive at hospitals unannounced. Passers-by or law enforcement personnel begin transporting victims to the nearest hospital, even if the nearest hospital is not intended for trauma care. This creates a need for transporting patients between facilities when emergency first-responder resources are likely already overwhelmed by the initial incident. Finally, resources must be reserved for salvageable victims in this setting. Care for patients with pulses must take priority, and only these patients should be allowed to consume surgical resources, intensive care beds, and blood products when there is a mass casualty incident.

CASE DISCUSSION

Abdominal Trauma in a Previously Healthy Patient

A 22-year-old, previously healthy, 70-kg man is brought to the emergency department (ED) at 9 am by his mother after fainting at home earlier that morning. The previous evening, he was involved in an altercation in a bar during which he was kicked repeatedly in the stomach. The patient is pale, tachycardic, and lethargic. His pulse is 140 beats/min, and his blood pressure is 60/34 mm Hg. A FAST (focused assessment with sonography for trauma) examination in the ED reveals free fluid in the abdomen. Two 18-gauge antecubital intravenous lines are placed, and a blood sample is sent to the blood bank for type and cross-matching. A massive transfusion protocol (MTP) is initiated. The patient is brought to the operating room within 16 min of his arrival in the ED.

What measures should be taken prior to induction of anesthesia?

The patient has life-threatening injuries. Although surgical intervention is necessary, the interval between anesthetic induction and surgical incision must be as short as possible. Avoiding hypothermia is critical. The operating room should be as warm as possible until the patient is draped. The trauma surgeons should be prepared to operate immediately if hemodynamic collapse occurs with anesthetic induction. This is why the skin must be prepared for incision from the patient's chin to his toes, with warm skin preparation solution prior to, and/or during, anesthetic induction. Delaying surgical incision for the placement of an arterial line or central venous access must not occur. Red blood cells and other blood products should be available prior to anesthetic induction.

Warm intravenous fluids are infused quickly to prevent hemodynamic collapse upon anesthetic induction. While the fluids are infusing, standard ASA monitors are applied while the patient is preoxygenated. The surgeons are gowning and gloving. Immediate release, non–cross-matched O-negative packed red blood cells (RBCs) are brought to the operating room. The room temperature is uncomfortably warm. Invasive hemodynamic monitoring catheters and ultrasound devices are present and immediately available.

What are the priorities of anesthetic induction and hemodynamic monitoring?

The patient is lethargic. Cerebral hypoperfusion, traumatic brain injury, or intoxication cannot be ruled out. The mechanism of injury is that of blunt trauma, obligating the need for cervical spinal cord immobilization until a more thorough neurological evaluation can occur. The anesthetic induction agent must be chosen to avoid hemodynamic collapse. Benzodiazepines, opioids, and propofol each attenuate sympathetic tone, and their administration may be life-threatening in this scenario. Since all trauma patients should be considered to have full stomachs, rapid sequence anesthetic induction/intubation is indicated. If sufficient staff is available, someone from the anesthesia or surgical team should be gowned and gloved, working next to the operating surgeons to place arterial and central venous lines, using ultrasound point-of-care assistance, if needed, at the time of surgical incision.

With the patient draped, the surgeons ready for incision, and the arrival of the uncrossmatched blood in the operating room, scopolamine, 0.4 mg, is injected intravenously followed immediately by succinylcholine, 100 mg, intravenously. With inline cervical spine immobilization maintained, the endotracheal tube is passed with the assistance of a video laryngoscope. Once endotracheal tube position is confirmed and secured, the surgeons initiate the incision and proceed with damage control surgical intervention. The surgeons make a full laparotomy incision while an anesthesia colleague places a left subclavian central venous catheter. Hemodynamic collapse occurs as blood spills from the surgical site. The arterial line is not yet in place, but central venous access via the subclavian vein is now present. The first MTP blood products arrive in the operating room.

What are the implications of damage control surgery (DCS) and damage control resuscitation (DCR)?

When confronted with hemodynamic instability during life-threatening hemorrhage, the surgeons intervene to stop the hemorrhage until the hemodynamic status can be stabilized and, in a case of abdominal trauma, to limit gastrointestinal contamination of the abdominal compartment. This represents DCS. In this case, they pack off the abdomen until sufficient blood-based resuscitation restores systolic blood pressures to 80 to 90 mm Hg, which allows the surgery to proceed.

DCR is an aggressive transfusion protocol utilized during life-threatening hemorrhage that seeks to mimic whole blood (ie, RBC, fresh frozen plasma [FFP], and platelet units in a ratio of 1:1:1). Emphasizing warmed blood product transfusion during hemorrhage reduces hypothermia and acidosis while attenuating trauma-induced coagulopathy (as long as intravenous crystalloid administration is kept to a minimum). Blood products in this scenario, with the exception of platelets, must be infused through a fluid warmer capable of delivering large volumes.

The surgeon packs the abdomen and compresses the aorta. Aortic compression is the most effective and prudent intervention in hemorrhage-related hemodynamic collapse; cardiopulmonary resuscitation (CPR) is not useful in blood loss scenarios. Blood products are administered through a rapid infusion device in a 1:1:1 ratio. An increased end-tidal carbon dioxide tracing is now observed, and the surgeon notes the aorta is now firmer. The noninvasive blood pressure cuff shows a systolic pressure of 82 mm Hg. The surgeon removes an abdominal pack and begins exploring the abdomen. Although DCR continues, surgical exploration is repeatedly interrupted due to hemodynamic instability. Eventually, a brachial artery monitoring line is placed with point-of-care ultrasound guidance.

What technology is available for more closely tailoring blood component administration in this situation?

DCR emphasizes blood product use during hemorrhage resuscitation. Experience with this lifesaving intervention suggests that blood product utilization can be more precise if functional coagulation tests (eg, thromboelastography [TEG] or rotational thromboelastometry [ROTEM]) are utilized. These technologies assess the functional status of clot formation, with results available within 5 min of sampling. Patterns of clot formation can guide the administration of platelets, fibrinogen, and plasma. Thrombolysis is also detected with this technology, providing evidence of the need for antithrombolytic therapies.

A blood gas sample demonstrates metabolic acidosis and hemoglobin of 7.0 g/dL. The functional coagulation study (TEG or ROTEM) demonstrates a hypercoagulable pattern. As a result, the anesthesiologist alters the transfusion ratios to 3 RBC:1 FFP:1 platelet units. The surgeon now indicates that the sources for bleeding—a ruptured spleen and lacerated kidney—are controlled. The anesthesiologist notifies the team that blood products will no longer need to be rapidly infused unless hemodynamic instability recurs.

Are there guidelines for the use of blood versus vasopressors?

The question of when to initiate vasopressors during trauma resuscitation has not been defined. So-called permissive hypotension during active surgical hemostasis and damage control resuscitation is optimal to prevent disruption of clot formation. Systolic blood pressures in the 80 to 90 mm Hg range reduce blood loss and transfusion needs. However, once the source of blood loss is surgically controlled, no guidelines exist as to when vasopressors should be initiated instead of continued transfusion of blood products.

As the surgeons continue assessing the abdominal cavity for any as yet undetected relevant trauma, the patient's systolic blood pressure gradually declines to 70 mm Hg. The patient's core temperature is 35.5°C, the blood gas shows an improvement of the metabolic acidosis, with a base excess of –4 mmol and hemoglobin of 10.0 g/dL. The TEG demonstrates normal coagulation patterns. Ionized calcium is within normal limits. The decision to initiate low-dose vasopressin and epinephrine infusions, rather than transfuse additional blood products, is made; the patient was otherwise healthy prior to this injury, and transfusion of additional blood products increases the risk of transfusion-associated circulatory overload (TACO). The patient's blood pressure and heart rate stabilize to within normal limits, the abdomen is temporarily closed, and he is transferred to the surgical intensive care unit while remaining intubated and sedated.

Summary

This typical trauma scenario broadly addresses the common resuscitation and management decisions required for major trauma resuscitation. At this time, applying these resuscitation concepts to intraoperative surgery-related hemorrhage is not supported. Unlike trauma, where the patient is typically hypotensive for an extended period of time (frequently more than an hour), intraoperative hemorrhage is typically recognized promptly and addressed rapidly. Such patients usually do not become profoundly acidotic prior to initiating resuscitation measures and transfusion. Unlike trauma coagulopathy, intraoperative coagulopathy in the setting of surgical hemorrhage is more likely dilutional rather than endothelium-derived (thrombolytic), as in the trauma setting. However, in response to hemodynamically significant acute intraoperative hemorrhage, the basic concepts of trauma resuscitation remain relevant: *Allow lower systolic blood pressures until the source for bleeding is identified and controlled, limit administration of intravenous crystalloids during hemorrhage in deference to administration of blood products, and utilize TEG or ROTEM to provide a functional assessment of clotting for the guidance of blood product administration.* These concepts are accepted and defendable interventions in nontrauma resuscitation, where research is ongoing to clarify best practices.

SUGGESTED READINGS

Adams SD, Holcomb JB. Geriatric trauma. *Curr Opin Crit Care.* 2015;21:520.

Allen CJ, Hannay WH, Murray CR, et al. Causes of death differ between elderly and adult falls. *J Trauma Acute Care Surg.* 2015;79:617.

Benz D, Balogh ZJ. Damage control surgery: current state and future directions. *Curr Opin Crit Care.* 2017;23:491.

Cannon JW, Mansoor A, Raja AS, et al. Damage control resuscitation in patients with severe traumatic hemorrhage: a practice management guideline from the Eastern Association for the Surgery of Trauma. *J Trauma Acute Care Surg.* 2017;82:605.

Cantle PM, Cotton BA. Balanced resuscitation in trauma management. *Surg Clin North Am.* 2017;97:999.

Clifford L, Qing J, Kor DJ, et al. Risk factors and clinical outcomes associated with perioperative transfusion-associated circulatory overload. *Anesthesiology.* 2017;126:409.

Curry N, Brohi K. Surgery in traumatic injury and perioperative considerations. *Semin Thromb Hemost.* 2020;46:73.

Dauer E, Goldberg A. What's new in trauma resuscitation? *Adv Surg.* 2019;53:221.

Holcomb JB, Tilley BC, Baraniuk S, et al. Transfusion of plasma, platelets and red blood cells in a 1:1:1 vs a 1:1:2 ratio and mortality in patients with severe trauma: the PROPPR randomized clinical trial. *JAMA.* 2015;313:471.

Kalkwarf KJ, Cotton BA. Resuscitation for hypovolemic shock. *Surg Clin North Am.* 2017;97:1307xs.

Leon M, Chavez L, Surani S. Abdominal compartment syndrome among surgical patients. *World J Gastrointest Surg.* 2021;13:330.

Mehta R, Chinthapalli K. Glasgow coma scale explained. *Br Med J.* 2019;365:l1296.

Moore EE, Moore HB, Kornblith LZ, et al. Trauma-induced coagulopathy. *Nat Rev Dis Primers.* 2021;7:30.

Newcombe VFJ, Chow A. The features of the typical traumatic brain injury patient in the ICU are changing: what will this mean for the intensivist? *Curr Opin Crit Care.* 2021;27:80.

Ramineni A, Roberts EA, Vora M, et al. Anesthesia considerations in neurological emergencies. *Neurol Clin.* 2021;39:319.

Savioli G, Ceresa IF, Caneva L, et al. Trauma-induced coagulopathy: overview of an emerging medical problem from pathophysiology to outcomes. *Medicines* (Basel). 2021;8:16.

Søvik S, Isachsen MS, Nordhuus KM, et al. Acute kidney injury in trauma patients admitted to the ICU: a systematic review and meta-analysis. *Intensive Care Med.* 2019;45:407.

Tisherman SA, Stein DM. ICU management of trauma patients. *Crit Care Med.* 2018;46:1991.

Wijayatilake DS, Jigajinni SV, Shrren PB. Traumatic brain injury: physiological targets for clinical practice in the prehospital setting and on the neuro-ICU. *Curr Opin Anesthesiol.* 2015;28:517-524.

Wray JP, Bridwell RE, Schauer SG, et al. The diamond of death: hypocalcemia in trauma and resuscitation. *Am J Emerg Med.* 2021;41:104.

CHAPTER

40

Maternal & Fetal Physiology & Anesthesia

Michael A. Frölich, MD, MS

KEY CONCEPTS

1. The minimum alveolar concentration (MAC) progressively decreases during pregnancy—at term, by as much as 40%—for all general anesthetic agents; MAC returns to normal by the third day after delivery.
2. Pregnant patients display enhanced sensitivity to local anesthetics during regional anesthesia and analgesia, and neural blockade occurs at reduced concentrations of local anesthetics; dose requirements may be reduced by as much as 30%.
3. Obstruction of the inferior vena cava by the enlarging uterus distends the epidural venous plexus and increases epidural blood volume.
4. Approximately 5% of women at term develop supine hypotension syndrome, which is characterized by hypotension associated with pallor, sweating, or nausea and vomiting.
5. The reduction in gastric motility and gastroesophageal sphincter tone places the parturient at high risk for regurgitation and pulmonary aspiration.
6. Ephedrine, which has considerable β-adrenergic activity, has traditionally been considered the vasopressor of choice for hypotension during pregnancy. However, clinical studies suggest that the α-adrenergic agonist phenylephrine is more effective in treating hypotension in pregnant patients and is associated with less fetal acidosis than ephedrine.
7. Volatile inhalational anesthetics decrease blood pressure and, potentially, uteroplacental blood flow. In concentrations of less than 1 MAC, however, their effects are generally minor, consisting of dose-dependent uterine relaxation and minor reductions in uterine blood flow.
8. The greatest strain on the parturient's heart occurs immediately after delivery, when intense uterine contraction and involution suddenly relieve inferior vena caval obstruction and increase cardiac output as much as 80% above late third-trimester values.
9. Current techniques employing dilute combinations of a local anesthetic (eg, bupivacaine, ≤0.125%) and an opioid (eg, fentanyl, ≤5 mcg/ml) for epidural or combined spinal–epidural (CSE) analgesia do not appear to prolong the first stage of labor or increase the likelihood of an operative delivery.

This chapter reviews the normal physiological changes associated with pregnancy, labor, and delivery. It concludes with a description of the physiological transition from fetal to neonatal life.

PHYSIOLOGICAL CHANGES DURING PREGNANCY

Pregnancy affects most organ systems (Table 40–1). Many of these physiological changes appear to be adaptive and useful to the mother in tolerating the stresses of pregnancy, labor, and delivery.

TABLE 40–1 Average maximum physiological changes associated with pregnancy.[1]

Parameter	Change
Neurological	
MAC	−40%
Respiratory	
Oxygen consumption	+20 to 50%
Airway resistance	−35%
FRC	−20%
Minute ventilation	+50%
Tidal volume	+40%
Respiratory rate	+15%
PaO_2	+10%
$PaCO_2$	−15%
HCO_3	−15%
Cardiovascular	
Blood volume	+35%
Plasma volume	+55%
Cardiac output	+40%
Stroke volume	+30%
Heart rate	+20%
Systolic blood pressure	−5%
Diastolic blood pressure	−15%
Peripheral resistance	−15%
Pulmonary resistance	−30%
Hematological	
Hemoglobin	−20%
Platelets	−10%
Clotting factors[2]	+30 to 250%
Renal	
GFR	+50%

[1]FRC, functional residual capacity; GFR, glomerular filtration rate; MAC, minimum alveolar concentration.

[2]Varies with each factor.

Central Nervous System Effects

1 **The minimum alveolar concentration (MAC) progressively decreases during pregnancy—at term, by as much as 40%—for all general anesthetic agents; MAC returns to normal by the third day after delivery.** Progesterone, which is sedating when given in pharmacological doses, increases up to 20 times normal at term and is at least partly responsible for this phenomenon. A surge in β-endorphin levels during labor and delivery also likely plays a major role.

2 **Pregnant patients display enhanced sensitivity to local anesthetics during regional anesthesia and analgesia, and neural blockade occurs at reduced concentrations of local anesthetics.** The term *minimum local analgesic concentration* (MLAC) is used in obstetric anesthesia to compare the relative potencies of local anesthetics and the effects of additives; MLAC is defined as the local analgesic concentration leading to satisfactory analgesia in 50% of patients (EC_{50}). Local anesthetic dose requirements during epidural anesthesia may be reduced as much as 30%, a phenomenon that appears to be hormonally mediated but may also be related to engorgement of the
3 epidural venous plexus. **Obstruction of the inferior vena cava by the enlarging uterus distends the epidural venous plexus and increases epidural blood volume. The latter has three major effects: (1) decreased spinal cerebrospinal fluid volume, (2) decreased potential volume of the epidural space, and (3) increased epidural (space) pressure.** The first two effects enhance the cephalad spread of local anesthetic solutions during spinal and epidural anesthesia (see Chapter 45). Bearing down during labor further accentuates all these effects. Positive (rather than the usual negative) epidural pressures have been recorded in parturients. Engorgement of the epidural veins also increases the likelihood of placing an epidural needle or catheter in a vein, resulting in an unintentional intravascular injection.

Respiratory Effects

Oxygen consumption and minute ventilation increase progressively during pregnancy. Tidal volume and, to a lesser extent, respiratory rate and inspiratory reserve volume also increase. By term, both oxygen consumption and minute ventilation have increased up to 50%. $PaCO_2$ decreases to 28 to 32 mm Hg; significant respiratory alkalosis is prevented by a compensatory decrease in plasma bicarbonate concentration. Hyperventilation may also increase PaO_2 slightly. Elevated levels of 2,3-diphosphoglycerate offset the effect of hyperventilation on hemoglobin's affinity for oxygen (see Chapter 23). The P_{50} for hemoglobin increases from 27 to 30 mm Hg; the combination of the latter with an increase in cardiac output (see next section on Cardiovascular Effects) enhances oxygen delivery to tissues.

The maternal respiratory pattern changes as the uterus enlarges. In the third trimester, the elevation of the diaphragm is compensated by an increase in the anteroposterior diameter of the chest; diaphragmatic motion, however, is not restricted. Both vital capacity and closing capacity are minimally affected, but functional residual capacity (FRC) decreases up to 20% at term; FRC returns to normal within 48 h after delivery. This decrease is principally due to a reduction in expiratory reserve volume as a result of larger than normal tidal volumes. Flow–volume loops are unaffected, and airway resistance decreases. Physiological dead space decreases but intrapulmonary shunting increases toward term. A chest film may show prominent vascular markings due to increased pulmonary blood volume and an elevated diaphragm. Pulmonary vasodilation prevents pulmonary pressures from rising.

The combination of decreased FRC and increased oxygen consumption promotes rapid oxygen desaturation during periods of apnea. Preoxygenation (denitrogenation) prior to induction of general anesthesia is therefore mandatory to avoid hypoxemia in pregnant patients. Closing volume exceeds FRC in some pregnant women at term when they lie supine. Under these conditions, atelectasis and hypoxemia readily occur. The decrease in FRC coupled with the increase in minute ventilation accelerates the uptake of all inhalational anesthetics. The reduction in dead space narrows the arterial end-tidal CO_2 gradient.

Engorgement of the respiratory mucosa during pregnancy predisposes the upper airways to trauma, bleeding, and obstruction. Gentle laryngoscopy and smaller endotracheal tubes (6–6.5 mm) should be employed during general anesthesia.

Cardiovascular Effects

Cardiac output and blood volume increase to meet increased maternal and fetal metabolic demands. In the first trimester, there is a substantial decrease in peripheral vascular resistance with a nadir during the middle of the second trimester and a subsequent plateau or slight increase for the remainder of the pregnancy. An increase (55%) in plasma volume in excess of an increase in red blood cell mass (45%) produces dilutional anemia and reduces blood viscosity. Hemoglobin concentration usually remains greater than 11 g/dL. Moreover, the reduction in hemoglobin concentration is offset by the increase in cardiac output and the rightward shift of the hemoglobin dissociation curve (see section on Respiratory Effects) to maintain oxygen delivery to tissues.

At term, blood volume has increased by 1000 to 1500 mL in most women, allowing them to easily tolerate the blood loss associated with delivery; total blood volume reaches 90 mL/kg. Average blood loss during vaginal delivery is 200 to 500 mL, compared with 800 to 1000 mL for a cesarean section. Blood volume does not return to normal until 1 to 2 weeks after delivery.

The increase in cardiac output (40% at term) is due to increases in both heart rate (20%) and stroke volume (30%). Cardiac chambers enlarge, and myocardial hypertrophy is often noted on echocardiography. Central venous, pulmonary artery, and pulmonary artery occlusion pressures remain unchanged. Most of these effects are observed in the first and, to a lesser extent, the second trimester. In the third trimester, cardiac output does not appreciably rise, except during labor. The greatest increases in cardiac output are seen during labor and immediately after delivery (see section on Effect of Labor on Maternal Physiology). Cardiac output often does not return to normal until 2 weeks after delivery.

Decreases in cardiac output can occur in the supine position after week 20 of pregnancy. Such decreases have been shown to be secondary to impeded venous return to the heart as the enlarging uterus compresses the inferior vena cava. 4 **Approximately 5% of women at term develop *supine hypotension syndrome* (aortocaval compression), which is characterized by hypotension associated with pallor, sweating, or nausea**

and vomiting. The cause of this syndrome appears to be compression of the inferior vena cava by the gravid uterus. *When combined with the hypotensive effects of regional or general anesthesia, aortocaval compression can readily produce fetal asphyxia. Turning the patient on her side typically restores venous return from the lower body and corrects the hypotension in such instances. This maneuver is conveniently accomplished by placing a wedge (>15°) under the right hip. The gravid uterus also compresses the aorta in most parturients when they are supine.* This latter effect decreases blood flow to the lower extremities and, more importantly, to the uteroplacental circulation. Uterine contraction reduces caval compression but exacerbates aortic compression.

Chronic partial caval obstruction in the third trimester predisposes to venous stasis, phlebitis, and edema in the lower extremities. Moreover, compression of the inferior vena cava below the diaphragm distends and increases blood flow through the paravertebral venous plexus (including the epidural veins), and to a minor degree, the abdominal wall.

Lastly, the elevation of the diaphragm shifts the heart's position in the chest, resulting in the appearance of an enlarged heart on a plain chest film and in left axis deviation and T wave changes on the electrocardiogram. Physical examination often reveals a grade I or II systolic ejection flow murmur and exaggerated splitting of the first heart sound (S_1); a third heart sound (S_3) may be audible. A few patients develop small, asymptomatic pericardial effusion.

Kidney & Gastrointestinal Effects

Renal plasma flow and the glomerular filtration rate increase during pregnancy; as a result, serum creatinine and blood urea nitrogen may decrease to as low as 0.5 mg/dL and 9 mg/dL, respectively. A decreased renal tubular threshold for glucose and amino acids is common and often results in mild glycosuria (1–10 g/d) or proteinuria (<300 mg/d), or both. Plasma osmolality decreases by 8 to 10 mOsm/kg.

5 **Gastroesophageal reflux and esophagitis are common during pregnancy. Gastric motility is reduced, and upward and anterior displacement of the stomach by the uterus promotes incompetence of the gastroesophageal sphincter. These factors place the parturient at high risk for regurgitation and pulmonary aspiration.** However, neither gastric acidity nor gastric volume changes significantly during pregnancy. Opioids and anticholinergics reduce lower esophageal sphincter pressure, may facilitate gastroesophageal reflux, and delay gastric emptying.

Hepatic Effects

Overall hepatic function and blood flow are unchanged; minor elevations in serum transaminases and lactic dehydrogenase levels may be observed in the third trimester. Mild elevations in serum alkaline phosphatase are due to its secretion by the placenta. A mild decrease in serum albumin is due to an expanded plasma volume, and as a result, colloid oncotic pressure is reduced. A 25% to 30% decrease in serum pseudocholinesterase activity is also present at term but rarely produces significant prolongation of muscle relaxation by succinylcholine. The metabolism of ester local anesthetics is not appreciably altered. Pseudocholinesterase activity may not return to normal until up to 6 weeks postpartum. High progesterone levels appear to inhibit the release of cholecystokinin, resulting in incomplete emptying of the gallbladder. The latter, together with altered bile acid composition, can predispose to the formation of cholesterol gallstones during pregnancy.

Hematological Effects

Pregnancy is associated with a hypercoagulable state that may be beneficial in limiting blood loss at delivery. Fibrinogen and concentrations of factors VII, VIII, IX, X, and XII all increase; only factor XI levels may decrease. Accelerated fibrinolysis can be observed late in the third trimester. In addition to the dilutional anemia (see the section on Cardiovascular Effects), leukocytosis (up to 21,000/μL) and a 10% decrease in platelet count may be encountered during the third trimester. Because of fetal utilization, iron and folate deficiency anemias readily develop if supplements of these nutrients are not taken.

Metabolic Effects

Complex metabolic and hormonal changes occur during pregnancy. Altered carbohydrate, fat, and protein metabolism favors fetal growth and development. These changes resemble starvation because blood glucose and amino acid levels are low and free fatty acid, ketone, and triglyceride levels are high. Nonetheless, pregnancy is a diabetogenic state; insulin levels steadily rise during pregnancy. Secretion of human placental lactogen, also called *human chorionic somatomammotropin*, by the placenta is probably responsible for the relative insulin resistance associated with pregnancy. Pancreatic beta cell hyperplasia occurs in response to an increased demand for insulin secretion.

Secretion of human chorionic gonadotropin and elevated levels of estrogens promote hypertrophy of the thyroid gland and increase thyroid-binding globulin; although thyroxine (T_4) and triiodothyronine (T_3) levels are elevated, free T_4, free T_3, and thyrotropin (thyroid-stimulating hormone) remain normal. Serum calcium levels decrease, but ionized calcium concentration remains normal.

Musculoskeletal Effects

Elevated levels of *relaxin*, a hormone secreted by the placenta and endometrium throughout pregnancy, help prepare for delivery by softening the cervix, inhibiting uterine contractions, and relaxing the pubic symphysis and pelvic joints. Ligamentous laxity of the spine increases the risk of back injury. The latter may contribute to the relatively frequent occurrence of back pain during pregnancy.

UTEROPLACENTAL CIRCULATION

A normal uteroplacental circulation (Figure 40–1) is critical in the development and maintenance of a healthy fetus. Uteroplacental insufficiency is an important cause of intrauterine fetal growth retardation and, when severe, can result in fetal demise. The integrity of this circulation is, in turn, dependent on both adequate uterine blood flow and normal placental function.

Uterine Blood Flow

At term, uterine blood flow represents about 10% of the cardiac output, or 600 to 700 mL/min (compared with 50 mL/min in the nonpregnant uterus). Eighty percent of uterine blood flow normally supplies the placenta; the remainder goes to the myometrium. Pregnancy maximally dilates the uterine vasculature so that autoregulation is absent but the uterine vasculature remains sensitive to α-adrenergic agonists. Uterine blood flow is not usually significantly affected by respiratory gas tensions, but extreme hypocapnia ($PaCO_2$ <20 mm Hg) can reduce uterine blood flow and causes fetal hypoxemia and acidosis.

Blood flow is directly proportional to the difference between uterine arterial and venous pressures but inversely proportionate to uterine vascular resistance. Although not under appreciable neural control, the uterine vasculature has α-adrenergic and possibly some β-adrenergic receptors.

Three major factors decrease uterine blood flow during pregnancy: (1) systemic hypotension, (2) uterine vasoconstriction, and (3) uterine contractions. Common causes of hypotension during pregnancy include aortocaval compression, hypovolemia, and sympathetic blockade following regional anesthesia. Stress-induced release of endogenous catecholamines (sympathoadrenal activation) during labor causes uterine arterial vasoconstriction. Any drug with α-adrenergic activity (eg, phenylephrine) is potentially capable of decreasing uterine
6 blood flow by vasoconstriction. Ephedrine, which has considerable β-adrenergic activity, has traditionally been considered the vasopressor of choice for hypotension during pregnancy. **However, clinical studies suggest that the α-adrenergic agonist phenylephrine is more effective in treating hypotension in pregnant patients and is associated with less fetal acidosis than ephedrine.**

Hypertensive disorders are often associated with decreased uterine blood flow due to generalized vasoconstriction. Uterine contractions decrease uterine blood flow by elevating uterine venous pressure and compressing arterial vessels as they traverse the myometrium. Hypertonic contractions during labor or during oxytocin infusions can critically compromise uterine blood flow.

Placental Function

The fetus is dependent on the placenta for respiratory gas exchange, nutrition, and waste elimination.

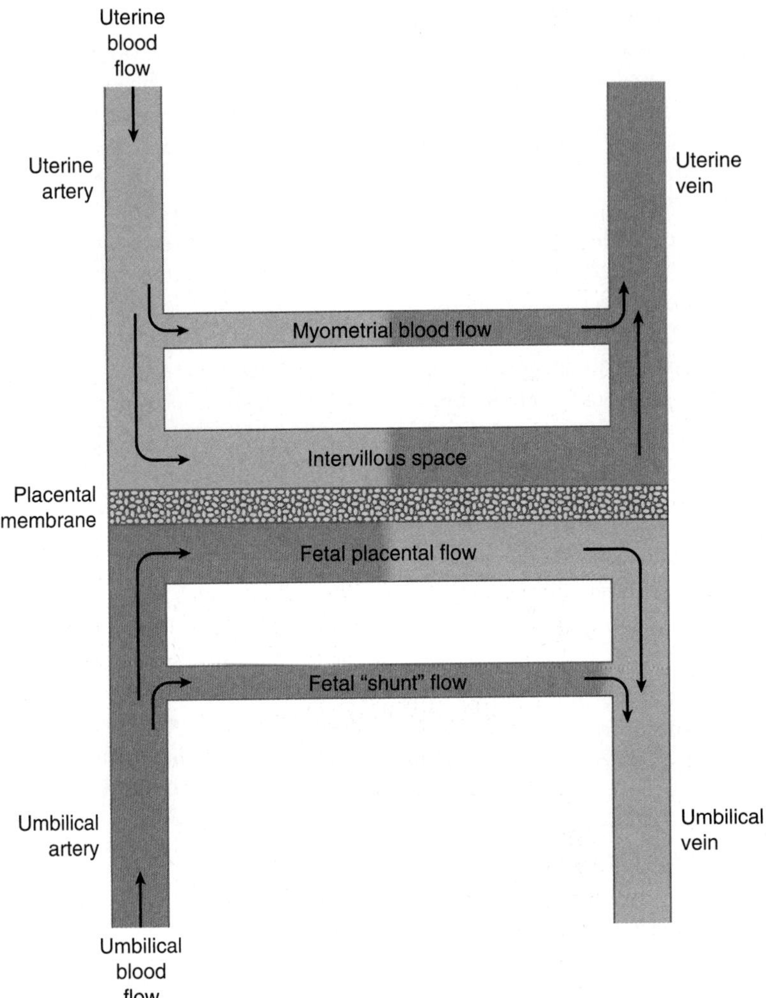

FIGURE 40–1 The uteroplacental circulation. (Reproduced with permission from Shnider S, Levinson G. *Anesthesia for Obstetrics.* 2nd ed. Philadelphia, PA: Williams & Wilkins; 1987.)

The placenta is formed by both maternal and fetal tissues and derives a blood supply from each. The resulting exchange membrane has a functional area of about 1.8 m^2.

A. Physiological Anatomy

The placenta (Figure 40–2) is composed of projections of fetal tissue (villi) that lie in maternal vascular spaces (intervillous spaces). As a result of this arrangement, the fetal capillaries within villi readily exchange substances with the maternal blood that bathes them. Maternal blood in the intervillous spaces is derived from spiral branches of the uterine artery and drains into the uterine veins. Fetal blood within villi is derived from the umbilical cord via two umbilical arteries and returns to the fetus via a single umbilical vein.

B. Placental Exchange

Placental exchange can occur by one of six mechanisms:

1. **Diffusion**—Respiratory gases and small ions are transported by diffusion. Most drugs used in anesthesia have molecular weights well

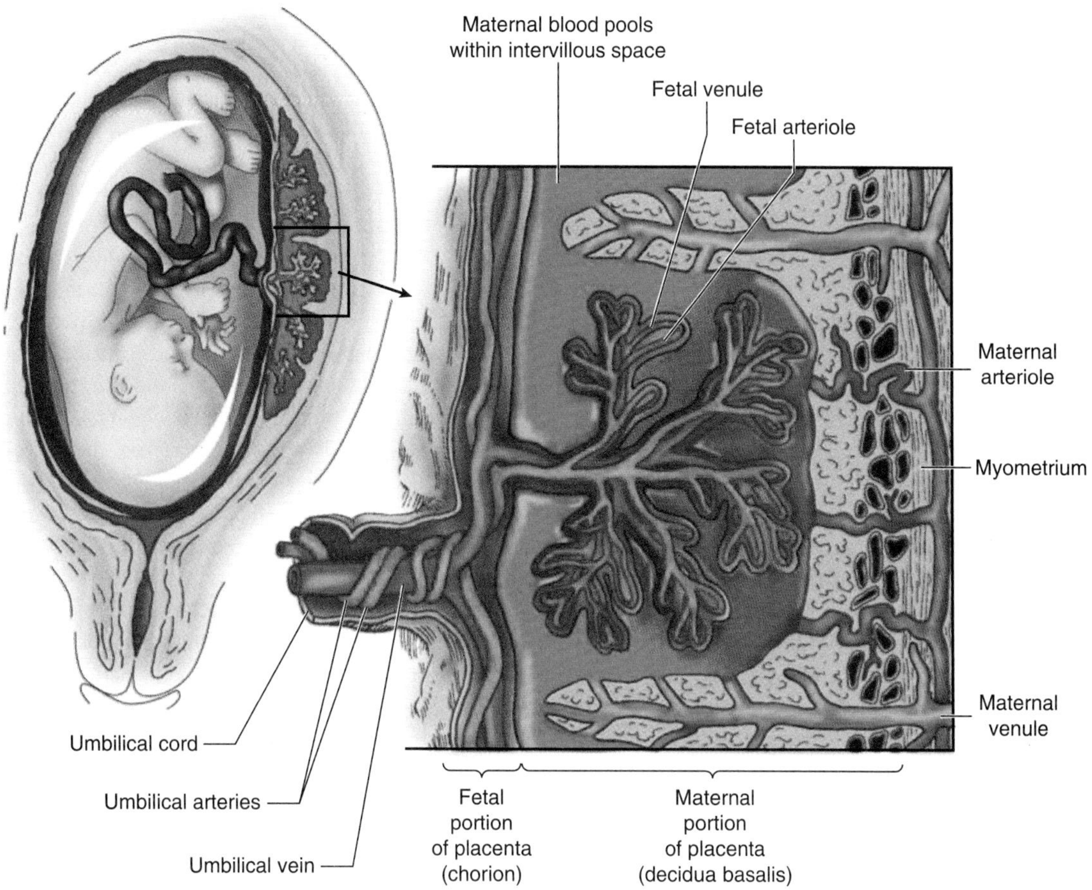

FIGURE 40–2 The placenta.

under 1000 and consequently can readily diffuse across the placenta.

2. **Osmotic and hydrostatic pressure (bulk flow)**—Water moves across by osmotic and hydrostatic pressures. Water enters the fetal circulation in quantities greater than any other substance.
3. **Facilitated diffusion**—Glucose enters the fetal circulation down the concentration gradient (no energy is consumed) facilitated by a specific transporter molecule.
4. **Active transport**—Amino acids, vitamin B_{12}, fatty acids, and some ions (calcium and phosphate) utilize this mechanism.
5. **Vesicular transport**—Large molecules, such as immunoglobulins, are transported by pinocytosis. Iron also enters the fetal circulation in this way, facilitated by ferritin and transferrin.
6. **Breaks**—Breaks in the placental membrane may permit the mixing of maternal and fetal blood. This probably underlies Rh sensitization (see Chapter 51). Rh sensitization occurs most commonly during delivery.

Respiratory Gas Exchange

At term, fetal oxygen consumption averages about 7 mL/min/kg of fetal body weight. Fortunately, because of multiple adaptive mechanisms, the normal fetus at term can survive 10 min or longer instead of the expected 2 min in a state of total oxygen deprivation. Partial or complete oxygen deprivation can result from umbilical cord compression, umbilical cord prolapse, placental abruption, severe maternal hypoxemia, or hypotension. Compensatory fetal mechanisms include redistribution of blood flow primarily to the brain, heart, placenta, and adrenal gland; decreased oxygen consumption; and anaerobic metabolism.

Transfer of oxygen across the placenta is dependent on the ratio of maternal uterine blood flow to fetal umbilical blood flow. The reserve for oxygen transfer is small even during normal pregnancy. Normal fetal blood from the placenta has a PaO_2 of only 30 to 35 mm Hg. To aid oxygen transfer, the fetal hemoglobin oxygen dissociation curve is shifted to the left such that fetal hemoglobin has a greater affinity for oxygen than does maternal hemoglobin (whose curve is already shifted to the right; see section on Respiratory Effects). In addition, fetal hemoglobin concentration is usually 15 g/dL (compared with approximately 12 g/dL in the mother).

Carbon dioxide readily diffuses across the placenta. Maternal hyperventilation (see section on Respiratory Effects) increases the gradient for the transfer of carbon dioxide from the fetus into the maternal circulation. Fetal hemoglobin has less affinity for carbon dioxide than do adult forms of hemoglobin. Carbon monoxide readily diffuses across the placenta, and fetal hemoglobin has a greater affinity for carbon monoxide than do adult forms.

Placental Transfer of Anesthetic Agents

Transfer of a drug across the placenta is reflected by the ratio of its fetal umbilical vein to maternal venous concentrations (UV/MV), whereas its uptake by fetal tissues can be correlated with the ratio of its fetal umbilical artery to umbilical vein concentrations (UA/UV). Fetal effects of drugs administered to parturients depend on multiple factors, including route of administration (oral, intramuscular, intravenous, epidural, or intrathecal), dose, timing of administration (both relative to delivery as well as contractions), and maturity of the fetal organs (brain and liver). Thus, a drug given hours before delivery or as a single intravenous bolus during a uterine contraction just prior to delivery (when uterine blood flow is maximally reduced) is unlikely to produce high fetal levels. Fortunately, current-anesthetic techniques for labor and delivery generally have minimal fetal effects despite the significant placental transfer of anesthetic agents and adjuncts.

All inhalational agents and most intravenous agents freely cross the placenta. Inhalational agents generally produce little fetal depression when they are given in limited doses (<1 MAC) and delivery occurs within 10 min of induction. Ketamine, propofol, and benzodiazepines readily cross the placenta and can be detected in the fetal circulation. Fortunately, when these agents are administered in usual induction doses, drug distribution, metabolism, and possibly placental uptake limit fetal effects. Although most opiates readily cross the placenta, their effects on neonates at delivery vary considerably. Newborns appear to be more sensitive to the respiratory depressant effect of morphine compared with other opioids. Although meperidine produces respiratory depression, peaking 1 to 3 h after administration, it produces less than morphine; butorphanol and nalbuphine produce even less respiratory depression but still may have significant neurobehavioral depressant effects. Midazolam, given as a single dose for maternal anxiolysis, has no measurable effect on the fetus. Although fentanyl readily crosses the placenta, it appears to have minimal neonatal effects unless larger intravenous doses (>1 mcg/kg) are given immediately before delivery. Epidural or intrathecal fentanyl, sufentanil, and, to a lesser extent, morphine generally produce minimal neonatal effects. Alfentanil causes neonatal depression similar to meperidine. Remifentanil also readily crosses the placenta and has the potential to produce respiratory depression in newborns. Fetal blood concentrations of remifentanil are generally about half those of the mother just prior to delivery. The UA/UV ratio is about 30%, suggesting a fairly rapid metabolism of remifentanil in the neonate. The highly ionized nature of muscle relaxants impedes placental transfer, resulting in minimal effects on the fetus. Based on its large molecular size and negative charge, sugammadex is not expected to cross the placenta in significant amounts.

Local anesthetics are weakly basic drugs that are principally bound to α_1-acid glycoprotein. Placental transfer depends on three factors: (1) pK_a (see Chapter 16), (2) maternal and fetal pH, and

(3) degree of protein binding. Except for chloroprocaine, fetal acidosis increases fetal-to-maternal drug ratios because the binding of hydrogen ions to the nonionized form causes trapping of the local anesthetic in the fetal circulation. Highly protein-bound agents diffuse slowly across the placenta; thus, greater protein binding of bupivacaine and ropivacaine, compared with that of lidocaine, likely accounts for their lower fetal blood levels. Chloroprocaine has the least placental transfer because it is rapidly hydrolyzed by plasma cholinesterase in the maternal circulation.

Most commonly used anesthetic adjuncts also readily cross the placenta. Thus, maternally administered ephedrine, β-adrenergic blockers (such as labetalol and esmolol), vasodilators, phenothiazines, antihistamines (H_1 and H_2), and metoclopramide are transferred to the fetus. Atropine and scopolamine, but not glycopyrrolate, cross the placenta; the latter's quaternary ammonium (ionized) structure results in only limited transfer.

Effect of Anesthetic Agents on Uteroplacental Blood Flow

Intravenous anesthetic agents have variable effects on uteroplacental blood flow. Propofol and barbiturates are typically associated with small reductions in uterine blood flow due to dose-dependent decreases in maternal blood pressure. A small induction dose, however, can produce greater reductions in blood flow as a result of sympathoadrenal activation (due to light anesthesia). Ketamine in doses of less than 1.5 mg/kg does not appreciably alter uteroplacental blood flow; its hypertensive effect typically counteracts any vasoconstriction. Uterine hypertonus may occur with ketamine at doses of more than 2 mg/kg. Etomidate likely has minimal effects, but its actions on uteroplacental circulation have not been well described.

7 **Volatile inhalational anesthetics decrease blood pressure and, potentially, uteroplacental blood flow. In concentrations of less than 1 MAC, however, their effects are generally minor, consisting of dose-dependent uterine relaxation and minor reductions in uterine blood flow.** Nitrous oxide has minimal effects on uterine blood flow when administered with a volatile agent. In animal studies, nitrous oxide alone can vasoconstrict the uterine arteries.

High blood levels of local anesthetics—particularly lidocaine—cause uterine arterial vasoconstriction. Such levels are seen only with unintentional intravascular injections and occasionally following paracervical blocks (in which the injection site is in close proximity to the uterine arteries), and local absorption or injection into these vessels cannot be ruled out). Spinal and epidural anesthesia typically do not decrease uterine blood flow except when arterial hypotension occurs. Moreover, uterine blood flow during labor may actually improve in preeclamptic patients following epidural anesthesia; a reduction in circulating endogenous catecholamines likely decreases uterine vasoconstriction. The addition of dilute concentrations of epinephrine to local anesthetic solutions does not appreciably alter uterine blood flow. Intravascular uptake of the epinephrine from the epidural space may result in only minor systemic β-adrenergic effects.

PHYSIOLOGY OF NORMAL LABOR

On average, labor commences 40 ± 2 weeks following the last menstrual period. The factors involved in the initiation of labor likely involve distention of the uterus, enhanced myometrial sensitivity to oxytocin, and altered prostaglandin synthesis by fetal membranes and decidual tissues. Although circulating oxytocin levels often do not increase at the beginning of labor, the number of myometrial oxytocin receptors rapidly increases. Several prodromal events usually precede true labor approximately 2 to 4 weeks before delivery: the fetal presenting part settles into the pelvis (*lightening*); patients develop uterine (*Braxton Hicks*) contractions that are characteristically irregular in frequency, duration, and intensity; and the cervix softens and thins out (*cervical effacement*). Approximately 1 week to 1 h before true labor, the cervical mucous plug (which is often bloody) breaks free (*bloody show*).

True labor begins when the sporadic Braxton Hicks contractions increase in strength (25–60 mm Hg), coordination, and frequency (15–20 min apart). Amniotic membranes may rupture spontaneously before or after the onset of true labor. Following progressive cervical dilation, the contractions propel

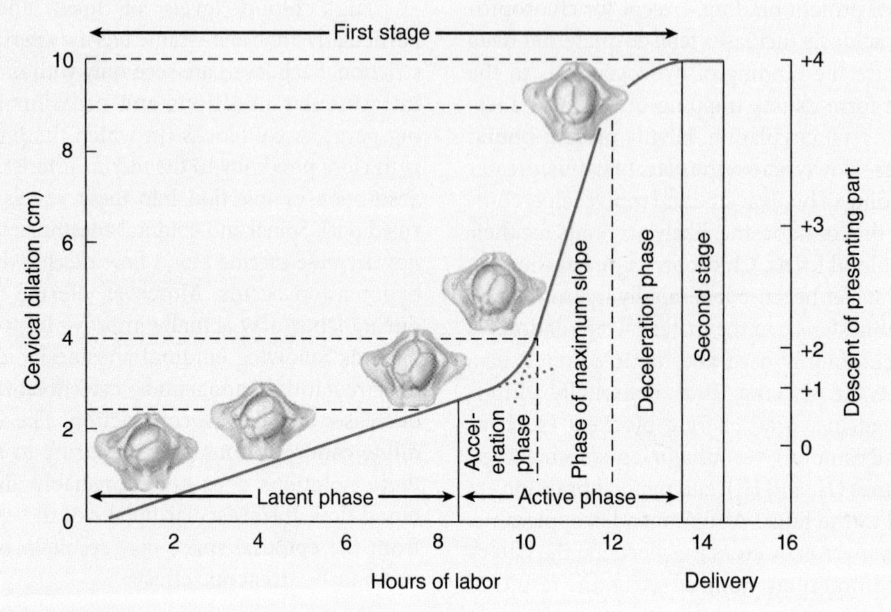

FIGURE 40–3 The course of normal labor. (Reproduced with permission from DeCherney AH, Pernoll ML. *Current Obstetric & Gynecologic Diagnosis & Treatment*, 9th ed. New York, NY: McGraw Hill; 2001.)

first the fetus and then the placenta through the pelvis and perineum. *By convention, labor is divided into three stages. The first stage is defined by the onset of true labor and ends with complete cervical dilation. The second stage begins with full cervical dilation, is characterized by fetal descent, and ends with complete delivery of the fetus. Finally, the third stage extends from the birth of the baby to the delivery of the placenta.*

Based on the rate of cervical dilation, the first stage is further divided into a slow *latent phase* followed by a faster *active phase* (Figure 40–3). The latent phase is characterized by progressive cervical effacement and minor dilation (2–4 cm). The subsequent active phase is characterized by more frequent contractions (3–5 min apart) and progressive cervical dilation up to 10 cm. The first stage usually lasts 8 to 12 h in nulliparous patients and about 5 to 8 h in multiparous patients.

Contractions during the second stage occur 1.5 to 2 min apart and last 1 to 1.5 min. Although contraction intensity does not appreciably change, the parturient, by bearing down, can greatly augment intrauterine pressure and facilitate expulsion of the fetus. The second stage usually lasts 15 to 120 min, and the third stage is typically 15 to 30 min.

The course of labor is monitored by uterine activity, cervical dilation, and fetal descent. Uterine activity refers to the frequency and magnitude of uterine contractions. The latter may be measured directly, with a catheter inserted through the cervix, or indirectly, with a tocodynamometer applied externally around the abdomen. Cervical dilation and fetal descent are assessed by pelvic examination. *Fetal station* refers to the level of descent (in centimeters) of the presenting part relative to the ischial spines (eg, −1 or +1).

Effect of Labor on Maternal Physiology

During intense painful contractions, maternal minute ventilation may increase up to 300%. Oxygen consumption also increases by an additional 60% above third-trimester values. With excessive hyperventilation, $PaCO_2$ may decrease below 20 mm Hg. Marked hypocapnia can cause periods of hypoventilation and transient maternal and fetal hypoxemia between contractions. Excessive maternal hyperventilation also reduces uterine blood flow and promotes fetal acidosis.

Each contraction places an additional burden on the heart by displacing 300 to 500 mL of blood from the uterus into the central circulation (analogous to an autotransfusion). Cardiac output rises 45% over
8 third-trimester values. **The greatest strain on the parturient's heart, however, occurs immediately after delivery, when intense uterine contraction and involution suddenly relieve inferior vena caval obstruction and increase cardiac output as much as 80% above late third-trimester values.**

Effect of Anesthetic Agents on Uterine Activity & Labor

A. Inhalational Agents

Sevoflurane, desflurane, isoflurane, and halothane depress uterine activity equally at equipotent doses; all cause dose-dependent uterine relaxation. Low doses (<0.75 MAC) of these agents, however, do not interfere with the effect of oxytocin on the uterus. Higher doses can result in uterine atony and increase blood loss at delivery. Nitrous oxide has minimal, if any, effects.

B. Parenteral Agents

Opioids minimally decrease the progression of labor; ketamine, in doses of less than 2 mg/kg, appears to have little effect.

C. Regional Anesthesia

The administration of epidural analgesia is usually based upon the patient's choice, and it is often utilized for patients with maternal or fetal factors that increase the likelihood of prolonged labor or cesarean delivery (Table 40–2). **Current evidence indicates
9 that dilute combinations of a local anesthetic (eg, bupivacaine, ≤0.125%) and an opioid (eg, fentanyl, ≤5 mcg/mL) for epidural or combined spinal–epidural (CSE) analgesia do not prolong labor or increase the likelihood of operative delivery.**

When greater concentrations of local anesthetic (eg, bupivacaine, 0.25%) are used for continuous epidural analgesia, the second stage of labor may be prolonged by approximately 15 to 30 min. Intense regional analgesia/anesthesia can remove the urge to bear down during the second stage (*Ferguson reflex*), and motor weakness can impair expulsive efforts, often prolonging the second stage of delivery. Use of dilute local anesthetic–opioid mixtures can preserve motor function and allow effective pushing. Intravenous fluid loading (crystalloid boluses) is often used to reduce the severity of hypotension following an epidural or subarachnoid injection, and the prophylactic infusion of phenylephrine started at the time of intrathecal local anesthetic injection is effective in preventing post-spinal hypotension. Fluid loading before a block in a euvolemic patient does not reduce the incidence of hypotension and has been shown to reduce endogenous oxytocin secretion from the pituitary and transiently decrease uterine activity. Some investigators mistakenly attribute neonatal or early childhood behavioral effects to epidural anesthesia when not properly accounting for difficult and prolonged labor.

TABLE 40–2 Factors that prolong labor, increase the likelihood of cesarean section, and often cause patients to request an epidural.

Primigravida
Prolonged labor
High parenteral analgesic requirements
Use of oxytocin
Large baby
Small pelvis
Fetal malpresentation

D. Vasopressors

Uterine muscle has both α and β receptors. α_1-Receptor stimulation causes uterine contraction, whereas β_2-receptor stimulation produces relaxation. In addition to causing uterine arterial constriction, large doses of α-adrenergic agents, such as phenylephrine, can produce tetanic uterine contractions. Small doses of phenylephrine (40 mcg) may increase uterine blood flow in normal parturients by raising arterial blood pressure. In contrast, ephedrine has little effect on uterine contractions.

E. Oxytocin

Oxytocin (Pitocin) is administered intravenously to induce or augment uterine contractions or to maintain uterine tone postpartum. It has a half-life of 3 to

5 min. Induction doses for labor are 0.5 to 8 mU/min. *Complications of oxytocin administration may include fetal distress due to hyperstimulation, uterine tetany, and, less commonly, maternal water retention (antidiuretic effect). Rapid intravenous infusion can cause transient systemic hypotension due to relaxation of vascular smooth muscle; reflex tachycardia may also occur.*

Uterine atony is the most common cause of severe postpartum hemorrhage. Immediate administration of oxytocin after delivery is a standard measure used to prevent this complication. Despite this practice, uterine atony complicates 4% to 6% of pregnancies. The concentration of volatile anesthetics should be reduced to 0.5 MAC in obstetric patients undergoing general anesthesia for cesarean delivery to avoid the uterine-relaxing effects of these drugs. Second-line oxytocics are methylergonovine (Methergine) and carboprost tromethamine (Hemabate).

F. Ergot Alkaloids

Methylergonovine causes intense and prolonged uterine contractions. It is therefore given only after delivery (postpartum) to treat uterine atony. Moreover, because it also constricts vascular smooth muscle and can cause severe hypertension if given as an intravenous bolus, it is usually administered only as a single 0.2 mg dose intramuscularly or in dilute form as an intravenous infusion over 10 minutes.

G. Prostaglandins

Carboprost tromethamine (Hemabate, prostaglandin $F_{2\alpha}$) is a synthetic analogue of prostaglandin $F_{2\alpha}$ that stimulates uterine contractions. It is often used to treat refractory postpartum hemorrhage. An initial dose of 0.25 mg intramuscularly may be repeated every 15 to 90 min to a maximum of 2 mg. Common side effects include nausea, vomiting, bronchoconstriction, and diarrhea. It is contraindicated in patients with asthma. Prostaglandin E_1 (Cytotec, rectal suppository) or E_2 (Dinoprostone, vaginal suppository) is sometimes administered and has no bronchoconstricting effect.

H. Magnesium

Magnesium is used in obstetrics both to stop premature labor (*tocolysis*) and prevent eclamptic seizures. It is usually administered as a 4-g intravenous loading dose over 20 min followed by a 2-g/h infusion. Therapeutic serum levels are considered to be 6 to 8 mg/dL. Serious side effects include hypotension, heart block, muscle weakness, and sedation. *Magnesium in these doses and concentrations intensifies neuromuscular blockade from nondepolarizing agents.*

I. β_2 Agonists

The β_2-adrenergic agonists ritodrine and terbutaline inhibit uterine contractions and are used to treat premature labor.

FETAL PHYSIOLOGY

The placenta, which receives nearly half the fetal cardiac output, is responsible for respiratory gas exchange. The fetal lungs receive little blood flow, and the pulmonary and systemic circulations are in parallel instead of in series, as in the adult (Figures 40–4 and 40–5). This arrangement is made possible by two cardiac shunts: the *foramen ovale* and the *ductus arteriosus*:

1. Well-oxygenated blood from the placenta (approximately 80% oxygen saturation) mixes with venous blood returning from the lower body (25% oxygen saturation) and flows via the inferior vena cava into the right atrium.
2. Right atrial anatomy preferentially directs blood flow from the inferior vena cava (67% oxygen saturation) through the foramen ovale into the left atrium.
3. Left atrial blood is then pumped by the left ventricle to the upper body (mainly the brain and the heart).
4. Poorly oxygenated blood from the upper body returns via the superior vena cava to the right atrium.
5. Right atrial anatomy preferentially directs flow from the superior vena cava into the right ventricle.
6. Right ventricular blood is pumped into the pulmonary artery.
7. Because of high pulmonary vascular resistance, 95% of the blood ejected from the right ventricle (60% oxygen saturation) is shunted across the ductus arteriosus, into the descending aorta, and back to the placenta and lower body.

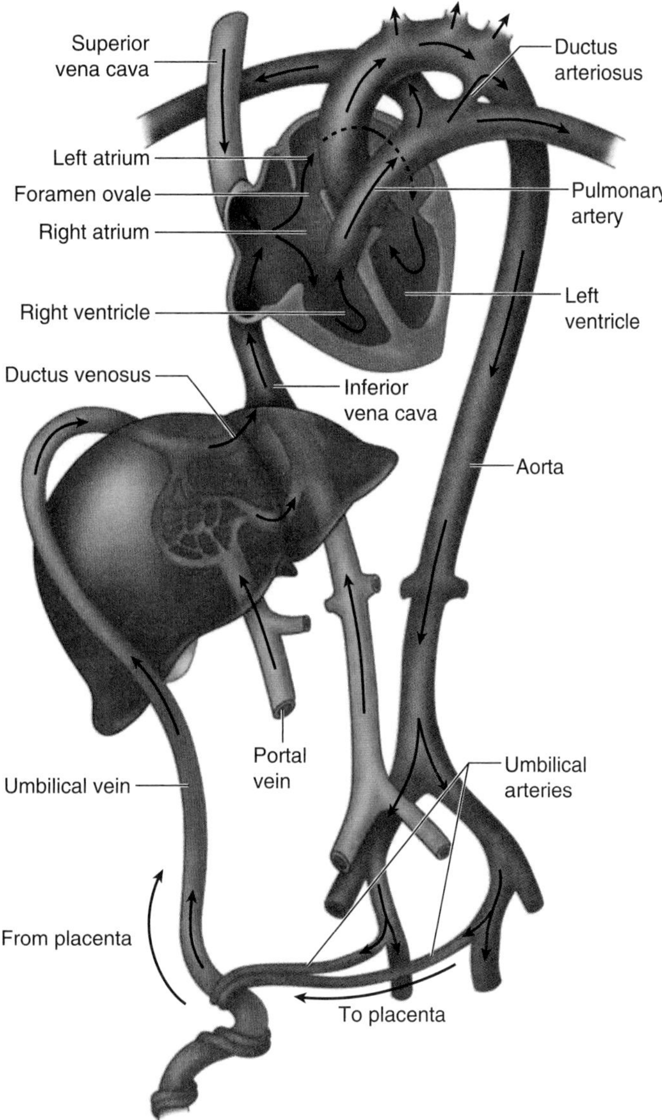

FIGURE 40–4 The fetal circulation before and after birth. (Reproduced with permission from Ganong WF. *Review of Medical Physiology,* 24th ed. New York, NY: McGraw Hill; 2012.)

The parallel circulation results in unequal ventricular flows; the right ventricle ejects two-thirds of the combined ventricular outputs, whereas the left ventricle ejects only one-third.

Up to 50% of the well-oxygenated blood in the umbilical vein can pass directly to the heart via the ductus venosus, bypassing the liver. The remainder of the blood flow from the placenta mixes with blood from the portal vein via the *portal sinus* and passes through the liver before reaching the heart. The latter may be important in allowing relatively rapid hepatic degradation of drugs (or toxins) that are absorbed from the maternal circulation.

In contrast to the fetal circulation, which is established very early during intrauterine life, maturation of the lungs lags behind. Extrauterine survival is not

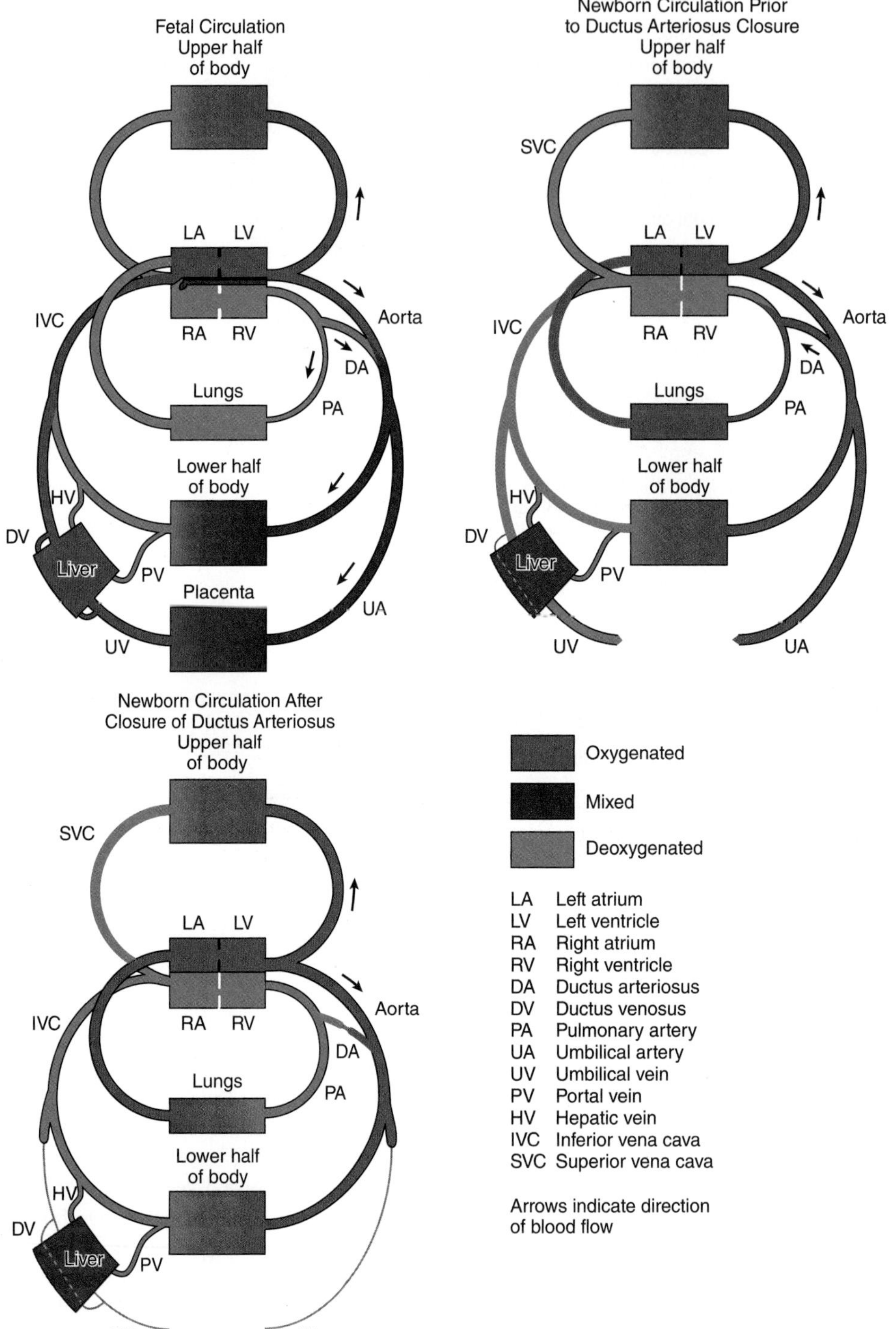

FIGURE 40–5 A schematic comparison of fetal and neonatal circulation. (Reproduced with permission from Danforth DN, Scott JR. *Obstetrics and Gynecology.* 5th ed. Philadelphia, PA: Lippincott Williams & Wilkins; 1986.)

possible until after 22 to 24 weeks of gestation, when pulmonary capillaries are formed and come to lie in close approximation to an immature alveolar epithelium. At 30 weeks, the cuboidal alveolar epithelium flattens out and begins to produce pulmonary surfactant. This substance provides alveolar stability and is necessary to maintain normal lung expansion after birth (see Chapter 23). Sufficient pulmonary surfactant is usually present after 34 weeks of gestation. Administration of glucocorticoids to the mother may accelerate fetal surfactant production.

PHYSIOLOGICAL TRANSITION OF THE FETUS AT BIRTH

The most profound adaptive changes at birth involve the circulatory and respiratory systems. Failure to make this transition successfully results in fetal death or permanent neurological damage.

At term, the fetal lungs are developed but contain about 90 mL of a plasma ultrafiltrate. During expulsion of the fetus at delivery, this fluid is normally squeezed from the lungs by the forces of the pelvic muscles and the vagina acting on the fetus (the *vaginal squeeze*). Any remaining fluid is reabsorbed by the pulmonary capillaries and lymphatics. Small (preterm) neonates and neonates delivered via cesarean section do not benefit from the vaginal squeeze and thus typically have greater difficulty in maintaining respirations (*transient tachypnea of the newborn*). Respiratory efforts are normally initiated within 30 s after birth and become sustained within 90 s. Mild hypoxia and acidosis as well as sensory stimulation—cord clamping, pain, touch, and noise—help initiate and sustain respirations, whereas the outward recoil of the chest at delivery aids in filling the lungs with air.

Lung expansion increases both alveolar and arterial oxygen tensions and decreases pulmonary vascular resistance. The increase in oxygen tension is a potent stimulus for pulmonary arterial vasodilation. The resultant increase in pulmonary blood flow and augmented flow to the left heart elevates left atrial pressure and functionally closes the foramen ovale. The increase in arterial oxygen tension also causes the ductus arteriosus to contract and functionally close. Other chemical mediators that may play a role in ductal closure include acetylcholine, bradykinin, and prostaglandins. The overall result is elimination of right-to-left shunting and establishment of the adult circulation (see Figure 40–5). Anatomic closure of the ductus arteriosus does not usually occur until about 2 to 3 weeks, whereas closure of the foramen ovale takes months, and may not occur at all.

Hypoxia or acidosis during the first few days of life can prevent or reverse these physiological changes, resulting in persistence of (or return to) the fetal circulation, or *persistent pulmonary hypertension of the newborn.* The right-to-left shunting promotes hypoxemia and acidosis, which in turn promotes more shunting (Figure 40–6). Right-to-left shunting may occur across the foramen ovale, the ductus arteriosus, or both.

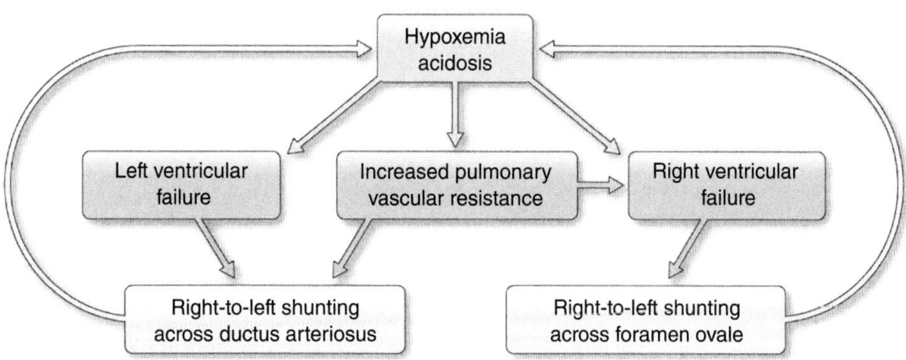

FIGURE 40–6 Pathophysiology of persistent pulmonary hypertension of the newborn (persistent fetal circulation).

CASE DISCUSSION

Postpartum Tubal Ligation

A 36-year-old woman is scheduled for bilateral tubal ligation 12 h after delivery of a healthy baby.

Is this patient still at increased risk for pulmonary aspiration?

Controversy exists over when the increased risk for pulmonary aspiration diminishes following pregnancy. Certainly, many factors contributing to delayed gastric emptying are alleviated shortly after delivery: mechanical distortion of the stomach is relieved, labor pains cease, and the circulating progesterone level rapidly declines. Gastric volume and acidity usually do not differ in pregnant compared with nonpregnant women, though 30% to 60% of pregnant patients have a gastric volume greater than 25 mL or a gastric fluid pH less than 2.5. In these parturients, gastric volume and gastric fluid pH (see section on Kidney & Gastrointestinal Effects) normalize within 24 h after delivery. Therefore, most clinicians still consider the immediate postpartum patient to be at increased risk for pulmonary aspiration and take appropriate precautions (see Chapters 17 and 41). It is not known when the risk returns to the level associated with elective surgical patients. Although some physiological changes associated with pregnancy may require up to 6 weeks for resolution, the increased risk of pulmonary aspiration probably returns to "normal" well before that time.

Other than aspiration risk, what factors determine the "optimal" time for postpartum sterilization?

The decision about when to perform postpartum tubal ligation (or laparoscopic fulguration) is complex and varies according to patient and obstetrician preferences as well as local practices. Factors influencing the decision include whether the patient had a vaginal or cesarean delivery and whether an anesthetic was administered for labor (epidural anesthesia) or delivery (epidural or general anesthesia).

Postpartum tubal ligation or fulguration may be (1) performed immediately following delivery of the baby and repair of the uterus during a cesarean section, (2) delayed 8 to 48 h following delivery to allow an elective fasting period, or (3) deferred until after the postpartum period (generally 6 weeks). Sterilization is technically easier to perform in the immediate postpartum period because of the enlargement of the uterus and tubes. Postpartum sterilizations following natural vaginal delivery are generally performed within 48 h of delivery.

What factors determine the selection of an anesthetic technique for postpartum sterilization?

When continuous epidural anesthesia is administered for labor and vaginal delivery, the epidural catheter may be left in place up to 48 h for subsequent tubal ligation. The delay allows a period of elective fasting. A T4–5 sensory level with regional anesthesia is usually necessary to ensure a pain-free anesthetic experience. Lower sensory levels (as low as T10) may be adequate but sometimes fail to prevent pain caused by surgical traction on the viscera.

When the patient has not had anesthesia for delivery, postpartum sterilization may be performed under either regional or general anesthesia. Because of the increased risk of pulmonary aspiration, regional anesthesia usually is preferred for bilateral tubal ligation via a mini-laparotomy. Many clinicians prefer spinal over epidural anesthesia in this setting because of its greater speed of onset, blockade density, and reliability (see Chapter 45). In addition, the incidence of postdural puncture headache is as low as 1% when a 25-gauge or smaller pencil-point needle is used. Dosage requirements for regional anesthesia generally return to normal within 24 to 36 h after delivery. Bupivacaine (8–12 mg) or lidocaine (60–75 mg) may be used for spinal anesthesia. For epidural anesthesia, 15 to 30 mL of lidocaine 1.5% to 2% or chloroprocaine 3% is most commonly used.

In contrast, when laparoscopic tubal fulguration is planned, general endotracheal anesthesia is preferred. Insufflation of gas during laparoscopy impairs pulmonary gas exchange and predisposes the patient to nausea, vomiting, and possibly pulmonary aspiration. Endotracheal intubation generally ensures adequate ventilation and protects the airway.

What considerations are important for postpartum patients undergoing general anesthesia?

Preoperative concerns include the persistently increased risk of pulmonary aspiration. Anemia is nearly always present as a result of the physiological effects of pregnancy combined with blood loss during and following delivery. Hemoglobin concentrations are usually greater than 9 g/dL, but levels as low as 7 g/dL are generally considered safe. Fortunately, sterilization procedures are rarely associated with significant blood loss.

The risk of pulmonary aspiration is diminished by a minimum of 8 h of fasting, premedication with an H_2 blocker (ranitidine), a clear antacid (sodium citrate), or metoclopramide (see Chapters 17 and 41). In addition, induction of anesthesia should employ a rapid-sequence technique prior to endotracheal intubation, and the patient should be extubated only when she is awake and protective airway reflexes have returned. Decreased plasma cholinesterase levels persist after delivery (see section on Hepatic Effects), modestly prolonging the effect of succinylcholine. The duration of rocuronium but not atracurium (or cisatracurium) has also been reported to be prolonged in postpartum women. Excessive concentrations of volatile agents should be avoided because of the at least theoretical risk of increasing uterine blood loss or inducing postpartum hemorrhage secondary to uterine relaxation. Intravenous opioids may be used to supplement inhalational agents. Intravenous drugs administered intraoperatively (other than meperidine and, to a lesser extent, morphine and hydromorphone) to mothers who are breastfeeding appear to have minimal if any effects on their neonates. There are no data regarding ketamine. With these few exceptions, current recommendations support immediate postanesthesia breastfeeding. The advice of some anesthetists to "pump and dump" breast milk for 24 h before resuming breastfeeding is outdated.

SUGGESTED READINGS

Butwick AJ, McDonnell N. Antepartum and postpartum anemia: a narrative review. *Int J Obstet Anesth.* 2021;102985.

Chestnut DH, Wong CA, Tsen LC, et al. *Chestnut's Obstetric Anesthesia: Principals and Practice.* 6th ed. Mosby; 2019.

Cunningham F, Leveno KJ, Tsen LC, et al. *Williams Obstetrics.* 25th ed. McGraw-Hill Education; 2018.

Dalal PG, Bosak J, Berlin C. Safety of the breast-feeding infant after maternal anesthesia. *Paediatr Anaesth.* 2014;24:359.

Hussey H, Hussey P, Meng ML. Peripartum considerations for women with cardiac disease. *Curr Opin Anaesthesiol.* 2021;34:218.

Lim G, Facco FL, Nathan N, Waters JH, Wong CA, Eltzschig HK. A review of the impact of obstetric anesthesia on maternal and neonatal outcomes. *Anesthesiology.* 2018;129:192.

Suresh M. *Shnider and Levinson's Anesthesia for Obstetrics.* 5th ed. Lippincott Williams & Wilkins; 2013.

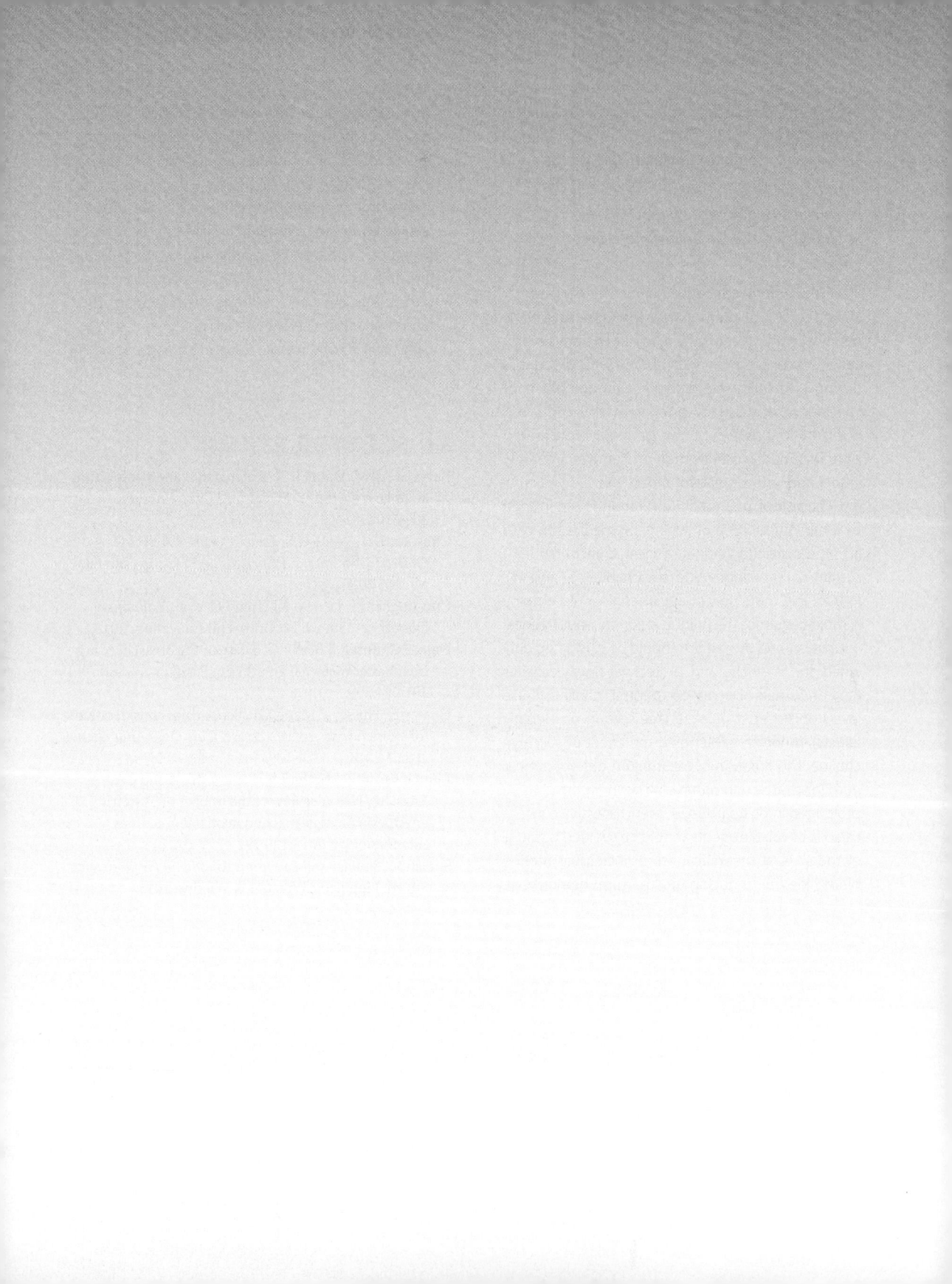

CHAPTER 41

Obstetric Anesthesia

Michael A. Frölich, MD, MS

KEY CONCEPTS

1. According to the U.S. Centers for Disease Control and Prevention, the leading causes of pregnancy-related death in the United States in 2017 were cardiovascular diseases (14%), infection/sepsis (13%), cardiomyopathy (12%), hemorrhage (11%), embolism (10%), stroke (8%), and hypertensive disorders of pregnancy (7%). Other pregnancy-related deaths were due to amniotic fluid embolism (6%), homicide (3%), unintentional injury (3%), and autoimmune disease (2%). Only 0.4% of maternal deaths were anesthesia related.
2. Regardless of the time of last oral intake, all obstetric patients are considered to have a full stomach and be at risk for pulmonary aspiration.
3. Nearly all parenteral opioid analgesics and sedatives readily cross the placenta and can affect the fetus. Regional anesthetic techniques are preferred for management of labor pain.
4. Using a local anesthetic–opioid mixture for lumbar epidural analgesia during labor significantly reduces drug requirements when compared with using either agent alone.
5. Analgesia during labor requires neural blockade at the T10–L1 sensory level in the first stage of labor and at the T10–S4 sensory level in the second stage.
6. Continuous lumbar epidural analgesia is the most versatile and most commonly employed technique because it can be used for pain relief for the first stage of labor as well as analgesia/anesthesia for subsequent vaginal delivery or cesarean section.
7. Epidural analgesia does not increase the rate of operative delivery and has little if any effect on labor progress when dilute mixtures of a local anesthetic and an opioid are used.
8. Unintentional intravascular or intrathecal placement of an epidural needle or catheter is possible even when needle or catheter aspiration does not yield blood or cerebrospinal fluid.
9. Hypotension is a common side effect of regional anesthetic techniques and can be treated with intravenous boluses of phenylephrine (40–120 mcg), supplemental oxygen, left uterine displacement, and an intravenous fluid bolus to prevent fetal compromise.
10. Techniques using combined spinal–epidural (CSE) analgesia and anesthesia may especially benefit patients with severe pain early in labor and those who receive analgesia/anesthesia immediately prior to delivery.
11. Spinal or epidural anesthesia is preferred to general anesthesia for cesarean section

—Continued next page

Continued—

because regional anesthesia is associated with less hemodynamic fluctuation, more gradual resolution of analgesia during anesthetic recovery, and lower maternal mortality.

12 Continuous epidural anesthesia allows better control over the sensory level than "single-shot" spinal anesthesia. Conversely, spinal anesthesia has a more rapid, predictable onset; may produce a more dense (more complete) block; and lacks the potential for serious systemic drug toxicity because of the smaller dose of local anesthetic employed.

13 The risk of systemic local anesthetic toxicity during epidural analgesia and anesthesia is minimized by slowly administering dilute solutions for labor pain and by fractionating the total dose administered for cesarean section into 5-mL increments.

14 Maternal hemorrhage is a common cause of maternal morbidity. Causes for antepartum hemorrhage include placenta previa, abruptio placentae, and uterine rupture. Common causes of postpartum hemorrhage include uterine atony, a retained placenta, obstetric lacerations, uterine inversion, and the use of tocolytic agents prior to delivery.

15 Intrauterine asphyxia during labor is the most common cause of neonatal depression. The benefit of continuous fetal heart rate monitoring throughout labor is controversial, but it is routinely used in combination with other fetal surveillance methods to guide the clinical management of parturients.

This chapter focuses on the practice of obstetric anesthesia. Techniques for analgesia and anesthesia during labor, vaginal delivery, and cesarean section are presented. The chapter concludes with a review of neonatal resuscitation.

ANESTHETIC RISK IN OBSTETRIC PATIENTS

Although most women of childbearing age would be considered to be at minimal operative risk, pregnancy, certain maternal–fetal factors, and preexisting medical conditions significantly increase surgical and obstetric risks.

Maternal Mortality

Maternal mortality is usually presented as the number of women who die while pregnant or within 42 days of pregnancy termination after excluding accidents and unrelated causes. This number is often indexed to the total number of live births. The maternal mortality index has decreased nearly 100-fold since 1900. In the United States, the maternal mortality rate was 17.4 deaths per 100,000 live births in 2018. The world average was 211 deaths per 100,000 live births in 2017. Of all maternal deaths worldwide, 99% occur in Africa, Asia, Latin America, and the Caribbean.

1 **In the United States, overall mortality risk is greater for women older than 40 years, Black women, and women who do not receive prenatal care. According to the U.S. Centers for Disease Control and Prevention, the leading causes of pregnancy-related death in the US in 2017 were cardiovascular diseases (14%), infection/sepsis (13%), cardiomyopathy (12%), hemorrhage (11%), embolism (10%), stroke (8%), and hypertensive disorders of pregnancy (7%). Other pregnancy-related deaths were due to amniotic fluid embolism (6%), homicide (3%), unintentional injury (3%), and autoimmune disease (2%). A variety of other conditions account for the remaining causes of maternal death, but only 0.4% were anesthesia related.** The most significant differences in pregnancy-related deaths by race were in the preeclampsia and eclampsia (12% Black, 5% White) and mental health conditions (1% Black, 11% White).

TABLE 41–1 Incidence of severe obstetric morbidity.[1]

Morbidity	Incidence per 1000
Severe hemorrhage	6.7
Severe preeclampsia	3.9
HELLP syndrome[2]	0.5
Severe sepsis	0.4
Eclampsia	0.2
Uterine rupture	0.2

[1]Note thromboembolic disease was excluded.

[2]HELLP syndrome consists of hemolysis, elevated liver enzymes, and low platelet count.

Data from Waterstone M, Bewley S, Wolfe C. Incidence and predictors of severe obstetric morbidity: Case-control study. *BMJ.* 2001 May 5; 322(7294):1089-1093.

Severe obstetric morbidity may be a more useful measure of peripartum outcome than maternal mortality. Data from the United Kingdom suggest that the incidence of severe obstetric morbidity is 12 per 1000 deliveries, 100 times more common than mortality. Risk factors include age greater than 34 years, non-White ethnicity, multiple pregnancies, history of hypertension, previous postpartum hemorrhage, and emergency cesarean delivery. Table 41–1 lists the estimated incidence of the most common causes of severe morbidity (not mortality); thromboembolic disease was deliberately excluded because of the difficulty in making the diagnosis in nonfatal cases. *By far the most common morbidities encountered in obstetrics are severe hemorrhage and severe preeclampsia.*

Anesthetic Mortality

Data collected between 1985 and 1990 suggested a maternal mortality rate of 32 deaths per 1,000,000 live births due to general anesthesia and 1.9 deaths per 1,000,000 live births due to regional anesthesia. More recent data between 2006 and 2010 suggest a lower overall maternal mortality from anesthesia (an estimated 0.9% of pregnancy-related deaths) with an even lower estimated percentage (0.4%) from 2014 to 2017, possibly due to greater use of regional anesthesia for labor and cesarean delivery. Most deaths occur during or after cesarean section. Moreover, the risk of an adverse outcome is much greater with emergency than elective cesarean sections.

Obstetric Anesthesia Closed Claims

Obstetric anesthesia care accounts for approximately 3% of the American Society of Anesthesiologists (ASA) Closed Claims database claims in the years 2000 to 2012. A comparison of obstetric anesthesia claims from 2000 to 2012 with 1993 to 1999 claims shows no significant change in the number of cesarean delivery–related closed claims. Payments on behalf of anesthesiologists occurred with delays in care, miscommunication in the level of urgency of the cesarean delivery, concerns over the management of a difficult intubation or high block, or lapses in care or record keeping.

General Approach to the Obstetric Patient

All patients entering the obstetric suite may require anesthesia services. Patients requiring anesthetic care for labor or a cesarean section should undergo a focused preanesthetic evaluation as early as possible, which should include maternal health, medical and surgical histories, anesthesia and anesthesia-related obstetric history, vital signs, airway assessment, and back examination for potential regional anesthesia. Obesity is becoming far more prevalent in the United States and is associated with an increased risk of almost all pregnancy complications: gestational hypertension, preeclampsia, gestational diabetes mellitus, delivery of large-for-gestational-age infants, and a higher incidence of congenital defects. Because obesity affects many aspects of obstetric anesthesia care, documentation of the patient's body mass index is an important aspect of the preanesthetic evaluation.

2 **Regardless of the time of last oral intake, all obstetric patients are considered to have a full stomach and to be at risk for pulmonary aspiration.** Because the duration of labor is often prolonged, guidelines usually allow small amounts of oral clear liquid during uncomplicated labor. The minimum fasting period for elective cesarean section remains

controversial but is typically recommended to be 6 h for light meals and 8 h for heavy meals. Prophylactic administration of a clear antacid (15–30 mL of 0.3 M sodium citrate orally) every 30 min prior to a cesarean section may help maintain gastric pH greater than 2.5 and may decrease the likelihood of severe aspiration pneumonitis. An H_2-blocking drug (eg, ranitidine, 100–150 mg orally or 50 mg intravenously) or metoclopramide, 10 mg orally or intravenously, should also be considered for high-risk patients and for those expected to receive general anesthesia. H_2 blockers reduce both gastric volume and pH but have no effect on the gastric contents already present. Metoclopramide accelerates gastric emptying, decreases gastric volume, and increases lower esophageal sphincter tone. The supine position should be avoided unless a left uterine displacement device (>15° wedge) is placed under the right hip to avoid hypotension.

Anesthesia for Labor & Vaginal Delivery

PAIN PATHWAYS DURING LABOR

The pain of labor arises from contraction of the myometrium against the resistance of the cervix and perineum, progressive dilation of the cervix and lower uterine segment, and stretching and compression of pelvic and perineal structures. Discomfort during the first stage of labor is primarily visceral pain resulting from uterine contractions and cervical dilation. It is usually initially confined to the T11–T12 dermatomes during the latent phase but eventually involves the T10–L1 dermatomes as labor enters the active phase. The visceral afferent fibers responsible for labor pain travel with sympathetic nerve fibers first to the uterovaginal plexus, then through the inferior hypogastric plexus, before entering the spinal cord with the T10–L1 nerve roots. The pain is initially perceived in the lower abdomen but may increasingly be referred to the lumbosacral area, gluteal region, and thighs as labor progresses. Pain intensity also increases with progressive cervical dilation and with increasing intensity and frequency of uterine contractions. Nulliparous women typically experience greater pain during the first stage of labor than multiparous women.

The onset of perineal pain at the end of the first stage signals the beginning of fetal descent and the second stage of labor. Stretching and compression of pelvic and perineal structures intensify the pain. Sensory innervation of the perineum is provided by the pudendal nerves (S2–4), so pain during the second stage of labor involves the T10–S4 dermatomes.

PSYCHOLOGICAL & NONPHARMACOLOGICAL ANALGESIC TECHNIQUES

Psychological analgesic techniques include those of Bradley, Dick-Read, Lamaze, and LeBoyer. Patient education and positive conditioning about the birthing process are central to such techniques. Pain during labor tends to be accentuated by fear of the unknown or by previous unpleasant experiences. The Lamaze technique, one of the most popular, coaches the parturient to take a deep breath at the beginning of each contraction, followed by rapid, shallow breathing for the duration of the contraction. The parturient also concentrates on an object in the room and attempts to focus her thoughts away from the pain. Less common nonpharmacological techniques include hypnosis, transcutaneous electrical nerve stimulation, biofeedback, and acupuncture. The success of all these techniques varies considerably from patient to patient, and many patients require additional forms of analgesia.

PARENTERAL AGENTS

3 **Nearly all parenteral opioid analgesics and sedatives readily cross the placenta and can affect the fetus. Concern regarding fetal depression limits the use of these agents to the early stages of labor or to situations in which regional anesthetic techniques are not available or appropriate.** Central nervous system (CNS) depression in the neonate may be manifested by a prolonged time to sustained respirations, respiratory acidosis, or an abnormal neurobehavioral examination. Moreover, loss of beat-to-beat

variability in the fetal heart rate (seen with most CNS depressants) and decreased fetal movements (due to sedation of the fetus) complicate the evaluation of fetal well-being during labor. Long-term fetal heart rate variability is affected more than short-term variability. The degree and significance of these effects depend on the specific agent, the dose, the time elapsed between its administration and delivery, and fetal maturity. Premature neonates exhibit the greatest sensitivity. In addition to maternal respiratory depression, opioids can also induce maternal nausea and vomiting and delay maternal gastric emptying.

Meperidine, a commonly used opioid, can be given in doses of 10 to 25 mg intravenously or 25 to 50 mg intramuscularly, usually up to a total of 100 mg. Maximal maternal and fetal respiratory depression is seen in 10 to 20 min following intravenous administration and in 1 to 3 h following intramuscular administration. Consequently, meperidine is usually administered early in labor when delivery is not expected for at least 4 h. Intravenous fentanyl, 25 to 100 mcg/h, has also been used for labor analgesia. Fentanyl in 25 to 100 mcg doses has a 3- to 10-min analgesic onset, initially lasts about 60 min, and lasts longer following multiple doses. However, maternal respiratory depression outlasts the analgesia. Lower doses of fentanyl may be associated with little or no neonatal respiratory depression and are reported to have no effect on Apgar scores. A substantial body of evidence supports the use of the ultra-short-acting opioid remifentanil for labor analgesia. Evidence suggests remifentanil is equally or more efficacious than other parenteral opioids or inhalational alternatives, though it does not provide the degree of pain relief offered by neuraxial analgesia. A popular patient-controlled analgesia setting for remifentanil administration is a 40-mcg bolus with a 2-min lockout. Careful one-on-one patient monitoring is mandatory. Agents with mixed agonist–antagonist activity (butorphanol, 1–2 mg, and nalbuphine, 10–20 mg intravenously or intramuscularly) are also effective and are associated with little or no cumulative respiratory depression, but excessive sedation with repeat doses can be problematic.

Promethazine (25–50 mg intramuscularly) and hydroxyzine (50–100 mg intramuscularly) can be useful alone or in combination with opioids. Both drugs reduce anxiety, opioid requirements, and the incidence of nausea but do not add appreciably to neonatal depression. A significant disadvantage of hydroxyzine is pain at the injection site following intramuscular administration. Nonsteroidal anti-inflammatory agents, such as ketorolac, are not recommended as antepartum therapy because they suppress uterine contractions and promote closure of the fetal ductus arteriosus.

Small doses (up to 2 mg intravenously) of midazolam may be administered in combination with a small dose of fentanyl (up to 100 mcg intravenously) in healthy parturients at term to facilitate the analgesic effect of neuraxial blockade. At this dose, maternal amnesia has not been observed. Chronic administration of the longer-acting benzodiazepine diazepam has been associated with fetal depression.

Low-dose intravenous ketamine is a powerful analgesic. In doses of 10 to 15 mg intravenously, good analgesia can be obtained in 2 to 5 min without loss of consciousness. Large boluses of ketamine (>1 mg/kg) can be associated with hypertonic uterine contractions. Low-dose ketamine is most useful just prior to delivery or as an adjuvant to regional anesthesia (see Chapter 9).

Inhalation of nitrous oxide–oxygen remains in common use for relief of mild labor pain. As previously noted, nitrous oxide has minimal effects on uterine blood flow or uterine contractions.

PUDENDAL NERVE BLOCK

Pudendal nerve blocks are often combined with perineal infiltration of local anesthetic to provide perineal anesthesia during the second stage of labor when other forms of anesthesia are not employed or prove to be inadequate. Paracervical plexus blocks are no longer used because of their association with a relatively high rate of fetal bradycardia; the close proximity of the injection site to the uterine artery may result in uterine arterial vasoconstriction, uteroplacental insufficiency, and increased levels of the local anesthetic in the fetal blood.

During a pudendal nerve block, a special needle (Koback) or guide (Iowa trumpet) is used to place the needle transvaginally underneath the ischial spine on each side; the needle is advanced 1 to 1.5 cm through the sacrospinous ligament, and 10 mL of 1% lidocaine or 2% chloroprocaine is injected following negative needle aspiration. The needle guide is used to limit the depth of injection and protect the fetus and vagina from the needle. Other potential complications include intravascular injection, retroperitoneal hematoma, and retropsoas or subgluteal abscess.

REGIONAL ANESTHETIC TECHNIQUES

Epidural or intrathecal techniques, alone or in combination, are currently the most popular methods of pain relief during labor and delivery. They can provide excellent analgesia while allowing the mother to be awake and cooperative during labor. Although spinal opioids or local anesthetics alone can provide adequate analgesia, techniques that combine the two have proved to be the most satisfactory in most parturients. **Moreover, the synergy between opioids and local anesthetics decreases dose requirements and provides excellent analgesia with few maternal side effects and little or no neonatal depression.**

4

1. Spinal Opioids Alone

Opioids may be given intrathecally as a single injection or intermittently via an epidural or intrathecal catheter (Table 41–2). Relatively large doses are required for analgesia during labor when epidural or intrathecal opioids are used alone. For example, the ED_{50} during labor is 124 mcg for epidural fentanyl and 21 mcg for epidural sufentanil. The higher doses may be associated with a high risk of side effects, most importantly respiratory depression. For this reason, combinations of local anesthetics and opioids are most commonly used (see later discussion). Pure opioid techniques are most useful for high-risk patients who may not tolerate the functional sympathectomy associated with spinal or epidural anesthesia (see Chapter 45). This group includes patients with hypovolemia or significant cardiovascular disease such as moderate to severe aortic stenosis, tetralogy of Fallot, Eisenmenger syndrome, or pulmonary hypertension. With the exception of meperidine, which has local anesthetic properties, spinal opioids alone do not produce motor blockade or sympathectomy. Thus, they do not impair the ability of the parturient to "push." Disadvantages include incomplete analgesia, lack of perineal relaxation, and potential side effects such as pruritus, nausea, vomiting, sedation, and respiratory depression. Side effects may be ameliorated with low doses of naloxone (0.1–0.2 mg/h intravenously).

TABLE 41–2 Spinal opioid dosages for labor and delivery.

Agent	Intrathecal	Epidural
Morphine	0.1–0.5 mg	5 mg
Meperidine	10–15 mg	50–100 mg
Fentanyl	10–25 mcg	50–150 mcg
Sufentanil	3–10 mcg	10–20 mcg

Intrathecal Opioids

Intrathecal morphine in doses of 0.1 to 0.3 mg may produce satisfactory and prolonged (4–6 h) analgesia during the first stage of labor. Unfortunately, the onset of analgesia is slow (45–60 min), and these doses may not be sufficient in many patients. However, higher doses are associated with a relatively high incidence of side effects. Morphine is therefore rarely used alone. The combination of morphine, 0.1 to 0.25 mg, and fentanyl, 12.5 mcg (or sufentanil, 5 mcg), may result in a more rapid onset of analgesia (5 min). Intermittent boluses of 10 to 15 mg of meperidine, 12.5 to 25 mcg of fentanyl, or 3 to 10 mcg of sufentanil via an intrathecal catheter can also provide satisfactory analgesia for labor. Early reports of fetal bradycardia following intrathecal opioid injections (eg, sufentanil) have not been confirmed by subsequent studies. Hypotension following administration of intrathecal opioids for labor may be due to the resultant analgesia and decreased circulating catecholamine levels.

Epidural Opioids

Relatively large doses (≥7.5 mg) of epidural morphine are required for satisfactory labor analgesia but are not recommended because of the increased risk of delayed respiratory depression and because the resultant analgesia is effective only in the early first stage of labor. Onset may take 30 to 60 min, but analgesia lasts up to 12 to 24 h (as does the risk of delayed respiratory depression). Epidural meperidine, 50 to 100 mg, provides good but relatively brief analgesia (1 to 3 h). Epidural fentanyl, 50 to 150 mcg, or sufentanil, 10 to 20 mcg, usually produces analgesia within 5 to 10 min with few side effects, but it has a short duration (1–2 h). Although "single-shot" epidural opioids do not appear to cause significant neonatal depression, caution should be exercised following repeated administrations. Combinations of a lower dose of morphine, 2.5 mg, with fentanyl, 25 to 50 mcg (or sufentanil, 7.5–10 mcg), may result in more rapid onset and prolongation of analgesia (4–5 h) with fewer side effects.

2. Local Anesthetic/Local Anesthetic–Opioid Mixtures

Epidural and spinal (intrathecal) analgesia more commonly utilizes local anesthetics either alone or
5 with opioids for labor and delivery. **Analgesia during the first stage of labor requires neural blockade at the T10–L1 sensory level, whereas pain relief during the second stage of labor requires**
6 **neural blockade at T10–S4. Programmed intermittent epidural bolus (PIEB) epidural analgesia and continuous epidural analgesia are the most effective methods for labor pain relief. These techniques can be used for pain relief for the first stage of labor as well as analgesia/anesthesia for subsequent vaginal delivery or cesarean section, if necessary.** "Single-shot" epidural, spinal, or combined spinal epidural analgesia may be appropriate when pain relief is initiated just prior to vaginal delivery (the second stage). Obstetric caudal injections have largely been abandoned because of less versatility; although effective for perineal analgesia/anesthesia, they require large volumes of local anesthetic to anesthetize upper lumbar and lower thoracic dermatomes. They have also been associated with early paralysis of the pelvic muscles that may interfere with normal rotation of the fetal head and with a small risk of accidental puncture of the fetus.

Absolute contraindications to regional anesthesia include patient refusal, infection at the injection site, coagulopathy, marked hypovolemia, and true allergies to the chosen local anesthetic. The patient's inability to cooperate may prevent successful regional anesthesia. Full anticoagulation markedly increases the risk of neuraxial anesthesia. Regional anesthesia should generally not be performed within 4 to 6 h of a subcutaneous dose of unfractionated heparin or within 10 to 12 h of administration of low-molecular-weight heparin (LMWH). Thrombocytopenia or concomitant administration of an antiplatelet agent increases the risk of spinal hematoma. *Vaginal birth after cesarean* (VBAC) delivery is not a contraindication to regional anesthesia during labor. Concern that anesthesia may mask pain associated with uterine rupture during VBAC may not be justified because not all dehiscences cause pain even without epidural anesthesia; moreover, changes in uterine tone and contraction pattern may be more reliable signs.

When performing any regional block, appropriate equipment and supplies for resuscitation must be immediately available, including oxygen, suction, a mask with a positive-pressure device for ventilation, a functioning laryngoscope and blades, endotracheal tubes (6 or 6.5 mm), oral and nasal airways, intravenous fluids, ephedrine, atropine, propofol, and succinylcholine. The ability to monitor blood pressure and heart rate is mandatory. A pulse oximeter and capnograph must be immediately available, and immediate availability of equipment such as a video laryngoscope or an intubating laryngeal mask airway device for use with a difficult airway is advisable.

Lumbar Epidural Analgesia

Epidural analgesia for labor may be administered in early labor after the patient has been evaluated by
7 her obstetrician. **Epidural analgesia does not increase the rate of operative delivery and has little if any effect on the progress of labor when dilute mixtures of a local anesthetic and an opioid are used. Concerns that regional analgesia will increase the likelihood of oxytocin augmentation, operative (eg, forceps) delivery, or cesarean section are unjustified.** Recent reports concerning an association of epidural analgesia and autism spectrum disorders are misleading as they do not consider the duration of labor and other important intrapartum risk factors that may relate to the

development of a child. It is often advantageous to place an epidural catheter early in labor when the patient is less uncomfortable and can be positioned more easily. Moreover, should an urgent or emergency cesarean section become necessary, the presence of a functioning epidural catheter makes it possible to avoid general anesthesia.

A. Technique

Parturients may be positioned on their sides or in the sitting position for the procedure. The sitting position often makes it easier to identify the midline and spine, particularly in obese patients. When epidural anesthesia is being given for vaginal delivery (second stage of labor), the sitting position may promote sacral spread.

Identification of the epidural space can be difficult, and unintentional dural puncture will sometimes occur even in experienced hands; the incidence of "wet taps" in obstetric patients is 0.25% to 9%, depending on clinician experience. Many practitioners add a compressible air bubble to the saline syringe and bounce the plunger to ensure that it moves freely and does not stick to the syringe wall (Figure 41–1A and C). Most clinicians advocate the midline approach, whereas a minority favors the paramedian approach. For the placement of a lumbar epidural catheter in the obstetric patient, most anesthesiologists advance the epidural needle with the left hand, which is braced against the patient's back, while applying continuous pressure to the plunger of a glass syringe filled with sterile saline (Figure 41–1A and C). Alternatively, some make use of the "wings" of the Weiss epidural needle by advancing it with both hands a few millimeters at a

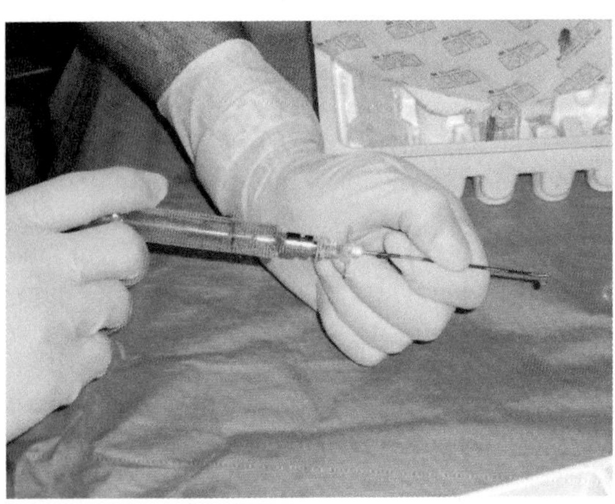
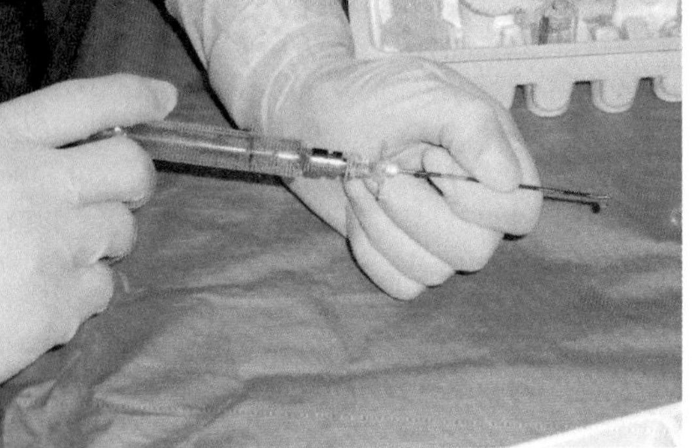
A

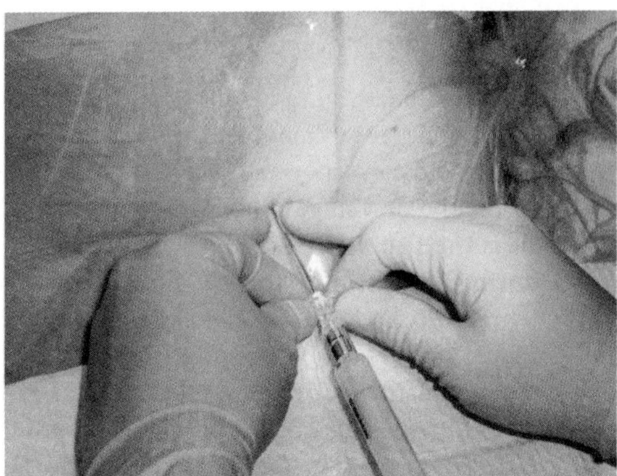
B

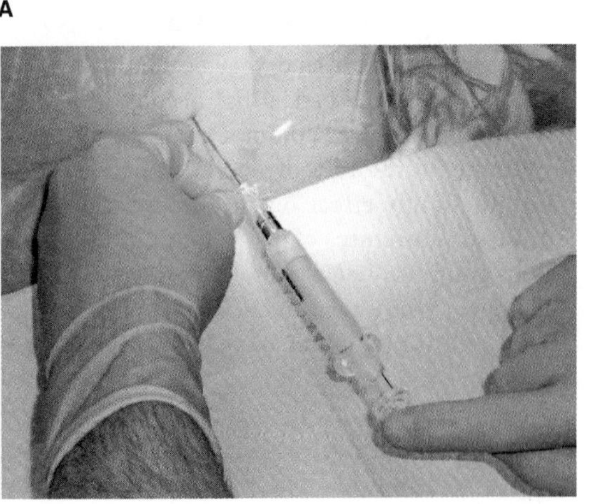
C

FIGURE 41–1 **A**: One-handed needle advancement; continuous pressure technique. The operator applies continuous pressure to the plunger of a loss-of-resistance syringe filled with saline and an air bubble while advancing the needle with the left hand braced against the patient's back. **B**: Bimanual needle advancement; intermittent pressure technique. The operator advances the loss-of-resistance syringe with both hands 2 to 3 mm at a time while appreciating the resistance encountered by the needle. **C**: In between bimanual advancements of the needle, the operator tests the tissue resistance of the needle tip by bouncing the plunger of the air-filled loss-of-resistance syringe. Many practitioners add a compressible air bubble to a saline-filled syringe and bounce the plunger to ensure that the plunger is moving freely and not sticking to the syringe barrel wall.

time (Figure 41–1B). A change of tissue resistance is then tested continuously using tactile feedback when advancing the needle and by intermittently applying pressure to the air-filled loss-of-resistance syringe. The latter technique allows for precise control of needle advancement and may allow a better distinction of various tissue densities. If air is used for detecting loss of resistance, the amount injected should be limited; injection of larger volumes of air (>2–3 mL) in the epidural space has been associated with patchy or unilateral analgesia and headache. The average depth of the lumbar epidural space in obstetric patients is 6 cm from the skin. Insertion of the epidural catheter at the L3–4 or L4–5 interspace is generally optimal for achieving a T10–S5 neural blockade. Ultrasound guidance has recently been offered as a tool in assisting with the placement of an epidural catheter. This technique allows the practitioner to judge the depth of the epidural space and estimate the best angle of needle insertion. The potential benefit of this technique is most obvious in obese patients with poor anatomic landmarks. However, the technique is highly user dependent, and few practitioners have adopted it.

If an unintentional dural puncture occurs, the anesthetist has two choices: (1) place the epidural catheter in the subarachnoid space for continuous spinal (intrathecal) analgesia and anesthesia (see discussion that follows) or (2) remove the needle and attempt placement at another spinal level. The intrathecally placed epidural catheter may be used as a continuous spinal anesthetic. If used in this fashion, an infusion of 0.0625% to 0.125% bupivacaine with fentanyl, 2 to 3 mcg/mL starting at 1–3 mL/h, is a typical choice.

B. Choice of Epidural Catheter

Many clinicians advocate the use of a multi-orifice catheter instead of a single-orifice catheter for obstetric anesthesia. Use of a multi-orifice catheter may be associated with fewer unilateral blocks and greatly reduces the incidence of false-negative aspiration when assessing for intravascular or intrathecal catheter placement. Advancing a multi-orifice catheter 4 to 6 cm into the epidural space appears to be optimal for obtaining adequate sensory levels. A single-orifice catheter need only be advanced 3 to 5 cm into the epidural space. Shorter insertion lengths in the epidural space (<5 cm) may favor dislodgment of the catheter out of the epidural space in obese patients following flexion/extension movements of the spine. Longer epidural insertion lengths in the epidural space may increase the risk of unilateral analgesia, epidural vein insertion, or catheter knots. Spiral wire-reinforced catheters are very resistant to kinking. A spiral or spring tip, particularly when used without a stylet, is associated with a reduced incidence of, and less intense, paresthesia.

C. Choice of Local Anesthetic Solutions

The addition of opioids to local anesthetic solutions for epidural anesthesia has dramatically changed the practice of obstetric anesthesia. The synergy between epidural opioids and local anesthetic solutions reflects separate sites of action: opioid receptors and neuronal axons, respectively. When the two are combined, very low concentrations of both local anesthetic and opioid can be used with excellent effect. In addition, the incidence of adverse side effects, such as hypotension and drug toxicity, is reduced. Although local anesthetics can be used alone, there is rarely a reason to do so. Moreover, when an opioid is omitted, the greater concentration of local anesthetic required (eg, bupivacaine, 0.25%, and ropivacaine, 0.2%) for adequate analgesia can impair the parturient's ability to push effectively as labor progresses. The most common local anesthetic/opioid combination used for labor analgesia is bupivacaine or ropivacaine in concentrations of 0.0625% to 0.125% with either fentanyl, 2 to 3 mcg/mL, or sufentanil, 0.3 to 0.5 mcg/mL. In general, the lower the concentration of the local anesthetic, the greater the concentration of opioid that is required. Very dilute local anesthetic mixtures (0.0625%) generally do not produce motor blockade and may allow some patients to ambulate ("walking" or "mobile" epidural). The long duration of action of bupivacaine makes it a popular agent for labor. Ropivacaine may be preferable because of its reduced potential for cardiotoxicity (see Chapter 16). At equianalgesic doses, ropivacaine and bupivacaine appear to produce the same degree of motor block.

The effect of epinephrine-containing solutions on the course of labor is somewhat controversial. Many clinicians use epinephrine-containing solutions only for intravascular test doses because of concern that the solutions may slow the progression of labor or adversely affect the fetus; others use only very dilute concentrations of epinephrine such as 1:800,000 or 1:400,000. However, studies comparing these various agents have failed to find any differences in neonatal Apgar scores, acid–base status, or neurobehavioral evaluations.

D. Epidural Activation for the First Stage of Labor

Initial epidural injections may be done either before or after the catheter is placed. Administration through the needle can facilitate catheter placement, whereas administration through the catheter provides assurance that the catheter is functioning properly. The following sequence is suggested for epidural activation:

1. Test for unintentional subarachnoid or intravascular placement of the needle or catheter using a 3-mL test dose of a local anesthetic with 1:200,000 epinephrine. Many clinicians test with lidocaine 1.5% because it results in less toxicity following unintentional intravascular injection and more rapid onset of spinal anesthesia following unintentional intrathecal injection than with bupivacaine or ropivacaine. The test dose should be injected between contractions to help reduce false-positive signs of an intravascular injection (ie, tachycardia due to a painful contraction).
2. If after 5 min signs of intravascular or intrathecal injection are absent, with the patient supine and left uterine displacement, administer 10 mL of the local anesthetic–opioid mixture in 5-mL increments, waiting 1 to 2 min between doses, to achieve a T10–L1 sensory level. The initial bolus is usually composed of 0.1% to 0.2% ropivacaine or 0.0625% to 0.125% bupivacaine combined with either 50 to 100 mcg of fentanyl or 10 to 20 mcg of sufentanil.
3. Monitor with frequent assessment of vital signs for 20 to 30 min or until the patient is stable. Pulse oximetry should be used. Oxygen is administered via a face mask if a significant decrease in blood pressure or oxygen saturation occurs.
4. Repeat steps 2 and 3 when pain recurs until the first stage of labor is completed. Alternatively, a continuous epidural infusion technique may be employed using bupivacaine or ropivacaine in concentrations of 0.0625% to 0.125% with either fentanyl, 1 to 5 mcg/mL, or sufentanil, 0.2 to 0.5 mcg/mL, at a rate of 10 mL/h, which subsequently is adjusted to the patient's analgesic requirements (range: 5–15 mL/h). A third choice would be to use **patient-controlled epidural analgesia** (PCEA). Some studies suggest that total drug requirements may be less and patient satisfaction greater with PCEA when compared with other epidural analgesia techniques. Traditional PCEA settings are typically a 5-mL bolus dose with a 5 to 10 min lockout and 0 to 12 mL/h basal rate; a 1-h limit of 15 to 25 mL is typically used. Recent evidence also suggests that compared with an epidural baseline infusion, programmed intermittent bolus techniques (eg, 6 mL bupivacaine 0.0625% every 30 min without baseline infusion) may improve patient satisfaction. Migration of the epidural catheter into a blood vessel during a continuous infusion technique may be heralded by loss of effective analgesia; a high index of suspicion is required because overt signs of systemic toxicity may be absent. Erosion of the catheter through the dura results in a slowly progressive motor blockade of the lower extremities and a rising sensory blockade level.

E. Epidural Administration During the Second Stage of Labor

Epidural analgesia administration for the second stage of labor should extend the block to include the S2–4 dermatomes. Whether a catheter is already in place or epidural anesthesia is just being initiated, the following steps should be undertaken:

1. If the patient does not already have a catheter in place, establish epidural space access while the patient is in a sitting position. A patient who already has an epidural catheter in place should be placed in a semiupright or sitting position prior to injection.

2. Give a 3-mL test dose of local anesthetic (eg, lidocaine 1.5%) with 1:200,000 epinephrine. As previously noted, the injection should be completed between contractions.
3. If, after 5 min, signs of intravascular or intrathecal injection are absent, administer 10 to 15 mL of additional local anesthetic–opioid mixture at a rate no faster than 5 mL every 1 to 2 min.
4. Lay the patient supine with left uterine displacement and monitor vital signs every 1 to 2 min for the first 15 min, then every 5 min thereafter.

F. Prevention of Unintentional Intravascular and Intrathecal Injections

Safe administration of epidural analgesia and anesthesia is dependent on avoiding unintentional intrathecal or intravascular injection. 8 **Unintentional intravascular or intrathecal placement of an epidural needle or catheter is possible even when aspiration fails to yield blood or cerebrospinal fluid (CSF).** The incidence of unintentional intravascular or intrathecal placement of an epidural catheter is 5% to 15% and 0.5% to 2.5%, respectively. Even a properly placed catheter can subsequently erode into an epidural vein or an intrathecal position. This possibility should be considered each time local anesthetic is injected through an epidural catheter—each dose should be considered a test dose.

Test doses of lidocaine (45–60 mg), bupivacaine (7.5–10 mg), ropivacaine (6–8 mg), or chloroprocaine (100 mg) can be given to exclude unintentional intrathecal placement. Signs of sensory and motor blockade usually become apparent within 2 to 3 min and 3 to 5 min, respectively, if the injection is intrathecal.

In patients not receiving β-adrenergic antagonists, the intravascular injection of a local anesthetic solution with 15 to 20 mcg of epinephrine consistently increases the heart rate by 20 to 30 beats/min within 30 to 60 s if the epidural catheter or needle tip is intravascular. This technique is not always reliable in parturients because they often have marked spontaneous baseline variations in heart rate with contractions. Alternative methods of detecting unintentional intravascular catheter placement are based on eliciting signs of CNS toxicity, including tinnitus, dizziness, perioral numbness, or metallic taste. The use of dilute local anesthetic solutions and slow injection rates of no more than 5 mL at a time may also enhance the detection of unintentional intravascular injections before catastrophic complications develop.

G. Management of Complications

9 **1. Hypotension—Generally defined as a greater than 20% decrease in the patient's baseline systolic blood pressure or a systolic blood pressure less than 100 mm Hg, hypotension is a common side effect of neuraxial anesthesia. It is primarily due to decreased sympathetic tone and is greatly accentuated by aortocaval compression or an upright or semiupright position. Treatment should consist of intravenous boluses of phenylephrine (40–120 mcg), supplemental oxygen, left uterine displacement, and an intravenous fluid bolus.** Although the routine use of a crystalloid fluid bolus prior to dosing an epidural catheter is not effective in the prevention of hypotension, ensuring proper intravenous hydration of the pregnant patient is important. The use of the head-down (Trendelenburg) position is controversial because of its potentially detrimental effects on pulmonary gas exchange.

2. Unintentional intravascular injection—Early recognition of intravascular injection facilitated by the use of small, repeated doses of local anesthetic instead of a large bolus may prevent more serious local anesthetic toxicity, such as seizures or cardiovascular collapse. Intravascular injections of toxic doses of lidocaine or chloroprocaine usually present as seizures. Propofol, 20 to 50 mg, will terminate seizure activity. Maintenance of a patent airway and adequate oxygenation are critical; however, administration of succinylcholine and endotracheal intubation are rarely necessary. Intravascular injections of bupivacaine can cause rapid cardiovascular collapse as well as seizure activity. Cardiac resuscitation may be exceedingly difficult and is aggravated by acidosis and hypoxia. An immediate infusion of 20% Intralipid combined with incremental doses of epinephrine has shown efficacy in reversing bupivacaine-induced cardiac toxicity. Amiodarone is the agent of choice for treating local anesthetic–induced ventricular arrhythmias.

3. Unintentional intrathecal injection—Even when dural puncture is recognized immediately after injection of local anesthetic, attempted aspiration of the local anesthetic will usually be unsuccessful. The patient should be placed supine with left uterine displacement. Head elevation accentuates the adverse effects of hypotension on cerebral blood flow and should be avoided. Hypotension must be treated promptly with phenylephrine and intravenous fluids. Moderate to profound hypotension may require the administration of epinephrine (10–50 mcg) or vasopressin (0.4–2.0 units intravenously). A high spinal level can also result in diaphragm and intercostal muscle paralysis, which necessitates intubation and ventilation with 100% oxygen. Delayed onset of a very high and often patchy or unilateral block may be due to unrecognized subdural injection (see Chapter 45), which is managed similarly.

4. Postdural puncture headache (PDPH)—There are many causes of headache after regional anesthesia in obstetrics. Caffeine-withdrawal and migraine headaches are not uncommon. Unintended dural puncture with a large epidural needle will commonly result in a PDPH as a consequence of decreased intracranial pressure with compensatory cerebral vasodilation (see Chapter 45). Bed rest, hydration, oral analgesics, and caffeine sodium benzoate (500 mg added to 1000 mL intravenous fluids administered at 200 mL/h) may be effective in patients with mild headaches and as a temporary treatment. Intravenous gabapentin, hydrocortisone, and oral theophylline have been shown to be successful in some studies. Patients with moderate to severe headaches usually require an epidural blood patch (10–20 mL; see Chapter 45). Prophylactic epidural blood patches are not recommended as 25% to 50% of patients may not require a blood patch following dural puncture. Delaying a blood patch for 24 h increases its efficacy, though supine bed rest for 24 h while awaiting the epidural blood patch is uncomfortable, inconvenient, and impractical for the new mother. Intracranial subdural hematoma has been reported as a rare complication 1 to 6 weeks following unintentional dural puncture in obstetric patients.

5. Maternal fever—Maternal fever is often interpreted as chorioamnionitis and may trigger an evaluation for neonatal sepsis. Contrary to reports by some authors, there is no clear evidence that epidural anesthesia affects maternal temperature or that neonatal sepsis is increased with epidural analgesia. An elevation in maternal temperature is associated with a high body mass index and with nulliparity in women and prolonged labor.

Combined Spinal & Epidural & Dural Puncture Epidural Analgesia

10 **Techniques using *combined spinal and epidural* (CSE) analgesia and anesthesia may especially benefit patients with severe pain early in labor and those who receive analgesia/anesthesia immediately prior to delivery.** Intrathecal opioid and local anesthetic are injected through the spinal needle, after which the spinal needle is withdrawn and an epidural catheter is placed via the epidural needle. The intrathecal drugs provide essentially immediate pain control and have minimal effects on the early progress of labor, whereas the epidural catheter provides a route for subsequent analgesia for labor and delivery or anesthesia for cesarean section. The addition of a small dose of local anesthetic agent to the intrathecal opioid injection greatly potentiates the opioid efficacy and can significantly reduce opioid requirements. Thus, many clinicians will inject preservative-free bupivacaine, 2.5 mg, or ropivacaine, 3 to 4 mg, with intrathecal opioid for analgesia in the first stage of labor. Typical intrathecal opioid doses for CSE are fentanyl, 10 to 12.5 mcg, or sufentanil, 5 mcg. Some studies suggest that CSE techniques may be associated with greater patient satisfaction and lower incidence of PDPH than epidural analgesia alone. The **dural puncture epidural** (DPE) technique is a modification of the CSE technique, where a dural perforation is created by a spinal needle but intrathecal medication administration is withheld. The DPE technique may improve labor analgesia quality with fewer side effects. With both the CSE and the DPE technique, a 24- to 27-gauge pencil-point spinal needle (Whitacre, Sprotte, or Gertie Marx) is used to minimize the incidence of PDPH.

For CSE techniques, the spinal and epidural needles may be placed at separate interspaces, but most clinicians use a needle-through-needle technique at the same interspace. The use of saline for identification of the epidural space may potentially cause confusion of saline for CSF. With the needle-through-needle technique, the epidural needle is placed in the epidural space, and a long spinal needle is then introduced through it and advanced farther into the subarachnoid space. After the intrathecal injection and withdrawal of the spinal needle, the epidural catheter is threaded into position, and the epidural needle is withdrawn. The risk of advancing the epidural catheter through the dural hole created by the spinal needle is negligible when a 25-gauge or smaller spinal needle is used. The epidural catheter, however, should be aspirated carefully prior to use, and local anesthetic should always be given slowly and in small increments to avoid unintentional intrathecal injections, as with all epidural analgesia and anesthesia techniques. Moreover, epidural drugs should be titrated carefully because the dural hole may facilitate the entry of epidural drugs into intrathecal space and thereby potentiate their effects.

Spinal Anesthesia

Spinal anesthesia given just prior to delivery—also known as a *saddle block*—provides profound anesthesia for operative vaginal delivery. Use of a 22-gauge or smaller, pencil-point spinal needle (Whitacre, Sprotte, or Gertie Marx) decreases the likelihood of PDPH. Hyperbaric tetracaine, 3–4 mg, bupivacaine, 2.5–5 mg, or lidocaine, 20–40 mg, usually provides excellent perineal anesthesia. The addition of fentanyl, 12.5–25 mcg, or sufentanil, 5–7.5 mcg, significantly potentiates the block. A T10 sensory level can be obtained with slightly larger amounts of local anesthetic. Three minutes after intrathecal injection of the hyperbaric solution, the patient is placed in the lithotomy position with left uterine displacement.

GENERAL ANESTHESIA

Because of the increased risk of aspiration, general anesthesia for vaginal delivery is avoided except for a true emergency. If an epidural catheter is already in place and time permits, rapid-onset regional anesthesia can be obtained with alkalinized lidocaine 2% or chloroprocaine 3%. Table 41–3 lists indications for general anesthesia during vaginal delivery. These indications are rare, and most include the need for urgent uterine relaxation.

TABLE 41–3 Indications for general anesthesia during vaginal delivery.

Fetal distress during the second stage
Tetanic uterine contractions
Breech extraction
Version and extraction
Manual removal of a retained placenta
Replacement of an inverted uterus

Anesthesia for Cesarean Section

Common indications for cesarean section are listed in Table 41–4. The choice of anesthesia for cesarean section is determined by multiple factors, including the indication for operative delivery, its urgency, patient and obstetrician preferences, and the skills of the anesthetist. In a given country, cesarean section rates may vary as much as twofold between

TABLE 41–4 Major indications for cesarean section.

Labor unsafe for mother and fetus
Increased risk of uterine rupture
Previous classic cesarean section
Previous extensive myomectomy or uterine reconstruction
Increased risk of maternal hemorrhage
Central or partial placenta previa
Abruptio placentae
Previous vaginal reconstruction
Dystocia
Abnormal fetopelvic relations
Fetopelvic disproportion
Abnormal fetal presentation
Transverse or oblique lie
Breech presentation
Dysfunctional uterine activity
Immediate or emergent delivery necessary
Fetal distress
Umbilical cord prolapse with fetal bradycardia
Maternal hemorrhage
Genital herpes with ruptured membranes
Impending maternal death

institutions. In some countries, cesarean delivery is seen as preferable to labor, and rates are much greater than those in the United States, where rates vary between 15% and 35% from hospital to hospital. In the United States, most elective cesarean sections are performed under spinal anesthesia.
11 **Regional anesthesia has become the preferred technique because general anesthesia is associated with a greater risk of maternal morbidity and mortality, greater hemodynamic fluctuation during anesthetic induction, and the need for additional analgesia during anesthetic recovery. Deaths associated with general anesthesia are generally related to airway problems, such as inability to intubate, inability to ventilate, or aspiration pneumonitis.** However, most of the studies showing a greater risk of general anesthesia were conducted before the arrival of video laryngoscopy and other advanced airway techniques. Deaths associated with regional anesthesia are generally related to the excessive dermatomal spread of blockade or to local anesthetic toxicity.

Additional advantages of regional anesthesia include (1) less neonatal exposure to potentially depressant drugs, (2) a decreased risk of maternal pulmonary aspiration, (3) an awake mother who can experience the birth of her child, and (4) the option of using spinal opioids for postoperative pain relief.
12 **Continuous epidural anesthesia allows better continuing control over the sensory level than "single-shot" spinal anesthesia techniques. Conversely, spinal anesthesia has a more rapid, predictable onset; may produce a denser (more complete) block; and lacks the potential for serious systemic drug toxicity because of the smaller local anesthetic dose employed.** Regardless of the regional technique chosen, one must be prepared to administer a general anesthetic at any time during the procedure. Moreover, administration of a nonparticulate antacid within 30 min of anticipated surgery must be considered (see above).

General anesthesia offers a very rapid and reliable onset and control over the airway and ventilation, but it is associated with greater hemodynamic fluctuations when compared with neuraxial anesthesia because of the physiologic response to anesthesia induction and airway manipulation. These effects are of particular concern in pregnant patients with associated hypertensive disorders. Other disadvantages of general anesthesia are the risk of pulmonary aspiration, the potential inability to intubate or ventilate the patient, and drug-induced fetal depression. Present anesthetic techniques, however, limit the dose of intravenous agents such that fetal depression is usually not clinically significant with general anesthesia when delivery occurs within 10 min of induction of anesthesia. Regardless of the type of anesthesia, neonates delivered more than 3 min after uterine incision have lower Apgar scores and pH values.

REGIONAL ANESTHESIA

Cesarean section requires that dermatomes up to and including T4 be anesthetized. Because of the associated sympathetic blockade, patients should receive an appropriate amount of intravenous fluids to eliminate any preexisting hypovolemia. Prophylactic hydration in the normovolemic patient has not been proven effective in reducing hypotension associated with neuraxial techniques. Concomitant with local anesthetic injection, phenylephrine may be titrated to maintain blood pressure within 20% of baseline. An approximate 10% decrease in blood pressure is expected. Some studies suggest that phenylephrine produces less neonatal acidosis than ephedrine, though administration of ephedrine, 5 to 10 mg intravenously, may be necessary for the hypotensive patient with a reduced heart rate.

After spinal anesthetic injection, the patient is placed supine with left uterine displacement; supplemental oxygen (40–50%) is given; and blood pressure is measured every 1 to 2 min until it stabilizes. Hypotension following epidural anesthesia administration typically has a slower onset. Slight Trendelenburg positioning facilitates achieving a T4 sensory level and may also help prevent severe hypotension. However, extreme degrees of Trendelenburg may interfere with pulmonary gas exchange.

Spinal Anesthesia

The patient is usually placed in the lateral decubitus or sitting position, and a hyperbaric solution of intrathecal lidocaine (50 to 60 mg) or bupivacaine

(10 to 15 mg) is injected. Bupivacaine should be chosen if the obstetrician will not likely complete the surgery in 45 minutes or less. Use of a 22-gauge or smaller, pencil-point spinal needle (Whitacre, Sprotte, or Gertie Marx) decreases the incidence of PDPH. Adding fentanyl, 10 to 25 mcg, or sufentanil, 5 to 10 mcg, to the intrathecal local anesthetic solution enhances the intensity of the spinal block and prolongs its duration without adversely affecting neonatal outcome. The addition of preservative-free morphine, 0.1 to 0.3 mg, can prolong postoperative analgesia up to 24 h but requires monitoring for delayed postadministration respiratory depression. Regardless of the anesthetic agents used, considerable variability in the maximal dermatomal extent of anesthesia should be expected (see Chapter 45). In obese patients, a standard 3.5-in. (9-cm) spinal needle may not be long enough to reach the subarachnoid space. In such cases, longer spinal needles of 4.75 in. (12 cm) to 6 in. (15.2 cm) may be required. To prevent these longer needles from bending, some anesthesiologists prefer larger diameter needles, such as the 22-gauge Sprotte needle. Alternatively, a 2.5-in. (6.3-cm) 20-gauge Quincke-type spinal needle can be used as a long introducer and guide for a 25-gauge pencil-point spinal needle.

Continuous spinal anesthesia is also a reasonable option, especially for obese patients, following unintentional dural puncture sustained while attempting to place an epidural catheter for cesarean section. After the catheter is advanced 3 to 5 cm into the lumbar subarachnoid space and secured, it can be used to inject anesthetic agents; moreover, it allows later supplementation of anesthesia if necessary.

Epidural Anesthesia

Epidural anesthesia for cesarean section is typically performed using a catheter, which allows supplementation of anesthesia, if necessary, and provides an excellent route for postoperative opi-
13 oid administration. **After negative aspiration and a negative test dose, a total volume of 15 to 35 mL of local anesthetic is injected slowly in 5-mL increments to minimize the risk of systemic local anesthetic toxicity.** Lidocaine 2% (typically with 1:200,000 epinephrine) or chloroprocaine 3% is most commonly used in the United States. The addition of fentanyl, 50 to 100 mcg, or sufentanil, 10 to 20 mcg, greatly enhances analgesic intensity and prolongs its duration without adversely affecting neonatal outcome. Some practitioners also add sodium bicarbonate (7.5% or 8.4% solution) to local anesthetic solutions (1 mEq sodium bicarbonate/10 mL of lidocaine) to increase the concentration of the nonionized free base and produce faster onset and more rapid spread of epidural anesthesia. If pain develops as the sensory level recedes, additional local anesthetic is administered in 5-mL increments to maintain a T4 sensory level. "Patchy" anesthesia prior to delivery of the infant can be treated with 10 to 20 mg of intravenous ketamine in combination with 1 to 2 mg of midazolam or 30% nitrous oxide. After delivery, intravenous opioid supplementation may also be used, provided excessive sedation and loss of consciousness are avoided. Pain that remains intolerable in spite of a seemingly adequate sensory level and that proves unresponsive to these measures necessitates general anesthesia with endotracheal intubation. Nausea can be treated intravenously with a 5-HT_3-receptor antagonist, such as ondansetron, 4 mg.

Epidural morphine, 5 mg, at the end of surgery provides good to excellent pain relief postoperatively for 6 to 24 h. An increased incidence (3.5–30%) of recurrent herpes simplex labialis infection 2 to 5 days following epidural morphine administration has been reported. Postoperative analgesia can also be provided by continuous epidural infusions of fentanyl, 25 to 75 mcg/h, or sufentanil, 5 to 10 mcg/h, at a volume delivery rate of approximately 10 mL/h. Epidural butorphanol, 2 mg, can also provide effective postoperative pain relief, but marked somnolence is often a side effect.

Combined Spinal & Epidural Anesthesia

The technique for CSE is described in the earlier section on Combined Spinal & Epidural Analgesia for labor and vaginal delivery. For cesarean section, CSE combines the benefit of rapid, reliable, intense blockade of spinal anesthesia with the flexible utility of an epidural catheter. The catheter also allows supplementation of anesthesia and can be used for postoperative analgesia. As mentioned previously, drugs administered epidurally should be titrated carefully because the dural hole created by the spinal needle may facilitate the movement of epidural drugs into CSF and thereby potentiate their effects.

GENERAL ANESTHESIA

Pulmonary aspiration of gastric contents and failed endotracheal intubation are the major causes of maternal morbidity and mortality associated with general anesthesia. All patients should receive antacid prophylaxis against aspiration pneumonia with 0.3 M sodium citrate, 30 mL, 30 to 45 min prior to induction. Patients with additional risk factors predisposing them to aspiration should also receive intravenous ranitidine, 50 mg, or metoclopramide, 10 mg, or both, 1 to 2 h prior to induction of general anesthesia; such risk factors include morbid obesity, symptoms of gastroesophageal reflux, a potentially difficult airway, or emergency surgical delivery without an elective fasting period. Premedication with oral omeprazole, 40 mg, at night and in the morning, also appears to be highly effective in high-risk patients undergoing elective cesarean section. Although anticholinergics theoretically may reduce lower esophageal sphincter tone, premedication with glycopyrrolate, 0.1 mg, helps reduce airway secretions and should be considered in patients with a potentially difficult airway.

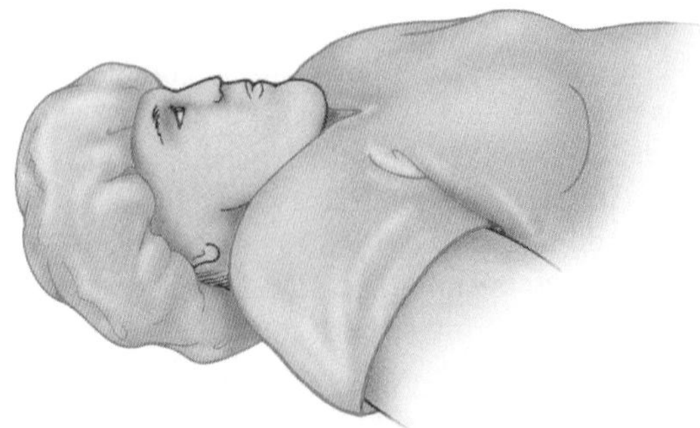

A

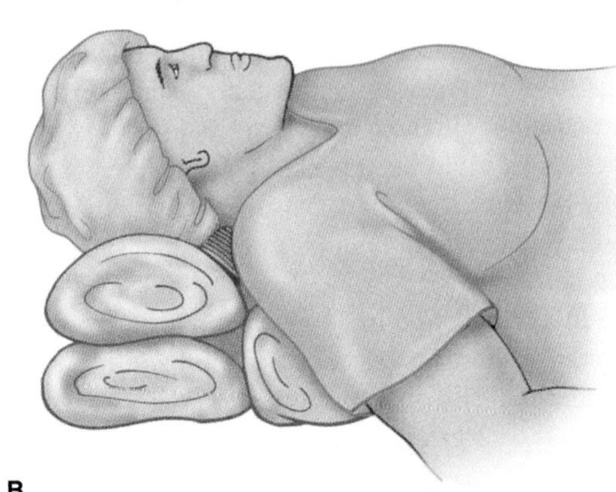

B

FIGURE 41–2 Optimal positioning for obese patients with a short neck. **A**: The normal supine position often prevents extension of the head and makes endotracheal intubation difficult. **B**: Elevation of the shoulder allows some neck flexion with more optimal extension of the head at the atlantooccipital joint, facilitating intubation.

Anticipation of a difficult endotracheal intubation may help reduce the likelihood of failed intubation. Examination of the neck, mandible, dentition, and oropharynx often helps predict which patients may have problems. Useful predictors of difficult intubation include Mallampati classification, short neck, receding mandible, prominent maxillary incisors, and history of difficult intubation (see Chapter 19). The higher incidence of failed intubation in pregnant relative to nonpregnant surgical patients may be due to airway edema, full dentition more likely found in young patients, or large breasts that can obstruct the handle of the laryngoscope in patients with short necks. Proper positioning of the head and neck may facilitate endotracheal intubation in obese patients: elevation of the shoulders, flexion of the cervical spine, and extension of the atlantooccipital joint (Figure 41–2). A variety of laryngoscope blades, a short laryngoscope handle, at least one extra stiletted endotracheal tube (6 mm), Magill forceps (for nasal intubation), a laryngeal mask airway (LMA), an intubating LMA (Fastrach), a fiberoptic bronchoscope, a video-assisted laryngoscope (GlideScope or Stortz CMAC), the capability for transtracheal jet ventilation, and possibly an esophageal–tracheal Combitube must be immediately available (see Chapter 19).

When a difficult airway is suspected, alternatives to the standard rapid-sequence induction with conventional laryngoscopy, such as regional anesthesia or awake fiberoptic techniques, should be considered. *We have found that video-assisted laryngoscopy has greatly reduced the likelihood of*

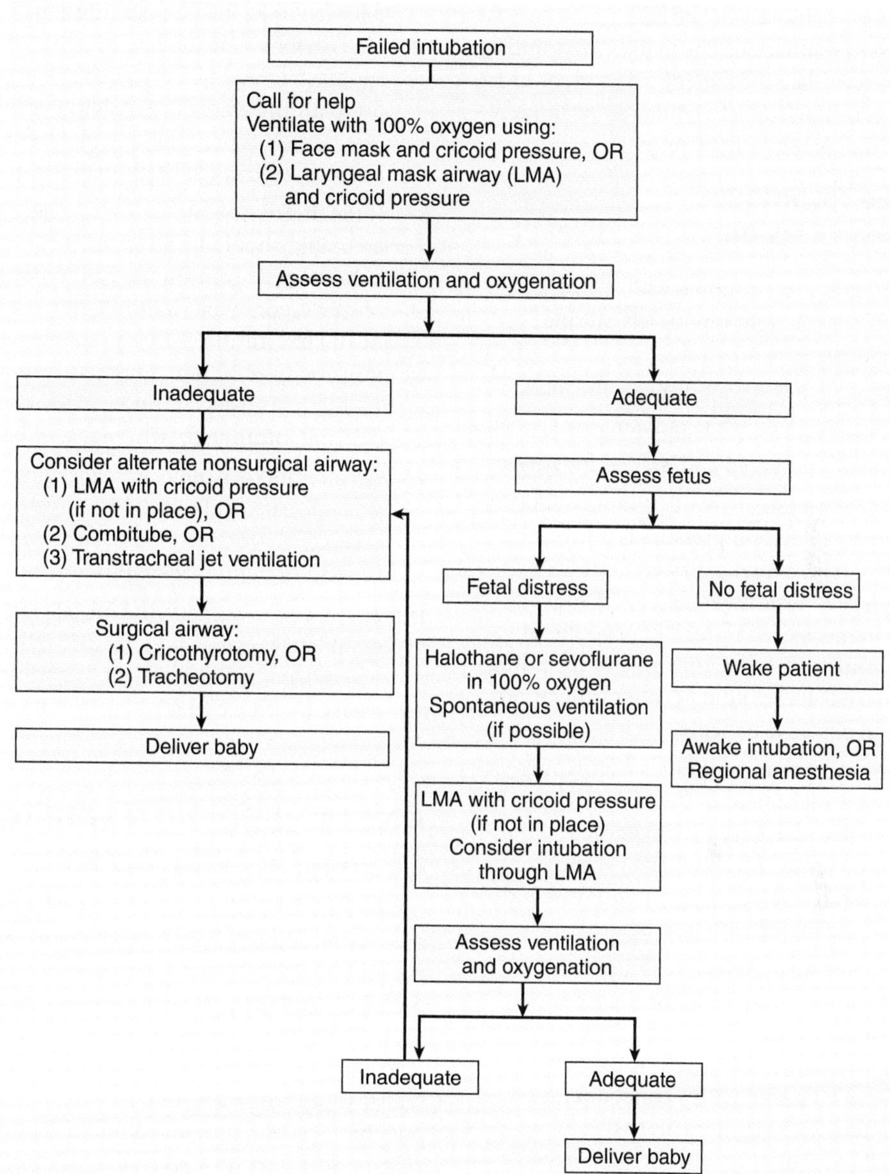

FIGURE 41–3 An algorithm for a difficult intubation in obstetric patients.

difficult or failed tracheal intubation at our institutions. Moreover, a clear plan should be formulated for a failed endotracheal intubation following induction of anesthesia (Figure 41–3). In the absence of fetal distress, the patient should be awakened, and an awake intubation with regional or topical local anesthesia should be initiated. In the presence of fetal distress, if spontaneous or positive-pressure ventilation by mask or LMA with cricoid pressure is possible, delivery of the fetus should be initiated. In such instances, a potent volatile agent with oxygen is employed for general anesthesia, but once the fetus is delivered, nitrous oxide may be added to reduce the concentration of the volatile agent; sevoflurane may be the best volatile agent because it may be least likely to depress ventilation. The inability to intubate the patient or ventilate the patient via mask or LMA will require transtracheal jet ventilation or immediate cricothyrotomy or tracheostomy.

Suggested Technique for Cesarean Section

1. The patient is placed supine with a wedge under the right hip for left uterine displacement.
2. Denitrogenation is accomplished with 100% oxygen for 3 to 5 min while monitors are applied.
3. The patient is prepared and draped for surgery.
4. When the surgeons are ready, a rapid-sequence induction with cricoid pressure is performed using propofol, 2 mg/kg, or ketamine, 1 to 2 mg/kg, and succinylcholine, 1.5 mg/kg. Ketamine is used instead of propofol in hypovolemic patients. Other agents, including methohexital and etomidate, offer little or no benefit in obstetric patients.
5. With few exceptions, surgery is begun only after proper placement of the endotracheal tube is confirmed. Excessive hyperventilation ($PaCO_2$ <25 mm Hg) should be avoided because it can reduce uterine blood flow and has been associated with fetal acidosis.
6. Fifty percent air in oxygen with up to 1 MAC expiratory volatile agent is used for maintenance of anesthesia until delivery of the infant. Thereafter, nitrous oxide up to 70% can be added with a concomitant reduction of the volatile agent to 0.75% MAC. The low dose of volatile agent helps ensure amnesia but is generally not enough to cause excessive uterine relaxation or prevent uterine contraction following oxytocin. A muscle relaxant of intermediate duration (cisatracurium, vecuronium, or rocuronium) is used for relaxation but may exhibit prolonged neuromuscular blockade in patients who are receiving magnesium sulfate.
7. For elective cesarean section, a slow 0.3 to 1 IU intravenous bolus of oxytocin over 1 min, followed by an intravenous infusion of 5 to 10 IU/h for 4 h, represents an evidence-based approach to dosing for women at low risk of postpartum hemorrhage. Additional intravenous agents, such as propofol, an opioid, or a benzodiazepine, can be given to ensure amnesia.
8. If the uterus does not contract readily, an opioid should be given and the halogenated agent should be discontinued. Methylergonovine (Methergine), 0.2 mg in 100 mL normal saline as an intravenous infusion over 10 min, may also be given. 15-Methylprostaglandin $F_{2\alpha}$ (Hemabate), 0.25 mg intramuscularly, may also be used.
9. An attempt to aspirate gastric contents via an oral gastric tube should be made prior to emergence from general anesthesia to decrease the risk of pulmonary aspiration.
10. At the end of surgery, the muscle relaxant is completely reversed, the gastric tube (if placed) is removed, and the patient is extubated when awake to reduce the risk of aspiration.

ANESTHESIA FOR EMERGENCY CESAREAN DELIVERY

Indications for emergency cesarean delivery include massive bleeding (placenta previa or accreta, abruptio placentae, or uterine rupture), umbilical cord prolapse, and severe fetal distress. A distinction must be made between a true emergency requiring immediate delivery (previously referred to as a "crash C-section") and one in which some delay is possible. Close communication with the obstetrician is necessary to determine whether the fetus, mother, or both are in immediate jeopardy.

The choice of anesthetic technique is determined by consideration for maternal safety (airway evaluation and aspiration risk), technical issues, and the anesthetist's personal expertise. Criteria leading to the diagnosis of nonreassuring fetal status should be reviewed because the fetal evaluation may be based on criteria with poor predictive accuracy and the fetal status may change. This information is required to choose the anesthetic technique that will produce the best outcome

TABLE 41–5 Signs of fetal distress.

Nonreassuring fetal heart rate pattern
Repetitive late decelerations
Loss of fetal beat-to-beat variability associated with late or deep decelerations
Sustained fetal heart rate <80 beats/min
Fetal scalp pH <7.20
Meconium-stained amniotic fluid
Intrauterine growth restriction

for both mother and fetus. Rapid institution of regional anesthesia is an option that is especially advocated for patients with a presumed difficult airway, high risk of aspiration, or both. This choice may be problematic in severely hypovolemic or hypotensive patients. If general anesthesia is chosen, adequate denitrogenation may be achieved rapidly with four maximal breaths of 100% oxygen while monitors are being applied. Ketamine, 1 mg/kg, may be substituted for propofol in hypotensive or hypovolemic patients. Having a video laryngoscope and other alternative airway equipment immediately available is essential.

Table 41–5 lists commonly accepted signs of *fetal distress*, an imprecise and poorly defined term. In most instances, the diagnosis is primarily based on the monitoring of fetal heart rate. Because worrisome fetal heart rate patterns have a relatively high incidence of false-positive results, careful interpretation of other parameters, such as fetal scalp pH or fetal pulse oximetry, may also be necessary. Moreover, continuation of fetal monitoring in the operating room may help avoid unnecessary induction of general anesthesia for fetal distress when additional time for the use of regional anesthesia is possible. In selected instances where immediate delivery is not absolutely mandatory, epidural anesthesia (with 3% chloroprocaine or alkalinized 2% lidocaine) or spinal anesthesia may be appropriate.

Anesthesia for the Complicated Pregnancy

UMBILICAL CORD PROLAPSE

Prolapse of the umbilical cord complicates 0.2% to 0.6% of deliveries. Umbilical cord compression following prolapse can rapidly lead to fetal asphyxia. Predisposing factors include excessive cord length, malpresentation, low birth weight, grand parity (more than five pregnancies), multiple gestations, and artificial rupture of membranes. The diagnosis is suspected after sudden fetal bradycardia or profound decelerations and is confirmed by physical examination. Treatment includes immediate steep Trendelenburg or knee–chest position and manual pushing of the presenting fetal part back up into the pelvis until immediate cesarean section under general anesthesia can be performed. If the fetus is not viable, vaginal delivery is allowed to continue.

DYSTOCIA & ABNORMAL FETAL PRESENTATIONS & POSITIONS

Primary Dysfunctional Labor

A *prolonged latent phase* by definition exceeds 20 h in a nulliparous parturient and 14 h in a multiparous patient. The cervix usually remains at 4 cm or less but is completely effaced. The etiology is likely ineffective contractions without a dominant myometrial pacemaker. Arrest of dilation is present when the cervix undergoes no further change after 2 h in the active phase of labor. A *protracted active phase* refers to slower than normal cervical dilation, defined as less than 1.2 cm/h in a nulliparous patient and less than 1.5 cm/h in a multiparous parturient. A *prolonged deceleration phase* occurs when cervical dilation slows markedly after 8 cm. The cervix becomes very edematous and appears to lose effacement. A *prolonged second stage* (*disorder of descent*) is defined as a descent of less than 1 cm/h and 2 cm/h in nulliparous and multiparous parturients, respectively. Failure of the head to descend 1 cm in station after adequate pushing is referred to as *arrest of descent*.

Oxytocin is usually the treatment of choice for uterine contractile abnormalities. The drug is given intravenously at 1 to 6 mU/min and increased in increments of 1 to 6 mU/min every 15 to 40 min, depending on the protocol. The use of amniotomy is controversial. Treatment is usually expectant management, as long as the fetus and mother are tolerating the prolonged labor. Operative vaginal or cesarean delivery is indicated when a trial of oxytocin is unsuccessful or when malpresentation or cephalopelvic disproportion is also present.

Breech Presentation

Breech presentations complicate 3% to 4% of deliveries and significantly increase both maternal and fetal morbidity and mortality rates. Breech presentations increase the incidence of cord prolapse more than tenfold. External cephalic version may be attempted after 34 weeks of gestation and prior to the onset of labor; however, the fetus may spontaneously return to the breech presentation before the onset of labor. Some obstetricians may administer a tocolytic agent at the same time. External version can be facilitated and its success rate improved by providing epidural analgesia with 2% lidocaine and fentanyl. Although an external version is successful in 75% of patients, it can cause placental abruption and umbilical cord compression, necessitating immediate cesarean section.

Because the shoulders or head can become trapped after vaginal delivery of the body, some obstetricians employ cesarean section for all breech presentations. If vaginal delivery is elected, manual or forceps-assisted partial breech extraction is usually necessary. The need for breech extraction does not appear to be increased when epidural anesthesia is used for labor—if labor is well established prior to epidural activation. Moreover, epidural anesthesia may decrease the likelihood of a trapped head because it relaxes the perineum. Nonetheless, the fetal head can become trapped in the uterus even during cesarean section under regional anesthesia; rapid induction of general endotracheal anesthesia and administration of a volatile agent may be attempted in such instances to relax the uterus. Alternatively, nitroglycerin, 50 to 100 mcg intravenously, can be administered.

Abnormal Vertex Presentations

When the fetal occiput fails to spontaneously rotate anteriorly, a persistent *occiput posterior presentation* results in a more prolonged and painful labor. Manual, vacuum, or forceps rotation is usually necessary but increases the likelihood of maternal and fetal injuries. Regional anesthesia can be used to provide perineal analgesia and pelvic relaxation, facilitating manual or forceps rotation followed by forceps delivery.

A *face presentation* occurs when the fetal head is hyperextended and generally requires cesarean section. A *compound presentation* occurs when an extremity enters the pelvis along with either the head or the buttocks. Vaginal delivery is usually still possible because the extremity often withdraws as the labor progresses.

Shoulder dystocia, or impaction of a shoulder against the pubic symphysis, complicates 0.2% to 2% of deliveries and is one of the major causes of birth injuries. Shoulder dystocias are often difficult to predict, and the most important risk factor is fetal macrosomia. Several obstetric maneuvers can be used to relieve shoulder dystocia, but a prolonged delay in the delivery could result in fetal asphyxia. Induction of general anesthesia may be necessary if an epidural catheter is not already in place.

MULTIPLE GESTATIONS

Multiple gestations account for approximately 1 in 150 births and are often complicated by breech presentation, prematurity, or both. Anesthesia may be necessary for version, extraction, or cesarean section. The second infant (and any subsequent ones) is often more depressed and asphyxiated than the first. Regional anesthesia provides effective pain relief during labor, minimizes the need for sedative and analgesic medication, and may shorten the interval between the birth of the first and second infants. Some studies suggest that the acid–base status of the second twin is improved when epidural anesthesia is used. Patients with multiple gestations are more prone to develop hypotension from aortocaval compression, particularly after regional anesthesia.

ANTEPARTUM HEMORRHAGE

14 **Maternal hemorrhage is one of the most common severe morbidities complicating obstetric anesthesia. Causes include uterine atony, placenta previa, abruptio placentae, and uterine rupture.**

Placenta Previa

A *placenta previa* is present if the placenta implants in advance of the fetal presenting part; this occurs in approximately 0.5% of pregnancies. It often occurs in patients who have had a previous cesarean section or uterine myomectomy. Other risk factors include multiparity, advanced maternal age, and a large placenta. An anterior-lying placenta previa increases the risk of excessive bleeding for cesarean section.

Placenta previa usually presents as painless vaginal bleeding, and although the bleeding often stops spontaneously, severe hemorrhage can occur at any time. The patient is usually treated with bed rest and observation when the gestation is less than 37 weeks in duration and the bleeding is mild to moderate. After 37 weeks of gestation, delivery is usually accomplished via cesarean section. Patients with low-lying placenta may rarely be allowed to deliver vaginally if the bleeding is mild.

Active bleeding or hemodynamic instability requires immediate cesarean section under general anesthesia. The patient should have two large-bore intravenous catheters in place; intravascular volume deficits must be replaced, and blood must be available for transfusion. The bleeding can continue after delivery because the placental implantation site in the lower uterine segment often does not contract as well as the rest of the uterus.

A history of a previous placenta previa or cesarean section increases the risk of abnormal placentation.

Abruptio Placentae

Premature separation of a normal placenta, *abruptio placentae*, complicates approximately 1% to 2% of pregnancies. Most abruptions are mild (grade I), but up to 25% are severe (grade III). Risk factors include hypertension, trauma, a short umbilical cord, multiparity, prolonged premature rupture of membranes, alcohol abuse, cocaine use, and an anatomically abnormal uterus. Patients usually experience painful vaginal bleeding and exhibit tenderness to palpation. Abdominal ultrasonography can help in the diagnosis. Factors in the choice between regional and general anesthesia include urgency for delivery, maternal hemodynamic stability, and presence of coagulopathy. Hemorrhage may remain concealed inside the uterus, contributing to underestimation of blood loss. Severe abruptio placentae can cause coagulopathy, particularly following fetal demise. Fibrinogen levels are mildly reduced (150–250 mg/dL) with moderate abruptions but are typically less than 150 mg/dL with fetal demise. The coagulopathy is thought to be due to activation of circulating plasminogen (fibrinolysis) and the release of tissue thromboplastins that precipitate disseminated intravascular coagulation (DIC). Platelet count and factors V and VIII are low, and fibrin split products are elevated. *Severe abruption is a life-threatening emergency that necessitates an emergency cesarean section. The need for massive blood transfusion, including the replacement of coagulation factors and platelets, should be anticipated.*

Uterine Rupture

Uterine rupture is relatively uncommon (1:1000–3000 deliveries) but can occur during labor as a result of (1) dehiscence of a scar from a previous (usually classic) cesarean section (such a trial of labor is termed *vaginal birth after cesarian* [VBAC]); extensive myomectomy or uterine reconstruction; (2) intrauterine manipulations or use of forceps (iatrogenic); or (3) spontaneous rupture following prolonged labor in patients with hypertonic contractions (particularly with oxytocin infusions), fetopelvic disproportion, or a very large, thin, and weakened uterus. Uterine rupture can present as frank hemorrhage, fetal distress, loss of uterine tone, hypotension with occult bleeding into the abdomen, or a combination of these. Even when epidural anesthesia is employed for labor, uterine rupture is often heralded by the abrupt onset of continuous abdominal pain and hypotension. Treatment requires volume resuscitation and immediate laparotomy, usually under general anesthesia. Ligation of the internal iliac (hypogastric) arteries, with or without hysterectomy, may be necessary to control hemorrhage.

PREMATURE RUPTURE OF MEMBRANES & CHORIOAMNIONITIS

Premature rupture of membranes (PROM) is present when leakage of amniotic fluid occurs before the onset of labor. Confirmation of this diagnosis frequently involves the *nitrazine test*: The mildly alkaline pH of amniotic fluid (>7.1) causes nitrazine paper to change color from orange to blue in contrast to normal vaginal secretions, which are acidic pH <6). PROM complicates 10% of all pregnancies and up to 35% of premature deliveries. Predisposing factors include a short cervix, prior history of PROM or preterm delivery, infection, multiple gestations, polyhydramnios, and smoking. Spontaneous labor commences within 24 h of ruptured membranes in 90% of patients. Management of PROM balances the risk of infection with the risk of fetal prematurity. Delivery is usually indicated sometime after 34 weeks of gestation. Preterm patients with a gestation of fewer than 34 weeks can be managed expectantly with prophylactic antibiotics, tocolytics, and two doses of glucocorticoid (to accelerate lung maturation) to await additional maturation of fetal organs. The longer the interval between rupture and the onset of labor, the greater the likelihood of chorioamnionitis. PROM also predisposes to placental abruption and postpartum endometritis.

Chorioamnionitis represents infection of the chorionic and amnionic membranes and may involve the placenta, uterus, umbilical cord, and fetus. It complicates up to 1% to 2% of pregnancies and is usually, but not always, associated with ruptured membranes. The contents of the amniotic cavity are normally sterile but become vulnerable to ascending bacterial infection from the vagina when the cervix dilates or the membranes rupture. Intraamniotic infections are less commonly caused by hematogenous spread of bacteria or retrograde seeding through the fallopian tubes. The principal maternal complications of chorioamnionitis are premature or dysfunctional labor, often leading to cesarean section, intraabdominal infection, septicemia, and postpartum hemorrhage. Fetal complications include acidosis, hypoxia, and septicemia.

Clinical signs of chorioamnionitis include fever (>38°C), maternal and fetal tachycardia, uterine tenderness, and foul-smelling or purulent amniotic fluid. Blood leukocyte count is useful only if markedly elevated because it normally increases during labor (normal average 15,000/μL). C-reactive protein levels are usually elevated (>2 mg/dL). Gram stain of amniotic fluid obtained by amniocentesis is helpful in ruling out infection.

The use of regional anesthesia in patients with chorioamnionitis is controversial because of the theoretical risk of promoting the development of meningitis or epidural abscess. However, evidence suggests that this risk is very low and that these concerns are likely unjustified. In the absence of overt signs of septicemia, thrombocytopenia, or coagulopathy, most clinicians offer regional anesthesia to patients with chorioamnionitis who have received antibiotic therapy.

PRETERM LABOR

Preterm labor by definition occurs between 20 and 37 weeks of gestation and is the most common complication of the third trimester. Approximately 8% of live-born infants in the United States are delivered before term. Important contributory maternal factors include extremes of age, inadequate prenatal care, unusual body habitus, increased physical activity, infections, prior preterm labor, multiple gestations, and other medical illnesses or complications during pregnancy.

Because of their small size and incomplete development, preterm infants—particularly those less than 30 weeks of gestational age or weighing less than 1500 g—experience a greater number of complications than term infants. PROM complicates one-third of premature deliveries; the combination of PROM and premature labor increases the likelihood of umbilical cord compression, resulting in fetal hypoxemia and asphyxia. Preterm infants with a breech presentation are particularly prone to prolapse of the umbilical cord during labor. Moreover, inadequate production of pulmonary surfactant frequently leads to *idiopathic respiratory distress syndrome* (hyaline membrane disease) after delivery since surfactant levels are generally adequate only after week 35 of gestation. In the past, fetal lung maturity (FLM) testing was used to determine whether the fetus's lungs were developed enough to allow for safe preterm or early-term delivery. In recent years, guidelines have shifted to state that there are other factors that should be used to determine whether to deliver a fetus, and FLM test results demonstrating mature lungs are not a rationale to proceed with delivery. These updated guidelines are based on several studies that have demonstrated worse outcomes with early-term births after FLM testing demonstrated lung maturity relative to outcomes seen with full-term births. Lastly, a soft, poorly calcified cranium predisposes these neonates to intracranial hemorrhage during vaginal delivery.

When preterm labor occurs before 35 weeks of gestation, bed rest and tocolytic therapy are usually initiated, with the goal of delaying birth to allow for the maternal administration of glucocorticoid (betamethasone) to enhance fetal lung maturity. Tocolytic therapy successfully delays birth by 48 hours in 75% of patients; however, little evidence exists that the eventual preterm delivery is prevented. The most commonly used tocolytics are the β_2-adrenergic agonist terbutaline and magnesium (6 g intravenously over 30 min followed by 2–4 g/h intravenously). Terbutaline, 2.5 to 5 mg orally every 4 to 6 h, may also have some β_1-adrenergic receptor activity, which accounts for some of its side effects. Maternal side effects include tachycardia, arrhythmias, myocardial ischemia, mild hypotension, hyperglycemia, hypokalemia, and, rarely, pulmonary edema. Other tocolytic agents include calcium channel blockers (nifedipine) and prostaglandin synthetase inhibitors. Fetal ductal constriction can occur after 32 weeks of gestation with the administration of nonsteroidal anti-inflammatory drugs (NSAIDs) such as indomethacin, but it is usually transient and resolves after discontinuation of the drug; NSAID-associated acute kidney injury in the fetus may cause oligohydramnios.

Anesthesia often becomes necessary when tocolytic therapy fails to arrest labor. The goal during vaginal delivery of a preterm fetus is a slow, controlled delivery with minimal pushing by the mother. An episiotomy and low forceps assistance are often employed. Spinal or epidural anesthesia promotes complete pelvic relaxation. Cesarean section is performed for fetal distress, breech presentation, intrauterine growth retardation, or failure of labor to progress. Residual effects from β-adrenergic agonists may complicate general anesthesia. Ketamine, ephedrine, and isoflurane should be used cautiously because of interaction with tocolytics. Hypokalemia is usually due to an intracellular uptake of potassium and rarely requires treatment; however, it may increase sensitivity to muscle relaxants. Magnesium therapy potentiates muscle relaxants and may predispose to hypotension secondary to vasodilation. Residual effects from tocolytics interfere with uterine contraction following delivery. Lastly, preterm newborns are often depressed at delivery and frequently need resuscitation; therefore, preparations for resuscitation should be completed prior to delivery.

HYPERTENSIVE DISORDERS

Hypertension during pregnancy can be classified as *pregnancy-induced hypertension* (PIH, often also referred to as *preeclampsia*), chronic hypertension that preceded pregnancy, or chronic hypertension with superimposed preeclampsia. *Preeclampsia is usually defined as a systolic blood pressure greater than 140 mm Hg or diastolic pressure greater than 90 mm Hg on two occasions at least 4 h apart after the 20th week of gestation in a woman with previously normal blood pressure.* Proteinuria (>300 mg/d or protein/creatinine ratio greater than 0.3) is not required for a diagnosis of preeclampsia but is present in approximately 75% of cases. When seizures occur, the syndrome is termed *eclampsia*. *HELLP syndrome* describes preeclampsia associated with *h*emolysis, *e*levated *l*iver enzymes, and a *l*ow *p*latelet count. In the United States, preeclampsia complicates approximately 7% to 10% of pregnancies; eclampsia is much less common, occurring in 1 of 10,000 to 15,000 pregnancies. Severe preeclampsia causes or contributes to 7% of maternal deaths and approximately 20% of perinatal deaths. Maternal deaths are usually due to stroke, pulmonary edema, hepatic necrosis or rupture, or a combination of these complications.

Pathophysiology & Manifestations

The pathophysiology of preeclampsia is related to vascular dysfunction of the placenta, resulting in abnormal prostaglandin metabolism. Patients with preeclampsia have elevated production of thromboxane A_2 (TXA_2) and decreased production of prostacyclin (PGI_2). TXA_2 is a potent vasoconstrictor and promoter of platelet aggregation, whereas PGI_2 is a potent vasodilator and inhibitor of platelet aggregation. Endothelial dysfunction may reduce the production of nitric oxide and increase the production of endothelin-1. The latter is also a potent vasoconstrictor and activator of platelets. Marked vascular reactivity and endothelial injury reduce placental perfusion and can lead to widespread systemic manifestations.

Severe preeclampsia substantially increases maternal and fetal morbidity and mortality. Features of severe preeclampsia include the standard features of preeclampsia in association with any of the following: blood pressure greater than 160/110 mm Hg, thrombocytopenia (<100,000/μL), proteinuria greater than 5 g/d, impaired liver function, progressive kidney insufficiency (serum creatinine concentration greater than 1.1 mg/d oliguria, pulmonary edema, and CNS signs or symptoms (headache or visual disturbances; Table 41–6*). Hepatic rupture may occur in patients with HELLP syndrome.*

Patients with severe preeclampsia or eclampsia have widely differing hemodynamic profiles. Most patients have low-normal cardiac filling pressures with increased systemic vascular resistance, but cardiac output may be reduced, normal, or increased.

TABLE 41–6 Complications of preeclampsia.

Neurological
Headache
Visual disturbances
Hyperexcitability
Seizures
Intracranial hemorrhage
Cerebral edema
Pulmonary
Upper airway edema
Pulmonary edema
Cardiovascular
Decreased intravascular volume
Increased arteriolar resistance
Hypertension
Heart failure
Hepatic
Impaired function
Elevated enzymes
Hematoma
Rupture
Renal
Proteinuria
Sodium retention
Decreased glomerular filtration
Kidney failure
Hematological
Coagulopathy
Thrombocytopenia
Platelet dysfunction
Prolonged partial thromboplastin time
Microangiopathic hemolysis

Treatment

Treatment of preeclampsia consists of bed rest, sedation, repeated doses of antihypertensive drugs (usually labetalol, 5–10 mg, or hydralazine, 5 mg intravenously), and magnesium sulfate (4 g loading followed by 1–3 g/h intravenously) to treat hyperreflexia and prevent convulsions. Therapeutic magnesium levels are 4 to 6 mEq/L. It is recommended that corticosteroids be given if the fetus is viable and 33 weeks of gestation or less.

Invasive arterial and central venous monitoring are indicated in patients with severe hypertension, pulmonary edema, refractory oliguria, or a combination of these; in such patients, an intravenous vasodilator infusion may be necessary. Definitive treatment of preeclampsia is delivery of the fetus and placenta.

Anesthetic Management

Standard anesthetic practices may be used for patients with mild preeclampsia. Spinal and epidural anesthesia are associated with similar decreases in arterial blood pressure in these patients. Patients with severe disease, however, are critically ill and require stabilization prior to administration of any anesthetic, including control of hypertension and correction of hypovolemia. *In the absence of coagulopathy, continuous epidural anesthesia is the first choice for most patients with preeclampsia during labor and vaginal delivery.* Moreover, continuous epidural anesthesia avoids the increased risk of a failed intubation due to severe edema of the upper airway.

A platelet count and coagulation profile should be checked prior to the institution of regional anesthesia in patients with severe preeclampsia. It has been recommended that regional anesthesia be avoided if the platelet count is less than 100,000/μL, but a platelet count as low as 50,000/μL may be acceptable in selected cases, particularly when the count has been stable and global coagulation, as measured by thrombelastography testing, is normal. Continuous epidural anesthesia decreases catecholamine secretion and improves uteroplacental perfusion by up to 75% in these patients, provided hypotension is avoided. Judicious fluid boluses may be required to correct hypovolemia. Goal-directed hemodynamic and fluid therapy utilizing arterial pulse wave contour analysis or other noninvasive cardiac function monitors such as echocardiography may be employed to guide fluid replacement. The use of an epinephrine-containing test dose for epidural anesthesia is controversial because of questionable reliability (see the earlier section, Prevention of Unintentional Intravascular and Intrathecal Injection) and the risk of exacerbating hypertension. Hypotension should be treated with smaller than usual doses of vasopressors because these patients tend to be very sensitive to these agents. Recent evidence suggests that spinal anesthesia does not, as previously thought, result in a more severe reduction of maternal blood pressure. Therefore, *both spinal and epidural anesthetics are reasonable choices for cesarean section in a preeclamptic patient.*

Intraarterial blood pressure monitoring is indicated in patients with severe hypertension during both general and regional anesthesia. Intravenous vasodilator infusions may be necessary to control blood pressure during general anesthesia. Intravenous labetalol (5–10-mg increments) can also be effective in controlling the hypertensive response to intubation and does not appear to alter placental blood flow. The short-term administration of intravenous nicardipine or clevidipine may be used to treat intraoperative hypertension. Because magnesium potentiates muscle relaxants, doses of nondepolarizing muscle relaxants should be reduced in patients receiving magnesium therapy and should be guided by a peripheral nerve stimulator. The patient with suspected magnesium toxicity, manifested by hyporeflexia, excessive sedation, blurred vision, respiratory compromise, and cardiac depression, can be treated with intravenous administration of calcium gluconate (1 g over 10 min).

HEART DISEASE

The marked cardiovascular changes associated with pregnancy, labor, and delivery often cause the 2% of parturients with heart disease to decompensate during this period. Although most pregnant patients with cardiac disorders have rheumatic heart disease, an increasing number of parturients are presenting with corrected or palliated congenital lesions. Anesthetic management is directed toward employing techniques that minimize the added stresses of labor and delivery, and specific management of the various lesions is discussed elsewhere. Most patients can be divided into one of two groups. Patients in the first group benefit from the reduced systemic vascular resistance caused by neuraxial analgesia and anesthesia techniques but usually not from excessive fluid administration. These patients include those with mitral or aortic insufficiency, chronic heart failure, or congenital lesions with left-to-right shunting. The induced sympathectomy from spinal or epidural techniques reduces both preload and afterload, relieves pulmonary congestion, and in some cases, increases cardiac output.

Patients in the second group do not benefit from a decrease in systemic vascular resistance. These patients include those with aortic stenosis, congenital lesions with right-to-left or bidirectional shunting, or primary pulmonary hypertension. Reductions in venous return (preload) or afterload are usually poorly tolerated. These patients are better managed with intraspinal opioids alone, systemic medications, pudendal nerve blocks, and, if necessary, general anesthesia.

AMNIOTIC FLUID EMBOLISM

Amniotic fluid embolism is a rare (1:20,000 deliveries) but often lethal complication (86% mortality rate in some series) that can occur during labor, vaginal delivery, cesarean section, or postpartum. Mortality may exceed 50% in the first hour. Entry of amniotic fluid into the maternal circulation can occur through any break in the uteroplacental membranes. Such breaks may occur during normal delivery or cesarean section or following placental abruption, placenta previa, or uterine rupture. In addition to the mechanical effects of fetal debris, various prostaglandins and leukotrienes in amniotic fluid appear to play an important role in the genesis of this syndrome. The alternate term *anaphylactoid syndrome of pregnancy* has been suggested to emphasize the systemic role of chemical mediators.

Patients typically present with sudden tachypnea, cyanosis, shock, and generalized bleeding. Three major pathophysiological manifestations are responsible: (1) acute pulmonary embolism, (2) DIC, and (3) uterine atony. Mental status changes, including seizures and pulmonary edema, may develop; the latter has both cardiogenic and noncardiogenic components. Acute left ventricular dysfunction is common. Although the diagnosis can be firmly established only by demonstrating fetal elements in the maternal circulation (usually at autopsy or less commonly by aspirating amniotic fluid from a central venous catheter), amniotic fluid embolism should always be suggested by sudden respiratory distress and circulatory collapse. The presentation may initially mimic acute pulmonary thromboembolism, venous air embolism, overwhelming septicemia, or hepatic rupture or cerebral hemorrhage in a patient with toxemia.

Treatment consists of cardiopulmonary resuscitation and supportive care. When cardiac arrest occurs prior to delivery of the fetus, the efficacy of closed-chest compressions may be marginal at best. Aortocaval compression impairs resuscitation in the supine position, whereas chest compressions are less effective in a lateral tilt position. Expeditious delivery appears to improve maternal and fetal outcomes, and immediate cesarean delivery should therefore be carried out. Once the patient is resuscitated, mechanical ventilation, fluid resuscitation, and inotropes are best provided under the guidance of invasive hemodynamic monitoring. Uterine atony is treated with oxytocin, methylergonovine, and prostaglandin $F_{2\alpha}$, whereas significant coagulopathies are treated with platelets and coagulation factors based on laboratory findings.

POSTPARTUM HEMORRHAGE

Postpartum hemorrhage is the leading cause of maternal mortality in developing countries, and it is diagnosed when postpartum blood loss exceeds 500 mL. Up to 4% of parturients may experience postpartum hemorrhage, which is often associated with a prolonged third stage of labor, preeclampsia, multiple gestations, and forceps delivery. Common causes include uterine atony, a retained placenta, obstetric lacerations, uterine inversion, and use of tocolytic agents prior to delivery. Atony is often associated with uterine overdistention (multiple gestation and polyhydramnios). Less commonly, a clotting defect may be responsible.

The anesthesia provider may be consulted to assist in venous access or fluid and blood resuscitation, as well as to provide anesthesia for careful examination of the vagina, cervix, and uterus. Perineal lacerations can usually be repaired with local anesthetic infiltration or pudendal nerve blocks. Residual anesthesia from prior epidural or spinal anesthesia facilitates examination of the patient; however, supplementation with an opioid, nitrous oxide, or both may be required. Induction of spinal or epidural anesthesia should be avoided in the presence of marked hypovolemia. General anesthesia is usually required for manual extraction of a retained placenta, reversion of an inverted uterus, or repair of a major laceration. Uterine atony should be treated with oxytocin (a slow 0.3–1 IU intravenous bolus of oxytocin over 1 min, followed by an infusion of 5–10 IU/h), methylergonovine (0.2 mg in 100 mL of normal saline administered over 10 min intravenously), and prostaglandin $F_{2\alpha}$ (0.25 mg intramuscularly). Emergency laparotomy and hysterectomy may be necessary in rare instances. Early ligation or embolization of the internal iliac (hypogastric) arteries may help avoid hysterectomy and reduce blood loss.

Fetal & Neonatal Resuscitation

FETAL RESUSCITATION

Resuscitation of the neonate starts during labor. Any compromise of the uteroplacental circulation readily

15 produces fetal asphyxia. **Intrauterine asphyxia during labor is the most common cause of neonatal depression. Fetal monitoring throughout labor is helpful in identifying which fetuses may be at risk, detecting fetal distress, and evaluating the effect of acute interventions.** These include correcting maternal hypotension with fluids or vasopressors, providing supplemental oxygen, and decreasing uterine contraction (stopping oxytocin or administering tocolytics). Some studies suggest that the normal fetus can compensate for up to 45 min of relative hypoxia, a period termed *fetal stress*; the latter is associated with a marked redistribution of blood flow primarily to the heart, brain, and adrenal glands. With time, however, progressive lactic acidosis and asphyxia produce increasing fetal distress that necessitates immediate delivery.

1. Fetal Heart Rate Monitoring

Monitoring of fetal heart rate (FHR) is presently the most useful technique in assessing fetal well-being, though alone it has a 35% to 50% false-positive rate of predicting fetal compromise. Because of this, the term *fetal distress* in the context of FHR monitoring has been largely replaced with *nonreassuring* FHR. A correct interpretation of heart rate patterns is crucial. Three parameters are evaluated: baseline heart rate, baseline variability, and the relationship to uterine contractions (deceleration patterns). Monitoring of heart rate is most accurate when fetal scalp electrodes are used, but this may require rupture of the membranes and is not without complications (eg, amnionitis or fetal injury). Based on concerns about a lack of consistency in interpretation and management of FHR, a three-tier FHR system was developed. **Category I** tracings are normal. **Category II** tracings are indeterminate and do not predict abnormal fetal acid–base status. **Category III** tracings are abnormal and include either absent baseline variability with recurrent late or variable decelerations or bradycardia or the presence of a sinusoidal pattern. They predict abnormal fetal acid–base status.

Baseline Heart Rate

The mature fetus normally has a baseline heart rate of 110 to 160 beats/min. An increased baseline heart rate may be due to prematurity, mild fetal hypoxia, chorioamnionitis, maternal fever, maternally administered drugs (anticholinergics or β-agonists), or, rarely, hyperthyroidism. A decreased baseline heart rate may be due to a postterm pregnancy, fetal heart block, or fetal asphyxia.

Baseline Variability

A healthy mature fetus normally displays a baseline beat-to-beat (R-wave to R-wave) variability that can be classified as *minimal* (<5 beats/min), *moderate* (6–25 beats/min), or *marked* (>25 beats/min). Baseline variability, which is best assessed with scalp electrodes, has become an important sign of fetal well-being and represents a normally functioning autonomic system. *Sustained decreased baseline variability is a prominent sign of fetal asphyxia.* CNS depressants (opioids, barbiturates, volatile anesthetics, benzodiazepines, or magnesium sulfate) and parasympatholytics (atropine) also decrease baseline variability, as do prematurity, fetal arrhythmias, and anencephaly. A sinusoidal pattern that resembles a smooth sine wave is associated with fetal depression (hypoxia, drugs, and anemia secondary to Rh isoimmunization).

Accelerations

Accelerations of FHR are defined as increases of 15 beats/min or more lasting for more than 15 s. Periodic accelerations in FHR reflect normal oxygenation and are usually related to fetal movements and responses to uterine pressure. Such accelerations are generally considered reassuring. By 32 weeks, fetuses display periodic increases in baseline heart rate that are associated with fetal movements. Normal fetuses have 15 to 40 accelerations/h, and the mechanism is thought to involve increases in catecholamine secretion with decreases in vagal tone. Accelerations diminish with fetal sleep, some drugs (opioids, magnesium, and atropine), as well as fetal hypoxia. Accelerations in response to fetal scalp or vibroacoustic stimulation are considered a reassuring sign of fetal well-being. *The absence of both baseline variability and accelerations is nonreassuring and may be an important sign of fetal compromise.*

Deceleration Patterns

A. Early (Type I) Decelerations

Early deceleration (usually 10–40 beats/min) (Figure 41–4A) is thought to be a vagal response to compression of the fetal head or stretching of the neck during uterine contractions. The heart rate forms a smooth mirror image of the contraction. Early decelerations are generally not associated with fetal distress and occur during the descent of the head.

B. Late (Type II) Decelerations

Late decelerations (Figure 41–4B) are associated with placental insufficiency and fetal compromise and are characterized by a decrease in heart rate at or following the peak of uterine contractions. Late decelerations may be subtle (as few as 5 beats/min) and are thought to represent the impact of decreased arterial oxygen tension on atrial chemoreceptors. Late decelerations with normal variability may be observed following acute insults (maternal hypotension or hypoxemia) and are usually reversible with treatment. Late decelerations with decreased variability are associated with prolonged asphyxia and may be an indication for fetal scalp sampling (see section on Other Monitoring). *Complete abolition of variability in this setting is an ominous sign signifying severe decompensation and the need for immediate delivery.*

C. Variable (Type III) Decelerations

The most common type of deceleration is *variable* (Figure 41–4C). These decelerations are variable in onset, duration, and magnitude (often >30 beats/min). They are typically abrupt in onset and are thought to be related to umbilical cord compression and acute intermittent decreases in umbilical blood flow. Variable decelerations are typically associated with fetal asphyxia when fetal heart rate declines to less than 60 beats/min, fetal bradycardia lasts more than 60 s, or recurrent bradycardia occurs in a pattern that persists for more than 30 min.

2. Other Monitoring

Other less commonly used monitors include fetal scalp pH measurements, scalp lactate concentration, fetal pulse oximetry, and fetal ST-segment analysis. Clinical experience is limited with all of these modalities except fetal scalp pH measurements. Unfortunately, fetal scalp pH measurement is associated with a small but significant incidence of false negatives and false positives. Fetal blood can be obtained and analyzed via a small scalp puncture once the membranes are ruptured. A fetal scalp pH higher than 7.20 is usually associated with a vigorous neonate, whereas a pH less than 7.20 is often, but not always, associated with a depressed neonate and necessitates prompt (typically operative) delivery. Because of wide overlap, fetal blood sampling can be interpreted correctly only in conjunction with heart rate monitoring.

3. Treatment of the Fetus

Treatment of intrauterine fetal asphyxia is aimed at preventing fetal demise or permanent neurological damage. All interventions are directed at restoring adequate uteroplacental circulation. Aortocaval compression, maternal hypoxemia or hypotension, or excessive uterine activity (during oxytocin infusions) must be corrected. Changes in maternal position, supplemental oxygen, and intravenous ephedrine or fluid, or adjustments in an oxytocin infusion often correct the problem. *Failure to relieve fetal stress, as well as progressive fetal acidosis and asphyxia, necessitate immediate delivery.*

NEONATAL RESUSCITATION

1. General Care of the Neonate

At least one qualified health care provider whose sole responsibility is to care for the neonate and who is capable of providing resuscitation should attend every delivery. As the head is delivered, the

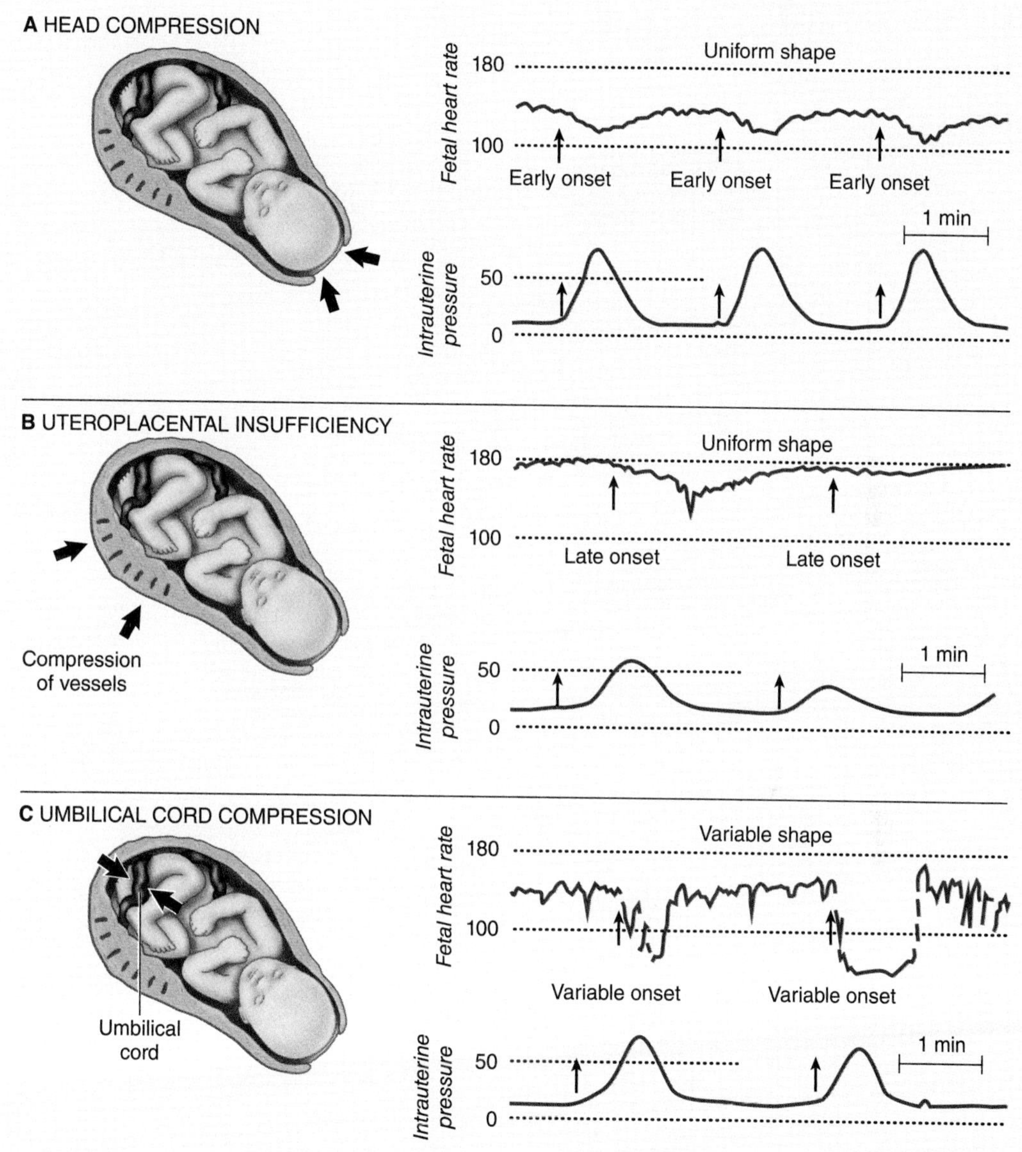

FIGURE 41–4 Periodic changes in fetal heart rate related to uterine contraction. **A**: Early (type I) decelerations. **B**: Late (type II) decelerations. **C**: Variable (type III) decelerations. (Reproduced with permission from Danforth DN, Scott JR. *Obstetrics and Gynecology.* 5th ed. Philadelphia, PA: Lippincott Williams & Wilkins; 1986.)

nose, mouth, and pharynx are suctioned with a bulb syringe. After the remainder of the body is delivered, the skin is dried with a sterile towel. Once the umbilical cord stops pulsating or neonatal breathing is initiated, the cord is clamped, and the neonate is placed in a radiant warmer with the bed tilted in a slight Trendelenburg position.

Neonatal evaluation and treatment are carried out simultaneously (Figure 41–5). If the neonate is obviously depressed, the cord is clamped early,

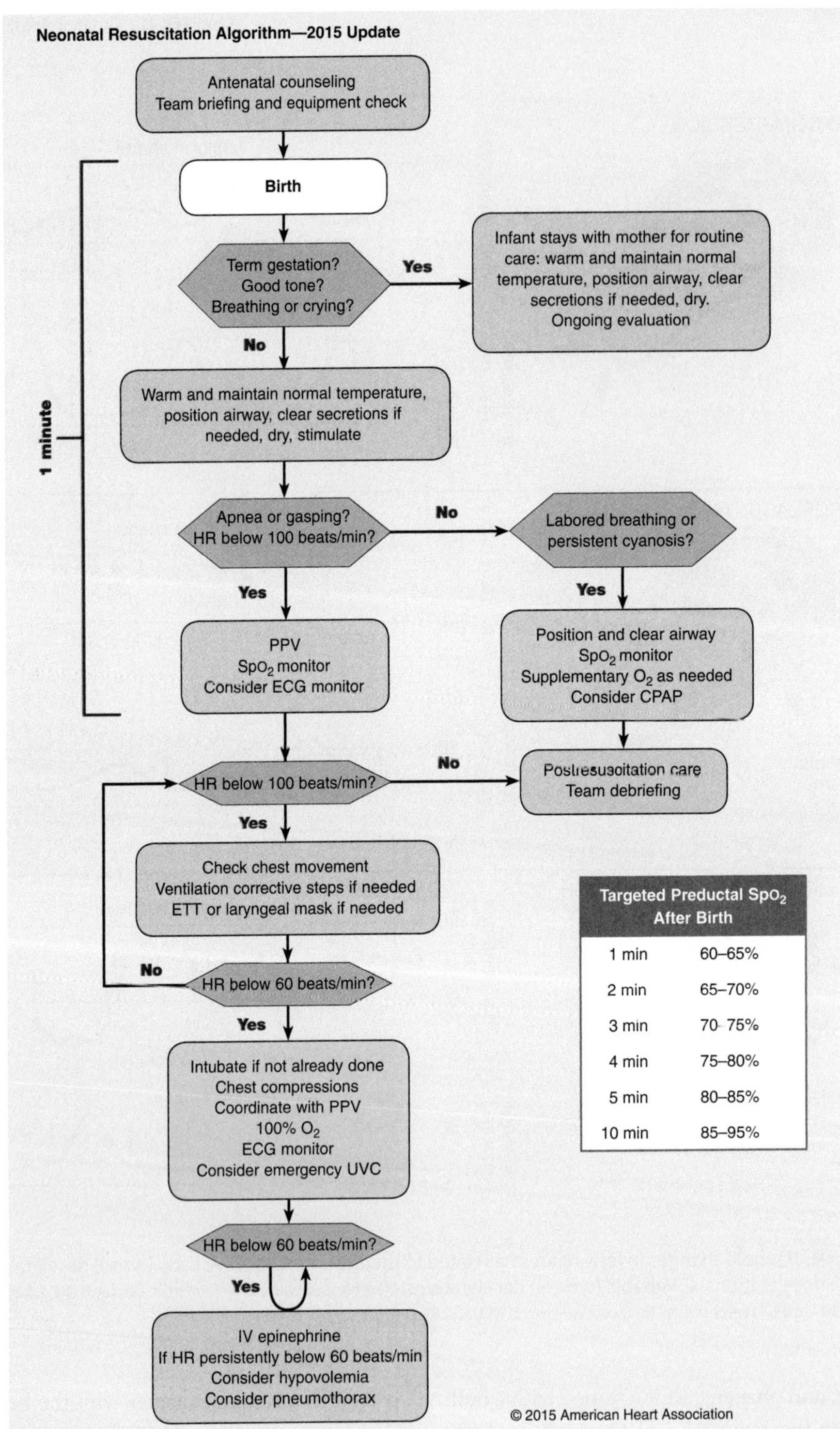

Targeted Preductal SpO_2 After Birth	
1 min	60–65%
2 min	65–70%
3 min	70–75%
4 min	75–80%
5 min	80–85%
10 min	85–95%

FIGURE 41–5 An algorithm for resuscitation of the newly born infant. CPAP, continuous positive airway pressure; ECG, electrocardiogram; ETT, endotracheal tube; HR, heart rate; IV, intravenous; PPV, positive pressure ventilation; UVC, umbilical venous catheter. (Reproduced with permission from Wyckoff MH, Aziz K, Escobedo MB, et al. Part 13: Neonatal Resuscitation: 2015 American Heart Association Guidelines Update for Cardiopulmonary Resuscitation and Emergency Cardiovascular Care. *Circulation.* 2015 Nov 3;132(18 Suppl 2):S543-S560.)

TABLE 41–7 Apgar score.

Sign	Points		
	0	1	2
Heart rate (beats/min)	Absent	<100	>100
Respiratory effort	Absent	Slow, irregular	Good, crying
Muscle tone	Flaccid	Some flexion	Active motion
Reflex irritability	No response	Grimace	Crying
Color	Blue or pale	Body pink, extremities blue	All pink

and resuscitation is initiated immediately. Breathing normally begins within 30 s and is sustained within 90 s. Respirations should be 30 to 60 breaths/min, and the heart rate should be 120 to 160 beats/min. Respirations are assessed by auscultation of the chest, whereas heart rate is determined by palpation of the pulse at the base of the umbilical cord or auscultation of the precordium. The neonate must be kept warm.

In addition to respirations and heart rate, color, tone, and reflex irritability should be evaluated. The Apgar score (Table 41–7), recorded at 1 min and again at 5 min after delivery, remains the most valuable assessment of the neonate. The 1-min score correlates with survival, whereas the 5-min score has a limited relationship to neurological outcome.

Neonates with Apgar scores of 8 to 10 are vigorous and may require only gentle stimulation (flicking the foot, rubbing the back, and additional drying). A catheter should first be gently passed through each nostril to rule out choanal atresia and then through the mouth to suction the stomach and rule out esophageal atresia.

2. Meconium-Stained Neonates

The presence or absence of meconium in the amniotic fluid (approximately 10% to 12% of deliveries) changes the immediate management of the neonate at birth. Fetal distress, particularly after 42 weeks of gestation, is often associated with the release of thick meconium into the amniotic fluid. Fetal gasping during stress results in the entry of a large amount of meconium-containing amniotic fluid into the lungs. When the neonate initiates respiration at birth, the meconium moves from the trachea and large airways down toward the periphery of the lung. *Thick or particulate meconium may obstruct small airways and cause severe respiratory distress in 15% of meconium-stained neonates. Moreover, these infants can develop persistent fetal circulation.*

Unless the neonate has absent or depressed respirations, thin watery meconium does not require suctioning beyond careful bulb suctioning of the oropharynx when the head emerges from the perineum (or from the uterus at cesarean section). When thick meconium is present in the amniotic fluid, however, some clinicians intubate and suction the trachea immediately after delivery but before the first breath is taken. However, recent evidence has challenged the benefit of tracheal suctioning even in the depressed infant. Tracheal suctioning of the thick meconium is accomplished by a special suctioning device attached to the endotracheal tube as the tube is withdrawn. If meconium is aspirated from the trachea, the procedure should be repeated until no meconium is obtained—but no more than three times, after which it is usually of no further benefit. The infant should then be given supplemental oxygen by face mask and observed closely. The stomach should also be suctioned to prevent passive regurgitation of any swallowed meconium. Newborns with meconium aspiration have an increased incidence of pneumothorax (10% compared with 1% for all vaginal deliveries).

3. Care of the Depressed Neonate

Approximately 6% of newborns require some form of advanced life support. Resuscitation of these depressed neonates, most of whom weigh less than 1500 g, requires two or more caregivers—one to manage the airway and ventilation and another to perform chest compressions, if necessary. A third caregiver greatly facilitates the placement of intravascular catheters and administration of fluids or drugs, or both. The anesthesia provider caring for the mother can render only brief assistance and only when it does not jeopardize the mother; other personnel are, therefore, usually responsible for neonatal resuscitation.

Because the most common cause of neonatal depression is intrauterine asphyxia, the emphasis in resuscitation is on respiration and oxygenation. Hypovolemia is also a contributing factor in a significant number of neonates. Factors associated with hypovolemia include early clamping of the umbilical cord, holding the neonate above the introitus prior to clamping, prematurity, maternal hemorrhage, placental transection during cesarean section, sepsis, and twin-to-twin transfusion.

Failure of the neonate to quickly respond to respiratory resuscitative efforts mandates vascular access and blood gas analysis; pneumothorax (1% incidence) and congenital anomalies of the airway, including tracheoesophageal fistula (1:3000–5000 live births), and congenital diaphragmatic hernia (1:2000–4000 live births) should be considered.

Grouping by the 1-min Apgar score greatly facilitates resuscitation: (1) mildly asphyxiated neonates (Apgar score of 5–7) usually need only stimulation while 100% oxygen is blown across the face; (2) moderately asphyxiated neonates (Apgar score of 3–4) require temporary assisted positive-pressure ventilation with mask and bag; and (3) severely depressed neonates (Apgar score of 0–2) should be immediately intubated, and chest compressions may be required.

Guidelines for Ventilation

Indications for positive-pressure ventilation of the neonate include (1) apnea, (2) gasping respirations, (3) persistent central cyanosis with 100% oxygen, and (4) a persistent heart rate less than 100 beats/min. Excessive flexion or extension of the neck can cause airway obstruction. A 1-inch-high towel under the shoulders may be helpful in maintaining proper head position. Assisted ventilation by bag and mask should be at a rate of 30 to 60 breaths/min with 100% oxygen. Initial breaths may require peak pressures of up to 40 cm H_2O, but pressures should not exceed 30 cm H_2O thereafter. Adequacy of ventilation should be checked by auscultation and chest excursions. Gastric decompression with an 8F tube often facilitates ventilation. If after 30 s the heart rate is greater than 100 beats/min and spontaneous ventilations become adequate, assisted ventilation is no longer necessary. *If the heart rate remains less than 60 beats/min or 60 to 80 beats/min without an increase in response to resuscitation, the neonate is intubated, and chest compressions are started.* If the heart rate is 60 to 80 beats/min and increasing, assisted ventilation is continued, and the neonate is observed. Failure of the heart rate to rise above 80 beats/min is an indication for chest compressions. Indications for endotracheal intubation also include ineffective or prolonged mask ventilation and the need to administer medications.

Intubation (Figure 41–6) is performed with a Miller 00, 0, or 1 laryngoscope blade, using a 2.5-, 3-, or 3.5-mm endotracheal tube (for neonates <1 kg, 1–2 kg, and >2 kg, respectively). Neonatal blades are also available for use with video-assisted laryngoscopy devices and should be available for neonatal

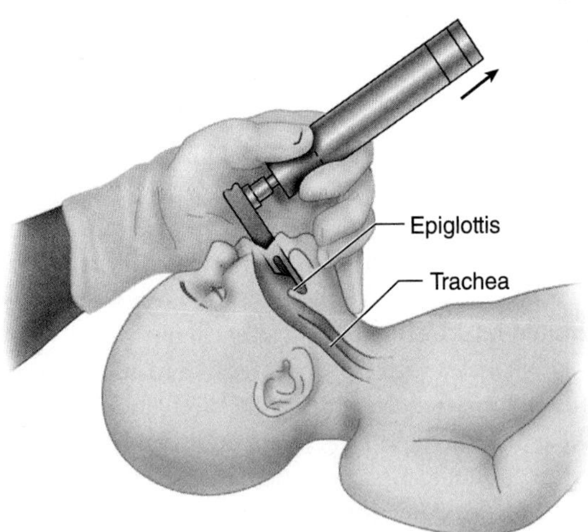

FIGURE 41–6 Intubation of the neonate. The head is placed in a neutral position, and the laryngoscope handle is held with the thumb and index finger as the chin is supported with the remaining fingers. Pressure applied over the hyoid bone with the little finger will bring the larynx into view. A straight blade such as a Miller 0 or 1 usually provides the best view.

intubation. Correct endotracheal tube size is indicated by a small leak with 20 cm H_2O pressure. Right endobronchial intubation should be excluded by chest auscultation. The correct depth of the endotracheal tube ("tip to lip") is usually 6 cm plus the weight in kilograms. Oxygen saturation can usually be measured by a pulse oximeter probe applied to the palm. Capnography should be used to confirm endotracheal intubation. Transcutaneous oxygen sensors are useful for measuring tissue oxygenation but require time for initial equilibration. Use of a laryngeal mask airway (LMA#1) has been reported in neonates weighing more than 2.5 kg and may be useful if endotracheal intubation is difficult (eg, Pierre Robin syndrome).

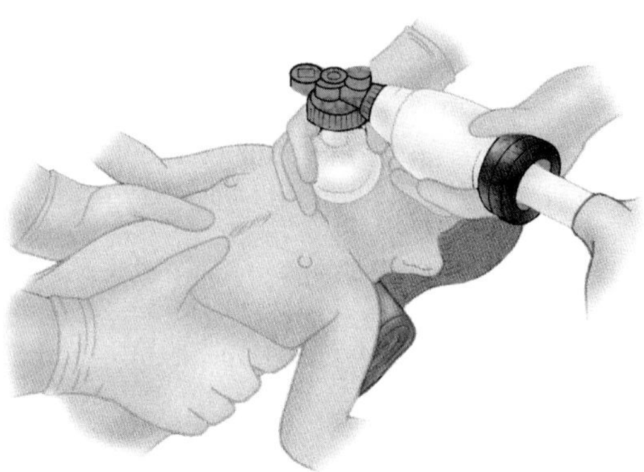

FIGURE 41–7 Chest compressions in the neonate. The neonate is held with both hands as each thumb is placed just beneath a line connecting the nipples and the remaining fingers encircle the chest. The sternum is compressed $^1/_3$ to ¾ in. (1 cm) at a rate of 120/min. (Reproduced with permission from Rudolph CD, Rudolph AM, Lister GE, et al. *Rudolph's Pediatrics*, 22nd ed. New York, NY: McGraw Hill; 2011.)

Guidelines for Chest Compressions

Indications for chest compressions are a heart rate that is less than 60 beats/min, or 60 to 80 beats/min and not rising after 30 s of adequate ventilation with 100% oxygen.

Cardiac compressions should be provided at a rate of 120/min. The two thumb/encircling hands technique (Figure 41–7) is generally preferred because it appears to generate higher peak systolic and coronary perfusion pressures. Alternatively, the two-finger technique can be used (Figure 41–8). The depth of compressions should be approximately one-third of the anterior–posterior diameter of the chest and sufficient to generate a palpable pulse.

Compressions should be interposed with ventilation in a 3:1 ratio, such that 90 compressions and 30 ventilations are given per minute. The heart rate should be checked periodically. Chest compressions should be stopped when the spontaneous heart rate exceeds 80 beats/min.

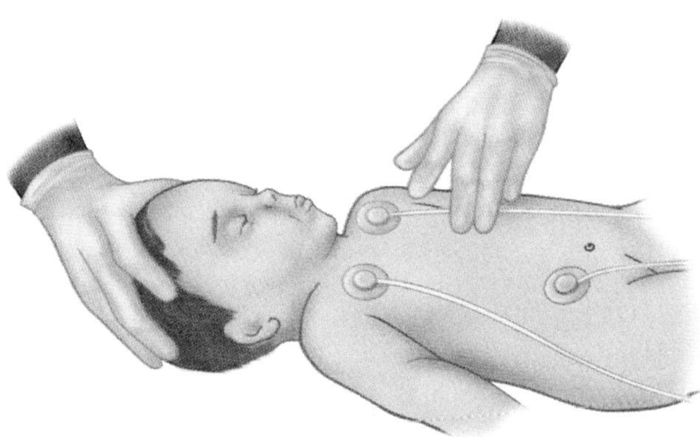

FIGURE 41–8 The alternative technique for neonatal chest compressions: two fingers are placed on the lower third of the sternum at right angles to the chest. The chest is compressed approximately 1 cm at a rate of 120/min.

Vascular Access

Cannulation of the umbilical vein with a 3.5F or 5F umbilical catheter is easiest and is the preferred technique. The tip of the catheter should be just below skin level and allow free backflow of blood; further advancement may result in the infusion of hypertonic solutions directly into the liver. A peripheral vein or even the endotracheal tube can be used as an alternate route for drug administration.

Cannulation of one of the two umbilical arteries allows measurement of blood pressure and facilitates blood gas measurements but may be more difficult. Specially designed umbilical artery catheters allow continuous PaO_2 or oxygen saturation monitoring as well as blood pressure. Care must be taken not to introduce any air into either the artery or the vein.

Volume Resuscitation

Nearly two-thirds of premature infants requiring resuscitation are hypovolemic at birth. Diagnosis is based on physical examination and a poor response to resuscitation. Neonatal blood pressure generally correlates with intravascular volume and should therefore routinely be measured. Normal blood pressure depends on birth weight and varies from 50/25 mm Hg for neonates weighing 1 to 2 kg to 70/40 mm Hg for those weighing over 3 kg. Low blood pressure and pallor suggest hypovolemia. Volume expansion may be accomplished with 10 mL/kg of lactated Ringer's injection, normal saline, or type O-negative blood cross-matched with maternal blood. Less common causes of hypotension include hypocalcemia, hypermagnesemia, and hypoglycemia.

Drug Therapy

A. Epinephrine

Epinephrine, 0.01 to 0.03 mg/kg (0.1–0.3 mL/kg of a 1:10,000 solution), should be given for asystole or a spontaneous heart rate less than 60 beats/min in spite of adequate ventilation and chest compressions. It may be repeated every 3 to 5 min. Epinephrine may be given in 1 mL of saline via the endotracheal tube when venous access is not available.

B. Naloxone

Naloxone, 0.1 mg/kg intravenously or 0.2 mg/kg intramuscularly, may be given to reverse the respiratory depressant effect of opioids given to the mother in the last 4 h of labor. *Withdrawal symptoms may be precipitated in babies of mothers who chronically consume opioids.*

C. Other Drugs

Other drugs may be indicated only in specific settings. Sodium bicarbonate (2 mEq/kg of a 0.5 mEq/mL 4.2% solution) should usually be given only for severe metabolic acidosis documented by blood gas measurements and when ventilation is adequate. It may also be administered during prolonged (>5 min) resuscitation—particularly if blood gas measurements are not readily available. The infusion rate should not exceed 1 mEq/kg/min to avoid hypertonicity and intracranial hemorrhage. As previously noted, to prevent hypertonicity-induced hepatic injury, the tip of the umbilical vein catheter should not be in the liver. Calcium gluconate 100 mg/kg ($CaCl_2$, 30 mg/kg) should be given only to neonates with documented hypocalcemia or those with suspected magnesium intoxication (from maternal magnesium therapy); these neonates are usually hypotensive, hypotonic, and appear vasodilated. Glucose (8 mg/kg/min of a 10% solution) is given only for documented hypoglycemia because hyperglycemia worsens hypoxic neurological deficits. Blood glucose should be measured because up to 10% of neonates may have hypoglycemia (glucose <35 mg/dL), particularly those delivered by cesarean section. Dopamine may be started at 5 mcg/kg/min to support arterial blood pressure. Lastly, surfactant may be given through the endotracheal tube to premature neonates with respiratory distress syndrome.

CASE DISCUSSION

Appendicitis in a Pregnant Woman

A 31-year-old woman with a 24-week gestation presents for an appendectomy.

How does pregnancy complicate the management of this patient?

Approximately 1% to 2% of pregnant patients require surgery during their pregnancy. The most common procedure during the first trimester is laparoscopy; appendectomy (1:1500 pregnancies) and cholecystectomy (1:2000–10,000 pregnancies) are the most commonly performed general surgical procedures. Cervical cerclage may be necessary for some patients for cervical incompetence. The physiological effects of pregnancy can alter the manifestations of the disease process and make diagnosis difficult. Patients may therefore present with advanced or complicated disease. The physiological changes associated with pregnancy (see Chapter 40) further predispose the patient to increased morbidity and mortality. Moreover, both the operation and the anesthesia can adversely affect the fetus.

What are the potentially detrimental effects of surgery and anesthesia on the fetus?

The procedure can have both immediate and long-term adverse effects on the fetus. Maternal hypotension, hypovolemia, severe anemia, hypoxemia, and marked increases in sympathetic tone can seriously compromise the transfer of oxygen and other nutrients across the uteroplacental circulation and promote intrauterine fetal asphyxia. The stress of the operative procedure and the underlying surgical disease process may also precipitate preterm labor, which often follows intraabdominal surgery near the uterus. Laparoscopy may be safely performed. Mild to moderate maternal hyperventilation and limiting both insufflation pressure and duration of the procedure limit the degree of fetal acidosis. Long-term detrimental effects relate to possible teratogenic effects on the developing fetus.

When is the fetus most sensitive to teratogenic influences?

Three stages of susceptibility are generally recognized. In the first 2 weeks of intrauterine life, teratogens have either a lethal effect or no effect on the embryo. The third to eighth weeks are the most critical period, when organogenesis takes place; drug exposure during this period can produce major developmental abnormalities. From the eighth week onward, organogenesis is complete, and organ growth takes place. Teratogen exposure during this last period usually results in only minor morphological abnormalities but can produce significant physiological abnormalities and growth retardation. Although the teratogenic influences of anesthetic agents have been extensively studied in animals, retrospective human studies have been inconclusive. Past concerns about the possible teratogenic effects of nitrous oxide and benzodiazepines do not appear to be justified. Nonetheless, exposure to all anesthetic agents should be kept to a minimum. We tend to administer only those agents that are required for the pregnant patient—and in our practice, nitrous oxide is never required, and benzodiazepines are rarely needed.

What would be the ideal anesthetic technique for this patient?

Toward the end of the second trimester (after 20–24 weeks of gestation), most of the major physiological changes associated with pregnancy have taken place. Regional anesthesia, when feasible, is preferable to general anesthesia to decrease the risks of pulmonary aspiration and failed intubation and to minimize drug exposure to the fetus. The patient should be maintained with left lateral uterine displacement when supine. Total drug exposure is least with spinal anesthesia. Moreover, spinal anesthesia may be preferable to epidural anesthesia because it is not associated with unintentional intravascular injection or the potential for accidental intrathecal injection of large epidural doses of local anesthetic. On the other hand, general anesthesia guarantees patient comfort and, when a volatile agent is used, may even suppress preterm labor (see Chapter 40). Nitrous oxide without concomitant administration of a halogenated anesthetic is reported to reduce uterine blood flow.

Although regional anesthesia is preferable in most instances, the choice between regional and general anesthesia must be individualized according to the patient, the anesthesiologist, and the type of surgery. Spinal anesthesia is usually satisfactory for open appendectomies, whereas general anesthesia is appropriate for laparoscopic procedures, including laparoscopic appendectomy.

Are any special monitors indicated perioperatively?

In addition to standard monitors, fetal heart rate and uterine activity should be monitored with a Doppler and tocodynamometer immediately prior to surgery and during anesthesia recovery in a woman who is 24 weeks or more pregnant. When regular organized uterine activity is detected, early treatment with a β-adrenergic agonist such as ritodrine usually aborts the preterm labor. Magnesium sulfate and oral or rectal indomethacin may also be used as tocolytics.

When should elective operations be performed during pregnancy?

All elective operations should be postponed until 6 weeks after delivery. Only emergency procedures that pose an immediate threat to the mother or fetus should be routinely performed. The timing of semielective or urgent procedures, such as those for cancer, valvular heart disease, or intracranial aneurysms, must be individualized and must balance the threat to maternal health versus fetal well-being. Controlled (deliberate) hypotensive anesthesia has been utilized to reduce blood loss during extensive cancer operations; nitroprusside, nitroglycerin, and hydralazine have been used during pregnancy without apparent fetal compromise. Nonetheless, large doses and prolonged infusions of nitroprusside should be avoided because the immature liver of the fetus may have a limited ability to metabolize the cyanide breakdown product. Cardiopulmonary bypass has been employed in pregnant patients successfully without adverse fetal outcomes. Elective use of circulatory arrest during pregnancy is not recommended.

GUIDELINES

Merchant RM, Topjian AA, Panchal AR, et al. Part 1: executive summary: 2020 American Heart Association guidelines for cardiopulmonary resuscitation and emergency cardiovascular care. *Circulation*. 2020;142:S337-357.

SUGGESTED READINGS

Davis N, Smoots A, Goodman D. Pregnancy-related deaths: data from 14 U.S. maternal mortality review committees, 2008–2017. Atlanta, GA: Centers for Disease Control and Prevention, U.S. Department of Health and Human Services; 2019.

Frölich MA, Esame A, Zhang K, et al. What factors affect intrapartum maternal temperature? A prospective cohort study: maternal intrapartum temperature. *Anesthesiology*. 2012;117:302.

Guglielminotti J, Wong CA, Friedman AM, Li G. Racial and ethnic disparities in death associated with severe maternal morbidity in the United States: failure to rescue. *Obstet Gynecol.* 2021;137:791.

Heesen M, Rijs K, Hilber N, et al. Ephedrine versus phenylephrine as a vasopressor for spinal anaesthesia-induced hypotension in parturients undergoing high-risk caesarean section: meta-analysis, meta-regression and trial sequential analysis. *Int J Obstet Anesth.* 2019;37:16.

Hussey H, Hussey P, Meng ML. Peripartum considerations for women with cardiac disease. *Curr Opin Anaesthesiol.* 2021;34:218.

Ngan Kee, Warwick D. A random-allocation graded dose–response study of norepinephrine and phenylephrine for treating hypotension during spinal anesthesia for cesarean delivery. *Anesthesiology.* 2017;127:934.

Peterson W, Tse B, Martin R, et al. Evaluating hemostatic thresholds for neuraxial anesthesia in adults with hemorrhagic disorders and tendencies: a scoping review. *Res Pract Thromb Haemost.* 2021;5:e12491.

Taskforce on Hypertension and Pregnancy. *Hypertension in Pregnancy*. Washington, DC: American College of Obstetricians and Gynecologists; 2013;122:1122.

Weiniger CF. Gerard W. Ostheimer lecture: what's new in obstetric anesthesia 2018. *Anesth Analg.* 2020;131:307.

CHAPTER

42

Pediatric Anesthesia

Seamas Dore, MD

KEY CONCEPTS

1. Neonates and infants have fewer and smaller alveoli, reducing lung compliance; in contrast, their cartilaginous rib cage makes their chest wall very compliant and increases airway resistance. Work of breathing is increased, and respiratory muscles more easily fatigue. These characteristics promote chest wall collapse during inspiration and relatively low residual lung volumes at expiration. The resulting decrease in functional residual capacity (FRC) limits oxygen reserves during periods of apnea (eg, intubation attempts) and predisposes neonates and infants to atelectasis and hypoxemia.

2. Compared with older children and adults, neonates and infants have a proportionately larger head and tongue, narrower nasal passages, an anterior and cephalad larynx, a longer epiglottis, and a shorter trachea and neck. These anatomic features make neonates and young infants obligate nasal breathers until about 5 months of age. The cricoid cartilage is the narrowest point of the airway in children younger than 5 years of age.

3. Cardiac stroke volume is relatively fixed by the immature, noncompliant left ventricle in neonates and infants. The cardiac output is therefore very sensitive to changes in heart rate.

4. Thin skin, low fat content, and a greater surface area relative to weight promote greater heat loss to the environment in neonates. Heat loss can be made worse by prolonged exposure to an inadequately warmed operating room environment, administration of room-temperature intravenous fluid and dehumidified anesthetic gases, and the effects of anesthetic agents on temperature regulation. Hypothermia has been associated with delayed awakening from anesthesia, cardiac arrhythmias, respiratory depression, increased pulmonary vascular resistance, and increased susceptibility to anesthetics and other agents.

5. Neonates, infants, and young children have relatively greater alveolar ventilation and reduced FRC compared with older children and adults. This greater minute ventilation-to-FRC ratio contributes to a rapid increase in alveolar anesthetic concentration that, combined with relatively greater blood flow to the brain, speeds inhalation induction.

6. The minimum alveolar concentration (MAC) for halogenated agents is greater in infants than in neonates and adults. In contrast to other agents, no increase in the MAC of sevoflurane can be demonstrated between neonates and infants. Sevoflurane appears to have a greater therapeutic index than halothane and is the preferred agent for inhaled induction in pediatric anesthesia.

7. Children are more susceptible than adults to cardiac arrhythmias, hyperkalemia, rhabdomyolysis, myoglobinemia, masseter

—Continued next page

Continued—

spasm, and malignant hyperthermia associated with succinylcholine. When a child experiences cardiac arrest following administration of succinylcholine, immediate treatment for hyperkalemia should be instituted.

8 Unlike adults, children may have profound bradycardia and sinus node arrest following the first dose of succinylcholine without atropine pretreatment.

9 A viral infection within 2 to 4 weeks before general anesthesia and endotracheal intubation appears to place the child at an increased risk for perioperative pulmonary complications, such as wheezing, laryngospasm, hypoxemia, and atelectasis.

10 Temperature must be closely monitored in pediatric patients because of their greater risk for malignant hyperthermia and greater susceptibility for intraoperative hypothermia or hyperthermia.

11 Meticulous attention to fluid intake and loss is required in younger pediatric patients because these patients have limited margins of error. A programmable infusion pump or a buret with a microdrip chamber is useful for accurate measurements. Drugs can be flushed through low dead-space tubing to minimize unnecessary fluid administration.

12 Laryngospasm can usually be avoided by extubating the patient either while awake or deeply anesthetized; both techniques have advocates. Extubation during the interval between these extremes, however, is generally recognized as more hazardous.

13 Patients with scoliosis due to muscular dystrophy are predisposed to malignant hypertension, cardiac arrhythmias, and untoward effects of succinylcholine (hyperkalemia, myoglobinuria, and sustained muscular contractures).

Pediatric anesthesia involves more than simply adjusting drug doses and equipment for smaller patients. Neonates (0–1 months), infants (1–12 months), toddlers (12–24 months), and young children (2–12 years of age) have differing anesthetic requirements. A safe anesthetic requires attention to the physiological, anatomic, and pharmacological characteristics of each group (Table 42–1). Risk is generally inversely proportional to age, and infants are at much greater risk of anesthetic morbidity and mortality than older children. In addition, pediatric patients are susceptible to illnesses that require unique surgical and anesthetic strategies.

ANATOMIC & PHYSIOLOGICAL DEVELOPMENT

Respiratory System

The transition from fetal to neonatal physiology is reviewed in Chapter 40. Compared with older children and adults, neonates and infants have weaker intercostal muscles and weaker diaphragms (due to a paucity of type I fibers). Consequently, they have less efficient ventilation, more pliable and coursing ribs, and protuberant abdomens. Alveoli are fully mature by about 8 years of age. The respiratory rate is increased in neonates and gradually falls to adult values by adolescence. Tidal volume and dead space per kilogram are nearly constant during
1 development. Neonates and infants have fewer and smaller alveoli, reducing lung compliance; in contrast, their cartilaginous rib cage makes their chest wall very compliant and increases airway resistance. Work of breathing is increased, and respiratory muscles fatigue more easily. These characteristics promote chest wall collapse during inspiration and relatively low residual lung volumes at expiration. The resulting decrease in functional residual capacity (FRC) limits oxygen reserves during periods of apnea (eg, intubation attempts) and predisposes

TABLE 42–1 Characteristics of neonates and infants that differentiate them from adult patients.

Physiological
Heart-rate-dependent cardiac output
Increased heart rate
Reduced blood pressure
Increased respiratory rate
Increased metabolic rate
Reduced lung compliance
Increased chest wall compliance
Reduced functional residual capacity
Increased ratio of body surface area to body weight
Increased total body water content
Anatomic
Noncompliant left ventricle
Residual fetal circulation
Difficult venous and arterial cannulation
Relatively larger head and tongue
Narrower nasal passages
Anterior and cephalad larynx
Relatively longer epiglottis
Shorter trachea and neck
More prominent adenoids and tonsils
Weaker intercostal and diaphragmatic muscles
Greater resistance to airflow
Pharmacological
Immature hepatic biotransformation
Decreased blood protein for drug binding
More rapid rise in FA/FI[1] and more rapid induction and recovery from inhaled anesthetics
Increased minimum alveolar concentration
Relatively larger volume of distribution for water-soluble drugs
Immature neuromuscular junction

[1]FA/FI, fractional alveolar concentration/fractional inspired concentration.

neonates and infants to atelectasis and hypoxemia. These effects of reduced FRC may be exaggerated by the relatively higher rate of oxygen consumption of neonates and infants, 6 to 8 mL/kg/min versus 3 to 4 mL/kg/min in adults. Moreover, hypoxic and hypercapnic ventilatory drives are not fully developed in neonates and infants. In contrast to adults, hypoxia and hypercapnia may depress respiration in these patients.

2 Neonates and infants have, compared with older children and adults, a proportionately larger head and tongue, narrower nasal passages, an anterior and cephalad larynx (the glottis is at a vertebral level of C4 versus C6 in adults), a longer epiglottis, and a shorter trachea and neck (Figure 42–1). These anatomic features make neonates and young infants obligate nasal breathers until about 5 months of age. **The cricoid cartilage is the narrowest point of the airway in children younger than 5 years of age; in adults, the narrowest point is the glottis (vocal cords).** One millimeter of mucosal edema will produce a greater decline in tracheal cross-sectional area and gas flow in children because of their smaller tracheal diameters.

Cardiovascular System

3 Cardiac stroke volume is relatively fixed by the immature, noncompliant left ventricle in neonates and infants. The cardiac output is therefore very sensitive to changes in heart rate (see Chapter 20). Although basal heart rate is greater in neonates and infants than in adults (Table 42–2), vagal stimulation, anesthetic overdose, or hypoxia can quickly trigger bradycardia with profound reductions in cardiac output. Sick infants undergoing emergency or prolonged surgery appear particularly prone to episodes of bradycardia that can lead to hypotension, asystole, and intraoperative death. The sympathetic nervous system and baroreceptor reflexes are not fully mature. The infant cardiovascular system displays a blunted response to exogenous catecholamines. The immature heart is more sensitive to depression by volatile anesthetics and to opioid-induced bradycardia. Infants are less able to respond to hypovolemia with compensatory vasoconstriction. Intravascular volume depletion in neonates and infants may be signaled by hypotension without tachycardia.

Metabolism & Temperature Regulation

Pediatric patients have a larger surface area per kilogram than adults (smaller body mass index). Metabolism and its associated parameters (oxygen consumption, CO_2 production, cardiac output, and

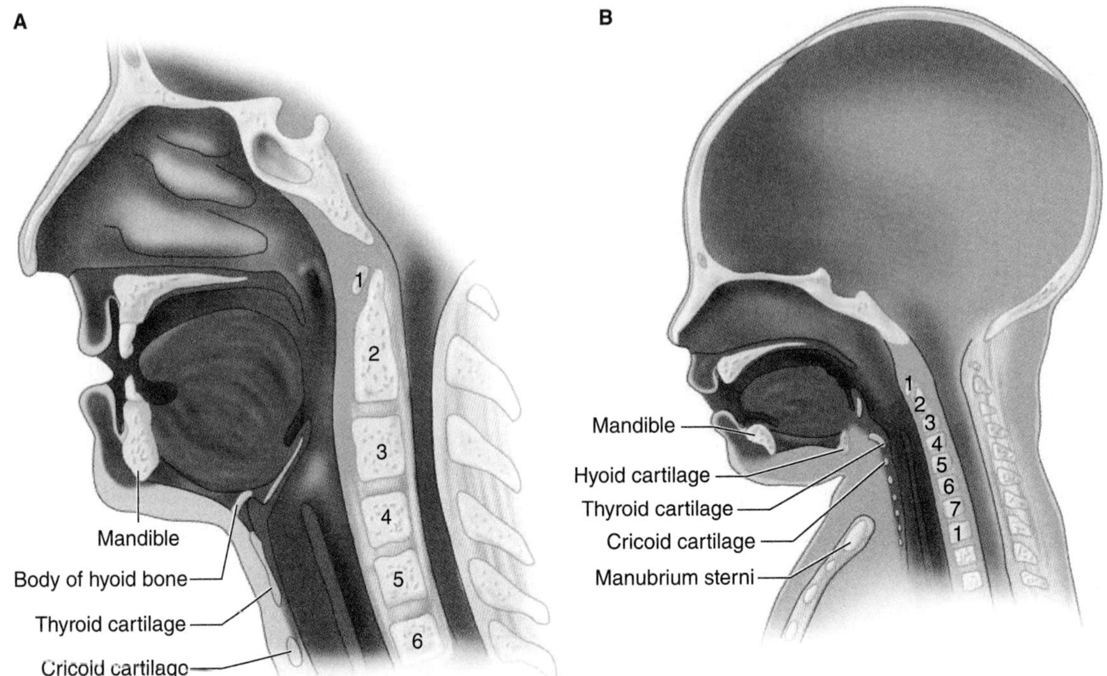

FIGURE 42–1 Sagittal section of the adult (**A**) and infant (**B**) airway. (Reproduced with permission from Snell RS, Katz J. *Clinical Anatomy for Anesthesiologists*. New York, NY: Appleton & Lange; 1988.)

alveolar ventilation) correlate better with surface area than with weight.

4 Thin skin, low fat content, and a greater surface area relative to weight promote greater heat loss to the environment in neonates. This problem can be made worse by prolonged exposure to an inadequately warmed operating room, administration of room temperature intravenous or irrigation fluid, and dehumidified anesthetic gases. Anesthetic agents impair temperature regulation (see Chapter 52). Even mild degrees of hypothermia can cause delayed awakening from anesthesia, cardiac arrhythmias, respiratory depression, increased pulmonary vascular resistance, and increased susceptibility to anesthetics, neuromuscular blockers, and other agents. Neonates produce heat by the metabolism of brown fat (*nonshivering thermogenesis*) and by shifting hepatic oxidative phosphorylation to a more thermogenic pathway. Yet the metabolism of brown fat is severely limited in premature infants and in sick neonates, who are deficient in fat stores. Furthermore, volatile anesthetics inhibit this process.

TABLE 42–2 Age-related changes in vital signs.[1]

Age	Respiratory Rate	Heart Rate	Arterial Blood Pressure	
			Systolic	*Diastolic*
Neonate	40	140	65	40
12 months	30	120	95	65
3 years	25	100	100	70
12 years	20	80	110	60

[1]Values are mean averages derived from numerous sources. Normal ranges may include measurements that deviate from these as much as 25–50%.

Kidney & Gastrointestinal Function

Kidney function usually approaches normal values (corrected for size) by 6 months of age, but this may be delayed until the child is 2 years old. Premature neonates often demonstrate renal immaturity with one or more of the following: decreased creatinine clearance, impaired sodium retention, impaired glucose excretion, impaired bicarbonate reabsorption, reduced diluting ability, and reduced concentrating ability. These abnormalities underscore the importance of appropriate fluid administration in neonates.

Neonates also have an increased likelihood of gastroesophageal reflux. The immature liver conjugates drugs and other molecules less readily.

Glucose Homeostasis

Neonates have relatively reduced glycogen stores, predisposing them to hypoglycemia. In general, neonates at greatest risk for hypoglycemia are premature or small for gestational age, are receiving total parenteral nutrition, or had mothers with diabetes.

PHARMACOLOGICAL DIFFERENCES

Pediatric drug dosing is typically adjusted on a per-kilogram basis for convenience (Table 42–3), though there are strong advocates for *allometric dosing*, in which adjustments for weight are not made in a linear fashion. In early childhood, a patient's weight can be approximated based on age in years:

$$50\text{th percentile weight (kg)} = (\text{Age} \times 2) + 9$$

In contrast to weight adjustment of drug dosing, allometric drug dose calculations take into account age-related physiological differences such as the disproportionately larger pediatric intravascular and extracellular fluid compartments, the immaturity of

TABLE 42–3 Pediatric drug dosages.

Drug	Comment	Dosage
Acetaminophen	Rectal PO IV (age >2 y) Maximum (per day)	40 mg/kg 10–20 mg/kg 15 mg/kg 60 mg/kg
Adenosine	Rapid IV bolus Repeat dose Maximum dose	0.1 mg/kg 0.2 mg/kg 12 mg
Albuterol	Nebulized	1.25–2.5 mg in 2 mL saline
Alfentanil	Anesthetic supplement (IV) Maintenance infusion	20–25 mcg/kg 1–3 mcg/kg/min
Aminophylline	Loading dose administered over 20 min (IV) Maintenance dose (therapeutic level: 10–20 mg/mL)	5–6 mg/kg 0.5–0.9 mg/kg/h
Amiodarone	Loading dose (IV) Repeat dose (slowly) Infusion Maximum dose	5 mg/kg 5 mg/kg 5–10 mcg/kg/min 20 mg/kg/day
Amoxicillin	PO	50 mg/kg
Ampicillin	IV	50 mg/kg
Ampicillin/sulbactam	IV	25–50 mg/kg
Atracurium	Intubation (IV)	0.5 mg/kg

(*continued*)

TABLE 42–3 Pediatric drug dosages. (Continued)

Drug	Comment	Dosage
Atropine	IV	0.01–0.02 mg/kg
	IM	0.02 mg/kg
	Minimum dose	0.1 mg
	Premedication (PO)	0.03–0.05 mg/kg
Bretylium	Loading dose (IV)	5 mg/kg
Caffeine	IV	10 mg/kg
Calcium chloride	IV (slowly)	5–20 mg/kg
Calcium gluconate	IV (slowly)	15–100 mg/kg
Cefazolin	IV	25 mg/kg
Cefotaxime	IV	25–50 mg/kg
Cefotetan	IV	20–40 mg/kg
Cefoxitin	IV	30–40 mg/kg
Ceftazidime	IV	30–50 mg/kg
Ceftriaxone	IV	25–50 mg/kg
Cefuroxime	IV	25 mg/kg
Chloral hydrate	PO	25–100 mg/kg
	Rectal	50 mg/kg
Cimetidine	IV or PO	5–10 mg/kg
Cisatracurium	Intubation (IV)	0.15 mg/kg
Clindamycin	IV	20 mg/kg
Dantrolene	Initial Dose (IV) rapid IV bolus, repeat PRN	2.5 mg/kg
	Typical Cumulative Dose	10 mg/kg
Desmopressin	IV	0.2–0.4 mcg/kg
Dexamethasone	IV	0.1–0.5 mg/kg
Dextrose	D25W or D50W (IV)	0.5–1 g/kg
Digoxin	IV	0.1–0.2 mg/kg
	Three divided doses over 24 h (IV)	15–30 mcg/kg
Diltiazem	IV over 2 min	0.25 mg/kg
Diphenhydramine	IV, IM, or PO	1 mg/kg
Dobutamine	Infusion	2–20 mcg/kg/min
Dolasetron	IV	0.35 mg/kg
Dopamine	Infusion	2–20 mcg/kg/min

(continued)

TABLE 42–3 Pediatric drug dosages. (Continued)

Drug	Comment	Dosage
Droperidol	IV	50–75 mcg/kg
Edrophonium	Depends on degree of paralysis (IV)	0.5–1 mg/kg
Ephedrine	IV	0.1–0.3 mg/kg
Epinephrine	IV bolus Endotracheal dose Infusion	10 mcg/kg 100 mcg/kg 0.05–1 mcg/kg/min
Epinephrine, 2.25% racemic	Nebulized	0.05 mL/kg in 3 mL saline
Esmolol	IV bolus IV infusion	100–500 mcg/kg 25–200 mcg/kg/min
Famotidine	IV	0.15 mg/kg
Fentanyl	Pain relief (IV) Pain relief (Intranasal) Premedication (Actiq PO) Anesthetic adjunct (IV) Maintenance infusion Main anesthetic (IV)	1–2 mcg/kg 2 mcg/kg 10–15 mcg/kg 1–5 mcg/kg 2–4 mcg/kg/h 50–100 mcg/kg
Flumazenil	IV	0.01 mg/kg
Fosphenytoin	IV	15–20 mg/kg
Furosemide	IV	0.2–1 mg/kg
Gentamicin	IV	2 mg/kg
Glucagon	IV	0.5–1 mg
Glucose	IV	0.5–1 g/kg
Glycopyrrolate	IV	0.01 mg/kg
Granisetron	IV	0.04 mg/kg
Heparin	IV (not for cardiac surgery) Cardiac surgery dose	100 units/kg 300–400 units/kg
Hydrocortisone	IV	1 mg/kg
Hydromorphone	IV	15–20 mcg/kg
Ibuprofen	PO	4–10 mg/kg
Imipenem	IV	15–25 mg/kg
Inamrinone	Loading (IV) Maintenance	1.5 mg/kg 5–10 mcg/kg/min

(continued)

TABLE 42–3 Pediatric drug dosages. (Continued)

Drug	Comment	Dosage
Insulin	Infusion	0.02–0.1 units/kg/h
Isoproterenol	Infusion	0.1–1 mcg/kg/min
Ketamine	Induction (IV) Induction (IM) Induction (per rectum) Maintenance infusion Premedication (PO) Sedation (IV)	1–2 mg/kg 6–10 mg/kg 10 mg/kg 25–75 mcg/kg/min 6–10 mg/kg 0.5–1 mg/kg
Ketorolac	IV	0.5–0.75 mg/kg
Labetalol	IV	0.25 mg/kg
Lidocaine	Loading Maintenance	1 mg/kg 20–50 mcg/kg/min
Magnesium sulphate	IV (slowly) Maximum single dose	25–50 mg/kg 2 g
Mannitol	IV	0.25–1 g/kg
Meperidine	Pain relief (IV)	0.2–0.5 mg/kg
Methohexital	Induction (IV) Induction (per rectum) Induction (IM)	1–2 mg/kg 25–30 mg/kg 10 mg/kg
Methylprednisolone	IV	2–4 mg/kg
Metoclopramide	IV	0.15 mg/kg
Metronidazole	IV	7.5 mg/kg
Midazolam	Premedication (PO) Maximum dose (PO) Sedation (IM) Sedation (IV)	0.5 mg/kg 20 mg 0.1–0.15 mg/kg 0.05 mg/kg
Milrinone	Loading (IV) Maintenance	50–75 mcg/kg 0.375–0.75 mcg/kg/min
Morphine	Pain relief (IV) Premedication (IM)	0.025–0.1 mg/kg 0.1 mg/kg
Naloxone	IV	0.01 mg/kg
Neostigmine	Depends on degree of paralysis (IV)	0.04–0.07 mg/kg
Nitroglycerin	IV	0.5–3 mcg/kg/min
Nitroprusside	Infusion	0.5–4 mcg/kg/min

(continued)

TABLE 42–3 Pediatric drug dosages. (Continued)

Drug	Comment	Dosage
Norepinephrine	Infusion	0.05–2 mcg/kg/min
Ondansetron	IV	0.1 mg/kg
Oxacillin	IV	50 mg/kg
Pancuronium	IV	0.1 mg/kg
Penicillin G	IV	50,000 units/kg
Pentobarbital	Premedication (IM)	1–2 mg/kg
Phenobarbital	Anticonvulsant dose (IV)	5–20 mg/kg
Phentolamine	IV	30 mcg/kg
Phenylephrine	IV	1–10 mcg/kg
Phenytoin	Slowly IV	5–20 mg/kg
Physostigmine	IV	0.01–0.03 mg/kg
Prednisone	PO	1 mg/kg
Procainamide	Loading dose (IV)	15 mg/kg
Propofol	Induction (IV) Maintenance infusion	2–3 mg/kg 60–250 mcg/kg/min
Propranolol	IV	10–25 mcg/kg
Prostaglandin E1	Infusion	0.05–0.1 mcg/kg/min
Protamine	IV	1 mg/100 units heparin
Ranitidine	IV	0.25–1.0 mg/kg
Remifentanil	IV bolus IV infusion	0.25–1 mcg/kg 0.05–2 mcg/kg/min
Rocuronium	Intubation (IV)	0.6–1.2 mg/kg
Sodium bicarbonate	IV	1 mEq/kg
Succinylcholine	Intubation (IV) Intubation (IM)	1–2mg/kg 4 mg/kg
Sugammadex[1]	Moderate block Deep block	2 mg/kg 4 mg/kg
Sufentanil	Premedication (intranasal) Anesthetic adjunct (IV) Maintenance infusion Main anesthetic (IV)	2 mcg/kg 0.5–1 mcg/kg 0.5–2 mcg/kg/h 10–15 mcg/kg

(continued)

TABLE 42–3 Pediatric drug dosages. (Continued)

Drug	Comment	Dosage
Thiopental	Induction (IV)	5–6 mg/kg
Trimethoprim/sulfamethoxazole	IV	4–5 mg/kg
Vancomycin	IV	20 mg/kg
Vecuronium	IV	0.1 mg/kg
Verapamil	IV	0.1–0.3 mg/kg

[1]This drug is not yet approved for pediatric administration.

hepatic biotransformation pathways, the increased organ blood flow, the decreased protein for drug binding, and the higher metabolic rate.

Neonates and infants have a proportionately greater total water content (70–75%) than adults (50–60%). Total body water content decreases while fat and muscle content increase with age. As a result, the volume of distribution for many intravenous drugs (eg, neuromuscular blockers) is disproportionately greater in neonates, infants, and young children, and the optimal dose (per kilogram) is usually greater than in older children and adults. A disproportionately smaller fat and muscle mass in neonates prolongs the clinical duration of action of lipid-soluble drugs such as propofol and fentanyl by delaying redistribution. Neonates also have a relatively decreased glomerular filtration rate, decreased hepatic blood flow, impaired renal tubular function, and immature hepatic enzyme systems. Increased intraabdominal pressure and abdominal surgery may further reduce hepatic blood flow. All these factors can impair renal drug handling, hepatic metabolism, and biliary excretion of drugs in neonates and young infants. Neonates also have decreased drug binding to proteins, notably for local anesthetics and many antibiotics. In the case of bupivacaine, an increase in free drug likely increases the risk of systemic toxicity.

Inhalational Anesthetics

5 Neonates, infants, and young children have relatively greater alveolar ventilation and reduced FRC compared with older children and adults. This greater minute ventilation-to-FRC ratio contributes to a rapid increase in alveolar anesthetic concentration that, combined with relatively greater blood flow to the brain, speeds inhalation induction. Furthermore, the blood/gas coefficients of volatile anesthetics are reduced in neonates compared with adults, contributing to faster induction times and increasing the risk of accidental overdosage.

6 The minimum alveolar concentration (MAC) for halogenated agents is greater in infants than in neonates and adults (Table 42–4). In contrast to other agents, no increase in the MAC of sevoflurane can be demonstrated between neonates and infants. Nitrous oxide does not appear to reduce the MAC of desflurane or sevoflurane in children to the same extent as it does for other agents.

The blood pressure of neonates and infants appears to be especially sensitive to volatile anesthetics. This clinical observation has been attributed to less well-developed compensatory mechanisms (eg, vasoconstriction, tachycardia)

TABLE 42–4 Approximate MAC[1] values for pediatric patients reported in % of an atmosphere.[2]

Agent	Neonates	Infants	Small Children	Adults
Halothane	0.90	1.1–1.2	0.9	0.75
Sevoflurane	3.2	3.2	2.5	2
Isoflurane	1.6	1.8–1.9	1.3–1.6	1.2
Desflurane	8–9	9–10	7–8	6

[1]MAC, minimum alveolar concentration.
[2]Values are derived from various sources.

and greater sensitivity of the immature myocardium to myocardial depressants. Halothane (now rarely used) sensitizes the heart to catecholamines; thus, the maximum recommended dose of epinephrine in local anesthetic solutions during halothane anesthesia is reduced. Cardiovascular depression, bradycardia, and arrhythmias are less frequent with sevoflurane than with halothane. Sevoflurane and halothane are less likely than other volatile agents to irritate the airway or cause breath holding or laryngospasm during induction (see Chapter 8). In general, volatile anesthetics appear to depress ventilation more in infants than in older children. Sevoflurane appears to produce the least respiratory depression. Halothane-induced hepatic dysfunction is much rarer in prepubertal children than adults. There are no reported instances of renal toxicity attributed to fluoride production during sevoflurane anesthesia in children. Sevoflurane is the preferred agent for inhaled induction in pediatric anesthesia.

Emergence is fast following sevoflurane or desflurane, but both agents are associated with agitation or delirium upon emergence, particularly in young children. Because of the latter, some clinicians switch to isoflurane for maintenance anesthesia following a sevoflurane induction (see later discussion).

Nonvolatile Anesthetics

After weight-adjustment of dosing, infants and young children require larger doses of propofol because of a larger volume of distribution compared with adults. Children also have a shorter elimination half-life and higher plasma clearance for propofol. Recovery from a single bolus is not appreciably different from that in adults; however, recovery following a continuous infusion may be more rapid. For the same reasons, children may require increased weight-adjusted rates of infusion for maintenance of anesthesia (up to 250 mcg/kg/min). Propofol is not recommended for prolonged sedation of critically ill pediatric patients in the intensive care unit (ICU) due to an association with mortality. This "propofol infusion syndrome" has been reported most often in critically ill children, but it has also been reported in adults undergoing long-term propofol sedation, particularly at increased doses (>5 mg/kg/h). Its essential features include rhabdomyolysis, metabolic acidosis, hemodynamic instability, hepatomegaly, and multiorgan failure.

Children require relatively larger doses of thiopental compared with adults. The elimination half-life is shorter and the plasma clearance is greater than in adults. In contrast, neonates appear to be more sensitive to barbiturates. Neonates have less protein binding, a longer half-life, and impaired clearance. The thiopental induction dose for neonates is 3 to 4 mg/kg compared with 5 to 6 mg/kg for infants.

Opioids appear to be more potent in neonates than in older children and adults. Morphine sulfate, particularly in repeated doses, should be used with caution in neonates because hepatic conjugation is reduced and renal clearance of morphine metabolites is decreased. The cytochrome P-450 pathways mature at the end of the neonatal period. Older children have relatively greater rates of biotransformation and elimination as a result of high hepatic blood flow. Remifentanil clearance is increased in neonates and infants, but elimination half-life is similar to adults. Neonates and infants may require slightly larger doses of ketamine than adults, but any difference, if present, is very small. Pharmacokinetic values are not significantly different from those of adults. Etomidate has not been well studied in patients younger than 10 years of age; its profile in old children is similar to that in adults. Midazolam has the fastest clearance of all the benzodiazepines, but its clearance is significantly reduced in neonates compared with older children.

Dexmedetomidine has been used widely for sedation and as a supplement to general anesthesia in children. In patients without an intravenous line, dexmedetomidine can be given intranasally (1–2 mcg/kg) for sedation.

Muscle Relaxants

For many reasons (including pharmacodynamic and case mix differences), muscle relaxants are less commonly used during induction of anesthesia in children than in adults. In North America, many children will have a laryngeal mask airway (LMA) or endotracheal tube placed after receiving an inhalation induction, placement of an intravenous catheter, and administration of various combinations of propofol, opioids, or lidocaine.

All muscle relaxants generally have a faster onset (up to 50% less delay) in pediatric patients because of shorter circulation times than in adults. In both children and adults, intravenous succinylcholine (1–1.5 mg/kg) has the fastest onset (see Chapter 11). Infants are given significantly larger doses of succinylcholine (2–3 mg/kg) than older children and adults because of the relatively larger volume of distribution (on a per kilogram basis). This discrepancy disappears if the dosage is based on body surface area. Table 42–5 lists commonly used muscle relaxants and their ED_{95} (the dose that produces 95% depression of evoked twitches). Infants require significantly smaller nondepolarizing muscle relaxant doses than older children (cisatracurium may possibly be an exception). Moreover, based on weight, older children require larger doses than adults for some neuromuscular blocking agents (eg, atracurium, see Chapter 11).

The response of neonates to nondepolarizing muscle relaxants is variable. Popular explanations for this include "immaturity of the neuromuscular junction" (in premature neonates), tending to increase sensitivity (unproven), counterbalanced by a disproportionately larger extracellular compartment, reducing drug concentrations (proven). The relative immaturity of neonatal hepatic function prolongs the persistence of drugs that depend primarily on hepatic metabolism (eg, rocuronium, vecuronium, pancuronium). Atracurium and cisatracurium do not depend on hepatic biotransformation and reliably behave as intermediate-acting muscle relaxants.

7 Children are more susceptible than adults to cardiac arrhythmias, hyperkalemia, rhabdomyolysis, myoglobinemia, masseter spasm, and malignant hyperthermia (see Chapter 52) associated with succinylcholine. When a child experiences cardiac arrest following administration of succinylcholine, immediate treatment for hyperkalemia should be instituted. Prolonged resuscitative efforts (potentially including cardiopulmonary bypass) may be required. Thus, succinylcholine is avoided for routine, elective paralysis for intubation in children and

8 adolescents. Children may have profound bradycardia and sinus node arrest following the first dose of succinylcholine without atropine pretreatment. Therefore, atropine (0.1 mg minimum) is customarily administered prior to succinylcholine in children. Generally accepted indications for intravenous succinylcholine in children include rapid sequence induction with a "full" stomach and laryngospasm that does not respond to positive-pressure ventilation. When rapid muscle relaxation is required prior to intravenous access (eg, with inhaled inductions in patients with full stomachs), intramuscular succinylcholine (4–6 mg/kg) with intramuscular atropine (0.02 mg/kg) can be used. Some clinicians advocate intralingual administration (2 mg/kg in the midline) as an alternate emergency route for succinylcholine.

Many clinicians consider rocuronium (0.6 mg/kg intravenously) the drug of choice (when an intravenous relaxant will be used) for routine intubation in pediatric patients because it has the fastest onset of nondepolarizing neuromuscular blocking agents (see Chapter 11). Larger doses of rocuronium (0.9–1.2 mg/kg) are preferred by many clinicians for rapid sequence induction if a prolonged duration (up to 90 min) is not a concern. Rocuronium is the only nondepolarizing neuromuscular blocker that has been adequately studied for intramuscular administration (1.0–1.5 mg/kg), but this approach requires 3 to 4 min for onset. Atracurium or cisatracurium may be preferred in young infants, particularly for short procedures, because these drugs consistently display short to intermediate duration.

TABLE 42–5 Approximate ED_{95} for muscle relaxants in infants and children.[1]

Agents	Infants ED_{95} (mg/kg)	Children ED_{95} (mg/kg)
Succinylcholine	0.7	0.4
Atracurium	0.25	0.35
Cisatracurium	0.05	0.06
Rocuronium	0.25	0.4
Vecuronium	0.05	0.08
Pancuronium	0.07	0.09

[1]Average values during nitrous oxide/oxygen anesthesia.

As with adults, the effect of muscle relaxants should be monitored with a peripheral nerve stimulator. Sensitivity varies significantly between patients. In the past, nondepolarizing blockade was typically reversed with neostigmine (0.03–0.07 mg/kg) or edrophonium (0.5–1 mg/kg) along with an anticholinergic agent (glycopyrrolate, 0.01 mg/kg, or atropine, 0.01–0.02 mg/kg). Currently, sugammadex, a specific antagonist for rocuronium and vecuronium, is the preferred reversal agent for these agents.

PEDIATRIC ANESTHETIC RISK

The Pediatric Perioperative Cardiac Arrest (POCA) Registry includes reports from millions of pediatric anesthetics administered since 1994. Case records of children experiencing cardiac arrests or death during or after recovery from anesthesia were investigated regarding any possible relationship with anesthesia. Anesthetic care was judged to have contributed to 150 arrests in 289 cases of cardiac arrest. Thus, the risk of cardiac arrest in pediatric anesthetic cases would appear to be approximately 1.4 in 10,000. Thirty-three percent of patients who experienced a cardiac arrest were classified as American Society of Anesthesiologists (ASA) physical status 1 or 2. Infants accounted for 55% of all anesthesia-related arrests in children, with those younger than 1 month of age having the greatest risk. After cardiac arrest, mortality was 26%. Six percent suffered permanent injury, but the majority (68%) had either no or only temporary injury. Mortality was 4% in patients classified as ASA physical status 1 and 2 compared with 37% in those with ASA physical status 3 to 5. As in adults, increased mortality risk is associated with ASA physical status 3 or greater and with emergency surgery.

Most cardiac arrests occurred during induction of anesthesia; bradycardia, hypotension, and a low SpO_2 frequently preceded arrest. Most arrests were judged to be medication related (Figure 42–2). Cardiovascular depression from halothane, alone or in combination with other drugs, was believed to be responsible for two-thirds of all medication-related arrests. Another 9% were due to intravascular injection of a local anesthetic, most often following negative aspiration before attempted caudal injection.

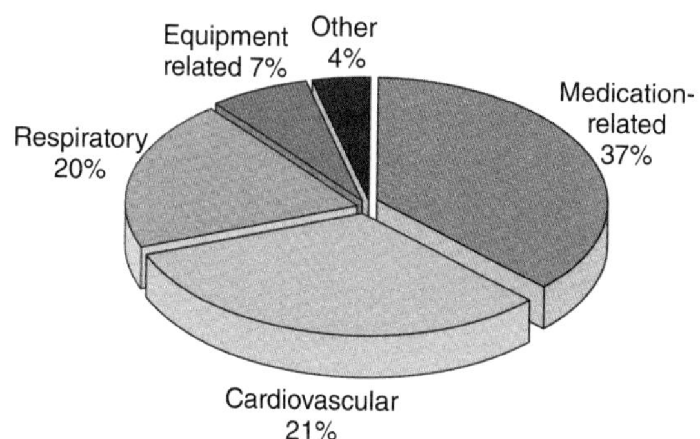

FIGURE 42–2 Mechanisms of cardiac arrest in pediatric patients, based on POCA Registry data.

Presumed cardiovascular mechanisms most often had no clear etiology; in more than 50% of those cases, the patient had congenital heart disease. Where a cardiovascular mechanism could be identified, it was most often related to hemorrhage, transfusion, or inadequate or inappropriate fluid therapy. These studies await replication in the modern, virtually "halothane-free" era in which regional techniques (and, presumably, the attendant risks) are markedly more prevalent.

Respiratory mechanisms of injury included laryngospasm, airway obstruction, and difficult intubation (in decreasing order). In most cases, the laryngospasm occurred during induction. Nearly all patients who experienced arrest in association with airway obstruction or difficult intubation had at least one major underlying disease.

The most common equipment-related cardiac arrests occurred during attempted central venous catheterization (eg, pneumothorax, hemothorax, or cardiac tamponade).

In recent years, increased scientific interest and public concern have focused on whether general anesthetic agents are toxic to the brains of infants and young children. The experimental data in animals have been consistently worrisome, but the clinical data currently available have not identified adverse outcomes comparable with those observed in animals. Progress in this area can be followed on the SmartTots website (www.smarttots.org), maintained by the International Anesthesia Research Society (see Chapter 8).

Children are at greater risk than adults of developing malignant hyperthermia. This complex and important topic is covered in depth in Chapter 52.

PEDIATRIC ANESTHETIC TECHNIQUES

Preoperative Considerations

A. Preoperative Interview

Depending on age, experiences, and maturity, children present with varying degrees of fright when faced with the prospect of procedures requiring anesthesia. Unlike adults, who are usually most concerned about the possibility of injury or death, children, when they verbalize their concerns, worry about pain and separation from their parents. Age-appropriate brochures and videos or tours can help prepare both children and parents. When time permits, one can demystify the process of anesthesia and surgery by explaining in age-appropriate terms what lies ahead. For example, the anesthesiologist might bring an anesthesia mask for the child to play with during the interview and describe it as something the astronauts use. In some centers, parents may be allowed to attend during preanesthetic preparations and induction of anesthesia. This can have a particularly calming influence on children undergoing repeated procedures (eg, administration of intrathecal chemotherapy). Unfortunately, outpatient and "same-day admit" surgery, coupled with a busy operating room schedule, often make it hard to adequately reassure parents and patients. Thus, premedication (discussed below) can be helpful. Some pediatric hospitals have induction rooms adjacent to their operating rooms to permit parental attendance and a quieter environment for anesthetic inductions.

B. Recent Upper Respiratory Tract Infection

Children frequently present for surgery with signs and symptoms—a runny nose with fever, cough, or sore throat—of a viral upper respiratory tract infection (URI). Attempts should be made to differentiate between an infectious cause of rhinorrhea and an
9 allergic or vasomotor cause. A viral infection within 2 to 4 weeks before general anesthesia and endotracheal intubation places the child at increased risk for perioperative pulmonary complications, including wheezing (10-fold), laryngospasm (5-fold), hypoxemia, and atelectasis. This is particularly likely if the child has a severe cough, high fever, or a family history of reactive airway disease. On the other hand, children can have mild URIs on a nearly monthly basis. It can become nearly impossible to schedule them for anesthesia at a time when they neither currently have, nor are recovering from, a URI. The decision to anesthetize children with URIs remains controversial and should be based on the severity of URI symptoms, the urgency of the surgery, and the presence of other coexisting illnesses. When anesthesia will be provided to a child with a URI, one may consider premedication with an anticholinergic or inhaled albuterol, avoiding intubation (if feasible) and humidifying inspired gases. A longer-than-usual stay in the postanesthesia recovery area may be required.

C. Laboratory Tests

Few, if any, preoperative laboratory tests are cost effective. Some pediatric centers require *no* preoperative laboratory tests in *healthy* children undergoing *minor* procedures. Obviously, this places responsibility on the anesthesiologist, surgeon, and pediatrician to correctly identify those patients who need preoperative testing for specific reasons.

Most asymptomatic patients with cardiac murmurs do not have significant cardiac pathology. Innocent murmurs may occur in more than 30% of normal children. These are typically soft, short systolic ejection murmurs that are best heard along the left upper or left lower sternal border and do not radiate. Innocent murmurs at the left upper sternal border typically are due to flow across the pulmonic valve (pulmonic ejection), whereas those at the lower left border typically are due to flow from the left ventricle to the aorta (Still's vibratory murmur). The pediatrician should carefully evaluate patients with a newly diagnosed murmur, particularly in infancy. Consultation with a pediatric cardiologist, echocardiography, or both should be obtained if the patient is symptomatic (eg, poor feeding, failure to thrive, easy fatigability). Murmurs that are loud, "harsh," holosystolic, diastolic, or radiate widely—or pulses that are either bounding or markedly diminished—require further evaluation and diagnosis.

D. Preoperative Fasting

Because children are more prone to dehydration than adults, their preoperative fluid restriction has always been more lenient. Several studies, however, have documented low gastric pH (<2.5) and relatively high residual volumes in pediatric patients scheduled for surgery, suggesting that children may be at a greater risk for aspiration than was previously thought. The incidence of aspiration is reported to be approximately 1:1000. *There is no evidence that prolonged fasting decreases the risk of aspiration.* In fact, several studies have demonstrated lower residual volumes and higher gastric pH in pediatric patients who received clear fluids a few hours before induction (see Chapter 53). The guideline on preoperative fasting produced by the American Society of Anesthesiologists specifies that infants may be fed breast milk up to 4 h before induction, and formula or liquids and a "light" meal may be given up to 6 h before induction. Clear fluids are offered until 2 h before induction. These recommendations are for healthy neonates, infants, and children without risk factors for decreased gastric emptying or aspiration. In any case, there is almost no clinical evidence for the recommendations.

E. Premedication

Sedative premedication is generally omitted for neonates and sick infants. Children who appear likely to exhibit uncontrollable separation anxiety may be given a sedative, such as midazolam (0.3–0.5 mg/kg, 15 mg maximum). The oral route is generally preferred because it is less traumatic than an intramuscular injection, but it requires 20 to 45 min for effect. Smaller doses of midazolam have been used in combination with oral ketamine (4–6 mg/kg) for inpatients. For uncooperative patients, intramuscular midazolam (0.1–0.15 mg/kg, 10 mg maximum) or ketamine (2–3 mg/kg) with atropine (0.02 mg/kg) may be helpful. Rectal midazolam (0.5–1 mg/kg, 20 mg maximum) or rectal methohexital (25–30 mg/kg of 10% solution) may also be administered in such cases while the child is in the parent's arms. Some clinicians administer dexmedetomidine (1–2 mcg/kg) or midazolam premedication intranasally. Fentanyl can also be administered as a lollipop (Actiq, 5–15 mcg/kg); however, fentanyl levels continue to rise intraoperatively and can contribute to postoperative analgesia.

In the past, young children routinely received anticholinergic drugs to prevent bradycardia. Atropine reduces the incidence of hypotension during induction in neonates and in infants younger than 3 months. Atropine can also prevent the accumulation of secretions that can block small airways and endotracheal tubes. Secretions can be particularly troublesome for children with URIs or those who have been given ketamine. Atropine may be administered orally (0.05 mg/kg), intramuscularly, or, occasionally, rectally. In current practice, most prefer to administer atropine intravenously during induction.

Monitoring

Monitoring requirements for infants and children are generally similar to those for adults with some minor modifications. Alarm limits (eg, for heart rate) should be appropriately adjusted. Smaller electrocardiographic electrode pads may be useful to avoid encroaching on surgical fields. Blood pressure cuffs must be properly sized and positioned. Noninvasive blood pressure monitors are reliable in infants and children. A precordial or esophageal stethoscope provides an inexpensive means of monitoring heart rate, the quality of heart sounds, and airway patency. Monitors may sometimes need to be first attached (or reattached) following induction of anesthesia in less cooperative patients.

Pulse oximetry and capnography assume an even more important role in infants and small children because hypoxemia and inadequate ventilation remain common causes of perioperative morbidity and mortality. In neonates, the pulse oximeter probe should preferably be placed on the right hand or earlobe to measure preductal oxygen saturation. As in adult patients, end-tidal CO_2 analysis allows assessment of the adequacy of ventilation, changes in cardiac output, confirmation of endotracheal tube placement, and early warning of malignant hyperthermia. Flow-through (mainstream) analyzers are usually less accurate in patients weighing less than 10 kg. Even with aspiration (sidestream) capnographs, the inspired (baseline) CO_2 can appear falsely elevated, and the expired (peak) CO_2 can be falsely low. The degree of error can be minimized by placing the sampling site as close as possible to the distal tip of the endotracheal tube, reducing the length of the sampling line and lowering gas-sampling flow rates (100–150 mL/min).

10 Temperature must be closely monitored in pediatric patients because of their greater risk for malignant hyperthermia and greater susceptibility for intraoperative hypothermia or hyperthermia. The risk of hypothermia can be reduced by maintaining a warm operating room environment (26°C or warmer), warming and humidifying inspired gases, using a warming blanket and warming lights, and warming all intravenous and irrigation fluids. These concerns, while important in all patients, are critically important in newborns. Care must be taken to prevent accidental burns and hyperthermia from overzealous warming efforts.

Invasive monitors (eg, arterial cannulation, central venous catheterization) demand expertise and judgment. Air bubbles must be removed from pressure tubing, and small volume flushes should be used to avoid air embolism, unintended heparinization, or fluid overload. The right radial artery is often chosen for cannulation in the neonate because its preductal location mirrors the oxygen content of the carotid and retinal arteries. A femoral artery catheter may be a suitable alternative in very small neonates. Left radial or right or left dorsalis pedis arteries are other alternatives. Critically ill neonates may retain an umbilical artery catheter. Internal jugular and subclavian approaches are often used for central lines. Ultrasonography should be used during placement of internal jugular catheters and provides useful information for arterial cannulation as well. Urinary output is an important (but neither sensitive nor specific) indicator of the adequacy of intravascular volume and cardiac output. Noninvasive monitors of stroke volume have only recently been tested in infants and young children.

Premature or small-for-gestational-age neonates, neonates who have received total parenteral nutrition, or neonates whose mothers have diabetes are prone to hypoglycemia. These infants should have frequent blood glucose measurements; levels below 30 mg/dL in the neonate, below 40 mg/dL in infants, and below 60 mg/dL in children (and below 80 mg/dL in adults) indicate hypoglycemia requiring immediate treatment. Blood sampling for arterial blood gases, hemoglobin, potassium, and ionized calcium concentration can be invaluable in critically ill patients undergoing major surgery or receiving transfusions.

Induction

General anesthesia is usually induced by an intravenous or inhalational technique. Induction with intramuscular ketamine (5–10 mg/kg) is reserved for specific situations, such as those involving combative, particularly mentally challenged, or autistic patients. Intravenous induction is usually preferred when the patient comes to the operating room with a functional intravenous catheter or will allow awake venous cannulation. Prior application of EMLA (*eutectic mixture of local anesthetic*) cream (see Chapter 16) may render intravenous cannulation less painful for the patient and less stressful for the parent and anesthesiologist. However, EMLA cream is neither a perfect nor a complete solution. Some children become anxious at the sight of a needle, particularly those who have had multiple needle punctures in the past, with or without EMLA. Furthermore, it can be difficult to anticipate in which extremity intravenous cannulation will prove to be successful. Finally, to be effective, EMLA cream must remain in contact with the skin for at least 30 to 60 min. Awake or sedated-awake intubation with topical anesthesia should be considered for emergency procedures in neonates and small infants when they are critically ill or a potentially difficult airway is present.

Intravenous Induction

The same induction sequence can be used as in adults: propofol (2–3 mg/kg) followed by a nondepolarizing muscle relaxant (eg, rocuronium, cisatracurium, atracurium), or succinylcholine. We routinely administer atropine prior to succinylcholine. The advantages of an intravenous technique include the availability of intravenous access if emergency drugs need to be administered and the rapidity of induction in the child at risk for aspiration. Alternatively (and very commonly in pediatric practice), intubation can be accomplished after the combination of propofol, lidocaine, and an opiate, with or without an inhaled agent, avoiding the need for a paralytic agent. Finally, paralytic agents are not needed for the placement of LMAs, which are commonly used in pediatric anesthesia.

Inhalational Induction

Most children do not arrive in the operating room with an intravenous line in place, and nearly all dread the prospect of being stuck with a needle. Fortunately, sevoflurane can render small children unconscious within minutes. We find this easier in children who have been sedated (most often with oral midazolam) prior to entering the operating room and who are sleepy enough to be anesthetized without ever knowing what has happened (*steal induction*). One can also insufflate the anesthetic gases over the face, place a drop of food flavoring on the inside of the mask (eg, oil of orange), and allow the child to sit during the early stages of induction. Specially contoured masks minimize dead space (see Figure 19–11).

There are many differences between adult and pediatric anatomy that influence mask ventilation and intubation. Equipment appropriate for age and size should be selected (Table 42–6). Neonates and most young infants are obligate nasal breathers and obstruct easily. Oral airways will help displace an oversized tongue; nasal airways, so useful in adults, can traumatize small nares or prominent adenoids in small children. Compression of submandibular soft tissues should be avoided during mask ventilation to prevent upper airway obstruction.

Typically, the child can be coaxed into breathing an odorless mixture of nitrous oxide (70%) and oxygen (30%). Sevoflurane (or halothane) can be added to the gas mixture in 0.5% increments every few breaths. As previously discussed, we favor sevoflurane in most situations. Desflurane and isoflurane are avoided for inhalation induction because they are pungent and associated with more coughing, breath-holding, and laryngospasm. We use a single (sometimes two) breath induction technique with sevoflurane (7–8% sevoflurane in 60% nitrous oxide) to speed the induction in cooperative patients. After an adequate depth of anesthesia has been achieved, an intravenous line can be started, and propofol and an opioid (or a muscle relaxant) can be administered to facilitate intubation. Patients typically pass through an excitement stage during which any stimulation can induce laryngospasm. Breath-holding must be distinguished from laryngospasm. Steady application of 10 cm of positive end-expiratory pressure will usually overcome laryngospasm.

TABLE 42–6 Sizing of airway equipment in children.

	Premature	Neonate	Infant	Toddler	Small Child	Large Child
Age	0–1 month	0–1 month	1–12 months	1–3 years	3–8 years	8–12 years
Weight (kg)	0.5–3	3–5	4–10	8–16	14–30	25–50
Tracheal (ET)[1] tube (mm i.d.)	2.5–3	3–3.5	3.5–4	4–4.5	4.5–5.5	5.5–6 (cuffed)
ET depth (cm at lips)	6–9	9–10	10–12	12–14	14–16	16–18
Suction catheter (F)	6	6	8	8	10	12
Laryngoscope blade	00	0	1	1.5	2	3
Mask size	00	0	0	1	2	3
Oral airway	000–00	00	0 (40 mm)	1 (50 mm)	2 (70 mm)	3 (80 mm)
Laryngeal mask airway (LMA#)	—	1	1	2	2.5	3

[1]ET, endotracheal tube.

Alternatively, the anesthesiologist can deepen the level of anesthesia by increasing the concentration of volatile anesthetic and place an LMA or intubate the patient under "deep" sevoflurane anesthesia. Because of the greater anesthetic depth required for tracheal intubation, the risk of cardiac depression, bradycardia, or laryngospasm occurring without intravenous access detracts from this latter technique. Intramuscular succinylcholine (4 mg/kg, not to exceed 150 mg) and atropine (0.02 mg/kg, not to exceed 0.4 mg) should be available if laryngospasm or bradycardia occurs before an intravenous line is established.

Positive-pressure ventilation during mask induction and prior to intubation sometimes causes gastric distention, with impairment of lung expansion. Suctioning with an orogastric or nasogastric tube will decompress the stomach, but it must be done without traumatizing fragile mucous membranes.

Intravenous Access

Intravenous cannulation in infants can be a vexing ordeal, particularly for infants who have spent weeks in a neonatal intensive care unit and have few intact veins. Even healthy 1-year-old children can prove a challenge because of extensive subcutaneous fat. Venous cannulation usually becomes easier after 2 years of age. The saphenous vein has a consistent location at the ankle, and an experienced practitioner can usually cannulate it even if it is not visible or palpable. Transillumination of the hands or ultrasonography will often reveal previously hidden cannulation sites. Twenty-four-gauge over-the-needle catheters are adequate in neonates and infants when blood transfusions are not anticipated. All air bubbles should be removed from the intravenous line to reduce the risk of paradoxical air embolism from occult patent foramen ovale. In emergency situations where intravenous access is impossible, fluids can be effectively infused through an 18-gauge needle inserted into the medullary sinusoids within the tibial bone. This intraosseous infusion can be used for all medications normally given intravenously, with almost as rapid results (see Chapter 55), and is considered part of the standard trauma resuscitation, advanced cardiac life support (ACLS), and pediatric advanced life support (PALS) protocols when intravenous access cannot be obtained.

Tracheal Intubation

One hundred percent oxygen should be administered prior to the obligatory period of apnea during intubation. The choice of muscle relaxant has been discussed earlier in this chapter. For awake intubations in neonates or infants, adequate preoxygenation and continued oxygen insufflation during laryngoscopy may help prevent hypoxemia.

The infant's prominent occiput tends to place the head in a flexed position prior to intubation. This is easily corrected by slightly elevating the shoulders on towels and placing the head on a doughnut-shaped pillow. In older children, prominent tonsillar tissue can obstruct visualization of the larynx. Straight laryngoscope blades aid intubation of the anterior larynx in neonates, infants, and young children (see Table 42–6). Endotracheal tubes that pass through the glottis may still impinge upon the cricoid cartilage, which is the narrowest point of the airway in children younger than 5 years of age. Mucosal trauma from trying to force a tube through the cricoid cartilage can cause postoperative edema, stridor, croup, and airway obstruction.

The appropriate diameter inside the endotracheal tube can be estimated by a formula based on age:

$$4 + \text{Age}/4 = \text{Tube diameter (in mm)}$$

For example, a 4-year-old child would be predicted to require a 5-mm uncuffed tube. This formula provides only a rough guideline, however. Exceptions include premature neonates (2.5–3 mm tube) and full-term neonates (3–3.5 mm tube). Alternatively, the practitioner can remember that a newborn takes a 2.5- or 3-mm tube and a 5-year-old takes a 5-mm tube. It should not be that difficult to identify which of the three sizes of tube between 3 and 5 mm is required in small children. In larger children, small (5–6 mm) cuffed tubes can be used either with or without the cuff inflated to minimize the need for precise sizing. Endotracheal tubes 0.5 mm larger and smaller than predicted should be readily available in or on the anesthetic cart. In the past, uncuffed endotracheal tubes were recommended for children aged 5 years or younger in the hope of decreasing the risk of postintubation croup. Currently, many anesthesiologists no longer use size 4.0 or larger uncuffed tubes. The leak test will minimize the likelihood that an excessively large tube has been inserted. Correct tube size and appropriate cuff inflation is confirmed by easy passage into the larynx and the development of a gas leak at 15 to 25 cm H_2O pressure. No leak indicates an oversized tube or overinflated cuff that should be replaced or deflated to prevent postoperative edema, whereas an excessive leak may preclude adequate ventilation and contaminate the operating room with anesthetic gases. As previously noted, many clinicians use a down-sized cuffed tube in younger patients at high risk for aspiration; minimal inflation of the cuff can stop any air leak. There is also a formula to estimate endotracheal length:

$$12 + \text{Age}/2 = \text{Length of tube (in cm)}$$

Again, this formula provides only a guideline, and the result must be confirmed by auscultation and clinical judgment. To avoid endobronchial intubation, the tip of the endotracheal tube should pass only 1 to 2 cm beyond an infant's glottis. Alternatively, one can intentionally advance the tip of the endotracheal tube into the right mainstem bronchus and then withdraw it until breath sounds are equal over both lung fields.

Maintenance

Ventilation is almost always controlled during anesthesia of neonates and infants when using a conventional semiclosed circle system. During spontaneous ventilation, even the low resistance of a circle system can become a significant obstacle for a sick neonate to overcome. Unidirectional valves, breathing tubes, and carbon dioxide absorbers account for most of this resistance. For patients weighing less than 10 kg, some anesthesiologists prefer the Mapleson D circuit or the Bain system because of their low resistance and light weight (see Chapter 3). Nonetheless, because breathing-circuit resistance is easily overcome by positive-pressure ventilation, the circle system can be safely used in patients of all ages if ventilation is controlled. Monitoring of airway pressure may provide early evidence of obstruction from a kinked endotracheal tube or accidental advancement of the tube into a mainstem bronchus.

Many anesthesia ventilators on older machines are designed for adult patients and cannot reliably provide the reduced tidal volumes and rapid rates required by neonates and infants. Unintentional delivery of large tidal volumes to a small child can generate excessive peak airway pressures and cause barotrauma. Pressure control ventilation, which is found on nearly all newer anesthesia ventilators, should be used for neonates, infants, and toddlers. Small tidal volumes can also be manually delivered with greater ease with a 1-L breathing bag than with a 3-L adult bag. For children less than 10 kg, adequate tidal volumes are achieved with peak inspiratory pressures of 15 to 18 cm H_2O. For larger children, the volume control ventilation may be used, and tidal volumes may be set at 6 to 8 mL/kg. Many spirometers are less accurate at lower tidal volumes. In addition, the gas lost in long, compliant adult breathing circuits becomes large relative to a child's small tidal volume. For this reason, pediatric breathing circuits are usually shorter, lighter, and stiffer (less compliant). Nevertheless, one should recall that the additional dead space contributed by the tube and circle system consists only of the volume of the distal limb of the Y-connector and that portion of the endotracheal tube that extends beyond (proximal to) the airway. In other words, the dead space is unchanged by switching from adult to pediatric breathing circuits. Condenser humidifiers or heat and moisture exchangers (HMEs) can add considerable dead space; depending on the size of the patient, either they should not be used, or an appropriately sized pediatric HME should be employed.

Anesthesia can be maintained in pediatric patients with the same agents as in adults. Some clinicians switch to isoflurane following a sevoflurane induction in the hope of reducing the likelihood of emergence agitation or postoperative delirium (see earlier discussion). Administration of an opioid (eg, fentanyl, 1–1.5 mcg/kg) or dexmedetomidine (0.5 mcg/kg, given slowly with heart rate monitoring) 15 to 20 min before the end of the procedure can reduce the incidence of emergence delirium and agitation if the surgical procedure is likely to produce postoperative pain. Although the MAC is greater in children than in adults (see Table 42–4), neonates may be particularly susceptible to the cardiac-depressing effects of general anesthetics and may not tolerate the concentrations of volatile agents required when the volatile agent alone is used to maintain good surgical operating conditions.

Perioperative Fluid Requirements

11 Meticulous attention to fluid intake and loss is required in younger pediatric patients because these patients have limited margins for error. A programmable infusion pump or a buret with a microdrip chamber are useful for accurate measurements. Drugs can be flushed through low-dead-space tubing to minimize unnecessary fluid. Fluid overload is diagnosed by prominent veins, flushed skin, increased blood pressure, decreased serum sodium, and a loss of the folds in the upper eyelids.

Fluid therapy can be divided into maintenance, deficit, and replacement requirements.

A. Maintenance Fluid Requirements

Maintenance requirements for pediatric patients can be determined by the "4:2:1 rule": 4 mL/kg/h for the first 10 kg of weight, 2 mL/kg/h for the second 10 kg, and 1 mL/kg/h for each remaining kilogram. The choice of maintenance fluid remains controversial. A solution such as D_5½ NS with 20 mEq/L of potassium chloride provides adequate dextrose and electrolytes at these maintenance infusion rates. D_5¼ NS may be a better choice in neonates because of their limited ability to handle sodium loads. Children up to the age of 8 years require 6 mg/kg/min of glucose to maintain euglycemia (40–125 mg/dL); premature neonates require 6–8 mg/kg/min. Euglycemia is normally well maintained in older children and adults by hepatic glycogenolysis and gluconeogenesis despite the administration of glucose-free solutions. Both hypoglycemia and hyperglycemia should be avoided; however, the amount of hepatic glucose production is widely variable during major surgery and critical illness. Thus, glucose infusion rates during longer surgeries, particularly in neonates and infants, should be adjusted based on blood glucose measurements.

B. Deficits

In addition to a maintenance infusion, any preoperative fluid deficits must be replaced. For example, if a 5-kg infant has not received oral or intravenous fluids for 4 h prior to surgery, a deficit of 80 mL has accrued (5 kg × 4 mL/kg/h × 4 h). In contrast to adults, infants respond to dehydration with decreased blood pressure and without increased heart rate. Preoperative fluid deficits are often administered with hourly maintenance requirements in aliquots of 50% in the first hour and 25% in the second and third hours. In the example above, a total of 60 mL would be given in the first hour (80/2 + 20) and 40 mL in the second and third hours (80/4 + 20). Bolus administration of dextrose-containing solutions should be avoided to prevent hyperglycemia. Preoperative fluid deficits are usually replaced with a balanced salt solution (eg, lactated Ringer's injection) or ½ normal saline. Normal saline has the disadvantage of promoting hyperchloremic acidosis.

C. Replacement Requirements

Replacement can be subdivided into blood loss and third-space loss.

1. Blood loss—The blood volume of premature neonates (100 mL/kg), full-term neonates (85–90 mL/kg), and infants (80 mL/kg) is proportionately larger than that of adults (65–75 mL/kg). An initial hematocrit of 55% in the healthy full-term neonate gradually falls to as low as 30% in the 3-month-old infant before rising to 35% by 6 months. Hemoglobin (Hb) type is also changing during this period: from a 75% concentration of HbF (greater oxygen affinity, reduced PaO_2, poor tissue unloading) at birth to almost 100% HbA (reduced oxygen affinity, high PaO_2, good tissue unloading) by 6 months.

Blood loss has been typically replaced with non–glucose-containing crystalloid (eg, 3 mL of lactated Ringer's injection for each milliliter of blood lost) or colloid solutions (eg, 1 mL of 5% albumin for each milliliter of blood lost) until the patient's hematocrit reaches a predetermined lower limit. In recent years, there has been increased emphasis on avoiding excessive fluid administration; thus blood loss is now commonly replaced by either colloid (eg, albumin) or packed red blood cells. In premature and sick neonates, the target hematocrit (for transfusion) may be as great as 40%, whereas in healthy older children, a hematocrit of 20% to 26% is generally well tolerated. Because of their small intravascular volume, neonates and infants are at an increased risk for electrolyte disturbances (eg, hyperglycemia, hyperkalemia, hypocalcemia) that can accompany rapid blood transfusion. Dosing of packed red blood cell transfusions is discussed in Chapter 51. Platelets and fresh frozen plasma, 10 to 15 mL/kg, should be given when blood loss exceeds one to two blood volumes. Recent practice, particularly with blood loss from trauma, favors "earlier" administration of plasma and platelets as part of a massive transfusion protocol. One unit of platelets per 10 kg weight raises the platelet count by about 50,000/μL. The pediatric dose of cryoprecipitate is 1 unit/10 kg weight.

2. "Third-space" loss—These losses are impossible to measure and must be estimated by the extent of the surgical procedure. In recent years, some investigators have questioned the very existence of the third space, and some have asserted that the third space exists as a consequence of excessive fluid administration.

One popular fluid administration guideline is 0 to 2 mL/kg/h for relatively atraumatic surgery (eg, strabismus correction where there should be *no* third-space loss) and up to 6 to 10 mL/kg/h for traumatic procedures (eg, abdominal abscess). Third-space loss is usually replaced with lactated Ringer's injection (see Chapter 49). It is safe to say that all issues relating to the third space have never been more controversial.

Regional Anesthesia & Analgesia

The primary uses of regional techniques in pediatric anesthesia have been to supplement and reduce general anesthetic requirements and to provide better postoperative pain relief. Blocks range in complexity from relatively simple peripheral nerve blocks (eg, penile block, ilioinguinal block); to brachial plexus, sciatic nerve, femoral nerve, and transversus abdominis plane (TAP) blocks; to major conduction blocks (eg, spinal or epidural techniques). Regional blocks in children (as in adults) are often facilitated by ultrasound guidance, less commonly with nerve stimulation.

Caudal blocks have proved useful following a variety of surgeries, including circumcision, inguinal herniorrhaphy, hypospadias repair, anal surgery, clubfoot repair, and other subumbilical procedures. Contraindications include infection around the sacral hiatus, coagulopathy, or anatomic abnormalities. The patient is usually lightly anesthetized or sedated and placed in the lateral position.

For pediatric caudal anesthesia, a short-bevel 22-gauge needle can be used. If the loss-of-resistance technique is used, the glass syringe should be filled with saline, not air, because of the latter's possible association with air embolism. After the characteristic pop that signals penetration of the sacrococcygeal membrane, the needle angle of approach is reduced, and the needle is advanced only a few more millimeters to avoid entering the dural sac or the anterior body of the sacrum. Aspiration is used to check for blood or cerebrospinal fluid; local anesthetic can then be slowly injected; failure of a 2-mL test dose of local anesthetic with epinephrine (1:200,000) to produce tachycardia helps exclude intravascular placement.

Many anesthetic agents have been used for caudal anesthesia in pediatric patients, with 0.125% to 0.25% bupivacaine or 0.2% ropivacaine being the most common. Ropivacaine appears to have less cardiac toxicity than bupivacaine when compared milligram to milligram. The addition of epinephrine to caudal solutions tends to increase the degree of motor block. Clonidine, either by itself or combined with local anesthetics, has also been widely used. Morphine sulfate (25 mcg/kg) or hydromorphone (6 mcg/kg) may be added to the local anesthetic solution to prolong postoperative analgesia for inpatients, but it will increase the risk of delayed postoperative respiratory depression. The volume of local anesthetic required depends on the level of blockade desired, ranging from 0.5 mL/kg for a sacral block to 1.25 mL/kg for a midthoracic block. Single-shot injections generally last 4 to 12 h. Placement of 20-gauge caudal catheters with continuous infusion of local anesthetic (eg, 0.125% bupivacaine or 0.1% ropivacaine at 0.2–0.4 mg/kg/h) or an opioid (eg, fentanyl, 2 mcg/mL at 0.6 mcg/kg/h) allows prolonged anesthesia and postoperative analgesia. Complications are rare but include local anesthetic toxicity from increased blood concentrations (eg, seizures, hypotension, arrhythmias), spinal blockade, and respiratory depression. Urinary retention is not a problem following single-dose caudal anesthesia.

Lumbar and thoracic epidural catheters can be placed in anesthetized children using the standard loss-of-resistance technique and either a midline or paramedian approach. In small children, caudal epidural catheters have been passed into a thoracic position with the tip localized radiographically.

Unilateral transversus abdominis plane (TAP) blocks are commonly used to provide analgesia after hernia repair. Bilateral TAP blocks can be used to provide effective postoperative analgesia after abdominal surgery with a lower midline incision. Rectus sheath blocks can be used for a midline incision in the upper abdomen.

Spinal anesthesia has been used in some centers for infraumbilical procedures in neonates and infants. Infants and children typically have minimal hypotension from sympathectomy. Intravenous access can be established (conveniently in the foot) after the spinal anesthetic has been administered. This technique has become more widely used for neonates and infants as the potential risk of neurotoxicity from general anesthesia has received greater attention.

Many children will not tolerate placement of nerve blocks or nerve block catheters while awake; however, most peripheral block techniques can be performed safely in anesthetized children. When the area of operation is the upper extremity, we recommend those brachial plexus procedures that can most readily be performed using ultrasound guidance, specifically axillary, supraclavicular, and infraclavicular blocks. We suggest that interscalene block be performed in anesthetized patients only by those with experience and skill with ultrasound guidance and only for procedures where other block techniques would be less effective (eg, upper shoulder procedures) because of the reported rare occurrence of accidental intramedullary injections when interscalene blocks were performed in anesthetized adults. Single-shot and continuous femoral, adductor canal, and sciatic blocks are easily performed in children using ultrasound guidance. The latter can be performed using either a gluteal or a popliteal approach.

A wide variety of other terminal nerve blocks (eg, digital nerve, median nerve, occipital nerve, etc) are easily performed to reduce postoperative pain in children.

Sedation for Procedures In & Out of the Operating Room

Sedation is often requested for pediatric patients inside and outside the operating room for nonsurgical procedures. Cooperation and motionlessness may be required for imaging studies, bronchoscopy, gastrointestinal endoscopy, cardiac catheterization, dressing changes, and minor procedures (eg, casting and bone marrow aspiration). Requirements vary depending on the patient and the procedure, ranging from anxiolysis (minimal sedation) to conscious sedation (moderate sedation and analgesia), to deep sedation/analgesia, and finally to general anesthesia. Anesthesiologists are held to the same standards whether they provide moderate or deep sedation or they provide general anesthesia. This includes preoperative preparation (eg, fasting), assessment, monitoring, and postoperative care. Airway obstruction and hypoventilation are the most commonly encountered problems associated with moderate or deep sedation. Cardiovascular depression is a risk with deep sedation or general anesthesia.

Table 42–3 includes doses of sedative-hypnotic drugs. One of the sedatives commonly used by nonanesthesia personnel in the past was chloral hydrate, 25 to 100 mg/kg orally or rectally. It has a slow onset of up to 60 min and a long half-life (8–11 h) that results in prolonged somnolence. Chloral hydrate is a poor choice given its propensity for producing cardiac arrhythmias at the larger doses needed for moderate sedation. Midazolam, 0.5 mg/kg orally or 0.1 to 0.15 mg/kg intravenously, is particularly useful because its effects can be readily reversed with flumazenil. Doses should be reduced whenever more than one agent is used because of the potential for synergistic respiratory and cardiovascular depression.

Propofol is by far the most useful sedative-hypnotic drug, though the drug is not approved for sedation of pediatric ICU patients and is not approved for administration by anyone other than those trained in the administration of general anesthesia.

In countries other than the United States, propofol is often administered using the Diprifusor, a computer-controlled infusion pump that maintains a constant target site concentration. Supplemental oxygen and close monitoring of the airway, ventilation, and other vital signs are mandatory (as with other agents). An LMA is usually well tolerated at higher propofol doses.

For imaging studies, intranasal dexmedetomidine has also proven useful, especially with infants who do not have or need intravenous access.

Emergence & Recovery

Pediatric patients are particularly vulnerable to two common postanesthetic complications: laryngospasm and postintubation croup. As with adult patients, postoperative pain requires close, careful attention. Pediatric anesthesia practice varies widely, particularly in regard to extubation following a general anesthetic. In some pediatric hospitals, all children who will be extubated after a general anesthetic arrive in the postanesthesia care unit (PACU) with the tube or LMA still in place. They are subsequently extubated by the PACU nurse when defined criteria are reached. In other centers, nearly all children are extubated in the operating room before arriving in the PACU. High quality and safety are reported at centers following either protocol.

A. Laryngospasm

Laryngospasm is a forceful, involuntary spasm of the laryngeal musculature caused by stimulation of the superior laryngeal nerve (see Chapter 19). It may occur at induction, emergence, or any time in between without an endotracheal tube. Presumably, it can also occur when a tube is in place, but its occurrence will not be recognized. Laryngospasm is more common in young pediatric patients (almost 1 in 50 anesthet-
12 ics) than in adults and is most common in infants 1 to 3 months old. Laryngospasm at the end of a procedure can usually be avoided by extubating the patient either while awake (opening the eyes) or while deeply anesthetized (spontaneously breathing but not swallowing or coughing); both techniques have advocates, and despite strong opinions, evidence is lacking as to which is the better approach. Extubation during the interval between these extremes, however, is generally recognized as more hazardous. Recent URI or exposure to secondhand tobacco smoke predisposes children to laryngospasm on emergence. Treatment of laryngospasm includes gentle positive-pressure ventilation, forward jaw thrust, deepening of the anesthetic with intravenous propofol, intravenous lidocaine (1–1.5 mg/kg), or paralysis with intravenous succinylcholine (0.5–1 mg/kg) or rocuronium (0.4 mg/kg) and controlled ventilation. Intramuscular succinylcholine (4–6 mg/kg) with atropine remains an acceptable alternative in patients without intravenous access and in whom conservative measures have failed. Laryngospasm is usually an immediate postoperative event but may occur in the recovery room as the patient wakes up and chokes on pharyngeal secretions. For this reason, recovering somnolent pediatric patients should be positioned in the lateral position so that oral secretions pool and drain away from the vocal cords. When the child begins to regain consciousness, having the parents at the bedside may reduce their anxiety.

B. Postintubation Croup

Croup is due to glottic or tracheal edema. Because the narrowest part of the pediatric airway is the cricoid cartilage, this is the most susceptible area. Croup is less common with properly sized endotracheal tubes that are small enough to allow a slight gas leak at 10 to 25 cm H_2O. Postintubation croup is associated with early childhood (age 1–4 years), repeated intubation attempts, overly large endotracheal tubes, prolonged surgery, head and neck procedures, and excessive movement of the tube (eg, coughing with the tube in place, moving the patient's head). Intravenous dexamethasone (0.25–0.5 mg/kg) may prevent the formation of edema, and inhalation of nebulized racemic epinephrine (0.25–0.5 mL of a 2.25% solution in 2.5 mL normal saline) is often an effective treatment. Although postintubation croup occurs later than laryngospasm, it will almost always appear within 3 h after extubation.

C. Postoperative Pain Management

Pain in pediatric patients has received considerable attention in recent years, and over that time, the use of regional anesthetic and analgesic techniques (as previously above) has greatly increased. Commonly used parenteral opioids include fentanyl (1–2 mcg/kg), morphine (0.05–0.1 mg/kg), and hydromorphone (15 mcg/kg). A multimodal technique incorporating ketorolac (0.5–0.75 mg/kg) and intravenous dexmedetomidine will reduce opioid requirements. Oral, rectal, or intravenous acetaminophen will also reduce opioid requirements and can be a helpful substitute for ketorolac.

Patient-controlled analgesia (see Chapter 48) can also be successfully used in patients as young as 5 years old, depending on their maturity and on preoperative preparation. Commonly used opioids include morphine and hydromorphone. With a 10-min lockout interval, the recommended interval dose is either morphine, 20 mcg/kg, or hydromorphone, 5 mcg/kg. As with adults, continuous infusions increase the risk of respiratory depression; typical continuous infusion doses are morphine, 0 to 12 mcg/kg/h, or hydromorphone, 0 to 3 mcg/kg/h. The subcutaneous route may be used with morphine. Nurse-controlled and parent-controlled analgesia remain controversial but widely used techniques for pain control in children.

As with adults, epidural infusions for postoperative analgesia often consist of a local anesthetic combined with an opioid. Bupivacaine, 0.1% to 0.125%, or ropivacaine, 0.1% to 0.2%, are often combined with fentanyl, 2 to 2.5 mcg/mL (or equivalent concentrations of morphine or hydromorphone). Recommended infusion rates depend on the size of the patient, the final drug concentration, and the location of the epidural catheter and range from 0.1 to 0.4 mL/kg/h. Local anesthetic infusions can also be used with continuous nerve block techniques, but this is less common than in adults.

Anesthetic Considerations in Specific Pediatric Conditions

PREMATURITY

Pathophysiology

Prematurity is defined as birth before 37 weeks of gestation. This is in contrast to *small for gestational age*, which describes an infant (full-term or premature) whose age-adjusted weight is less than the fifth percentile. The multiple medical problems of premature neonates are usually due to immaturity of major organ systems or to intrauterine asphyxia. Pulmonary complications include hyaline membrane disease, apneic spells, and bronchopulmonary dysplasia. Exogenous pulmonary surfactant has proved to be an effective treatment for respiratory distress syndrome in premature infants. A patent ductus arteriosus leads to shunting and may possibly lead to pulmonary edema and congestive heart failure. Persistent hypoxia or shock may result in ischemic gut and necrotizing enterocolitis. Prematurity increases susceptibility to infection, hypothermia, intracranial hemorrhage, and kernicterus. Premature neonates also have an increased incidence of congenital anomalies.

Anesthetic Considerations

The small size (often <1000 g) and fragile medical condition of premature neonates demand that special attention be paid to airway control, fluid management, and temperature regulation. The problem of *retinopathy of prematurity*, a fibrovascular proliferation overlying the retina that may lead to progressive visual loss, deserves special consideration. Recent evidence suggests that fluctuating oxygen levels may be more damaging than increased oxygen tension. Moreover, other major risk factors, such as respiratory distress, apnea, mechanical ventilation, hypoxia, hypercarbia, acidosis, heart disease, bradycardia, infection, parenteral nutrition, anemia, and multiple blood transfusions, must be present. Nonetheless, oxygenation should be continuously monitored (typically with pulse oximetry), with particular attention given to infants younger than 44 weeks post conception. Normal PaO_2 is 60 to 80 mm Hg in neonates. Excessive inspired oxygen concentrations are avoided by blending oxygen with air. Excessive inspired oxygen tensions can also predispose these patients to chronic lung disease.

Premature neonates have reduced anesthetic requirements. Opioid-based anesthetics are often favored over pure volatile anesthetic-based techniques because of the perceived tendency of the latter to cause myocardial depression.

Premature infants whose age is less than 50 (some authorities would say 60) weeks post conception at the time of surgery are prone to postoperative episodes of obstructive and central apnea for up to 24 h. In fact, even full-term infants can experience rare apneic spells following general anesthesia. **Risk factors for postanesthetic apnea include a low gestational age at birth, anemia (<30%), hypothermia, sepsis, and neurological abnormalities**. The risk of postanesthetic apnea may be decreased by intravenous administration of caffeine (10 mg/kg) or aminophylline.

Thus, elective (particularly outpatient) procedures should be deferred until the preterm infant reaches the age of at least 50 weeks post conception. A 6-month symptom-free interval has been suggested for infants with a history of apneic episodes or bronchopulmonary dysplasia. If surgery must be performed earlier, monitoring with pulse oximetry for 12 to 24 h postoperatively is mandatory for infants less than 50 weeks post conception; infants between 50 and 60 weeks conception should be closely observed in the postanesthesia recovery unit for at least 2 h.

Sick, premature neonates often receive multiple transfusions of blood during their stay in the intensive care nursery. Their immunocompromised status predisposes them to cytomegalovirus infection following transfusion. Preventive measures include transfusing only with leukocyte-reduced red blood cells.

INTESTINAL MALROTATION & VOLVULUS

Pathophysiology

Malrotation of the intestines is a developmental abnormality that permits spontaneous abnormal rotation of the midgut around the mesentery (superior mesenteric artery). The incidence of malrotation is estimated to be about 1:500 live births. Most patients with malrotation of the midgut present during infancy with symptoms of bowel obstruction. Coiling of the duodenum with the ascending colon can produce complete or partial duodenal obstruction. The most serious complication of malrotation, a midgut volvulus, can rapidly compromise intestinal blood supply causing infarction. Midgut volvulus is a true surgical emergency that most commonly occurs in infancy, with up to one-third occurring in the first week of life. The mortality rate is high (up to 25%). Typical symptoms are bilious vomiting, progressive abdominal distention and tenderness, metabolic acidosis, and hemodynamic instability. Bloody diarrhea may be indicative of bowel infarction. Upper gastrointestinal imaging confirms the diagnosis.

Anesthetic Considerations

Surgery provides the only definitive treatment of malrotation and midgut volvulus. If an obstruction is present but obvious volvulus has not yet occurred, preoperative preparation may include stabilization of any coexisting conditions, insertion of a nasogastric (or orogastric tube) to decompress the stomach, broad-spectrum antibiotics, and fluid and electrolyte replacement before prompt transport to the operating room.

These patients are at increased risk for pulmonary aspiration. Depending on the size of the patient, rapid sequence induction (or awake intubation) should be employed. Patients with volvulus are usually hypovolemic and acidotic and may be prone to hypotension. Postoperative ventilation will often be necessary, making an opioid-based anesthetic a reasonable choice. Fluid resuscitation, likely including blood products, with correction of acidosis is usually necessary. Arterial and central venous lines are helpful. Surgical treatment includes reducing the volvulus, freeing the obstruction, and resecting any obviously necrotic bowel. Bowel edema can complicate abdominal closure and has the potential to produce an abdominal compartment syndrome. The latter can impair ventilation, hinder venous return, and produce acute kidney injury; delayed fascial closure may be necessary. A second-look laparotomy may be required 24 to 48 h later to ensure viability of the remaining bowel and close the abdomen.

CONGENITAL DIAPHRAGMATIC HERNIA

Pathophysiology

During fetal development, the gut can herniate into the thorax through one of three diaphragmatic defects: the left or right posterolateral foramina of Bochdalek or the anterior foramen of Morgagni. The reported incidence of diaphragmatic hernia is 1 in

3000 to 5000 live births. Left-sided herniation is the most common type (90%). Hallmarks of **diaphragmatic herniation** include hypoxemia, a scaphoid abdomen, and evidence of bowel in the thorax by auscultation or imaging. Congenital diaphragmatic hernia is often diagnosed antenatally during a routine obstetric ultrasound examination. A reduction in alveoli and bronchioli (pulmonary hypoplasia) and malrotation of the intestines are almost always present. The ipsilateral lung is particularly impaired, and the herniated gut can compress and retard the maturation of both lungs. Diaphragmatic hernia, often accompanied by marked pulmonary hypertension, is associated with 40% to 50% mortality. Cardiopulmonary compromise is primarily due to pulmonary hypoplasia and pulmonary hypertension rather than to the mass effect of the herniated viscera.

Treatment is aimed at immediate stabilization with sedation, paralysis, and moderate hyperventilation. Pressure-limited ventilation is used. Some centers employ permissive hypercapnia (postductal $PaCO_2$ <65 mm Hg) and accept mild hypoxemia (preductal SpO_2 >85%) in an effort to reduce pulmonary barotrauma. High-frequency oscillatory ventilation (HFOV) can improve ventilation and oxygenation with less barotrauma. Inhaled nitric oxide may be used to lower pulmonary artery pressures, but it does not appear to improve survival. If the pulmonary hypertension stabilizes and there is little right-to-left shunting, early surgical repair may be undertaken. If the patient fails to stabilize, venoarterial extracorporeal membrane oxygenation (ECMO) may be undertaken. Treatment with prenatal intrauterine surgery has not improved outcomes.

Anesthetic Considerations

Gastric distention must be minimized by placement of a nasogastric tube and avoidance of high levels of positive-pressure ventilation. The neonate is preoxygenated and typically intubated without the aid of muscle relaxants. Anesthesia is maintained with low concentrations of volatile agents or opioids, muscle relaxants, and oxygen-enriched air. Hypoxia and expansion of air in the bowel contraindicate the use of nitrous oxide. If possible, peak inspiratory airway pressures should be less than 30 cm H_2O. **A sudden fall in lung compliance, blood pressure, or oxygenation may signal a contralateral (usually right-sided) pneumothorax and necessitate the placement of a chest tube.** Arterial blood gases are monitored by sampling a preductal artery if an umbilical artery catheter is not already in place. Surgical repair is performed via a subcostal incision of the affected side; the bowel is reduced into the abdomen, and the diaphragm is closed. Aggressive attempts at expansion of the ipsilateral lung following surgical decompression are detrimental. The extent of pulmonary hypoplasia and the presence of other congenital defects determine the prognosis.

TRACHEOESOPHAGEAL FISTULA

Pathophysiology

There are several types of tracheoesophageal fistulae (Figure 42–3). The most common (type IIIB) is the combination of an upper esophagus that ends in a blind pouch and a lower esophagus that connects to the trachea. Breathing results in gastric distention, whereas feeding leads to choking, coughing, and cyanosis (three Cs). The diagnosis is suspected by failure to pass a catheter into the stomach and confirmed by visualization of the catheter coiled in a blind, upper esophageal pouch. Aspiration pneumonia and the coexistence of other congenital anomalies (eg, cardiac) are common. These may include the association of *v*ertebral defects, *a*nal atresia, *t*racheoesophageal fistula with *e*sophageal atresia, and *r*adial dysplasia, known as *VATER syndrome*. The VACTERL variant also includes *c*ardiac and *l*imb anomalies. Preoperative management is directed at identifying all congenital anomalies and preventing aspiration pneumonia. This may include maintaining the patient in a head-up position, using an oral-esophageal tube, and avoiding feedings. Gastrostomy sometimes may be performed under local anesthesia. Definitive surgical treatment is usually postponed until any pneumonia clears or improves with antibiotic therapy.

Anesthetic Considerations

These neonates tend to have copious pharyngeal secretions that require frequent suctioning before

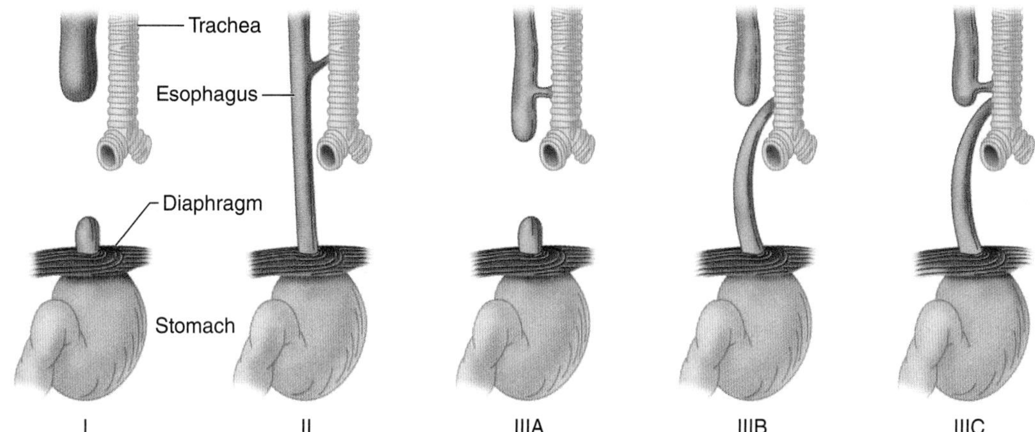

FIGURE 42–3 Of the five types of tracheoesophageal fistula, type IIIB represents 90% of cases.

and during surgery. Positive-pressure ventilation is avoided prior to intubation as the resulting gastric distention may interfere with lung expansion. Intubation is often performed awake and without muscle relaxants. These neonates are often dehydrated and malnourished due to poor oral intake.

The key to successful management is ensuring that the endotracheal tube is positioned correctly. Ideally, the tip of the tube lies distal to the fistula and proximal to the carina so that anesthetic gases pass into the lungs instead of the stomach. This is impossible if the fistula connects to the carina or a mainstem bronchus. In these situations, intermittent venting of a gastrostomy tube may permit positive-pressure ventilation without excessive gastric distention. Suctioning of the gastrostomy tube and upper esophageal pouch tube helps prevent aspiration pneumonia. Surgical division of the fistula and esophageal anastomosis is performed via a right extrapleural thoracotomy with the patient in the left lateral position. A precordial stethoscope should be placed in the dependent (left) axilla since obstruction of the mainstem bronchus during surgical retraction is not uncommon. A drop in oxygen saturation indicates that the retracted lung needs to be reexpanded. Surgical retraction can also compress the great vessels, trachea, heart, and vagus nerve. Blood pressure should be continuously monitored with an arterial line. These infants often require ventilation with 100% oxygen. Blood should be immediately available for transfusion. Postoperative complications include gastroesophageal reflux, aspiration pneumonia, tracheal compression, and anastomotic leakage. Most patients must remain intubated and receive positive-pressure ventilation in the immediate postoperative period. Neck extension and instrumentation (eg, suctioning) of the esophagus may disrupt the surgical repair and should be avoided.

GASTROSCHISIS & OMPHALOCELE

Pathophysiology

Gastroschisis and omphalocele are congenital disorders characterized by defects in the abdominal wall that allow external herniation of viscera. Omphaloceles occur at the base of the umbilicus, have a hernia sac, and are often associated with other congenital anomalies such as trisomy 21, diaphragmatic hernia, and cardiac and bladder malformations. In contrast, the gastroschisis defect is usually lateral to the umbilicus, does not have a hernia sac, and is often an isolated finding. Antenatal diagnosis by ultrasound can be followed by elective cesarean section at 38 weeks and immediate surgical repair. Perioperative management focuses on preventing hypothermia, infection, and dehydration. These problems are usually more serious in gastroschisis, as the protective hernial sac is absent.

Anesthetic Considerations

The stomach is decompressed with a nasogastric tube before induction. Intubation can be accomplished with the patient awake or anesthetized and with or without muscle relaxation. Nitrous oxide should be avoided. Muscle relaxation is required for replacing the bowel into the abdominal cavity. A one-stage closure (primary repair) is often not advisable as it can cause abdominal compartment syndrome. A staged closure with a temporary Silastic "silo" may be necessary, followed by a second procedure a few days later for complete closure. Suggested criteria for a staged closure include intragastric or intravesical pressure greater than 20 cm H_2O, peak inspiratory pressure greater than 35 cm H_2O, or an end-tidal CO_2 greater than 50 mm Hg. The neonate remains intubated after the procedure and is weaned from the ventilator over the next 1 to 2 days in the intensive care nursery.

HYPERTROPHIC PYLORIC STENOSIS

Pathophysiology

Hypertrophic pyloric stenosis impedes emptying of gastric contents. **Persistent vomiting depletes potassium, chloride, hydrogen, and sodium ions, causing hypochloremic metabolic alkalosis**. Initially, the kidney tries to compensate for the alkalosis by excreting sodium bicarbonate in the urine. Later, as hyponatremia and dehydration worsen, the kidneys must conserve sodium even at the expense of hydrogen ion excretion (*paradoxic aciduria*). Correction of the volume and ion deficits and metabolic alkalosis is an indication for hydration with a sodium chloride (rather than lactated Ringer's) solution supplemented with potassium chloride.

Anesthetic Considerations

Surgery should be delayed until fluid and electrolyte abnormalities have been corrected. Operation for correction of pyloric stenosis is never an emergency. The stomach should be emptied with a nasogastric or orogastric tube; the tube should be suctioned with the patient in the supine and lateral positions. Diagnosis often requires contrast radiography, and all contrast media must be suctioned from the stomach before induction. Techniques for intubation and induction vary, but in all cases, the patient's increased risk of aspiration must be considered. Experienced clinicians have variously advocated awake intubation, rapid sequence intravenous induction, and even careful inhalation induction in selected patients. Pyloromyotomy typically is a short procedure that may require muscle relaxation. These neonates may be at increased risk for respiratory depression and hypoventilation in the recovery room because of persistent metabolic (measurable in arterial blood) or cerebrospinal fluid alkalosis (despite neutral arterial pH).

INFECTIOUS CROUP, FOREIGN BODY ASPIRATION, & ACUTE EPIGLOTTITIS

Pathophysiology

Croup is obstruction of the airway characterized by a barking cough. One type of croup, postintubation croup, has already been discussed. Another type is due to viral infection. **Infectious croup** usually follows a viral URI in children aged 3 months to 3 years. The airway *below* the epiglottis is involved (laryngotracheobronchitis). Infectious croup progresses slowly and rarely requires intubation. **Foreign body aspiration** is typically encountered in children aged 6 months to 5 years. Commonly aspirated objects include peanuts, coins, small batteries, screws, nails, tacks, and small pieces of toys. Onset is typically acute, and the obstruction may be supraglottic, glottic, or subglottic. Stridor is prominent with the first two, whereas wheezing is more common with the latter. A clear history of aspiration may be absent. Morbidity and mortality in infants and children due to aspiration or swallowing of button batteries has increased markedly over the past two decades because of larger battery diameter, increasing the likelihood of airway obstruction or esophageal impaction, and increased battery current and voltage secondary to the change in lithium battery composition, leading to rapid and severe tissue burns. Aspiration or swallowing of a button battery is an emergency requiring immediate removal of the battery. **Acute epiglottitis** is a bacterial infection (most commonly *Haemophilus influenzae* type B) classically affecting 2- to 6-year-old children but also occasionally appearing in older children and adults. It rapidly progresses from a sore throat to dysphagia and complete airway obstruction. The term *supraglottitis* has been suggested because the inflammation typically involves all supraglottic structures. Endotracheal intubation and antibiotic therapy can be lifesaving. Epiglottitis has increasingly become a disease of adults because of the widespread use of *H. influenzae* vaccines in children.

Anesthetic Considerations

Patients with croup are managed conservatively with oxygen and mist therapy. Nebulized racemic epinephrine and intravenous dexamethasone (0.25–0.5 mg/kg) are used. Indications for intubation include progressive intercostal retractions, obvious respiratory fatigue, and central cyanosis.

Anesthetic management of a foreign body aspiration is challenging, particularly with supraglottic and glottic obstruction. Minor manipulation of the airway can convert partial into complete obstruction. Experts recommend careful inhalational induction for a supraglottic object and gentle upper airway endoscopy to remove the object, secure the airway, or both. When the object is subglottic, a rapid-sequence or inhalational induction is usually followed by rigid bronchoscopy by the surgeon or endotracheal intubation and flexible bronchoscopy. Surgical preferences may vary according to the size of the patient and the nature and location of the foreign body. Close cooperation between the surgeon and anesthesiologist is essential.

Children with impending airway obstruction from epiglottitis present in the operating room for definitive diagnosis by laryngoscopy followed by intubation. A preoperative lateral neck radiograph may show a characteristic thumblike epiglottic shadow, which is very specific but often absent. The radiograph is also helpful in revealing other causes of obstruction, such as foreign bodies.

Rapid onset and progression of stridor, drooling, hoarseness, tachypnea, chest retractions, and a preference for the upright position are predictive of airway obstruction. Total obstruction can occur at any moment, and preparations for a possible tracheostomy must be made prior to induction of general anesthesia. Laryngoscopy should not be performed before the induction of anesthesia because of the increased risk of laryngospasm. In most cases, an inhalational induction is performed with the patient in the sitting position, using a volatile anesthetic and oxygen. Oral intubation with an endotracheal tube one-half to one size smaller than usual is attempted as soon as an adequate depth of anesthesia is established. The oral tube may be replaced with a well-secured nasal endotracheal tube at the end of the procedure, as the latter is better tolerated in the postoperative period. If intubation is impossible, rigid either an emergency bronchoscopy or an emergency surgical airway are required.

TONSILLECTOMY & ADENOIDECTOMY

Pathophysiology

Lymphoid hyperplasia can lead to upper airway obstruction, obligate mouth breathing, and even pulmonary hypertension with cor pulmonale. Although these extremes of pathology are unusual, all children undergoing tonsillectomy or adenoidectomy should be considered to be at increased risk for perioperative airway problems.

Anesthetic Considerations

Surgery should be postponed if there is evidence of acute infection or suspicion of a clotting abnormality. Administration of an anticholinergic agent will decrease pharyngeal secretions. A history of airway obstruction or apnea suggests an inhalational induction without paralysis until the ability to ventilate with positive pressure is established. A reinforced or preformed endotracheal tube (eg, RAE tube) may decrease the risk of kinking by the surgeon's self-retaining mouth gag. Blood transfusion is rarely necessary, but one must be wary of occult blood loss. Extubation should be preceded by gentle inspection and suctioning of the pharynx. Although deep extubation decreases the chance of laryngospasm and may prevent blood clot dislodgment from coughing, awake extubation is generally preferred to reduce the likelihood of aspiration. Postoperative vomiting is common, and gastric suctioning is usually performed prior to extubation. One must be alert in the recovery room for postoperative bleeding, signs of which may include restlessness, pallor, tachycardia, or hypotension. If reoperation is necessary to control bleeding, intravascular volume must first be restored unless airway obstruction is present or imminent. Evacuation of stomach contents with a nasogastric tube is followed by a rapid-sequence induction. Because of the possibility of bleeding and airway obstruction, children younger than 3 years old may be hospitalized for the first postoperative night. Sleep apnea and recent infection increase the risk of postoperative complications and may necessitate admission.

MYRINGOTOMY & INSERTION OF TYMPANOSTOMY TUBES

Pathophysiology

Children presenting for myringotomy and insertion of tympanostomy tubes have a long history of URIs that have spread through the eustachian tube, causing repeated episodes of otitis media. Causative organisms are usually bacterial and include pneumococcus, *H. influenzae*, *Streptococcus*, and *Mycoplasma pneumoniae*. Myringotomy, a radial incision in the tympanic membrane, releases any fluid that has accumulated in the middle ear. Tympanostomy tubes provide long-term drainage. Because of the chronic and recurring nature of this illness, it is not surprising that these patients often have symptoms of a URI on the day of scheduled surgery.

Anesthetic Considerations

These are typically very short (10–15 min) outpatient procedures. Inhalational induction is a common technique. Unlike tympanoplasty surgery, nitrous oxide diffusion into the middle ear is not a concern during myringotomy because of the brief period of anesthetic exposure before the middle ear is vented. Because most of these patients are otherwise healthy and there is no blood loss, intravenous access is usually not necessary. Ventilation with a face mask or LMA minimizes the risk of perioperative respiratory complications (eg, laryngospasm) associated with intubation.

TRISOMY 21 SYNDROME (DOWN SYNDROME)

Pathophysiology

An additional chromosome 21—part or whole—results in the most common pattern of congenital human malformation: Down syndrome. Characteristic abnormalities of interest to the anesthesiologist include a short neck, atlantooccipital instability, irregular dentition, mental retardation, hypotonia, and a large tongue. Associated abnormalities include congenital heart disease in 40% of patients (particularly endocardial cushion and ventricular septal defects), subglottic stenosis, tracheoesophageal fistula, chronic pulmonary infections, and seizures. These neonates are often premature and small for their gestational age. Later in life, many patients with Down syndrome undergo multiple procedures requiring general anesthesia.

Anesthetic Considerations

Because of anatomic differences, these patients often have difficult airways, particularly during infancy. The size of the endotracheal tube required is typically smaller than that predicted by age. Respiratory complications such as postoperative stridor and apnea are common. Neck flexion during laryngoscopy and intubation may result in atlanto-occipital dislocation because of the congenital laxity of these ligaments. The possibility of associated congenital diseases must always be considered. As in all pediatric patients, care must be taken to avoid air bubbles in the intravenous line because of possible right-to-left shunts and paradoxical air emboli.

CYSTIC FIBROSIS

Pathophysiology

Cystic fibrosis is a genetic disease of the exocrine glands primarily affecting the pulmonary and gastrointestinal systems. Abnormally thick and viscous secretions coupled with decreased ciliary activity lead to pneumonia, wheezing, and bronchiectasis. Pulmonary function studies reveal increased residual volume and airway resistance with decreased vital capacity and expiratory flow rate. Malabsorption syndrome may lead to dehydration and electrolyte abnormalities.

Anesthetic Considerations

Anticholinergic drugs have been used without ill effects, and the choice of whether to use them appears to be inconsequential. Induction with inhalational anesthetics may be prolonged in patients with severe pulmonary disease. Intubation should not be performed until the patient is deeply anesthetized to avoid coughing and stimulation of mucus secretions. The patient's lungs should be suctioned during general anesthesia and before extubation to minimize the accumulation of secretions. The outcome is favorably influenced by preoperative and postoperative respiratory therapy that includes bronchodilators, incentive spirometry, postural drainage, and pathogen-specific antibiotic therapy.

SCOLIOSIS

Pathophysiology

Scoliosis is lateral rotation and curvature of the vertebrae and a deformity of the rib cage. It can have many etiologies, including idiopathic, congenital, neuromuscular, and traumatic. Scoliosis can affect cardiac and respiratory function. Elevated pulmonary vascular resistance from chronic hypoxia causes pulmonary hypertension and right ventricular hypertrophy. Respiratory abnormalities include reduced lung volumes and chest wall compliance. PaO_2 is reduced as a result of ventilation/perfusion mismatching, whereas an increased $PaCO_2$ signals severe disease.

Anesthetic Considerations

Preoperative evaluation may include pulmonary function tests, arterial blood gases, and electrocardiography. Corrective surgery is complicated by prone positioning and the possibility of major blood loss and paraplegia. Spinal cord function can be assessed by neurophysiological monitoring (somatosensory and motor evoked potentials, see Chapters 6 and 26) or by awakening the patient intraoperatively to test lower limb muscle strength. Patients with severe respiratory disease may remain intubated postoperatively. 13 Patients with scoliosis due to muscular dystrophy are predisposed to malignant hyperthermia, cardiac arrhythmias, and untoward effects of succinylcholine (hyperkalemia, myoglobinuria, and sustained muscular contractures).

GUIDELINES

American Academy of Pediatrics—Section on Anesthesiology. Critical elements for the pediatric perioperative anesthesia environment. *Pediatrics.* 2015;136:1200.

Green SM, Leroy PL, Roback MG, et al; International Committee for the Advancement of Procedural Sedation. An international multidisciplinary consensus statement on fasting before procedural sedation in adults and children. *Anaesthesia.* 2020;75:374.

Ivani G, Suresh S, Ecoffey C, et al. The European Society of Regional Anaesthesia and Pain Therapy and the American Society of Regional Anesthesia and Pain Medicine joint committee practice advisory on controversial topics in pediatric regional anesthesia. *Reg Anesth Pain Med.* 2015;40:526.

SUGGESTED READINGS

Adler AC, Matisoff AJ, DiNardo JA, Miller-Hance WC. Point-of-care ultrasound in pediatric anesthesia: perioperative considerations. *Curr Opin Anaesthesiol.* 2020;33:343.

Boric K, Dosenovic S, Jelicic Kadic A, et al. Interventions for postoperative pain in children: an overview of systematic reviews. *Paediatr Anaesth.* 2017;27:893.

Cravero JP, Havidich JE. Pediatric sedation—evolution and revolution. *Paediatr Anaesth.* 2011;21:800.

Kramer RE, Lerner DG, Lin T, et al; North American Society for Pediatric Gastroenterology, Hepatology, and Nutrition Endoscopy Committee. Management of ingested foreign bodies in children: a clinical report of the NASPGHAN Endoscopy Committee. *J Pediatr Gastroenterol Nutr.* 2015;60:562.

Mitchell MC, Farid I. Anesthesia for common pediatric emergency surgeries. *Surg Clin North Am.* 2017;97:223.

Morray JP. Cardiac arrest in anesthetized children: recent advances and challenges for the future. *Paediatr Anaesth.* 2011;21:722.

Suresh S, Ecoffey C, Bosenberg A, et al. The European Society of Regional Anaesthesia and Pain Therapy/American Society of Regional Anesthesia and Pain Medicine Recommendations on Local Anesthetics and Adjuvants Dosage in Pediatric Regional Anesthesia. *Reg Anesth Pain Med.* 2018;43:211.

Vanlinthout LE, Geniets B, Driessen JJ, et al. Neuromuscular-blocking agents for tracheal intubation in pediatric patients (0-12 years): a systematic review and meta-analysis. *Paediatr Anaesth.* 2020;30:401.

Vargas A, Sawardekar A, Suresh S. Updates on pediatric regional anesthesia safety data. *Curr Opin Anaesthesiol.* 2019;32:649.

Zuppa AF, Curley MAQ. Sedation analgesia and neuromuscular blockade in pediatric critical care: overview and current landscape. *Pediatr Clin North Am.* 2017;64:1103.

WEBSITE

Smart Tots. http://www.smarttots.org/.

CHAPTER 43

Geriatric Anesthesia

KEY CONCEPTS

1. In the absence of coexisting disease, resting systolic cardiac function seems to be preserved, even in octogenarians. Increased vagal tone and decreased sensitivity of adrenergic receptors lead to a decline in heart rate.
2. Older adult patients undergoing echocardiographic evaluation for surgery have an increased incidence of diastolic dysfunction compared with younger patients.
3. Diminished cardiac reserve in many older adult patients may be manifested as exaggerated decreases in blood pressure during induction of general anesthesia. A prolonged circulation time delays the onset of intravenous drugs but speeds induction with inhalational agents.
4. Aging decreases the elasticity of lung tissue, allowing overdistention of alveoli and collapse of small airways. Residual volume and the functional residual capacity increase with aging. Airway collapse increases residual volume and closing capacity. Even in normal persons, closing capacity exceeds functional residual capacity at age 45 years in the supine position and age 65 years in the sitting position.
5. The neuroendocrine response to stress seems to be largely preserved or, at most, only slightly decreased in healthy older adult patients. Aging is associated with a decreasing response to β-adrenergic agents.
6. Impairment of Na^+ handling, concentrating ability, and diluting capacity predispose older adult patients to both dehydration and fluid overload.
7. Liver mass and hepatic blood flow decline with aging. Hepatic function declines in proportion to the decrease in liver mass.
8. Aging produces both pharmacokinetic and pharmacodynamic changes. Disease-related changes and wide variations among individuals in similar populations prevent convenient generalizations.
9. The principal pharmacodynamic change associated with aging is a reduced anesthetic requirement, represented by a reduced minimum alveolar concentration (MAC).
10. Older adult patients display a lower dose requirement for propofol, etomidate, opioids, benzodiazepines, and barbiturates.

The older adult patient typically presents for surgery with several chronic medical conditions, in addition to any acute surgical illness. Age is not a contraindication to anesthesia and surgery; however, perioperative morbidity and mortality are greater in older adults than younger surgical patients.

TABLE 43–1 Similarities between older adult people and infants, compared with the general population.

Decreased ability to increase heart rate in response to hypovolemia, hypotension, or hypoxia
Decreased lung compliance
Decreased arterial oxygen tension
Impaired ability to cough
Decreased renal tubular function
Increased susceptibility to hypothermia

As with pediatric patients, optimal anesthetic management of older adult patients depends upon an understanding of the normal changes in physiology, anatomy, pharmacokinetics, and pharmacodynamics that accompany aging. In fact, there are many similarities between older adult patients and pediatric patients (Table 43–1). Individual genetic polymorphisms and lifestyle choices can modulate the inflammatory response to surgery and anesthesia. Consequently, chronologic age may not fully reflect an individual patient's physical condition. The relatively increased incidence of serious physiological abnormalities in older adult patients demands careful preoperative evaluation.

Older adult patients are frequently treated with β-blockers. Chronically administered β-blockers should be continued perioperatively to avoid hypertension, tachycardia, and myocardial injury from β-blocker withdrawal. Because older adult patients frequently take multiple drugs for multiple conditions, they often benefit from an evaluation before the day of surgery, even when scheduled for outpatient surgery. A careful review of patients' medication lists can reveal the routine use of oral hypoglycemic agents, angiotensin-converting enzyme inhibitors or angiotensin receptor blockers, antiplatelet agents, statins, and anticoagulants. Patients with type 2 diabetes who are taking SGLT-2 inhibitors and who are undergoing surgery or hospitalized for major illness are at risk for diabetic ketoacidosis, including euglycemic diabetic ketoacidosis (see Chapter 35). Patients anticipating surgery should be instructed to discontinue these medications at least 3 (canagliflozin, dapagliflozin, or empagliflozin) or 4 days (ertugliflozin) before scheduled surgery to minimize the risk of postoperative diabetic ketoacidosis. Blood glucose levels should be appropriately monitored and managed until normal oral intake has resumed following serious illness or surgery, at which time the SGLT-2 medication can be resumed. Preoperative laboratory studies should be guided by patient condition and history. Patients who have cardiac stents requiring antiplatelet therapy present particularly vexing problems. Their management should be closely coordinated among the surgeon, cardiologist, and anesthesiologist and adhere to appropriate management guidelines (see Chapter 21). At no time should one discontinue antiplatelet/anticoagulant therapy without discussing the plan with the patient's primary physicians.

PREOPERATIVE ASSESSMENT

To promote quality improvement in geriatric surgical care, extensive best practice guidelines have been issued by the American College of Surgeons National Surgical Quality Improvement Program (NSQIP) and the American Geriatrics Society (AGS). These guidelines provide a systematic approach to perioperative geriatric care. In particular, they require the care team to confirm that the patient's wishes regarding treatment preferences and advanced directives are understood and documented. A checklist to ensure optimal preoperative assessment in the geriatric surgical patient is suggested (Table 43–2).

A cognitive assessment such as the Mini-Cog examination is recommended for patients who do not have a history of dementia or cognitive impairment (Figure 43–1). Depression screening should also be conducted. Frailty, reflecting a decrease in functional reserve capacity and an inability to respond to the physiological challenges presented by the stress of surgery, can be assessed using one of several scoring systems. A simple scoring system from Makary et al is presented in Table 43–3.

An optimal preoperative assessment provides the care team with the information needed to identify patients at greater risk for adverse outcomes and enact strategies to mitigate those risks where possible. Moreover, such assessment permits realistic discussions of likely patient outcomes when considering surgical interventions.

TABLE 43–2 Checklist for the optimal preoperative assessment of the geriatric surgical patient.

In addition to conducting a complete history and physical examination of the patient, the following assessments are strongly recommended:

- ☐ Assess the patient's **cognitive ability** and **capacity** to understand the anticipated surgery.
- ☐ Screen the patient for **depression**.
- ☐ Identify the patient's risk factors for developing postoperative **delirium**.
- ☐ Screen for **alcohol** and other **substance abuse/dependence**.
- ☐ Perform a preoperative **cardiac** evaluation according to the American College of Cardiology/American Heart Association algorithm for patients undergoing noncardiac surgery.
- ☐ Identify the patient's risk factors for postoperative **pulmonary** complications, and implement appropriate strategies for prevention.
- ☐ Document **functional status** and history of **falls**.
- ☐ Determine baseline **frailty** score.
- ☐ Assess patient's **nutritional status,** and consider preoperative interventions if the patient is at severe nutritional risk.
- ☐ Take an accurate and detailed **medication history,** and consider appropriate perioperative adjustments. Monitor for **polypharmacy**.
- ☐ Determine the patient's **treatment goals** and **expectations** in the context of the possible treatment outcomes.
- ☐ Determine patient's **family** and **social support system**.
- ☐ Order appropriate preoperative **diagnostic tests** focused on older adult patients.

Reproduced with permission from Chow W, Rosenthal R, Merkow R, et al. Optimal preoperative assessment of the geriatric surgical patient: A best practice guideline from the American College of Surgeons National Surgical Quality Improvement Program and the American Geriatrics Society. *J Am Coll Surg*. 2012 Oct;215(4):453-466.

Age-Related Anatomic & Physiological Changes

CARDIOVASCULAR SYSTEM

Cardiovascular diseases are more prevalent in the geriatric population than the general population. Still, it is important to distinguish between changes in physiology that accompany normal aging and changes in physiology from diseases common in the geriatric population (Table 43–4). For example, atherosclerosis is pathological—it is not present in healthy older adult patients. On the other hand, a reduction in arterial elasticity caused by fibrosis of the media is part of the normal aging process. Changes in the cardiovascular system that accompany aging include decreased vascular and myocardial compliance and autonomic responsiveness. In addition to myocardial fibrosis, calcification of the valves can occur. Older adult patients with systolic murmurs should be suspected of having

1 aortic stenosis. However, in the absence of coexisting disease, resting systolic cardiac function seems to be preserved, even in octogenarians. Functional capacity of less than 4 metabolic equivalents (METS) is associated with potential adverse outcomes (see Chapter 21). Increased vagal tone and decreased sensitivity of adrenergic receptors lead to a decline in heart rate; maximal heart rate declines by approximately 1 beat/min per year of age over 50. Fibrosis of the conduction system and loss of sinoatrial node cells increase the incidence of arrhythmias, particularly atrial fibrillation and flutter. Preoperative risk assessment and evaluation of the patient with cardiac disease have been discussed in Chapters 18, 20, and 21. Age per se does not mandate any particular battery of tests or evaluative tools, though there is a long tradition of routinely requesting tests such as a 12-lead electrocardiogram in patients who are older than a defined age. Additionally, the NSQIP/AGS guidelines recommend that hemoglobin, kidney function tests, and albumin be determined (Table 43–5).

Some older adults will present for surgery with previously undetected conditions that require intervention, such as arrhythmias, congestive heart failure, or myocardial ischemia. Cardiovascular evaluation should be guided by American Heart Association or other relevant national or international guidelines.

2 Older adult patients undergoing echocardiographic evaluation for surgery have an increased incidence of diastolic dysfunction compared with younger patients. Diastolic dysfunction prevents the ventricle from optimally relaxing and consequently inhibits diastolic ventricular filling. The ventricle becomes less compliant, and filling

Mini-Cog©

Instructions for Administration & Scoring

ID: __________ Date: ______________

Step 1: Three Word Registration

Look directly at person and say, "Please listen carefully. I am going to say three words that I want you to repeat back to me now and try to remember. The words are [select a list of words from the versions below]. Please say them for me now." If the person is unable to repeat the words after three attempts, move on to Step 2 (clock drawing).

The following and other word lists have been used in one or more clinical studies.[1-3] For repeated administrations, use of an alternative word list is recommended.

Version 1	Version 2	Version 3	Version 4	Version 5	Version 6
Banana	Leader	Village	River	Captain	Daughter
Sunrise	Season	Kitchen	Nation	Garden	Heaven
Chair	Table	Baby	Finger	Picture	Mountain

Step 2: Clock Drawing

Say: "Next, I want you to draw a clock for me. First, put in all of the numbers where they go." When that is completed, say: "Now, set the hands to 10 past 11."

Use preprinted circle (see next page) for this exercise. Repeat instructions as needed as this is not a memory test. Move to Step 3 if the clock is not complete within three minutes.

Step 3: Three Word Recall

Ask the person to recall the three words you stated in Step 1. Say: "What were the three words I asked you to remember?" Record the word list version number and the person's answers below.

Word List Version: ________ Person's Answers: ______________ ______________ ______________

Scoring

Word Recall: _____ (0-3 points)	1 point for each word spontaneously recalled without cueing.
Clock Draw: _____ (0 or 2 points)	Normal clock = 2 points. A normal clock has all numbers placed in the correct sequence and approximately correct position (e.g., 12, 3, 6 and 9 are in anchor positions) with no missing or duplicate numbers. Hands are pointing to the 11 and 2 (11:10). Hand length is not scored. Inability or refusal to draw a clock (abnormal) = 0 points.
Total Score: _____ (0-5 points)	Total score = Word Recall score + Clock Draw score. A cut point of <3 on the Mini-Cog™ has been validated for dementia screening, but many individuals with clinically meaningful cognitive impairment will score higher. When greater sensitivity is desired, a cut point of <4 is recommended as it may indicate a need for further evaluation of cognitive status.

FIGURE 43–1 Cognitive assessment with the Mini-Cog: 3-item recall, clock draw, and interpretation. (Mini-Cog™ © S. Borson. All rights reserved. Reprinted with permission of the author solely for clinical and educational purposes. May not be modified or used for commercial, marketing, or research purposes without permission of the author (soob@uw.edu). v. 01.19.16.)

Clock Drawing

ID:__________ Date:______________

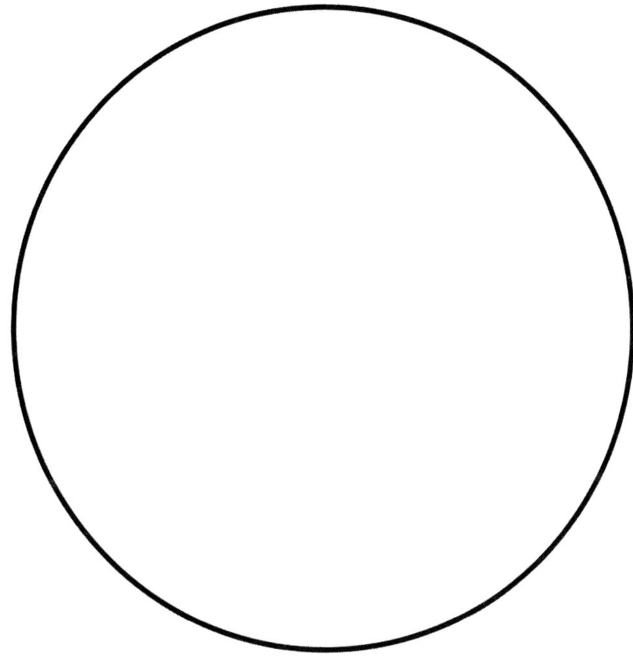

References

1. Borson S, Scanlan JM, Chen PJ et al. The Mini-Cog as a screen for dementia: Validation in a population based sample. J Am Geriatr Soc 2003;51:1451–1454.

2. Borson S, Scanlan JM, Watanabe J et al. Improving identification of cognitive impairment in primary care. Int J Geriatr Psychiatry 2006;21: 349–355.

3. Lessig M, Scanlan J et al. Time that tells: Critical clock-drawing errors for dementia screening. Int Psychogeriatr. 2008 June; 20(3): 459–470.

FIGURE 43–1 *(Continued)*

pressures are increased. Diastolic dysfunction is *not* equivalent to diastolic heart failure. In some patients with symptoms of heart failure, systolic ventricular function can be well preserved, despite congestion secondary to severe diastolic dysfunction. But in most instances, diastolic heart failure coexists with systolic dysfunction.

Echocardiography is used to assess diastolic dysfunction. A ratio of greater than 15 between the peak E velocity of transmitral diastolic filling and the E′ tissue Doppler velocity is associated with elevated left ventricular end-diastolic pressure and diastolic dysfunction. Conversely, a ratio of less than 8 is consistent with normal diastolic function (Figure 43–2).

TABLE 43–3 Frailty score (operational definition).[1]

Criteria	Definition
Shrinkage	Unintentional weight loss ≥10 past year
Weakness	Decreased grip strength
Exhaustion	Self-reported poor energy and endurance
Low physical activity	Low weekly energy expenditure
Slowness	Slow walking

[1]The patient receives 1 point for each criterion met: 0–1, not frail; 2–3, intermediate frail (pre-frail); 4–5, frail.

Data from Makary MA, Segev DL, Pronovost PJ, et al. Frailty as a predictor of surgical outcomes in older patients. *J Am Coll Surg*. 2010 Jun;210(6):901-908.

Marked diastolic dysfunction may be seen with systemic hypertension, coronary artery disease, cardiomyopathies, and valvular heart disease (particularly aortic stenosis), all of which are more common in older than younger patients. Patients may be asymptomatic or report exercise intolerance, dyspnea, cough, or fatigue. Diastolic dysfunction results in relatively large increases in ventricular end-diastolic pressure, with small changes of left ventricular volume; the atrial contribution to ventricular filling becomes even more important than in younger patients. Atrial enlargement predisposes patients to atrial fibrillation and flutter. Patients are at increased risk of developing congestive heart failure. The older adult patient with diastolic dysfunction may poorly tolerate perioperative fluid administration, resulting in elevated left ventricular end-diastolic pressure and pulmonary congestion.

3 Diminished cardiac reserve in many older adult patients may be manifested as exaggerated decreases in blood pressure during induction of general anesthesia. A prolonged circulation time delays the onset of intravenous drugs but speeds induction with inhalational agents. Like infants, older adult patients have less ability to respond to hypovolemia, hypotension, or hypoxia with an increase in heart rate. Ultimately, cardiovascular diseases, including heart failure, stroke, arrhythmias, and hypertension, and frailty contribute to an increased risk of morbidity and mortality and increased cost of care in older adult patients.

RESPIRATORY SYSTEM

4 Aging decreases the elasticity of lung tissue, allowing overdistention of alveoli and the collapse of small airways. Residual volume and functional residual capacity increase with aging. Airway collapse increases residual volume and closing capacity. Even in normal persons, closing capacity exceeds functional residual capacity at age 45 years in the supine position and age 65 years in the sitting position. When this happens, some airways close during part of normal tidal breathing, resulting in a mismatch of ventilation and perfusion. The additive effect of these changes variably decreases arterial oxygen tension. Both anatomic and physiological dead space increase. Other pulmonary effects of aging are summarized in Table 43–4.

Decreased respiratory muscle function/mass, a less compliant chest wall, and intrinsic changes in lung function can increase the work of breathing and make it more difficult for older adult patients to muster a respiratory reserve in settings of acute illness (eg, infection). Many patients also present with obstructive or restrictive lung diseases. In patients who have no intrinsic pulmonary disease, gas exchange is unaffected by aging.

Measures to prevent perioperative hypoxia in older adult patients include a longer preoxygenation period prior to induction, increased inspired oxygen concentrations during anesthesia, positive end-expiratory pressure, and pulmonary toilet. Aspiration pneumonia is a potentially life-threatening complication in older adult patients. Ventilatory impairment in the recovery room is more common in older adult patients than younger patients. Factors associated with an increased risk of postoperative pulmonary complications include older age, chronic obstructive pulmonary disease, sleep apnea, malnutrition, and abdominal or thoracic surgical incisions.

METABOLIC & ENDOCRINE FUNCTION

Basal and maximal oxygen consumption decline with age. After reaching peak weight at about age 60 years, most men and women begin losing weight;

TABLE 43–4 Age-related physiological changes and common diseases of older adults.

Normal Physiological Changes	Common Pathophysiology
Cardiovascular	Atherosclerosis
Decreased arterial elasticity	Coronary artery disease
Elevated afterload	Essential hypertension
Elevated systolic blood pressure	Congestive heart failure
Left ventricular hypertrophy	Cardiac arrhythmias
Decreased adrenergic activity	Aortic stenosis
Decreased resting heart rate	
Decreased maximal heart rate	
Decreased baroreceptor reflex	
Respiratory	Emphysema
Decreased pulmonary elasticity	Chronic bronchitis
Decreased alveolar surface area	Pneumonia
Increased residual volume	
Increased closing capacity	
Ventilation/perfusion mismatching	
Decreased arterial oxygen tension	
Increased chest wall rigidity	
Decreased muscle strength	
Decreased cough	
Decreased maximal breathing capacity	
Blunted response to hypercapnia and hypoxia	
Renal	Diabetic nephropathy
Decreased renal blood flow	Hypertensive nephropathy
Decreased renal plasma flow	Prostatic obstruction
Decreased glomerular filtration rate	Congestive heart failure
Decreased renal mass	
Decreased tubular function	
Impaired sodium handling	
Decreased concentrating ability	
Decreased diluting capacity	
Impaired fluid handling	
Decreased drug excretion	
Decreased renin–aldosterone responsiveness	
Impaired potassium excretion	

the average older adult man and woman weigh less than their younger counterparts. Heat production decreases, heat loss increases, and hypothalamic temperature-regulating centers may reset at a lower level.

Diabetes affects approximately 15% of patients older than age 70 years. Its impact on numerous organ systems can complicate perioperative management. Diabetic neuropathy and autonomic dysfunction are particular problems for the older adult.

Increasing insulin resistance leads to a progressive decrease in the ability to avoid hyperglycemia with glucose loads. Institutions typically have their own protocols on how to manage increased

TABLE 43–5 Preoperative tests recommended for all geriatric surgical patients.

Preoperative Tests	Indications
Hemoglobin	Recommended for all geriatric surgical patients, especially those: Undergoing operations with anticipated clinically significant blood loss or transfusion requirement. With suspected or known severe anemia
Renal function tests (blood urea nitrogen, creatinine)	Recommended for all geriatric surgical patients, especially those: Undergoing major surgery[1] With diabetes, hypertension, cardiovascular disease, or who use medications that affect renal function ACE inhibitors, NSAID[2]
Serum albumin	Recommended for all geriatric surgical patients, especially those: With known liver disease, multiple serious chronic illnesses, and recent major illness Undergoing major surgery Likely to have malnutrition

[1]Major surgery includes cardiac, vascular, thoracic, and abdominal operations.

[2]ACE, angiotensin-converting enzyme; NSAID, nonsteroidal anti-inflammatory drug.

Reproduced with permission from Chow W, Rosenthal R, Merkow R, et al. Optimal preoperative assessment of the geriatric surgical patient: A best practice guideline from the American College of Surgeons National Surgical Quality Improvement Program and the American Geriatrics Society. *J Am Coll Surg.* 2012 Oct;215(4):453-466.

blood glucose perioperatively, and these protocols reflect the changing consensus about appropriate blood glucose targets. Attempts to maintain blood glucose within a strictly normal range during surgery, anesthesia, or critical illness may lead to hypoglycemia and adverse outcomes. Anesthesia practitioners are advised to be aware of changing performance benchmarks related to this measure.

5 The neuroendocrine response to stress seems to be largely preserved or, at most, only slightly decreased in healthy older adult patients. Aging is associated with a decreasing response to β-adrenergic agents.

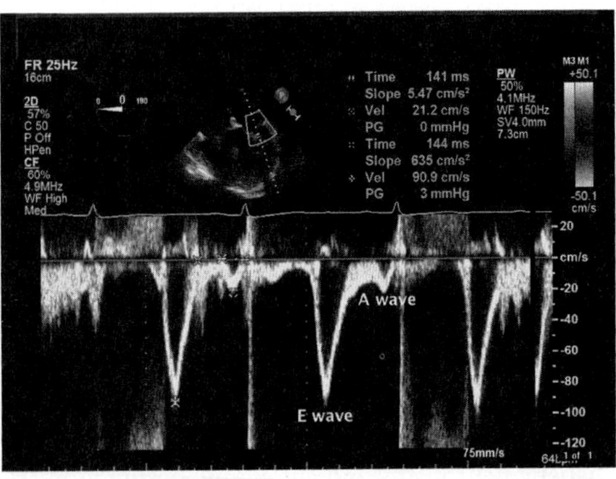

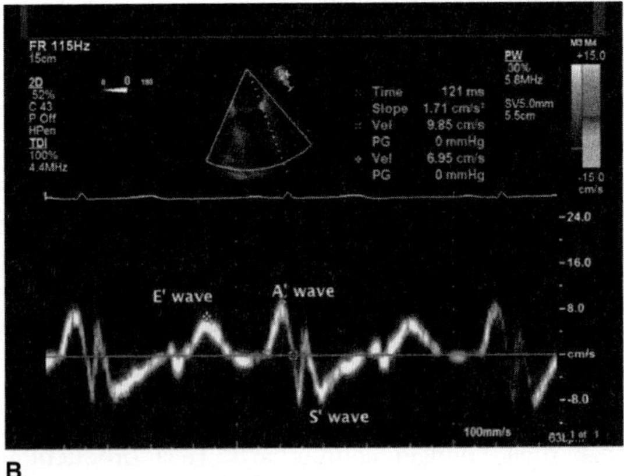

FIGURE 43–2 **A**: In this Doppler study of diastolic inflow, the E wave is seen with a peak velocity of 90.9 cm/s. This Doppler study reflects the velocity of blood as it fills the left ventricle early in diastole. **B**: In tissue Doppler, the velocity of the movement of the lateral annulus of the mitral valve is measured. The E′ wave in this image is 6.95 cm/s. This corresponds to the movement of the myocardium during diastole. (Reproduced with permission from Wasnick J, Hillel Z, Kramer D, et al. *Cardiac Anesthesia & Transesophageal Echocardiography.* New York, NY: McGraw Hill; 2011.)

KIDNEY FUNCTION

Kidney blood flow and kidney mass (eg, glomerular number and tubular length) decrease with age. Kidney function, as determined by glomerular filtration rate and creatinine clearance, is reduced (see Table 43–4). The serum creatinine concentration is unchanged because of a decrease in muscle mass and creatinine production, whereas blood urea nitrogen gradually
6 increases with aging. Impairment of Na^+ handling, concentrating ability, and diluting capacity predispose older adult patients to both dehydration and fluid overload. The response to antidiuretic hormone and aldosterone is reduced. The ability to reabsorb glucose is decreased. The combination of reduced kidney blood flow and decreased nephron mass in older adult patients increases the risk of acute kidney failure in the postoperative period, particularly when patients are exposed to nephrotoxic drugs and techniques.

As kidney function declines, so does the kidney's ability to excrete drugs. The decreased capacity to handle water and electrolyte loads makes proper fluid management more critical; older adult patients are more predisposed to developing hypokalemia and hyperkalemia. This is further complicated by the common use of diuretics in the older adult population. The search is ongoing for drugs that might protect the kidney perioperatively, as well as for specific genetic profiles of patients at greater risk of perioperative kidney injury.

GASTROINTESTINAL FUNCTION

7 Liver mass and hepatic blood flow decline with aging. Hepatic function declines in proportion to the decrease in liver mass. Thus, the rate of biotransformation and albumin production decreases. Plasma cholinesterase levels are reduced in older adult men. Malnutrition is associated with adverse surgical outcomes. Nutritional screening should be a part of preoperative assessment. NSQIP/AGS guidelines, in particular, note a severe nutritional risk is present when:

1. Body mass index (BMI) is less than 18.5 kg/m^2
2. Serum albumin is less than 3 g/dL
3. Unintended weight loss is greater than 10% within 6 months

NERVOUS SYSTEM

Brain mass decreases with age; neuronal loss is prominent in the cerebral cortex, particularly the frontal lobes. Cerebral blood flow also decreases about 10% to 20% in proportion to neuronal losses. It remains tightly coupled to metabolic rate, and autoregulation is intact. Neurons lose the complexity of their dendritic tree and the number of synapses. The synthesis of neurotransmitters is reduced. Serotonergic, adrenergic, and γ-aminobutyric acid (GABA) binding sites are also reduced. Astrocytes and microglial cells increase in number.

Dosage requirements for general (minimum alveolar concentration [MAC]) anesthetics are reduced. Administration of a given volume of epidural local anesthetic tends to result in more extensive spread in older adult patients. A longer duration of action should be expected from a given dose of spinal local anesthetic.

Currently, much work is being done to determine whether surgery and anesthesia harm the brain in some manner. Unlike delirium, which is a clinical diagnosis of a confusional state, postoperative cognitive dysfunction (POCD) is diagnosed by neurobehavioral testing. Up to 30% of older adult patients can demonstrate abnormal neurobehavioral testing within the first week after an operation; however, such testing may identify dysfunction already present in these individuals prior to any surgery or anesthesia exposure. Ultimately, the question remains unanswered as to whether general anesthetic agents in and of themselves result in neurotoxicity in the aged (or infant) brain. It is also possible that side effects of illness (eg, inflammation) and the neuroendocrine stress response contribute to perioperative brain injury in some manner, independent of anesthesia. In one study, 20% of older adult patients presenting for elective total joint arthroplasty demonstrated preoperative cognitive impairment; furthermore, POCD was independent of the type of anesthesia or surgery at 3 months postoperatively. Postoperative delirium is common in older adult patients, especially those with preoperative impairment. Frailty is common in older adult patients awaiting surgery and predicts postoperative delirium. Delirium has a particularly frequent incidence following hip surgery. Factors associated with postoperative

TABLE 43–6 Predisposing and precipitating factors for delirium after surgery.

	Precipitating Factors	
Predisposing Factors, Preoperative	**Intraoperative**	**Postoperative**
Demographics	Type of operation	Early complications of operation
Increasing age	Hip fracture	Low hematocrit
Male gender	Cardiac surgery	Cardiogenic shock
Comorbidities	Vascular surgery	Hypoxemia
Impaired cognition	Complexity of operation	Prolonged intubation
Dementia	Operation time	Sedation management
Mild cognitive impairment	Shock/hypotension	Pain
Preoperative memory complaint	Arrhythmia	Later complications of operation
Atherosclerosis	Decreased cardiac output	Low albumin
Intracranial stenosis	Emergency surgery	Abnormal electrolytes
Carotid stenosis	Operative factors	Iatrogenic complications
Peripheral vascular disease	Intraoperative temperature	Pain
Prior stroke/transient ischemic attack	Benzodiazepine administration	Infection
Diabetes	Propofol administration	Liver failure
Hypertension	Blood transfusion	Renal failure
Atrial fibrillation	Anesthesia factors	Sleep–wake disturbance
Low albumin	Type of anesthesia	Alcohol withdrawal
Electrolyte abnormalities	Duration of anesthesia	
Psychiatric disease	Cognitively active medications	
Anxiety		
Depression		
Benzodiazepine use		
Function		
Impaired functional status		
Sensory impairment		
Lifestyle factors		
Alcohol use		
Sleep deprivation		
Smoking		

Reproduced with permission from Rudoph J, Marcantonio E. Postoperative delirium: acute change with long term implications. *Anesth Analg.* 2011 May;112(5):1202-1211.

delirium in the older adult and ways to avoid it are presented in Tables 43–6 and 43–7.

The AGS has developed guidelines for the prevention and treatment of postoperative delirium in older adults. These guidelines suggest that nonopioid analgesia techniques be employed where possible to reduce the likelihood of postoperative delirium. Additionally, they recommend avoidance of meperidine, drugs with anticholinergic effects, and benzodiazepines. Studies are unclear whether increased depth of general anesthesia is associated with postoperative delirium.

Older adult patients often take more time to recover from the central nervous system effects of general anesthesia, especially if they were confused or disoriented preoperatively. This is important in outpatient surgery when the lack of a home health caregiver may necessitate patients to assume a higher level of self-care. In the absence of disease, perioperative decreases in cognitive function are normally small. Short-term memory seems to be most affected. Continued physical and intellectual activity seems to have a positive effect on the preservation of cognitive functions.

TABLE 43–7 Prevention of delirium after surgery.

Module	Postoperative Intervention
Cognitive stimulation	Orientation (clock, calendar, orientation board) Avoid cognitively active medications
Improve sensory input	Glasses Hearing aids/amplifiers
Mobilization	Early mobilization and rehabilitation
Avoidance of psychoactive medication	Elimination of unnecessary medications Pain management protocol
Fluid and nutrition	Fluid management Electrolyte monitoring and repletion Adequate nutrition protocol
Avoidance of hospital complications	Bowel protocol Early removal of urinary catheters Adequate central nervous system O_2 delivery, including supplemental O_2 and transfusion for very low hematocrit Postoperative complication monitoring protocol

Reproduced with permission from Rudoph J, Marcantonio E. Postoperative delirium: acute change with long term implications. *Anesth Analg.* 2011 May;112(5):1202-1211.

The etiology of POCD is likely multifactorial and includes drug effects, pain, underlying brain dysfunction, hypothermia, and metabolic disturbances. Older adult patients are particularly sensitive to centrally acting anticholinergic agents, such as scopolamine and atropine. Some patients experience prolonged or permanent POCD after surgery and anesthesia. Some studies suggest that POCD can be detected in 10% to 15% of patients older than age 60 years up to 3 months following major surgery. In some settings (eg, following cardiac and major orthopedic procedures), intraoperative arterial emboli may be contributory. Animal studies suggest that anesthesia without surgery can impair learning for weeks, particularly in older animals. Older adult inpatients seem to have a greater risk of POCD than older adult outpatients.

Increasingly, the term *perioperative neurocognitive disorders* has been employed to describe both pre- and postoperative cognitive dysfunction. The exact mechanism of cognitive decline is unclear. Theories concerning anesthetic neurotoxicity in adults are discussed in Chapter 28. Some have suggested that monitoring the depth of anesthesia with the bispectral index may be useful to reduce the incidence of cognitive decline. Other investigations have looked to blunt the inflammatory response to surgery to somehow mitigate perioperative cognitive dysfunction. Likewise, studies are ongoing to identify biomarkers of perioperative neuronal injury.

MUSCULOSKELETAL SYSTEM

Muscle mass is reduced in older adult patients. With aging, skin atrophies and is more susceptible to trauma from the removal of adhesive tape, electrocautery pads, and electrocardiographic electrodes. Veins are often frail and easily ruptured by intravenous cannulas. Arthritic joints may interfere with positioning or regional anesthesia. Degenerative cervical spine disease can limit neck extension, potentially making intubation difficult.

Age-Related Pharmacological Changes

8 Aging produces both pharmacokinetic (the relationship between drug dose and plasma concentration) and pharmacodynamic (the relationship between plasma concentration and clinical effect) changes. Disease-related changes and wide variations among individuals in similar populations prevent generalizations.

A progressive decrease in muscle mass and increase in body fat (particularly in older women) results in decreased total body water. The reduced volume of distribution for water-soluble drugs can lead to greater plasma concentrations; conversely, an increased volume of distribution for lipid-soluble drugs could theoretically reduce their plasma concentration. Any change in volume of distribution sufficient to significantly change concentrations will influence the elimination time. Because kidney and liver function declines with age, reductions in clearance prolong the duration of action of many drugs.

Distribution and elimination are also affected by any altered plasma protein concentrations. Albumin binds acidic drugs (eg, barbiturates, benzodiazepines, opioid agonists). α_1-Acid glycoprotein binds basic drugs (eg, local anesthetics). Concentrations of these binding proteins may vary depending upon diseases associated with aging.

9 The principal pharmacodynamic change associated with aging is a reduced anesthetic requirement, represented by a reduced MAC. Careful titration of anesthetic agents helps avoid adverse side effects and unexpected, prolonged duration; short-acting intravenous agents, such as propofol, remifentanil, and succinylcholine, may be particularly useful in older adult patients. Drugs that are not significantly dependent on liver or kidney function or blood flow, such as inhalation anesthetics, atracurium, or cisatracurium, are useful.

INHALATIONAL ANESTHETICS

The MAC for inhalational agents is reduced by 4% per decade of age over 40 years. Anesthetics reduce the connectivity of different parts of the brain, leading to loss of consciousness. Functional connectivity patterns in the brain are affected by aging, and these changes may contribute to the increased sensitivity to anesthetics in the older adult. The onset of inhalation anesthesia is faster if cardiac output is depressed, whereas it is delayed if there is a significant ventilation/perfusion abnormality. Recovery from anesthesia with a volatile anesthetic may be prolonged because of an increased volume of distribution (increased body fat) and decreased pulmonary gas exchange. Decreased liver function is of less importance, as modern inhalational agents undergo little metabolism. Modern agents that are rapidly eliminated (eg, sevoflurane or desflurane) are good choices for speeding emergence in the older adult patient.

NONVOLATILE ANESTHETIC AGENTS

In general, older adult patients display a lower dose requirement for propofol, etomidate, opioids, benzodiazepines, and barbiturates. The typical octogenarian will require a smaller induction dose of propofol than that required by a 20-year-old patient.

Although propofol may be close to an ideal induction agent in older adult patients because of its rapid elimination, it is more likely to cause apnea and hypotension than in younger patients. Both pharmacokinetic and pharmacodynamic factors are responsible for this enhanced sensitivity. Older adult patients require nearly 50% lower blood levels of propofol for anesthesia than do younger patients. Moreover, both the rapidly equilibrating peripheral compartment volume and the systemic clearance for propofol are significantly reduced in older adult patients. The initial volume of distribution for etomidate significantly decreases with aging: lower doses are required to achieve the same electroencephalographic endpoint in older adult patients (compared with young patients).

Enhanced sensitivity to fentanyl, alfentanil, and sufentanil is primarily pharmacodynamic. Pharmacokinetics for these opioids are not significantly affected by age. Dose requirements for the same EEG endpoint using fentanyl and alfentanil are 50% lower in older adult patients.

Aging increases the volume of distribution for all benzodiazepines due to relatively increased fat, effectively prolonging their elimination half-lives. Enhanced pharmacodynamic sensitivity to benzodiazepines is also observed. Midazolam requirements are generally 50% less in older adult patients, and its elimination half-life is prolonged by about 50%.

Anticholinergic drugs and benzodiazepines are associated with an increased risk of postoperative delirium. Conversely, a single bolus of ketamine (0.5 mg/kg) has been suggested in one trial to reduce the incidence of delirium. Use of sedative and antinausea agents with anticholinergic and antidopaminergic properties may produce adverse effects in patients with Parkinson disease.

MUSCLE RELAXANTS

10 The response to succinylcholine is not altered by aging. Decreased cardiac output and reduced muscle blood flow, however, may cause up to a twofold prolongation in the onset of neuromuscular blockade in older adult patients. Recovery from

nondepolarizing muscle relaxants that depend on kidney excretion (eg, pancuronium) may be delayed due to decreased drug clearance. Likewise, decreased hepatic excretion from a loss of liver mass prolongs the elimination half-life and duration of action of rocuronium and vecuronium. The pharmacological profiles of atracurium and cisatracurium are not significantly affected by age.

CASE DISCUSSION

The Older Adult Patient with a Fractured Hip

An 86-year-old patient is scheduled for open reduction and internal fixation of a subtrochanteric fracture of the femur.

How should this patient be evaluated for the risk of perioperative morbidity?

Anesthetic risk correlates much better with the presence of coexisting disease than chronological age. Therefore, preanesthetic evaluation should concentrate on the identification of age-related diseases (see Table 43–4) and an estimation of physiological reserve. There is a tremendous physiological difference between a patient who walks three blocks to a grocery store on a regular basis and one who is bedridden, even though both may be the same age. Obviously, any condition that may be amenable to preoperative therapy (eg, bronchodilator administration) must be identified and addressed. On the other hand, lengthy delays may compromise surgical repair and greatly increase the likelihood of mortality in the older adult patient with a femur fracture.

What factors might influence the choice between regional and general anesthesia?

Advanced age is not a contraindication for either regional or general anesthesia. Each technique, however, has its advantages and disadvantages in the older adult population. For hip surgery, regional anesthesia can be achieved with a spinal or epidural block extending to the T10 sensory level. Both of these blocks require patient cooperation and the ability to lie still for the duration of the surgery. A paramedian approach may be helpful when optimal positioning is not possible. Unless regional anesthesia is accompanied by heavy sedation, postoperative confusion and disorientation may be less troublesome than after general anesthesia. Cardiovascular changes are usually limited to a decrease in arterial blood pressure as sympathetic block is established. Although this decrease can be treated with fluid loading, a patient with borderline heart function may develop congestive heart failure when the block dissipates and sympathetic tone returns. Vasoconstrictors can be used to support the blood pressure during periods of sympathetic blockade. Reduced peripheral vascular resistance can result in profound hypotension and cardiac arrest in patients with aortic stenosis, a common valvular lesion in the older adult population. Likewise, patients can become profoundly hypotensive secondary to reduced peripheral vascular resistance accompanying neuraxial anesthesia. Invasive arterial pressure monitoring is at times useful when taking the older adult patient to surgery. Monitors of hemodynamic function using pulse contour analysis that estimate stroke volume variation in addition to transesophageal echocardiography can all be employed to guide fluid therapy. The benefits of transesophageal echocardiography must be considered in the context of the risks of esophageal rupture and mediastinitis in the older adult.

Are there any specific advantages or disadvantages to a regional technique in older adult patients having hip surgery?

A major advantage in regional anesthesia—particularly for hip surgery—is a lower incidence of postoperative thromboembolism. This is presumably due to peripheral vasodilation and maintenance of venous blood flow in the lower extremities. Many anesthesiologists believe that regional anesthesia maintains respiratory function better than general anesthesia. Unless the anesthetic level involves the intercostal musculature, ventilation and the cough reflex are well maintained. Studies conflict as to whether regional anesthesia offers a mortality advantage in the management of surgical treatment for fractures of the hip.

Technical problems associated with regional anesthesia in the older adult include obscured landmarks as a result of degeneration of the vertebral column and the difficulty of obtaining adequate patient positioning secondary to pain related to the fracture. A hypobaric or isobaric solution can be injected intrathecally to avoid having the patient lie on the fracture. Postdural puncture headache is less of a problem in the older adult population.

If the patient refuses regional anesthesia, is general anesthesia acceptable?

General anesthesia is an acceptable alternative to neuraxial techniques. One advantage is that the patient can be induced in bed and moved to the operating room table after intubation, avoiding the pain of positioning.

What specific factors should be considered during induction and maintenance of general anesthesia with this patient?

It is important to remember that because a subtrochanteric fracture can be associated with more than 1 L of occult blood loss, induction with propofol may lead to an exaggerated decrease in arterial blood pressure. Initial hypotension may be replaced by hypertension and tachycardia during laryngoscopy and intubation. This "roller-coaster" variation in blood pressure increases the risk of myocardial ischemia. Older adult patients often have reduced vascular compliance and wide pulse pressures, leading to dramatic swings in both systolic and diastolic blood pressure during anesthesia.

Intraoperative paralysis with a nondepolarizing muscle relaxant improves surgical conditions and allows maintenance of a lighter plane of anesthesia. Reduced anesthetic depth, as guided by processed electroencephalographic monitors, may possibly result in a reduced incidence of postoperative delirium, though this remains controversial.

SUGGESTED READINGS

Akhtar S. Pharmacological consideration in the older adult. *Curr Opin Anesthesiol.* 2018;31:11.

Akhtar S, Ramachandran R. Geriatric pharmacology. *Anesthesiol Clin.* 2015;33:457.

Alvis B, Hughes C. Physiology considerations in geriatric patients. *Anesthesiol Clin.* 2015;33:447.

American Geriatrics Society Expert Panel on Postoperative Delirium in Older Adults. American Geriatrics Society abstracted clinical practice guideline for postoperative delirium in older adults. *J Am Geriatr Soc.* 2015;63:142.

Berger M, Nadler J, Browndyke J, et al. Postoperative cognitive dysfunction: minding the gaps in our knowledge of a common postoperative problem in the older adult. *Anesthesiol Clin.* 2015;33:517.

Chow W, Rosenthal R, Merkow R, et al. Optimal preoperative assessment of the geriatric surgical patient: a best practice guideline from the American College of Surgeons National Surgical Quality Improvement Program and the American Geriatrics Society. *J Am Coll Surg.* 2012;215:453.

Costa-Martins I, Carreteiro J, Santos A, et al. Post-operative delirium in older hip fracture patients: a new onset or was it already there? *Eur Geriatr Med.* 2021;12:777.

Dalton A, Zafirova Z. Preoperative management of the geriatric patient: frailty and cognitive impairment assessment. *Anesthesiol Clin.* 2018;36:599.

Evered L, Scott D, Silbert B. Cognitive decline associated with anesthesia and surgery in the older adult: does this contribute to dementia prevalence? *Curr Opin Psychiatry.* 2017;20:220.

Evered LA, Silbert BS. Postoperative cognitive dysfunction and noncardiac surgery. *Anesth Analg.* 2018;127:496.

Evered L, Silbert B, Knopman DS, et al; Nomenclature Consensus Working Group. Recommendations for the nomenclature of cognitive change associated with anaesthesia and surgery-2018. *Anesth Analg.* 2018;127:1189.

Evered LA, Vitug S, Scott DA, Silbert B. Preoperative frailty predicts postoperative neurocognitive disorders after total hip joint replacement surgery. *Anesth Analg.* 2020;131:1582.

Guay J, Parker MJ, Gajendragadkar PR, Kopp S. Anaesthesia for hip fracture surgery in adults. Cochrane Database Syst Rev. 2016 Feb;2: CD000521.

Khan KT, Hemati K, Donovan AL. Geriatric physiology and the frailty syndrome. *Anesthesiol Clin.* 2019;37:453.

Murthy S, Hepner D, Cooper Z, et al. Controversies in anaesthesia for noncardiac surgery in older adults. *Br J Anaesth.* 2015;115(suppl 2):ii15.

Nakhaie M, Tsai M. Preoperative assessment of geriatric patients. *Anesthesiol Clin.* 2015;33:471.

Peden CJ, Miller TR, Deiner SG, Eckenhoff RG, Fleisher LA; Members of the Perioperative Brain Health Expert Panel. Improving perioperative brain health: an expert consensus review of key actions for the perioperative care team. *Br J Anaesth.* 2021;126:423.

Safavynia SA, Goldstein PA. The role of neuroinflammation in postoperative cognitive dysfunction: moving from hypothesis to treatment. *Front Psychiatry.* 2019;9:752.

Sillner AY, McConeghy RO, Madrigal C, Culley DJ, Arora RC, Rudolph JL. The association of a frailty index and incident delirium in older hospitalized patients: an observational cohort study. *Clin Interv Aging.* 2020;15:2053.

Soffin EM, Gibbons MM, Wick EC, et al. Evidence review conducted for the Agency for Healthcare Research and Quality Safety Program for Improving Surgical Care and Recovery: focus on anesthesiology for hip fracture surgery. *Anesth Analg.* 2019;128:1107.

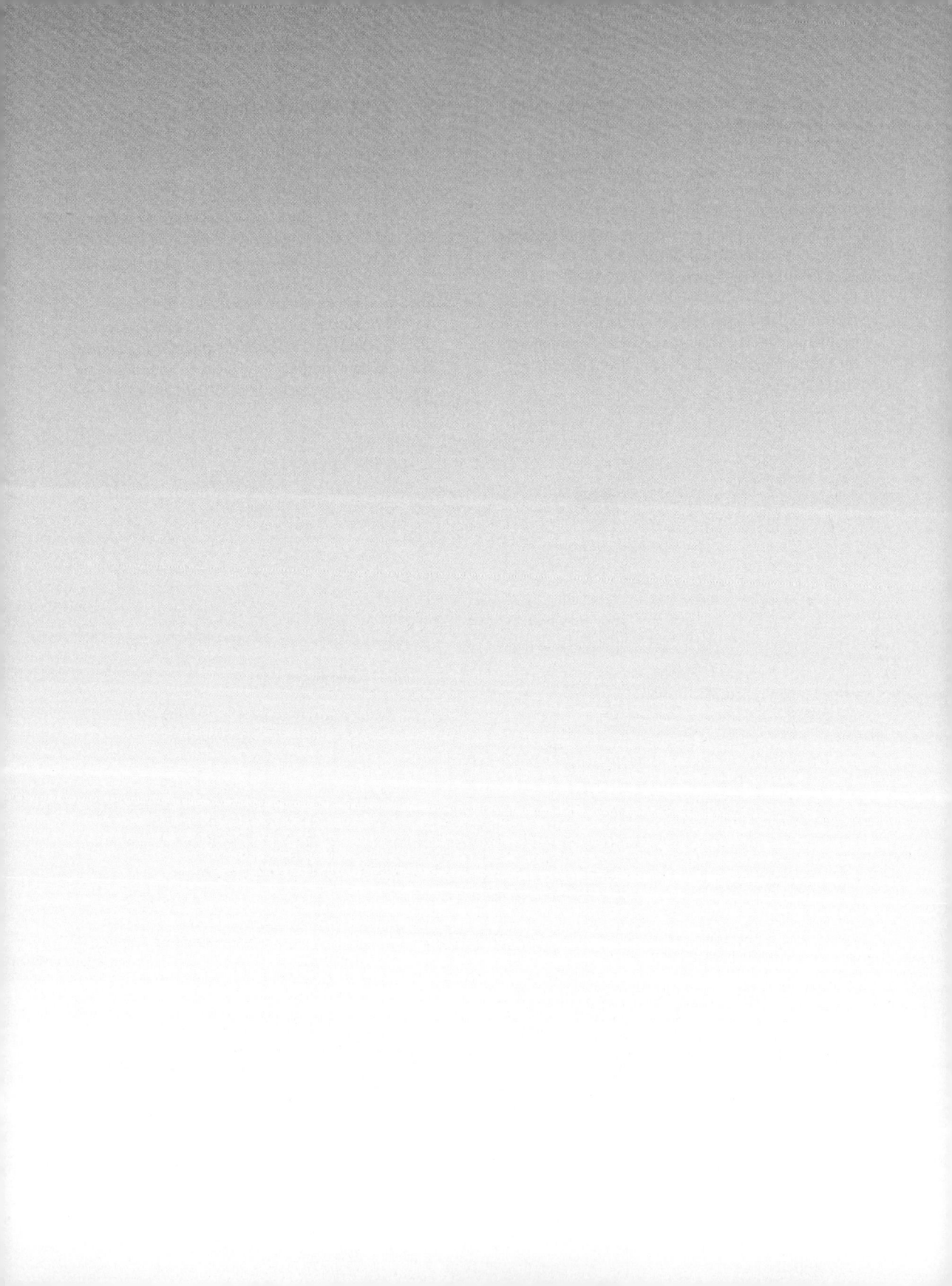

CHAPTER 44

Ambulatory & Non–Operating Room Anesthesia

KEY CONCEPTS

1. Non–operating room anesthesia requires the anesthesia provider to work in remote locations in a hospital, where ease of access to the patient and anesthesia equipment may be limited; furthermore, the support staff at these locations may be unfamiliar with the requirements for safe anesthetic delivery.
2. Anesthesia providers should confirm that both the infrastructure and operational policies are consistent with acceptable anesthesia practice standards before providing anesthesia in such settings.
3. In general, ambulatory procedures should be of a complexity and duration such that one could reasonably assume that the patient will make an expeditious recovery and not require postprocedure hospital admission.
4. Factors considered in selecting patients for ambulatory procedures include systemic illnesses and their current management, airway management problems, sleep apnea, morbid obesity, previous adverse anesthesia outcomes (eg, malignant hyperthermia), allergies, and the patient's social network (eg, availability of someone to be responsive to the patient for 24 h).

Outpatient/ambulatory anesthesia is the subspecialty of anesthesiology that deals with the preoperative, intraoperative, and postoperative anesthetic care of patients undergoing elective, same-day surgical procedures. Patients undergoing ambulatory surgery rarely require admission to a hospital and are fit enough to be discharged from the surgical facility less than 24 hours after the procedure.

Non–operating room anesthesia (NORA; also referred to as *out of the operating room anesthesia*) encompasses both inpatients and ambulatory surgery patients who undergo anesthesia in settings outside of a traditional operating room. These patients can vary greatly, ranging from claustrophobic individuals in need of anesthesia for magnetic resonance imaging (MRI) procedures to critically ill septic patients undergoing endoscopic retrograde cholangiopancreatography in the endoscopy suite.

1 NORA requires the anesthesia provider to work in remote locations in a hospital, where ease of access to the patient and anesthesia equipment may be limited; furthermore, the support staff at these locations may be unfamiliar with the requirements for safe anesthetic delivery.

Office-based anesthesia refers to the delivery of anesthesia in a practitioner's office that has a procedural suite. Office-based anesthesia is frequently administered to patients undergoing cosmetic surgery or dental procedures.

Although anesthetic techniques may be similar for inpatients, ambulatory surgery center patients,

out of the operating room patients, and office-based anesthesia patients, these patients have differing needs. Thus, there are guidelines and statements from the American Society of Anesthesiologists (ASA) that pertain to these different locations. All of these recommendations should be reviewed at the ASA website (www.asahq.org/For-Healthcare-Professionals/Standards-Guidelines-and-Statements.aspx) as they are subject to change and modification. Accreditation agencies, such as The Joint Commission (TJC), the Accreditation Association for Ambulatory Healthcare, and the American Association for the Accreditation of Ambulatory Surgical Facilities, engage in various inspections and reviews to ensure that facilities meet acceptable
2 standards for the procedural services provided. Anesthesia providers should confirm that the operational infrastructure and policies are consistent with acceptable anesthesia practice standards before providing anesthesia in such settings.

CANDIDATES FOR AMBULATORY & OFFICE-BASED ANESTHESIA

Patients with multiple comorbid conditions now present for ambulatory procedures. Each patient must be considered in the context of their comorbidities, the type of surgery to be performed, and
3 the expected response to anesthesia. In general, ambulatory procedures should be of a complexity and duration such that one could reasonably assume that the patient will not require postprocedure hospital admission. ASA physical status and a thorough medical history are crucial in the initial screening of patients selected for ambulatory or office-based procedures. The initial screen can often be accomplished by telephone and can identify those patients who will benefit from being seen and examined prior to the day of surgery and also those patients who are inappropriate for ambulatory surgery. ASA 4 and 5 patients would not generally be candidates for ambulatory surgery. ASA 3 patients with diabetes, hypertension, and stable coronary artery disease should not be precluded from an ambulatory procedure provided that their diseases are well controlled. Ultimately, the surgeon and anesthesia provider must identify patients for whom an ambulatory or office-based setting is likely to provide benefits (eg, convenience, reduced costs and charges) that outweigh risks (eg, the lack of immediate availability of all hospital services, such as a cardiac catheterization laboratory, emergency cardiovascular stents, assistance with airway rescue, rapid consultation).

4 Factors considered in selecting patients for ambulatory procedures include systemic illnesses and their current management, airway management problems, sleep apnea, morbid obesity, previous adverse anesthesia outcomes (eg, malignant hyperthermia), allergies, and the availability of someone to attend to the patient for 24 h. Patients with difficult airways should probably not be candidates for office-based procedures; however, they may be appropriately cared for in a well-equipped and fully staffed ambulatory surgery center. Important considerations for such patients include the availability of difficult airway equipment, such as an intubating laryngeal mask airway and videolaryngoscope, the availability of additional experienced anesthesia providers, and someone capable of performing emergency tracheostomy/cricothyroidotomy. If there are concerns regarding the ability to manage the airway in an ambulatory surgery setting, the patient will be better served in a hospital setting.

Similarly, patients with unstable comorbid conditions, such as decompensated congestive heart failure or uncontrolled hypertension, may benefit from having their procedure performed in a hospital rather than a freestanding facility. The hospital-based ambulatory surgery center provides such patients with both the availability of a hospital's resources and the convenience of being an ambulatory patient. Should their condition warrant additional care, hospital admission is possible; however, such flexibility comes with the increased costs associated with hospital care.

Procedures suitable for ambulatory surgery should have a minimal risk of perioperative hemorrhage, airway compromise, and no particular requirement for specialized postoperative care. Based on risk identification, the anesthesiologist should be able to reduce the likelihood of unforeseen adverse events. Although current evidence-based medicine can provide recommendations for some high-risk ambulatory issues, evidence is lacking for most such situations.

SPECIFIC PATIENT CONDITIONS & AMBULATORY SURGERY

Obesity & Obstructive Sleep Apnea

Obesity is associated with many concomitant disease states, such as hypertension, diabetes, hyperlipidemia, the combination of the preceding three disease states (metabolic syndrome), and obstructive sleep apnea (OSA). The physiological derangements that accompany these conditions include changes in oxygen demand, carbon dioxide production, alveolar ventilation, and cardiac output. There is no precise "cutoff" body mass index (BMI) for patients who may or may not undergo ambulatory surgery. However, Joshi and colleagues suggest that patients with a BMI less than 40 kg/m^2 tolerate ambulatory surgery adequately, assuming control of comorbidities. Conversely, patients with a BMI greater than 50 kg/m^2 are thought to be at greater risk in the ambulatory surgical care environment. Patients with obesity and OSA are at increased risk of postoperative respiratory complications, such as prolonged airway obstruction and apnea, particularly if they will receive opioids postoperatively. Scores for predicting the probability of these complications can aid in the preoperative assessment and referral to a hospital setting (Tables 44–1 and 44–2). However, the ASA guidelines note that the literature is insufficient to offer guidance as to which OSA patients can be safely managed on an inpatient versus an outpatient basis. Although a sleep study is the standard way to diagnose sleep apnea, many patients with OSA have never been identified as having OSA. Consequently, an anesthesiologist may be the first physician to detect the presence or risk of sleep apnea. Preoperative initiation of continuous positive airway pressure (CPAP) may reduce the incidence of postoperative cardiac complications, according to ASA guidelines. Avoidance of respiratory depressants to the degree possible through the use of opioid-sparing multimodal analgesia, neuraxial, and regional anesthetic techniques is likewise suggested when appropriate (opioid-sparing strategies are also of key importance in minimizing the risk of postoperative nausea and vomiting). In addition to the usual discharge criteria, the ASA also recommends that patients at increased risk from OSA not be discharged to an unmonitored setting until they no longer are at risk for perioperative respiratory depression. Other ASA recommendations include:

- Return of room air oxygen saturation to baseline level prior to discharge
- Observation of respiratory function when unstimulated, such as when sleeping
- Consideration of CPAP or noninvasive positive-pressure ventilation (NIPPV) if frequent airway obstruction or hypoxemia develops postoperatively
- A possible prolonged period of postoperative observation to ensure that patients with OSA are not at increased risk from postoperative respiratory depression compared with non-OSA patients undergoing similar procedures

The literature is insufficient to offer guidance regarding an appropriate time to discharge patients with OSA from the surgical facility.

The Society for Ambulatory Anesthesia has issued its own consensus statement regarding the management of OSA perioperatively (Table 44–3). This statement recommends the use of the STOP-Bang criteria for preoperative OSA screening. Additionally, the consensus statement provides a decision tree to assist in determining which known and presumed OSA patients are candidates for ambulatory surgery (Figure 44–1). The Society of Anesthesia and Sleep Medicine has also issued guidelines to assist in the screening for OSA. Their recommendations are summarized in Table 44–4. The 2018 recommendations include:

- Patients with OSA should be considered at risk for a difficult airway, including both intubation and ventilation. Difficult airway precautions should be taken in patients with obstructive sleep apnea.

TABLE 44–1 Identification and assessment of obstructive sleep apnea: example.[1]

A. Clinical signs and symptoms suggesting the possibility of OSA
   1. Predisposing physical characteristics
      a. BMI 35 kg/m^2 [95th percentile for age and gender][2]
      b. Neck circumference 17 inches (men) or 16 inches (women)
      c. Craniofacial abnormalities affecting the airway
      d. Anatomical nasal obstruction
      e. Tonsils nearly touching or touching in the midline
   2. History of apparent airway obstruction during sleep (two or more of the following are present; if patient lives alone or sleep is not observed by another person, then only one of the following needs to be present)
      a. Snoring (loud enough to be heard through closed door)
      b. Frequent snoring
      c. Observed pauses in breathing during sleep
      d. Awakens from sleep with choking sensation
      e. Frequent arousals from sleep
      f. [Intermittent vocalization during sleep][2]
      g. [Parental report of restless sleep, difficulty breathing, or struggling respiratory efforts during sleep][3]
   3. Somnolence (one or more of the following is present)
      a. Frequent somnolence or fatigue despite adequate "sleep"
      b. Falls asleep easily in a nonstimulating environment (eg, watching TV, reading, riding in or driving a car) despite adequate "sleep"
      c. [Parent or teacher comments that child appears sleepy during the day, is easily distracted, is overly aggressive, or has difficulty concentrating][3]
      d. [Child often difficult to arouse at usual awakening time][2]

If a patient has signs or symptoms in two or more of the above categories, there is a significant probability that he or she has OSA. The severity of OSA may be determined by sleep study (see below). If a sleep study is not available, such patients should be treated as though they have moderate sleep apnea unless one or more of the signs or symptoms above is severely abnormal (eg, markedly increased BMI or neck circumference, respiratory pauses that are frightening to the observer, patient regularly falls asleep within minutes after being left unstimulated), in which case they should be treated as though they have severe sleep apnea.

B. If a sleep study has been done, the results should be used to determine the perioperative anesthetic management of a patient. However, because sleep laboratories differ in their criteria for detecting episodes of apnea and hypopnea, the Task Force believes that the sleep laboratory's assessment (none, mild, moderate, or severe) should take precedence over the actual AHI (the number of episodes of sleep-disordered breathing per hour). If the overall severity is not indicated, it may be determined by using the table below:

Severity of OSA	Adult AHI	Pediatric AHI
None	0–5	0
Mild OSA	6–20	1–5
Moderate OSA	21–40	6–10
Severe OSA	>40	>10

[1]AHI, apnea-hypopnea index; BMI, body mass index; OSA, obstructive sleep apnea; TV, television.

[2]Items in brackets refer to pediatric patients.

Reproduced with permission from Gross JB, Bachenberg KL, Benumof JL, et al. Practice guidelines for the perioperative management of patients with obstructive sleep apnea: A report by the American Society of Anesthesiologists Task Force on Perioperative Management of patients with obstructive sleep apnea. *Anesthesiology.* 2006 May;104(5):1081.

- Neuromuscular blockade may increase the risk of postoperative respiratory failure in OSA patients.
- Opioids may likewise contribute to an increased risk for respiratory complications in this population.
- Patients with OSA receiving propofol for procedural sedation may be at increased risk for hypoxia.

Perioperative complications associated with OSA are increasingly the subject of malpractice litigation. Difficult airway management and

TABLE 44–2 Obstructive sleep apnea scoring system: example.[1,2]

	Points
A. Severity of sleep apnea based on sleep study (or clinical indicators if sleep study not available). Point score _______ (0–3)[1,2]	
Severity of OSA (Table 44–1)	
None	0
Mild	1
Moderate	2
Severe	3
B. Invasiveness of surgery and anesthesia. Point score _______ (0–3)	
Type of surgery and anesthesia	
Superficial surgery under local or peripheral nerve block anesthesia without sedation	0
Superficial surgery with moderate sedation or general anesthesia	1
Peripheral surgery with spinal or epidural anesthesia (with no more than moderate sedation)	1
Peripheral surgery with general anesthesia	2
Airway surgery with moderate sedation	2
Major surgery, general anesthesia	3
Airway surgery, general anesthesia	3
C. Requirement for postoperative opioids. Point score _______ (0–3)	
Opioid requirement	
None	0
Low-dose oral opioids	1
High-dose oral opioids, parenteral or neuraxial opioids	3
D. Estimation of perioperative risk. Overall score = the score for A plus the greater of the score for either B or C. Point score _______ (0–6)[3,4]	

[1]A scoring system similar to this table may be used to estimate whether a patient is at increased perioperative risk of complications from obstructive sleep apnea (OSA). This example, which has not been clinically validated, is meant only as a guide, and clinical judgment should be used to assess the risk of an individual patient.

[2]One point may be subtracted if a patient has been on continuous positive airway pressure (CPAP) or noninvasive positive-pressure ventilation (NIPPV) before surgery and will be using the appliance consistently during the postoperative period.

[3]One point should be added if a patient with mild or moderate OSA also has a resting arterial carbon dioxide tension ($PaCO_2$) greater than 50 mm Hg.

[4]Patients with score of 4 may be at increased perioperative risk from OSA; patients with a score or 5 or 6 may be at significantly increased perioperative risk from OSA.

Reproduced with permission from Gross JB, Bachenberg KL, Benumof JL, et al. Practice guidelines for the perioperative management of patients with obstructive sleep apnea: A report by the American Society of Anesthesiologists Task Force on Perioperative Management of patients with obstructive sleep apnea. *Anesthesiology.* 2006 May;104(5):1081-1093.

TABLE 44–3 STOP–Bang questionnaire for screening patients to determine the risk of obstructive sleep apnea.[1]

S = Snoring. Do you snore loudly (louder than talking or loud enough to be heard through closed doors)?
T = Tiredness. Do you often feel tired, fatigued, or sleepy during daytime?
O = Observed apnea. Has anyone observed you stop breathing during your sleep?
P = Pressure. Do you have or are you being treated for high blood pressure?
B = BMI >35 kg/m^2
A = Age >50 years
N = Neck circumference >40 cm
G = Male gender

[1]Fewer than 3 questions positive: low risk of OSA; 3 or more questions positive: high risk of OSA; 5 to 8 questions positive: high probability of moderate-to-severe OSA.

Data from Chung F, Yegneswaran B, Liao P, et al. STOP questionnaire: A tool to screen patients for obstructive sleep apnea. *Anesthesiology.* 2008 May;108(5):812-821.

cardiopulmonary arrest associated with death or brain injury are often the basis of such claims.

Cardiac Conditions

Patients present for ambulatory procedures with a variety of cardiac conditions treated both pharmacologically and mechanically (eg, cardiac resynchronization therapy, implantable cardioverter-defibrillators [ICDs], stents). Anesthesia staff working in ambulatory settings likely will encounter large numbers of such patients who, despite a substantial cardiac history, are now medically stable. Patients with stents are likely to be receiving antiplatelet regimens. As always, these agents should not be discontinued unless a discussion has occurred between the patient, cardiologist, and surgeon regarding both the necessity of surgery and the risk of discontinuation of antiplatelet therapy. Likewise, β-blockers should be continued perioperatively. Angiotensin-converting enzyme inhibitors and angiotensin receptor blockers may contribute to transient hypotension with anesthesia induction, but their continuation or discontinuation perioperatively remains controversial as patients so treated likely will need to have intraoperative hypotension or postoperative hypertension, or both, corrected in either case.

The ASA provided updated guidelines on the management of cardiac implantable electronic

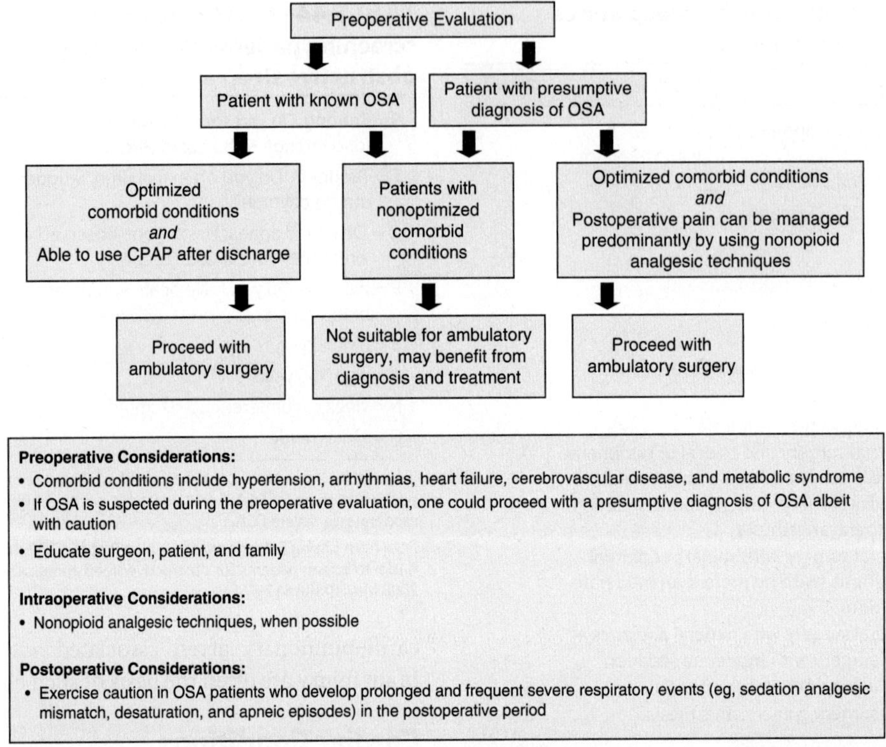

FIGURE 44–1 Decision making in preoperative selection of a patient with obstructive sleep apnea (OSA) scheduled for ambulatory surgery. CPAP, continuous positive airway pressure. (Reproduced with permission from Joshi G, Ankichetty S, Gan T, Chung F. Society for Ambulatory Anesthesia consensus statement on preoperative selection of adult patients with obstructive sleep apnea scheduled for ambulatory surgery. *Anesth Analg.* 2012 Nov;115(5):1060-1068.)

devices in 2020. These guidelines suggest that if electromagnetic interference is likely to occur through the use of electrosurgery, the antitachycardia functions should be suspended while the patient remains in a monitored environment. The guidelines also suggest that if monopolar electrosurgery is planned above the umbilicus, the pacing function in a pacemaker-dependent patient should be set to asynchronous mode. They also suggest using bipolar electrosurgery where possible. If monopolar electrosurgery is to be employed, the dispersive pad should be positioned in such a manner to prevent current from passing near the device or leads. The ASA guidelines suggest interrogation of the device postoperatively when:

- Emergency surgery occurred without an opportunity to evaluate the device.
- There is suspicion that the antitachycardia function is disabled.
- Antitachycardia therapy was observed or suspected.
- There is concern for cardiac implantable electronic device malfunction (ie, significant electromagnetic interference occurred in close proximity to the cardiac implantable device, an invasive procedure was performed in close proximity to the cardiac implantable electronic device generator or lead, or large fluid shifts occurred.

An external defibrillator should always be available whenever the ICD's antitachycardia features are suspended.

TABLE 44-4 Society of Anesthesia and Sleep Medicine recommendations for obstructive sleep apnea.

- ☐ **Patients with obstructive sleep apnea (OSA) undergoing procedures under anesthesia are at increased risk for perioperative complications compared with patients without the disease diagnosis.** Identifying patients at high risk for OSA before surgery for targeted perioperative precautions and interventions may help reduce perioperative patient complications.
- ☐ **Screening tools help risk stratify patients with suspected OSA with reasonable accuracy.** Practice groups should consider making OSA screening part of standard preanesthetic evaluation.
- ☐ **There is insufficient evidence in the current literature to support canceling or delaying surgery for a formal diagnosis (laboratory or home polysomnography) in patients with suspected OSA,** unless there is evidence of an associated significant or uncontrolled systemic disease or additional problems with ventilation or gas exchange.
- ☐ The patient and the health care team should be aware that both diagnosed OSA (whether treated, partially treated, or untreated) and suspected OSA may be associated with increased postoperative morbidity.
- ☐ If available, consideration should be given to obtaining results of the sleep study and, where applicable, the patient's recommended positive airway pressure (PAP) setting before surgery.
- ☐ If resources allow, facilities should consider having PAP equipment for perioperative use or have patients bring their own PAP equipment with them to the surgical facility.
- ☐ **Additional evaluation to allow preoperative cardiopulmonary optimization should be considered in patients with diagnosed, partially treated/untreated, and suspected OSA where there is indication of an associated significant or uncontrolled systemic disease or additional problems with ventilation or gas exchange such as: (i) hypoventilation syndromes, (ii) severe pulmonary hypertension, and (iii) resting hypoxemia in the absence of other cardiopulmonary disease.**
- ☐ **Where management of comorbid conditions has been optimized, patients with diagnosed, partially treated/untreated OSA, or suspected OSA may proceed to surgery provided strategies for mitigation of postoperative complications are implemented.**
- ☐ The risks and benefits of the decision to proceed with or delay surgery include consultation and discussion with the surgeon and the patient.
- ☐ **The use of PAP therapy in previously undiagnosed but suspected OSA patients should be considered case by case.** Because of the lack of evidence from randomized controlled trials, we cannot recommend its routine use.
- ☐ **Continued use of PAP therapy at previously prescribed settings is recommended during periods of sleep while hospitalized, both preoperatively and postoperatively.** Adjustments may need to be made to the settings to account for perioperative changes such as facial swelling, upper airway edema, fluid shifts, pharmacotherapy, and respiratory function.

Reproduced with permission from Chung F, Memtsoudis S, Ramachandran S, et al. Society of Anesthesia and Sleep Medicine guidelines on preoperative screening and assessment of adult patients with obstructive sleep apnea. *Anesth Analg.* 2016 Aug;123(2):452-473.

Glucose Control

In a consensus statement on perioperative glucose control, the Society for Ambulatory Anesthesia found insufficient evidence to make strong recommendations about glucose management in ambulatory patients, and thus management suggestions parallel those of the inpatient population with a target intraoperative blood glucose concentration of less than 180 mg/dL.

Malignant Hyperthermia

Patients with a history of malignant hyperthermia can safely be given nontriggering anesthetics and discharged as ambulatory patients. Prophylactic dantrolene should not be administered.

INTRAOPERATIVE CONSIDERATIONS

Intraoperative management in the ambulatory patient undergoing surgery is aimed at providing rapid emergence, good postprocedure analgesia, minimal risk of postoperative nausea and vomiting (PONV), and rapid return of fitness for discharge while also providing acceptable operating conditions. Often these goals compete with one another. Although inhalational anesthesia with sevoflurane may speed emergence, compared with total intravenous anesthesia (TIVA), the likelihood of PONV may be greater if an additional prophylactic drug is not administered. Numerous studies have shown how regional anesthesia can speed discharge time, compared with general anesthetics, in the ambulatory population—in part, by potentially reducing the incidence of PONV and the need for opioid analgesia. Nitrous oxide increases the likelihood of PONV, but this effect can be overcome by adding a prophylactic antiemetic agent. Likewise, multimodal perioperative analgesia can be approached using a variety of drugs, including local anesthetics, acetaminophen, and nonsteroidal anti-inflammatory agents (NSAIDs) to reduce the use of opioids, which contribute to PONV risk.

Thromboembolism remains a risk after ambulatory and office-based surgery, as with inpatient surgery. Pneumatic compression devices and pharmacological thromboprophylaxis should be used in patients at increased risk. During monitored anesthesia care, supplemental oxygen can contribute to the risk of operating room fires by creating an oxygen-rich environment that facilitates ignition by cautery devices. During head and neck surgery, anesthesia providers must be especially vigilant not to create a potential fire hazard. When oxygen is administered via a nasal cannula or face mask, the minimal amount of supplemental oxygen should be delivered, if any, and tenting of the drapes around the patient's head should be prevented.

POSTANESTHESIA RECOVERY & DISCHARGE

Managing a patient's emergence, postoperative pain, and PONV is critical to expediting discharge. A standardized plan to handle complications, such as postoperative pain and PONV, should be in place preoperatively to streamline management as much as possible.

The entire anesthetic experience of the ambulatory surgery patient should be focused on patient safety, minimizing complications, especially postoperative pain and PONV, and facilitating readiness for discharge. Multimodal approaches are advised; see Chapter 17 for a discussion of PONV prophylaxis and management. Use of a combination of agents (eg, ondansetron and dexamethasone) has shown greater efficacy than monotherapy (eg, ondansetron alone) in patients at high risk for PONV. Likewise, analgesia regimens that minimize or avoid opioid use reduce the risk of PONV.

Pain management is centered on the combined use of regional techniques, opioids, and NSAIDs (multimodal analgesia). Gabapentinoids (gabapentin, pregabalin) may have beneficial effects as part of a multimodal pain regimen. Likewise, oral, rectal, or intravenous acetaminophen or NSAIDs, or both, can be useful in the ambulatory setting.

DISCHARGE CRITERIA

Scoring systems have been devised to assess home readiness after ambulatory surgery and to facilitate timely and safe postanesthesia care unit (PACU) discharge. The Aldrete scoring system, which includes activity, respiration, circulation, consciousness, and oxygen saturation, helps guide recovery from the PACU in the ambulatory surgery unit. Scoring systems and guidelines that standardize patient discharge from the ambulatory surgery center to home are also available (Tables 44–5 through 44–8).

Criteria for discharge generally require that the patient:

- Be alert and oriented to time and place
- Have stable vital signs
- Have pain controlled by oral analgesics, liposomal bupivacaine, or peripheral nerve block

TABLE 44–5 Stages of recovery.

Stage of Recovery	Clinical Definition
Early recovery	Awakening and recovery of vital reflexes
Intermediate recovery	Immediate clinical recovery Home readiness
Late recovery	Full recovery Psychological recovery

Data from Steward DJ, Volgyesi G. Stabilometry: A new tool for measuring recovery following general anaesthesia. *Can Anaesth Soc J.* 1978 Jan;25(1):4-6.

TABLE 44–6 The modified Aldrete scoring system for determining when patients are ready for discharge from the postanesthesia care unit.[1,2]

Activity: able to move voluntarily or on command	
4 extremities	2
2 extremities	1
0 extremities	0
Respiration	
Able to deep breathe and cough freely	2
Dyspnea, shallow or limited breathing	1
Apneic	0
Circulation	
BP ± 20 mm of preanesthetic level	2
BP ± 20–50 mm of preanesthesia level	1
BP ± 50 mm of preanesthesia level	0
Consciousness	
Fully awake	2
Arousable on calling	1
Not responding	0
O_2 saturation	
Able to maintain O_2 saturation >92% on room air	2
Needs O_2 inhalation to maintain O_2 saturation >90%	1
O_2 saturation <90% even with O_2 supplementation	0

[1]BP, blood pressure.

[2]A score ≥9 was required for discharge.

Reproduced with permission from Aldrete AL. The post anesthesia recovery score revisited (letter). *Clin Anesth.* 1995 Feb;7(1):89-91.

- Have nausea or emesis controlled
- Be able to walk without dizziness
- Have no unexpected bleeding from the operative site
- Be able to take oral fluids and void
- Have discharge instructions and prescriptions from the surgeon and anesthesiologist
- Accept readiness for discharge
- Be accompanied by a responsible adult escort

Increasingly, patients are not being required to drink or void before discharge from ambulatory surgery centers (ASCs). Such patients require plans and instructions for follow-up care to provide for possible rehydration and bladder catheterization if required.

TABLE 44–7 Guidelines for safe discharge after ambulator surgery.

Vital signs must have been stable for at least 1 h
The patient must be
Oriented to person, place, and time
Able to retain orally administered fluids
Able to void
Able to dress
Able to walk without assistance
The patient must not have
More than minimal nausea and vomiting
Excessive pain
Bleeding
The patient must be discharged by both the person who administered anesthesia and the person who performed surgery, or by their designates. Written instructions for the postoperative period at home, including a contact place and person, must be reinforced.
The patient must have a responsible, "vested" adult escort them home and stay with them at home.

Reproduced with permission from Korttila K. Recovery from outpatient anaesthesia, factors affecting outcome. *Anaesthesia.* 1995 Oct;50(suppl):22-28.

UNANTICIPATED HOSPITAL ADMISSION FOLLOWING AMBULATORY SURGERY

Occasionally, an ambulatory surgery patient may require transfer to a nearby hospital. Some surgical complications cannot be repaired in the ambulatory operating suite. *Inadequately controlled pain and postoperative nausea and vomiting are the two most frequent causes of unplanned hospital admission from ASCs and from office surgery practices.* Accreditation agencies mandate that office-based operating rooms have appropriate emergency equipment, drugs, and protocols for patient transfer to a nearby hospital. In addition to advanced cardiac life support medications, dantrolene and intravenous lipid emulsion should be available to treat malignant hyperthermia and local anesthetic systemic toxicity, respectively. Additionally, surgeons operating in an office-based practice must have admitting privileges at a nearby hospital or arrangements with an accepting physician to provide for patient transfer.

TABLE 44–8 Postanesthesia discharge scoring system (PADS) for determining home-readiness.[1,2]

Vital signs	
Vital signs must be stable and consistent with age and preoperative baseline	
BP and pulse within 20% of preoperative baseline	2
BP and pulse 20%–40% of preoperative baseline	1
BP and pulse >40% of preoperative baseline	0
Activity level	
Patient must be able to ambulate at preoperative level	
Steady gait, no dizziness, or meets preoperative level	2
Requires assistance	1
Unable to ambulate	0
Nausea and vomiting	
The patient should have minimal nausea and vomiting before discharge	
Minimal: successfully treated with PO medication	2
Moderate: successfully treated with IM medication	1
Severe: continues after repeated treatment	0
Pain	
The patient should have minimal or no pain before discharge	
The level of pain that the patient has should be acceptable to the patient	
Pain should be controllable by oral analgesics	
The location, type, and intensity of pain should be consistent with anticipated postoperative discomfort	
Acceptability	
Yes	2
No	1
Surgical bleeding	
Postoperative bleeding should be consistent with expected blood loss for the procedure	
Minimal: does not require dressing change	2
Moderate: up to two dressing changes required	1
Severe: more than three dressing changes required	0

[1]BP, blood pressure; IM, intramuscular; PO, per os.

[2]Maximal score = 10; patients scoring ≥9 are fit for discharge.

Reproduced with permission from Marshall SI, Chung F. Assessment of "home readiness": Discharge criteria and postdischarge complications. *Curr Opin Anesthiol.* 1997 Dec;10(6):445-450.

NON–OPERATING ROOM ANESTHESIA

Off-site anesthesia (non–operating room anesthesia, NORA) encompasses all sedation/anesthesia provided by anesthesiology services outside of the operating room environment. Our experience has been that requests for these services in remote locations have been steadily increasing, and in some hospitals today, more anesthetics are routinely administered for procedures off-site than in the operating room suite. We and others assign "block time" for such procedures just as we do for the various surgeons and surgical services. We and other institutions have constructed procedural suites where bronchoscopy, gastrointestinal endoscopy, and other procedures can be performed in a centralized area for increased safety and efficiency. The same basic standards for anesthesia care must be met, regardless of the location. Furthermore, the challenges of unfamiliar environments that are far removed from the surgical suite require advance planning for the off-site anesthesia provider.

In contrast to patients undergoing office-based or ambulatory surgery center procedures, NORA patients are frequently among the sickest of inpatients. Often such locations as the endoscopy suite, cardiac catheterization laboratory, electrophysiology laboratory, radiology suite, or radiotherapy unit were constructed without the anticipation that anesthesia services would be provided there. Consequently, anesthesia workspace is routinely constrained, and access to the patient is limited. Moreover, the procedural physicians and ancillary staff in these areas often fail to understand what is required to safely deliver anesthesia (hence the frequent request to "give them a squirt" of propofol) and do not know how to assist the anesthesia provider(s) when difficulty arises. As noted in the ASA guidelines, the standard of care for NORA is the same as in the operating room (Table 44–9)—and patients expect this!

Basic principles for assessing and mitigating the risk of NORA can be broadly classified into three categories: patient factors, environmental issues, and procedure-related aspects. Patient factors include comorbidity, airway assessment, fasting status, and monitoring. Environmental issues include anesthesia equipment, emergency equipment, and magnetic

TABLE 44–9 American Society of Anesthesiologists guidelines for non–operating room anesthetizing locations.

Reliable O_2 source with backup	Sufficient space for anesthesia personnel, equipment
Suction apparatus	Emergency cart, defibrillator, drugs, etc
Waste gas scavenging	Reliable means for two-way communication
Adequate monitoring equipment	Applicable facility, safety codes met
Safe electrical outlets	Appropriate postanesthesia management
Adequate illumination, battery backup	

Data from American Society of Anesthesiologists guidelines for non-operating room anesthetizing locations (2008). Committee of Origin: Standards and Practice Parameters (approved by the ASA House of Delegates on October 15, 2003 and amended on October 22, 2008.

and radiation hazards. Procedure-related aspects include duration, level of discomfort, patient position, and surgical support.

The ASA Closed Claims Database has demonstrated that claims related to NORA care have a greater severity of injury than closed claims related to operating room anesthesia care. Monitored anesthesia care was the primary technique in more than half of the claims reviewed. Many of these closed claims arose from injuries related to inadequate oxygenation/ventilation during endoscopy.

Increasingly, personnel in the endoscopy suite and the emergency department who are not qualified anesthesia providers provide sedation with a variety of agents. In fact, some reports indicate that non–anesthesia providers administer sedation and analgesia for almost 40% of the procedures performed in the United States. The ASA guidelines and the Joint Commission have described the continuum of depth of sedation, ranging from minimal sedation to general anesthesia (Table 44–10). The Centers for Medicare and Medicaid Services has mandated that all sedation in a hospital be under the direction of a physician—generally, the anesthesia service chief. Consequently, anesthesiologists must not only from time to time provide anesthesia in non–operating room settings, but they must also develop policies and quality assurance review mechanisms for non–anesthesia providers to safely and legally provide sedation. Such policies should be focused on assuring that those providing or directing sedation have the necessary skills to rescue the patient should mild or moderate sedation unintentionally progress to deep sedation or general anesthesia.

Risks associated with sedation/analgesia are highlighted in Table 44–11. Sedation providers should know how to reverse benzodiazepines and opioids and provide bag/mask airway support and be facile in the use of airway adjuvants. A mechanism to ensure the timely arrival of anesthesia personnel capable of airway rescue must likewise be incorporated into such policies.

TABLE 44–10 Continuum of depth of sedation/analgesia/anesthesia.

Level	Type	Responsiveness	Airway	Spontaneous Ventilation	Cardiovascular Function
1	Minimal	Normal to verbal stimulation	Unaffected	Unaffected	Unaffected
2	Moderate	Purposeful response to verbal or tactile stimulation	No intervention required	Adequate	Usually maintained
3	Deep	Purposeful after repeated or painful stimulus	Intervention may be required	May be inadequate	Usually maintained
4	General anesthesia	Unarousable to painful stimulus	Intervention often required	Often inadequate	May be impaired

Data from American Society of Anesthesiologists.

TABLE 44–11 Complications associated with sedation and analgesia.

Airway
Airway obstruction
Aspiration
Regurgitation
Dental/soft tissue injury
Respiratory
Respiratory depression
Hypoxemia
Hypercarbia
Apnea
Cardiovascular
Hypotension
Cardiac arrhythmias
Neurological
Deeper level of sedation
Unresponsiveness
Other
Undesirable patient movement
Drug interactions
Adverse reactions
Unanticipated admission

Data from American Society of Anesthesiologists.

TABLE 44–12 Common locations for non–operating room anesthesia.[1]

Radiology
Neurointerventional radiology
Vascular radiology
MRI/CT
PET scan
Endoscopy Suite
Gastrointestinal suite
Bronchoscopy
Intensive Care Unit
Tracheostomy, percutaneous gastrostomy
Intracranial and other catheter placement
Abdominal/pelvic explorations
Invasive Cardiology Suite
Cardiac catheterization lab
Cardioversion
Electrophysiology suite
Radiation Therapy
Emergency Medicine Suite
Psychiatry
Electroconvulsive therapy suite
Urology
Lithotripsy
Dental Surgery

[1]CT, computed tomography; MRI, magnetic resonance imaging; PET, positron emission tomography.

Data from American Society of Anesthesiologists.

SPECIAL CONSIDERATIONS IN & OUT OF OPERATING ROOM LOCATIONS

Anesthesia services are requested at various locations throughout the hospital facility; some of these are delineated in Table 44–12. Postprocedure disposition (whether discharge or admission) needs appropriate coordination by the anesthesiologist for postanesthesia care or safe transport from the remote unit, or both.

Patients presenting to the gastrointestinal endoscopy suite include healthy individuals for routine diagnostic screenings, as well as patients with fulminant cholangitis, sepsis, or gastrointestinal hemorrhage or obstruction. As always, the patient's current illness and comorbidities, as well as the specific diagnostic/therapeutic procedure, determine both the anesthetic techniques (sedation or general anesthesia) and the monitoring required.

Patients undergoing cardiac catheterization are routinely sedated by cardiologists without the involvement of an anesthesiologist. Occasionally, a patient with significant comorbidities (eg, morbid obesity) requires the presence of a qualified anesthesia provider. General anesthesia is sometimes required for placement of aortic stents, which are increasingly performed by cardiologists in the cardiac catheterization laboratory. Specially built hybrid surgical suites enable both open and catheter-based vascular repairs. Increasingly, patients for transcatheter aortic valve replacement (TAVR) are managed with local anesthesia and sedation rather than general anesthesia. Institutional protocols and patient characteristics determine the anesthetic/sedation management of these patients. General anesthesia is frequently administered to patients in the neurointerventional suite for treatment of cerebral aneurysms and ischemic strokes.

Patients requiring electrophysiology procedures for catheter-mediated arrhythmia ablation often need general anesthesia or deep sedation. Such patients may have heart failure, leading to potential hemodynamic difficulties perioperatively. Sudden hypotension can herald the development of pericardial tamponade secondary to catheter perforation of the heart. As rhythm inducibility can be affected by anesthetic agents, most electrophysiology units have established their own protocols for anesthesia or sedation management, depending upon which rhythms are to be ablated. Other patients require sedation for the placement of ICDs. Once placed, the device will be tested by inducing ventricular fibrillation. During testing, deeper levels of sedation are required, as the defibrillation shock can be frightening and very uncomfortable. Likewise, anesthesia staff are called upon to provide anesthesia for cardioversion of patients in atrial fibrillation. These patients usually have associated cardiac diseases and require brief intravenous anesthetics to facilitate cardioversion. Oftentimes, a transesophageal echocardiogram must be performed prior to cardioversion to rule out clot in the left atrial appendage. In such cases, anesthesia staff may also provide sedation for this procedure. Determination as to whether a patient needs sedation or general anesthesia with or without intubation is dependent upon routine patient assessment.

Children and some adults (ie, those who are claustrophobic, developmentally disabled, or have conditions that prevent them from remaining still or lying flat) require anesthesia or sedation for MRI and computed tomography (CT) imaging. Additionally, painful CT-guided biopsies or ablative procedures may require anesthesia management. The anesthetic technique is dependent upon the procedure and patient comorbidities.

MRI creates numerous problems for anesthesia staff. First, all ferromagnetic materials must be excluded from the area of the magnet. Most institutions have policies and training protocols to prevent catastrophes (eg, oxygen tanks flying into the scanner). Second, all anesthetic equipment must be compatible with the magnet in use. Third, patients must be free of implants that could interact with the magnet, such as pacemakers, vascular clips, ICDs, and infusion pumps. As with all NORA, the exact choice of technique is dependent upon the patient's comorbidities. Both deep sedation and general anesthesia approaches with intubation or supraglottic airways can be used, depending on practitioner preference and patient requirements.

Patients often require general anesthesia and tight blood pressure control to facilitate coiling and embolization of cerebral aneurysms, arteriovenous malformations, or stenting and clot removal for acute strokes. Patients taken to the radiology suite for relief of portal hypertension (see Chapters 33 and 34) via the creation of a transjugular intrahepatic portosystemic shunt (TIPS) are frequently hypovolemic with profound ascites and are at risk of esophageal variceal bleeding and aspiration. General anesthesia with intubation is preferred for management of the TIPS procedure.

Anesthesia for electroconvulsive therapy is often provided in a separate suite in the psychiatry unit or a monitored area in the hospital (eg, PACU). Patient comorbidity, drug interactions with various psychotropic medications, multiple anesthetic procedures, and effects of anesthetic agents on the quality of electroconvulsive therapy also need to be considered (see Chapter 28).

Anesthesia providers are at times called to deliver anesthesia in the intensive care unit (ICU) for bedside tracheostomy, emergency chest and abdominal exploration, or gastrointestinal endoscopic procedures in patients considered too critically ill to tolerate transport to the operating room. In most of these cases, the anesthesia staff generally employ the ICU ventilator and monitors. Intravenous agents are typically used along with muscle relaxants. When anesthesia for bedside tracheostomy is performed, it is important that the endotracheal tube not be withdrawn from the trachea until end-tidal CO_2 is measured from the newly placed tracheostomy tube.

CASE DISCUSSION

Acute Hypoxia After TIPS Procedure in the Radiology Suite

A 58-year-old woman with decompensated cryptogenic cirrhosis and refractory ascites, currently on the liver transplant list, is scheduled for an urgent TIPS procedure.

What does a TIPS procedure entail? What are its indications and contraindications?

TIPS (transjugular intrahepatic portosystemic shunt) involves the passage of a catheter, usually inserted through the internal jugular vein and directed into the liver, which creates a low-resistance conduit between a portal vein and a hepatic vein by deployment of an intrahepatic expandable stent. Hemodynamically, this allows immediate decompression of portal hypertension by partial or complete diversion of portal flow from hepatic sinusoids into the inferior vena cava and the systemic circulation.

Indications for the TIPS procedure include variceal bleeding not controlled by endoscopic or medical therapy, intractable ascites, hepatic hydrothorax, Budd–Chiari syndrome, hepatorenal syndrome, hepatopulmonary syndrome, and bridge to liver transplantation. Some contraindications of TIPS are primary prevention of variceal hemorrhage, congestive heart failure, severe pulmonary hypertension and tricuspid regurgitation, severe hepatic failure, hepatocellular carcinoma, active intrahepatic or systemic infection, and severe coagulopathy or thrombocytopenia.

What are the anesthetic strategies for TIPS? What are some preoperative and intraoperative concerns in these patients?

TIPS can be performed under moderate sedation, monitored anesthesia care, or general anesthesia. Given the usual need for long immobilization, potential risk of aspiration, and significant comorbidity, general anesthesia is often the recommended anesthetic plan.

Preoperative considerations include risk of aspiration, gastrointestinal bleeding, decreased functional residual capacity from ascites, pleural effusions, coagulopathy, thrombocytopenia, and hepatic encephalopathy. Intraoperative considerations should include careful hemodynamic monitoring (usually via arterial catheter) and frequent measurement of blood gases, electrolytes, and coagulation parameters. Altered pharmacokinetics of anesthetic agents from liver failure should also be kept in mind.

The patient is induced with etomidate, fentanyl, and succinylcholine, using rapid sequence induction; atraumatic intubation is accomplished uneventfully. Prior to placement of the TIPS, the radiologist evacuates approximately 8 L of ascitic fluid.

What are your concerns about this paracentesis? How would you balance these hemodynamic fluid shifts?

Large volume paracentesis is believed to be a relatively safe and effective procedure; however, it can lead to paracentesis-induced circulatory dysfunction characterized by a marked activation of the renin–angiotensin axis, as well as accentuation of the arteriolar vasodilation that is present in cirrhotic patients. Administration of albumin may mitigate the hemodynamic effects of large volume paracentesis.

GUIDELINES

American Society of Anesthesiologists Task Force on Perioperative Management of Patients with Cardiac Implantable Electronic Devices. Practice advisory for the perioperative management of patients with cardiac implantable electronic devices: pacemakers and implantable cardioverter-defibrillators 2020. *Anesthesiology.* 2020;132:225.

American Society of Anesthesiologists Task Force on Perioperative Management of Patients with Obstructive Sleep Apnea. Practice guidelines for the perioperative management of patients with obstructive sleep apnea. *Anesthesiology.* 2014;120:268.

Chung F, Memtsoudis S, Ramachandran S, et al. Society of Anesthesia and Sleep Medicine guidelines on preoperative screening and assessment of adult patients with obstructive sleep apnea. *Anesth Analg.* 2016;123:452.

Joshi G, Ankichetty S, Gan T, Chung F. Society for Ambulatory Anesthesia consensus statement on preoperative selection of adult patients with obstructive sleep apnea scheduled for ambulatory surgery. *Anesth Analg.* 2012;115:1060.

Joshi G, Chung F, Vann M, et al. Society for Ambulatory Anesthesia consensus statement on perioperative blood glucose management in diabetic patients undergoing ambulatory surgery. *Anesth Analg.* 2010;111:1378.

Memtsoudis SG, Cozowicz C, Nagappa M, et al. Society of Anesthesia and Sleep Medicine guideline on intraoperative management of adult patients with obstructive sleep apnea. *Anesth Analg.* 2018;127:967.

SUGGESTED READINGS

Balciscueta I, Barberà F, Lorenzo J, Martínez S, Sebastián M, Balciscueta Z. Ambulatory laparoscopic cholecystectomy: systematic review and meta-analysis of predictors of failure. *Surgery.* 2021;170:373.

Chang B, Urman RD. Non-operating room anesthesia: the principles of patient assessment and preparation. *Anesthesiol Clin.* 2016;34:223.

Dziadzko M, Aubrun F. Management of postdischarge nausea and vomiting. *Best Pract Res Clin Anaesthesiol.* 2020;34:771.

Elvir-Lazo O, White P. The role of multimodal analgesia in pain management after ambulatory surgery. *Curr Opin Anesthesiol.* 2010;23:697.

Fouladpour N, Jesudoss R, Bolden N, et al. Perioperative complications in obstructive sleep apnea patients undergoing surgery; a review of the legal literature. *Anesth Analg.* 2016;122:145.

Gerstein NS, Young A, Schulman PM, Stecker EC, Jessel PM. Sedation in the electrophysiology laboratory: a multidisciplinary review. *J Am Heart Assoc.* 2016;5:e003629.

Metzner J, Domino K. Risks of anesthesia or sedation outside the operating room: the role of the anesthesia care provider. *Curr Opin Anaesthesiol.* 2010;23:523.

Okocha O, Gerlach RM, Sweitzer B. Preoperative evaluation for ambulatory anesthesia: what, when, and how? *Anesthesiol Clin.* 2019;37:195.

Roberts JD. Ambulatory anesthesia for the cardiac catheterization and electrophysiology laboratories. *Anesthesiol Clin.* 2014;32:381.

Rubin D. Anesthesia for ambulatory diagnostic and therapeutic radiology procedures. *Anesthesiol Clin.* 2014;32:371.

Shapiro F, Punwani N, Rosenberg N, et al. Office-based anesthesia: safety and outcomes. *Anesth Analg.* 2014;119:276.

Smith I, Jackson I. Beta-blockers, calcium channel blockers, angiotensin-converting enzyme inhibitors and angiotensin receptor blockers: should they be stopped or not before ambulatory anaesthesia? *Curr Opin Anesthesiol.* 2010;23:687.

White P, Tang J, Wender R, et al. The effects of oral ibuprofen and celecoxib in preventing pain, improving recovery outcomes and patient satisfaction after ambulatory surgery. *Anesth Analg.* 2011;112:323.

CHAPTER 45

Spinal, Epidural, & Caudal Blocks

KEY CONCEPTS

1. Neuraxial anesthesia greatly expands the anesthesiologists' armamentarium, in many cases providing alternatives to general anesthesia. Neuraxial anesthesia may also be used simultaneously with general anesthesia or afterward for postoperative analgesia. Neuraxial blocks can be performed as a single injection or with a catheter to allow intermittent boluses or continuous infusions.
2. Performing a lumbar (subarachnoid) spinal puncture below L1 in an adult (L3 in a child) usually avoids potential needle trauma to the spinal cord.
3. The principal site of action for neuraxial blockade is believed to be the nerve root, at least during the initial onset of block.
4. Differential blockade typically results in sympathetic blockade (judged by temperature sensitivity) that may be two segments or more cephalad than the sensory block (pain, light touch), which, in turn, is usually several segments more cephalad than the motor blockade.
5. Interruption of efferent autonomic transmission at the spinal nerve roots during neuraxial blocks produces sympathetic blockade.
6. Neuraxial blocks typically produce variable decreases in blood pressure that may be accompanied by a decrease in heart rate.
7. Deleterious cardiovascular effects should be anticipated and steps undertaken to minimize the degree of hypotension. However, volume loading with 10 to 20 mL/kg of intravenous fluid in a healthy patient before initiation of the block has been shown repeatedly to fail to prevent hypotension (in the absence of preexisting hypovolemia).
8. Excessive or symptomatic bradycardia should be treated with atropine, and hypotension should be treated with vasopressors.
9. Major contraindications to neuraxial anesthesia include lack of consent, coagulation abnormalities, severe hypovolemia, elevated intracranial pressure, and infection at the site of injection.
10. For epidural anesthesia, a sudden loss of resistance (to injection of air or saline) is encountered as the needle passes through the ligamentum flavum and enters the epidural space. For spinal anesthesia, the needle is advanced through the

—*Continued next page*

Continued—

epidural space and penetrates the dura–subarachnoid membranes, as signaled by freely flowing cerebrospinal fluid.

11 Continuous epidural anesthesia is a neuraxial technique offering a range of applications wider than single-dose spinal anesthesia. An epidural block can be performed at the lumbar, thoracic, or cervical level.

12 Epidural techniques are widely used for surgical anesthesia, obstetric analgesia, postoperative pain control, and chronic pain management.

13 Epidural anesthesia is slower in onset (10–20 min) and may not be as dense as spinal anesthesia, a feature that can be useful clinically.

14 The quantity (volume and concentration) of local anesthetic needed for epidural anesthesia is larger than that needed for spinal anesthesia. Toxic side effects are almost guaranteed if a "full epidural dose" is injected intrathecally or intravascularly.

15 Caudal epidural anesthesia is a common regional technique in pediatric patients.

Spinal, caudal, and epidural blocks were first used for surgical procedures at the turn of the twentieth century. These central blocks were widely used worldwide until reports of permanent neurological injury appeared, most prominently in the United Kingdom. However, a large-scale epidemiological study conducted in the 1950s proved that complications were rare when these blocks were performed skillfully, with attention to asepsis, and when newer, safer local anesthetics were used. Today, neuraxial blocks are routinely employed for labor analgesia, cesarian delivery, orthopedic surgery, perioperative analgesia, and chronic pain management. However, as is true for all medical procedures, they are associated with complications, and much literature has examined the incidence of complications following neuraxial blocks in patients with different disease states.

1 *Neuraxial anesthesia*, the collective term for spinal, caudal, and epidural anesthesia, greatly expands the anesthesiologists' armamentarium, in many cases providing alternatives to general anesthesia. Neuraxial anesthesia may be used simultaneously with general anesthesia or afterward for postoperative analgesia. Neuraxial blocks can be performed as a single injection or with a catheter to allow intermittent boluses or continuous infusions.

Adverse reactions and complications associated with neuraxial anesthesia range from self-limited back soreness to debilitating permanent neurological deficits and even death. The anesthesia practitioner must therefore be thoroughly familiar with the relevant anatomy and the pharmacology and toxic dosages of the agents employed. The anesthesia practitioner must diligently employ sterile techniques and quickly address physiological derangements arising from neuraxial techniques.

THE ROLE OF NEURAXIAL ANESTHESIA IN ANESTHETIC PRACTICE

Some studies suggest that postoperative morbidity may be reduced when neuraxial blockade is used either alone or in combination with general anesthesia. Some less convincing studies suggest that neuraxial blocks are associated with reduced perioperative mortality. Neuraxial blocks may reduce the incidence of venous thrombosis and pulmonary embolism, cardiac complications in high-risk patients, bleeding and transfusion requirements, vascular graft occlusion, and pneumonia and respiratory depression following upper abdominal or thoracic surgery in patients with chronic lung disease. Neuraxial blocks may also allow the earlier return of gastrointestinal function following surgery. Proposed mechanisms (in addition to precluding the need for larger doses of systemic anesthetics and opioids) include reducing the hypercoagulable state associated with surgery, increasing tissue blood flow, improving oxygenation from decreased splinting, enhancing peristalsis, and suppressing the neuroendocrine stress response to surgery. Reduction of systemic opioid administration may decrease the incidence of atelectasis, hypoventilation, and aspiration pneumonia and reduce the duration of ileus. Postoperative epidural analgesia may also significantly reduce both the need for mechanical ventilation and its duration after major abdominal or thoracic surgery.

Neuraxial versus General Anesthesia in The Sick Older Adult Patient

Anesthesia providers are all too familiar with situations in which a consultant "clears" a sick older adult patient with significant cardiac disease for surgery "under spinal anesthesia." A spinal anesthetic with little or no intravenous sedation may reduce the likelihood of postoperative delirium or cognitive dysfunction, which are sometimes seen in the older adult population. Unfortunately, many patients will require some sedation during the procedure, either for comfort or to facilitate cooperation. Is spinal anesthesia always safer in a patient with severe coronary artery disease or with a decreased ejection fraction? Ideally, an anesthetic technique should produce neither hypotension (which decreases myocardial perfusion pressure) nor hypertension and tachycardia (which increase myocardial oxygen consumption). Spinal anesthesia may produce both hypotension and bradycardia. Administration of large intravenous volumes may lead to fluid overload in the older adult patient with diastolic dysfunction, especially after the sympathetic block resolves postoperatively. General anesthesia, on the other hand, also poses potential problems for patients with cardiac compromise. Most general anesthetics are cardiac depressants, and many cause vasodilation. Deep anesthesia can readily cause hypotension, whereas light anesthesia relative to the level of stimulation causes hypertension and tachycardia. Research is ongoing to discern if neuraxial techniques offer survival and other benefits to patients compared with general anesthetics for major operations such as open reduction and internal fixation of femoral neck fractures. To date, the results are conflicting. A 2018 cohort study utilizing Canadian data demonstrated that hospitals in which 20% to 25% of hip fracture patients are managed with neuraxial anesthesia have improved survival rates. Of course, this association may reflect overall improved processes (with prompt surgical repairs) in hospitals where staff are particularly adroit at providing neuraxial anesthesia to the hip fracture population. Nonetheless, a 2017 meta-analysis failed to demonstrate a survival benefit from neuraxial anesthesia in patients undergoing major truncal or lower limb surgery. Indeed, this review suggested that general anesthesia may protect against myocardial infarction compared with neuraxial anesthesia. Nevertheless, reduced pulmonary complications, intensive care unit admissions, thromboembolic events, and surgical site infections were noted in patients who were provided neuraxial anesthesia alone or in combination with a general anesthetic.

The Obstetric Patient

Currently, epidural anesthesia is widely used for analgesia in women in labor and during vaginal delivery. Cesarean delivery is most commonly performed under spinal or epidural anesthesia. Both blocks allow a mother to remain awake and experience the birth of her child. Large population studies in Great Britain and the United States have shown that regional anesthesia for cesarean delivery is associated with less maternal morbidity and mortality than is general anesthesia. This may have been largely due to a reduction in the incidence of pulmonary aspiration and failed intubation when neuraxial anesthesia is employed. Fortunately, the increased availability of video laryngoscopes may also reduce the incidence of adverse outcomes related to airway difficulties associated with general anesthesia for cesarean delivery.

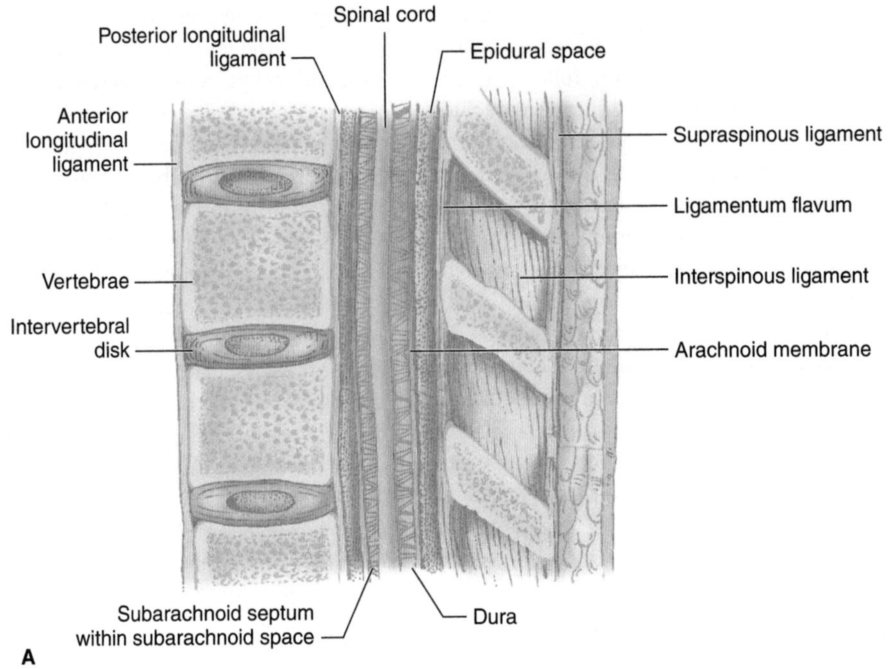

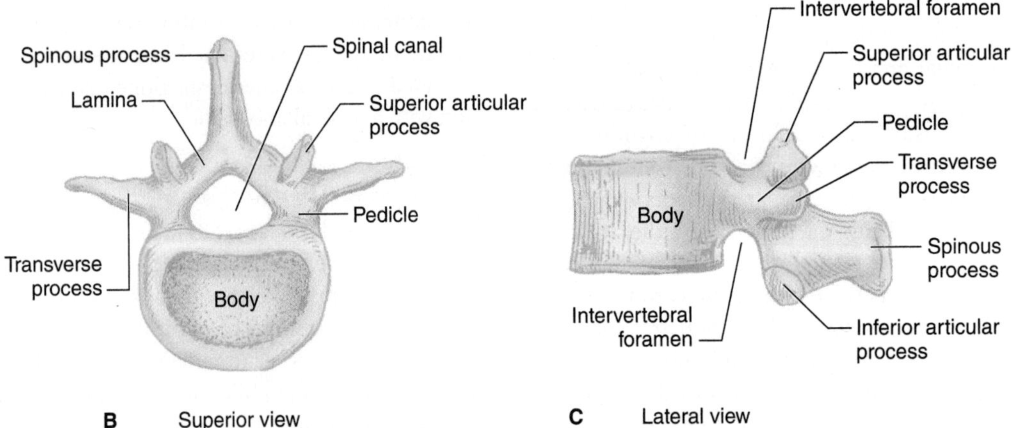

FIGURE 45–1 **A:** Sagittal section through lumbar vertebrae. **B, C:** Common features of vertebrae.

Anatomy

THE VERTEBRAL COLUMN

The spine is composed of the vertebral bones and intervertebral disks (Figure 45–1). There are 7 cervical (C), 12 thoracic (T), and 5 lumbar (L) vertebrae (Figure 45–2). The sacrum is a fusion of 5 sacral (S) vertebrae, and there are small rudimentary coccygeal vertebrae. The spine as a whole provides structural support for the body, protection for the spinal cord and nerves, and allows a degree of mobility in several spatial planes. At each vertebral level, paired spinal nerves exit the central nervous system (see Figure 45–2).

Vertebrae differ in shape and size at various levels. The first cervical vertebra, the *atlas*, lacks a

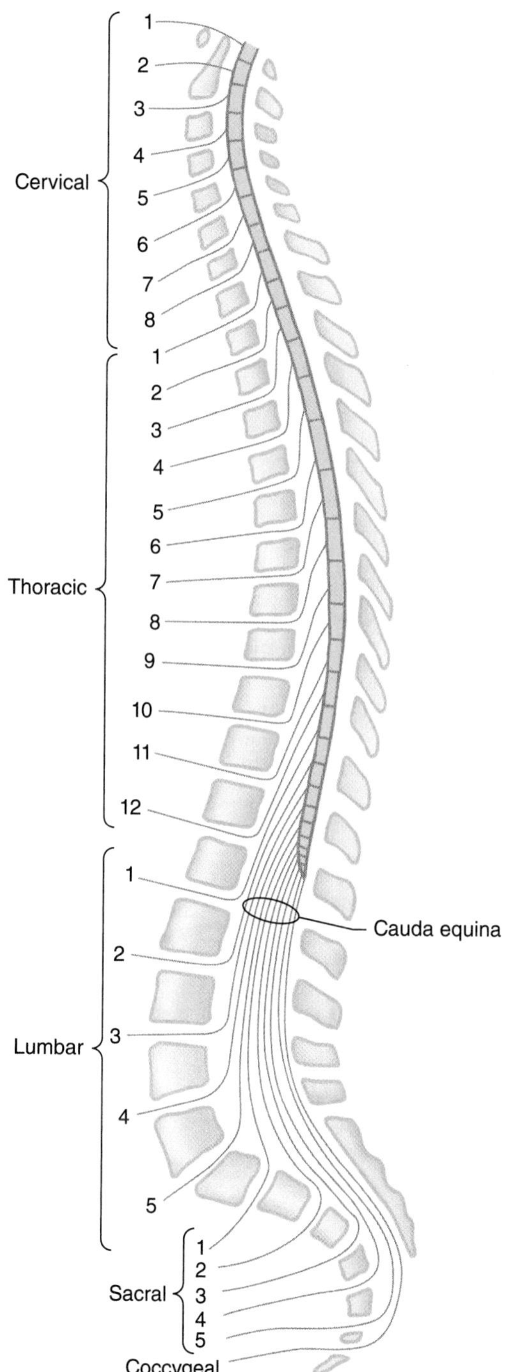

FIGURE 45–2 The vertebral column. (Adapted with permission from Waxman SG. *Correlative Neuroanatomy,* 24th ed. New York, NY: McGraw Hill; 2000.)

body and has unique articulations with the base of the skull and with the second vertebra. The second vertebra, called the *axis*, consequently has atypical articulating surfaces as well. All 12 thoracic vertebrae articulate with their corresponding ribs. Lumbar vertebrae have a large anterior cylindrical vertebral body. A hollow ring is defined anteriorly by the vertebral body, laterally by the *pedicles* and *transverse processes,* and posteriorly by the *laminae* and *spinous processes* (see Figures 45–1B and C). The laminae extend between the transverse processes and the spinous processes, and the pedicle extends between the vertebral body and the transverse processes. When stacked vertically, the hollow rings become the spinal canal in which the spinal cord and its coverings sit. The individual vertebral bodies are connected by the *intervertebral disks.* There are four small synovial joints at each vertebra, two articulating with the vertebra above it and two with the vertebra below. These are the *facet joints*, which are adjacent to the transverse processes (see Figure 45–1C). The pedicles are notched superiorly and inferiorly, and these notches form the intervertebral foramina from which the spinal nerves exit. Sacral vertebrae normally fuse into one large bone, the sacrum, but each one retains discrete anterior and posterior intervertebral foramina. The laminae of S5 and all or part of S4 normally do not fuse, leaving a caudal opening to the spinal canal, the sacral hiatus (Figure 45–3).

The spinal column normally forms a double C, being convex anteriorly in the cervical and lumbar regions (see Figure 45–2). Ligamentous elements provide structural support and, together with supporting muscles, help maintain the unique shape. Ventrally, the vertebral bodies and intervertebral disks are connected and supported by the anterior and posterior longitudinal ligaments (see Figure 45–1A). Dorsally, the *ligamentum flavum, interspinous ligament,* and *supraspinous ligament* provide additional stability. In the midline approach, a needle passes through these three dorsal ligaments and through an oval space between the bony lamina and spinous processes of adjacent vertebrae (Figure 45–4).

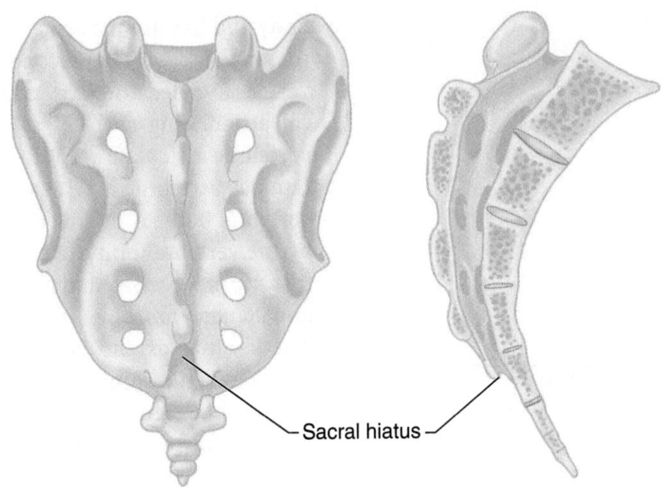

FIGURE 45–3 Posterior and sagittal views of the sacrum and coccyx.

THE SPINAL CORD

The spinal canal contains the spinal cord with its coverings (the meninges), fatty tissue, and a venous plexus (Figure 45–5). The meninges are composed of three layers: the *pia mater*, the *arachnoid mater*, and the *dura mater*; all are contiguous with their cranial counterparts (Figure 45–6). The pia mater is adherent to the spinal cord, whereas the arachnoid mater is usually adherent to the thicker and denser

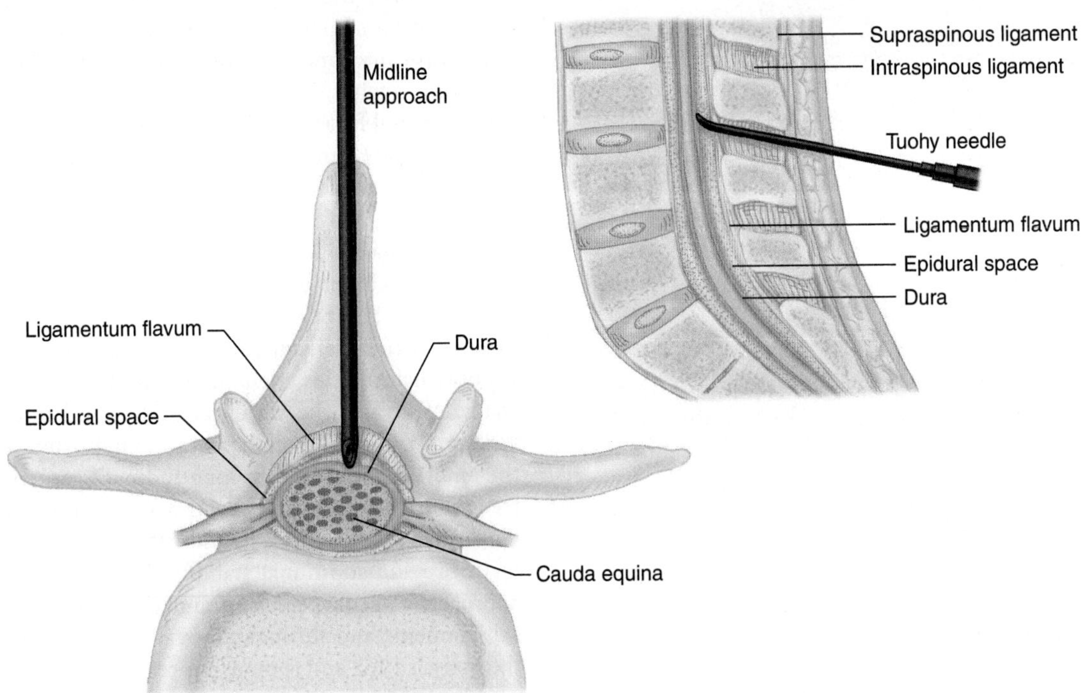

FIGURE 45–4 Lumbar epidural anesthesia; midline approach.

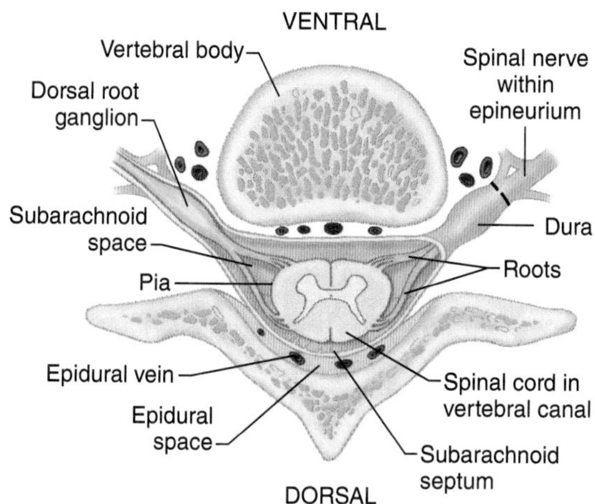

FIGURE 45–5 Exit of the spinal nerves. (Adapted with permission from Waxman SG. *Correlative Neuroanatomy,* 24th ed. New York, NY: McGraw Hill; 2000.)

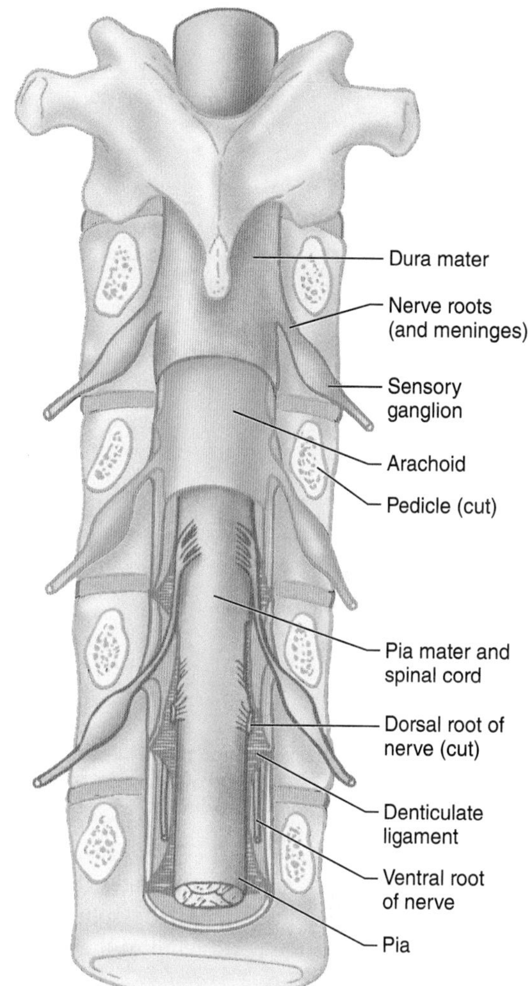

FIGURE 45–6 The spinal cord.

dura mater. Cerebrospinal fluid (CSF) is contained between the pia and arachnoid maters in the subarachnoid space. The spinal *subdural space* is generally a poorly demarcated, potential space that exists between the dura and arachnoid membranes. In comparison, the *epidural space* is a better-defined potential space bounded by the dura and the ligamentum flavum (see Figures 45–1 and 45–5).

The spinal cord normally extends from the foramen magnum to the level of L1 in adults (Figure 45–7). In children, the spinal cord ends at L3 and moves up with age. The anterior and posterior nerve roots at each spinal level join one another and exit the intervertebral foramina, forming spinal nerves from C1 to S5 (see Figure 45–2). At the cervical level, the nerves arise above their respective vertebrae but, starting at T1, exit below their vertebrae. As a result, there are eight cervical nerve roots but only seven cervical vertebrae. The cervical and upper thoracic nerve roots emerge from the spinal cord and exit the vertebral foramina nearly at the same level (see Figure 45–2). But, because the spinal cord normally ends at L1, lower nerve roots course some distance before exiting the intervertebral foramina. These lower spinal nerves form the *cauda equina* ("horse's tail"; see Figure 45–2). 2 Therefore, performing a lumbar (subarachnoid) puncture below L1 in an adult (L3 in a child) usually avoids potential needle trauma to the spinal cord; damage to the cauda equina is unlikely as these nerve roots float in the dural sac below L1 and tend to be pushed away (rather than pierced) by an advancing needle.

A *dural sheath* invests most nerve roots for a small distance, even after they exit the spinal canal (see Figure 45–5). Nerve blocks close to the intervertebral foramen therefore carry a risk of subdural or subarachnoid injection. The dural sac and the subarachnoid and subdural spaces usually extend to S2 in adults and often to S3 in children, important considerations in avoiding accidental dural puncture during caudal anesthesia. An extension of the

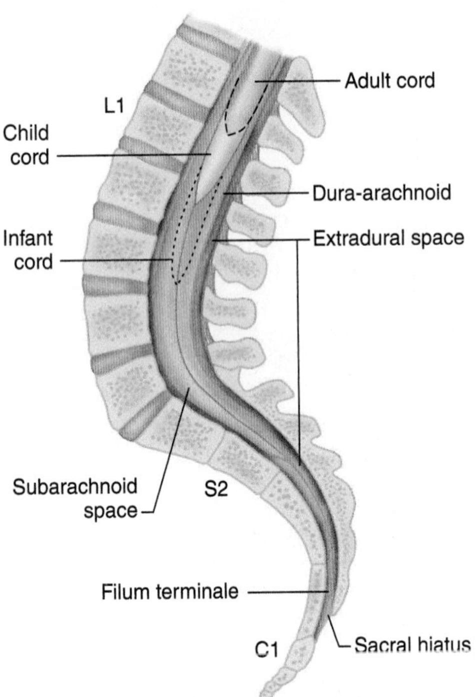

FIGURE 45–7 Sagittal view through the lumbar vertebrae and sacrum. Note the end of the spinal cord rises with development from approximately L3 to L1. The dural sac normally ends at S2.

pia mater, the *filum terminale*, penetrates the dura and attaches the terminal end of the spinal cord (*conus medullaris*) to the periosteum of the coccyx (see Figure 45–7).

The blood supply to the spinal cord and nerve roots is derived from a single anterior spinal artery and paired posterior spinal arteries (Figure 45–8). The anterior spinal artery is formed from the vertebral artery at the base of the skull and courses down along the anterior surface of the cord. The anterior spinal artery supplies the anterior two-thirds of the cord, whereas the two posterior spinal arteries supply the posterior one-third. The posterior spinal arteries arise from the posterior inferior cerebellar arteries and course down along the dorsal surface of the cord medial to the dorsal nerve roots. The anterior and posterior spinal arteries receive additional blood flow from the intercostal arteries in the thorax and the lumbar arteries in the abdomen. One of these radicular arteries is typically large, the *artery of Adamkiewicz*,

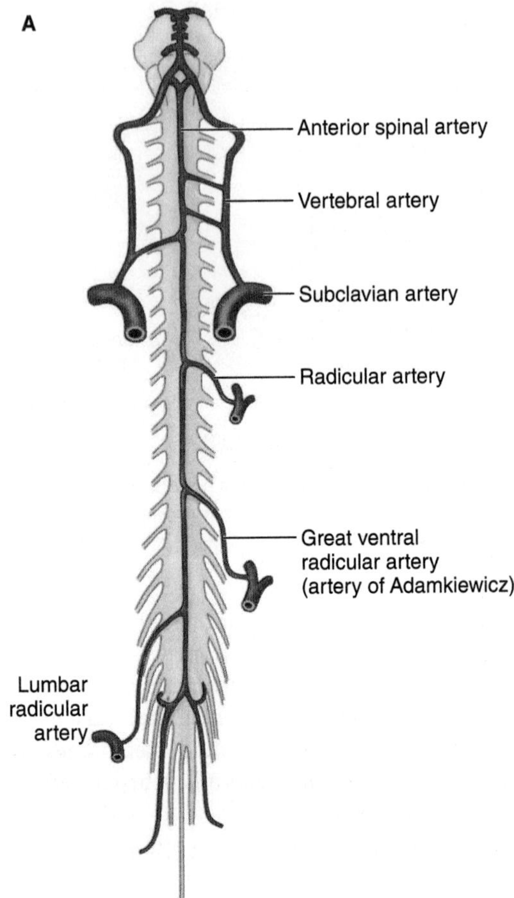

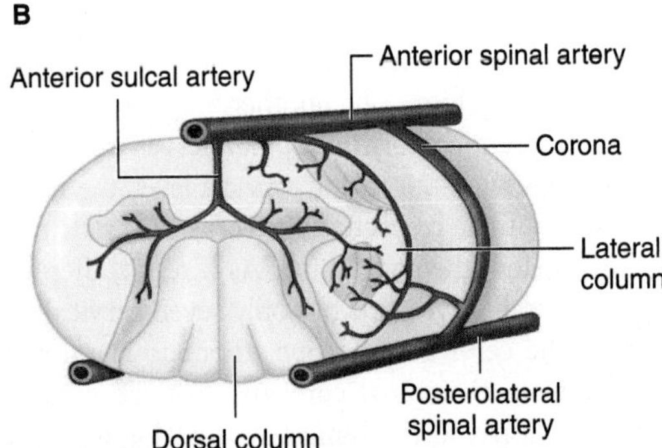

FIGURE 45–8 Arterial supply to the spinal cord. **A**: Anterior view showing principal sources of blood supply. **B**: Cross-sectional view through the spinal cord showing paired posterior spinal arteries and a single anterior spinal artery. (Adapted with permission from Waxman SG. *Correlative Neuroanatomy*, 24th ed. New York, NY: McGraw Hill; 2000.)

or *arteria radicularis magna*, arising from the aorta (see Figure 45–8A). It is typically unilateral and nearly always arises on the left side, providing the major blood supply to the anterior, lower two-thirds of the spinal cord. Injury to this artery can result in *anterior spinal artery syndrome* (see Chapter 22).

Mechanism of Action

3 The principal site of action for neuraxial blockade is believed to be the nerve root, at least during the initial onset of block. Local anesthetics may also have actions on structures within the spinal cord during epidural and spinal anesthesia. Local anesthetic is injected into CSF (spinal anesthesia) or the epidural space (epidural and caudal anesthesia) and bathes the nerve root in the subarachnoid space or epidural space, respectively. Direct injection of local anesthetic into CSF for spinal anesthesia allows a relatively small dose and volume of local anesthetic to achieve dense sensory and motor blockade. In contrast, neuraxial block is achieved only with much larger volumes and quantities of local anesthetic molecules during epidural and caudal anesthesia. The injection site (spinal level) for epidural anesthesia is ideally located at the midpoint of the dermatomes that must be anesthetized. Blockade of neural transmission (conduction) in the posterior nerve root fibers interrupts somatic and visceral sensation, whereas blockade of anterior nerve root fibers prevents efferent motor and autonomic outflow.

SOMATIC BLOCKADE

Neuraxial blocks provide excellent operating conditions by interrupting the afferent transmission of painful stimuli and abolishing the efferent impulses responsible for skeletal muscle tone. Sensory blockade interrupts both somatic and visceral painful stimuli. The mechanism of action of local anesthetic agents is discussed in Chapter 16. Smaller and myelinated fibers are generally more easily blocked than larger and unmyelinated ones. The size and character of the fiber types, and the fact that the concentration of local anesthetic decreases with increasing distance from the level of injection, explains the phenomenon of *differential blockade* during neuraxial anesthesia.
4 Differential blockade typically results in sympathetic blockade (judged by temperature sensitivity) that may be two segments or more cephalad than the sensory block (pain, light touch), which, in turn, is usually several segments more cephalad than the motor blockade.

AUTONOMIC BLOCKADE

5 Interruption of efferent autonomic transmission at the spinal nerve roots during neuraxial blocks produces sympathetic blockade. Sympathetic outflow from the spinal cord may be described as *thoracolumbar*, whereas parasympathetic outflow is *craniosacral*. Sympathetic preganglionic nerve fibers (small, myelinated B fibers) exit the spinal cord with the spinal nerves from T1–L2 and may course many levels up or down the sympathetic chain before synapsing with a postganglionic cell in a sympathetic ganglion. In contrast, parasympathetic preganglionic fibers exit the spinal cord with the cranial and sacral nerves. Neuraxial anesthesia does not block the vagus nerve (tenth cranial nerve). The physiological responses to neuraxial blockade therefore result from decreased sympathetic tone or unopposed parasympathetic tone, or both.

Cardiovascular Manifestations

6 Neuraxial blocks produce variable decreases in blood pressure that may be accompanied by a decrease in heart rate. These effects generally increase with more cephalad dermatomal levels and more extensive sympathectomy. Vasomotor tone is primarily determined by sympathetic fibers arising from T5 to L1, innervating arterial and venous smooth muscle. Blocking these nerves causes vasodilation of the venous capacitance vessels and pooling of blood in the viscera and lower extremities, thereby decreasing the effective circulating blood volume and often decreasing cardiac output. Arterial vasodilation may also decrease systemic vascular resistance. The effects of arterial vasodilation may be minimized by compensatory vasoconstriction above the level of the block, particularly when the extent of sensory anesthesia is limited to the lower thoracic dermatomes. A high sympathetic block not only prevents

compensatory vasoconstriction but may also block the sympathetic cardiac accelerator fibers that arise at T1 to T4. Profound hypotension may result from arterial dilation and venous pooling combined with bradycardia. These effects are exaggerated if venous pooling is further augmented by a head-up position or by the weight of a gravid uterus on the vena cava. Unopposed vagal tone may explain the sudden bradycardia, complete heart block, or cardiac arrest occasionally seen with spinal anesthesia.

7 Deleterious cardiovascular effects can be anticipated, and steps should be undertaken to minimize the degree of hypotension. However, the formerly common practice of volume loading with 10 to 20 mL/kg of intravenous fluid in a healthy patient before initiation of the block has been shown repeatedly to fail to prevent hypotension (in the absence of preexisting hypovolemia). Left uterine displacement in the third trimester of pregnancy helps minimize physical obstruction to venous return in some patients. Despite these efforts, hypotension may still occur and should be treated promptly. Autotransfusion may be accomplished by placing the patient in a head-down position. A bolus of intravenous fluid (5–10 mL/kg) may be helpful in patients who have adequate cardiac and renal function to be able to "handle" the fluid load
8 after the block wears off. Excessive or symptomatic bradycardia should be treated with atropine, and hypotension should be treated with vasopressors. Direct α-adrenergic agonists (such as phenylephrine) primarily produce vasoconstriction, increasing systemic vascular resistance, and may reflexively increase bradycardia. The "mixed" agent ephedrine has direct and indirect β-adrenergic effects that increase heart rate and contractility, and indirect α-adrenergic effects that also produce vasoconstriction. Phenylephrine is the preferred agent for hypotension during neuraxial blocks in obstetrical patients. Norepinephrine has also been suggested to restore blood pressure following neuraxial anesthesia-induced hypotension. Some investigators have suggested that ondansetron, a 5-HT receptor antagonist, can mitigate spinal anesthesia-induced hypotension by blunting the Bezold–Jarisch reflex, which is influenced by serotonin release secondary to decreased venous return during spinal anesthesia.

Pulmonary Manifestations

Alterations in pulmonary physiology are usually minimal with neuraxial blocks because the diaphragm is innervated by the phrenic nerve, with fibers originating from C3 to C5. Even with high thoracic levels, tidal volume is unchanged; there is only a small decrease in vital capacity, which results from a loss of the abdominal muscles' contribution to forced expiration.

Patients with severe chronic lung disease may rely upon accessory muscles of respiration (intercostal and abdominal muscles) to actively inspire or exhale. High levels of neural blockade will impair these muscles. Similarly, effective coughing and clearing of secretions require these muscles for expiration. For these reasons, neuraxial blocks should be used with caution in patients with limited respiratory reserve. These deleterious effects need to be weighed against the advantages of avoiding airway instrumentation and positive-pressure ventilation. For surgical procedures above the umbilicus, a purely regional technique may not be the best choice in patients with severe lung disease. On the other hand, these patients may benefit from the effects of thoracic epidural analgesia (using diluted local anesthetics and opioids) or intrathecal opioids in the postoperative period, particularly following upper abdominal or thoracic surgery. Some evidence suggests that postoperative thoracic epidural analgesia in high-risk patients can improve pulmonary outcomes by decreasing the incidence of pneumonia and respiratory failure, improving oxygenation, and decreasing the duration of mechanical ventilatory support.

Gastrointestinal Manifestations

Neuraxial block–induced sympathectomy allows vagal "dominance" with a small, contracted gut and active peristalsis. This can improve operative conditions during intestinal surgery when used as an adjunct to general anesthesia. Postoperative epidural analgesia with local anesthetics and minimal systemic opioids hastens the return of gastrointestinal function after open abdominal procedures.

Hepatic blood flow will decrease with reductions in mean arterial pressure from any anesthetic technique, including neuraxial anesthesia.

Urinary Tract Manifestations

Renal blood flow is maintained through autoregulation, and there is little effect of neuraxial anesthesia on kidney function with normal systemic blood pressures. Neuraxial anesthesia at the lumbar and sacral levels blocks both sympathetic and parasympathetic control of bladder function. Loss of autonomic bladder control results in urinary retention until the block wears off. If no urinary catheter is placed perioperatively, it is prudent to use the local anesthetic of the shortest duration sufficient for the surgical procedure and to administer the minimal safe volume of intravenous fluid. Patients with a history of urinary retention should be checked for bladder distention after neuraxial anesthesia.

Metabolic & Endocrine Manifestations

Surgical trauma produces a systemic *neuroendocrine stress response* via activation of somatic and visceral afferent nerve fibers, in addition to a localized inflammatory response. This systemic response includes increased concentrations of adrenocorticotropic hormone, cortisol, epinephrine, norepinephrine, and vasopressin levels, as well as activation of the renin–angiotensin–aldosterone system. Clinical manifestations include intraoperative and postoperative hypertension, tachycardia, hyperglycemia, protein catabolism, suppressed immune responses, and altered renal function. Neuraxial blockade can partially suppress (during major invasive abdominal or thoracic surgery) or totally block (during lower extremity surgery) the neuroendocrine stress response. Neuraxial block should precede incision and continue postoperatively to maximize this blunting of the neuroendocrine stress response.

Clinical Considerations Common to Spinal & Epidural Blocks

Indications

Neuraxial blocks may be used alone or in conjunction with general anesthesia for many procedures below the neck. As a primary anesthetic, neuraxial blocks have proved most useful in lower abdominal, inguinal, urogenital, rectal, and lower extremity surgery. Lumbar spinal surgery may also be performed under spinal anesthesia. Upper abdominal procedures (eg, gastrectomy) have been performed with spinal or epidural anesthesia, but because it can be difficult to safely achieve a sensory level adequate for patient comfort, these techniques are less commonly used.

If a neuraxial anesthetic is being considered, the risks and benefits must be discussed with the patient, and informed consent should be obtained. The patient must be mentally prepared for neuraxial anesthesia, and neuraxial anesthesia must be appropriate for the type of surgery. Patients should understand that they will have little or no lower extremity motor function until the block resolves. Procedures that require maneuvers that might compromise respiratory function (eg, pneumoperitoneum or pneumothorax) or operations that are unusually long are typically performed with general anesthesia, with or without neuraxial blockade.

Contraindications

9 Major contraindications to neuraxial anesthesia include lack of consent, coagulation abnormalities, severe hypovolemia, elevated intracranial pressure (particularly with an intracranial mass), and infection at the site of injection. Other relative contraindications include severe aortic or mitral stenosis and severe left ventricular outflow obstruction (hypertrophic obstructive cardiomyopathy); however, with close monitoring and control of the anesthetic level, neuraxial anesthesia can be performed safely in patients with stenotic valvular heart disease, particularly if the extensive dermatomal spread of anesthesia is not required (eg, "saddle" block spinal anesthetics).

Relative and controversial contraindications are also shown in Table 45–1. Inspection and palpation of the back can reveal surgical scars, scoliosis, skin lesions, and whether or not the spinous processes can be identified. Although preoperative screening tests are not required in healthy patients undergoing neuraxial blockade, appropriate testing should be performed if the clinical history suggests a coagulation abnormality. Neuraxial anesthesia in the presence of sepsis or bacteremia could theoretically predispose patients to seeding of the infectious agents into the epidural or subarachnoid space.

TABLE 45–1 Contraindications to neuraxial blockade.

Absolute
Infection at the site of injection
Lack of consent
Coagulopathy or other bleeding diathesis
Severe hypovolemia
Increased intracranial pressure
Relative
Sepsis
Uncooperative patient
Preexisting neurological deficits
Demyelinating lesions
Stenotic valvular heart lesions
Left ventricular outflow obstruction (hypertrophic obstructive cardiomyopathy)
Severe spinal deformity
Controversial
Prior back surgery at the site of injection
Complicated surgery
Prolonged operation
Major blood loss
Maneuvers that compromise respiration

Patients with preexisting neurological deficits or demyelinating diseases may report worsening symptoms following a neuraxial block. It may be impossible to discern the effects or complications of the block from preexisting deficits or unrelated exacerbation of preexisting disease. For these reasons, some risk-averse practitioners avoid neuraxial anesthesia in such patients. A preoperative neurological examination should thoroughly document any deficits. In a retrospective study examining the records of 567 patients with preexisting neuropathies, two of the patients developed new or worsening neuropathy following neuraxial anesthesia. Although this finding indicates a relatively low risk of further injury, study investigators suggest that an injured nerve is vulnerable to additional injury, increasing the likelihood of poor neurological outcomes. However, a history of preexisting neurological deficits or demyelinating disease is at best a relative contraindication, and the balance of perioperative risks in this patient population may favor neuraxial anesthesia in select patients.

Regional anesthesia requires at least some degree of patient cooperation. This may be difficult or impossible for patients with dementia, psychosis, or emotional instability. The decision must be individualized. Unsedated young children may not be suitable for pure regional techniques; however, regional anesthesia is frequently used with general anesthesia in children.

Neuraxial Blockade in the Setting of Anticoagulants & Antiplatelet Agents

Whether a block should be performed in the setting of anticoagulants and antiplatelet agents can be problematic. The American Society of Regional Anesthesia and Pain Medicine (ASRA) has issued guidelines on this subject. Because guidelines are frequently revised and updated, practitioners are advised to seek the most recent edition. Fortunately, the incidence of epidural hematoma is reported to be infrequent (1 in 150,000 epidurals). The use of anticoagulant and antiplatelet medications continues to increase, placing an ever-larger number of patients at potential risk of epidural hematomas. However, because of the rarity of epidural hematomas, most guidelines are based on expert opinion and case series reviews, as clinical trials are not feasible.

A. Oral Anticoagulants

If neuraxial anesthesia is to be used in patients receiving warfarin therapy, a normal prothrombin time and international normalized ratio usually will be documented prior to the block, unless the drug has been discontinued for weeks. Anesthesia staff should always consult with the patient's primary physicians whenever considering the discontinuation of antiplatelet or antithrombotic therapy. New agents such as the direct thrombin inhibitor dabigatran and the factor X_a inhibitors rivaroxaban and apixaban are increasingly encountered by anesthesia providers (Figure 45–9).

Recommendations related to anti–factor Xa agents include:

- Rivaroxaban should be discontinued 72 hours before a neuraxial block. If a block is considered less than 72 hours after discontinuation of rivaroxaban, one can

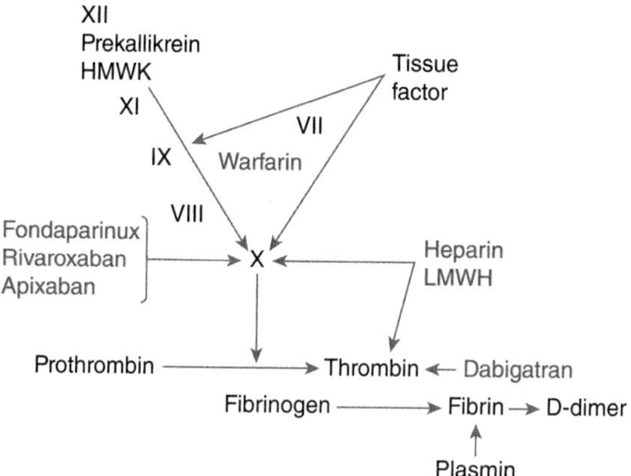

FIGURE 45–9 Sites of action of anticoagulant drugs. Clotting factors are indicated by Roman numerals. Warfarin reduces the production of factors VII, IX, X, and prothrombin. Heparin and LMWH inhibit factor Xa and thrombin. Fondaparinux, rivaroxaban, and apixaban are direct factor Xa inhibitors. Dabigatran is a direct thrombin inhibitor. HMWK, high-molecular-weight kininogen; LMWH, low-molecular-weight heparin. (Reproduced with permission from Benzon H, Avram M, Green D, Bonow R. New oral anticoagulants and regional anesthesia. *Br J Anaesth*. 2013 Dec;111(Suppl 1):i96-i113.)

check anti–factor Xa activity; however, an acceptable level of activity has not been determined. Neuraxial catheters should be removed 6 hours before the first postoperative dose. Should rivaroxaban be administered before catheter removal, 22 to 26 hours should elapse before catheter removal, or an anti–factor Xa assay should be assessed before catheter removal.

- Apixaban recommendations are similar to those for rivaroxaban, except they suggest waiting 26 to 30 hours for catheter removal in the event that a postoperative dose has been inadvertently administered.
- Edoxaban recommendations are similar; however, the guidelines suggest that catheter removal be held for 20 to 28 hours or an anti–factor Xa assay be completed.
- Betrixaban should be discontinued 3 days before neuraxial block, and neuraxial block should not be performed in patients with a creatinine clearance of less than 30 mL/min. Neuraxial catheters should be removed 5 hours before resumption of betrixaban postoperatively. In the event that the catheter remains in place and a dose is given, the guidelines suggest waiting 72 hours before catheter removal.

Dabigatran is a direct thrombin inhibitor. Because dabigatran is dependent on kidney function, recommendations may be adjusted based upon patient status (eg, kidney function is reliably determined, and the patient is not older than 65 years of age, hypertensive, or on antiplatelet medications). These recommendations include:

- Dabigatran should be discontinued 72 hours prior to neuraxial anesthesia in patients with creatinine clearance greater than 80 mL/min. Monitoring the direct thrombin time or ecarin clotting time is suggested if neuraxial anesthesia is considered less than 72 hours since the discontinuation of therapy. However, an acceptable level of dabigatran activity has not been determined.
- A 96-hour discontinuation period is suggested prior to neuraxial anesthesia in patients with a creatinine clearance of 50 to 79 mL/min and 120 hours for patients with a creatinine clearance of 30 to 49 mL/min. Neuraxial anesthesia is not recommended for patients taking dabigatran with a creatinine clearance of less than 30 mL/min.
- Catheters should be removed 6 hours before resuming dabigatran therapy. In the event of dosing a patient with dabigatran in the presence of an indwelling catheter, 34 to 36 hours should elapse before catheter removal.

Thrombin clotting time assays can be used to detect the effects of dabigatran. Likewise, factor Xa inhibitors can be assessed through assays of factor Xa inhibition. Anesthesia providers planning neuraxial procedures should consult closely with the patient's primary providers to discern if suspension of anticoagulation can be done safely when considering a neuraxial technique. Bridging therapy with heparin can be considered during the time that oral anticoagulation is suspended if there is increased thrombotic risk.

B. Antiplatelet Drugs

By themselves, aspirin and other nonsteroidal anti-inflammatory drugs (NSAIDs) do not increase the risk of spinal hematoma from neuraxial anesthesia procedures or epidural catheter removal. This assumes a normal patient with a normal coagulation profile who is not receiving other medications that might affect clotting mechanisms. In contrast, more potent agents should be stopped, and neuraxial blockade should generally be administered only after their effects have worn off. The waiting period depends on the specific agent: for ticlopidine, it is 10 days; clopidogrel, 5 to 7 days; prasugrel, 7 to 10 days; ticagrelor, 5 to 7 days; abciximab, 24 to 48 h; and eptifibatide, 4 to 8 h. Neuraxial techniques should be avoided in patients receiving antiplatelet medications until platelet function has been recovered. Metabolites of clopidogrel and prasugrel block the P2Y12 receptor, impeding platelet aggregation. Ticagrelor directly inhibits the P2Y12 receptor. Both prasugrel and ticagrelor have greater platelet inhibition compared with clopidogrel. In patients with a recently placed cardiac stent, discontinuation of antiplatelet therapy can result in stent thrombosis and acute ST-segment elevation myocardial infarction. The risks versus the benefits of a neuraxial technique should be discussed with the patient and the patient's primary physicians.

Resumption of antiplatelet medications may occur at the time of catheter removal with thienopyridine therapy (ticlopidine, clopidogrel, prasugrel) unless a loading dose is to be administered. In the latter case, drug therapy should resume 6 hours after catheter removal. A similar recommendation is offered for ticagrelor.

Guidelines suggest that dipyridamole be discontinued 24 hours before neuraxial block and that it be resumed 6 hours after catheter removal.

C. Standard (Unfractionated) Heparin

Low-dose subcutaneous (SC) heparin prophylaxis is not a contraindication to neuraxial anesthesia or epidural catheter removal. Guidelines suggest that neuraxial anesthesia occur 4 to 6 h after dosing with 5000 units of subcutaneous heparin. Additional delays are indicated for patients receiving higher dose SC thromboprophylaxis. Catheter removal should occur 4 to 6 hours following low-dose SC heparin administration. In patients who are to receive systemic heparin intraoperatively, blocks may be performed 1 h or more before heparin administration. A bloody epidural or spinal catheter placement does not necessarily require cancellation of surgery, but discussion of the risks with the surgeon and careful postoperative monitoring is needed. Removal of an epidural catheter should occur 1 h before or 2 to 4 h after subsequent heparin dosing. The patient's coagulation status should be assessed before the catheter is removed.

Neuraxial anesthesia should be avoided in patients on therapeutic doses of intravenous heparin and with increased partial thromboplastin time. If the patient is started on heparin after the placement of an epidural catheter, the catheter should be removed only after discontinuation or interruption of heparin infusion and evaluation of the coagulation status. The risk of spinal hematoma is unclear in the setting of the anticoagulation required for cardiac surgery, and we have used epidural techniques for pain control after such procedures as off-pump coronary bypass only in the rare instances where the anticipated benefits exceed the perceived risks. Prompt diagnosis and evacuation of symptomatic epidural hematomas increase the likelihood that neurologic function will be preserved.

D. Low-Molecular-Weight Heparin (LMWH)

A number of cases of spinal hematoma were reported associated with neuraxial anesthesia after patients began receiving LMWH, enoxaparin (Lovenox), in the United States in 1993. **Many of these cases involved intraoperative or early postoperative LMWH use, and several patients were receiving concomitant antiplatelet medication**. Guidelines include:

- Heparin-induced thrombocytopenia can occur during LMWH therapy, and as such, a platelet count should be obtained in patients receiving LMWH for longer than 4 days prior to neuraxial block.
- LMWH therapy should be delayed in the event of a bloody neuraxial block for 24 hours in consultation with the surgeon.

- Neuraxial block should occur 12 hours after LMWH administration.
- In patients receiving higher doses of LMWH (eg, enoxaparin 1 mg/kg every 12 hours), neuraxial block should be delayed for 24 hours. Anti–factor Xa activity should be checked in older adult patients and those with reduced kidney function.
- Twice-daily LMWH therapy should be initiated postoperatively no earlier than 12 hours after neuraxial block. Catheters should be removed before LMWH therapy. LMWH should be administered 4 hours after catheter removal.
- Single daily dosing of LMWH therapy should start no sooner than 12 hours after needle placement for neuraxial block, and the second dose should occur no sooner than 24 hours after the first dose. Indwelling neuraxial catheters can be maintained, assuming no other hemostasis-altering medications are administered. Catheter removal should occur 12 hours after the last dose of LMWH, and subsequent dosing should not occur until 4 hours after catheter removal.

The anti–factor Xa agent fondaparinux is suggested for use as thromboprophylaxis in the setting of neuraxial anesthesia only if performed under the conditions used in clinical trials, such as a single pass of the needle, atraumatic placement of the block, and avoidance of indwelling catheters. If these conditions are not feasible, alternative thromboprophylaxis methods should be considered.

E. Fibrinolytic or Thrombolytic Therapy

Neuraxial anesthesia should not be performed if a patient has received fibrinolytic or thrombolytic therapy.

The American Society of Regional Anesthesia and Pain Medicine (ASRA) has developed a smartphone application (ASRA Coags Regional app) to assist in the perioperative management of patients taking drugs that affect coagulation. We strongly urge regional anesthesia practitioners to utilize this resource.

F. Considerations for Obstetric Anesthesia

The Society for Obstetric Anesthesia and Perinatology has prepared a consensus statement regarding the thromboprophylaxis management of pregnant and postpartum patients. It provides decision aids to guide the management of neuraxial anesthesia in urgent and emergency conditions (Figures 45–10 and 45–11).

Although the incidence of hematoma formation following neuraxial anesthesia is low, there is an expanding armamentarium of anticoagulant and antiplatelet medications employed in clinical practice. Consequently, practitioners are strongly advised to continually review current recommendations from the various organizations.

Awake or Asleep?

When used in conjunction with general anesthesia, should lumbar neuraxial anesthesia be performed after induction of general anesthesia? This is controversial. The major arguments for having the patient asleep are that (1) most patients, if given a choice, would prefer to be asleep and (2) the possibility of sudden patient movement causing injury is markedly diminished. The major argument in favor of neuraxial blockade administration only while the patient is still awake is that the patient can alert the clinician to paresthesia and pain on injection in this circumstance, both of which have been associated with postoperative neurological deficits. Although many clinicians are comfortable performing lumbar epidural or spinal puncture in anesthetized or deeply sedated adults, there is greater consensus, though not unanimous opinion, that thoracic and cervical punctures should, except under unusual circumstances, only be performed in awake, responsive patients. Pediatric neuraxial blocks, particularly caudal and epidural blocks, are usually performed under general anesthesia.

Technical Considerations

Neuraxial blocks must be performed only in a facility in which all the equipment and drugs needed for intubation, resuscitation, and general anesthesia are immediately available. Regional anesthesia is greatly facilitated by adequate patient preparation and

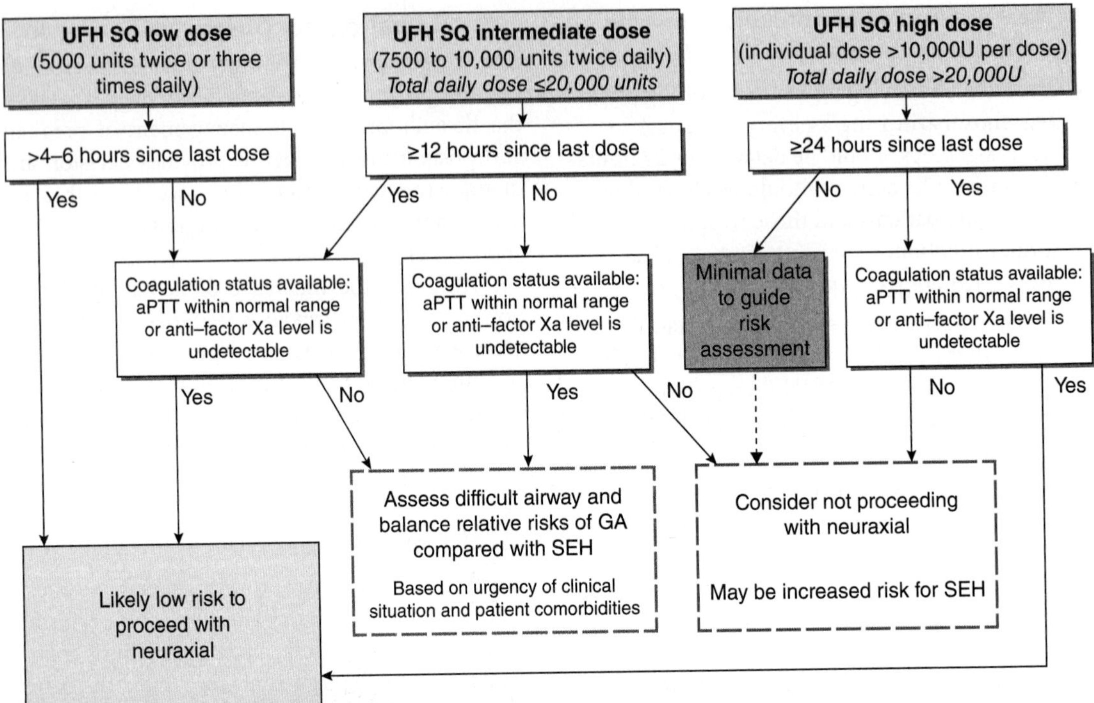

FIGURE 45–10 Decision aid for urgent or emergency neuraxial procedures in the obstetric patient receiving UFH. *Assume normal renal function, body weight >40 kg and no other contraindications to neuraxial anesthesia. aPTT, activated partial thromboplastin time; GA, general anesthesia; SEH, spinal epidural hematoma; SQ, subcutaneous; UFH, unfractionated heparin. Note: This SOAP consensus statement is not intended to set out a legal standard of care and does not replace medical care or the judgment of the responsible medical professional considering all the circumstances presented by an individual patient. (Reproduced with permission from Leffert L, Butwick A, Carvalho B, et al: The Society for Obstetric Anesthesia and Perinatology Consensus Statement on the Anesthetic Management of Pregnant and Postpartum Women Receiving Thromboprophylaxis or Higher Dose Anticoagulants, *Anesth Analg.* 2018 Mar;126(3):928-944.)

premedication. The patient should be told what to expect so as to minimize anxiety. This is particularly important in situations in which premedication is not used, as is typically the case in obstetric anesthesia. Supplemental oxygen via a face mask or nasal cannula may be required to avoid hypoxemia when sedation is used. Minimum monitoring requirements include blood pressure and pulse oximetry for labor analgesia. Monitoring for blocks administered for surgical anesthesia is the same as that for general anesthesia.

Surface Anatomy

Spinous processes are usually palpable and help define the midline. Ultrasound can be used when landmarks are not palpable (Figure 45–12). Ultrasound is less useful in patients with easily identified landmarks. The spinous processes of the cervical and lumbar spine are nearly horizontal, whereas those in the thoracic spine slant in a caudal direction and can overlap significantly (see Figure 45–2). Therefore, when performing a lumbar or cervical epidural block (with maximum spinal flexion), the needle is directed with only a slight cephalad angle, if at all, whereas for a thoracic block, the needle must be angled significantly more cephalad to enter the thoracic epidural space. In the cervical area, the first palpable spinous process is that of C2, but the most prominent one is that of C7 (*vertebra prominens*). With the arms at the side, the spinous process of T7 is usually at the same level as the inferior angle of the scapulae (Figure 45–13). A line drawn between

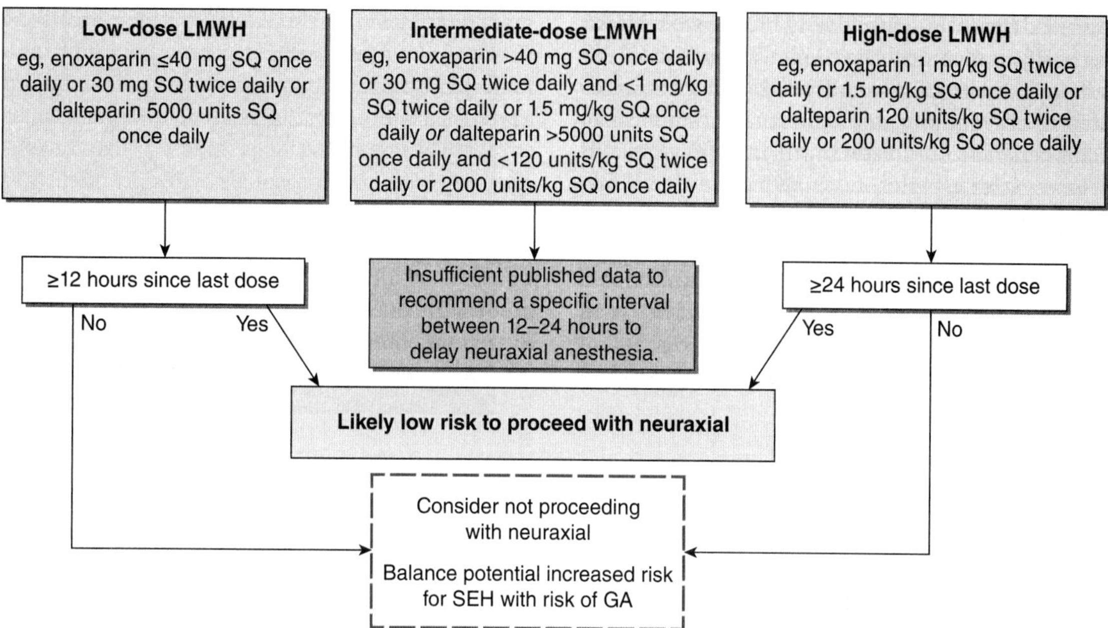

FIGURE 45–11 Decision aid for urgent or emergency neuraxial procedures in the obstetric patient receiving LMWH. *Assume normal renal function, body weight >40 kg, and no other contraindications to neuraxial anesthesia. GA, general anesthesia; LMWH, low molecular weight heparin; SEH, spinal epidural hematoma; SQ, subcutaneous. Note: This SOAP consensus statement is not intended to set out a legal standard of care and does not replace medical care or the judgment of the responsible medical professional considering all the circumstances presented by an individual patient. (Reproduced with permission from Leffert L, Butwick A, Carvalho B, et al: The Society for Obstetric Anesthesia and Perinatology Consensus Statement on the Anesthetic Management of Pregnant and Postpartum Women Receiving Thromboprophylaxis or Higher Dose Anticoagulants, *Anesth Analg.* 2018 Mar;126(3):928-944.)

the highest points of both iliac crests (*Tuffier's line*) usually crosses either the body of L4 or the L4–L5 interspace. Counting spinous processes up or down from these reference points identifies other spinal levels. A line connecting the posterior superior iliac spine crosses the S2 posterior foramina. In slender persons, the sacrum is easily palpable, and the sacral hiatus is felt as a depression just above or between the gluteal clefts and above the coccyx, defining the point of entry for caudal blocks.

Patient Positioning

A. Sitting Position

The anatomic midline is often easier to identify when the patient is sitting than when the patient is in the lateral decubitus position (Figure 45–14). This is particularly true with obese patients. Patients sit with their elbows resting on their thighs or a bedside table, or they can hug a pillow. Flexion of the spine (arching the back "like an angry cat") maximizes the "target" area between adjacent spinous processes and brings the spine closer to the skin surface (Figure 45–15).

B. Lateral Decubitus

Many clinicians prefer the lateral position for neuraxial blocks (Figure 45–16). Patients lie on their side with their knees flexed and pulled high against the abdomen or chest, assuming a "fetal position." An assistant can help the patient assume and hold this position.

C. Buie's (Jackknife) Position

This position may be used for anorectal procedures utilizing an isobaric or hypobaric anesthetic

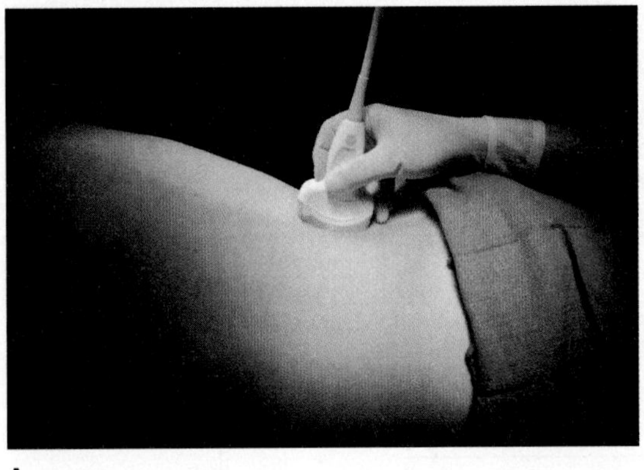

A

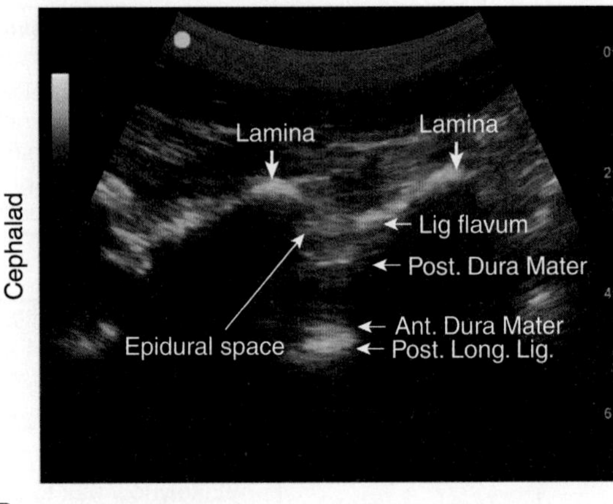

B

FIGURE 45–12 **A**: Transducer position to image paramedian epidural space at the lumbar spine, longitudinal view. **B**: Corresponding ultrasound image. Ant. Dura Mater, anterior dura mater; Lig. Flavum, ligamentum flavum; Post. Dura Mater, posterior dura mater; Post. Long. Lig., posterior longitudinal ligament. (Reproduced with permission from Hadzic, A. *Peripheral Nerve Blocks and Anatomy for Ultrasound-Guided Regional Anesthesia*, 2nd ed. New York, NY: McGraw Hill; 2012.)

solution (see later discussion). The advantage is that the block is done in the same position as the operative procedure so the patient does not have to be moved following the block. The disadvantage is that CSF will not freely flow through the needle, so correct subarachnoid needle tip placement will need to be confirmed by CSF aspiration. A prone

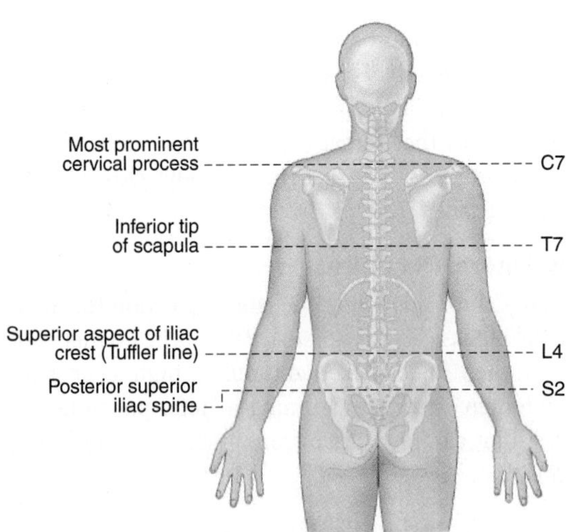

FIGURE 45–13 Surface landmarks for identifying spinal levels.

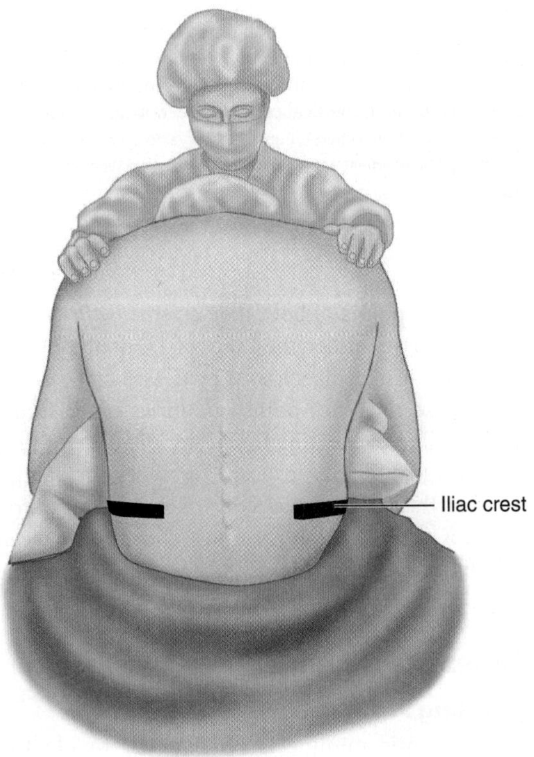

FIGURE 45–14 Sitting position for neuraxial blockade. Note an assistant helps in obtaining maximal spinal flexion.

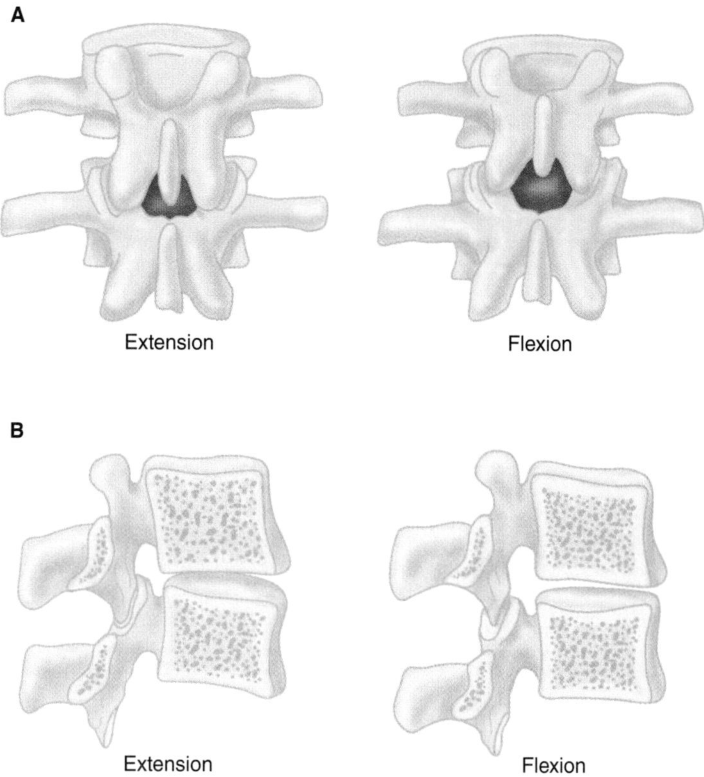

FIGURE 45–15 The effect of flexion on adjacent vertebrae. **A**: Posterior view. **B**: Lateral view. Note the target area (interlaminar foramen) for neuraxial blocks increases in size with flexion.

position is typically used when fluoroscopic guidance is required.

Anatomic Approach

A. Midline Approach

The spine is palpated, and the patient's body is positioned so that a needle passed parallel to the floor will stay midline as it courses deeper (see Figure 45–4). A sterile field is established with an appropriate antibacterial solution. A fenestrated sterile drape is applied. After the preparation solution has dried, the depression between the spinous processes of the vertebrae above and below the level to be used is palpated; this will be the needle entry site. A skin wheal is raised at the level of the chosen interspace with a local anesthetic using a small (25-gauge) needle. A longer needle can be used for deeper local anesthetic infiltration.

Next, the procedure needle is introduced in the midline. As the spinous processes course caudad from their origin at the spine, the needle will be directed slightly cephalad. The subcutaneous tissues offer little resistance to the needle. As the needle courses deeper, it will enter the supraspinous and interspinous ligaments, felt as an increase in tissue resistance. The needle also feels more firmly implanted in the back (like "an arrow in a target"). If bone is contacted superficially, a midline needle is likely hitting the lower spinous process. Contact with bone at a deeper level usually indicates that the needle is in the midline and hitting the upper spinous process or that it is lateral to the midline and hitting a lamina. In either case, the needle must be redirected. As the needle penetrates the ligamentum flavum, an obvious increase in resistance is encountered. At this point, the procedures for spinal and epidural anesthesia differ.

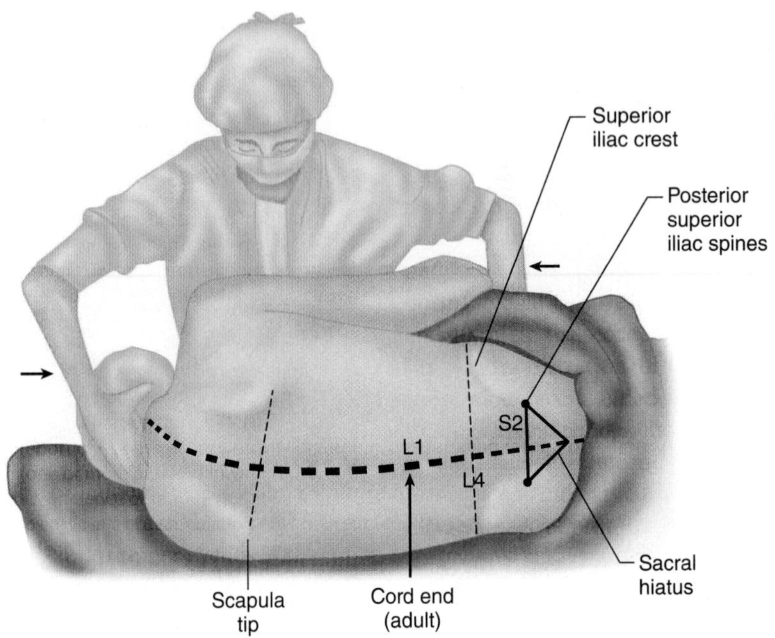

FIGURE 45–16 Lateral decubitus position for neuraxial blockade. Note again the assistant helping to provide maximal spine flexion.

10 For epidural anesthesia, a sudden loss of resistance (to injection of air or saline) is encountered as the needle passes through the ligamentum flavum and enters the epidural space. For spinal anesthesia, the needle is advanced through the epidural space and penetrates the dura–subarachnoid membranes, as signaled by freely flowing CSF.

B. Paramedian Approach

The paramedian technique may be selected, particularly if epidural or subarachnoid block is difficult, particularly in patients who cannot be positioned easily (eg, severe arthritis, kyphoscoliosis, or prior spine surgery) (Figure 45–17). Many clinicians routinely use the paramedian approach for thoracic epidural puncture. After skin preparation and sterile draping (as previously described), the skin wheal for a paramedian approach is raised 2 cm lateral to the inferior aspect of the superior spinous process of the desired level. Because this approach is lateral to most of the interspinous ligaments and penetrates the paraspinous muscles, the needle may encounter little resistance initially and may not seem to be in firm tissue. The needle is directed and advanced at a 10° to 25° angle toward the midline. If bone is encountered at a shallow depth with the paramedian approach, the needle is likely in contact with the medial part of the lower lamina and should be redirected mostly upward and perhaps slightly more laterally. On the other hand, if bone is encountered deeply, the needle is usually in contact with the lateral part of the lower lamina and should be redirected only slightly craniad, more toward the midline (Figure 45–18).

C. Assessing Level of Blockade

With knowledge of the sensory dermatomes (see Appendix), the extent of sensory block can be assessed by a blunted needle or a piece of ice.

D. Ultrasound- or Fluoroscopy-Guided Neuraxial Blockade

Although it has not, as of yet, transformed the practice of neuraxial blockade in the same manner as it has for other procedures, ultrasound guidance can facilitate neuraxial blockade in patients with poorly palpable landmarks. As with other uses of ultrasound, specific training is required for practitioners

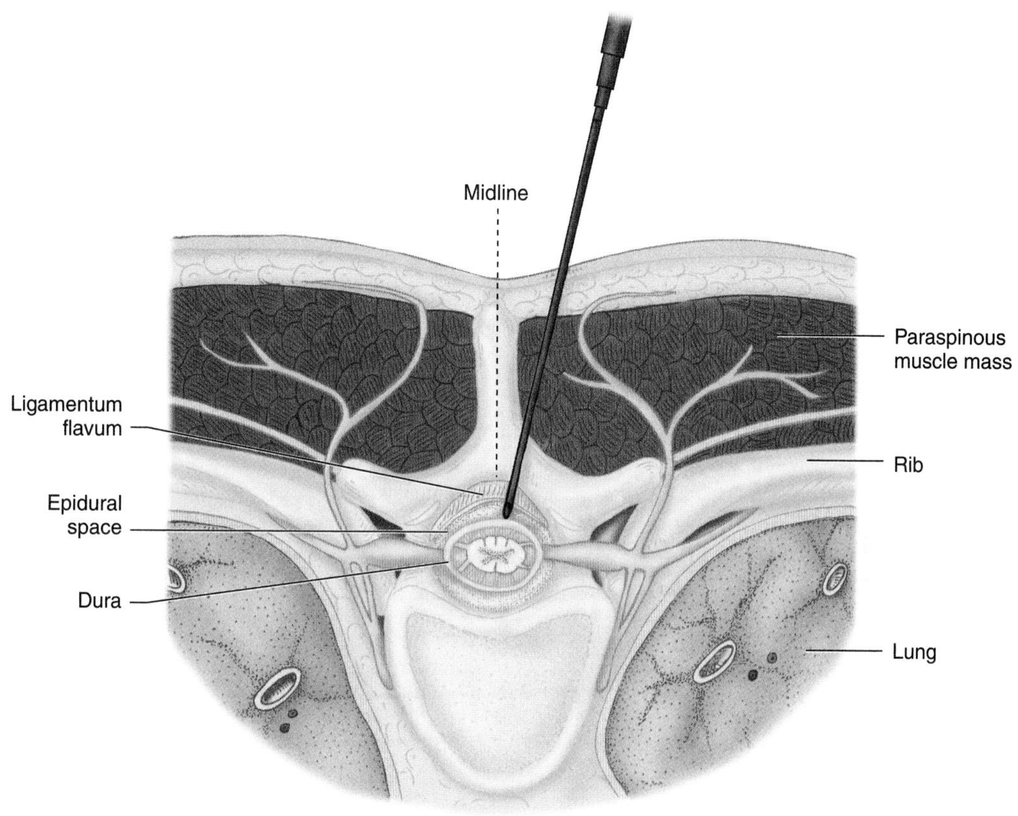

FIGURE 45–17 Paramedian approach.

to identify the landmarks and interspaces necessary for neuraxial blockade correctly. Some clinicians routinely use fluoroscopy to perform thoracic epidural procedures, which allows them to confirm correct placement with radiocontrast dye.

Spinal Needles

Spinal needles are commercially available in an array of sizes, lengths, and bevel and tip designs (Figure 45–19). All should have a tightly fitting, removable stylet that completely occludes the lumen to avoid tracking epithelial cells into the subarachnoid space. Broadly, they can be divided into either sharp (cutting)-tipped or blunt-tipped needles. The Quincke needle is a cutting needle with end injection. The introduction of blunt tip (pencil-point) needles has markedly decreased the incidence of postdural puncture headache. The Whitacre and other pencil-point needles have rounded points and side injection. The Sprotte is a side-injection needle with a long opening. It has the advantage of more vigorous CSF flow when compared with similar gauge needles. However, this can lead to a failed block if the distal part of the opening is subarachnoid (with freely flowing CSF), the proximal part is not past the dura, and the full dose of medication is not delivered intrathecally. In general, the smaller the gauge needle (along with the use of a blunt-tipped needle), the lower the incidence of headache.

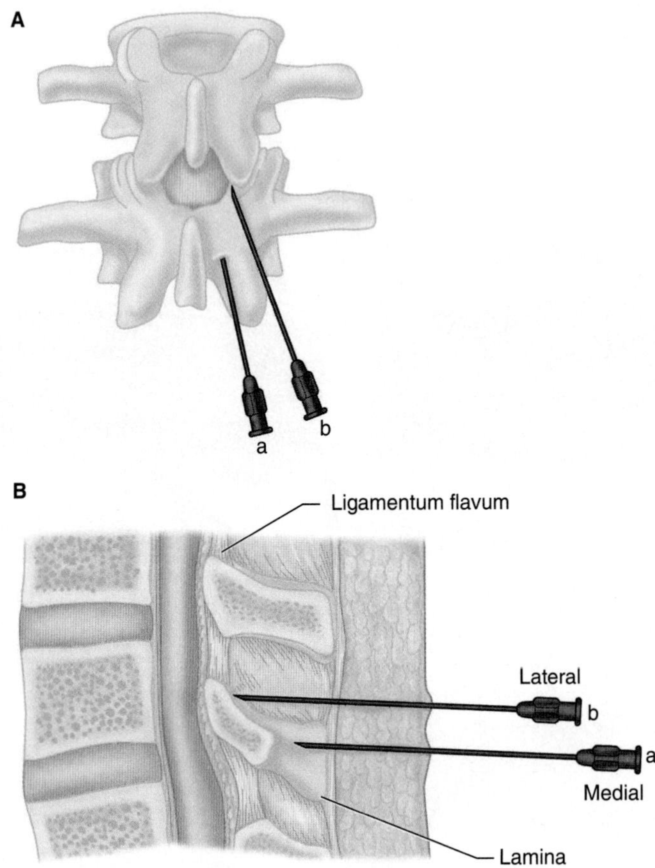

FIGURE 45–18 Paramedian approach. A needle that encounters bone at a shallow depth (a) is usually hitting the medial lamina, whereas one that encounters bone deeply (b) is farther lateral from the midline. **A**: Posterior view. **B**: Parasagittal view.

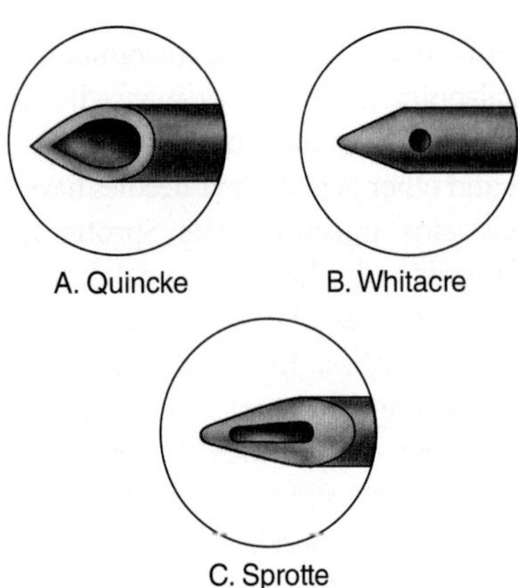

FIGURE 45–19 Spinal needles.

Spinal Catheters

Larger catheters designed for epidural use are frequently employed for continuous spinal anesthesia following accidental dural puncture during the performance of epidural anesthesia. Catheters must be carefully labeled as being subarachnoid, as opposed to epidural, to avoid the potential for excessive dosing.

Specific Technique for Spinal Anesthesia

The midline or paramedian approaches, with the patient positioned in the lateral decubitus, sitting, or prone positions, can be used for spinal anesthesia.

As previously discussed, the needle is advanced from the skin through the deeper structures until two "pops" are felt. The first is penetration of the ligamentum flavum, and the second is penetration of the dura–arachnoid membrane. Successful dural puncture is confirmed by withdrawing the stylet to verify the free flow of CSF. With small-gauge needles (<25 gauge), aspiration may be necessary to detect CSF. If free flow occurs initially but CSF cannot be aspirated after attaching the syringe, the needle likely will have moved. Persistent paresthesia or pain with injection of drugs should prompt the clinician to withdraw and redirect the needle.

Factors Influencing Level of Spinal Block

Table 45–2 lists factors that have been shown to affect the level of neural blockade following spinal anesthesia. The most important determinants are the baricity of the local anesthetic solution, the position of the patient during and immediately after injection, and drug dosage. In general, the larger the dosage or more cephalad the site of injection, the more cephalad the level of anesthesia that will be obtained. Moreover, migration of the local anesthetic cephalad in CSF depends on its density relative to CSF (*baricity*). CSF has a specific gravity of 1.003 to 1.008 at 37°C. Table 45–3 lists the specific gravity of anesthetic solutions. A *hyperbaric* solution of local anesthetic is denser (heavier) than CSF, whereas a *hypobaric* solution is less dense (lighter) than CSF. The local anesthetic solutions can be made hyperbaric by the addition of glucose or hypobaric by the addition of sterile water or fentanyl. Thus, with the patient in a head-down position, a hyperbaric solution spreads cephalad, and a hypobaric anesthetic solution moves caudad. A head-up position causes a hyperbaric solution to settle caudad and a hypobaric solution to ascend cephalad. Similarly, when a patient remains in a lateral position, a hyperbaric spinal solution will have a greater effect on the dependent (down) side, whereas a hypobaric solution will achieve a higher level on the nondependent (up) side. An *isobaric* solution tends to remain at the level of injection. Anesthetic agents lacking glucose may be mixed with CSF (at least 1:1) to make their solutions isobaric. Other factors affecting the level of neural blockade include the level of injection and the patient's height and vertebral column anatomy. The direction of the needle bevel or injection port may also play a role; higher levels of anesthesia are achieved if the injection is directed cephalad than if the point of injection is oriented laterally or caudad.

Hyperbaric solutions tend to move to the most dependent area of the spine (normally T4–T8 in the supine position).

With normal spinal anatomy, the apex of the thoracolumbar curvature is T4 (Figure 45–20).

TABLE 45–2 Factors affecting the dermatomal spread of spinal anesthesia.

Most important factors
Baricity of anesthetic solution
Position of the patient
During injection
Immediately after injection
Drug dosage
Site of injection
Other factors
Age
Cerebrospinal fluid
Curvature of the spine
Drug volume
Intraabdominal pressure
Needle direction
Patient height
Pregnancy

TABLE 45–3 Specific gravities of some spinal anesthetic agents.

Agent	Specific Gravity
Bupivacaine	
0.5% in 8.25% dextrose	1.0227–1.0278
0.5% plain	0.9990–1.0058
Lidocaine	
2% plain	1.0004–1.0066
5% in 7.5% dextrose	1.0262–1.0333
Tetracaine	
0.5% in water	0.9977–0.9997
0.5% in D_5W	1.0133–1.0203

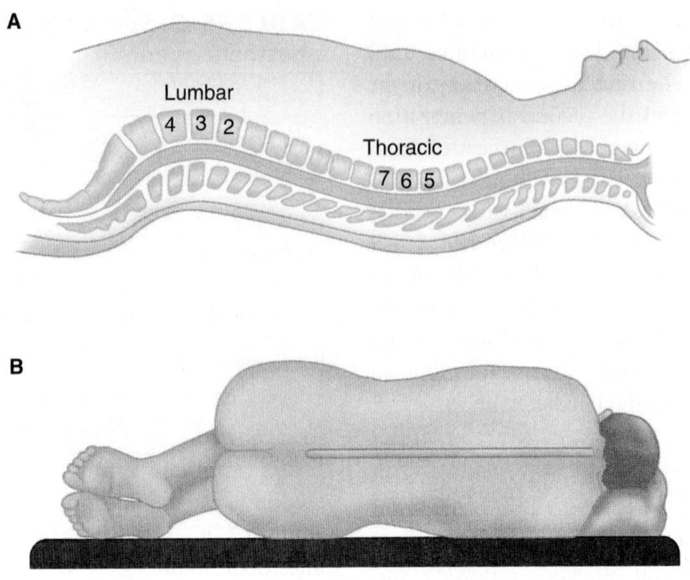

FIGURE 45–20 The position of the spinal canal in the supine position (**A**) and lateral decubitus position (**B**). Note the lowest point is usually between T5 and T7, where a hyperbaric solution tends to settle once the patient is placed supine.

In the supine position, this should limit a hyperbaric solution to produce a level of anesthesia at or below T4. Abnormal curvatures of the spine, such as scoliosis and kyphoscoliosis, have multiple effects on spinal anesthesia. Placing the block becomes more difficult because of the rotation and angulation of the vertebral bodies and spinous processes. Finding the midline and the interlaminar space may be difficult. The paramedian approach to lumbar puncture may be preferable in patients with severe scoliosis and kyphoscoliosis. Reviewing radiographs of the spine before attempting the block may be useful. Spinal curvature affects the ultimate level by changing the contour of the subarachnoid space. Previous spinal surgery can similarly result in technical difficulties in placing a block. Correctly identifying the interspinous and interlaminar spaces may be difficult at the levels of previous laminectomy or spinal fusion. The paramedian approach may be easier, or a level above the surgical site can be chosen. The block may be incomplete or the level may be different than anticipated as a result of postsurgical anatomic changes.

Lumbar CSF volume inversely correlates with the dermatomal spread of spinal anesthesia. Increased intraabdominal pressure or other conditions that cause engorgement of the epidural veins, thus decreasing CSF volume, are associated with greater dermatomal spread for a given volume of injectate. This would include conditions such as pregnancy, ascites, and large abdominal tumors. In these clinical situations, higher levels of anesthesia are achieved with a given dose of local anesthetic than would otherwise be expected. For spinal anesthesia on a term parturient, some clinicians reduce the dosage of anesthetic by one-third compared with a nonpregnant patient, particularly when the block will be initiated with the patient in the lateral position. Age-related decreases in CSF volume are likely responsible for the higher anesthetic levels achieved in the elderly for a given dosage of spinal anesthetic. Severe kyphosis or kyphoscoliosis can also be associated with a decreased volume of CSF and often results in a higher-than-expected level, particularly with a hypobaric technique or rapid injection.

Spinal Anesthetic Agents

Many local anesthetics have been used for spinal anesthesia in the past, but only a few are currently in use (Table 45–4). Only preservative-free local anesthetic solutions are used. The addition of

TABLE 45–4 Dosages, uses, and duration of commonly used spinal anesthetics.[1]

Drug	Preparation	Dose (mg)	Procedures	Duration (h) Plain	Duration (h) Epinephrine
2-chloroprocaine	1%, 2%, 3%	30–60	Ambulatory, T8	1–2	Not recommended (flu-like symptoms)
Lidocaine	2%	40–50	Ambulatory, T8	1–2	Only modest effect, not recommended
Mepivacaine[2]	1.5%	30 (T9)	Ambulatory surgery, knee scope, TURP	1–2	Not recommended
		45 (T6)[3]		1.5–3	
		60 (T5)		2–3.5	
Bupivacaine	0.5%	7.5	Ambulatory lower limb	1–2	
		10	THA, TKA, femur ORIF	2	
		15		3	4–5
Bupivacaine	0.75% in 8.25% dextrose	4–10	Perineum, lower limbs[4]	1.5–2	1.5–2.5
		12–14	Lower abdomen		
		12–18	Upper abdomen		
Ropivacaine	0.5%, 0.75%	15–17.5	T10 level	2–3	Does not prolong block
		18–22.5	T8 level	3–4	
	1% + 10% dextrose (equal volumes D_{10} and ropivacaine)	18–22.5	T4 level	1.5–2	
Tetracaine	1% + 10% dextrose (0.5% hyperbaric)	4–8	Perineum/lower extremities	1.5–2	3.5–4
		10–12	Lower abdomen		
		10–16	Upper abdomen		

Adjuvant	Dose (mcg)	Duration (h)	Comments/Side Effects
Fentanyl	10–25	1–2	Itching; nausea; urinary retention; sedation; ileus; respiratory depression (delayed with morphine—↓ dose with older adults or patients with sleep apnea)
Sufentanil	1.25–5	1	
Morphine	125–250	4–24	
Epinephrine	100–200		Prolongs nerve exposure to local anesthetic + α-adrenergic modulation
Phenylephrine	1000–2000		Hypotension. Prolongs tetracaine but not bupivacaine. Extends tetracaine better than epinephrine does. May cause TNS
Clonidine	15–150		Hypotension. Sedation. Prolongs motor and sensory block

[1]THA, total hip arthroplasty; TKA, total knee arthroplasty; TNS, transient neurological symptoms; TURP, transurethral resection of the prostate; ORIF, open reduction and internal fixation.

[2]Used as an alternative to lidocaine, but TNS also occurs with mepivacaine.

[3]Each change of 15 mg prolongs or hastens ambulatory milestones by 20 to 30 min. Fentanyl, 10 mcg, extends surgical block but not ambulatory recovery times and should probably be added if using 30-mg dose to ensure adequate duration.

[4]Very low dose (4–5 mg) works well for ambulatory, unilateral, knee surgery. Keep patient lateral, affected side down, for 6 min after block.

Reproduced with permission from Atchabahian A, Gupta R: *The Anesthesia Guide.* New York, NY: McGraw Hill; 2013.

vasoconstrictors (α-adrenergic agonists, epinephrine [0.1–0.2 mg]) and opioids enhance the quality or prolong the duration of spinal anesthesia, or both. Vasoconstrictors seem to delay the uptake of local anesthetics from CSF and may have weak spinal analgesic properties. Opioids and clonidine can likewise be added to spinal anesthetics to improve both the quality and duration of the subarachnoid block.

Until very recently in North America, hyperbaric spinal anesthesia was more commonly used than hypobaric or isobaric techniques. The level of anesthesia is then dependent on the patient's position during and immediately following the injection. In the sitting position, a "saddle block" can be achieved by keeping the patient sitting for 3 to 5 min following injection so that only the lower lumbar nerves and sacral nerves are blocked. If the patient is moved from a sitting position to a supine position immediately after injection, the agent will move more cephalad to the dependent region defined by the thoracolumbar curve. Hyperbaric anesthetics injected intrathecally with the patient in a lateral decubitus position can be used for unilateral lower extremity procedures. The patient is placed laterally, with the extremity to be operated on in a dependent position. If the patient is kept in this position for about 5 min following injection, the block will tend to be denser and achieve a higher level on the operative, dependent side.

If regional anesthesia is chosen for surgical procedures involving hip or lower extremity fracture, hypobaric or isobaric spinal anesthesia can be useful because the patient need not lie on the fractured extremity.

Epidural Anesthesia

11 Continuous epidural anesthesia is a neuraxial technique offering a range of applications wider than single-dose spinal anesthesia. An epidural block can be performed at the lumbar, thoracic, or cervical level. Sacral epidural anesthesia is referred to as a *caudal block* and is described at the end of this chapter.

12 Epidural techniques are widely used for surgical anesthesia, obstetric analgesia, postoperative pain control, and chronic pain management. Epidurals can be used as a single-shot technique or with a catheter that allows intermittent boluses or continuous infusion, or both. The motor block can range from none to complete. All of these variables are controlled by the choice of drug, concentration, dosage, and level of injection.

The epidural space surrounds the dura mater posteriorly, laterally, and anteriorly. Nerve roots travel in this space as they exit laterally through the foramen and course outward to become peripheral nerves. Other contents of the lumbar epidural space include fatty connective tissue, lymphatics, and a rich venous (Batson) plexus. Fluoroscopic studies have demonstrated the presence of septa or connective tissue bands within the epidural space, possibly explaining the occasional one-sided epidural
13 block. Epidural anesthesia is slower in onset (10–20 min) and may not be as dense as spinal anesthesia, a feature that can be useful clinically. For example, by using relatively dilute concentrations of a local anesthetic combined with an opioid, an epidural provides analgesia without motor block. This is commonly employed for labor and postoperative analgesia. Moreover, a segmental block is possible because the anesthetic can be confined close to the level at which it was injected. A segmental block is characterized by a well-defined band of anesthesia at certain nerve roots, leaving nerve roots above *and* below unblocked. This can be seen with a thoracic epidural that provides upper abdominal anesthesia while sparing cervical and lumbar nerve roots.

Epidural anesthesia is most often performed in the thoracic and lumbar regions. Midline (see Figure 45–4) or paramedian approaches (see Figure 45–17) can be used. Because the spinal cord typically terminates at the L1 level, there is an extra measure of safety in performing the block in the lower lumbar interspaces, particularly if an accidental dural puncture occurs (see "Complications," later).

Thoracic epidural blocks are technically more difficult to accomplish than are lumbar blocks because of greater angulation and the overlapping of the spinous processes at the vertebral level (Figure 45–21). Moreover, the potential risk of spinal cord injury with an accidental dural puncture, though exceedingly small with good technique, may be greater than that at the lumbar level. Thoracic epidural blocks can be accomplished with either a midline or paramedian approach.

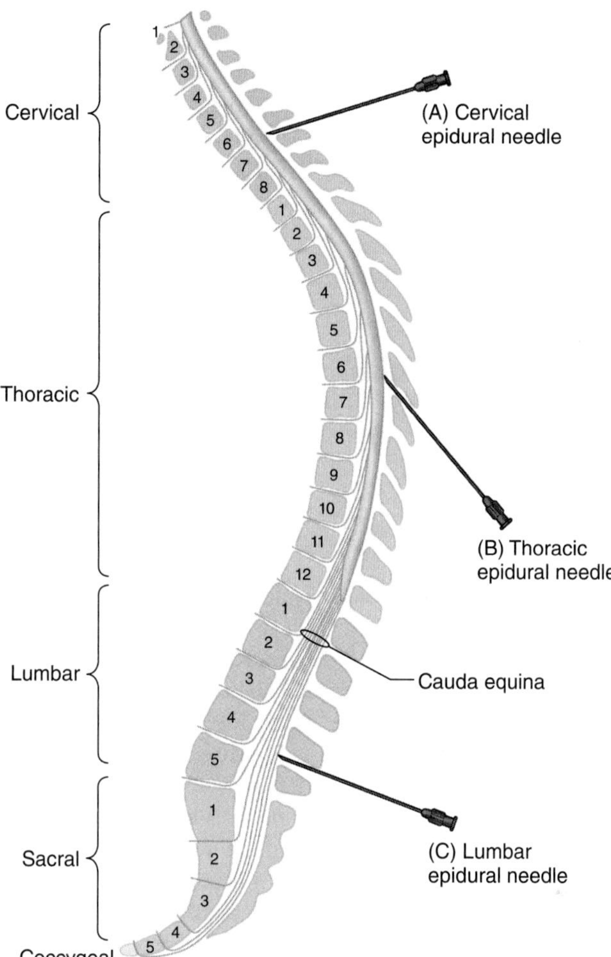

FIGURE 45–21 Angulation of the epidural needle at the cervical (**A**), thoracic (**B**), and lumbar (**C**) levels. Note that an acute angulation (30–50°) is required for a thoracic epidural block, whereas only a slight cephalad orientation is usually required for cervical and lumbar epidural blocks.

The thoracic epidural technique is more commonly used for postoperative analgesia than as a primary anesthetic. Single-shot or catheter techniques are used for the management of chronic pain. Infusions via an epidural catheter are useful for providing prolonged durations of analgesia and may obviate or shorten postoperative ventilation in patients with underlying lung disease and following chest surgery.

Cervical epidural blocks are usually performed with the patient sitting, with the neck flexed, using the midline approach. They are used most often for the management of acute and chronic pain.

Epidural Needles

The standard epidural needle is typically 17 to 18 gauge, 3 or 3.5 inches long, and has a blunt bevel with a gentle curve of 15° to 30° at the tip. The Tuohy needle is most commonly used (Figure 45–22). The blunt, curved tip theoretically helps to push away the dura after passing through the ligamentum flavum instead of penetrating it. Straight needles without a curved tip (Crawford needles) may have a greater incidence of dural puncture. Needle modifications include winged hubs and introducer devices set into the hub designed for guiding catheter placement.

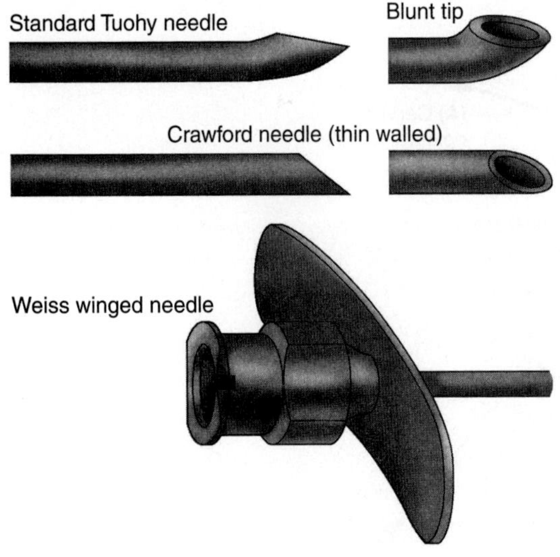

FIGURE 45–22 Epidural needles.

Epidural Catheters

Placing a catheter into the epidural space allows for continuous infusion or intermittent bolus techniques. In addition to extending the duration of the block, catheter techniques may allow a lower total dose of anesthetic to be used.

Epidural catheters are useful for intraoperative epidural anesthesia and postoperative analgesia. Typically, a 19- or 20-gauge catheter is introduced through a 17- or 18-gauge epidural needle. When using a curved tipped needle, the bevel opening is directed either cephalad or caudad, and the catheter is advanced 2 to 6 cm into the epidural space. The shorter the distance the catheter is advanced, the more likely it is to become dislodged. Conversely, the further the catheter is advanced, the greater the chance of a unilateral block (due to the catheter tip either exiting the epidural space via an intervertebral foramen or coursing into the anterolateral recesses of the epidural space), "knotting," and or penetration of an epidural vein. After the catheter is advanced to the desired depth, the needle is removed, and the catheter is left in place. The catheter can be taped or otherwise secured along the back. Catheters that will remain in place for prolonged times (eg, >1 week) may be tunneled under the skin. Catheters have either a single port at the distal end or multiple side ports close to a closed tip. Some have a stylet for easier insertion or to help steer the catheter passage in the epidural space with fluoroscopic guidance. Spiral wire-reinforced catheters are very resistant to kinking. The spiral or spring tip is associated with fewer, less intense paresthesia and may be associated with a lower incidence of inadvertent intravascular perforation.

Specific Techniques for Epidural Anesthesia

Using the midline or paramedian approaches detailed previously, the anesthesia provider passes the epidural needle through the skin and the ligamentum flavum. The needle must stop short of piercing the dura. Two techniques make it possible to determine when the tip of the needle has entered the (potential) epidural space: the "loss of resistance" and "hanging drop" techniques.

The loss of resistance technique is preferred by most clinicians. The needle is advanced through the subcutaneous tissues with the stylet in place until the interspinous ligament is entered, as noted by an increase in tissue resistance. The stylet or introducer is removed, and a glass syringe is filled with saline or air is attached to the hub of the needle. If the tip of the needle is within the ligament, gentle attempts at injection are met with resistance, and injection is not possible. The needle is then slowly advanced, millimeter by millimeter, with either continuous or rapidly repeating attempts at injection. As the tip of the needle just enters the epidural space, there is a sudden loss of resistance, and injection is now easy.

Once the interspinous ligament has been entered and the stylet has been removed, the hanging drop technique requires that the hub of the needle be filled with solution so that a drop hangs from its outside opening. The needle is then slowly advanced deeper. As long as the tip of the needle remains within the ligamentous structures, the drop remains "hanging." However, as the tip of the needle enters the epidural space, it creates negative pressure, and the drop of fluid is sucked into the needle. If the needle becomes plugged, the drop will not be drawn into the hub of the needle, and accidental dural puncture may occur. Some clinicians prefer to use this technique for the paramedian approach and for cervical epidurals. Experienced "epiduralists" will generally have sensed the "give" in their hands as the epidural needle tip passes through the ligamentum flavum, and rely on either the loss of resistance or hanging drop as confirmation (rather than as the primary test) that the needle has entered the epidural space.

Activating an Epidural

14 The quantity (volume and concentration) of local anesthetic needed for epidural anesthesia is larger than that needed for spinal anesthesia. Toxic side effects are almost guaranteed if a "full epidural dose" is injected intrathecally or intravascularly. Safeguards against toxic epidural side effects include test dosing and incremental dosing. These safeguards apply whether the injection is through the needle or through an epidural catheter.

Test doses are designed to detect both subarachnoid and intravascular injection. The classic test dose combines local anesthetic and epinephrine, typically 3 mL of 1.5% lidocaine with 1:200,000 epinephrine (0.005 mg/mL). The 45 mg of lidocaine, if injected intrathecally, will produce spinal anesthesia that should be rapidly apparent. Some clinicians have suggested the use of lower test doses of local anesthetic because an unintended injection of 45 mg of intrathecal lidocaine can be difficult to manage in areas such as labor rooms. The 15-mcg dose of epinephrine, if injected intravascularly, should produce a noticeable increase in heart rate (20% or more), with or without hypertension. Unfortunately, epinephrine as a marker of intravenous injection is not ideal. False positives (a uterine contraction causing pain or an increase in heart rate coincident to test dosing) and false negatives (bradycardia and exaggerated hypertension in response to epinephrine in patients taking β-blockers) can occur. **Simply aspirating prior to injection is insufficient to avoid accidental intravenous injection**; most experienced practitioners have encountered false-negative aspirations through both a needle and a catheter.

Incremental dosing is a very effective method of avoiding serious complications ("each dose is a test dose"). If aspiration is negative, a fraction of the total intended local anesthetic dose is injected, typically 5 mL. This dose should be large enough to produce mild symptoms (tinnitus or metallic taste) or signs (slurred speech, altered mentation) of intravascular injection to occur but small enough to avoid seizures or cardiovascular compromise. This is particularly important for labor epidurals that are to be used for cesarean delivery. If the initial labor epidural bolus was delivered through the needle and the catheter was then inserted, it may be erroneously assumed that the catheter is well positioned because the patient is still comfortable from the initial bolus. If the catheter was inserted into a blood vessel, or if after initial successful placement it has since migrated intravascularly, systemic toxicity will likely result if the full anesthetic dose is injected. Catheters can migrate intrathecally or intravascularly from an initially correct epidural position at any time after placement, but migration is most likely to occur with movement of the patient.

If a clinician uses an initial test dose, is diligent about aspirating prior to each injection, and always uses incremental dosing, major systemic toxic side effects and total spinal anesthesia from accidental intrathecal injections will be rare. Rescue lipid emulsion (20% Intralipid 1.5 mL/kg) must be available whenever epidural blocks are performed in the event of local anesthetic systemic toxicity.

Factors Affecting Level of Block

Factors affecting the level of epidural anesthesia may not be as predictable as with spinal anesthesia. In adults, 1 to 2 mL of local anesthetic per segment to be blocked is a generally accepted guideline. For example, to achieve a T4 sensory level from an L4–L5 injection would require about 12 to 24 mL. For segmental or analgesic blocks, less volume is needed.

The dose required to achieve the same level of anesthesia decreases with age. This is probably a result of age-related decreases in the size or compliance of the epidural space. Although there is little correlation between body weight and epidural dosage requirements, patient height affects the extent of cephalad spread. Thus, shorter patients may require only 1 mL of local anesthetic per segment to be blocked, whereas taller patients generally require 2 mL per segment. Although less dramatic than with hyperbaric or hypobaric spinal anesthesia, the spread of epidural local anesthetics tends to be partially affected by gravity. The lateral decubitus, Trendelenburg, and reverse Trendelenburg positions can be used to help achieve blockade in the desired dermatomes.

Additives to the local anesthetic, particularly opioids, tend to have a greater effect on the quality ("density") of epidural anesthesia than on the duration of the block. Epinephrine in concentrations of 5 mcg/mL prolongs the effect of epidural lidocaine, mepivacaine, and chloroprocaine more than that of bupivacaine, levobupivacaine, or ropivacaine. In addition to prolonging the duration and improving the quality of the block, epinephrine delays vascular absorption and reduces peak systemic blood levels of all epidurally administered local anesthetics.

Epidural Anesthetic Agents

The epidural agent is chosen based on the desired clinical effect, whether it is to be used as a primary anesthetic, supplementation of general anesthesia, or analgesia. The anticipated duration of the procedure may call for a short- or long-acting single shot anesthetic or the insertion of a catheter (Table 45–5). Commonly used short- to intermediate-acting agents for surgical anesthesia include chloroprocaine, lidocaine, and mepivacaine. Longer-acting agents include bupivacaine, levobupivacaine, and ropivacaine.

Following the initial 1 to 2 mL per segment bolus (in fractionated doses), repeat doses delivered through an epidural catheter are done on a fixed time interval (either as a bolus or continuous infusion), based on the practitioner's experience with the agent, or only re-dosed when the block demonstrates some degree of regression. Once regression in sensory level has occurred, one-third to one-half of the initial activation dose can generally safely be reinjected in incremental doses.

It should be noted that chloroprocaine, an ester with rapid onset, short duration, and extremely low systemic toxicity, may interfere with the analgesic effects of epidural opioids. Previous chloroprocaine formulations with preservatives, specifically bisulfite and ethylenediaminetetraacetic acid (EDTA), produced cauda equina syndrome when accidentally injected in a large volume intrathecally. Bisulfite preparations of chloroprocaine were believed to be associated with neurotoxicity, whereas EDTA formulations were associated with severe back pain (presumably due to localized hypocalcemia). Most current preparations of chloroprocaine are preservative-free and without these complications, and at least one formulation is approved for spinal anesthesia.

Surgical anesthesia is obtained with a 0.5% bupivacaine formulation. The 0.75% formulation of

TABLE 45–5 Agents for epidural anesthesia.

Agent	Concentration	Onset	Sensory Block	Motor Block
Chloroprocaine	2%	Fast	Analgesic	Mild to moderate
	3%	Fast	Dense	Dense
Lidocaine	≤1%	Intermediate	Analgesic	Minimal
	1.5%	Intermediate	Dense	Mild to moderate
	2%	Intermediate	Dense	Dense
Mepivacaine	1%	Intermediate	Analgesic	Minimal
	2–3%	Intermediate	Dense	Dense
Bupivacaine	≤0.25%	Slow	Analgesic	Minimal
	0.5%	Slow	Dense	Mild to moderate
	0.75%	Slow	Dense	Moderate to dense
Ropivacaine	0.2%	Slow	Analgesic	Minimal
	0.5%	Slow	Dense	Mild to moderate
	0.75–1.0%	Slow	Dense	Moderate to dense

bupivacaine is no longer used in obstetrics because its use in cesarean delivery was associated with reports of cardiac arrest after accidental intravenous injection. Very dilute concentrations of bupivacaine (eg, 0.0625%) are commonly combined with fentanyl and used for labor analgesia and for postoperative pain management. Compared with bupivacaine, ropivacaine may produce less motor block at similar concentrations while maintaining a satisfactory sensory block.

Local Anesthetic pH Adjustment

Local anesthetic solutions have an acidic pH for chemical stability and bacteriostasis. Local anesthetic solutions that are formulated with epinephrine by the manufacturer are more acidic than the "plain" solutions that do not contain epinephrine. Because they are weak bases, they exist primarily in the ionic form in commercial preparations. The onset of neural block requires permeation of lipid barriers by the uncharged form of the local anesthetic. Increasing the pH of the solutions increases the fraction of the uncharged form of the local anesthetic. The addition of sodium bicarbonate (1 mEq/10 mL of local anesthetic) to the local anesthetic solution immediately before injection may therefore accelerate the onset of the neural blockade. Sodium bicarbonate is typically not added to bupivacaine, which precipitates above a pH of 6.8.

Failed Epidural Blocks

Unlike spinal anesthesia, in which the procedural endpoint is usually very clear (free-flowing CSF), the onset is very fast, and the technique has a very high success rate, epidural anesthesia is dependent on the detection of a more subjective loss of resistance (or hanging drop). Also, the onset of epidural anesthesia is slower, and the more variable anatomy of the epidural space and less predictable spread of local anesthetic make epidural anesthesia inherently less predictable than spinal anesthesia.

Misplaced injections of local anesthetic can occur in a number of situations. In some patients, the spinal ligaments are soft, and either good resistance is never appreciated, or a false loss of resistance is encountered. Similarly, entry into the paraspinous muscles during an off-center midline approach may cause a false loss of resistance. Other causes of failed epidural anesthesia (such as intrathecal, subdural, and intravenous injection) are discussed in a later section of this chapter on complications.

A unilateral block can occur if the medication is delivered through a catheter that has either exited the epidural space or coursed laterally. The chance of this occurring increases as longer lengths of catheter are threaded into the epidural space. When unilateral block occurs, the problem may be overcome by withdrawing the catheter 1 to 2 cm and reinjecting it with the patient turned with the unblocked side down. Segmental sparing, which may be due to septations within the epidural space, may also be corrected by injecting additional local anesthetic with the unblocked segment positioned down. The large size of the L5, S1, and S2 nerve roots may delay adequate penetration of local anesthetic and is thought to be responsible for sacral sparing. The latter is particularly a problem for surgery on the knee, ankle, or foot; in such cases, elevating the head of the bed and reinjecting the catheter with additional anesthetic solution can sometimes achieve a more intense block of these large nerve roots. Patients may report visceral pain despite a seemingly good epidural block. In some cases (eg, traction on the inguinal ligament and spermatic cord), a high thoracic sensory level may alleviate the pain; in other cases (traction on the peritoneum), intravenous supplementation with opioids or other agents may be necessary. Visceral afferent fibers that travel with the vagus nerve may be responsible.

Caudal Anesthesia

15 Caudal epidural anesthesia is a common regional technique in pediatric patients. It may also be used for anorectal surgery in adults. The caudal space is the sacral portion of the epidural space. Caudal anesthesia involves needle or catheter penetration of the sacrococcygeal ligament covering the sacral hiatus that is created by the unfused S4 and S5 laminae. The hiatus may be felt as a groove or notch above the coccyx and between two bony prominences, the *sacral cornua*

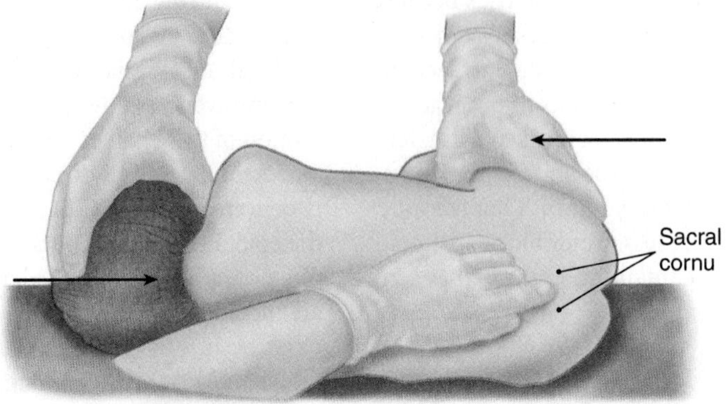

FIGURE 45–23 Positioning an anesthetized child for caudal block and palpation for the sacral hiatus. An assistant gently helps flex the spine.

(see Figure 45–3). Its anatomy is very easily appreciated in infants and children (Figure 45–23). The posterior superior iliac spines and the sacral hiatus define an equilateral triangle (see Figure 45–16). Calcification of the sacrococcygeal ligament may make caudal anesthesia difficult or impossible in older adults. As previously noted, the dural sac extends to the first sacral vertebra in adults and to about the third sacral vertebra in infants, making accidental intrathecal injection a common concern in infants.

In children, caudal anesthesia is typically combined with general anesthesia for intraoperative supplementation and postoperative analgesia. It is commonly used for procedures below the diaphragm, including urogenital, rectal, inguinal, and lower extremity surgery. Pediatric caudal blocks are most commonly performed after the induction of general anesthesia. However, regional techniques are increasingly used for surgical anesthesia in infants and young children because of concerns about the possible neurotoxic effects of general anesthesia in that population. The patient is placed in the lateral or prone position with one or both hips flexed, and the sacral hiatus is palpated. After sterile skin preparation, a needle or intravenous catheter (18–23 gauge) is advanced at a 45° angle cephalad until a pop is felt as the needle pierces the sacrococcygeal ligament. The angle of the needle is then flattened and advanced (Figure 45–24). Aspiration for blood and CSF is performed, and, if negative, the injection can proceed. Some clinicians recommend test dosing as with other epidural techniques, though many simply rely on incremental dosing with frequent aspiration. Tachycardia (if epinephrine is used) or increasing size of the T waves on electrocardiography may indicate intravascular injection. Complications are fortunately infrequent but include total spinal and intravenous injection, causing seizure or cardiac arrest. Ultrasound has also been employed in the performance of caudal blocks.

A dosage of 0.5 to 1.0 mL/kg of 0.125% to 0.25% bupivacaine (or ropivacaine), with or without epinephrine, can be used. Opioids may also be added (eg, 30–40 mcg/kg of morphine). Clonidine is often included as well. The analgesic effects of the block may extend for hours into the postoperative period.

For adults undergoing anorectal procedures, caudal anesthesia can provide dense sacral sensory blockade with limited cephalad spread. Furthermore, the injection can be given with the patient in the prone jackknife position, which is the same position used for surgery (Figure 45–25). A dose of 15 to 20 mL of 1.5% to 2.0% lidocaine, with or without epinephrine, is usually effective. Fentanyl, 50 to 100 mcg, may also be added. This technique should be avoided in patients with pilonidal cysts because the needle may pass through the cyst track and can potentially introduce bacteria into the caudal epidural space.

TABLE 45–7 Incidence of serious complications from spinal and epidural anesthesia.

Technique	Cardiac Arrest	Death	Seizure	Cauda Equina Syndrome	Paraplegia	Radiculopathy
Spinal (*n* = 40,640)	26	6	0	5	0	19
Epidural (*n* = 30,413)	3	0	4	0	1	5

Data from Auroy Y, Narchi P, Messiah A, et al. Serious complications related to regional anesthesia: Results of a prospective survey in France. *Anesthesiology.* 1997 Sep;87(3):479-486.

the block extends to cranial nerves, as a "total spinal." These conditions can also occur following attempted epidural or caudal anesthesia if there is accidental intrathecal injection (see later discussion). Apnea is more often the result of severe sustained hypotension and medullary hypoperfusion than a response to phrenic nerve paralysis from anesthesia of C3 to C5 roots. Anterior spinal artery syndrome has been reported following neuraxial anesthesia, presumably due to prolonged severe hypotension combined with an increase in intraspinal pressure.

Treatment of an excessively high neuraxial block involves maintaining adequate arterial oxygenation and ventilation and supporting the circulation. When respiratory insufficiency becomes evident, in addition to supplemental oxygen and assisted ventilation, intubation and mechanical ventilation may be necessary. Hypotension can be treated with intravenous vasopressors and rapid administration of intravenous fluids. Bradycardia can be treated early with atropine. Ephedrine or epinephrine can also increase heart rate and arterial blood pressure.

B. Cardiac Arrest During Spinal Anesthesia

Examination of data from the ASA Closed Claim Project identified several cases of cardiac arrest during spinal anesthesia. Because many of these cases predated the routine use of pulse oximetry, oversedation and unrecognized hypoventilation and hypoxia may have contributed. However, large prospective studies continue to report a relatively high incidence (perhaps as high as 1:1500) of cardiac arrest in patients having received a spinal anesthetic. Many of these cardiac arrests were preceded by bradycardia, and many occurred in young, healthy patients. Prompt drug treatment of hypovolemia, hypotension, and bradycardia is strongly recommended to prevent this from occurring.

C. Urinary Retention

Local anesthetic block of S2 to S4 root fibers decreases urinary bladder tone and inhibits the voiding reflex. Epidural opioids can also interfere with normal voiding.

Complications Associated with Needle or Catheter Insertion

A. Inadequate Anesthesia or Analgesia

As with other regional anesthesia techniques, neuraxial blocks are associated with a low but measurable failure rate that is usually inversely proportional to the clinician's experience. Failure may still occur even when CSF is obtained during spinal anesthesia. Movement of the needle during injection, incomplete entry of the needle opening into the subarachnoid space, subdural injection, or injection of the local anesthetic solution into a nerve root sleeve may be responsible. Causes for failed epidural blocks were discussed earlier (see "Failed Epidural Blocks").

B. Intravascular Injection

Accidental intravascular injection of the local anesthetic for epidural and caudal anesthesia can produce very high serum drug levels and local anesthetic systemic toxicity (LAST), which may affect the central nervous system (seizure and unconsciousness) and the cardiovascular system (hypotension, arrhythmias, depressed contractility, asystole). Because the dosage of medication for spinal anesthesia is relatively small, LAST is seen after epidural and caudal (but not spinal) blocks. Local anesthetic may be injected directly into an epidural vein through a needle or later through a catheter that has entered a vein. The incidence of intravascular injection can be minimized by carefully aspirating the needle (or catheter) before every injection, using a test dose, always injecting local anesthetic in incremental doses, and close observation for early signs of intravascular injection (tinnitus, lingual sensations). When administering fractionated doses of epidural local anesthetic, one must always remember the clinical adage, "every dose is a test dose." Advanced cardiac life support should be initiated if cardiac arrest occurs. Lipid emulsion, 20% 1.5-mL/kg bolus, should be given, followed by a 0.25-mL/kg infusion. Lipid emulsion provides a reservoir in the blood to collect and transfer local anesthetic away from the heart and brain. Incremental 1-mcg/kg doses of epinephrine should be administered rather than larger 10-mcg/kg doses. Should cardiac function not be restored, additional lipid emulsion can be administered up to 10 mL/kg. Cardiopulmonary bypass can be used should the patient fail to respond to resuscitative efforts. Local anesthetics vary in their propensity to produce severe cardiac toxicity. The rank order of local anesthetic potency at producing seizures and cardiac toxicity is the same as the rank order for potency at nerve blocks. Chloroprocaine has relatively low potency and also is metabolized very rapidly; lidocaine and mepivacaine are intermediate in potency and toxicity; and levobupivacaine, ropivacaine, bupivacaine, and tetracaine are most potent and the most toxic.

C. Total Spinal Anesthesia

Total spinal anesthesia can occur following attempted epidural or caudal anesthesia if there is accidental intrathecal injection. Onset is usually rapid because the amount of anesthetic required for epidural and caudal anesthesia is 5 to 10 times that required for spinal anesthesia. Careful aspiration, use of a test dose, and incremental injection techniques (remember, "every dose is a test dose") during epidural and caudal anesthesia can help avoid this complication.

D. Subdural Injection

Because of the larger amount of local anesthetic administered, accidental subdural injection of local anesthetic during attempted epidural anesthesia is much more serious than during attempted spinal anesthesia. A subdural injection of epidural doses of local anesthetic produces a clinical presentation similar to that of high spinal anesthesia, with the exception that the onset may be delayed for 15 to 30 min and the block may be "patchy." The spinal subdural space is a potential space between the dura and the arachnoid that extends intracranially, so local anesthetic injected into the spinal subdural space can ascend to higher levels than when injected into the epidural space. As with high spinal anesthesia, treatment is supportive and may require intubation, mechanical ventilation, and cardiovascular support. The effects generally last from one to several hours.

E. Backache

As a needle passes through skin, subcutaneous tissues, muscle, and ligaments, it causes varying degrees of tissue trauma. Bruising and a localized inflammatory response with or without reflex muscle spasm may be responsible for postoperative backache. One should remember that up to 25% to 30% of patients receiving general anesthesia also report backache postoperatively, and a significant percentage of the general population has chronic back pain. Postoperative back soreness or ache is usually mild and self-limited, though it may last for a number of weeks. If treatment is sought, acetaminophen or NSAIDs should suffice. Although backache is usually benign, it may be an important clinical sign of much more serious complications, such as epidural hematoma and abscess (see later discussion).

F. Postdural Puncture Headache

Any breach of the dura may result in a postdural puncture headache (PDPH). This may follow a diagnostic lumbar puncture, a myelogram, a spinal anesthetic, or an epidural "wet tap" in which the epidural needle passed through the epidural space and entered the subarachnoid space. Similarly, an epidural catheter might puncture the dura at any time and result in PDPH. An epidural wet tap is usually immediately recognized as CSF pouring from the epidural needle or aspirated from an epidural catheter. However, PDPH can follow a seemingly uncomplicated epidural anesthetic and may be the result of just the tip of the needle scratching through the dura. Typically, PDPH is bilateral, frontal, retroorbital, or occipital and extends into the neck. It may be throbbing or constant and associated with photophobia and nausea. The hallmark of PDPH is its association with body position. The pain is aggravated by sitting or standing and relieved or decreased by lying down flat. The onset of headache is usually 12 to 72 h following the procedure; however, it may be seen almost immediately.

PDPH is believed to result from leakage of CSF from a dural defect and subsequent intracranial hypotension. Loss of CSF at a rate faster than it can be produced causes traction on structures supporting the brain, particularly the meninges, dura, and tentorium. Increased traction on blood vessels and cranial nerves may also contribute to the pain. Traction on the cranial nerves may occasionally cause diplopia (usually the sixth cranial nerve) and tinnitus. Subdural hematoma can occur following a tear of the intracerebral veins secondary to intracranial hypotension due to CSF loss. The incidence of PDPH is strongly related to needle size, needle type, and patient population. The larger the needle, the greater the likelihood that PDPH will occur. Cutting-point needles are associated with a higher incidence of PDPH than pencil-point needles of the same gauge. Factors that increase the risk of PDPH include young age, female sex, and pregnancy. The greatest risk, then, would be expected following an accidental dural puncture with a large epidural needle in a young pregnant woman (perhaps as high as 20%–50%). The lowest incidence would be expected in an older adult man using a 27-gauge pencil-point needle (<1%). Studies of obstetric patients undergoing spinal anesthesia for cesarean delivery with small-gauge pencil-point needles have shown rates as low as 3% or 4%.

Conservative treatment of PDPH involves recumbent positioning, analgesics, intravenous or oral fluid administration, and caffeine. Keeping the patient supine will decrease the hydrostatic pressure, driving fluid out of the dural hole and minimizing the headache. Analgesic medication may range from acetaminophen to NSAIDs and opioids. Hydration and caffeine work to stimulate the production of CSF. Caffeine further helps by vasoconstricting intracranial vessels, as cerebral vasodilation is thought to be a response to intracranial hypotension secondary to the CSF leak. Stool softeners and a soft diet are used to minimize Valsalva straining. Sphenopalatine ganglion block has been suggested as an approach to dural puncture headache. Local anesthetic is applied via swabs inserted into the posterior nasal pharynx. Headache may persist for days, despite conservative therapy.

An epidural blood patch is an effective and frequently used treatment for PDPH. It involves injecting 15 to 20 mL of autologous blood into the epidural space at, or one interspace below, the level of the dural puncture. It is believed to stop further leakage of CSF by either mass effect or coagulation. Headache resolution is usually immediate and complete, but it may take several hours as CSF production slowly rebuilds intracranial pressure. Approximately 90% of patients will respond to a single blood patch, and 90% of initial nonresponders will obtain relief from a second injection. We do not recommend prophylactic blood patching after a wet tap. Not all patients will develop PDPH following a wet tap, and in any case, prophylaxis has not proven terribly effective. When evaluating patients with presumed PDPH, other sources of headache, including migraine, caffeine withdrawal, meningeal infection, and subarachnoid hemorrhage, should be considered in the differential diagnosis.

G. Neurological Injury

Perhaps no complication is more perplexing or distressing than persistent neurological deficits following an apparently routine neuraxial block. An epidural hematoma or abscess must be ruled out. Either nerve roots or spinal cord may be injured. The latter may be avoided if the neuraxial blockade is performed below the termination of the conus (L1 in adults and L3 in children). Postoperative peripheral neuropathies may be due to direct physical trauma to nerve roots. Although most resolve spontaneously, some are permanent. Any sustained paresthesia during neuraxial anesthesia/analgesia should alert the clinician to redirect the needle. Injections should be immediately stopped and the needle withdrawn if the injection is associated with pain. Direct injection into the spinal cord can cause paraplegia. Damage to the conus medullaris may cause isolated sacral nerve dysfunction. Not all neurological deficits that are reported after a regional anesthetic are the direct result of the block procedure. Postpartum neurological deficits, including lateral femoral cutaneous neuropathy and foot drop, were recognized as complications before the era of routine obstetric epidural anesthesia/analgesia.

H. Spinal or Epidural Hematoma

Needle or catheter trauma to epidural veins often causes minor bleeding in the spinal canal, though this usually has no consequences. The incidence of spinal hematomas has been estimated to be about 1:150,000 for epidural blocks and 1:220,000 for spinal anesthetics. The vast majority of reported cases have occurred in patients with abnormal coagulation secondary to either disease or drugs. Some hematomas have occurred immediately following the removal of an epidural catheter. Thus, both insertion and removal of an epidural catheter can lead to epidural hematoma formation.

Diagnosis and treatment must be prompt if permanent neurological sequelae secondary to neuronal ischemia are to be avoided. The onset of symptoms is typically more sudden than with epidural abscess. **Symptoms include sharp back and leg pain with motor weakness or sphincter dysfunction, or both**. When hematoma is suspected, magnetic resonance (MR) or computed tomography (CT) imaging and neurosurgical consultation must be obtained immediately. In many cases, good neurological recovery has occurred in patients who have undergone prompt surgical decompression.

Neuraxial anesthesia should be avoided in patients with coagulopathy, significant thrombocytopenia, platelet dysfunction, or those who have received fibrinolytic or thrombolytic therapy. Practice guidelines should be reviewed when considering neuraxial anesthesia in such patients, and the risk versus benefit of these techniques should be weighed and delineated in the informed consent process.

I. Meningitis and Arachnoiditis

Infection of the subarachnoid space can follow neuraxial blocks as the result of contamination of the equipment or injected solutions or as a result of organisms tracked in from the skin. Indwelling catheters may become colonized with skin organisms.

Strict sterile technique must be employed. Careful attention is particularly warranted in the labor room, where family members are often curious to see what is being done to mitigate the parturient's pain. If hospital policy permits their presence during epidural placement, such individuals should be advised to avoid contaminating the tray. Family members should also wear a mask to prevent contamination of the epidural tray with oral flora.

J. Epidural Abscess

Spinal epidural abscess (EA) is a rare but potentially devastating complication of neuraxial anesthesia. The reported incidence varies widely, from 1:6500 to 1:500,000 epidurals. Most reported anesthesia-related cases involve epidural catheters. In one reported series, there was a mean of 5 days from catheter insertion to the development of symptoms, though presentation can be delayed for weeks.

There are four classic clinical stages of EA, though progression and time course can vary. Initially, symptoms include back pain that is intensified by percussion over the spine. Second, nerve root or radicular pain develops. The third stage is marked by motor or sensory deficits or sphincter dysfunction. Paraplegia or paralysis marks the fourth stage. Ideally, the diagnosis is made in the early stages. Prognosis has consistently been shown to correlate with the degree of neurological dysfunction at the time the diagnosis is made. Back pain and fever after epidural anesthesia should alert the clinician to consider EA. Radicular pain or neurological deficit heightens the urgency to investigate. Once EA is suspected, the catheter should be removed (if still present) and the tip cultured. The injection site is examined for evidence of infection; if pus is expressed, it is sent for culture. Blood cultures should be obtained. If suspicion is high and cultures have been obtained, anti-*Staphylococcus* coverage can be instituted, as the most common organisms causing EA are *Staphylococcus aureus* and *S. epidermidis*. MR or CT imaging should be performed to confirm or rule out the diagnosis. We recommend prompt consultation with specialists in neurosurgical and infectious disease. In addition to antibiotics, treatment of EA usually involves decompression (laminectomy), though percutaneous drainage with fluoroscopic or

CT guidance has been used. Suggested strategies for guarding against the occurrence of EA include (1) minimizing catheter manipulations and maintaining a closed system when possible; (2) using a micropore (0.22-μm) bacterial filter; and (3) removing an epidural catheter or at least changing the catheter, filter, and solution after a defined time interval (eg, some clinicians replace or remove all epidurals after 4 days).

K. Sheering of an Epidural Catheter

There is a risk of neuraxial catheters sheering and breaking off inside of tissues if they are withdrawn through the needle. If a catheter must be withdrawn while the needle remains in situ, both must be carefully withdrawn *together*. If a catheter breaks off within the epidural space, many experts suggest leaving it and observing the patient. If, however, the breakage occurs in superficial tissues, the catheter should be surgically removed.

Complications Associated with Drug Toxicity

A. Local Anesthetic Systemic Toxicity

Absorption of excessive amounts of local anesthetics can produce toxic blood levels (see "Intravascular Injection"). Excessive absorption from epidural or caudal blocks is rare when appropriate doses of local anesthetic are used.

B. Transient Neurological Symptoms

First described in 1993, **transient neurological symptoms** (TNS), also referred to as *transient radicular irritation* (TRI), are characterized by back pain radiating to the legs without sensory or motor deficits, occurring after the resolution of spinal anesthesia and resolving spontaneously within several days. It is most commonly associated with hyperbaric lidocaine (incidence up to 12%), but it has also been reported with tetracaine (2%), bupivacaine (1%), mepivacaine, prilocaine, procaine, and subarachnoid ropivacaine. There are also case reports of TNS following epidural anesthesia. The incidence of this syndrome is greatest among outpatients, particularly men undergoing surgery in the lithotomy position, and least among inpatients undergoing surgery in positions other than lithotomy.

CASE DISCUSSION

Neuraxial Anesthesia for Cystoscopy & Ureteral Stent Placement

A 56-year-old man presents for cystoscopy and stent placement for a large kidney stone. The patient has a long history of spinal problems and has undergone fusion of the cervical spine (C3–C6) and laminectomy with fusion of the lower lumbar spine (L3–L5). On examination, he has no neck flexion or extension and has a Mallampati class IV airway.

What types of anesthesia are appropriate for this patient?

Cystoscopy and stent placement usually require general or neuraxial anesthesia. Selection of the type of anesthesia, as always, should be based on patient preference after informed consent. This patient presents potential difficulties for both general and regional anesthesia. The limited excursion of the cervical spine, together with the anatomy of a class IV airway, makes difficulty in intubation and possibly ventilation almost certain. Induction of general anesthesia would be safest after the airway is secured with an awake fiberoptic intubation.

Regional anesthesia also presents a problem in that the patient has had previous back surgery in the lumbar area, where neuraxial anesthesia is most commonly performed. Postoperative distortion of the anatomy makes the block technically challenging and may increase the likelihood of a failure, inadvertent dural puncture during epidural anesthesia, paresthesia, and unpredictable spread of the local anesthetics.

If the patient chooses to have neuraxial anesthesia, would spinal or epidural anesthesia be more appropriate?

The associated sympathectomy and subsequent drop in blood pressure are more gradual after epidural anesthesia than that following spinal anesthesia. With either type of anesthesia, significant hypotension should be treated with vasoconstrictors and fluids, and bradycardia should be treated with anticholinergics.

After an explanation of the options, the patient seems to understand the risks of both types of anesthesia and desires epidural anesthesia. Placement of an epidural catheter is attempted at the L1 to L2 interspace, but accidental dural puncture occurs. What options are now available?

Options include injecting a spinal dose of local anesthetic through the epidural needle to induce spinal anesthesia, passing an epidural catheter into the subarachnoid space to perform a continuous spinal anesthetic, or proceeding with an awake fiberoptic intubation in advance of general anesthesia. If a spinal dose of local anesthetic is to be injected, the syringe and needle should be kept in place for a few moments to prevent significant back leakage of anesthetic through the large dural hole. Threading an epidural catheter through the needle into the subarachnoid space allows subsequent redosing and may reduce the incidence of dural puncture headache. When a catheter is advanced in the subarachnoid space well below L2, it should not be advanced more than 2 to 3 cm to avoid injury to the cauda equina.

How might a dural puncture affect subsequent epidural or spinal anesthesia?

A potential hazard of epidural anesthesia at a level adjacent to a large dural puncture is the possibility that some local anesthetic might pass through the dural puncture into the subarachnoid space. This could result in a higher than expected level of sensory and motor blockade.

GUIDELINES

American Society of Regional Anesthesia and Pain Medicine. ASRA guideline apps. https://www.asra.com/page/150/asra-apps.

Leffert L, Butwick A, Carvalho B, et al; members of the SOAP VTE Taskforce. The Society for Obstetric Anesthesia and Perinatology consensus statement on the anesthetic management of pregnant and postpartum women receiving thromboprophylaxis or higher dose anticoagulants. *Anesth Analg.* 2018;126:928.

SUGGESTED READINGS

Benzon H, Asher Y, Hartrick C. Back pain and neuraxial anesthesia. *Anesth Analg* 2016;122:2047.

Cappelleri G, Fanelli A. Use of direct oral anticoagulants with regional anesthesia in orthopedic patients. *J Clin Anesth.* 2016;32:224.

Chin KJ, Karmakar M, Peng P. Ultrasonography of the adult thoracic and lumbar spine for central neuraxial blockade. *Anesthesiology.* 2011;114:1459.

Fettiplace MR, Weinberg G. The mechanisms underlying lipid resuscitation therapy. *Reg Anesth Pain Med.* 2018;43:138.

Forster J. Short-acting spinal anesthesia in the ambulatory setting. *Curr Opin Anesthesiol.* 2014;27:597.

Gaiser RR. Postdural puncture headache: an evidence-based approach. *Anesthesiol Clin* 2017;35:157.

Goeller J, Bhalla T, Tobias J. Combined use of neuraxial and general anesthesia during major abdominal procedures in neonates and infants. *Pediatr Anesth.* 2014;24:553.

Guay J, Suresh S, Kopp S. The use of ultrasound guidance for perioperative neuraxial and peripheral nerve blocks in children. *Cochrane Database Syst Rev.* 2016:CD011436.

Gupta R, McEvoy M. Initial experience of the American Society of Regional Anesthesia and Pain Medicine coags regional smartphone application. *Reg Anesth Pain Med.* 2016;41:334.

Hadzic A. *Hadzic's Textbook of Regional Anesthesia and Acute Pain Management.* 2nd ed. McGraw-Hill; 2017.

Hampl K, Stenfeldt T, Wulf H. Spinal anesthesia revisited: toxicity of new and old drugs and compounds. *Curr Opin Anesthesiol.* 2014;27:549.

Hebl J, Horlocker T, Kopp S, et al. Neuraxial blockade in patients with preexisting spinal stenosis, lumbar disk disease, or prior spine surgery: efficacy and neurologic complications. *Anesth Analg.* 2010;111:1511.

Heesen M, Klimek M, Hoeks SE, Rossaint R. Prevention of spinal anesthesia-induced hypotension during cesarean delivery by 5-hydroxytryptamine-3 receptor antagonists: a systematic review and meta-analysis and meta-regression. *Anesth Analg.* 2016;123:977.

Horlocker TT, Vandermeulen E, Kopp SL, Gogarten W, Leffert LR, Benzon HT. Regional anesthesia in the patient receiving antithrombotic or thrombolytic therapy: American Society of Regional Anesthesia and Pain Medicine evidence-based guidelines (fourth edition). *Reg Anesth Pain Med.* 2018;43:263.

Johnson R, Kopp S, Burkle C, et al. Neuraxial vs general anesthesia for total hip and total knee arthroplasty: a systematic review of comparative effectiveness research. *Br J Anaesth.* 2016;116:163.

Kocarev M, Khalid F, Khatoon F, Fernando R. Neuraxial labor analgesia: a focused narrative review of the 2017 literature. *Curr Opin Anaesthesiol.* 2018;31:251.

Lee JE, George RB, Habib AS. Spinal-induced hypotension: incidence, mechanisms, prophylaxis, and management: summarizing 20 years of research. *Best Pract Res Clin Anaesthesiol.* 2017;31:57.

Lee LA, Posner KL, Domino KB, et al. Injuries associated with regional anesthesia in the 1980s and 1990s: a closed claims analysis. *Anesthesiology.* 2004;101:143.

Lees D, Frawley G, Taghavi K, Mirjalili S. A review of the surface and internal anatomy of the caudal canal in children. *Pediatr Anesth.* 2014;24:799.

Leffert LR, Dubois HM, Butwick AJ, Carvalho B, Houle TT, Landau R. Neuraxial anesthesia in obstetric patients receiving thromboprophylaxis with unfractionated or low-molecular-weight heparin: a systematic review of spinal epidural hematoma. *Anesth Analg.* 2017;125:223.

Marhofer P, Keplinger M, Klug W, Metzelder M. Awake caudals and epidurals should be used more frequently in neonates and infants. *Pediatr Anesth.* 2015;25:93.

Narouze S, Benzon H, Provenzano D, et al. Interventional spine and pain procedures in patients on antiplatelet and anticoagulant medications: guidelines from the American Society of Regional Anesthesia and Pain Medicine, the European Society of Regional Anaesthesia and Pain Therapy, the American Academy of Pain Medicine, the International Neuromodulation Society, the North American Neuromodulation Society, and the World Institute of Pain. *Reg Anesth Pain Med.* 2015;40:182.

Neal J, Kopp S, Pasternak J, et al. Anatomy and pathophysiology of spinal cord injury associated with regional anesthesia and pain medicine. *Reg Anesth Pain Med.* 2015;40:506.

Neuman M, Rosenbaum P, Ludwig J, et al. Anesthesia technique, mortality, and length of stay after hip fracture surgery. *JAMA.* 2014;311:2508.

Peralta F, Devroe S. Any news on the postdural puncture headache front? *Best Pract Res Clin Anaesthesiol.* 2017;31:35.

Perlas A, Chaparro LE, Chin KJ. Lumbar neuraxial ultrasound for spinal and epidural anesthesia: a systematic review and meta-analysis. *Reg Anesth Pain Med.* 2016;41:251.

Sachs A, Smiley R. Post dural puncture headache: the worst common complication in obstetric anesthesia. *Sem Perinatol.* 2014;38:386.

Vasques F, Behr A, Weinberg G, et al. A review of local anesthetic systemic toxicity cases since publication of the American Society of Regional Anesthesia recommendations: to whom it may concern. *Reg Anesth Pain Med.* 2015;40:698.

Volk T, Kubulus C. New oral anticoagulants and neuraxial regional anesthesia. *Curr Opin Anesthesiol.* 2015;28:605.

Wiegele M, Marhofer P, Longqvist P. Caudal epidural blocks in paediatric patients: a review and practical considerations. *Br J Anaesth* 2019;122:509.

CHAPTER

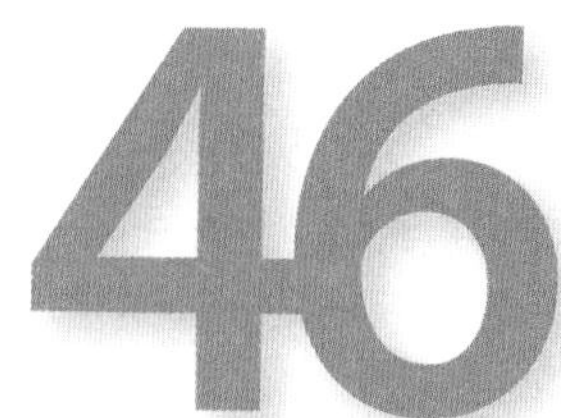

Peripheral Nerve Blocks

John J. Finneran IV, MD and
Brian M. Ilfeld, MD, MS (Clinical Investigation)

KEY CONCEPTS

1. In addition to potent analgesia, regional anesthesia may lead to reductions in the stress response, systemic analgesic requirements, opioid-related side effects, general anesthesia requirements, and, possibly, the development of chronic postoperative pain. Regional analgesia may accelerate postoperative convalescence.

2. Regional anesthetics must be administered in an area where standard anesthetic monitors, supplemental oxygen, and resuscitative medications and equipment are immediately available.

3. Over the past decade, *fascial plane blocks* have become a popular alternative to conventional peripheral nerve blocks or thoracic epidural analgesia. These blocks rely on depositing a large volume of local anesthetic into fascial planes in which target nerves are contained.

4. Local anesthetic may be deposited at any point along the brachial plexus, depending on the desired block effects: interscalene for shoulder and proximal humerus surgical procedures; and supraclavicular, infraclavicular, or axillary for surgeries distal to the mid-humerus.

5. A properly performed interscalene block almost invariably blocks the ipsilateral phrenic nerve, so careful consideration must be given to patients with severe pulmonary disease or preexisting contralateral phrenic nerve palsy. Bilateral interscalene blocks are always contraindicated.

6. Brachial plexus block at the level of the cords provides excellent anesthesia for procedures at or distal to the elbow. The upper arm and shoulder are not anesthetized with this approach. As with other brachial plexus blocks, the intercostobrachial nerve (T2 dermatome) is spared.

7. The axillary, musculocutaneous, and medial brachial cutaneous nerves branch from the brachial plexus proximal to where local anesthetic is deposited for an axillary brachial plexus block and thus are usually spared from blockade. The musculocutaneous nerve can be independently blocked to anesthetize the lateral forearm.

8. Often it is necessary to anesthetize a single terminal nerve, either for minor surgical procedures with a limited field or as a supplement to an incomplete brachial plexus block. Terminal nerves may be anesthetized anywhere along their course.

9. Intravenous regional anesthesia, also called a *Bier block*, can provide intense surgical anesthesia for relatively short (45–60 min) surgical procedures on an extremity.

10. A femoral nerve block alone will seldom provide adequate surgical anesthesia, but it is often used to provide postoperative analgesia for hip, thigh, knee, and ankle procedures.

—*Continued next page*

Continued—

11 Patients with continuous adductor canal catheters are able to ambulate further on the first day following total knee arthroplasty than patients with either femoral block (limited by weakness) or no block (limited by pain).

12 Blockade of the sciatic nerve may occur anywhere along its course and is indicated for surgical procedures involving the posterior thigh, knee, lower leg, ankle, and foot.

13 Popliteal nerve blocks provide excellent coverage for foot and ankle surgery while sparing much of the hamstring muscles, allowing lifting of the foot with knee flexion and thus facilitating ambulation. All sciatic nerve blocks fail to provide complete anesthesia for the leg and ankle, as the medial leg and ankle are innervated by the saphenous nerve. When a saphenous (or femoral) block is added, complete anesthesia below the knee is provided.

14 A complete ankle block requires a series of five nerve blocks, but the process may be streamlined to minimize needle insertions. All five injections are required to anesthetize the entire foot; however, surgical procedures may not require that all terminal nerves be blocked.

15 The superficial cervical plexus block targets the cutaneous branches of the cervical plexus, while the deep cervical plexus block targets the C2 to C4 nerve roots as they emerge from the vertebral foramina. Randomized trials have failed to find a difference in the quality of surgical anesthesia yielded by either technique, and hemidiaphragmatic paralysis may occur with either.

16 Intercostal blocks result in the highest blood levels of local anesthetic per local anesthetic dose injected of any nerve block procedure, and if multiple blocks will be performed, care must be taken to avoid toxic systemic levels of local anesthetic.

17 The thoracic paravertebral space is defined posteriorly by the superior costotransverse ligament, anterolaterally by the parietal pleura, medially by the vertebrae and the intervertebral foramina, and inferiorly and superiorly by the heads of the ribs.

18 The subcostal (T12), ilioinguinal (L1), and iliohypogastric (L1) nerves are targeted in the transversus abdominus plane (TAP) block, providing anesthesia to the ipsilateral lower abdomen below the umbilicus.

An understanding of regional anesthesia anatomy and techniques is required of a well-rounded anesthesiologist. Although anatomic relationships have not changed over time, our ability to identify them has improved. From the paresthesia-seeking techniques described by Winnie to the popularization of the nerve stimulator and the introduction of ultrasound guidance, anesthesiologists and their patients have benefitted from evolving and improving techniques. The field of regional anesthesia has accordingly expanded to one that addresses not only the intraoperative concerns of the anesthesiologist but also longer-term perioperative pain management and acceleration of convalescence.

1 In addition to potent analgesia, regional anesthesia may lead to reductions in the stress response, systemic analgesic requirements, opioid-related side effects, general anesthesia requirements, and, possibly, the development of chronic postoperative pain.

PATIENT SELECTION

The selection of a regional anesthetic technique is a process that begins with a thorough history and physical examination. As with any medical procedure, a risk–benefit analysis must be performed. The risk–benefit ratio often favors regional anesthesia in patients with multiple comorbidities for whom a general anesthetic carries a greater risk. In addition, patients intolerant of opioids (eg, those with obstructive sleep apnea or at high risk for nausea) may benefit from the opioid-sparing effects of a regional analgesic. Patients who will likely have prolonged postoperative pain and those with chronic pain or opioid tolerance may receive optimal analgesia with a continuous peripheral nerve block (perineural local anesthetic infusion).

A comprehensive knowledge of regional anatomy and an understanding of the planned surgical procedure are important for selection of the appropriate regional anesthetic technique. If possible, advanced discussion of various considerations (tourniquet placement, skin or bone autograft harvesting, projected surgical duration) should be undertaken with the surgical team. Also, knowing the anticipated course of recovery and anticipated level of postoperative pain will often influence specific decisions regarding a regional anesthetic technique (eg, single injection versus continuous nerve block).

RISKS & CONTRAINDICATIONS

Patient understanding and cooperation are key to the success and safety of every regional anesthetic procedure; patients who cannot remain still for a procedure may be at increased risk. Examples include pediatric patients and some developmentally delayed individuals, as well as patients with dementia or movement disorders. For such patients, the risks of performing the block under deep sedation or general anesthesia must be weighed against the benefit of the nerve block. Bleeding disorders and pharmacological anticoagulation heighten the risk of local hematoma or hemorrhage, and this risk must be balanced against the possible benefits of regional blockade. Specific peripheral nerve block locations warranting the most concern are posterior lumbar plexus and paravertebral blocks owing to their relative proximity to the retroperitoneal space and neuraxis, respectively. Additionally, paravertebral blocks, intercostal nerve blocks, and supraclavicular brachial plexus blocks carry a risk of pneumothorax.

Placement of a block needle through a site of infection can theoretically track infectious material deeper into the body, where it poses a risk to the target nerve and surrounding structures. Therefore, the presence of local infection is a relative contraindication to performing a peripheral nerve block. Indwelling perineural catheters can serve as a nidus of infection; however, the risk in patients with systemic infection remains unknown. The bacterial colonization rate of indwelling catheters increases with the duration of therapy, and these patients must be monitored for signs and symptoms of infection. However, there is no specific time point when a catheter should be removed if it continues to provide benefit and no infection concerns are present.

Although nerve injury is always a possibility with a regional anesthetic, some patients are at increased risk. Individuals with a preexisting nerve condition (eg, peripheral neuropathy or previous nerve injury) may have a higher incidence of complications, including prolonged or permanent sensorimotor block. Persistent neuropathic symptoms are more common after brachial plexus blocks and distal upper extremity blocks compared with lower extremity or truncal blocks. The precise mechanisms have yet to be clearly defined but may involve local ischemia from high injection pressure or vasoconstrictors, the neurotoxic effect of local anesthetics, or direct trauma to nerve tissue. The most common symptoms include minor paresthesia and subjectively decreased sensation. Patient reassurance and intermittent follow-up are important as these symptoms usually resolve spontaneously. If more concerning symptoms are present (eg, persistent motor deficit, absent sensation, or severe pain), a neurology consultation and nerve conduction studies may be warranted. Close communication with the surgical team is paramount in making such decisions.

Other risks associated with regional anesthesia include systemic local anesthetic toxicity from intravascular injection or perivascular absorption. In the event of a systemic local anesthetic toxic reaction, seizure activity and cardiovascular collapse may occur. Supportive measures must begin immediately. In the case of cardiovascular collapse, one must call for assistance (perhaps by a "code blue"), initiate cardiopulmonary resuscitation, administer incremental doses of epinephrine, infuse intravenous lipid emulsion, and, if all else fails, prepare for cardiopulmonary bypass. Importantly, it should be noted that there are several additional differences from standard Advanced Cardiac Life Support resuscitative measures for a patient with cardiovascular collapse secondary to local anesthetic systemic toxicity. These include reduction in epinephrine dose and avoidance of lidocaine as an antiarrhythmic, β-blockers, calcium channel blockers, and vasopressin.

Site-specific risks should also be considered for each individual patient. In a patient with severe pulmonary compromise or hemidiaphragmatic paralysis, for example, a contralateral interscalene or cervical plexus block with resultant phrenic nerve block could be catastrophic.

CHOICE OF LOCAL ANESTHETIC

The decision about which local anesthetic to employ for a particular nerve block depends on the desired onset, duration, and relative blockade of sensory and motor fibers. Potential for systemic toxicity should be considered, as well as site-specific risks. A detailed discussion of local anesthetics is provided elsewhere (see Chapter 16).

PREPARATION

2 Regional anesthetics must be administered in an area where standard anesthetic monitors, supplemental oxygen, and resuscitative medications and equipment are immediately available. Patients should be monitored with pulse oximetry, noninvasive blood pressure, and electrocardiography; measurement of end-tidal carbon dioxide (CO_2) and the fraction of inspired oxygen (Fio_2) should also be available. Positioning should be ergonomically favorable for the practitioner and comfortable for the patient. Intravenous premedication may be employed to allay anxiety and minimize discomfort. A relatively short-acting benzodiazepine and opioid are most often used and should be titrated for comfort while ensuring that patients can respond to verbal cues. Sterile technique should be strictly observed.

BLOCK TECHNIQUES

Field Block Technique

A *field block* is a local anesthetic injection that targets terminal cutaneous nerves (Figure 46–1). Field blocks are used commonly by surgeons to minimize incisional pain and may be used as a supplementary technique or as a sole anesthetic for minor, superficial procedures. Anesthesiologists often use field blocks to anesthetize the superficial cervical plexus for procedures involving the neck or shoulder; the intercostobrachial nerve for surgery involving the medial upper extremity proximal to the elbow (in combination with a brachial plexus nerve block); and the subcutaneous nerves innervating the foot and ankle as part of an "ankle block" as described later in this chapter. Field blocks may be undesirable in cases where they obscure or distort the operative anatomy or where local tissue acidosis from infection prevents effective local anesthetic function.

Paresthesia Technique

Formerly the mainstay of regional anesthesia, this technique is now rarely taught for nerve localization. With anatomic relationships and surface landmarks as a guide, a block needle is advanced toward the target nerve or plexus. Paresthesia (abnormal sensation) is elicited in the area of sensory distribution when a needle makes direct contact with a sensory nerve. With more modern nerve localization techniques, paresthesia is generally avoided. If paresthesia occurs, the needle should be redirected. Paresthesia occurring during injection may indicate an intraneural location of the needle tip.

Nerve Stimulation Technique

For this technique, an insulated needle concentrates electrical current at the needle tip, while a wire attached to the needle hub connects to a nerve stimulator—a battery-powered machine that emits a small amount (0–5 mA) of electric current at a set frequency (usually 1 or 2 Hz). A grounding electrode is attached to the patient to complete the circuit (Figure 46–2). When the insulated needle tip is placed in proximity to a motor nerve, specific muscle contractions are induced, and local anesthetic is injected. Although it is common to

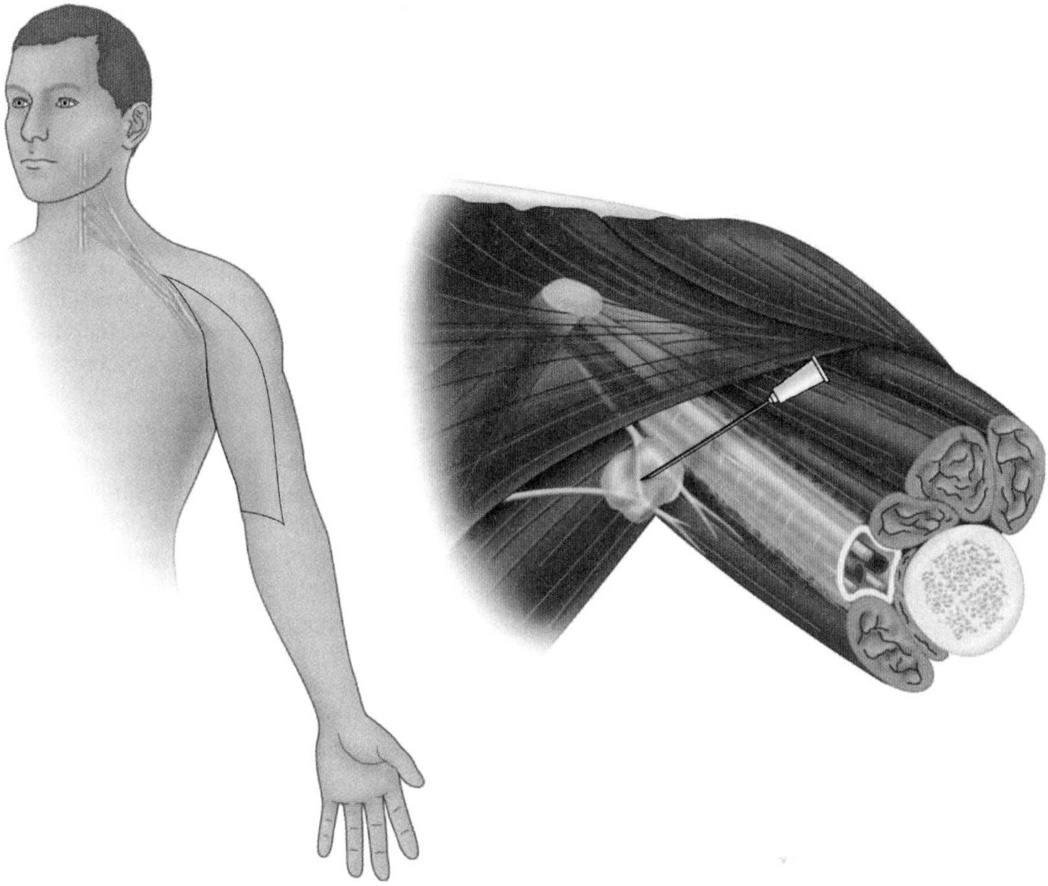

FIGURE 46–1 A field block targets terminal cutaneous nerves, such as the intercostobrachial nerve.

redirect the block needle until muscle contractions occur at a current less than 0.5 mA, there is scant evidence to support this specific current in all cases. Similarly, although some have suggested that muscle contraction with current less than 0.2 mA implies intraneural needle placement, there is little evidence to support this specific cutoff. Nonetheless, most practitioners inject local anesthetic when current between 0.2 and 0.5 mA results in a motor response. For most blocks using this technique in adults, 30 to 40 mL of anesthetic is usually injected with gentle aspiration between divided doses.

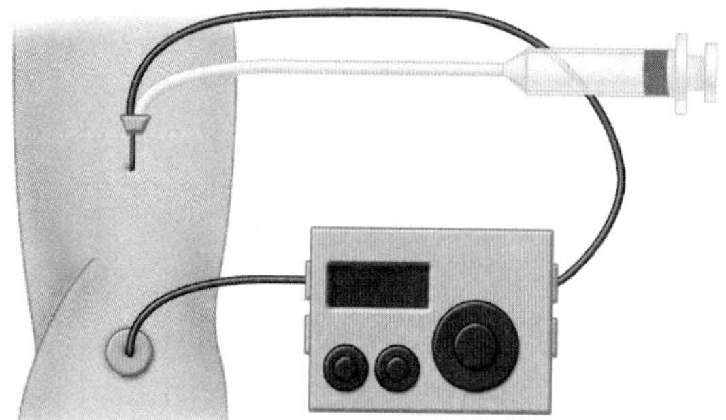

FIGURE 46–2 A nerve stimulator delivers a small amount of electrical current to the block needle to facilitate nerve localization.

Ultrasound Technique

Ultrasound imaging has overwhelmingly become the dominant modality taught for nerve localization and needle guidance in recent years. Therefore, ultrasound-guided techniques will be the primary focus of this chapter. Ultrasound may be used either alone or combined with other modalities such as nerve stimulation. Ultrasound uses high-frequency (1–20 MHz) sound waves emitted from piezoelectric crystals that are reflected to different degrees by tissues of different densities, thereby returning a signal to the transducer. Depending on the amplitude and timing of signals received, the piezoelectric elements deform to create an electronic voltage that is converted into a two-dimensional grayscale image. The degree of efficiency with which sound passes through or is reflected by a substance determines its echogenicity. Structures and substances through which sound passes easily are described as *hypoechoic* and appear dark or black on the ultrasound screen. In contrast, structures reflecting more sound waves appear brighter or white and are termed *hyperechoic.*

The optimal transducer varies depending upon the depth of the target nerve and approach angle of the needle relative to the transducer (Figure 46–3). High-frequency transducers provide a high-resolution picture with a relatively clear image but offer poor tissue penetration and are therefore used predominantly for more superficial nerves. Low-frequency transducers provide an image of poorer quality but have better tissue penetration and are therefore used for deeper structures. Transducers with a *linear array* offer an undistorted image and are therefore often the first choice among practitioners. However, when a steep needle trajectory relative to the long axis of the transducer is required, linear array transducers will poorly visualize the needle. For deeper target nerves that require a more acute angle between the needle and the transducer, a *curved array* (*curvilinear*) transducer will maximize returning ultrasound waves, providing the optimal needle image (see Figure 46–3). Nerves are best imaged in cross-section, where they have a characteristic honeycomb appearance (*short-axis*). Needle insertion can pass either parallel (*in-plane*) or not parallel (*out-of-plane*) to the plane of the ultrasound waves (Figure 46–4). In-plane technique is more frequently utilized as the entire shaft of the needle can be visualized as it approaches the target nerve and navigates surrounding structures. Unlike nerve stimulation alone, ultrasound guidance allows for a variable volume of local anesthetic to be injected, with the final amount determined by what is observed under direct ultrasound visualization. Generally, the goal will be a circumferential spread around the target nerve, and

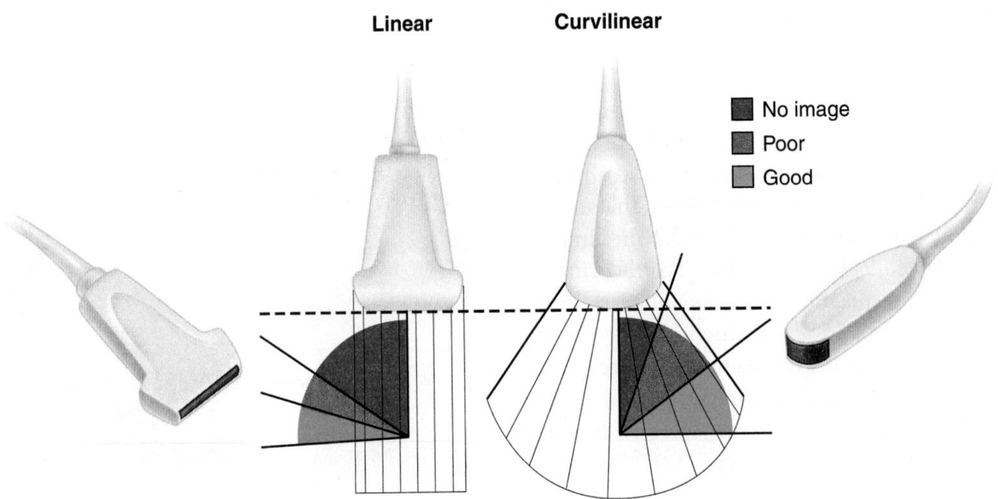

FIGURE 46–3 A linear probe offers higher resolution with less penetration. A curvilinear probe provides better penetration with lower resolution.

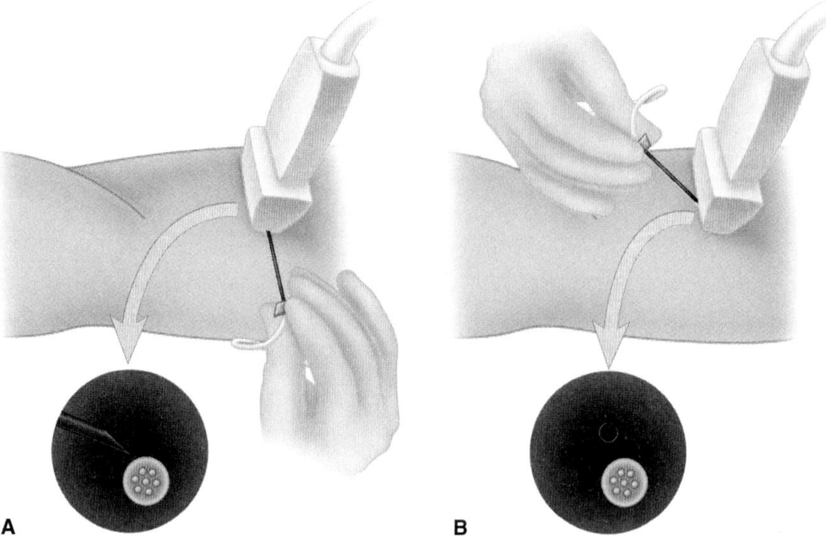

FIGURE 46–4 *In-plane* (**A**) and *out-of-plane* (**B**) ultrasound approaches.

this technique usually results in a smaller injected volume (10–30 mL) of local anesthetic.

Continuous Peripheral Nerve Blocks

Also termed *perineural local anesthetic infusion*, continuous peripheral nerve blocks involve the placement of a percutaneous catheter adjacent to a peripheral nerve, followed by local anesthetic administration to prolong a nerve block (Figure 46–5). Potential advantages most frequently include reductions in resting and dynamic pain, supplemental analgesic requirements, opioid-related side effects, and sleep disturbance. In some cases, patient satisfaction, ambulation, and functioning may be improved, accelerated resumption of passive joint range-of-motion realized, and reduced time until discharge readiness as well as actual discharge from the hospital or rehabilitation center achieved. Recent evidence suggests that continuous sciatic, femoral, and paravertebral perineural local anesthetic infusions in the immediate postoperative period may decrease the risk of persistent ("chronic") postsurgical pain.

There are many types of perineural catheters, including nonstimulating and stimulating, flexible and relatively rigid, and through-the-needle, over-the-needle, and suture-catheters. Currently, there is little evidence that a single design results in superior effects. Long-acting local anesthetics (eg, ropivacaine or bupivacaine) are nearly exclusively used for infusions since they provide a more favorable sensory to motor block ratio. Dilute local anesthetic (eg, 0.1–0.2% ropivacaine or bupivacaine) is often infused with the aim of minimizing induced motor block; however, evidence suggests that the total drug mass (dose)—and not concentration—determines block effects. Unlike *single-injection* peripheral nerve blocks, no adjuvant added to a perineural local anesthetic *infusion* has been demonstrated to be beneficial. The local anesthetic may be administered exclusively as bolus doses (patient controlled or automated) or a basal infusion, and a combination of these methods is frequently utilized. Continuous peripheral nerve blocks may be provided on an ambulatory basis using a small, portable infusion pump (Figure 46–6).

As with all medical procedures, there are potential risks associated with continuous peripheral nerve blocks. Therefore, these infusions are usually reserved for patients having procedures expected to result in postoperative pain that is difficult to control

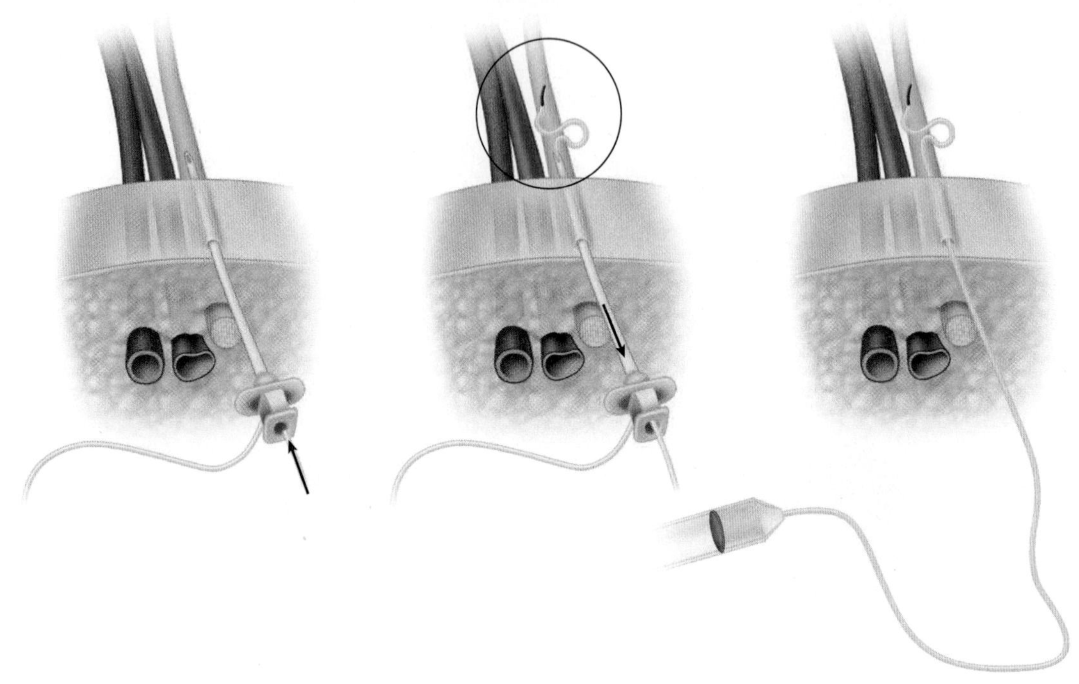

FIGURE 46–5 Placement of a percutaneous catheter adjacent to a peripheral nerve.

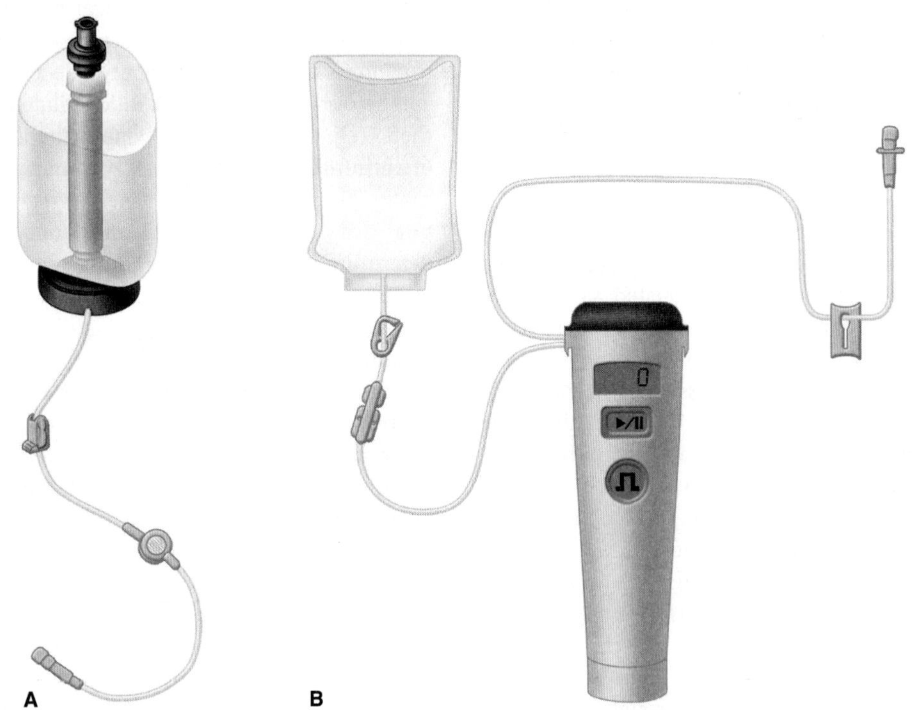

FIGURE 46–6 Elastomeric (**A**) and electronic (**B**) portable infusion pumps.

with oral analgesics and that will not resolve in less time than the duration of a single-injection peripheral nerve block. Serious complications, which are relatively rare, include systemic local anesthetic toxicity, catheter retention, nerve injury, and infection. In addition, a perineural infusion affecting the femoral nerve (including fascial plane blocks whose effect is primarily mediated by femoral nerve blockade) increases the risk of falling, though to what degree and by what specific mechanism (eg, sensory, motor, or proprioception deficits) remain unknown.

Fascial Plane Blocks

3 Over the past decade, *fascial plane blocks* have become a popular alternative to conventional lower extremity peripheral nerve blocks or thoracic epidural analgesia. These blocks rely on depositing a large volume of local anesthetic into fascial planes in which target nerves are contained. Fascial plane blocks have advantages and disadvantages compared with their respective conventional nerve block alternatives. Often, multiple nerves or dermatomes can be anesthetized by a single injection to a fascial plane that would require multiple injections to cover individual nerves or dermatomes using conventional nerve blocks. Fascial plane blocks are also generally more superficial than conventional nerve or epidural blocks. Both of these factors contribute to the potentially increased safety of fascial plane blocks. However, since fascial plane blocks usually require a large volume, the concentration of local anesthetic is generally decreased, reducing the likelihood that the block will provide surgical anesthesia. Further, since fascial plane blocks do not target individual nerves, the likelihood of successfully blocking the target nerve is diminished when compared with direct injection of local anesthetic around a nerve. For these reasons, fascial plane blocks are better used when one's goal is analgesia rather than anesthesia.

UPPER EXTREMITY PERIPHERAL NERVE BLOCKS

Brachial Plexus Anatomy

The brachial plexus is formed by the union of the anterior primary divisions (*ventral rami*) of the fifth through the eighth cervical spinal nerves (C5–C8) and the first thoracic spinal nerve (T1). Contributions from C4 and T2 are generally minor or absent. As the nerve roots leave the intervertebral foramina, they converge, successively forming *trunks*, *divisions*, *cords*, *branches*, and then finally terminal nerves. The three distinct **trunks** formed between the anterior and middle scalene muscles are termed *superior*, *middle*, and *inferior* based on their vertical orientation. As the trunks pass over the lateral border of the first rib and under the clavicle, each trunk divides into *anterior* and *posterior* **divisions**. As the brachial plexus emerges below the clavicle, the fibers combine again to form three **cords** that are named according to their relationship to the axillary artery: *lateral*, *medial*, and *posterior*. At the lateral border of the pectoralis minor muscle, each cord gives off a large branch before ending as a major terminal nerve. The lateral cord gives off the lateral branch of the median nerve and terminates as the musculocutaneous nerve; the medial cord gives off the medial branch of the median nerve and terminates as the ulnar nerve; and the posterior cord gives off the axillary nerve and terminates as the radial nerve.
4 Local anesthetic may be deposited at any point along the brachial plexus, depending on the desired block effects (Figure 46–7): interscalene for shoulder and proximal humerus surgical procedures; and supraclavicular, infraclavicular, and axillary for surgeries distal to the mid-humerus.

Interscalene Block

An interscalene brachial plexus block is indicated for procedures involving the shoulder and upper arm (Figure 46–8). Roots C5 to C7 are most densely blocked with this approach, and the ulnar nerve originating from C8 and T1 is usually spared. Therefore, interscalene blocks are not appropriate for surgery at or distal to the elbow. For complete surgical anesthesia of the shoulder as well as postoperative analgesia following clavicle surgical reduction and fixation, the supraclavicular nerve (cutaneous branch of C3 and C4) may need to be supplemented with a cervical plexus block.

Contraindications to an interscalene block include local infection, severe coagulopathy, local anesthetic
5 allergy, and patient refusal. A properly performed

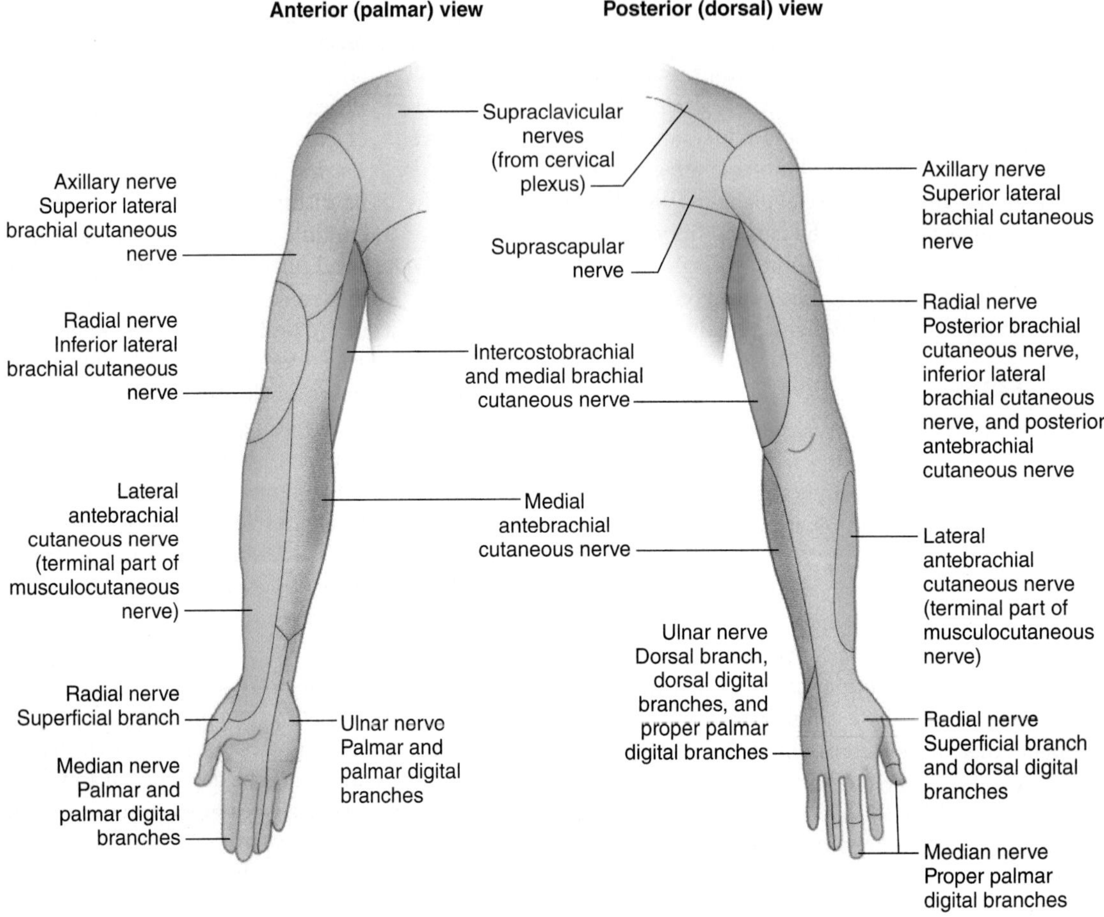

FIGURE 46–7 The location of local anesthetic deposition along the brachial plexus depends on the desired effects of the block.

interscalene block almost invariably blocks the ipsilateral phrenic nerve (completely with nerve stimulation techniques, but less so with certain low-volume ultrasound-guided techniques), so careful consideration must be given to patients with severe pulmonary disease or preexisting contralateral phrenic nerve palsy. Bilateral interscalene blocks are absolutely contraindicated. Hemidiaphragmatic paresis may result in dyspnea, hypercapnia, and hypoxemia. Horner syndrome (myosis, ptosis, and anhidrosis) frequently results from proximal tracking of local anesthetic and blockade of sympathetic fibers to the cervicothoracic ganglion. Recurrent laryngeal nerve involvement often induces hoarseness. In a patient with contralateral vocal cord paralysis, respiratory distress may ensue. Other site-specific risks include vertebral artery injection (suspect if immediate seizure activity is observed), spinal or epidural injection, and pneumothorax; however, these complications have primarily been reported with non–ultrasound-guided blocks. As little as 1 mL of local anesthetic delivered into the vertebral artery may induce a seizure. Similarly, intrathecal, subdural, and epidural local anesthetic spread is possible; and injection into the spinal cord resulting in a cervical syrinx has been reported. Lastly, pneumothorax is possible because of the close proximity of the apical pleura.

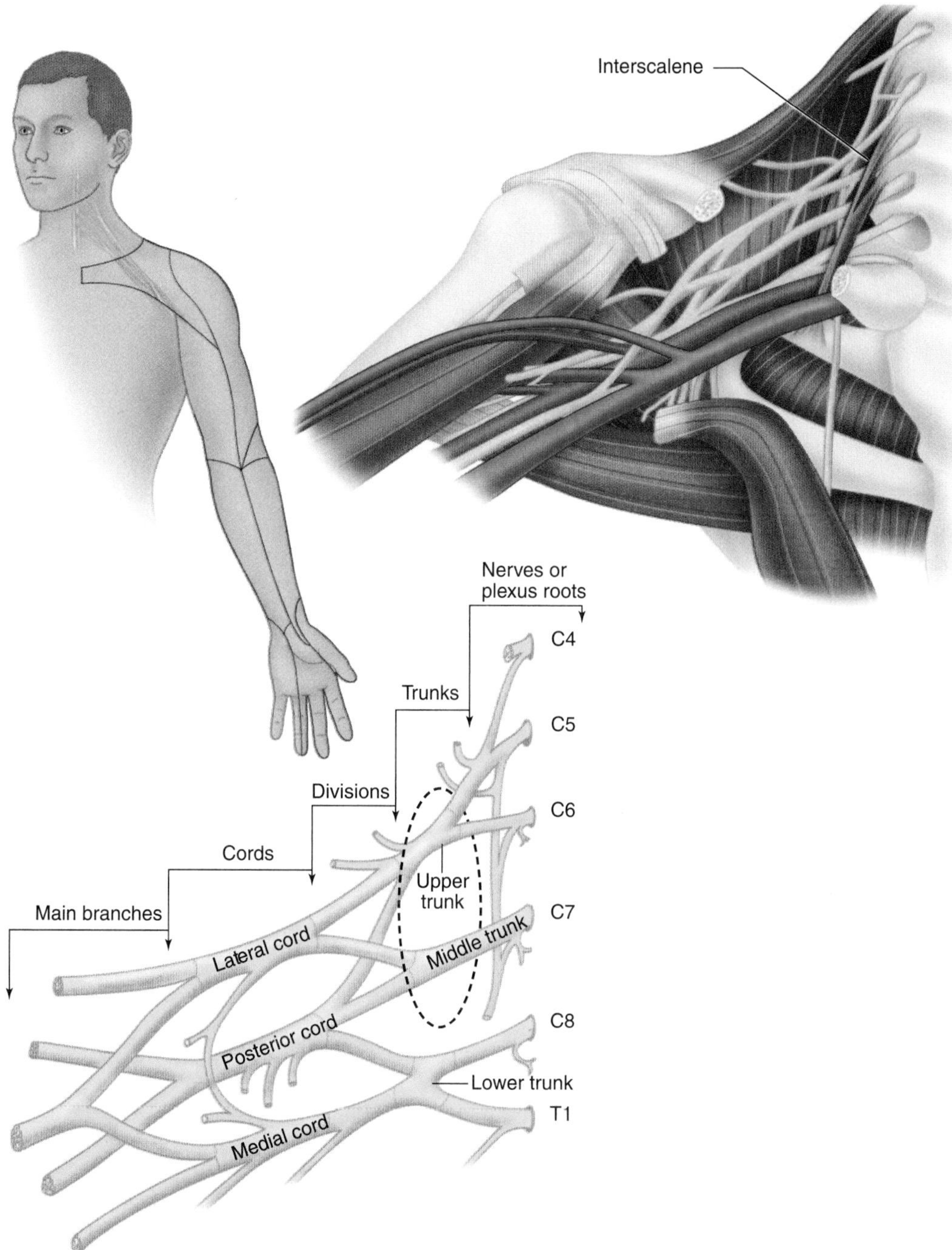

FIGURE 46–8 An interscalene block is appropriate for shoulder and proximal humerus procedures. The ventral rami of C5–C8 and T1 form the brachial plexus.

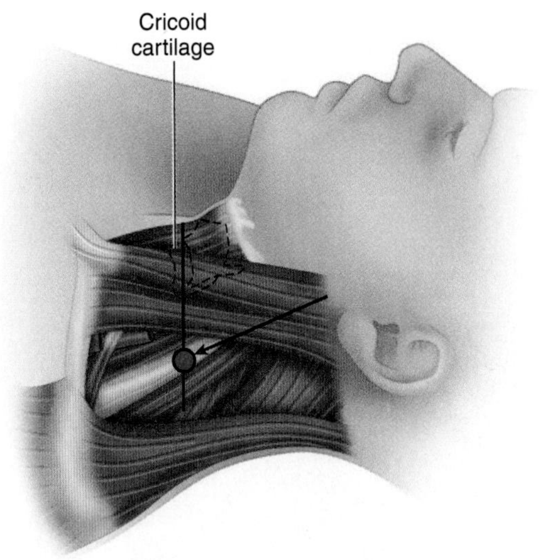

FIGURE 46–9 The brachial plexus passes between the anterior and middle scalene muscles at the level of the cricoid cartilage, or the C6 vertebra.

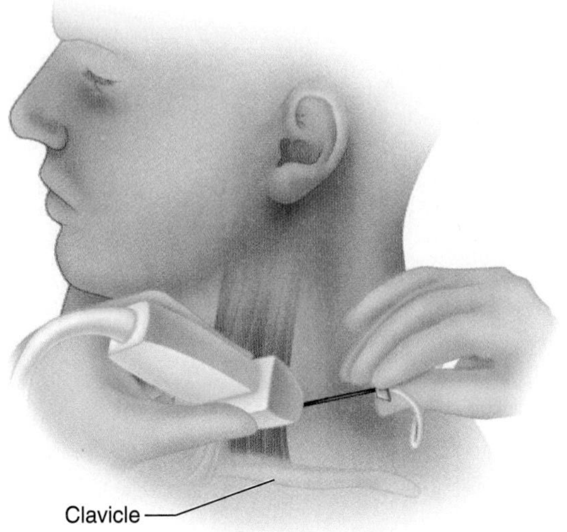

FIGURE 46–10 Interscalene block positioning.

The brachial plexus passes between the anterior and middle scalene muscles at the level of the cricoid cartilage, or C6 (Figure 46–9). Palpation of the interscalene groove is usually accomplished with the patient supine and the head rotated 30° or less to the contralateral side. The external jugular vein often crosses the interscalene groove at the level of the cricoid cartilage. Having the patient lift and turn the head against resistance often helps delineate the anatomy. If surgical anesthesia is desired for the entire shoulder, the intercostobrachial (T2) and supraclavicular (C3 and C4) must usually be anesthetized separately. Continuous interscalene blocks provide potent analgesia following shoulder surgery.

A needle in-plane technique is generally used, and an insulated needle attached to a nerve stimulator can be used to confirm the accuracy of the targeted structure. After identification of the sternocleidomastoid muscle and interscalene groove at the approximate level of C6, a high-frequency linear transducer is placed perpendicular to the course of the interscalene muscles (short axis; Figure 46–10). The brachial plexus and anterior and middle scalene muscles should be visualized in cross-section (Figure 46–11). The brachial plexus at this level appears most commonly as three hypoechoic circles with hyperechoic borders. These circles generally correspond to either nerve roots of C5, C6, and C7; C5 and two rootlets of C6 (C6 A and B); or, rarely, the upper, middle, and lower trunks. Tracing these structures proximally is not necessary, but it can be done to determine their true anatomic identities. As the interscalene block is used for shoulder analgesia, the primary target for local anesthetic should be between the two most superficial nerves (most commonly C5 and C6). The carotid artery and internal jugular vein may be seen lying anterior to the anterior scalene muscle; the sternocleidomastoid is visible superficially as it tapers to form its posterior edge.

Using an in-plane technique, the anesthetist inserts the needle just posterolateral to the ultrasound transducer in a direction exactly parallel to the ultrasound beam and advances it in an anteromedial direction. It may be helpful to have the patient turn slightly laterally with the surgical side up to facilitate manipulation of the needle. Alternatively, folded towels or blankets under the head and operative shoulder may create a space for the operator's hands while manipulating the needle. The needle is advanced through the middle scalene muscle until it has passed through the fascia anteriorly into the interscalene groove. The needle tip and shaft should be visualized during the entire block procedure.

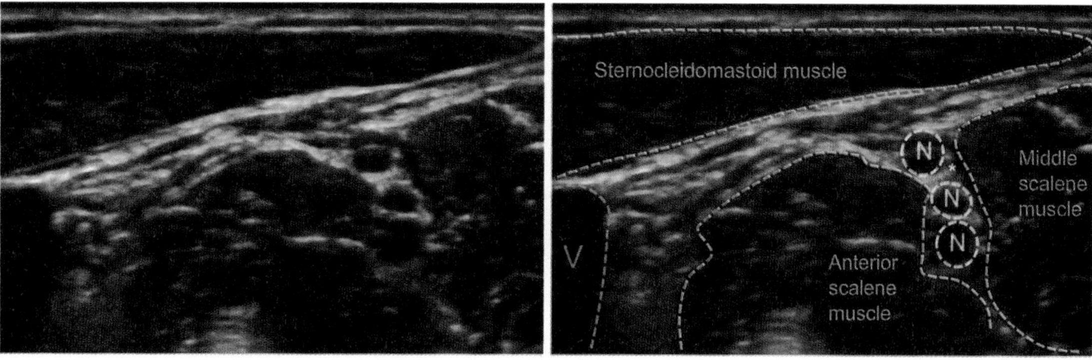

FIGURE 46–11 Interscalene block. N, brachial plexus nerve roots in cross-section; V, internal jugular vein; asterisk indicates target location for local anesthetic.

Depending on visualized spread relative to the target nerve(s), a lower volume (10 mL) may be employed for postoperative analgesia, whereas a larger volume (20–30 mL) is commonly used for surgical anesthesia. As the volume used increases, so does the likelihood of incidental phrenic nerve blockade.

Supraclavicular Block

Once described as the "spinal of the arm" due to its relatively rapid onset and reliability, a supraclavicular block offers dense anesthesia of the brachial plexus for surgical procedures at or distal to the elbow (Figure 46–12). Historically, the supraclavicular block fell out of favor due to the relatively increased incidence of pneumothorax that occurred with paresthesia and nerve stimulator techniques. It has seen a resurgence in recent years with the use of ultrasound guidance, which may significantly reduce (but not eliminate) the risk of pneumothorax. The supraclavicular block does not reliably anesthetize the suprascapular nerve. Thus, the supraclavicular block is not ideal for shoulder surgery unless combined with a suprascapular nerve block. Sparing of distal branches, most commonly the ulnar nerve, may occur. This can be avoided by carefully tracing the plexus cephalad and caudad with ultrasound to identify the lower trunk and ensure it is anesthetized. Supraclavicular perineural catheters provide inferior analgesia compared with infraclavicular perineural catheter infusion and are more often displaced with movement.

The precautions taken with patient selection for an interscalene block should be exercised with a supraclavicular block, as well. Nearly half of patients undergoing supraclavicular block will experience ipsilateral phrenic nerve palsy, although ultrasound guidance may decrease this incidence by facilitating reduced local anesthetic volume. Horner syndrome and recurrent laryngeal nerve palsy may also occur. Risks of pneumothorax and subclavian artery puncture remain, although they are theoretically less likely with ultrasound guidance.

The patient should be positioned supine with the head turned 30° toward the contralateral side. A linear, high-frequency transducer is placed in the supraclavicular fossa superior to the clavicle and angled slightly toward the thorax (Figure 46–13). The subclavian artery is easily identified. The brachial plexus appears as multiple hypoechoic disks (sometimes referred to as a cluster of grapes), just superficial and posterolateral to the subclavian artery (Figure 46–14). Anatomic variability exists; however, these most frequently are the anterior and posterior divisions of each trunk. The first rib should also be identified as a hyperechoic line just deep to the artery. Pleura may be identified adjacent to the rib and can be distinguished from bone by its movement with breathing.

The block needle is inserted posterolateral to the transducer in an anteromedial direction, parallel to the ultrasound beam. The needle is advanced medially toward the subclavian artery

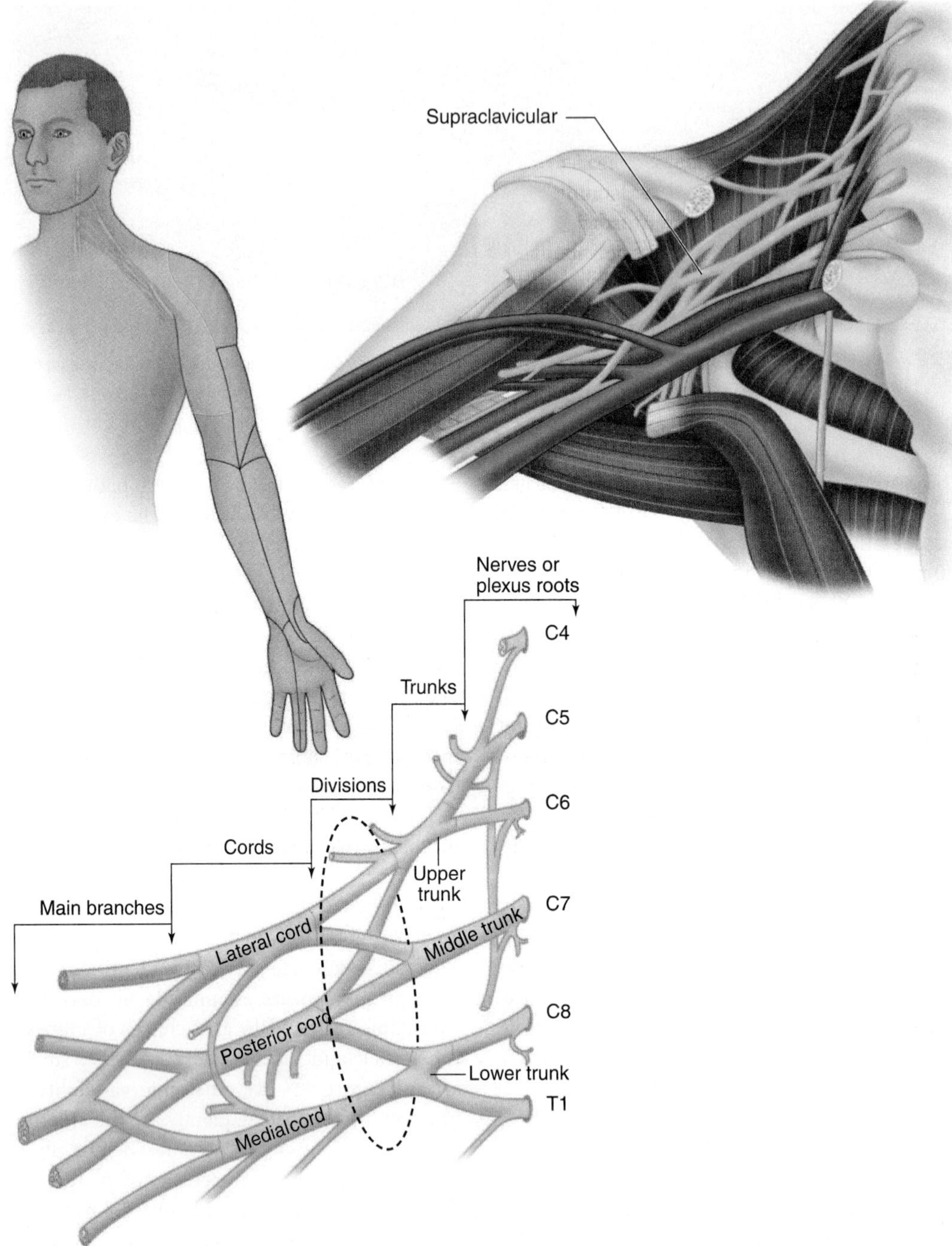

FIGURE 46–12 A supraclavicular block can provide dense anesthesia for procedures at or distal to the elbow. Light blue shading indicates regions of variable blockade; purple shading indicates regions of more reliable blockade.

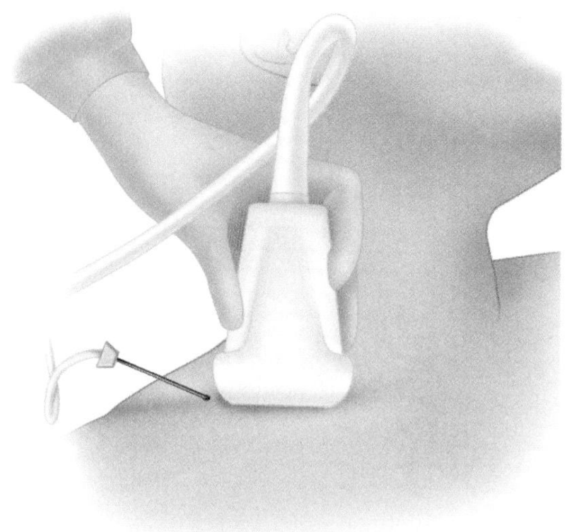

FIGURE 46–13 Supraclavicular block positioning.

until the tip is visualized near the brachial plexus, just lateral and superficial to the artery. Local anesthetic spread should be visualized surrounding the plexus after careful aspiration and incremental injection, which often requires injections in multiple locations with a highly variable volume (20–30 mL). Recent evidence suggests that the most important injection location is the "corner pocket" between the artery, plexus, and first rib. Reports have also suggested confining local anesthetic to this location reduces the incidence of phrenic nerve block while still providing surgical anesthesia to the upper extremity.

Infraclavicular Block

As the brachial plexus traverses beyond the first rib and into the axilla, the cords are named for their positions relative to the axillary artery: *medial*, *lateral*, and *posterior*.

6 Brachial plexus block at the level of the cords provides excellent anesthesia for procedures at, or distal to, the elbow (Figure 46–15). The upper arm and shoulder will not be fully anesthetized with this approach. As with other brachial plexus blocks, the intercostobrachial nerve (T2 dermatome) is spared. Site-specific risks of the infraclavicular approach include vascular puncture and pneumothorax, though they are less common than with supraclavicular block. It is prudent to consider an alternative approach for patients with an indwelling vascular catheter in the ipsilateral subclavian region and for patients with an ipsilateral transvenous pacemaker.

With the patient in the supine position, a high-frequency linear or small curvilinear ultrasound probe is placed in the parasagittal plane over a point 2 cm medial and 2 cm caudad to the coracoid process (Figure 46–16). The use of a high-frequency linear probe will provide a higher resolution image of the target nerves; however, a small curvilinear probe will better visualize the needle because of the

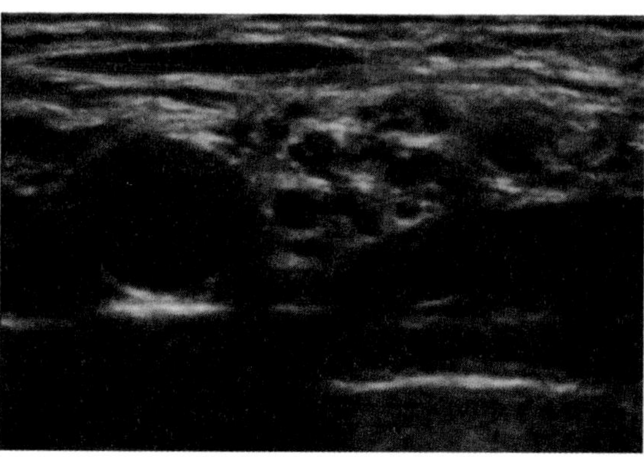

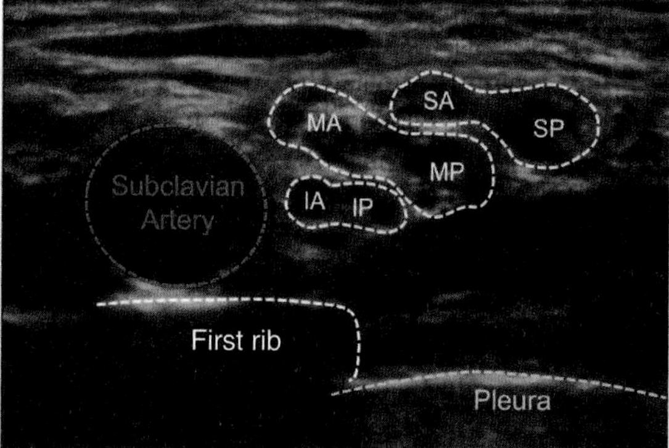

FIGURE 46–14 Supraclavicular brachial plexus block. IA, anterior division of inferior trunk; IP, posterior division of inferior trunk; MA, anterior division of middle trunk; MP, posterior division of middle trunk; SA, anterior division of superior trunk; SP, posterior division of superior trunk.

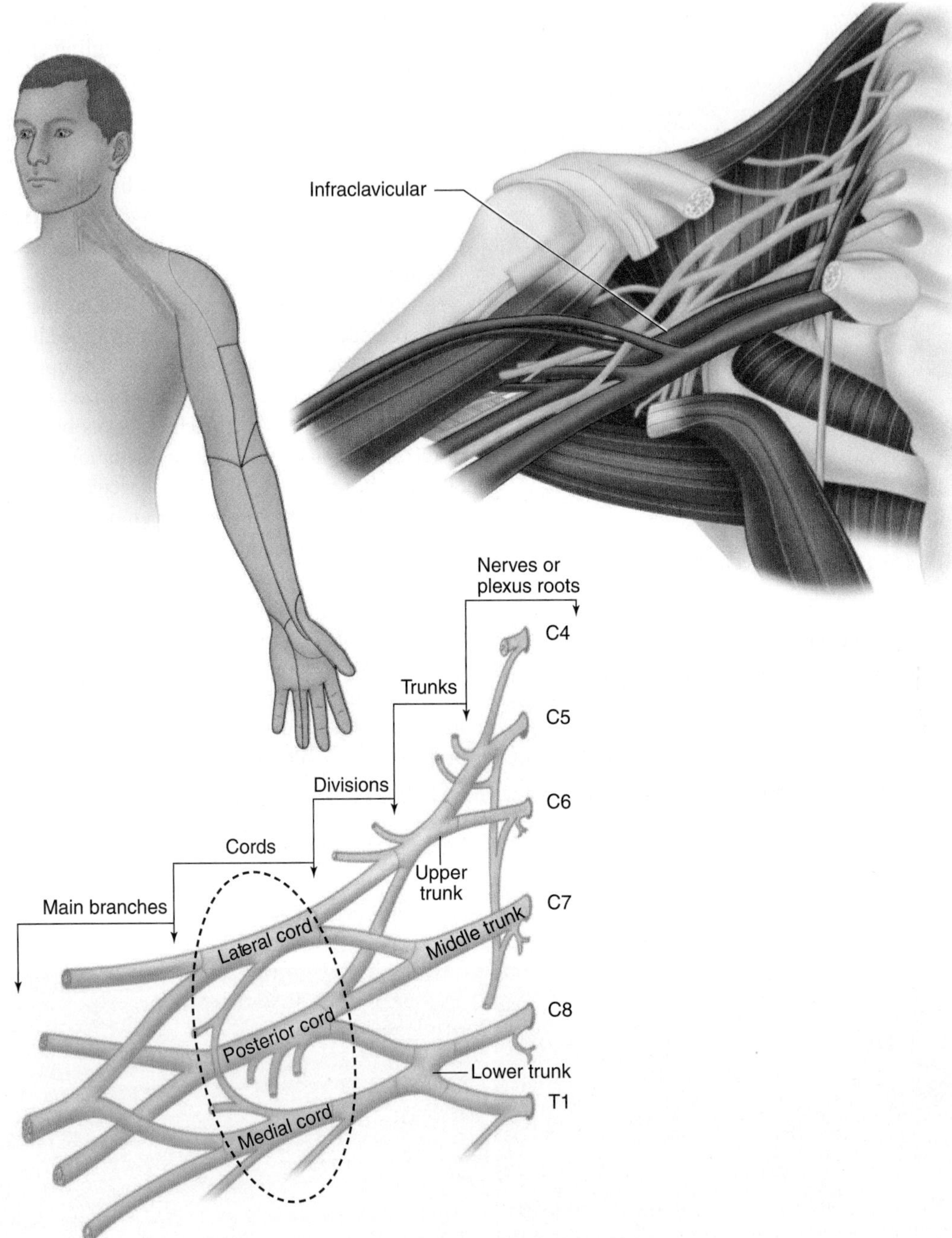

FIGURE 46–15 Infraclavicular block coverage and anatomy. Light blue shading indicates regions of variable blockade; purple shading indicates regions of more reliable blockade.

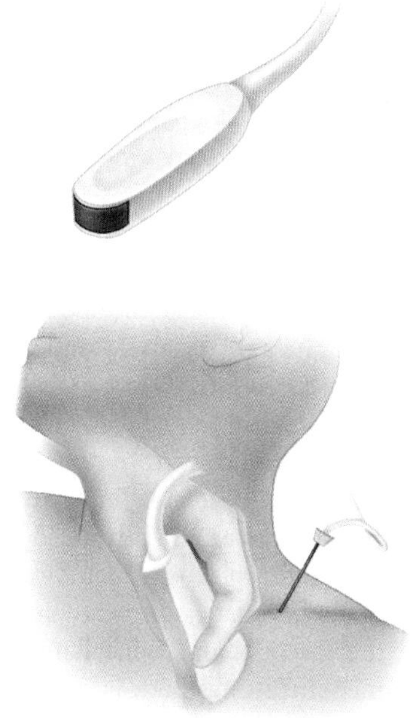

FIGURE 46–16 Infraclavicular block positioning.

steep angle, especially in larger patients. Abducting the arm 90° dramatically improves visualization of the axillary artery and brachial plexus. For patients with elbow or radius fractures, a splint may make this positioning difficult or impossible. In such cases, consider discussing the removal of the splint with the surgical team prior to the block (the splint will soon be removed in the operating room anyway). Supplementary opioid or ketamine analgesia may be required to accomplish this positioning in patients with fractures.

The axillary artery and vein are identified in cross-section (Figure 46–17). The medial, lateral, and posterior cords appear as hyperechoic bundles positioned caudad, cephalad, and posterior to the artery, respectively. A long (10-cm) needle is inserted 1 to 3 cm cephalad to the transducer. Optimal needle positioning is between the axillary artery and the posterior cord, where a single 30-mL injection is as effective as individual cord injections. Insertion of a perineural catheter should be in the same location

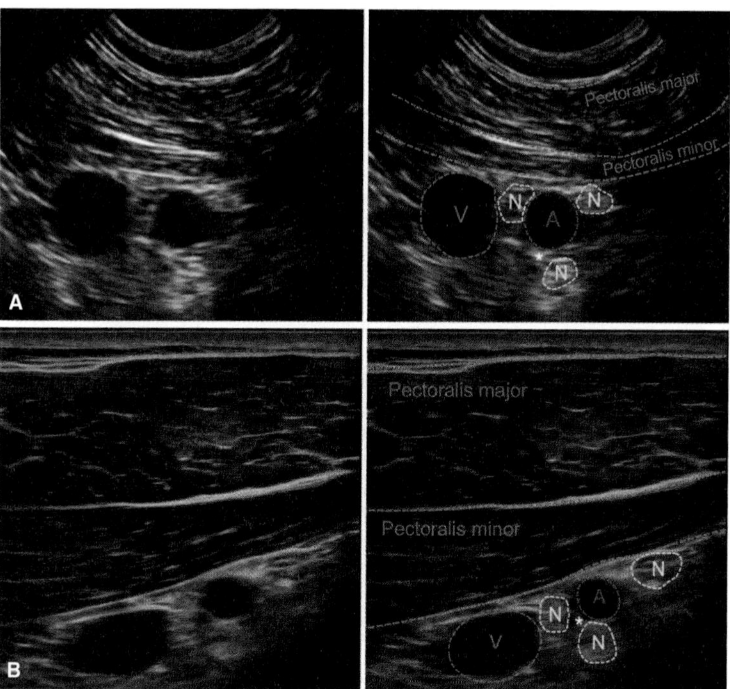

FIGURE 46–17 Infraclavicular block with (A) Small curvilinear probe and (B) High frequency linear probe: A, axillary artery; N, medial, lateral, and posterior cords of the brachial plexus; V, axillary vein; asterisk indicates the location of local anesthetic deposition.

posterior to the axillary artery. Infraclavicular perineural infusion has been shown to provide analgesia superior to that of both supraclavicular and axillary infusions.

Axillary Block

At the lateral border of the pectoralis minor muscle, the cords of the brachial plexus form large terminal branches oriented around the axillary artery 7 (Figure 46–18). The axillary, musculocutaneous, and medial brachial cutaneous nerves branch from the brachial plexus proximal to where local anesthetic is deposited for an axillary brachial plexus block and thus are usually spared from blockade (Figure 46–19). At this level, the major terminal nerves often are separated by fascia; therefore, multiple injections (5–10 mL each) may be required to reliably produce anesthesia of the arm distal to the elbow (Figure 46–20).

There are few contraindications to axillary brachial plexus blocks. Local infection, neuropathy, and bleeding risk must be considered. Because the axilla is highly vascularized, there is a risk of local anesthetic uptake through small veins traumatized by needle placement. The axilla is also a suboptimal site for perineural catheter placement because of greatly inferior analgesia relative to that of infraclavicular infusion, as well as theoretically increased risks of infection and catheter dislodgement.

The patient should be positioned supine, with the arm abducted 90° or the operative hand placed behind the head. The head is turned toward the contralateral side. The axillary artery pulse should be palpated, and its location should be marked as a reference point. The axillary artery and vein(s) are visualized in cross-section with a high-frequency linear array ultrasound transducer. The brachial plexus can be identified surrounding the artery (Figure 46–21). The needle is inserted superior (lateral) to the transducer and advanced inferiorly (medially) toward the plexus under direct visualization. The nerves must be targeted individually because of the fascial separations between them, and 5 to 10 mL of local anesthetic is injected around each nerve. The musculocutaneous nerve can be visualized either between the two heads of the coracobrachialis or between the coracobrachialis and biceps brachii muscles, and this nerve eventually terminates as the lateral antebrachial cutaneous nerve. Therefore, the musculocutaneous nerve

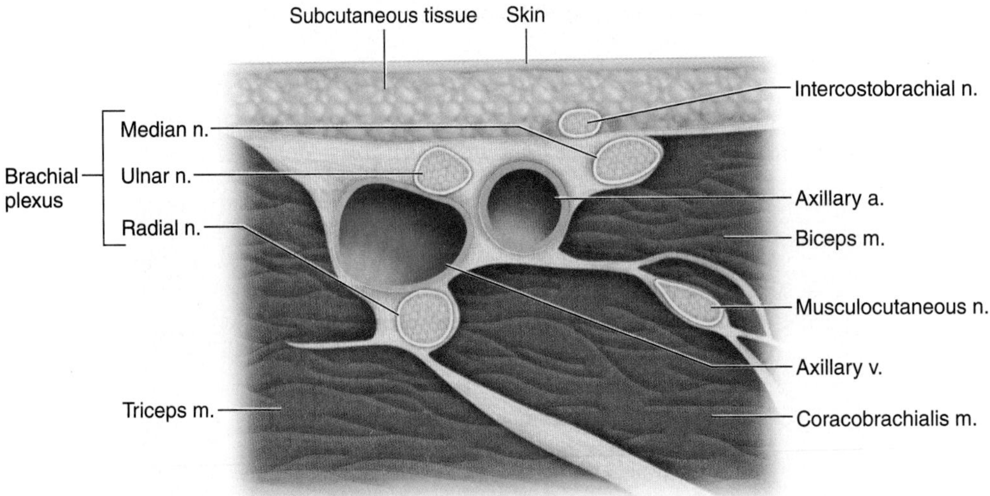

FIGURE 46–18 Positioning of terminal nerves about the axillary artery (variations are common). a., artery; m., muscle; n., nerve; v. vein.

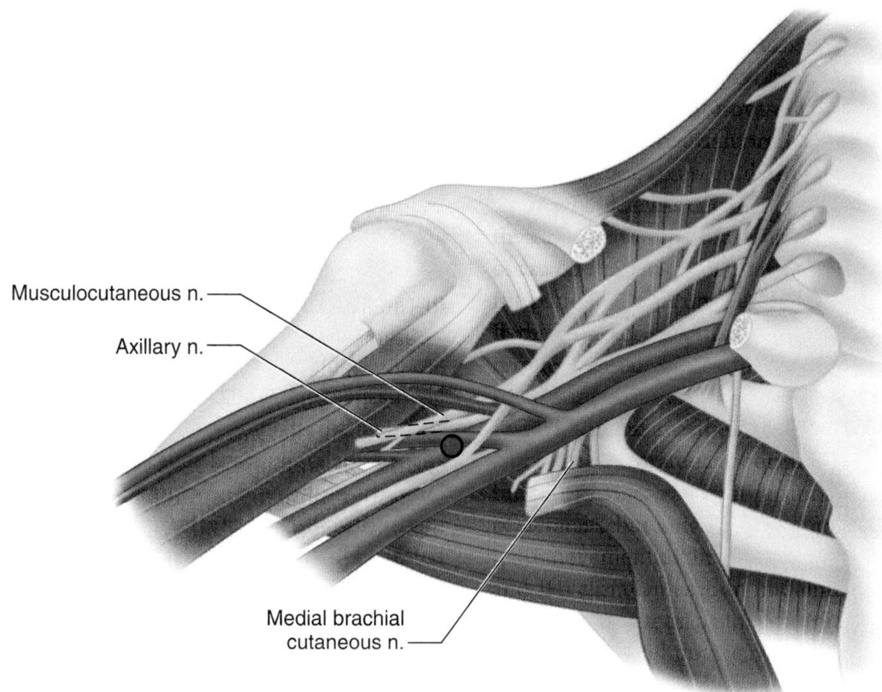

FIGURE 46–19 Axillary block. The axillary, musculocutaneous, and medial brachial cutaneous nerves are usually spared with an axillary approach. Red dot indicates target for local anesthetic. n., nerve.

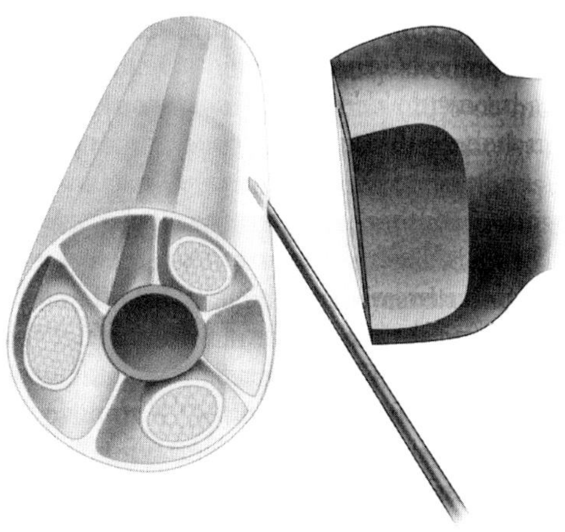

FIGURE 46–20 A multiple injection technique is more effective for the axillary nerve block because of fascial separation between nerves.

must also be anesthetized if the surgery involves the lateral forearm.

Blocks of the Terminal Nerves

8 It is often necessary to anesthetize a single terminal nerve, either for minor surgical procedures with a limited field or as a supplement to an incomplete brachial plexus block. Terminal nerves may be anesthetized anywhere along their course.

A. Suprascapular Nerve Block

The suprascapular nerve is a proximal branch of the brachial plexus, originating from the upper trunk. This nerve provides the primary innervation to the glenohumeral joint and therefore must be anesthetized for analgesia following shoulder surgery. After branching from the upper trunk, the nerve passes deep to the omohyoid muscle and then through the suprascapular notch and into the supraspinous fossa

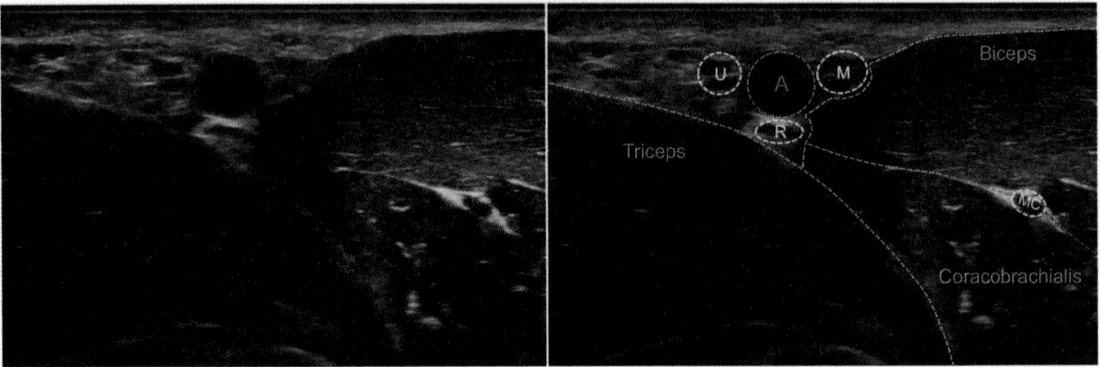

FIGURE 46–21 Axillary brachial plexus block. A, axillary artery; M, median nerve; MC, musculocutaneous nerve; R, radial nerve; U, ulnar nerve.

prior to innervating muscles of the rotator cuff and the glenohumeral joint (Figure 46–22).

The suprascapular nerve can be blocked by a variety of techniques, including landmark-based, fluoroscopy, nerve stimulation, and ultrasound guidance. When combined with an infraclavicular nerve block, shoulder analgesia can be accomplished while minimizing the risk of hemidiaphragmatic paralysis associated with an interscalene nerve block. With an ultrasound-guided approach, the nerve can be localized anteriorly as it courses deep to the omohyoid muscle or posteriorly as it runs in the supraspinous fossa (Figure 46–23). At either location, 5 to 10 mL of local anesthetic should be sufficient to block the nerve.

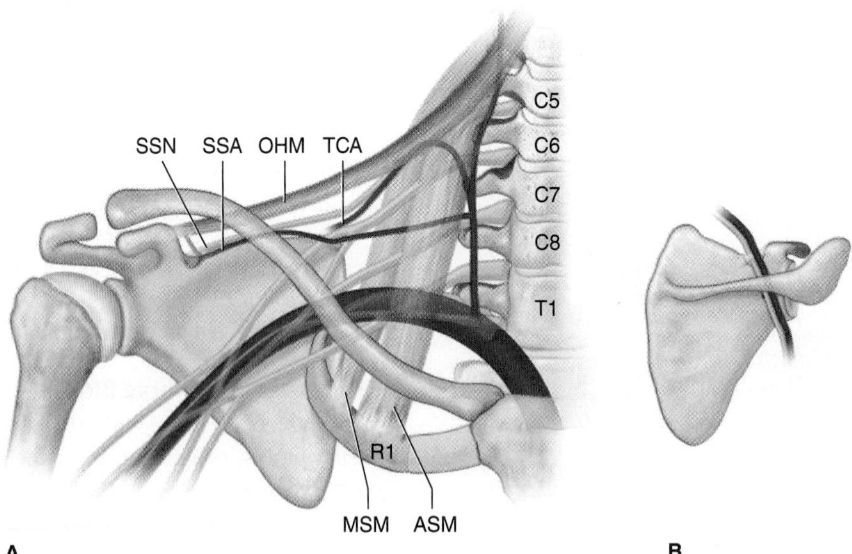

FIGURE 46–22 Suprascapular nerve course. **(A)** Suprascapular nerve course in anterior shoulder: SSN, suprascapular nerve; SSA. suprascapular artery, OHM, omohyoid muscle; TCA, transverse cervical artery, MSM, middle scalene muscle; ASM, anterior scalene muscle; **(B)** Suprascapular nerve course in posterior shoulder.

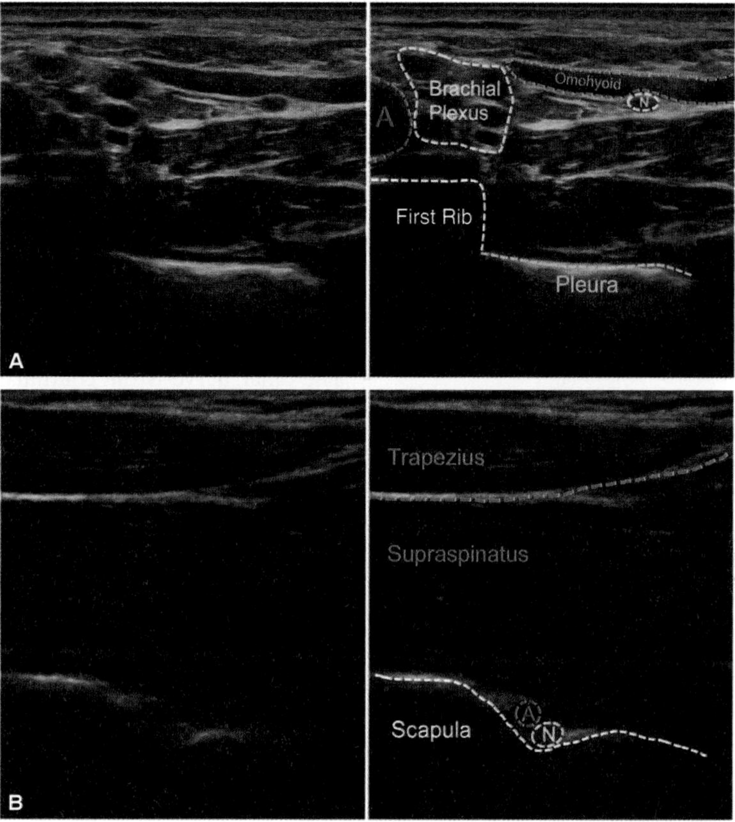

FIGURE 46–23 Suprascapular nerve block performed (**A**) proximally deep to the omohyoid muscle and (**B**) distally in the supraspinous fossa. A, suprascapular artery; N, suprascapular nerve.

B. Median Nerve Block

The median nerve is derived from the lateral and medial cords of the brachial plexus. It enters the arm and runs just medial to the brachial artery (Figure 46–24). As it enters the antecubital space, it lies medial to the brachial artery near the insertion of the biceps tendon. Just distal to this point, it gives off numerous motor branches to the wrist and finger flexors and follows the interosseous membrane to the wrist. At the level of the proximal wrist flexion crease, it lies directly deep to the palmaris longus tendon in the carpal tunnel. The median nerve provides the primary motor innervation to the muscles in the anterior forearm responsible for flexing the fingers and wrist (with some contribution from the ulnar nerve) as well as to the thenar muscles. It supplies sensory innervation to the hand, as seen in Figure 46–25. Isolated block of the median nerve may be required for minor procedures in the lateral palm or on the palmar aspect of the first three and a half fingers, used in combination with other distal nerve blocks to anesthetize all or part of the hand or performed as a rescue block if a brachial plexus block fails to anesthetize this area of the hand.

The median nerve may be blocked with ultrasound guidance at any point in the forearm. However, it is most easily visualized and blocked at the level of the mid-forearm, where it is sandwiched between the muscle bellies of the flexor digitorum profundus and flexor digitorum superficialis muscles (Figure 46–26). At this location, the tendons of these muscles may be easily confused with the nerve;

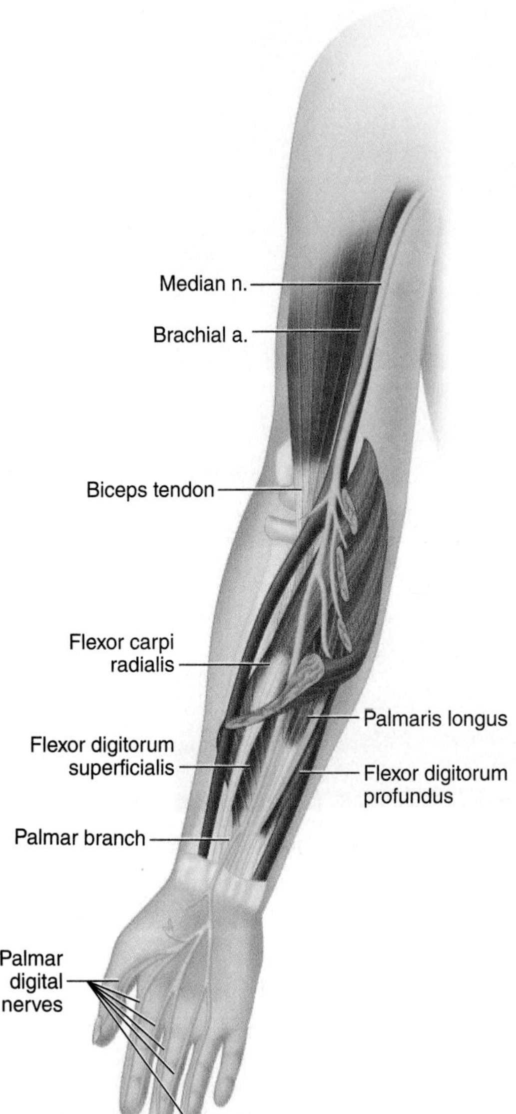

FIGURE 46–24 Median nerve course.

however, scanning proximally with the probe will reveal that the tendons merge with the surrounding muscle while the nerve remains a constant. A short 22-gauge needle is inserted on the ulnar aspect of the ultrasound in an ulnar-to-radial direction, and local anesthetic (4–8 mL) is deposited circumferentially around the nerve.

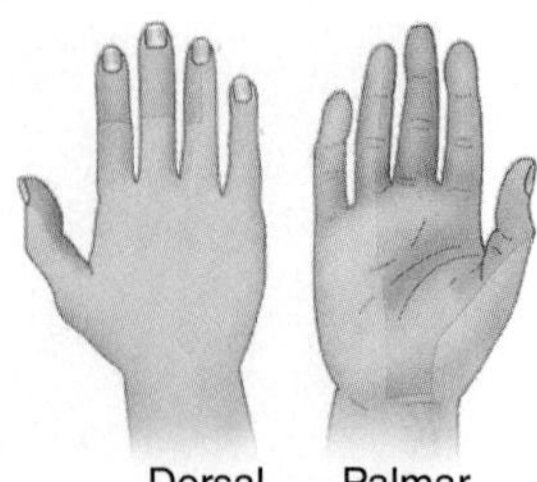

FIGURE 46–25 Median nerve sensory distribution.

C. Ulnar Nerve Block

The ulnar nerve is the continuation of the medial cord of the brachial plexus and maintains a position medial to the axillary and brachial arteries in the upper arm (Figure 46–27). At the distal third of the humerus, the nerve moves more medially and passes under the arcuate ligament of the medial epicondyle. The nerve is frequently palpable just proximal to the medial epicondyle, and compression in this location results in cubital tunnel syndrome. In the mid-forearm, the nerve lies between the flexor digitorum profundus, flexor digitorum superficialis, and the flexor carpi ulnaris. At the wrist, it is lateral to the flexor carpi ulnaris tendon and medial to the ulnar artery. The ulnar nerve supplies motor innervation to the intrinsic muscles of the hand (except the thenar muscles) and contributes to flexion of the wrist. The sensory distribution of the ulnar nerve is seen in Figure 46–28.

Indications for ulnar nerve block are similar to those described for the median nerve. The nerve is most easily identified in the distal third of the forearm, where it runs parallel to the ulnar artery. Palpation for the pulse of the artery can help determine transducer placement. After the nerve is identified in cross-section, it should be traced proximally to a point where it is no longer directly adjacent to the artery to avoid accidental intravascular injection. As with median nerve block, a short 22-gauge needle is inserted on the ulnar aspect of the ultrasound and advanced in an ulnar-to-radial direction. Local anesthetic (4–8 mL) is deposited circumferentially around the nerve (Figure 46–29).

D. Radial Nerve Block

The radial nerve—the terminal branch of the posterior cord of the brachial plexus—courses posterior

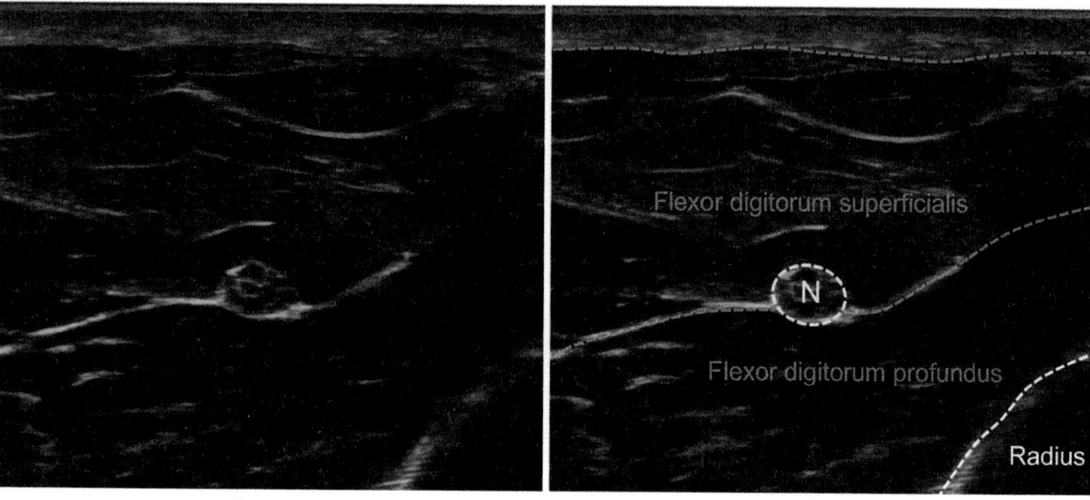

FIGURE 46–26 Median nerve block. N, median nerve.

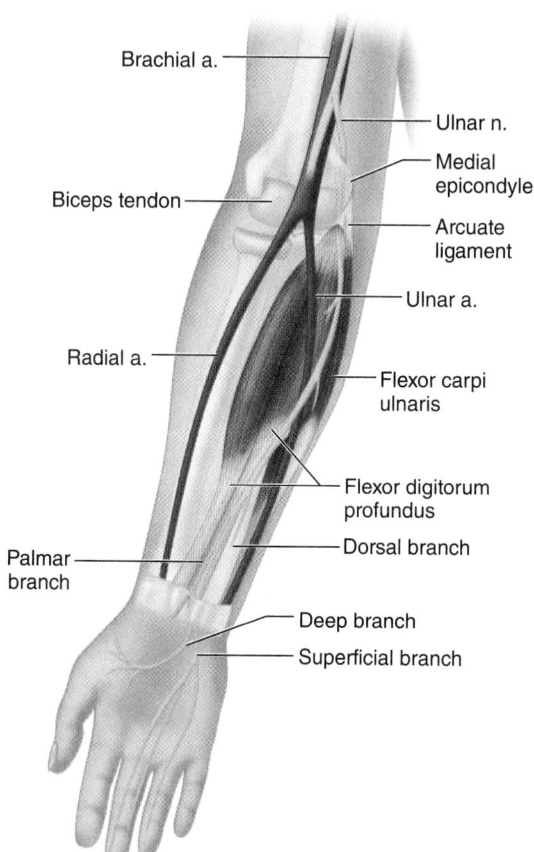

FIGURE 46–27 Ulnar nerve course. a., artery; n., nerve.

to the humerus, innervating the triceps muscle and entering the spiral groove of the humerus before it moves laterally at the elbow (Figure 46–30). This anatomic relationship should be of particular importance to the regional anesthesiologist as humeral fractures in this location (or surgical fixation of such fractures) may result in nerve entrapment or laceration. Terminal sensory branches include the lateral cutaneous nerve of the arm and the posterior cutaneous nerve of the forearm. After exiting the spiral groove, the nerve travels posterior to the lateral epicondyle and deep to the brachioradialis muscle. At this location, the radial nerve separates into superficial and deep branches. The deep branch remains close to the periosteum and innervates the extensor muscles of the forearm. The superficial branch

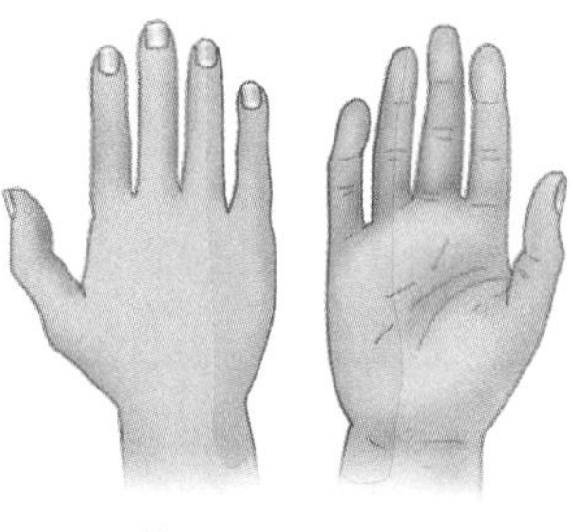

FIGURE 46–28 Ulnar nerve sensory distribution.

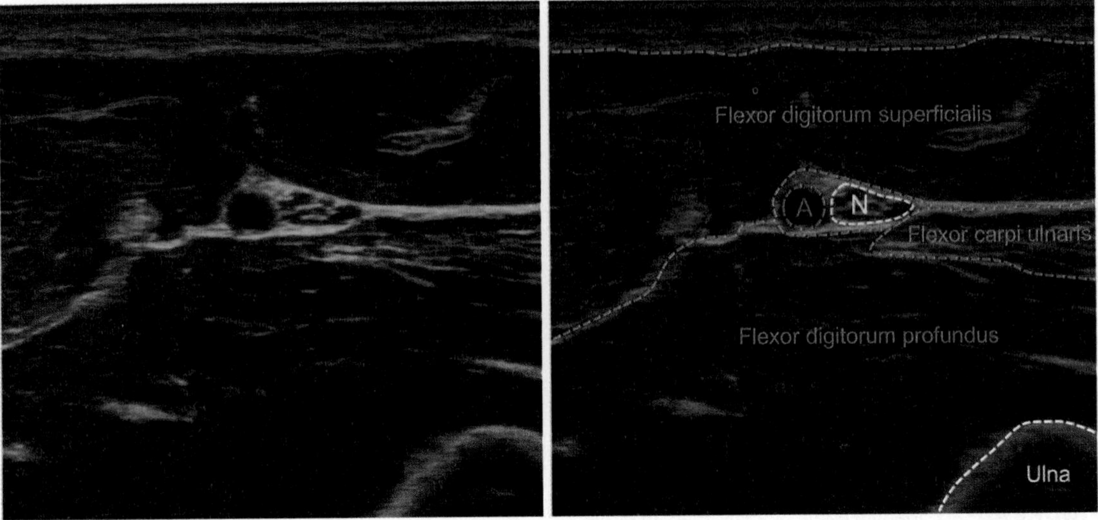

FIGURE 46–29 Ulnar nerve block. A, ulnar artery; N, ulnar nerve.

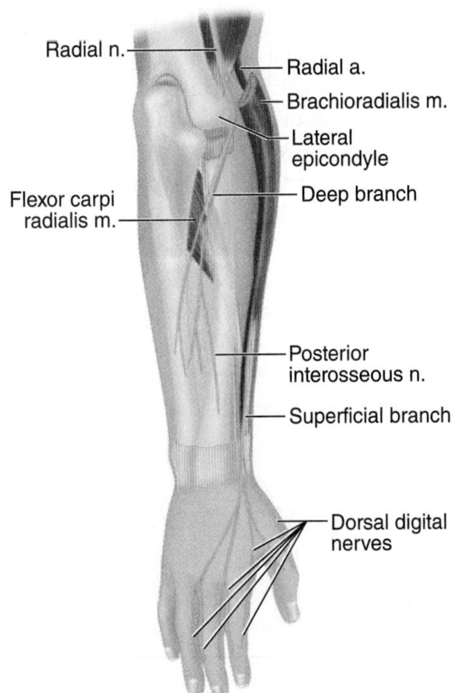

FIGURE 46–30 Radial nerve course. a., artery; m., muscle; n., nerve.

follows the radial artery, emerging from underneath thc brachioradialis, and crosses the "anatomic snuff box" to innervate the radial aspects of the dorsal wrist and the dorsal aspect of the lateral three digits and half of the fourth (Figure 46–31).

The radial nerve is most easily visualized on ultrasound as a structure consisting of two hypoechoic circles with hyperechoic borders immediately deep to the brachioradialis muscle in the forearm 2 to 3 cm distal to the lateral epicondyle. The nerve's characteristic appearance at the location has led to it frequently being referred to as "snake's eyes"

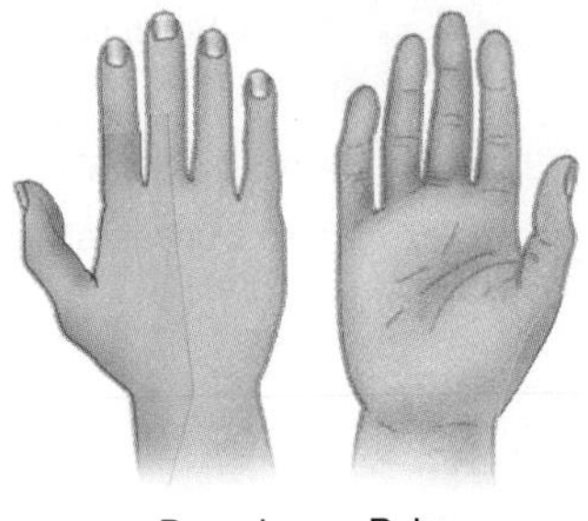

FIGURE 46–31 Radial nerve sensory distribution.

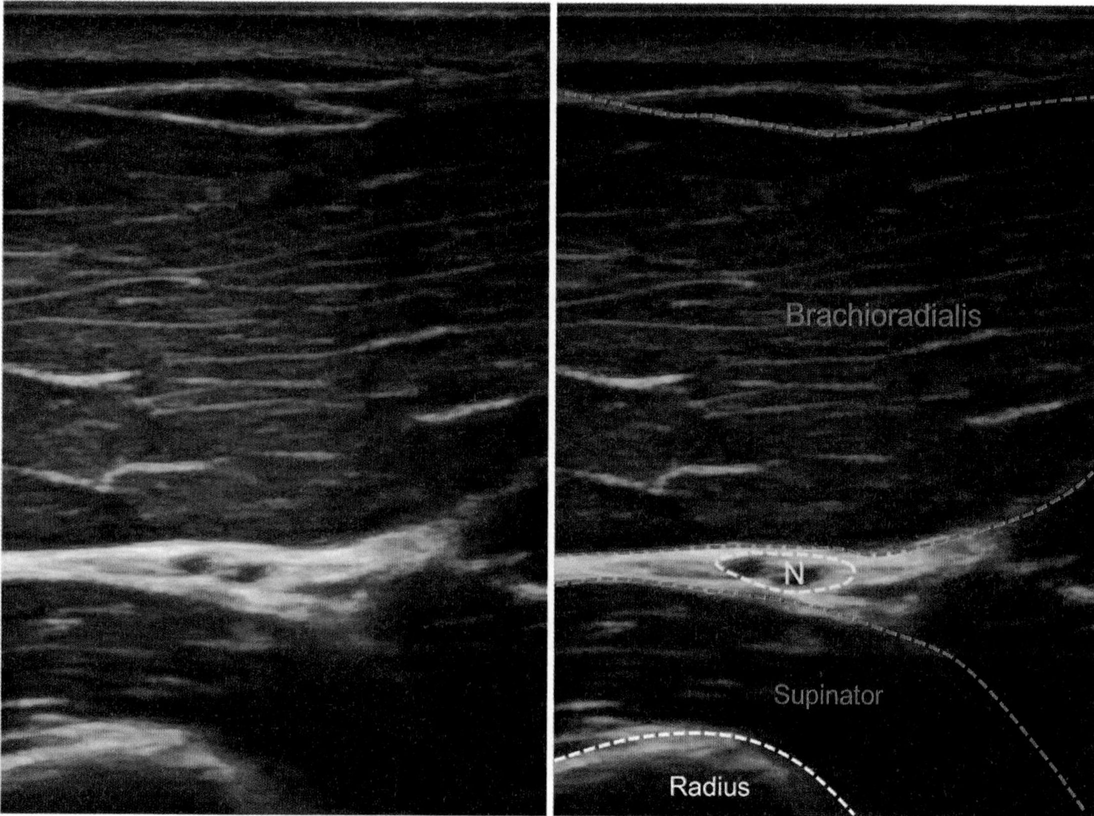

FIGURE 46–32 Radial nerve block. N, radial nerve.

(Figure 46–32). A short 22-gauge needle is inserted on the anterior side of the probe and advanced posteriorly. After piercing through the fascia of the brachioradialis, 4 to 8 mL of local anesthetic is injected to provide circumferential coverage of the nerve. The nerve may also be blocked using ultrasound as far proximally as the distal arm where it is visualized, leaving the spiral groove of the humerus or distally as far as the distal forearm where the superficial branch runs parallel to the radial artery.

Alternatively, local anesthetic can be injected as a field block in the dorsal subcutaneous tissue proximal to the base of the thumb and index finger.

E. Musculocutaneous Nerve Block

Blocking the musculocutaneous nerve is essential to complete the anesthesia for the forearm and wrist when performing an axillary brachial plexus block. The musculocutaneous nerve is the terminal branch of the lateral cord of the brachial plexus and the most proximal of the major nerves to emerge from the plexus (Figure 46–33). This nerve innervates the coracobrachialis and biceps muscles then distally terminates as the lateral antebrachial cutaneous nerve, supplying sensory input to the lateral aspect of the forearm and wrist.

To target the musculocutaneous nerve following an ultrasound-guided axillary block, the needle is redirected laterally (see Figure 46–21) toward the musculocutaneous nerve lying between the heads of the coracobrachialis muscle or between the coracobrachialis and the biceps brachii muscles. After advancing the needle toward the nerve, 4 to 8 mL of local anesthetic is injected around the nerve.

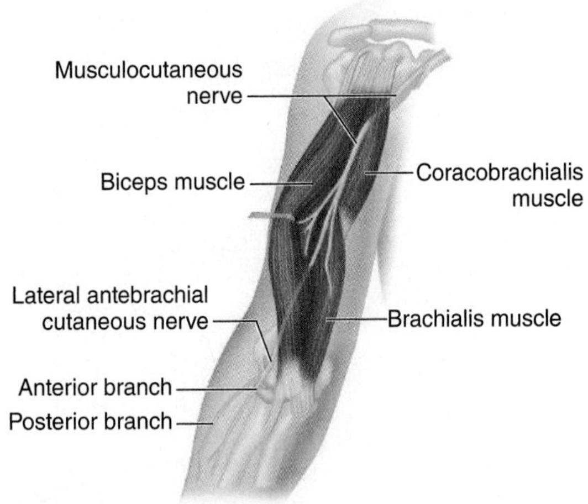

FIGURE 46–33 Musculocutaneous nerve course.

F. Digital Nerve Blocks

Digital nerve blocks are used for minor surgeries on the fingers or as a supplement to incomplete brachial plexus or terminal nerve blocks. Sensory innervation of each finger is provided by four small digital nerves that enter each digit at its base in each of the four corners (Figure 46–34). A small-gauge needle is inserted at the medial and lateral aspects of the base of the selected digit, and 2 to 3 mL of local anesthetic is injected. The addition of a vasoconstrictor (epinephrine) to the local anesthetic reduces blood flow to the digit; however, there are no case reports of necrosis following the use of epinephrine with lidocaine or other modern local anesthetics. Nevertheless, it seems prudent to include epinephrine only as a *surgical* decision to avoid the need for a tourniquet.

F. Intercostobrachial Nerve Block

The *intercostobrachial nerve* originates in the upper thorax (T2) and becomes superficial on the medial upper arm. It supplies cutaneous innervation to the medial aspect of the proximal arm and is *not* anesthetized with a brachial plexus block (Figure 46–35). Given that this location is frequently the site of a tourniquet during upper extremity surgeries, intercostobrachial nerve block is frequently performed as a supplement to brachial plexus blockade for awake upper extremity surgery under regional anesthesia. The patient should be supine with the arm abducted and externally rotated. Starting at the

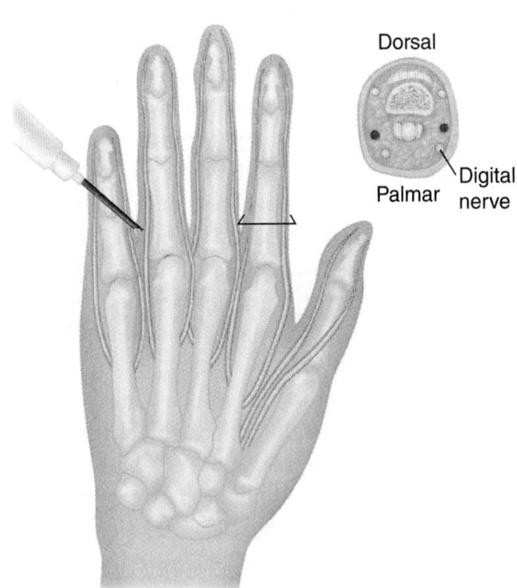

FIGURE 46–34 Sensory innervation of the fingers is provided by the digital nerves.

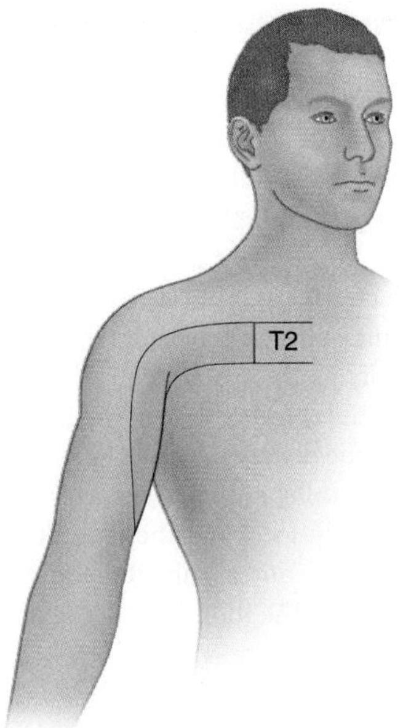

FIGURE 46–35 Intercostobrachial nerve cutaneous innervation.

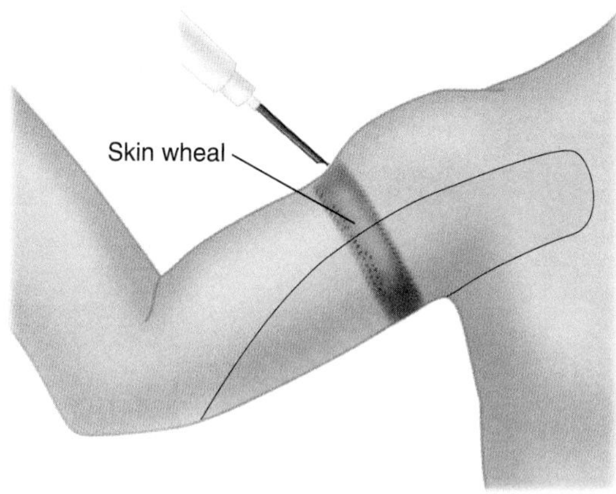

FIGURE 46–36 Intercostobrachial nerve block.

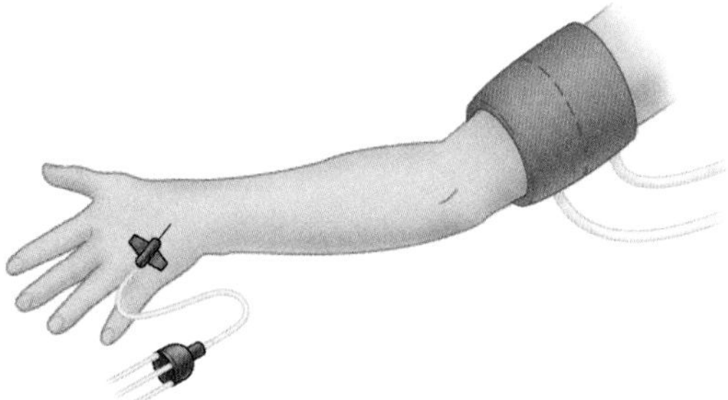

FIGURE 46–37 Intravenous regional anesthesia provides surgical anesthesia for procedures of short duration.

deltoid prominence and proceeding posteriorly, the anesthesia provider performs a field block in a linear fashion using 5 mL of local anesthetic, extending to the most posterior aspect of the medial arm (Figure 46–36).

Intravenous Regional Anesthesia

9 Intravenous regional anesthesia, also called a *Bier block*, eponymously named after Augustus Karl Gustav Bier, can provide surgical anesthesia for relatively short (45–60 min) and superficial surgical procedures on an extremity (eg, carpal tunnel release). An intravenous catheter is usually inserted on the dorsum of the hand (or foot), and a double pneumatic tourniquet is placed on the forearm or arm or below the knee or on the thigh. The extremity is elevated for passive exsanguination and then actively exsanguinated by tightly wrapping an Esmarch elastic bandage from a distal to proximal direction. For providers with limited experience wrapping an Esmarch bandage, consider allowing the surgeon to do this task as this will also provide the surgical exsanguination. Failure to properly exsanguinate the extremity will interfere with both the anesthetic and surgery. The proximal tourniquet (closer to the patient's heart) is inflated, the Esmarch bandage removed, and 0.5% lidocaine (30-40 mL for a forearm or ankle, 50 mL for an arm or below the knee, and 100 mL for a thigh tourniquet) injected over 2 to 3 min through the catheter, which is subsequently removed (Figure 46–37). If sedation is not administered prior to local anesthetic infiltration, this may cause discomfort. Anesthesia is usually established after 5 to 10 min. Tourniquet pain usually develops after 20 to 30 min, at which time the distal tourniquet is inflated and the proximal tourniquet subsequently deflated. Patients usually tolerate the distal tourniquet for an additional 15 to 20 min because it is inflated over an anesthetized area. Even for surgical procedures of very short duration, the tourniquet *must* be left inflated for a total of at least 15 to 20 min to avoid a rapid intravenous bolus of local anesthetic resulting in systemic toxicity. Slow deflation is also recommended to provide an additional margin of safety. Lidocaine is almost exclusively used as the anesthetic for intravenous regional anesthesia, and bupivacaine and ropivacaine are absolutely contraindicated because of the potential for cardiac toxicity.

LOWER EXTREMITY PERIPHERAL NERVE BLOCKS

Lumbar & Sacral Plexus Anatomy

The *lumbosacral plexus* provides innervation to the lower extremities (Figure 46–38). The lumbar plexus is formed by the ventral rami of L1 to L4, with occasional contribution from T12. It lies within the psoas muscle, with branches descending into the proximal thigh. Three major nerves from the lumbar plexus make contributions to the lower limb: the *femoral* (L2–4), *lateral femoral cutaneous* (L2–3),

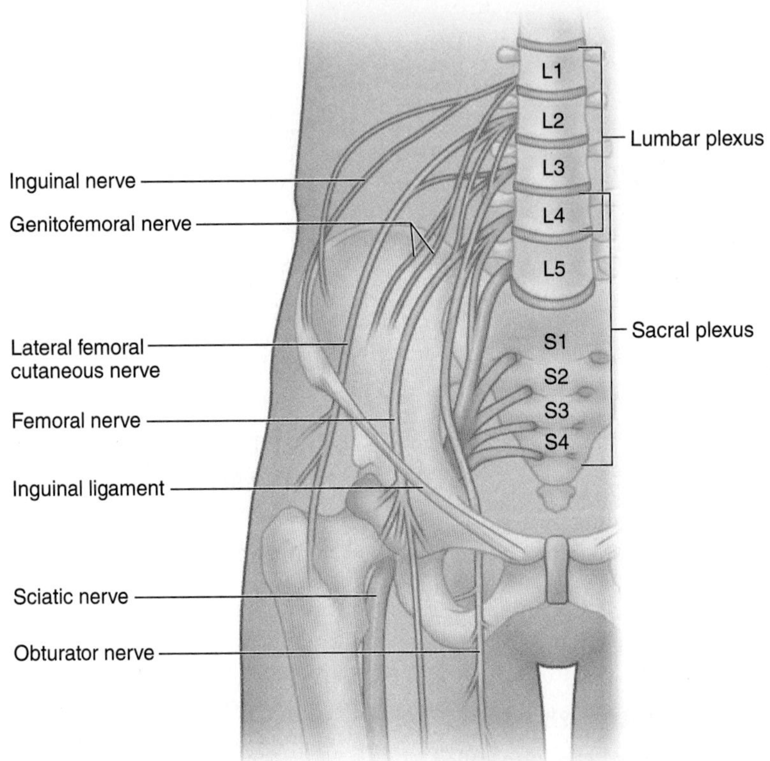

FIGURE 46–38 The ventral rami of L1 to L5 and S1 to S4 form the lumbosacral plexus, which provides innervation to the lower extremities.

and *obturator* (L2–4). These provide motor and sensory innervation to the anterior portion of the thigh and sensory innervation to the medial leg. The sacral plexus arises from L4 to L5 and S1 to S4. The posterior thigh and most of the leg and foot are supplied by the *tibial* and *peroneal* portions of the sciatic nerve. The *posterior femoral cutaneous nerve* (S1–S3) provides sensory innervation to the posterior thigh; it travels with the sciatic nerve as it emerges around the piriformis muscle.

Femoral Nerve Block

10 The femoral nerve innervates the main hip flexors and knee extensors and provides much of the sensory innervation of the hip and thigh (Figure 46–40). Its most medial branch is the *saphenous nerve*, which innervates much of the skin of the medial leg and ankle joint. A femoral nerve block alone will seldom provide adequate surgical anesthesia, but it is often used to provide postoperative analgesia for hip, thigh, knee, and ankle (via the saphenous nerve) procedures (see Figure 46–39). Femoral nerve blocks have a relatively low rate of complications and few contraindications. Local infection, previous vascular grafting, and local adenopathy should be carefully considered in patient selection. Additionally, all providers and the patient should be informed that weight bearing on the affected leg will not be possible until block resolution. As it provides the sole motor innervation to the quadriceps, blocking the femoral nerve will result in the knee "buckling" if weight bearing is attempted.

Lower Extremity Blocks and Indications	
Indication	**Blocks**
Hip	
Acetabulum ORIF	Suprainguinal fascia iliaca, femoral nerve block (strongly consider neuraxial)
Hip arthroplasty, fracture, ORIF	Suprainguinal fascia iliaca, femoral nerve block, infrainguinal fascia iliaca (strongly weight fall risk)
Hip arthroscopy	Suprainguinal fascia iliaca (potential fall risk), pericapsular nerve group block
Thigh	
Femoral shaft ORIF	Femoral nerve block, infrainguinal fascia iliaca, suprainguinal fascia iliaca
Distal femur ORIF	Femoral nerve block, infrainguinal fascia iliaca, (+/– subgluteal sciatic block)
Skin graft harvest from thigh	Femoral (anterior) or LFCN (lateral), infrainguinal fascia iliaca
Above knee amputation	Femoral + subgluteal sciatic nerve blocks (strongly consider continuous blocks)
Knee	
Knee arthroplasty	Adductor canal block (lumbar plexus + subgluteal sciatic for surgical anesthetic)
Knee arthroscopy	Adductor canal block
Patellar ORIF or tendon repair	Femoral block (assuming a knee immobilizer will be used)
Anterior cruciate ligament reconstruction	AC block (consider addition of subgluteal sciatic if hamstring autograft planned)
Tibial plateau ORIF	Subgluteal sciatic nerve block (lateral hardware) vs femoral nerve block (medial hardware); Consider performing block on POD 1 if concern for compartment syndrome is high. **Always discuss compartment syndrome risk with surgeon.**
Leg	
Tibial shaft ORIF or intramedullary nail	Sciatic nerve block (+/– adductor canal block if nail is placed anterograde through the knee). Consider performing block on POD 1 if concern for compartment syndrome is high.
Below knee amputation	Sciatic + adductor canal (or femoral) nerve blocks
Ankle and Foot	
Ankle arthroplasty, fusion or ORIF	Sciatic and subsartorial saphenous nerve blocks
Metatarsal ORIF	Sciatic block (+ distal saphenous block for first) metatarsal)
Hallux valgus deformity correction	Sciatic block + distal saphenous block
Transmetatarsal amputation	Sciatic block + distal saphenous block
Toe amputation	Ankle block

FIGURE 46–39 Lower extremity blocks and indications. LFCN, lateral femoral cutaneous nerve; ORIF, open reduction and internal fixation; POD 1, postoperative day one.

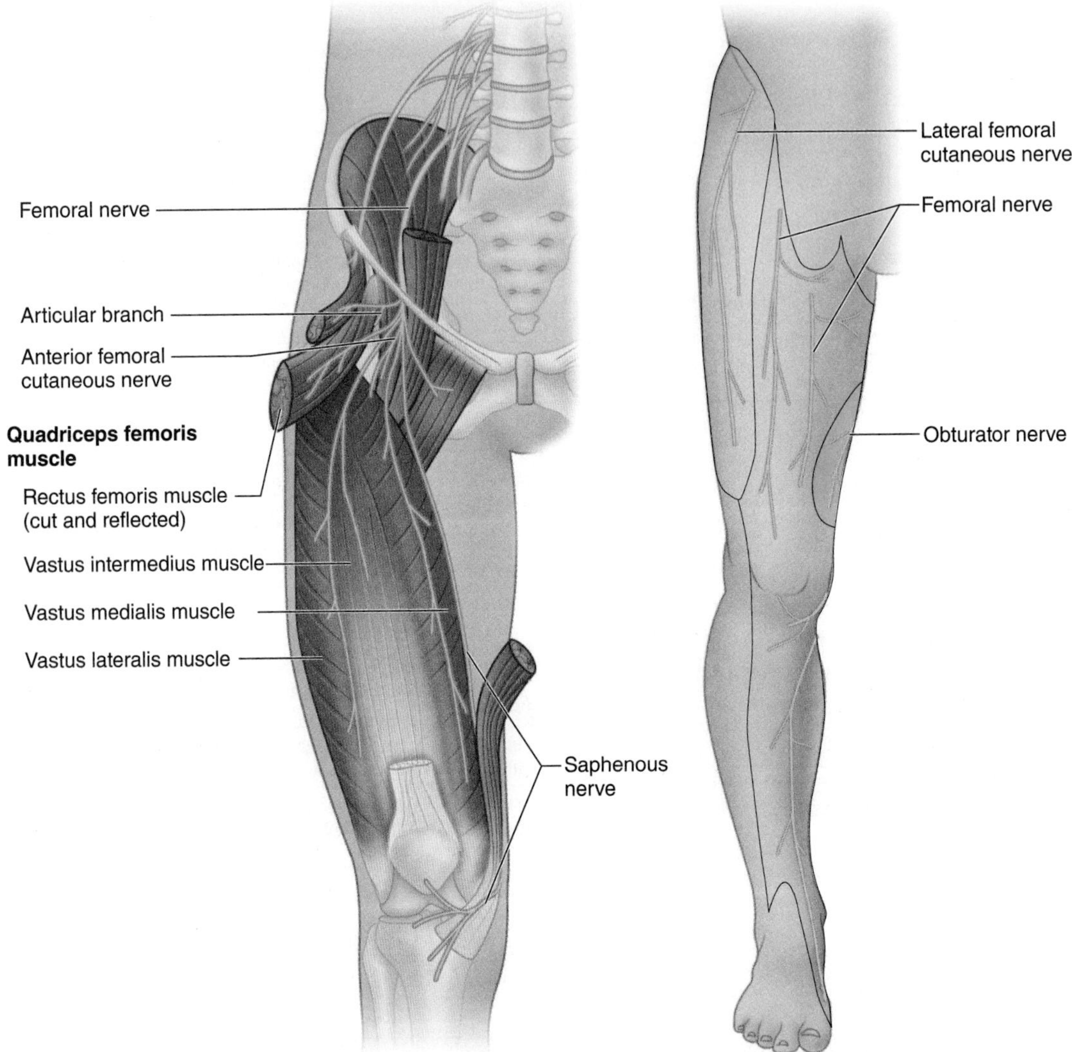

FIGURE 46–40 The femoral nerve provides sensory innervation to the hip and thigh, and to the medial leg via its terminal branch, the saphenous nerve.

A high-frequency linear ultrasound transducer is placed over the area of the inguinal crease, and the femoral artery and femoral vein are visualized in cross-section with the overlying fascia iliaca (Figure 46–41). Just lateral to the artery and deep to the fascia iliaca, the femoral nerve appears in cross-section as a spindle-shaped structure with a "honeycomb" texture (Figure 46–42). Because ultrasound waves traverse fluid-filled structures more easily than solid tissue, there may be an area of artificial brightness deep to the femoral artery. Novice providers may mistake this artifact for the femoral nerve.

Using an in-plane technique, the block needle is inserted parallel to the ultrasound transducer just lateral to the outer edge. The needle is advanced through the sartorius muscle, deep to the fascia

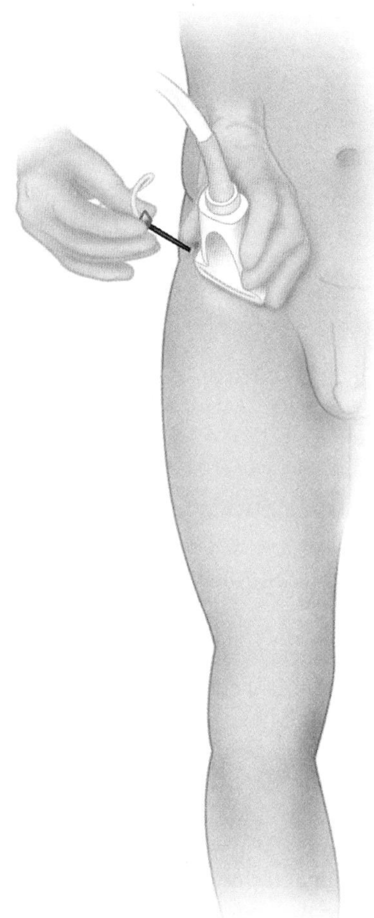

FIGURE 46–41 Femoral nerve block positioning.

iliaca, until it is visualized just lateral to the femoral nerve. Local anesthetic is injected while observing its hypoechoic spread deep to the fascia iliaca and around the nerve. When performing a continuous femoral nerve block, placing the catheter superficial to the nerve will produce less motor blockade but no decrease in analgesia compared with placing the catheter deep into the nerve.

Fascia Iliaca Plane Block

The goal of a *fascia iliaca plane block* is similar to that of a femoral nerve block (analgesia of the hip, thigh, and knee), but the approach is slightly different. As a plane block, the fascia iliaca block depends on infiltrating a large volume of local anesthetic under the fascia iliaca with spread to the terminal branches of the lumbar plexus. A blind technique relying on feeling two "pops" as the needle traversed the fascia lata and fascia iliaca was historically used and provided a relatively reliable level of anesthesia. However, ultrasound-guided techniques have become the preferred method for performing fascia iliaca blocks. The fascia iliaca block may be performed with either a conventional *infrainguinal* or newer *suprainguinal* technique (Figure 46–43).

Infrainguinal Fascia Iliaca Block

The *infrainguinal fascia iliaca block* is similar to the landmark-based block. The femoral vessels and fascia iliaca are identified in the same manner as an ultrasound-guided femoral nerve block. The fascia

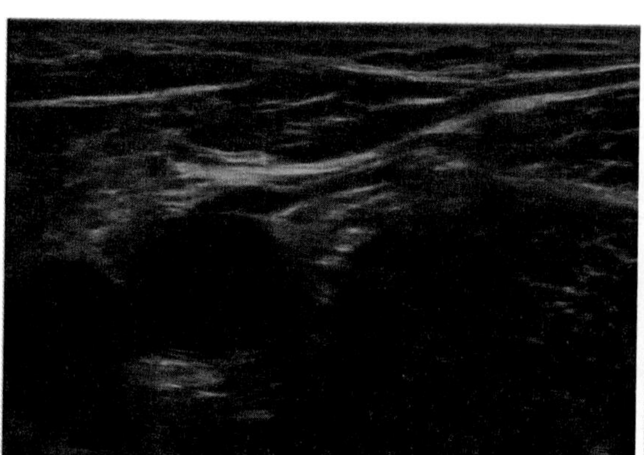

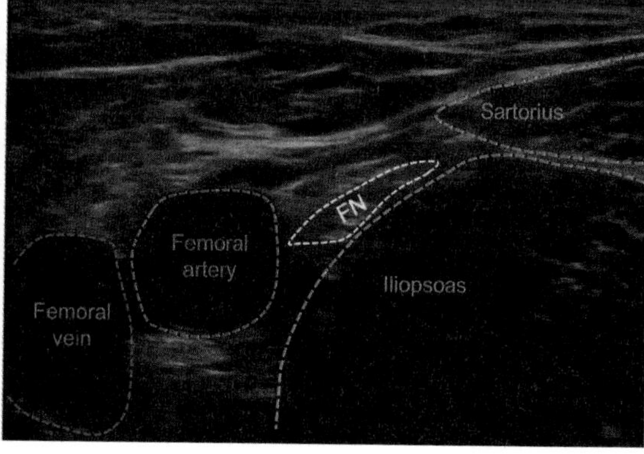

FIGURE 46–42 Femoral nerve block. FN, femoral nerve.

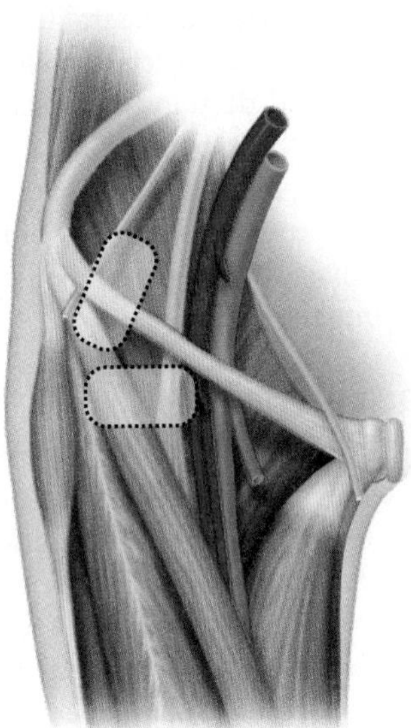

FIGURE 46–43 Ultrasound probe orientation for suprainguinal and infrainguinal fascia iliaca blocks.

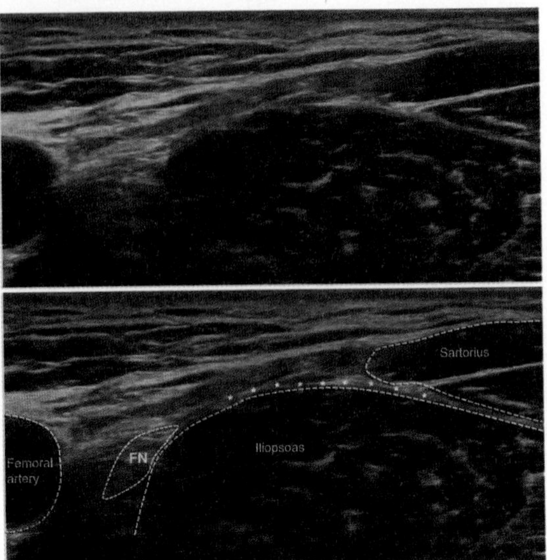

FIGURE 46–44 Infrainguinal fascia iliaca block. FN, femoral nerve; asterisk denotes target area of fascia iliaca for local anesthetic.

is then traced laterally until the sartorius muscle is visualized. The block needle enters the skin lateral to the ultrasound transducer and should pierce the fascia in a location corresponding roughly to the lateral third of the inguinal ligament. A large volume of local anesthetic (30–50 mL) is infiltrated with spread underneath the fascia iliaca visualized on ultrasound. This block usually anesthetizes both the femoral nerve and lateral femoral cutaneous nerves because the local anesthetic is deposited under the fascia iliaca between the two nerves that run in the same plane between the fascia and underlying muscles (Figure 46–44). Despite the historical name of this block as the "3-in-1 block," the obturator nerve is rarely, if ever, successfully anesthetized using this technique.

Suprainguinal Fascia Iliaca Block

The *suprainguinal fascia iliaca block* is a modification of the infrainguinal technique. By moving the local anesthetic target cephalad to the inguinal ligament, the goal of this block is to confine the spread of local anesthetic to the bowl of the pelvis. In this location, the terminal nerves of the lumbar plexus lie closer in proximity to one another, and the femoral, lateral femoral cutaneous, and obturator nerves may be more reliably blocked compared to the infrainguinal technique. Additionally, as these nerves are blocked at a more proximal location compared with the infrainguinal technique, there may be a greater chance of anesthetizing the articular branches to the hip.

A linear transducer is placed in a parasagittal orientation with a slight oblique rotation at a point just medial to the anterior superior iliac spine (see Figure 46–43) over and roughly perpendicular to the inguinal ligament. The fascia iliaca is identified as a hyperechoic line on the superficial border of the iliacus muscle, and the internal oblique and sartorius muscles meet at the inguinal ligament (often referred to as a "bow tie.") The block needle enters either at the level of the inguinal ligament or just caudad to the ligament and is advanced to puncture through the fascia iliaca (Figure 46–45). A large volume of local anesthetic (50–60 mL) is injected with spread visualized between the fascia iliaca and iliacus muscle.

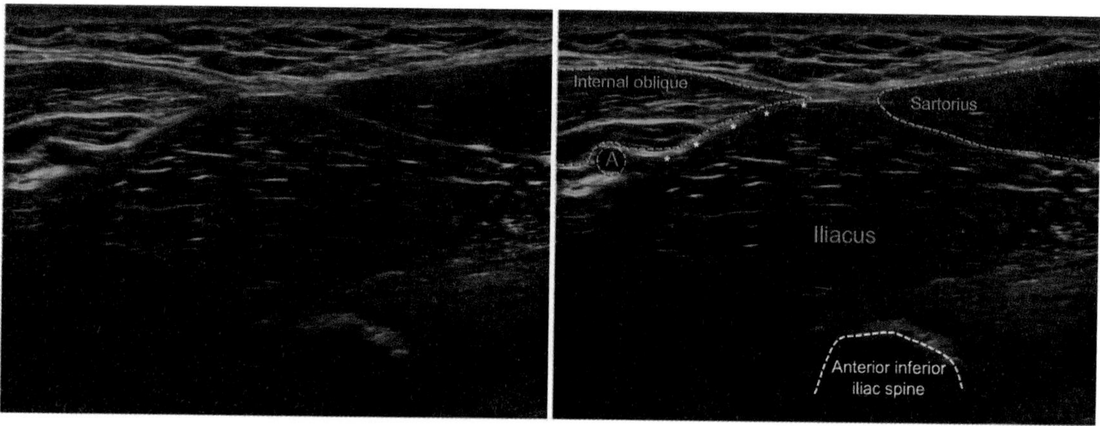

FIGURE 46–45 Suprainguinal fascia iliaca block. A, deep circumflex iliac artery; asterisk represents target area of fascia iliaca for local anesthetic.

Lateral Femoral Cutaneous Nerve Block

The *lateral femoral cutaneous nerve* provides sensory innervation to the lateral thigh (see Figure 46–40). It may be anesthetized as a supplement to a femoral nerve block or as an isolated block for limited anesthesia of the lateral thigh. As there are few vital structures in proximity to the lateral femoral cutaneous nerve, and complications with this block are exceedingly rare. The lateral femoral cutaneous nerve (L2–L3) departs from the lumbar plexus, traverses laterally from the psoas muscle, and courses anterolaterally along the iliacus muscle (see Figure 46–38). It emerges inferior and medial to the anterior superior iliac spine (ASIS) to supply the cutaneous sensory innervation of the lateral thigh. As a nerve with no motor component, it is an excellent target to provide analgesia to a split-thickness skin graft donor site. The blocked area can then be marked preoperatively so the surgeon may harvest from this location.

The patient is positioned supine, and a linear ultrasound transducer is used to identify the sartorius muscle just distal to the inguinal ligament (Figure 46–46). The nerve is identified in the short axis in the intermuscular space between the posterior border of the sartorius muscle and the anterior border of the tensor fasciae latae muscle (Figure 46–47). A short 22-gauge block needle is inserted lateral to the probe and advanced to the intermuscular plane between the sartorius and tensor fasciae latae muscles. Local anesthetic (5–10 mL) is infiltrated in this plane under ultrasound visualization.

Obturator Nerve Block

A block of the *obturator nerve* is usually required for complete anesthesia of the knee and is often performed in combination with femoral and sciatic nerve blocks for this purpose. Obturator nerve block may also be performed to prevent adductor muscle spasms during transurethral bladder resection if a nondepolarizing muscle relaxant is not used. The obturator nerve contributes sensory branches to the hip and knee joints, a variable degree of sensation to the medial thigh, and motor innervation to the adductors of the hip (Figure 46–48).

In the medial thigh, the obturator nerve splits into an anterior and posterior branch. A linear transducer is placed on the medial thigh approximately 1 to 2 cm distal to the inguinal crease, and the adductors longus, brevis, and magnus muscles are identified. The nerves are visualized as slender, fusiform structures with the anterior branch between the adductor longus and adductor brevis muscles and the posterior branch between the adductor brevis and adductor magnus muscles (Figure 46–49).

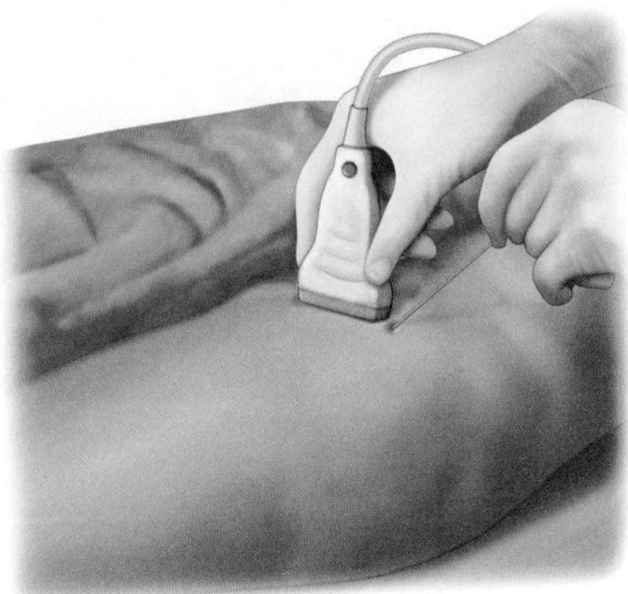

FIGURE 46–46 Lateral femoral cutaneous nerve block positioning

Local anesthetic (8–10 mL) is injected between the muscle layers to anesthetize both branches of the nerve.

Posterior Lumbar Plexus (Psoas Compartment) Block

Posterior lumbar plexus blocks are useful for surgical procedures involving areas innervated by the femoral, lateral femoral cutaneous, and obturator nerves (Figure 46–50). These include procedures on the hip, knee, and anterior thigh. Complete anesthesia of the knee can be attained in combination with a proximal sciatic nerve block. The lumbar plexus is in close proximity to multiple sensitive structures (Figure 46–51), and reaching it requires a long needle. Hence, the posterior lumbar plexus block has one of the highest complication rates of any peripheral nerve block; risks include retroperitoneal hematoma, intravascular local anesthetic injection

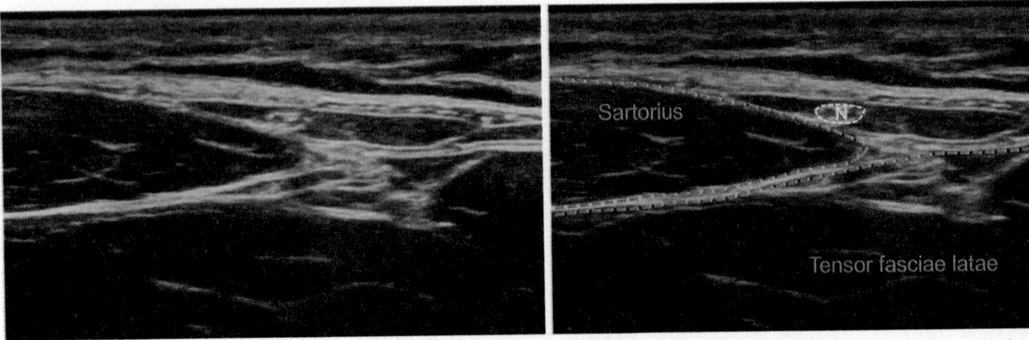

FIGURE 46–47 Lateral femoral cutaneous nerve block. N, lateral femoral cutaneous nerve.

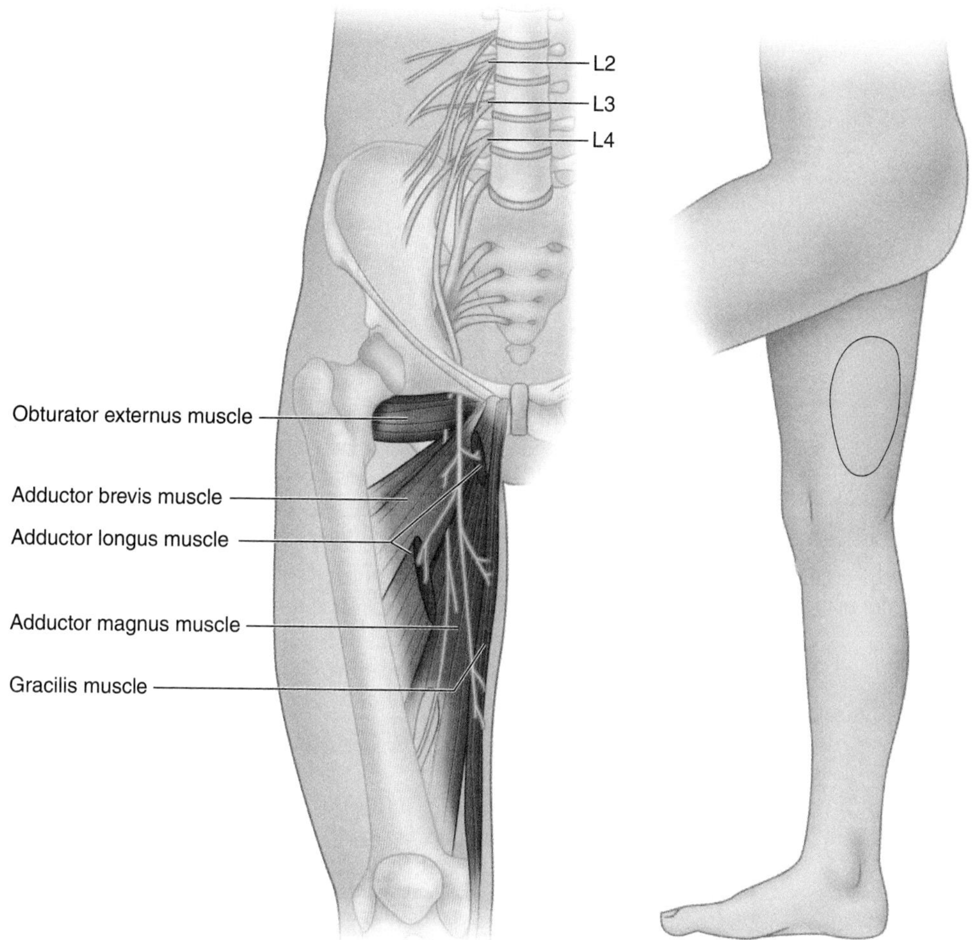

FIGURE 46–48 Obturator nerve innervation.

with toxicity, intrathecal and epidural injections, and renal capsular puncture.

Lumbar nerve roots emerge from the vertebral foramina into the body of the psoas muscle and travel within the muscle compartment before exiting as terminal nerves (see Figure 46–38). The posterior lumbar plexus blocks deposit local anesthetic within the body of the psoas muscle. The patient is positioned in lateral decubitus for a landmark-based technique and lateral, sitting, or prone for an ultrasound-guided technique. If positioned lateral decubitus, the side to be blocked is in the nondependent position (Figure 46–52).

A. Landmark-Based Technique

The midline is palpated, and the spinous processes are identified if possible. A line is first drawn through the lumbar spinous processes, and both iliac crests are identified and connected with a line to approximate the level of L4. The posterior superior iliac spine is then palpated, and a line is drawn cephalad, parallel to the first line. A long (10- to 15-cm) insulated needle is inserted at the point of intersection between the transverse (intercrestal) line and the intersection of the lateral and middle thirds of the two sagittal lines. A large curvilinear ultrasound probe can be used to estimate the depth of the transverse process,

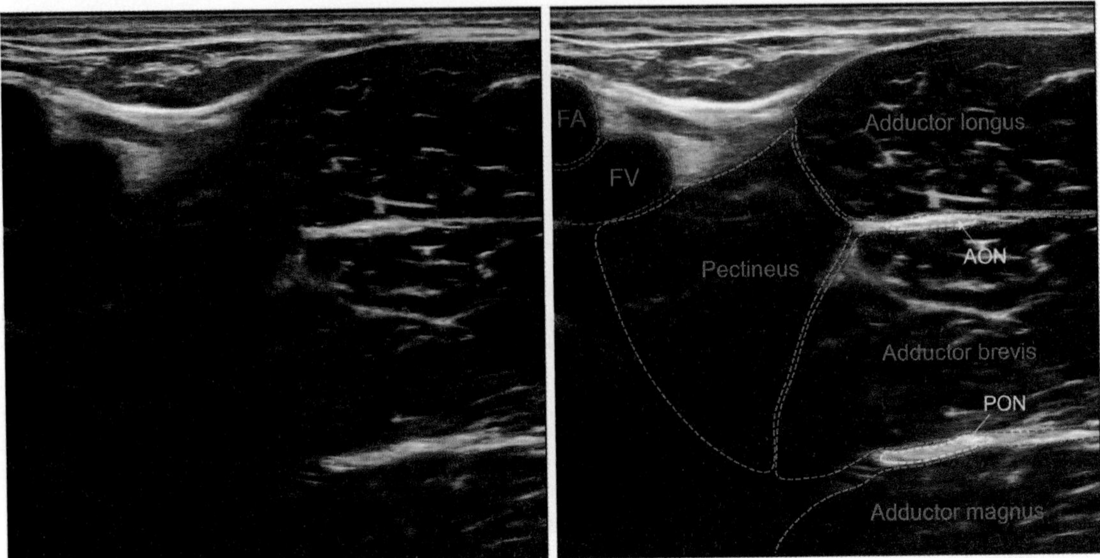

FIGURE 46–49 Obturator nerve block. AON, anterior branch of the obturator nerve; FA, femoral artery; FV, femoral vein; PON, posterior branch of the obturator nerve.

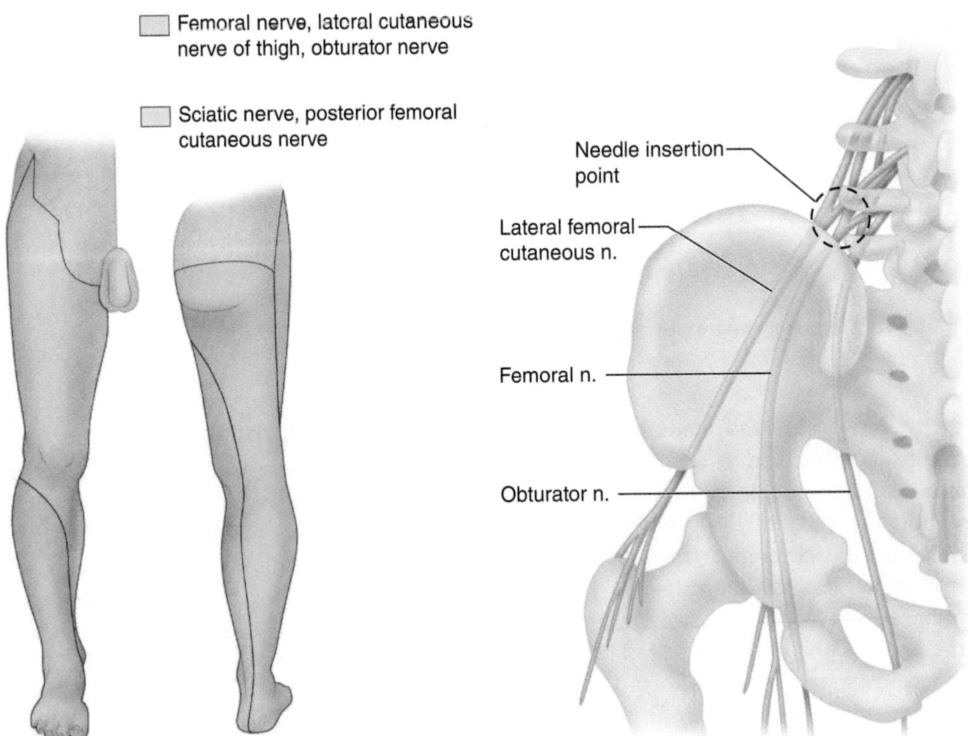

FIGURE 46–50 Lumbar plexus blocks provide anesthesia to the femoral, lateral femoral cutaneous, and obturator nerves. n., nerve.

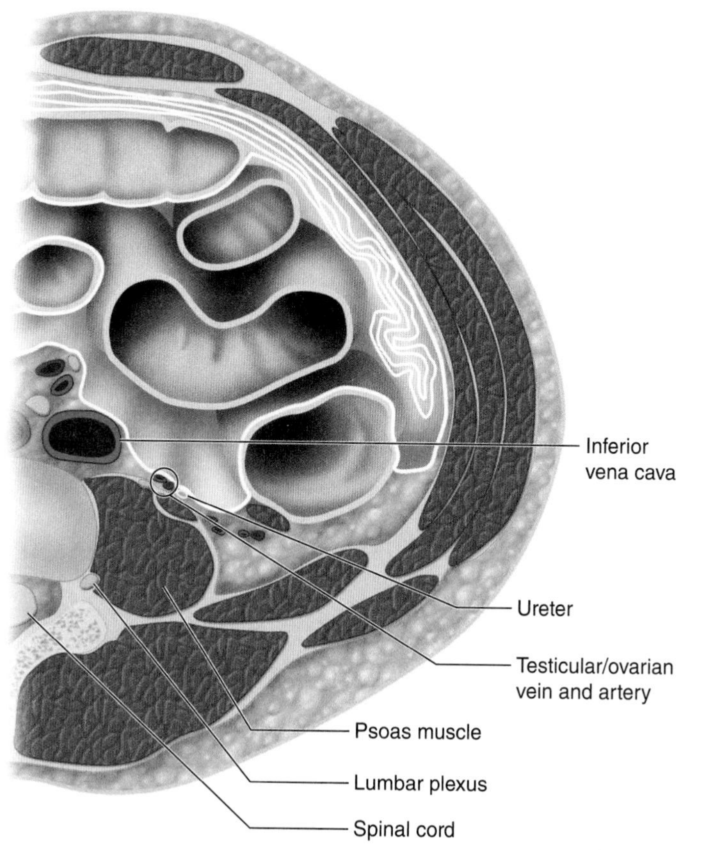

FIGURE 46–51 The lumbar plexus lies in close proximity to many vital structures.

and this has been suggested to improve both success and safety. The needle is advanced in an anterior direction until a femoral motor response is elicited (quadriceps contraction). If the transverse process is contacted, the needle should be withdrawn slightly and "walked off" the transverse process in a caudad direction, maintaining the needle in the parasagittal plane. The needle should never be inserted more than 3 cm past the depth at which the transverse process was originally contacted to avoid exiting the psoas muscle anteriorly. Local anesthetic volumes greater than 20 mL will increase the risk of bilateral spread and contralateral limb involvement.

B. Ultrasound-Guided Technique

A large curvilinear probe is used due to the depth of the target and placed in the midsagittal plane to identify the lumbar spinous processes. The probe is then moved laterally toward the operative side to visualize the transverse processes of the second, third, and fourth lumbar vertebrae or "trident sign." The psoas muscle is visible between the acoustic shadows of the transverse processes with the classic striated appearance of muscle, and the lumbar plexus is visible as a hyperechoic density in the posterior part of the muscle (Figure 46–53). As with the landmark-based technique, a long needle is required. The block needle is advanced in an in-plane fashion between the L3 and L4 transverse processes, and local anesthetic (20 mL) is injected in the plane containing the nerve roots of the lumbar plexus.

Adductor Canal Block

The *adductor canal block* is used for analgesia of the knee and medial leg; single injection or continuous techniques can be used. The quadriceps muscles are

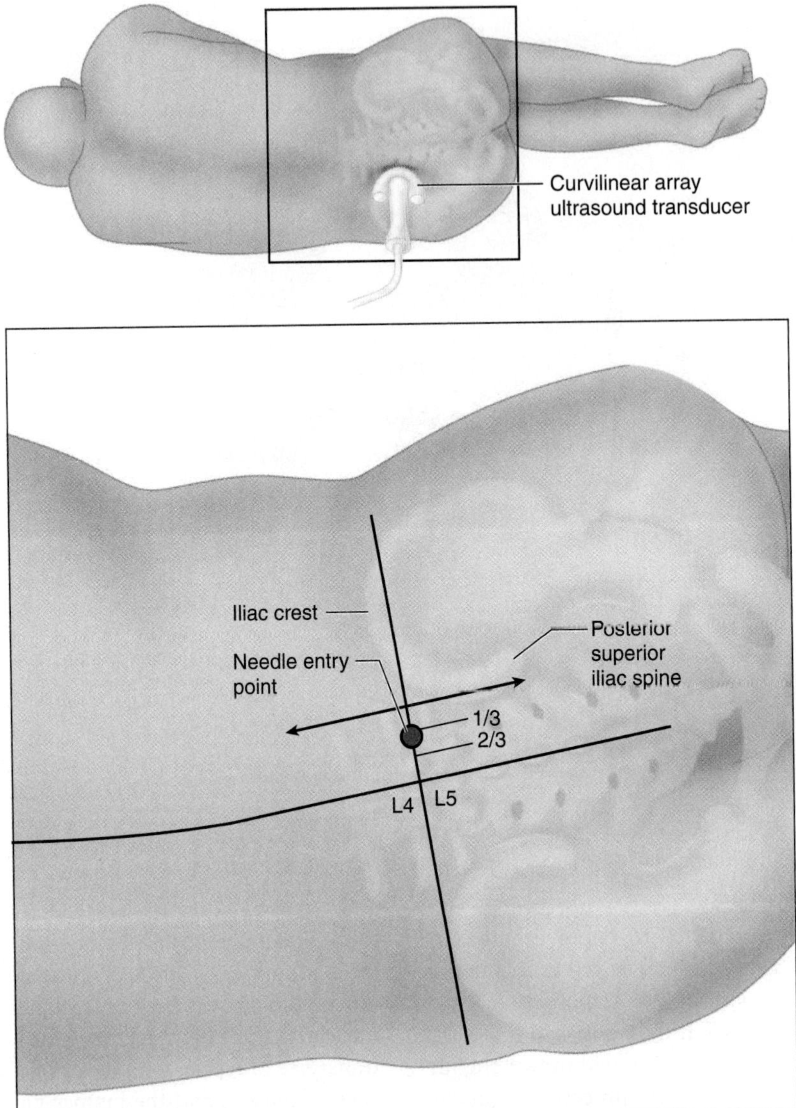

FIGURE 46–52 Patient positioning, surface landmarks, and ultrasound probe orientation for posterior lumbar plexus block.

affected to a lesser degree by an adductor canal block than by a femoral block, which may facilitate ambu-
11 lation following knee surgery. In fact, patients with continuous adductor canal catheters are able to ambulate further on the first day following total knee arthroplasty than patients with either femoral block (limited by weakness) or no block (limited by pain). Bounded by the sartorius muscle medially, the vastus medialis anteriorly, and the adductor muscles posteriorly, the adductor canal contains several nerves that provide sensory innervation to the knee. Most notable is the saphenous nerve, though this block may affect the posterior division of the obturator nerve and the nerve to the vastus medialis as well.

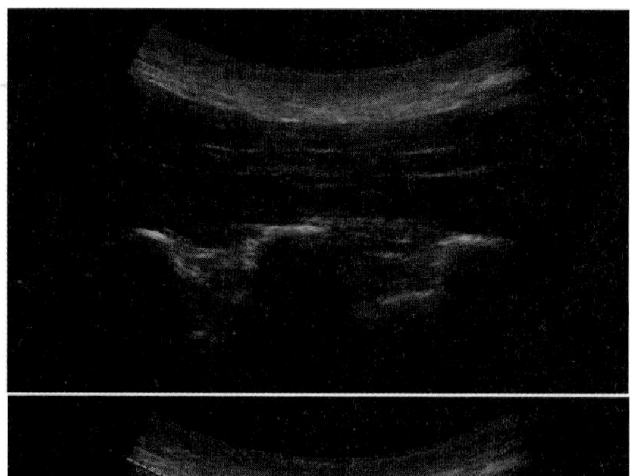

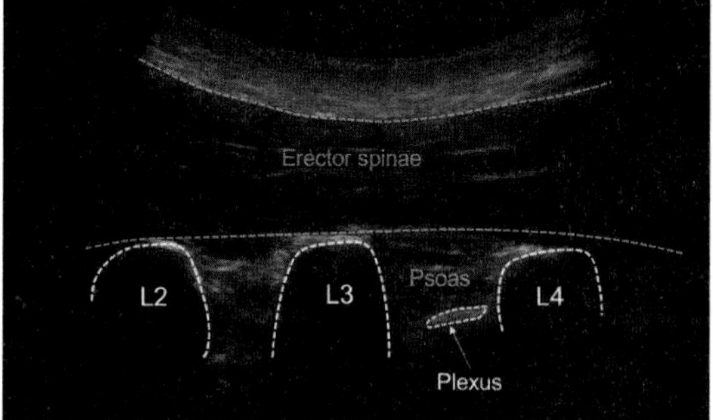

FIGURE 46–53 Posterior lumbar plexus block. L2, L3, L4, transverse processes of the second, third, and fourth lumbar vertebrae.

The patient is positioned supine with the knee slightly bent and the leg externally rotated. A high-frequency linear transducer is positioned in a transverse orientation over the medial thigh, halfway between the ASIS and the superior patellar pole (Figure 46–54). The femoral artery and vein are visualized deep to the sartorius muscle, and the saphenous nerve lies just anterior to the vessels (Figure 46–55). The block needle is placed 2 to 3 cm lateral to the transducer and advanced in-plane to the triangular space deep to the sartorius muscle and anterior to the artery. After careful aspiration for nonappearance of blood, 15 to 20 mL of local anesthetic is injected.

Saphenous Nerve Block

The saphenous nerve is the most medial branch of the femoral nerve and innervates the skin over the medial leg and the ankle joint (see Figure 46–40). Therefore, this block is used mainly in conjunction with a sciatic nerve block to provide complete anesthesia/analgesia below the knee.

A. Ultrasound-Guided Subsartorial Technique

The saphenous nerve may be accessed proximal to the knee, just deep to the sartorius muscle. A high-frequency linear probe is used to identify the junction between the sartorius and vastus medialis muscles in cross-section distal to the adductor canal. A block needle is inserted from medial to lateral, and 5 to 10 mL of local anesthetic is deposited within this fascial plane (Figure 46–56). The nerve is often visible between the sartorius and vastus medialis muscles and, if so, should be targeted with the local anesthetic. If the nerve is not visible, hydrodissecting this plane with local anesthetic also produces a reliable block of the saphenous nerve.

B. Proximal Landmark-Based Technique

A short block needle is inserted 2 cm distal to the tibial tuberosity and directed medially, infiltrating 5 to 10 mL of local anesthetic as the needle passes toward the posterior aspect of the leg (Figure 46–57).

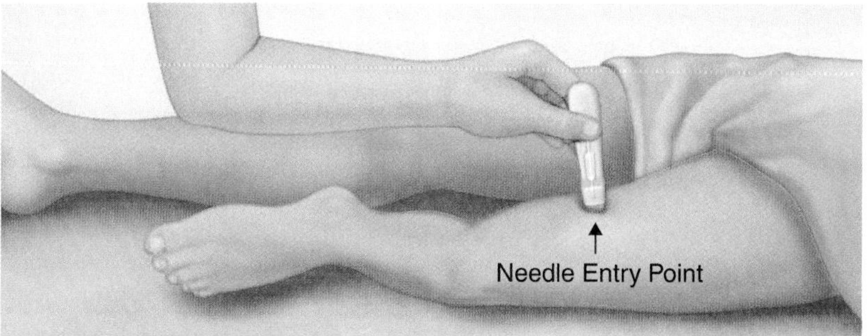

FIGURE 46–54 Positioning for adductor canal block. The patient is positioned supine with the leg externally rotated. A high-frequency linear transducer is placed in a transverse orientation at the mid-thigh.

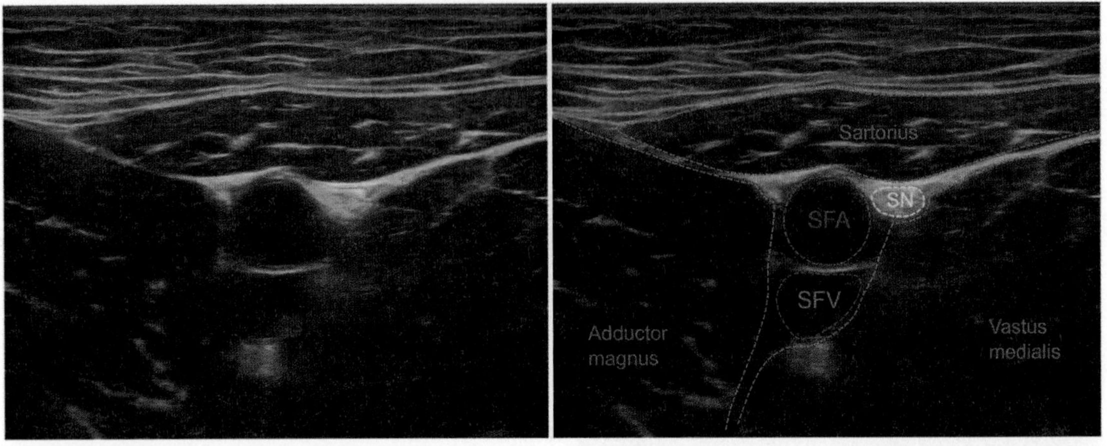

FIGURE 46–55 Adductor canal block. SFA, superficial femoral artery; SFV, superficial femoral vein; SN, saphenous nerve.

Ultrasound may be used to identify the saphenous vein near the tibial tuberosity and facilitate a *perivascular technique* with infiltration about the vein.

C. Distal Saphenous Technique

The medial malleolus is identified, infiltrating 5 mL of local anesthetic in a line running medially around the ankle (see "Ankle Block," below).

Sciatic Nerve Block

The sciatic nerve originates from the lumbosacral trunk and is composed of nerve roots L4 to L5 and S1 to S3 (Figure 46–58). The nerve exits the pelvis via the greater sciatic foramen and travels in the posterior thigh before bifurcating into the tibial and common peroneal nerves in the popliteal fossa. The sciatic nerve provides the sensory innervation to the posterior knee and the entire leg, ankle, and foot, with the exception of the medial leg and ankle, which is innervated by the saphenous nerve. It is responsible for innervating the hamstring muscles and all motor innervation distal to the knee. Blockade of the 12 sciatic nerve may occur anywhere along its course and is indicated for surgical procedures involving the posterior thigh, knee, lower leg, and foot (see Figure 46–39). The posterior femoral

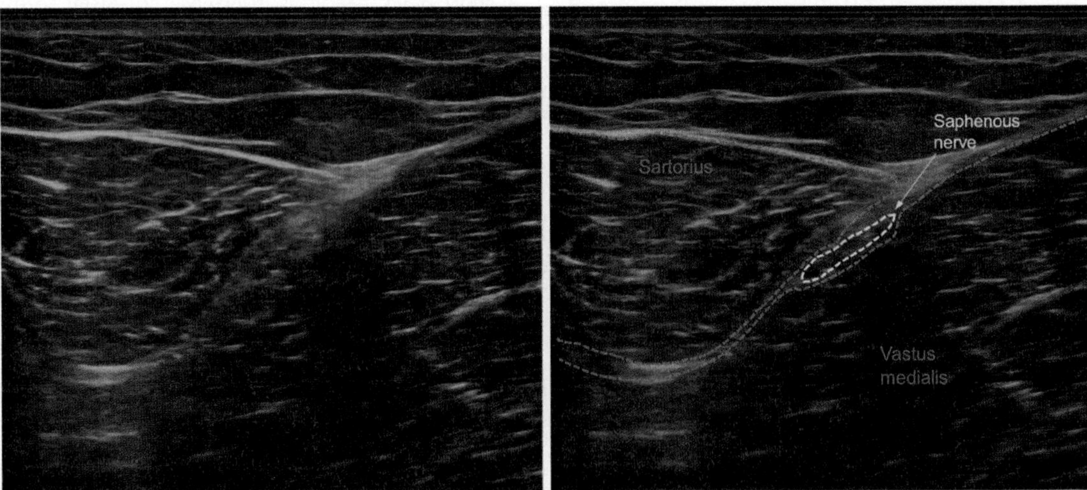

FIGURE 46–56 Subsartorial saphenous nerve block.

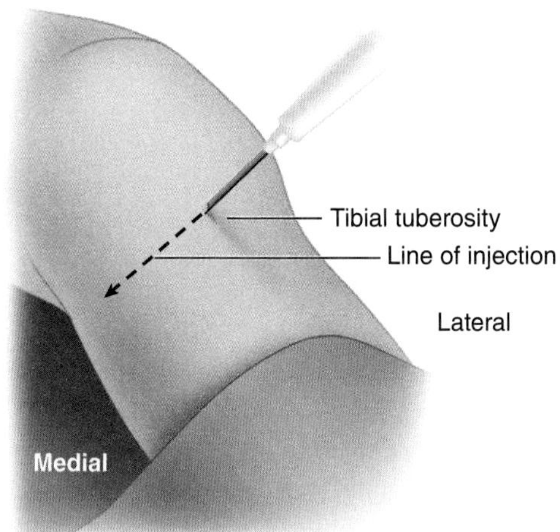

FIGURE 46–57 Proximal landmark-based saphenous nerve block.

cutaneous nerve, responsible for sensory innervation to the posterior thigh and into the popliteal fossa, is variably anesthetized as well, depending on the approach. More cephalad blocks increase the likelihood of posterior femoral cutaneous nerve coverage.

Parasacral Block

The parasacral block is a true block of the sacral plexus, arising from L4 to S4 (see Figure 46–38) and the only peripheral block that reliably anesthetizes all the terminal branches of the plexus, including the posterior femoral cutaneous nerve (PFCN). The sciatic nerve blocks described below anesthetize the PFCN to varying degrees, as will be described. The patient is positioned in the lateral decubitus position with the operative side up, and a vertical line is drawn between the posterior superior iliac spine and ischial tuberosity. A long stimulating block needle is inserted 6 cm inferior to the posterior superior iliac spine along this line with a parasagittal orientation perpendicular to the body axis. The needle is advanced until a motor response in the leg or foot is elicited, usually occurring at a depth of approximately 7 cm. Great care should be taken when performing the block because injury to the pelvic viscera is a potential risk.

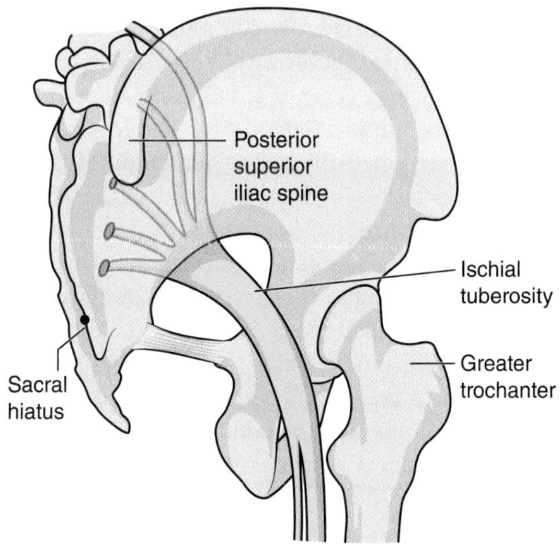

FIGURE 46–58 Proximal sciatic nerve anatomy.

A. Subgluteal Approach

A subgluteal approach to the sciatic nerve is just distal to the classic nerve stimulator–based "Labat approach," which had the disadvantage of being a very deep block where the sciatic nerve is closer in proximity to the pelvic viscera and poorly visualized with ultrasound. The subgluteal approach is useful when coverage of the posterior knee and PFCN are required (though the PFCN is less frequently anesthetized in comparison to the parasacral block). This approach is preferred if combining with femoral nerve or lumbar plexus block for knee surgeries (eg, tibial plateau fracture operative fixation, knee arthroplasty, below the knee amputation). If ambulation is desired within the local anesthetic duration, consider a popliteal approach (see next section) that will not affect the hamstring muscles to the same degree, allowing knee flexion to lift the foot with the use of crutches.

The patient is positioned in Sim's position (Figure 46–59) or prone, and a large curvilinear (linear may be sufficient for very thin individuals) ultrasound transducer is placed over the midpoint between the ischial tuberosity and the greater trochanter in a transverse orientation. Both bony structures should be visible in the ultrasound field simultaneously. Gluteal muscles are identified superficially, along with the fascial layer defining their deep border. The triangular sciatic nerve should be visible in cross-section just deep to this layer in a

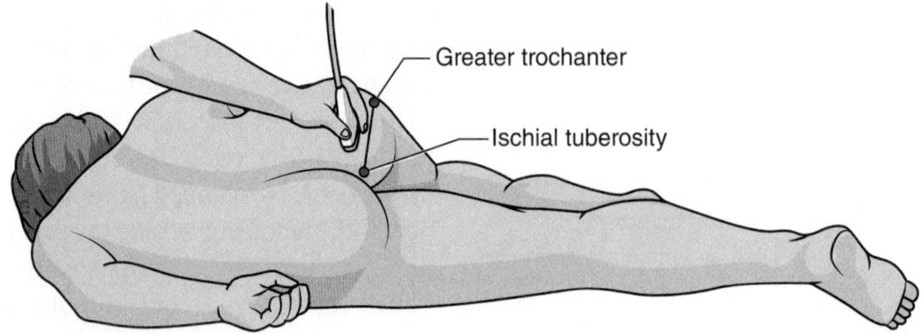

FIGURE 46–59 Patient, ultrasound transducer, and needle positioning for proximal sciatic nerve block.

location approximately midway between the ischial tuberosity and the greater trochanter, superficial to the quadratus femoris muscle (Figure 46–60).

The block needle is inserted just lateral to the ultrasound transducer near the greater trochanter. It is advanced through the field of the ultrasound beam until the tip is visible deep to the gluteus maximus, next to the sciatic nerve, and local anesthetic spread around the nerve should be observed. Nerve stimulation may be a useful supplement to ultrasound guidance for subgluteal sciatic nerve blocks, especially in obese patients or those who have undergone amputation resulting in altered anatomic relationships.

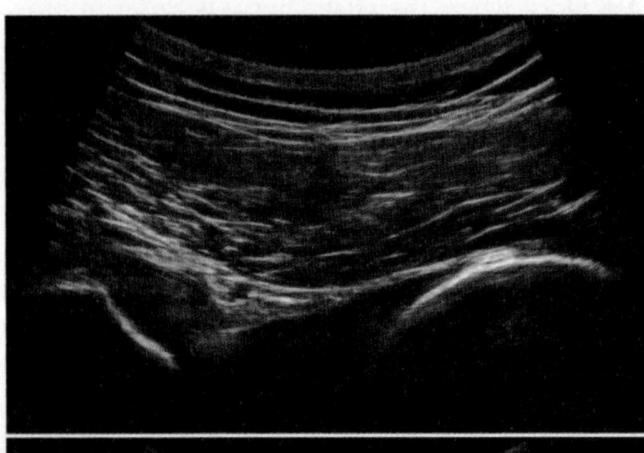

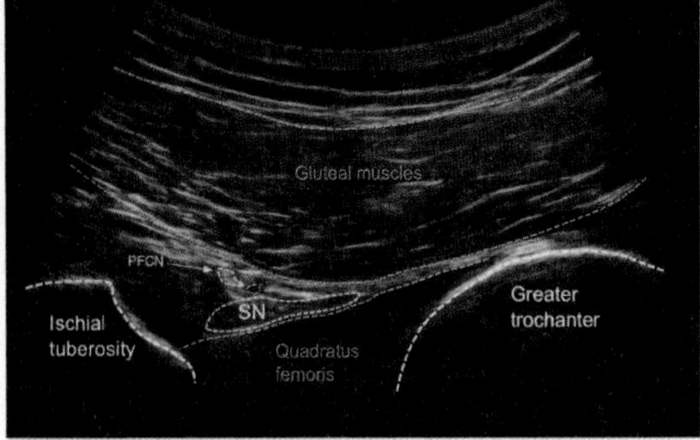

FIGURE 46–60 Subgluteal sciatic nerve block. PFCN, posterior femoral cutaneous nerve; SN, sciatic nerve; red and blue circles outline the inferior gluteal artery and vein, respectively.

B. Popliteal Approach

13 *Popliteal nerve blocks* provide excellent coverage for foot and ankle surgery while sparing much of the hamstring motor function, allowing lifting of the foot with knee flexion and thus facilitating ambulation. All sciatic nerve blocks fail to provide complete anesthesia for the cutaneous medial leg and ankle joint capsule, but when a saphenous (or femoral) block is added, complete anesthesia below the knee is provided. The major site-specific risk of a popliteal block is vascular puncture, owing to the sciatic nerve's proximity to the popliteal vessels at this location.

The sciatic nerve divides into the tibial and common peroneal nerves within or just proximal to the popliteal fossa (Figure 46–61). The upper popliteal fossa is bounded laterally by the biceps femoris tendon and medially by the semitendinosus and semimembranosus tendons. Cephalad to the flexion crease of the knee, the popliteal artery is immediately lateral to the semitendinosus tendon. The popliteal vein is lateral to the artery, and the tibial and common peroneal nerves are just superficial and lateral to the vein and medial to the biceps tendon, 2 to 6 cm deep to the skin. The tibial nerve continues deep behind the gastrocnemius muscle, and the common peroneal nerve exits the popliteal fossa between the head and neck of the fibula to supply the lower leg.

With the patient in the prone position, the apex of the popliteal fossa is identified (Figure 46–62). Using

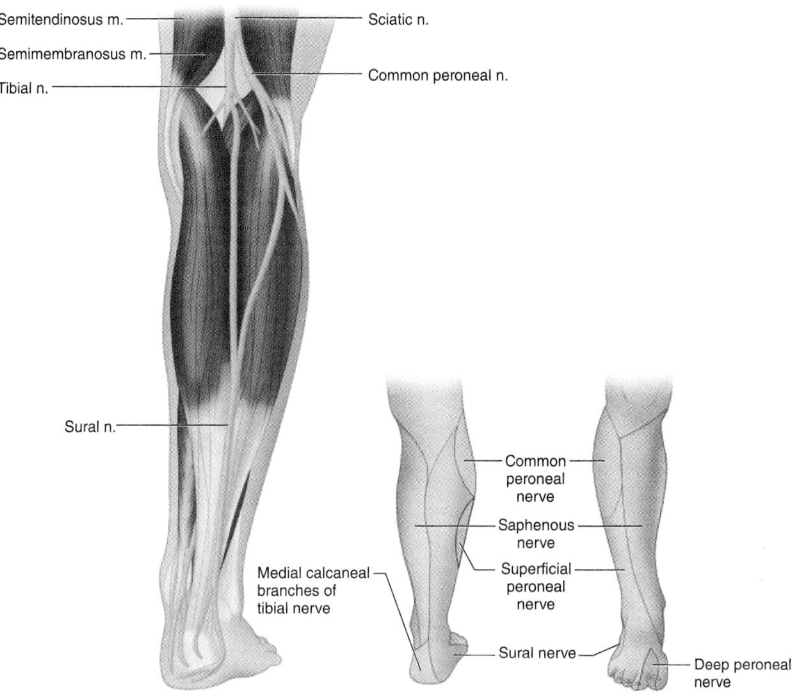

FIGURE 46–61 The sciatic nerve divides into tibial and peroneal branches just proximal to the popliteal fossa and provides sensory innervation to much of the lower leg.

a high-frequency linear ultrasound transducer placed in a transverse orientation, the femur, biceps femoris muscle, popliteal vessels, and sciatic nerve or branches are identified in cross-section (Figure 46–63). The nerve is usually superficial and lateral to the vessels and is often located in close relationship to the biceps femoris muscle abutting its medial edge.

The block needle is inserted using in-plane technique, lateral to the ultrasound transducer, and traversing the biceps femoris muscle. The needle is advanced in the ultrasound plane, and its deep or superficial approach to the nerve is visualized.

If surgical anesthesia is desired, local anesthetic should be seen surrounding all sides of the nerve, which usually requires multiple needle tip redirections with incremental injections. For analgesia alone, a single injection of local anesthetic deep or superficial to the nerve is acceptable. Injection within the paraneural sheath (*subparaneural block*) hastens onset and reduces the necessary volume to achieve a surgical block. However, care must be taken when using this technique to avoid intrafascicular injection as this may result in irreversible axonal injury. If surgical anesthesia is not required, there is limited benefit to a subparaneural block. Similarly, the subparaneural technique confers no benefit for continuous popliteal sciatic nerve blocks aside from those mentioned for single-injection blocks.

Ultrasound-guided popliteal sciatic blocks may be performed with the patient in the lateral or supine positions (the latter with leg up-raised on several pillows), but this makes the procedures more technically challenging.

Ankle Block

For surgical procedures of the foot, an ankle block is a fast, low-technology, low-risk means of providing anesthesia. Excessive injectate volume and the use of vasoconstrictors such as epinephrine must be avoided to minimize the risk of ischemic complications. Since this block includes five separate injections, it is often uncomfortable for patients, and adequate sedation and analgesia premedication is especially important.

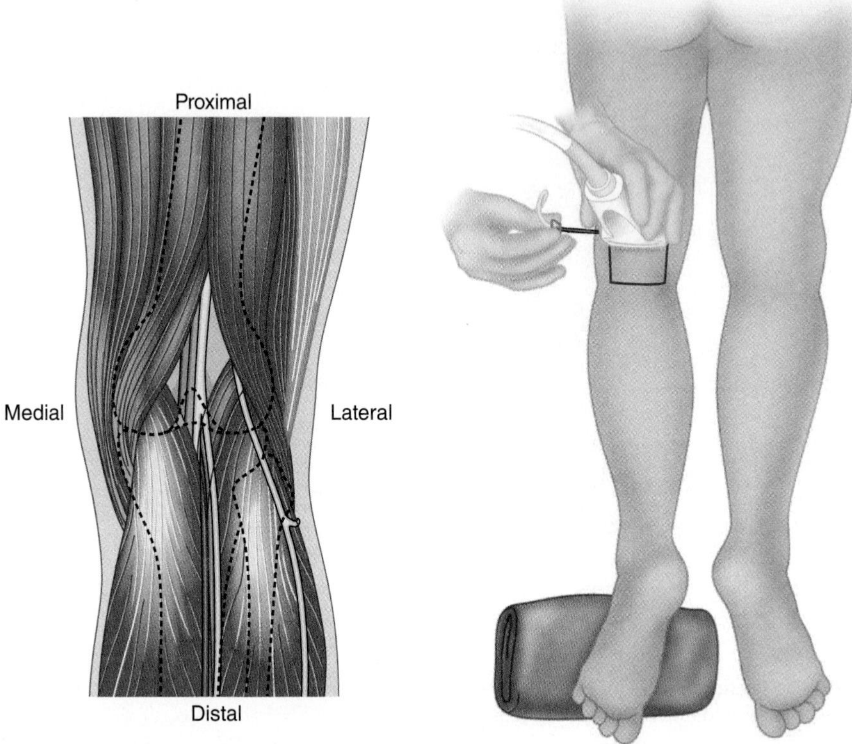

FIGURE 46–62 (**A**) Anatomy of the sciatic nerve in the popliteal fossa and (**B**) patient positioning, probe, and needle orientation for popliteal sciatic nerve block.

Five nerves supply sensation to the foot (Figure 46–64). The *saphenous nerve* is a terminal branch of the femoral nerve and the only innervation of the foot that is not a branch of the sciatic nerve. It supplies cutaneous sensation to the anteromedial foot and is most consistently located just anterior to the medial malleolus. The *deep peroneal nerve* runs in the anterior compartment of the leg after branching off the common peroneal nerve, entering the ankle between the extensor hallucis longus and the extensor digitorum longus tendons (Figure 46–65), just lateral to the dorsalis pedis artery. It provides innervation to the toe extensors and sensation to the first dorsal web space. The *superficial peroneal nerve*, also a branch of the common peroneal nerve, descends toward the ankle in the lateral compartment, giving off motor branches to the muscles of foot eversion. It enters the ankle just superficial to the extensor digitorum longus and extensor retinaculum and provides cutaneous sensation to the dorsum of the foot and toes (except the first webspace). The *tibial nerve* traverses the leg on the deep surface of the soleus muscle and enters the foot posterior to the medial malleolus, branching into calcaneal, lateral plantar, and medial plantar nerves. It is located behind the posterior tibial artery at the level of the medial malleolus and provides sensory innervation to the heel, the medial sole, and part of the lateral sole of the foot, as well as the tips of the toes. The *sural nerve* is a branch of the tibial nerve and enters the foot between the Achilles tendon and the lateral malleolus to provide sensation to the lateral foot.

14 A complete ankle block requires a series of five nerve blocks, but the process may be streamlined to minimize needle insertions (Figure 46–66). All five injections are required to anesthetize the

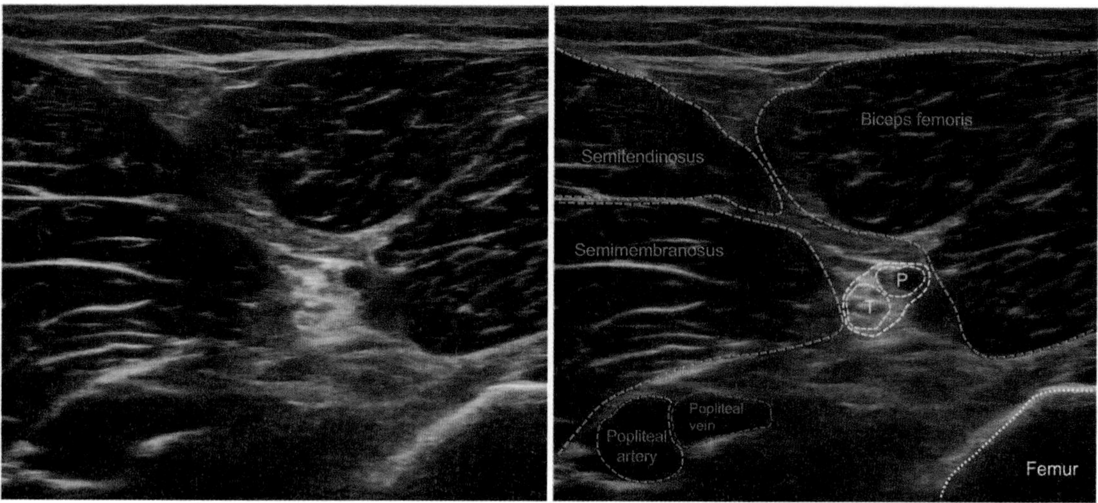

FIGURE 46–63 Popliteal sciatic nerve block. P, common peroneal nerve; T, tibial nerve.

entire foot; however, surgical procedures rarely require that all terminal nerves be blocked. In addition, unlike a sciatic nerve block, an ankle block provides no analgesia for (below-the-knee) tourniquet pain, nor does it allow for perineural catheter insertion. The groove between the extensor hallucis longus and extensor digitorum longus tendons is identified to block the deep peroneal nerve. The dorsalis pedis pulse is often palpable here. A short, small-gauge block needle is inserted perpendicular to the skin just lateral to the pulse, bone is contacted, and 5 mL of local anesthetic is infiltrated as the needle is withdrawn. From this insertion site, a subcutaneous wheal of 5 mL of local anesthetic is extended toward the lateral malleolus to target the superficial peroneal nerve. The needle is withdrawn and redirected from the same location in a medial direction, infiltrating 5 mL of local anesthetic toward the medial malleolus to target the saphenous nerve. The posterior tibial nerve may be located by identifying the posterior tibial artery pulse behind the medial malleolus. A short, small-gauge block needle is inserted just posterior to the artery and 5 mL of local anesthetic is distributed in the pocket deep to

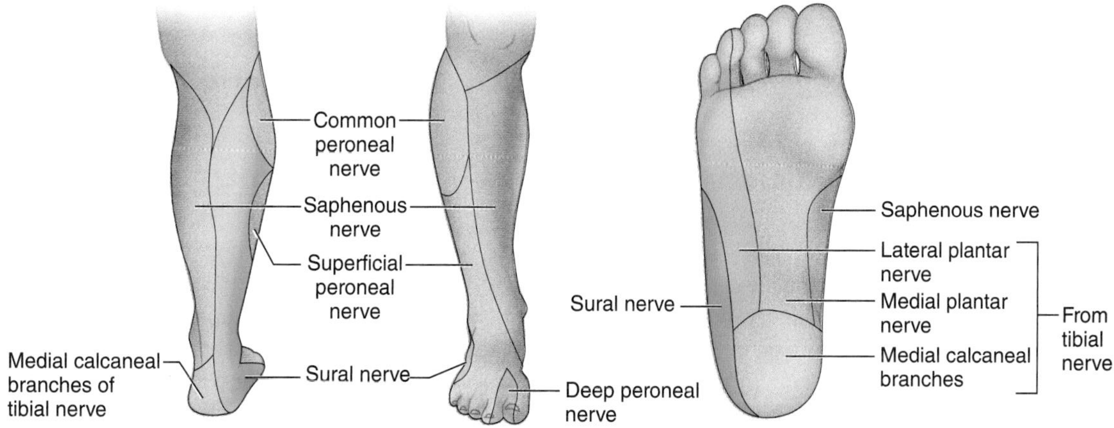

FIGURE 46–64 Cutaneous innervation of the foot.

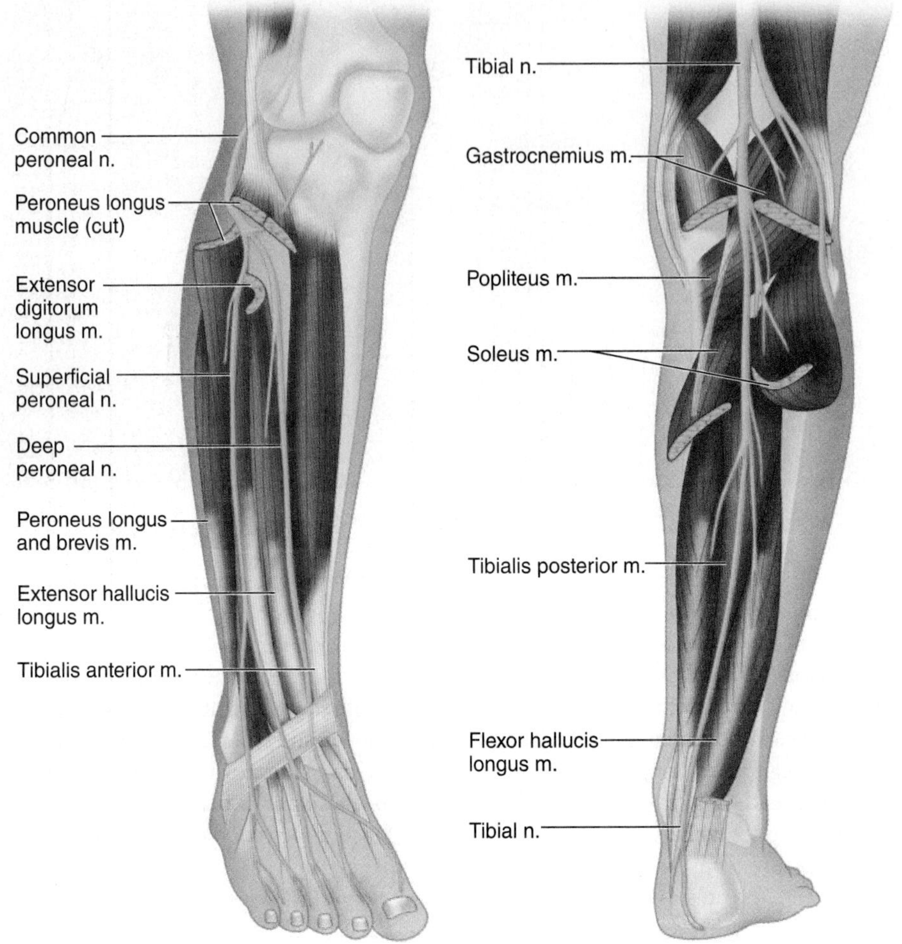

FIGURE 46–65 Tibial and common peroneal nerve courses. m., muscle; n., nerve.

the flexor retinaculum. Five mL of local anesthetic is injected subcutaneously posterior to the lateral malleolus to target the sural nerve.

Pericapsular Nerve Group Block

The pericapsular nerve group (PENG) block is a recently described fascial plane block for hip analgesia targeting the articular branches of the femoral and obturator nerves as they innervate the anterior hip joint capsule. This block offers the exciting possibility of hip analgesia without motor blockade. As of this writing, there is only evidence from case series to support its use; however, clinical trials are ongoing. These may eventually demonstrate this block to be a useful motor-sparing alternative for analgesia related to hip fractures, arthroplasty, and arthroscopy.

PERIPHERAL NERVE BLOCKS OF THE NECK

Cervical Plexus Block

The cervical plexus is formed from the anterior rami of the first four cervical vertebrae (C1–C4) in the neck just lateral to the transverse processes of the vertebrae (Figure 46–67). The plexus has four cutaneous branches (lesser occipital, greater auricular, transverse cervical, and supraclavicular nerves) and three

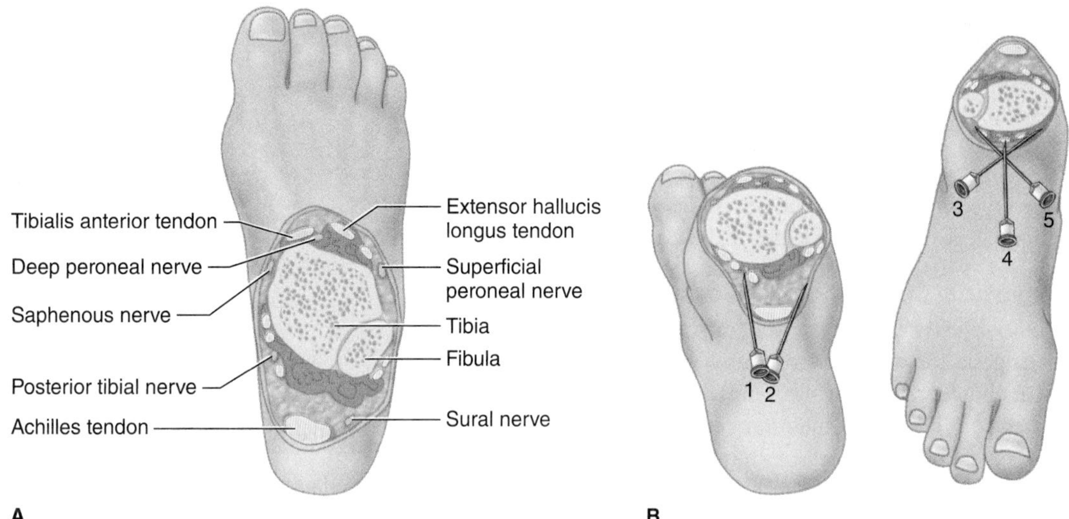

FIGURE 46–66 Needle placement for ankle block: 1 – tibial block; 2 – sural block; 3 – saphenous block; 4 – deep peroneal block; 5 – superficial peroneal block.

main motor branches (phrenic and ansa cervicalis nerves and an unnamed branch to the posterior neck muscles). It supplies sensation to the jaw, neck, occiput, and areas of the chest and shoulder, and blockade is indicated for unilateral neck surgery (eg, carotid endarterectomy) or as a supplement to interscalene block for clavicle or shoulder anesthesia/analgesia. The cervical plexus may be blocked with either a

15 *superficial* or *deep* technique. The *superficial cervical plexus block* targets the cutaneous branches of the plexus, while the *deep cervical plexus block* targets the nerve roots as they emerge from

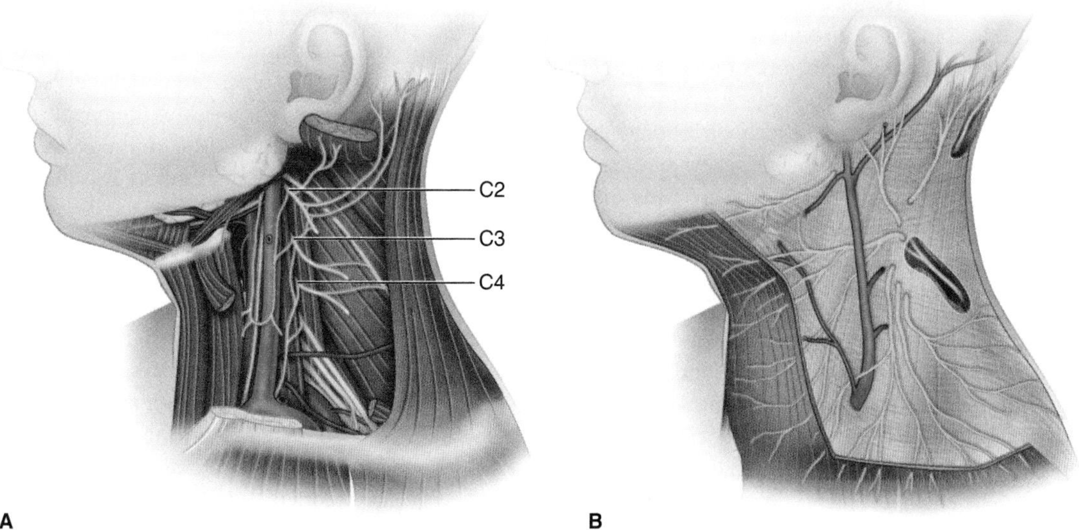

FIGURE 46–67 (**A**) Deep and (**B**) superficial anatomy of the cervical plexus.

the vertebral foramina. Although the latter may theoretically provide better analgesia to the deeper structures of the neck, randomized trials have failed to find a difference in the quality of surgical anesthesia yielded by either technique. Hemidiaphragmatic paralysis may occur with both deep and superficial blocks; thus, the same precautions discussed above for interscalene blocks apply to cervical plexus blocks.

A. Superficial Cervical Plexus Block

The *superficial cervical plexus block* provides cutaneous analgesia for surgical procedures on the neck, anterior shoulder, and clavicle. This technique takes advantage of the curious anatomic relationship that all the cutaneous branches of the cervical plexus coalesce at a point just posterior to the sternocleidomastoid roughly halfway between its origin on the clavicle and insertion on the mastoid process (see Figure 46–67B). The cutaneous nerves all emerge from this point to innervate the skin covering the jaw, neck, occiput, and medial shoulder.

1. Landmark-based approach—The patient is positioned supine with the head turned away from the side to be blocked. It is helpful to identify, so as to avoid, the external jugular vein. The sternocleidomastoid muscle is identified by asking the patient to turn the head against resistance to the operative side, and its posterior edge is marked. At a point approximately halfway between the mastoid and clavicle, a short block needle is inserted, directed cephalad toward the mastoid process, and 5 to 10 mL of local anesthetic is injected in a subcutaneous plane. The needle is turned and advanced in a caudad direction, maintaining a path along the posterior border of the sternocleidomastoid muscle. An additional 5 to 10 mL of local anesthetic is infiltrated subcutaneously. A dilute concentration of local anesthetic (eg, 0.25% bupivacaine) is appropriate, as this is essentially a field block.

2. Ultrasound-Guided Approach—The patient is positioned in the same way as for the landmark technique, and a high-frequency linear probe is placed in transverse orientation on the sternocleidomastoid muscle at the halfway point between the mastoid and clavicle. The cutaneous nerves of the cervical plexus can be identified as round, hypoechoic structures in the fascial plane deep to the sternocleidomastoid

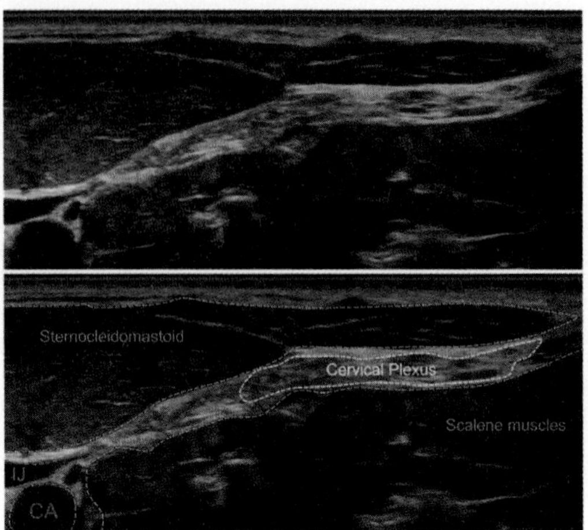

FIGURE 46–68 Ultrasound-guided superficial cervical plexus block. CA, carotid artery.

(Figure 46–68). A short block needle is inserted on the posterior side of the transducer and directed toward this plane. Local anesthetic (5–10 mL) is injected, and the plane should be hydrodissected by this injection.

B. Deep Cervical Plexus Block

The *deep cervical plexus block* anesthetizes the nerve roots of the cervical plexus as they emerge from the vertebral foramina. This should, at least theoretically, provide a denser block to the deeper structures of the neck. However, in randomized clinical trials, the deep block has not been found to be more effective in providing surgical anesthesia for carotid endarterectomy. As this block targets the nerve roots near the foramina, there is a risk of the needle passing through the foramen resulting in the epidural or intrathecal spread of local anesthetic. This risk may be reduced with the use of in-plane needle localization. The vertebral artery passes close to the target nerves as well, and even a very small dose of local anesthetic injected into the artery will be carried directly to the brain and likely result in a seizure.

Positioning for the deep block is similar to the superficial block. With the use of a small curvilinear ultrasound probe placed on the lateral neck in transverse orientation, the transverse process of the sixth cervical vertebra (C6) is identified by its prominent anterior tubercle at approximately the level of the cricoid cartilage. The transverse processes of

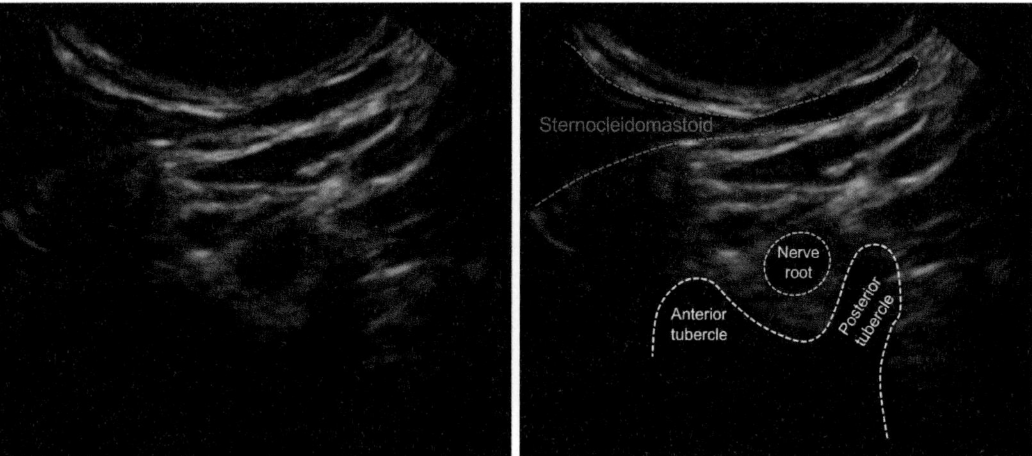

FIGURE 46–69 Ultrasound-guided deep cervical plexus block.

C5 through C2 are identified in sequence by scanning cephalad in a line toward the mastoid process. At each level from C2 through C4, a small gauge block needle is inserted immediately posterior to the ultrasound probe and advanced to a point adjacent to the nerve root (Figure 46–69). After careful aspiration for blood, 5 mL of local anesthetic is injected with spread visualized around the nerve root. The C1 nerve root cannot be reached directly but should be anesthetized by spread from the injection at C2.

PERIPHERAL NERVE BLOCKS OF THE TRUNK

Neuraxial anesthesia is the gold standard for anesthesia and analgesia of the thorax, abdomen, and pelvis. Neuraxial techniques anesthetize the chest, abdominal, and pelvic walls as well as the visceral organs contained within. However, epidural and spinal anesthesia techniques have many limitations. Neuraxial anesthetics cannot be administered to anticoagulated patients, nor can they be used to provide analgesia for outpatient surgeries. Further, these techniques are associated with risks of injury to the spinal cord or nerve roots, hematoma resulting in spinal cord or nerve root ischemia, profound hypotension, and epidural or meningeal infection.

Given the limitations of neuraxial analgesia, numerous techniques have been devised to provide truncal analgesia in patients who are poor candidates for spinal or epidural anesthesia (Figure 46–70). The paravertebral block was one of the first such techniques and offers many of the advantages associated with epidural analgesia; however, the risks of paravertebral block include significant hypotension and pneumothorax. Intercostal blocks provide a dense block to a single thoracic dermatome, yet they are also associated with pneumothorax and require the block to be performed at every dermatomal level that is to be anesthetized. In recent years, there has been a strong interest in the regional anesthesia community to devise new fascial plane blocks to provide analgesia to the chest, abdominal, and pelvic walls that can be administered as a single injection to each side, have a relatively long duration of action, and are associated with minimal risks and side effects. This trend mirrors the evolution of surgical techniques over the same time period, as surgical procedures have become less invasive and same-day discharge has become more common.

Intercostal Block

Intercostal blocks provide analgesia following thoracic and upper abdominal surgery and relief of pain associated with rib fractures, herpes zoster, and cancer. These blocks require individual injections delivered at each of the intercostal nerves that innervate the dermatomes to be anesthetized. 16 Intercostal blocks result in the highest blood levels of local anesthetic per local anesthetic dose injected of any nerve block procedure, and if

Truck Blocks and Indications	
Indication	**Blocks**
Thoracic	
Breast surgery	Paravertebral (T2–T6), serratus anterior plane, pectoralis, erector spinae plane
Thoracotomy and video assisted thoracoscopic surgery (VATS)	Paravertebral, intercostal, erector spinae plane (strongly consider neuraxial)
Rib or sternal fractures	Paravertebral, intercostal, serratus anterior plane, pectoralis, erector spinae plane (strongly consider neuraxial if incentive spirometry is still limited by pain following block)
Abdominal and Pelvic	
Ventral hernia repair	Paravertebral (T7–T11), rectus sheath
Exploratory laparotomy	Rectus sheath, (strongly consider neuraxial)
Laparoscopic abdominal surgery	Transversus abdominis plane, erector spinae plane, quadratus lumborum
Inguinal hernia repair	Transversus abdominis plane, paravertebral (T9–T11)
Cesarean section	Quadratus lumborum, transversus abdominis plane (vs administration of neuraxial opioids)
Laparoscopic gynecologic surgery	Quadratus lumborum, transversus abdominis plane
Open gynecologic surgery	Quadratus lumborum, transversus abdominis plane (consider neuraxial)
Abdominal penetrating injuries	Rectus sheath, transversus abdominis plane, paravertebral (strongly consider neuraxial if patient has extensive visceral injuries)

FIGURE 46–70 Truncal blocks for various indications.

multiple blocks will be performed, care must be taken to avoid toxic levels of local anesthetic. The intercostal block has one of the highest complication rates of any peripheral nerve block due to the close proximity of the intercostal artery and vein (intravascular local anesthetic injection) and the underlying pleura (pneumothorax). In addition, duration is impressively short due to the high vascular flow and the high rate of local anesthetic uptake and removal from the local tissues, and placement of a perineural catheter is tenuous, at best. With the advent of ultrasound guidance and fascial plane blocks for thoracoabdominal analgesia, intercostal nerve blocks have largely been replaced by other blocks requiring only a single injection to cover a large area of the chest wall.

The intercostal nerves arise from the dorsal and ventral rami of the thoracic spinal nerves. They exit from the spine at the intervertebral foramen and enter a groove on the underside of the corresponding rib, running with the intercostal artery and vein. The nerve is generally the most inferior structure in the neurovascular bundle between the internal and innermost intercostal muscles (Figure 46–71). Each nerve provides sensory innervation to its corresponding dermatome, with branches emerging over the length of the nerve.

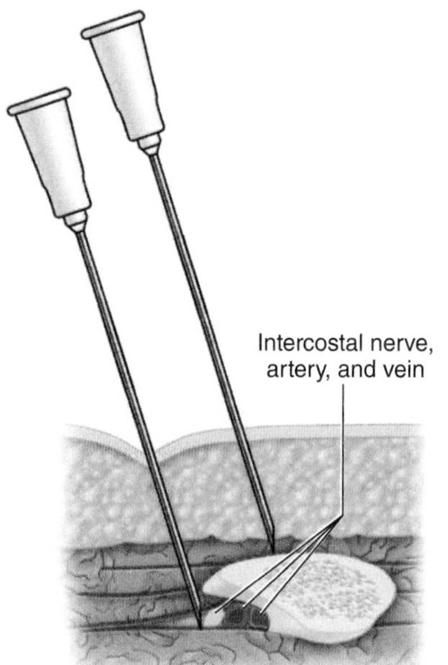

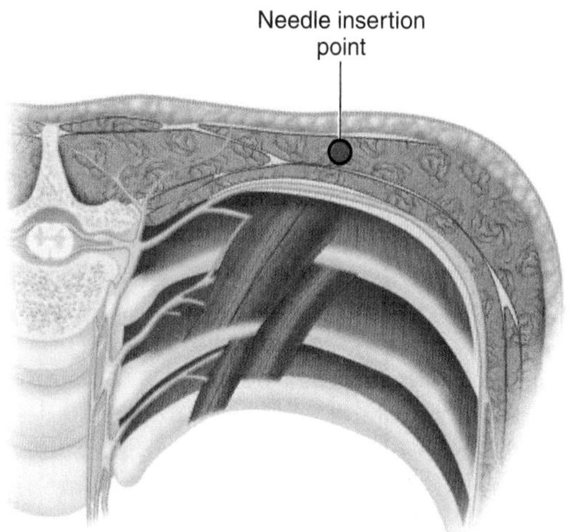

FIGURE 46–71 Anatomy and needle positioning for intercostal nerve block.

With the patient in the lateral decubitus, supine, or prone position, the level of each rib in the mid and posterior axillary line is palpated and marked. A small-gauge needle is inserted at the inferior edge of each of the selected ribs, bone is contacted, and the needle is then "walked off" inferiorly (see Figure 46–71). The needle is advanced approximately 0.25 cm. Following aspiration, observing for blood or air, 3 to 5 mL of local anesthetic is injected at each desired level. Ultrasound guidance can also be used and may allow for multiple levels to be reached via a single skin entry point by redirecting a long block needle (Figure 46–72).

Paravertebral Block

Paravertebral blocks provide surgical anesthesia or postoperative analgesia for procedures involving the thoracic or abdominal wall, mastectomy, inguinal or abdominal hernia repair, and more invasive unilateral

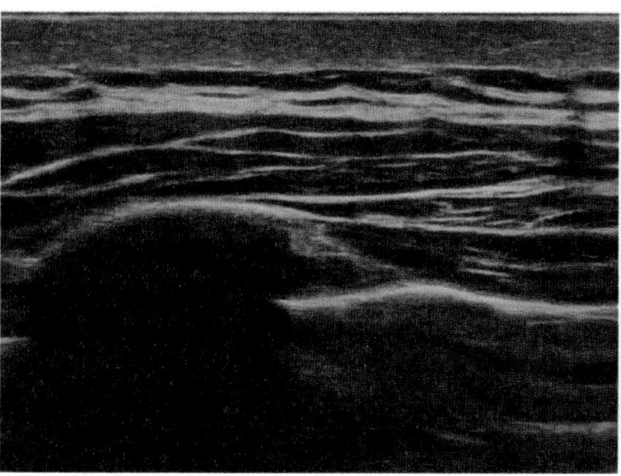

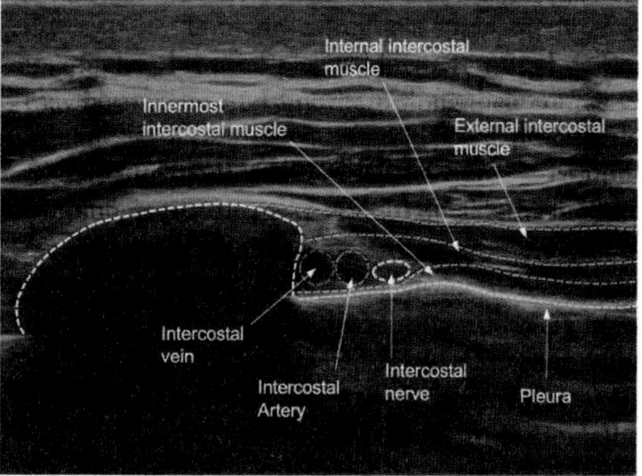

FIGURE 46–72 Ultrasound-guided intercostal nerve block.

abdominal procedures such as open nephrectomy or cholecystectomy. Paravertebral blocks usually cover one to two dermatomes above and below the level of the injection. Therefore, multiple injections delivered at various vertebral levels may be required depending on the area of body wall to be anesthetized. For example, a simple mastectomy would require coverage of dermatomes T2 to T6, and paravertebral blocks at the T3 and T5 levels should provide coverage. For axillary node dissection, an additional injection at T2 should be performed to cover the C7 through T2 dermatomes. For inguinal hernia repair, blocks should be performed to provide coverage from T10 through L2. Ventral hernias require bilateral injections corresponding to the level of the surgical site. The major complication of thoracic paravertebral injections is pneumothorax, whereas retroperitoneal structures may be at risk with lumbar-level injections. Hypotension and bradycardia secondary to sympathectomy can be observed with multilevel thoracic blocks. Unlike the intercostal approach, long-acting local anesthetic will have a nearly 24-hour duration, and perineural catheter insertion is an option (though local anesthetic spread from a single catheter to multiple levels is variable).

Each spinal nerve emerges from the intervertebral foramina and divides into two rami: a larger *anterior ramus*, which innervates the muscles and skin over the anterolateral body wall and limbs, and a smaller *posterior ramus*, which reflects posteriorly and innervates the skin and muscles of the back and neck

17 (Figure 46–73). The thoracic paravertebral space is defined posteriorly by the superior costotransverse ligament, anterolaterally by the

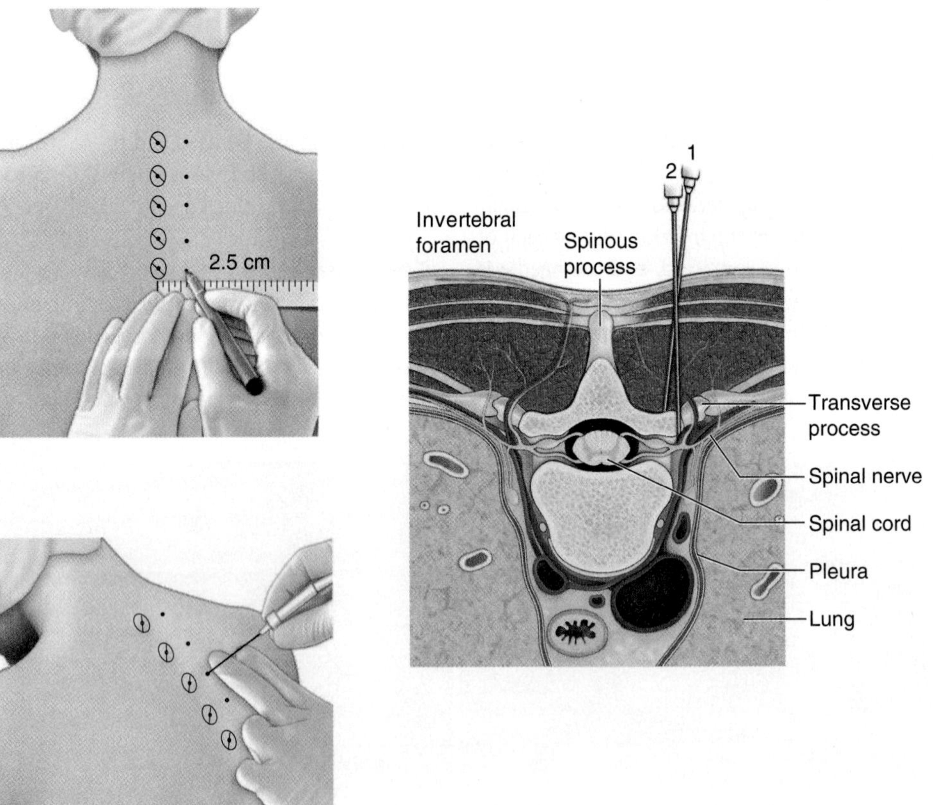

FIGURE 46–73 Paravertebral anatomy and traditional approach. Surface anatomy. Spinous processes are identified by circles and needle insertion sites for transverse processes are identified by dots. Needle is first inserted perpendicular to the plane of the skin to contact the transverse process (1), then redirected caudally (2) and advanced 1 cm.

parietal pleura, medially by the vertebrae and the intervertebral foramina, and inferiorly and superiorly by the heads of the ribs.

With the patient seated and vertebral column flexed, each spinous process is palpated, counting from the prominent C7 for thoracic blocks, and the iliac crests as a reference for lumbar levels. From the midpoint of the superior aspect of each spinous process, a point 2.5 cm laterally is measured and marked. In the thorax, the target nerve is located lateral to the spinous process *above* it because of the steep angulation of thoracic spinous processes (eg, the T4 nerve root is located lateral to the spinous process of T3). If an ultrasound-guided approach is used, the transverse processes may alternatively be numbered by counting down from the first rib (T1) or up from the twelfth rib (T12).

A. Landmark-Based Technique

A 20-gauge Tuohy needle is inserted at each point and advanced perpendicular to the skin (see Figure 46–73). Upon contact with the transverse process, the needle is withdrawn slightly and redirected caudad an additional 1 cm. A "pop" or loss of resistance may be felt as the needle passes through the costotransverse ligament. Some practitioners use a loss-of-resistance syringe to guide placement; others prefer the use of a nerve stimulator with chest wall motion for the endpoint. Five mL of local anesthetic is injected at each level. The difficulty with this technique is that the depth of the transverse process is simply estimated; thus, the risk of pneumothorax is relatively high. Using ultrasound to gauge transverse process depth prior to needle insertion theoretically decreases the risk of pneumothorax

B. Ultrasound-Guided Technique

An ultrasound transducer with a large curvilinear array is used, and the beam is oriented in a parasagittal or transverse plane. The transverse process, head of the rib, costotransverse ligament, and pleura are identified. The paravertebral space may be approached from a caudad-to-cephalad direction with a parasagittal ultrasound orientation (Figure 46–74) or a lateral-to-medial direction with a transverse ultrasound orientation (Figure 46–75). It is helpful to visualize the needle in-plane as it passes through the costotransverse ligament and observe a downward displacement of the pleura as local anesthetic is injected. Five to 10 mL of local anesthetic is injected at each level.

Erector Spinae Plane Block

The *erector spinae plane (ESP) block* is emerging as a useful alternative to paravertebral block for surgery involving the thoracoabdominal wall, and it can provide analgesia for rib fractures. It was first described as an analgesic therapy for chest wall neuropathic pain in 2016, and its popularity has increased dramatically

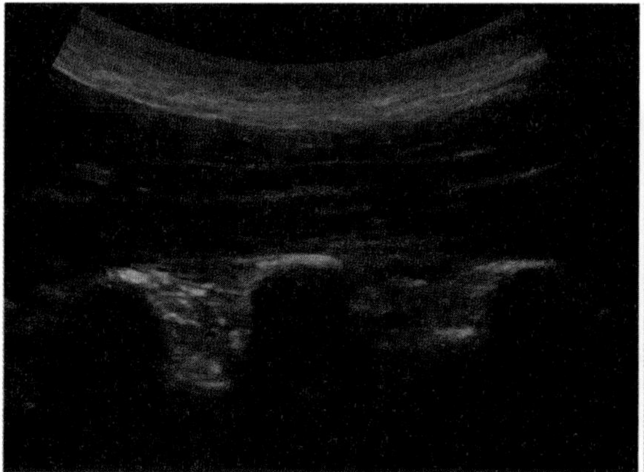

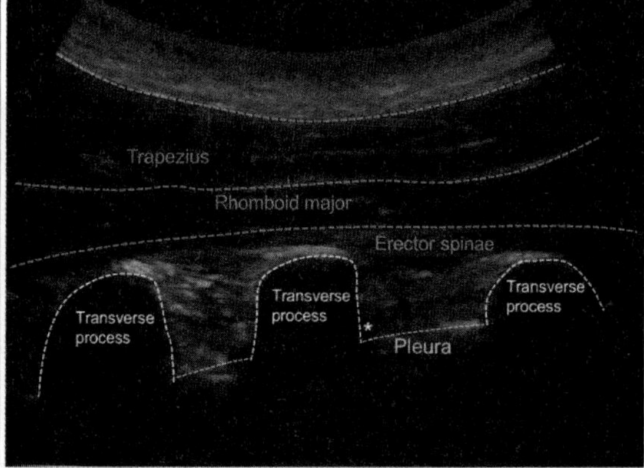

FIGURE 46–74 Paravertebral block using parasagittal ultrasound-guided technique. Asterisk indicates local anesthetic target. Pleura should be pushed in an anterior direction with local anesthetic injection.

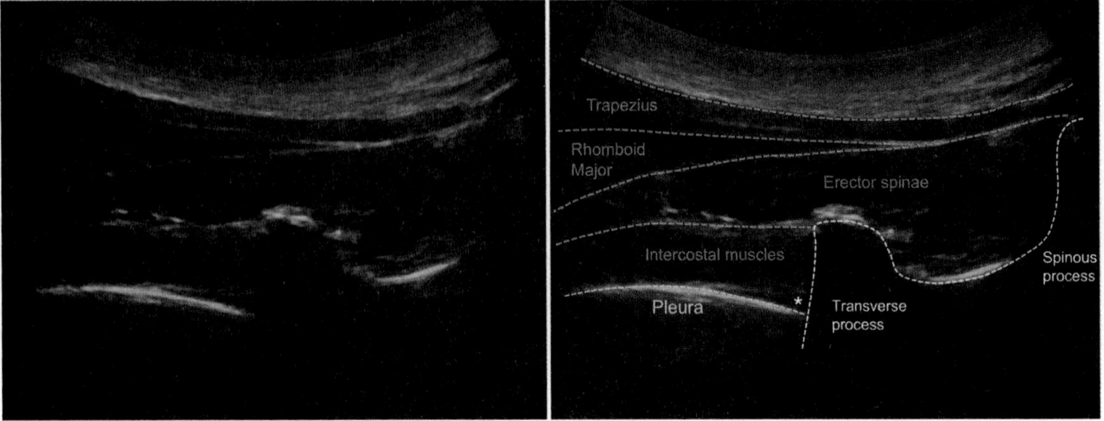

FIGURE 46–75 Paravertebral block using transverse ultrasound-guided technique. Asterisk indicates local anesthetic target.

over the subsequent years. The underlying mechanism for this fascial plane block has not been fully elucidated; however, it may be that local anesthetic diffuses to the paravertebral space. Although randomized trials have found the ESP block to provide inferior analgesia compared with the paravertebral block, the simplicity of the technique may make this a preferable option for chest or abdominal wall analgesia in the hands of nonexpert providers or in settings not well equipped to manage the potential complications associated with paravertebral blocks. However, it must be noted that pneumothorax has been reported as a complication of this block.

The erector spinae group consists of three muscles, the iliocostalis, the longissimus, and the spinalis, which function together to straighten and rotate the axial skeleton. In the high thoracic region, the muscles lie deep to the trapezius and rhomboid muscles, while in the low thoracic region, they are deep to the latissimus dorsi muscle. The objective of the erector spinae plane block is to deposit a large volume of local anesthetic in the plane deep to the erector spinae muscles, between the muscle and transverse process.

A linear or large curvilinear ultrasound probe is placed on the back in a parasagittal orientation, and the trapezius, rhomboid, and erector spinae muscles are visualized superficial to the transverse processes (see Figure 46–74). A long block needle is inserted either caudad to the probe and directed superiorly or cephalad to the probe and directed inferiorly. The needle is guided in an in-plane fashion to contact the transverse process. Local anesthetic is injected and should be seen spreading deep to the erector spinae over several spinal levels above and below the injection level. As this is a fascial plane block and the goal is to cover many dermatomes with a single injection, a large volume (30–50 mL) is used.

Pecs I/II Block

The *pectoralis nerve* or *Pecs block* is another less invasive alternative to paravertebral block for surgery involving the chest wall. The Pecs I block was first described in 2011 as a fascia plane block targeting the medial and lateral pectoral nerves in the plane between the pectoralis major and minor muscles, hence the name *pectoralis nerve block*. The block is achieved by depositing local anesthetic in the plane between the pectoralis major and pectoralis minor muscles at the level of the third rib. The following year, the Pecs II or modified Pecs block was described targeting the intercostobrachial, the third through sixth intercostals, and the long thoracic nerves, in addition to those blocked by the Pecs I, by adding an injection between the pectoralis minor and serratus anterior muscles.

A high-frequency linear transducer is placed at the mid-clavicular line with an oblique orientation to the parasagittal plane (Figure 46–76A). The pectoralis major, pectoralis minor, and axillary vessels are identified. Tracing the muscles toward their insertion, the serratus anterior muscle may then be identified deep to the pectoralis muscles and superficial to the third and fourth ribs (Figure 46–76B). A needle is inserted lateral to the transducer and advanced in-plane to target the interfascial plane between the pectoralis major and minor muscles. After injection of 10 to 15 mL of local anesthetic in this plane with spread visualized between the muscles (Pecs I), the needle is advanced through the pectoralis minor to inject another 10 to 15 mL of local anesthetic between the pectoralis minor and serratus anterior muscles.

Serratus Anterior Plane Block

The *serratus anterior plane (SAP) block* is a further modification of the pectoralis nerve block, moving the injection target for local anesthetic proximally to the plane between the serratus anterior and latissimus dorsi muscles. This is the approximate location where the lateral cutaneous branches of the intercostal nerves pierce the serratus anterior muscle, and the block aims to anesthetize the hemithorax via these branches. Similar to the ESP and

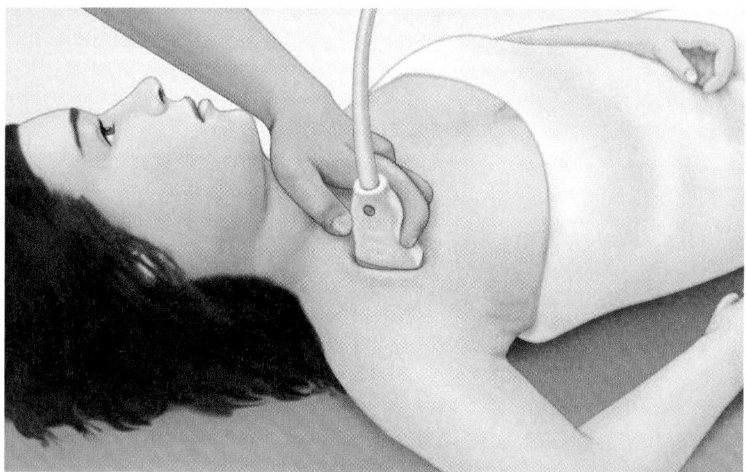

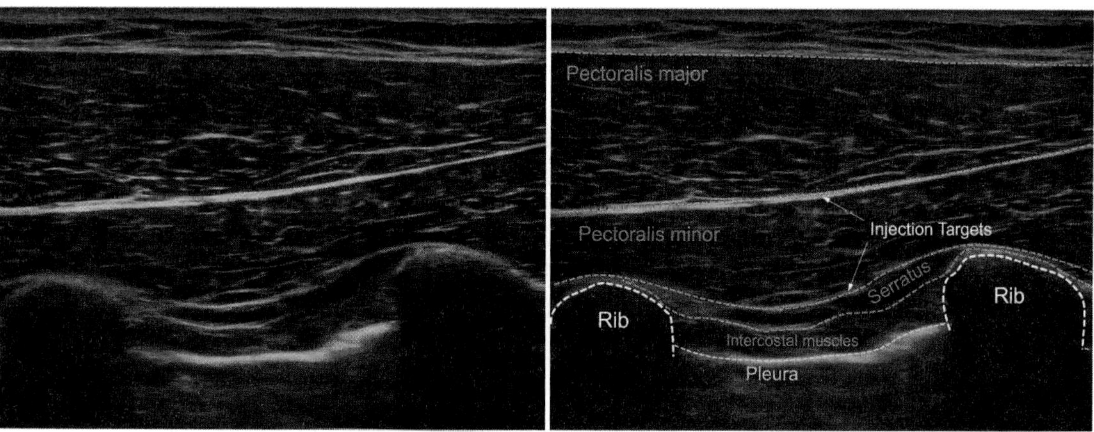

B

FIGURE 46–76 (**A**) Patient and ultrasound transducer positioning for pectoralis nerve block (PECS II) and (**B**) PECS II imaging: arrows indicate local anesthetic targets.

Pecs blocks, the SAP block is a more superficial alternative to the paravertebral block for unilateral chest wall anesthesia/analgesia. However, further studies are needed to compare these novel chest wall blocks against each other as well as the paravertebral block.

The patient is placed prone with the ipsilateral shoulder abducted and the arm resting behind the head. A linear ultrasound transducer is placed on the chest in sagittal orientation, and the ribs are counted down to the level of the fourth or fifth rib (Figure 46–77A). Maintaining these ribs in

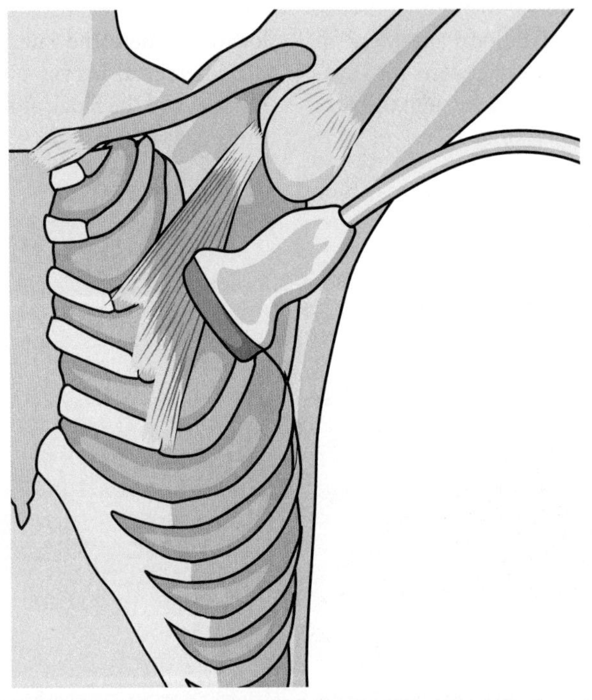

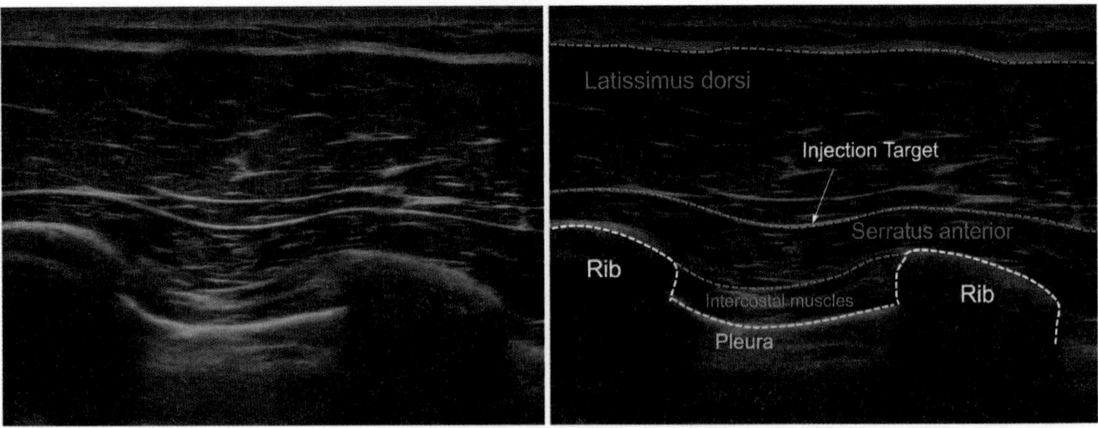

FIGURE 46–77 (**A**) Positioning for serratus anterior plane (SAP) block and (**B**) SAP block imaging: arrow indicates local anesthetic target.

cross-section, the anesthesia provider moves the probe laterally to the midaxillary line, eventually producing a nearly coronal orientation of the ultrasound probe. The serratus anterior muscle is identified directly superficial to the ribs in the midaxillary position, and the latissimus dorsi muscle is identified superficial to the serratus at this location. The block needle is inserted on the superomedial side of the probe and directed inferolaterally toward the plane between the latissimus dorsi (superficial) and serratus anterior (deep) muscles (Figure 46–77B). Local anesthetic is injected to hydrodissect this plane, and 20 to 30 mL can be deposited. Even in obese individuals, the target depth should be no more than 1 to 3 cm. Care must be taken to avoid going too deep and injuring the pleura.

Transversus Abdominis Plane Block

The *transversus abdominis plane* (TAP) block is most often used to provide surgical anesthesia for minor, superficial procedures on the lower abdominal wall or postoperative analgesia for procedures below the umbilicus. For inguinal hernia surgeries, intravenous or local supplementation may be necessary to provide anesthesia during peritoneal traction. Potential complications include violation of the peritoneum with or without bowel perforation, and the use of ultrasound is highly recommended to minimize this risk.

18 The *subcostal* (T12), *ilioinguinal* (L1), and *iliohypogastric* (L1) nerves are targeted in the TAP block, providing anesthesia to the ipsilateral lower abdomen below the umbilicus (Figure 46–78).

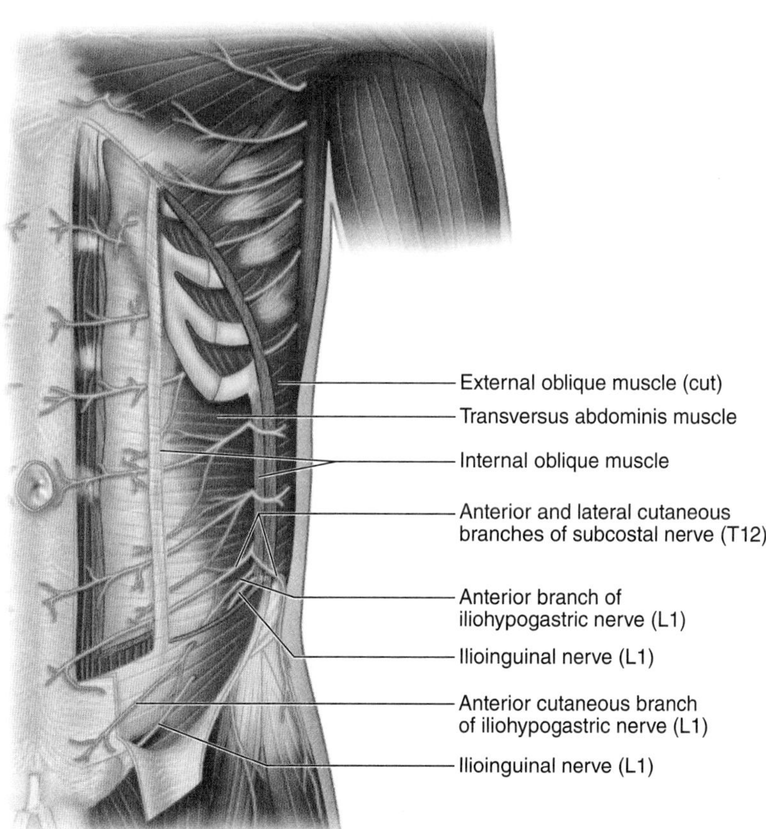

FIGURE 46–78 Transversus abdominis plane (TAP) block anatomy.

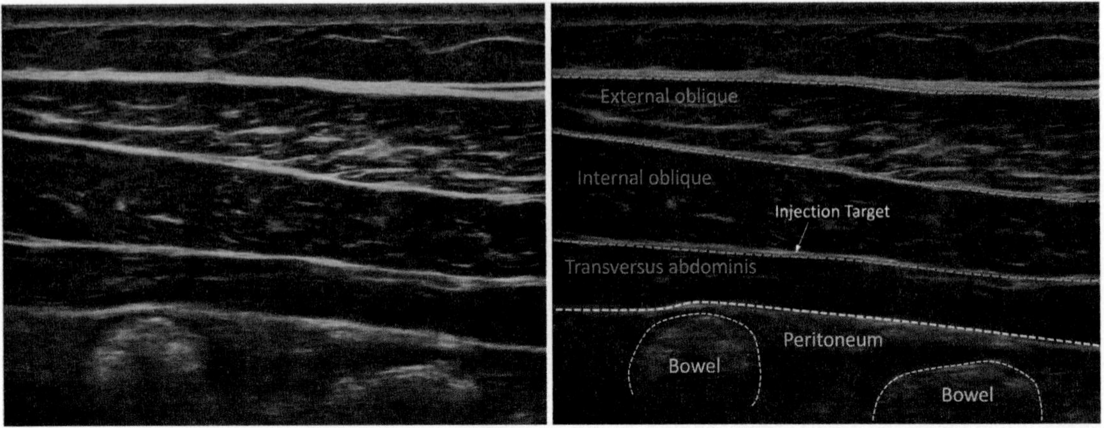

FIGURE 46–79 Transversus abdominis plane (TAP) block.

For part of their course, these three nerves travel in the muscle plane between the internal oblique and transversus abdominis muscles. Needle placement should be between the two fascial layers of these muscles, with local anesthetic filling the transversus abdominis plane. The patient is ideally positioned in lateral decubitus, but if mobility is limited, the block may be performed in the supine position.

With a linear (or curvilinear for very obese patients) array transducer oriented parallel to the inguinal ligament, the layers of the *external oblique*, *internal oblique*, and *transversus abdominis* muscles are identified just superior to the ASIS (Figure 46–79). Muscles appear as striated hypoechoic structures with hyperechoic layers of fascia at their borders. The block needle is inserted in-plane just lateral (posterior) to the transducer and advanced, as tactile feedback from fascial planes is noted, to the hyperechoic effacement of the deep border of the internal oblique and the superficial border of transversus abdominis. As with other fascial plane blocks, a large volume of local anesthetic is used. Approximately 30 mL of local anesthetic is injected, observing for an elliptical separation between the two fascial layers.

Rectus Sheath Block

The *rectus sheath* block is an ultrasound-guided abdominal field block targeting the anterior cutaneous branches of the seventh through the twelfth intercostal nerves as they pierce the rectus abdominis (Figure 46–80A). Local anesthetic is deposited deep to the rectus abdominis muscles bilaterally, producing an elliptical, midline block distribution extending from the xiphoid process to the symphysis pubis. Single-injection rectus sheath blocks will produce surgical anesthesia for superficial procedures in the midline abdominal wall (eg, umbilical hernia repair); however, no analgesia will be provided to visceral structures. Bilateral continuous rectus sheath blocks offer a less invasive alternative to thoracic epidural infusions for analgesia following midline laparotomy incisions.

With the patient supine, a linear ultrasound probe is placed over the midline of the abdomen in a transverse orientation. The hyperechoic linea alba is found at the midline between the rectus muscles on either side. Scanning laterally, the rectus abdominis muscle is seen as a spindle-shaped, hypoechoic muscle with hyperechoic fascia superficial and deep to the muscle, comprising the rectus sheath. The block needle should enter from the lateral side of the transducer, taking a shallow angle relative to the probe to avoid piercing too deep if the patient moves suddenly. The needle is advanced through the rectus muscle to its deep surface, and 20 mL of local anesthetic is injected to hydrodissect the rectus sheath from the underlying transversalis fascia (Figure 46–80B).

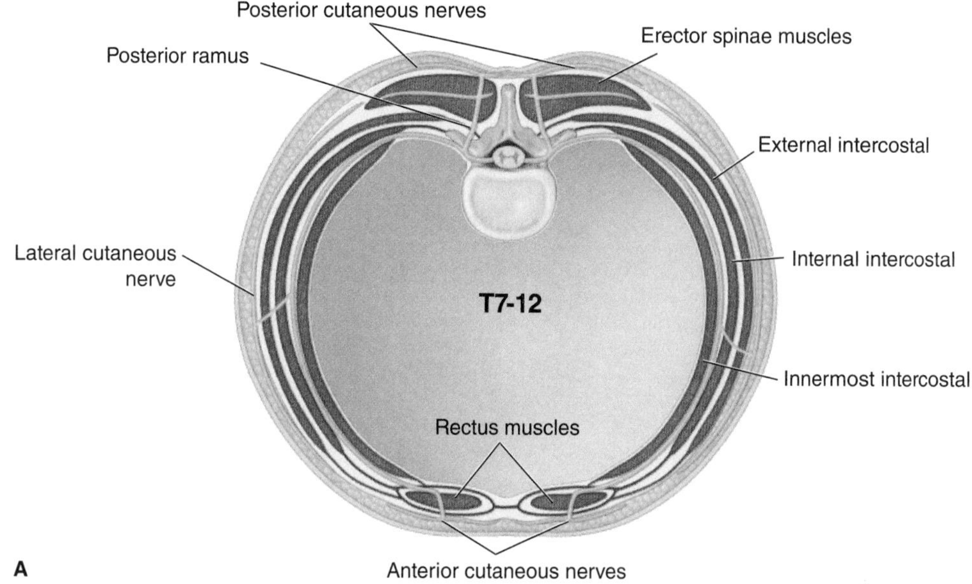

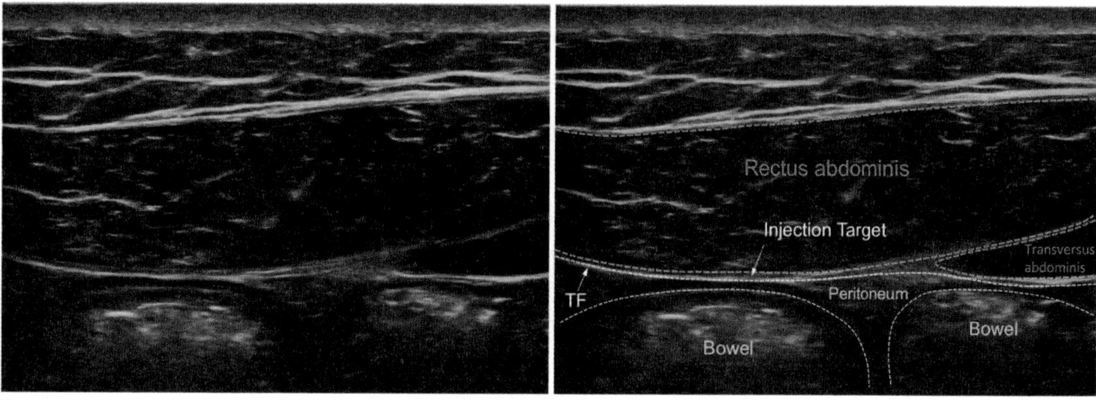

FIGURE 46–80 (**A**) Course of the intercostal nerves and the anterior cutaneous branches, local anesthetic is deposited deep to the rectus abdominis muscle to anesthetize the anterior cutaneous branches (**B**) Rectus sheath block. TF, transversalis fascia; arrow indicates local anesthetic target.

Quadratus Lumborum Blocks

The *quadratus lumborum* (QL) blocks are a recently described group of blocks targeting local anesthetic to various surfaces of the quadratus lumborum muscle (Figure 46–81A) to anesthetize the lower thoracic and lumbar regions. Three distinct blocks have been described, targeting the lateral surface (type 1), posterior surface (type 2), and anterior aspect between the quadratus and psoas muscles (transmuscular). As of the time of the writing of this chapter, there are little clinical data comparing the three techniques. The vast majority of publications related to the various QL blocks at this time are in the form of case series or cadaver studies, but clinical trials have demonstrated benefit following cesarean section and laparoscopic gynecologic surgery. Differing mechanisms of action have been proposed for each of the techniques based on evidence from cadaveric studies; however,

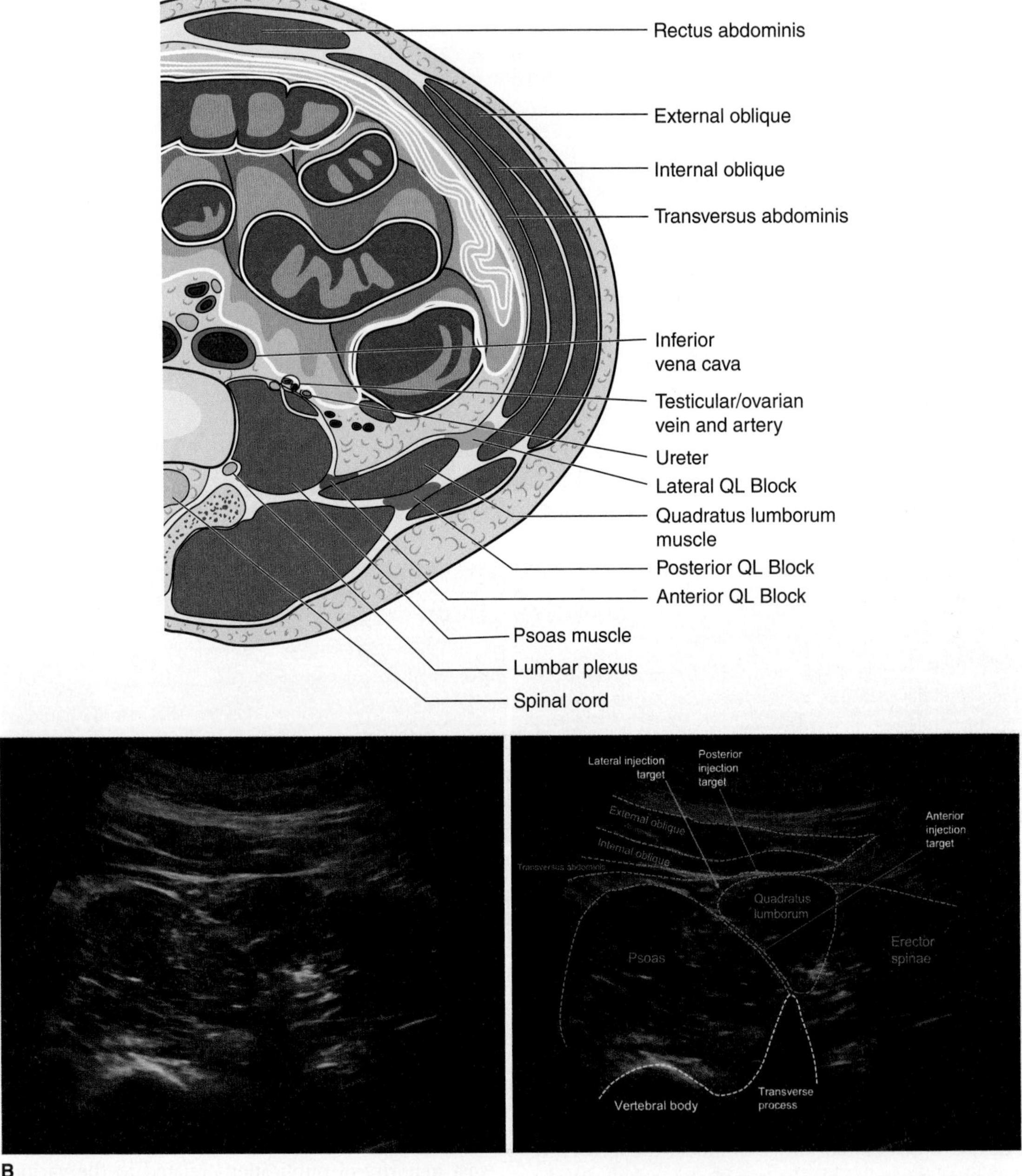

FIGURE 46–81 (**A**) Anatomy of the quadratus lumborum (QL) block (**B**) QL block. Blue arrow, posterior QL block approach; green arrow lateral QL block approach; purple arrow, anterior QL block approach.

discussion of each of these mechanisms is beyond the scope of this chapter.

A. Type 1 Quadratus Lumborum Block

The *Type 1 quadratus lumborum block* (QL1), also referred to as the *lateral quadratus lumborum block*, targets local anesthetic to the lateral aspect of the quadratus lumborum muscle deep to the posterior aponeurosis of the transversus abdominis muscle. The patient is positioned supine or lateral with a linear or large curvilinear ultrasound probe in transverse orientation placed in the midaxillary line. The block needle is inserted anterolateral to the transducer and advanced to puncture through the posterior aponeurosis of the transversus abdominis muscle and inject local anesthetic (20–30 mL) on the lateral aspect of the quadratus lumborum muscle.

B. Type 2 Quadratus Lumborum Block

The *Type 2 quadratus lumborum block* (QL2), also referred to as the *posterior quadratus lumborum block*, targets local anesthetic to the posterior aspect of the quadratus lumborum muscle, between this muscle and the overlying erector spinae muscle group. With the patient in the lateral decubitus position, a linear or curvilinear ultrasound probe is placed in transverse orientation in the midaxillary line and then moved posteriorly to identify the border between the quadratus lumborum and erector spinae muscles. The block needle is inserted on the lateral aspect of the ultrasound probe and advanced in-plane to this fascial layer. Local anesthetic (20–30 mL) is injected to hydrodissect this fascial plane.

C. Transmuscular Quadratus Lumborum Block

The *transmuscular quadratus lumborum block*, also referred to as the *anterior quadratus lumborum block*, requires the block needle to traverse the muscle belly of the quadratus lumborum and targets local anesthetic to the anterior aspect of the quadratus lumborum muscle, where it borders the psoas muscle. The patient is positioned lateral or prone, and a large curvilinear probe is placed in the midaxillary line and then moved posteriorly to identify the quadratus lumborum, erector spinae, and psoas muscles. The block needle is inserted on the posteromedial side of the ultrasound transducer and sequentially pierces the erector spinae and quadratus lumborum muscles to reach the border between the anterior aspect of the quadratus lumborum and the psoas muscle. Injection of local anesthetic (20–30 mL) should spread between these two muscles.

SUGGESTED READINGS

Chin KJ, McDonnell JG, Carvalho B, Sharkey A, Pawa Amit, Gadsden J. Essentials of our current understanding: abdominal wall blocks. *Reg Anesth Pain Med* 2017;42:133.

Hadzic A, ed. *Peripheral Nerve Blocks and Anatomy for Ultrasound-Guided Regional Anesthesia*. 2nd ed. McGraw-Hill; 2012.

Hebl JR, Lennon RL, eds. *Mayo Clinic Atlas of Regional Anesthesia and Ultrasound-Guided Nerve Blockade*. Oxford University Press; 2010.

Ilfeld BM. Continuous peripheral nerve blocks: an update of the published evidence and comparison with novel alternative analgesic modalities. *Anesth Analg*. 2017;124:308.

Kang RA, Chung YH, Ko JS, Yang MK, Choi DH. Reduced hemidiaphragmatic paresis with a "corner pocket" technique for supraclavicular brachial plexus block: single-center, observer-blinded, randomized controlled trial. *Reg Anesth Pain Med*. 2018;43:720.

Perlas A, Chan VW, Simons M. Brachial plexus examination and localization using ultrasound and electrical stimulation: a volunteer study. *Anesthesiology*. 2003;99:429.

Sites BD, Brull R, Chan VW, et al. Artifacts and pitfall errors associated with ultrasound-guided regional anesthesia. Part I: understanding the basic principles of ultrasound physics and machine operations. *Reg Anesth Pain Med*. 2007;32:412.

Sites BD, Brull R, Chan VW, et al. Artifacts and pitfall errors associated with ultrasound-guided regional anesthesia. Part II: A pictorial approach to understanding and avoidance. *Reg Anesth Pain Med*. 2007;32:419.

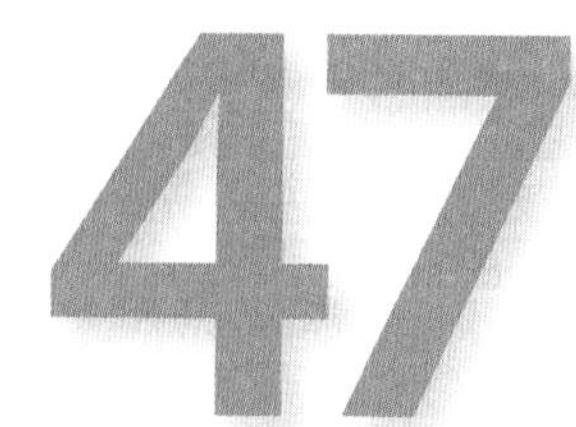

CHAPTER 47

Chronic Pain Management

Bruce M. Vrooman, MD, MS, and Kimberly M. Youngren, MD

KEY CONCEPTS

1. Pain may be classified according to pathophysiology (eg, nociceptive or neuropathic pain), etiology (eg, arthritis or cancer pain), or the affected area (eg, headache or low back pain).
2. *Nociceptive* pain is caused by activation or sensitization of peripheral *nociceptors*, specialized receptors that transduce noxious stimuli. *Neuropathic* pain is the result of injury or acquired abnormalities of peripheral or central neural structures.
3. *Acute pain* is caused by noxious stimulation due to injury, a disease process, or the abnormal function of muscle or viscera. It is almost always nociceptive.
4. *Chronic pain* is pain that persists beyond the usual course of an acute disease or after a reasonable time for healing to occur, typically 1 to 6 months. Chronic pain may be nociceptive, neuropathic, or mixed.
5. *Modulation* of pain occurs peripherally at the nociceptor, in the spinal cord, or in supraspinal structures. Modulation can either inhibit (suppress) or facilitate (intensify) pain.
6. At least three mechanisms are responsible for *central sensitization* in the spinal cord: (1) wind-up and sensitization of second-order wide dynamic range neurons; (2) dorsal horn neuron receptor field expansion; and (3) hyperexcitability of flexion reflexes.
7. Chronic pain may be caused by a combination of peripheral, central, and psychological mechanisms.
8. Moderate to severe acute pain, regardless of site, can affect the function of nearly every organ and may adversely influence perioperative recovery and outcomes.
9. The evaluation of any patient with pain should include several key components, including location, onset, and quality of pain; any alleviating or exacerbating factors; and a pain history, including previous therapies and changes in symptoms over time.
10. Psychosocial evaluation is useful whenever medical evaluation fails to reveal an apparent cause for pain, pain intensity is disproportionate to disease or injury, or psychological or social issues are apparent.
11. Myofascial pain syndromes are common disorders characterized by aching muscle pain, muscle spasm, stiffness, weakness, and, occasionally, autonomic dysfunction.
12. Ninety percent of disc herniations occur at L5–S1 or L4–L5. Symptoms usually develop following flexion injuries or heavy lifting and may be associated with bulging, protrusion, or extrusion of the disc.

—Continued next page

Continued—

13. Back pain caused by spinal stenosis usually radiates into the buttocks, thighs, and legs. Termed *pseudoclaudication* or *neurogenic claudication,* this pain is characteristically worse with exercise and relieved by rest, particularly sitting with the spine flexed.

14. Diabetic neuropathy produces the most common type of neuropathic pain.

15. *Complex regional pain syndrome* (CRPS) is a neuropathic pain disorder with significant autonomic features that is usually subdivided into two variants: *CRPS 1,* formerly known as *reflex sympathetic dystrophy* (RSD), and *CRPS 2,* formerly known as *causalgia.* The major difference between the two is the absence or presence, respectively, of documented nerve injury.

16. *Trigeminal neuralgia* (*tic douloureux*) is classically unilateral and usually located in the V2 or V3 distribution of the trigeminal nerve. It has an electric shock quality, with episodes lasting from seconds to minutes, and is often provoked by contact with a discrete trigger.

17. Antidepressants are most useful for patients with neuropathic pain and demonstrate an analgesic effect that occurs at a dose lower than needed for antidepressant activity.

18. Anticonvulsant medications are useful for patients with neuropathic pain, especially trigeminal neuralgia and diabetic neuropathy.

19. Patients who experience *opioid tolerance* require escalating doses of opioid to maintain the same analgesic effect. *Physical dependence* manifests in opioid *withdrawal* when the opioid medication is either abruptly discontinued or the dose is abruptly and significantly decreased. *Psychological dependence,* characterized by behavioral changes focusing on drug craving, is rare in patients with cancer.

20. Complications of stellate block include intravascular and subarachnoid injection, hematoma, pneumothorax, epidural anesthesia, brachial plexus block, hoarseness due to blockade of the recurrent laryngeal nerve, and, rarely, osteomyelitis or mediastinitis.

21. *Ganglion impar block* is effective for patients with visceral or sympathetically maintained pain in the perineal area.

22. Neurolytic blocks are indicated for patients with severe, intractable cancer pain in whom more conventional therapy proves inadequate or conventional analgesic modalities are accompanied by unacceptable side effects.

23. Spinal cord stimulation may be most effective for neuropathic pain; accepted indications include sympathetically mediated pain, spinal cord lesions with localized segmental pain, phantom limb pain, ischemic lower extremity pain due to peripheral vascular disease, adhesive arachnoiditis, peripheral neuropathies, postthoracotomy pain, intercostal neuralgia, postherpetic neuralgia, angina, visceral abdominal pain, and visceral pelvic pain.

24. Patients with pathological or osteoporotic vertebral compression fracture may benefit from vertebral augmentation with polymethylmethacrylate cement. *Vertebroplasty* involves injection of the cement through the trocar needle. *Kyphoplasty* involves inflation of a balloon inserted through a percutaneously placed trocar needle, with subsequent injection of cement.

25. Acupuncture can be a useful adjunct for patients with chronic pain, particularly that associated with chronic musculoskeletal disorders and headaches.

Pain is the most common symptom that prompts patients to see a physician, and the symptom may have a wide variety of causes, ranging from relatively benign conditions to acute injury, myocardial ischemia, degenerative changes, or malignancy. In most cases, after a diagnosis is made, conservative measures are prescribed, and the patient responds successfully. In others, referral to a pain medicine specialist for evaluation and treatment improves outcomes and conserves health care resources, and in some, surgery will be indicated. In still other situations, pain persists, and patients develop chronic pain, the cause of which remains obscure after preliminary investigations have excluded serious and life-threatening illnesses and, if warranted, surgical intervention has either failed to relieve pain or has produced a new pain syndrome.

The term *pain management* in a general sense applies to the entire discipline of anesthesiology, but its modern usage more specifically involves management of pain throughout the perioperative period as well as nonsurgical pain in both inpatient and outpatient settings. Pain medicine practice may be broadly divided into *acute* and *chronic* pain management. The former primarily deals with patients recovering from surgery or with acute medical conditions in a hospital or ambulatory surgery center setting (see Chapter 48), whereas the latter includes patients almost always seen in the outpatient setting. Unfortunately, this distinction is artificial and considerable overlap exists; a good example is the patient with cancer who frequently requires short- and long-term pain management in both inpatient and outpatient settings.

The contemporary practice of pain management is not limited to anesthesiologists but is often team-based and includes other physicians (physiatrists, surgeons, internists, oncologists, psychiatrists, neurologists) and nonphysicians (nurses, psychologists, physical therapists, acupuncturists, hypnotists). The most effective approaches are multidisciplinary, in which the patient is evaluated by one or more physicians who conduct an initial examination, make a diagnosis, and formulate a treatment plan, typically using the services and resources of other health care providers.

Anesthesiologists trained in pain management are in a unique position to coordinate multidisciplinary pain management centers because of their broad training in dealing with a wide variety of patients from surgical, obstetric, pediatric, and medical subspecialties and their expertise in clinical pharmacology and applied neuroanatomy, including the use of peripheral and central nerve blocks.

DEFINITIONS & CLASSIFICATION OF PAIN

Like other conscious sensations, normal pain perception depends on specialized neurons that function as receptors, detecting a noxious stimulus and then transducing and conducting it to the central nervous system. Sensation is often described as either *protopathic* (noxious) or *epicritic* (nonnoxious). Epicritic sensations (light touch, pressure, proprioception, and temperature discrimination) are characterized by low-threshold receptors and are generally conducted by large myelinated nerve fibers. In contrast, protopathic sensations (pain) are detected by high-threshold receptors (also called *nociceptors*) and conducted by smaller myelinated (Aδ) and unmyelinated (C) nerve fibers.

What Is Pain?

Pain is not just a sensory modality but an experience. The International Association for the Study of Pain defines pain as **an unpleasant sensory and emotional experience associated with, or resembling that associated with, actual or potential tissue damage.** This definition recognizes the interplay between the objective, physiological sensory aspects of pain and its subjective, emotional, and psychological components.

The response to pain can be highly variable among different individuals as well as in the same person at different times. There are differences related to both gender and age in pain perception, experiences, and coping strategies. Brain activation and brain imaging patterns differ between genders, with some of these differences decreasing with age and disappearing entirely after age 40.

The term *nociception* is derived from *noci* (Latin for harm or injury) and is used to describe neural responses to traumatic or noxious stimuli. All nociception produces pain, but not all pain results from nociception. Many patients experience pain in the absence of noxious stimuli. It is therefore clinically useful to divide pain into one of two categories: (1) *acute pain*, which is primarily due to nociception, and (2) *chronic pain*, which may or may not be due to nociception and in which psychological and behavioral factors often play a major role. Table 47–1 lists terms frequently used in describing pain.

TABLE 47–1 Terms used in pain management.

Term	Description
Allodynia	Perception of an ordinarily nonnoxious stimulus as pain
Analgesia	Absence of pain perception
Anesthesia	Absence of all sensation
Anesthesia dolorosa	Pain in an area that lacks sensation
Dysesthesia	Unpleasant or abnormal sensation with or without a stimulus
Hypalgesia (hypoalgesia)	Diminished response to noxious stimulation (eg, pinprick)
Hyperalgesia	Increased response to noxious stimulation
Hyperesthesia	Increased response to mild stimulation
Hyperpathia	Presence of hyperesthesia, allodynia, and hyperalgesia usually associated with overreaction, and persistence of the sensation after the stimulus
Hypesthesia (hypoesthesia)	Reduced cutaneous sensation (eg, light touch, pressure, temperature)
Neuralgia	Pain in the distribution of a nerve or a group of nerves
Paresthesia	Abnormal sensation perceived without an apparent stimulus
Radiculopathy	Functional abnormality of one or more nerve roots

1 Pain may also be classified according to pathophysiology (eg, nociceptive or neuropathic pain), etiology (eg, arthritis or cancer pain), or the affected area (eg, headache or low back pain). Such classifications are useful in the selection of treat-
2 ment modalities and drug therapy. *Nociceptive* pain is caused by activation or sensitization of peripheral *nociceptors*, specialized receptors that transduce noxious stimuli. *Neuropathic* pain is the result of injury or acquired abnormalities of peripheral or central neural structures.

A. Acute Pain

3 *Acute pain* is caused by noxious stimulation due to injury, a disease process, or the abnormal function of muscle or viscera. It is almost always nociceptive. Nociceptive pain serves to detect, localize, and limit tissue damage. Four physiological processes are involved: *transduction, transmission, modulation*, and *perception*. Acute pain is typically associated with a systemic neuroendocrine stress response that is proportional to the pain's intensity. The most common causes of acute pain include trauma, surgery, and labor (obstetric), as well as pain associated with acute medical illnesses, such as myocardial infarction, pancreatitis, and renal calculi. Most forms of acute pain resolve spontaneously or with treatment in a few days or weeks. When pain fails to resolve because of either abnormal healing or inadequate treatment, it becomes *chronic*. Two types of acute (nociceptive) pain—*somatic* and *visceral*—are differentiated based on origin and features.

1. Somatic pain—Somatic pain can be further classified as superficial or deep. Superficial somatic pain is due to nociceptive input from skin, subcutaneous tissues, and mucous membranes. It is characteristically well localized and described as a sharp, pricking, throbbing, or burning sensation.

Deep somatic pain arises from muscles, tendons, joints, or bones. In contrast to superficial somatic pain, it usually has a dull, aching quality and is less well localized. An additional feature is that both the intensity and duration of the stimulus affect the degree of localization. For example, pain following brief minor trauma to the elbow joint is localized to the elbow, but severe or sustained trauma often causes pain in the whole arm.

2. Visceral pain—Visceral acute pain is due to a disease process or abnormal function involving an internal organ or its covering (eg, parietal pleura, pericardium, or peritoneum). Four subtypes are described: (1) true localized visceral pain, (2) localized parietal pain, (3) referred visceral pain, and (4) referred parietal pain. True visceral pain is dull, diffuse, and usually midline. It is frequently associated with abnormal autonomic activity causing nausea, vomiting, sweating, and changes in blood pressure and heart rate. Parietal pain is typically sharp and often described as a stabbing sensation that is either localized to the area around the organ or referred to a distant site (Table 47–2). The phenomenon of visceral or parietal pain referred to cutaneous areas results from patterns of embryological development and migration of tissues and the convergence of visceral and somatic afferent input into the central nervous system. Thus, pain involving the peritoneum or pleura over the central diaphragm is frequently referred to the neck and shoulder, whereas pain involving the parietal surfaces of the peripheral diaphragm is referred to the chest or upper abdominal wall.

TABLE 47–2 Patterns of referred pain.

Location	Cutaneous Dermatome
Central diaphragm	C4
Lungs	T2–T6
Aorta	T1–L2
Heart	T1–T4
Esophagus	T3–T8
Pancreas and spleen	T5–T10
Stomach, liver, and gallbladder	T6–T9
Adrenals	T8–L1
Small intestine	T9–T11
Colon	T10–L1
Kidney, ovaries, and testes	T10–L1
Ureters	T10–T12
Uterus	T11–L2
Bladder and prostate	S2–S4
Urethra and rectum	S2–S4

B. Chronic Pain

4 *Chronic pain* persists beyond the usual course of an acute disease or after a reasonable time for healing to occur, typically 1 to 6 months. Chronic pain may be *nociceptive, neuropathic,* or *mixed.* Psychological mechanisms or environmental factors, or both, frequently play a major role. Patients with chronic pain often have attenuated or absent neuroendocrine stress responses related to the pain and prominent sleep and mood disturbances. Neuropathic pain is classically paroxysmal and lancinating, has a burning quality, and is associated with *hyperpathia*—an uncomfortable or painful response to a normally innocuous stimulus. When it is also associated with loss of sensory input (eg, amputation) into the central nervous system, it is termed *deafferentation pain.* When the sympathetic system plays a major role, it is often termed *sympathetically maintained pain.*

The most common forms of chronic pain include those associated with musculoskeletal disorders, chronic visceral disorders, lesions of peripheral nerves, nerve roots, or dorsal root ganglia (including diabetic neuropathy, causalgia, phantom limb pain, and postherpetic neuralgia), lesions of the central nervous system (stroke, spinal cord injury, multiple sclerosis), and cancer pain. The pain of most musculoskeletal disorders (eg, rheumatoid arthritis and osteoarthritis) is primarily nociceptive, whereas pain associated with peripheral or central neural disorders is primarily neuropathic. The pain associated with some disorders, such as cancer and chronic back pain (particularly after surgery), is often mixed.

Anatomy & Physiology of Nociception

PAIN PATHWAYS

Pain is conducted along three neuronal pathways that transmit noxious stimuli from the periphery to the cerebral cortex (Figure 47–1). The cell bodies of

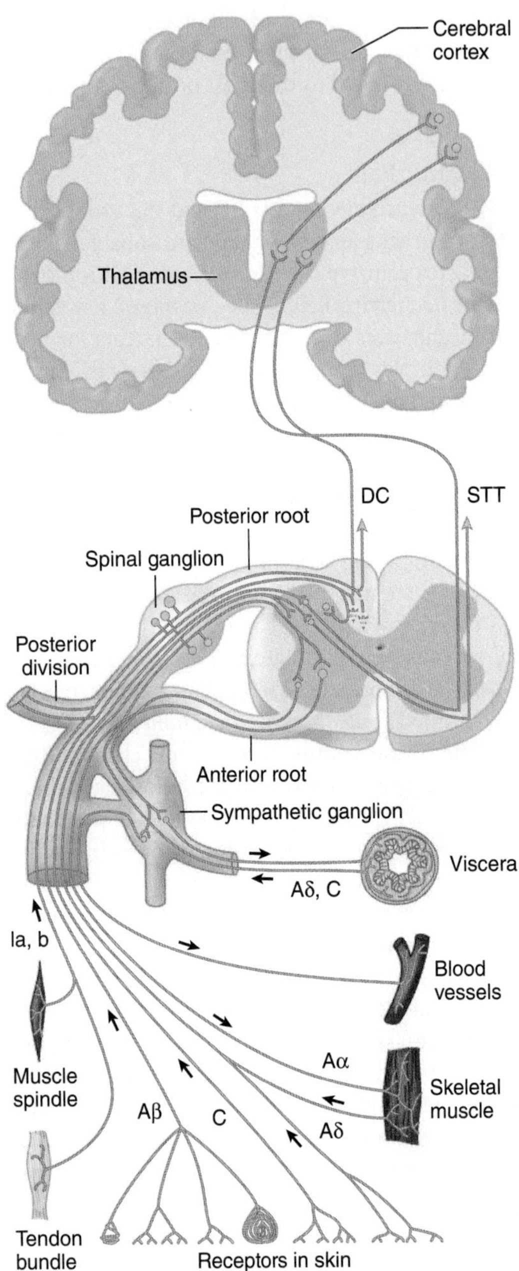

FIGURE 47–1 Pain pathways. DC, dorsal column; STT, spinothalamic tracts.

primary afferent neurons are located in the dorsal root ganglia, which lie in the vertebral foramina at each spinal cord level. Each neuron has a single axon that bifurcates, sending one end to the peripheral tissues it innervates and the other into the *dorsal horn* of the spinal cord. In the dorsal horn, the primary afferent neuron synapses with a second-order neuron whose axon crosses the midline and ascends in the contralateral *spinothalamic tract* to reach the thalamus. Second-order neurons synapse in thalamic nuclei with third-order neurons, which in turn send projections through the internal capsule and corona radiata to the postcentral gyrus of the cerebral cortex (Figure 47–2).

First-Order Neurons

The majority of first-order neurons send the proximal end of their axons into the spinal cord via the dorsal (sensory) spinal root at each cervical, thoracic, lumbar, and sacral level. Some unmyelinated afferent (C) fibers have been shown to enter the spinal cord via the ventral nerve (motor) root, accounting for observations that some patients continue to feel pain even after transection of the dorsal nerve root (rhizotomy) and report pain following ventral root stimulation. Once in the dorsal horn, in addition to synapsing with second-order neurons, the axons of first-order neurons may synapse with interneurons, sympathetic neurons, and ventral horn motor neurons.

Pain fibers originating from the head are carried by the trigeminal (V), facial (VII), glossopharyngeal (IX), and vagal (X) nerves. The Gasserian ganglion contains the cell bodies of sensory fibers in the ophthalmic, maxillary, and mandibular divisions of the trigeminal nerve. Cell bodies of first-order afferent neurons of the facial nerve are located in the geniculate ganglion; those of the glossopharyngeal nerve lie in its superior and petrosal ganglia; and those of the vagal nerve are located in the jugular ganglion (somatic) and the ganglion nodosum (visceral). The proximal axonal processes of the first-order neurons in these ganglia reach the brainstem nuclei via their respective cranial nerves, where they synapse with second-order neurons in brainstem nuclei.

SECOND-ORDER NEURONS

Afferent fibers segregate according to size as they enter the spinal cord, with large, myelinated fibers becoming medial and small, unmyelinated fibers becoming lateral. Pain fibers may ascend or descend

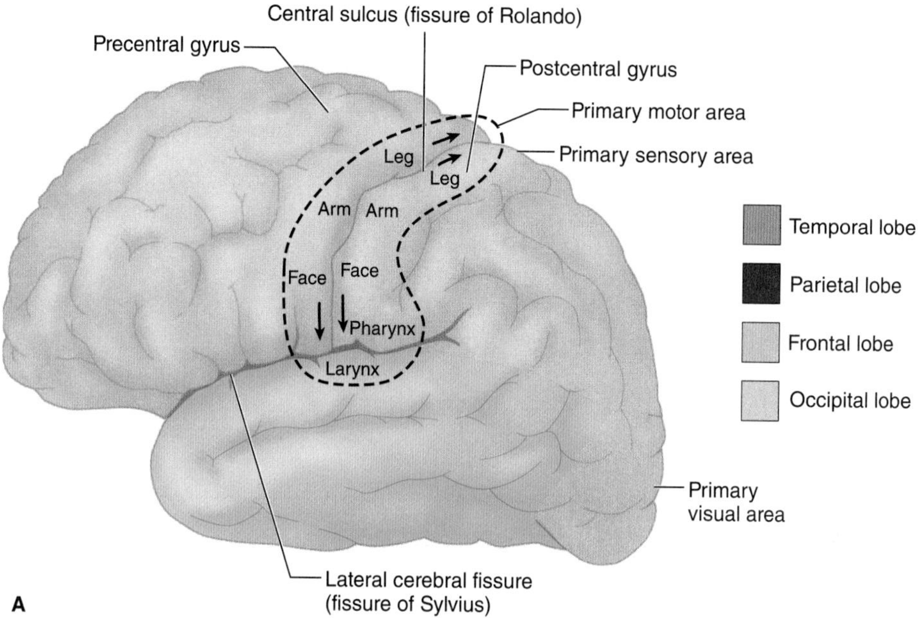

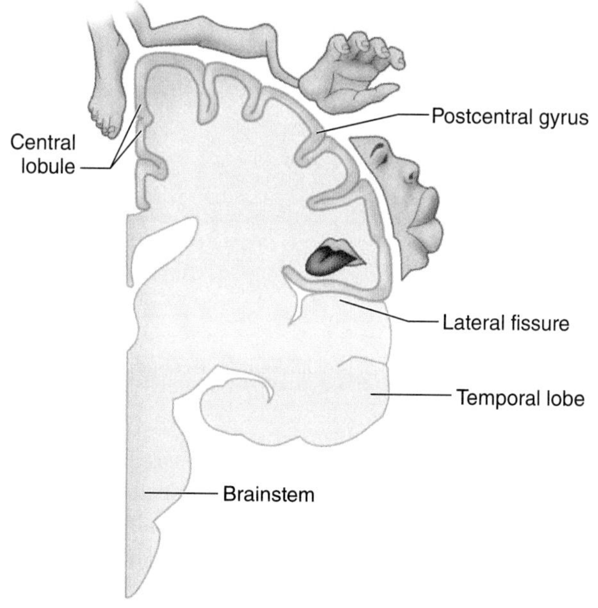

FIGURE 47–2 Lateral (**A**) and coronal (**B**) views of the brain show the location of the primary sensory cortex. Note the cortical representation of body parts, the sensory homunculus (**B**).

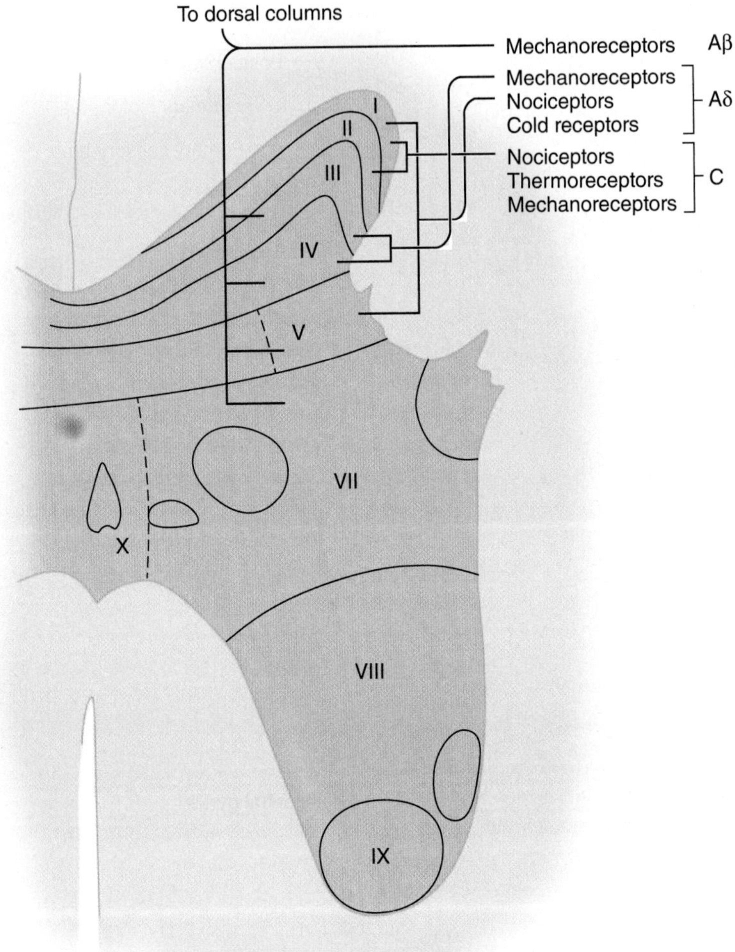

FIGURE 47–3 Rexed spinal cord laminae. Note the termination of the different types of primary afferent neurons.

one to three spinal cord segments in the *Lissauer tract* before synapsing with second-order neurons in the gray matter of the ipsilateral dorsal horn. In many instances, they communicate with second-order neurons through interneurons.

Spinal cord gray matter was divided by Rexed into ten laminae (Figure 47–3 and Table 47–3). The first six laminae, which make up the *dorsal horn*, receive all afferent neural activity and represent the principal site of modulation of pain by ascending and descending neural pathways. Second-order neurons are either *nociceptive-specific* or *wide dynamic range* (WDR) neurons. Nociceptive-specific neurons serve only noxious stimuli, but WDR neurons also receive nonnoxious afferent input from Aβ, Aδ, and C fibers. Nociceptive-specific neurons are arranged somatotopically in lamina I and have discrete, somatic receptive fields; they are normally silent and respond only to high-threshold noxious stimulation, poorly encoding stimulus intensity. WDR neurons are the most prevalent cell type in the dorsal horn. Although they are found throughout the dorsal horn,

TABLE 47–3 Spinal cord laminae.

Lamina	Predominant Function	Input	Name
I	Somatic nociception thermoreception	Aδ, C	Marginal layer
II	Somatic nociception thermoreception	C, Aδ	Substantia gelatinosa
III	Somatic mechanoreception	Aβ, Aδ	Nucleus proprius
IV	Mechanoreception	Aβ, Aδ	Nucleus proprius
V	Visceral and somatic nociception and mechanoreception	Aβ, Aδ, (C)	Nucleus proprius WDR neurons[1]
VI	Mechanoreception	Aβ	Nucleus proprius
VII	Sympathetic		Intermediolateral column
VIII		Aβ	Motor horn
IX	Motor	Aβ	Motor horn
X		Aβ, (Aδ)	Central canal

[1]WDR, wide dynamic range.

WDR neurons are most abundant in lamina V. During repeated stimulation, WDR neurons characteristically increase their firing rate exponentially in a graded fashion (*wind-up*), even with the same stimulus intensity. They have large receptive fields compared with nociceptive-specific neurons.

Most nociceptive C fibers send collaterals to, or terminate on, second-order neurons in laminae I and II, and, to a lesser extent, in lamina V. In contrast, nociceptive Aδ fibers synapse mainly in laminae I and V, and, to a lesser degree, in lamina X. Lamina I responds primarily to noxious (nociceptive) stimuli from cutaneous and deep somatic tissues. Lamina II, also called the *substantia gelatinosa*, contains many interneurons and plays a major role in processing and modulating nociceptive input from cutaneous nociceptors. It is a major site of action for opioids. Laminae III and IV primarily receive nonnociceptive sensory input. Laminae VIII and IX make up the *anterior (motor) horn*. Lamina VII is the *intermediolateral column* and contains the cell bodies of preganglionic sympathetic neurons.

Visceral afferents terminate primarily in lamina V and, to a lesser extent, in lamina I. These two laminae represent points of central convergence between somatic and visceral inputs. Lamina V responds to both noxious and nonnoxious sensory input and receives both visceral and somatic pain afferents. The phenomenon of convergence between visceral and somatic sensory input is manifested clinically as *referred pain* (see Table 47–2). Compared with somatic fibers, visceral nociceptive fibers are fewer in number, more widely distributed, proportionately activate a larger number of spinal neurons, and are not organized somatotopically.

A. The Spinothalamic Tract

The axons of most second-order neurons cross the midline close to their dermatomal level of origin (at the anterior commissure) to the contralateral side of the spinal cord before they form the *spinothalamic tract* and send their fibers to the thalamus, the reticular formation, the nucleus raphe magnus, and the periaqueductal gray. The spinothalamic tract, which is classically considered the major pain pathway, lies anterolaterally in the white matter of the spinal cord (Figure 47–4). This ascending tract can be divided into a *lateral* and a *medial* tract. The lateral spinothalamic (neospinothalamic) tract projects mainly to the ventral posterolateral nucleus of the thalamus and carries discriminative aspects of pain, such as location, intensity, and duration. The medial spinothalamic (paleospinothalamic) tract projects to the medial thalamus and is responsible for mediating the

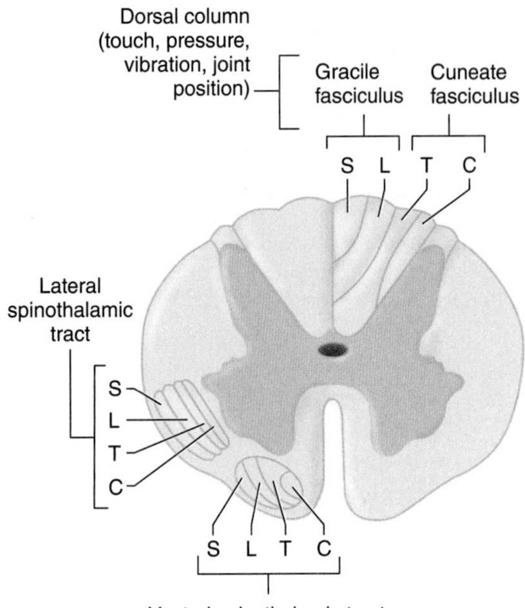

FIGURE 47–4 A cross-section of the spinal cord showing the spinothalamic and other ascending sensory pathways. Note the spatial distribution of fibers from different spinal levels: cervical (C), lumbar (L), sacral (S), and thoracic (T).

autonomic and unpleasant emotional perceptions of pain. Some spinothalamic fibers also project to the periaqueductal gray and thus may be an important link between the ascending and descending pathways. Collateral fibers also project to the reticular activating system and the hypothalamus; these are likely responsible for the arousal response to pain.

B. Alternate Pain Pathways

As with epicritic sensation, pain fibers ascend diffusely, ipsilaterally, and contralaterally; some patients continue to perceive pain following ablation of the contralateral spinothalamic tract, and therefore other ascending pain pathways are also important. The spinoreticular tract is thought to mediate arousal and autonomic responses to pain. The spinomesencephalic tract may be important in activating antinociceptive, descending pathways because it has some projections to the periaqueductal gray. The spinohypothalamic and spinotelencephalic tracts activate the hypothalamus and evoke emotional behavior. The spinocervical tract ascends uncrossed to the lateral cervical nucleus, which relays the fibers to the contralateral thalamus; this tract is likely a major alternative pathway for pain. Lastly, some fibers in the dorsal columns (which mainly carry light touch and proprioception) are responsive to pain; they ascend medially and ipsilaterally.

C. Integration with the Sympathetic and Motor Systems

Somatic and visceral afferents are fully integrated with the skeletal motor and sympathetic systems in the spinal cord, brainstem, and higher centers. Afferent dorsal horn neurons synapse both directly and indirectly with anterior horn motor neurons. These synapses are responsible for the reflex muscle activity—whether normal or abnormal—that is associated with pain. In a similar fashion, synapses between afferent nociceptive neurons and sympathetic neurons in the intermediolateral column result in reflex sympathetically mediated vasoconstriction, smooth muscle spasm, and the release of catecholamines, both locally and from the adrenal medulla.

Third-Order Neurons

Third-order neurons are located in the thalamus and send fibers to somatosensory areas I and II in the postcentral gyrus of the parietal cortex and the superior wall of the Sylvian fissure, respectively. Perception and discrete localization of pain take place in these cortical areas. Although most neurons from the lateral thalamic nuclei project to the primary somatosensory cortex, neurons from the intralaminar and medial nuclei project to the anterior cingulate gyrus and are likely involved in mediating the suffering and emotional components of pain.

PHYSIOLOGY OF NOCICEPTION

1. Nociceptors

Nociceptors are characterized by a high threshold for activation and encode the intensity of stimulation by increasing their discharge rates in a graded fashion. Following repeated stimulation, they characteristically display delayed adaptation, sensitization, and afterdischarges.

Noxious sensations can often be broken down into two components: a fast, sharp, and well-localized sensation ("first pain"), which is conducted with a short latency (0.1 s) by Aδ fibers (tested by pinprick); and a slower onset, duller, and often poorly localized sensation ("second pain"), which is conducted by C fibers. In contrast to well-localized *epicritic* sensation, which may be transduced by specialized end organs on the afferent neuron (eg, Pacinian corpuscle for touch), less well-localized *protopathic* sensation is transduced mainly by free nerve endings *nociceptors* that sense heat and mechanical and chemical tissue damage. Nociceptor types include (1) *mechanonociceptors,* which respond to pinch and pinprick, (2) *silent nociceptors,* which respond only in the presence of inflammation, and (3) *polymodal* mechanoheat nociceptors. The last are the most prevalent and respond to excessive pressure, extremes of temperature (>42°C and <40°C), and noxious substances such as bradykinin, histamine, serotonin, H+, K+, some prostaglandins, capsaicin, and possibly adenosine triphosphate. At least two nociceptor receptors (containing ion channels in nerve endings) have been identified, TRPV1 and TRPV2. Both respond to high temperatures. Capsaicin stimulates the TRPV1 receptor. Polymodal nociceptors are slow to adapt to strong pressure and display heat sensitization.

Cutaneous Nociceptors

Nociceptors are present in both somatic and visceral tissues. Primary afferent neurons reach tissues by traveling along spinal somatic, sympathetic, or parasympathetic nerves. Somatic nociceptors include those in skin (cutaneous) and deep tissues (muscle, tendons, fascia, bone), whereas visceral nociceptors include those in internal organs. The cornea and tooth pulp are unique in that they are almost exclusively innervated by nociceptive Aδ and C fibers.

Deep Somatic Nociceptors

Deep somatic nociceptors are less sensitive to noxious stimuli than cutaneous nociceptors but are easily sensitized by inflammation. The pain arising from them is characteristically dull and poorly localized. Specific nociceptors exist in muscles and joint capsules, and they respond to mechanical, thermal, and chemical stimuli.

Visceral Nociceptors

Visceral organs are generally insensitive tissues that mostly contain silent nociceptors. Some organs appear to have specific nociceptors, such as the heart, lung, testis, and bile ducts. Most other organs, such as the intestines, are innervated by polymodal nociceptors that respond to smooth muscle spasm, ischemia, and inflammation. These receptors generally do not respond to the cutting, burning, or crushing that occurs during surgery. A few organs, such as the brain, lack nociceptors altogether; however, the brain's meningeal coverings do contain nociceptors.

Like somatic nociceptors, those in the viscera are the free nerve endings of primary afferent neurons whose cell bodies lie in the dorsal horn. These afferent nerve fibers, however, frequently travel with efferent sympathetic nerve fibers to reach the viscera. Afferent activity from these neurons enters the spinal cord between T1 and L2. Nociceptive C fibers from the esophagus, larynx, and trachea travel with the vagus nerve to enter the nucleus solitarius in the brainstem. Afferent pain fibers from the bladder, prostate, rectum, cervix and urethra, and genitalia are transmitted into the spinal cord via parasympathetic nerves at the level of the S2 to S4 nerve roots. Though relatively few compared with somatic pain fibers, fibers from primary visceral afferent neurons enter the cord and synapse more diffusely with single fibers, often synapsing with multiple dermatomal levels and often crossing to the contralateral dorsal horn.

2. Chemical Mediators of Pain

Several neuropeptides (eg, *substance P* and *calcitonin gene-related peptide* [CGRP]) and excitatory amino acids (eg, glutamate) function as neurotransmitters for afferent neurons subserving pain (Table 47–4). Many, if not most, of these neurons contain more than one neurotransmitter, all of which are simultaneously released.

Substance P is an 11-amino-acid peptide that is synthesized and released by first-order neurons both peripherally and in the dorsal horn. Also found in other parts of the nervous system and the intestines,

TABLE 47–4 Major neurotransmitters mediating or modulating pain.

Neurotransmitter	Receptor[1]	Effect on Nociception
Substance P	Neurokinin–1	Excitatory
Calcitonin gene-related peptide		Excitatory
Glutamate	NMDA, AMPA, kainate, quisqualate	Excitatory
Aspartate	NMDA, AMPA, kainate, quisqualate	Excitatory
Adenosine triphosphate (ATP)	P_1, P_2	Excitatory
Somatostatin		Inhibitory
Acetylcholine	Muscarinic	Inhibitory
Enkephalins	μ, δ, κ	Inhibitory
β-Endorphin	μ, δ, κ	Inhibitory
Norepinephrine	α_2	Inhibitory
Adenosine	A_1	Inhibitory
Serotonin	5-HT_1 (5-HT_3)	Inhibitory
γ-Aminobutyric acid (GABA)	A, B	Inhibitory
Glycine		Inhibitory

[1]AMPA, 2-(aminomethyl)phenylacetic acid; NMDA, *N*-methyl-D-aspartate; 5-HT, 5-hydroxytryptamine.

it facilitates transmission in pain pathways via neurokinin-1 receptor activation. In the periphery, substance P neurons send collaterals that are closely associated with blood vessels, sweat glands, hair follicles, and mast cells in the dermis. Substance P sensitizes nociceptors, degranulates histamine from mast cells and serotonin from platelets, and is a potent vasodilator and chemoattractant for leukocytes. Substance P–releasing neurons also innervate the viscera and send collateral fibers to paravertebral sympathetic ganglia. Intense stimulation of viscera, therefore, can cause direct postganglionic sympathetic discharge.

Both opioid and α_2-adrenergic receptors have been described on or near the terminals of unmyelinated peripheral nerves. Although their physiological role is not clear, the latter may explain the observed analgesia of peripherally applied opioids, particularly in the presence of inflammation.

3. Modulation of Pain

5 *Modulation* of pain occurs peripherally at the nociceptor, in the spinal cord, and in supraspinal structures. Modulation can either inhibit (suppress) or facilitate (intensify) pain.

Peripheral Modulation of Pain

Nociceptors and their neurons display *sensitization* following repeated stimulation. Sensitization may be manifested as an enhanced response to noxious stimulation or a newly acquired responsiveness to a wider range of stimuli, including nonnoxious stimuli.

A. Primary Hyperalgesia

Sensitization of nociceptors results in a decrease in threshold, an increase in the frequency response to the same stimulus intensity, a decrease in response latency, and spontaneous firing even after cessation of the stimulus (after discharges). Such sensitization, termed *primary hyperalgesia*, commonly occurs with injury or following the application of heat and is mediated by the release of noxious substances from damaged tissues. Histamine is released from mast cells, basophils, and platelets, whereas serotonin is released from mast cells and platelets. Bradykinin released from tissues following activation of factor XII activates free nerve endings via specific B_1 and B_2 receptors.

Prostaglandins are produced following tissue damage by the action of phospholipase A_2 on phospholipids released from cell membranes to form arachidonic acid (Figure 47–5). The cyclooxygenase (COX) pathway then converts the latter into endoperoxides, which in turn are transformed into prostacyclin, prostaglandins, and thromboxanes. The lipoxygenase pathway converts arachidonic acid into hydroperoxy compounds, which are subsequently converted into leukotrienes. Acetylsalicylic acid (aspirin), nonsteroidal anti-inflammatory

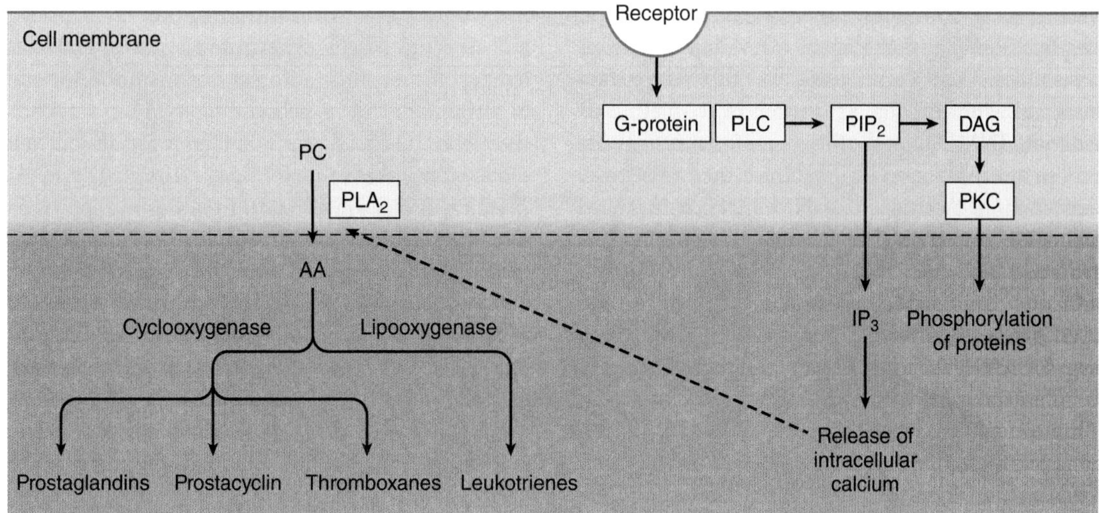

FIGURE 47–5 Phospholipase C (PLC) catalyzes the hydrolysis of phosphatidylinositol 4,5-bisphosphate (PIP2) to produce inositol triphosphate (IP3) and diacylglycerol (DAG). Protein kinase C (PKC) is also important. Phospholipase A_2 (PLA_2) catalyzes the conversion of phosphatidylcholine (PC) to arachidonic acid (AA).

drugs (NSAIDs), and likely also acetaminophen produce analgesia by inhibition of COX. The analgesic effect of corticosteroids is likely the result of inhibition of prostaglandin production through blockade of phospholipase A_2 activation.

B. Secondary Hyperalgesia

Neurogenic inflammation, also called *secondary hyperalgesia*, plays an important role in peripheral sensitization following injury. It is manifested by the *triple response of Lewis*: a red flush around the site of injury (*flare*), local tissue edema, and sensitization to noxious stimuli. Secondary hyperalgesia is primarily due to the antidromic release of substance P (and probably CGRP). Substance P degranulates histamine and 5-HT, vasodilates blood vessels, causes tissue edema, and induces the formation of leukotrienes. The neural origin of this response is supported by the following findings: (1) it can be produced by electrical stimulation of a sensory nerve, (2) it is not observed in denervated skin, and (3) it is diminished by injection of a local anesthetic. *Capsaicin* applied topically in a gel, cream, or patch depletes substance P, diminishes neurogenic inflammation, and is useful for some patients with postherpetic neuralgia.

Central Modulation of Pain

A. Facilitation

6 At least three mechanisms are responsible for the phenomenon of *central sensitization* in the spinal cord:

1. Wind-up and sensitization of second-order neurons. WDR neurons increase their frequency of discharge with the same repetitive stimuli and exhibit prolonged discharge, even after afferent C fiber input has stopped.
2. Receptive field expansion. Dorsal horn neurons increase their receptive fields such that adjacent neurons become responsive to stimuli (whether noxious or not) to which they were previously unresponsive.
3. Hyperexcitability of flexion reflexes. Enhancement of flexion reflexes is observed both ipsilaterally and contralaterally.

Neurochemical mediators of central sensitization include substance P, CGRP, vasoactive intestinal peptide (VIP), cholecystokinin (CCK), angiotensin, and galanin, as well as the excitatory amino acids L-glutamate and L-aspartate. These substances trigger changes in membrane excitability by interacting with G protein–coupled membrane receptors on neurons (see Figure 47–5).

L-Glutamate and L-aspartate play important roles in wind-up, via activation of *N*-methyl-D-aspartate (NMDA) and other receptor mechanisms and in the induction and maintenance of central sensitization. Activation of NMDA receptors also induces nitric oxide synthetase, increasing the formation of nitric oxide. Both prostaglandins and nitric oxide facilitate the release of excitatory amino acids in the spinal cord. Thus, COX inhibitors such as acetylsalicylic acid (ASA) and NSAIDs have important analgesic actions in the spinal cord.

B. Inhibition

Transmission of nociceptive input in the spinal cord can be inhibited by segmental activity in the cord itself, as well as by descending neural activity from supraspinal centers.

1. Segmental inhibition—Activation of large afferent fibers subserving sensation inhibits WDR neuron and spinothalamic tract activity. Moreover, activation of noxious stimuli in noncontiguous parts of the body inhibits WDR neurons at other levels, which may explain why pain in one part of the body inhibits pain in other parts. These two phenomena support a "gate" theory for pain processing in the spinal cord, as initially hypothesized by Melzack and Wall.

Glycine and γ-aminobutyric acid (GABA) are amino acids that function as inhibitory neurotransmitters and likely play an important role in segmental inhibition of pain in the spinal cord. Antagonism of glycine and GABA results in powerful facilitation of WDR neurons and produces allodynia and hyperesthesia. There are two subtypes of GABA receptors: $GABA_A$, for which muscimol is an agonist, and $GABA_B$, for which baclofen is an agonist. Segmental inhibition appears to be mediated by $GABA_B$ receptor activity. The $GABA_A$ receptor, which is activated by benzodiazepines, includes a Cl^- channel. Activation of glycine receptors also increases Cl^- conductance across neuronal cell membranes. Adenosine also modulates nociceptive activity in the dorsal horn. At least two receptors are known: A_1, which inhibits adenyl cyclase, and A_2, which stimulates adenyl cyclase. The A_1 receptor mediates adenosine's antinociceptive action.

2. Supraspinal inhibition—Several supraspinal structures send fibers down the spinal cord to inhibit pain in the dorsal horn. Important sites of origin for these descending pathways include the periaqueductal gray, reticular formation, and nucleus raphe magnus (NRM). Stimulation of the periaqueductal gray area in the midbrain produces widespread analgesia in humans. Axons from these tracts act presynaptically on primary afferent neurons and postsynaptically on second-order neurons (or interneurons). These pathways mediate their antinociceptive action via α_2-adrenergic, serotonergic, and opiate (μ, δ, and κ) receptor mechanisms. These pathways explain the analgesic efficacy of antidepressants that block the reuptake of catecholamines and serotonin.

Inhibitory adrenergic pathways originate primarily from the periaqueductal gray area and the reticular formation. Norepinephrine mediates this action via activation of presynaptic or postsynaptic α_2 receptors. At least part of the descending inhibition from the periaqueductal gray is relayed first to the NRM and medullary reticular formation; serotonergic fibers from the NRM then relay the inhibition to dorsal horn neurons via the dorsolateral funiculus.

The *endogenous opiate system* (primarily the NRM and reticular formation) acts via methionine enkephalin, leucine enkephalin, and β-endorphin, all of which are antagonized by naloxone. These opioids act presynaptically to hyperpolarize primary afferent neurons and inhibit the release of substance P; they also appear to cause some postsynaptic inhibition. Exogenous opioids primarily act postsynaptically on the second-order neurons or interneurons in the substantia gelatinosa.

PATHOPHYSIOLOGY OF CHRONIC PAIN

7 **Chronic pain may be caused by a combination of peripheral, central, and psychological mechanisms.** Sensitization of nociceptors plays a major role in the origin of pain associated with peripheral mechanisms, such as chronic musculoskeletal and visceral disorders.

TABLE 47–5 Mechanisms of neuropathic pain.

Spontaneous self-sustaining neuronal activity in the primary afferent neuron (such as a neuroma)
Marked mechanosensitivity associated with chronic nerve compression
Short-circuits between pain fibers and other types of fibers following demyelination, resulting in activation of nociceptive fibers by nonnoxious stimuli at the site of injury (ephaptic transmission)
Functional reorganization of receptive fields in dorsal horn neurons such that sensory input from surrounding intact nerves emphasizes or intensifies any input from the area of injury
Spontaneous electrical activity in dorsal horn cells or thalamic nuclei
Release of segmental inhibition in the spinal cord
Loss of descending inhibitory influences that are dependent on normal sensory input
Lesions of the thalamus or other supraspinal structures

Neuropathic pain involves peripheral–central and central neural mechanisms that are complex and generally associated with partial or complete lesions of peripheral nerves, dorsal root ganglia, nerve roots, or more central structures (Table 47–5). Peripheral mechanisms include spontaneous discharges, sensitization of receptors (to mechanical, thermal, and chemical stimuli), and upregulation of adrenergic receptors. Neural inflammation may also be present. Systemic administration of local anesthetics and anticonvulsants suppresses the spontaneous firing of sensitized or traumatized neurons, and this laboratory observation is reinforced by the clinical efficacy of agents such as lidocaine, mexiletine, and carbamazepine in many patients with neuropathic pain. Central mechanisms include loss of segmental inhibition, wind-up of WDR neurons, spontaneous discharges in deafferentated neurons, and reorganization of neural connections.

The sympathetic nervous system appears to play a major role in some patients with chronic pain. The efficacy of sympathetic nerve blocks in some of these patients supports the concept of sympathetically maintained pain. Painful disorders that often respond to sympathetic blocks include complex regional pain syndrome, deafferentation syndromes due to nerve avulsion or amputations,

TABLE 47–6 Psychological mechanisms or environmental factors associated with chronic pain.

Psychophysiological mechanisms in which emotional factors act as the initiating cause (eg, tension headaches)
Learned or operant behavior in which chronic behavior patterns are rewarded (eg, by attention of a spouse) following an often minor injury
Psychopathology such as major affective disorders (depression), schizophrenia, and somatization disorders (conversion hysteria) in which the patient has an abnormal preoccupation with bodily functions
Pure psychogenic mechanisms (somatoform pain disorder), in which suffering is experienced despite absence of nociceptive input

and postherpetic neuralgia. However, the simplistic theory of heightened sympathetic activity resulting in vasoconstriction, edema, and hyperalgesia fails to account for the warm skin and erythema observed in some patients. Similarly, clinical and experimental observations do not satisfactorily support the theory of aberrant (*ephaptic*) transmission between pain fibers and adjacent demyelinated sympathetic fibers.

Psychological mechanisms or environmental factors are rarely the sole mechanisms for chronic pain but are commonly seen in combination with other mechanisms (Table 47–6).

SYSTEMIC RESPONSES TO PAIN

Systemic Responses to Acute Pain

Acute pain is typically associated with a systemic neuroendocrine stress response that is proportional to pain intensity. The pain pathways mediating the afferent limb of this response are discussed above. The efferent limb is mediated by the sympathetic nervous and endocrine systems. Sympathetic activation increases efferent sympathetic tone to all viscera and releases catecholamines from the adrenal medulla. The hormonal response results from increased sym-

pathetic tone and from hypothalamically mediated reflexes. *Moderate to severe acute pain,*

regardless of site, may adversely affect perioperative recovery and outcomes.

A. Cardiovascular Effects

Cardiovascular effects of acute pain often include hypertension, tachycardia, enhanced myocardial irritability, and increased systemic vascular resistance. Cardiac output increases in most normal patients but may decrease in patients with compromised ventricular function. Because of the increase in myocardial oxygen demand, pain can worsen or precipitate myocardial ischemia.

B. Respiratory Effects

An increase in total body oxygen consumption and carbon dioxide production promotes an increase in minute ventilation. The latter increases the work of breathing, particularly in patients with underlying lung disease. Pain due to abdominal or thoracic incisions further compromises pulmonary function because of guarding (splinting). Decreased movement of the chest wall reduces tidal volume and functional residual capacity, promoting atelectasis, intrapulmonary shunting, hypoxemia, and, less commonly, hypoventilation. Reductions in vital capacity impair coughing and clearing of secretions.

C. Gastrointestinal and Urinary Effects

Enhanced sympathetic tone increases sphincter tone and decreases intestinal and urinary bladder motility, promoting ileus and urinary retention. Hypersecretion of gastric acid can promote stress ulceration. Nausea, vomiting, and constipation are common. In addition, systemic opioids used to treat postoperative pain (and also administered as a component of the operative anesthetic) are a common cause of postoperative ileus and urinary retention.

D. Endocrine Effects

Stress increases the release of catabolic hormones (catecholamines, cortisol, glucagon) and inhibits the release of anabolic hormones (insulin and testosterone). Patients develop a negative nitrogen balance, carbohydrate intolerance, and increased lipolysis. The increase in cortisol, renin, angiotensin, aldosterone, and antidiuretic hormone results in sodium retention, water retention, and secondary expansion of the extracellular space.

E. Hematological Effects

The neuroendocrine stress response to acute pain may increase platelet adhesiveness, reduce fibrinolysis, and promote a hypercoagulable state.

F. Immune Effects

The neuroendocrine stress response produces leukocytosis and may predispose patients to infection. Worsening carbohydrate intolerance with sustained hyperglycemia also increases the risk of infection. Stress-related immunodepression may enhance tumor growth and metastasis.

G. Psychological Effects

Anxiety and sleep disturbances are common reactions to acute pain. Depression is common with prolonged pain. Some patients react with frustration and anger that may be directed at family, friends, and medical staff.

Systemic Responses to Chronic Pain

The neuroendocrine stress response in the setting of chronic pain is generally observed only in patients with severe recurring pain due to peripheral (nociceptive) mechanisms and in patients with prominent central mechanisms such as pain associated with paraplegia. Sleep and affective disturbances, particularly depression, are often prominent in patients with chronic pain, and many such patients also experience significant changes in appetite and increased stress related to social relationships.

Evaluation of the Patient with Chronic Pain

9 **The evaluation of any patient with pain should include several key components, including location, onset, and quality of pain; any alleviating or exacerbating factors; and pain history, including previous therapies and changes in symptoms over time. Chronic pain usually includes a psychological component that should be addressed.**

Questionnaires, diagrams, and pain scales are useful tools that help patients adequately describe the characteristics of their pain and how it affects their quality of life. Information gathered during the history and physical examination can help distinguish pain location, type, and systemic sequelae, if any. Imaging studies such as plain radiographs, computed tomography (CT), magnetic resonance imaging (MRI), and bone scans can often help delineate physiological causes. A comprehensive evaluation is needed prior to determining appropriate treatment options.

PAIN MEASUREMENT

Pain is a subjective experience that is influenced by psychological, social, cultural, and other variables. Clear definitions are necessary, as pain may be described in terms of tissue destruction or bodily or emotional reaction.

The numerical rating scale, Wong-Baker FACES rating scale, visual analog scale (VAS), and McGill Pain Questionnaire (MPQ) are most commonly used. In the numerical scale, 0 corresponds to no pain, and 10 is intended to reflect the worst possible pain. The Wong-Baker FACES pain scale, designed for children 3 years of age and older, is useful in patients with whom communication may be difficult. The patient is asked to point to various facial expressions ranging from a smiling face (no pain) to an extremely unhappy one that expresses the worst possible pain. The VAS is a 10-cm horizontal line labeled "no pain" at one end and "worst pain imaginable" on the other end. The patient is asked to mark on this line where the intensity of the pain lies. The distance from "no pain" to the patient's mark numerically quantifies the pain. The VAS is a simple and efficient method that correlates well with other reliable methods.

The MPQ is a checklist of words describing symptoms. Unlike other pain rating methods that assume pain is one-dimensional and describe intensity but not quality, the MPQ attempts to define the pain in three major dimensions: (1) sensory–discriminative (nociceptive pathways), (2) motivational–affective (reticular and limbic structures), and (3) cognitive–evaluative (cerebral cortex). It contains 20 sets of descriptive words that are divided into four major groups: 10 sensory, 5 affective, 1 evaluative, and 4 miscellaneous. The patient selects the sets that apply to their pain and circles the words in each set that best describe the pain.

PSYCHOSOCIAL EVALUATION

10 **Psychosocial evaluation is useful whenever medical evaluation fails to reveal an apparent cause for pain, when pain intensity, characteristics, or duration are disproportionate to disease or injury, or when psychological or social issues, or both, are apparent.** These types of evaluations help clarify the role of behavioral factors. The most commonly used psychological tests are the Minnesota Multiphasic Personality Inventory (MMPI) and the Beck Depression Inventory. The MMPI is used primarily to confirm clinical impressions about the role of psychological factors; it cannot reliably distinguish between "organic" and "functional" pain. Depression is very common in patients with chronic pain. It is often difficult to determine the relative contribution of depression to the suffering associated with pain. The Beck Depression Inventory is a useful test for identifying patients with major depression.

Several tests have been developed to assess functional limitations or impairment (disability) and quality of life. These include the Multidimensional Pain Inventory (MPI), Medical Outcomes Survey 36-Item Short Form (SF-36), Pain Disability Index (PDI), and Oswestry Disability Index (ODI).

Emotional disorders are commonly associated with reports of chronic pain, and chronic pain often results in varying degrees of psychological distress. Both the pain and emotional distress need to be treated. Table 47–7 lists emotional disorders in which treatment should be primarily directed at the emotional disorder.

ELECTROMYOGRAPHY & NERVE CONDUCTION STUDIES

Electromyography and **nerve conduction studies** complement one another and are useful for confirming the diagnosis of entrapment syndromes,

TABLE 47–7 Emotional and related disorders commonly associated with chronic pain.

Disorder	Brief Description
Somatization disorder	Physical symptoms of a medical condition that cannot be explained, resulting in involuntary distress and physical impairment
Conversion disorder	Symptoms of voluntary motor or sensory deficits that suggest a medical condition; symptoms cannot be medically explained but are associated with psychological factors and are not intentionally feigned
Hypochondriasis	Prolonged (>6 months) preoccupation with the fear of having a serious illness despite adequate medical evaluation and reassurance
Malingering	Intentional production of physical or psychological symptoms that is motivated by external incentives (eg, avoiding work or financial compensation)
Substance-related disorders	Habitual misuse of prescribed or illicit substances that often precedes and drives complaints of pain and drug-seeking behavior

radicular syndromes, neural trauma, and polyneuropathies. They can often distinguish between neurogenic and myogenic disorders. Patterns of abnormalities can localize a lesion to the spinal cord, nerve root, limb plexus, or peripheral nerve. In addition, they may also be useful in clarifying the contribution of "organic" disorders when psychogenic pain or a "functional" syndrome is suspected.

Electromyography employs needle electrodes to record potentials in individual muscles. Muscle potentials are recorded first while the muscle is at rest and then as the patient is asked to move the muscle. Abnormal findings suggestive of denervation include persistent insertion potentials, the presence of positive sharp waves, fibrillations, or fasciculation potentials. Abnormalities in muscles produce changes in amplitude and duration as well as polyphasic action potentials. Peripheral nerve conduction studies employ supramaximal stimulations of motor or mixed sensorimotor nerve, whereas complex motor action potentials are recorded over the appropriate muscle. The time between the stimulation and the onset of the muscle potential (latency) is a measurement of the fastest conducting motor fibers in the nerve. The amplitude of the recorded potential indicates the number of functional motor units, whereas its duration reflects the range of conduction velocities in the nerve. Conduction velocity can be obtained by stimulating the nerve from two points and comparing the latencies. When a pure sensory nerve is evaluated, the nerve is stimulated while action potentials are recorded either proximally or distally (antidromic conduction).

Nerve conduction studies distinguish between mononeuropathies (due to trauma, compression, or entrapment) and polyneuropathies. The latter includes acute or chronic neuropathies that are widespread and symmetrical (eg, related to diabetes, alcohol abuse, malnutrition, toxins, or drugs such as chemotherapeutic agents) or that are focal but random (eg, mononeuropathy multiplex).

Selected Pain Syndromes

ENTRAPMENT SYNDROMES

Neural compression may occur wherever a nerve courses through an anatomically narrowed passage, and *entrapment neuropathies* can involve sensory, motor, or mixed nerves. Genetic factors and repetitive macrotrauma or microtrauma are likely involved, and adjacent tenosynovitis is often responsible. Table 47–8 lists the most commonly recognized entrapment syndromes. When a sensory nerve is involved, patients report pain and numbness in its distribution distal to the site of entrapment; occasionally, a patient may report pain referred proximal to the site of entrapment. Entrapment of the sciatic nerve can mimic a herniated intervertebral disc. Entrapment of a motor nerve produces weakness in the muscles it innervates. Even entrapments of "pure" motor nerves can produce a vague pain that may be mediated by afferent fibers from muscles and joints. The diagnosis can usually be confirmed by electromyography and nerve conduction studies. Neural blockade of the nerve with local anesthetic,

TABLE 47–8 Entrapment neuropathies.

Nerve	Entrapment Site	Location of Pain
Cranial nerves VII, IX, and X	Styloid process or stylohyoid ligament	Ipsilateral tonsil, base of tongue, temporomandibular joint, and ear (Eagle syndrome)
Brachial plexus	Scalenus anticus muscle or a cervical rib	Ulnar side of arm and forearm (scalenus anticus syndrome)
Suprascapular nerve	Suprascapular notch	Posterior and lateral shoulder
Median nerve	Pronator teres muscle	Proximal forearm and palmar surface of the first three digits (pronator syndrome)
Median nerve	Carpal tunnel	Palmar surface of the first three digits (carpal tunnel syndrome)
Ulnar nerve	Cubital fossa (elbow)	Fourth and fifth digits of the hand (cubital tunnel syndrome)
Ulnar nerve	Guyon's canal (wrist)	Fourth and fifth digits of the hand
Lateral femoral cutaneous nerve	Anterior iliac spine under the inguinal ligament	Anterolateral thigh (meralgia paresthetica)
Obturator nerve	Obturator canal	Upper medial thigh
Saphenous nerve	Subsartorial tunnel (adductor canal)	Medial calf
Sciatic nerve	Sciatic notch	Buttock and leg (piriformis syndrome)
Common peroneal nerve	Fibular neck	Lateral distal leg and foot
Deep peroneal nerve	Anterior tarsal tunnel	Big toe or foot
Superficial peroneal nerve	Deep fascia above the ankle	Anterior ankle and dorsum of foot
Posterior tibial nerve	Posterior tarsal tunnel	Undersurface of foot (tarsal tunnel syndrome)
Interdigital nerve	Deep transverse tarsal ligament	Between toes and foot (Morton neuroma)

with or without corticosteroid, may be diagnostic and may provide temporary pain relief. Treatment is usually symptomatic, with oral analgesics and temporary immobilization, but it may eventually include operative decompression. The development of complex regional pain syndrome may respond to sympathetic blocks.

MYOFASCIAL PAIN

11 *Myofascial pain syndromes* are common disorders characterized by aching muscle pain, muscle spasm, stiffness, weakness, and, occasionally, by autonomic dysfunction. Patients have discrete areas (*trigger points*) of marked tenderness in one or more muscles or the associated connective tissue. Palpation of the involved muscles may reveal tight, ropy bands over trigger points. Signs of autonomic dysfunction (vasoconstriction or piloerection) in the overlying muscles may be present. The pain characteristically radiates in a fixed pattern that does not follow dermatomes.

Gross trauma or repetitive microtrauma may play a major role in initiating myofascial pain syndromes. Trigger points develop following acute injury; stimulation of these active trigger points produces pain, and the ensuing muscle spasm sustains the pain. When the acute episode subsides, the trigger points become *latent* (tender but not pain producing), only to be reactivated at a later time by subsequent stress. The pathophysiology is poorly understood.

The diagnosis of a myofascial pain syndrome is suggested by the character of the pain and by palpation of discrete trigger points that reproduce it. Common syndromes produce trigger points in the levator scapulae, masseter, quadratus lumborum, and gluteus medius muscles. The latter two syndromes produce low back pain and should be considered in all patients with back pain; moreover, gluteal trigger points can mimic S1 radiculopathy.

Although myofascial pain may spontaneously resolve without sequelae, many patients continue to have latent trigger points. When trigger points are active, treatment is directed at regaining muscle length and elasticity. Analgesia may be provided utilizing local anesthetic (1–3 mL) trigger point injections. Topical cooling with either an ethyl chloride or fluorocarbon (fluoromethane) spray can also induce reflex muscle relaxation, facilitating massage ("stretch and spray") and ultrasound therapy. Physical therapy is important in establishing and maintaining normal range of motion for affected muscles, and biofeedback may be helpful.

FIBROMYALGIA

The American College of Rheumatology has identified three criteria that, if met, suggest the diagnosis of *fibromyalgia*:

1. Widespread Pain Index (WPI) score of 7 or higher and a Symptom Severity (SS) Scale score of 5 or higher, or a WPI score of 3 to 6 and an SS Scale score of 9 or higher.
2. Symptoms remain at a similar level for at least 3 months.
3. Absence of another disorder that would otherwise explain the pain.

Treatment of fibromyalgia may include cardiovascular conditioning, strength training, improving sleep hygiene, cognitive-behavioral therapy, tai chi, patient education, and pharmacotherapy. Medications approved by the U.S. Food and Drug Administration (FDA) for the treatment of fibromyalgia include pregabalin (Lyrica), duloxetine (Cymbalta), and milnacipran (Savella). The use of low-dose naltrexone is currently being investigated.

LOW BACK PAIN & RELATED SYNDROMES

Back pain is a common complaint and a major cause of disability. Lumbosacral strain, degenerative disc disease, and myofascial syndromes are the most common causes. Low back pain, with or without associated leg pain, may also have congenital, traumatic, degenerative, inflammatory, infectious, metabolic, psychological, or neoplastic causes. Moreover, back pain can be due to disease processes in the abdomen and pelvis, particularly those affecting retroperitoneal structures (pancreas, kidneys, ureters, aorta), the uterus and adnexa, the prostate, or the rectosigmoid colon. Disorders of the hip can also mimic back disorders. A positive *Patrick's sign* (or *Patrick's test*)—that is, the elicitation of pain in the hip or sacroiliac joint when the examiner places the ipsilateral heel of the supine patient on the contralateral knee and presses down on the ipsilateral knee—helps identify back pain due to hip or sacroiliac joint disorders. This sign is also referred to by the acronym FABERE (sign) because the movement of the leg involves *f*lexion, *ab*duction, *e*xternal *r*otation, and *e*xtension.

1. Applied Anatomy of the Back

The back can be described in terms of *anterior* and *posterior* elements. The anterior elements consist of cylindrical vertebral bodies interconnected by intervertebral discs and supported by anterior and posterior longitudinal ligaments. The posterior elements are bony arches extending from each vertebral body, consisting of two pedicles, two transverse processes, two laminae, and a spinous process. The transverse and spinous processes provide points of attachment for the muscles that move and protect the spinal column. Adjacent vertebrae also articulate posteriorly by two gliding facet joints.

Spinal structures are innervated by the sinuvertebral branches and posterior rami of spinal nerves.

The sinuvertebral nerve arises before each spinal nerve divides into anterior and posterior rami and reenters the intervertebral foramen to innervate the posterior longitudinal ligament, the posterior annulus fibrosus, periosteum, dura, and epidural vessels. Paraspinal structures are supplied by the posterior primary ramus. Each facet joint is innervated by the *medial branch* of the posterior primary rami of the spinal nerves above and below the joint.

As lumbar spinal nerve roots exit the dural sac, they travel down 1 to 2 cm laterally before exiting through their respective intervertebral foramina; thus, for example, the L5 nerve root leaves the dural sac at the level of the L4–L5 disc (where it is more likely to be compressed) but leaves the spinal canal beneath the L5 pedicle opposite the L5–S1 disc.

2. Paravertebral Muscle & Lumbosacral Joint Sprain/Strain

Approximately 80% to 90% of low back pain reports arise from sprain or strain associated with lifting heavy objects, falls, or sudden abnormal movements of the spine. The term *sprain* is generally used when the pain is related to a well-defined acute injury, whereas *strain* is used when the pain is more chronic and is likely related to repetitive minor injuries.

Injury to paravertebral muscles and ligaments results in reflex muscle spasm, which may or may not be associated with trigger points. The pain is usually dull and aching and occasionally radiates down the buttocks or hips. Sprain is a self-limited benign process that resolves in 1 to 2 weeks. Symptomatic treatment consists of rest and oral analgesics.

The sacroiliac joint is particularly vulnerable to rotational injuries. It is one of the largest joints in the body and functions to transfer weight from the upper body to the lower extremities. Acute or chronic injury can cause *subluxation* (slippage) of the joint. Pain originating from this joint is characteristically located along the posterior ilium and radiates down the hips and posterior thigh to the knees. The diagnosis is suggested by tenderness on palpation, particularly on the medial aspect of the posterior superior iliac spine, and by pain with compression of the joints. Pain relief following injection of the joint with local anesthetic (3 mL) is diagnostic and may also be therapeutic. Injection of intraarticular steroid medication may be considered. For potentially longer duration of analgesia, radiofrequency ablation may be performed at the dorsal ramus of L5 as well as the lateral branches of the S1, S2, and S3 nerves if the patient initially responded well to local anesthetic injections of the sacroiliac joint or to diagnostic injections of these nerves.

3. Buttock Pain

Buttock pain may arise from several different factors and can be quite debilitating. *Coccydynia* may result from trauma to the coccyx or surrounding ligaments. It may resolve by means of physical therapy, coccygeal nerve blocks to the lateral aspects of the coccyx, or ablative or neuromodulatory procedures. *Piriformis syndrome* presents as pain in the buttock, which can be accompanied by numbness and tingling in the distribution of the sciatic nerve. The nerve may or may not be entrapped. Injection of local anesthetic into the belly of this muscle or into trigger points located at the origin and insertion of the muscle may help relieve the pain. Spinal stenosis and disc disease can also produce buttock pain.

4. Degenerative Disc Disease

Intervertebral discs bear at least one-third of the weight of the spinal column. Their central portion, the *nucleus pulposus*, is composed of gelatinous material early in life. This material degenerates and becomes fibrotic with advancing age and following trauma. The nucleus pulposus is ringed by the *annulus fibrosus*, which is thinnest posteriorly and bounded superiorly and inferiorly by cartilaginous plates. *Discogenic pain* may be due to one of two major mechanisms: (1) protrusion or extrusion of the nucleus pulposus posteriorly or (2) loss of disc height, resulting in the reactive formation of bony spurs (osteophytes) from the rims of the vertebral bodies above and below the disc. Degenerative disc disease most commonly affects the lumbar spine because it is subjected to the greatest motion and because the posterior longitudinal ligament is thinnest at L2–L5. Factors such as increased body weight and cigarette smoking may play a role in the development of lumbar disc disease. The role of the disc in producing chronic back pain is not clearly understood. In patients with persistent axial low back pain, the history and physical examination may provide clues. There may be an element of discogenic pain if the patient has discomfort when sitting or standing, or when maintaining a certain position for an extended period of time.

Discography is a procedure that is sometimes used to try to provide some objective evidence of the role of a given disc in producing a patient's back pain. The opening pressure can be assessed via a needle inserted into the disc, and a subsequent injection of radiocontrast material typically produces increased pressure that may reproduce the patient's pain and may provide radiographic identification of anatomic abnormalities within the disc (eg, a rent or tear). If the pain produced with injection is similar to that which the patient experiences on a daily basis, it is deemed *concordant* pain. If not, it is deemed *discordant*. In some circumstances, the pressure in the disc following injection is not significantly higher than the opening pressure, and this may be due to the presence of a fissure in the disc that tracks to the epidural space. Treatment options for discogenic pain include conservative therapy, steroid injections into the disc, heating the posterior annulus of the disc by way of radiofrequency ablation, surgical removal of herniated disc fragments, and surgical fusion with bone graft or hardware placement. Each option has shown mixed degrees of success. The evaluation and treatment of discogenic pain is an area of significant controversy and ongoing research. In the presence of axial low back pain with degenerative changes along the vertebral body endplate, consideration may be given to intraosseous basivertebral nerve radiofrequency ablation for what is considered *vertebrogenic* pain. This transpedicular procedure may obviate the need for a diagnostic discography procedure and has been supported in recent clinical trials. **Figures 47–6A, B, and C** illustrate the basivertebral nerve radiofrequency procedure.

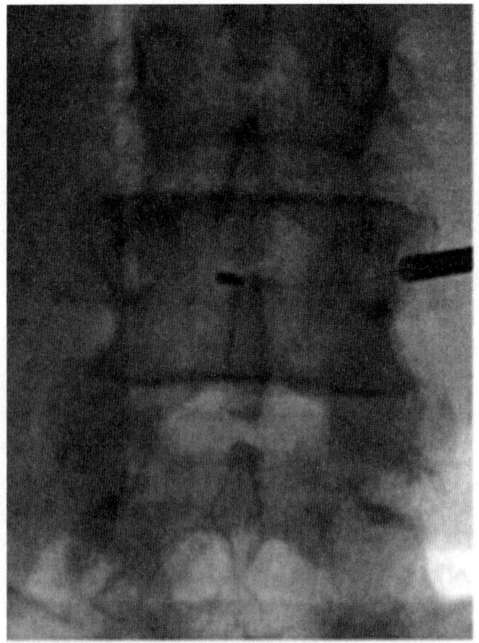

A

FIGURE 47–6A Basivertebral nerve radiofrequency ablation. In the anterior/posterior fluoroscopic image above, a trochar has been advanced through the right pedicle of the L4 vertebra, and a curvilinear probe has been advanced beyond the midline, 1 cm anterior to the central posterior aspect of the vertebral body and in the distribution of the basivertebral nerve.

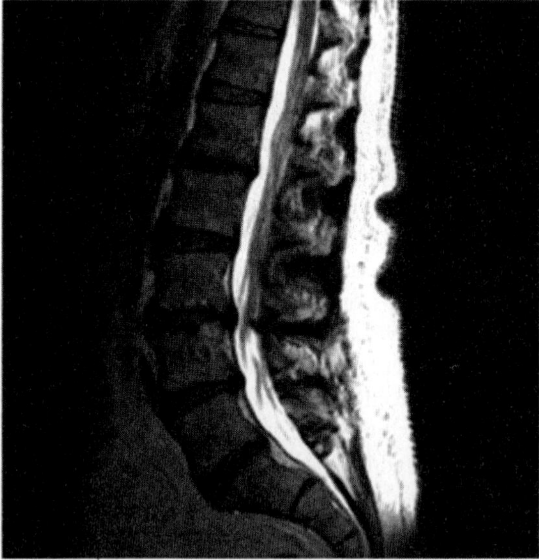

B

FIGURE 47–6B Basivertebral nerve radiofrequency ablation. In the subsequent sagittal view of postprocedure T2-weighted magnetic resonance imaging, the 1-cm spherical lesions from this two-level radiofrequency ablation procedure can be seen at L3 and L4, with degenerative (Modic) changes appreciated at the inferior end-plate of L3 and the superior end-plate of L4.

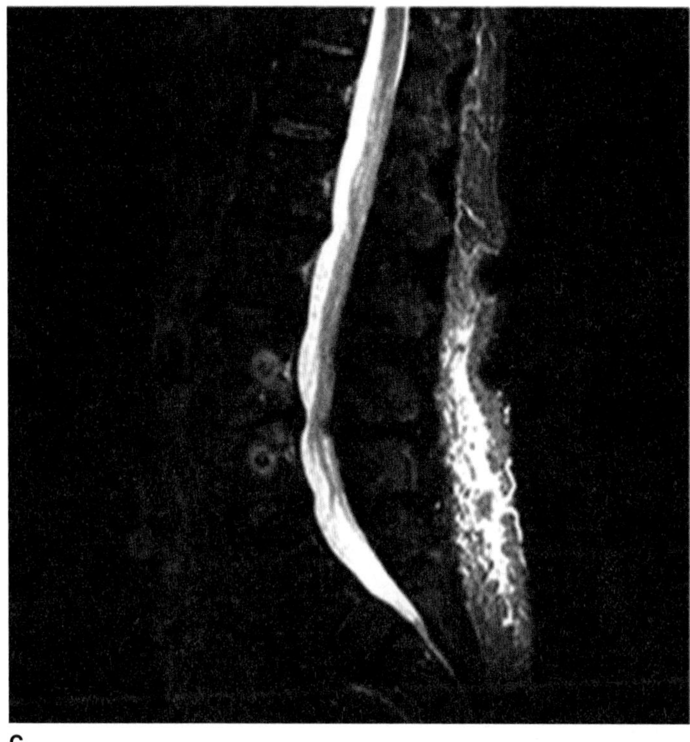

FIGURE 47–6C Basivertebral nerve radiofrequency ablation. The corresponding short tau inversion recovery (STIR) magnetic resonance imaging reveals active inflammatory changes in the respective end-plates of L3 and L4, indicative of active vertebral degeneration. A STIR sequence is a magnetic resonance imaging technique that suppresses signal from fat and enhances signal from neoplastic and inflammatory tissue.

Herniated (Prolapsed) Intervertebral Disc

Weakness and degeneration of the annulus fibrosus and posterior longitudinal ligament can allow herniation of the nucleus pulposus posteriorly into the spinal canal. 12 **Ninety percent of disc herniations occur at L5–S1 or L4–L5. Symptoms usually develop following flexion injuries or heavy lifting and may be associated with bulging, protrusion, or extrusion of the disc.** Disc herniations usually occur posterolaterally and often result in compression of adjacent nerve roots, producing pain that radiates along the corresponding dermatome (*radiculopathy*, or *radicular pain*). *Sciatica* describes pain along the sciatic nerve due to compression of the lower lumbar nerve roots. When disc material is extruded through the annulus fibrosus and posterior longitudinal ligament, free fragments can become wedged in the spinal canal or the intervertebral foramina. Less commonly, a large disc bulges or large fragments extrude posteriorly, compressing the cauda equina in the dural sac; in these instances, patients can experience bilateral pain, urinary retention, or, less commonly, fecal incontinence.

Pain associated with disc disease is aggravated by bending, lifting, prolonged sitting, or anything that increases intraabdominal pressure, such as sneezing, coughing, or straining. It is usually relieved by lying down. Numbness or weakness is indicative of radiculopathy (Table 47–9). Bulging of the disc through the posterior longitudinal ligament can also produce low back pain that radiates to the hips or buttocks. *Straight leg-raising tests* may be used to assess nerve root compression. With the patient supine and the knee fully extended, the leg on the affected side is raised, and the angle at which

TABLE 47–9 Lumbar disc radiculopathies.

	Disk Level		
	L3–L4 (L4 Nerve)	*L4–L5 (L5 Nerve)*	*L5–S1 (S1 Nerve)*
Pain distribution	Anterolateral thigh, anteromedial calf to the ankle	Lateral thigh, anterolateral calf, medial dorsum of foot, especially between the first and second toes	Gluteal region, posterior thigh, posterolateral calf, lateral dorsum and undersurface of the foot, particularly between fourth and fifth toes
Weakness	Quadriceps femoris	Dorsiflexion of the foot	Plantar flexion of foot
Reflex affected	Knee	None	Ankle

the pain develops is noted; dorsiflexion of the ankle with the leg raised typically exacerbates the pain by further stretching the lumbosacral plexus. Pain while raising the contralateral leg is an even more reliable sign of nerve compression.

MRI evaluation of the spine has increased dramatically in the past decade in association with a severalfold increase in back surgeries—without improved patient outcome. The American Pain Society's clinical practice guidelines for low back pain do not recommend routine imaging or other diagnostic tests for patients with nonspecific low back pain. Up to 30% to 40% of asymptomatic persons have abnormalities of spinal structures on CT or MRI. In addition, the patient's awareness of their imaging abnormalities may influence self-perception of health and functional ability.

Imaging studies and other tests should be obtained when severe or progressive neurological deficits are present or when serious underlying conditions are suspected. CT myelography is the most sensitive test for evaluating subtle neural compression. Discography may be considered when the pain pattern does not match the clinical findings. A centrally herniated disc will usually cause pain at the lower level, and a laterally protruded disc will cause pain at the same level as the disc. For example, a centrally located disc herniation at L4–L5 may compress the L5 nerve root, whereas a laterally located disc herniation at this level may compress the L4 nerve root.

The natural course of herniated disc disorders is generally benign, and the duration of pain is usually less than 2 months. Over 75% of patients treated nonsurgically, even those with radiculopathy, progress to complete or near-complete pain relief. The goals of treatment should therefore be to alleviate pain and to rehabilitate the patient to return to a maximally functional quality of life and employment (if employed). Acute back pain due to a herniated disc can be initially managed with modification of activity and with medications such as NSAIDs and acetaminophen. A short course of opioids may be considered for patients with severe pain. After the acute symptoms subside, the patient can be referred to a physical therapist for instruction on exercises to improve lower back health. Patients who smoke tobacco should be advised to stop smoking, not only for the obvious health benefits but also because nicotine may further compromise blood flow to the relatively avascular intervertebral disc. Percutaneous disc decompression involving extraction of a small amount of nucleus pulposus may help decompress the nerve root. For patients with acute-onset weakness correlating with the level of the disc herniation, surgical management should be considered.

When symptoms persist beyond 3 months, the pain may be considered chronic and may require a multidisciplinary approach. Physical therapy continues to be a very important component of rehabilitation. NSAIDs and antidepressants are also helpful, and percutaneous interventions may be considered. Of note, back supports should be discouraged because they may weaken paraspinal muscles.

Spinal Stenosis

Spinal stenosis is a disease of advancing age. Degeneration of the nucleus pulposus reduces disc height and leads to osteophyte formation (*spondylosis*) at

the endplates of adjoining vertebral bodies. In conjunction with facet joint hypertrophy and ligamentum flavum hypertrophy and calcification, this process leads to progressive narrowing of the neural foramina and spinal canal. Neural compression may cause radiculopathy that mimics a herniated disc. Extensive osteophyte formation may compress multiple nerve roots and cause bilateral
13 pain. The back pain usually radiates into the buttocks, thighs, and legs. It is characteristically worse with exercise and relieved by rest, particularly sitting with the spine flexed (*shopping cart sign*). The terms *pseudoclaudication* and *neurogenic claudication* are used to describe such pain that develops with prolonged standing or ambulation. The diagnosis is suggested by the clinical presentation and is confirmed by MRI, CT, or myelography. Electromyography and nerve conduction studies may be useful in evaluating the degree of neurological compromise.

Patients with mild to moderate stenosis and radicular symptoms may obtain benefit from epidural steroid injections via a transforaminal, interlaminar, or caudal approach, which may help these individuals tolerate physical therapy. Those with moderate to severe stenosis may be candidates for the minimally invasive lumbar decompression (MILD) procedure, which involves percutaneously sculpting the lamina and ligamentum flavum to reduce central canal compression. Severe, multilevel symptoms may warrant surgical decompression.

5. Facet Syndrome

Degenerative changes in the facet (zygapophyseal) joints may also produce back pain. Pain may be near the midline; radiate to the gluteal region, thigh, and knee; and be associated with muscle spasm. Hyperextension and lateral rotation of the spine usually exacerbate the pain. The diagnosis may be confirmed if pain relief is obtained following intraarticular injection of local anesthetic solution into affected joints or by blockade of the medial branch of the posterior division (ramus) of the spinal nerves that innervate them. Long-term studies suggest that medial branch nerve blocks are more effective than facet joint injections. Medial branch rhizotomy may provide long-term analgesia for patients with facet joint disease.

6. Cervical Pain

Although most spine-related pain due to disc disease, spinal stenosis, or degenerative changes in the zygapophyseal joints is felt in the low back and lower extremities, patients may have cervical pain attributed to these processes. *A key anatomic difference is that the cervical nerve roots, unlike those in the thoracic and lumbar spine, exit the foramina above the vertebral bodies for which they are named.* This occurs until the level of C7, where the extra cervical nerve roots, C8, exit below the pedicles of C7, thus transitioning to the nomenclature of the thoracic- and lumbar-level vertebral bodies and nerve root denominations. The clinical examination may help identify the nerve root that is affected with confirmation by a selective nerve root block. Risks inherent with percutaneous cervical procedures include accidental intravascular injection of local anesthetic or steroid. *Particulate steroid injections in the neck have been associated with devastating outcomes and must be avoided.*

For primarily axial pain in the neck with extension into the head or to the shoulders, cervical medial branch blocks may clarify the diagnosis. Long-term analgesia may be obtained with radiofrequency ablation of the medial branches innervating the zygapophyseal joints.

7. Congenital Abnormalities

Congenital abnormalities of the back may be asymptomatic and remain occult for many years. Abnormal spinal mechanics can make the patient prone to back pain, and in some instances, progressive deformities. Relatively common anomalies include sacralization of L5 (the vertebral body is fused to the sacrum), lumbarization of S1 (it functions as a sixth lumbar vertebra), *spondylolysis* (disruption of the pars interarticularis), *spondylolisthesis* (displacement anteriorly of one vertebral body on the next due to disruption of the posterior elements, usually the pars interarticularis), and *spondyloptosis* (subluxation of one vertebral body on another resulting in one body in front of the next). These diagnoses are made with radiographic imaging studies. Spinal fusion may be necessary for patients with progressive symptoms and spinal instability.

8. Tumors

A wide range of benign and malignant tumors may lead to back pain. When diagnosed by imaging alone, these tumors will be managed by neurosurgeons, radiotherapists, and/or oncologists, not by pain specialists.

9. Infection

Bacterial infections of the spine usually begin as discitis before progressing to osteomyelitis and can be due to pyogenic as well as tuberculous organisms. Patients may present with chronic back pain without fever or leukocytosis (eg, spinal tuberculosis). Those with acute discitis, osteomyelitis, or epidural abscess present with acute pain, fever, leukocytosis, elevated sedimentation rate, and elevated C-reactive protein, warranting immediate initiation of antibiotics. Urgent surgical intervention is indicated when the patient also experiences acute weakness.

10. Arthritides

Ankylosing spondylitis is a familial disorder that is associated with the HLA-B27 antigen. It typically presents as low back pain associated with early morning stiffness in a young male patient. The pain has an insidious onset and may initially improve with activity. After a few months to years, the pain gradually intensifies and is associated with progressively restricted movement of the spine. Diagnosis may be difficult early in the disease, but radiographic evidence of sacroiliitis is usually present. As the disease progresses, the spine develops a characteristic "bamboo-like" radiographic appearance. Some patients develop arthritis of the hips and shoulders, as well as extraarticular inflammatory manifestations. Treatment is primarily directed at the functional preservation of posture. NSAIDs are effective analgesics that reduce early morning stiffness. Anti–tumor necrosis factor-α agents, including infliximab (Remicade), etanercept (Enbrel), adalimumab (Humira), and golimumab (Simponi), decrease the progression of ankylosing spondylitis when administered early in the course of therapy. However, patients treated with these medications may be at increased risk for infection and development of lymphoma.

Patients with Reiter syndrome, psoriatic arthritis, or inflammatory bowel disease may also present with low back pain, but extraspinal manifestations are usually more prominent. Rheumatoid arthritis usually spares the spine except for the zygapophyseal joints of the cervical spine.

NEUROPATHIC PAIN

Neuropathic pain tends to be paroxysmal and sometimes lancinating with a burning quality, and it is usually accompanied by hyperpathia. It is associated with diabetic neuropathy, causalgia, phantom limbs, postherpetic neuralgia, stroke, spinal cord injury, and multiple sclerosis. Cancer pain and chronic low back pain may also have prominent neuropathic components. Mechanisms of neuropathic pain are reviewed earlier in this chapter.

Neuropathic pain is often difficult to treat, and multiple therapeutic modalities may be needed. Treatment options include anticonvulsants (eg, gabapentin, pregabalin), antidepressants (tricyclic antidepressants or serotonin-norepinephrine reuptake inhibitors), antiarrhythmics (mexiletine), α_2-adrenergic agonists (clonidine), topical agents (lidocaine or capsaicin), and analgesics (NSAIDs and opioids). Of note, tricyclic antidepressants may have significant anticholinergic side effects that may limit their tolerability; secondary amines, such as nortriptyline or desipramine, may have fewer or less severe anticholinergic side effects than tertiary amines such as amitriptyline or imipramine. Sympathetic blocks are effective in selected disorders (see later discussion). Spinal cord stimulation may be effective for patients who do not tolerate or respond to other treatments. Spinal opioids may be effective and appropriate for selected patients.

Diabetic Neuropathy

14 *Diabetic neuropathy* is the most common type of neuropathic pain and is a major cause of morbidity and disability. Its pathophysiology may be related to microangiopathy and to abnormal glycation of proteins as a consequence of chronic

hyperglycemia. Diabetic neuropathy may be generalized, symmetric, focal, or multifocal, affecting peripheral (sensory or motor), cranial, or autonomic nerves.

The most common diabetic neuropathy syndrome is *peripheral polyneuropathy*, which results in symmetric numbness ("stocking-and-glove" distribution), paresthesia, dysesthesia, and pain. The pain varies in intensity, may be severe, and is often worst at night. Loss of proprioception may lead to gait disturbances, and sensory deficits can lead to repetitive traumatic injuries. Isolated mononeuropathies affecting individual nerves may lead to wrist or foot drop or to cranial nerve palsy. Mononeuropathies typically have a sudden onset and are self-limiting, lasting a few weeks. Autonomic neuropathy typically affects the gastrointestinal tract, causing diarrhea, delayed gastric emptying, and esophageal motility disorders. Orthostatic hypotension and other forms of autonomic dysfunction are common.

Treatment of diabetic neuropathy is symptomatic and directed at optimal glycemic control to slow progression. Acetaminophen and NSAIDs are usually ineffective for moderate to severe pain, and risks associated with opioids limit their use. Adjuvant drugs play a major role. The combination of an antiepileptic drug and a tricyclic antidepressant may be particularly effective.

Sympathetically Maintained & Sympathetically Independent Pain

15 ***Complex regional pain syndrome* (CRPS) is a neuropathic pain disorder with significant autonomic features that is usually subdivided into two variants: *CRPS 1*, formerly known as *reflex sympathetic dystrophy* (RSD), and *CRPS 2*, formerly known as *causalgia*. The major difference between the two is the absence or presence, respectively, of documented nerve injury.** Signs, symptoms, pathophysiology, and response to treatment are quite similar. Previously, this condition was thought to represent sympathetically maintained pain, but there is recent evidence that in some cases the pain may be sympathetically independent.

CRPS is a largely underdiagnosed condition affecting at least 50,000 patients a year in the United States alone. It affects individuals from childhood to late adulthood and may occur more commonly in females. Patients frequently present with burning neuropathic pain accompanied by hyperalgesia and allodynia. The autonomic nervous system may be involved, exemplified by alterations in sweating (sudomotor changes), color, and skin temperature, and by trophic changes in the skin, hair, or nails. Decreases in strength and range of motion in the affected extremity may be present. CRPS 2 may develop after minimal injury, though the most common initiating events are surgery, fractures, crush injuries, and sprains.

The pathophysiology of CRPS 1 and 2 probably involves both the sympathetic nervous system and the central nervous system. There may be changes in the cutaneous innervation after a nerve injury, along with changes in central and peripheral sensitization. Genetic, inflammatory, and psychological factors may all play roles. Causalgia (which means burning pain), first identified by Weir Mitchell in injured veterans of the American Civil War, typically follows gunshot injuries or other major trauma to large nerves. The pain often has an immediate onset and is associated with allodynia, hyperpathia, and vasomotor and sudomotor dysfunction. It is exacerbated by factors that increase sympathetic tone, such as fear, anxiety, light, noise, or touch. The syndrome has a variable duration that can range from days to months or may be permanent. Causalgia commonly affects the brachial plexus, particularly the median nerve, and the tibial division of the sciatic nerve in the lower extremity.

Patients with CRPS often respond to sympathetic blocks, but a multidisciplinary therapeutic approach must be utilized to avoid long-term functional and psychological disability. Some patients recover spontaneously, but if CRPS is left untreated, other patients can progress to severe and irreversible functional disability. Sympathetic blocks and intravenous regional sympatholytic blockade are equally effective; these blocks should be continued until either a cure is achieved or the therapeutic response plateaus. The blocks facilitate physical therapy, which plays a central role and typically consists of active movement without weights and desensitization therapy. Many patients require a series of three to seven blocks. The likelihood of a cure is greater (>90%) if treatment is initiated within 1 month of symptom onset and appears to decrease over time with therapeutic delay.

Some patients benefit from transcutaneous electrical nerve stimulation (TENS) therapy. Spinal cord stimulation can be particularly effective in both acute and chronic settings. In the acute phase of treatment, there is increasing interest in placing tunneled epidural catheters for infusion therapy, or percutaneous electrodes for extended trials of spinal cord stimulation, in order to help patients tolerate physical therapy. Many patients benefit from surgical implantation of peripheral nerve stimulators placed directly on larger injured nerves.

For sympathetically maintained pain, oral α-adrenergic blockers, such as the nonselective phenoxybenzamine or the α_1-selective prazosin, may be beneficial. Orthostatic hypotension may occur with these agents, and dosage should be increased gradually. Anticonvulsant and antidepressant medications may also be beneficial.

Surgical sympathectomy in patients with chronic symptoms frequently results in only transient relief and, in some cases, a new, alternate pain syndrome. Patients with pain refractory to prior medical or procedural therapies may respond to intravenous ketamine infusions in a monitored setting.

ACUTE HERPES ZOSTER & POSTHERPETIC NEURALGIA

The varicella-zoster virus (VZV) infects dorsal root ganglia during an initial childhood chickenpox infection, where it remains latent until reactivation. Acute herpes zoster, which represents VZV reactivation, manifests as an erythematous vesicular rash (*shingles*) in a dermatomal distribution that is usually associated with severe pain. Dermatomes T3–L3 are most commonly affected. The pain often precedes the rash by 48 to 72 h, and the rash usually lasts 1 to 2 weeks. Herpes zoster may occur at any age but is most common in older adults and immunocompromised individuals. Approximately one in three people will develop herpes zoster during their lifetime. It is typically a self-limited disorder in younger, healthy patients (<50 years old). Treatment is primarily supportive, consisting of oral analgesics and oral acyclovir, famciclovir, ganciclovir, or valacyclovir. Antiviral therapy reduces the duration of the rash and speeds healing. Immunocompromised patients with disseminated infection (nondermatomal distribution of vesicles) require intravenous acyclovir therapy.

The incidence of severe, radicular pain following resolution of acute herpes zoster, a condition termed *postherpetic neuralgia* (PHN), is estimated to be 50% in patients older than 50 years of age. PHN is often debilitating and can be very difficult to treat, frequently lasting months to years. An oral course of corticosteroids during acute zoster may decrease the incidence of PHN but remains controversial and may increase the likelihood of viral dissemination in immunocompromised patients. Sympathetic blocks performed during the acute episode of herpes zoster often produce excellent analgesia and may decrease the incidence of PHN, though this is controversial. Some studies suggest that when sympathetic blocks are initiated within 2 months of the rash, PHN resolves in up to 80% of patients. Once the neuralgia is well established, however, sympathetic blocks, like other treatments, are generally ineffective. Antidepressants, anticonvulsants, and TENS may be useful in some patients. Tricyclic antidepressants may be particularly effective, though their use is often limited by anticholinergic side effects. Application of a transdermal lidocaine 5% patch (Lidoderm) over the most painful area may help relieve symptoms, presumably by decreasing peripheral sensitization of nerve endings and receptors. Application of capsaicin cream or a transdermal capsaicin 8% patch (Qutenza) may be helpful; however, Qutenza must be administered in a monitored setting. Administration of EMLA (*e*utectic *m*ixture of *l*ocal *a*nesthetic) cream 1 h before application of the transdermal capsaicin patch may decrease the incidence and severity of pain from the capsaicin in the patch. Epidural steroid injections have not been proven to prevent postherpetic neuralgia. The optimal management of herpes zoster and PHN is *prevention*, and zoster vaccine (Shingrix) is strongly recommended for all immunocompetent individuals 50 years of age or older who have no contraindications.

HEADACHE

Headache affects nearly everyone at some time in life. In the vast majority of cases, headaches are not of sufficient severity or frequency for the individual to seek medical attention and do not reflect a serious underlying disorder. However, as with other reports of pain, the possibility of a medically important underlying disorder should always be considered. The practitioner should solicit other associated symptoms or clinical findings that suggest serious underlying pathology. Table 47–10 lists important causes of headache. There is significant variability in clinical presentation and overlap in the symptoms of the major headache syndromes, particularly between tension and migraine headaches.

TABLE 47–10 Classification of headaches.

Classic headache syndromes
Migraine
Tension
Cluster
Vascular disorders
Temporal arteritis
Stroke
Venous thrombosis
Neuralgias
Trigeminal
Glossopharyngeal
Occipital
Intracranial pathology
Tumor
Cerebrospinal fluid leak
Pseudomotor cerebri
Meningitis
Aneurysm
Eye disorders
Glaucoma
Optic neuritis
Sinus disease
Allergic
Bacterial
Temporomandibular joint disease
Dental disorders
Drug-induced
Acute ingestion
Withdrawal (eg, caffeine and alcohol)
Systemic disorders
Infections
Viral (eg, influenza)
Bacterial
Fungal
Metabolic
Hypoglycemia
Hypoxemia
Hypercarbia
Trauma
Miscellaneous
Cold stimulus (swallowing cold liquid)

Tension Headache

Tension headaches are classically described as tight, bandlike pain or discomfort that is often associated with neck muscle tightness. The headache may be frontal, temporal, or occipital and is more often bilateral than unilateral. Intensity typically builds gradually and fluctuates, lasting hours to days. They may be associated with emotional stress or depression. Treatment is symptomatic and most commonly consists of NSAIDs or acetaminophen, or both, with caffeine often combined with both of these agents in a single medication.

Migraine Headache

Migraine headaches are typically described as throbbing or pounding and are often associated with photophobia, scotoma, nausea and vomiting, and localized transient neurological dysfunction (aura). The latter may be sensory, motor, visual, or olfactory. *Classic migraines* by definition are preceded by an aura, whereas *common migraines* are not. The pain lasts 4 to 72 h and is usually unilateral, but it can be bilateral with a frontotemporal location. Migraines primarily affect children (both sexes equally) and young adults (predominantly females). A family history is often present. Provocation by odors, certain foods (eg, red wine), menses, and sleep deprivation is common. Sleep characteristically relieves the headache. The pathophysiology is complex and may include vasomotor, autonomic (serotonergic brainstem systems), and trigeminal nucleus dysfunction. Treatment is both abortive and prophylactic. Rapid abortive treatment includes oxygen, sumatriptan (6 mg subcutaneously), dihydroergotamine

(1 mg intramuscularly or subcutaneously), intravenous lidocaine (100 mg), nasal butorphanol (1–2 mg), and sphenopalatine ganglion block. Other abortive options include zolmitriptan or sumatriptan nasal spray, dihydroergotamine nasal spray, or an oral serotonin 5-HT1B/1D-receptor agonist (almotriptan, frovatriptan, naratriptan, rizatriptan, eletriptan, or sumatriptan). Prophylactic treatment may include β-adrenergic blockers, calcium channel blockers, valproic acid, amitriptyline, and onabotulinumtoxinA (Botox) injections. In 2018, the FDA approved a new class of preventative migraine medications consisting of erenumab (Aimovig), fremanezumab (Ajovy), and galcanezumab (Emgality), all targeting CGRP.

Cluster Headache

Cluster headaches are classically unilateral and periorbital, occurring in clusters of one to three attacks a day over a 4- to 8-week period. The pain is described as a burning or drilling sensation that may awaken the patient from sleep. Each episode lasts 30 to 120 min. Remissions lasting a year at a time are common. Red eye, tearing, nasal stuffiness, ptosis, and Horner syndrome are classic findings. The headaches are typically episodic but can become chronic without remissions. Cluster headaches primarily affect males (90%). Abortive treatments include oxygen and sphenopalatine block. Lithium, a short course of steroid medication, and verapamil may be used for prophylaxis.

Temporal Arteritis

Temporal arteritis is an inflammatory disorder of extracranial arteries. The headache can be bilateral or unilateral and is located in the temporal area in at least 50% of patients. The pain develops over a few hours, is usually dull in quality but may be lancinating at times, and is often worse at night and in cold weather. Scalp tenderness is usually present. Temporal arteritis is often accompanied by polymyalgia rheumatica, fever, and weight loss. It is a relatively common disorder of older patients (>55 years), with an incidence of about 1 in 10,000 per year and a slight female predominance. Early diagnosis and treatment with steroids is important because progression can lead to blindness through involvement of the ophthalmic artery.

Trigeminal Neuralgia

16 **Trigeminal neuralgia (*tic douloureux*) is classically unilateral and usually located in the V2 or V3 distribution of the trigeminal nerve. It has an electric shock quality, with episodes lasting from seconds to minutes, and is often provoked by contact with a discrete trigger.** Facial muscle spasm may be present. Middle-aged and older adults are affected, with a 2:1 female-to-male ratio. Common causes of trigeminal neuralgia include compression of the nerve by the superior cerebellar artery as it exits the brainstem, multiple sclerosis, and cerebellopontine angle tumor. The drug of choice for treatment is carbamazepine, though it carries a risk of agranulocytosis. Phenytoin or baclofen may be added, particularly if patients do not tolerate sufficient doses of carbamazepine. More invasive treatments for patients who do not respond to drug therapy include glycerol injection, radiofrequency ablation, balloon compression of the Gasserian ganglion, and microvascular decompression of the trigeminal nerve.

ABDOMINAL PAIN

Chronic abdominal pain has a variety of causes, and it is useful to distinguish between *somatosensory*, *visceral*, and *centralized* pain origins. A differential epidural block may help in elucidating the primary source, but it is time consuming and may be difficult to interpret, and thus is uncommonly used. When it is thought that a patient may have abdominal pain originating from the abdominal wall, a transversus abdominis plane (TAP) block with ultrasound guidance may be both diagnostic and therapeutic (see Chapter 46). If no relief is obtained for the duration of the local anesthetic, the pain may have a visceral or central origin. Anterior cutaneous abdominal nerve block as well as trigger point injections of the abdominal wall are treatment options for patients with somatosensory abdominal wall pain. Visceral pain may best respond to a celiac or splanchnic nerve block and possibly to subsequent splanchnic

TABLE 47–11 Selected oral nonopioid analgesics.

Analgesic	Onset (h)	Dose (mg)	Dosing Interval (h)	Maximum Daily Dosage (mg)
Salicylates				
Acetylsalicylic acid (aspirin)	0.5–1.0	500–1000	4	3600–6000
Diflunisal (Dolobid)	1–2	500–1000	8–12	1500
Choline magnesium trisalicylate (Trilisate)	1–2	500–1000	12	2000–3000
p-Aminophenols				
Acetaminophen (Tylenol, others)	0.5	500–1000	4	1200–4000
Proprionic acids				
Ibuprofen (Motrin, others)	0.5	400	4–6	3200
Naproxen (Naprosyn)	1	250–500	12	1500
Naproxen sodium (Anaprox)	1–2	275–550	6–8	1375
Indoles				
Indomethacin (Indocin)	0.5	25–50	8–12	150–200
Ketorolac (Toradol)	0.5–1	10	4–6	40
COX-2 Inhibitors				
Celecoxib (Celebrex)	3	100–200	12	400

radiofrequency ablation. Patients with pain that is primarily of a central origin may respond to multidisciplinary therapy, including counseling and biofeedback training.

CANCER-RELATED PAIN

Cancer-related pain may be due to the primary cancer lesion itself, metastatic disease, complications such as neural compression or infection, or treatment such as surgery, chemotherapy, or radiation therapy. In addition, the cancer patient may have acute or chronic pain that is entirely unrelated to the cancer. The pain manager must therefore have a thorough understanding of the nature of the cancer, its stage, the presence of metastatic disease, and treatments.

Most cancer pain can be managed with oral analgesics. The World Health Organization recommends a progressive, three-step approach: (1) nonopioid analgesics such as aspirin, acetaminophen, or an NSAID for mild pain, (2) "weak" oral opioids such as codeine or oxycodone for moderate pain, and (3) stronger opioids such as morphine or hydromorphone for severe pain (Tables 47–11 and 47–12). Parenteral therapy is necessary when patients have refractory pain, cannot take medication orally, or have poor enteral absorption. Regardless of the agent selected, in most instances drug therapy should be provided on a fixed time schedule rather than as needed, with additional short-acting medication available for *breakthrough pain*. Adjuvant drug therapy, including antidepressants and anticonvulsants, may be used to both increase analgesia quality and decrease opioid-related side effects (Tables 47–13 and 47–14). Intrathecal drug delivery systems may improve analgesia and, via a drug-sparing effect, also help decrease side effects associated with oral or intravenous agents. Numerous intrathecal agents have been studied, and opioids have been utilized both alone and in combination with other medications. Ziconotide is a direct-acting N-type calcium-channel blocker that may be helpful for refractory pain or as a first-line agent. It is administered intrathecally and acts by decreasing the release of substance P from the presynaptic nerve terminal in the dorsal horn of the spinal cord.

TABLE 47–12 Oral opioids.

Opioid	Onset (h)	Relative Potency	Initial Dose (mg)	Dosing Interval (h)
Codeine	0.25–1.0	20	30–60	4
Hydromorphone (Dilaudid)	0.3–0.5	0.6	2–4	4
Hydrocodone[1]	0.5–1.0	3	5–7.5	4–6
Oxycodone[2] (OxyFast, Roxicodone)	0.5	3	5–10	6
Levorphanol (Levo-Dromoran)	1–2	0.4	4	6–8
Methadone (Dolophine)	0.5–1.0	1	20	6–8
Propoxyphene (Darvon)[3]	1–2	30	100	6
Tramadol (Rybix, Ryzolt, Ultram)	1–2	30	50	4–6
Morphine solution[4] (Roxanol)	0.5–1	1	10	3–4
Morphine sustained-release[4] (MS Contin, Oramorph SR)	1	1	15	8–12
(Kadian)	1	1	10–20	12–24
(Avinza)	1	1	30	24

[1]Preparations also contain acetaminophen (Hycet, Lorcet, Lortab, Norco, Vicodin, others).
[2]Preparations may contain acetaminophen (Percocet) or aspirin (Percodan).
[3]Some preparations contain acetaminophen (Darvocet).
[4]Used primarily for cancer pain.

Dose-dependent side effects include auditory hallucinations and worsening of preexisting depression or psychosis. It does not lead to significant withdrawal symptoms if abruptly discontinued.

Surgery, radiation therapy, chemotherapy, and comprehensive palliative care may prolong survivorship for patients with cancer. However, survivorship may be accompanied by therapy-related acute or chronic pain, including radiation fibrosis or chemotherapy-induced peripheral neuropathy, or both.

Interventional Therapies

Interventional therapy options for cancer pain include pharmacological treatment, nerve blocks with local anesthetics and steroid or a neurolytic solution, radiofrequency ablation, neuromodulatory techniques, or multidisciplinary treatment (psychological interventions, physical or occupational therapy, or modalities such as acupuncture).

PHARMACOLOGICAL INTERVENTIONS

Pharmacological interventions in pain management include acetaminophen, cyclooxygenase (COX) inhibitors, antidepressants, neuroleptic agents, anticonvulsants, corticosteroids, systemic administration of local anesthetics, and opioids.

Acetaminophen

Acetaminophen (paracetamol) is an oral analgesic and antipyretic agent that is also available as an intravenous preparation (Ofirmev). It inhibits prostaglandin synthesis but lacks significant anti-inflammatory activity. Acetaminophen has few side effects but is hepatotoxic at high doses. The recommended adult maximum daily limit is 3000 mg/d, reduced from a previously recommended limit of 4000 mg/d. Isoniazid, zidovudine, barbiturates, and alcohol consumption may potentiate acetaminophen toxicity.

TABLE 47–13 Selected antidepressants.

Drug	Norepinephrine Reuptake Inhibition	Serotonin Reuptake Inhibition	Sedation	Antimuscarinic Activity	Orthostatic Hypotension	Half-Life (h)	Daily Dose (mg)
Amitriptyline (Elavil)	++	++++	High	High	Moderate	30–40	25–300
Bupropion (Wellbutrin)	+	+	Low	Low	Low	11–14	300–450
Citalopram (Celexa)	0	+++	Low	Low	Low	35	20–40
Clomipramine (Anafranil)	+++	+++	High	Moderate	Moderate	20–80	75–300
Desipramine (Norpramin)	+++	0	Low	Low	Low	12–50	50–300
Doxepin (Sinequan)	+	++	High	High	Moderate	8–24	75–400
Escitalopram	0	+++	Low	Low	Low	27–32	10–20
Fluoxetine (Prozac)	0	+++	Low	Low	Low	160–200	20–80
Imipramine (Tofranil)	++	+++	Moderate	Moderate	High	6–20	75–400
Nefazodone (Serzone)	0	+	Low	Low	Low	2–4	300–600
Nortriptyline (Pamelor)	++	+++	Moderate	Moderate	Low	15–90	40–150
Paroxetine (Paxil)	0	+++	Low	Low	Low	31	20–40
Sertraline (Zoloft)	0	+++	Low	Low	Low	26	50–200
Trazodone (Desyrel)	0	++	High	Low	Moderate	3–9	150–400
Venlafaxine (Effexor)	+	+++	Low	Low	Low	5–11	75–375

Nonsteroidal Anti-inflammatory Drugs (NSAIDs)

Nonopioid oral analgesics include salicylates, acetaminophen, and NSAIDs (see Table 47–11). NSAIDs inhibit prostaglandin synthesis by inhibiting cyclooxygenase (COX) activity. Prostaglandins sensitize and amplify nociceptive input, and blockade of their synthesis results in the analgesic, antipyretic, and anti-inflammatory properties characteristic of NSAIDs. At least two types of COX are recognized. COX-1 is found throughout body tissues, with functions including promotion of gastric

TABLE 47–14 Anticonvulsants possibly useful in pain management.

Anticonvulsant	Half-Life (h)	Daily Dose (mg)	Therapeutic Level[1] (mcg/mL)
Carbamazepine (Tegretol)	10–20	200–1200	4–12
Clonazepam (Klonopin)	40–30	1–40	0.01–0.08
Gabapentin (Neurontin)	5–7	900–4000	>2
Lamotrigine (Lamictal)	24	25–400	2–20
Phenytoin (Dilantin)	22	200–600	10–20
Pregabalin (Lyrica)	6	150–600	2.8–8.2
Topiramate (Topamax)	20–30	25–200	Unknown
Valproic acid (Depakene)	6–16	750–1250	50–100

[1]Efficacy in pain management may not correlate with blood level.

mucus production, which protects the stomach lining, and stimulation of thromboxane A_2 production in platelets, which induces platelet aggregation. COX-2 is induced primarily with inflammation. COX inhibitors likely have important peripheral and central nervous system actions. Their analgesic action is limited by side effects and toxicity at higher doses, especially peptic ulceration and kidney failure. Selective COX-2 inhibitors, such as celecoxib (Celebrex), have a lower risk of peptic ulceration but are associated with an increased risk of thrombotic events, including myocardial infarction. The COX-2 inhibitor rofecoxib (Vioxx) has been taken off the market in the United States for this reason. Some types of pain, particularly pain that follows orthopedic and gynecological surgery, respond very well to COX inhibitors.

All of the nonopioid oral analgesic agents are well absorbed enterally. Food delays absorption but otherwise has no effect on bioavailability. Because most of these agents are highly protein bound (>80%), they can displace other highly bound drugs such as warfarin. All undergo hepatic metabolism and are excreted by the kidney. Dosages should therefore be reduced, or alternative medications selected, in patients with hepatic or kidney impairment.

The most common side effects of aspirin (acetylsalicylic acid, ASA) and other NSAIDs are stomach upset, heartburn, nausea, and ulceration of the gastric mucosa. Diclofenac (Voltaren, Cambia, Cataflam) is available as both an oral preparation and a topical gel or patch that may be less likely to contribute to gastric distress.

Other side effects of NSAIDs include dizziness, headache, and drowsiness. With the exception of selective COX-2 inhibitors, all COX inhibitors decrease platelet aggregation. Aspirin irreversibly inhibits platelet aggregation for 1 to 2 weeks, whereas the antiplatelet effect of other NSAIDs is reversible and lasts approximately five elimination half-lives (24–96 h). This inhibition of platelet aggregation does not appreciably increase the incidence of postoperative hemorrhage following most outpatient procedures. NSAIDs may exacerbate bronchospasm in patients with the triad of nasal polyps, rhinitis, and asthma. ASA should not be used in children with varicella or influenza infections because it may precipitate Reye syndrome. NSAIDs may cause acute kidney injury, particularly in patients with underlying kidney dysfunction.

Antidepressants

17 Antidepressants are most useful for patients with neuropathic pain and demonstrate an analgesic effect that occurs at a dose lower than that needed for antidepressant activity. Both of these actions are due to blockade of presynaptic reuptake of serotonin, norepinephrine, or both. Older tricyclic agents appear to be more effective analgesics than selective serotonin reuptake inhibitors (SSRIs). Serotonin and norepinephrine reuptake inhibitors (SNRIs) may provide the most favorable balance between analgesic efficacy and side effects. Antidepressants potentiate the action of opioids and frequently help normalize sleep patterns.

All antidepressant medications undergo extensive first-pass hepatic metabolism and are highly protein bound. Most are highly lipophilic and have large volumes of distribution. Elimination half-lives of most of these medications vary between 1 and 4 days, and many have active metabolites. Available agents differ in their side effects (see Table 47–13), which include antimuscarinic effects (dry mouth, impaired visual accommodation, urinary retention, constipation), antihistaminic effects (sedation and increased gastric pH), α-adrenergic blockade (orthostatic hypotension), and a quinidine-like effect (atrioventricular block, QT prolongation, torsades de pointes).

Serotonin and Norepinephrine Reuptake Inhibitors

The SNRIs milnacipran (Ixel, Savella, Dalcipran, Toledomin) and duloxetine (Cymbalta) have been approved in the United States for the treatment of fibromyalgia. Milnacipran has an elimination half-life of 8 h, is minimally metabolized by the liver, and is primarily excreted unchanged in the urine. Duloxetine is also useful in the treatment of neuropathic pain and depression. It has a half-life of 12 h, is metabolized by the liver, and most of its metabolites are excreted in the urine.

Absolute and relative contraindications for the use of SNRIs include known hypersensitivity, usage of other drugs that act on the central nervous system (including monoamine oxidase inhibitors), hepatic and kidney impairment, uncontrolled narrow-angle glaucoma, and suicidal ideation. Common side effects include nausea, headache, dizziness, constipation, insomnia, hyperhidrosis, hot flashes, vomiting, palpitations, dry mouth, and hypertension.

Neuroleptics

Neuroleptic medications may occasionally be useful for patients with refractory neuropathic pain and may be most helpful in patients with marked agitation or psychotic symptoms. The most commonly used agents are fluphenazine (Prolixin), haloperidol (Haldol), chlorpromazine (Thorazine, Largactil), and perphenazine (Trilafon). Their therapeutic action appears to be due to blockade of dopaminergic receptors in mesolimbic sites. Unfortunately, the same action in nigrostriatal pathways can produce undesirable extrapyramidal side effects, such as mask-like facies, a festinating gait, cogwheel rigidity, and bradykinesia. Some patients also develop acute dystonic reactions such as oculogyric crisis and torticollis. Long-term side effects include akathisia (extreme restlessness) and tardive dyskinesia (involuntary choreoathetoid movements of the tongue, lip smacking, and truncal instability). Like antidepressants, many of these drugs also have antihistaminic, antimuscarinic, and α-adrenergic–blocking effects.

Antispasmodics & Muscle Relaxants

Antispasmodics may be helpful for patients with musculoskeletal sprain and pain associated with spasm or contractures. Tizanidine (Zanaflex) is a centrally acting α_2-adrenergic agonist used in the treatment of muscle spasm in conditions such as multiple sclerosis, low back pain, and spastic diplegia. Cyclobenzaprine (Flexeril) also may be effective for these conditions. Its precise mechanism of action is unknown.

Baclofen (Gablofen, Lioresal), a $GABA_B$ receptor agonist, is particularly effective in the treatment of muscle spasm associated with multiple sclerosis or spinal cord injury when administered by continuous intrathecal drug infusion. Abrupt discontinuation of this medication has been associated with fever, altered mental status, pronounced muscle spasticity or rigidity, rhabdomyolysis, and death.

Corticosteroids

Glucocorticoids are extensively used in pain management for their anti-inflammatory and possibly analgesic actions. They may be given topically, orally, or parenterally (intravenously, subcutaneously, intrabursally, intraarticularly, or epidurally). Table 47–15 lists the most commonly used agents, which differ in potency, relative glucocorticoid and mineralocorticoid activities, and duration of action. Large doses or prolonged administration result in significant side effects. Excess glucocorticoid activity can produce hypertension, hyperglycemia, increased susceptibility to infection, peptic ulcers, osteoporosis, aseptic necrosis of the femoral head, proximal myopathy, cataracts, and, rarely, psychosis. Patients with diabetes may have elevated blood glucose levels after corticosteroid injections. Patients

TABLE 47–15 Selected corticosteroids.

Drug	Routes Given[1]	Glucocorticoid Activity	Mineralocorticoid Activity	Equivalent Dose (mg)	Half-Life (h)
Hydrocortisone	O, I, T	1	1	20	8–12
Prednisone	O	4	0.8	5	12–36
Prednisolone	O, I	4	0.8	5	12–36
Methylprednisolone (Depo-Medrol, Solu-Medrol)	O, I, T	5	0.5	4	12–36
Triamcinolone (Aristocort)	O, I, T	5	0.5	4	12–36
Betamethasone (Celestone)	O, I, T	25	0	0.75	36–72
Dexamethasone (Decadron)	O, I, T	25	0	0.75	36–72

[1]O, oral; I, injectable; T, topical.

Data from Goodman LS, Gilman AG. *The Pharmacologic Basis of Therapeutics*. 8th ed. New York, NY: Pergamon, 1990.

can also develop the physical features characteristic of Cushing syndrome. Excess mineralocorticoid activity causes sodium retention and hypokalemia and may precipitate congestive heart failure.

Many corticosteroid preparations are suspensions rather than solutions, and the relative particulate size of a given glucocorticoid suspension may affect the risk of neural damage due to arterial occlusion when accidental arterial injection occurs. Dexamethasone is the preferred corticosteroid for injection procedures involving relatively vascular areas such as the head and neck region because of the relatively small size of its suspension particles.

Anticonvulsants

18 Anticonvulsant medications are useful for patients with neuropathic pain, especially trigeminal neuralgia and diabetic neuropathy, because they can suppress the spontaneous neural discharges that play a major role in these disorders. The most commonly utilized agents are phenytoin (Dilantin), carbamazepine (Tegretol), valproic acid (Depakene, Stavzor), clonazepam (Klonopin), and gabapentin (Neurontin) (see Table 47–14). Pregabalin (Lyrica) has been approved for the treatment of diabetic peripheral neuropathy and fibromyalgia and is widely prescribed for all forms of neuropathic pain. Lamotrigine (Lamictal) and topiramate (Topamax) may also be effective. All are highly protein bound and have relatively long half-lives. Carbamazepine (Carbatrol, Equetro, Tegretol) has a slow and unpredictable absorption, which requires monitoring of blood levels for optimal efficacy. Phenytoin (Dilantin, Phenytek) may be effective but is associated with the side effect of gum hyperplasia. Levetiracetam (Keppra) and oxcarbazepine (Trileptal) have been used as adjuvant pain therapies. Gabapentin and pregabalin may also be effective adjuvants for the treatment of acute postoperative pain.

Local Anesthetics

Systemic infusion of local anesthetic medication produces sedation and central analgesia and is occasionally used in the treatment of patients with neuropathic pain. The resultant analgesia may outlast the pharmacokinetic profile of the local anesthetic and break the so-called pain cycle. Lidocaine and procaine are the most commonly used agents. They are given either as a slow bolus or by continuous infusion. Lidocaine is given by infusion over 5 to 30 min for a total of 1 to 5 mg/kg. Procaine, 200 to 400 mg, can be given intravenously over the course of 1 to 2 h. Monitoring by qualified medical personnel should include electrocardiography, blood pressure, respiration, pulse oximetry, and mental status, and full resuscitation equipment must be immediately available. Signs of toxicity, such as tinnitus, slurring of speech, excessive sedation, or nystagmus, necessitate slowing or discontinuing the infusion to avoid the progression to seizures. Patients who do not respond satisfactorily to anticonvulsants but respond to intravenous local anesthetics may benefit from chronic oral antiarrhythmic therapy. Mexiletine (Mexitil, 150–300 mg every 6–8 h) is a class 1B antiarrhythmic that is commonly used and generally well tolerated.

Topical lidocaine preparations in concentrations up to 5% may be helpful in the treatment of some neuropathic pain conditions. A 5% lidocaine transdermal patch (Lidoderm) containing 700 mg of lidocaine has been approved for the treatment of PHN. One to three patches may be applied to dry, intact skin, alternating 12 h on, then 12 h off.

α_2-Adrenergic Agonists

The primary effect of α_2-adrenergic agonists is the activation of descending inhibitory pathways in the spinal cord dorsal horn. Epidural and intrathecal α_2-adrenergic agonists are particularly effective in the treatment of neuropathic pain and opioid tolerance. Clonidine (Catapres), a direct-acting α_2-adrenergic agonist, is effective as an adjunctive medication in the treatment of severe pain. The oral dosage is 0.1 to 0.3 mg twice daily; a transdermal patch (0.1–0.3 mg/d) is also available and is usually applied for 7 d. When used in combination with a local anesthetic or opioid in an epidural or intrathecal infusion, clonidine may contribute to a synergistic or prolonged analgesic effect, or both, especially for neuropathic pain.

Opioids

The most commonly prescribed oral opioid agents are codeine, oxycodone, and hydrocodone. They are easily absorbed, but hepatic first-pass metabolism limits systemic delivery. Like other opioids, they undergo hepatic biotransformation and conjugation before renal elimination. Codeine is transformed by the liver into morphine. The side effects of orally administered opioids are similar to those of systemic opioids. When prescribed on a fixed schedule, stool softeners or laxatives are often indicated. Tramadol (Ultram, Rybix, Ryzolt) is a synthetic oral opioid that also blocks neuronal reuptake of norepinephrine and serotonin. It appears to have the same efficacy as the combination of codeine and acetaminophen but is associated with significantly less respiratory depression and has little effect on gastric emptying. Tramadol is contraindicated in patients taking SSRIs, SNRIs, and monoamine oxidase inhibitors (MAOIs) because of the risk of serotonin syndrome.

Moderate to severe cancer pain may be treated with an immediate-release oral morphine preparation (MSIR, Roxanol), which has an effective half-life of 2 to 4 h. Once the patient's daily requirements are determined, the same dose can be given in the form of a sustained-release morphine preparation (MS Contin, Oramorph SR, Kadian, Avinza, and others), which is dosed every 8 to 24 h. The immediate-release preparation is then used only as needed for breakthrough pain. Oral transmucosal fentanyl lozenges (Actiq, 200–1600 mcg) can also be used for breakthrough pain but are very expensive. Excessive sedation can be treated with dextroamphetamine (Dexedrine, ProCentra) or methylphenidate (Ritalin), 5 mg in the morning and 5 mg in the early afternoon. Most patients taking chronic opioid medications require a stool softener. Nausea may be treated with transdermal scopolamine, oral meclizine, or metoclopramide. Hydromorphone (Dilaudid) is an excellent alternative to morphine, particularly in older adult patients because of fewer side effects, and in patients with impaired kidney function. Methadone (Dolophine) has a half-life of 15 to 30 h, but its clinical duration is shorter and quite variable (usually 6–8 h). Naloxone may also be prescribed for potential opioid-induced respiratory depression. 19 **Patients who experience *opioid tolerance* require escalating doses of opioid to maintain the same analgesic effect. *Physical dependence* manifests in opioid *withdrawal* symptoms when the opioid medication is abruptly discontinued or the dose is abruptly and significantly decreased. *Psychological dependence*, characterized by behavioral changes focusing on drug craving, is rare in cancer patients.** The development of opioid tolerance is highly variable but results in some desirable effects such as decreased opioid-related sedation, nausea, and respiratory depression. Unfortunately, despite tolerance, many patients continue to suffer from constipation. Physical dependence occurs in all patients receiving large doses of opioids for extended periods. Opioid withdrawal phenomena can be precipitated by the administration of opioid antagonists. Concomitant use of peripheral opioid antagonists that do not cross the blood–brain barrier, such as methylnaltrexone (Relistor) and alvimopan (Entereg), may help reduce systemic opioid side effects without significantly affecting analgesia.

Tapentadol (Nucynta), a μ-opioid receptor agonist that also has norepinephrine reuptake inhibition properties, has been introduced for the management of acute and chronic pain. This opioid may be associated with less nausea and vomiting and less constipation. It should not be used concomitantly with MAOIs, SSRIs, or SNRIs because of the risk of serotonin syndrome.

A. Parenteral Opioid Administration

Intravenous, intraspinal (epidural or intrathecal), or transdermal routes of opioid administration may be utilized when the patient fails to adequately respond to or is unable to tolerate oral regimens. However, when the patient's pain increases significantly or changes markedly in quality, it is equally important to reevaluate the patient for adequacy of pain diagnosis and for the potential of disease progression. In patients with cancer, adjunctive treatments such as surgery, radiation, chemotherapy, hormonal therapy, and neurolysis may be helpful. Intramuscular opioid administration is rarely optimal because of variability in systemic absorption and resultant delay and variation in clinical effect.

B. Intravenous Opioid Therapy

Parenteral opioid therapy is usually best accomplished by intermittent or continuous intravenous infusion, or both, but can also be given subcutaneously. Contemporary portable infusion devices have patient-controlled analgesia (PCA) capability, allowing the patient to self-treat for breakthrough pain.

C. Spinal Opioid Therapy

The use of intraspinal opioids is an excellent alternative for patients obtaining poor relief with other analgesic techniques or who experience unacceptable side effects. Epidural and intrathecal opioids offer pain relief with substantially lower total doses of opioid and fewer systemic side effects. When compared with intermittent boluses, continuous intraspinal infusion techniques reduce drug requirements, minimize side effects, and decrease the likelihood of intrathecal or epidural catheter occlusion. Myoclonic activity may be occasionally observed with intrathecal morphine or hydromorphone.

Epidural or intrathecal catheters can be placed percutaneously or surgically implanted to provide long-term effective pain relief. Epidural catheters can be attached to lightweight external pumps that can be worn by ambulatory patients. A temporary catheter must be inserted first to confirm the efficacy of the technique. Correct placement of the permanent catheter should be confirmed using fluoroscopy with contrast dye. Completely implantable intrathecal catheters with externally programmable pumps can also be used for continuous infusion (Figure 47–7). The reservoir of the implanted pump (Figure 47–8) is periodically refilled percutaneously. Implantable systems are most appropriate for patients with a life expectancy of several months or longer, whereas tunneled epidural catheters are appropriate for patients expected to live only weeks. An inflammatory mass (granuloma) at the tip of the intrathecal catheter may form and reduce efficacy.

The most frequently encountered problem associated with intrathecal opioids is tolerance, which is usually, but not always, a slowly developing phenomenon. Adjuvant therapy may be used to address this problem and may include intermittent local anesthetics or a mixture of opioids with local anesthetics (bupivacaine or ropivacaine 2–24 mg/d), clonidine (2–4 mcg/kg/h or 48–800 mcg/d, respectively), or the GABA agonist baclofen. Clonidine is particularly useful for neuropathic pain. In high doses, it is more likely to be associated with hypotension and bradycardia.

Complications of spinal opioid therapy include local skin infection, intrathecal pump pocket infection, meningitis, other infections, and death or permanent injury related to pump programming, pump refill, or drug dilution errors. Superficial infections can be reduced by the use of a silver-impregnated cuff close to the exit site. Other complications of spinal opioid therapy include epidural hematoma, which may become clinically apparent either immediately following catheter placement or several

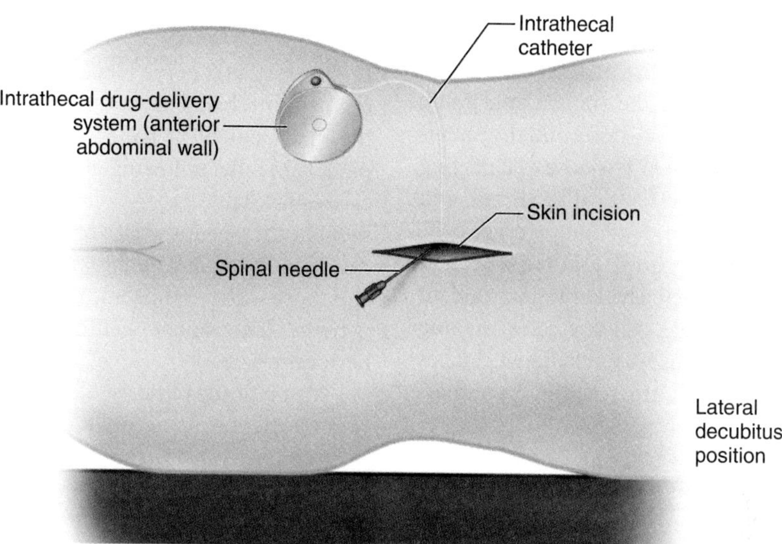

FIGURE 47–7 Placement of an implanted intrathecal drug delivery system. With the patient in the right lateral decubitus position, access to the intrathecal space and to the anterior abdominal wall is optimized. After the posterior incision is made, a needle is advanced through the incision into the intrathecal space, and a catheter is advanced through the needle into the posterior intrathecal space. After the proximal catheter end is anchored, the distal end of the catheter is tunneled around the flank, beneath the costal margin and to the anterolateral aspect of the abdominal wall.

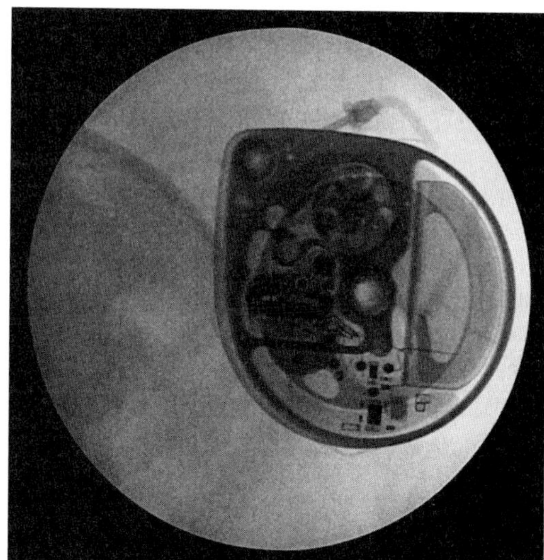

FIGURE 47–8 Fluoroscopic image showing an intrathecal drug pump implanted in the anterolateral abdomen wall. The catheter connecting the pump to the intrathecal space is tunneled around the flank.

days later, and respiratory depression. Respiratory depression secondary to spinal opioid overdose can be treated by decreasing the pump infusion rate to its lowest setting and initiating a naloxone intravenous infusion.

D. Transdermal Fentanyl

Transdermal fentanyl (Duragesic patch) is an alternative to sustained-release oral morphine and oxycodone preparations, particularly when oral medication is not possible. Currently available patches are constructed as a drug reservoir that is separated from the skin by a microporous rate-limiting membrane and an adhesive polymer. A very large quantity of fentanyl (10 mg) provides a large force for transdermal diffusion. Transdermal fentanyl patches are available in 25, 50, 75, and 100 mcg/h sizes that provide drug delivery for 2 to 3 days. The largest patch is equivalent to 60 mg/d of intravenous morphine. The major obstacle to fentanyl absorption through the skin is the stratum corneum. Because the dermis acts as a secondary reservoir, fentanyl absorption continues for several hours after the patch is removed. The transdermal route avoids hepatic first-pass metabolism.

Major disadvantages of the transdermal route are its slow rate of drug delivery onset and the inability to rapidly change dosage in response to changing opioid requirements. Blood fentanyl levels rise and reach a plateau in 12 to 40 h, providing average concentrations of 1, 1.5, and 2 ng/mL for the 50, 75, and 100 mcg/h patches, respectively. Large interpatient variability results in actual delivery rates ranging from 50 to 200 mcg/h. Transdermal fentanyl patches are often diverted for illicit use, resulting in numerous accidental fatalities.

E. Opioid Risks and the Opioid Abuse Crisis

Opioid medications have been identified as having greater risks to patients than were previously considered, including dependence, addiction, overdose, endocrine changes, immunological compromise, hyperalgesia, and respiratory depression that may be life threatening. The efficacy and appropriateness of opioid treatment for chronic benign pain have increasingly come into question as well, as risks may outweigh potential or real benefits. In 2016 the U.S. Centers for Disease Control and Prevention published guidelines for prescribing opioids for chronic pain to help mitigate risks (see Guidelines at the end of this chapter).

Botulinum Toxin (Botox)

OnabotulinumtoxinA (Botox) injection has been increasingly utilized in the treatment of pain syndromes. Studies support its use in the treatment of conditions associated with involuntary muscle contraction (eg, focal dystonia and spasticity), and it is approved by the U.S. FDA for prophylactic treatment of chronic migraine headache. This toxin blocks acetylcholine released at the synapse in motor nerve endings but not sensory nerve fibers. Proposed mechanisms of analgesia include improved local blood flow, relief of muscle spasms, and release of muscular compression of nerve fibers

PROCEDURAL THERAPY

1. Diagnostic & Therapeutic Blocks

Local anesthetic nerve blocks are useful in delineating pain mechanisms, and they play a major role in the management of patients with acute or chronic pain. Pain relief following diagnostic nerve blockade carries favorable prognostic implications for a subsequent therapeutic series of blocks. This technique can identify patients exhibiting a placebo response and those with psychogenic mechanisms. In selected patients, "permanent" neurolytic nerve blocks may be appropriate.

The efficacy of nerve blocks is due to interruption of afferent nociceptive activity, which may be in addition to, or in combination with, blockade of afferent and efferent limbs of abnormal reflex activity involving sympathetic nerve fibers and skeletal muscle innervation. The pain relief frequently outlasts the known pharmacological duration of the agent employed by hours or up to several weeks. The selection of the type of block depends on the location of pain, its presumed mechanism, and the experience and skill of the treating physician. Local anesthetic solutions may be infiltrated locally or injected at specific peripheral nerve, somatic plexus, sympathetic ganglia, or nerve root sites, or they may be administered epidurally or intrathecally.

Ultrasound-Guided Procedures

The use of ultrasound in interventional pain medicine has increased dramatically over the past two decades due to its utility in precisely visualizing vascular, neural, and other anatomic structures, its role as an alternative to the use of fluoroscopy and radiocontrast agents, and progressive improvements in technology leading to better visual images and simplicity of use. Procedures that may benefit from ultrasound guidance include trigger point injections, nerve blocks, and joint injections.

Fluoroscopy

Fluoroscopy is useful for visualizing bony structures and observing the spread of radiopaque contrast agents. Fluoroscopy with contrast agent may be used to minimize the risk of intravascular injection of therapeutic agents. Care should be taken to avoid excessive radiation dosage and to employ appropriate radiation shielding, given the risks of ionizing radiation to the patient and to the health care team.

2. Somatic Nerve Blocks

Trigeminal Nerve Block

A. Indications

The two principal indications for trigeminal nerve block are trigeminal neuralgia and intractable facial cancer pain. Depending on the site of pain, these blocks may be performed on the Gasserian ganglion itself, on one of the major divisions (ophthalmic, maxillary, or mandibular), or on one of their smaller nerve branches.

B. Anatomy

The rootlets of cranial nerve V arise from the brainstem and join one another to form a crescent-shaped sensory (Gasserian) ganglion in *Meckel's cave*. Most of the ganglion is invested with a dural sleeve. The three subdivisions of the trigeminal nerve arise from the ganglia and exit the cranium separately (Figure 47–9A).

C. Technique

1. Gasserian ganglion block—Fluoroscopic guidance is mandatory for the performance of this procedure (Figure 47–9B). An 8- to 10-cm 22-gauge needle is inserted approximately 3 cm lateral to the angle of the mouth at the level of the upper second molar. The needle is then advanced posteromedially and angled superiorly to bring it into alignment with the pupil in the anterior plane and with the mid-zygomatic arch in the lateral plane. Without entering the mouth, the needle should pass between the mandibular ramus and the maxilla and lateral to the pterygoid process to enter the cranium through the foramen ovale. After a negative aspiration for cerebrospinal fluid and blood, local anesthetic is injected.

2. Blocks of the ophthalmic nerve and its branches—In this procedure, to avoid denervation-related keratitis, only the supraorbital branch is blocked in most cases (Figure 47–9C); the ophthalmic division itself is not blocked. The nerve is easily located and blocked with local anesthetic at the *supraorbital notch,* which is located on the supraorbital ridge above the pupil. The supratrochlear branch can also be blocked with local anesthetic at the superior medial corner of the orbital ridge.

3. Blocks of the maxillary nerve and its branches—With the patient's mouth slightly opened, an 8- to 10-cm 22-gauge needle is inserted between the zygomatic arch and the notch of the mandible (Figure 47–9D). After contact with the lateral pterygoid plate at about 4-cm depth (position 1 in Figure), the needle is partially withdrawn and angled slightly superiorly and anteriorly to pass into the pterygopalatine fossa (position 2). Local anesthetic is injected once paresthesia is elicited. Both the maxillary nerve and the sphenopalatine (pterygopalatine) ganglia are usually anesthetized by this technique. The sphenopalatine ganglion (and anterior ethmoid nerves) can be anesthetized transmucosally with topical anesthetic applied through the nose; several cotton applicators soaked with local anesthetic (cocaine or lidocaine) are inserted along the medial wall of the nasal cavity into the area of the sphenopalatine recess. The sphenopalatine ganglion blockade may be helpful for patients with chronic nasal pain, cluster headache, or Sluder neuralgia.

The infraorbital branch of cranial nerve V passes through the infraorbital foramen, where it can be blocked with local anesthetic. This foramen is approximately 1 cm below the orbit and is usually located with a needle inserted about 2 cm lateral to the nasal ala and directed superiorly, posteriorly, and slightly laterally.

4. Blocks of the mandibular nerve and its branches—With the patient's mouth slightly opened (Figure 47–9E), an 8- to 10-cm 22-gauge needle is inserted between the zygomatic arch and the mandibular notch. After contact with the lateral pterygoid plate (position 1 in figure), the needle is partially withdrawn and angled slightly superiorly and posteriorly toward the ear (position 2). Local anesthetic is injected once paresthesia is elicited.

The lingual and inferior alveolar branches of the mandibular nerve may be blocked intraorally utilizing a 10-cm 22-gauge needle (Figure 47–9F).

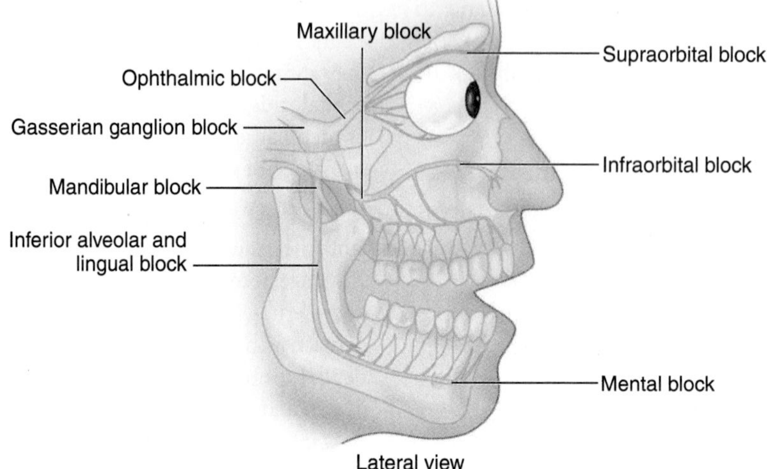

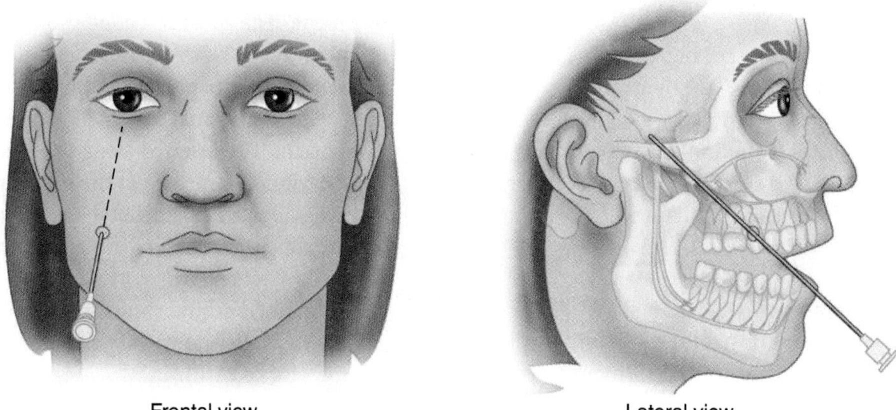

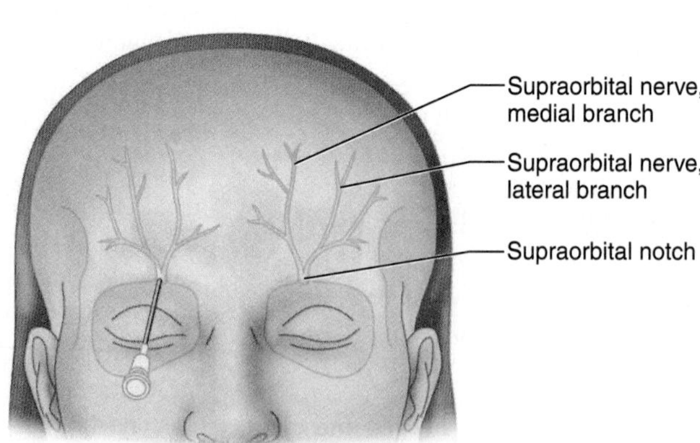

FIGURE 47–9 A-F Trigeminal nerve blocks.

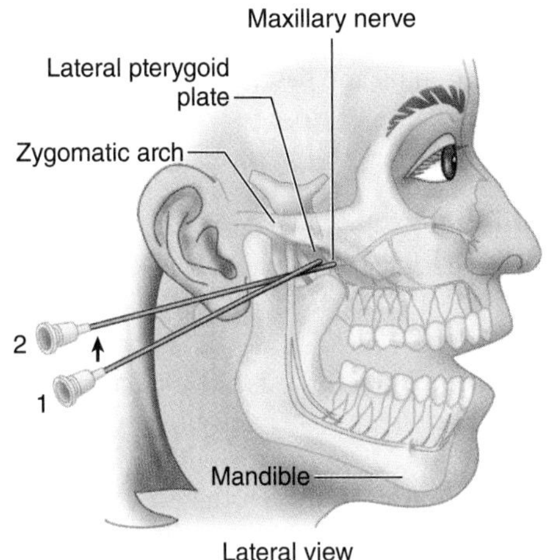

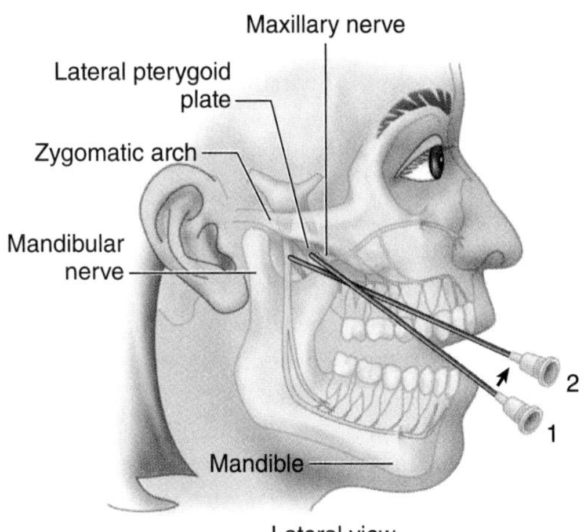

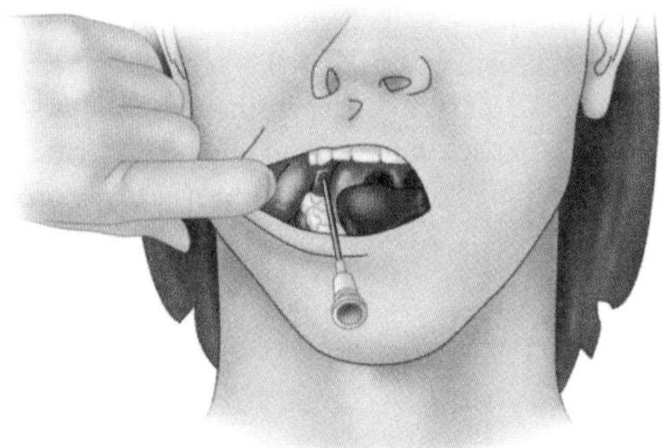

F: Lingual and inferior alveolar nerve block
Frontal view

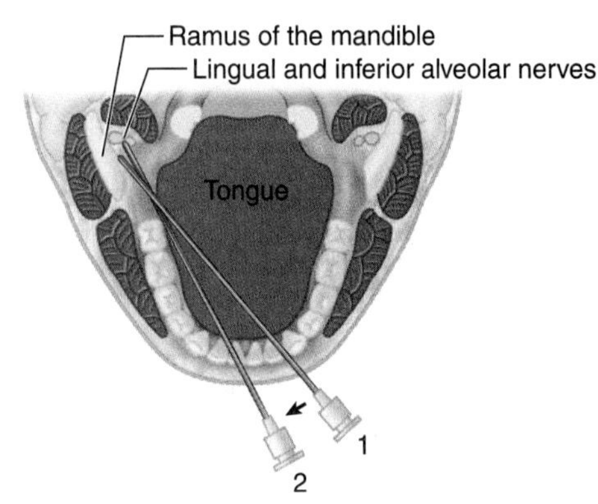

FIGURE 47–9 *(Continued)*

The patient is asked to open the mouth maximally, and the coronoid notch is palpated with the index finger of the nonoperative hand. The needle is then introduced at the same level (approximately 1 cm above the surface of the last molar), medial to the finger but lateral to the pterygomandibular plica (position 1 in figure). It is advanced posteriorly 1.5 to 2 cm along the medial side of the mandibular ramus, making contact with the bone (position 2). Both nerves are usually blocked following injection of local anesthetic.

The terminal portion of the inferior alveolar nerve may be blocked as it emerges from the mental foramen at the mid-mandible just beneath the corner of the mouth. Local anesthetic is injected once paresthesia is elicited or the needle is felt to enter the foramen.

D. Complications

Complications of a Gasserian ganglion block include accidental intravascular injection, subarachnoid injection, Horner syndrome, and motor block of the muscles of mastication. The potential for serious hemorrhage is greatest for blockade of the maxillary nerve. The facial nerve may be unintentionally blocked during blocks of the mandibular division.

Facial Nerve Block

A. Indications

Blockade of the facial nerve is occasionally indicated to relieve spastic contraction of the facial muscles, treat herpes zoster involving the facial nerve, and facilitate certain surgical procedures involving the eye.

B. Anatomy

The facial nerve can be blocked where it exits the cranium through the stylomastoid foramen. A small sensory component supplies special sensation (taste) to the anterior two-thirds of the tongue and general sensation to the tympanic membrane, external auditory meatus, soft palate, and part of the pharynx.

C. Technique

The entry point is just anterior to the mastoid process, beneath the external auditory meatus, and at the midpoint of the mandibular ramus. The nerve is approximately 1 to 2 cm deep and is blocked with local anesthetic just below the stylomastoid process.

D. Complications

If the needle is inserted too deeply past the level of the styloid bone, the glossopharyngeal and vagal nerves may also be blocked. *Careful aspiration is necessary because of the proximity of the facial nerve to the carotid artery and the internal jugular vein.*

Glossopharyngeal Block

A. Indications

Glossopharyngeal nerve block may be used for patients with pain due to cancer involving the base of the tongue, the epiglottis, or the palatine tonsils. It can also be used to distinguish glossopharyngeal neuralgia from trigeminal and geniculate neuralgia.

B. Anatomy

The nerve exits from the cranium via the jugular foramen medial to the styloid process and courses anteromedially to supply the posterior third of the tongue, pharyngeal muscles, and mucosa. The vagus and spinal accessory nerves also exit the cranium via the jugular foramen and descend alongside the glossopharyngeal nerve in close proximity to the internal jugular vein.

C. Technique

The block is performed using a 5-cm 22-gauge needle inserted just posterior to the angle of the mandible (Figure 47–10). The nerve is approximately 3 to 4 cm deep; therefore, use of a nerve stimulator facilitates correct placement of the needle. An alternative approach is from a point over the styloid process, midway between the mastoid process and the angle of the mandible; the nerve is located just anteriorly.

D. Complications

Complications include dysphagia and vagal blockade resulting in ipsilateral vocal cord paralysis and tachycardia. Block of the accessory nerve and hypoglossal nerves causes ipsilateral paralysis of the trapezius muscle and the tongue, respectively. Careful aspiration is necessary to prevent intravascular injection.

Occipital Nerve Block

A. Indications

Occipital nerve block is useful diagnostically and therapeutically in patients with occipital headaches and neuralgias.

B. Anatomy

The *greater occipital nerve* is derived from the dorsal primary rami of the C2 and C3 spinal nerves, whereas the *lesser occipital nerve* arises from the ventral rami of the same roots.

C. Technique

The greater occipital nerve is blocked approximately 3 cm lateral to the occipital prominence at the level of the superior nuchal line (Figure 47–11); the nerve is just medial to the occipital artery, which is often palpable. The lesser occipital nerve is blocked 2 to 3 cm more laterally along the nuchal ridge. Ultrasound guidance may be employed to help identify

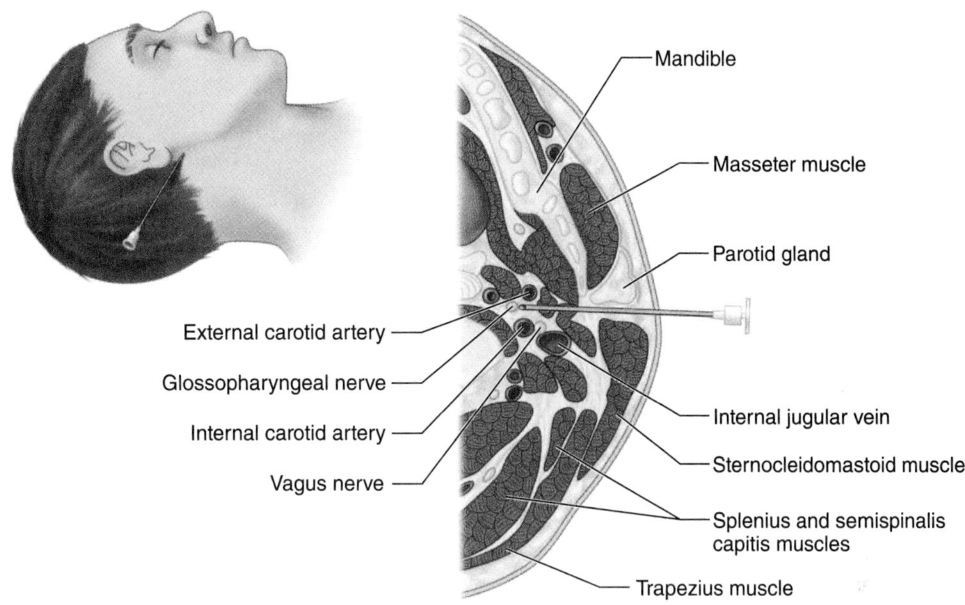

FIGURE 47–10 Glossopharyngeal nerve block.

the nerves. For patients who have responded well, but temporarily, to occipital nerve blocks, implantation of an occipital nerve stimulator may provide prolonged relief.

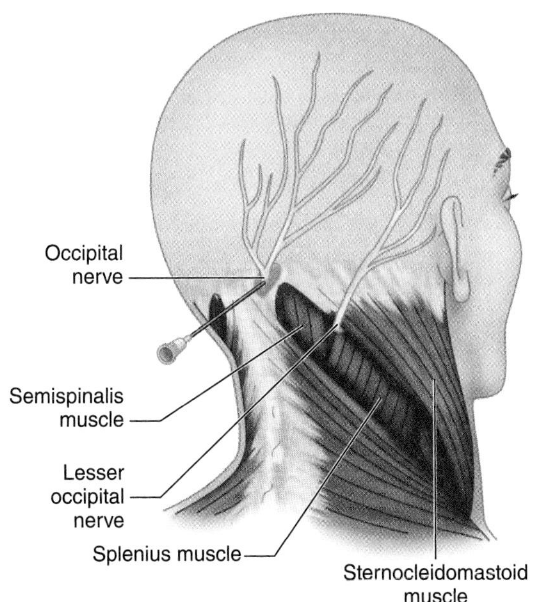

FIGURE 47–11 Occipital nerve blocks.

D. Complications

Rarely, intravascular injections may occur.

Suprascapular Nerve Block

A. Indications

This block is useful for painful conditions arising from the shoulder, including arthritis, bursitis, and myofascial pain.

B. Anatomy

The suprascapular nerve is the major sensory nerve of the shoulder joint. It arises from the brachial plexus (C4–C6) and passes over the upper border of the scapula in the suprascapular notch to enter the suprascapular fossa.

C. Technique

The nerve is blocked at the *suprascapular notch,* which is located at the junction of the lateral and middle thirds of the superior scapular border (Figure 47–12). Correct placement of the needle is determined by paresthesia, ultrasound, or nerve stimulator use.

D. Complications

Pneumothorax is possible if the needle is advanced too far anteriorly. Paralysis of the supraspinatus and

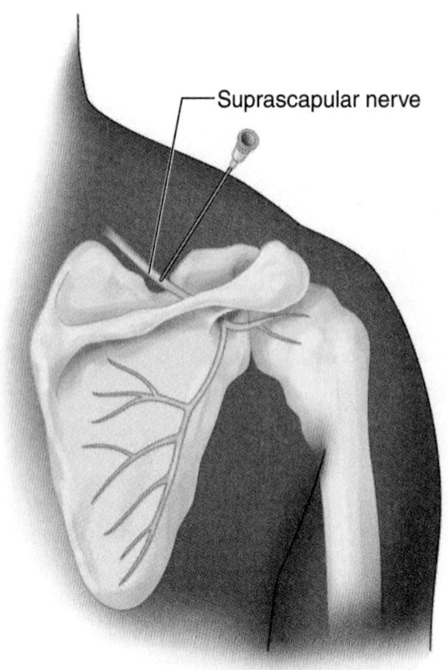

FIGURE 47–12 Suprascapular nerve block.

infraspinatus muscles will result in impaired shoulder abduction.

Cervical Paravertebral Nerve Blocks

A. Indications

Cervical paravertebral nerve blocks can be useful diagnostically and therapeutically for patients with cervical disc displacement, cervical foraminal stenosis, or cancer-related pain originating from the cervical spine or shoulder.

B. Anatomy

The cervical spinal nerves lie in the sulcus of the transverse process of their respective vertebral levels. *As noted earlier in this chapter, unlike thoracic and lumbar nerve roots, those in the cervical spine exit the foramina above the vertebral bodies for which they are named.*

C. Technique

The lateral approach is most commonly used to block C2–C7 (Figure 47–13). Patients are asked to turn the head to the opposite side while in a sitting or supine position. A line is then drawn between the mastoid process and the tubercle of the C6 transverse process (*Chassaignac tubercle*). A series of injections are made with a 5-cm 22-gauge needle along a second parallel line 0.5 cm posterior to the first line. In the case of diagnostic blocks, a smaller injectate volume may be helpful to minimize local anesthetic spread to adjacent structures and thereby increase block specificity. Because the transverse process of C2 is usually difficult to palpate, the injection for this level is placed 1.5 cm beneath the mastoid process. The other transverse processes are usually interspaced 1.5 cm apart and are 2.5 to 3 cm deep. Fluoroscopy is useful in identifying specific vertebral levels during diagnostic blocks, and this block may also be performed with ultrasound guidance.

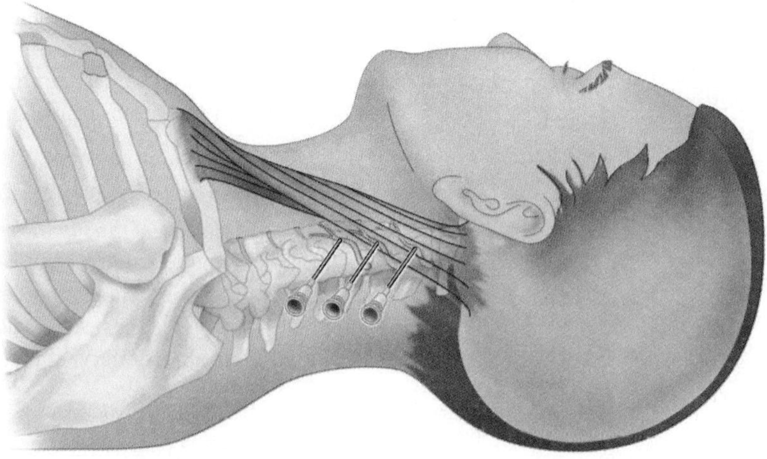

FIGURE 47–13 Cervical paravertebral nerve block.

D. Complications

Unintentional intrathecal or epidural anesthesia at this level rapidly causes respiratory paralysis and hypotension. Injection of even small volumes of local anesthetic into the vertebral artery causes unconsciousness and seizures. Other complications include Horner syndrome and blockade of the recurrent laryngeal and phrenic nerves.

Embolic cerebrovascular and spinal cord complications have resulted from injection of particulate steroid with this block. Particulate steroid must not be used with cervical paravertebral nerve blocks because of possible anomalous vertebral artery anatomy in this region.

Thoracic Paravertebral Nerve Block

This technique may be used to block the upper thoracic dermatome segments because the scapula interferes with the intercostal technique at these levels. Unlike an intercostal nerve block, a thoracic paravertebral nerve block anesthetizes both the dorsal and ventral rami of spinal nerves. It is therefore useful in patients with pain originating from the thoracic spine, thoracic cage, or abdominal wall, including compression fractures, proximal rib fractures, and acute herpes zoster (shingles). This block is also frequently utilized for intraoperative anesthesia and for postoperative pain management in breast surgery and is described in detail in Chapter 46.

Lumbar Paravertebral Nerve Blocks

A. Indications

Lumbar paravertebral nerve blocks may be useful in evaluating pain due to disorders involving the lumbar spine or spinal nerves.

B. Anatomy

The lumbar spinal nerves enter the *psoas compartment* after exiting the intervertebral foramina beneath the pedicles and transverse processes. This compartment is formed by the psoas fascia anteriorly, the quadratus lumborum fascia posteriorly, and the vertebral bodies medially.

C. Technique

The approach to lumbar spinal nerves is essentially the same as for thoracic paravertebral blockade (Figure 47–14). An 8-cm 22-gauge needle is usually used, and radiographic confirmation of the correct level is helpful. For diagnostic blocks, only 2 mL of local anesthetic is injected at any one level because larger volumes may block more than one level. Larger volumes of local anesthetic are used for therapeutic blocks or to produce complete somatic and sympathetic block of the lumbar nerves.

D. Complications

Complications are primarily those of unintentional intrathecal or epidural anesthesia. Patients may

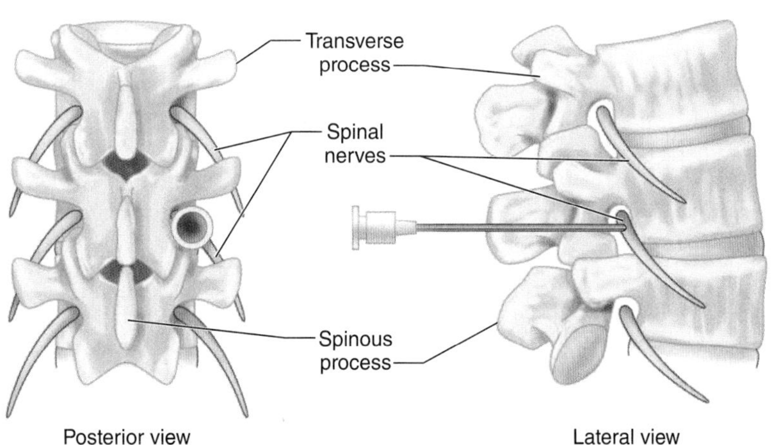

FIGURE 47–14 Lumbar paravertebral nerve blocks.

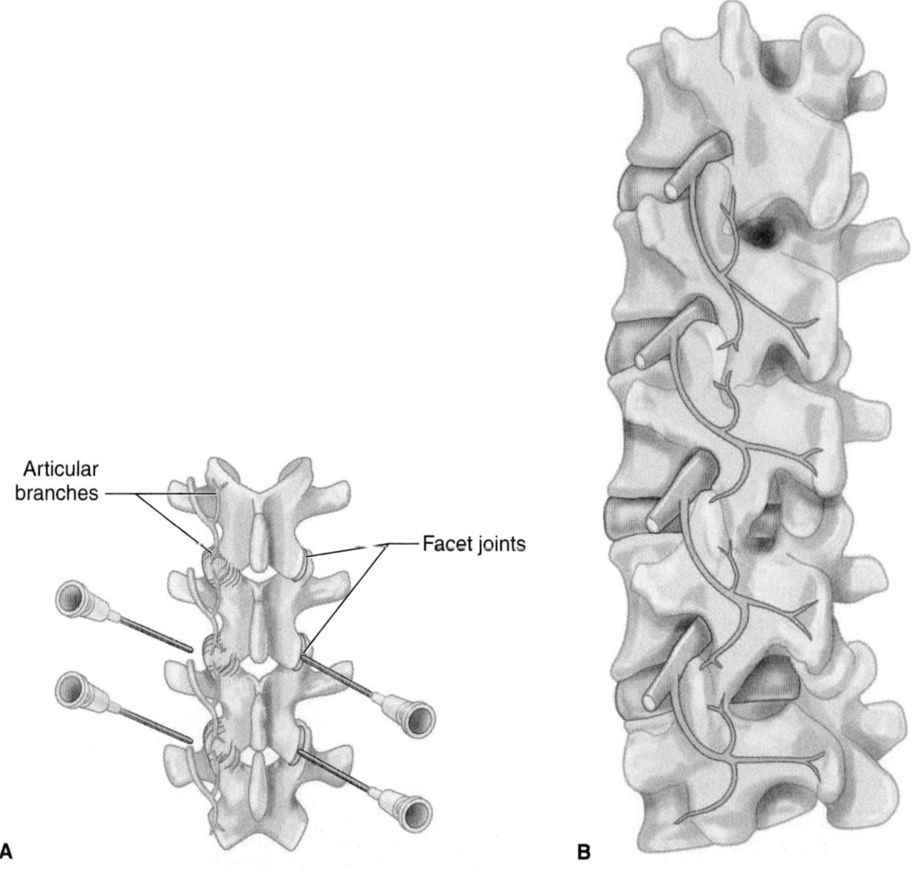

FIGURE 47–15 Lumbar medial branch nerve and facet blocks. **A**: Posterior view; **B**: 30° oblique posterior view.

experience paresthesia if inadvertent nerve contact occurs during needle placement. Some physicians advocate the use of a blunt-tipped needle to (theoretically) decrease the risk of accidental intraneural injection. Digital subtraction angiography with radiopaque contrast may lessen the risk of intravascular injection of local anesthetic or steroid medication.

Cervical, Thoracic, & Lumbar Medial Branch Blocks

A. Indications

These blocks may be utilized in patients with back pain to assess the contribution of lumbar facet (zygapophyscal) joint disease. Corticosteroids are commonly injected with the local anesthetic when the intraarticular technique is chosen. The cervical, thoracic, or lumbar facet joints may be injected for diagnostic and potentially therapeutic purposes.

B. Anatomy

Each facet joint is innervated by the medial branches of the posterior primary division of the spinal nerves above and below the joint (Figure 47–15). Thus, every joint is supplied by two or more adjacent spinal nerves. Each medial branch crosses the upper border of the lower transverse process running in a groove between the root of the transverse process and the superior articular process.

C. Technique

These blocks are performed under fluoroscopic guidance with the patient in a prone position or the lateral position for cervical procedures. A posterior–anterior

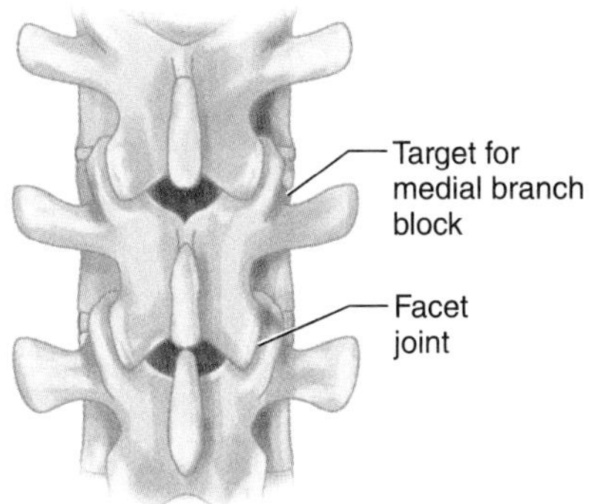

FIGURE 47–16 Anatomy of the lumbar facet joint and location for blocking the medial branch of the posterior primary division of the lumbar spinal nerves above and below the joint.

view facilitates visualization of the spine for lumbar medial branch blocks. A 10-cm 22-gauge needle is inserted 3 to 4 cm lateral to the spinous process at the desired level and directed anteriorly toward the junction of the transverse process and the superior articular process to block the medial branch of the posterior division of the spinal nerve (Figures 47–16 through 47–18).

Alternatively, local anesthetic with or without corticosteroid may be directly injected into the facet joint. Positioning the patient prone and using an oblique fluoroscopic view facilitates identification of the joint space. Correct placement of the needle may be confirmed by injecting radiopaque contrast prior to injection of local anesthetic. Total injection volumes should ideally be limited to less than 1 mL to prevent rupture of the joint capsule.

D. Complications

Injection into a dural sleeve results in a subarachnoid block, whereas injection near the spinal nerve root results in sensory and motor block at that level. Because the joint normally has a small volume, larger injections can cause rupture of the joint capsule.

If a patient achieves improved pain control after a diagnostic block, they may be considered for radiofrequency ablation of the medial branch. There is debate about whether a second, confirmatory diagnostic block should be performed prior to radiofrequency ablation. Injection of steroid may be considered before or after radiofrequency ablation to theoretically decrease the chance for postprocedural neuritis.

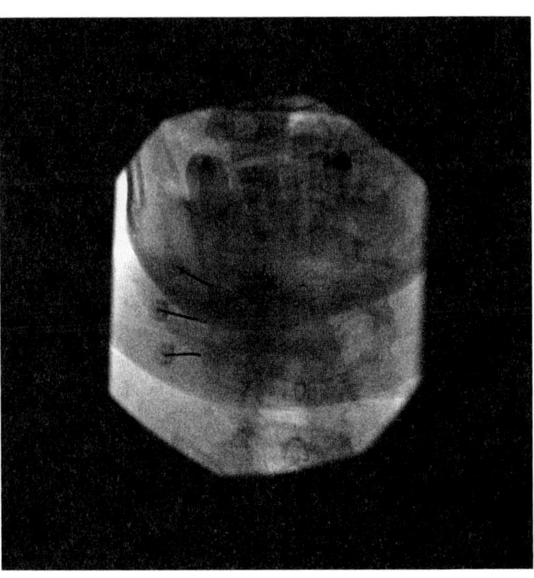

A

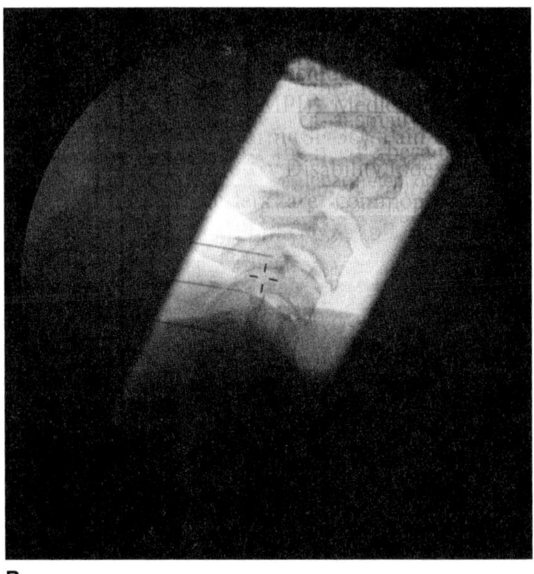

B

FIGURE 47–17 Fluoroscopic image of a cervical medial branch blockade. **A**: Anteroposterior view; **B**: Lateral view. The lateral view reveals the needles at C4, C5, and C6 advanced toward the trapezoid of the articular pillar at each level. Note the "waist" of the vertebrae. Spinal needles may be advanced to come into contact with the medial branch of the nerve.

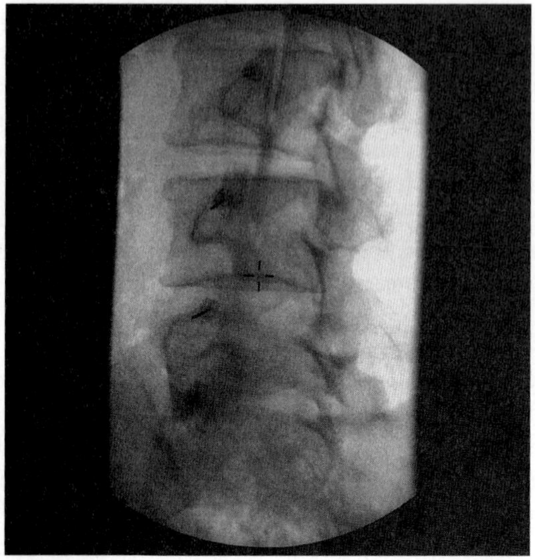

FIGURE 47–18 Left lumbar medial branch blockade, oblique view.

Trans-Sacral Nerve Block

A. Indications

This technique is useful in the diagnosis and treatment of pelvic and perineal pain. In addition, blockade of the S1 spinal root can help define its role in back pain.

B. Anatomy

The five paired sacral spinal nerves and one pair of coccygeal nerves descend in the sacral canal, and each nerve then exits through its respective intervertebral foramen. The S5 and coccygeal nerves exit through the sacral hiatus.

C. Technique

While the patient is prone, the sacral foramina are identified with a needle along a line drawn 1.5 cm medial to the posterior superior iliac spine and 1.5 cm lateral to the ipsilateral sacral cornu (Figure 47–19). Correct positioning requires entry of the needle into the posterior sacral foramen and usually produces paresthesia. The S1 nerve root is usually 1.5 cm above the level of the posterior superior iliac spine along this imaginary line. Blockade of the S5 and coccygeal nerves can be accomplished by injection at the sacral hiatus.

D. Complications

Complications are rare but include nerve damage and intravascular injection.

Pudendal Nerve Block

A. Indications

Pudendal nerve block is useful in evaluating patients with perineal somatosensory pain.

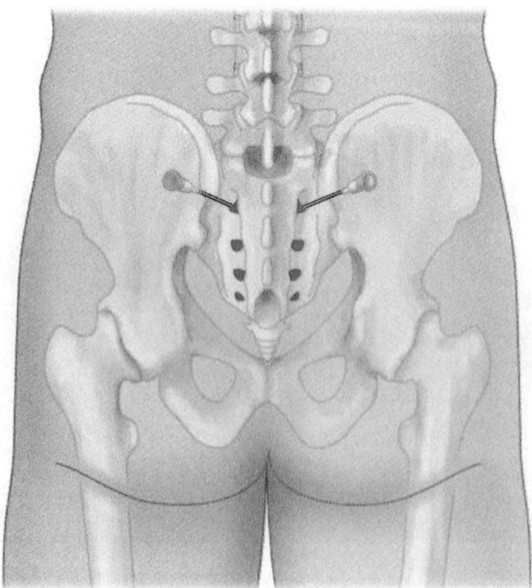

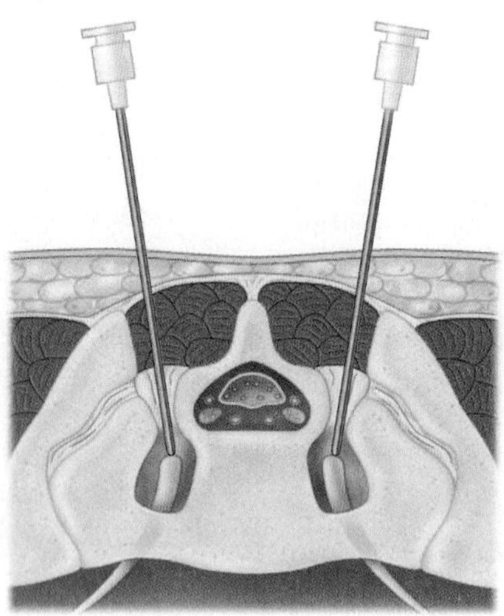

FIGURE 47–19 Trans-sacral nerve block.

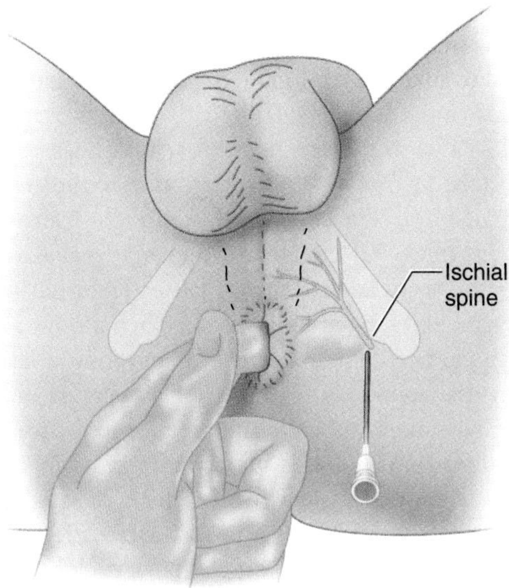

FIGURE 47–20 Pudendal nerve block.

B. Anatomy

The pudendal nerve arises from S2–S4 and courses between the sacrospinous and the sacrotuberous ligaments to reach the perineum.

C. Technique

This block is usually performed transperineally with the patient in the lithotomy position (Figure 47–20), though it may be performed via a posterior approach in the prone position. Injection of anesthetic is carried out percutaneously just posterior to the ischial spine at the attachment of the sacrospinous ligament. The ischial spine can be palpated transrectally or transvaginally. Alternatively, this procedure may be performed in the prone position with a 22-gauge needle directed toward the base of the ischial spine. Patients should be advised that they may have numbness of the genitalia for several hours after this procedure is performed.

D. Complications

Potential complications include unintentional sciatic blockade and intravascular injection.

3. Sympathetic Nerve Blocks

Sympathetic blockade can be accomplished by a variety of techniques, including intrathecal, epidural, and paravertebral blocks. Unfortunately, these approaches usually block both somatic and sympathetic fibers. Problems with differential spinal and epidural techniques are discussed later in this section. The following techniques specifically block sympathetic fibers and can be used to define the role of the sympathetic system in a patient's pain and possibly also provide long-term pain relief. The most common indications for sympathetic nerve blocks include reflex sympathetic dystrophy, visceral pain, acute herpetic neuralgia, postherpetic pain, and peripheral vascular disease. Isolated sympathetic blockade to a region is characterized by loss of sympathetic tone, as evidenced by increased cutaneous blood flow and cutaneous temperature, and by unaltered somatic sensation. Other tests include loss of the skin conductance (sympathogalvanic reflex) and sweat response (ninhydrin, cobalt blue, or starch tests) following a painful stimulus.

Cervicothoracic (Stellate) Block

A. Indications

This block is often used for patients with head, neck, arm, and upper chest pain. It is commonly referred to as a *stellate block* or *stellate ganglion block*, and it usually blocks the upper thoracic as well as all cervical ganglia. Injection of larger volumes of anesthetic often extends the block to the T5 ganglia. Stellate ganglion blocks have also been used for posttraumatic stress disorder, severe vasomotor symptoms associated with menopause, vasospastic disorders of the upper extremity, and refractory ventricular tachycardia.

B. Anatomy

Sympathetic innervation of the head, neck, and most of the arm is derived from four cervical ganglia, the largest being the stellate ganglion. The latter usually represents a fusion of the lower cervical and first thoracic ganglia. Some sympathetic innervation of the arm (T1) as well as innervation of all of the thoracic viscera derives from the five upper thoracic ganglia. The sympathetic supply to the arm in some individuals may also originate from T2–T3 via anatomically distinct nerves (*Kuntz nerves*) that join the brachial plexus high in the axilla. These nerves may be missed by a stellate block but not by an axillary block. The point of injection is at the level of the stellate ganglion, which lies posterior to the origin of the vertebral artery from the subclavian artery, anterior to the longus colli muscle and the first rib, anterolateral to the prevertebral fascia, and medial to the scalene muscles.

C. Technique

The paratracheal technique is most commonly used (Figure 47–21), though an oblique or posterior approach may also be taken. With the patient's head extended, a 4- to 5-cm 22-gauge needle is inserted at the medial edge of the sternocleidomastoid muscle just below the level of the cricoid cartilage at the level of the transverse process of C6 (Chassaignac tubercle) or C7 (3–5 cm above the clavicle). The nonoperative hand should be used to retract the muscle together with the carotid sheath prior to needle insertion. The needle is advanced to the transverse process and withdrawn 2 to 3 mm prior to injection. Aspiration must be carried out in two planes before a 1-mL test dose is used to exclude unintentional intravascular injection into the vertebral or subclavian arteries or subarachnoid injection into a dural sleeve. A total of 5 to 10 mL of local anesthetic may be injected. Fluoroscopy or ultrasound may be used to visualize the anatomy and decrease the risk of inadvertent intravascular injection.

For an ultrasound-guided approach, the patient is placed in the supine position with the neck extended and rotated to the contralateral side. A linear probe is placed in transverse orientation over the cricoid cartilage and moved laterally until the transverse process of C6 (Chassaignac tubercle) is visualized in addition to the adjacent carotid artery, internal jugular vein, and longus colli muscle. Then a 4- to 5-cm 22-gauge needle is inserted in-plane from a lateral to medial approach, with the target being medial to the Chassaignac tubercle and anterior to the prevertebral fascia. C6 level is preferred to avoid inadvertent vertebral artery puncture, which is possible at C7. A test dose of 1 mL of local anesthetic should be injected after negative aspiration to exclude unintentional intravascular or subarachnoid injection and ensure filling of local anesthetic in the expected plane. Next, an additional 4 to 5 mL of local anesthetic may be injected.

Correct placement of the needle is usually followed promptly by an increase in the skin temperature of the ipsilateral arm and the onset of *Horner syndrome*. The latter consists of ipsilateral ptosis, meiosis, enophthalmos, nasal congestion, and anhydrosis of the neck and face.

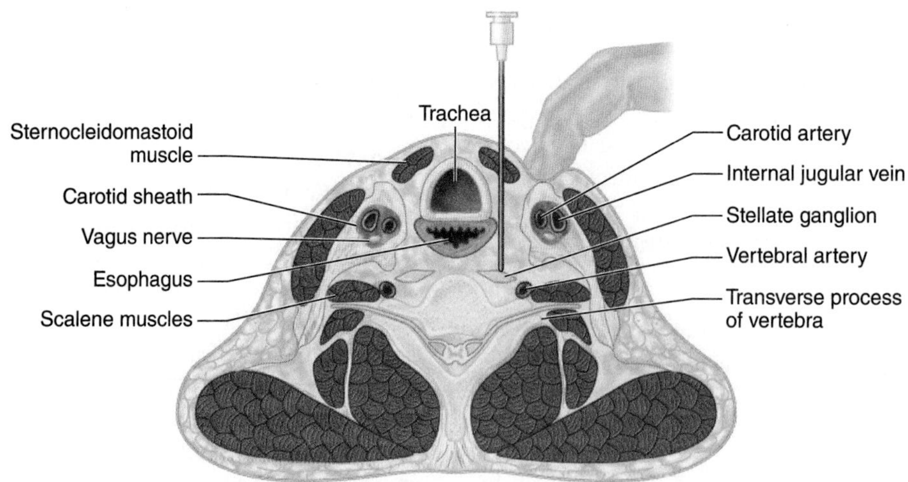

FIGURE 47–21 Stellate block.

D. Complications

20 **In addition to intravascular and subarachnoid injection, other complications of stellate block include hematoma, pneumothorax, epidural anesthesia, brachial plexus block, hoarseness due to blockade of the recurrent laryngeal nerve, and, rarely, osteomyelitis or mediastinitis following esophageal puncture, particularly if a left-sided approach is taken.** The posterior approach may have the highest incidence of pneumothorax.

Thoracic Sympathetic Chain Block

The thoracic sympathetic ganglia lie just lateral to the vertebral bodies and anterior to the spinal nerve roots, but this block is generally not used because of a significant risk of pneumothorax.

Splanchnic Nerve Block

Three groups of splanchnic nerves (greater, lesser, and least) arise from the lower seven thoracic sympathetic ganglia on each side and descend alongside the vertebral bodies to communicate with the celiac ganglia. *Although similar to celiac plexus block (see below), the splanchnic nerve block may be preferred because it is less likely to block the lumbar sympathetic chain and because it requires less anesthetic.*

The needle is inserted 6 to 7 cm from the midline at the lower end of the T11 spinous process and advanced under fluoroscopic guidance to the anterolateral surface of T12. Ten mL of local anesthetic is injected on each side. The needle should maintain contact with the vertebral body at all times to avoid a pneumothorax. Other complications may include hypotension and possible injury to the azygos vein on the right or to the hemiazygos vein and the thoracic duct on the left.

If a patient's pain lessens after a splanchnic nerve block, the procedure may be repeated to ensure that this result was not due to placebo effect. In addition, if the patient obtained pain relief from the initial block, he or she may subsequently benefit from radiofrequency ablation of the splanchnic nerves at T11 and T12, with potentially longer duration of analgesia. Performing the procedure on one side initially and then the other side on a subsequent day is advised because of the risk of pneumothorax.

Celiac Plexus Block

A. Indications

A celiac plexus block is indicated for patients with pain arising from the abdominal viscera, particularly cancers.

B. Anatomy

The celiac ganglia vary in number (one to five), form, and position. They are generally clustered at the level of the body of L1, posterior to the vena cava on the right, just lateral to the aorta on the left, and posterior to the pancreas.

C. Technique

The patient is placed in a prone position, and a 15-cm 22-gauge needle is used to inject 15 to 20 mL of local anesthetic (Figure 47–22). Each needle is inserted 7 to 8 cm from the midline at the inferior edge of the spinous process of L1 and advanced under Fluoroscopic guidance toward the midline. The needle passes under the edge of the 12th rib and should be positioned anterior to the body of L1 in the lateral radiographic view and close to the midline overlying the same vertebral body in the anteroposterior view. When CT guidance is used, the tip of the needle should come to lie anterolateral to the aorta at a level between the celiac and superior mesenteric arteries.

The celiac plexus block may be performed from multiple approaches, including the posterior retrocrural approach, posterior anterocrural approach, posterior transaortic approach, or anterior approach. These blocks may be facilitated with fluoroscopic, CT, or ultrasound guidance.

D. Complications

The most common complication is postural hypotension from block of visceral sympathetic innervation and resultant vasodilation. For this reason, patients should be adequately hydrated intravenously prior to this block, and precautions should be taken to minimize the risk of orthostatic lightheadedness or syncope. Accidental intravascular injection into the vena cava is more likely to produce a severe systemic reaction than accidental intraaortic injection. Other, less common complications include pneumothorax,

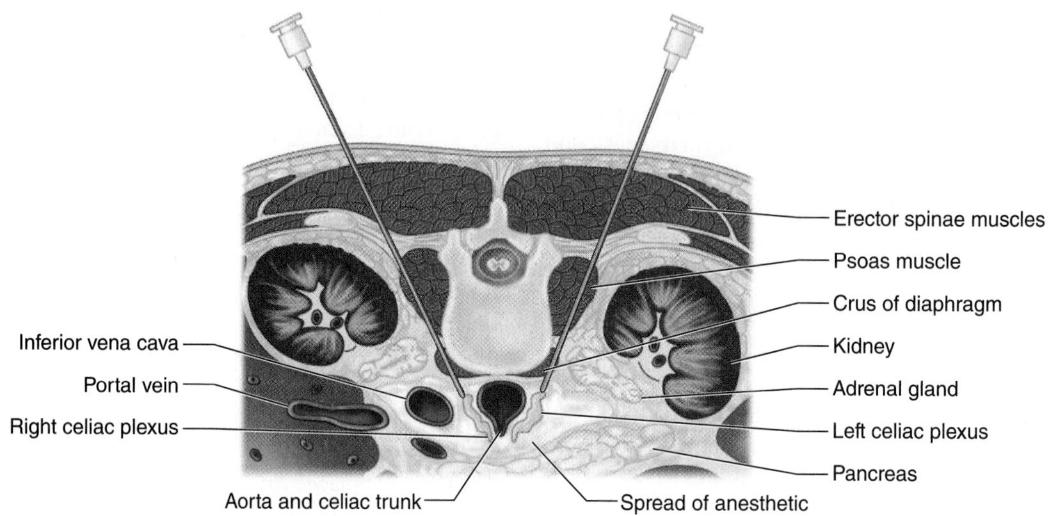

FIGURE 47–22 Celiac plexus block.

retroperitoneal hemorrhage, injury to the kidneys or pancreas, sexual dysfunction, or, rarely, paraplegia (due to spasm of, or injury to, the lumbar artery of Adamkiewicz). Blocking the sympathetic chain may result in relatively unopposed parasympathetic activity that may lead to increased gastrointestinal motility and diarrhea. Back pain is another common side effect of a celiac plexus block.

Lumbar Sympathetic Block

A. Indications

Lumbar sympathetic block may be indicated for painful conditions involving the pelvis or the lower extremities and possibly for some patients with peripheral vascular disease.

B. Anatomy

The lumbar sympathetic chain contains three to five ganglia and is a continuation of the thoracic chain. It also supplies sympathetic fibers to the pelvic plexus and ganglia. The lumbar sympathetic chain ganglia are in a more anteromedial position to the vertebral bodies than the thoracic ganglia and are anterior to the psoas muscle and fascia. The lumbar chain is usually posterior to the vena cava on the right but is just lateral to the aorta on the left.

C. Technique

A single-needle technique at the L3 level on either side is most commonly employed with the patient either prone or in a lateral position (Figure 47–23). The needle is inserted at the upper edge of the spinous process and is directed above or just lateral to the transverse process of the vertebrae (depending on the distance from the midline). Fluoroscopic or ultrasound guidance is often used.

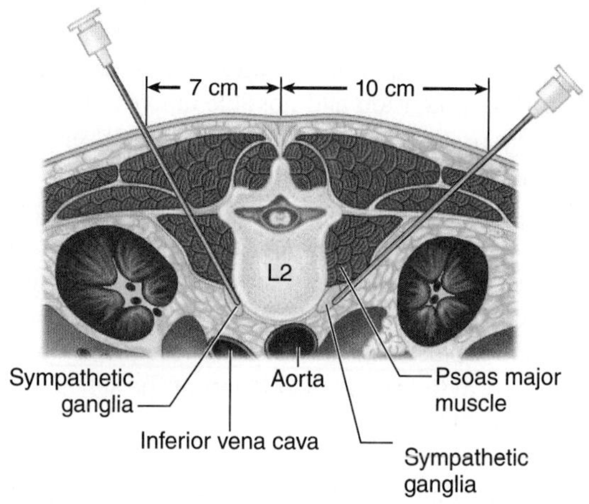

FIGURE 47–23 Lumbar sympathetic block.

D. Complications

Complications include intravascular injection into the vena cava, aorta, or lumbar vessels and somatic nerve block of the lumbar plexus. In particular, the genitofemoral nerve may be blocked.

Superior Hypogastric Plexus Block

A. Indications

This procedure is indicated for pelvic pain that is unresponsive to lumbar or caudal epidural blocks. The hypogastric plexus contains visceral sensory fibers that bypass the lower spinal cord. This block is often appropriate for patients with cancer of the cervix, uterus, bladder, prostate, or rectum and may also be effective for some women with chronic noncancer pelvic pain.

B. Anatomy

The hypogastric plexus contains not only postganglionic fibers derived from the lumbar sympathetic chain but also visceral sensory fibers from the cervix, uterus, bladder, prostate, and rectum. The superior hypogastric plexus usually lies just to the left of the midline at the L5 vertebral body and beneath the bifurcation of the aorta. The fibers of this plexus divide into left and right branches and descend to the pelvic organs via the left and right inferior hypogastric and pelvic plexuses. The inferior hypogastric plexus additionally receives preganglionic parasympathetic fibers from the S2–S4 spinal nerve roots.

C. Technique

The patient is positioned prone, and a 15-cm needle is inserted approximately 7 cm lateral to the L4–L5 spinal interspace. The needle is directed medially and caudally under fluoroscopic or ultrasound guidance so that it passes by the transverse process of L5. In its final position, the needle should lie anterior to the intervertebral disc between L5 and S1 and within 1 cm of the vertebral bodies in the anteroposterior view. When fluoroscopy is used, injection of radiopaque contrast confirms that the needle is correctly positioned in the retroperitoneal space, and 8 to 10 mL of local anesthetic is then injected. The superior hypogastric plexus block may also be performed using a transdiscal approach, though this technique is associated with the risk of discitis.

D. Complications

Complications include intravascular injection and transient bowel and bladder dysfunction.

Ganglion Impar Block

A. Indications

***Ganglion impar block* is effective for patients with visceral or sympathetically maintained pain in the perineal area.**

B. Anatomy

The ganglion impar (*ganglion of Walther*) is the most caudal part of the sympathetic trunks. The two lowest pelvic sympathetic ganglia often fuse forming one ganglion in the midline just anterior to the coccyx.

C. Technique

The patient may be positioned in the prone, lateral decubitus, or lithotomy position. A 22-gauge needle is advanced through the sacrococcygeal ligament and the rudimentary disc into a position just anterior to the coccyx. This procedure can be facilitated with fluoroscopy or ultrasound. Radiofrequency ablation, or in some cases a neurolytic injection, may provide longer duration of analgesia for this sympathetically mediated pain.

D. Complications

Intravascular injection and transient bowel or bladder dysfunction are possible. Alternative approaches involve placement of the needle through the anococcygeal ligament, though these have a higher risk of rectal perforation.

Intravenous Regional Block

A *Bier block* (see Chapter 46) utilizing local anesthetic solution with or without adjuvants can be used to interrupt sympathetic innervation to an extremity. A total volume of 50 mL of 0.5% lidocaine is typically injected, either alone or in combination with clonidine (150 mcg) and, in some cases, ketorolac (15–30 mg). This technique is described in Chapter 46.

4. Epidural Injections

Epidural steroid injections (Figure 47–24) are used for symptomatic relief of radicular pain associated

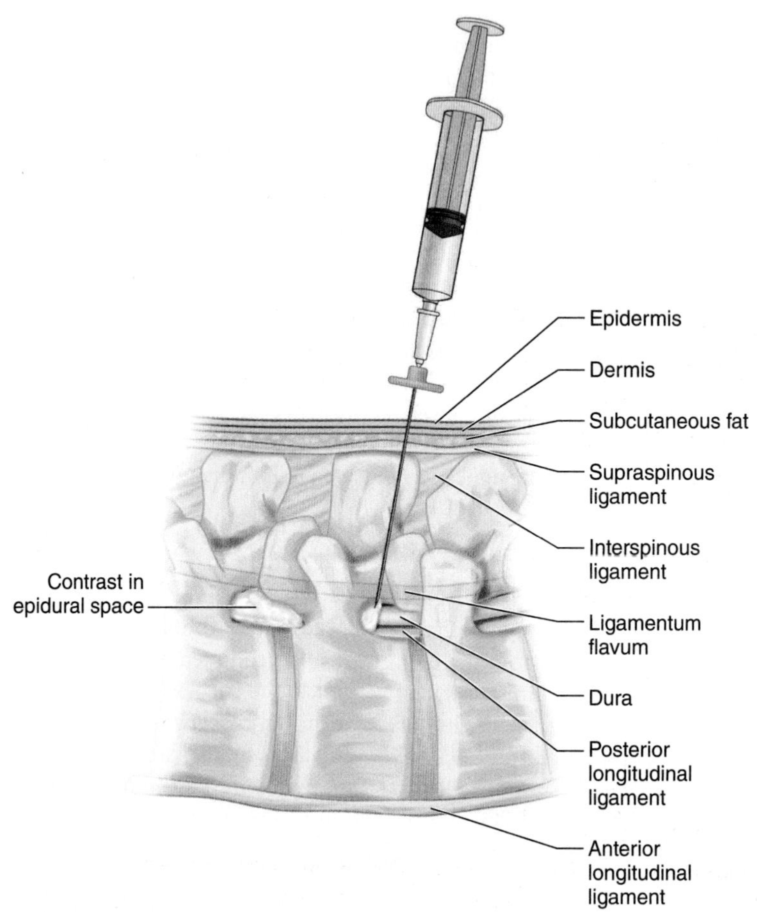

FIGURE 47–24 Epidural injection.

with nerve root compression. Pathological studies often demonstrate local inflammatory changes following disc herniation, and clinical improvement appears to be correlated with resolution of resultant nerve root edema. Epidural steroid injections are clearly superior to local anesthetics alone. They are most effective when given within 2 weeks of pain onset but appear to be of little benefit in the absence of neural compression or irritation. Long-term studies have failed to show any persistent benefit after 3 months, and these injections may change the time course of pain relief without changing long-term outcomes.

The two most commonly used agents are methylprednisolone acetate (40–80 mg) and triamcinolone diacetate (40–80 mg). Dexamethasone is being used with increased frequency because of its smaller particulate size (smaller than an erythrocyte). Intravascular injection of steroid suspension with larger particulate size may lead to embolic complications. The steroid may be injected with diluent (saline) or local anesthetic in volumes of 6 to 10 mL or 10 to 20 mL for lumbar and caudal injections, respectively. Simultaneous injection of opioids offers no added benefit and may significantly increase risks. The epidural needle should be cleared of the steroid prior to its withdrawal to prevent formation of a fistula tract or skin discoloration. Injection of local anesthetic along with the steroid can be helpful if the patient has significant muscle spasm, but it is associated with

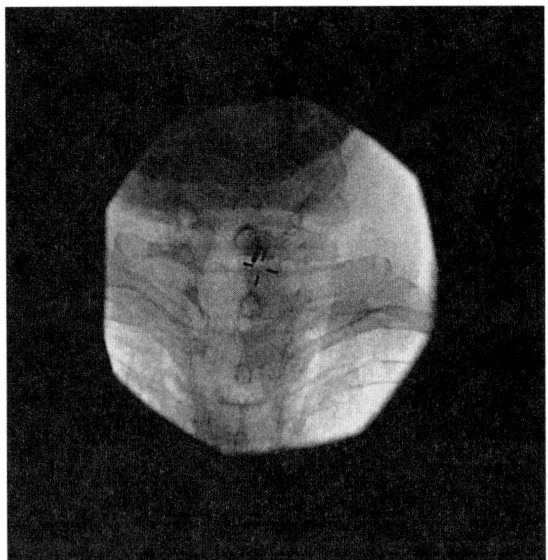

FIGURE 47–25 Fluoroscopic image of a C7–T1 epidural steroid injection; anteroposterior view. Note the Tuohy needle advanced just to the right of midline for treatment of degenerative disc disease and right radicular pain.

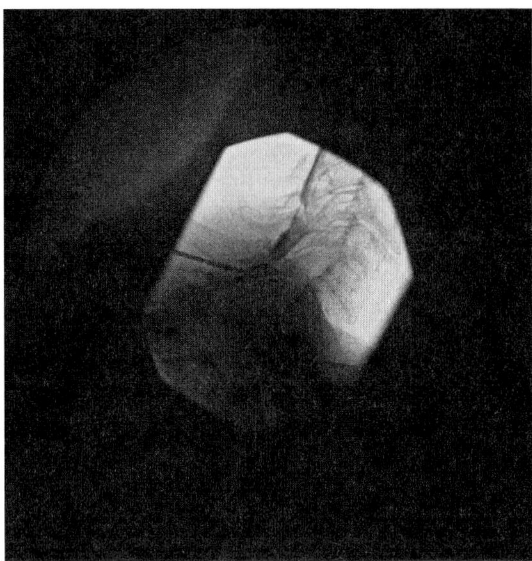

FIGURE 47–26 Fluoroscopic image of a C7–T1 epidural steroid injection with contrast; lateral view. Note radiopaque contrast confirmation of the needle in the epidural space. Live fluoroscopy is used to minimize the risk of inadvertent intravascular injection.

risks of intrathecal or subdural injection, resulting in lower extremity weakness and risk of patient fall, and intravascular injection. The presenting pain is often transiently intensified following injection, and the local anesthetic provides immediate pain relief until the steroidal anti-inflammatory effects take place, usually within 12 to 48 h.

Epidural steroid injections may be most effective when the injection is at the site of injury. Only a single injection is given if complete pain relief is achieved. If there is a good but temporary response, a second injection may be given 2 to 4 weeks later. Larger or more frequent doses increase the risk of adrenal suppression and systemic side effects. Most pain practitioners utilize fluoroscopy for epidural injection and confirm correct placement with injection of radiopaque contrast (Figures 47–25 through 47–27). A *transforaminal epidural steroid injection* (TFESI) may be more effective than the standard interlaminar epidural technique, especially for radicular pain. The needle is directed under fluoroscopic guidance into the foramen of the affected nerve root; contrast is then injected to confirm spread into the epidural

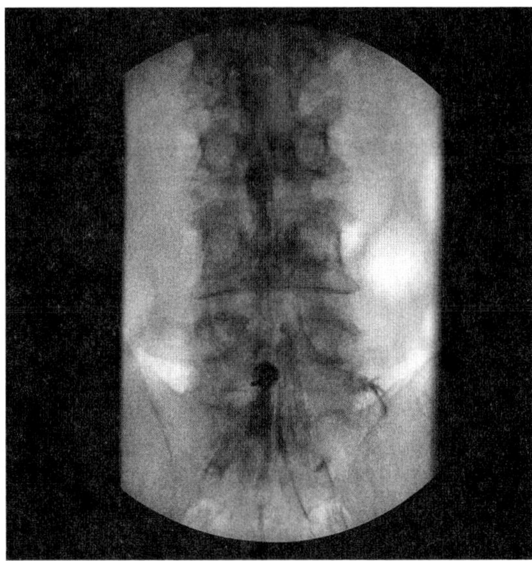

FIGURE 47–27 Lumbar epidural steroid injection, anteroposterior view. The epidural injection of contrast followed by local anesthetic and steroid solution results in spread at multiple levels of the epidural space and through the neuroforamen.

space and absence of intravascular injection prior to steroid injection. This technique differs from a *selective nerve root block* (SNRB) in two important ways; with an SNRB, the needle does not enter the foramen, and the injected solution tracks along the nerve but not into the epidural space. The SNRB may be helpful as a diagnostic procedure for the surgeon who is considering a foraminotomy at a particular affected level based upon imaging, clinical presentation, and the results of the SNRB. TFESI may be particularly effective for the treatment of radicular pain. However, a parasagittal interlaminar technique may yield similar results with a more technically straightforward approach.

Caudal epidural steroid injections may be used in patients with previous back surgery when scarring and anatomic distortion make lumbar epidural injections more difficult. Unfortunately, migration of the steroid to the site of injury may not be optimal because of anatomic distortion of the epidural space. The use of a stylet-guided catheter to direct the injection more precisely within the sacral and epidural canal may improve outcomes. However, above the level of S2, there is a risk of thecal perforation with a stylet-guided catheter. Intrathecal steroid injections are not recommended because the ethylene glycol preservative in the suspension has been implicated in arachnoiditis following unintentional subarachnoid injections.

5. Radiofrequency Ablation & Cryoneurolysis

Percutaneous *radiofrequency ablation* (RFA) relies on the heat produced by current flow from an active electrode that is incorporated at the tip of a special needle. The needle is positioned using fluoroscopic guidance. Electrical stimulation (2 Hz for motor responses, 50 Hz for sensory responses) and impedance measurement via the electrode prior to ablation also help confirm correct electrode positioning. Depending on the location of the block, the heating temperature generated at the electrode is precisely controlled (60–90°C for 1–3 min) to ablate the nerve without causing excessive collateral tissue damage. RFA is commonly used for trigeminal rhizotomy and medial branch (facet) rhizotomy. It has also been used for dorsal root rhizotomy and lumbar sympathectomy, and it may be effective for medial branches of the spinal nerves that innervate facet joints. Pain relief is usually limited to 3 to 12 months due to nerve regeneration after RFA. The lesion from thermal RFA is typically ovoid in shape and dependent upon factors such as the gauge of the needle, the temperature of the needle tip, and the duration of the heating procedure. Cooling the RFA needle with a sterile water system may decrease the charring associated with thermal lesioning and extend the spread of the lesion while heating at lower temperatures. Pulsed radiofrequency at 42°C is also being evaluated for various pain conditions.

Cryoneurolysis may produce temporary analgesia (*cryoanalgesia*) for weeks to months by freezing and thawing tissue. The temperature at the tip of a cryoprobe rapidly drops as carbon dioxide or nitrous oxide gas at high pressure is allowed to expand. The probe tip, which can achieve temperatures of –50°C to –70°C, is introduced via a 12- to 16-gauge catheter. Electrical stimulation (2–5 Hz for motor responses and 50–100 Hz for sensory responses) helps confirm correct positioning of the probe. Two or more 2-min cycles of freezing and thawing are usually administered. Cryoneurolysis is most commonly used to achieve long-term blockade of peripheral nerves and may be particularly useful for postthoracotomy pain. Patients often have neuropathic pain following thoracotomy or similar surgery. Diagnostic intercostal nerve blocks using a local anesthetic may be helpful to identify the nerve(s) that may be contributing to chronic thoracic or abdominal pain, and intercostal nerve blocks may also be utilized for longer term analgesia. The principal risks of intercostal nerve blocks are pneumothorax and local anesthetic toxicity. RFA of the intercostal nerves may be helpful as a palliative therapy for intercostal neuralgia, though there is a risk of deafferentation pain after this procedure.

6. Chemical Neurolysis

***Neurolytic blocks* are indicated for patients with severe, intractable cancer pain in whom**

more conventional therapy proves inadequate or conventional analgesic modalities are accompanied by unacceptable side effects. The most common chemical neurolytic techniques utilized for cancer patients are celiac plexus, lumbar sympathetic chain, hypogastric plexus, and ganglion impar blocks. Chemical neurolysis may also occasionally be used in patients with refractory benign neuralgia and, rarely, in patients with peripheral vascular disease. These blocks can be associated with considerable morbidity (loss of motor and sensory function), so patients must be selected carefully and only after thorough consideration of alternative analgesic modalities. Moreover, although the initial result may be excellent, the original pain may recur, or new deafferentation or central pain may develop in a majority of patients within weeks to months.

Temporary destruction of nerve fibers or ganglia can be accomplished by injection of alcohol or phenol. These neurolytic agents are not selective, affecting visceral, sensory, and motor fibers equally. Ethyl alcohol 50% to 100% causes extraction of membrane phospholipids and precipitation of lipoproteins in axons and Schwann cells, whereas phenol 6% to 12% coagulates proteins. Alcohol causes severe pain on injection; thus, local anesthetic is usually administered first. For peripheral nerve blocks, alcohol may be given undiluted, but for sympathetic blocks in which large volumes are injected, it is given in a 1:1 mixture with bupivacaine. Phenol is usually painless when injected either as a 6% or an 8% aqueous solution or in glycerol; a 12% phenol solution can be prepared in radiopaque contrast solution.

Neurolytic Techniques

Neurolytic celiac plexus or splanchnic nerve blocks may be effective for painful intraabdominal neoplasms, especially pancreatic cancer. Lumbar sympathetic, hypogastric plexus, or ganglion impar neurolytic blocks can be used for pain secondary to pelvic neoplasms. Neurolytic saddle block can provide pain relief for patients with refractory pain from pelvic malignancy; however, bowel and bladder dysfunction should be expected. Neurolytic intercostal blocks can be helpful for patients with painful rib metastases. Additional neurodestructive procedures, such as pituitary adenolysis and cordotomy, may be useful in end-of-life palliative care.

When considering any neurolytic technique, at least one diagnostic block with a local anesthetic solution alone should be performed initially to confirm the pain pathway(s) involved and to assess the potential efficacy and morbidity of the planned neurolysis. Local anesthetic solution should again be injected immediately prior to the neurolytic agent under fluoroscopic guidance. Following injection of any neurolytic agent, the needle must be cleared with air or saline prior to withdrawal to prevent damage to superficial structures.

Many clinicians prefer alcohol for celiac plexus block and phenol for lumbar sympathetic block. For subarachnoid neurolytic techniques, very small amounts of neurolytic agent (0.1 mL) are injected. Alcohol is hypobaric, whereas phenol in glycerin is hyperbaric. The patient undergoing subarachnoid neurolysis is carefully positioned so that the solution travels to the appropriate level and is confined to the dorsal horn region following subarachnoid administration.

Patients with cancer frequently receive anticoagulation therapy if they are at elevated risk for venous thromboembolic phenomena. When such a patient has discontinued anticoagulant medication in preparation for a diagnostic local anesthetic block, it may be more practical to obtain consent for a neurolytic procedure in advance and to follow the diagnostic block immediately with chemical neurolysis if the diagnostic procedure has resulted in pain relief.

7. Differential Neural Blockade

Pharmacological or anatomic differential neural blockade has been advocated as a method of distinguishing somatic, sympathetic, and psychogenic pain mechanisms. The procedure is controversial owing to the challenges of interpreting the data and the inability to define exactly which nerve fibers or pathways are blocked, and it is rarely used. Theoretically, the pharmacological approach relies on the differential sensitivity of nerve fibers to local anesthetics. Preganglionic sympathetic (B) fibers are reported to be most sensitive, closely followed by pain (Aδ) fibers, somatosensory (Aβ) fibers, motor fibers (Aα), and, finally, C fibers. By using different concentrations of local anesthetic, it may be possible to selectively block certain types of fibers while preserving the function of others. The challenge is that the critical concentration needed to block sympathetic fibers can vary considerably between patients, and conduction block by local anesthetics is dependent not only on fiber size but also on the duration of contact, length of nerve exposed to the anesthetic, and frequency of impulses conducted. Many clinicians have therefore abandoned the use of pharmacological differential neural blocks in favor of anatomic differential blockade.

Stellate ganglion blocks can be used to selectively block sympathetic fibers to the head, neck, and arm. Celiac plexus, hypogastric plexus, and lumbar paravertebral sympathetic blocks can be used for sympathetic blocks of the abdomen, pelvis, and leg, respectively. Selective nerve root, intercostal, cervical plexus, brachial plexus, or lumbosacral plexus blocks may be used for somatic nerve blockade.

Differential epidural blocks may be used for thoracic pain when the techniques for sympathetic blockade carry a significant risk of pneumothorax (Table 47–16). After each epidural injection, the patient is evaluated for pain relief, signs of sympathetic blockade (eg, a decrease in blood pressure), sensation to pinprick and light touch, and motor function. If the pain disappears after the saline injection, the patient either has psychogenic pain (usually a profound, long-lasting effect) or is displaying a placebo effect (usually short lasting). If pain relief coincides with isolated signs of sympathetic blockade, it is likely mediated by sympathetic fibers. If pain relief only follows somatosensory blockade, it is likely mediated by somatic fibers. Lastly, if the pain persists even after signs of motor blockade, the pain is either central (supraspinal) or psychogenic.

TABLE 47–16 Solutions for differential epidural blockade.

Solution	Epidural[1]
Placebo	Saline
Sympatholytic	0.5% lidocaine
Somatic	1% lidocaine
All fibers	2% lidocaine

[1]Chloroprocaine may be used instead.

The differential epidural block carries the risk of any neuraxial block and the possibility of hypotension and blocking cardiac accelerator fibers at T1–T4. The level should not extend above the T5 dermatome due to these risks. Following catheter insertion, injections should be administered with the patient in a monitored setting for the remainder of the procedure.

Although differential epidural blockade has limitations, it may be helpful to identify primarily centralized pain when a patient continues to have a significant level of pain despite multilevel dermatomal blockade of the painful region. It is unlikely that a subsequent nerve block would help treat the painful condition.

When it is thought that a patient may have abdominal pain from the anterior abdominal wall, a TAP block may be performed using ultrasound guidance. This may offer potential short- or long-term relief and can be considered as an alternative to differential epidural blockade. If no relief is obtained, the pain may have a visceral origin or a central cause. Visceral pain may best respond to a celiac or splanchnic nerve block and possibly to subsequent splanchnic RFA or chemical neurolysis. Patients with pain that is primarily of a central origin may respond to multidisciplinary therapy, including counseling and biofeedback training.

8. Neuromodulation

Electrical stimulation of the nervous system can produce analgesia in patients with acute and chronic pain. Current may be applied transcutaneously, epidurally, or by electrodes implanted into the central nervous system.

Transcutaneous Electrical Nerve Stimulation

Transcutaneous electrical nerve stimulation (TENS) is thought to produce analgesia by stimulating large afferent fibers. It may have a role for patients with mild to moderate acute pain and those with chronic low back pain, arthritis, and neuropathic pain. The gate theory of pain processing suggests that the afferent input from large epicritic fibers competes with that from the smaller pain fibers. An alternative theory proposes that at high rates of stimulation, TENS causes conduction block in small afferent pain fibers.

With conventional TENS, electrodes are applied to the same dermatome as the pain and are stimulated periodically by direct current from a generator (usually for 30 min several times a day). A current of 10 to 30 mA with a pulse width of 50 to 80 μs is applied at a frequency of 80 to 100 Hz. Some patients whose pain is refractory to conventional TENS respond to low-frequency TENS (acupuncture-like TENS), which employs stimuli with a pulse width greater than 200 μs at frequencies less than 10 Hz (for 5–15 min). Unlike conventional TENS, low-frequency stimulation is at least partly reversed by naloxone, suggesting a role for endogenous opioids. This technique is also called *dorsal column stimulation* because it was originally thought to produce analgesia by directly stimulating large Aβ fibers in the dorsal columns of the spinal cord.

Spinal Cord Stimulation

23 ***Spinal cord stimulation*** **(SCS) may be effective for neuropathic pain, including sympathetically mediated pain, spinal cord lesions with localized segmental pain, phantom limb pain, ischemic lower extremity pain due to peripheral vascular disease, adhesive arachnoiditis, peripheral neuropathies, post-thoracotomy pain, intercostal neuralgia, postherpetic neuralgia, angina, visceral abdominal pain, and visceral pelvic pain. Patients with persisting pain after back surgery, which is typically a mixed nociceptive–neuropathic disorder, also appear to benefit from SCS.**

Temporary electrodes are initially placed in the posterior epidural space and connected to an external electrical pulse generator to evaluate efficacy in a 5- to 7-day trial (Figures 47–28 and 47–29). The trial may be extended, particularly if it allows a patient, such as one with CRPS, to tolerate more aggressive physical therapy. If a favorable response is obtained, a fully implantable system is inserted. Unfortunately, the effectiveness of the technique decreases with time in some patients.

Dorsal root ganglion (DRG) stimulation has been shown to be an effective therapy and alternative to SCS to help treat CRPS in the lower extremities and improve tolerance of physical therapy (Figure 47–30).

Complications of SCS and DRG stimulation include infection, lead migration, and lead breakage.

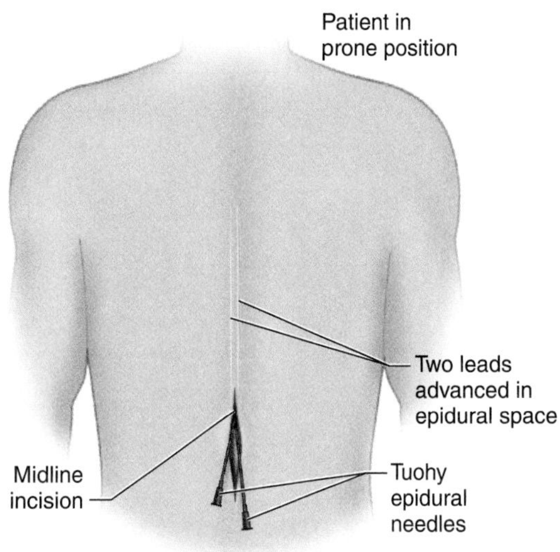

FIGURE 47–28 Patient positioning for insertion of a spinal cord stimulator (SCS) with fluoroscopic guidance.

Peripheral Nerve Stimulation

Peripheral nerve stimulation (PNS) differs from SCS in that leads are placed in close anatomic proximity to an injured peripheral nerve. The leads may be placed percutaneously, with or without ultrasound guidance, or surgically under direct vision of the nerve. Occipital nerve stimulators are one form of peripheral nerve stimulator that may be helpful in treating occipital neuralgia and migraine headache (Figure 47–31). The use of PNS has expanded in recent years, with the development of less invasive implantable and removable leads with external, rather than implanted, pulse generators.

Deep Brain Stimulation

Deep brain stimulation (DBS) is used for intractable cancer pain and for intractable nonmalignant neuropathic pain. Electrodes are implanted stereotactically into the periaqueductal and periventricular gray areas for nociceptive pain, usually in patients with cancer or chronic low back pain. For neuropathic pain, the electrodes are frequently implanted into the ventral posterolateral and ventral posteromedial thalamic nuclei. DBS may also be helpful for patients with movement disorders, headache, and neuropsychiatric disorders. The most serious

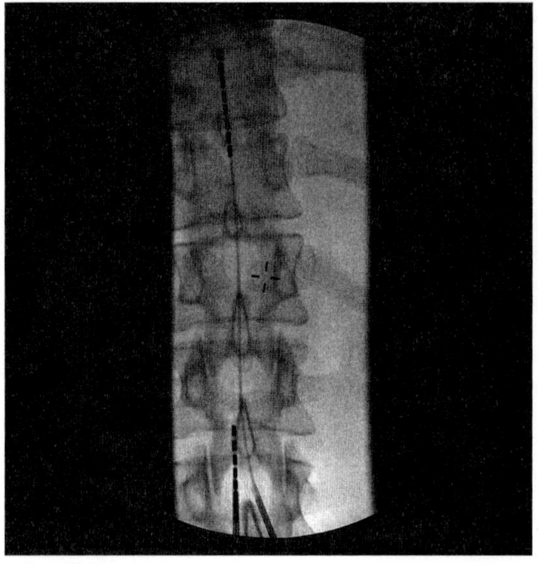
A

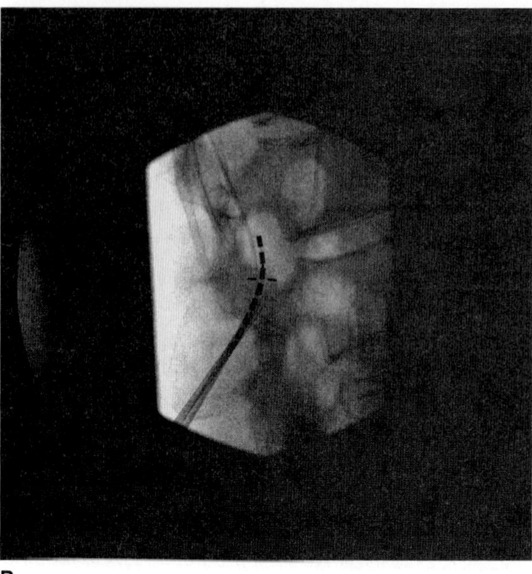
B

FIGURE 47–29 Two-lead SCS placement. **A**: Anteroposterior view. The right contact lead has been advanced to its final position at the top of T10. The left lead is advanced through the Tuohy needle. **B**: Lateral view. The first lead is in position, with the left lead entering the epidural space.

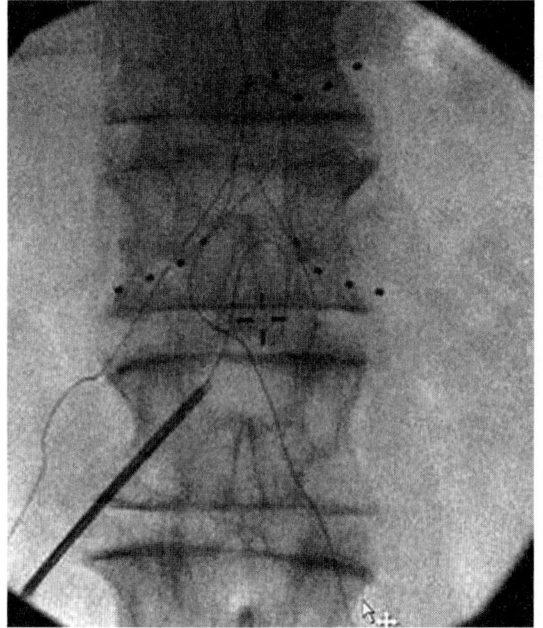
A

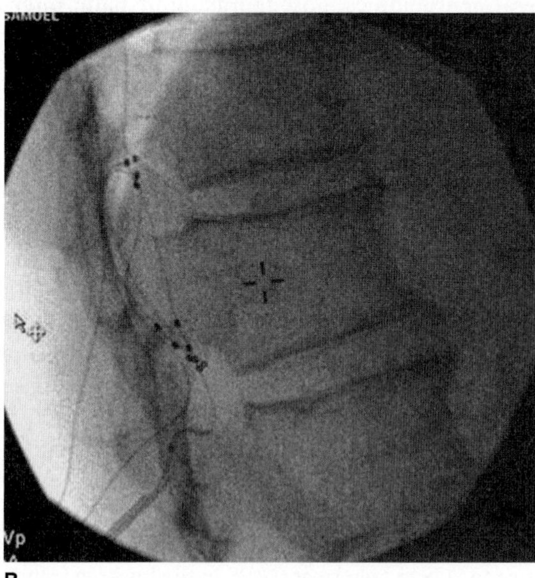
B

FIGURE 47–30 Dorsal root ganglion (DRG) stimulation. **A**: Anteroposterior view. Dorsal root ganglion stimulation at right T11 and bilateral T12. Note Tuohy needle entry into the lateral aspect of the epidural space one level below the stimulator exiting the contralateral foramen. **B**: Lateral view reveals one dorsal root ganglion stimulator at T11 and two at T12.

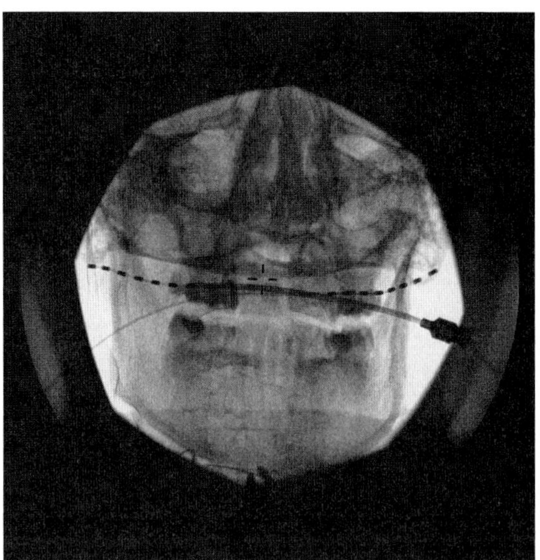

FIGURE 47–31 Occipital nerve stimulator placement, anteroposterior view. Following the placement of a right occipital nerve stimulator lead below the nuchal ridge, a left occipital nerve stimulator lead has been advanced through the introducer needle.

complications are intracranial hemorrhage and infection.

9. Vertebral Augmentation

24 **Patients with pathological or osteoporotic vertebral compression fractures may benefit from *vertebral augmentation* with polymethylmethacrylate (PMMA) cement. *Vertebroplasty* involves injection of the cement through the trocar needle. *Kyphoplasty* involves inflation of a balloon inserted through a percutaneously placed trocar needle, with subsequent injection of cement** (Figure 47–32). Anteroposterior and lateral fluoroscopic views facilitate optimal placement of the cement. For patients with a sacral insufficiency fracture, *cement sacroplasty* may help stabilize the fracture. Risks of vertebral augmentation include direct nerve injury (due to placement of the trocar needle), hemorrhage, cement extravasation, and embolic events.

Kiva VCF vertebral augmentation has become available as an alternative approach to increase vertebral height after a recent compression fracture. The Kiva procedure involves placing a coil into the vertebral body over which a polyetheretherketone (PEEK) implant may be inserted. PMMA cement may be injected subsequently into the PEEK implant (Figure 47–33)

MULTIDISCIPLINARY TREATMENT

Psychological Interventions

Psychological techniques, including cognitive therapy, behavioral therapy, biofeedback, relaxation techniques, and hypnosis, are widely used as part of a multidisciplinary approach to pain control. Cognitive interventions are based on the assumption that a patient's attitude toward pain can influence the perception of pain. Maladaptive

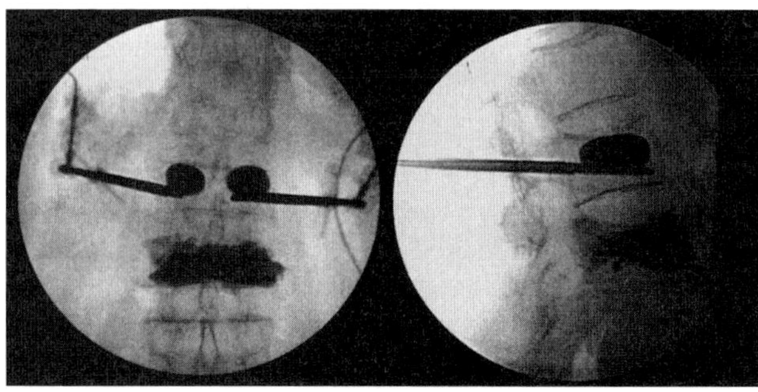

A B

FIGURE 47–32 Kyphoplasty. **A**: Anteroposterior view reveals inflation of balloons at L2 prior to deflation and subsequent injection of polymethylmethacrylate (PMMA) at that level. Previously injected PMMA can be seen at L3 into the cavity created by bilateral balloon inflation and deflation. **B**: Lateral view. The balloons are inflated above the introducers at L2. The previously injected PMMA can be seen in the L3 vertebral body.

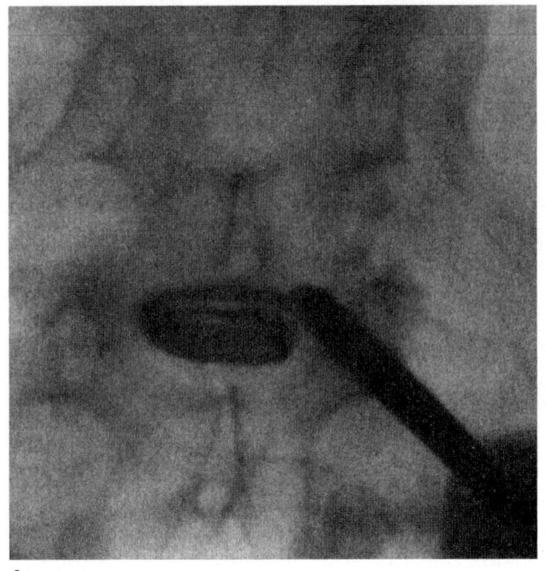

A

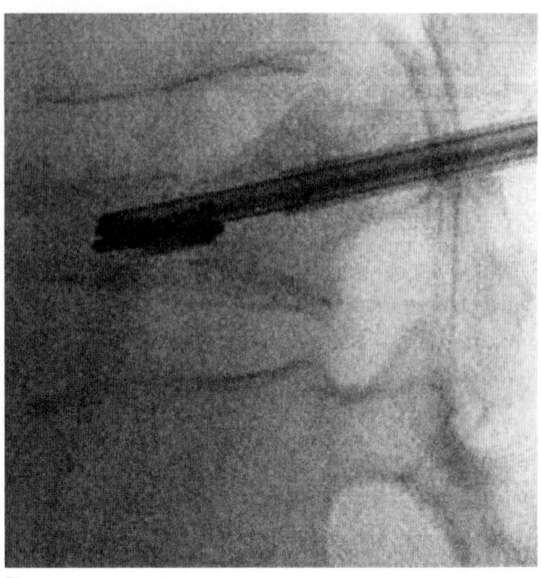

B

FIGURE 47–33 Kiva vertebral compression fracture (KCF) system for vertebral augmentation. **A**: Anteroposterior view reveals appropriate width of coil to allow for subsequent polyetheretherketone (PEEK) implant deployment. **B**: Lateral view reveals advancing coil to create a cavity and allow for advancing and deployment of a PEEK implant and subsequent injection of PMMA.

attitudes contribute to suffering and disability. Pain coping skills are taught either individually or in group therapy. The most common techniques include *attention diversion* and *imagery*. *Behavioral (operant) therapy* is based on the premise that behavior in patients with chronic pain is determined by consequences of the behavior. Positive reinforcers (such as attention from a spouse) tend to enable or intensify the pain, whereas negative reinforcers reduce pain. The therapist's role is to guide behavior modification with the aid of family members and medical providers to nurture negative reinforcers and minimize positive reinforcers.

Relaxation techniques teach the patient to alter the arousal response and the increase in sympathetic tone associated with pain. The most commonly employed technique is a progressive muscle relaxation exercise. *Biofeedback* and *hypnosis* are closely related interventions. All forms of biofeedback are based on the principle that patients can be taught to control involuntary physiological parameters. Once proficient in the technique, the patient may be able to induce a relaxation response and more effectively apply coping skills to control physiological factors (eg, muscle tension) that worsen pain. The most commonly utilized physiological parameters in biofeedback are muscle tension (electromyographic biofeedback) and temperature (thermal biofeedback). The effectiveness of hypnosis varies considerably among individuals. Hypnotic techniques teach patients to alter pain perception by having them focus on other sensations, localize the pain to another site, and dissociate themselves from a painful experience through imagery. Patients with chronic headaches and musculoskeletal disorders benefit most from these relaxation techniques.

Physical Therapy

Heat and cold can provide pain relief by alleviating muscle spasm. In addition, heat decreases joint stiffness and increases blood flow, and cold vasoconstricts and can reduce tissue edema. The analgesic action of heat and cold may at least partially be explained by the gate theory of pain processing.

Superficial heating modalities include conductive (hot packs, paraffin baths, fluidotherapy), convective (hydrotherapy), and radiant (infrared) techniques. Techniques for application of deep heat include ultrasound as well as shortwave and microwave diathermy. These modalities are more effective for pain involving deep joints and muscles. Cold is most effective for pain associated with acute injuries and edema, and it can also relieve muscle spasm. Application may take the form of cold packs, ice massage, or vapocoolant sprays (ethyl chloride or fluoromethane).

Exercise should be part of any rehabilitation program for chronic pain. A graded exercise program prevents joint stiffness, muscle atrophy, and contractures, all of which can contribute to the patient's pain and functional disabilities. McKenzie exercises are particularly helpful for patients with lumbar disc displacement. Patients may state that physical therapy has not helped in the past; however, the efficacy of previous physical therapy techniques should be assessed, and the appropriateness of current physical therapy sessions and of the home exercise program should also be evaluated. By facilitating increased range of motion and providing constant resistance, aquatherapy may be particularly helpful for patients who may not be able to tolerate other forms of therapy.

Acupuncture

25 **Acupuncture can be a useful adjunct for patients with chronic pain, particularly that associated with chronic musculoskeletal disorders and headaches.** The technique involves the insertion of needles into discrete, anatomically defined points, called *meridians*. Stimulation of the needle after insertion takes the form of twirling or of application of a mild electrical current. Insertion points appear to be unrelated to the conventional anatomy of the nervous system. Although the scientific literature concerning the mechanism of action and role of acupuncture in pain management is controversial, some studies suggest that acupuncture stimulates the release of endogenous opioids, as its effects can be antagonized by naloxone.

GUIDELINES

Benzon HT, Maus TP, Kang HR, et al. The use of contrast agents in interventional pain procedures: a multispecialty and multisociety practice advisory on nephrogenic systemic fibrosis, gadolinium deposition in the brain, encephalopathy after unintentional intrathecal gadolinium injection, and hypersensitivity reactions. *Anesth Analg.* 2021;133:535.

Cohen SP, Bhaskar A, Bhatia A, et al. Consensus practice guidelines on interventions for lumbar facet joint pain from a multispecialty, international working group. *Reg Anesth Pain Med.* 2020;45:424.

Deer TR, Pope JE, Hyek SM, et al. The Polyanalgesic Consensus Conference (PACC): recommendations on intrathecal drug infusion systems best practices and guidelines. *Neuromodulation.* 2017;20:96.

Dowell D, Haegerich TM, Chou R. CDC guidelines for prescribing opioids for chronic pain—United States, 2016. *MMWR Recomm Rep.* 2016;65:1.

Narouze S, Benzon HT, Provenzano D, et al. Interventional spine and pain procedures in patients on antiplatelet and anticoagulant medications (second edition): guidelines From the American Society of Regional Anesthesia and Pain Medicine, the European Society of Regional Anaesthesia and Pain Therapy, the American Academy of Pain Medicine, the International Neuromodulation Society, the North American Neuromodulation Society, and the World Institute of Pain. *Reg Anesth Pain Med.* 2018;43:225.

Rathmell JP, Benzon HT, Dreyfuss T, et al. Safeguards to prevent neurologic complications after epidural steroid injections: consensus opinions from a multidisciplinary working group and national organizations. *Anesthesiology.* 2015;122:974.

Van Boxem K, Rijsdijk M, Hans G, et al. Safe use of epidural corticosteroid injections: recommendations of the WIP Benelux Work Group. *Pain Pract.* 2019;19:61.

SUGGESTED READINGS

Abd-Elsayed A, Karri J, Michael A, et al. Intrathecal drug delivery for chronic pain syndromes: a review of considerations in practice management. *Pain Physician.* 2020;23:E591.

Cheng J, Chen SL, Zimmerman N, et al. A new radiofrequency ablation procedure to treat sacroiliac joint pain. *Pain Physician.* 2016;19:603.

Cohen I, Lema MJ. What's new in chronic pain pathophysiology. *Can J Pain.* 2020;4:13.

Culp C, Kim HK, Abdi S. Ketamine use for cancer and chronic pain management. *Front Pharmacol.* 2021;11:599721.

Davis T, Loudermilk E, Depalma M, et al. Prospective, multicenter, randomized, crossover clinical trial comparing the safety and effectiveness of cooled radiofrequency ablation with corticosteroid injection in the management of knee pain from osteoarthritis. *Reg Anesth Pain Med.* 2018;43:84.

Deer TR, Esposito MF, McRoberts WP, et al. A systematic literature review of peripheral nerve stimulation therapies for the treatment of pain. *Pain Medicine.* 2020;21:1590.

Deer TR, Levy RM, Kramer J, et al. Dorsal root ganglion stimulation yielded higher treatment success rate for complex regional pain syndrome and causalgia at 3 and 12 months: a randomized comparative trial. *Pain.* 2017;158:669.

Desai MJ, Kapural L, Petersohn JD, et al. A prospective, randomized, multicenter, open-label clinical trial comparing intradiscal biacuplasty to conventional medical management for discogenic lumbar back pain. *Spine.* 2016;41:1065.

Encinosa W, Bernard D, Selden TM. Opioid and non-opioid analgesic prescribing before and after the CDC's 2016 opioid guideline. *Int J Health Econ Manag.* 2021:1.

Gilmore CA, Ilfeld BM, Rosenow JM, et al. Percutaneous 60-day peripheral nerve stimulation implant provides sustained relief of chronic pain following amputation: 12-month follow-up of a randomized, double-blind, placebo-controlled trial. *Reg Anesth Pain Med.* 2020;45:44.

Kapural L, Yu C, Doust MW, et al. Comparison of 10-kHz high-frequency and traditional low-frequency spinal cord stimulation for the treatment of chronic back and leg pain: 24-month results from a multicenter, randomized, controlled pivotal trial. *Neurosurgery.* 2016;79:667.

Khalil JG, Smuck M, Koreckij T, et al. A prospective, randomized, multicenter study of intraosseous basivertebral nerve ablation for the treatment of chronic low back pain. *Spine.* 2019;19:1620.

Long Y, Yi W, Yang D. Advances in vertebral augmentation systems for osteoporotic vertebral compression fractures. *Pain Res Manag.* 2020;2020:3947368.

Meng L, Tseng CH, Shivkumar K, Ajijola O. Efficacy of stellate ganglion blockade in managing electrical storm: a systematic review. *JACC Clin Electrophysiol.* 2017;3:942.

Ni Y, Yang L, Han R, et al. Implantable peripheral nerve stimulation for trigeminal neuropathic pain: a systematic review and meta-analysis. *Neuromodulation.* 2021;24:983.

Niraj G, Kamel Y. Ultrasound-guided subcostal TAP block with depot steroids in the management of chronic abdominal pain secondary to chronic pancreatitis: a three-year prospective audit in 54 patients. *Pain Medicine.* 2020;21:118.

Otten LA, Bornemann R, Jansen TR, et al. Comparison of balloon kyphoplasty with the new Kiva VCF system for the treatment of vertebral compression fractures. *Pain Physician.* 2013;16:E505.

Provenzano DA, Watson TW, Somers DL, et al. The interaction between the composition of preinjected fluids and duration of radiofrequency on lesion size. *Reg Anesth Pain Med.* 2015;40:112.

Smuck M, Khalil J, Barrette K, et al; INTRACEPT Trial Investigators. Prospective, randomized, multicenter study of intraosseous basivertebral nerve ablation for the treatment of chronic low back pain: 12-month results. *Reg Anesth Pain Med.* 2021;46:683.

Strand NH, D'Souza R, Wie C, et al. Mechanism of action of peripheral nerve stimulation. *Curr Pain Headache Rep.* 2021;25:47.

Suri H, Ailani J. Cluster headache: a review and update in treatment. *Curr Neurol Neurosci Rep.* 2021;21:31.

Toljan K, Vrooman B. Low-dose naltrexone (LDN)—review of therapeutic utilization. *Medical Sciences.* 2018;6:82.

Vrooman B, Kapural L, Sarwar S, et al. Lidocaine 5% patch for treatment of acute pain after robotic cardiac surgery and prevention of persistent incisional pain: a randomized, placebo-controlled, double-blind trial. *Pain Medicine.* 2015;16:1610.

CHAPTER 48

Enhanced Recovery Protocols & Optimization of Perioperative Outcomes

Gabriele Baldini, MD, MSc

KEY CONCEPTS

1. A well-functioning enhanced recovery program (ERP) uses evidence-based practices to ensure continuity of care, decrease variation in clinical management, minimize organ dysfunction, decrease postoperative complications, and accelerate convalescence. Adherence to ERP pathways is associated with better postoperative outcomes, accelerated convalescence, and lower costs.
2. The perioperative surgical home (PSH) is defined by interdisciplinary, team-based global management of the surgical patient throughout the surgical care continuum. PSH management begins following the initial surgical diagnosis and patient preparation and ends when the patient is returned to the care of their primary health care provider after full recovery. It includes several perioperative enhanced recovery program (ERP) elements that are adapted to the local clinical care environment.
3. Persistent postsurgical pain (chronic pain that continues beyond the typical healing period of 1 to 2 months following surgery or well past the normal period for postoperative follow-up) is increasingly acknowledged as a common and vexing problem following surgery.
4. The magnitude of the surgical stress response is related to the intensity of the surgical stimulus, hypothermia, and psychological stress. It can be moderated by perioperative interventions, including neural blockade and reduction in procedural invasiveness.
5. Neuraxial blockade of nociceptive stimuli by epidural and spinal local anesthetics blunts the metabolic, inflammatory, and neuroendocrine stress response to surgery. In major open abdominal and thoracic procedures, thoracic epidural blockade with local anesthetic provides excellent analgesia, facilitates mobilization, and decreases the incidence and severity of ileus.
6. Epidural blockade using a solution of local anesthetic and low-dose opioid provides better postoperative analgesia at rest and with movement than systemic opioids. By sparing opioid use and minimizing the incidence of systemic opioid-related side effects, epidural analgesia facilitates both earlier mobilization and earlier resumption of oral nutrition, expediting exercise activity and attenuating loss of body mass.
7. Peripheral nerve blocks (PNBs) with local anesthetics (single-shot or continuous infusion) block afferent nociceptive pathways and are an excellent way to minimize the need for systemic opioids and thereby reduce the incidence of opioid-related side effects.

—Continued next page

Continued—

8 Lidocaine (intravenous bolus of 100 mg or 1.5–2 mg/kg, followed by continuous intravenous infusion of 1.5–3 mg/kg/h or 2–3 mg/min) has analgesic, antihyperalgesic, and anti-inflammatory properties.

9 Multimodal analgesia combines different classes of medications that have different (*multimodal*) pharmacological mechanisms of action, resulting in additive or synergistic effects to reduce postoperative pain and its sequelae.

10 The addition of nonsteroidal anti-inflammatory drugs (NSAIDs) to systemic opioid analgesia diminishes postoperative pain intensity, reduces opioid requirements, and decreases opioid-related side effects such as postoperative nausea and vomiting (PONV), sedation, and urinary retention. However, NSAIDs may increase the risk of gastrointestinal and wound bleeding, adversely impact kidney function, and impair wound healing.

11 Opioid administration by patient-controlled analgesia provides better pain control, greater patient satisfaction, and fewer opioid side effects when compared with nurse-administered on-request (PRN) parenteral opioid administration.

12 Single-shot and continuous peripheral nerve blockade is frequently utilized for fast-track ambulatory and inpatient orthopedic surgery and can accelerate recovery from surgery and improve analgesia and patient satisfaction.

13 Postoperative ileus delays postoperative resumption of enteral feeding, is often a source of considerable patient discomfort, and is one of the most common causes of prolonged postoperative hospital length of stay and preventable hospitalization costs. Nasogastric tubes should be discouraged whenever possible or used for only a very short period of time, even with gastrointestinal surgery. The opioid-sparing effects of multimodal analgesia shorten the duration of postoperative ileus or may preempt it entirely.

14 Because either excessive, or excessively restricted, perioperative fluid therapy increases the incidence and severity of postoperative ileus, a goal-directed fluid administration strategy may be beneficial, especially in patients undergoing major surgery associated with large fluid shifts or patients at high risk of developing postoperative gastrointestinal complications.

Evolution of Enhanced Recovery Programs

Advances in surgical and anesthetic management have progressively decreased risk-adjusted perioperative mortality and morbidity. Continued improvement in perioperative outcomes, including accelerated postoperative convalescence and decreased perioperative complications, depends upon the continued evolution of integrated, multidisciplinary team approaches to perioperative care. The goal of team-based care is to combine individual evidence-based elements of perioperative care (eg, analgesic regimens, nutritional interventions, physical therapy), each of which may have modest benefits when used in isolation, into a tightly coordinated effort that has significant synergistic, beneficial effects upon surgical outcomes (the *theory of aggregation of marginal gains*).

Such coordinated, multidisciplinary perioperative care programs are termed *enhanced recovery programs* (ERPs), *fast-track surgery*, or *enhanced recovery after surgery* (ERAS) (Figure 48–1). 1

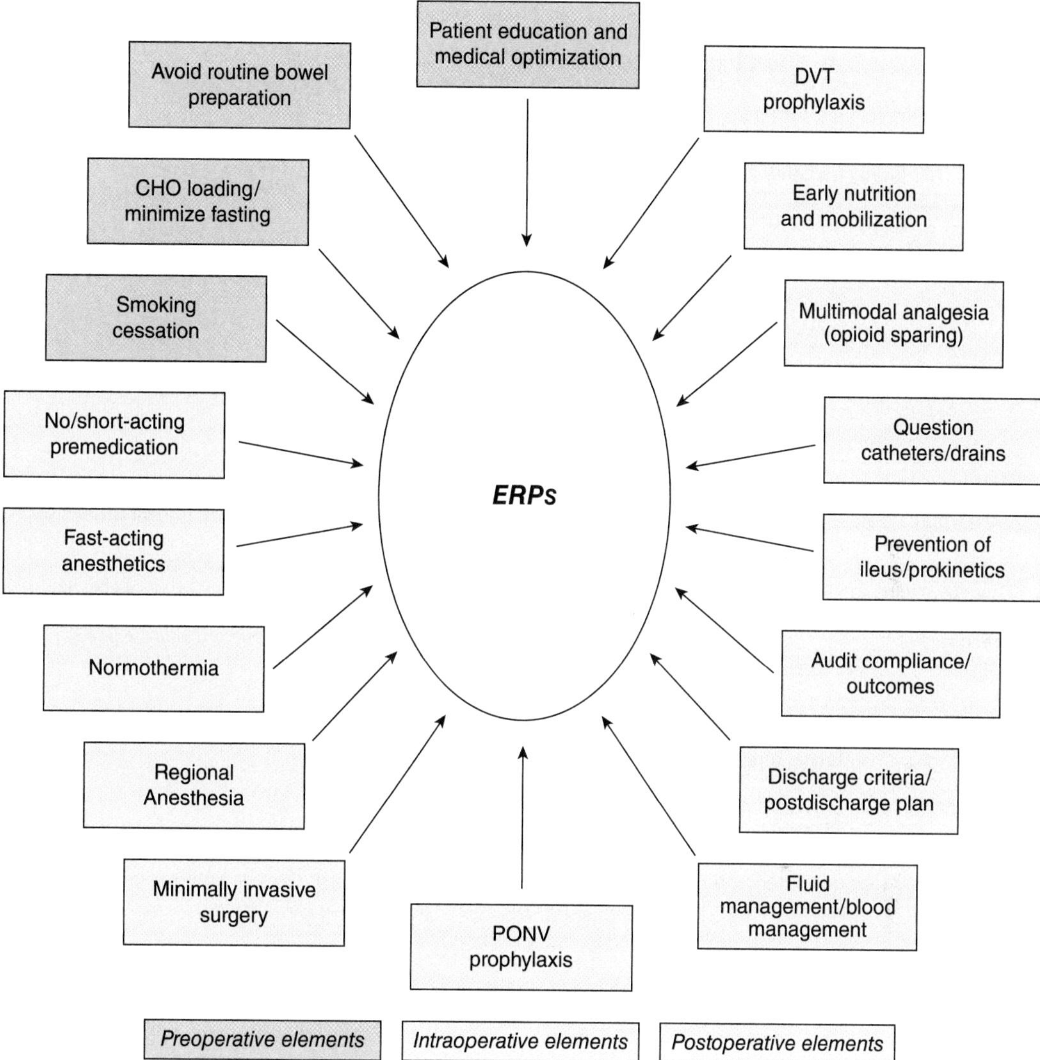

FIGURE 48–1 Perioperative elements contributing to enhanced recovery after surgery (ERAS). CHO, carbohydrate; DVT, deep vein thrombosis; PONV, postoperative nausea and vomiting. (Reproduced with permission from Fearon KC, Ljungqvist O, Von Meyenfeldt M, et al. Enhanced recovery after surgery: A consensus review of clinical care for patients undergoing colonic resection. *Clin Nutr.* 2005 June;24(3):466-477.)

A well-functioning ERP uses evidence-based practices that ensure continuity of care, decrease variation in clinical management, minimize organ dysfunction, decrease postoperative complications, and accelerate convalescence (Figure 48–2). The success of ERPs relies upon the additive or synergistic effects of the interventions included in these programs. Adherence to ERP pathways is associated with better postoperative outcomes, accelerated convalescence, and lower costs.

Assessing outcomes following ERP adoption is critical. Hospital length of stay is a commonly used measure of success, though in many health care systems, the timing of hospital discharge is more influenced by administrative and organizational issues than by discrete surgical and medical milestones in

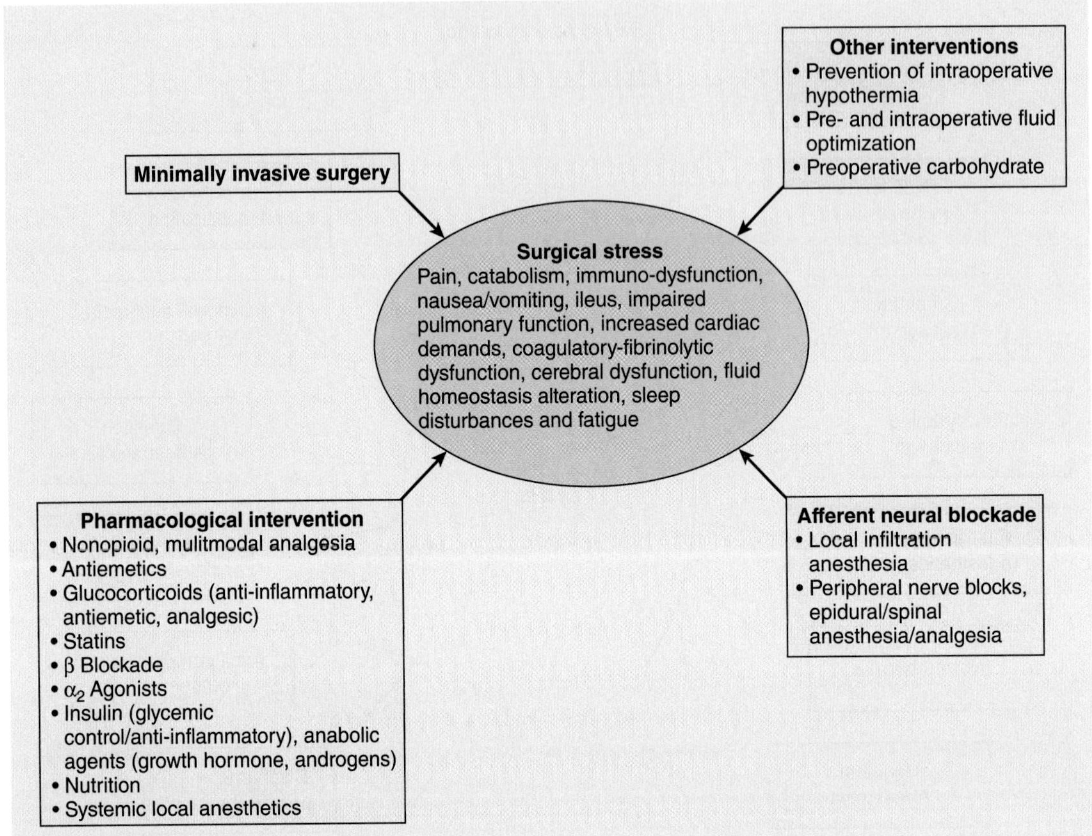

FIGURE 48–2 Multimodal interventions to attenuate the surgical stress response. (Reproduced with permission from Kehlet H, Wilmore DW. Evidence-based surgical care and the evolution of fast-track surgery. *Ann Surg.* 2008 Aug;248(2):189-198.)

the patient's postoperative recovery. Little research has been undertaken to define the process of postoperative recovery, and there is only limited consensus as to outcome measures that confirm that postoperative recovery has been accomplished for a given surgical disease. Other measures of successful implementation of ERPs include reduced rates of hospital readmission and reduced rates and severity of perioperative complications. Promising data suggest that ERPs may improve oncologic outcomes after surgery.

Anesthetic interventions that reduce pain, facilitate earlier postoperative mobilization, and allow earlier resumption of oral feeding accelerate the pace of perioperative recovery. In this context, the anesthesia provider must not only provide ideal anesthetic management throughout the procedure but must also help improve overall perioperative care. These goals are achieved through optimizing the patient's preoperative medical condition, avoiding prolonged fasting, moderating the adverse effects of the intraoperative neuroendocrine stress response, and providing multimodal pain and symptom management to accelerate postoperative recovery.

Initially developed for patients undergoing colorectal and cardiac surgery, ERPs have also been developed for patients undergoing most other forms of major surgery. Many ERP guidelines and consensus statements are available from the various surgical specialty societies.

2 The *perioperative surgical home (PSH)* has been defined as a "patient-centered, innovative model of delivering health care during the entire patient surgical/procedural experience; from the time of the decision for surgery until the patient has recovered and returned to the care of his or her patient-centered medical home or primary health care provider." The PSH "provides coordination of care throughout all of the clinical microsystems of care." PSH programs can be considered an evolution of ERPs because they include several perioperative ERP elements but are adapted to the local clinical environment. Anesthesiologists often play a pivotal, coordinating role in the PSH, integrating perioperative medical, anesthetic, and surgical care provided to surgical patients. Accordingly, anesthesiology residency and fellowship programs must expand their curricula to include these broad issues.

3 *Persistent postsurgical pain* (chronic pain that continues beyond the typical healing period of 1–2 months following surgery) is increasingly acknowledged as a common and vexing problem following surgery. The incidence of persistent postsurgical pain may exceed 30% after some operations, especially amputations, thoracotomy, mastectomy, and inguinal herniorrhaphy. Although the cause is unclear, several risk factors have been identified (Figure 48–3). Multimodal perioperative pain control is often suggested as a fundamental preemptive strategy to reduce the incidence of persistent postsurgical pain (see Chapter 47).

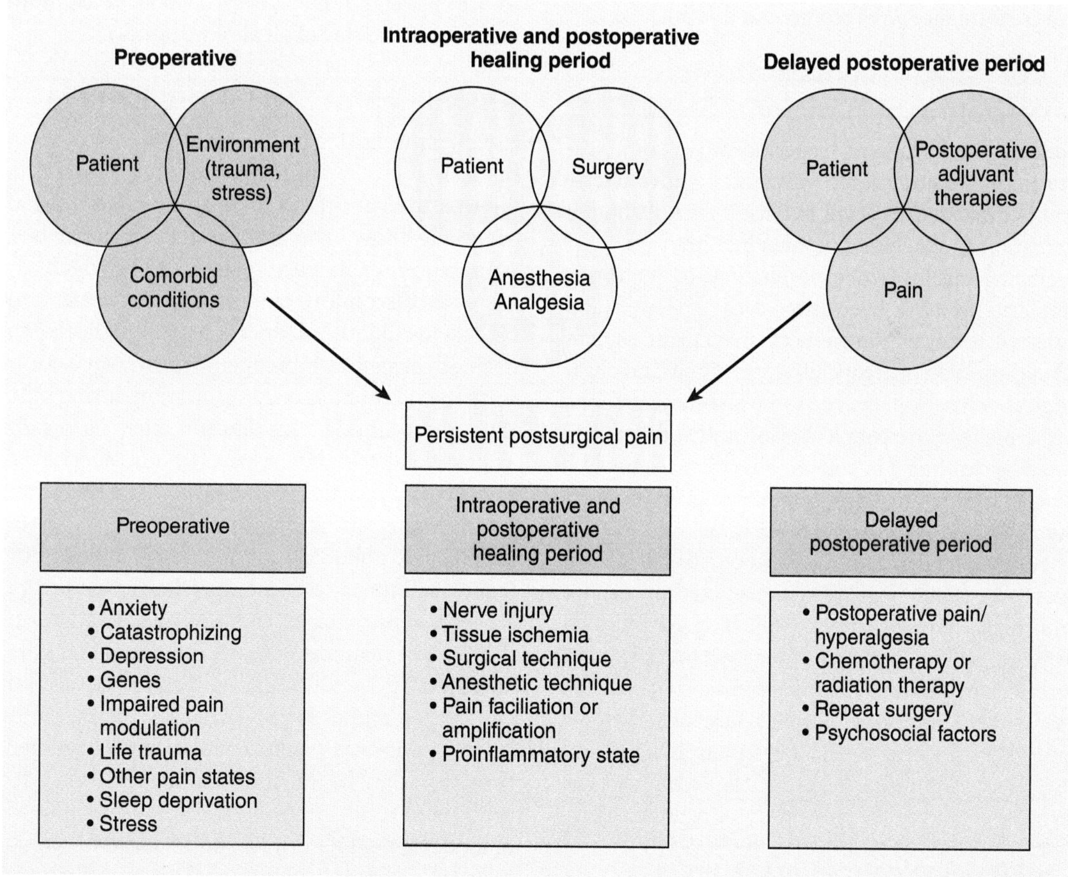

FIGURE 48–3 Risk factors for persistent postsurgical pain. (Reproduced with permission from Wu CL, Raja SN. Treatment of acute postoperative pain. *Lancet.* 2011;377(9784):2215-2225.)

Anesthetic Management–Related Factors Contributing to Enhanced Recovery

PREOPERATIVE PERIOD

Patient Education

The patient and family must cooperate and actively participate if an ERP is to be effective. Preoperative teaching must use plain language and avoid medical jargon. Well-designed print, video, and online materials presented in the patient's native language are useful to introduce ERPs. Smartphone text messaging and patient navigation apps are often utilized to help organize and coordinate the patient's perioperative care continuum and to assess care quality and care team performance. We recommend this practice.

Preoperative Risk Assessment & Optimization of Functional Status

Reducing the likelihood of perioperative complications improves surgical recovery. Preoperative assessment is discussed in detail in Chapter 18. Although international guidelines evaluating the risk for developing cardiovascular, respiratory, or metabolic complications have been extensively reviewed and published, less attention has been given to assessment and optimization of preoperative functional and physiological status. Nonetheless, some recommendations can be made. For example, perioperative β-blockers should be continued in patients already receiving this therapy. Perioperative statins appear to decrease postoperative cardiovascular complications and should not be abruptly discontinued perioperatively. Several procedure-specific scoring systems based on patient comorbidity, type of surgery, and biochemical data are being used to predict postoperative mortality and morbidity. In addition, risk-adjusted scoring systems, such as the American College of Surgeons National Surgical Quality Improvement Program (NSQIP) and the Society of Thoracic Surgeons National Database, can be used to compare outcomes among institutions.

Smoking & Alcohol Cessation

Preoperative evaluation of surgical risk and optimization of medical comorbidities provides an opportunity to modify habits that may negatively impact the patient's short- and long-term health and quality of life. Smoking, drug abuse, and excessive alcohol use are risk factors for postoperative complications. Perioperative interventions can reduce risks of complications, accelerate surgical recovery, and reduce perioperative costs. A recent meta-analysis found that preoperative smoking cessation, for any type of surgery, reduced postoperative complications by 41%, especially those related to wound healing and the lungs. Intense preoperative smoking cessation programs of 3 to 4 weeks' duration that include pharmacological interventions (eg, nicotine replacement therapy) and patient counseling produce better results than brief and isolated preoperative smoking cessation interventions. Many psychological and pharmacological strategies are also available to help patients stop excessive alcohol consumption and reduce the risk of alcohol withdrawal.

Guidelines for Food & Fluid Intake

Preoperative fasting and surgical stress induce insulin resistance. Furthermore, patients who are not allowed to drink fluids after an overnight fast and especially those who receive a mechanical bowel preparation experience dehydration, which may increase discomfort and cause drowsiness and orthostatic lightheadedness. Although fasting has been advocated as a preoperative strategy to minimize the risk of pulmonary aspiration during induction of anesthesia, this benefit must be weighed against the detrimental aspects of this practice.

Research suggests that avoiding preoperative fasting and ensuring adequate hydration and energy supply may moderate postoperative insulin resistance. Preliminary evidence has shown that preoperative administration of carbohydrate (CHO) drinks (eg, 50 g of maltodextrin 2–3 h before induction of anesthesia) is safe and reduces insulin resistance, hunger, fatigue, and postoperative nausea and vomiting (PONV). Moreover, CHO drinks positively influence the recovery of bowel and immune function. However, these results have been achieved mainly with maltodextrin CHO drinks and in surgeries provoking a strong stress response, such as open abdominal surgery. In contrast, recent data show that preoperative maltodextrins do not attenuate insulin resistance in patients undergoing minimally invasive surgery. It should also be noted that administering simple CHO drinks does not trigger the same reduction in insulin resistance observed with maltodextrin. It is important to educate patients to drink preoperative CHO over a short time, as sipping these beverages over hours does not induce a sufficient insulin response to reduce insulin resistance.

Contemporary fasting guidelines in the United States and elsewhere allow clear fluids up to 2 h prior to induction of anesthesia in patients at low risk for pulmonary aspiration (see Chapter 18). The safety of allowing clear fluids, CHO drinks, or both 2 h before induction of anesthesia has been demonstrated by magnetic resonance imaging studies in healthy volunteers. Residual gastric volume 2 h after 400 mL of oral carbohydrate (12.5% maltodextrins) was found to be similar to the residual gastric volume following an overnight fast (mean volume 21 mL). The safety of this practice has been tested in patients with uncomplicated type 2 diabetes mellitus, without evidence of worsened risk of aspiration. Despite several clinical trials demonstrating that prolonged fasting impairs postoperative recovery, compliance with evidence-based fasting guidelines unfortunately remains low, as physicians continue to order *nil per os* (NPO) after midnight.

INTRAOPERATIVE PERIOD

Antithrombotic Prophylaxis

Antithrombotic prophylaxis reduces perioperative venous thromboembolism risk and related morbidity and mortality. Both pneumatic compression devices and anticoagulant medications are now commonly used. Because neuraxial anesthesia techniques are commonly employed, the appropriate timing of antithrombotic agents in these cases is critically important to minimize the risk of epidural hematoma. International recommendations on the management of anticoagulated patients receiving regional anesthesia are discussed in Chapter 45.

Antibiotic Prophylaxis

Appropriate selection and timing of preoperative antibiotic prophylaxis reduce the risk of surgical site infections. Antibiotics should be administered intravenously within 1 h before skin incision and, based on their plasma half-life and estimated blood loss, should be repeated during lengthy surgeries to ensure adequate tissue concentrations persist. Recent data from large national databases have demonstrated that administration of oral antibiotics 24 h prior to colorectal surgery in patients receiving mechanical bowel preparation (MBP) reduces the risk of surgical site infections when compared with patients receiving MBP alone or those not receiving MBP. Antibiotic prophylaxis for surgical site infections should be discontinued within 24 h following an operation, except for cardiothoracic patients, who (according to current guidelines) may receive antibiotics for 48 h after an operation.

Strategies to Minimize the Surgical Stress Response

The surgical stress response is characterized by neuroendocrine, metabolic, inflammatory, and immunological changes initiated by the physiological trespass of the surgical incision and subsequent invasive procedures. The stress response can adversely affect organ function and perioperative outcomes and may include induction of a catabolic state as well as a transient, but reversible, state of insulin resistance, characterized by decreased peripheral glucose uptake and increased endogenous glucose production. 4 The magnitude of the surgical stress response is related to the intensity of surgical stimulus, hypothermia, and psychological stress. It can be moderated by perioperative interventions, including maintenance of normothermia, neural blockade, and reduction in procedural invasiveness. Much recent effort has focused on developing surgical and anesthetic techniques that reduce the surgical stress response, with the goal of lowering the risk of perioperative organ dysfunction and perioperative complications. An overview of several techniques that have proved effective in ERP protocols follows.

A. Minimally Invasive Surgery

It is well established that minimally invasive surgical procedures are associated with significantly less surgical stress than corresponding "open" procedures. Published data highlight the safety of minimally invasive procedures in the hands of adequately trained and experienced surgeons. Moreover, a longer-term salutary impact is achieved when laparoscopic techniques are included in ERPs. For example, laparoscopic procedures are associated with a reduced incidence of surgical complications, especially surgical site infections, when compared with the same procedures performed in "open" fashion. A laparoscopic approach is also associated with less postoperative surgical pain, better postoperative respiratory function, and less morbidity in older adult postoperative patients. Advancements in surgical care over the past two decades, such as robotic surgery, natural orifice specimen extraction during laparoscopic surgery, endoscopic surgical approaches, and minimally invasive orthopedic surgery, have further moderated the stress of surgery, and we expect such progress to continue.

B. Regional Anesthesia/Analgesia Techniques

A variety of fast-track surgical procedures have taken advantage of the beneficial clinical and metabolic effects of regional anesthesia/analgesia techniques
5 (Table 48–1). Neuraxial blockade of nociceptive stimuli by epidural and spinal local anesthetics blunts metabolic, inflammatory, and neuroendocrine stress responses to surgery. In major open abdominal and thoracic procedures, thoracic epidural blockade with local anesthetic is a recommended anesthetic component of a postoperative ERP, providing excellent analgesia, facilitating mobilization and physical therapy, and decreasing the incidence and severity of ileus. However, the advantages of epidural blockade in such cases are not as clear when minimally invasive surgical techniques are used, and in certain cases, epidural blockade may delay recovery and prolong hospital stay. Lumbar epidural anesthesia/analgesia should be discouraged for abdominal surgery because it often does not provide adequate segmental analgesia for an abdominal incision. In addition, it frequently causes urinary retention and lower limb sensory and motor blockade, increasing the need for urinary drainage catheters (with accompanying increased risk of urinary tract infection), delaying mobilization and recovery, and increasing the risk of falls.

6 Epidural blockade using a solution of local anesthetic and low-dose opioid provides better postoperative analgesia at rest and with movement than systemic opioids (Figure 48–4 and Table 48–2). By sparing opioid use and minimizing the incidence of systemic opioid-related side effects, epidural analgesia facilitates both earlier mobilization and earlier resumption of oral nutrition, expediting exercise activity and attenuating loss of body mass. It minimizes postoperative insulin resistance by attenuating the postoperative hyperglycemic response and by facilitating the utilization of exogenous glucose, thereby preventing postoperative loss of amino acids and conserving lean body mass.

If spinal anesthesia is used for fast-track (and especially ambulatory) surgery, consideration must be given to potential delayed recovery due to persisting motor blockade. The use of smaller doses of intrathecal local anesthetics (lidocaine, 30–40 mg; bupivacaine, 3–10 mg; or ropivacaine, 5–10 mg) with lipophilic intrathecal opioids (fentanyl, 10–25 mcg, or sufentanil, 5–10 mcg) can prolong postoperative analgesia and minimize motor block without delaying recovery from anesthesia. The introduction of ultra-short-acting intrathecal agents such as 2-chloroprocaine (still controversial at present) may further speed the fast-track process. Spinal opioids are associated with side effects such as nausea, pruritus, and postoperative urinary retention. Adjuvants such as clonidine are effective alternatives to intrathecal opioids, with the goal of avoiding opioid side effects that may delay hospital discharge. For example, intrathecal clonidine added to spinal local anesthetic provides effective analgesia with less urinary retention than intrathecal morphine. In a recent study, lower cortisol and glucose levels were observed in colorectal patients receiving spinal anesthesia with intrathecal local anesthetic and morphine compared with patients receiving systemic opioids; however, the inflammatory response did not differ between the two analgesic techniques. Further studies are needed to define the safety and efficacy of regional anesthesia techniques in fast-track cardiac surgery, where currently available studies have yielded contradictory findings.

7 Peripheral nerve blocks (PNBs) with local anesthetics (single-shot or continuous infusion) block afferent nociceptive pathways and are an excellent way to minimize the need for

TABLE 48–1 Enhanced recovery programs that incorporate regional anesthesia/analgesia techniques.[1]

Type of Surgery	Incision	Regional Anesthesia /Analgesia Techniques	Length of Stay
Colorectal resection	Laparotomy, laparoscopy	TEA, intrathecal analgesia, pre-peritoneal wound infusion of ropivacaine, intraperitoneal local anesthetic, intravenous lidocaine, TAP block	2–4 d
Hernia repair	Open	Local infiltration, INB, TAP block	2-4 h
Gastrectomy	Laparotomy, laparoscopy	TEA, wound infusion of local anesthetic, TAP block (subcostal)	3–4 d
Thoracic surgery	Thoracotomy	TEA, ICB	1–4 d
Esophageal surgery	Laparotomy	TEA	3–5 d
Open aortic surgery	Laparotomy	TEA	3–5 d
Liver surgery	Laparotomy	TEA, intrathecal analgesia, wound infusion of local anesthetic	4 d
Pancreaticoduodenectomy	Laparotomy, laparoscopy	TEA, wound infusion of local anesthetic, TAP block	5–8 d
Nephrectomy	Laparotomy, laparoscopy	TEA	2–4 d
Hysterectomy	Laparotomy, laparoscopy	TAP	1–2 d
Radical cystectomy	Laparotomy	TEA, wound infusion of local anesthetic	5–7 d
Arthroplasty (hip, knee)	Open	CPNB (femoral and sciatic), high-volume periarticular infiltration	1–3 d

[1]CPNB, continuous peripheral nerve block; ICB, intercostal block; INB, ilioinguinal nerve block; TAP, transversus abdominus plane block; TEA, thoracic epidural analgesia.

systemic opioids and thereby reduce the incidence of opioid-related side effects and facilitate recovery (see Chapter 46). The choice of local anesthetic, dosage, and concentration should be made with the goal of avoiding prolonged motor blockade and delayed mobilization and discharge.

C. Intravenous Lidocaine Infusion

8 Lidocaine (intravenous bolus of 100 mg or 1.5–2 mg/kg, followed by continuous intravenous infusion of 1.5–3 mg/kg/h or 2–3 mg/min) has analgesic, antihyperalgesic, and anti-inflammatory properties. In patients undergoing colorectal and radical retropubic prostate surgeries, intravenous lidocaine reduces requirements for opioids and general anesthetic agents, provides satisfactory analgesia, facilitates the early return of bowel function, and accelerates hospital discharge. Although lidocaine infusion potentially may replace neuraxial blockade and regional anesthesia in some circumstances, more studies are needed to confirm the efficacy of this technique in the context of ERPs. The most effective dose

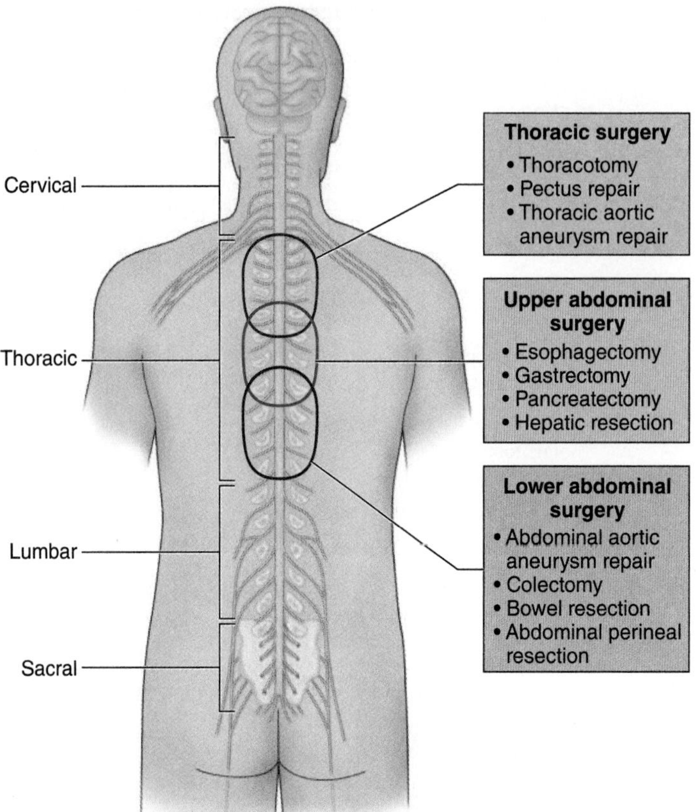

FIGURE 48–4 Optimal regions for placing an epidural catheter in the adult spine when administering epidural anesthesia/analgesia for thoracic and abdominal procedures. (Reproduced with permission from Manion SC, Brennan TJ. Thoracic epidural analgesia and acute pain management. *Anesthesiology.* 2011 July;115(1):181-188.)

and duration of infusion for various surgical procedures remain to be determined; even a short duration of lidocaine infusion may have benefit.

D. β-Blockade Therapy

β-Blockers blunt the sympathetic response during laryngoscopy and intubation and attenuate the surgical stress-induced increase in circulating catecholamines. They also have been shown to prevent adverse perioperative cardiovascular events in at-risk patients undergoing noncardiac surgery and to help maintain hemodynamic stability during the intraoperative period and during emergence from anesthesia. They possess anticatabolic properties, which may be explained by reduced energy requirements associated with decreased adrenergic stimulation. Intravenous esmolol reduces the requirement of volatile anesthetic agents and decreases minimum alveolar concentration values; it has also been shown to reduce postoperative pain intensity, opioid consumption, and PONV. A positive protein balance has been reported in critically ill patients when β-blockade is combined with parenteral nutrition. However, the precise role of β-blockers as adjuvant analgesics in the context of ERPs remains undetermined. In addition, there is unequivocal evidence that β-blocker therapy should not be initiated for prophylaxis against cardiac events in the perioperative period because of increased mortality and increased risk of stroke associated with this strategy.

TABLE 48–2 Options for composition of thoracic epidural infusion analgesia solutions.

Local Anesthetic	Opioid	Advantages	Disadvantages
Bupivacaine, 0.125%	None	↓ Nausea/Vomiting ↓ Pruritus ↓ Sedation ↓ Respiratory depression	↑ Hypotension ↑ Motor blockage
Bupivacaine, 0.1%	Hydromorphone, 5–10 mcg/mL or Fentanyl, 2–5 mcg/mL	↓ Both hemodynamic and opioid side effects	—
Bupivacaine, 0.05%	Hydromorphone, 5–10 mcg/mL or Fentanyl, 2–5 mcg/mL	↓ Both hemodynamic and opioid side effects	—
Bupivacaine, 0.05%	Hydromorphone, 20 mcg/mL or Fentanyl, 5–10 mcg/mL	↓ Both hemodynamic and opioid side effects	—
None	Hydromorphone, 20–40 mcg/mL	↓ Hypotension ↓ Motor blockade	↑ Nausea/Vomiting ↑ Pruritus ↑ Sedation ↑ Respiratory depression

Reproduced with permission from Manion SC, Brennan TJ. Thoracic epidural analgesia and acute pain management. *Anesthesiology.* 2011 July;115(1):181.

E. α_2-Agonist Therapy

Both clonidine and dexmedetomidine have anesthetic and analgesic properties. Clonidine decreases postoperative pain, reduces opioid consumption and opioid-related side effects, and prolongs neuraxial and peripheral nerve local anesthetic blockade. Both have been associated with hypotension and bradycardia. In patients undergoing cardiovascular fast-track surgery, spinal morphine with clonidine decreases extubation time, provides effective analgesia, and improves the quality of recovery. The role of dexmedetomidine in ERP pathways has not been extensively studied.

Use of Short-Acting Intravenous & Inhalation Agents

A. Intravenous Anesthetics

Intravenous propofol is the deep sedation and general anesthesia induction agent of choice for most surgical procedures. Propofol total intravenous anesthesia (TIVA) is often used as part of a multimodal regimen for patients at high risk for PONV.

B. Inhalational Anesthetics

When compared with other volatile anesthetic agents, desflurane and sevoflurane may shorten anesthesia emergence, reduce postanesthesia care unit (PACU) length of stay, and decrease recovery-associated costs. There is controversial evidence that avoidance of deep general anesthesia by use of bispectral index (BIS) monitoring may improve outcomes, including a reduction of the incidence of postoperative delirium and cognitive dysfunction. Nitrous oxide, because of its anesthetic- and analgesic-sparing effects, rapid pharmacokinetic profile, and low cost, is sometimes administered with other inhalation agents. However, routine administration of nitrous oxide has declined over the past three decades because it may cause bowel distention and impair the laparoscopic surgeon's view of anatomic structures and may increase the risk of PONV (see Chapter 8).

C. Opioids

Short-acting opioids such as fentanyl, alfentanil, and remifentanil are commonly used during fast-track surgery in combination with inhalation agents or propofol and with regional or local anesthesia/analgesia techniques. However, intraoperative administration of remifentanil to patients who will experience extensive postoperative pain has been associated with opioid-induced hyperalgesia, acute opioid tolerance, and increased analgesic requirements during the postoperative period. There is increasing evidence that the use of opioids should be minimized in all phases of the perioperative course as part of a multimodal analgesia technique to reduce opioid side effects and optimize recovery. Opioid-free anesthesia has been shown to reduce PONV and postoperative opioid use when compared with opioid-based anesthesia and may be an attractive alternative technique, especially in patients at high risk for PONV, sleep apnea, or respiratory depression. However, a recent multicenter randomized controlled trial (prematurely interrupted due to safety concerns in patients receiving dexmedetomidine) has shown that replacing intraoperative opioids with dexmedetomidine infusion during noncardiac surgery increases the risk of bradycardia, hypoxia, and prolonged recovery room length of stay, despite an observed reduction in PONV and opioid consumption.

Maintenance of Normothermia

The inhibitory effects of anesthetic agents on thermoregulation, exposure to the relatively cool operating room environment, and intraoperative heat loss can lead to hypothermia in all patients undergoing surgical procedures. The duration and extent of the surgical procedure directly correlate with hypothermia risk. Perioperative hypothermia increases cardiovascular morbidity and wound infection risk by increasing sympathetic discharge and inhibiting cellular immune response. A decrease in core body temperature of 1.9°C triples the incidence of surgical wound infection. The risk of bleeding and blood transfusion requirement is also increased with hypothermia. Furthermore, by impairing the metabolism of many anesthetic agents, hypothermia may significantly prolong anesthesia recovery (see Chapter 52).

Maintenance of Adequate Tissue Oxygenation

Surgical stress leads to impaired pulmonary function and peripheral vasoconstriction, resulting in arterial and local tissue hypoxemia, respectively. Perioperative hypoxia can increase cardiovascular and cerebral complications, and many strategies should be adopted during the perioperative period to prevent its development.

Maintenance of adequate perioperative oxygenation by oxygen supplementation has been associated with the improvement of some clinically relevant outcomes. Early trials showed that intraoperative and postoperative (for 2 h) inspired oxygen concentrations greater than 60% increases arterial and subcutaneous oxygen tension and may decrease the rate of wound infection and lower the incidence of PONV without increasing potential complications associated with high inspired oxygen fraction, such as atelectasis and hypercapnia. However, evidence remains inconclusive to recommend routine use of high oxygen fractions, as one of the latest meta-analyses could not refute a 20% increase in mortality. Regional anesthesia techniques decrease vascular resistance and may improve peripheral tissue perfusion and oxygenation and lessen the risk of deep venous thrombosis. Finally, early mobilization and avoidance of bedrest improves postoperative central and peripheral tissue oxygenation and may also lessen the risk of deep venous thrombosis.

Postoperative Nausea & Vomiting Prophylaxis

PONV is a frequent complication that delays early feeding and postoperative recovery. The risk of PONV can be easily stratified before surgery to facilitate adequate preemptive strategies. Preemptive strategies minimizing the risk of PONV are strongly advocated for any type of surgery, and consensus guidelines for prevention and management of PONV are available in current literature (see Chapters 17 and 56).

Goal-Directed Fluid & Hemodynamic Therapy

There is increasing evidence that perioperative fluid administration affects patient outcome following major surgery, with the quantity of fluid administered—either too restrictive or too liberal—being associated with increased incidence of postoperative complications. Observational studies reveal large variations in practitioners' fluid management strategies. Most attention is focused on avoiding hypovolemia, whereas excessively liberal fluid administration and its attendant adverse effects, though more difficult to observe in the operating room, are probably more common. Fluid overload, especially of crystalloid, has been associated with reduced tissue oxygenation, anastomotic leakage, pulmonary edema, pneumonia, wound infection, postoperative ileus, and prolonged hospitalization. Furthermore, excess fluids commonly increase body weight by 3 to 6 kg and may impair postoperative mobilization. The largest multicenter randomized controlled trial to date comparing restrictive fluid therapy (≤5 mL/kg/h) with more liberal fluid therapy (8 mL/kg/h) using isotonic crystalloid solutions (the RELIEF trial) found that acute kidney injury occurred more frequently in patients treated with restrictive fluid therapy. Notably, despite patients in the liberal fluid therapy group receiving more fluids, their 24-h weight gain was below 2 kg, and postoperative outcomes were no worse. Based on these results, fluid therapy in patients undergoing major noncardiac surgery should aim to achieve a positive fluid balance of 1 to 2 L at the end of surgery by infusing isotonic, balanced, crystalloid solutions.

The concept of goal-directed fluid therapy (GDFT) is based on optimization of hemodynamic measures such as heart rate, blood pressure, stroke volume, pulse pressure variation, and stroke volume variation obtained by noninvasive cardiac output devices such as pulse-contour arterial waveform analysis, transesophageal echocardiography, or esophageal Doppler (see Chapter 5). GDFT aims to avoid both hypovolemia and fluid excess, and it is the optimal approach for fluid administration in high-risk surgical patients.

The type of fluid infused is also important: isotonic, balanced crystalloid should be used to replace extracellular losses, whereas iso-oncotic colloids are commonly used to replace physiologically important blood losses (Table 48–3).

TABLE 48–3 Physiologically based first-line fluid replacement for goal-directed therapy.

Physiological Requirement	Replace with	Amount
Extracellular		
Insensible perspiration	Crystalloids[1]	
Closed abdomen		0.5 mL/kg/h
Open abdomen		1 mL/kg/h
Urine production	Crystalloids	Measured output[3]
Intravascular		
Blood loss	Colloids[2]	Estimated losses
Further preload deficit	Colloids	According to clinical estimation[4]

[1]Crystalloids should be given in an isotonic balanced form.
[2]Colloids should be given in an iso-oncotic form in balanced solutions.
[3]First-line approach in healthy kidneys.
[4]If possible, use extended monitoring (eg, PiCCO system, esophageal Doppler).

Reproduced with permission from Chappell D, Jacob M. Influence of non-ventilatory options on postoperative outcome. *Best Pract Res Clin Anaesthesiol.* 2010 June;24(2):267-281.

POSTOPERATIVE PERIOD

Immediate Postoperative Care

A. Strategies to Minimize Postoperative Shivering

The primary cause of postoperative shivering is perioperative hypothermia, though other, nonthermoregulatory mechanisms may be involved. Postoperative shivering can greatly increase oxygen consumption, catecholamine release, cardiac output, heart rate, blood pressure, and intracranial and intraocular pressure. This increases cardiovascular morbidity, especially in older adult patients, and increases PACU length of stay and perioperative cost. Shivering is uncommon in older adult and hypoxic patients; the efficacy of thermoregulation decreases with aging, and hypoxia can directly inhibit shivering. Many drugs, notably meperidine, clonidine, and tramadol, can be used to reduce postoperative shivering; however, prevention via strategies intended to minimize thermal loss is optimal (see Chapter 52).

B. PONV Treatment

Pharmacological treatment of PONV should be promptly initiated once medical or surgical causes of PONV have been ruled out (see Chapters 17 and 56).

C. Multimodal Analgesia

9 Multimodal analgesia combines different classes of medications that have different (*multimodal*) pharmacological mechanisms of action, resulting in additive or synergistic effects to reduce postoperative pain and its sequelae. Such an approach can achieve desired analgesic effects while reducing analgesic dosage and associated side effects. Multimodal pain management often includes the utilization of regional analgesic techniques, including local anesthetic wound infusion, epidural/intrathecal analgesia, or single-shot/continuous peripheral nerve blockade. Multimodal analgesia is routinely utilized in ERPs to improve postoperative outcomes. Discussion here focuses on principal analgesic interventions used in perioperative multimodal analgesia regimens.

10 **1. NSAIDs**—The addition of nonsteroidal anti-inflammatory drugs (NSAIDs) to systemic opioid analgesia diminishes postoperative pain intensity, reduces opioid requirements, and decreases opioid-related side effects such as PONV, sedation, and urinary retention. However, NSAIDs may increase the risk of gastrointestinal and wound bleeding, decrease kidney function, and impair wound healing. It is controversial as to whether NSAIDs may have a detrimental effect on gastrointestinal tract anastomotic healing and increase the risk of anastomotic leak.

Perioperative administration of selective cyclooxygenase-2 (COX-2) inhibitor NSAIDs likewise reduces postoperative pain and decreases both opioid consumption and opioid-related side effects. Although their use reduces the incidence of NSAID-related platelet dysfunction and gastrointestinal bleeding, the potential adverse effects of COX-2 inhibitors on kidney function remain controversial. Concerns have also been raised, primarily with rofecoxib and valdecoxib, regarding COX-2 safety for patients undergoing cardiovascular surgery. Increased cardiovascular risk associated with the perioperative use of celecoxib or valdecoxib in patients with minimal cardiovascular risk factors and undergoing nonvascular surgery is unproven. Further studies are needed to establish the analgesic efficacy and safety of COX-2 inhibitors, their clinical impact on postoperative outcomes, and their precise role in ERPs.

2. Acetaminophen (paracetamol)—Oral, rectal, or parenteral acetaminophen is a common component of multimodal analgesia. Acetaminophen's analgesic effect is 20% to 30% less than that of NSAIDs, but its pharmacological profile is safer. Analgesic efficacy improves when the drug is administered together with NSAIDs, and it significantly reduces pain intensity and spares opioid consumption after orthopedic and abdominal surgery. However, acetaminophen may not reduce opioid-related side effects. Routine administration of acetaminophen in combination with regional anesthesia and analgesia techniques may allow NSAIDs to be reserved for control of breakthrough pain, thus limiting the potential for NSAID-related side effects.

3. Gabapentinoids—Oral gabapentin and pregabalin given as a single dose preoperatively may decrease postoperative pain and opioid consumption in the first 24 h following surgery. There is debate about the dose and duration of perioperative use of these drugs and whether they may potentially alter the incidence of chronic pain after surgery. Common side effects include sedation and dizziness, especially in older adult patients, which may increase the risk of patient falls.

4. *N*-methyl-D-aspartate (NMDA) receptor antagonists—Ketamine: Perioperative low-dose ketamine (bolus, infusion) has been associated with significant reduction in pain, opioid consumption, and PONV. Ketamine has also been shown to be of particular benefit in patients on chronic opioids.

Magnesium: Magnesium may also reduce postoperative pain and opioid consumption, although the optimal dosing is uncertain. Side effects include hypotension and potentiation of neuromuscular blockade.

5. Intravenous lidocaine—Intravenous lidocaine infusion analgesia has recently increased in popularity because there is good evidence to support its use as a component of multimodal analgesia. In major abdominal surgery, it is associated with the faster return of bowel function and decreased hospital length of stay. Continuous cardiovascular monitoring is frequently advocated for patients receiving intravenous lidocaine, and therefore its use is currently limited to settings such as the PACU, ICU, or a monitored hospital ward. However, several centers have developed and implemented perioperative protocols to safely use intravenous lidocaine on surgical wards without continuous cardiovascular monitoring.

6. Opioids—Despite the increasing use of new, nonopioid analgesic medications and adjuvants and of regional anesthesia and analgesia techniques intended to minimize opioid requirements and opioid-related side effects (Table 48–4), the use of systemic opioids remains a cornerstone in the management of surgical pain. Parenteral opioids are frequently prescribed in the postoperative period
11 during the transitional phase to oral analgesia. Opioid administration by patient-controlled analgesia (PCA) provides better pain control, greater patient satisfaction, and fewer opioid side effects when compared with nurse-administered, on-request (PRN) parenteral opioid administration. Oral administration of opioids, such as oxycodone or hydrocodone, in combination with NSAIDs or acetaminophen, or both, is common in the perioperative period.

7. Epidural analgesia—In addition to providing excellent analgesia, epidural blockade blunts the neuroendocrine stress response associated with surgery, decreases postoperative morbidity, attenuates catabolism, and accelerates postoperative functional recovery. Compared with systemic opioid analgesia, thoracic epidural analgesia provides better static and dynamic pain relief. However, these benefits have mainly been observed in patients undergoing open abdominal and thoracic surgery; its usefulness in patients undergoing minimally invasive abdominal and thoracic surgery is questionable, as recent trials have suggested it may actually prolong in-hospital recovery in such cases. Long-acting local anesthetics such as ropivacaine (0.2%), bupivacaine (0.0625–0.125%), and levobupivacaine (0.1–0.125%) are commonly administered together with lipophilic opioids by continuous epidural infusion or by patient-controlled epidural analgesia (PCEA). As previously noted, administering low doses of local anesthetic via thoracic epidural infusion instead of lumbar levels avoids lower extremity motor blockade that may delay postoperative mobilization and recovery and will increase the risk of patient falls. Adding opioids to epidural local anesthetics improves the quality of postoperative analgesia without delaying recovery of bowel function.

8. Paravertebral nerve blocks—Paravertebral and other truncal nerve blocks provide similar parietal analgesia to epidural blockade but without the risk of epidural-related side effects. However, they have been poorly studied in the context of ERPs.

12 **9. Peripheral nerve blockade**—Single-shot and continuous peripheral nerve blockade is frequently utilized for fast-track ambulatory and inpatient orthopedic surgery, and it can accelerate recovery from surgery and improve both analgesia and patient satisfaction (see Chapters 38 and 46). For some procedures, blocking multiple nerves can provide analgesic benefits superior to blockade of a single nerve. The opioid-sparing effect of nerve blocks minimizes the risk of systemic opioid-related side effects. Appropriate patient selection and strict adherence to institutional clinical pathways help ensure the success of peripheral nerve blockade as a fast-track orthopedic analgesia technique and also help minimize its risks.

Advances in ultrasound imaging technology and techniques have accelerated interest in abdominal and chest wall blockade, facilitating the selective localization of specific nerves and the direct deposition of local anesthetic solutions in proximity to the compartments where specific nerves are located (see Chapters 38 and 46).

Single-shot perineural administration of liposomal bupivacaine has been used recently to extend the analgesic duration of peripheral nerve blocks to up to 72 h after surgery. However, preliminary studies have not consistently shown expected benefits, and the role of liposomal local anesthetic preparations in postoperative analgesia and ERPs has, therefore, yet to be precisely defined.

10. High-volume local anesthetic infiltration analgesia and wound infusion—High-volume

TABLE 48–4 Analgesic adjuvants in the perioperative period.[1,2]

Adjuvant	Type of Surgery or Clinical Setting	Analgesic Efficacy as Adjuvant	Dosages Used (Boluses, CI)	Administration			Monitoring
				Route	*Timing*	*Postoperative Duration*	
Lidocaine	Tonsillectomy Cardiac Abdominal (laparotomy, laparoscopic) Thoracotomy Hysterectomy Laparoscopic prostatectomy Orthopedic	– + + + + + –	1.5 mg/kg, *followed by* 1.5–2 mg/kg/h CI (Intra, until skin closure), *and then* 1 mg/kg/h CI (Post)	IV	Pre,[3] Intra, Peri	30 min–48 h	Signs of local anesthetic toxicity (CNS cardiovascular)
Ketamine	Cardiac Thoracotomy Abdominal Gynecological Orthopedic Spine Chronic use of opioids Preventing chronic pain OIH	+ + + – – +/– + +/– +/–	0.5–1 mg/kg, *followed by* 2–10 mcg/kg/min CI	IV	Pre, Post (PCA[4]), Peri	4–72 h	CNS[5] (level of sedation, nystagmus hallucinations), cardiovascular
Gabapentinoids Gabapentin	Cholecystectomy Hysterectomy Spine Hip arthroplasty Preventing chronic pain	– + + – +/–	300–1200 mg	PO	Pre,[6] Post		CNS[5] (level of sedation, somnolence, dizziness), leg edema
Pregabalin	Hysterectomy Laparoscopic cholecystectomy Preventing chronic pain	+ – +/–	75–300 mg	PO	Pre, Post		
$MgSO_4$	Cardiac Cholecystectomy Lower limb orthopedic Gynecological Ambulatory	+ + + + +	30–50 mg/kg, *followed by* 8–15 mg/kg/h CI	IV	Pre, Intra		CNS (somnolence), neuromuscular function, respiratory depression, cardiovascular (bradycardia)

Steroids	Hip arthroplasty Breast Laparoscopic cholecystectomy	+ + +	Dexamethasone: 8–16 mg Methylprednisolone: 125 mg	IV	Pre	Glycemia, GI bleeding, wound healing
α_2-Agonist Clonidine	PO Abdominal Total knee arthroplasty Hysterectomy Prostatectomy IV Cholecystectomy Abdominal Spine	 – + + – – + +	PO 3–5 mcg/kg IV 150 mcg	PO, IV	Pre,[7] Intra, Post (PCA[8])	CNS[5] (level of sedation), cardiovascular (hypotension, bradycardia)
Dexmedetomidine	Thoracotomy Abdominal Hysterectomy Bariatric	+ + + +	Loading dose 0.5–1 mcg/kg, *followed by* 0.2–0.4 mcg/kg/h CI	IV	Pre, Intra, Post (PCA[9])	

[1]Efficacy of these agents as adjuvant analgesics has been demonstrated by a reduction of pain or opioid consumption, or both; or opioid side effects; or all three.

[2]CI, continuous infusion; CNS, central nervous system; GI, gastrointestinal; Intra, intraoperative period; IV, intravenous; OIH, opioid-induced hyperalgesia; PCA, patient-controlled analgesia; Peri, preoperative, intraoperative, and postoperative periods; PO, oral; Post, postoperative period; Pre, preoperative period during induction.

[3]Bolus, or 30 min before induction of anesthesia.

[4]As a 1-mg demand dose, lockout time 7 min.

[5]Psychotomimetic side effects are dose-dependent.

[6]Single dose, 1–2.5 h before surgery.

[7]Given PO 60–90 min before surgery.

[8]As a 20-mcg demand dose, lockout time 5 min.

[9]As a 5-mcg demand dose, lockout time 5 min.

local anesthetic infiltration analgesia with a mixture of local anesthetic and epinephrine, with or without systemic NSAIDs, has recently gained popularity in patients undergoing total hip and knee replacements, and it is currently replacing peripheral nerve blocks in many institutions, especially in the context of an ERP (see Chapter 38). However, supporting evidence demonstrating that this technique is superior to peripheral nerve blockade is currently lacking. Moreover, its impact on metabolic and inflammatory responses and on non–analgesic-related outcomes remains unknown. The impact of peripheral nerve blocks and rehabilitation therapy on functional outcomes also remains incompletely studied.

Local anesthetic wound infusions can be used to improve postoperative pain control and reduce the necessity for opioids, especially in patients undergoing open abdominal surgery and in whom epidural analgesia is contraindicated. The analgesic efficacy of local anesthetic wound infusion has also been established for multiple other surgical procedures. Inconsistent results from wound infusion may be secondary to type, concentration, and dose of local anesthetic employed; catheter placement; and mode of local anesthetic delivery.

11. Intraperitoneal instillation and nebulization of local anesthetic—Instillation and nebulization of intraperitoneal local anesthetic decreases pain intensity and decreases opioid consumption following open abdominal and laparoscopic surgery. However, the precise roles of these techniques in multimodal management remain to be determined.

Strategies to Facilitate Recovery on the Surgical Unit

A. Organization of Multidisciplinary Surgical Care

The multidisciplinary aspect of postoperative care should bring together the surgeon, anesthesia care team, nurses, nutritionist, physiotherapist, pharmacist, consultants, and case manager/social worker in an interdisciplinary team effort to optimize each patient's care based upon standardized, procedure-specific protocols. Comfortable chairs and walkers should be made readily available near each patient bed to encourage patients to sit, stand, and walk and to minimize the risk of patient falls. Routine bed rest after surgery should be avoided. Patients should be encouraged to sit in a chair the afternoon or evening following surgery, with ambulation starting the same or next day. If patients are unable to get out of bed, they should be instructed and encouraged to perform physical and deep breathing exercises in their beds.

B. Optimization of Analgesia to Facilitate Functional Recovery

A well-organized, well-trained, acute pain service (APS) utilizing procedure-specific clinical protocols to optimally manage analgesia and related side effects helps drive ERPs. The quality of pain relief and symptom control heavily influences postoperative recovery; optimal mobilization and dietary intake depend upon adequate analgesia with minimal analgesic-related side effects. The surgeon and the APS must identify and employ optimal analgesic techniques tailored to the patient and specific surgical procedure, and the quality of analgesia and risk of analgesic-related side effects must be closely and continuously assessed. The goal is not to achieve "zero pain" but to make patients reasonably comfortable while walking and performing physiotherapy, with minimal side effects such as lightheadedness, sedation, nausea and vomiting, urinary retention, ileus, and leg weakness. *It should be noted that opioid-related PONV is the most common cause of unplanned hospital admission following ambulatory surgery and opioid-related ileus is one of the most common causes of extended hospital length of stay. Both of these problems significantly increase perioperative costs.*

C. Strategies to Minimize Postoperative Ileus

13 Postoperative ileus delays postoperative resumption of enteral feeding, is often a source of considerable patient discomfort, and is one of the most common causes of prolonged postoperative hospital length of stay and preventable hospitalization costs. Because early enteral nutrition is associated with decreased postoperative morbidity, *interventions* and *strategies aimed at minimizing the risk and severity of postoperative ileus are essential for patients in an ERP.* Four main mechanisms

contribute to ileus: sympathetic inhibitory reflexes, local inflammation initiated by the operative procedure, intraoperatively and postoperatively administered systemic opioids, and bowel edema caused by administration of excess intravenous fluid. *Nasogastric tubes, frequently inserted after abdominal surgery, do not speed the recovery of bowel function and may increase pulmonary morbidity by increasing the risk of aspiration. Therefore, nasogastric tubes should be discouraged whenever possible or used for only a very short period of time, even with gastrointestinal surgery.*

Multimodal analgesia with minimal or nonopioid analgesia techniques shorten the duration of postoperative ileus or may preempt it entirely. Minimally invasive surgical techniques are associated with less surgical stress and inflammation than open procedures, resulting in a more rapid return of bowel function. For open abdominal procedures, thoracic epidural local anesthetic infusions not only provide superior analgesia but also speed the recovery of bowel function by suppressing inhibitory sympathetic spinal cord reflexes that promote the development and severity of postoperative ileus. Epidural analgesia does not appear to have the same impact following laparoscopic procedures. Laxatives such as milk of magnesia and bisacodyl reduce postoperative ileus duration. Prokinetic medications such as metoclopramide are ineffective. Neostigmine increases peristalsis but may also increase the incidence of PONV.

By stimulating gastrointestinal reflexes (sham feeding), postoperative chewing gum has been proposed as a safe and low-cost intervention to accelerate the recovery of bowel function. However, the results of a recent multicenter randomized controlled trial do not support the implementation of chewing gum to improve postoperative outcomes if it is implemented in the context of an ERP. Peripheral opioid μ-receptor antagonists methylnaltrexone (Relistor) and alvimopan (Entereg) minimize the adverse effects of opioids on bowel function without antagonizing systemic opioid analgesia because of their limited ability to cross the blood–brain barrier. In laparotomy patients receiving high-dose intravenous morphine analgesia, alvimopan decreases the duration of postoperative ileus by 16 to 18 h, decreases the incidence of nasogastric tube reinsertion, shortens hospital length of stay, and lowers hospital readmission rates, especially in patients undergoing bowel resection. Nevertheless, recovery of postoperative bowel function in such alvimopan-treated, high-dose systemic morphine analgesia patients remains slower than that of patients utilizing opioid-sparing, multimodal ERPs. A recent meta-analysis demonstrated that the benefits of alvimopan are more evident in patients undergoing open surgery than in patients undergoing minimally invasive surgery and treated with an ERP.

Excessive perioperative fluid administration commonly causes bowel mucosal edema and delays the postoperative return of bowel function. Because 14 either excessive, or excessively restricted, perioperative fluid therapy increases the incidence and severity of postoperative ileus, a goal-directed fluid administration strategy may be beneficial, especially for patients undergoing major surgery associated with large fluid shifts and for patients at high risk of developing postoperative gastrointestinal complications (see Chapter 51).

Issues in the Implementation of Enhanced Recovery Programs

The success of ERPs depends upon the ability and willingness of perioperative team stakeholders to reach evidence-based interdisciplinary consensus. Many traditional aspects of perioperative care, such as use of drains, dietary and activity restrictions, excessive or excessively restrictive fluid management, and bedrest lack evidence basis. These measures must be extensively scrutinized and revised in ERPs. Patient involvement and patient and family expectations are fundamentally important but frequently overlooked aspects of these programs. New surgical techniques, such as transverse incisions or minimally invasive surgery, may require surgeons to acquire and perfect new skills. Similarly, the emphasis on thoracic epidural blockade or peripheral nerve blocks, pharmacological modulation of the neuroendocrine stress response to surgery, goal-directed fluid and hemodynamic therapy, and integral involvement of a well-organized and managed APS requires a substantial expansion of the traditional roles of anesthesiologists and of the anesthesia care team. Aggressive analgesia and symptom management, early ambulation and physiotherapy, early feeding, and early removal or total avoidance of urinary drainage catheters represent significant changes to the traditional ways that postoperative patients have been cared for in the past. Successful implementation of such innovations requires a well-organized, well-led, highly trained, highly motivated nursing staff.

Although there are published studies of successful ERPs, there are no "off-the-shelf" protocols with universal application: Local differences in goals, expertise, experience, resources, and politics markedly influence the development, implementation, and management of ERPs for each institution or health care system. Every ERP should be regarded as a continuous quality improvement exercise. Each family of similar surgical procedures requires a standardized interdisciplinary clinical protocol or pathway, with specialized input from a team with experience in caring for those patients. Such an interdisciplinary team should include representation from surgery, anesthesiology, nursing, pharmacy, physiotherapy, nutrition, and administration, and it should be responsible not only for each clinical protocol's creation but also for continuously monitoring its efficacy and cost and for instituting continuous improvement-related protocol modifications and provider feedback as indicated by outcomes data (Figure 48–5).

Optimal perioperative care requires the anesthesia provider to be an integral part of the perioperative surgical care team leadership and management. The skill sets of the anesthesiologist and anesthesia care team are essential for the success of ERPs and have potential benefits for surgical

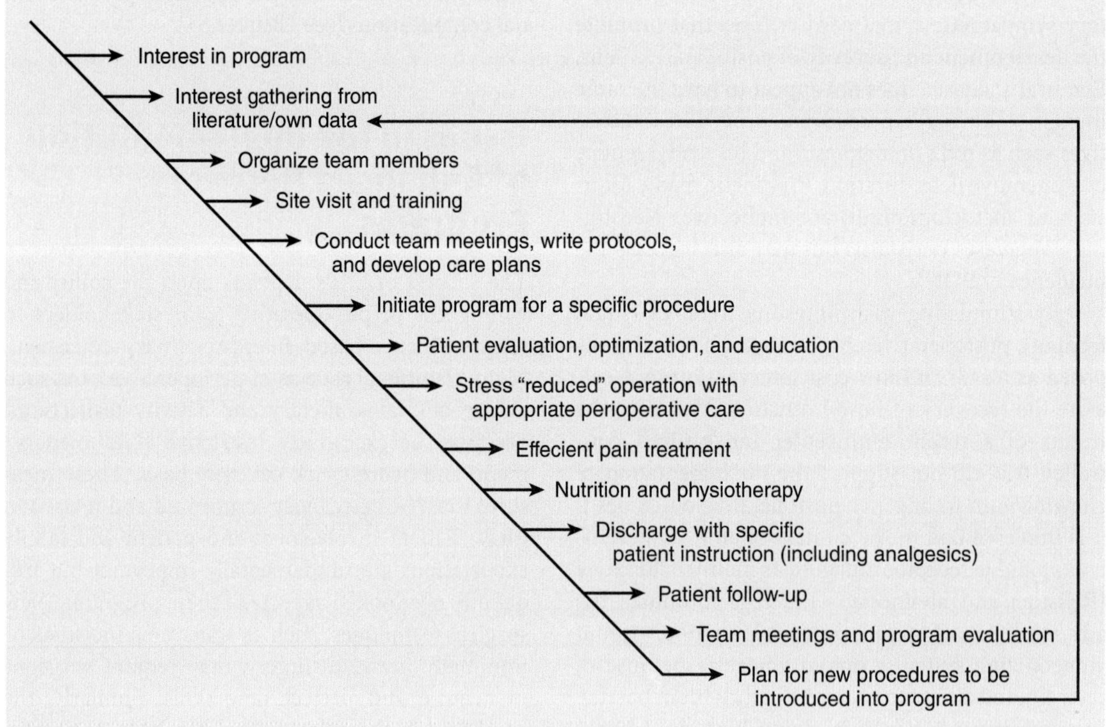

FIGURE 48–5 Stepwise process for initiating and implementing an enhanced recovery program. (Reproduced with permission from Kehlet H, Wilmore DW. Evidence-based surgical care and the evolution of fast-track surgery. *Ann Surg.* 2008 Aug;248(2):189-198.)

care delivery on a global basis, from initial surgical diagnosis, preoperative evaluation, and presurgical preparation through postoperative recovery and return of the patient to their primary health care provider. The perioperative surgical home concept represents an accumulation of developments derived from ambulatory, minimally invasive, fast-track, enhanced recovery, and interdisciplinary, team-based surgical care and allows both quality- and cost-related variables to be analyzed and optimized from the patient's perspective (eg, incidence and severity of perioperative complications, hospital length of stay, hospital readmission rate, return to work, return to chemotherapy). By optimizing these many variables, the PSH contributes a higher value surgical experience to the patient. This requires new standards for clinical education and training.

GUIDELINES & CONSENSUS STATEMENTS

Bratzler DW, Dellinger EP, Olsen KM, et al. Clinical practice guidelines for antimicrobial prophylaxis in surgery. *Am J Health Syst Pharm*. 2013;70:195.

Enhanced Recovery Society Guidelines: https://erassociety.org/guidelines/list-of-guidelines/. Accessed June 1, 2021.

Holubar SD, Hedrick T, Gupta R, et al. American Society for Enhanced Recovery (ASER) and Perioperative Quality Initiative (POQI) joint consensus statement on prevention of postoperative infection within an enhanced recovery pathway for elective colorectal surgery. *Perioper Med (Lond)*. 2017;6:4.

McEvoy MD, Scott MJ, Gordon DB, et al. American Society for Enhanced Recovery (ASER) and Perioperative Quality Initiative (POQI) joint consensus statement on optimal analgesia within an enhanced recovery pathway for colorectal surgery: Part 1—from the preoperative period to PACU. *Perioper Med (Lond)*. 2017;6:8.

Moonesinghe SR, Grocott MPW, Bennett-Guerrero E, et al. American Society for Enhanced Recovery (ASER) and Perioperative Quality Initiative (POQI) joint consensus statement on measurement to maintain and improve quality of enhanced recovery pathways for elective colorectal surgery. *Perioper Med (Lond)*. 2017;6:6.

Scott MJ, McEvoy MD, Gordon DB, et al. American Society for Enhanced Recovery (ASER) and Perioperative Quality Initiative (POQI) joint consensus statement on optimal analgesia within an enhanced recovery pathway for colorectal surgery: Part 2—from PACU to the transition home. *Perioper Med (Lond)*. 2017;6:7.

Thiele RH, Raghunathan K, Brudney C, et al. American Society for Enhanced Recovery (ASER) and Perioperative Quality Initiative (POQI) joint consensus statement on perioperative fluid management within an enhanced recovery pathway for colorectal surgery. *Periop Med (Lond)*. 2016;5:24.

SUGGESTED READINGS

Aarts M-A, Okrainec A, Glicksman A, et al. Adoption of enhanced recovery after surgery (ERAS) strategies for colorectal surgery at academic teaching hospitals and impact on total length of hospital stay. *Surg Endosc*. 2012;26:442.

Aldecoa C, Bettelli G, Bilotta F, et al. European Society of Anaesthesiology evidence-based and consensus-based guideline on postoperative delirium. *Eur J Anaesthesiol*. 2017;34:192.

Alhasashemi M, Hamad R, El-Kefraoui C, et al. The association of alvimopan treatment with postoperative outcomes after abdominal surgery: a systematic review across different surgical procedures and contexts of perioperative care. *Surgery*. 2021;169:934.

Alvis BD, Amsler RG, Leisy PJ, et al. Effects of an anesthesia perioperative surgical home for total knee and hip arthroplasty at a Veterans Affairs Hospital: a quality improvement before-and-after cohort study. *Can J Anaesth*. 2021;68:367.

Amir A, Jolin S, Amberg S, Nordstrom S. Implementation of Pecs I and Pecs II blocks as part of opioid-sparing approach to breast surgery. *Reg Anesth Pain Med*. 2016;41:544.

Baldini G. Perioperative smoking and alcohol cessation. In: Ljungqvist O, Nader F, Urman RD, eds. *Enhanced Recovery After Surgery*. Springer; 2020.

Beloeil H, Garot M, Lebuffe G, et al. Balanced opioid-free anesthesia with dexmedetomidine *versus* balanced anesthesia with remifentanil for major or intermediate noncardiac surgery: the Postoperative and Opioid-free Anesthesia (POFA) randomized clinical trial. *Anesthesiology*. 2021;134:541.

Carli F, Kehlet H, Baldini G, et al. Evidence basis for regional anesthesia in multidisciplinary fast-track surgical care pathways. *Reg Anesth Pain Med*. 2011;36:63.

Day AR, Smith RV, Scott MJ, et al. Randomized clinical trial investigating the stress response from two different methods of analgesia after laparoscopic colorectal surgery. *Br J Surg*. 2015;102:1473.

de Leede EM, van Leersum NJ, Kroon HM. Multicentre randomized clinical trial of the effect of chewing gum after abdominal surgery. *Br J Surg* 2018;105:820.

Fiore JF Jr, Castelino T, Pecorelli N, et al. Ensuring early mobilization within an enhanced recovery program for colorectal surgery: a randomized controlled trial. *Ann Surg*. 2016;666:223.

Foo I, Macfarlane AJR, Srivastava D, et al. The use of intravenous lidocaine for postoperative pain and recovery: international consensus statement on efficacy and safety. *Anaesthesia*. 2021;76:238.

Gillis C, Carli F. Promoting perioperative metabolic and nutritional care. *Anesthesiology*. 2015;123:1455.

Gómez-Izquierdo JC, Trainito A, Mirzakandov D, et al. Goal-directed fluid therapy does not reduce primary postoperative ileus after elective laparoscopic colorectal surgery: a randomized controlled trial. *Anesthesiology*. 2017;127:36.

Hamilton TW, Athanassoglou V, Mellon S, et al. Liposomal bupivacaine infiltration at the surgical site for the management of postoperative pain. *Cochrane Database Syst Rev*. 2017;(2):CD011419.

Hubner M, Blanc C, Roulin D, et al. Randomized clinical trial on epidural versus patient-controlled analgesia for laparoscopic colorectal surgery within an enhanced recovery pathway. *Ann Surg*. 2015;261:648.

Ji YD, Harris JA, Gibson LE, et al. The efficacy of liposomal bupivacaine for opioid and pain reduction: a systematic review of randomized clinical trials. *J Surg Res*. 2021;264:510.

Joshi GP, Kehlet H. Meta-analyses of gabapentinoids for pain management after knee arthroplasty: a caveat emptor? A narrative review. *Acta Anaesthesiol Scand*. 2021;65:865.

Kain ZN, Vakharia S, Garson L. The perioperative surgical home as a future perioperative practice model. *Anesth Analg*. 2014;118:1126.

Levy BF, Scott MJ, Fawcett W, et al. Randomized clinical trial of epidural, spinal or patient-controlled analgesia for patients undergoing laparoscopic colorectal surgery. *Br J Surg*. 2011;98:1068.

Ljungqvist O, Scott M, Fearon KC. Enhanced recovery after surgery: a review. *JAMA Surg*. 2017;152:292.

Miller TE, Roche AM, Mythen M. Fluid management and goal-directed therapy as an adjunct to enhanced recovery after surgery (ERAS). *Can J Anesthesia*. 2015;62:158.

Myles P, Bellomo R, Corcoran T et al. Restrictive versus liberal fluid therapy for major abdominal surgery. *N Engl J Med*. 2018;378:2263.

Nicklas J, Diener O, Leistenschneider M et al. Personalised haemodynamic management targeting baseline cardiac index in high-risk patients undergoing major abdominal surgery: a randomised single-centre clinical trial. *Br J Anaesth* 2020;125:122.

Odor PM, Bampoe S, Gilhooly D, Creagh-Brown B, Moonesinghe SR. Perioperative interventions for prevention of postoperative pulmonary complications: systematic review and meta-analysis. *BMJ*. 2020;368:m540.

Pecorelli N, Hershorn O, Baldini G, et al. Impact of adherence to care pathway interventions on recovery following bowel resection within an established enhanced recovery program. *Surg Endosc*. 2017;31:1760.

Shanthanna H, Ladha KS, Kehlet H, et al. Perioperative opioid administration. *Anesthesiology*. 2021;134:645.

Smith MD, McCall J, Plank L, et al. Preoperative carbohydrate treatment for enhancing recovery after elective surgery. *Cochrane Database Syst Rev*. 2014;(8):CD009161.

Terkawi AS, Mavridis D, Sessler DI, et al. Pain management modalities after total knee arthroplasty: a network meta-analysis of 170 randomized controlled trials. *Anesthesiology*. 2017;126:923.

Wetterslev J, Meyhoff CS, Jørgensen LN, Gluud C, Lindschou J, Rasmussen LS. The effects of high perioperative inspiratory oxygen fraction for adult surgical patients. *Cochrane Database Syst Rev*. 2015;2015:CD008884.

Ziemann-Gimmel P, Goldfarb AA, Koppman J, et al. Opioid-free total intravenous anaesthesia reduces postoperative nausea and vomiting in bariatric surgery beyond triple prophylaxis. *Br J Anaesth*. 2014;112:906.

CHAPTER 49

Management of Patients with Fluid & Electrolyte Disturbances

KEY CONCEPTS

1. Osmotic pressure is generally dependent only on the number of nondiffusible solute particles. This is because the average kinetic energy of particles in solution is similar regardless of their mass.
2. Potassium is the most important determinant of intracellular osmotic pressure, whereas sodium is the most important determinant of extracellular osmotic pressure.
3. Fluid exchange between the intracellular and interstitial spaces is governed by the osmotic forces created by differences in nondiffusible solute concentrations.
4. Serious manifestations of hyponatremia are generally associated with plasma sodium concentrations less than 120 mEq/L.
5. Excessively rapid correction of hyponatremia has been associated with demyelinating lesions in the pons (*central pontine myelinolysis*) and more generally in both pontine and extrapontine central nervous system structures (*osmotic demyelination syndrome*), resulting in both temporary and permanent neurological sequelae.
6. A major hazard of increased extracellular volume is impaired gas exchange caused by pulmonary interstitial edema, alveolar edema, or large collections of pleural or ascitic fluid.
7. Intravenous replacement of potassium chloride is usually reserved for patients with, or at risk for, significant cardiac manifestations or severe muscle weakness. The goal of intravenous therapy is to remove the patient from immediate danger, not to correct the entire potassium deficit.
8. Because of its lethal potential, hyperkalemia exceeding 6 mEq/L should always be corrected.
9. Symptomatic hypercalcemia requires rapid treatment. The most effective initial treatment is rehydration followed by brisk diuresis (urinary output 200–300 mL/h) using an intravenous saline infusion and a loop diuretic to accelerate calcium excretion.
10. Symptomatic hypocalcemia is a medical emergency and should be treated immediately with intravenous calcium chloride (3–5 mL of a 10% solution) or calcium gluconate (10–20 mL of a 10% solution).
11. Some patients with severe hypophosphatemia may require mechanical ventilation postoperatively because of muscle weakness.
12. Severe hypermagnesemia can lead to respiratory and cardiac arrest.
13. Isolated hypomagnesemia should be corrected before elective procedures because of its potential for causing cardiac arrhythmias.

Fluid and electrolyte disturbances are common in the perioperative period. Moreover, large volumes of intravenous fluids and blood components are often required to correct fluid deficits and compensate for blood loss during surgery. Major disturbances in fluid and electrolyte balance can rapidly alter cardiovascular, neurological, and neuromuscular functions, so anesthesia providers must have a clear understanding of normal water and electrolyte physiology. This chapter examines the body's fluid compartments and common water and electrolyte derangements, their treatment, and anesthetic implications. Acid–base disorders and intravenous fluid and blood therapy are discussed in Chapters 50 and 51.

Nomenclature of Solutions

The system of international units (SI) has still not gained universal acceptance in clinical practice, and many older expressions of concentration remain in common use. Thus, for example, the quantity of a solute in a solution may be expressed in grams, moles, or equivalents. To complicate matters further, the concentration of a solution may be expressed either as quantity of solute per volume of solution or quantity of solute per weight of solvent.

MOLARITY, MOLALITY, & EQUIVALENCY

One *mole* (mol) of a substance represents 6.02×10^{23} molecules. *Molarity* is the standard SI unit of concentration that expresses the number of moles of solute per *liter of solution* (mol/L, or M). *Molality* is an alternative term that expresses moles of solute per *kilogram of solvent*. Equivalency is also commonly used for substances that ionize: The number of equivalents of an ion in solution is the number of moles multiplied by its charge (valence). Thus, a 1 M solution of $MgCl_2$ yields 2 equivalents of magnesium per liter and 2 equivalents of chloride per liter.

OSMOLARITY, OSMOLALITY, & TONICITY

Osmosis is the net movement of water across a semipermeable membrane as a result of a difference in nondiffusible solute concentrations across the membrane. *Osmotic pressure* is the pressure that must be applied to the side with more solute to prevent a net movement of water across the membrane to dilute the solute.

1 **Osmotic pressure is generally dependent only on the number of nondiffusible solute particles. This is because the average kinetic energy of particles in solution is similar regardless of their mass.** One *osmole* (Osm) equals 1 mol of nondissociable substances. For substances that ionize, however, each mole results in *n* Osm, where *n* is the number of ionic species produced. Thus, 1 mol of a highly ionized substance such as NaCl dissolved in solution should produce 2 Osm; in reality, ionic interaction between the cation and anion reduces the effective activity of each such that NaCl behaves as if it is only 75% ionized. A difference of 1 mOsm/L between two solutions results in an osmotic pressure of 19.3 mm Hg. The osmolarity of a solution is equal to the number of osmoles per *liter* of solution, whereas its osmolality equals the number of osmoles per *kilogram* of solvent. *Tonicity*, a term that is often used interchangeably with osmolarity and osmolality, refers to the effect a solution has on cell volume. An *isotonic* solution has no effect on cell volume, whereas *hypotonic* and *hypertonic* solutions increase and decrease cell volume, respectively.

Fluid Compartments

Body water is distributed between two major fluid compartments separated by cell membranes: intracellular fluid (ICF) and extracellular fluid (ECF). The latter can be further subdivided into intravascular and interstitial compartments. The interstitium includes all fluid that is both outside cells and outside the vascular endothelium. The relative contributions of each compartment to total body water (TBW) and body weight are delineated in Table 49–1.

TABLE 49–1 Body fluid compartments (based on an average 70-kg man).

Compartment	Fluid as Percent Body Weight (%)	Total Body Water (%)	Fluid Volume (L)
Intracellular	40	67	28
Extracellular			
Interstitial	15	25	10.5
Intravascular	5	8	3.5
Total	60	100	42

The volume of fluid (water) within each compartment is determined by its solute composition and concentrations (Table 49–2). Differences in solute concentrations are largely due to the characteristics of the physical barriers that separate compartments. *The osmotic forces created by "trapped" solutes govern the distribution of water between compartments and ultimately each compartment's volume.*

INTRACELLULAR FLUID

The outer membrane of cells plays an important role in regulating intracellular volume and composition. A membrane-bound adenosine triphosphate (ATP)–dependent pump exchanges Na^+ for K^+ in a 3:2 ratio. Because cell membranes are relatively impermeable to sodium ions and, to a lesser extent, potassium ions, potassium is concentrated intracellularly, whereas sodium is concentrated extracellularly.

2 As a result, **potassium is the most important determinant of intracellular osmotic pressure, whereas sodium is the most important determinant of extracellular osmotic pressure.**

The impermeability of cell membranes to most proteins results in a high intracellular protein concentration. Because proteins act as nondiffusible solutes (anions), the unequal exchange ratio of 3 Na^+ for 2 K^+ by the cell membrane pump is critical in preventing relative intracellular hyperosmolality. Interference with Na^+–K^+-ATPase activity, as occurs during ischemia or hypoxia, results in the progressive swelling of cells.

EXTRACELLULAR FLUID

The principal function of ECF is to provide a medium for the delivery of cell nutrients and electrolytes and for the removal of cellular waste products. Maintenance of normal extracellular volume—particularly the circulating component (intravascular volume)—is critical. For the reasons described

TABLE 49–2 The composition of fluid compartments.

	Gram-Molecular Weight	Intracellular (mEq/L)	Extracellular	
			Intravascular (mEq/L)	*Interstitial (mEq/L)*
Sodium	23.0	10	145	142
Potassium	39.1	140	4	4
Calcium	40.1	<1	3	3
Magnesium	24.3	50	2	2
Chloride	35.5	4	105	110
Bicarbonate	61.0	10	24	28
Phosphorus	31.0[1]	75	2	2
Protein (g/dL)		16	7	2

[1]PO_4^{3-} is 95 g.

earlier, sodium is quantitatively the most important extracellular cation and the major determinant of extracellular osmotic pressure and volume. *Changes in ECF volume are therefore related to changes in total body sodium content.* The latter is a function of sodium intake, renal sodium excretion, and extrarenal sodium losses (see later discussion).

Interstitial Fluid

Very little interstitial fluid is normally in the form of free fluid. Most interstitial water is in chemical association with extracellular proteoglycans, forming a gel. Interstitial fluid pressure is generally thought to be negative (approximately –5 mm Hg). Increases in extracellular volume are normally proportionately reflected in intravascular and interstitial volume. However, as interstitial fluid volume progressively increases, interstitial pressure also rises and eventually becomes positive. When the latter occurs, free fluid in the interstitial gel matrix increases rapidly, and the result is an expansion only of the interstitial fluid compartment (Figure 49–1). In this way, the interstitial compartment acts as an overflow reservoir for the intravascular compartment, as seen clinically in tissue edema.

Because only small quantities of plasma proteins can normally cross capillary clefts, the protein content of interstitial fluid is relatively low (2 g/dL). Protein entering the interstitial space is returned to the vascular system via the lymphatic system.

Intravascular Fluid

Intravascular fluid, commonly referred to as *plasma*, is restricted to the intravascular space by the vascular endothelium. Most electrolytes (small ions) freely pass between plasma and the interstitium, resulting in nearly identical electrolyte composition. However, the tight intercellular junctions between adjacent endothelial cells impede the passage of plasma proteins to outside the intravascular compartment. As a result, plasma proteins (mainly albumin) are the only osmotically active solutes in fluid not normally exchanged between plasma and interstitial fluid.

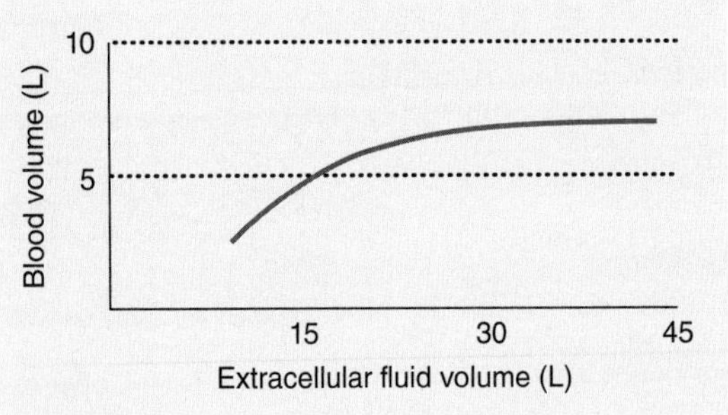

FIGURE 49–1 The relationship between blood volume and extracellular fluid volume. (Modified with permission from Guyton AC. *Textbook of Medical Physiology,* 7th ed. Philadelphia, PA: WB Saunders; 1986.)

EXCHANGE BETWEEN FLUID COMPARTMENTS

Diffusion results from the random movement of molecules due to their kinetic energy and is responsible for most fluid and solute exchange between compartments. The rate of diffusion of a substance across a membrane depends upon (1) the permeability of that substance through that membrane; (2) the concentration difference for that substance between the two sides; (3) the pressure difference between either side because pressure imparts greater kinetic energy; and (4) the electrical potential across the membrane for charged substances.

Diffusion Through Cell Membranes

Diffusion between interstitial fluid and ICF may take place by one of several mechanisms: (1) directly through the lipid bilayer of the cell membrane, (2) through ion channels within the membrane, or (3) by reversible binding to a carrier protein that can traverse the membrane (*facilitated diffusion*). Oxygen, carbon dioxide (CO_2), water, and lipid-soluble molecules penetrate the cell membrane directly. Cations such as Na^+, K^+, and Ca^{2+} penetrate the lipid membrane poorly and can diffuse only through specific ion channels. Passage through these channels is dependent on membrane voltage and, in some cases, the binding of ligands (such as acetylcholine) to membrane receptors. The diffusion of glucose and amino acids is aided by membrane-bound carrier proteins.

3 **Fluid exchange between the intracellular and interstitial spaces is governed by the osmotic forces created by differences in nondiffusible solute concentrations.** Changes in osmolality between intracellular and interstitial compartments result in a

net water movement from the relatively hypoosmolar compartment to the relatively hyperosmolar compartment.

Diffusion Through Capillary Endothelium

Capillary walls are typically 0.5 μm thick and consist of a single layer of endothelial cells with their basement membrane. Intercellular clefts, 6 to 7 nm wide, separate each cell from its neighbors. Oxygen, CO_2, water, and lipid-soluble substances can penetrate directly through both sides of the endothelial cell membrane. Only low-molecular-weight, water-soluble substances such as sodium, chloride, potassium, and glucose readily cross intercellular clefts. High-molecular-weight substances such as plasma proteins penetrate the endothelial clefts poorly, with the exception of the liver and the lungs, where the clefts are larger.

Fluid exchange across capillary walls differs from that across cell membranes in that it is governed by differences in hydrostatic pressures in addition to osmotic forces (Figure 49–2). These forces are operative on both arterial and venous ends of capillaries, with a tendency for fluid to move out of capillaries at the arterial end and back into capillaries at the venous end. Moreover, the magnitude of these forces differs among the various tissue beds. Arterial capillary pressure is determined by precapillary sphincter tone. Thus, capillaries that require high pressure, such as glomeruli, have low precapillary sphincter tone, whereas the normally low-pressure capillaries of muscle have high precapillary sphincter tone. Normally, all but 10% of the fluid filtered is reabsorbed back into capillaries. What is not reabsorbed (about 2 mL/min) enters the interstitial fluid and is then returned by lymphatic flow to the intravascular compartment.

Disorders of Water Balance

The human body at birth is approximately 75% water by weight. By 1 month, this value decreases to 65%, and by adulthood, it increases to 60% for men and 50% for women. The higher fat content in women decreases water content. For the same reason, obesity and advanced age further decrease water content.

NORMAL WATER BALANCE

The normal adult daily water intake averages 2500 mL, which includes approximately 300 mL as a byproduct of the metabolism of energy substrates. Daily water loss averages 2500 mL and is typically accounted for by 1500 mL in urine, 400 mL in respiratory tract evaporation, 400 mL in skin evaporation, 100 mL in sweat, and 100 mL in feces. Evaporative loss is very important in thermoregulation because this mechanism normally accounts for 20% to 25% of heat loss.

Both ICF and ECF osmolalities are tightly regulated to maintain normal water content in tissues. Changes in water content and cell volume may induce significant impairment of function, especially in the brain (see later discussion).

RELATIONSHIP OF PLASMA SODIUM CONCENTRATION, EXTRACELLULAR OSMOLALITY, & INTRACELLULAR OSMOLALITY

The osmolality of ECF is equal to the sum of the concentrations of all dissolved solutes. Because Na^+ and its anions account for nearly 90% of these solutes, the following approximation is valid:

$$\text{Plasma osmolality} = 2 \times \text{Plasma sodium concentration}$$

Moreover, because ICF and ECF are in osmotic equilibrium, plasma sodium concentration $[Na^+]_{plasma}$ generally reflects total body osmolality:

$$\text{Total body osmolality} = \frac{\text{Extracellular solutes} + \text{Intracellur solutes}}{\text{TBW}}$$

Because sodium and potassium are the major intra- and extracellular solutes, respectively:

$$\text{Total body osmolality} = \frac{(Na^+_{\text{extracellular}} \times 2) + (K^+_{\text{intracellular}} \times 2)}{\text{TBW}}$$

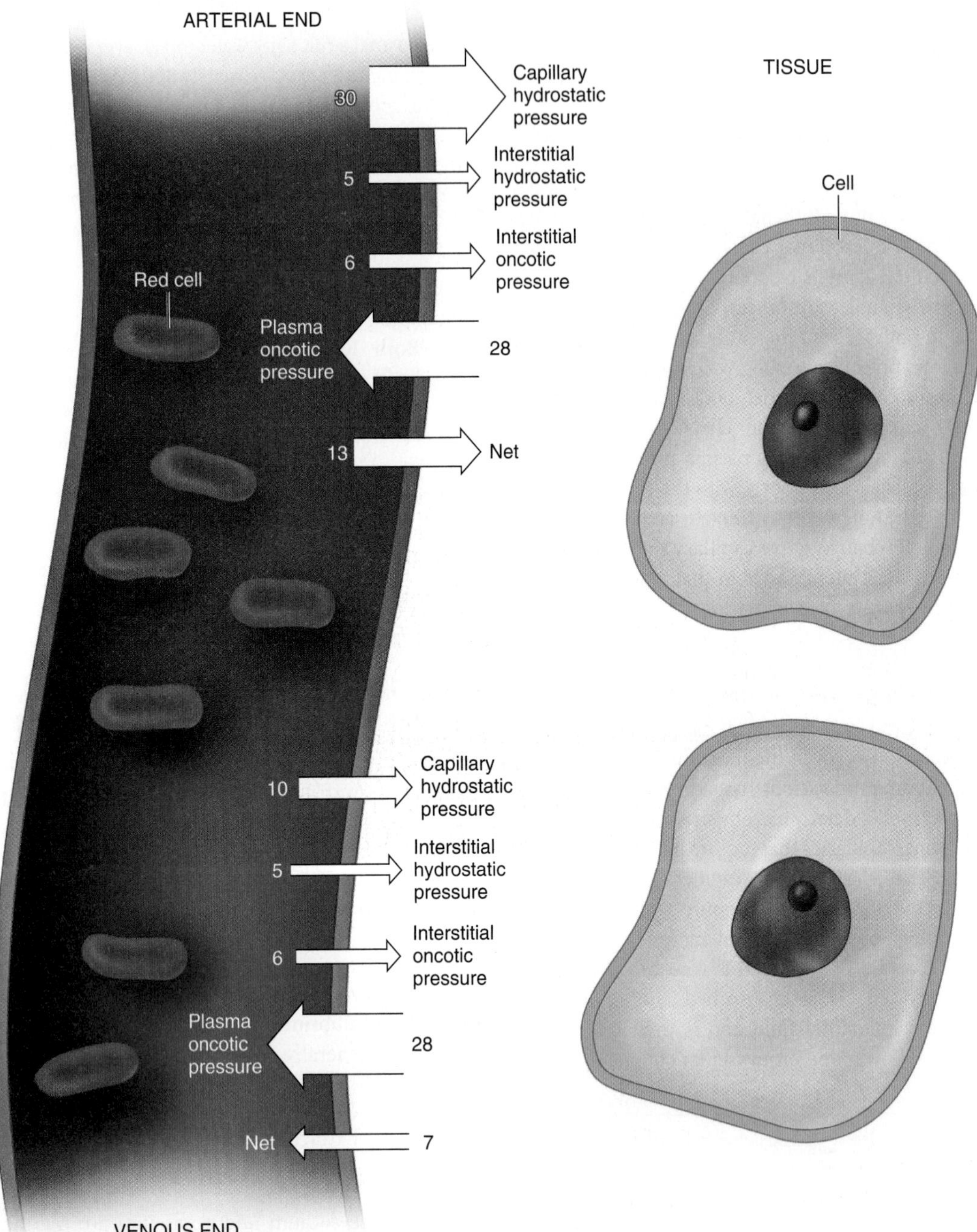

FIGURE 49–2 Capillary fluid exchange. The numbers in this figure are in mm Hg and indicate the pressure gradient for the respective pressures. "Net" refers to the net pressure at either end of the capillary (ie, 13 mm Hg at the arterial and 7 mm Hg at the venous end of the capillary).

Combining the two approximations:

$$[\text{Na}^+]_{\text{plasma}} \approx \frac{(\text{Na}^+_{\text{extracellular}} \times 2)+(\text{K}^+_{\text{intracellular}} \times 2)}{\text{TBW}}$$

Based on these principles, the effect of isotonic, hypotonic, and hypertonic fluid loads on compartmental water content and plasma osmolality can be calculated (Table 49–3). The potential importance of intracellular potassium concentration is readily apparent from this equation. Thus, *significant potassium losses may contribute to hyponatremia.*

In pathologic states, glucose and, to a much lesser extent, urea can contribute significantly to extracellular osmolality. A more accurate approximation of plasma osmolality is therefore given by the following equation:

Plasma osmolality (mOsm/kg)

$$= [\text{Na}^+] \times 2 + \frac{\text{BUN}}{2.8} + \frac{\text{Glucose}}{18}$$

where [Na⁺] is expressed as mEq/L and blood urea nitrogen (BUN) and glucose as mg/dL. Urea is an ineffective osmole because it readily permeates cell membranes and is therefore frequently omitted from this calculation:

$$\text{Effective plasma osmolality} = [\text{Na}^+] \times 2 + \frac{\text{Glucose}}{18}$$

Plasma osmolality normally varies between 280 and 290 mOsm/L. Plasma sodium concentration decreases approximately 1 mEq/L for every 62 mg/dL increase in glucose concentration. A discrepancy between the measured and calculated osmolality is referred to as an *osmolal gap*. Significant osmolal gaps indicate a high concentration of an abnormal osmotically active molecule in plasma such as ethanol, mannitol, methanol, ethylene glycol, or isopropyl alcohol. Osmolal gaps may also be seen in patients with chronic kidney disease (attributed to retention of small solutes), patients with ketoacidosis (as a result of a high concentration of ketone bodies), and those receiving large amounts of glycine (as during transurethral resection of the prostate). Lastly, osmolal gaps may also be present in patients with marked hyperlipidemia or hyperproteinemia. In such instances, the protein or lipid part of plasma

TABLE 49–3 Effect of different fluid loads on extracellular and intracellular water contents.[1]

A. Normal

Total body solute = 280 mOsm/kg × 42 kg = 11,760 mOsm
Intracellular solute = 280 mOsm/kg × 25 kg = 7000 mOsm
Extracellular solute = 280 mOsm/kg × 17 kg = 4760 mOsm
Extracellular sodium concentration = 280 ÷ 2 = 140 mEq/L

	Intracellular	Extracellular
Osmolality		
Volume (L)	25	17
Net water gain	0	0

B. Isotonic load: 2 L of Isotonic saline (NaCl)

Total body solute = 280 mOsm/kg × 44 kg = 12,320 mOsm
Intracellular solute = 280 mOsm/kg × 25 kg = 7000 mOsm
Extracellular solute = 280 mOsm/kg × 19 kg = 5320 mOsm

	Intracellular	Extracellular
Osmolality	280	280
Volume (L)	25	19
Net water gain	0	2

Net effect: Fluid remains in extracellular compartment.

C. Free water (hypotonic) load: 2 L water

New body water = 42 + 2 = 44 kg
New body osmolality = 11,760 mOsm ÷ 44 kg = 267 mOsm/kg
New intracellular volume = 7000 mOsm ÷ 267 mOsm/kg = 26.2 kg
New extracellular sodium concentration = 267 ÷ 2 = 133 mEq/L

	Intracellular	Extracellular
Osmolality	267.0	267.0
Volume (L)	26.2	17.8
Net water gain	+1.2	+0.8

Net effect: Fluid distributes between both compartments.

D. Hypertonic load: 600 mEq NaCl (no water)

Total body solute = 11,760 + 600 = 12,360 mOsm/kg
New body osmolality = 12,360 mOsm/kg ÷ 42 kg = 294 mOsm
New extracellular solute = 600 + 4760 = 5360 mOsm
New extracellular volume = 5360 mOsm ÷ 294 mOsm/kg = 18.2 kg
New intracellular volume = 42 – 18.2 = 23.8 kg
New extracellular sodium concentration = 294 ÷ 2 = 147 mEq/L

	Intracellular	Extracellular
Osmolality	294.0	294.0
Volume (L)	23.8	18.2
Net water gain	–1.2	+1.2

Net effect: An intracellular to extracellular movement of water.

[1]Based on a 70-kg adult man.

contributes significantly to plasma volume; although plasma [Na^+] is decreased, [Na^+] in the water phase of plasma (true plasma osmolality) remains normal. The water phase of plasma is normally only 93% of its volume; the remaining 7% consists of plasma lipids and proteins.

CONTROL OF PLASMA OSMOLALITY

Plasma osmolality is closely regulated by the hypothalamus, which controls both the secretion of antidiuretic hormone (ADH) and the thirst mechanism. Plasma osmolality is therefore maintained within relatively narrow limits by control of both water intake and water excretion.

Secretion of Antidiuretic Hormone

Specialized neurons in the hypothalamus are sensitive to changes in extracellular osmolality. When ECF osmolality increases, these cells shrink and cause ADH release from the posterior pituitary. ADH markedly increases water reabsorption in renal collecting tubules (see Chapter 30), which reduces plasma osmolality back to normal. Conversely, a decrease in extracellular osmolality causes osmoreceptors to swell and suppresses the release of ADH. Decreased ADH secretion allows water diuresis, which increases osmolality to normal. Peak diuresis occurs once circulating ADH is metabolized (90–120 minutes). With complete suppression of ADH secretion, the kidneys can excrete up to 10 to 20 L of water per day.

Nonosmotic Release of Antidiuretic Hormone

Carotid baroreceptors (volume receptors), as well as low-pressure volume receptors in the atria, vena cavae, and pulmonary arteries, also influence ADH release. A fall in wall tension results in a reflex increase of ADH secretion from the posterior pituitary. An increased stretch of these receptors not only suppresses ADH secretion, but the increased atrial volume receptor stretch also increases secretion of *atrial natriuretic peptide* (ANP; see later discussion), which promotes renal excretion of sodium and water. Increased sympathetic activity associated with conditions such as pain, emotional stress, and hypoxia also promotes ADH release.

Thirst

Activation of osmoreceptors in the lateral preoptic area of the hypothalamus neurons by increases in ECF osmolality induces thirst, stimulating the individual to drink water. Conversely, hypoosmolality suppresses thirst. *Thirst is the major defense mechanism against hyperosmolality and hypernatremia* because it is the only mechanism that increases water intake.

HYPEROSMOLALITY & HYPERNATREMIA

Hyperosmolality occurs whenever total body solute content increases relative to TBW and is usually, but not always, associated with hypernatremia ([Na^+] > 145 mEq/L). Hyperosmolality without hypernatremia may be seen during marked hyperglycemia or following the accumulation of abnormal osmotically active substances in plasma (see earlier discussion). In the latter two instances, plasma sodium concentration may actually decrease as water is drawn from the intracellular to the extracellular compartment. For every 100 mg/dL increase in plasma glucose concentration, plasma sodium decreases approximately 1.6 mEq/L.

Hypernatremic patients may be hypovolemic, euvolemic, or hypervolemic (Table 49–4). However, *hypernatremia is nearly always the result of either a relative loss of water in excess of sodium (hypotonic fluid loss) or the retention of large quantities of sodium.* Even when kidney concentrating ability is impaired, thirst is normally highly effective in preventing hypernatremia. Hypernatremia is therefore most commonly seen in debilitated patients who are unable to drink, the very aged, the very young, and patients with altered consciousness. Much of the total body sodium is stored in the skin, bone, and cartilage, which serves as a reservoir for the rest of the body, and patients with dysnatremias may have a low, normal, or high total body sodium content (Figure 49–3).

TABLE 49–4 Differential diagnosis of hypernatremia.

Hypovolemic hypernatremia
Body fluid loss (eg, burns, sweating)
Diuretic use
Gastrointestinal loss (eg, vomiting, diarrhea, fistulas)
Heat injury
Osmotic diuresis (eg, hyperosmolar nonketotic coma, enteral feeding)
Postobstructive diuresis
Euvolemic hypernatremia
Central diabetes insipidus
Nephrogenic diabetes insipidus
Fever
Hyperventilation/mechanical ventilation
Hypodipsia
Medications (eg, amphotericin aminoglycosides, lithium, phenytoin)
Sickle cell disease
Suprasellar and infrasellar tumors
Hypervolemic hypernatremia
Cushing syndrome
Hemodialysis
Hyperaldosteronism
Iatrogenic (eg, salt tablet or salt water ingestion, saline infusions, saline enemas, intravenous bicarbonate, enteral feedings)

Data from Braun MM, Barstow CH, Pyzocha NJ. Diagnosis and management of sodium disorders: Hyponatremia and hypernatremia. *Am Fam Phys.* 2015 Mar 1;91(5):299-307.

Hypernatremia & Low Total Body Sodium Content

These patients have lost both sodium and water, but the water loss is in relative excess to that of the sodium loss. Hypotonic losses can be renal (osmotic diuresis) or extrarenal (diarrhea or sweat). In either case, patients usually manifest signs of hypovolemia (see Chapter 51). Urinary sodium concentration is generally greater than 20 mEq/L with renal losses and less than 10 mEq/L with extrarenal losses.

Hypernatremia & Normal Total Body Sodium Content

This group of patients generally manifests signs of water loss without overt hypovolemia unless the water loss is massive. Total body sodium content is generally normal. Nearly pure water losses can occur via the skin, respiratory tract, or kidneys. Occasionally, transient hypernatremia is observed with the movement of water into cells following exercise, seizures, or rhabdomyolysis. *The most common cause of hypernatremia in conscious patients with normal total body sodium content is diabetes insipidus.* Diabetes insipidus (DI) is characterized by marked impairment in renal concentrating ability that is due

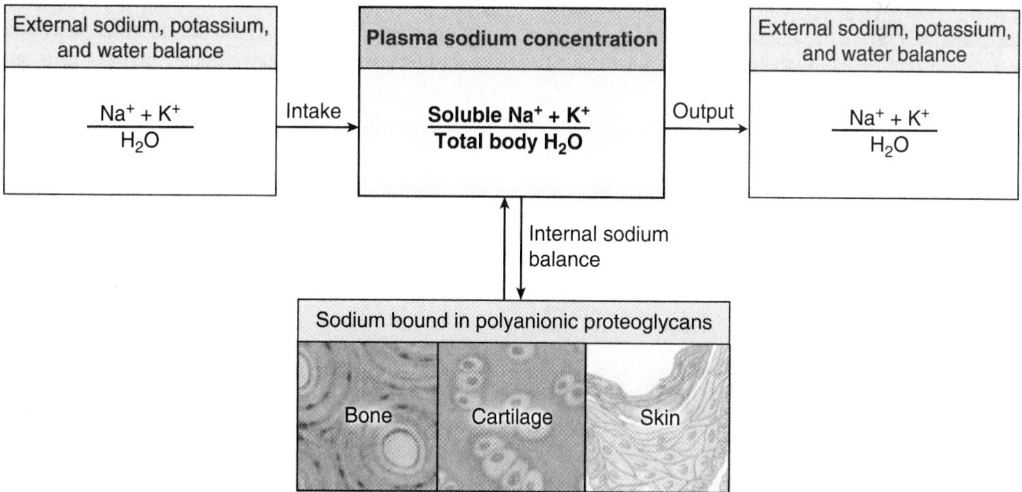

FIGURE 49–3 Solute and water balance and the plasma sodium concentration. Plasma sodium concentration is determined according to the ratio of sodium and potassium to total body water. This concentration is altered by net external intake/output balances of sodium, potassium, and water and by internal exchanges between sodium that is free in solution and sodium that is bound to polyanionic proteoglycans in bone, cartilage, and skin. (Reproduced with permission from Sterns RH. Disorders of plasma sodium—Causes, consequences, and correction. *N Engl J Med.* 2015 Jan 1;372(1):55-65.)

either to decreased ADH secretion (*central DI*) or failure of the renal tubules to respond normally to circulating ADH (*nephrogenic DI*). Rarely, *essential hypernatremia* may be encountered in patients with central nervous system disorders. These patients appear to have "reset" osmoreceptors that function at a higher baseline osmolality.

A. Central Diabetes Insipidus

Lesions in or around the hypothalamus and the pituitary stalk frequently produce DI. DI often develops with brain death. Transient DI is also commonly seen following neurosurgical procedures and head trauma. The diagnosis is suggested by a history of polydipsia, polyuria (often >6 L/d), and the absence of hyperglycemia. In the perioperative setting, the diagnosis of DI is suggested by marked polyuria without glycosuria and a urinary osmolality lower than plasma osmolality. The absence of thirst in unconscious individuals leads to marked water losses and can rapidly produce hypovolemia. The diagnosis of central DI is confirmed by an increase in urinary osmolality following the administration of exogenous ADH. Aqueous vasopressin (5–10 units subcutaneously or intramuscularly every 4–6 hours) is the treatment of choice for acute central DI. Vasopressin in oil (0.3 mL intramuscularly every day) is longer lasting but is more likely to cause water intoxication. Desmopressin (DDAVP), a synthetic analog of ADH with a 12- to 24-hour duration of action, is available as an intranasal preparation (10–40 mcg/day either as a single daily dose or divided into two doses) that can be used in both ambulatory and perioperative settings.

B. Nephrogenic Diabetes Insipidus

Nephrogenic DI can be congenital but is more commonly secondary to other disorders, including chronic kidney disease, hypokalemia, hypercalcemia, sickle cell disease, and hyperproteinemia. Nephrogenic DI can also be secondary to the side effects of some drugs (amphotericin B, lithium, demeclocycline, ifosfamide, mannitol). ADH secretion in nephrogenic DI is normal, but the kidneys fail to respond to ADH, and urinary concentrating ability is therefore impaired. The diagnosis is confirmed by the failure of the kidneys to produce hypertonic urine following the administration of exogenous ADH. Treatment is generally directed at the underlying illness and ensuring an adequate fluid intake. Volume depletion by a thiazide diuretic can paradoxically decrease urinary output by reducing water delivery to collecting tubules. Sodium and protein restriction can similarly reduce urinary output.

Hypernatremia & Increased Total Body Sodium Content

This condition most commonly results from the administration of large quantities of hypertonic saline solutions (3% NaCl or 7.5% $NaHCO_3$). Patients with primary hyperaldosteronism and Cushing syndrome may also have elevations in serum sodium concentration along with signs of increased sodium retention.

Clinical Manifestations of Hypernatremia

Neurological manifestations predominate in patients with symptomatic hypernatremia, and restlessness, lethargy, and hyperreflexia can progress to seizures, coma, and ultimately death. Symptoms correlate more closely with the rate of movement of water out of brain cells than with the absolute level of hypernatremia. Rapid decreases in brain volume can rupture cerebral veins and result in focal intracerebral or subarachnoid hemorrhage. Seizures and serious neurological damage are common, particularly in children with acute hypernatremia when plasma [Na^+] exceeds 158 mEq/L. Chronic hypernatremia is usually better tolerated than the acute form. After 24 to 48 hours, intracellular osmolality begins to rise as a result of increases in intracellular inositol and amino acid concentrations, and brain intracellular water content slowly returns to normal.

Treatment of Hypernatremia

The treatment of hypernatremia is aimed at restoring plasma osmolality to normal and correcting the underlying cause. Water deficits should generally be corrected over 48 hours because rapid correction (or overcorrection) can cause cerebral edema. Enteral free water administration is preferable when feasible, but a hypotonic intravenous solution

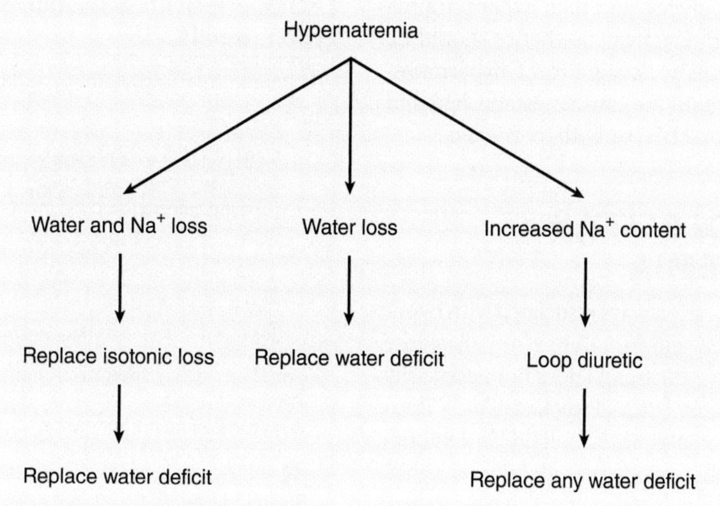

FIGURE 49–4 Algorithm for the treatment of hypernatremia.

such as 5% dextrose in water can also be used (see later discussion). Abnormalities in extracellular volume must also be corrected (Figure 49–4). Hypernatremic patients with decreased total body sodium should be given isotonic fluids to restore plasma volume to normal *before* treatment with a hypotonic solution. Hypernatremic patients with increased total body sodium should be treated with a loop diuretic along with intravenous 5% dextrose in water. The treatment of DI is discussed in the preceding section.

Rapid correction of hypernatremia can result in seizures, brain edema, permanent neurological damage, and even death. Serial Na^+ osmolalities should be obtained during treatment. In general, decreases in plasma sodium concentration should not proceed at a rate faster than 0.5 mEq/L/h.

Example: A 70-kg man is found to have a plasma [Na^+] of 160 mEq/L. What is his water deficit?

If one assumes that hypernatremia in this case represents water loss only, then total body osmoles are unchanged. Thus, assuming a normal [Na^+] of 140 mEq/L and TBW content that is 60% of body weight:

$$\text{Normal TBW} \times 140 = \text{Present TBW} \times [Na^+]_{plasma} \text{ or}$$
$$(70 \times 0.6) \times 140 = \text{Present TBW} \times 160$$

Solving the equation:

Present TBW = 36.7 L

$$\text{Water deficit} = \text{Normal TBW} - \text{Present TBW or}$$
$$(70 \times 0.6) - 36.7 = 5.3 \text{ L}$$

To replace this deficit over 48 hours, it is necessary to administer 5.3 L of enteral free water in small amounts over 48 hours, or, 5% dextrose in water intravenously, 5300 mL over 48 hours, or 110 mL/h.

Note that this method ignores any coexisting isotonic fluid deficits, which, if present, should be replaced with an isotonic solution.

Anesthetic Considerations

Hypernatremia has been demonstrated to increase the minimum alveolar concentration for inhalation anesthetics in animal studies, but its clinical significance is more closely related to the associated fluid deficits. Hypovolemia accentuates any vasodilation or cardiac depression from anesthetic agents and predisposes to hypotension and hypoperfusion of tissues. Decreases in the volume of distribution for drugs necessitate dose reductions for most intravenous agents, whereas decreases in cardiac output enhance the uptake of inhalation anesthetics.

Even mild serum sodium elevation is associated with increased perioperative morbidity, mortality, and hospital length of stay, and thus hypernatremia must not be ignored. Elective anesthetics should be postponed in patients with significant hypernatremia (>150 mEq/L) until the cause is established and total body sodium or TBW, or both, corrected.

HYPOOSMOLALITY & HYPONATREMIA

Hypoosmolality is nearly always associated with hyponatremia ([Na^+] <135 mEq/L). Table 49–5 lists rare instances in which hyponatremia does not necessarily reflect hypoosmolality (*pseudohyponatremia*). Routine measurement of plasma osmolality in hyponatremic patients rapidly excludes pseudohyponatremia.

Hyponatremia invariably reflects water retention from either an absolute increase in TBW or a loss of sodium in relative excess to loss of water. The kidneys' normal capacity to produce dilute urine with an osmolality as low as 40 mOsm/kg (specific gravity 1.001) allows them to excrete over 10 L of free water per day if necessary. Because of this tremendous reserve, hyponatremia is nearly always the result of a defect in urinary diluting capacity (urinary osmolality >100 mOsm/kg or specific gravity >1.003—ie, the limited ability of the kidneys to excrete free water). Rare instances of hyponatremia without an abnormality in renal-diluting capacity (urinary osmolality <100 mOsm/kg) are generally attributed to primary polydipsia or reset osmoreceptors; the latter two conditions can be differentiated by water restriction.

TABLE 49–5 Causes of pseudohyponatremia.

Hyponatremia with a normal plasma osmolality
Asymptomatic
Marked hyperlipidemia
Marked hyperproteinemia
Symptomatic
Marked glycine absorption during transurethral surgery
Hyponatremia with an elevated plasma osmolality
Hyperglycemia
Administration of mannitol

Adapted with permission from Rose RD. *Clinical Physiology of Acid-Base and Electrolyte Disorders,* 3rd ed. New York, NY: McGraw Hill; 1989.

TABLE 49–6 Classification of hypoosmolal hyponatremia.

Decreased total body sodium content
Renal
Diuretics
Mineralocorticoid deficiency
Salt-losing nephropathies
Osmotic diuresis (glucose, mannitol)
Renal tubular acidosis
Extrarenal
Vomiting
Diarrhea
Integumentary loss (sweating, burns)
Normal total body sodium content
Primary polydipsia
Syndrome of inappropriate antidiuretic hormone
Glucocorticoid deficiency
Hypothyroidism
Drug-induced
Increased total body sodium content
Congestive heart failure
Cirrhosis
Nephrotic syndrome

Clinically, hyponatremia is best classified according to total body sodium content (Table 49–6). Hyponatremia associated with transurethral resection of the prostate is discussed in Chapter 32.

Hyponatremia & Low Total Body Sodium

Progressive losses of both sodium and water eventually lead to extracellular volume depletion. As the intravascular volume deficit approaches 5% to 10%, nonosmotic ADH secretion is activated (see earlier discussion). With further volume depletion, the stimuli for nonosmotic ADH release overcome any hyponatremia-induced suppression of ADH, and preservation of circulatory volume takes place at the expense of plasma osmolality.

Fluid losses resulting in hyponatremia may be renal or extrarenal in origin. Renal losses are most commonly related to thiazide diuretics and result in a urinary [Na^+] greater than 20 mEq/L. Extrarenal losses are typically gastrointestinal and usually are associated with a urinary [Na^+] of less than 10 mEq/L. A major exception to the latter is hyponatremia due to vomiting, which can result in a urinary [Na^+] greater than

20 mEq/L. In this situation, renal compensation for the associated metabolic alkalosis results in bicarbonaturia, with concomitant excretion of Na^+ with HCO_3 to maintain electrical neutrality in the urine; urinary chloride concentration, however, is usually less than 10 mEq/L.

Hyponatremia & Increased Total Body Sodium

Edematous disorders are characterized by an increase in both total body sodium and TBW. When the increase in TBW is relatively greater than the increase in total body sodium, hyponatremia occurs. Edematous disorders include congestive heart failure, cirrhosis, kidney failure, and nephrotic syndrome. Hyponatremia in these settings results from progressive impairment of renal free water excretion and generally parallels underlying disease severity. Pathophysiological mechanisms include nonosmotic ADH release and decreased delivery of fluid to nephron distal diluting segments (see Chapter 30).

Hyponatremia with Normal Total Body Sodium

Hyponatremia in the absence of edema or hypovolemia may be seen with glucocorticoid insufficiency, hypothyroidism, drug therapy, and the syndrome of inappropriate antidiuretic hormone secretion (SIADH, also referred to as the *syndrome of inappropriate antidiuresis* [SIAD]; Table 49–7). The hyponatremia associated with adrenal hypofunction may be due to co-secretion of ADH with corticotropin-releasing factor (CRF). Diagnosis of SIADH requires exclusion of other causes of hyponatremia and the absence of hypovolemia, edema, and adrenal, renal, or thyroid disease. Various malignant tumors, pulmonary diseases, and central nervous system disorders are commonly associated with SIADH. In most such instances, plasma ADH concentration is not elevated but is inadequately suppressed relative to the degree of hypoosmolality in plasma; urine osmolality is usually greater than 100 mOsm/kg, and urine sodium concentration is greater than 40 mEq/L.

Cerebral salt wasting (CSW) is a syndrome of inappropriate renal sodium wasting and hyponatremia with polyuria and hypovolemia that may be seen with intracranial disease, including brain tumors, subarachnoid hemorrhage, subdural hematoma, meningitis, and head trauma. Proposed mechanisms for this disorder include excess secretion of natriuretic peptides and altered sympathetic stimulation to the kidney. Both SIADH and CSW are characterized by elevated urine sodium concentration, low serum osmolality, and high urine osmolality. However, patients with SIADH are usually euvolemic or mildly hypervolemic, whereas patients with CSW are hypovolemic, and thus treatments for these two disorders are very different. The treatment

TABLE 49–7 Causes of SIADH.[1]

Pulmonary disease
Pneumonia
Tuberculosis
Abscess
Asthma
Malignancy
Lung
Gastrointestinal
Genitourinary
CNS disease
Hemorrhage
Hematoma
Infection
Tumors
Drugs
Stimulate AVP release
Chlorpropamide
Clofibrate
Carbamazepine
Vincristine
SSRIs
MDMA
Ifosfamide
Antipsychotics
Opioids
Potentiate action of AVP
Chlorpropamide
NSAIDs
Cyclophosphamide
AVP analogues
Desmopressin
Oxytocin
Vasopressin

[1]AVP, arginine vasopressin; CNS, central nervous system; MDMA, 3,4-methylenedioxy-*N*-methamphetamine; NSAIDs, nonsteroidal anti-inflammatory drugs; SIADH, syndrome of inappropriate secretion of antidiuretic hormone; SSRIs, selective serotonin reuptake inhibitors.

Adapted with permission from Buffington MA, Abreo K. Hyponatremia: A review. *J Intens Care Med.* 2016 May;31(4):223-236.

of SIADH is free water restriction, and the treatment of CSW is volume and sodium replacement with normal or hypertonic saline.

Clinical Manifestations of Hyponatremia

Symptoms of hyponatremia are primarily neurological and result from an increase in intracellular water. Their severity is generally related to the rapidity with which extracellular hypoosmolality develops. Patients with mild to moderate hyponatremia ([Na^+] >125 mEq/L) are frequently asymptomatic. Early symptoms are typically nonspecific and may include anorexia, nausea, and weakness. Progressive cerebral edema, however, results in lethargy, confusion, seizures, coma, and finally death. 4 **Serious manifestations of hyponatremia are generally associated with plasma sodium concentrations less than 120 mEq/L.**

Patients with slowly developing or chronic hyponatremia are generally less symptomatic, probably because the gradual compensatory loss of intracellular solutes (primarily Na^+, K^+, and organic osmolytes) restores cell volume to near normal. Neurological symptoms in patients with chronic hyponatremia may be related more closely to changes in cell membrane potential (due to a low extracellular [Na^+]) than to changes in cell volume.

Treatment of Hyponatremia

As with hypernatremia, the treatment of hyponatremia (Figure 49–5) is directed at correcting both the underlying disorder as well as the plasma [Na^+]. *Isotonic saline is generally the treatment of choice for hyponatremic patients with decreased total body sodium content.* Once the ECF deficit is corrected, spontaneous water diuresis returns plasma [Na^+] to normal. *Conversely, water restriction is the primary treatment for hyponatremic patients with normal or increased total body sodium.* More specific treatments such as hormone replacement in patients with adrenal or thyroid hypofunction and measures aimed at improving cardiac output in patients with heart failure may also be indicated. Demeclocycline (Declomycin, Declostatin), a tetracycline antibiotic that antagonizes ADH activity at the renal tubules, is often used as an adjunct in the treatment of SIADH when water restriction alone is insufficient.

Acute, symptomatic hyponatremia requires prompt treatment. In such instances, correction of plasma [Na^+] to greater than 125 mEq/L is usually sufficient to alleviate symptoms and signs. The amount of NaCl necessary to raise plasma [Na^+] to the desired value, the Na^+ deficit, can be estimated by the following formula:

$$Na^+ \text{ deficit} = \text{TBW} \times (\text{Desired } [Na^+] - \text{Present } [Na^+])$$

5 **Excessively rapid correction of hyponatremia has been associated with demyelinating lesions in the pons (*central pontine myelinolysis*) and more generally in both pontine and extrapontine central nervous system structures (*osmotic demyelination syndrome*), resulting in both temporary and permanent neurological sequelae. The rapidity with which hyponatremia is corrected should be tailored to the severity of symptoms.** The following correction rates have been suggested: for mild symptoms, 0.5 mEq/L/h or less; for moderate symptoms, 1 mEq/L/h or less; and for severe symptoms, 1.5 mEq/L/h or less.

Example: An 80-kg woman is lethargic and is found to have plasma [Na^+] of 118 mEq/L. How much NaCl must be given to raise her plasma [Na^+] to 130 mEq/L?

$$Na^+ \text{ deficit} = \text{TBW} \times (130 - 118) \text{ mEq}$$

TBW is approximately 50% of body weight in females:

$$Na^+ \text{ deficit} = 80 \text{ kg} \times 0.5 \times (130 - 118) \text{ mEq} = 480 \text{ mEq}$$

Because normal (isotonic) saline contains 154 mEq/L, the patient should receive 480 mEq ÷ 154 mEq/L, or 3.12 L of normal saline. For a correction rate of 0.5 mEq/L/h, this amount of saline should be given over 24 hours (130 mL/h).

Note that this calculation does not take into account any coexisting isotonic fluid deficits, which, if present, should also be replaced. More rapid correction of hyponatremia can be achieved by giving a loop diuretic to induce water diuresis while replacing urinary Na^+ losses with isotonic saline. Even more rapid corrections can be achieved with intravenous hypertonic saline (3% NaCl). Hypertonic saline may

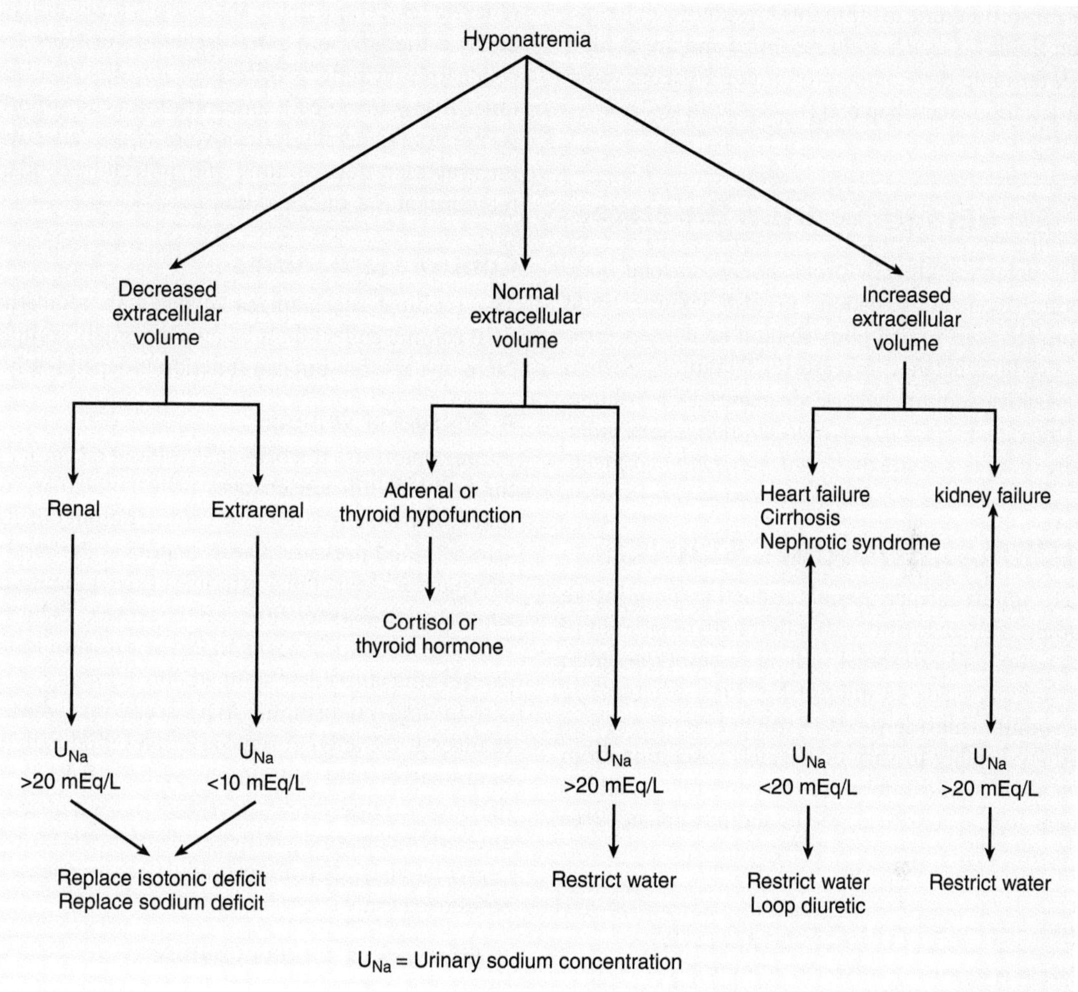

FIGURE 49–5 Algorithm for the treatment of hyponatremia.

be indicated in markedly symptomatic patients with plasma [Na^+] less than 110 mEq/L. Three percent NaCl should be administered with caution because it can precipitate pulmonary edema, hypokalemia, hyperchloremic metabolic acidosis, and transient hypotension; bleeding associated with prolongation of the prothrombin time and activated partial thromboplastin time has been reported.

Anesthetic Considerations

Hyponatremia is the most common electrolyte disorder, and SIADH is its most common cause. Hyponatremia, in association with its underlying disorder(s), increases perioperative morbidity and mortality as well as hospital length of stay and costs. A plasma sodium concentration greater than 130 mEq/L is usually considered safe for patients undergoing general anesthesia. In most circumstances, plasma [Na^+] should be corrected to greater than 130 mEq/L for elective procedures, even in the absence of neurological symptoms. Lower concentrations may result in significant cerebral edema that can be manifested intraoperatively as a decrease in minimum alveolar concentration or postoperatively as agitation, confusion, or somnolence. Patients undergoing transurethral resection of the prostate can absorb significant amounts of water from irrigation fluids (as much as 20 mL/min) and are at high risk for rapid development of profound acute water intoxication (see Chapter 32).

Disorders of Sodium Balance

ECF volume is directly proportionate to total body sodium content. Variations in ECF volume result from changes in total body sodium content. A positive sodium balance increases ECF volume, whereas a negative sodium balance decreases ECF volume. *Extracellular (plasma)* Na^+ *concentration is more indicative of water balance than total body sodium content.*

NORMAL SODIUM BALANCE

Net sodium balance is equal to total sodium intake (adults average 170 mEq/d) minus both renal sodium excretion and extrarenal sodium losses. (One gram of sodium yields 43 mEq of Na^+ ions, whereas 1 g of sodium chloride yields 17 mEq of Na^+ ions.) The kidneys' ability to vary urinary Na^+ excretion from less than 1 mEq/L to more than 100 mEq/L allows them to play a critical role in sodium balance (see Chapter 30).

REGULATION OF SODIUM BALANCE & EXTRACELLULAR FLUID VOLUME

Because of the relationship between ECF volume and total body sodium content, regulation of one is intimately tied to the other. This regulation is achieved via sensors that detect changes in the most important component of ECF, namely, the "effective" intravascular volume. The latter correlates more closely with the rate of perfusion in renal capillaries than with measurable intravascular fluid (plasma) volume. Indeed, with edematous disorders (heart failure, cirrhosis, and kidney failure), "effective" intravascular volume can be independent of the measurable plasma volume, ECF volume, or cardiac output.

ECF volume and total body sodium content are ultimately controlled by appropriate adjustments in renal Na^+ excretion. In the absence of kidney disease, diuretic therapy, and renal ischemia, urinary Na^+ concentration reflects "effective" intravascular volume. A low urine Na^+ concentration (<10 mEq/L) is therefore generally indicative of a low "effective" intravascular fluid volume and reflects secondary retention of Na^+ by the kidneys.

Control Mechanisms

The multiple mechanisms involved in regulating ECF volume and sodium balance normally complement one another but can function independently.

A. Sensors of Volume

Baroreceptors are the principal volume receptors in the body. Significant changes in intravascular volume (preload) affect not only cardiac output but also arterial blood pressure. Baroreceptors at the carotid sinus and afferent renal arterioles (juxtaglomerular apparatus) indirectly function as sensors of intravascular volume. Changes in blood pressure at the carotid sinus modulate sympathetic nervous system activity and nonosmotic ADH secretion, whereas changes at the afferent renal arterioles modulate the renin–angiotensin–aldosterone system (RAAS). As previously noted, stretch receptors in both atria are affected by changes in intravascular volume, and the degree of atrial distention modulates the release of atrial natriuretic hormone and ADH.

B. Effectors of Volume Change

Regardless of the mechanism, effectors of volume change ultimately alter urinary Na^+ excretion. *Decreases in "effective" intravascular volume decrease urinary* Na^+ *excretion, whereas increases in the "effective" intravascular volume increase urinary* Na^+ *excretion.* These mechanisms include the following:

1. **Renin–angiotensin–aldosterone**—Renin secretion increases the formation of angiotensin II. The latter increases the secretion of aldosterone and has a direct effect on enhancing Na^+ reabsorption in the proximal renal tubules. Angiotensin II is also a potent direct vasoconstrictor, and it potentiates the actions of norepinephrine. Secretion of aldosterone enhances Na^+ reabsorption in the distal nephron (see Chapter 30) and is a major determinant of urinary Na^+ excretion.

2. **Atrial natriuretic peptide (ANP)**—This peptide is normally released from both right and left atrial cells in response to atrial distention. ANP appears to have two major actions: arterial vasodilation and increased urinary sodium and water excretion in the renal collecting tubules. Na^+-mediated afferent arteriolar dilation and efferent arteriolar constriction can also increase glomerular filtration rate (GFR). Other effects include the inhibition of both renin and aldosterone secretion and antagonism of ADH.
3. **Brain natriuretic peptide (BNP)**—ANP, BNP, and C-type natriuretic peptide are structurally related peptides. BNP is released by the cardiac ventricles in response to increased ventricular volume and pressure, including ventricular overdistention, and also by the brain in response to increased blood pressure. BNP levels are usually approximately 20% of ANP levels, but in congestive heart failure, BNP levels may exceed those of ANP.
4. **Sympathetic nervous system activity**—Enhanced sympathetic activity increases Na^+ reabsorption in the proximal renal tubules, resulting in Na^+ retention, and increases renal vasoconstriction, which reduces renal blood flow (see Chapter 30). Conversely, stimulation of left atrial stretch receptors results in decreases in renal sympathetic tone and increases in renal blood flow (*cardiorenal reflex*) and glomerular filtration.
5. **Glomerular filtration rate and plasma sodium concentration**—The amount of Na^+ filtered in the kidneys is directly proportionate to the product of the GFR and plasma Na^+ concentration. Because GFR is usually proportionate to intravascular volume, intravascular volume expansion can increase Na^+ excretion. Conversely, intravascular volume depletion decreases Na^+ excretion. Similarly, even small elevations of blood pressure can result in a relatively large increase in urinary Na^+ excretion because of the resultant increase in renal blood flow and glomerular filtration rate. Blood pressure–induced diuresis (*pressure natriuresis*) appears to be independent of any known humorally or neurally mediated mechanism.
6. **Tubuloglomerular balance**—Despite wide variations in the amount of Na^+ filtered in nephrons, Na^+ reabsorption in the proximal renal tubules is normally controlled within narrow limits. Factors considered to be responsible for tubuloglomerular balance include the rate of renal tubular flow and changes in peritubular capillary hydrostatic and oncotic pressures.
7. **Antidiuretic hormone**—Although ADH secretion normally has little effect on Na^+ excretion, nonosmotic secretion of this hormone (see above) can play an important part in maintaining extracellular volume with moderate to severe decreases in the "effective" intravascular volume.

Extracellular Osmoregulation versus Volume Regulation

Osmoregulation protects the normal ratio of solutes to water, whereas extracellular volume regulation preserves absolute solute and water content (Table 49–8). As noted previously, *volume regulation generally takes precedence over osmoregulation.*

Anesthetic Implications

Problems related to altered sodium balance (*dysnatremia*) result from its direct manifestations as well as those of the underlying disorder(s). Although patients with disorders of sodium balance may be euvolemic, they usually present with either hypovolemia (sodium deficit) or hypervolemia (sodium excess); (see **Tables 49–4** and **49–6**). Both disturbances should be corrected before elective surgical procedures. Cardiac, liver, and kidney function should also be carefully evaluated in the presence of sodium excess (typically manifested as tissue edema).

Hypovolemic patients are sensitive to the vasodilating and negative inotropic effects of vapor anesthetics, propofol, and drug-induced histamine release. Dosage requirements for other drugs may be reduced to compensate for decreases in their volume of distribution. Hypovolemic patients are particularly sensitive to sympathetic blockade from spinal or epidural anesthesia. If general anesthesia must be administered before adequate correction

TABLE 49–8 Osmoregulation versus volume regulation.

	Volume Regulation	Osmoregulation
Purpose	Control extracellular volume	Control extracellular osmolality
Mechanism	Vary renal Na^+ excretion	Vary water intake Vary renal water excretion
Sensors	Afferent renal arterioles Carotid baroreceptors Atrial stretch receptors	Hypothalamic osmoreceptors
Effectors	Renin-angiotensin-aldosterone Sympathetic nervous system Tubuloglomerular balance Renal pressure natriuresis Atrial natriuretic peptide Antidiuretic hormone Brain natriuretic peptide	Thirst Antidiuretic hormone

Adapted with permission from Rose RD. *Clinical Physiology of Acid-Base and Electrolyte Disorders,* 3rd ed. New York, NY: McGraw Hill; 1989.

of hypovolemia, etomidate or ketamine may be the induction agent of choice.

Hypervolemia may be corrected preoperatively with diuretics. **A major hazard of increased extracellular volume is impaired gas exchange due to pulmonary interstitial edema, alveolar edema, or large collections of pleural or ascitic fluid.**

6

Disorders of Potassium Balance

Potassium plays a major role in regulating membrane potential as well as in carbohydrate and protein synthesis (see later discussion). Intracellular potassium concentration is estimated to be 140 mEq/L, whereas normal extracellular potassium concentration is approximately 4 mEq/L.

NORMAL POTASSIUM BALANCE

Dietary potassium intake averages 80 mEq/d in adults (range, 40–140 mEq/d). About 70 mEq of that amount is normally excreted in urine, whereas the remaining 10 mEq is lost through the gastrointestinal tract.

Renal excretion of potassium can vary from as little as 5 mEq/L to over 100 mEq/L. Nearly all the potassium filtered in glomeruli is normally reabsorbed in the proximal tubule and the loop of Henle. As a component of the RAAS, the aldosterone is secreted by the adrenal cortex in response to stimulation by angiotensin II. Acting on mineralocorticoid receptors in the distal tubules and collecting ducts of the kidney, aldosterone promotes sodium resorption directly coupled to potassium secretion. Aldosterone also directly influences potassium balance through its influence on kidney reabsorption/loss of sodium and the resultant regulatory influence on kidney water reabsorption/loss and blood volume and blood pressure (see earlier discussion and Chapter 30). *Mineralocorticoid receptor antagonists* (MRAs) block the sodium retention/potassium loss effects of aldosterone. The *potassium-sparing* diuretics spironolactone and eplerenone are MRAs that exemplify these effects by promoting sodium and water loss along with potassium retention. Amiloride and triamterene also antagonize the sodium retention/potassium loss effects of aldosterone but do so by blocking sodium channels in renal collecting tubule epithelial cells.

REGULATION OF EXTRACELLULAR POTASSIUM CONCENTRATION

Extracellular potassium concentration is determined by cell membrane Na^+–K^+-ATPase activity and plasma [K^+] and is influenced by the balance of total body potassium intake and excretion. Cell membrane Na^+–K^+-ATPase activity regulates the distribution of potassium between cells and ECF, whereas plasma [K^+], nephron Na^+ load, and aldosterone are the major determinants of urinary potassium excretion.

INTERCOMPARTMENTAL SHIFTS OF POTASSIUM

Intercompartmental shifts of potassium are known to occur following changes in extracellular pH (see Chapter 50), circulating insulin levels, circulating catecholamine activity, and plasma osmolality. Insulin and catecholamines directly affect Na^+–K^+-ATPase activity and decrease plasma [K^+]. Exercise may transiently increase plasma [K^+] as a result of the release of K^+ by muscle cells; the increase in plasma [K^+] (0.3–2 mEq/L) is proportionate to the intensity and duration of muscle activity. Intercompartmental potassium shifts are also likely to be responsible for changes in plasma [K^+] in syndromes of *periodic paralysis* (see Chapter 29).

Because the ICF may buffer up to 60% of an acid load (see Chapter 50), changes in extracellular hydrogen ion concentration (pH) directly affect extracellular [K^+]. In the setting of acidosis, extracellular hydrogen ions enter cells, displacing intracellular potassium ions; the resultant movement of potassium ions out of cells maintains electrical balance but increases extracellular and plasma [K^+]. Conversely, during alkalosis, extracellular potassium ions move into cells to balance the movement of hydrogen ions out of cells; as a result, plasma [K^+] decreases. Although the relationship is variable, a useful rule of thumb is that plasma potassium concentration changes approximately 0.6 mEq/L per 0.1-unit change in arterial pH (range 0.2–1.2 mEq/L per 0.1 unit).

Changes in circulating insulin levels can directly alter plasma [K^+] independent of that hormone's effect on glucose transport. Insulin enhances the activity of membrane-bound Na^+–K^+-ATPase, increasing cellular uptake of potassium in the liver and in skeletal muscle.

Sympathetic stimulation increases intracellular uptake of potassium by enhancing Na^+–K^+-ATPase activity through activation of β_2-adrenergic receptors. Plasma [K^+] often decreases following the administration of β_2-adrenergic agonists as a result of the uptake of potassium by muscle and the liver. In contrast, α-adrenergic activity may impair the intracellular movement of K^+.

Acute increases in plasma osmolality (hypernatremia, hyperglycemia, or mannitol administration) may increase plasma [K^+] (about 0.6 mEq/L per 10 mOsm/L). In such instances, the movement of water out of cells (down its osmotic gradient) is accompanied by the movement of K^+ out of cells.

Hypothermia has been reported to lower plasma [K^+] as a result of cellular uptake. Rewarming reverses this shift and may result in transient hyperkalemia if potassium was given during the hypothermia.

Urinary Excretion of Potassium

Urinary potassium excretion generally parallels its extracellular concentration (see preceding discussion). Extracellular [K^+] is a major determinant of aldosterone secretion from the adrenal gland: hyperkalemia stimulates aldosterone secretion, whereas hypokalemia suppresses aldosterone secretion. Renal tubular flow in the distal nephron may also be an important determinant of urinary potassium excretion because high tubular flow rates (as during osmotic diuresis) increase potassium secretion by keeping the capillary to renal tubular gradient for potassium secretion high. Conversely, slow tubular flow rates increase [K^+] in tubular fluid and decrease the gradient for K^+ secretion, thereby decreasing renal potassium excretion.

HYPOKALEMIA

Hypokalemia, defined as plasma [K^+] less than 3.5 mEq/L, can occur as a result of (1) an intercompartmental shift of K^+, (2) increased potassium loss, or (3) an inadequate potassium intake (Table 49–9). Plasma potassium concentration typically correlates poorly with the total potassium deficit. A decrease in plasma [K^+] from 4 mEq/L to 3 mEq/L usually represents a 100- to 200 mEq total body deficit, whereas plasma [K^+] below 3 mEq/L can represent a deficit of 200 mEq to 400 mEq.

TABLE 49–9 Major causes of hypokalemia.

Excess renal loss
Mineralocorticoid excess
Primary hyperaldosteronism (Conn syndrome)
Glucocorticoid-remediable hyperaldosteronism
Renin excess
Renovascular hypertension
Bartter syndrome
Liddle syndrome
Diuresis
Chronic metabolic alkalosis
Antibiotics
Carbenicillin
Gentamicin
Amphotericin B
Renal tubular acidosis
Distal, gradient-limited
Proximal
Ureterosigmoidostomy
Gastrointestinal losses
Vomiting
Diarrhea, particularly secretory diarrheas
ECF → ICF shifts
Acute alkalosis
Hypokalemic periodic paralysis
Barium ingestion
Insulin therapy
Vitamin B_{12} therapy
Thyrotoxicosis (rarely)
Inadequate intake

Hypokalemia due to the Intracellular Movement of Potassium

Hypokalemia due to the intracellular movement of potassium occurs with alkalosis, insulin administration, β_2-adrenergic agonists, and hypothermia and during attacks of hypokalemic periodic paralysis. Cellular K^+ uptake by red blood cells and platelets also accounts for the hypokalemia seen in patients recently treated with folate or vitamin B_{12} for megaloblastic anemia.

Hypokalemia due to Increased Potassium Losses

Excessive potassium loss is usually either renal or gastrointestinal. Renal wasting of potassium is most commonly the result of diuresis or enhanced mineralocorticoid activity. Other renal causes include hypomagnesemia, renal tubular acidosis (see Chapter 30), ketoacidosis, salt-wasting nephropathies, and some drug therapies (eg, amphotericin B). Increased gastrointestinal loss of potassium is most commonly due to nasogastric suctioning or persistent vomiting or diarrhea. Other gastrointestinal causes include losses from fistulae, laxative abuse, villous adenomas, and pancreatic tumors secreting vasoactive intestinal peptide.

Chronically increased sweat formation occasionally causes hypokalemia when potassium intake is limited. Dialysis with a low-potassium-containing dialysate solution can also cause hypokalemia. Uremic patients may actually have a total body potassium deficit (primarily intracellular) despite a normal or even high plasma concentration; the absence of hypokalemia in these instances is probably due to acidosis-induced intercompartmental shifts. Dialysis in these patients unmasks the total body potassium deficit and often results in hypokalemia.

Urinary [K^+] less than 20 mEq/L is generally indicative of increased extrarenal K^+ losses, whereas concentrations greater than 20 mEq/L suggest renal wasting of K^+.

Hypokalemia due to Decreased Potassium Intake

Because of the kidney's ability to decrease urinary potassium excretion to as little as 5 to 20 mEq/L, marked reductions in potassium intake are required to produce hypokalemia. Low potassium intake, however, often accentuates the effects of increased potassium loss.

Clinical Manifestations of Hypokalemia

Hypokalemia can produce widespread organ dysfunction (Table 49–10). Most patients are asymptomatic until plasma [K^+] falls below 3 mEq/L. Cardiovascular effects are most clinically significant and include an abnormal electrocardiogram (ECG; Figure 49–6), arrhythmias, decreased cardiac contractility, and labile arterial blood pressure due to autonomic dysfunction. *ECG manifestations are primarily due to delayed ventricular repolarization and include T-wave flattening and inversion, an increasingly prominent U wave, ST-segment depression, increased P-wave amplitude, and prolongation of the*

TABLE 49–10 Effects of hypokalemia.

Cardiovascular
Electrocardiographic changes/arrhythmias
Myocardial dysfunction
Neuromuscular
Skeletal muscle weakness
Tetany
Rhabdomyolysis
Ileus
Renal
Polyuria (nephrogenic diabetes insipidus)
Increased ammonia production
Increased bicarbonate reabsorption
Hormonal
Decreased insulin secretion
Decreased aldosterone secretion
Metabolic
Negative nitrogen balance
Encephalopathy in patients with liver disease

Adapted with permission from Schrier RW. *Renal and Electrolyte Disorders.* 3rd ed. Philadelphia, PA: Little, Brown and Company; 1986.

P–R interval. Increased myocardial cell automaticity and delayed repolarization promote both atrial and ventricular arrhythmias.

Neuromuscular effects of hypokalemia include skeletal muscle weakness, hyporeflexia, muscle cramping, ileus, and, rarely, flaccid paralysis or rhabdomyolysis. Hypokalemia induced by diuretics is often associated with metabolic alkalosis; as the kidneys absorb sodium to compensate for intravascular volume depletion, and in the presence of diuretic-induced hypochloremia, bicarbonate is absorbed, and potassium is excreted. The end result is hypokalemia and hypochloremic metabolic alkalosis. Kidney dysfunction is seen due to impaired concentrating ability (resistance to ADH, resulting in polyuria) and increased production of ammonia, resulting in impairment of urinary acidification. Increased ammonia production represents intracellular acidosis; hydrogen ions move intracellularly to compensate for intracellular potassium losses. The resulting metabolic alkalosis, together with increased ammonia production, can precipitate encephalopathy in patients with advanced liver disease.

Treatment of Hypokalemia

The treatment of hypokalemia depends on the presence and severity of any associated organ dysfunction. Significant ECG changes such as ST-segment changes or arrhythmias mandate continuous ECG monitoring, particularly during intravenous K^+ replacement. Digoxin sensitizes the heart to changes in potassium ion concentration.

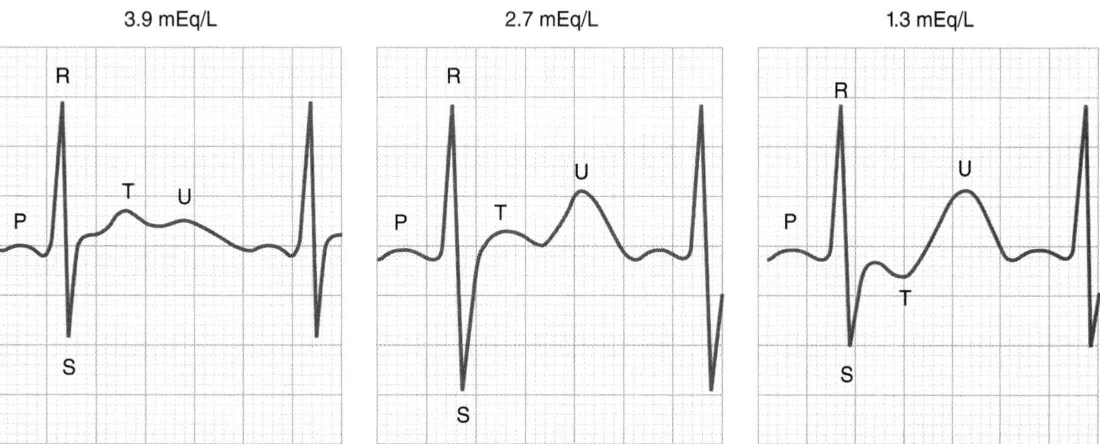

FIGURE 49–6 Electrocardiographic effects of acute hypokalemia. Note the progressive flattening of the T wave, an increasingly prominent U wave, increased amplitude of the P wave, prolongation of the P–R interval, and ST-segment depression.

In most circumstances, the safest method by which to correct a potassium deficit is oral replacement over several days (60–80 mEq/d). **Intravenous replacement of potassium chloride is usually reserved for patients with, or at risk for, significant cardiac manifestations or severe muscle weakness. The goal of intravenous therapy is to remove the patient from immediate danger, not to correct the entire potassium deficit.** Because of potassium's irritative effect on peripheral veins, peripheral intravenous replacement should not exceed 8 mEq/h. More rapid intravenous potassium replacement (10–20 mEq/h) requires central venous administration and close ECG monitoring. Intravenous replacement should generally not exceed 240 mEq/d. Dextrose-containing solutions should be avoided in cases of hypokalemia because the resulting hyperglycemia and secondary insulin secretion may worsen the low plasma [K^+].

7

Potassium chloride is the preferred potassium salt when a metabolic alkalosis is also present because it also corrects the chloride deficit discussed earlier. Potassium bicarbonate or equivalent (K^+ acetate or K^+ citrate) may be used in patients with metabolic acidosis. Potassium phosphate is a suitable alternative with concomitant hypophosphatemia (eg, diabetic ketoacidosis).

Anesthetic Considerations

Hypokalemia is a common preoperative finding. The decision to proceed with elective surgery is often based on plasma [K^+] no lower than 3 mEq/L. The decision, however, should also be based on the rate at which the hypokalemia developed as well as the presence or absence of secondary organ dysfunction. In general, chronic mild hypokalemia (3–3.5 mEq/L) without ECG changes does not increase anesthetic risk. *The exception is the rare patient receiving digoxin who risks developing digoxin toxicity from the hypokalemia; plasma [K+] values above 4 mEq/L are desirable in such patients.*

The intraoperative management of hypokalemia requires vigilant ECG monitoring. Intravenous potassium should be given if atrial or ventricular arrhythmias develop. Glucose-free intravenous solutions should be used and hyperventilation avoided to prevent further decreases in plasma [K^+]. Increased sensitivity to neuromuscular blockers (NMBs) may occur.

HYPERKALEMIA

Hyperkalemia exists when plasma [K^+] exceeds 5.5 mEq/L, and it rarely occurs in normal individuals because of the kidney's capability to excrete large potassium loads. When potassium intake is increased slowly, the kidneys can excrete as much as 500 mEq of K^+ per day. The sympathetic nervous system and insulin secretion also play important roles in preventing acute increases in plasma [K^+] following acquired potassium loads.

Hyperkalemia can result from (1) an intercompartmental shift of potassium ions, (2) decreased urinary excretion of potassium, or, rarely, (3) an increased potassium intake or increased release from a formerly ischemic organ (Table 49–11).

TABLE 49–11 Causes of hyperkalemia.

Pseudohyperkalemia
Red cell hemolysis
Marked leukocytosis/thrombocytosis
Intercompartmental shifts
Acidosis
Hypertonicity
Rhabdomyolysis
Excessive exercise
Periodic paralysis
Succinylcholine
Decreased renal potassium excretion
Kidney failure
Decreased mineralocorticoid activity and impaired Na^+ reabsorption
Acquired immunodeficiency syndrome
Potassium-sparing diuretics
Spironolactone
Eplerenone
Amiloride
Triamterene
ACE[1] inhibitors
Nonsteroidal anti-inflammatory drugs
Pentamidine
Trimethoprim
Enhanced Cl^- reabsorption
Gordon syndrome
Cyclosporine
Increased potassium intake
Salt substitutes

[1]ACE, angiotensin-converting enzyme.

Measurements of plasma potassium concentration can be spuriously elevated if red cells hemolyze in a blood specimen. In vitro release of potassium from blood specimen leukocytes can also falsely indicate increased levels in the measured plasma [K^+] when the leukocyte count exceeds 70,000 × 10^9/L. A similar release of potassium from platelets may occur when the platelet count exceeds 1,000,000 × 10^9/L.

Hyperkalemia due to Extracellular Movement of Potassium

Movement of K^+ out of cells can be seen with acidosis, cell lysis following chemotherapy, hemolysis, rhabdomyolysis, massive tissue trauma, hyperosmolality, digitalis overdosage, hyperkalemic periodic paralysis, and with administration of succinylcholine, β_2-adrenergic blockers, and arginine hydrochloride. The average increase in plasma [K^+] of 0.5 mEq/L following succinylcholine administration can be exaggerated in patients with large burns, severe muscle trauma, or muscle denervation. Succinylcholine should be avoided in these settings.

Hyperkalemia due to Decreased Renal Excretion of Potassium

Decreased renal excretion of potassium can result from (1) marked reductions in glomerular filtration, (2) decreased aldosterone activity, or (3) a defect in potassium secretion in the distal nephron.

Glomerular filtration rates less than 5 mL/min are nearly always associated with hyperkalemia. Patients with lesser degrees of kidney impairment can also readily develop hyperkalemia when faced with increased potassium loads (dietary, catabolic, or iatrogenic). Uremia may also impair Na^+–K^+-ATPase activity.

Hyperkalemia due to decreased aldosterone activity can result from a primary defect in adrenal hormone synthesis or a defect in the RAAS. Patients with primary adrenal insufficiency (Addison disease) and those with isolated 21-hydroxylase adrenal enzyme deficiency have marked impairment of aldosterone synthesis. Patients with the syndrome of isolated hypoaldosteronism (also called *hyporeninemic hypoaldosteronism* or type IV renal tubular acidosis) are usually patients with diabetes with kidney impairment; they have an impaired ability to increase aldosterone secretion in response to hyperkalemia. These patients develop hyperkalemia when they increase their potassium intake or when given potassium-sparing diuretics. They also often have varying degrees of Na^+ wasting and hyperchloremic metabolic acidosis.

Drugs interfering with the RAAS have the potential to cause hyperkalemia, particularly in the presence of kidney disease. Nonsteroidal anti-inflammatory drugs (NSAIDs) inhibit prostaglandin-mediated renin release. Angiotensin-converting enzyme (ACE) inhibitors and angiotensin receptor blockers (ARBs) interfere with angiotensin II–mediated release of aldosterone. Heparin used in thromboprophylaxis regimens may cause hyperkalemia (*heparin-induced hyperkalemia* [HIH]) by interfering with aldosterone secretion and antagonizing the activity of angiotensin II receptors. Potassium-sparing diuretics antagonize aldosterone activity in the kidney, impairing potassium excretion (see earlier discussion).

Decreased renal excretion of potassium may also occur as a result of an intrinsic or acquired defect in the distal nephron's ability to secrete potassium. Such defects may occur even in the presence of normal kidney function and are characteristically unresponsive to mineralocorticoid therapy. The kidneys of patients with *pseudohypoaldosteronism* display intrinsic resistance to aldosterone. Acquired defects have been associated with systemic lupus erythematosus, sickle cell anemia, obstructive uropathies, and cyclosporine nephropathy in transplanted kidneys.

Hyperkalemia due to Increased Potassium Intake

Increased potassium loads rarely cause hyperkalemia in normal individuals unless large amounts are given rapidly and intravenously. Hyperkalemia, however, may be seen when potassium intake is increased in patients receiving β-blockers or in patients with impaired kidney function. Unrecognized sources of potassium include potassium penicillin, sodium substitutes (primarily potassium salts), and transfusion of stored whole blood. The plasma [K^+] in a unit of whole blood can increase to 30 mEq/L after 21 days of storage. The risk of hyperkalemia from multiple transfusions (*transfusion-associated hyperkalemia*) is reduced, though not eliminated, by minimizing the volume of plasma given through the use of packed red blood cell transfusions or by using washed red blood cells (see Chapter 51).

Clinical Manifestations of Hyperkalemia

The most important effects of hyperkalemia are on skeletal and cardiac muscle. Skeletal muscle weakness is generally not seen until plasma [K^+] is greater than 8 mEq/L. Cardiac manifestations (Figure 49–7) are primarily due to delayed depolarization and are consistently present when plasma [K^+] is greater than 7 mEq/L. ECG changes characteristically progress sequentially from symmetrically peaked T waves (often with a shortened QT interval) → widening of the QRS complex → prolongation of the P–R interval → loss of the P wave → loss of R-wave amplitude → ST-segment depression (occasionally elevation) → an ECG that resembles a sine wave, before progressing to ventricular fibrillation and asystole. Contractility may be relatively well preserved until late in the course of progressive hyperkalemia. Hypocalcemia, hyponatremia, and acidosis accentuate the cardiac effects of hyperkalemia.

Treatment of Hyperkalemia

Because of its lethal potential, hyperkalemia exceeding 6 mEq/L should always be corrected. Treatment is directed to reversal of cardiac manifestations and skeletal muscle weakness and to the restoration of normal plasma [K^+]. The therapeutic modalities employed depend on the cause of hyperkalemia and the severity of manifestations. Hyperkalemia associated with hypoaldosteronism can be treated with mineralocorticoid replacement. Drugs contributing to hyperkalemia should be discontinued, and sources of increased potassium intake should be reduced or stopped.

Calcium salts (5–10 mL of 10% calcium gluconate or 3–5 mL of 10% calcium chloride) partially antagonize the cardiac effects of hyperkalemia and are useful in symptomatic patients with marked hyperkalemia. Calcium salt effects are rapid but short lived. Care must be exercised in administering calcium salts to patients taking digoxin because calcium potentiates digoxin toxicity.

An intravenous infusion of glucose and insulin (30–50 g of glucose with 10 units of insulin) promotes cellular uptake of potassium and lowers plasma [K^+], but it may take up to 1 hour for peak effect. When metabolic acidosis is present, intravenous sodium bicarbonate promotes cellular uptake of potassium and decreases plasma [K^+] within

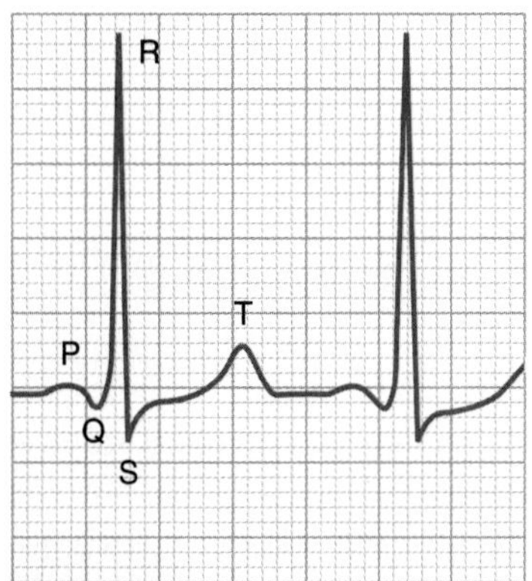

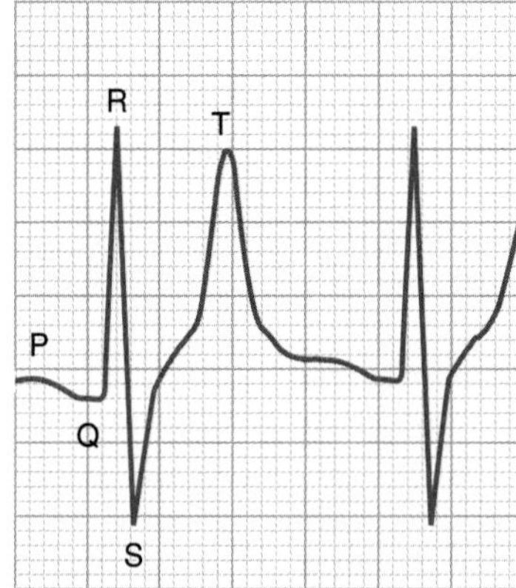

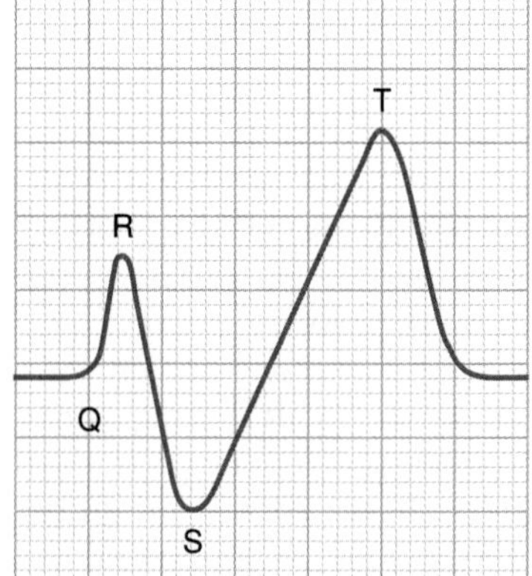

FIGURE 49–7 Electrocardiographic effects of hyperkalemia. Electrocardiographic changes characteristically progress from symmetrically peaked T waves, often with a shortened QT interval, to widening of the QRS complex, prolongation of the P–R interval, loss of the P wave, loss of R-wave amplitude, and ST-segment depression (occasionally elevation)—to an ECG that resembles a sine wave—before final progression into ventricular fibrillation or asystole.

15 minutes. β-Agonists promote cellular uptake of potassium and may be useful in acute hyperkalemia associated with massive transfusions; low-dose epinephrine infusion often rapidly decreases plasma [K^+] and provides inotropic support in this setting.

The ultimate goal of urgent or emergency treatment of hyperkalemia is the reduction of total body potassium. Forced diuresis with a loop diuretic is an effective treatment of acute hyperkalemia in patients with adequate kidney function, and dialysis is the definitive urgent or emergency therapeutic modality for patients with impaired kidney function. Elimination of excess potassium can also be accomplished with oral or rectal administration of the nonabsorbable cation-exchange resin, sodium polystyrene sulfonate (SPS, Kayexalate). However, the safety and efficacy of SPS have been repeatedly questioned, and a U.S. Food and Drug Administration (FDA) black box warning cautions its use in patients with abnormal bowel function because of the risk of intestinal necrosis in such circumstances. SPS should not be utilized to treat urgent or emergency hyperkalemia because the onset of its effect takes several hours.

Patiromer, a nonabsorbed cation exchange polymer that binds potassium in exchange for calcium in the gastrointestinal tract, is approved by the FDA as an effective treatment for chronic hyperkalemia. Like SPS, it should not be used to treat urgent or emergency hyperkalemia because of its delayed onset of action.

Anesthetic Considerations

Elective surgery should not be undertaken in patients with significant hyperkalemia. Anesthetic management of hyperkalemic perioperative patients is directed at both lowering the plasma potassium concentration and preventing any further increases, with the treatment approach dependent upon situational acuity. The ECG should be carefully monitored. Succinylcholine is contraindicated, as is the use of potassium-containing intravenous solutions. The avoidance of metabolic or respiratory acidosis is critical to prevent further increases in plasma [K^+]. Ventilation should be controlled under general anesthesia, and mild hyperventilation may be desirable. Lastly, neuromuscular function should be monitored closely as hyperkalemia can accentuate the effects of NMBs.

Disorders of Calcium Balance

Although 98% of total body calcium is in bone, maintenance of a normal extracellular calcium concentration is critical to homeostasis. Calcium ions are involved in nearly all essential biological functions, including muscle contraction, the release of neurotransmitters and hormones, blood coagulation, and bone metabolism, and abnormalities in calcium balance can result in profound physiological derangements.

NORMAL CALCIUM BALANCE

Calcium intake in adults averages 600 to 800 mg/d, and calcium absorption occurs primarily in the proximal small bowel. Calcium is also secreted into the intestinal tract, a phenomenon that appears to be constant and independent of absorption. Up to 80% of the daily calcium intake is normally lost in feces.

The kidneys are responsible for most calcium excretion. Renal calcium excretion averages 100 mg/d but may vary from as low as 50 mg/d to more than 300 mg/d. Normally, 98% of the filterable calcium is reabsorbed. Calcium reabsorption parallels that of sodium in the proximal renal tubules and the ascending loop of Henle. In the distal tubules, however, calcium reabsorption is dependent on parathyroid hormone (PTH) secretion, whereas sodium reabsorption is dependent on aldosterone secretion. Increased PTH levels enhance distal calcium reabsorption and thereby decrease urinary calcium excretion.

Plasma Calcium Concentration

The normal plasma calcium concentration is 8.5 to 10.5 mg/dL (2.1–2.6 mmol/L). Approximately 50% is in the free, ionized form, 40% is protein bound (mainly to albumin), and 10% is complexed with anions such as citrate and amino acids. The free, ionized calcium concentration ([Ca^{2+}]) is physiologically most important. Plasma [Ca^{2+}] is normally 4.75 to 5.3 mg/dL (1.19–1.33 mmol/L). Changes in plasma albumin concentration affect the total, but not ionized, calcium concentration: For each increase or decrease of 1 g/dL in albumin, the total plasma calcium concentration increases or decreases approximately 0.8 to 1.0 mg/dL, respectively.

Changes in plasma pH directly affect the degree of protein binding and thus ionized calcium concentration. Ionized calcium increases approximately 0.16 mg/dL for each decrease of 0.1 unit in plasma pH and decreases by the same amount for each 0.1 unit increase in pH.

Regulation of Extracellular Ionized Calcium Concentration

Calcium normally enters ECF by either absorption from the intestinal tract or resorption of bone; only 0.5% to 1% of calcium in bone is exchangeable with ECF. In contrast, calcium normally leaves the extracellular compartment by (1) deposition into bone, (2) urinary excretion, (3) secretion into the intestinal tract, and (4) sweat formation. Extracellular [Ca^{2+}] is closely regulated by three hormones—PTH, vitamin D, and calcitonin—that act primarily on bone, the distal renal tubules, and the small bowel. Hormonal control of calcium by the PTH–vitamin D axis is described in Chapter 35.

HYPERCALCEMIA

Hypercalcemia can occur as a result of a variety of disorders (Table 49–12). In *primary hyperparathyroidism*, secretion of PTH is inappropriately increased in relation to [Ca^{2+}]. In contrast, in *secondary hyperparathyroidism* (eg, chronic kidney failure or malabsorption syndromes), PTH levels are elevated in response to chronic hypocalcemia. Prolonged secondary hyperparathyroidism, however, can occasionally result in the autonomous secretion of PTH, resulting in a normal or elevated [Ca^{2+}] (*tertiary hyperparathyroidism*).

TABLE 49–12 Causes of hypercalcemia.

Hyperparathyroidism
Malignancy
Excessive vitamin D intake
Paget disease of bone
Granulomatous disorders (sarcoidosis, tuberculosis)
Chronic immobilization
Milk-alkali syndrome
Adrenal insufficiency
Drug-induced
Thiazide diuretics
Lithium

Patients with cancer can present with hypercalcemia whether or not bone metastases are present. This is most often due to direct bony destruction, secretion of humoral mediators of hypercalcemia (PTH-like substances, cytokines, prostaglandins), or both. Hypercalcemia due to increased turnover of calcium from bone can also be encountered in patients with benign conditions such as Paget disease and chronic immobilization. Increased gastrointestinal absorption of calcium can lead to hypercalcemia in patients with *milk-alkali syndrome* (marked increase in calcium intake), excessive vitamin D intake, or granulomatous disease (enhanced sensitivity to vitamin D).

Clinical Manifestations of Hypercalcemia

Hypercalcemia often produces anorexia, nausea, vomiting, weakness, and polyuria. Ataxia, irritability, lethargy, or confusion can rapidly progress to coma. Hypertension is often present initially before hypovolemia supervenes. ECG signs include a shortened ST segment and shortened QT interval. Hypercalcemia increases cardiac sensitivity to digitalis. Hypercalcemia may promote pancreatitis, peptic ulcer disease, and kidney failure.

Treatment of Hypercalcemia

9 **Symptomatic hypercalcemia requires rapid treatment. The most effective initial treatment is rehydration followed by brisk diuresis (urinary output 200–300 mL/h) using an intravenous saline infusion and a loop diuretic to accelerate calcium excretion.** Premature diuretic therapy before rehydration may aggravate hypercalcemia by exacerbating volume depletion. Renal loss of potassium and magnesium usually occurs during diuresis, mandating

close laboratory monitoring and intravenous replacement as necessary. Although hydration and diuresis may remove the potential risk of cardiovascular and neurological complications of hypercalcemia, the serum calcium level usually remains elevated above normal. Additional therapy with a bisphosphonate or calcitonin may be required to further lower the serum calcium level. Severe hypercalcemia (>15 mg/dL) usually requires additional therapy after saline hydration and furosemide. Bisphosphonates or calcitonin are the preferred agents. Intravenous administration of pamidronate (Aredia) or etidronate (Didronel) is often used in this setting. Hemodialysis is very effective in correcting severe hypercalcemia and may be necessary in the presence of kidney or heart failure. Additional treatment depends on the underlying cause of the hypercalcemia and may include glucocorticoids in the setting of vitamin D–induced hypercalcemia, such as granulomatous disease states.

It is necessary to look for the underlying etiology and direct appropriate treatment toward the cause of the hypercalcemia once any critical hypercalcemia threat has been addressed. *Approximately 90% of all hypercalcemia is due to either malignancy or hyperparathyroidism. The best laboratory test for discriminating between these two main categories of hypercalcemia is the PTH assay.* The serum PTH concentration is usually suppressed in malignancy states and elevated in hyperparathyroidism.

Anesthetic Considerations

Significant hypercalcemia is a medical emergency and should be corrected before any elective anesthetic is administered. Ionized calcium levels should be monitored closely. If surgery must be performed, saline diuresis should be continued intraoperatively with care to avoid hypovolemia; appropriate goal-directed hemodynamic and fluid management therapy (see Chapter 51) should be used, especially for patients with cardiac or kidney impairment. Serial measurements of $[K^+]$ and $[Mg^{2+}]$ are obtained in anticipation of diuresis-related hypokalemia and hypomagnesemia. Responses to anesthetic agents and NMBs are not predictable. Ventilation should be controlled under general anesthesia. Acidosis should be avoided so as to not worsen the elevated plasma $[Ca^{2+}]$.

HYPOCALCEMIA

Hypocalcemia should be diagnosed only on the basis of the plasma ionized calcium concentration. When direct measurements of plasma $[Ca^{2+}]$ are not available, the total calcium concentration must be corrected for decreases in plasma albumin concentration (see earlier discussion). Causes of hypocalcemia are listed in Table 49–13.

Hypocalcemia due to hypoparathyroidism is a relatively common cause of symptomatic hypocalcemia. Hypoparathyroidism may be surgical (see Chapter 37), idiopathic, part of multiple endocrine defects (most often with adrenal insufficiency), or associated with hypomagnesemia. Magnesium deficiency may impair the secretion of PTH and antagonize the effects of PTH on bone. Sepsis is often accompanied by suppressed PTH release, resulting in hypocalcemia. Hyperphosphatemia (see later discussion) is also a relatively common cause of hypocalcemia, particularly in patients with chronic kidney failure. Hypocalcemia due to vitamin D deficiency may be the result of a markedly reduced intake (nutritional), vitamin D malabsorption, or abnormal vitamin D metabolism.

Chelation of calcium ions with the citrate ions in blood preservatives is an important cause of perioperative hypocalcemia in transfused patients;

TABLE 49–13 Causes of hypocalcemia.

Hypoparathyroidism
Pseudohypoparathyroidism
Vitamin D deficiency
Nutritional
Malabsorption
Postsurgical (gastrectomy, short bowel)
Inflammatory bowel disease
Altered vitamin D metabolism
Hyperphosphatemia
Precipitation of calcium
Pancreatitis
Rhabdomyolysis
Fat embolism
Chelation of calcium
Multiple rapid red blood transfusions or rapid infusion of large amounts of albumin

similar transient decreases in [Ca^{2+}] are also possible following rapid infusions of large volumes of albumin. Hypocalcemia following acute pancreatitis is thought to be due to the precipitation of calcium with fats (soaps) following the release of lipolytic enzymes and fat necrosis; hypocalcemia following fat embolism may have a similar basis. Hypocalcemia following rhabdomyolysis results from the precipitation of calcium in injured muscle tissue or from the forced diuresis used to preempt acute kidney injury in this condition, or both.

Tumor lysis syndrome, another cause of hypocalcemia, is the result of rapid destruction of malignant cells from chemotherapy or radiation therapy and may have an incidence as high as 25% in the treatment of some cancers. It is the most common oncologic emergency and is the result of the rapid shift of potassium, phosphorus, and nucleic acid material into the extracellular space, overwhelming normal homeostatic mechanisms that would otherwise compensate. Acute kidney injury or failure secondary to acute uric acid nephropathy due to the metabolism of released nucleic acids degrades or abolishes the kidney's ability to excrete potassium and phosphate. Hyperphosphatemia promotes phosphate chelation with calcium, resulting in acute hypocalcemia. It also results in renal calcium–phosphate salt deposition, further promoting acute kidney injury or failure. The acute hypocalcemia and hyperkalemia of tumor lysis syndrome may result in muscle weakness, tetany, cardiac arrhythmia, seizures, and death.

Less common causes of hypocalcemia include calcitonin-secreting medullary carcinomas of the thyroid, osteoblastic metastatic disease (breast and prostate cancer), and *pseudohypoparathyroidism* (familial unresponsiveness to PTH). Transient hypocalcemia may be seen after heparin, protamine, or glucagon administration.

Clinical Manifestations of Hypocalcemia

Manifestations of hypocalcemia include paresthesia, confusion, laryngeal stridor (laryngospasm), carpopedal spasm (Trousseau sign), masseter spasm (Chvostek sign), and seizures. Biliary colic and bronchospasm have also been described. ECG may reveal cardiac irritability or QT interval prolongation, which may not correlate in severity with the degree of hypocalcemia. Decreased cardiac contractility may result in heart failure, hypotension, or both. Decreased responsiveness to digoxin and β-adrenergic agonists may also occur.

Treatment of Hypocalcemia

10 **Symptomatic hypocalcemia is a medical emergency and should be treated immediately with intravenous calcium chloride (3–5 mL of a 10% solution) or calcium gluconate (10–20 mL of a 10% solution).** Ten mL of 10% $CaCl_2$ contains 272 mg of Ca^{2+}, whereas 10 mL of 10% calcium gluconate contains 93 mg of Ca^{2+}. Intravenous calcium should not be given with bicarbonate- or phosphate-containing solutions to avoid precipitation. Serial ionized calcium monitoring is mandatory. Repeat intravenous boluses or a continuous infusion (Ca^{2+} 1–2 mg/kg/h) may be necessary. Plasma magnesium concentration should be checked to exclude hypomagnesemia. In chronic hypocalcemia, oral calcium ($CaCO_3$) and vitamin D replacement are usually adequate.

Anesthetic Considerations

Significant hypocalcemia should be corrected preoperatively. Serial ionized calcium levels should be monitored intraoperatively in patients with a history of hypocalcemia. Alkalosis should be avoided to prevent further decreases in [Ca^{2+}]. Intravenous calcium may be necessary following rapid transfusions of citrated blood products or large volumes of albumin solutions (see Chapter 51). Potentiation of the negative inotropic effects of anesthetics should be expected. Responses to NMBs are inconsistent and require nerve stimulator monitoring.

Disorders of Phosphorus Balance

Phosphorus is an important intracellular constituent. Its presence is required for the synthesis of phospholipids and phosphoproteins in cell membranes and intracellular organelles, phosphonucleotides involved in protein synthesis and reproduction, and ATP used for the storage of energy. Only 0.1% of total body phosphorus is in ECF, with 85% in bone and 15% in intracellular fluid.

NORMAL PHOSPHORUS BALANCE

Phosphorus intake averages 800 to 1500 mg/d in adults, and 80% of that amount is normally absorbed in the proximal small bowel. Vitamin D increases the intestinal absorption of phosphorus. The kidneys are the major route for phosphorus excretion and are responsible for regulating total body phosphorus content. Urinary excretion of phosphorus depends on both intake and plasma concentration. Secretion of PTH promotes urinary phosphorus excretion by inhibiting proximal tubular reabsorption. The latter effect may be offset by the PTH-induced release of phosphate from bone.

Plasma Phosphorus Concentration

Plasma phosphorus exists in both organic and inorganic forms. Organic phosphorus is mainly in the form of phospholipids. Of the inorganic phosphorus fraction, 80% is filterable in the kidneys, and 20% is protein bound. Most inorganic phosphorus is in the form of $H_2PO_4^-$ and HPO_4^{2-} in a 1:4 ratio. By convention, plasma phosphorus is measured as milligrams of elemental phosphorus. Normal plasma phosphorus concentration is 2.5 to 4.5 mg/dL (0.8–1.45 mmol/L) in adults and up to 6 mg/dL in children. Plasma phosphorus concentration is usually measured during fasting because recent carbohydrate intake transiently decreases plasma phosphorus concentration. Hypophosphatemia increases vitamin D production, whereas hyperphosphatemia depresses it. The latter plays an important role in the genesis of secondary hyperparathyroidism in patients with chronic kidney disease (see Chapter 31).

HYPERPHOSPHATEMIA

Hyperphosphatemia may be seen with increased phosphorus intake (abuse of phosphate laxatives or excessive potassium phosphate administration), decreased phosphorus excretion (chronic kidney disease), or tumor lysis syndrome (see earlier discussion).

Clinical Manifestations of Hyperphosphatemia

Although hyperphosphatemia per se does not appear to be directly responsible for any functional disturbances, significant hyperphosphatemia may produce hypocalcemia via phosphate chelation with plasma [Ca^{2+}] and may also produce acute kidney injury via parenchymal and tubular deposits of calcium phosphate salts. Hyperphosphatemia is associated with increased mortality in patients with chronic kidney disease and kidney failure, and it is managed in this patient population by dietary restriction, use of phosphate binders, dialysis, or a combination of these methods.

Treatment of Hyperphosphatemia

Hyperphosphatemia is generally treated with phosphate-binding antacids such as aluminum hydroxide or aluminum carbonate.

Anesthetic Considerations

Although specific interactions between hyperphosphatemia and anesthesia have not been described, kidney function should be assessed, and hypocalcemia should be excluded.

HYPOPHOSPHATEMIA

Hypophosphatemia is usually the result of either a negative phosphorus balance or cellular uptake of extracellular phosphorus (an intercompartmental shift). Intercompartmental shifts of phosphorus can occur during alkalosis and following carbohydrate ingestion or insulin administration. Large doses of aluminum- or magnesium-containing antacids, severe burns, insufficient phosphorus supplementation during total parenteral nutrition, diabetic ketoacidosis, alcohol withdrawal, and prolonged respiratory alkalosis can each produce negative phosphorus balance and lead to severe hypophosphatemia (<0.3 mmol/dL or <1.0 mg/dL). In contrast to respiratory alkalosis, metabolic alkalosis rarely leads to severe hypophosphatemia.

Clinical Manifestations of Hypophosphatemia

Mild to moderate hypophosphatemia (1.5–2.5 mg/dL) is generally asymptomatic. In contrast, severe hypophosphatemia (<1.0 mg/dL) is associated with increased morbidity and mortality in critically ill patients. Cardiomyopathy, impaired oxygen delivery (decreased 2,3-diphosphoglycerate levels), hemolysis, impaired leukocyte function, platelet dysfunction, encephalopathy, arrhythmia, skeletal myopathy, respiratory failure, rhabdomyolysis, skeletal demineralization, metabolic acidosis, and hepatic dysfunction have all been associated with severe hypophosphatemia. However, at this time, it is uncertain whether hypophosphatemia is a direct and independent contributor to these major morbidities or to mortality or if it is merely a marker of illness severity.

Treatment of Hypophosphatemia

Oral phosphorus replacement is generally preferable to parenteral replacement because of the increased risk of phosphate precipitation with calcium, resulting in hypocalcemia, and also because of the increased risks of hyperphosphatemia, hypomagnesemia, and hypotension. Accordingly, intravenous replacement therapy is usually reserved for instances of symptomatic hypophosphatemia and extremely low phosphate levels (<0.32 mmol/L). In situations where oral phosphate replacement is utilized, vitamin D is required for intestinal phosphate absorption.

Anesthetic Considerations

Anesthetic management of patients with hypophosphatemia requires familiarity with its potential complications (see earlier discussion). Hyperglycemia and respiratory alkalosis should be avoided to prevent further decreases in plasma phosphorus concentration. Neuromuscular function must be carefully monitored when NMBs are given. **Some**

11 **patients with severe hypophosphatemia may require mechanical ventilation postoperatively because of muscle weakness.**

Disorders of Magnesium Balance

Magnesium functions as a cofactor in many enzyme pathways. Only 1% to 2% of total body magnesium stores is present in the ECF compartment, with 67% contained in bone and the remaining 31% in intracellular fluid. Magnesium decreases anesthetic requirements, attenuates nociception, blunts the cardiovascular response to laryngoscopy and intubation, and potentiates NMBs. Suggested mechanisms of action include altering central nervous system neurotransmitter release, moderating adrenal medullary catecholamine release, and antagonizing the effect of calcium on vascular smooth muscle. Magnesium impairs the calcium-mediated presynaptic release of acetylcholine and may also decrease motor end-plate sensitivity to acetylcholine and alter myocyte membrane potential.

In addition to the treatment of magnesium deficiency, magnesium is used to treat preeclampsia and eclampsia, torsades de pointes, and digoxin-induced cardiac tachyarrhythmias.

NORMAL MAGNESIUM BALANCE

Magnesium intake averages 20 to 30 mEq/d (240–370 mg/d) in adults. Of that amount, only 30% to 40% is absorbed, mainly in the distal small bowel. Renal excretion is the primary route for elimination, averaging 6 to 12 mEq/d. Magnesium reabsorption by the kidneys is very efficient. Twenty-five percent of filtered magnesium is reabsorbed in the proximal tubule, and 50% to 60% is reabsorbed in the thick ascending limb of the loop of Henle. Factors known to increase magnesium reabsorption in the kidneys include hypomagnesemia, PTH, hypocalcemia, ECF depletion, and metabolic alkalosis. Factors known to increase renal excretion include hypermagnesemia, acute volume expansion, aldosterone, hypercalcemia, ketoacidosis, diuretics, phosphate depletion, and alcohol ingestion.

Plasma Magnesium Concentration

Plasma [Mg^{2+}] is closely regulated between 1.7 and 2.1 mEq/L (0.7–1 mmol/L or 1.7–2.4 mg/dL) through interaction of the gastrointestinal tract (absorption), bone (storage), and kidneys (excretion). Approximately 50% to 60% of plasma magnesium is unbound and diffusible.

HYPERMAGNESEMIA

Increases in plasma [Mg^{2+}] are nearly always due to excessive intake (magnesium-containing antacids or laxatives: magnesium hydroxide, Milk of Magnesia), kidney impairment (GFR <30 mL/min), or both. Less common causes include adrenal insufficiency, hypothyroidism, rhabdomyolysis, and lithium administration. Magnesium sulfate therapy for preeclampsia and eclampsia can result in maternal and fetal hypermagnesemia.

Clinical Manifestations of Hypermagnesemia

Symptomatic hypermagnesemia typically presents with neurological, neuromuscular, and cardiac manifestations, including hyporeflexia, sedation, muscle weakness, and respiratory depression. Vasodilation, bradycardia, and myocardial depression may cause hypotension. ECG signs may include prolongation of the P–R interval and widening of the QRS complex.

Severe hypermagnesemia can lead to respiratory and cardiac arrest.

Treatment of Hypermagnesemia

With relatively mild hypermagnesemia, all that is usually necessary is to discontinue source(s) of magnesium intake (most often antacids or laxatives). In cases of relatively high [Mg^{2+}], and especially in the presence of clinical signs of magnesium toxicity, intravenous calcium can temporarily antagonize most of the effects of clinical toxicity. Forced diuresis with a loop diuretic and intravenous fluid replacement enhances urinary magnesium excretion in patients with adequate kidney function. When diuretic administration with intravenous infusion is used to enhance magnesium excretion in urgent or emergency cases of magnesium toxicity, serial measurements of [Ca^{2+}] and [Mg^{2+}] should be obtained, a urinary catheter is required, and goal-directed hemodynamic and fluid management should be considered. Dialysis will be necessary for patients with significant kidney impairment or kidney failure. Ventilatory or circulatory support, or both, may be necessary.

Anesthetic Considerations

Hypermagnesemia requires close monitoring of the ECG, blood pressure, and neuromuscular function. Potentiation of the vasodilatory and negative inotropic properties of anesthetics should be expected. Dosages of nondepolarizing NMBs should be reduced.

HYPOMAGNESEMIA

Hypomagnesemia is a common problem, particularly in critically ill patients, and is often associated with deficiencies of other intracellular components such as potassium and phosphorus. It is commonly found in patients undergoing major cardiothoracic or abdominal operations, and its incidence among patients in intensive care units may exceed 50%. Deficiencies of magnesium are generally the result of inadequate intake, reduced gastrointestinal absorption, increased renal excretion, or a combination of these factors (Table 49–14). Drugs that cause renal wasting of magnesium include ethanol, theophylline, diuretics, cisplatin, aminoglycosides, cyclosporine, amphotericin B, pentamidine, and granulocyte colony-stimulating factor. Hypomagnesemia has also been associated with long-term proton pump inhibitor (PPI) therapy, with such cases ascribed to the impaired intestinal absorption of magnesium. However, the prevalence of hypomagnesemia among patients with chronic use of PPIs is probably less than 1%. Unless patients receive intraoperative supplementation, hypomagnesemia is common after cardiopulmonary bypass because of hemodilution and the frequent use of albumin, transfusion, and other magnesium-lowering constituents in the priming solution.

Clinical Manifestations of Hypomagnesemia

Most patients with hypomagnesemia are asymptomatic, but weakness, fasciculation, paresthesia, confusion, ataxia, and seizures may be encountered.

TABLE 49–14 Causes of hypomagnesemia.

Inadequate intake
Nutritional
Reduced gastrointestinal absorption
Malabsorption syndromes
Small bowel or biliary fistulas
Prolonged nasogastric suctioning
Severe vomiting or diarrhea
Chronic laxative abuse
Chronic proton pump inhibitor (PPI) use
Increased renal losses
Diuresis
Diabetic ketoacidosis
Hyperparathyroidism
Hyperaldosteronism
Hypophosphatemia
Nephrotoxic drugs
Postobstructive diuresis
Multifactorial
Chronic alcoholism
Protein–calorie malnutrition
Hyperthyroidism
Pancreatitis
Burns

Hypomagnesemia is frequently associated with both hypocalcemia (impaired PTH secretion) and hypokalemia (due to renal K^+ wasting). Cardiac manifestations include arrhythmias and potentiation of digoxin toxicity; both are worsened by hypokalemia. Hypomagnesemia is associated with an increased incidence of atrial fibrillation. Prolongation of the P–R and QT intervals may also be present.

Treatment of Hypomagnesemia

Asymptomatic hypomagnesemia can be treated orally or intramuscularly. Serious manifestations such as seizures should be treated with intravenous magnesium sulfate, 1 to 2 g (8–16 mEq or 4–8 mmol) given over 10 to 60 minutes.

Anesthetic Considerations

Although no specific anesthetic interactions are described, coexistent electrolyte disturbances such as hypokalemia, hypophosphatemia, and hypocalcemia are often present and should be corrected before

surgery. **Isolated hypomagnesemia should be corrected before elective procedures because of its potential to cause arrhythmias.** Moreover, magnesium appears to have intrinsic antiarrhythmic properties and possibly cerebral protective effects (see Chapter 26). It is frequently administered preemptively in patients undergoing cardiac surgery.

CASE DISCUSSION

Electrolyte Abnormalities Following Urinary Diversion

A 70-year-old man with carcinoma of the bladder presents for a radical cystectomy and ileal loop urinary diversion. He weighs 70 kg and has a 20-year history of hypertension. Preoperative laboratory measurements revealed normal plasma electrolyte concentrations and a BUN of 20 mg/dL with a serum creatinine of 1.5 mg/dL. The operation lasts 4 hours and is performed under general anesthesia. The estimated blood loss is 900 mL. Fluid replacement consists of 3500 mL of lactated Ringer's injection and 750 mL of 5% albumin.

One hour after admission to the postanesthesia care unit, the patient is awake, his blood pressure is 130/70 mm Hg, and he appears to be breathing well (18 breaths/min, Fio_2 = 0.4). Urinary output has been only 20 mL in the last hour. Laboratory measurements are as follows: Hb, 10.4 g/dL; plasma Na^+, 133 mEq/L; K^+, 3.8 mEq/L; Cl^-, 104 mEq/L; total CO_2, 20 mmol/L; Pao_2, 156 mm Hg; arterial blood pH, 7.29; $Paco_2$, 38 mm Hg; and calculated HCO_3^-, 18 mEq/L. (See Table 49–15 for normal ranges or common electrolytes.)

What is the most likely explanation for the hyponatremia?

Multiple factors tend to promote hyponatremia postoperatively, including nonosmotic ADH secretion due to surgical stress, hypovolemia, or pain; large evaporative and functional fluid losses (tissue sequestration); and the administration of hypotonic intravenous fluids. Hyponatremia is particularly common postoperatively in patients who have received relatively large amounts of lactated Ringer's injection ([Na^+] 130 mEq/L); the

TABLE 49–15 Normal physiologic ranges of common electrolytes and effects of excess or deficit.

Electrolyte	Normal Values (mmol/L)	Effect of Excess	Effect of Deficit
Cation			
Sodium	136–145	Cerebral hemorrhage and venous thrombosis, altered mental status, seizures and coma. Cerebral edema if corrected too quickly	Neuromuscular excitability (eg, hyperreflexia), altered mental status, lethargy, irritability, seizures and coma. Demyelination syndromes if corrected too quickly.
Potassium	3.5–5.0	Peaked T-waves, widened QRS, ventricular arrhythmias, cardiac arrest. Flaccid paralysis (especially in hyperkalemic familial periodic paralysis)	Depressed ST segments, biphasic T waves, prominent U waves/tachyarrhythmias. Muscle weakness, tetany and cramping, rhabdomyolysis, ileus, respiratory failure, polyuria with secondary polydipsia
Calcium	Total: 2.10–2.60, ionized: 1.10–1.35	Neurological (headache, fatigue, apathy, confusion), gastrointestinal (pain, constipation, vomiting), renal (polyuria, nephrolithiasis, kidney failure) cardiovascular (arrhythmias, short QT interval and atrioventricular or bundle branch block) and skeletal (pain, arthralgia)	Tetany, diffuse encephalopathy, seizures, hyperreflexia, laryngospasm, dehydration secondary to hypercalcemic nephrogenic diabetes insipidus
Magnesium	0.6–1.2	Prolonged PR interval, widened QRS, hyporeflexia, respiratory depression, cardiac arrest	Muscle weakness, tetany, hyperreflexia, seizures, cardiac arrhythmias. Often associated with hypocalcemia and hypokalemia
Anion			
Chloride	95–105	Possible acute renal impairment	Unknown/related to associated abnormality
Phosphate	0.8–1.5	Symptoms of acute hypocalcaemia, acute tubular necrosis, ectopic calcification	Below 0.32 mmol/L: respiratory muscle dysfunction, left shift of oxyhemoglobin dissociation curve, myocardial dysfunction, arrhythmias, myopathy, encephalopathy, irritability, seizures, coma, rhabdomyolysis, hemolytic anemia

Reproduced with permission from Tan SC, Freebairn R. Electrolyte disorders in the critically ill. *Anaesth Intens Care Med.* 2017 Mar;18(3):133-137.

postoperative plasma [Na^+] generally approaches 130 mEq/L in such patients. (Fluid replacement in this patient was appropriate considering basic maintenance requirements, blood loss, and the additional fluid losses usually associated with this type of surgery.)

Why is the patient hyperchloremic and acidotic (normal arterial blood pH is 7.35–7.45)?

Operations for supravesical urinary diversion utilize a segment of bowel (ileum, ileocecal segment, jejunum, or sigmoid colon) that is made to function as a conduit or reservoir. The simplest and most common procedure utilizes an isolated loop of ileum as a conduit: the proximal end is anastomosed to the ureters, and the distal end is brought through the skin, forming a stoma.

Whenever urine comes in contact with bowel mucosa, the potential for significant fluid and electrolyte exchange exists. The ileum actively absorbs chloride in exchange for bicarbonate and sodium in exchange for potassium or hydrogen ions. When chloride absorption exceeds sodium absorption, plasma chloride concentration increases, whereas plasma bicarbonate concentration decreases, and hyperchloremic metabolic acidosis is established. In addition, the colon absorbs NH^{4+} directly from urine; the latter may also be produced by urea-splitting bacteria. Hypokalemia results if significant amounts of Na^+ are exchanged for K^+. Potassium losses through the conduit are increased by high urinary sodium concentrations. Moreover, a potassium deficit may be present—even in the absence of hypokalemia—because the movement of K^+ out of cells (secondary to the acidosis) can prevent an appreciable decrease in extracellular plasma [K^+].

Are there any factors that tend to increase the likelihood of hyperchloremic metabolic acidosis following urinary diversion?

The longer the urine is in contact with bowel, the greater the chance that hyperchloremia and acidosis will occur. Mechanical problems such as poor emptying or redundancy of a conduit—along with hypovolemia—thus predispose to hyperchloremic metabolic acidosis. Preexisting kidney disease also appears to be a major risk factor and probably represents an inability to compensate for the excessive bicarbonate losses.

What treatment, if any, is required for this patient?

The ileal loop should be irrigated with saline to exclude partial obstruction and ensure the free drainage of urine. Hypovolemia should be considered and treated based on goal-directed hemodynamic and fluid therapy or the response to a fluid challenge (see Chapter 51). A mild to moderate systemic acidosis (arterial pH >7.25) is generally well tolerated by most patients. Moreover, hyperchloremic metabolic acidosis following ileal conduits is often transient and usually due to urinary stasis. Persistent or more severe acidosis requires treatment with sodium bicarbonate. Potassium replacement may also be required if hypokalemia is present.

Are electrolyte abnormalities seen with other types of urinary diversion?

Procedures employing bowel as a conduit (ileal or colonic) are less likely to result in hyperchloremic metabolic acidosis than those in which bowel functions as a reservoir. The incidence of hyperchloremic metabolic acidosis approaches 80% following ureterosigmoidostomies.

WEBSITES

Endotext (free source of endocrine information) www.endotext.org (accessed June 21, 2021)

SUGGESTED READINGS

Al Dhaybi O, Bakris G. Mineralocorticoid antagonists in chronic kidney disease. *Curr Opin Nephrol Hypertens.* 2017;26:50.

Awad S, Allison SP, Lobo DN. The history of 0.9% saline. *Clin Nutr.* 2008;27:179.

Ball SG, Iqbal Z. Diagnosis and treatment of hyponatraemia. *Best Pract Res Clin Endocrinol Metabol.* 2016;30:161.

Bernardi M, Zaccherini G. Approach and management of dysnatremias in cirrhosis. *Hepatol Int.* 2018;12:487.

Buffington MA, Abreo K. Hyponatremia: a review. *J Intensive Care Med.* 2016;31:223.

Campese VM, Adenuga G. Electrophysiological and clinical consequences of hyperkalemia. *Kidney Int Suppl.* 2016;6:16.

Clase CM, Carrero J-J, Ellison DH, et al. Potassium homeostasis and management of dyskalemia in kidney diseases: conclusions from a Kidney Disease: Improving Global Outcomes (KDIGO) controversies conference. *Kidney Int.* 2020;97:42.

Cuesta M, Thompson CJ. The syndrome of inappropriate antidiuresis (SIAD). *Best Pract Res Clin Endocrinol Metabol.* 2016;30:175.

El-Sharkawy AM, Sahota O, Maughan RJ, et al. The pathophysiology of fluid and electrolyte balance in the older adult surgical patient. *Clin Nutr*. 2014;33:6.

Epstein M, Lifschitz MD. Potassium homeostasis and dyskalemias: The respective roles of renal, extrarenal, and gut sensors in potassium handling. *Kidney Int Suppl*. 2016;6:7.

Fairley JL, Zhang L, Glassford NJ, et al. Magnesium status and magnesium therapy in cardiac surgery: a systematic review and meta-analysis focusing on arrhythmia prevention. *J Crit Care*. 2017;42:69.

Filippatos TD, Liamis G, Christopoulou F, et al. Ten common pitfalls in the evaluation of patients with hyponatremia. *Eur J Internal Med*. 2016;29:22.

Findakly D, Luther RD 3rd, Wang J. Tumor lysis syndrome in solid tumors: a comprehensive literature review, new insights, and novel strategies to improve outcomes. *Cureus*. 2020;12:e8355.

Giordano M, Ciarambino T, Lo Priore E, et al. Serum sodium correction rate and the outcome in severe hyponatremia. *Am J Emerg Med*. 2017;35:1691.

Joergensen D, Tazmini K, Jacobsen D. Acute dysnatremias—a dangerous and overlooked clinical problem. *Scand J Trauma Resusc Emerg Med*. 2019;27:58.

Kovesdy CP. Updates in hyperkalemia: outcomes and therapeutic strategies. *Rev Endocr Metab Disord*. 2017;18:41.

Krummel T, Prinz E, Metten M-A, et al. Prognosis of patients with severe hyponatraemia is related to not only to hyponatraemia but also to comorbidities and to medical management: results of an observational retrospective study. *BMC Nephrol*. 2016;17:159.

Lepage L, Desforges K, Lafrance J-P. New drugs to prevent and treat hyperkalemia. *Curr Opin Nephrol Hypertens*. 2016;25:524.

Liamis G, Filippatos TD, Elisaf MS. Electrolyte disorders associated with the use of anticancer drugs. *Eur J Pharmacol*. 2016;777:78.

Lippi G, South AM, Henry BM. Electrolyte imbalances in patients with severe coronavirus disease 2019 (COVID-19). *Ann Clin Biochem*. 2020;57:262.

Muhsin SA, Mount DB. Diagnosis and treatment of hypernatremia. *Best Pract Res Clin. Endocrinol Metab*. 2016;30:189.

Palmer BF, Clegg DJ. Physiology and pathophysiology of potassium homeostasis: core curriculum 2019. *Am J Kidney Dis*. 2019;74:682.

Patel S, Rauf A, Khan H, et al. Renin–angiotensin–aldosterone (RAAS): the ubiquitous system for homeostasis and pathologies. *Biomed Pharmacother*. 2017;94:317.

Pepe J, Colangelo L, Biamonte F, et al. Diagnosis and management of hypocalcemia. *Endocrine*. 2020;69:485.

Robertson GL. Diabetes insipidus: differential diagnosis and management. *Best Pract Res Clin Endocrinol Metabol*. 2016;30:205.

Rossignole P, Legrand M, Kosiborod M, et al. Emergency management of severe hyperkalemia: guideline for best practice and opportunities for the future. *Pharmacol Res*. 2016;113:585.

Sarwar CMS, Papadimitriou L, Pitt B, et al. Hyperkalemia in heart failure. *J Am Coll Cardiol*. 2016;68:1575.

Schaefer JA, Gales MA. Potassium-binding agents to facilitate renin–angiotensin–aldosterone system inhibitor therapy. *Ann Pharmacother*. 2016;50:502.

Srinutta T, Chewcharat A, Takkavatakarn K, et al. Proton pump inhibitors and hypomagnesemia. A meta-analysis of observational studies. *Medicine*. 2019;98:e17788.

Sterns RH. Disorders of plasma sodium—causes, consequences, and correction. *N Engl J Med*. 2015;372:55.

Tan SC, Freebairn R. Electrolyte disorders in the critically ill. *Anaesth Intens Care Med*. 2017;18:133.

Tinawi M. New trends in the utilization of intravenous fluids. *Cureus*. 2021;13:e14619.

Van Laecke S. Hypomagnesemia and hypermagnesemia. *Acta Clin Belg*. 2019;74:41.

Vu BN, De Castro AM, Shottland D, et al. Patiromer. The first potassium binder approved in over 50 years. *Cardiol In Rev*. 2016;24:316.

Weir MR. Current and future treatment options for managing hyperkalemia. *Kidney Int Suppl*. 2016;6:29.

Weir MR, Bakris GL, Bushinksky DA, et al. Patiromer in patients with kidney disease and hyperkalemia receiving RAAS inhibitors. *N Engl J Med*. 2015;372:211.

Yamada S, Inaba M. Potassium metabolism and management in patients with CKD. *Nutrients*. 2021;13:1751.

Zhu CY, Surgeon C, Yeh MW. Diagnosis and management of primary hyperparathyroidism. *J Am Med Assoc*. 2020;323:1186.

CHAPTER

50

Acid–Base Management

KEY CONCEPTS

1. The strong ion difference, $PaCO_2$, and total weak acid concentration best explain acid–base balance in physiological systems.
2. The bicarbonate buffer is effective against metabolic, but not respiratory, acid–base disturbances.
3. In contrast to the bicarbonate buffer, hemoglobin is capable of buffering both carbonic (CO_2) and noncarbonic (nonvolatile) acids.
4. As a general rule, $PaCO_2$ can be expected to increase 0.25 to 1 mm Hg for each 1 mEq/L increase in $[HCO_3^-]$.
5. The renal response to acidemia is threefold: (1) increased reabsorption of filtered $[HCO_3^-]$, (2) increased excretion of titratable acids, and (3) increased production of ammonia.
6. With chronic respiratory acidosis, plasma $[HCO_3^-]$ increases approximately 4 mEq/L for each 10 mm Hg increase in $PaCO_2$ above 40 mm Hg.
7. Diarrhea is a common cause of hyperchloremic metabolic acidosis.
8. The distinction between acute and chronic respiratory alkalosis is not always made because the compensatory response to chronic respiratory alkalosis is quite variable: Plasma $[HCO_3^-]$ decreases 2 to 5 mEq/L for each 10 mm Hg decrease in $PaCO_2$ below 40 mm Hg.
9. Vomiting or continuous loss of gastric fluid by gastric drainage (nasogastric suctioning) can result in marked metabolic alkalosis, extracellular volume depletion, and hypokalemia.
10. The combination of alkalemia and hypokalemia can precipitate severe atrial and ventricular arrhythmias.
11. Changes in temperature affect $PaCO_2$, PaO_2 and pH. Both $PaCO_2$ and PaO_2 decrease during hypothermia, but pH increases because temperature does not appreciably alter $[HCO_3^-]$ and the dissociation of water decreases (decreasing H^+ and increasing pH).

Nearly all biochemical reactions in the body depend on the maintenance of a physiological hydrogen ion concentration, and abnormal hydrogen ion concentrations are associated with widespread organ dysfunction. Disorders of this regulation—usually referred to as *acid–base balance*—are of prime importance in critical illness. Changes in ventilation and perfusion, as well as infusion of electrolyte-containing solutions, are common during anesthesia and can rapidly alter acid–base balance.

Our understanding of acid–base balance is evolving. In the past, we focused on the concentration of hydrogen ions [H^+], carbon dioxide (CO_2) balance, and the base excess/deficit. We now understand that 1 the *strong ion difference* (SID), $PaCO_2$ and *total weak acid concentration* (A_{TOT}) best explain acid–base balance in physiological systems.

This chapter examines acid–base physiology and the perioperative care implications of common disturbances. Clinical measurements of blood gases and their interpretation are reviewed.

Definitions

ACID–BASE CHEMISTRY

Hydrogen Ion Concentration & pH

In an aqueous solution, water molecules reversibly dissociate into hydrogen and hydroxide ions:

$$H_2O \leftrightarrow H^+ + OH^-$$

This process is described by the dissociation constant, K_W:

$$K_W = [H^+] + [OH^-] = 10^{-14}$$

The concentration of water is omitted from the denominator of this expression because it does not vary appreciably and is already included in the constant. Therefore, given [H^+] or [OH^-], the concentration of the other ion can be readily calculated.

Example: If [H^+] = 10^{-8} nEq/L, then [OH^-] = $10^{-14} \div 10^{-8} = 10^{-6}$ nEq/L.

Arterial [H^+] is normally 40 nEq/L, or 40×10^{-9} mol/L. Hydrogen ion concentration is more commonly expressed as pH, which is defined as the negative logarithm (base 10) of [H^+] (Figure 50–1). Normal arterial pH is therefore $-\log(40 \times 10^{-9}) = 7.40$. Hydrogen ion concentrations between 16 and 160 nEq/L (pH 6.8–7.8) are compatible with life.

Like most dissociation constants, K_W is affected by changes in temperature. Thus, the electroneutrality point for water occurs at a pH of 7.0 at 25°C, but at about a pH of 6.8 at 37°C; temperature-related changes may be important during hypothermia (see Chapter 22).

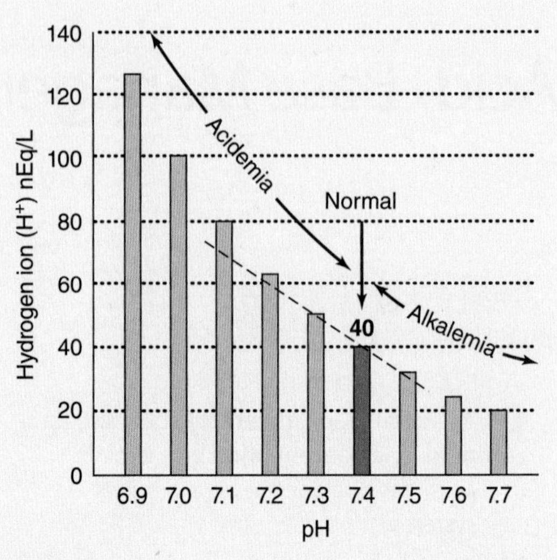

FIGURE 50–1 The relationship between pH and [H^+]. Note that between a pH of 7.10 and 7.50, the relationship between pH and [H^+] is nearly linear. (Reproduced with permission from Narins RG, Emmett M. Simple and mixed acid–base disorders: A practical approach. *Medicine.* 1980 May;59(3):161-187.)

Because physiological fluids are complex aqueous solutions, SID, the $PaCO_2$, and A_{TOT} are other factors that affect the dissociation of water into H^+ and OH^-.

Acids & Bases

An *acid* is usually defined as a chemical species that can act as a proton (H^+) donor, whereas a *base* is a species that can act as a proton acceptor (Brönsted–Lowry definitions). In physiological solutions, it is probably better to use the Arrhenius definitions: An acid is a compound that contains hydrogen and reacts with water to form hydrogen ions. A base is a compound that produces hydroxide ions in water. Using these definitions, the SID becomes important because other ions in solutions (cations and anions) will affect the dissociation constant for water and, therefore, the hydrogen ion concentration. A *strong acid* is a substance that readily and almost irreversibly gives up an H^+ and increases [H^+], whereas a *strong base* avidly binds H^+ and decreases [H^+]. In contrast, *weak acids* reversibly donate H^+, whereas *weak bases* reversibly bind H^+; both weak acids and bases tend to have less of an effect on [H^+] (for a given concentration of the parent compound) than do strong acids and bases. *Biological compounds are either weak acids or weak bases.*

For a solution containing the weak acid HA, where

$$HA \leftrightarrow H^+ + A^-$$

a dissociation constant, *K*, can be defined as follows:

$$K = \frac{[H^+][A^-]}{[HA]} \quad \text{or} \quad [H^+] = \frac{K[HA]}{[A^-]}$$

The negative logarithmic form of the latter equation is called the *Henderson–Hasselbalch equation*:

$$pH = pK + \log\left(\frac{[A^-]}{[HA]}\right)$$

From this equation, it is apparent that the pH of this solution is related to the ratio of the dissociated anion to the undissociated acid.

This approach works well with pure water: The concentration of $[H^+]$ must equal $[OH^-]$. But physiological solutions are far more complex. Even in such a complex solution, the $[H^+]$ can be predicted using three variables: the SID, the $PaCO_2$, and A_{TOT}.

Strong Ion Difference

The SID is the sum of all the strong, completely, or almost completely dissociated cations (Na^+, K^+, Ca^{2+}, Mg^{2+}) minus the strong anions (eg, Cl^-, lactate$^-$; Figure 50–2). Although we can calculate the SID, because the laws of electroneutrality must be observed, if there is a SID other unmeasured ions must be present. $PaCO_2$ is an independent variable, assuming ventilation is ongoing. The conjugate base of HA is A^- and is composed mostly of phosphates and proteins that do not change independently of the other two variables. A^- plus AH is an independent variable because its value is not determined by any other variable. Note that $[H^+]$ is not a strong ion (water does not completely dissociate), but it can, does, and must change in response to any change in SID, $PaCO_2$, or A_{TOT} to comply with the laws of electroneutrality and conservation of mass. Hydrogen ions are created or consumed based on changes in the dissociation of water.

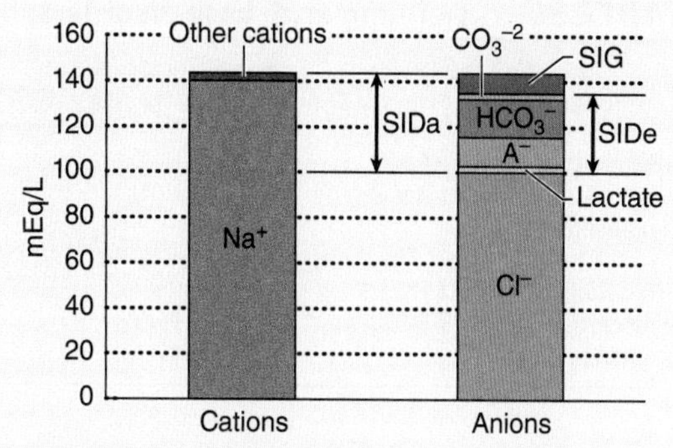

FIGURE 50–2 The strong ion difference (SID). SIDa, apparent strong ion difference; SIDe, effective strong ion difference. The strong ion gap (SIG) is the difference between SIDa and SIDe and represents the anion gap. (Reproduced with permission from Greenbaum J, Nirmalan M. Acid-base balance: Stewart's physiochemical approach. *Curr Anaesth Crit Care.* 2005 June; 16(3):133-135.)

Conjugate Pairs & Buffers

As previously discussed, when the weak acid HA is in solution, HA can act as an acid by donating an H^+, and A^- can act as a base by taking up H^+. A^- is therefore often referred to as the *conjugate base* of HA. A similar concept can be applied to weak bases. Consider the weak base B, where

$$B + H^+ \leftrightarrow BH^+$$

BH^+ is therefore the conjugate acid of B.

A *buffer* is a solution that contains a weak acid and its conjugate base or a weak base and its conjugate acid (conjugate pairs). Buffers minimize any change in $[H^+]$ by readily accepting or giving up hydrogen ions. It is readily apparent that buffers are most efficient in minimizing changes in the $[H^+]$ of a solution (ie, $[A^-] = [HA]$) when pH = p*K*. Moreover, the conjugate pair must be present in significant quantities in solution to act as an effective buffer.

CLINICAL DISORDERS

A clear understanding of acid–base disorders and compensatory physiological responses requires precise terminology (Table 50–1). The suffix "-osis" is used here to denote any pathological process that alters arterial pH. Thus, any disorder that tends to reduce pH to a less than normal value is an *acidosis*, whereas one tending to increase pH is termed an *alkalosis*.

TABLE 50–1 Defining acid–base disorders.

Disorder	Primary Change	Compensatory Response
Respiratory Acidosis Alkalosis	↑ $PaCO_2$ ↓ $PaCO_2$	↑ HCO_3– ↓ HCO_3–
Metabolic Acidosis Alkalosis	↓ HCO_3– ↑ HCO_3–	↓ $PaCO_2$ ↑ $PaCO_2$

If the disorder primarily affects [HCO_3^-], it is termed *metabolic*. If the disorder primarily affects $PaCO_2$ it is termed *respiratory*. Secondary compensatory responses (discussed in the next section) should be referred to as just that and not as an "-osis." For example, one might refer to a metabolic acidosis with respiratory compensation.

When only one pathological process occurs by itself, the acid–base disorder is considered to be *simple* (Figure 50–3). The presence of two or more primary processes indicates a *mixed* acid–base disorder.

The suffix "-emia" is used to denote the net effect of all primary processes and compensatory physiological responses (described next) on arterial blood pH. Because arterial blood pH is normally between 7.35 and 7.45 in adults, the term *acidemia* signifies a pH less than 7.35, whereas *alkalemia* signifies a pH greater than 7.45.

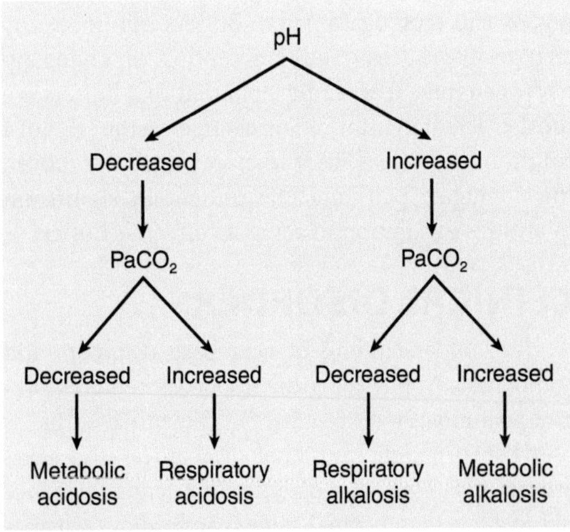

FIGURE 50–3 Diagnosis of simple acid–base disorders.

Compensatory Mechanisms

Physiological responses to changes in [H^+] are characterized by three phases: (1) immediate chemical buffering, (2) respiratory compensation (whenever possible), and (3) a slower but more effective renal compensatory response that may nearly normalize arterial pH even if the underlying pathological process remains present.

BODY BUFFERS

Physiologically important buffers in humans include bicarbonate (H_2CO_3/HCO_3^-), hemoglobin (HbH/Hb^-), other intracellular proteins (PrH/Pr^-), phosphates ($H_2PO_4^-/HPO_4^{2-}$), and ammonia (NH_3/NH_4^+). The effectiveness of these buffers in the various fluid compartments is related to their concentration. Bicarbonate is the most important buffer in the extracellular fluid compartment. Hemoglobin, though restricted inside red blood cells, also functions as an important buffer in blood. Other proteins probably play a major role in buffering the intracellular fluid compartment. Phosphate and ammonium ions are important urinary buffers.

Buffering of the extracellular compartment can also be accomplished by the exchange of extracellular H^+ for Na^+ and Ca^{2+} ions from bone and by the exchange of extracellular H^+ for intracellular K^+. Acid loads can demineralize bone and release alkaline compounds ($CaCO_3$ and $CaHPO_4$). Alkaline loads ($NaHCO_3$) increase the deposition of carbonate in bone.

Buffering by plasma bicarbonate is almost immediate, whereas that due to interstitial bicarbonate requires 15 to 20 min. In contrast, buffering by intracellular proteins and bone is slower (2–4 h). Up to 50% to 60% of acid loads may ultimately be buffered by bone and intracellular buffers.

The Bicarbonate Buffer

Although in the strictest sense, the bicarbonate buffer consists of H_2CO_3 and HCO_3^-, arterial CO_2 tension ($PaCO_2$) may be substituted for H_2CO_3 because:

$$H_2O + CO_2 \leftrightarrow H_2CO_3 \leftrightarrow H^+ + HCO_3^-$$

This hydration of CO_2 is catalyzed by carbonic anhydrase. If adjustments are made in the dissociation constant for the bicarbonate buffer and if the solubility coefficient for CO_2 (0.03 mEq/L) is taken into consideration, the Henderson–Hasselbalch equation for bicarbonate can be written as follows:

$$pH = pK' + \left(\frac{[HCO_3^-]}{0.03\ PaCO_2}\right)$$

where $pK' = 6.1$.

Note that its pK' is well removed from the normal arterial pH of 7.40, which means that bicarbonate would not be expected to be an efficient extracellular buffer (see earlier discussion). The bicarbonate system is, however, important for two reasons: (1) Bicarbonate (HCO_3^-) is present in relatively high concentrations in extracellular fluid, and (2) more importantly, $PaCO_2$ and plasma $[HCO_3^-]$ are closely regulated by the lungs and the kidneys, respectively. The ability of these two organs to alter the $[HCO_3^-]/PaCO_2$ ratio allows them to exert important influences on arterial pH.

A simplified and more practical derivation of the Henderson–Hasselbalch equation for the bicarbonate buffer is as follows:

$$[H^+] = 24 \times \frac{PaCO_2}{[HCO_3^-]}$$

This equation is very useful clinically because pH can be readily converted to $[H^+]$ (Table 50–2). Note that below 7.40, $[H^+]$ increases 1.25 nEq/L for each 0.01 decrease in pH; above 7.40, $[H^+]$ decreases 0.8 nEq/L for each 0.01 increase in pH.

Example: If arterial pH = 7.28 and $PaCO_2$ = 24 mm Hg, what should the plasma $[HCO_3^-]$ be?

$$[H^+] = 40 + [(40 - 28) \times 1.25] = 55\ nEq/L$$

Therefore,

$$55 = 24 \times \frac{24}{[HCO_3^-]} \quad \text{and}$$

$$[HCO_3^-] = \frac{(24 \times 24)}{55} = 10.5\ mEq/L$$

It should be emphasized that the bicarbonate buffer is effective against metabolic, but not respiratory, acid–base disturbances. If 3 mEq/L of a strong nonvolatile acid, such as HCl, is added to extracellular fluid, the following reaction takes place:

$$3\ mEq/L\ of\ H^+\ 24\ mEq/L\ of\ HCO_3^- \rightarrow H_2CO_3 + H_2O + 3\ mEq/L\ of\ CO_2 + 21\ mEq/L\ of\ HCO_3^-$$

Note that HCO_3^- reacts with H^+ to produce CO_2. Moreover, the CO_2 generated is normally eliminated by the lungs such that $PaCO_2$ does not change. Consequently, $[H^+] = 24 \times 40 \div 21 = 45.7$ nEq/L, and pH = 7.34. Furthermore, the decrease in $[HCO_3^-]$ reflects the amount of nonvolatile acid added.

In contrast, an increase in CO_2 tension (volatile acid) has a minimal effect on $[HCO_3]$. If, for example, $PaCO_2$ increases from 40 to 80 mm Hg, the dissolved CO_2 increases only from 1.2 mEq/L to 2.2 mEq/L. Moreover, the equilibrium constant for the hydration of CO_2 is such that an increase of this magnitude minimally drives the reaction to the left:

$$H_2O + CO_2 \leftrightarrow H_2CO_3 \leftrightarrow H^+ + HCO_3^-$$

If the valid assumption is made that $[HCO_3^-]$ does not appreciably change, then

$$[H^+] = \frac{(24 \times 80)}{24} = 80\ nEq/L \quad \text{and} \quad pH = 7.10$$

TABLE 50–2 The relationship between pH and [H⁺].

pH	$[H^+]$ nEq/L
6.80	158
6.90	126
7.00	100
7.10	79
7.20	63
7.30	50
7.40	40
7.50	32
7.60	25
7.70	20

$[H^+]$ therefore increases by 40 nEq/L, and because HCO_3^- is produced in a 1:1 ratio with H^+, $[HCO_3^-]$ also increases by 40 nEq/L. Thus, extracellular $[HCO_3^-]$ increases negligibly, from 24 mEq/L to 24.000040 mEq/L. Therefore, **the bicarbonate buffer is not effective against increases in $PaCO_2$, and changes in $[HCO_3^-]$ do not reflect the severity of a respiratory acidosis.**

Hemoglobin as a Buffer

Hemoglobin is rich in histidine, which is an effective buffer from pH 5.7 to 7.7 (pK_a 6.8). **Hemoglobin is the most important noncarbonic buffer in intravascular fluid.** Simplistically, hemoglobin may be thought of as existing in red blood cells in equilibrium as a weak acid (HHb) and a potassium salt
3 (KHb). **In contrast to the bicarbonate buffer, hemoglobin is capable of buffering both carbonic (CO_2) and noncarbonic (nonvolatile) acids:**

$$H^+ + KHb \leftrightarrow HHb + K^+ \text{ and}$$
$$H_2CO_3 + KHb \leftrightarrow HHb + HCO_3^-$$

RESPIRATORY COMPENSATION

Changes in alveolar ventilation responsible for the respiratory compensation of $PaCO_2$ are mediated by chemoreceptors within the brainstem and the carotid and aortic bodies (see Chapter 23). These receptors respond to changes in cerebrospinal spinal fluid pH. Minute ventilation increases 1 to 4 L/min for every (acute) 1 mm Hg increase in $PaCO_2$. In fact, the lungs are responsible for eliminating the approximately 15,000 to 20,000 mEq of CO_2 produced every day as a byproduct of carbohydrate and fat metabolism. Respiratory compensatory responses are also important in defending against marked changes in pH during metabolic disturbances.

Respiratory Compensation During Metabolic Acidosis

Decreases in arterial blood pH stimulate medullary respiratory centers. The resulting increase in alveolar ventilation lowers $PaCO_2$ and tends to restore arterial pH toward normal. The respiratory response to lower the $PaCO_2$ occurs rapidly but may not reach a predictably steady state until 12 to 24 h; pH is never completely restored to normal. $PaCO_2$ normally decreases 1 to 1.5 mm Hg below 40 mm Hg for every 1 mEq/L decrease in plasma $[HCO_3^-]$.

Respiratory Compensation During Metabolic Alkalosis

Increases in arterial blood pH depress respiratory centers. The resulting alveolar hypoventilation tends to elevate $PaCO_2$ and restore arterial pH toward normal. The respiratory response to metabolic alkalosis is generally less predictable than the respiratory response to metabolic acidosis. Hypoxemia, as a result of progressive hypoventilation, eventually activates oxygen-sensitive chemoreceptors; the latter stimulates ventilation and limits the compensatory respiratory response. Consequently, $PaCO_2$ usually does not increase above 55 mm Hg in response to
4 metabolic alkalosis. As a general rule, $PaCO_2$ can be expected to increase 0.25 to 1 mm Hg for each 1 mEq/L increase in $[HCO_3^-]$.

RENAL COMPENSATION

The ability of the kidneys to control the amount of HCO_3^- reabsorbed from filtered tubular fluid, form new HCO_3^-, and eliminate H^+ in the form of acids and ammonium ions (see Chapter 30) allows them to exert a major influence on pH during both metabolic and respiratory acid–base disturbances. The kidneys are responsible for eliminating the approximately 1 mEq/kg per day of sulfuric acid, phosphoric acid, uric acid, and incompletely oxidized organic acids that are normally produced by the metabolism of dietary and endogenous proteins, nucleoproteins, and organic phosphates (from phosphoproteins and phospholipids). Incomplete metabolism of fatty acids and glucose produces keto acids and lactic acid. Endogenous bases are produced during the metabolism of some anionic amino acids (eg, glutamate and aspartate) and other organic compounds (eg, citrate, acetate, and lactate), but the quantity is insufficient to offset the endogenous acid production.

Renal Compensation During Acidosis

5 **The renal response to acidemia is threefold: (1) increased reabsorption of the filtered HCO_3, (2) increased excretion of acids, and (3) increased production of ammonia.** Although these mechanisms are probably activated immediately, their effects are generally not appreciable for 12 to 24 h and may not be maximal for up to 5 days.

A. Increased Reabsorption of HCO_3^-

Bicarbonate reabsorption is shown in Figure 50–4. CO_2 within renal tubular cells combines with water in the presence of carbonic anhydrase. The carbonic acid (H_2CO_3) formed rapidly dissociates into H^+ and HCO_3^-. Bicarbonate ion then enters the bloodstream while the H^+ is secreted into the renal tubule, where it reacts with filtered HCO_3^- to form H_2CO_3. Carbonic anhydrase associated with the luminal brush border catalyzes the dissociation of H_2CO_3 into CO_2 and H_2O. The CO_2 thus formed can diffuse back into the renal tubular cell to replace the CO_2 originally consumed. The proximal tubules normally reabsorb 80% to 90% of the filtered bicarbonate load along with sodium, whereas the distal tubules are responsible for the remaining 10% to 20%. Unlike the proximal H^+ pump, the H^+ pump in the distal tubule is not necessarily linked to sodium reabsorption and is capable of generating steep H^+ gradients between tubular fluid and tubular cells. Urinary pH can decrease to as low as 4.4 (compared with a pH of 7.40 in plasma).

B. Increased Excretion of Acids

After all of the HCO_3^- in tubular fluid is reclaimed, the H^+ secreted into the tubular lumen can combine with HPO_4^{2-} to form $H_2PO_4^-$ (Figure 50–5); the latter is not readily reabsorbed because of its charge and is therefore eliminated in urine. The net result is that H^+ is excreted from the body as $H_2PO_4^-$ and the HCO_3^- that is generated in the process can enter

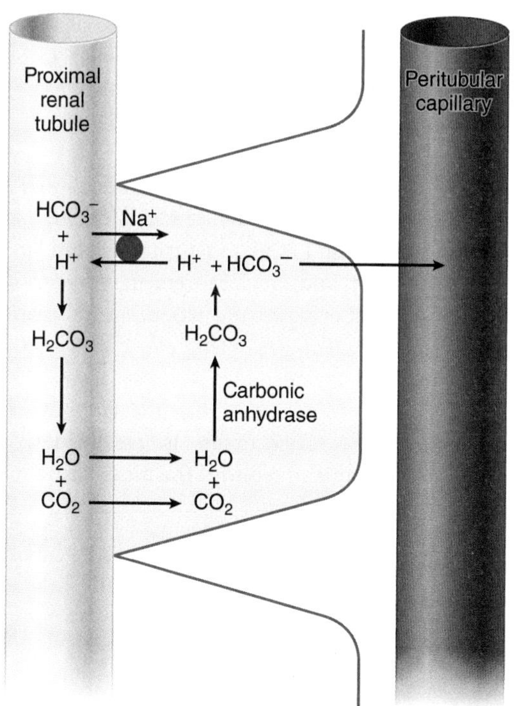

FIGURE 50–4 Reclamation of filtered HCO_3^- by the proximal renal tubules.

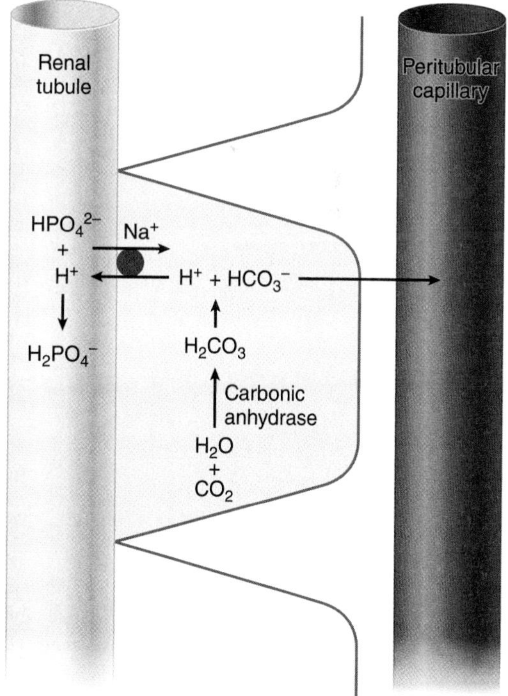

FIGURE 50–5 Formation of a titratable acid in urine.

the bloodstream. With a p*K* of 6.8, the $H_2PO_4^-$/HPO_4^{2-} pair is normally an ideal urinary buffer. When urinary pH approaches 4.4, however, all of the phosphate reaching the distal tubule is in the $H_2PO_4^-$ form; HPO_4^{2-} ions are no longer available for eliminating H^+.

C. Increased Formation of Ammonia

After complete reabsorption of HCO_3^- and consumption of the phosphate buffer, the NH_3/NH_4^+ pair becomes the most important urinary buffer (Figure 50–6). Deamination of glutamine within the mitochondria of proximal tubular cells is the principal source of NH_3 production in the kidneys. Acidemia markedly increases renal NH_3 production. The ammonia formed is then able to passively cross the cell's luminal membrane, enter the tubular fluid, and react with H^+ to form NH_4^+. Unlike NH_3, NH_4^+ does not readily penetrate the luminal membrane and is therefore trapped within the tubules. Thus, the excretion of NH_4^+ in urine effectively eliminates H^+.

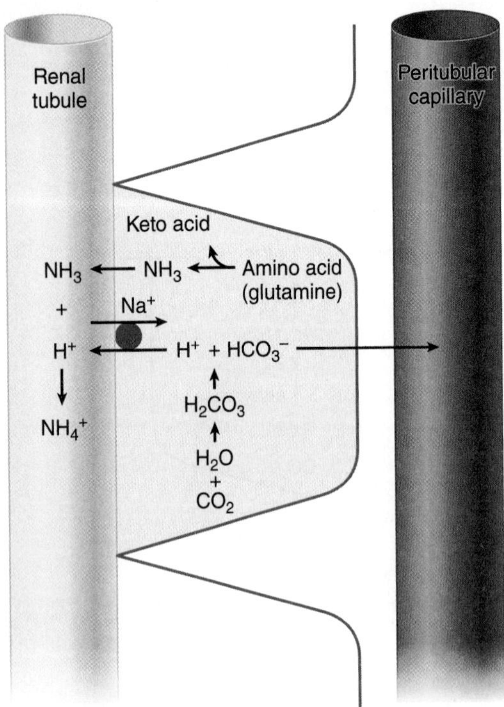

FIGURE 50–6 Formation of ammonia in urine.

Renal Compensation During Alkalosis

The tremendous amount of HCO_3^- normally filtered (and normally subsequently reabsorbed) allows the kidneys to rapidly excrete large amounts of bicarbonate, if necessary (see Chapter 49). As a result, the kidneys are highly effective in protecting against metabolic alkalosis, which therefore generally occurs only in association with concomitant sodium deficiency or mineralocorticoid excess. Sodium depletion decreases extracellular fluid volume and enhances Na^+ reabsorption in the proximal tubule. The Na^+ ion is brought across with a Cl^- ion to maintain neutrality. As Cl^- ions decrease in number (<10 mEq/L of urine), HCO_3^- must be reabsorbed. Increased H^+ secretion in exchange for augmented Na^+ reabsorption favors HCO_3^- formation with metabolic alkalosis. Similarly, increased mineralocorticoid activity augments aldosterone-mediated Na^+ reabsorption in exchange for H^+ secretion in the distal tubules. The resulting increase in HCO_3^- formation can initiate or propagate metabolic alkalosis. Metabolic alkalosis is commonly associated with increased mineralocorticoid activity, even in the absence of sodium and chloride depletion.

Base Excess

Base excess is defined as the amount of acid or base (expressed in mEq/L) that must be added for blood pH to return to 7.40 and $PaCO_2$ to return to 40 mm Hg at full O_2 saturation and 37°C. Moreover, it adjusts for noncarbonic buffering in the blood. Simplistically, *base excess represents the metabolic component of an acid–base disturbance. A positive value indicates metabolic alkalosis, whereas a negative value reveals metabolic acidosis.* Base excess is usually derived from a nomogram and requires the measurement of hemoglobin concentration.

Acidosis

PHYSIOLOGICAL EFFECTS OF ACIDEMIA

Biochemical reactions are very sensitive to changes in [H^+]. [H^+] is strictly regulated (36–43 nmol/L), as H^+ ions have high charge densities and "large" electric fields that can affect the strength of hydrogen bonds that are present on most physiological molecules. The overall effects of acidemia represent the balance between the direct biochemical effects of H+ and the effects of acidemia-induced sympathoadrenal activation. With severe acidosis (pH <7.20), direct cardiac and smooth muscle depression reduces cardiac contractility and peripheral vascular resistance, resulting in progressive hypotension. Severe acidosis can lead to tissue hypoxia, despite a rightward shift in hemoglobin affinity for oxygen. Both cardiac and vascular smooth muscle become less responsive to endogenous and exogenous catecholamines, and the ventricular fibrillation threshold is decreased. The movement of K^+ out of cells in exchange for increased extracellular H^+ results in hyperkalemia that is also potentially lethal. *Plasma [K+] increases approximately 0.6 mEq/L for each 0.10 decrease in pH.*

Central nervous system depression is more prominent with respiratory acidosis than with metabolic acidosis. This effect is often termed *CO_2 narcosis.* Unlike CO_2, H^+ ions do not readily penetrate the blood–brain barrier.

RESPIRATORY ACIDOSIS

Respiratory acidosis is defined as a primary increase in $PaCO_2$. This increase drives the reaction

$$H_2O + CO_2 \leftrightarrow H_2CO_3 \leftrightarrow H^+ + HCO_3^-$$

to the right, leading to an increase in $[H^+]$ and a decrease in arterial pH. For the reasons described previously, $[HCO_3^-]$ is minimally affected.

$PaCO_2$ represents the balance between CO_2 production and CO_2 elimination:

$$PaCO_2 = \frac{CO_2 \text{ production}}{\text{Alveolar ventilation}}$$

CO_2 is a byproduct of fat and carbohydrate metabolism—and muscle activity, body temperature, and thyroid hormone activity can all have major influences on CO_2 production. Nevertheless, CO_2 production does not appreciably vary under most circumstances, and respiratory acidosis is usually the result of alveolar hypoventilation (Table 50–3). In patients with a limited capacity to increase alveolar ventilation, however, increased CO_2 production (eg, malignant hyperthermia, status epilepticus, thyroid storm, neuroleptic malignant syndrome, serotonin syndrome) can precipitate respiratory acidosis.

TABLE 50–3 Differential diagnosis of respiratory acidosis.

Alveolar hypoventilation
Central nervous system depression
Drug-induced
Sleep disorders
Obesity hypoventilation (Pickwickian) syndrome
Cerebral ischemia
Cerebral trauma
Neuromuscular disorders
Myopathies
Neuropathies
Chest wall abnormalities
Flail chest
Kyphoscoliosis
Pleural abnormalities
Pneumothorax
Pleural effusion
Airway obstruction
Upper airway
Foreign body
Tumor
Laryngospasm
Sleep disorders
Lower airway
Severe asthma
Chronic obstructive pulmonary disease
Tumor
Parenchymal lung disease
Pulmonary edema
Cardiogenic
Noncardiogenic
Pulmonary emboli
Pneumonia
Aspiration
Interstitial lung disease
Ventilator malfunction
Increased CO_2 production
Large caloric loads
Malignant hyperthermia
Intensive shivering
Prolonged seizure activity
Thyroid storm
Extensive thermal injury (burns)

Acute Respiratory Acidosis

The compensatory response to acute (6–12 h) elevations in $PaCO_2$ is limited. Buffering is primarily provided by hemoglobin and the exchange of extracellular H^+ for Na^+ and K^+ from bone and the intracellular fluid compartment (see earlier discussion). The renal response to retain more bicarbonate is acutely very limited. As a result, plasma $[HCO_3^-]$ increases only about 1 mEq/L for each 10 mm Hg increase in $PaCO_2$ above 40 mm Hg.

Chronic Respiratory Acidosis

Renal compensation in respiratory acidosis is appreciable only after 12 to 24 h and may not be maximal
6 until 3 to 5 days have elapsed. With chronic respiratory acidosis, plasma $[HCO_3^-]$ increases approximately 4 mEq/L for each 10 mm Hg increase in $PaCO_2$ above 40 mm Hg.

Treatment of Respiratory Acidosis

Respiratory acidosis is treated by reversing the imbalance between CO_2 production and alveolar ventilation. In most instances, this is accomplished by increasing alveolar ventilation. Measures aimed at reducing CO_2 production are useful only in specific instances (eg, dantrolene for malignant hyperthermia, muscle paralysis for status epilepticus, antithyroid medication for thyroid storm, reduced caloric intake in patients receiving excessive enteral or parenteral nutrition). Measures aimed at improving alveolar ventilation (in addition to controlled mechanical ventilation) include bronchodilation, reversal of narcosis, and improving lung compliance via diuresis. Severe acidosis (pH <7.20), CO_2 narcosis, and respiratory muscle fatigue are indications for mechanical ventilation. An increased inspired oxygen concentration is also usually necessary because coexistent hypoxemia is common. Intravenous $NaHCO_3$ is rarely necessary unless pH is less than 7.10 and HCO_3^- is less than 15 mEq/L. Sodium bicarbonate therapy, especially when administered as a bolus, will transiently increase $PaCO_2$:

$$H^+ + HCO_3^- \leftrightarrow CO_2 + H_2O$$

Buffers that do not produce CO_2, such as Carbicarb or tromethamine (THAM), are theoretically attractive alternatives; however, there is almost no evidence that they have greater efficacy than bicarbonate. Carbicarb is a mixture of 0.3 M sodium bicarbonate and 0.3 M sodium carbonate; buffering by this mixture mainly produces sodium bicarbonate instead of CO_2. Tromethamine has the added advantage of lacking sodium and may be a more effective intracellular buffer. Neither Carbicarb nor tromethamine is currently available for clinical use in the United States.

Patients with chronic respiratory acidosis require special consideration. When such patients develop acute ventilatory failure, the goal of therapy should be to return $PaCO_2$ to the patient's "normal" baseline. Normalizing the patient's $PaCO_2$ to 40 mm Hg produces the equivalent of a respiratory alkalosis (see later discussion). Oxygen therapy must also be carefully controlled because the respiratory drive in these patients may be dependent on hypoxemia, not $PaCO_2$. *"Normalization" of $PaCO_2$ or relative hyperoxia can precipitate severe hypoventilation in such cases.*

METABOLIC ACIDOSIS

Metabolic acidosis is defined as a primary decrease in $[HCO_3^-]$. Pathological processes can initiate metabolic acidosis by one of three mechanisms: (1) consumption of HCO_3^- by a strong nonvolatile acid, (2) renal or gastrointestinal wasting of bicarbonate, or (3) rapid dilution of the extracellular fluid compartment with a bicarbonate-free fluid.

A fall in plasma $[HCO_3^-]$ without a proportionate reduction in $PaCO_2$ decreases arterial pH. The pulmonary compensatory response in a simple metabolic acidosis (see preceding discussion) characteristically does not reduce $PaCO_2$ to a level that completely normalizes pH but nevertheless can produce marked hyperventilation (*Kussmaul respiration*).

Table 50–4 lists disorders that can cause metabolic acidosis. Note that differential diagnosis of metabolic acidosis may be facilitated by a calculation of the *anion gap*.

The Anion Gap

The anion gap in plasma is most commonly defined as the difference between the major measured cations and the major measured anions:

$$\text{Anion gap} = \text{Major plasma cations} - \text{Major plasma anions}$$

Or

$$\text{Anion gap} = ([Na^+] - ([Cl^-] + [HCO_3^-])$$

TABLE 50–4 Differential diagnosis of metabolic acidosis.

Increased anion gap
- Increased production of endogenous nonvolatile acids
  - Kidney failure
  - Ketoacidosis
    - Diabetic
    - Starvation
  - Lactic acidosis
  - Mixed
    - Nonketotic hyperosmolar coma
    - Alcoholic
  - Inborn errors of metabolism
- Ingestion of toxin
  - Salicylate
  - Methanol
  - Ethylene glycol
  - Paraldehyde
  - Toluene
  - Sulfur
  - Rhabdomyolysis

Normal anion gap (hyperchloremic)
- Increased gastrointestinal losses of HCO_3^-
  - Diarrhea
  - Anion exchange resins (cholestyramine)
  - Ingestion of $CaCl_2$, $MgCl_2$
  - Fistulas (pancreatic, biliary, or small bowel)
  - Ureterosigmoidostomy or obstructed ileal loop
- Increased renal losses of HCO_3^-
  - Renal tubular acidosis
  - Carbonic anhydrase inhibitors
  - Hypoaldosteronism
- Dilutional
  - Large amount of bicarbonate-free fluids (eg, 0.9% NaCl)
- Total parenteral nutrition (Cl– salts of amino acids)
- Increased intake of chloride-containing acids
  - Ammonium chloride
  - Lysine hydrochloride
  - Arginine hydrochloride

Some practitioners also include plasma K^+ in the calculation. Using normal values,

$$\text{Anion gap} = 140 - (104 + 24) = 12 \text{ mEq/L}$$
$$(\text{Normal range} = 7 - 14 \text{ mEq/L})$$

In reality, an anion gap cannot exist because electroneutrality must be maintained in the body; the sum of all anions must equal the sum of all cations. Therefore,

$$\text{Anion gap} = \text{Unmeasured anions} - \text{Unmeasured cations}$$

"Unmeasured cations" include K^+, Ca^{2+}, and Mg^{2+}, whereas "unmeasured anions" include all organic anions (including plasma proteins), phosphates, and sulfates. Plasma albumin normally accounts for the largest fraction of the anion gap (approximately 11 mEq/L). The anion gap decreases by 2.5 mEq/L for every 1 g/dL reduction in plasma albumin concentration. *Any process that increases "unmeasured anions" or decreases "unmeasured cations" will increase the anion gap. Conversely, any process that decreases "unmeasured anions" or increases "unmeasured cations" will decrease the anion gap.*

Mild elevations of plasma anion gap up to 20 mEq/L may not be helpful diagnostically during acidosis, but values greater than 30 mEq/L usually indicate the presence of a high anion gap acidosis. Metabolic alkalosis can also produce a high anion gap because of extracellular volume depletion, an increased charge on albumin, and a compensatory increase in lactate production. A low plasma anion gap may be encountered with hypoalbuminemia, bromide or lithium intoxication, and multiple myeloma.

High Anion Gap Metabolic Acidosis

Metabolic acidosis with an increased anion gap is characterized by an increase in relatively strong nonvolatile acids. These acids dissociate into H^+ and their respective anions; the H^+ consumes HCO_3^- to produce CO_2, whereas their anions (conjugate bases) accumulate and take the place of HCO_3^- in extracellular fluid (hence the anion gap increases). Nonvolatile acids can be endogenously produced or ingested.

A. Failure to Excrete Endogenous Nonvolatile Acids

Endogenously produced organic acids are normally eliminated by the kidneys in urine (as described earlier). Glomerular filtration rates below 20 mL/min (kidney injury or failure) typically result in progressive metabolic acidosis from the accumulation of these acids.

B. Increased Endogenous Nonvolatile Acid Production

Severe tissue hypoxia following hypoxemia, hypoperfusion (ischemia), or an inability to utilize oxygen (cyanide poisoning) can result in lactic acidosis. Lactic acid is the end product of the anaerobic metabolism of glucose (glycolysis) and can rapidly accumulate under these conditions. Decreased utilization of lactate by the liver and, to a lesser extent, by the kidneys is less commonly responsible for lactic acidosis; causes include hypoperfusion, alcoholism, and liver disease. Lactate levels can be readily measured and are normally 0.3 to 1.3 mEq/L. Acidosis resulting from D-lactic acid, which is not recognized by α-lactate dehydrogenase (and not measured by routine assays), may be encountered in patients with short bowel syndromes; D-lactic acid is formed by colonic bacteria from dietary glucose and starch and is absorbed systemically.

An absolute or relative lack of insulin can result in hyperglycemia and progressive ketoacidosis from the accumulation of β-hydroxybutyric and acetoacetic acids (diabetic ketoacidosis). Ketoacidosis may also be seen following starvation or alcoholic binges. The pathophysiology of the acidosis often associated with severe alcoholic intoxication and nonketotic hyperosmolar coma is complex and may represent a buildup of lactic, keto, or other unknown acids.

Some inborn errors of metabolism, such as maple syrup urine disease, methylmalonic aciduria, propionic acidemia, and isovaleric acidemia, produce a high anion gap metabolic acidosis as a result of an accumulation of abnormal amino acids.

C. Ingestion of Exogenous Nonvolatile Acids

Ingestion of large amounts of salicylates may result in metabolic acidosis. Salicylic acid and other acid intermediates rapidly accumulate and produce a high anion gap acidosis. Because salicylates also produce direct respiratory stimulation, most adults develop mixed metabolic acidosis with superimposed respiratory alkalosis. Ingestion of methanol (methyl alcohol) frequently produces acidosis and retinitis. Symptoms are typically delayed until the slow oxidation of methanol by alcohol dehydrogenase produces formic acid, which is highly toxic to the retina. The high anion gap represents the accumulation of many organic acids, including acetic acid. The toxicity of ethylene glycol is also the result of the action of alcohol dehydrogenase to produce glycolic acid. Glycolic acid, the principal cause of the acidosis, is further metabolized to form oxalic acid, which may be deposited in the renal tubules and produce acute kidney injury.

Normal Anion Gap Metabolic Acidosis

Metabolic acidosis associated with a normal anion gap is typically characterized by hyperchloremia. Plasma [Cl^-] increases to take the place of the HCO_3^- ions that are lost. *Hyperchloremic metabolic acidosis* most commonly results from abnormal gastrointestinal or renal losses of HCO_3^-, or from excessive intravenous administration of 0.9% NaCl solution.

Calculation of the anion gap in urine can be helpful in diagnosing a normal anion gap acidosis.

$$\text{Urine anion gap} = ([Na^+] + [K^+]) - [Cl^-]$$

The urine anion gap is normally positive or close to zero. The principal unmeasured urinary cation is normally NH_4^+, which should increase (along with Cl^-) during a metabolic acidosis; the latter results in a negative urinary anion gap. Impairment of H^+ or NH_4^+ secretion, as occurs in kidney failure or renal tubular acidosis (discussed below), results in a positive urine anion gap despite systemic acidosis.

A. Increased Gastrointestinal Loss of HCO_3^-

7 Diarrhea is a common cause of hyperchloremic metabolic acidosis. Diarrheal fluid contains 20 to 50 mEq/L of HCO_3^-. Small bowel, biliary, and pancreatic fluids are all rich in HCO_3^-. Loss of large volumes of these fluids can lead to hyperchloremic metabolic acidosis. Patients with ureterosigmoidostomies and those with ileal loop neobladders that are too long or that become partially obstructed frequently develop hyperchloremic metabolic acidosis. The ingestion of chloride-containing anion-exchange resins (cholestyramine) or large amounts of calcium or magnesium chloride can result in increased absorption of chloride and loss of bicarbonate ions. The nonabsorbable resins bind bicarbonate ions, whereas calcium and magnesium combine with bicarbonate to form insoluble salts within the intestines.

B. Increased Renal Loss of HCO_3^-

Renal wasting of HCO_3^- can occur as a result of failure to reabsorb filtered HCO_3^- or to secrete adequate amounts of H^+ in the form of titratable acid or ammonium ion. These defects are encountered in patients taking carbonic anhydrase inhibitors, such as acetazolamide, and in those with renal tubular acidosis.

Renal tubular acidosis (RTA) is a disease of systemic acidosis resulting from inadequate renal compensation for systemic acid production. The kidneys are unable to adequately acidify the urine, and urinary pH is inappropriately high relative to the systemic acidemia. Kidney function is otherwise normal. RTA involves a defect in distal renal tubular H^+ secretion (type 1 RTA), proximal renal tubular reabsorption of filtered HCO_3^- (type 2 RTA), or both (type 3 RTA). Type 4 RTA is the result of hypoaldosteronism or renal insensitivity to aldosterone.

C. Other Causes of Hyperchloremic Acidosis

Dilutional hyperchloremic acidosis may occur when extracellular volume is rapidly expanded with a bicarbonate-free, chloride-rich fluid such as normal saline. Plasma [HCO_3^-] decreases in proportion to the amount of fluid infused as extracellular HCO_3^- is diluted, and this fall in [HCO_3^-] is compensated by a rise in [Cl^-]. This is a reason we prefer balanced salt solutions over 0.9% saline for fluid resuscitation. Amino acid infusions (parenteral hyperalimentation) contain organic cations in excess of organic anions and can produce hyperchloremic metabolic acidosis because chloride is commonly used as the anion for the cationic amino acids. Lastly, the administration of excessive quantities of chloride-containing acids, such as ammonium chloride or arginine hydrochloride (usually given to treat a metabolic alkalosis), can cause hyperchloremic metabolic acidosis.

Treatment of Metabolic Acidosis

Several general measures can be undertaken to control the severity of acidemia until the underlying processes are corrected. Any respiratory component of the acidemia should be corrected. Respiration should be controlled, if necessary; a $PaCO_2$ in the low 30s may be desirable to partially return pH to normal. If arterial blood pH remains below 7.20, alkali therapy, usually in the form of a 7.5% $NaHCO_3$ solution, may be necessary. $PaCO_2$ may transiently rise as HCO_3^- is consumed by acids, emphasizing the need to control ventilation in severe acidemia. The amount of $NaHCO_3$ given is decided empirically as a fixed dose (1 mEq/kg) or is derived from the base excess and the calculated bicarbonate space (discussed next). In either case, serial blood gas measurements are mandatory to avoid complications (eg, overshoot alkalosis and sodium overload) and to guide further therapy. Increasing arterial pH above 7.25 is usually sufficient to overcome the adverse physiological effects of the acidemia. Profound or refractory acidemia may require acute hemodialysis with a bicarbonate dialysate.

The routine use of large amounts of $NaHCO_3$ in treating cardiac arrest and low flow states, especially when not guided by laboratory analysis, is not recommended. Paradoxical intracellular acidosis may occur, particularly when CO_2 elimination is impaired, because the CO_2 formed readily enters cells, but the bicarbonate ion does not. Alternate buffers that do not produce CO_2, such as Carbicarb or tromethamine (THAM), may be theoretically preferable but are unproven clinically.

Specific therapy for diabetic ketoacidosis includes replacement of the existing fluid deficit resulting from a hyperglycemic osmotic diuresis first, as well as insulin, potassium, phosphate, and magnesium. The treatment of lactic acidosis should be directed first at restoring adequate oxygenation and tissue perfusion. Alkalinization of the urine with $NaHCO_3$ to a pH greater than 7.0 increases the elimination of salicylate following salicylate poisoning. Treatment options for ethanol or ethylene glycol intoxication include ethanol infusion or fomepizole administration, which competitively inhibit alcohol dehydrogenase, and hemodialysis or hemofiltration.

Bicarbonate Space

The *bicarbonate space* is defined as the volume to which HCO_3^- will distribute when administered intravenously. Although this theoretically should equal the extracellular fluid space (approximately 25% of body weight), in reality, it ranges anywhere between 25% and 60% of body weight, depending on the severity and duration of the acidosis. This variation is at least partly related to the amount of intracellular and bone buffering that has taken place.

Example: Calculate the amount of $NaHCO_3$ necessary to correct a base deficit (BD) of −10 mEq/L for a 70-kg man with an estimated HCO_3^- space of 30%:

$$NaHCO_3 = BD \times 30\% \times \text{body weight in L}$$
$$NaHCO_3 = -10 \text{ mEq/L} \times 30\% \times 70 \text{ L} = 210 \text{ mEq}$$

In practice, only 50% of the calculated dose (eg, 105 mEq) is usually infused, after which another blood gas is measured.

ANESTHETIC CONSIDERATIONS IN PATIENTS WITH ACIDOSIS

Acidemia can potentiate the depressant effects of most sedatives and anesthetic agents on the central nervous and circulatory systems. Because most opioids are weak bases, acidosis can increase the fraction of the drug in the nonionized form and facilitate opioid penetration into the brain, potentiating its sedative effect. The circulatory depressant effects of both volatile and intravenous anesthetics can also be exaggerated. Moreover, any agent that rapidly decreases sympathetic tone can potentially allow unopposed circulatory depression in the setting of acidosis. Halothane is more arrhythmogenic in the presence of acidosis. Succinylcholine should generally be avoided in acidotic patients with hyperkalemia to prevent further increases in plasma [K^+].

Alkalosis

PHYSIOLOGICAL EFFECTS OF ALKALOSIS

Alkalosis increases the affinity of hemoglobin for oxygen and shifts the oxygen dissociation curve to the left, making it more difficult for hemoglobin to give up oxygen to tissues. The movement of H^+ out of cells in exchange for the movement of extracellular K^+ into cells can produce hypokalemia. Alkalosis increases the number of anionic binding sites for Ca^{2+} on plasma proteins and can therefore decrease ionized plasma [Ca^{2+}], leading to circulatory depression and neuromuscular irritability. Respiratory alkalosis reduces cerebral blood flow. In the lungs, respiratory alkalosis increases bronchial smooth muscle tone (bronchoconstriction) but decreases pulmonary vascular resistance.

RESPIRATORY ALKALOSIS

Respiratory alkalosis is defined as a primary decrease in $PaCO_2$. The mechanism is usually an inappropriate increase in alveolar ventilation relative to CO_2 production. Table 50–5 lists the most common causes of respiratory alkalosis. The distinction between acute and chronic respiratory alkalosis is not always made because the compensatory response to chronic respiratory alkalosis is quite variable: Plasma [HCO_3^-] usually decreases 2 to 5 mEq/L for each 10 mm Hg decrease in $PaCO_2$ below 40 mm Hg.

8

TABLE 50–5 Differential diagnosis of respiratory alkalosis.

Central stimulation
Pain
Anxiety
Ischemia
Stroke
Tumor
Infection
Fever
Drug-induced
Salicylates
Progesterone (pregnancy)
Analeptics (doxapram)
Peripheral stimulation
Hypoxemia
High altitude
Pulmonary disease
Congestive heart failure
Noncardiogenic pulmonary edema
Asthma
Pulmonary embolism
Severe anemia
Unknown mechanism
Sepsis
Metabolic encephalopathies
Iatrogenic
Ventilator-induced

Treatment of Respiratory Alkalosis

Correction of the underlying process is the only treatment for respiratory alkalosis. For severe alkalemia (arterial pH >7.60), intravenous hydrochloric acid, arginine chloride, or ammonium chloride may be indicated (see later discussion).

METABOLIC ALKALOSIS

Metabolic alkalosis is defined as a primary increase in plasma [HCO_3^-]. Most cases of metabolic alkalosis can be divided into (1) those associated with NaCl deficiency and extracellular fluid depletion, often described as *chloride-sensitive*, and (2) those associated with enhanced mineralocorticoid activity, commonly referred to as *chloride-resistant* (Table 50–6).

TABLE 50–6 Differential diagnosis of metabolic alkalosis.

Chloride-sensitive
Gastrointestinal
Vomiting
Gastric drainage
Chloride diarrhea
Villous adenoma
Renal
Diuretics
Posthypercapnic
Low chloride intake
Sweat
Cystic fibrosis
Chloride-resistant
Increased mineralocorticoid activity
Primary hyperaldosteronism
Edematous disorders (secondary hyperaldosteronism)
Cushing syndrome
Licorice ingestion
Bartter syndrome
Severe hypokalemia
Miscellaneous
Massive blood transfusion
Acetate-containing colloid solutions
Alkaline administration with renal insufficiency
Alkali therapy
Combined antacid and cation-exchange resin therapy
Hypercalcemia
Milk-alkali syndrome
Bone metastases
Sodium penicillins
Glucose feeding after starvation

Chloride-Sensitive Metabolic Alkalosis

Depletion of extracellular fluid causes the renal tubules to avidly reabsorb Na^+. Because not enough Cl^- is available to accompany all of the Na^+ ions reabsorbed, increased H^+ secretion must take place to maintain electroneutrality. In effect, HCO_3^- ions that might otherwise have been excreted are reabsorbed, resulting in metabolic alkalosis. Physiologically, maintenance of extracellular fluid volume is therefore given priority over acid–base balance. Because secretion of K^+ ion can also maintain electroneutrality, potassium secretion is also enhanced. Moreover, hypokalemia augments H^+ secretion (and HCO_3^- reabsorption) and will also propagate metabolic alkalosis. Indeed, severe hypokalemia alone can cause alkalosis. Urinary chloride concentrations during a chloride-sensitive metabolic alkalosis are characteristically low (<10 mEq/L).

Diuretic therapy is the most common cause of chloride-sensitive metabolic alkalosis. Diuretics, such as furosemide, ethacrynic acid, and thiazides, increase Na^+, Cl^-, and K^+ excretion, resulting in NaCl depletion, hypokalemia, and usually mild metabolic alkalosis. Loss of gastric fluid is also a common cause of chloride-sensitive metabolic alkalosis. 9 **Vomiting or continuous loss of gastric fluid by gastric drainage (nasogastric suctioning) can result in marked metabolic alkalosis, extracellular volume depletion, and hypokalemia.** Gastric secretions contain 25 to 100 mEq/L of H^+, 40 to 160 mEq/L of Na^+, about 15 mEq/L of K^+, and about 200 mEq/L of Cl^-. Rapid normalization of $PaCO_2$ after plasma [HCO_3^-] has risen in chronic respiratory acidosis results in metabolic alkalosis (*posthypercapnic alkalosis*; see the previous section). Infants being fed formulas containing Na^+ without chloride readily develop metabolic alkalosis because of the increased H^+ (or K^+) secretion that must accompany sodium absorption.

Chloride-Resistant Metabolic Alkalosis

Increased mineralocorticoid activity commonly results in metabolic alkalosis, even when it is not associated with extracellular volume depletion. Inappropriate increases in mineralocorticoid activity cause sodium retention and expansion of extracellular fluid volume. Increased H^+ and K^+ secretion take place to balance enhanced mineralocorticoid-mediated sodium reabsorption, resulting in metabolic alkalosis and hypokalemia. Urinary chloride concentrations are typically greater than 20 mEq/L in such cases.

Other Causes of Metabolic Alkalosis

Metabolic alkalosis is rarely encountered in patients given even large doses of $NaHCO_3$ unless renal excretion of HCO_3^- is impaired. The administration of large amounts of blood products and some plasma protein–containing colloid solutions frequently results in metabolic alkalosis because citrate, lactate, and acetate contained in these fluids are converted by the liver into HCO_3^-. Patients receiving high doses of sodium penicillin (particularly carbenicillin) can develop metabolic alkalosis. Because penicillins act as nonabsorbable anions in the renal tubules, increased H^+ (or K^+) secretion must accompany sodium absorption. Hypercalcemia that results from nonparathyroid causes (milk-alkali syndrome and bone metastases) is also often associated with metabolic alkalosis.

Treatment of Metabolic Alkalosis

As with other acid–base disorders, correction of metabolic alkalosis is never complete until the underlying disorder is corrected. When ventilation is controlled, any respiratory component contributing to alkalemia should be corrected by decreasing minute ventilation to normalize $PaCO_2$. The treatment of choice for chloride-sensitive metabolic alkalosis is the administration of intravenous saline (NaCl) and potassium (KCl). H_2-blocker therapy is useful when excessive loss of gastric fluid is a factor. Acetazolamide may also be useful in edematous patients. Alkalosis associated with primary increases in mineralocorticoid activity readily responds to aldosterone antagonists (spironolactone). When arterial blood pH is greater than 7.60, treatment with intravenous hydrochloric acid (0.1 mol/L), ammonium chloride (0.1 mol/L), arginine hydrochloride, or hemodialysis should be considered.

ANESTHETIC CONSIDERATIONS IN PATIENTS WITH ALKALEMIA

Cerebral ischemia can occur from a marked reduction in cerebral blood flow during respiratory alkalosis, particularly during hypotension. **The combination of alkalemia and hypokalemia can precipitate severe cardiac arrhythmias.** Reports of the effects of alkalemia on neuromuscular blockers are inconsistent.

10

DIAGNOSIS OF ACID–BASE DISORDERS

Interpretation of acid–base status from analysis of blood gases requires a systematic approach. A recommended approach follows (see Figure 50–3):

1. Examine arterial pH: Is acidemia or alkalemia present?
2. Examine $PaCO_2$: Is the change in $PaCO_2$ consistent with a respiratory component?
3. If the change in $PaCO_2$ does not explain the change in arterial pH, does the change in $[HCO_3^-]$ indicate a metabolic component?
4. Make a tentative diagnosis (see Table 50–1).
5. Compare the change in $[HCO_3^-]$ with the change in $PaCO_2$. Does a compensatory response exist (Table 50–7)? Because arterial pH is related to the ratio of $PaCO_2$ to $[HCO_3^-]$, both respiratory and renal compensatory mechanisms are always such that $PaCO_2$ and $[HCO_3^-]$ change in the same direction. A change in opposite directions implies a mixed acid–base disorder.
6. If the compensatory response is more or less than expected, by definition, a mixed acid–base disorder exists.
7. Calculate the plasma anion gap in the case of metabolic acidosis.
8. Measure the urinary chloride concentration in the case of metabolic alkalosis.

TABLE 50–7 Normal compensatory responses in acid–base disturbances.

Disturbance	Response	Expected Change
Respiratory acidosis		
Acute	↑ $[HCO_3-]$	1 mEq/L/10 mm Hg increase in $PaCO_2$
Chronic	↑ $[HCO_3-]$	4 mEq/L/10 mm Hg increase in $PaCO_2$
Respiratory alkalosis		
Acute	↓ $[HCO_3-]$	2 mEq/L/10 mm Hg decrease in $PaCO_2$
Chronic	↓ $[HCO_3-]$	4 mEq/L/10 mm Hg decrease in $PaCO_2$
Metabolic acidosis	↓ $PaCO_2$	1.2 × the decrease in $[HCO_3-]$
Metabolic alkalosis	↑ $PaCO_2$	0.7 × the increase in $[HCO_3-]$

An alternative approach that is rapid, though less precise, is to correlate changes in pH with changes in CO_2 or HCO_3. For a respiratory disturbance, every 10 mm Hg change in CO_2 should change arterial pH by approximately 0.08 in the opposite direction. During metabolic disturbances, every 6 mEq change in HCO_3 also changes arterial pH by 0.1 in the same direction. If the change in pH is greater or less than predicted, a mixed acid–base disorder is likely to be present.

MEASUREMENT OF BLOOD GAS TENSIONS & pH

Values obtained by routine blood gas measurement include oxygen and carbon dioxide tensions (PaO_2 and $PaCO_2$), pH, $[HCO_3^-]$, base excess, hemoglobin, and the percentage oxygen saturation of hemoglobin. As a rule, only PaO_2, $PaCO_2$, and pH are measured. Hemoglobin and percentage oxygen saturation are measured with a co-oximeter. $[HCO_3^-]$ is derived using the Henderson–Hasselbalch equation and base excess from the Siggaard–Andersen nomogram.

Sample Source & Collection

Arterial blood samples are most commonly used clinically, though capillary or venous blood can be used if the limitations of such samples are recognized. Oxygen tension in venous blood (normally 40 mm Hg) reflects tissue extraction, not pulmonary function. Venous $PaCO_2$ is usually 4 to 6 mm Hg higher than $PaCO_2$. Consequently, venous blood pH is usually 0.05 lower than arterial blood pH. Despite these limitations, venous blood is often useful in determining acid–base status. Capillary blood represents a mixture of arterial and venous blood, and the values obtained reflect this fact. Samples are usually collected in heparin-coated syringes and should be analyzed as soon as possible. Air bubbles should be eliminated, and the sample should be capped and placed on ice to prevent significant uptake of gas from blood cells or loss of gases to the atmosphere. Although heparin is highly acidic, excessive heparin in the sample syringe usually lowers pH only minimally but decreases $PaCO_2$ in direct proportion to the percentage of dilution and has a variable effect on PaO_2.

Temperature Correction

11 Changes in temperature affect $PaCO_2$, PaO_2, and pH. Decreases in temperature lower the partial pressure of a gas in solution—even though the total gas content does not change—because gas solubility is inversely proportionate to temperature. Both $PaCO_2$ and PaO_2 therefore decrease during hypothermia, but pH increases because temperature does not appreciably alter $[HCO_3^-]$ and the dissociation of water decreases (decreasing H^+ and increasing pH). Because blood gas tensions and pH are always measured at 37°C, controversy exists over whether to correct the measured values to the patient's actual temperature. "Normal" values at temperatures other than 37°C are not known. Many clinicians use the measurements at 37°C directly (*α-stat*), regardless of the patient's actual temperature (see Chapter 22).

CASE DISCUSSION

A Complex Acid–Base Disturbance

A 1-month-old male infant with an anorectal malformation undergoes anoplasty. Postoperatively, he is found to be in congestive heart failure resulting from coarctation of the aorta. He is noted to have tachypnea, decreased urinary

output, poor peripheral perfusion, hepatomegaly, and cardiomegaly. Following tracheal intubation, the infant is placed on a ventilator (pressure support ventilation, fraction of inspired oxygen [Fio_2] = 1.0). Initial arterial blood gas, hemoglobin, and electrolyte measurements are as follows:

$PaCO_2$ = 11 mm

pH = 7.47

PaO_2 = 209 mm Hg

Calculated [HCO_3^-] = 7.7 mEq/L

Base deficit (BD) = –14.6 mEq/L

Hemoglobin (Hb) = 9.5 g/Dl

[Na^+] = 135 mEq/L

[Cl^-] = 95 mEq/L

[K^+] = 5.5 mEq/L

[Total CO_2] = 8 mEq/L

Note that the [total CO_2] normally measured with electrolytes includes both plasma [HCO_3^-] and dissolved CO_2 in plasma.

What is the acid–base disturbance?

Using the approach described earlier, the patient clearly has an alkalosis (pH >7.45), which is at least partly respiratory in origin ($PaCO_2$ <40 mm Hg). Because $PaCO_2$ has decreased by nearly 30 mm Hg, we would expect [HCO_3^-] to be 18 mEq/L:

$$(40 - 10) \times \frac{2\,\text{mEq/L}}{10} = 6\ \text{mEq/L below 24 mEq/L}$$

In fact, the patient's [HCO_3^-] is nearly 10 mEq/L less than that! The patient therefore also has a mixed acid–base disturbance: primary respiratory alkalosis and primary metabolic acidosis. Note that the difference between the patient's [HCO_3^-] and the [HCO_3^-] expected for a pure respiratory alkalosis roughly corresponds to the base excess.

What are the likely causes of these disturbances?

The respiratory alkalosis is probably the result of congestive heart failure, whereas the metabolic acidosis results from lactic acidosis secondary to poor perfusion. The latter is suggested by the calculated plasma anion gap:

$$\text{Anion gap} = 135 - (95 + 8) = 32\ \text{mEq/L}$$

The lactate level was in fact measured and found to be elevated at 14.4 mEq/L. It is probable that fluid overload precipitated the congestive heart failure.

What treatment is indicated?

Treatment should be directed at the primary process (ie, the congestive heart failure). The patient was treated with diuresis and inotropes.

Following diuresis, the patient's tachypnea has improved, but perfusion still seems to be poor. Repeat laboratory measurements are as follows (Fio_2 = 0.5):

$PaCO_2$ = 23 mm Hg

pH = 7.52

PaO_2 = 136 mm Hg

Calculated [HCO_3^-] = 18 mEq/L

BD = –3.0 mEq/L

Hb = 10.3 g/dL

[Na^+] = 137 mEq/L

[Cl^-] = 92 mEq/L

[K^+] = 3.9 mEq/L

[Total CO_2] = 18.5 mEq/L

What is the acid–base disturbance?

Respiratory alkalosis is still present, whereas the BD has improved. Note that the hemoglobin concentration has increased slightly but [K^+] has decreased as a result of the diuresis. With the new $PaCO_2$, the expected [HCO_3^-] should be 20.6 mEq/L:

$$(40 - 10) \times \frac{2\,\text{mEq/L}}{10} = 3.4\ \text{mEq/L below 24 mEq/L}$$

Therefore, the patient still has metabolic acidosis because the [HCO_3^-] is 2 mEq/L less. Note again that this difference is close to the given BD and that the anion gap is still high:

$$\text{Anion gap} = 137 - (92 + 18) = 27$$

The repeat lactate measurement is now 13.2 mEq/L.

The high anion gap and lactate level explain why the patient is still not doing well and indicate that a new process is masking the severity of the metabolic acidosis (which is essentially unchanged).

Given the clinical course, it is likely that the patient now has a triple acid–base disorder: respiratory alkalosis, metabolic acidosis, and now metabolic alkalosis. The latter probably resulted from hypovolemia secondary to excessive diuresis (chloride-sensitive metabolic alkalosis). Note also that the metabolic alkalosis is nearly equal in magnitude to the metabolic acidosis.

The patient was subsequently given packed red blood cells in saline, and within 24 h, all three disorders began to improve:

$PaCO_2$ = 35 mm Hg

pH = 7.51

PaO_2 = 124 mm Hg

Calculated $[HCO_3^-]$ = 26.8 mEq/L

Base excess = +5.0 mEq/L

Hb = 15 g/dL

$[Na^+]$ = 136 mEq/L

$[Cl^-]$ = 91 mEq/L

$[K^+]$ = 3.2 mEq/L

[Total CO_2] = 27 mEq/L

Lactate = 2.7 mEq/L

Outcome

The respiratory alkalosis and the metabolic acidosis have now resolved, and the metabolic alkalosis is now most prominent.

Intravenous KCl replacement and a small amount of saline were judiciously given, followed by complete resolution of metabolic alkalosis. The patient subsequently underwent surgical correction of the coarctation.

SUGGESTED READINGS

Ayers P, Dixon C, Mays A. Acid-base disorders: learning the basics. *Nutr Clin Pract.* 2015;30:14.

Dhondup T, Qian Q. Electrolyte and acid-base disorders in chronic kidney disease and end-stage kidney failure. *Blood Purif.* 2017;43:179.

Dzierba AL, Abraham P. A practical approach to understanding acid-base abnormalities in critical illness. *J Pharm Pract.* 2011;24:17.

Filis C, Vasileiadis I, Koutsoukou A. Hyperchloraemia in sepsis. *Ann Intensive Care.* 2018;8:43.

Kilic O, Gultekin Y, Yazici S. The impact of intravenous fluid therapy on acid-base status of critically ill adults: a Stewart approach-based perspective. *Int J Nephrol Renovasc Dis.* 2020;13:219.

Kimura S, Shabsigh M, Morimatsu H. Traditional approach versus Stewart approach for acid-base disorders: inconsistent evidence. *SAGE Open Med.* 2018;6:2050312118801255.

Kraut JA, Madias NE. Metabolic acidosis: pathophysiology, diagnosis, and management. *Nature Rev Nephrol.* 2010;6:274.

Seifter JL, Chang H-Y. Disorders of acid-base balance: new perspectives. *Kidney Dis.* 2016;2:170.

Yessayan L, Yee J, Finak S, et al. Continuous renal replacement therapy for the management of acid-base and electrolyte imbalances in acute kidney injury. *Adv Chron Kidney Dis.* 2016;23:203.

CHAPTER

51 Fluid Management & Blood Component Therapy

KEY CONCEPTS

1. While the intravascular half-life of a crystalloid solution is 20 to 30 min, most colloid solutions have intravascular half-lives between 3 and 6 h.
2. Patients with a normal hematocrit should generally be transfused only after losses greater than 10% to 20% of their blood volume. The timing of transfusion initiation is based on the patient's procedure, comorbid conditions, and rate of blood loss.
3. The most severe transfusion reactions are due to ABO incompatibility; naturally acquired antibodies can react against the transfused foreign antigens, activate complement, and result in intravascular hemolysis.
4. In anesthetized patients, an acute hemolytic reaction is manifested by a rise in temperature, unexplained tachycardia, hypotension, hemoglobinuria, diffuse oozing in the surgical field, or a combination of these findings.
5. Allogeneic transfusion of blood products may diminish immunoresponsiveness and promote inflammation.
6. Immunocompromised and immunosuppressed patients (eg, premature infants, organ transplant recipients, patients with cancer) are particularly susceptible to severe transfusion-related cytomegalovirus (CMV) infections. Ideally, such patients should receive only CMV-negative units.
7. The most common cause of nonsurgical bleeding following massive blood transfusion is dilutional thrombocytopenia.
8. Clinically important hypocalcemia, causing cardiac depression, will not occur in most normal patients unless the transfusion rate exceeds 1 unit every 5 min, and intravenous calcium salts should rarely be required in the absence of measured hypocalcemia.
9. Once normal tissue perfusion is restored, any metabolic acidosis typically resolves and metabolic alkalosis commonly occurs as citrate and lactate contained in transfusions and resuscitation fluids are converted to bicarbonate by the liver.

Almost all patients undergoing surgical procedures require venous access for administration of intravenous fluids and medication, and some patients will require transfusion of blood components. The anesthesia provider should be able to assess intravascular fluid, electrolyte, and blood components with sufficient accuracy to correct existing abnormalities and replace ongoing losses. Errors in fluid and electrolyte replacement or transfusion may result in morbidity or death.

Evaluation of Intravascular Volume

Intravascular volume can be estimated using patient history, physical examination, and laboratory analysis, often with the aid of sophisticated hemodynamic monitoring techniques. Regardless of the method employed, serial evaluations are necessary to confirm initial impressions and to guide fluid, electrolyte, and blood component therapy. All parameters are indirect, nonspecific measures of volume; therefore, reliance upon one parameter may lead to erroneous conclusions.

PATIENT HISTORY

The patient history may reveal recent oral intake, persistent vomiting or diarrhea, gastric suction, significant blood loss or wound drainage, intravenous fluid and blood administration, and recent dialysis if the patient has kidney failure.

PHYSICAL EXAMINATION

Indications of hypovolemia include abnormal skin turgor, dehydration of mucous membranes, thready peripheral pulses, increased resting heart rate, decreased blood pressure, decreased urine output, or orthostatic heart rate and blood pressure changes from the supine to sitting or standing positions (Table 51–1). Unfortunately, medications administered during anesthesia, as well as the neuroendocrine stress response to surgery and anesthesia, frequently alter these signs and render them unreliable in the immediate postoperative period. Intraoperatively, in addition to heart rate and blood pressure, the fullness of a peripheral pulse, urinary flow rate, and indirect signs, such as the blood pressure response to positive-pressure ventilation and to vasodilating or negative inotropic effects of anesthetics, are often used for guidance.

Pitting edema—presacral in the bedridden patient or pretibial in the ambulatory patient—and increased urinary flow are signs of excess extracellular water and likely hypervolemia in patients with normal cardiac, liver, and kidney function. Late signs of hypervolemia in settings such as congestive heart failure may include tachycardia, tachypnea, elevated jugular pulse pressure, lung crackles, wheezing, cyanosis, and pink, frothy pulmonary secretions.

LABORATORY EVALUATION

Several laboratory measurements may be used as indicators of intravascular volume and adequacy of tissue perfusion, including serial hematocrits, arterial blood pH, urinary specific gravity or osmolality, urinary sodium or chloride concentration, serum sodium, and

TABLE 51–1 Signs of fluid loss (hypovolemia).

	Fluid Loss (Expressed as Percentage of Body Weight)		
Sign	*5%*	*10%*	*15%*
Mucous membranes	Dry	Very dry	Parched
Sensorium	Normal	Lethargic	Obtunded
Orthostatic changes In heart rate In blood pressure	None	Present	Marked >15 bpm ↑[1] >10 mm Hg ↓
Urinary flow rate	Mildly decreased	Decreased	Markedly decreased
Pulse rate	Normal or increased	Increased >100 bpm	Markedly increased >120 bpm
Blood pressure	Normal	Mildly decreased with respiratory variation	Decreased

[1]bpm, beats per minute.

the blood urea nitrogen (BUN)-to-serum creatinine ratio. However, these measurements are only indirect indices of intravascular volume. Moreover, they are affected by many perioperative factors and often cannot be relied upon intraoperatively. Laboratory signs of dehydration may include increasing hematocrit and hemoglobin, progressive metabolic acidosis (including lactic acidosis), urinary specific gravity greater than 1.010, urinary sodium less than 10 mEq/L, urinary osmolality greater than 450 mOsm/L, hypernatremia, and BUN-to-creatinine ratio greater than 10:1. The hemoglobin and hematocrit are usually unchanged in patients with acute hypovolemia secondary to acute blood loss because there is insufficient time for extravascular fluid to shift into the intravascular space. Ultrasonography can reveal a nearly collapsed vena cava or incompletely filled cardiac chambers. Radiographic indicators of volume overload include increased pulmonary vascular and interstitial markings (*Kerley "B" lines*), diffuse alveolar infiltrates, or both.

HEMODYNAMIC MEASUREMENTS

Hemodynamic monitoring is discussed in Chapter 5. Central venous pressure (CVP) monitoring has been used when volume status is difficult to assess by other means or when rapid or major alterations are expected. However, single CVP readings do not provide an accurate or reliable indication of volume status.

Pulmonary artery pressure monitoring has been used in settings where CVP readings do not correlate with the clinical assessment or when the patient has primary or secondary right ventricular dysfunction; the latter is usually due to pulmonary or left ventricular disease, respectively. Pulmonary artery occlusion pressure (PAOP) readings of less than 8 mm Hg may indicate hypovolemia in patients with normal left ventricular compliance; however, values less than 15 mm Hg may be associated with relative hypovolemia in patients with poor ventricular compliance. PAOP measurements greater than 18 mm Hg are elevated and may imply left ventricular volume overload. The normal relationship between PAOP and left ventricular end-diastolic volume is altered by the presence of mitral valve disease, severe aortic stenosis, or a left atrial myxoma or thrombus, as well as by increased thoracic and pulmonary airway pressures (see Chapters 5, 20, 21, and 22). All PAOP measurements should be obtained at end expiration and interpreted in the context of the clinical setting. Finally, one should recognize that multiple studies have failed to show that pulmonary artery pressure monitoring leads to improved outcomes in critically ill patients and that echocardiography provides a much more accurate and less invasive estimate of cardiac filling and function.

Intravascular volume status may be difficult to assess, and noninvasive assessments using arterial pulse contour analysis and estimation of stroke volume variation (eg, LIDCOunity, Vigileo FloTrak), esophageal Doppler, transesophageal echocardiography, transthoracic echocardiography) should be considered when an accurate determination of hemodynamic and fluid status is important. Stroke volume variation (SVV) is calculated as follows:

$$SVV = SV_{max} - SV_{min}/SV_{mean}$$

The maximum, minimum, and mean SV are calculated for a set period of time by the various measuring devices. During spontaneous ventilation, the blood pressure decreases on inspiration. During positive pressure ventilation, the opposite occurs. Normal SVV is less than 10% to 15% for patients on controlled ventilation. Patients with greater degrees of SVV are likely to be responsive to fluid therapy. In addition to providing a better assessment of volume and hemodynamic status than that obtained with CVP monitoring, these noninvasive modalities avoid multiple risks associated with central venous and pulmonary artery catheters. Consequently, we rarely employ pulmonary artery catheters to guide hemodynamic therapy.

Intravenous Fluids

Intravenous fluid therapy may consist of infusions of crystalloids, colloids, or a combination of both. Crystalloid solutions are aqueous solutions of ions (salts) with or without glucose, whereas colloid solutions also contain high-molecular-weight substances such as proteins or large glucose polymers.

Colloid solutions help maintain plasma colloid oncotic pressure (see Chapter 49) and for the most part remain intravascular, whereas crystalloid solutions rapidly equilibrate with and distribute throughout the entire extracellular fluid space.

Longstanding controversy remains regarding the use of colloid versus crystalloid fluids for surgical patients. Proponents of colloids justifiably argue that by maintaining plasma oncotic pressure, colloids are more efficient (ie, a smaller volume of colloids than crystalloids is required to produce the same effect) in restoring normal intravascular volume and cardiac output. Crystalloid proponents, on the other hand, maintain that the crystalloid solutions are equally effective when given in appropriate amounts and are much less expensive. Concerns that colloids may enhance the formation of pulmonary edema fluid in patients with increased pulmonary capillary permeability are unfounded (see Chapter 23). Several generalizations can be made:

1. Crystalloids, when given in sufficient amounts, are just as effective as colloids in restoring intravascular volume.
2. Replacing an intravascular volume deficit with crystalloids generally requires three to four times the volume needed when using colloids.
3. Surgical patients may have an extracellular fluid deficit that exceeds the intravascular deficit.
4. Severe intravascular fluid deficits can be more rapidly corrected using colloid solutions.
5. The rapid administration of large volumes of crystalloids (>4–5 L) often leads to tissue edema.

Tissue edema secondary to excessive fluid administration can impair oxygen transport, tissue healing, and return of bowel function following surgery and may increase the risk of surgical site infection.

CRYSTALLOID SOLUTIONS

Crystalloids are often considered as the initial resuscitation fluid in patients with hemorrhagic and septic shock, in burn patients, in patients with head injury (to maintain cerebral perfusion pressure), and in patients undergoing plasmapheresis and liver resection. Colloids may be included in resuscitation efforts following initial administration of crystalloid solutions depending upon anesthesia provider preferences and institutional protocols.

A wide variety of solutions is available, and choice is according to the type of fluid loss being replaced. For losses primarily involving water, replacement is with hypotonic solutions, and if losses involve both water and electrolytes, replacement is with isotonic electrolyte solutions. Glucose is provided in some solutions to maintain tonicity or prevent ketosis and hypoglycemia due to fasting or because of tradition. Children are prone to developing hypoglycemia (serum glucose <50 mg/dL) following 4- to 8-hour fasts.

Because most intraoperative fluid losses are isotonic, isotonic crystalloid solutions such as normal saline or *balanced* electrolyte solutions (low-[Cl^-] crystalloids, which have preserved ionic "balance" by replacing Cl^- with lactate, gluconate, or acetate) such as lactated Ringer's solution or PlasmaLyte are most commonly used for replacement (Table 51–2). **Normal saline, when given in large volumes, produces hyperchloremic metabolic acidosis because of its high chloride content and lack of bicarbonate** (see Chapter 50). **In addition, chloride-rich crystalloids such as normal saline may contribute to perioperative acute kidney injury. Therefore, we prefer balanced salt solutions for most perioperative uses.** Normal saline is the preferred solution to correct hypochloremic metabolic alkalosis and for diluting packed red blood cells (PRBCs) prior to transfusion. Five percent dextrose in water (D_5W) is used for the replacement of pure water deficits and as a maintenance fluid for patients on sodium restriction. Hypertonic 3% saline is sometimes employed in therapy for severe, symptomatic hyponatremia (see Chapter 49). Hypotonic solutions must be administered slowly to avoid inducing hemolysis.

COLLOID SOLUTIONS

The osmotic activity of high-molecular-weight substances in colloids tends to maintain these solutions
1 intravascularly. While the intravascular half-life of a crystalloid solution is 20 to 30 min, most colloid solutions have intravascular half-lives between 3 and 6 h. The relatively greater cost

TABLE 51–2 Composition of plasma, 0.9% saline, and commonly used balanced crystalloids.

	Human Plasma	0.9% Sodium Chloride	Hartmann's	Ringer's Lactate	Ringer's Acetate	Plasma-Lyte 148	Plasma-Lyte A pH 7.4	Sterofundin/ Ringerfundin
Osmolarity (mOsm/L)	275–295	308	278	273	276	295	295	309
pH	7.35–7.45	4.5–7.0	5.0–7.0	6.0–7.5	6.0–8.0	4.0–8.0	7.4	5.1–5.9
Sodium (mmol/L)	135–145	154	131	130	130	140	140	145
Chloride (mmol/L)	94–111	154	111	109	112	98	98	127
Potassium (mmol/L)	3.5–5.3	0	5	4	5	5	5	4
Calcium (mmol/L)	2.2–2.6	0	2	1.4	1	0	0	2.5
Magnesium (mmol/L)	0.8–1.0	0	0	0	1	1.5	1.5	1
Bicarbonate (mmol/L)	24–32							
Acetate (mmol/L)	1	0	0	0	27	27	27	24
Lactate (mmol/L)	1–2	0	29	28	0	0	0	0
Gluconate (mmol/L)	0	0	0	0	0	23	23	0
Maleate (mmol/L)	0	0		0		0	0	5
Na:Cl ratio	1.21:1 to 1.54:1	1:1	1.18:1	1.19:1	1.16:1	1.43:1	1.43:1	1.14:1

Reproduced with permission from Lobo DN, Awad S. Should chloride-rich crystalloids remain the mainstay of fluid resuscitation to prevent "pre-renal" acute kidney injury?: Con. *Kidney Int.* 2014 Dec;86(6):1096-1105.

and occasional complications associated with colloids may limit their use. Generally accepted indications for colloids include (1) fluid resuscitation in patients with severe intravascular fluid deficits (eg, hemorrhagic shock) prior to the arrival of blood for transfusion and (2) fluid resuscitation in the presence of severe hypoalbuminemia or conditions associated with large protein losses such as burns. For burn patients, colloids are not included in most initial resuscitation protocols, but they may be considered following initial resuscitation with more extensive burn injuries during subsequent operative procedures.

Many clinicians also use colloid solutions in conjunction with crystalloids when fluid replacement needs exceed 3 to 4 L prior to blood transfusion. It should be noted that colloid solutions are prepared in normal saline (Cl^- 145–154 mEq/L) and thus can also cause hyperchloremic metabolic acidosis (see earlier discussion). Some clinicians suggest that during anesthesia, maintenance (and other) fluid requirements be provided with crystalloid solutions and blood loss be replaced on a milliliter-per-milliliter basis with colloid solutions (including blood products).

Several colloid solutions are generally available. All are derived from either plasma proteins or synthetic glucose polymers and are supplied in isotonic electrolyte solutions.

Blood-derived colloids include albumin (5% and 25% solutions) and plasma protein fraction (5% solution, eg, Plasmanate). Both are heated to 60°C for at least 10 h to minimize the risk of transmitting hepatitis and other viral diseases. Plasma protein fraction contains α- and β-globulins in addition to albumin and has occasionally resulted in hypotensive allergic reactions, especially with rapid (> 10 mL/min) infusion. Synthetic colloids include gelatins and dextrose starches. *Gelatins* (eg, Gelofusine) are associated with histamine-mediated allergic reactions and are not available in the United States. *Dextran* is a complex polysaccharide available as dextran 70 (Macrodex) and dextran 40 (Rheomacrodex), which have average molecular weights of 70,000 and 40,000, respectively. Dextran is used as a volume expander but also reduces blood viscosity, von Willebrand factor antigen, platelet adhesion, and RBC aggregation. Because of these latter properties, dextrans are used to improve microcirculatory flow and decrease the risk of thrombus formation after microvascular surgery. Infusions exceeding 20 mL/kg per day can interfere with blood typing, may prolong bleeding time, and have been associated with bleeding complications. Dextran has been associated with acute kidney injury and failure and should not be administered to patients with a history of kidney disease or to those at risk for acute kidney injury (eg, older adult or critically ill patients). Anaphylactoid and anaphylactic reactions have been reported. Dextran 1 (Promit) acts as a hapten and binds circulating dextran antibodies and thus may be administered prior to dextran 40 or dextran 70 to prevent severe anaphylactic reactions.

Hetastarch (hydroxyethyl starch) is available in multiple formulations that are designated by concentration, molecular weight, the degree of starch substitution (on a molar basis), and the ratio of hydroxylation between the C2 and the C6 positions. Thus, in some countries, a wide variety of formulations are available with concentrations between 6% and 10%, molecular weights between 200 and 670, and degree of molar substitution between 0.4 and 0.7. Smaller starch molecules are eliminated by the kidneys, whereas large molecules must first be broken down by amylase. Hetastarch is highly effective as a plasma expander and is less expensive than albumin. Allergic reactions are rare, but anaphylactoid and anaphylactic reactions have been reported. Hetastarch can decrease von Willebrand factor antigen levels, may prolong the prothrombin time, and has been associated with hemorrhagic complications. It is potentially nephrotoxic and should not be administered to patients at risk for acute kidney injury, including older adult patients and patients who are critically ill or have a history of kidney disease. Its perioperative use in patients who are not critically ill or are not at increased risk of acute kidney injury remains controversial.

Perioperative Fluid Therapy

Perioperative fluid therapy aims to replace normal losses (maintenance requirements) and correct preexisting fluid deficits and surgical losses (including blood loss).

NORMAL MAINTENANCE REQUIREMENTS

In the absence of oral intake, fluid and electrolyte deficits can rapidly develop as a result of continued urine formation, gastrointestinal secretions, sweating, and insensible losses from the skin and lungs. Normal maintenance requirements can be estimated from Table 51–3.

PREEXISTING DEFICITS

Patients presenting for surgery after a traditional overnight fast without any fluid intake will have a preexisting deficit proportionate to the duration of the fast. The deficit can be estimated by multiplying the normal maintenance rate by the length of the fast. For the average 70-kg person fasting for 8 h, this amounts to (40 + 20 + 50) mL/h × 8 h, or 880 mL (Table 51–3). In fact, the real deficit is less as a result of renal conservation—after all, how many of us would feel the need to consume nearly 1 L of fluid

TABLE 51–3 Estimating maintenance fluid requirements.[1]

Weight	Rate
For the first 10 kg	4 mL/kg/h
For the next 10 kg	Add 2 mL/kg/h
For each kg above 20 kg	Add 1 mL/kg/h

[1]Example: What are the maintenance fluid requirements for a 25-kg child?

Answer: 40 + 20 + 5 = 65 mL/h.

TABLE 51–4 Electrolyte content of body fluids.

Fluid	Na^+ (mEq/L)	K^+ (mEq/L)	Cl^- (mEq/L)	HCO_3^- (mEq/L)
Sweat	30–50	5	45–55	
Saliva	2–40	10–30	6–30	30
Gastric juice				
High acidity	10–30	5–40	80–150	
Low acidity	70–140	5–40	55–95	5–25
Pancreatic secretions	115–180	5	55–95	60–110
Biliary secretions	130–160	5	90–120	30–40
Ileal fluid	40–135	5–30	20–90	20–30
Diarrheal stool	20–160	10–40	30–120	30–50

upon awakening after 8 h of sleep? Current anesthesia practice often allows oral fluids up to 2 h before an elective procedure, and the preoperative regimen may include carbohydrate fluid loading (see Chapters 18 and 48). Such patients will present for surgical or procedural care with essentially no fluid deficit, as will the hospitalized patient who has received preoperative intravenous maintenance fluids.

Abnormal fluid losses frequently contribute to preoperative deficits. Preoperative bleeding, vomiting, nasogastric suction, diuresis, and diarrhea are often contributory. Losses (actually, redistribution; see next section) due to fluid sequestration by traumatized or infected tissues, coagulopathy-related occult hematoma formation, or ascites can also be substantial. Increased insensible losses due to hyperventilation, fever, and sweating are often overlooked.

Ideally, deficits should be replaced preoperatively in surgical patients, and the fluids administered should be similar in composition to the fluids lost (Table 51–4).

SURGICAL FLUID LOSSES

Blood Loss

One of the most important, yet difficult, tasks in anesthesia is to estimate blood loss to guide fluid therapy and transfusion. These estimates may be complicated by occult bleeding into the wound, into a hollow viscus, or under the surgical drapes.

The most commonly used method for estimating blood loss is the measurement of blood in the surgical suction container and a visual estimation of the blood on surgical sponges ("4 by 4's") and laparotomy pads ("lap sponges"). A fully soaked "4 × 4" is generally considered to hold 10 mL of blood, whereas a soaked "lap" may hold 100 to 150 mL. More accurate estimates are obtained if sponges and laps are weighed before and after use, which is especially important during pediatric procedures. The use of irrigating solutions complicates estimates, and their volume should be subtracted. Serial hematocrits or hemoglobin concentrations reflect the ratio of RBCs to plasma, not necessarily blood loss, and rapid fluid shifts and intravenous replacement affect such measurements.

Other Fluid Losses

Many surgical procedures are associated with obligatory losses of fluids other than blood. Such losses are due mainly to evaporation and internal redistribution of body fluids. Evaporative losses are most significant with large wounds, especially burns, and are proportional to the surface area exposed and to the duration of the surgical procedure.

Internal redistribution of fluids—often called *third-spacing*—can cause massive fluid shifts and severe intravascular depletion in patients with peritonitis, burns, and similar situations characterized by inflamed or infected tissue. Traumatized, inflamed, or infected tissue can sequester large amounts of fluid in the interstitial space and can translocate fluid across serosal surfaces (ascites) or into the bowel lumen. Shifting of intravascular fluid into the interstitial space (edema) is especially important; protein-free fluid shift across an intact vascular barrier into the interstitial space is exacerbated by hypervolemia (water and sodium excess), and pathological alteration of the vascular barrier allows protein-rich fluid shift.

INTRAOPERATIVE FLUID REPLACEMENT

Intraoperative fluid therapy should supply basic fluid requirements and replace residual preoperative deficits as well as intraoperative losses (blood loss, fluid redistribution, evaporation). Selection of the type of intravenous solution may be guided by the surgical procedure and the expected blood loss. For minor procedures involving minimal or no blood loss, minimal or no fluid is often administered other than for drug delivery and for maintenance of intravenous line patency. For all other procedures, a balanced crystalloid such as lactated Ringer's solution or PlasmaLyte is generally used for maintenance requirements.

Goal-Directed Fluid Therapy

The concept of *goal-directed fluid therapy* (GDFT) arose from a 1983 study by Shoemaker and colleagues that demonstrated lower mortality in critically ill patients in whom tissue oxygen delivery was optimized through "physiological goals" related to cardiac output and fluid administration. The current concept of GDFT has many variations, but in general, it uses hemodynamic variables such as stroke volume, cardiac output, cardiac index, and mean arterial blood pressure to determine fluid volume adminstration responsiveness and guide fluid administration by bolus. Some anesthesiologists also incorporate the use of inotropes and vasopressors in their GDFT regimens. GDFT has been widely incorporated into enhanced recovery protocols, but studies of GDFT have been inconsistent to date, with some investigators reporting fewer postoperative complications and shorter hospital lengths of stay. Inconsistent reports of GDFT results may be due to inconsistent GDFT regimens or to the possibility that not all operations (eg, those with less physiological trespass, such as laparoscopic or robotic procedures) require GDFT.

Replacing Blood Loss

Ideally, blood loss should be replaced with sufficient crystalloid or colloid solutions to maintain normovolemia until the danger of anemia outweighs the risks of transfusion. At that point, further blood loss is replaced with transfusion of RBCs to maintain hemoglobin concentration (or hematocrit) at an acceptable level. There are no mandatory transfusion triggers. The point where the benefits of transfusion outweigh its risks must be considered on an individual basis.

Below a hemoglobin concentration of 7 g/dL, the resting cardiac output increases to maintain normal oxygen delivery. An increased hemoglobin concentration may be appropriate for older and sicker patients with cardiac or pulmonary disease, especially when there is clinical evidence (eg, a reduced mixed venous oxygen saturation and a persisting tachycardia) suggesting that a transfusion will be beneficial.

In settings other than massive trauma, most clinicians administer lactated Ringer's solution or PlasmaLyte in approximately three to four times the volume of the blood lost, or colloid in a volume equal to blood loss, until the transfusion trigger point is reached. At that time, blood is replaced unit-for-unit as it is lost with reconstituted PRBCs (see Chapter 39).

The transfusion point can be determined preoperatively from the hematocrit and by estimating
2 blood volume (Table 51–5). Patients with a normal hematocrit should generally be transfused only after losses greater than 10% to 20% of their blood volume. The timing of transfusion initiation is based on the patient's procedure, comorbid conditions, and rate of blood loss. The amount of blood loss necessary for the hematocrit to fall to 30% can be calculated as follows:

TABLE 51–5 Average blood volumes.

Age	Blood Volume
Neonates	
Premature	95 mL/kg
Full-term	85 mL/kg
Infants	80 mL/kg
Adults	
Men	75 mL/kg
Women	65 mL/kg

1. Estimate blood volume from **Table 51–5**.
2. Estimate the RBC volume (RBCV) at the preoperative hematocrit ($RBCV_{preop}$).
3. Estimate RBCV at a hematocrit of 30% ($RBCV_{30\%}$), assuming normal blood volume is maintained.
4. Calculate the RBCV lost when the hematocrit is 30%; $RBCV_{lost} = RBCV_{preop} - RBCV_{30\%}$.
5. Allowable blood loss = $RBCV_{lost} \times 3$.

Example: An 85-kg woman has a preoperative hematocrit of 35%. How much blood loss will decrease her hematocrit to 30%?

$$\text{Estimated blood volume} = 65 \text{ mL/kg} \times 85 \text{ kg} = 5525 \text{ mL.}$$
$$RBCV_{35\%} = 5525 \times 35\% = 1934 \text{ mL.}$$
$$RBCV_{30\%} = 5525 \times 30\% = 1658 \text{ mL.}$$
$$\text{Red cell loss at } 30\% = 1934 - 1658 = 276 \text{ mL.}$$
$$\text{Allowable blood loss} = 3 \times 276 \text{ mL} = 828 \text{ mL.}$$

Therefore, transfusion should be considered only when this patient's blood loss exceeds 800 mL. **Increasingly, transfusions are not recommended until the hematocrit decreases to 24% or less (hemoglobin <8.0 g/dL), but transfusion decisions must be made on an individualized basis and take into account the potential for further blood loss, rate of blood loss, and comorbid conditions (eg, cardiac disease).**

Clinical guidelines for commonly used transfusions include: (1) transfusing 1 unit of RBCs will increase hemoglobin 1 g/dL and the hematocrit 2% to 3% in adults, and (2) a 10-mL/kg transfusion of RBCs will increase hemoglobin concentration by 3 g/dL and the hematocrit by 10%.

Replacing Redistributive & Evaporative Losses

Because redistributive and evaporative losses are primarily related to wound size, extent of surgical dissection and manipulation, and procedural duration, procedures can be classified according to the degree of tissue trauma. These additional fluid losses can be replaced according to Table 51–6, based on whether tissue trauma is minimal, moderate, or severe. These values are only guidelines, and actual needs vary considerably from patient to patient. Fluid replacement can also be guided by a GDFT regimen.

Transfusion

BLOOD GROUPS

Human red cell membranes are estimated to contain at least 300 different antigenic determinants, and at least 20 separate blood group antigen systems are known. Fortunately, only the ABO and the Rh systems are important in most blood transfusions. Individuals often produce antibodies (alloantibodies) to the alleles they lack within each system. Such antibodies are responsible for the most serious reactions to transfusions. Antibodies may occur spontaneously or in response to sensitization from a previous transfusion or pregnancy.

The ABO System

ABO blood group typing is determined by the presence or absence of A or B RBC surface antigens: Type A blood has A RBC antigen, type B blood has B

TABLE 51–6 Redistribution and evaporative surgical fluid losses.

Degree of Tissue Trauma	Additional Fluid Requirement
Minimal (eg, herniorrhaphy)	0–2 mL/kg
Moderate (eg, open cholecystectomy)	2–4 mL/kg
Severe (eg, open bowel resection)	4–8 mL/kg

RBC antigen, type AB blood has both A and B RBC antigens, and type O blood has neither A nor B RBC antigen present. Almost all individuals not having A or B antigen "naturally" produce antibodies, mainly immunoglobulin (Ig) M, against those missing antigens within the first year of life.

The Rh System

There are approximately 46 Rhesus group red cell surface antigens, and patients with the D Rhesus antigen are considered *Rh-positive.* Approximately 85% of the white population and 92% of the black population has the D antigen, and individuals lacking this antigen are called *Rh-negative.* In contrast to the ABO groups, Rh-negative patients usually develop antibodies against the D antigen only after an Rh-positive transfusion or with pregnancy, in the situation of an Rh-negative mother delivering an Rh-positive baby.

Other RBC Antigen Systems

Other red cell antigen systems include Lewis, P, Ii, MNS, Kidd, Kell, Duffy, Lutheran, Xg, Sid, Cartright, YK, Ss, and Chido Rodgers. Fortunately, with some exceptions (Kell, Kidd, Duffy, and Ss), alloantibodies against these antigens rarely cause serious hemolytic reactions.

COMPATIBILITY TESTING

The purpose of compatibility testing is to predict and to prevent antigen–antibody reactions resulting from red cell transfusions.

ABO–Rh Testing

3 The most severe transfusion reactions are due to ABO incompatibility; naturally acquired antibodies can react against the transfused (foreign) antigens, activate complement, and result in intravascular hemolysis. The patient's red cells are tested with serum known to have antibodies against A and against B to determine blood type. Because of the almost universal prevalence of natural ABO antibodies, confirmation of blood type is then made by testing the patient's serum against red cells with a known antigen type.

The patient's red cells are also tested with anti-D antibodies to determine Rh status. If the subject is Rh-negative, the presence of anti-D antibody is checked by mixing the patient's serum against Rh-positive red cells. The probability of developing anti-D antibodies after a single exposure to the Rh antigen is 50% to 70%.

Antibody Screen

The purpose of this test is to detect in the serum the presence of the antibodies that are most commonly associated with non-ABO hemolytic reactions. The test (also known as the *indirect Coombs test*) requires 45 min and involves mixing the patient's serum with red cells of known antigenic composition; if specific antibodies are present, they will coat the red cell membrane, and subsequent addition of an antiglobulin antibody will result in red cell agglutination. Antibody screens are routinely done on all donor blood and are frequently done for a potential recipient instead of a *crossmatch* (described next).

Crossmatch

A crossmatch mimics the transfusion: Donor red cells are mixed with recipient serum. **Crossmatching serves three functions: (1) it confirms ABO and Rh typing, (2) it detects antibodies to the other blood group systems, and (3) it detects antibodies in low titers or those that do not agglutinate easily.**

Type & Crossmatch versus Type & Screen

In the situation of negative antibody screen without crossmatch, the incidence of serious hemolytic reaction with ABO- and Rh-compatible transfusion is less than 1:10,000. Crossmatching, however, assures optimal safety and detects the presence of less common antibodies not usually tested for in a screen. Because of the expense and time involved (45 min), crossmatches are often now performed before the need to transfuse only when the patient's antibody screen is positive, when the probability of transfusion is high, or when the patient is considered at risk for alloimmunization.

EMERGENCY TRANSFUSIONS

When a patient is exsanguinating, the urgent need to transfuse may arise prior to completion of a crossmatch, screen, or even blood typing. **If the patient's blood type is known, an abbreviated crossmatch, requiring less than 5 min, will confirm ABO compatibility. If the recipient's blood type and Rh status are not known with certainty and the transfusion must be started before determination, type O Rh-negative (*universal donor*) red cells may be used.** RBCs, fresh frozen plasma (FFP), and platelets are often transfused in a balanced ratio (1:1:1) in *massive transfusion protocols* and in trauma *damage control resuscitation* (see later discussion and Chapter 39).

BLOOD BANK PRACTICES

Blood donors are screened to exclude medical conditions that might adversely affect the donor or the recipient. Once the blood is collected, it is typed, screened for antibodies, and tested for hepatitis B, hepatitis C, syphilis, and human immunodeficiency virus. A preservative–anticoagulant solution is added. The most commonly used solution is **CPDA-1**, which contains citrate as an anticoagulant (citrate functions in this capacity by binding calcium), phosphate as a buffer, dextrose as a red cell energy source, and adenosine as a precursor for adenosine triphosphate (ATP) synthesis. CPDA-1-preserved blood can be stored for 35 days, after which the viability of the red cells rapidly decreases. Alternatively, the use of either AS-1 (Adsol) or AS-3 (Nutrice) extends the shelf-life to 6 weeks.

Nearly all units collected are separated into their component parts (ie, red cells, platelets, and plasma), and whole blood units are rarely available for transfusion in civilian practice. When centrifuged, 1 unit of whole blood yields approximately 250 mL of PRBCs with a hematocrit of 70%; following the addition of saline preservative, the volume of a unit of PRBCs often reaches 350 mL. Red cells are normally stored at 1°C to 6°C but may be frozen in a hypertonic glycerol solution for up to 10 years. The latter technique is usually reserved for storage of blood with rare phenotypes.

The supernatant is centrifuged to yield platelets and plasma. The unit of platelets obtained generally contains 50 to 70 mL of plasma and can be stored at 20°C to 24°C for 5 days. The remaining plasma supernatant is further processed and frozen to yield FFP; rapid freezing helps prevent inactivation of the labile coagulation factors V and VIII. Slow thawing of FFP yields a gelatinous precipitate (cryoprecipitate) that contains increased concentrations of factor VIII and fibrinogen. Once separated, cryoprecipitate can be refrozen for storage. One unit of blood yields about 200 mL of plasma, which is frozen for storage; once thawed, it must be transfused within 24 h. Most platelets are now obtained from donors by apheresis, and a single platelet apheresis unit is equivalent to the number of platelets derived from 6 to 8 units of whole blood.

The use of leukocyte-reduced (*leukoreduction*) blood products has been rapidly adopted by many countries, including the United States, to decrease the risk of transfusion-related febrile reactions, infections, and immunosuppression.

INTRAOPERATIVE TRANSFUSION PRACTICES

RBCs

Blood transfusions should usually be given as PRBCs, which allows optimal utilization of blood bank resources. Surgical patients require volume as well as red cells, and crystalloid or colloid can be infused simultaneously through a second intravenous line for volume replacement.

Prior to transfusion, each unit must be carefully checked against the blood bank slip and the recipient's identity bracelet. The transfusion tubing should contain a 170-μm filter to trap any clots or debris. Blood for intraoperative transfusion should be warmed to 37°C during infusion, especially when more than 2 to 3 units will be transfused; failure to do so can result in profound hypothermia. The additive effects of hypothermia and the typically low levels of 2,3-diphosphoglycerate (2,3-DPG) in stored blood can cause a marked leftward shift of the hemoglobin–oxygen dissociation curve (see Chapter 23) and, at least theoretically, promote tissue hypoxia.

FFP

FFP contains all plasma proteins, including most clotting factors. **Transfusion of FFP is indicated to treat isolated factor deficiencies, reverse warfarin therapy, and correct coagulopathy associated with liver disease.** Each unit of FFP generally increases the level of each clotting factor by 2% to 3% in adults. The initial therapeutic dose is usually 10 to 15 mL/kg. The goal is to achieve 30% of the normal coagulation factor concentration. Administration of FFP and platelets in treatment of coagulopathy is now often guided by point-of-care coagulation analysis, such as thromboelastography (TEG), rotational thromboelastometry (ROTEM), or Sonoclot, a practice we recommend.

FFP may also be used in patients who have received massive blood transfusions (see later discussion and Chapter 39) and continue to bleed following platelet transfusions. Patients with antithrombin III deficiency or thrombotic thrombocytopenic purpura also benefit from FFP transfusions.

Each unit of FFP carries the same infectious risk as a unit of whole blood. In addition, occasional patients may become sensitized to plasma proteins. ABO-compatible units are usually given but are not mandatory. As with red cells, FFP should generally be warmed to 37°C prior to transfusion.

Platelets

Platelet transfusions should be given to patients with bleeding associated with thrombocytopenia or dysfunctional platelets. Prophylactic platelet transfusions are also indicated in patients with platelet counts below 10,000 to 20,000 × 10^9/L because of an increased risk of spontaneous hemorrhage.

Platelet counts less than 50,000 × 10^9/L are associated with increased blood loss during surgery, and such patients often receive prophylactic platelet transfusions before surgery or invasive procedures. Vaginal delivery and minor surgical procedures may be performed in patients with normal platelet function and counts greater than 50,000 × 10^9/L. Administration of a single unit of platelets may be expected to increase the platelet count by 5000 to 10,000 × 10^9/L, and with administration of a platelet apheresis unit, by 30,000 to 60,000 × 10^9/L.

ABO-compatible platelet transfusions are desirable but not necessary. Transfused platelets generally survive only 1 to 7 days following transfusion. ABO compatibility may increase platelet survival. Rh sensitization can occur in Rh-negative recipients due to the presence of a few red cells in Rh-positive platelet units. Moreover, anti-A or anti-B antibodies in the 70 mL of plasma in each platelet unit can cause a hemolytic reaction against the recipient's red cells when a large number of ABO-incompatible platelet units is given. Administration of Rh immunoglobulin to Rh-negative individuals can protect against Rh sensitization following Rh-positive platelet transfusions.

Granulocyte Transfusions

Granulocyte transfusions, prepared by leukapheresis, may be indicated in neutropenic patients with bacterial infections not responding to antibiotics. Transfused granulocytes have a very short circulatory life span, so daily transfusions of 10^{10} granulocytes are usually required. Irradiation of these units decreases the incidence of graft-versus-host reactions, pulmonary endothelial damage, and other problems associated with transfusion of leukocytes (see next section), but may adversely affect granulocyte function. The availability of granulocyte colony-stimulating factor (G-CSF) and granulocyte-macrophage colony-stimulating factor (GM-CSF) has greatly reduced the need for granulocyte transfusions.

Indications for Procoagulant Transfusions

Blood products can be misused in surgical settings. The use of a transfusion algorithm, particularly for components such as plasma, platelets, and cryoprecipitate, and particularly when the algorithm is guided by appropriate laboratory testing, will reduce unnecessary transfusion of these precious, costly, and potentially dangerous resources (see Chapter 22). Following military experience, major civilian trauma care units commonly transfuse blood products in equal ratios early in the resuscitation of patients with severe trauma to preempt or correct trauma-induced coagulopathy. This balanced approach to transfusion of blood products, 1:1:1 (one unit of FFP and one unit of platelets with each unit of PRBCs), is termed *damage control resuscitation* (see Chapter 39). Based on studies of military trauma and also studies in elective cardiac and orthopedic surgery, tranexamic acid or epsilon aminocaproic acid are often administered prophylactically to reduce blood loss. Additionally, the use of coagulation factor concentrates (eg, prothrombin complex concentrate, recombinant factor VIIa) is incorporated into the treatment of perioperative coagulopathy and hemorrhage when the benefit outweighs any potential increased risk of thrombosis.

Complications of Blood Transfusion

IMMUNE COMPLICATIONS

Immune complications following blood transfusions are primarily due to sensitization of the recipient to donor red cells, white cells, platelets, or plasma proteins. Less commonly, the transfused cells or serum may mount an immune response against the recipient.

1. Hemolytic Reactions

Hemolytic reactions usually involve specific destruction of the transfused red cells by the recipient's antibodies. Less commonly, hemolysis of a recipient's red cells occurs as a result of transfusion of red cell antibodies. Incompatible units of platelet concentrates, FFP, clotting factor concentrates, or cryoprecipitate may contain small amounts of plasma with anti-A or anti-B (or both) alloantibodies. Transfusions of large volumes of such units can lead to intravascular hemolysis. Hemolytic reactions are commonly classified as either *acute* (intravascular) or *delayed* (extravascular).

Acute Hemolytic Reactions

Acute intravascular hemolysis is usually due to ABO blood incompatibility, and the reported frequency is approximately 1:38,000 transfusions. **The most common cause is misidentification of a patient, blood specimen, or transfusion unit, a risk that is not abolished with autologous blood transfusion.** These reactions are often severe and may occur after infusion of as little as 10 to 15 mL of ABO-incompatible blood. The risk of a fatal hemolytic reaction is about 1 in 100,000 transfusions. In awake patients, symptoms include chills, fever, nausea, and chest and flank pain.

4 **In anesthetized patients, an acute hemolytic reaction may be manifested by a rise in temperature, unexplained tachycardia, hypotension, hemoglobinuria, diffuse oozing in the surgical field, or a combination of these findings.** Disseminated intravascular coagulation, shock, and acute kidney failure can develop rapidly. The severity of a reaction often depends upon the volume of incompatible blood that has been administered.

Management of hemolytic reactions can be summarized as follows:

1. If a hemolytic reaction is suspected, the transfusion must be stopped immediately, and the blood bank must be notified.
2. The unit must be rechecked against the blood slip and the patient's identity bracelet.
3. Blood must be drawn to identify hemoglobin in plasma, repeat compatibility testing, and obtain coagulation studies and a platelet count.
4. A urinary bladder catheter should be inserted, and the urine should be tested for hemoglobin.
5. Forced diuresis should be initiated with mannitol, intravenous fluids, and a loop diuretic if necessary.

Hemolytic Reactions

A delayed hemolytic reaction—also called *extravascular hemolysis*—is generally mild and is caused by antibodies to non-D antigens of the Rh system or to foreign alleles in other systems such as the Kell, Duffy, or Kidd antigens. Following an ABO and Rh D-compatible transfusion, patients have a 1% to 1.6% chance of forming antibodies directed against foreign antigens in these other systems. By the time significant amounts of these antibodies have formed (weeks to months), the transfused red cells have been cleared from the circulation. Moreover, the titer of these antibodies subsequently decreases and may become undetectable. Reexposure to the same foreign antigen during a subsequent red cell transfusion, however, triggers an anamnestic antibody response against the foreign antigen. The hemolytic reaction is therefore typically delayed 2 to 21 days after transfusion, and symptoms are generally mild, consisting of malaise, jaundice, and fever. The patient's hematocrit typically fails to rise or rises only transiently, in spite of the transfusion and the absence of bleeding. The serum unconjugated bilirubin increases as a result of hemoglobin breakdown.

Diagnosis of delayed antibody-mediated hemolytic reactions may be facilitated by the antiglobulin (Coombs) test. The *direct Coombs* test detects the presence of antibodies on the membrane of red cells. In this setting, however, this test cannot distinguish between recipient antibodies coated on donor red cells and donor antibodies coated on recipient red cells. The latter requires a more detailed reexamination of pretransfusion specimens from both the patient and the donor.

The treatment of delayed hemolytic reactions is primarily supportive. The frequency of delayed hemolytic transfusion reactions is estimated to be approximately 1:12,000 transfusions. Pregnancy (exposure to fetal red cells) can also be responsible for the formation of alloantibodies to red cells.

2. Nonhemolytic Immune Reactions

Nonhemolytic immune reactions are due to sensitization of the recipient to the donor's white cells, platelets, or plasma proteins; the risk of these reactions may be minimized by the use of leukoreduced blood products.

Febrile Reactions

White cell or platelet sensitization is typically manifested as a febrile reaction. Such reactions are relatively common (1%–3% of transfusion episodes) and are characterized by an increase in temperature without evidence of hemolysis. Patients with a history of repeated febrile reactions should receive leukoreduced transfusions only.

Urticarial Reactions

Urticarial reactions are usually characterized by erythema, hives, and itching without fever. They are relatively common (1% of transfusions) and are thought to be due to sensitization of the patient to transfused plasma proteins. Urticarial reactions can be treated with antihistaminic drugs (H_1 and perhaps H_2 blockers) and steroids.

Anaphylactic Reactions

Anaphylactic reactions are rare (approximately 1:150,000 transfusions). These severe reactions may occur after only a few milliliters of blood has been given, typically in IgA-deficient patients with anti-IgA antibodies who receive IgA-containing blood transfusions. The prevalence of IgA deficiency is estimated to be 1:600 to 1:800 in the general population. Such reactions require treatment with epinephrine, fluids, corticosteroids, and H_1 and H_2 blockers. Patients with IgA deficiency should receive thoroughly washed PRBCs, deglycerolized frozen red cells, or IgA-free blood units.

Transfusion-Related Acute Lung Injury

Transfusion-related acute lung injury (TRALI) presents as acute hypoxia and noncardiac pulmonary edema occurring within 6 h of blood product transfusion. It may occur as frequently as 1:5000 transfused units and with transfusion of any blood component, but especially platelets and FFP. Treatment is similar to that for acute respiratory distress syndrome (see Chapter 58), with the important difference that TRALI may resolve within a few days with supportive therapy. The incidence of TRALI, until recently the leading cause of transfusion-related death, has markedly declined with the recognition that the presence of HLA antibodies in donor plasma is the principal TRALI risk factor and that this risk can be mitigated by accepting plasma and platelet donations only from males, or from females who either have never been pregnant or who have been tested and found to be anti-HLA negative (see Chapter 39).

Transfusion-Associated Circulatory Overload

Transfusion-associated circulatory overload (TACO) occurs when blood products are administered at an excessive rate, usually in a massive hemorrhage resuscitation scenario. This is most likely to occur when the provider continues to administer blood products without recognizing that the source of bleeding has been controlled. Communication between the team members resuscitating the patient with blood products and those attempting to control the hemorrhage is critical (see Chapter 39). *TACO has replaced TRALI as the leading transfusion-related risk for trauma patients.*

Graft-Versus-Host Disease

This type of reaction may be seen in immunocompromised patients. Cellular blood products contain lymphocytes capable of mounting an immune response against the compromised recipient. The use of special leukocyte filters alone does not reliably prevent graft-versus-host disease; irradiation of red cell, granulocyte, and platelet blood products effectively eliminates lymphocytes without altering the efficacy of such transfusions.

Post-Transfusion Purpura

Post-transfusion purpura is a potentially fatal thrombocytopenic disorder that occurs, rarely, following blood or platelet transfusion. It results from the development of platelet alloantibodies that destroy the patient's own platelets. The platelet count typically drops precipitously 5 to 10 days following transfusion. Treatment may include intravenous IgG and plasmapheresis.

Transfusion-Related Immunomodulation

5 Allogeneic transfusion of blood products may diminish immunoresponsiveness and promote inflammation. Post-transfusion immunosuppression is clearly evident in kidney transplant recipients, in whom preoperative blood transfusion improves graft survival. *Recent studies suggest that perioperative transfusion may increase the risk of postoperative bacterial infection, cancer recurrence, and mortality, all of which emphasize the need to avoid unnecessary blood product administration.*

INFECTIOUS COMPLICATIONS

Viral Infections

A. Hepatitis

The incidence of post-transfusion viral hepatitis varies greatly, from approximately 1:200,000 transfusions (for hepatitis B) to approximately 1:1,900,000 (for hepatitis C). Most acute cases are anicteric. Hepatitis C is the more serious infection; most cases progress to chronic hepatitis, with cirrhosis developing in 20% of chronic carriers and hepatocellular carcinoma developing in up to 5% of chronic carriers.

B. Acquired Immunodeficiency Syndrome (AIDS)

All blood is tested for the presence of anti-HIV-1 and anti-HIV-2 antibodies. The requirement for donor blood testing by the U.S. Food and Drug Administration (FDA) has decreased the risk of transfusion-transmitted HIV to approximately 1:1,900,000 transfusions.

C. Other Viral Infections

Cytomegalovirus (CMV) and Epstein–Barr virus usually cause asymptomatic or mild systemic illness. Some individuals infected with these viruses become asymptomatic infectious carriers; the white cells in blood units from such donors are capable of transmitting

6 either virus. Immunocompromised and immunosuppressed patients (eg, premature infants, organ transplant recipients, and cancer patients) are particularly susceptible to severe transfusion-related CMV infections. Ideally, such patients should receive only CMV-negative units. However, recent studies indicate that the risk of CMV transmission from transfusion of leukoreduced blood products is equivalent to CMV test-negative units. Human T-cell lymphotropic viruses 1 and 2 (HTLV-1 and HTLV-2) are leukemia and lymphoma viruses, respectively, that have been reported to be transmitted by blood transfusion; the former has also been associated with myelopathy. Parvovirus transmission has been reported following transfusion of coagulation factor concentrates and can result in transient aplastic crises in immunocompromised hosts. West Nile virus infection may result in encephalitis with a fatality rate of up to 10%, and transmission of this virus by transfusion has been reported. The risk of transfusion-transmitted COVID-19 infection from asymptomatic blood donors or from blood donors developing symptoms after a donation is believed to be very low at the time of this printing; however, COVID-19 is a relatively novel disease, and therefore the risk of

transfusion-related disease transmission is not precisely known at this time.

Parasitic Infections

Parasitic diseases that can be transmitted by transfusion include malaria, toxoplasmosis, and Chagas disease. Such cases are very rare in developed countries.

Bacterial Infections

Bacterial contamination of blood products is the second leading cause of transfusion-associated mortality. The prevalence of positive bacterial cultures in blood products ranges from 1:2000 for platelets to 1:7000 for PRBCs and may be due to donor bacteremia or to inadequate antisepsis during phlebotomy. The prevalence of sepsis due to blood transfusion ranges from 1:25,000 for platelets to 1:250,000 for PRBCs. Both gram-positive (*Staphylococcus*) and gram-negative (*Yersinia* and *Citrobacter*) bacteria can contaminate blood transfusions and transmit disease. Blood products should be administered over a period shorter than 4 h to avoid the possibility of bacterial contamination. Specific bacterial diseases rarely transmitted by blood transfusions from donors include syphilis, brucellosis, salmonellosis, yersiniosis, and various rickettsioses.

MASSIVE BLOOD TRANSFUSION

Massive transfusion is most often defined as the need to transfuse the patient's total estimated blood volume in less than 24 h, or one-half the patient's total estimated blood volume in 1 hour. For most adult patients, the total estimated blood volume is the equivalent of 10 to 20 units. The approach to massive transfusion (and to lesser degrees of transfusion) after trauma has been greatly influenced by recent military experience, in which outcomes have improved with concurrent transfusion of PRBCs, FFP, and platelets to avoid dilutional coagulopathy (see Chapter 39).

Coagulopathy

7 **The most common cause of nonsurgical bleeding following massive blood transfusion is dilutional thrombocytopenia**, though clinically significant dilution of coagulation factors may also occur. Point-of-care coagulation studies and platelet counts should guide platelet and FFP transfusion. Although most clinicians will be familiar with "routine" coagulation tests (eg, prothrombin time [PT], activated partial thromboplastin time [aPTT], international normalized ratio [INR], platelet count, fibrinogen), multiple studies show that viscoelastic analysis of whole blood clotting (thromboelastography, rotation thromboelastometry, or Sonoclot analysis) is more useful in resuscitation, liver transplantation, and cardiac surgery. We strongly recommend the use of this technology in these settings.

Citrate Toxicity

Calcium binding by the citrate preservative can rise in importance following transfusion of large volumes
8 of blood or blood products. Clinically important hypocalcemia, causing cardiac depression, will not occur in most normal patients unless the transfusion rate exceeds 1 unit every 5 min, and intravenous calcium salts should rarely be required in the absence of measured hypocalcemia. Because citrate metabolism is primarily hepatic, patients with liver disease or dysfunction (and possibly hypothermic patients) may develop hypocalcemia and require calcium infusion during massive transfusion, as may small children and others with relatively impaired parathyroid–vitamin D function.

Hypothermia

Massive blood transfusion is an absolute indication for warming all blood products and intravenous fluids to normal body temperature. Ventricular arrhythmias progressing to fibrillation often occur at temperatures close to 30°C, and hypothermia will hamper cardiac resuscitation. The customary use of rapid infusion devices with efficient heat transfer capability has decreased the incidence of transfusion-related hypothermia.

Acid–Base Balance

Although stored blood is acidic due to the citric acid anticoagulant and accumulation of red cell metabolites (carbon dioxide and lactic acid), metabolic acidosis due to transfusion is uncommon because citric acid and lactic acid are rapidly metabolized to bicarbonate by the normal liver. However, in the situation of massive blood transfusion, acid–base status is largely dependent upon tissue perfusion, rate of 9 blood transfusion, and citrate metabolism. Once normal tissue perfusion is restored, any metabolic acidosis typically resolves, and metabolic alkalosis commonly occurs as citrate and lactate contained in transfusions and resuscitation fluids are converted to bicarbonate by the liver.

Serum Potassium Concentration

The extracellular concentration of potassium in stored blood steadily increases with time, although the amount of extracellular potassium transfused with each unit is typically less than 4 mEq per unit. Hyperkalemia can develop regardless of the age of the blood when transfusion rates exceed 100 mL/min. The treatment of hyperkalemia is discussed in Chapter 49. Hypokalemia is commonly encountered postoperatively, particularly in association with metabolic alkalosis (see Chapters 49 and 50).

Alternative Strategies for Management of Blood Loss During Surgery

AUTOLOGOUS TRANSFUSION

Patients undergoing elective surgical procedures with a high probability for transfusion can donate their own blood for use during that surgery. The collection is usually started 4 to 5 weeks before the procedure. The patient is usually allowed to donate a unit as long as the hematocrit is at least 34% or hemoglobin at least 11 g/dL. A minimum of 72 h is required between donations to ensure plasma volume has returned to normal. With iron supplementation and erythropoietin therapy, at least 3 or 4 units can usually be collected before the operation. Autologous blood transfusions probably do not adversely affect survival in patients undergoing operations for cancer. Although autologous transfusions likely reduce the risk of infection and transfusion reactions, they are not risk free. Risks include immunologic reactions resulting from clerical errors in collection, labeling, and administration; bacterial contamination; and improper storage. Allergic reactions can occur when allergens (eg, ethylene oxide) dissolve into the blood from collection and storage equipment.

BLOOD SALVAGE & REINFUSION

This technique is used widely during cardiac, major vascular, and orthopedic surgery (see Chapter 22). The shed blood is aspirated intraoperatively into a reservoir and mixed with heparin. After a sufficient amount of blood is collected, the red cells are concentrated and washed to remove debris and anticoagulant and then reinfused into the patient. The concentrates obtained usually have hematocrits of 50% to 60%. To be used effectively, this technique requires blood losses greater than 1000 to 1500 mL. Contraindications to blood salvage and reinfusion include septic contamination of the wound and perhaps malignancy. Newer, simpler systems allow reinfusion of shed blood without centrifugation.

NORMOVOLEMIC HEMODILUTION

Acute normovolemic hemodilution relies on the premise that if the concentration of red cells is decreased, less red cell mass is lost when large amounts of blood are shed; moreover, cardiac output remains normal because intravascular volume is maintained. One or 2 units of blood are typically removed just prior to surgery from a large-bore intravenous catheter and replaced with crystalloid and colloids so that the patient remains normovolemic but has a hematocrit of 21% to 25%. The blood that is removed is stored in a CPD bag at room temperature (up to 6 h) to preserve platelet function; the blood is given back to the patient after the blood loss, or sooner if necessary. The use of normovolemic hemodilution is now rare because of progressive improvements in transfusion safety.

DONOR-DIRECTED TRANSFUSIONS

Patients can request donated blood from family members or friends known to be ABO compatible. Most blood banks discourage this practice and generally require donation at least 7 days before surgery to process the donated blood and confirm compatibility. Studies comparing the safety of donor-directed units with that of random donor units have found either no difference or that random units from blood banks are safer than directed units.

CASE DISCUSSION

A Patient with Sickle Cell Disease

A 24-year-old woman with a history of sickle cell anemia presents with abdominal pain and is scheduled for cholecystectomy.

What is sickle cell anemia?

Sickle cell anemia is a hereditary hemolytic anemia resulting from the formation of an abnormal hemoglobin (HbS). HbS differs structurally from the normal adult hemoglobin (HbA) only in the substitution of valine for glutamic acid at the sixth position of the β chain. Functionally, sickle hemoglobin has less affinity for oxygen (P_{50} = 31 mm Hg) as well as less solubility. Upon deoxygenation, HbS readily polymerizes and precipitates inside RBCs, causing them to sickle. Patients with sickle cell anemia produce variable amounts (2%–20%) of fetal hemoglobin (HbF), and it is likely that cells with large amounts of HbF are somewhat protected from sickling. The continuous destruction of irreversibly sickled cells leads to anemia, and hematocrits are typically 18% to 30% due to extravascular hemolysis. RBC survival is reduced to 10 to 15 days, compared with up to 120 days in normal individuals.

What is the difference between sickle cell anemia and sickle cell trait?

When the genetic defect for adult hemoglobin is present on both the maternally and paternally derived chromosomes, the patient is homozygous for HbS and has *sickle cell anemia* (HbSS). When only one chromosome has the sickle gene, the patient is heterozygous and has *sickle cell trait* (HbAS). Patients with the sickle trait produce variable amounts of HbA (55%–60%) and HbS (35%–40%). Unlike those with HbSS, they are generally not anemic, are asymptomatic, and have a normal life span. Sickling occurs only under extreme hypoxemia or in low-flow states. Sickling is particularly apt to occur in the renal medulla; indeed, many patients with the sickle trait have impaired renal concentrating ability. Patients with HbAS may have renal medullary, splenic, and pulmonary infarcts.

Sickle cell anemia is primarily a disease of individuals of Central African ancestry. Approximately 0.2% to 0.5% of Black Americans are homozygous for the sickle gene, and approximately 8% to 10% are heterozygous. Sickle cell anemia is found less commonly in patients of Mediterranean ancestry.

What is the pathophysiology?

Conditions favoring the formation of deoxyhemoglobin (eg, hypoxemia, acidosis, intracellular hypertonicity or dehydration, increased 2,3-DPG levels, increased temperature) can precipitate sickling in patients with HbSS. Hypothermia may also be detrimental because of associated vasoconstriction (see below). Intracellular polymerization of HbS distorts red cells and makes them less pliable and more "sticky," increasing blood viscosity. Sickling may initially be reversible but eventually becomes irreversible in some RBCs. The formation of red cell aggregates in capillaries can obstruct tissue microcirculation, and a vicious cycle is established in which circulatory stasis leads to localized hypoxia, which, in turn, causes more sickling.

With what symptoms do patients with sickle cell anemia usually present?

Patients with HbSS generally first develop symptoms in infancy, when levels of HbF decline. The disease is characterized by both acute episodic crises and chronic and progressive features (Table 51–7). Children display delayed growth and have recurrent infections. Recurrent splenic infarction leads to splenic atrophy and functional asplenism by adolescence. Patients may die from recurrent infections or kidney failure. Chronic abdominal, bone, and joint pain is typical and often complicated by repeated, acutely painful sickling crises, so patients frequently

TABLE 51–7 Manifestations of sickle cell anemia.

Neurological
Stroke
Subarachnoid hemorrhage
Coma
Seizures
Ocular
Vitreous hemorrhage
Retinal infarcts
Proliferative retinopathy
Retinal detachment
Pulmonary
Increased intrapulmonary shunting
Pleuritis
Recurrent pulmonary infections
Pulmonary infarcts
Cardiovascular
Congestive heart failure
Cor pulmonale
Pericarditis
Myocardial infarction
Gastrointestinal
Cholelithiasis (pigmented stones)
Cholecystitis
Hepatic infarcts
Hepatic abscesses
Hepatic fibrosis
Hematological
Anemia
Aplastic anemia
Recurrent infections
Splenic infarcts
Splenic sequestration
Functional asplenia
Genitourinary
Hematuria
Renal papillary necrosis
Impaired renal concentrating ability
Nephrotic syndrome
Renal insufficiency
Renal failure
Priapism
Skeletal
Synovitis
Arthritis
Aseptic necrosis of femoral head
Small bone infarcts in hand and feet (dactylitis)
Biconcave ("fishmouth") vertebrae
Osteomyelitis
Skin
Chronic ulcers

receive chronic opioid therapy. Because of issues related to analgesic tolerance and addiction, these patients often benefit from management by pain specialists. Crises are often precipitated by infection, cold weather, dehydration, or other forms of stress. Crises may be divided into three types:

1. **Vasoocclusive crises:** These acute episodes can result in micro- or macroinfarctions, depending on the vessels involved. Most painful crises are thought to be due to microinfarcts in various tissues. Clinically, they present as acute abdominal, chest, back, or joint pain. Differentiation between surgical and nonsurgical causes of abdominal pain is difficult. Most patients form pigmented gallstones by adulthood, and many present with acute cholecystitis. Vasoocclusive phenomena in larger vessels can produce thromboses resulting in splenic, cerebral, pulmonary, hepatic, renal, and, less commonly, myocardial infarctions.
2. **Aplastic crisis:** Profound anemia (Hb 2–3 g/dL) can rapidly occur when red cell production in the bone marrow is exhausted or suppressed. Infections and folate deficiency may play a major role. Some patients also develop leukopenia.
3. **Splenic sequestration crisis:** Sudden pooling of blood in the spleen can occur in infants and young children and can cause life-threatening hypotension. The mechanism is thought to be partial or complete occlusion of venous drainage from the spleen.

How is sickle cell anemia diagnosed?

RBCs from patients with sickle cell anemia readily sickle after the addition of an oxygen-consuming reagent (metabisulfite) or a hypertonic ionic solution (solubility test). Confirmation requires hemoglobin electrophoresis.

What would be the best way to prepare patients with sickle cell anemia for surgery?

Optimal preoperative preparation includes the following: patients should be well hydrated, infections should be controlled, and the hemoglobin concentration should be at an acceptable level.

Preoperative transfusion must be individualized for the patient and to the surgical procedure. Partial exchange transfusions before major surgical procedures are usually advocated, which decrease blood viscosity, increase blood oxygen-carrying capacity, and decrease the likelihood of sickling. The goal of such transfusions is generally to achieve a hematocrit of 35% to 40% with 40% to 50% normal hemoglobin (HbA). Chronic management of sickle cell disease has been revolutionized by the introduction of hydroxyurea.

Are there any special intraoperative considerations?

Conditions that might promote hemoglobin desaturation or low-flow states should be avoided. Every effort must be made to avoid hypothermia, hyperthermia, acidosis, and even mild degrees of hypoxemia, hypotension, or hypovolemia. Relatively generous hydration and a relatively high (>50%) inspired oxygen tension are important. The principal compensatory mechanism for impaired tissue oxygen delivery in these patients is increased cardiac output, which should be maintained intraoperatively. GDFT may be useful. Mild alkalosis may help avoid sickling, but even moderate degrees of respiratory alkalosis may have an adverse effect on cerebral blood flow. Tourniquet use, other than brief, should be avoided.

Are there any special postoperative considerations?

Most perioperative deaths occur in the postoperative period, and the same management principles applied intraoperatively should be used after surgery. Hypoxemia and pulmonary complications are major risk factors. Supplemental oxygen; optimal hemodynamic, fluid, and pain and symptom management; and pulmonary physiotherapy with early mobilization all help minimize the risk of these complications.

What is the pathophysiology of thalassemia?

Thalassemia is a hereditary defect in the production of one or more of the normal subunits of hemoglobin. Patients with thalassemia may be able to produce normal HbA but have reduced amounts of α- or β-chain production; the severity of this defect depends on the subunit affected and the degree to which hemoglobin production is affected. Symptoms range from absent to severe. Patients with α-thalassemia produce reduced amounts of the α subunit, whereas patients with β-thalassemia produce reduced amounts of the β subunit. The formation of hemoglobin with abnormal subunit composition can alter the red cell membrane and lead to variable degrees of hemolysis as well as ineffective hematopoiesis. The latter can result in hypertrophy of the bone marrow and often an abnormal skeleton. *Maxillary hypertrophy* may make tracheal intubation difficult. Thalassemias are most common in patients of Southeast Asian, African, Mediterranean, and Indian ancestry.

What is hemoglobin C disease?

Substitution of lysine for glutamic acid at position 6 on the β subunit results in hemoglobin C (HbC). Approximately 0.05% of Black Americans carry the gene for HbC. Patients homozygous for HbC generally have only mild hemolytic anemia and splenomegaly and rarely develop significant complications. The tendency for HbC to crystallize in hypertonic environments is probably responsible for the hemolysis and characteristically produces *target cells* on the peripheral blood smear.

What is the significance of the genotype HbSC?

Nearly 0.1% of Black Americans are simultaneously heterozygous for both HbS and HbC (HbSC). These patients generally have mild to moderate hemolytic anemia. Some patients occasionally have painful crises, splenic infarcts, and hepatic dysfunction. Eye manifestations similar to those associated with HbSS disease are particularly prominent. Women with HbSC have a high rate of complications during the third trimester of pregnancy and delivery.

What is hemoglobin E?

Hemoglobin E is the result of a single substitution on the β chain and is the second most common hemoglobin variant worldwide. It is most often encountered in patients from Southeast Asia. Although oxygen-binding affinity is normal, the substitution impairs the production of β chains (similar to β-thalassemia). Homozygous patients have marked microcytosis and prominent target cells, but usually they are not anemic and lack any other manifestations.

What is the hematologic significance of glucose-6-phosphate dehydrogenase (G6PD) deficiency?

RBCs are normally well protected against oxidizing agents. The sulfhydryl groups on hemoglobin are protected by reduced glutathione. The latter is regenerated by NADPH (reduced nicotinamide adenine dinucleotide phosphate), which itself is regenerated by glucose metabolism in the hexose monophosphate shunt. G6PD is a critical enzyme in this pathway. A defect in this pathway results in an inadequate amount of reduced glutathione, which can potentially result in the oxidation and precipitation of hemoglobin in red cells (seen as *Heinz bodies*) and hemolysis.

Abnormalities in G6PD are relatively common, with over 400 variants described. Clinical manifestations are variable, depending on the functional significance of the enzyme abnormality. Up to 15% of Black American males have the common, clinically significant A^- variant. A second variant is common in individuals of eastern Mediterranean ancestry, and a third is found in individuals of Chinese ancestry. Because the locus for the enzyme is on the X chromosome, abnormalities are X-linked traits, with males being primarily affected. G6PD activity decreases as RBCs age; therefore, aging red cells are most susceptible to oxidation. This decay is markedly accelerated in patients with the Mediterranean variant, but only moderately so in patients with the A^- variant.

Most patients with G6PD deficiency are not anemic but can develop hemolysis following stresses such as viral and bacterial infections or after the administration of certain drugs (Table 51–8). Hemolytic episodes can be precipitated by metabolic acidosis (eg, diabetic ketoacidosis) and may present with hemoglobinuria and hypotension. Such episodes are generally self-limited because only the older population of RBCs is destroyed. Mediterranean variants may be associated with chronic hemolytic anemia of varying severity and may include the classic feature of marked sensitivity to fava beans.

Management of G6PD deficiency is primarily preventive, avoiding factors known to promote or exacerbate hemolysis. Measures aimed at preserving kidney function (see above) are indicated in patients who develop hemoglobinuria.

TABLE 51–8 Drugs to avoid in patients with G6PD[1] deficiency.

Drugs that may cause hemolysis
Sulfonamides
Antimalarial drugs
Nitrofurantoin
Nalidixic acid
Probenecid
Aminosalicylic acid
Phenacetin
Acetanilid
Ascorbic acid (in large doses)
Vitamin K
Methylene blue
Quinine[2]
Quinidine[3]
Chloramphenicol
Penicillamine
Dimercaprol
Other drugs
Prilocaine
Nitroprusside

[1]G6PD, glucose-6-phosphate dehydrogenase.
[2]May be safe in patients with A^- variant.
[3]Should be avoided because of potential to cause methemoglobinemia.

SUGGESTED READINGS

Abboud MR. Standard management of sickle cell disease complications. *Hematol Oncol Stem Cel Ther.* 2020;13:85.

Abeysiri S, Chau M, Richards T. Perioperative anemia management. *Semin Thromb Hemost.* 2020;46:8.

Avery P, Morton S, Tucker H, et al. Whole blood transfusion versus component therapy in adult trauma patients with acute major haemorrhage. *Emerg Med J.* 2020;37:370.

Bariteau CM, Bochey P, Lindholm PF. Blood transfusion utilization in hospitalized COVID-19 patients. *Transfusion.* 2020;60:1919.

Boer C, Bossers SM, Koning NJ. Choice of fluid type: physiological concepts and perioperative indications. *Br J Anaesth.* 2018;120:384.

Bolcato M, Russo M, Trentino K, et al. Patient blood management: the best approach to transfusion medicine risk management. *Transfus Apher Sci.* 2020;59:102779.

Bulman J, Chacko B. What is the best fluid type for management of patients with an identified acute kidney injury? *Clin Nephrol.* 2019;91:269.

Cap AP, Beckett A, Benov A, et al. Whole blood transfusion. *Mil Medicine.* 2018;183 Suppl:44.

Cappy P, Candotti D, Sauvage V, et al. No evidence of SARS-CoV-2 transfusion transmission despite RNA detection in blood donors showing symptoms after donation. *Blood.* 2020;136:1888.

Cohen T, Haas T, Cushing MM. The strengths and weaknesses of viscoelastic testing compared to traditional coagulation testing. *Transfusion.* 2020;60 Suppl 6:S2.

DeLoughery TG. Transfusion replacement strategies in Jehovah's Witnesses and others who decline blood products. *Clin Adv Hematol Oncol.* 2020;18:826.

Fellahi JL, Futier E, Vaisse C, et al. Perioperative hemodynamic optimization: from guidelines to implementation-an experts' opinion paper. *Ann Intensive Care.* 2021;11:58.

Franchini M, Mannuccio Mannucci P. The never ending success story of tranexamic acid in acquired bleeding. *Haematologica.* 2020;105:1201.

Gordon D, Spiegel R. Fluid resuscitation: history, physiology, and modern fluid resuscitation strategies. *Emerg Med Clin North Am.* 2020;38:783.

Grottke O, Mallaiah S, Karkouti K, et al. Fibrinogen supplementation and its indications. *Semin Thromb Hemost.* 2020;46:38.

Harada M, Ko A, Barmparas G, et al. 10-Year trend in crystalloid resuscitation: reduced volume and lower mortality. *Int J Surg.* 2017;38:78.

Hervig TA, Doughty HA, Cardigan RA, et al. Re-introducing whole blood for transfusion: considerations for blood providers. *Vox Sang.* 2021;116:167.

Hoorn E. Intravenous fluids: balancing solutions. *J Nephrol.* 2017;30:385.

Joosten A, Coeckelenbergh S, Alexander B, et al. Hydroxyethyl starch for perioperative goal-directed fluid therapy in 2020: a narrative review. *BMC Anesthesiol.* 2020;20:209.

Lin SY, Chang YL, Yeh HC. Blood transfusion and risk of venous thromboembolism. A population-based cohort study. *Thromb Haemost.* 2020;120:156.

Lippi G, Favolaro EJ, Buoro S. Platelet transfusion thresholds: how low can we go in respect to platelet counting? *Semin Thromb Hemost.* 2020;46:238.

MacDonald N, Pearse RM. Are we close to the ideal intravenous fluid? *Br J Anaesth.* 2017;119:i63.

Makaryus R, Miller TE, Gan TJ. Current concepts of fluid management in enhanced recovery pathways. *Br J Anaesth.* 2018;120:376.

Malbrain MLNG, Langer T, Annane D, et al. Intravenous fluid therapy in the perioperative and critical care setting: executive summary of the International Fluid Academy (IFA). *Ann Intens Care.* 2020;10:64.

McSorley ST, Tham A, Dolan RD, et al. Perioperative blood transfusion is associated with postoperative systemic inflammatory response and poorer outcomes following surgery for colorectal cancer. *Ann Surg Oncol.* 2020;27:833.

Meneses E, Boneva D, McKenney M, Elkbuli A. Massive transfusion protocol in adult trauma population. *Am J Emerg Med.* 2020;38:2661.

Meyhoff TS, Møller MH, Hjortrup PB, et al. Lower vs higher fluid volumes during initial management of sepsis: a systematic review with meta-analysis and trial sequential analysis. *Chest.* 2020;157:1478.

Nederpelt CJ, Hechi EI, Kongkaewpaisan N, et al. Fresh frozen plasma-to-packed red blood cell ratio and mortality in traumatic hemorrhage: nationwide analysis of 4,427 patients. *J Am Coll Surg.* 2020;230:893.

Pau AK, Aberg J, Baker J, et al. Convalescent plasma for the treatment of COVID-19: perspectives of the National Institutes of Health COVID_19 Treatment Guidelines Panel. *Ann Intern Med.* 2021;174:93.

Prodger CF, Rampotas A, Estcourt LJ. Platelet transfusion: alloimmunization and refractoriness. *Semin Hematol.* 2020;57:92.

Puckett J, Pickering J, Palmer S, et al. Low versus standard urine output targets in patients undergoing major abdominal surgery. A randomized noninferiority trial. *Ann Surg*. 2017;265:874.

Rasmussen KC, Secher NH, Pedersen T. Effect of perioperative crystalloid or colloid fluid therapy on hemorrhage, coagulation competence, and outcome. A systematic review and stratified meta-analysis. *Medicine*. 2016;95:311(e4498).

Rollins KE, Lobo DN. Intraoperative goal-directed fluid therapy in elective major abdominal surgery: a meta-analysis of randomized controlled trials. *Ann Surg*. 2016;263:465.

Salinas Cisneros G, Thein SL. Recent advances in the treatment of sickle cell disease. *Front Physiol*. 2020;11:435.

Seifter J, Change HY. Extracellular acid-base balance and ion transport between body fluid compartments. *Physiology*. 2017;32:367.

Shah A, Stanworth SJ, Docherty AB. Restrictive blood transfusion—is less really more? *Anaesthesia*. 2020:75:433.

Shoemaker WC, Appel P, Bland R. Use of physiologic monitoring to predict outcome and to assist in clinical decisions in critically ill postoperative patients. *Am J Surg*. 1983;146:43.

Solves AP. Platelet transfusion: an update on challenges and outcomes. *J Blood Med*. 2020;11:19.

Thiele T, Greinacher A. Platelet Transfusion in perioperative medicine. *Semin Thromb Hemost*. 2020;46:50.

Tseng CH, Chen TT, Wu MY, et al. Resuscitation fluid types in sepsis, surgical, and trauma patients: a systematic review and sequential network meta-analyses. *Crit Care*. 2020;24:693.

Vlaar AP, Oczkowski S, de Bruin S, et al. Transfusion strategies in non-bleeding critically ill adults: a clinical practice guideline from the European Society of Intensive Care Medicine. *Intensive Care Med*. 2020;46:673.

Wang AS, Dhillon NK, Linaval NT, et al. The impact of IV electrolyte replacement on the fluid balance of critically ill surgical patients. *Am Surg*. 2019;85:1171.

Wise R, Faurie M, Mailbrain M, et al. Strategies for intravenous fluid resuscitation in trauma patients. *World J Surg*. 2017;41:1170.

Xu Y, Wang S, He L, et al. Hydroxyethyl starch 130/0.4 for volume replacement therapy in surgical patients: a systematic review and meta-analysis of randomized controlled trials. *Perioper Med* (Lond). 2021;10:16.

CHAPTER 52

Thermoregulation, Hypothermia, & Malignant Hyperthermia

KEY CONCEPTS

1. When there is no attempt to actively warm an anesthetized patient, core temperature usually decreases 1°C to 2°C during the first hour of general anesthesia (phase one), followed by a more gradual decline during the ensuing 3 to 4 h (phase two), eventually reaching a point of steady state.

2. In the normal, unanesthetized patient, the hypothalamus maintains core body temperature within very narrow tolerances, termed the *interthreshold range*, with the threshold for sweating and vasodilation at one extreme and the threshold for vasoconstriction and shivering at the other.

3. Anesthetics inhibit central thermoregulation by interfering with these hypothalamic reflex responses.

4. Postoperative hypothermia should be treated with a forced-air warming device, if available; alternatively, warming lights or heating blankets can be used to restore body temperature to normal.

5. Nearly 50% of patients who experience an episode of malignant hyperthermia (MH) have had at least one previous uneventful exposure to anesthesia, during which they received a recognized triggering agent. Why MH fails to occur after every exposure to a triggering agent is unclear.

6. The earliest signs of MH during anesthesia include muscle rigidity, tachycardia, unexplained hypercarbia, and increased temperature.

7. Susceptibility to MH may be increased in several musculoskeletal diseases. These include central-core disease, multi-minicore myopathy, and King–Denborough syndrome.

8. Treatment of an MH episode is directed at terminating the episode and treating complications such as hyperthermia and acidosis. The mortality rate for MH, even with prompt treatment, ranges from 5% to 30%. First and most importantly, the triggering agent must be stopped; second, dantrolene must be given immediately.

9. Dantrolene, a hydantoin derivative, directly interferes with muscle contraction by inhibiting calcium ion release from the sarcoplasmic reticulum. The dose is 2.5 mg/kg intravenously every 5 min until the episode is terminated (upper limit, 10 mg/kg). Dantrolene should be continued for 24 h after initial treatment.

10. Propofol, etomidate, benzodiazepines, ketamine, thiopental, methohexital, opiates, droperidol, nitrous oxide, nondepolarizing muscle relaxants, and all local anesthetics are safe for use in MH-susceptible patients.

THERMOREGULATION & HYPOTHERMIA

Anesthesia and surgery predispose patients to **hypothermia,** usually defined as a body temperature less than 36°C. Unintentional perioperative hypothermia is more common in patients at the extremes of age and in those undergoing abdominal surgery or procedures of long duration, especially with cold ambient operating room temperatures; it will occur in nearly every such patient unless steps are taken to prevent this complication.

Hypothermia (in the absence of shivering) reduces metabolic oxygen requirements and can be protective during cerebral or cardiac ischemia. **Nevertheless, hypothermia has multiple deleterious physiological effects (Table 52–1).** In fact, unintended perioperative hypothermia has been associated with an increased mortality rate.

Core temperature is normally the same as the central venous blood temperature (except during periods of relatively rapid temperature change as can occur during and after extracorporeal perfusion).

1 When there is no attempt to actively warm an anesthetized patient, core temperature usually decreases 1°C to 2°C during the first hour of general anesthesia (phase one), followed by a more gradual decline during the ensuing 3 to 4 h (phase two), eventually reaching a point of steady state (phase three). With general, epidural, or spinal anesthesia, most of the initial decrease in temperature during phase one is explained by redistribution of heat from warm "central" compartments (eg, abdomen, thorax) to cooler peripheral tissues (eg, arms, legs) from anesthetic-induced vasodilation. This initial heat loss can be greatly reduced by warming the patient preoperatively. Actual heat loss from the patient to the environment is a minor contributor.

TABLE 52–1 Deleterious effects of hypothermia.

Cardiac arrhythmias and ischemia
Increased peripheral vascular resistance
"Left shift" of the hemoglobin–oxygen saturation curve
Reversible coagulopathy (platelet dysfunction)
Increased postoperative protein catabolism and stress response
Altered mental status
Impaired renal function
Delayed drug metabolism
Impaired wound healing
Increased risk of infection

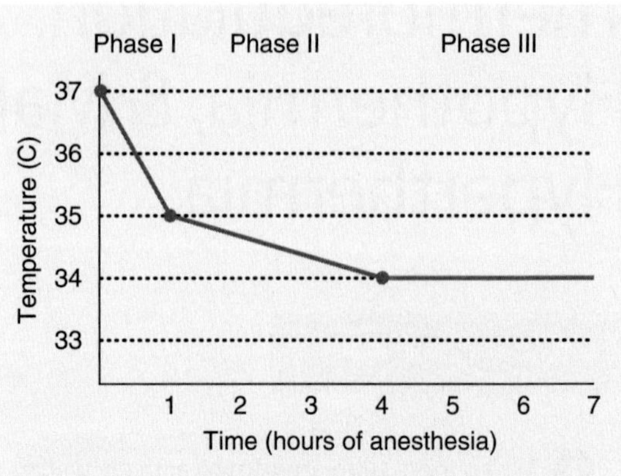

FIGURE 52–1 Unintentional hypothermia during general anesthesia follows a typical pattern: a steep drop in core temperature during the first hour (phase one, redistribution), followed by a gradual decline during the next 3 to 4 h (phase two, heat loss), eventually reaching a steady state (phase three).

Continuous heat loss to the environment is the primary driver for the slower decline during phase two. At steady state, heat loss equals metabolic heat production (Figure 52–1).

2 In the normal unanesthetized patient, the hypothalamus maintains core body temperature within very narrow tolerances, termed the *interthreshold range,* with the threshold for sweating and vasodilation at one extreme and the threshold for vasoconstriction and shivering at the other. Increasing core temperature a fraction of a degree induces sweating and vasodilation, whereas a minimally reduced core temperature triggers vasoconstriction and shivering. 3 Anesthetic agents inhibit central thermoregulation by interfering with these hypothalamic reflex responses. For example, isoflurane produces a concentration-dependent decrease in the threshold temperature that triggers vasoconstriction (3°C decrease for each percent of inhaled isoflurane). Both general and neuraxial anesthetics increase the interthreshold range, albeit by different mechanisms. Spinal and epidural anesthetics, like general anesthetics, lead to

hypothermia by causing vasodilation and internal redistribution of heat. The thermoregulatory impairment from conduction anesthesia that allows continued heat loss is likely also due to altered perception by the hypothalamus of temperature in the anesthetized dermatomes.

Preoperative Considerations

Prewarming the patient for half an hour with convective, forced-air warming blankets reduces the phase one decline in core temperature by reducing the central–peripheral temperature gradient.

Intraoperative Considerations

A cold ambient temperature in the operating room, prolonged exposure of a large wound, and the use of large amounts of room-temperature intravenous fluids or high flows of unhumidified gases can contribute to hypothermia. Methods to minimize phase two heat loss during anesthesia include the use of forced-air warming blankets and warm-water blankets, heated humidification of inspired gases, warming of intravenous fluids, and increasing ambient operating room temperature. Passive insulators such as heated cotton blankets or so-called space blankets have limited utility unless the entire body is covered.

Postoperative Considerations

Shivering can occur in postanesthesia care units (PACUs) or critical care units as a result of actual hypothermia or neurological aftereffects of general anesthetic agents. Shivering is also common immediately postpartum. Shivering in such instances represents the body's effort to increase heat production and raise body temperature and may be associated with intense vasoconstriction. Emergence from even brief general anesthesia is sometimes also associated with shivering. Although shivering can be part of nonspecific neurological signs (posturing, clonus, the Babinski sign) sometimes observed during emergence, shivering is typically associated with hypothermia, longer durations of surgery, and the use of greater concentrations of volatile anesthetics. Occasionally, shivering is intense enough to cause hyperthermia (38°C–39°C) and metabolic acidosis, both of which promptly resolve when the shivering stops. Both spinal and epidural anesthesia lower the shivering threshold and vasoconstrictive response to hypothermia; shivering may also be encountered in the PACU following regional anesthesia. Other causes of shivering should be excluded, such as sepsis, drug allergy, or a transfusion reaction. Intense shivering may increase oxygen consumption, carbon dioxide (CO_2) production, and cardiac output. These physiological effects are often poorly tolerated by patients with preexisting cardiac or pulmonary impairment.

Postoperative shivering may increase oxygen consumption as much as fivefold, decrease arterial oxygen saturation, and be associated with an increased risk of myocardial ischemia. Although postoperative shivering can be effectively treated with small intravenous doses of meperidine (12.5–25 mg) in adults, the better option is to reduce the likelihood of shivering by maintaining normothermia. Shivering in intubated and mechanically ventilated patients can also be controlled with sedation and a muscle relaxant pending normothermia and dissipation of all effects of anesthesia.

4 Postoperative hypothermia should be treated with a forced-air warming device, if available; alternatively, warming lights or heating blankets can be used. In addition to an increased incidence of myocardial ischemia, hypothermia has been associated with arrhythmias, hypertension, impaired hemostasis and increased transfusion requirements, increased incidence of surgical site infections, prolonged PACU stay, and increased duration of muscle relaxant effects, the last of which can be especially harmful to the recently extubated patient.

MALIGNANT HYPERTHERMIA

Malignant hyperthermia (MH) is a rare (1:15,000 in pediatric patients and 1:40,000 in adult patients) genetic hypermetabolic muscle disease, the characteristic phenotypical signs and symptoms of which most commonly appear with exposure to inhaled general anesthetics or succinylcholine (triggering agents). MH may occasionally present more than an hour after emergence from an anesthetic and rarely may occur without exposure to known triggering agents. Most cases have been reported in young males; almost none have been reported in infants, and few have been reported in the older adult population. Nevertheless, all ages and both sexes may be affected. The incidence of MH susceptibility varies greatly from country to country and even among different geographic localities within the same country, reflecting varying gene pools. The upper Midwest appears to have the greatest prevalence of MH susceptibility in the United States.

Pathophysiology

A halogenated anesthetic agent alone may trigger an episode of MH (Table 52–2). In many of the early reported cases, both succinylcholine and a halogenated anesthetic agent were used, and so-called masseter muscle rigidity was observed. However, succinylcholine is less frequently used in modern practice, and about half of the cases in the past decade were associated with a volatile anesthetic as the only triggering agent. Whether succinylcholine is a trigger in the absence of a volatile agent is now controversial.

5 Nearly 50% of patients who experience an episode of MH have had at least one previous uneventful exposure to anesthesia, during which they received a recognized triggering agent. Why MH fails to occur after every exposure to a triggering agent is unclear. Investigations into the biochemical causes of MH susceptibility reveal an uncontrolled increase in intracellular calcium in skeletal muscle. The sudden release of calcium from the sarcoplasmic reticulum removes the inhibition of troponin, resulting in sustained muscle contraction. Markedly increased adenosine triphosphatase activity results in an uncontrolled hypermetabolic state with greatly increased oxygen consumption and CO_2 production, producing severe lactic acidosis and hyperthermia.

Most patients with an episode of MH have relatives who have had a similar episode or who have an abnormal halothane–caffeine contracture test (see later discussion). The complexity of genetic inheritance patterns in families reflects the fact that MH can be associated with a variety of different mutations. The major focus of investigations into the genetic mechanisms of MH has been on the gene for the ryanodine (Ryr_1) receptor, located on chromosome 19. Ryr_1 is a calcium channel responsible for calcium release from the sarcoplasmic reticulum, and it plays an important role in muscle depolarization. Most families in which there is susceptibility to MH harbor one of the known mutations of Ryr_1.

TABLE 52–2 Drugs known to trigger malignant hyperthermia.

Inhaled general anesthetics
Ether
Halothane
Methoxyflurane
Enflurane
Isoflurane
Desflurane
Sevoflurane
Depolarizing muscle relaxant
Succinylcholine

Clinical Manifestations

6 The earliest signs of MH during anesthesia include muscle rigidity, tachycardia, unexplained hypercarbia, and increased temperature (Table 52–3). Two or more of these signs greatly

TABLE 52–3 Signs of malignant hyperthermia.

Markedly increased metabolism
Increased carbon dioxide production
Increased oxygen consumption
Reduced mixed venous oxygen tension
Metabolic acidosis
Cyanosis
Mottling
Increased sympathetic activity
Tachycardia
Hypertension
Arrhythmias
Muscle damage
Masseter spasm
Generalized rigidity
Increased serum creatine kinase
Hyperkalemia
Hypernatremia
Hyperphosphatemia
Myoglobinemia
Myoglobinuria
Hyperthermia
Fever
Sweating

increase the likelihood that the clinical signs are the result of MH. The hypercarbia (due to increased CO_2 production) results in tachypnea when the patient is breathing spontaneously. Overactivity of the sympathetic nervous system produces tachyarrhythmias, hypertension, and mottled cyanosis. Hyperthermia may be an early sign, and when it occurs, core temperature can rise as much as 1°C every 5 min. Generalized muscle rigidity is not always present. Hypertension may be rapidly followed by hypotension and cardiac depression. Dark-colored urine typically identifies myoglobinuria.

Laboratory testing typically reveals mixed metabolic and respiratory acidosis with a marked base deficit, hyperkalemia, hypermagnesemia, and reduced mixed-venous oxygen saturation. Some case reports describe isolated respiratory acidosis early in the course of an episode of MH. Serum ionized calcium concentration is variable: It may initially increase and then later decrease. Patients typically have increased serum myoglobin, creatine kinase (CK), lactic dehydrogenase, and aldolase levels. When peak serum CK levels (the maximum is usually measured 12–18 h after anesthesia) exceed 20,000 IU/L, the diagnosis is strongly suspected. It should be noted that succinylcholine administration to some patients without MH may cause serum myoglobin and CK levels to increase markedly.

Much of the problem in diagnosing MH arises from its variable presentation. An unanticipated doubling or tripling of end-tidal CO_2 (in the absence of a ventilatory change) is an early and sensitive indicator of MH. If the patient survives the initial presentation, acute kidney failure and disseminated intravascular coagulation (DIC) can rapidly ensue. Other complications of MH include cerebral edema with seizures and hepatic failure. Most MH deaths from DIC and organ failure arise from delayed or no treatment with dantrolene.

7 Susceptibility to MH may be increased in several musculoskeletal diseases, including central-core disease, multi-minicore myopathy, and King–Denborough syndrome. Duchenne and other muscular dystrophies, nonspecific myopathies, heatstroke, and osteogenesis imperfecta have been associated with MH-like symptoms in some reports; however, their association with MH is controversial. Other possible clues to susceptibility include a family history of anesthetic complications or a history of unexplained fevers or muscular cramps. There are several reports of MH episodes occurring in patients with a history of exercise-induced rhabdomyolysis. Prior uneventful anesthetics and the absence of a positive family history are notoriously unreliable predictors of lack of susceptibility to MH. Any patient who develops masseter muscle rigidity during induction of anesthesia should be considered potentially susceptible to MH.

Intraoperative Considerations

8 Treatment of an MH episode is directed at terminating the episode and treating complications such as hyperthermia and acidosis. The mortality rate for MH, even with prompt treatment, ranges from 5% to 30%. Table 52–4 illustrates a standard protocol for the management of MH.

A. Acute Treatment Measures

First and most importantly, volatile agents and succinylcholine must be discontinued immediately. Even trace amounts of anesthetics released from soda lime, breathing tubes, and breathing bags may be detrimental. The patient should be hyperventilated

TABLE 52–4 Protocol for immediate treatment of malignant hyperthermia.

1. Discontinue volatile anesthetic and succinylcholine. Notify the surgeon. Call for help.
2. Mix dantrolene sodium with sterile distilled water, and administer 2.5 mg/kg intravenously as soon as possible.
3. Administer bicarbonate for metabolic acidosis.
4. Institute cooling measures (lavage, cooling blanket, cold intravenous solutions).
5. Treat severe hyperkalemia with dextrose, 25–50 g intravenously, and regular insulin, 10–20 units intravenously (adult dose).
6. Administer antiarrhythmic agents if needed despite correction of hyperkalemia and acidosis.
7. Monitor end-tidal CO_2 tension, electrolytes, blood gases, creatine kinase, serum myoglobin, core temperature, urinary output and color, and coagulation status.
8. If necessary, consult on-call physicians at the 24-hour MHAUS hotline, **1-800-644-9737**.

Data from the MHAUS protocol available at https://www.mhaus.org/healthcare-professionals/mhaus-recommendations/.

with 100% oxygen to counteract the effects of uncontrolled CO_2 production and increased oxygen consumption.

B. Dantrolene Therapy

The mainstay of therapy for MH is the immediate administration of intravenous dantrolene. Its safety and efficacy mandate its immediate use in this 9 potentially life-threatening situation. Dantrolene interferes with muscle contraction by binding the Ryr_1 receptor channel and inhibiting calcium ion release from the sarcoplasmic reticulum. The dose is 2.5 mg/kg intravenously every 5 min until the episode is terminated (upper limit, 10 mg/kg). "Conventional" dantrolene is packaged as 20 mg of lyophilized powder to be dissolved in 60 mL of sterile water, and thus reconstitution of the initial dose can be unavoidably time consuming. A new, more costly formulation is available in which 250 mg can be reconstituted in 5 mL, making it an attractive option for the "initial" dose of dantrolene given as an emergency treatment when MH is first diagnosed (Table 52–5). The effective half-life of dantrolene is about 6 h.

After initial control of symptoms, 1 mg/kg of dantrolene intravenously is recommended every 6 h for 24 to 48 h to prevent relapse (MH can recur within 24 h of an initial episode). Dantrolene is also used to decrease temperature in patients with thyroid "storm" and neuroleptic malignant syndrome. When given chronically for spastic disorders, it has been associated with hepatic dysfunction. The most serious complication following acute administration is generalized muscle weakness, possibly with respiratory insufficiency or aspiration pneumonia. Dantrolene can cause phlebitis and should be given through a central venous line if one is available. Following administration of dantrolene, most patients revert to normal acid–base status promptly and require no further pharmacological treatment.

TABLE 52–5 Dantrolene formulations.

Revonto	Ryanodex
One vial contains 20 mg	One vial contains 250 mg
Mix with 60 mL sterile water	Mix with 5 mL sterile water
Contains 3000 mg mannitol	Contains 125 mg mannitol
Solution pH ~9.5	Solution pH ~10.3
Shelf life 3 y	Shelf life 2 y
Cost $62/vial[1]	Cost $2581/vial[1]
Remains on formulary for subsequent treatment doses	Formulary restriction limiting use to initial dose

Personal Communication from Rodney Stiltner, VCU Health System, Richmond, VA; 23 Apr 2018.

C. Correction of Acid–Base/Electrolyte Imbalances

Persisting metabolic acidosis should be treated with intravenous sodium bicarbonate, recognizing that this treatment will worsen the hypercarbia. Hyperkalemia should be treated with glucose, insulin, and diuresis. There is no useful role for intravenous calcium salts in the treatment of MH. Antiarrhythmic agents, vasopressors, and inotropes should be administered if indicated. Calcium channel blockers should not be given to patients receiving dantrolene because this combination appears to promote hyperkalemia. Furosemide may be used to establish diuresis and prevent acute kidney failure, which may develop as a consequence of myoglobinuria. Dantrolene contains a considerable amount of mannitol (3 g per 20-mg bottle); thus, furosemide or bumetanide should be used in preference to mannitol for diuresis.

D. Cooling the Patient

If fever is present, cooling measures should be instituted immediately. Surface cooling with ice packs over major arteries, cold air convection, and cooling blankets are used. Iced saline lavage of the stomach and any open body cavities (eg, in patients undergoing abdominal surgery) should also be instituted. The use of hypothermic cardiopulmonary bypass may be appropriate if other measures fail.

E. Management of the Patient with Isolated Masseter Muscle Rigidity

Masseter muscle rigidity, or trismus, is a forceful contraction of the jaw musculature that prevents full mouth opening. This must be distinguished from incomplete jaw relaxation due to inadequate dosing or inadequate delay after dosing of muscle relaxants. Both myotonia and MH can cause masseter spasm.

The two disorders can be differentiated by the medical history, neurological examination, and electromyography. The historical incidence of masseter muscle rigidity following administration of succinylcholine with halothane to pediatric patients was 1% or more; fortunately, only a small fraction of these patients actually developed MH. Isolated masseter muscle rigidity is now of mostly historical interest given the rare combination of halothane and succinylcholine in current pediatric practice. With masseter muscle spasm but no other sign of MH, most anesthesiologists would allow surgery to proceed using nontriggering anesthetic agents. Elevated serum CK levels after an episode of masseter muscle rigidity may indicate an underlying myopathy.

Postoperative Considerations

A. Confirmation of the Diagnosis

Patients who have survived an unequivocal episode of MH are considered susceptible. If the diagnosis remains in doubt postoperatively, testing is indicated. Baseline CK may be elevated chronically in 50% to 70% of people at risk for MH but is not diagnostic. A halothane-caffeine contracture test will require that a fresh biopsy specimen of living skeletal muscle be exposed to a caffeine, halothane, or combination caffeine–halothane bath. The halothane–caffeine contracture test may have a 10% to 20% false-positive rate, but the false-negative rate is close to zero. Very few centers worldwide perform this test. Genetic testing of patients and first-degree relatives is the more common and much more convenient current approach.

Both European and North American MH registries have been established to help physicians identify and treat patients with suspected MH, as well as provide standardization for diagnosis and testing. The Malignant Hyperthermia Association of the United States (MHAUS, telephone 1-800-986-4287) operates a 24-hour hotline (1-800-644-9737) and a website (http://www.mhaus.org). This website has a frequently updated section on the genetic testing and diagnosis of patients suspected of having MH.

1. Differential diagnosis—Several disorders may superficially resemble MH (Table 52–6). However, MH is associated with greater degrees of metabolic acidosis and venous desaturation than any of these other conditions. In current practice, the most common condition confused with MH is hypercarbia from CO_2 insufflation for laparoscopy. This condition can result in an unexpected increase in end-tidal CO_2 with accompanying tachycardia. Surgery and anesthesia can precipitate thyroid storm in patients with undiagnosed or poorly controlled hyperthyroidism. The signs of thyroid storm include tachycardia, tachyarrhythmias (particularly atrial fibrillation), hyperthermia (often ≥40°C), hypotension, and in some cases, congestive heart failure. In contrast to MH, hypokalemia is very common in thyroid storm. Unlike typical MH, thyroid storm generally develops postoperatively (see Chapter 35). Pheochromocytoma is associated with dramatic increases in heart rate and blood pressure but not with an increase in CO_2 production, end-tidal CO_2, or temperature (see Chapter 35). Cardiac arrhythmias or ischemia may also be prominent. Rarely, such patients may have hyperthermia (>38°C) from catecholamine-mediated increases in metabolic rate together with decreased heat elimination from intense vasoconstriction. Sepsis shares several characteristics with MH, including fever, tachypnea, tachycardia, and metabolic acidosis (see Chapter 57). Sepsis can be difficult to diagnose if there is no obvious primary site of infection.

TABLE 52–6 Differential diagnosis of hyperthermia in the intraoperative and immediate postoperative periods.

Malignant hyperthermia
Neuroleptic malignant syndrome
Thyroid storm
Pheochromocytoma
Drug-induced hyperthermia
Serotonin syndrome
Iatrogenic hyperthermia
Brainstem/hypothalamic injury
Sepsis
Transfusion reaction

Less commonly, drug-induced hyperthermia may be encountered in the perioperative period. In these cases, the drugs appear to markedly increase serotonin activity in the brain, causing hyperthermia, confusion, shivering, diaphoresis, hyperreflexia, and myoclonus. Drug combinations associated with this *serotonin syndrome* include monoamine oxidase inhibitors (MAOIs) and meperidine, and MAOIs and selective serotonin reuptake inhibitors (SSRIs). Hyperthermia can also be caused by some illicit drugs, including 3,4-methylenedioxymethamphetamine (MDMA or "ecstasy"), cocaine, amphetamines, phencyclidine (PCP), and lysergic acid diethylamide (LSD).

Iatrogenic hyperthermia is also a possibility, particularly in pediatric patients. Common sources of excessive heat in the operating room include humidifiers on ventilators, warming blankets, heat lamps, and increased ambient temperature. Injuries to the brainstem, hypothalamus, or nearby regions can be associated with marked hyperthermia.

2. Neuroleptic malignant syndrome—Neuroleptic malignant syndrome (NMS) is characterized by hyperthermia, muscle rigidity with extrapyramidal signs (dyskinesia), altered consciousness, and autonomic lability in patients receiving antidopaminergic agents. The syndrome is caused by an imbalance of neurotransmitters in the central nervous system. It can occur either during drug therapy with antidopaminergic agents (eg, phenothiazines, butyrophenones, thioxanthenes, metoclopramide) or less commonly following the withdrawal of dopaminergic agonists (levodopa or amantadine) in patients with Parkinson disease. Thus, NMS appears to involve abnormal central dopaminergic activity, as opposed to altered peripheral calcium release seen in MH; nondepolarizing relaxants reverse the rigidity of NMS, but not the rigidity associated with MH.

NMS does not appear to be inherited and typically takes hours to weeks to develop; most episodes develop within 2 weeks of a dose adjustment. Hyperthermia generally tends to be mild and appears to be proportional to the amount of rigidity. Autonomic dysfunction results in tachycardia, labile blood pressure, diaphoresis, increased secretions, and urinary incontinence. Muscle rigidity can produce dyspnea and respiratory distress and, together with the increased secretions, can promote aspiration pneumonia. CK levels are typically elevated; some patients may develop rhabdomyolysis resulting in myoglobinemia, myoglobinuria, and acute kidney failure.

Mild forms of NMS promptly resolve after withdrawal of the causative drug (or reinstitution of antiparkinsonian therapy). Initial treatment of more severe forms of NMS should include oxygen therapy and endotracheal intubation for respiratory distress or altered consciousness. Marked muscle rigidity can be controlled with muscle paralysis, dantrolene, or a dopaminergic agonist (amantadine, bromocriptine, levodopa), depending on the severity and acuity of the syndrome. Resolution of the muscle rigidity usually decreases body temperature.

This syndrome is considered a separate entity from MH; nevertheless, some clinicians believe that NMS may predispose patients to MH and recommend that patients with NMS should not receive succinylcholine or a volatile anesthetic. In contrast to patients with NMS, patients susceptible to MH can safely receive phenothiazines.

B. Prophylaxis, Postanesthesia Care, and Discharge

10 Propofol, etomidate, benzodiazepines, ketamine, thiopental, methohexital, opiates, droperidol, nitrous oxide, nondepolarizing muscle relaxants, and all local anesthetics are safe for use in MH-susceptible patients. An adequate supply of dantrolene should always be available wherever general anesthesia is provided. Prophylactic administration of intravenous dantrolene to susceptible patients is not appropriate if a nontriggering anesthetic is administered.

For MH-susceptible patients, the consensus is that the vaporizers should be removed from the anesthesia workstation (or fixed in an "off" position) and the machine should be flushed with 10 L/min of fresh gas (air or oxygen) for at least 5 min. This step should reduce concentrations of volatile anesthetics to less than 1 part per million. Additionally, the CO_2 absorbent and circle system (or other anesthetic circuit) hoses should be changed. **Manufacturers of modern anesthesia machines make differing recommendations (based on the design of their machine) for how to prepare their machines to manage MH-susceptible patients. We strongly**

recommend that the reader review the specific recommendations for the anesthesia machine(s) at their hospital.

MH-susceptible patients who have undergone an uneventful procedure with a nontriggering anesthetic can be discharged from the PACU or ambulatory surgery unit when they meet standard criteria. There are no reported cases of MH-susceptible patients experiencing MH after receiving a nontriggering anesthetic during uneventful surgery.

SUGGESTED READINGS

Arrich J, Holzer M, Havel C, Müllner M, Herkner H. Hypothermia for neuroprotection in adults after cardiopulmonary resuscitation. *Cochrane Database Syst Rev*. 2016;(2):CD004128.

Baldo BA, Rose MA The anaesthetist, opioid analgesic drugs, and serotonin toxicity: a mechanistic and clinical review. *Br J Anaesth*. 2020;124:44.

Campbell G, Alderson P, Smith AF, Warttig S. Warming of intravenous and irrigation fluids for preventing inadvertent perioperative hypothermia. *Cochrane Database Syst Rev*. 2015;(4):CD009891.

De Wel B, Claes KG. Malignant hyperthermia: still an issue for neuromuscular disease? *Curr Opin Neurol*. 2018;31:628.

Dietrich WD, Bramlett HM. Therapeutic hypothermia and targeted temperature management in traumatic brain injury: clinical challenges for successful translation. *Brain Res*. 2016;1640(Pt A):94.

Ellinas H. Albrecht MA. Malignant hyperthermia update. *Anesthesiol Clin*. 2020;38:165.

Galvin IM, Levy R, Boyd JG, Day AG, Wallace MC. Cooling for cerebral protection during brain surgery. *Cochrane Database Syst Rev*. 2015;(1):CD006638.

Maryansky A, Rose JC, Rosenblatt MA, et al. Postoperative hyperthermia and hemodynamic instability in a suspected malignant hyperthermia-susceptible patient: a case report. *Anesth Analg Prac*. 2021;15:e01314.

Sessler DI. Perioperative temperature monitoring. *Anesthesiology*. 2021;134:111.

Sessler DI. Perioperative thermoregulation and heat balance. *Lancet*. 2016;387:2655.

Van Rensburg R, Decloedt EH. An approach to the pharmacotherapy of neuroleptic malignant syndrome. *Psychopharmacol Bull*. 2019;49:84.

WEBSITES

Association of Anaesthetists of Great Britain & Ireland. http://www.aagbi.org/

Malignant Hyperthermia Association of the United States. http://www.mhaus.org/

CHAPTER 53

Nutrition in Perioperative & Critical Care

KEY CONCEPTS

1 The fit, previously well-nourished patient undergoing elective surgery could be fasted for up to a week postoperatively without apparent adverse effect on outcomes, provided that fluid and electrolyte needs are met. On the other hand, it is well established in multiple studies that malnourished patients benefit from nutritional repletion via either enteral or parenteral routes prior to surgery.

2 The indications for total parenteral nutrition (TPN) are narrow, including those patients who cannot absorb enteral solutions (eg, small bowel obstruction, short gut syndrome); partial parenteral nutrition may be indicated to supplement enteral nutrition (EN) when EN cannot fully provide for nutritional needs.

3 TPN will generally require a venous access line with its catheter tip in the superior vena cava. The line or port through which the TPN solution will be infused should be dedicated to this purpose, if at all possible, and strict aseptic techniques should be employed for insertion and care of the catheter.

4 In a patient with critical illness, discontinuing an EN infusion may require multiple potentially dangerous adjustments in insulin infusions and maintenance of intravenous fluid rates. Meanwhile, the evidence is sparse that EN infusions delivered through an appropriately sited gastrointestinal feeding tube increase the risk of aspiration pneumonitis.

5 Regardless of whether the TPN infusion is continued, reduced, replaced with 10% dextrose, or stopped, blood glucose monitoring will be needed during all but short, minor surgical procedures.

Issues related to nutrition tend to be far removed from the usual concerns of the surgical anesthesiologist, other than those related to whether the patient listed for elective surgery has fasted for whatever interval one's institution or colleagues insist upon (this highly controversial issue is also considered in Chapter 19). On the other hand, appropriate nutritional support has been recognized to be of key importance for favorable outcomes in patients with critical illness, a large fraction of whom will require procedural services. Severe malnutrition causes widespread organ dysfunction and increases the risk of perioperative morbidity and mortality. Nutritional repletion may improve wound healing, restore immune competence, and reduce morbidity and mortality rates in critically ill patients. Nutritional support is a key element of an enhanced recovery program (these issues are dealt with in Chapter 48).

This chapter cannot provide a complete review of nutrition for the patient undergoing surgery or with critical illness but rather offers the framework for providing basic nutritional support in such patients. We consider, for example, whether enteral nutrition (EN) or parenteral nutrition (PN) will best meet the needs of an individual patient. This chapter also briefly reviews the conditions under which the ongoing nutritional needs of patients may come into conflict with anesthetic preferences and dogmas, such as the duration that patients must not receive EN before undergoing general anesthesia.

BASIC NUTRITIONAL NEEDS

Maintenance of normal body mass, composition, structure, and function requires intake of water, energy substrates, and specific nutrients. Ions and compounds that cannot be synthesized from other nutrients are characterized as "essential." Relatively few essential nutrients are required to form the thousands of compounds that make up the body. Known essential nutrients include 8 to 10 amino acids, 2 fatty acids, 13 vitamins, and approximately 16 minerals.

Energy is normally derived from dietary or endogenous carbohydrates, fats, and protein. Metabolic breakdown of these substrates yields the adenosine triphosphate required for normal cellular function. Dietary fats and carbohydrates normally supply most of the body's energy requirements. Dietary proteins provide amino acids for protein synthesis; however, when their supply exceeds requirements, amino acids also function as energy substrates. The metabolic pathways of carbohydrate, fat, and amino acid substrates overlap, such that some interconversions can occur (see Figure 33–4). Excess amino acids can be converted to carbohydrate or fatty acid precursors. Excess carbohydrates are stored as glycogen in the liver and skeletal muscle. When glycogen stores are saturated (200–400 g in adults), excess carbohydrate is converted to fatty acids and stored as triglycerides, primarily in fat cells.

During starvation, the protein content of essential tissues is spared. As blood glucose concentration begins to fall during fasting, insulin secretion decreases, and counterregulatory hormones (eg, glucagon) increase. Hepatic and, to a lesser extent, renal glycogenolysis and gluconeogenesis are enhanced. As glycogen supplies are depleted (within 24 h), gluconeogenesis from amino acids becomes increasingly important. Only neural tissue, renal medullary cells, and erythrocytes continue to utilize glucose—in effect, sparing tissue proteins. Lipolysis is enhanced, and fats become the principal energy source. Glycerol from triglycerides enters the glycolytic pathway, and fatty acids are broken down to acetyl coenzyme A (acetyl-CoA). Excess acetyl-CoA results in the formation of ketone bodies (ketosis). Some fatty acids can contribute to gluconeogenesis. If starvation is prolonged, the brain, kidneys, and muscles will also begin to utilize ketone bodies efficiently.

1 The previously well-nourished patient undergoing elective surgery *could* be fasted for up to a week postoperatively, provided fluid and electrolyte needs are met. Whether early postoperative nutritional support influences outcomes likely depends on the extent of preoperative malnutrition, the number of nutrient deficiencies, and the severity of the illness, injury, or surgical procedure. The optimal timing and amount of nutrition support following acute illness remain unknown. On the other hand, malnourished patients, including those experiencing sarcopenia associated with COVID-19, likely benefit from nutritional repletion before and after surgery.

Modern surgical practice has evolved to an expectation of an accelerated ("enhanced") recovery. Enhanced recovery programs generally include early enteral feeding, even in patients undergoing surgery on the gastrointestinal tract, so prolonged periods of postoperative starvation are no longer common practice. Such protocols often specify a carbohydrate drink the night before surgery and again shortly before the operation. Previously well-nourished patients should receive nutritional support after no more than 5 days of postsurgical starvation, and those with ongoing critical illness or severe malnutrition should be given nutritional support immediately. The healing of wounds requires energy, protein, lipids, electrolytes, trace elements, and vitamins. Depletion of any of these substrates may delay wound healing and predispose to complications, such as infection. Nutrient depletion may also delay optimal muscle function, which is important for supporting increased respiratory demands and early mobilization of the patient.

The resting metabolic rate can be measured (but often inaccurately) using indirect calorimetry (known as a metabolic cart) or by estimating energy expenditure using standard nomograms (such as the

Harris–Benedict equation) to approximate the daily energy requirements. Alternatively, a simple and practical approach assumes that patients require 25 to 30 kcal/kg daily. The weight is usually taken as the ideal body weight or adjusted body weight. Thus, obese patients require an estimation of ideal body weight to prevent overfeeding. One determines the daily requirements to ensure that patients are not unnecessarily overfed, recognizing that nutritional requirements can increase greatly above basal levels with certain conditions (eg, burns).

HOW TO FEED THE PATIENT

After total parenteral nutrition (TPN) was established as a feasible approach for feeding patients lacking a functional gut, physicians extended the practice of TPN to many circumstances where "logic" or "clinical experience" suggested that it would be better than EN. In the past, one such indication was acute pancreatitis: In the 1970s, many clinicians thought that a period of TPN would put the gut and pancreas at "rest," allowing for weight gain and resolution of pain. Unfortunately, both "logic" and "clinical experience" were incorrect. Now, the worldwide consensus expressed in clinical practice guidelines is that patients with acute pancreatitis (and indeed all others with functioning guts) will have worse outcomes if TPN is provided rather than EN. **2** Today, the indications for TPN are narrow and include patients who cannot absorb enteral solutions (eg, small bowel obstruction, short gut syndrome).

Partial PN may be indicated to supplement EN when EN cannot fully provide for nutritional needs. In the latter circumstance, recent evidence supports delaying supplemental PN in previously well-nourished patients. Earlier initiation of supplemental PN in previously well-nourished patients, as had been supported in some European guidelines, resulted in worse outcomes in a large randomized clinical trial; however, smaller randomized clinical trials have suggested findings to the contrary. The divergent results from these trials may be associated with the type of parenteral formulations being used, the types of patients being studied, the timing of PN administration, and treatment in the control groups. Thus, further studies are needed to better define patients who may benefit from PN, as well as the optimal timing of nutritional support and formulations for feeding. In short, EN should be the primary mode of nutritional support, and PN should be used when EN is not indicated, not tolerated, or not sufficient.

There was a time when nearly every physician who took care of critically ill patients was in the position of frequently ordering TPN for patients. This is no longer the case, given that EN is now so much more widely employed. As a consequence, many hospitals and health systems insist that a nutrition support team take responsibility for those rarer patients who will receive TPN.

In general, patients with critical illness should undergo whatever initial hemodynamic resuscitation they require before initiation of nutritional support (either EN or PN). Absorption, distribution, and metabolism of nutrients require tissue blood flow, oxygen, and carbon dioxide removal. Adequate tissue blood flow requires an adequately resuscitated patient. Patients with critical illness who require EN will usually require the placement of a feeding tube. Feeding tubes may be placed into the stomach in patients with adequate gastric emptying and a low risk of aspiration. In patients with delayed gastric emptying or those at high risk of aspiration, feeding tubes are best placed into the small intestine. Ideally, the tip of such tubes will be sited within the small intestine, either by the transpyloric placement of a nasoenteral tube or directly into the jejunum (via a percutaneous route) during abdominal surgery, reducing the likelihood of gastric distention and regurgitation. Patients who are unable to eat but require EN over long periods of time will often undergo percutaneous endoscopic placement of gastrostomy (PEG) tubes (the tips of such tubes can be sited distal to the pylorus). One should confirm that the tips of all feeding tubes are appropriately located before initiating feeds to reduce the likelihood that EN solutions will be accidentally infused, say, into the tracheobronchial tree or abdominal cavity.

3 TPN will generally require that a venous access line be placed with the catheter tip in the superior vena cava. PN can be given through a peripheral intravenous catheter but will require larger volumes of fluid (to accommodate the requirement for reduced osmolarity) and will carry an increased risk of phlebitis. The catheter or port through which the TPN solution will be infused should be dedicated to this purpose, if at all possible, and strict aseptic techniques should be employed for insertion and care of the catheter.

COMPLICATIONS OF NUTRITIONAL SUPPORT

Diarrhea is a common problem with EN and may be related to either hyperosmolarity of the solution or lactose intolerance. Gastric distention is another complication that increases the risk of regurgitation and pulmonary aspiration; the use of duodenal or jejunostomy tubes should decrease the likelihood of gastric distention. Complications of TPN are either metabolic or related to central venous access (Table 53–1). Bloodstream infections associated with central and peripheral venous lines remain a major concern, particularly in patients with critical illness and immunocompromised states.

Overfeeding with excess amounts of glucose can increase energy requirements and production of carbon dioxide; the respiratory quotient can be greater than 1 because of lipogenesis. Overfeeding can lead to reversible cholestatic jaundice. Mild elevations of serum transaminases and alkaline phosphatase may reflect fatty infiltration of the liver as a result of overfeeding.

TABLE 53–1 Complications of total parenteral nutrition.

Catheter-related complications
Pneumothorax
Hemothorax
Chylothorax
Hydrothorax
Air embolism
Cardiac tamponade
Thrombosis of central vein
Bloodstream infection
Metabolic complications
Azotemia
Hepatic dysfunction
Cholestasis
Hyperglycemia
Hyperosmolar coma
Diabetic ketoacidosis
Excessive carbon dioxide production
Hypoglycemia (due to interruption of infusion)
Metabolic acidosis or alkalosis
Hypernatremia
Hyperkalemia
Hypokalemia
Hypocalcemia
Hypophosphatemia
Hyperlipidemia
Pancreatitis
Fat embolism syndrome
Anemia
Iron
Vitamin D, K, or B_{12} deficiency
Essential fatty acid deficiency
Hypervitaminosis A
Hypervitaminosis D

SPECIFIC NUTRIENTS

Certain nutrients have been associated with improved outcomes. Surgery and anesthesia are well-recognized inducers of inflammation, producing changes in local (near the wound) and plasma concentrations of neurohormones, cytokines, and other mediators. Many investigators have hypothesized that adverse neurohormonal and inflammatory responses to surgery and anesthesia can be ameliorated through specific diets. Several clinical trials (and a recent meta-analysis) suggest that the addition of "immunomodulating" nutrients (specifically arginine and "fish" oil) to EN may reduce the risk of infection and reduce the length of hospital stay in high-risk surgical patients. Similarly, current guidelines for perioperative PN also advocate the inclusion of n-3 fatty acids. There is some evidence that inclusion of long-chain n-3 polyunsaturated fatty acids (n-3 PUFAs), long-chain monounsaturated fatty acids (found in olive oil), or medium-chain fatty acids may be preferable to the use of solutions (such as soybean-derived lipids) that are rich in longer chain n-6 PUFA. However, such solutions (although widely available outside of the United States) are not approved for use in the United States.

In the past, it was customary to individualize TPN solutions for each patient. There is little evidence that this is necessary, except in patients who cannot handle a sodium load (eg, those with severe heart failure). Adjustments may also be made in patients requiring renal replacement therapy; however, in most cases, this is not necessary. Similarly, except in patients who are already suffering from hepatic encephalopathy, most patients with liver disease can safely receive standard amino acid solutions. Thus, most patients receiving EN and PN can be safely managed with standardized, "off-the-shelf" nutritional formulations. Both EN and PN standardized formulations are available in ready-to-use formats that decrease preparation times, reduce contamination risks during formulation, and are associated with lower costs and similar outcomes to compounded solutions.

ENTERAL NUTRITION & *NIL PER OS* RULES PRIOR TO ELECTIVE SURGERY

Long before the recognition by Mendelsohn of the problem posed by aspiration pneumonitis, anesthesiologists were reluctant to anesthetize patients scheduled for elective surgery if they had not been fasted overnight. Over time, the standard duration of no solid food *per os* has steadily declined, particularly in infants and young children. 4 In a patient with critical illness, discontinuing an EN infusion may require multiple potentially dangerous adjustments in insulin infusions and intravenous fluid rates. Meanwhile, the evidence is sparse that EN infusions delivered through an appropriately sited gastrointestinal feeding tube increase the risk of aspiration pneumonitis. It is also relatively easy to empty the stomach immediately prior to anesthesia and surgery using 5 to 10 min of intermittent suction through a nasogastric tube. Therefore, current guidelines and current published evidence support continuing EN infusions (particularly when they are delivered distal to the pylorus) perioperatively and intraoperatively. Similarly, allowing preoperative patients to consume clear liquids, as desired, up to the time of surgery seems to have no influence on the risk of adverse outcomes from aspiration pneumonitis. Moreover, there is abundant evidence that administering a preoperative carbohydrate "load" to nondiabetic patients shortly before surgery will have the salutary metabolic effect of increasing plasma insulin concentrations, decreasing postoperative insulin resistance, reducing the likelihood of hemodynamic instability, and reducing the likelihood of postoperative nausea or vomiting (see Chapter 48). Such preoperative carbohydrate loading is not nearly as commonplace as we believe it should be.

TPN & SURGERY

Patients who receive TPN often require surgical procedures. Metabolic abnormalities are relatively common and, ideally, should be corrected preoperatively. For example, hypophosphatemia is a serious and often unrecognized complication that can contribute to postoperative muscle weakness and respiratory failure.

When TPN infusions are abruptly stopped or decreased perioperatively, hypoglycemia may develop. Frequent measurements of blood glucose concentration are therefore required in such instances during general anesthesia. Conversely, if the TPN solution is continued unchanged, excessive hyperglycemia resulting in hyperosmolar nonketotic coma or ketoacidosis (in patients with diabetes) is also possible. The neuroendocrine stress response to surgery frequently aggravates glucose intolerance. 5 Regardless of whether the TPN infusion is continued, reduced, replaced with 10% dextrose, or stopped, blood glucose monitoring will be needed during all but short, minor surgical procedures.

GUIDELINES

American Dietetic Association. Critical illness evidence-based nutrition practice guideline. http://www.guidelines.gov/content.aspx?id=12818&search=ada+critical+illness+nutrition

American Society for Parenteral and Enteral Nutrition. http://www.nutritioncare.org/Guidelines_and_Clinical_Resources/Clinical_Guidelines/

European Society for Clinical Nutrition and Metabolism. http://www.espen.org/education/espen-guidelines

SUGGESTED READINGS

De Waele E, Jakubowski JR, Stocker R, Wischmeyer PE. Review of evolution and current status of protein requirements and provision in acute illness and critical care. *Clin Nutr.* 2021;40:2958.

Escuro AA, Hummell AC. Enteral formulas in nutrition support practice: is there a better choice for your patient? *Nutr Clin Pract.* 2016;31:709.

Fukatsu K. Role of nutrition in gastroenterological surgery. *Ann Gastroenterol Surg.* 2019;3:160.

Magee G, Zaloga GP, Turpin RS, Sanon M. A retrospective, observational study of patient outcomes for critically ill patients receiving parenteral nutrition. *Value Health.* 2014;17:328.

Marcotte E, Chand B. Management and prevention of surgical and nutritional complications after bariatric surgery. *Surg Clin North Am.* 2016;96:843.

Patkova A, Joskova V, Havel E, et al. Energy, protein, carbohydrate, and lipid intakes and their effects on morbidity and mortality in critically ill adult patients: a systematic review. *Adv Nutr.* 2017;8:624.

Reintam Blaser A, Starkopf J, Alhazzani W, et al; ESICM Working Group on Gastrointestinal Function. Early enteral nutrition in critically ill patients: ESICM clinical practice guidelines. *Intensive Care Med.* 2017;43:380.

Sandrucci S, Cotogni P, De Zolt Ponte B Impact of artificial nutrition on postoperative complications. *Healthcare* (Basel). 2020;8:559.

Scott M, Martindale R. Perioperative nutrition: a high-impact, low-risk, low-cost intervention. *Anesth Analg.* 2018;126:1803.

Weimann A, Braga M, Carli F, et al. ESPEN guideline: clinical nutrition in surgery. *Clin Nutr.* 2017;36:623.

Wischmeyer PE, Carli F, Evans DC, et al; Perioperative Quality Initiative (POQI) 2 Workgroup. American Society for Enhanced Recovery and Perioperative Quality Initiative joint consensus statement on nutrition screening and therapy within a surgical enhanced recovery pathway. *Anesth Analg.* 2018;126:1883.

Yao H, He C, Deng L, Liao G. Enteral versus parenteral nutrition in critically ill patients with severe pancreatitis: a meta-analysis. *Eur J Clin Nutr.* 2018;72:66.

Yeung SE, Hilkewich L, Gillis C, Heine JA, Fenton TR. Protein intakes are associated with reduced length of stay: a comparison between Enhanced Recovery After Surgery (ERAS) and conventional care after elective colorectal surgery. *Am J Clin Nutr.* 2017;106:44.

Zaloga GP. Parenteral nutrition in adult inpatients with functioning gastrointestinal tracts: Assessment of outcomes. *Lancet.* 2006;367:1101.

CHAPTER

54

Anesthetic Complications

KEY CONCEPTS

1. The likelihood of anesthetic complications will never be zero. All anesthesia practitioners, irrespective of their experience, abilities, diligence, and best intentions, will participate in anesthetics that are associated with patient injury.
2. Malpractice occurs when four requirements have been met: (1) the practitioner must have a duty to the patient; (2) there must have been a breach of duty (deviation from the standard of care); (3) the patient (plaintiff) must have suffered an injury; and (4) the proximate cause of the injury must have been the practitioner's deviation from the standard of care.
3. Anesthetic mishaps can be categorized as preventable or unpreventable. Of the preventable incidents, most involve human error, as opposed to equipment malfunctions.
4. The relative decrease in death attributed to respiratory rather than cardiovascular damaging events has been attributed to the increased use of pulse oximetry and capnometry.
5. Many anesthetic fatalities occur only after a series of coincidental circumstances, misjudgments, and technical errors combine (mishap chain).
6. Despite differing mechanisms, anaphylactic and anaphylactoid reactions are typically clinically indistinguishable and equally life threatening.
7. True anaphylaxis due to anesthetic agents is rare; anaphylactoid reactions are much more common.
8. Patients with spina bifida, spinal cord injury, and congenital abnormalities of the genitourinary tract have a markedly increased incidence of latex allergy. The incidence of latex anaphylaxis in children is estimated to be 1 in 10,000.
9. There is no clear evidence that exposure to trace amounts of anesthetic agents presents a health hazard to operating room personnel; however, the U.S. Occupational Health and Safety Administration continues to set maximum acceptable trace concentrations of less than 25 ppm for nitrous oxide and 0.5 ppm for halogenated anesthetics (2 ppm if the halogenated agent is used alone).
10. Hollow (hypodermic) needles pose a greater risk than do solid (surgical) needles because of the potentially larger inoculum. The use of gloves, needleless systems, and protected needle devices may decrease the incidence of some (but not all) types of injury.
11. Anesthesiology is a high-risk medical specialty for substance abuse.
12. The three most important methods of minimizing radiation doses are limiting total exposure time during procedures, using proper barriers, and maximizing one's distance from the source of radiation.

1 The likelihood of anesthetic complications will never be zero. All anesthesia practitioners, irrespective of their experience, abilities, diligence, and best intentions, will participate in anesthetics that are associated with patient injury. Moreover, unexpected adverse perioperative outcomes can lead to litigation, even if those outcomes did not directly arise from anesthetic mismanagement. This chapter reviews management approaches for complications secondary to anesthesia and discusses medical malpractice and legal issues from an American (U.S.) perspective. Readers based in other countries may not find this section to be as relevant to their practices.

LITIGATION & ANESTHETIC COMPLICATIONS

All anesthesia practitioners will have patients with adverse outcomes, and in the United States, most anesthesiologists will at some point in their career be involved to one degree or another in malpractice litigation. Consequently, anesthesia practitioners should expect litigation to be a part of their professional lives, and they should maintain adequate professional liability insurance with coverage appropriate for the community in which they practice.

When unexpected events occur, anesthesia practitioners must generate an appropriate differential diagnosis, seek any necessary consultation, and execute a treatment plan to mitigate (to the greatest degree possible) any patient injury. Appropriate, contemporaneous documentation in the patient record is critically important as adverse outcomes will be reviewed by quality assurance and performance improvement authorities. Deviations from acceptable practice will likely be noted in the practitioner's quality assurance file. Should an adverse outcome lead to litigation, the medical record documents the practitioner's actions at the time of the incident. Years may pass before litigation proceeds to the point where the anesthesia provider is asked about the case in question. Although memories fade, a clear and complete anesthesia record can provide evidence that a complication was recognized and appropriately treated.

It is often difficult to predict which cases will be pursued by plaintiffs! Litigation may ensue when it is clear (at least to the defense team) that the anesthesia care conformed to standards, and, conversely, a suit may not be filed when there is obvious anesthesia culpability. That said, anesthetics that are followed by unexpected death, paralysis, or brain injury of young, economically productive individuals are particularly attractive to plaintiff's lawyers. When a patient has an unexpectedly poor outcome, one should expect litigation irrespective of one's "positive" relationship with the patient or the injured patient's family or guardians.

2 Malpractice occurs when four requirements are met: (1) the practitioner must have a duty to the patient; (2) there must have been a breach of duty (deviation from the standard of care); (3) the patient (plaintiff) must have suffered an injury; and (4) the proximate cause of the injury must have been the practitioner's deviation from the standard of care. A duty is established when the practitioner has an obligation to provide care (physician–patient relationship). The practitioner's failure to execute that duty constitutes a breach of duty. Injuries can be physical, emotional, or financial. Causation is established if, but for the breach of duty, the patient would not have experienced the injury. When a claim is meritorious, the tort system attempts to compensate the injured patient or family members, or both, by awarding them monetary damages. Being sued is extremely stressful, regardless of the perceived "merits" of the claim.

Preparation for defense begins before an injury has occurred. The patient grants informed consent following a discussion of the risks and benefits of the anesthesia options that are available and reasonable. Informed consent does not consist of handing the patient a form to sign. Informed consent requires that the patient understand the choices being presented. As previously noted, appropriate documentation of patient care activities, differential diagnoses, and therapeutic interventions helps provide a defensible record of the care that was provided, resistant to the passage of time and the stress of the litigation experience.

When an adverse outcome occurs, the hospital or practice risk management group, or both, must be immediately notified. Likewise, one's liability insurance carrier should be notified of the possibility of a claim for damages. Some policies have a clause that disallows the practitioner from admitting errors to patients and families. Consequently, it is important to know and obey the institution's and insurer's approach to adverse outcomes. Nevertheless, most risk managers advocate a frank and honest disclosure of adverse events to patients or approved family members. It is possible to express sorrow about an adverse outcome without admitting "guilt." It may be helpful to have such discussions while accompanied by risk management personnel or a departmental leader.

It must never be forgotten that the tort system is designed to be adversarial. Unfortunately, this makes every patient a potential courtroom adversary. Malpractice insurers will hire a legal defense firm to represent the anesthesia practitioner involved. Typically, multiple practitioners and the hospitals in which they work will be named to involve the maximal number of insurance policies that might pay in the event of a plaintiff's victory and to ensure that the defendants cannot choose to attribute "blame" for the adverse event to whichever person or entity was not named in the suit. In some systems (usually when everyone in a health system is insured by the same carrier), all of the named entities are represented by one defense team. More commonly, various insurers and attorneys represent specific practitioners and institutional providers. In this instance, those involved may deflect and diffuse blame from themselves and focus blame on others also named in the action. *Discovery* is the process by which the plaintiff's attorneys access the medical records and depose witnesses under oath to establish the elements of the case: duty, breach, injury, and causation. False testimony can lead to criminal charges of perjury. One should not discuss elements of any case with anyone other than a risk manager, insurer, or attorney because other conversations are not protected from discovery.

Oftentimes, expediency and financial risk exposure will argue for settlement of the case. The practitioner may or may not be able to participate in this decision depending upon the insurance policy. Settled cases are reported to the National Practitioner Data Bank and become a part of the practitioner's record. Moreover, malpractice suits, settlements, and judgments must be reported to hospital authorities as part of the credentialing process. When applying for licensure or hospital appointment, all such actions must be reported. Failure to do so can lead to adverse consequences.

For a medical defendant, the litigation process begins with the delivery of a summons indicating that an action is pending. Once delivered, the anesthesia defendant must contact their malpractice insurer/risk management department, who will appoint legal counsel. Counsel for both the plaintiff and defense will identify "independent expert consultants" to review the cases. These consultants are paid for their time and expenses and can arrive at dramatically different assessments of the case materials. Following review by expert consultants, the plaintiff's counsel may depose the principal actors involved in the case. Providing testimony will be stressful. Generally, one should follow the advice of one's attorney, who will prepare the practitioner in advance for the deposition and be present during the deposition. Oftentimes, the plaintiff's attorneys will attempt to anger or confuse the deponent, hoping to provoke a response favorable to the claim. Most defense attorneys will advise their clients to answer questions as literally and simply as possible without offering extraneous commentary. Should the plaintiff's attorney become abusive or misleading, the defense attorney will object for the record. However, depositions, also known as "examinations before trial," are not held in front of a judge (only the attorneys, the deponent, the court reporter[s], and sometimes a videographer are present).

Following discovery, the insurers, plaintiffs, and defense attorneys will "value" the case and attempt to monetize the damages. Items, such as pain and suffering, loss of consortium with spouses, lost wages, and many other factors, are included in determining what the injury is worth. Also during this period, the defense attorney may petition the court to grant defendants a "summary judgment," dismissing the defendant from the case if there is no evidence of malpractice elicited during the discovery process. At times, the plaintiff's attorneys will dismiss the suit against certain named individuals after they have testified, particularly when their testimony implicates other named defendants.

Settlement negotiations will occur in nearly every action. Juries are unpredictable, and both parties are often hesitant to take a case to trial. There are expenses associated with litigation, and both plaintiff and defense attorneys will try to avoid uncertainties.

Many anesthesia providers will not want to settle a case because the settlement must be reported. Nonetheless, an award in excess of the insurance policy maximum may (depending on the jurisdiction) place the personal assets of the defendant providers at risk. One should remember that an adverse judgment may arise from a case in which most anesthesiologists would find the care to meet acceptable standards!

When a case proceeds to trial, the first step is jury selection in the process of *voir dire*—from the French—"to see, to say." In this process, attorneys for the plaintiff and defendant will use various profiling techniques to attempt to identify (and remove) jurors who are less likely to be sympathetic to their case, while keeping the jurors deemed most likely to favor their side. Each attorney is able to strike a certain number of jurors from the pool. The jurors will be questioned about such matters as their educational level, history of litigation themselves, professions, and so forth.

Following empanelment, the case is presented to the jury. Each attorney attempts to educate the jurors—who usually have limited knowledge of health care (physicians and nurses will usually be struck from the jury)—as to the standard of care for a particular procedure and how the defendants did or did not breach their duty to the patient to uphold those standards. Expert witnesses will attempt to define what the standard of care is for the community, and the plaintiff and defendant will present experts with views that are favorable to their respective cause. The attorneys will attempt to discredit the opponent's experts and challenge their opinions. Exhibits are often used to explain to the jury what should or should not have happened and why the injuries for which damages are being sought were caused by the practitioner's negligence.

After the attorneys conclude their closing remarks, the judge will "charge" the jurors with their duty and will delineate what they can consider in making their judgment. Once a case is in the hands of a jury, anything can happen. Many cases will settle during the course of the trial, as neither party wishes to be subject to the arbitrary decisions of an unpredictable jury. Should the case not settle, the jurors will reach a verdict. When a jury determines that the defendants were negligent and negligence was the cause of the plaintiff's injuries, the jury will determine an appropriate award. If the award is so egregiously large that it is inconsistent with awards for similar injuries, the judge may reduce its amount. Of course, following any verdict, there are numerous appeals that may be filed. It is important to note that appeals typically do not relate to the medical aspects of the case but are filed because the trial process itself was somehow flawed.

Unfortunately, a malpractice action can take years to reach a conclusion. Consultation with a mental health professional may be appropriate for the defendant when the litigation process results in stress and depression.

Determining what constitutes the "standard of care" is increasingly complicated. In the United States, the definition of "standard of care" is made separately by each state. The standard of care is *not* necessarily "best practices" or even the care that another physician would prefer. Generally, the standard of care is met when a patient receives care that other reasonable physicians in similar circumstances would regard as adequate. The American Society of Anesthesiologists (ASA) has published standards, and these provide a basic framework for routine anesthetic practice (eg, monitoring). Increasingly, a myriad of "guidelines" have been developed by multiple specialty societies to identify best practices in accordance with assessments of the evidence in the literature. The increasing number of guidelines proffered by the numerous anesthesia and other societies and their frequent updating can make it difficult for clinicians to stay abreast of the changing nature of practice. This is a particular problem when two societies produce conflicting guidelines on the same topic using the same data. Likewise, the information upon which guidelines are based can range from randomized clinical trials to the opinion of "experts" in the field. Consequently, guidelines do not hold the same weight as standards. Guidelines produced by reputable societies will generally include an appropriate disclaimer based on the level of evidence used to generate the guideline. Nonetheless, plaintiff's attorneys will attempt to use guidelines to establish a "standard of care," when, in fact, clinical guidelines are prepared to assist in guiding the delivery of therapy. However, if deviation from guidelines is required for good patient care, the rationale for such actions should be documented on the anesthesia record, as plaintiff's attorneys may attempt to use the guideline as a *de facto* standard of care.

ADVERSE ANESTHETIC OUTCOMES

Incidence

There are several reasons why it is difficult to accurately measure the incidence of adverse anesthesia-related outcomes. First, it is often difficult to determine whether a poor outcome arises from the patient's underlying disease, the surgical procedure, or the anesthetic management. In some cases, all three factors contribute to a poor outcome. Clinically important measurable outcomes are relatively rare after elective anesthetics. For example, death is a clear endpoint, and perioperative deaths do occur with some regularity. But, because deaths attributable to anesthesia are much rarer, a very large series of patients must be studied to assemble conclusions that have statistical significance. Nonetheless, many studies have attempted to determine the incidence of complications due to anesthesia. Unfortunately, studies vary in criteria for defining an anesthesia-related adverse outcome and are limited by retrospective analysis.

Perioperative mortality is usually defined as death within 48 h of surgery. It is clear that most perioperative fatalities are due to the patient's preoperative disease or the surgical procedure. In a study conducted between 1948 and 1952, anesthesia mortality in the United States was approximately 5100 deaths per year or 3.3 deaths per 100,000 population. A review of cause of death files in the United States showed that the rate of anesthesia-related deaths was 1.1 out of 1,000,000 population or 1 anesthetic death per 100,000 procedures between 1999 and 2005 (Figure 54–1). These results suggest a 97% decrease in anesthesia mortality since the 1940s. However, a 2002 study reported an estimated rate of 1 death per 13,000 anesthetics. Due to differences in methodology, there are discrepancies in the literature as to how well anesthesiology is doing in achieving safe practice. In a 2008 study of 815,077 patients (ASA class 1, 2, or 3) who underwent elective surgery at U.S. Department of Veterans Affairs hospitals, the

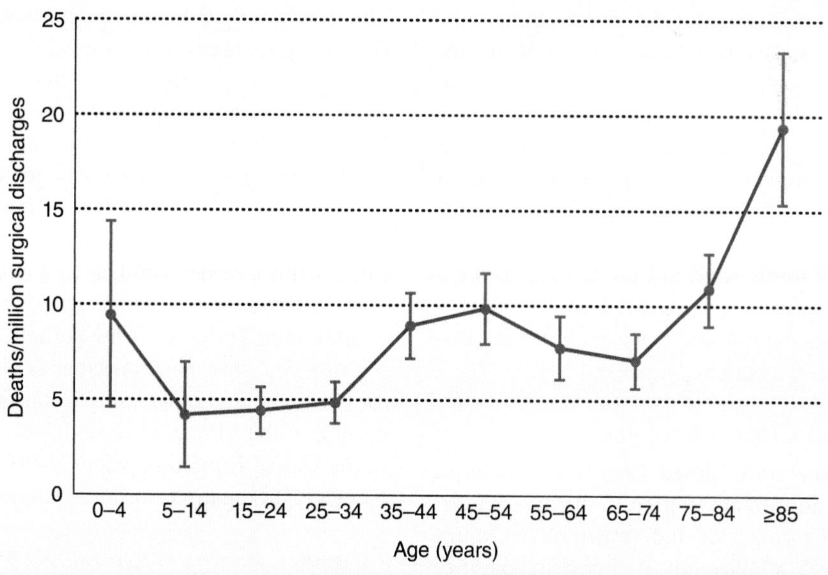

FIGURE 54–1 Annual in-hospital anesthesia-related deaths rates per million hospital surgical discharges and 95% confidence intervals by age, United States, 1999-2005. (Reproduced with permission from Li G, Warner M, Lang B, et al. Epidemiology of anesthesia-related mortality in the United States 1999–2005. Anesthesiology. 2009.) Apr;110(4):759-765.

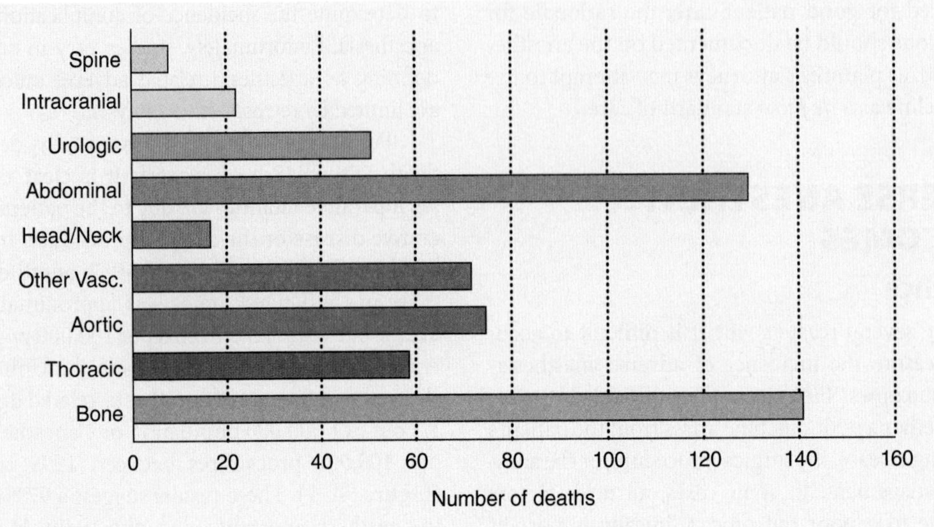

FIGURE 54–2 Total number of deaths by type of surgery in Veterans Affairs hospitals. Vasc., vascular. (Reproduced with permission from Bishop M, Souders J, Peterson C, et al. Factors associated with unanticipated day of surgery deaths in Department of Veterans Affairs hospitals. *Anesth Analg.* 2008 Dec;107(6):1924-1935.)

mortality rate was 0.08% on the day of surgery. The strongest association with perioperative death was the type of surgery (Figure 54–2). Other preoperative factors associated with increased risk of death included dyspnea, reduced albumin concentrations, increased bilirubin, and increased creatinine concentrations. A subsequent review of the 88 deaths that occurred on the surgical day noted that 13 of the patients might have benefitted from better anesthesia care, and estimates suggest that death might have been prevented by better anesthesia practice in 1 of 13,900 cases. Additionally, this study reported that the immediate postsurgical period tended to be the time of unexpected mortality. Indeed, often missed opportunities for improved anesthetic care occur following complications when "failure to rescue" contributes to patient demise.

ASA Closed Claims Project

The goal of the ASA Closed Claims Project is to identify common events leading to claims in anesthesia, patterns of injury, and strategies for injury prevention. It is a collection of closed malpractice claims that provides a "snapshot" of anesthesia liability rather than a study of the incidence of anesthetic complications because only events that lead to the filing of a malpractice claim are considered. The Closed Claims Project consists of trained physicians who review claims against physician anesthesiologists represented by some U.S. malpractice insurers. The number of claims in the database continues to rise each year as new claims are closed and reported. The claims are grouped according to specific damaging events and complication type. Closed Claims Project analyses have been reported for airway injury, nerve injury, awareness, and so forth. These analyses provide insights into the circumstances that result in claims; however, the incidence of a complication cannot be determined from closed claim data because we know neither the actual incidence of the complication (some with the complication may not file suit) nor how many anesthetics were performed for which the particular complication might possibly develop. Other similar analyses have been performed in the United Kingdom, where National Health Service (NHS) Litigation Authority claims are reviewed.

Causes

Anesthetic mishaps can be categorized as preventable or unpreventable. Examples of the

TABLE 54–1 Human errors that may lead to preventable anesthetic accidents.

Unrecognized breathing circuit disconnection
Mistaken drug administration
Airway mismanagement
Anesthesia machine misuse
Fluid mismanagement
Intravenous line disconnection

latter include fatal idiosyncratic drug reactions or any poor outcome that occurs despite proper management. However, studies of anesthetic-related deaths or near misses suggest that many accidents are preventable. Of these preventable incidents, most involve human error (Table 54–1), as opposed to equipment malfunctions (Table 54–2). Unfortunately, some rate of human error is inevitable. During the 1990s, the top three causes for claims in the ASA Closed Claims Project were death (22%), nerve injury (18%), and brain damage (9%). In a 2009 report based on an analysis of NHS litigation records, anesthesia-related claims accounted for 2.5% of total claims filed and 2.4% of the value of all NHS claims. Moreover, regional and obstetrical anesthesia were responsible for 44% and 29%, respectively, of anesthesia-related claims filed. The authors of the latter study noted that there are two ways to examine data related to patient harm: critical incident and closed claim analyses. Clinical (or critical) incident data consider events that either cause harm or result in a "near-miss." Comparison between clinical incident datasets and closed claims analyses demonstrates that not all critical events generate claims and that claims may be filed in the absence of negligent care. Consequently, closed claims reports must always be considered in this context.

TABLE 54–2 Equipment malfunctions that may lead to preventable anesthetic accidents.

Breathing circuit
Monitoring device
Ventilator
Anesthesia machine
Laryngoscope

Situational awareness errors are thought to contribute greatly to patient injury. Situational awareness consists of three elements:

- **Perception** or detection of relevant information
- **Comprehension** or the ability to use perceived information to arrive at a diagnosis
- **Projection** or the ability to predict the patient's clinical course and mitigate any potential harm

A review of closed claims suggests that situational awareness errors contributed to three-fourths of claims for death and brain injury from 2002 to 2013.

MORTALITY & BRAIN INJURY

Trends in anesthesia-related death and brain damage have been tracked for many years. In a Closed Claims Project report examining claims in the period between 1975 and 2000, there were 6750 claims (Figure 54–3A and B), 2613 of which were for brain injury or death. The proportion of claims for brain injury or death was 56% in 1975 but decreased to 27% by 2000. The primary pathological mechanisms by which these outcomes occurred were related to cardiovascular or respiratory problems. Early in the study period, respiratory-related damaging events were responsible for more than 50% of brain injury/death claims, whereas cardiovascular-related damaging events were responsible for 27% of such claims; however, by the late 1980s, the percentage of damaging events related to respiratory issues had decreased, with both respiratory and cardiovascular events being equally likely to contribute to severe brain injury or death. Respiratory damaging events included difficult airway, esophageal intubation, and unexpected extubation. Cardiovascular damaging events were usually multifactorial. Closed claims reviewers found that anesthesia care was substandard in 64% of claims in which respiratory complications contributed to brain injury or death but in only 28% of cases in which the primary mechanism of patient injury was cardiovascular in nature. Esophageal intubation, premature extubation, and inadequate ventilation

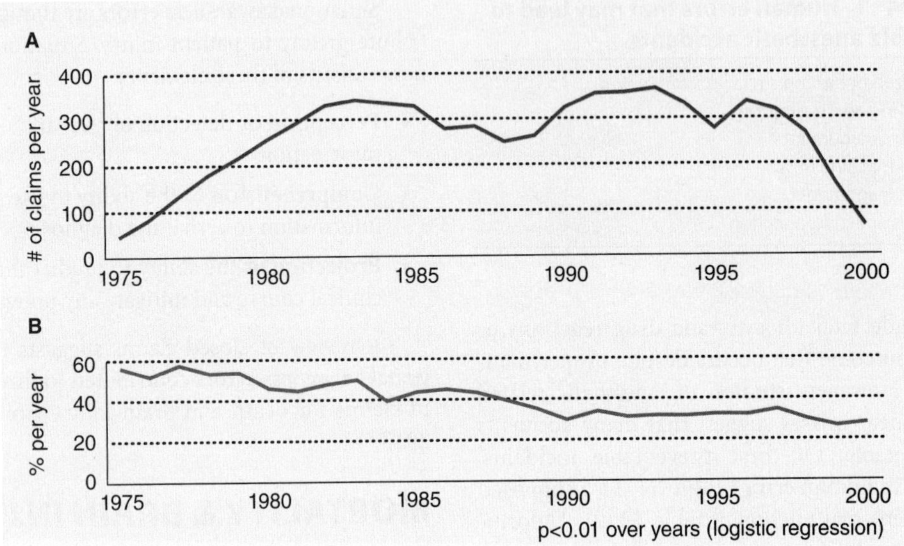

FIGURE 54–3 **A**: The total number of claims by the year of injury. Retrospective data collection began in 1985. Data in this analysis include data collected through December 2003. **B**: Claims for death or permanent brain damage as a percentage of total claims per year by year of injury. (Reproduced with permission from Cheney FW, Domino KB, Caplan RA, Posner KL. Nerve injury associated with anesthesia: A closed claims analysis. *Anesthesiology.* 1999 Apr; 90(4):1062-1069.)

were the primary mechanisms by which less than optimal anesthetic care was thought to have contributed to patient injury related to respiratory events. 4 The relative decrease in causes of death being attributed to respiratory rather cardiovascular damaging events during the review period was attributed to the increased use of pulse oximetry and capnometry. Nevertheless, failure to correctly interpret capnographic readings contributes to failure to detect esophageal intubations. A 2019 review of difficult tracheal intubation claims notes that clinical judgment failures were common and that delays persist in securing a surgical airway in the "can't intubate, can't ventilate" scenario.

A 2010 study examining the NHS Litigation Authority dataset noted that airway-related claims led to higher awards and poorer outcomes than did non–airway-related claims. Indeed, airway manipulation and central venous catheterization claims in this database were most associated with patient death. Trauma to the airway also generates significant claims if esophageal or tracheal rupture occurs. Postintubation mediastinitis should always be considered whenever there are repeated unsuccessful airway manipulations because early intervention presents the best opportunity to mitigate any injuries incurred.

VASCULAR CANNULATION

Claims related to central venous access in the ASA database were associated with patient death 47% of the time and represented 1.7% of the 6449 claims reviewed. Complications secondary to guidewire or catheter embolism, tamponade, bloodstream infections, carotid artery puncture, hemothorax, and pneumothorax all contributed to patient injury. Although guidewire and catheter embolisms typically were associated with less severe patient injuries, these complications were generally attributed to substandard care. Tamponade following line placement often led to a claim for patient death. The authors of a 2004 closed claims analysis recommended reviewing the chest radiograph following line placement and repositioning lines found in the heart or at an acute angle to reduce the likelihood of vascular perforation and tamponade. Brain damage and stroke are associated with claims secondary to carotid cannulation. Multiple confirmatory methods including

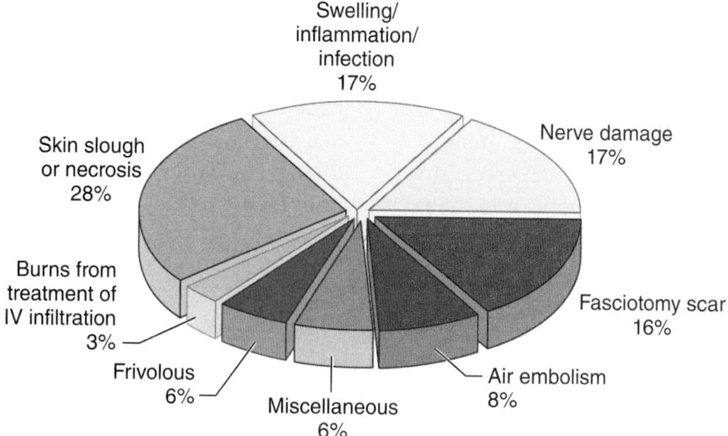

FIGURE 54–4 Injuries related to IV catheters (n = 127). (Reproduced with permission from Bhananker S, Liau D, Kooner P, et al. Liability related to peripheral venous and arterial catheterization: A closed claims analysis. *Anesth Analg.* 2009 July;109(1):124-129.)

ultrasound should be used to ensure that the internal jugular and not the carotid artery is cannulated.

Claims related to peripheral vascular cannulation in the ASA database accounted for 2% of 6849 claims, 91% of which were for complications secondary to the extravasation of fluids or drugs from peripheral intravenous catheters that resulted in extremity injury (Figure 54–4). Air embolisms, infections, and vascular insufficiency secondary to arterial spasm or thrombosis also resulted in claims. Of interest, intravenous catheter claims in patients who had undergone cardiac surgery formed the largest cohort of claims related to peripheral intravenous catheters, most likely due to the usual practice of tucking the arms alongside the patient during the procedure, placing them out of view of the anesthesia providers. Radial artery catheters seem to generate few closed claims; however, femoral artery catheters can lead to greater complications and potentially increased liability exposure.

OBSTETRIC ANESTHESIA

Both critical incident and closed claims analyses have been reported regarding complications and mortality related to obstetrical anesthesia.

In a study reviewing anesthesia-related maternal mortality in the United States using the Pregnancy Mortality Surveillance System, which collects data on all reported deaths causally related to pregnancy, 86 of the 5946 pregnancy-related deaths reported to the Centers for Disease Control and Prevention were thought to be anesthesia related or approximately 1.6% of total pregnancy related-deaths in the period 1991 to 2002. The anesthesia mortality rate in this period was 1.2 per million live births, compared with 2.9 per million live births in the period 1979 to 1990. The decline in anesthesia-related maternal mortality may be secondary to the decreased use of general anesthesia in parturients, reduced doses of bupivacaine in epidurals, improved airway management protocols and devices, and greater use of incremental (rather than bolus) dosing of epidural catheters.

In a 2009 study examining the epidemiology of anesthesia-related complications in labor and delivery in New York State from 2002 to 2005, an anesthesia-related complication was reported in 4438 of 957,471 deliveries (0.5%). The incidence of complications was increased in patients undergoing cesarean section, those living in rural areas, and those with other medical conditions. Complications of neuraxial anesthesia (eg, postdural puncture headache) were most common, followed by systemic complications, including aspiration or cardiac events. Other reported problems were related to anesthetic dose administration and unintended overdosages.

ASA Closed Claims Project analyses were reported in 2009 for the period 1990 to 2003.

Four hundred twenty-six claims from this period were compared with 190 claims in the database prior to 1990. After 1990, the proportion of claims for maternal or fetal demise was lower than that recorded prior to 1990. After 1990, the number of claims for maternal nerve injury increased. In the review of claims in which anesthesia was thought to have contributed to the adverse outcome, anesthesia delay, poor communication, and substandard care were thought to have resulted in poor newborn outcomes. Prolonged attempts to secure neuraxial blockade in the setting of emergency cesarean section can contribute to adverse fetal outcomes. Additionally, the closed claims review indicated that poor communication between the obstetrician and the anesthesiologist regarding the urgency of newborn delivery was likewise thought to have contributed to newborn demise and neonatal brain injury.

Maternal death claims were secondary to airway difficulty, maternal hemorrhage, and high neuraxial blockade. The most common claim associated with obstetrical anesthesia was related to nerve injury following regional anesthesia. Nerve injury can be secondary to neuraxial anesthesia and analgesia, but it can also result from obstetrical causes. Retained epidural catheter fragments also constitute a source for obstetrical anesthesia-related claims. Early neurological consultation to identify the source of nerve injury is suggested to discern if the injury could be secondary to obstetrical rather than anesthesia interventions. A 2019 closed claims review identifies high neuraxial block, embolic events, and failed intubation as the causes of maternal death or brain injury most likely to result in a claim being paid.

REGIONAL ANESTHESIA

In a closed claims analysis, peripheral nerve blocks were involved in 159 of the 6894 claims analyzed. Peripheral nerve block claims were for death (8%), permanent injuries (36%), and temporary injuries (56%). The brachial plexus was the most common location for nerve injury. In addition to ocular injury, cardiac arrest following retrobulbar block contributed to anesthesiology claims. Cardiac arrest and epidural hematomas are two of the more common damaging events leading to severe injuries related to regional anesthesia. Neuraxial hematomas in both obstetrical and nonobstetrical patients were associated with coagulopathy (either intrinsic to the patient or secondary to medical interventions). In one study, cardiac arrest related to neuraxial anesthesia contributed to roughly one-third of the death or brain damage claims in both obstetrical and nonobstetrical patients. Accidental intravenous injection and local anesthesia toxicity also contributed to claims for brain injury or death.

Nerve injuries constitute the third most common source of anesthesia litigation. A retrospective review of patient records and a claims database showed that 112 of 380,680 patients (0.03%) experienced perioperative nerve injury. Patients with hypertension and diabetes and those who were smokers were at increased risk of developing perioperative nerve injury. Perioperative nerve injuries may result from compression, stretch, ischemia, other traumatic events, and unknown causes. Improper positioning can lead to nerve compression, ischemia, and injury; however, not every nerve injury is the result of improper positioning. The care received by patients with ulnar nerve injury was rarely judged to be inadequate in the ASA Closed Claims database. Even awake patients undergoing spinal anesthesia have been reported to experience upper extremity injury. Moreover, many peripheral nerve injuries do not become manifest until more than 48 h after anesthesia and surgery, suggesting that some nerve damage that occurs in surgical patients may arise from events taking place after the patient leaves the operating room setting.

A 2018 closed claim review of peripheral nerve injury following general anesthesia could not detect an etiology in nearly 50% of cases and found that in 91% of cases, the anesthesia care was appropriate. Ischemia, inflammation, genetic predisposition, and the "double crush" phenomenon may all contribute to the development of perioperative neuropathy following general anesthesia.

PEDIATRIC ANESTHESIA

In a 2007 study reviewing 532 claims in pediatric patients younger than 16 years of age in the ASA Closed Claims database from 1973 to 2000 (Figure 54–5), a decrease in the proportion of claims

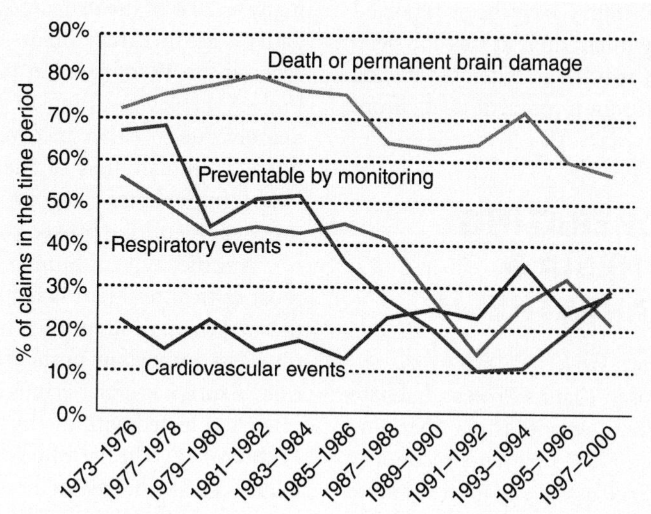

FIGURE 54–5 Trends over time. Outcome, type of event, and prevention by better monitoring. Years are grouped for illustration. (Reproduced with permission from Jimenez N, Posner K, Cheney F, et al. An update on pediatric anesthesia liability: A closed claims analysis. *Anesth Analg.* 2007 Jan;104(1):147-129.)

for death and brain damage was noted over the three decades. Likewise, the percentage of claims related to respiratory events also was reduced. Compared with before 1990, the percentage of claims secondary to respiratory events decreased during the years 1990 to 2000, accounting for only 23% of claims in the latter study years compared with 51% of claims in the 1970s. Moreover, the percentage of claims that could be avoided by better monitoring decreased from 63% in the 1970s to 16% in the 1990s. Death and brain damage constitute the major complications for which claims are filed. In the 1990s, cardiovascular events joined respiratory complications in sharing the primary causes of pediatric anesthesia litigation. In the previously mentioned study, better monitoring and newer airway management techniques may have reduced the incidence of respiratory events leading to litigation-generating complications in the latter years of the review period. Additionally, the possibility of a claim being filed secondary to death or brain injury is greater in children who are in ASA classes 3, 4, or 5.

In a review of the Pediatric Perioperative Cardiac Arrest Registry, which collects information from about 80 North American institutions that provide pediatric anesthesia, 193 arrests were reported in children between 1998 and 2004. During the study period, 18% of the arrests were "drug related," compared with 37% of all arrests during the years 1994 to 1997. Cardiovascular arrests occurred most often (41%), with hypovolemia and hyperkalemia being the most common causes. Respiratory arrests (27%) were most commonly associated with laryngospasm. Central venous catheter placement with resultant vascular injury also contributed to some perioperative arrests. Arrests from cardiovascular causes occurred most frequently during surgery, whereas arrests from respiratory causes tended to occur after surgery.

A review of data from the Pediatric Perioperative Cardiac Arrest Registry with a focus on children with congenital heart disease found that such children were more likely to arrest perioperatively secondary to a cardiovascular cause. In particular, children with a single ventricle were at increased risk of perioperative arrest. Children with aortic stenosis and cardiomyopathy were similarly found to be at increased risk of cardiac arrest perioperatively.

Increasingly, obese children present for anesthesia and surgery. These children are at particular risk for obstructive sleep apnea, increased sensitivity to opioids, and respiratory arrest. In particular, death and neurological injury have been reported following tonsillectomy in children at risk for sleep apnea. At-risk children require an extended period of postoperative monitoring to prevent death from perioperative apnea.

OUT OF THE OPERATING ROOM ANESTHESIA & MONITORED ANESTHESIA CARE

Review of the ASA Closed Claims Project database indicates that anesthesia at remote (non–operating room) locations poses a risk to patients secondary to hypoventilation and excessive sedation. Remote location anesthesia care was more likely than operating room anesthesia care to involve a claim for death (54% vs 29%, respectively). The endoscopy suite and cardiac catheterization laboratory were the most frequent locations from which claims were generated. Monitored anesthesia care (MAC) was the most common technique employed in these claims. Overwhelmingly, adverse respiratory events were most frequently responsible for the injury.

An analysis of the ASA Closed Claims Project database focusing on MAC likewise revealed that oversedation and respiratory arrest frequently led to claims. Claims for burn injuries suffered in operating room fires were also found in the database. Supplemental oxygen, draping, pooling of flammable antiseptic preparatory solutions, and surgical cautery combine to produce the potential for operating room fires (see Chapter 2).

EQUIPMENT PROBLEMS

"Equipment problems" is probably a misnomer; the ASA Closed Claims Project review of 72 claims involving gas delivery systems found that equipment *misuse* was three times more common than equipment *malfunction*. Anesthesia gas delivery claims have decreased in recent years, accounting for just 1% of claims in the new millennium. Provider equipment misuse was associated with severe patient injuries.

Errors in drug administration also typically involve human error. It has been suggested that as many as 20% of the drug doses given to hospitalized patients are incorrect. Errors in drug administration account for 4% of cases in the ASA Closed Claims Project. Errors resulting in claims were most frequently due to either incorrect dosage or unintentional administration of the wrong drug (syringe swap). In the latter category, accidental administration of epinephrine proved particularly dangerous.

Another type of human error occurs when the most critical problem is ignored because the anesthesia provider's attention is inappropriately focused on a less important problem or an incorrect solution (*fixation error*). Serious anesthetic mishaps are often associated with distractions and other factors (Table 54–3). The harmful impact of most equipment failures can be decreased or avoided when the problem is identified during the mandatory preoperative anesthesia workstation inspection and checkout. 5 Many anesthetic fatalities occur only after a series of coincidental circumstances, misjudgments, and technical errors combine (*mishap chain*).

Prevention

Drug syringes and ampules in the workspace should be restricted to those needed for the current patient to minimize errors in drug administration. Drugs should be consistently diluted to the same concentration in the same way for each use, and they should be clearly labeled. Computer systems for scanning bar-coded drug labels may help to reduce

TABLE 54–3 Factors associated with human errors and equipment misuse.

Factor	Example
Inadequate preparation	No machine checkout or preoperative evaluation; haste and carelessness; production pressure
Inadequate experience and training	Unfamiliarity with anesthetic technique or equipment
Environmental limitations	Inability to visualize surgical field: poor communication with surgeons
Physical and emotional factors	Fatigue; distraction caused by personal problems

medication errors. The conduct of all anesthetics should follow a predictable pattern by which the anesthetist actively surveys the monitors, the surgical field, and the patient on a recurrent basis. In particular, patient positioning should be frequently reassessed to avoid the possibility of nerve compression or stretch injuries. Increasingly, protocols or algorithms, or both, are provided in anesthetizing locations to ensure compliance with preprocedural checklists, standardize responses to adverse events, and minimize errors related to transfer of patient care between clinicians. According to a 2018 retrospective cohort study, handover of anesthesia care between providers is associated with a greater incidence of adverse postoperative events compared with cases where no intraoperative handover occurred. Consequently, efforts to minimize the number of handovers of care and standardize the process for necessary handovers are key elements of quality patient management.

AIRWAY INJURY

The daily insertion of endotracheal tubes (particularly with stylets), laryngeal mask airways, oral/nasal airways, gastric tubes, transesophageal echocardiogram (TEE) probes, esophageal (bougie) dilators, and emergency airways all involve the risk of airway damage. Common patient reports, such as sore throat and dysphagia, are usually self-limiting, but they may also be nonspecific symptoms of more ominous complications.

The most common persisting airway injury is dental trauma. In a retrospective study of 600,000 surgical cases, the incidence of injury requiring dental intervention and repair was approximately 1 in 4500. In most cases, laryngoscopy and endotracheal intubation were involved, and the upper incisors were the most frequently injured. Major risk factors for dental trauma included tracheal intubation, preexisting poor dentition, and patient characteristics associated with difficult airway management (including limited neck motion, previous head and neck surgery, craniofacial abnormalities, and a history of difficult intubation).

Laryngeal injuries included vocal cord paralysis, granuloma, and arytenoid dislocation. Most tracheal injuries were associated with emergency surgical tracheotomy, but a few were related to endotracheal intubation. Some injuries occurred during seemingly easy, routine intubations. Proposed mechanisms include excessive tube movement in the trachea and excessive cuff inflation, leading to pressure necrosis. Esophageal perforations contributed to death in 5 of 13 patients reviewed. Esophageal perforation often presents with delayed-onset subcutaneous emphysema or pneumothorax, unexpected febrile state, and sepsis. Pharyngoesophageal perforation is associated with difficult intubation, age over 60 years, and female gender. As in tracheal perforation, signs and symptoms are often delayed in onset. Initial sore throat, cervical pain, and cough progress to fever, dysphagia, and dyspnea, as mediastinitis, abscess, or pneumonia develop. Mortality rates of up to 50% have been reported after esophageal perforation, with better outcomes attributable to rapid detection and treatment.

Minimizing the risk of airway injury begins with the preoperative assessment. Documentation of current dentition (including dental work) should be included. The ASA algorithm for difficult airway management is a useful guide to have immediately available in every anesthetizing location.

PERIPHERAL NERVE INJURY

The most commonly injured peripheral nerve is the ulnar nerve (Figure 54–6). In a retrospective study of over 1 million patients, ulnar neuropathy (persisting for more than 3 months) occurred in approximately 1 in 2700 patients. Of interest, initial symptoms were most frequently noted more than 24 h after a surgical procedure. Risk factors included male gender, hospital stay greater than 14 days, and very thin or obese body habitus. More than 50% of these patients regained full sensory and motor function within 1 year. Anesthetic technique was not implicated as a risk factor; 25% of patients with ulnar neuropathy underwent monitored care or lower extremity regional technique. Many ulnar neuropathies occurred despite notation of extra padding over the elbow area.

The Role of Positioning

External pressure on a nerve may compromise its perfusion and disrupt its cellular integrity, resulting

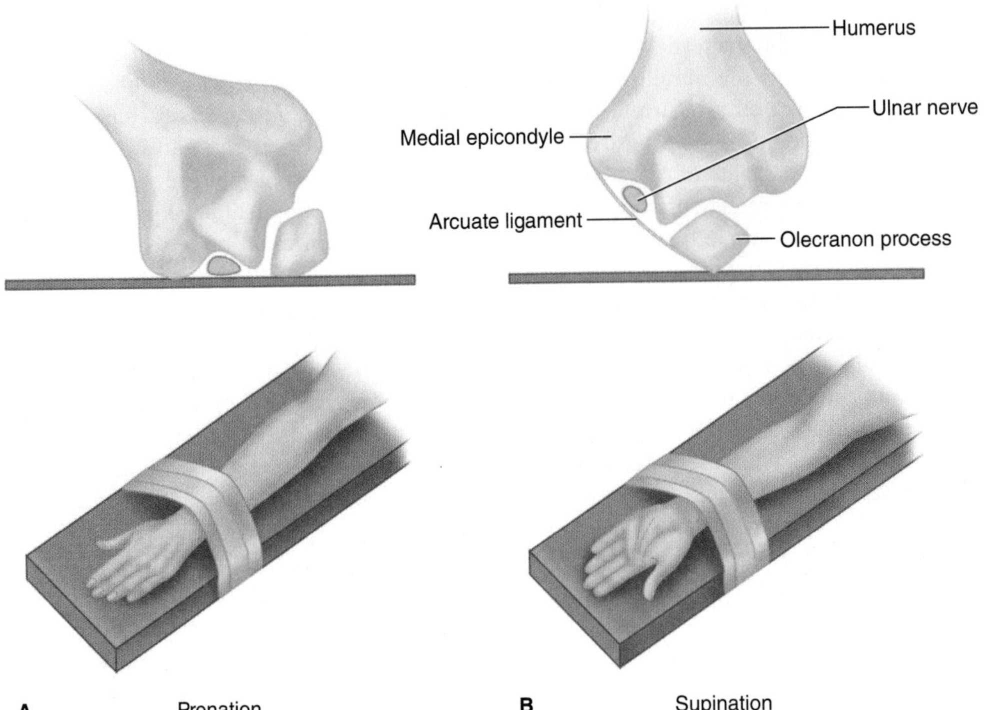

FIGURE 54–6 A: Pronation of the forearm can cause external compression of the ulnar nerve in the cubital tunnel. B: Forearm supination avoids this problem. (Modified with permission from Wadsworth TG. The cubital tunnel and the external compression syndrome. *Anesth Analg.* 1974 Mar-April;53(2):303-308.)

in edema, ischemia, and necrosis. Pressure injuries are particularly likely when nerves pass through closed compartments or take a superficial course (eg, the peroneal nerve around the fibula). Postoperative lower extremity neuropathies, particularly those involving the peroneal nerve, have been associated with the lithotomy position with extreme degrees (high) or prolonged (greater than 2 h) durations. Other risk factors for postoperative lower extremity neuropathy include hypotension, thin body habitus, older age, vascular disease, diabetes, and cigarette smoking. An axillary (chest) "roll" is commonly used to reduce pressure on the inferior shoulder and brachial plexus of patients in the lateral decubitus position. This roll should be located caudad to the axilla to prevent direct pressure on the brachial plexus and should be large enough to relieve any pressure from the mattress on the lower shoulder.

The data are convincing that some postoperative peripheral nerve injuries are not preventable. The risk of peripheral neuropathy should be included in discussions leading to informed consent. When reasonable, patients with contractures (or other causes of limited flexibility) can be positioned before induction of anesthesia to check for feasibility and discomfort. Final positioning should be evaluated prior to draping. In most circumstances, the head and neck should be kept in a neutral position. Shoulder braces to support patients maintained in a steep Trendelenburg position should be avoided if possible (as should steep Trendelenburg position itself, if possible), and shoulder abduction and lateral rotation should be minimized. The upper extremities should not be extended to greater than 90°. (There should be no continuous external compression on the knee, ankle, or heel.) Although injuries may still occur, additional padding may be helpful in vulnerable areas. Documentation should include information on positioning, including the presence of padding. Finally, patients who report sensory or motor dysfunction in the postoperative period should be reassured that this is usually a temporary condition, and motor and sensory function should be documented. When symptoms persist for more than 24 h, the patient should be referred to a neurologist, physiatrist, or hand surgeon who is knowledgeable about perioperative nerve damage for evaluation. Physiological testing, such as nerve conduction and electromyographic studies, can be useful to document whether nerve damage is a new or chronic condition. In the latter case, fibrillations will be observed in chronically denervated muscles. Fibrillations should not be present in the first few days after an acute nerve injury.

Complications Related to Positioning

Changes of body position have physiological consequences that can be exaggerated in disease states. General and regional anesthesia may limit the cardiovascular response to such a change. Even positions that are safe for short periods may eventually lead to complications in persons who are not able to move in response to pain. Regional and general anesthesia abolish protective reflexes and predispose patients to injury.

Many complications, including air embolism, blindness from sustained pressure on the globe, and finger amputation following a crush injury, can be caused by improper patient positioning (Table 54–4). These complications are best prevented by evaluating the patient's postural limitations during the preanesthetic visit; padding pressure points, susceptible nerves, and any area of the body that will *possibly* be in contact with the operating table or its attachments; avoiding flexion or extension of a joint to its limit; having an awake patient assume the position to ensure comfort; and understanding the potential complications of each position. Monitors must often be disconnected during patient repositioning, making this a time of greater risk for unrecognized hemodynamic derangement or hypoventilation.

Compartment syndromes can result from hemorrhage into a closed space following a vascular puncture or prolonged venous outflow obstruction,

TABLE 54–4 Complications associated with patient positioning.

Complication	Position	Prevention
Venous air embolism	Sitting, prone, reverse Trendelenburg	Maintain adequate venous pressure; ligate "open" veins
Alopecia	Supine, lithotomy, Trendelenburg	Avoid prolonged hypotension, padding, and occasional head turning
Backache	Any	Lumbar support, padding, and slight hip flexion
Extremity compartment syndromes	Especially lithotomy	Maintain perfusion pressure and avoid external compression
Corneal abrasion	Any, but especially prone	Taping or lubricating eye
Digit amputation	Any	Check for protruding digits before changing table configuration
Nerve palsies		
Brachial plexus	Any	Avoid stretching or direct compression at neck, shoulder, or axilla
Common peroneal	Lithotomy, lateral decubitus	Avoid sustained pressure on lateral aspect of upper fibula
Radial	Any	Avoid compression of lateral humerus
Ulnar	Any	Avoid sustained pressure on ulnar groove
Retinal ischemia	Prone, sitting	Avoid pressure on globe
Skin necrosis	Any	Avoid sustained pressure over bony prominences

particularly when associated with hypotension. In severe cases, this may lead to muscle necrosis, myoglobinuria, and kidney damage, unless the pressure within the extremity compartment is relieved by surgical decompression (fasciotomy) or in the abdominal compartment by laparotomy.

AWARENESS UNDER GENERAL ANESTHESIA

A continuing series of media reports have imprinted the fear of awareness under general anesthesia in the psyche of the general population. Accounts of recall and helplessness while paralyzed have made unconsciousness a primary concern of patients undergoing general anesthesia. When unintended intraoperative awareness does occur, patients may exhibit symptoms ranging from mild anxiety to posttraumatic stress disorder (eg, sleep disturbances, nightmares, social difficulties).

Although the incidence is difficult to measure, approximately 2% of the closed claims in the ASA Closed Claims Project database relate to awareness under anesthesia. Analysis of the NHS Litigation Authority database from 1995 to 2007 revealed that 19 of 93 relevant claims were for "awake paralysis." Clearly, awareness is of great concern to patients and may lead to litigation. Certain types of surgeries are most frequently associated with awareness, including those for major trauma, obstetrics, and major cardiac procedures. In some instances, awareness may result from the reduced depth of anesthesia that can be tolerated by the patient. In early studies, recall rates for intraoperative events during major trauma surgery have been reported to be as frequent as 43%; the incidence of awareness during cardiac surgery and cesarean sections is 1.5% and 0.4%, respectively. As of 1999, the ASA Closed Claims Project reported 79 awareness claims; approximately 20% of the claims were for awake paralysis, and the remainder of the claims were for recall under general anesthesia. Most claims for awake paralysis were thought to be due to errors in drug labeling and administration, such as administering paralytics before inducing anesthesia. Since the 1999 review, another 71 cases have appeared in the database. Claims for recall were more likely in women undergoing general anesthesia without a volatile agent. Patients with long-term substance abuse may have increased anesthesia requirements that if not met can lead to awareness.

Other specific causes of awareness include inadequate inhalational anesthetic delivery (eg, from vaporizer malfunction) and medication errors. Some patients may report awareness when, in fact, they received monitored anesthesia care or regional anesthesia with moderate sedation; thus, anesthetists should make sure that patients have appropriate expectations when regional or local techniques are employed. Likewise, patients requesting regional or local anesthesia because they want to "see it all" or "stay in control" often can become irate when sedation dulls their memory of the perioperative experience. In all cases, candid discussion between anesthesia staff and the patient is necessary to avoid unrealistic expectations.

Some clinicians routinely discuss the possibility of intraoperative recall and the steps that will be taken to minimize it as part of the informed consent for general anesthesia. This makes particular sense for those procedures in which recall is more likely. It is advisable to also remind patients who are undergoing monitored anesthesia care with sedation that awareness is expected. Volatile anesthetics should be administered at a level consistent with amnesia. If this is not possible, benzodiazepines (or scopolamine, or both) can be administered. Movement of a patient may indicate inadequate anesthetic depth. Documentation should include end-tidal concentrations of anesthetic gases (when available) and dosages of amnesic drugs. Use of a bispectral index scale (BIS) monitor or similar monitors may be helpful, though randomized clinical trials have failed to demonstrate a reduced incidence of awareness with the use of BIS when compared with appropriate concentrations of volatile agents. Finally, if there is evidence of intraoperative awareness during postoperative rounds, the practitioner should obtain a detailed account of the experience, answer patient questions, be very empathetic, and refer the patient for psychological counseling if appropriate. Most patients reporting awareness are dissatisfied with the manner in which their concerns are addressed, according to a report of the North American Anaesthesia Awareness Registry.

EYE INJURY

A wide range of perioperative eye injuries from simple corneal abrasion to blindness have been reported. Corneal abrasion is by far the most common and transient eye injury. The ASA Closed Claims Project identified a small number of claims for abrasion, in which the cause was rarely identified (20%) and the incidence of permanent injury was low (16%). It also identified a subset of claims for blindness that resulted from patient movement during ophthalmological surgery. These cases occurred in patients receiving either general anesthesia or monitored anesthesia care.

Although the cause of corneal abrasion may not be obvious, securely closing the eyelids with tape or a clear adhesive bandage after loss of consciousness (but prior to intubation) and avoiding direct contact between eyes and oxygen masks, drapes, lines, and pillows (particularly during monitored anesthesia care, in transport, and in nonsupine positions) can help minimize the possibility of injury. Adequate anesthetic depth (and, in most cases, paralysis) should be maintained to prevent movement during ophthalmological surgery under general anesthesia. In patients scheduled for MAC, the patient must understand that movement under monitored care is hazardous and, thus, that only minimal sedation may be administered to ensure that he or she can cooperate. Vigilance must be maintained regarding patients' propensity to want to rub their eyes following emergence from anesthesia, especially in response to blurred vision secondary to residual eye lubrication ointment. Initial treatment consists of topical anesthetic agents, antibiotic prophylaxis, and lubricant eye drops. Most corneal abrasions heal with 72 h. Ophthalmology consultation is indicated if healing is delayed or symptoms worsen.

Postoperative vision loss is most commonly reported after cardiopulmonary bypass, radical neck dissection, and spinal surgeries in the prone position, and symptoms range from decreased visual acuity to complete blindness. Ischemic optic neuropathy (ION) is now the most common cause of postoperative vision loss. Both preoperative and intraoperative factors may be contributory. Many of the case reports implicate preexisting hypertension, diabetes, coronary artery disease, and smoking, suggesting that preoperative vascular abnormalities may play a role. Intraoperative deliberate hypotension and anemia have also been implicated in spine surgery, perhaps because of their potential to reduce oxygen delivery. Finally, prolonged surgical time in positions that compromise venous outflow (prone, head down, compressed abdomen) has also been found to be a factor in spine surgery. Symptoms are usually present immediately upon awakening from anesthesia but have been reported up to 12 days postoperatively. Analysis of case records submitted to the ASA Postoperative Vision Loss Registry revealed that vision loss was secondary to ION in 83 of 93 cases. Instrumentation of the spine was associated with ION when surgery lasted more than 6 h and blood loss was more than 1 L. ION can occur in patients whose eyes are free of pressure secondary to the use of pin fixation, indicating that direct pressure on the eye is not required to produce ION. Cortical blindness can likewise occur perioperatively in association with profound hypoperfusion or embolic loads. Recovery from cortical blindness is more likely than from other causes of perioperative vision loss. Increased venous pressure in patients in the Trendelenburg position may reduce blood flow to the optic nerve.

It is difficult to formulate recommendations to prevent this complication because risk factors for ION are often unavoidable. Steps that might be taken include (1) limiting the degree and duration of controlled (deliberate) hypotension, (2) transfusing severely anemic patients who seem to be at risk of ION, and (3) discussing with the surgeon the possibility of staged operations in high-risk patients to limit prolonged procedures.

Of note, postoperative vision loss can be caused by other mechanisms as well, including angle-closure glaucoma, embolic phenomenon to the cortex or retina, or posterior reversible encephalopathy syndrome (PRES). The latter is related to cerebral edema in the parieto-occipital regions. Immediate evaluation is advised in such circumstances.

TABLE 54–6 Clinical manifestations of anaphylaxis.

Organ System	Signs and Symptoms
Cardiovascular	Hypotension,[1] tachycardia, arrhythmias
Pulmonary	Bronchospasm,[1] cough, dyspnea, pulmonary edema, laryngeal edema, hypoxia
Dermatological	Urticaria,[1] facial edema, pruritus

[1]Key signs during general anesthesia.

6 sulfate) or activate complement. Despite differing mechanisms, anaphylactic and anaphylactoid reactions typically are clinically indistinguishable and equally life threatening. Table 54–7 lists common causes of anaphylactic and anaphylactoid reactions.

Serum tryptase measurement is helpful in confirming the diagnosis of an anaphylactic reaction. Treatment must be immediate and tailored to the severity of the reaction (Table 54–8).

TABLE 54–8 Treatment of anaphylactic and anaphylactoid reactions.

Discontinue drug administration
Administer 100% oxygen
Epinephrine (0.01–0.5 mg IV or IM)[1]
Consider intubation
Intravenous fluid bolus
Diphenhydramine (50–75 mg IV)
Ranitidine (150 mg IV)
Hydrocortisone (up to 200 mg IV) or methylprednisolone (1–2 mg/kg)

[1]The dose and route of epinephrine depend on the severity of the reaction. An infusion of 1–5 mcg/min may be necessary in adults.

3. Allergic Reactions to Anesthetic Agents

7 True anaphylaxis due to anesthetic agents is rare; anaphylactoid reactions are much more common. Risk factors associated with hypersensitivity to anesthetics include female gender, atopic

TABLE 54–7 Causes of anaphylactic and anaphylactoid reactions.

Anaphylactic reactions against polypeptides	Venoms (Hymenoptera, fire ant, snake, jellyfish)
	Airborne allergens (pollen, molds, danders)
	Foods (peanuts, milk, egg, seafood, grain)
	Enzymes (trypsin, streptokinase, chymopapain, asparaginase)
	Heterologous serum (tetanus antitoxin, antilymphocyte globulin, antivenin)
	Human proteins (insulin, corticotropin, vasopressin, serum and seminal proteins)
	Latex
Anaphylactic reactions against hapten carrier	Antibiotics (penicillin, cephalosporins, sulfonamides)
	Disinfectants (ethylene oxide, chlorhexidine)
	Local anesthetics (procaine)
Anaphylactoid reactions	Polyionic solutions (radiocontrast medium, polymyxin B)
	Opioids (morphine, meperidine)
	Hypnotics (propofol, thiopental)
	Muscle relaxants (rocuronium, succinylcholine, cisatracurium)
	Synthetic membranes (dialysis)
	Nonsteroidal antiinflammatory drugs
	Preservatives (sulfites, benzoates)
	Protamine
	Dextran
	Steroids
	Exercise
	Idiopathic

Adapted with permission from Bochner BS, Lichtenstein LM. Anaphylaxis. *N Engl J Med.* 1991 June 20;324(25):1785-1790.

history, preexisting allergies, and previous anesthetic exposures. An estimated 1 in 6500 patients has an allergic reaction to a muscle relaxant. In many instances, the patient had no previous exposure to the agent. Investigators opine that over-the-counter drugs, cosmetics, and food products, many of which contain tertiary or quaternary ammonium ions, can sensitize susceptible individuals.

The incidence of anaphylaxis for propofol and thiopental is 1 in 60,000 and 1 in 30,000, respectively. Allergic reactions to etomidate, ketamine, and benzodiazepines are exceedingly rare. True anaphylactic reactions due to opioids are far less common than nonimmune histamine release. Similarly, anaphylactic reactions to local anesthetics are much less common than vasovagal reactions, toxic reactions to accidental intravenous injections, and side effects from absorbed or intravenously injected epinephrine. IgE-mediated reactions to certain ester-type local anesthetics (eg, procaine and benzocaine), however, are well described secondary to a reaction to the metabolite, para-aminobenzoic acid. In contrast, true anaphylaxis due to amide-type local anesthetics is very rare; in some instances, the preservative (paraben or methylparaben) was believed to be responsible for an apparent anaphylactoid reaction to a local anesthetic. Moreover, the cross-reactivity between amide-type local anesthetics seems to be low. Volatile anesthetics are not likely to initiate anaphylaxis.

4. Latex Allergy

The severity of allergic reactions to latex-containing products ranges from mild contact dermatitis to life-threatening anaphylaxis. Latex allergy associated with anaphylaxis during anesthesia is now much rarer due to the removal of latex-containing products from the medical environment. Most serious reactions seem to involve a direct IgE-mediated immune response to polypeptides in natural latex, though some cases of contact dermatitis may be due to a type IV sensitivity reaction to chemicals introduced in the manufacturing process. Nonetheless, a relationship between the occurrence of contact dermatitis and the probability of future anaphylaxis has been suggested. Chronic exposure to latex and a history of atopy increases the risk of sensitization. Health care workers and patients undergoing frequent procedures with latex items (eg, repeated urinary bladder catheterization, barium enema examinations) should therefore be considered at increased risk.
8 Patients with spina bifida, spinal cord injury, and congenital abnormalities of the genitourinary tract have a markedly increased incidence of latex allergy. The incidence of latex anaphylaxis in children is estimated to be 1 in 10,000. A history of allergic symptoms to latex should be sought in all patients during the preanesthetic interview. Foods that cross-react with latex include mango, kiwi, chestnut, avocado, passion fruit, and banana. Interleukin (IL)-18 and IL-13 single nucleotide polymorphisms may affect the sensitivity of individuals to latex and promote allergic responses.

Anaphylactic reactions to latex may be confused with reactions to other substances (eg, drugs, blood products) because the onset of symptoms can be delayed for more than 1 h after initial exposure. Treatment is the same as for other forms of anaphylactic reactions. Preventing a reaction in sensitized patients includes pharmacological prophylaxis and absolute avoidance of latex. Preoperative administration of H_1 and H_2 histamine antagonists and steroids may provide some protection, though their use is controversial. Although most pieces of anesthetic equipment are now latex-free, some may still contain latex. Manufacturers of latex-containing medical products must label their products accordingly. **Only devices specifically known not to contain latex (eg, polyvinyl or neoprene gloves, silicone endotracheal tubes or laryngeal masks, plastic face masks) can be used in latex-allergic patients.**

5. Allergies to Antibiotics

Many true drug allergies in surgical patients are due to antibiotics, mainly β-lactam antibiotics, such as penicillins and cephalosporins. Although 1% to 4% of β-lactam administrations result in allergic reactions, only 0.004% to 0.015% of these reactions result in anaphylaxis. Up to 2% of the general population is allergic to penicillin, but only 0.01% of penicillin administrations result in anaphylaxis. Cephalosporin cross-sensitivity in patients with penicillin allergy is estimated to be 2% to 7%, but a history of an anaphylactic reaction to penicillin increases the cross-reactivity rate up to 50%. However, these figures likely exaggerate the cross-reactivity between penicillin IgE-mediated allergic reactions and some cephalosporins that differ structurally from penicillin (cefazolin). Moreover, the risk of the alternative to cephalosporin in patients allergic to penicillin (often vancomycin) may present a greater risk to the patient than the cephalosporin! Sulfonamide allergy is also relatively common in surgical patients. Sulfa drugs include sulfonamide antibiotics, furosemide, hydrochlorothiazide, and captopril. Fortunately, the frequency of cross-reactivity among these agents is low.

Like cephalosporins, vancomycin is commonly used for antibiotic prophylaxis in surgical patients. Vancomycin is associated with a reaction (the "red man" or "red neck" syndrome) that consists of intense pruritus, flushing, and erythema of the head and upper torso in addition to arterial hypotension. Isolated systemic hypotension seems to be primarily mediated by histamine release because pretreatment with H_1 and H_2 antihistamines can prevent hypotension, even with rapid rates of vancomycin administration. Vancomycin can also produce true anaphylactic or anaphylactoid reactions. Protamine commonly causes vasodilatory hypotension and less commonly presents as an anaphylactoid reaction with pulmonary hypertension and systemic hypotension.

Immunological mechanisms are associated with other perioperative pathologies. Transfusion-related lung injury may be secondary to the activity of antibodies in the donor plasma, producing a hypersensitivity reaction that leads to lung infiltrates and hypoxemia (see Chapter 51). IgG antibody formation directed at heparin–PF4 complexes results in platelet activation, thrombosis, and heparin-induced thrombocytopenia.

QUALITY MANAGEMENT

Risk management and continuous quality improvement programs at the departmental level may reduce anesthetic morbidity and mortality rates and decrease perioperative costs by addressing monitoring standards, equipment, practice guidelines, continuing education, care variation and quality of care, and staffing and "system" issues. Specific responsibilities of peer review committees include identifying and preventing potential problems, formulating and periodically revising departmental policies, ensuring the availability of properly functioning anesthetic equipment, enforcing standards required for clinical privileges, and evaluating the appropriateness and quality of patient care. A quality improvement system impartially and continuously reviews complications, compliance with standards, and quality indicators (see Chapter 59).

Health care purchasers seek maximal health care value.

$$\text{Value} = \frac{\text{Quality}}{\text{Cost}}$$

Consequently, anesthesia providers must consistently deliver high-quality results while minimizing expenses. To achieve value, hospitals and providers alike have looked to adopt principles of continuous improvement borrowed from industry. Adapting the work of W. Edwards Deming, health care organizations often employ the PDSA (Plan-Do-Study-Act) cycle to promote ongoing improvement, standardize results, and reduce waste (Figure 54–9). So-called *lean* management strategies are used to achieve maximal health care value by continually attempting to improve processes to minimize variability so as to ensure optimal results with minimal waste.

OCCUPATIONAL HAZARDS IN ANESTHESIOLOGY

Anesthesia providers spend much of their workday exposed to anesthetic gases, low-dose ionizing radiation, electromagnetic fields, blood products, and workplace stress. Each of these can contribute to negative health effects. A 2000 paper compared the mortality risks of anesthesiologists and internists. Death from heart disease or cancer did not differ between the groups; however, anesthesiologists had an increased rate of suicide and illicit drug-related death (Table 54–9). Anesthesiologists also had a greater chance of death from external causes, such as boating, bicycling, and aeronautical accidents compared with internists. Nevertheless, both anesthesiologists and

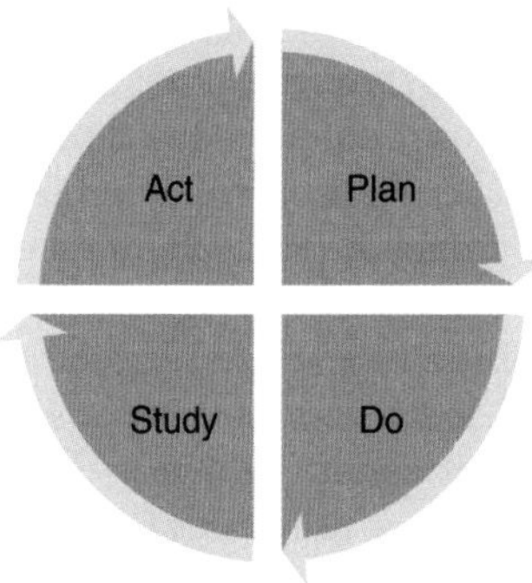

FIGURE 54–9 Plan-Do-Study-Act (PDSA) cycle for improvement. (Reproduced with permission from Moriates C, Arora V, Shah N: *Understanding Value-Based Healthcare.* New York, NY: McGraw Hill; 2015.)

internists had lower mortality than the general population, likely due to their higher socioeconomic status. Anesthesiologists' access to parenteral opioids possibly contributes to a more than twofold greater risk for drug-related deaths compared with that of internists.

1. Chronic Exposure to Anesthetic Gases

9 There is no clear evidence that exposure to trace amounts of anesthetics presents a health hazard to operating room personnel. However, because previous studies examining this issue have yielded flawed but conflicting results, the U.S. Occupational Health and Safety Administration (OSHA) continues to set maximum acceptable trace concentrations of less than 25 ppm for nitrous oxide and 0.5 ppm for halogenated anesthetics (2 ppm if the halogenated agent is used alone). Achieving these minuscule concentrations depends on efficient scavenging equipment, adequate operating room ventilation, and conscientious anesthetic technique. Most people cannot detect the odor of volatile agents at a concentration of less than 30 ppm. If there is no functioning scavenging system, operating room anesthetic gas concentrations may reach 3000 ppm for nitrous oxide and 50 ppm for volatile agents.

2. Infectious Diseases

Hospital workers are exposed to many infectious diseases prevalent in the community (eg, respiratory viral infections, rubella, tuberculosis, and, currently, SARS-CoV-2). Herpetic whitlow is an infection of the finger with herpes simplex virus type 1 or 2 and usually involves direct contact of previously traumatized skin with contaminated oral secretions. Prevention involves wearing gloves when contacting oral secretions.

Viral DNA has been identified in the smoke plume generated during laser treatment of condylomata. The theoretical possibility of viral transmission from this source can be minimized by

TABLE 54–9 Relative rate ratios for drug and suicide deaths comparing anesthesiologists with internists before and after January 1, 1987.[1]

		Anesthesiologists (*N*)	Internists (*N*)	RR[2]	95% CI
All drug-related deaths	<1987	36	14	2.65	1.42–4.91
	≥1987	55	19	2.87	1.71–4.84
Drug-related suicides	<1987	16	11	1.48	0.69–3.20
	≥1987	32	11	2.88	1.45–5.71
Suicides	<1987	41	33	1.25	0.79–1.97
	≥1987	62	38	1.60	1.07–2.39

[1]CI, confidence interval.

[2]Relative ratio (RR) of anesthesiologists compared with internists for that time period, RR is adjusted for age, gender, and race.

Reproduced with permission from Alexander B, Checkoway H, Nagahama S, Domino K. Cause-specific mortality risks of anesthesiologists. *Anesthesiology.* 2000 Oct;93(4):922-930.

using smoke evacuators, gloves, and properly fitted, appropriate, OSHA-approved masks.

Also concerning is the potential of acquiring serious blood-borne infections, such as hepatitis B, hepatitis C, or human immunodeficiency virus (HIV). Although parenteral transmission of these diseases can occur following mucous membrane, cutaneous, or percutaneous exposure to infected body fluids, accidental injury with a needle contaminated with infected blood represents the most common occupational mechanism. The risk of transmission can be estimated if three factors are known: the prevalence of the infection within the patient population, the incidence of exposure (eg, frequency of needlestick), and the rate of seroconversion after a single exposure. The seroconversion rate after a specific exposure depends on several factors, including the infectivity of the organism, the stage of the patient's disease (extent of viremia), the size of the inoculum, and the immune status of the health care provider. Rates of seroconversion following a single needlestick are estimated to range
10 between 0.3% and 30%. Hollow (hypodermic) needles pose a greater risk than do solid (surgical) needles because of the potentially larger inoculum. The use of gloves and needleless systems or protected needle devices may decrease the incidence of some (but not all) types of injury.

The initial management of needlesticks involves cleaning the wound and notifying the appropriate authority within the health care facility. After an exposure, anesthesia providers should report to their institution's emergency or employee health department for appropriate counseling on postexposure prophylaxis options. All operating room staff should be made aware of the institution's employee health notification pathway for needlestick and other injuries.

Fulminant hepatitis B (1% of acute infections) carries a 60% mortality rate. Chronic active hepatitis (<5% of all cases) is associated with an increased incidence of hepatic cirrhosis and hepatocellular carcinoma. Transmission of the virus is primarily through contact with blood products or body fluids. The diagnosis is confirmed by detection of hepatitis B surface antigen (HBsAg). Uncomplicated recovery is signaled by the disappearance of HBsAg and the appearance of antibodies to the surface antigen (anti-HBs). A hepatitis B vaccine is available and is strongly recommended prophylactically for anesthesia personnel. The appearance of anti-HBs after a three-dose regimen indicates successful immunization.

Hepatitis C is another important occupational hazard in anesthesiology. Many of these infections lead to chronic hepatitis, which, although often asymptomatic, can progress to liver failure and death. It is now possible to cure hepatitis C with antiviral drug regimens.

Anesthesia personnel seem to be at low risk for the occupational contraction of HIV. Universal contact precautions should be routinely employed to mitigate the risk of transmission of infectious diseases to anesthesia providers.

COVID-19 remains a concern for health care workers, especially those engaged in aerosolizing procedures such as intubation or those caring for a coughing patient. At the time of this writing, vaccination is underway. Nevertheless, the appearance of SARS-CoV-2 variants and the uncertain ability of current vaccines to prevent serious illness or death from variants underscores the need for practitioners to remain vigilant in wearing personal protective equipment and maintaining basic personal hygiene practices such as hand washing and the use of hand sanitizers.

3. Substance Abuse

11 Anesthesiology is a high-risk medical specialty for substance abuse. Reasons for this include the stress of anesthetic practice and the easy availability of drugs with addiction potential (potentially attracting people at risk of addiction to the field). The likelihood of developing substance abuse is increased by coexisting personal problems.

The voluntary use of nonprescribed mood-altering pharmaceuticals is a disease. If untreated, substance abuse often leads to death from drug overdose—intentional or unintentional. One of the greatest challenges in treating drug abuse is identifying the afflicted individual, as denial is a consistent feature. Unfortunately, changes evident to an outside observer are often both vague and late: reduced involvement in social activities, subtle changes in appearance, extreme mood swings, and altered work habits. Options related to routine and for-cause workplace drug testing can be explored with a certified medical review officer (MRO). Treatment begins with careful, well-planned intervention. Those inexperienced in this area should consult with an addiction specialist or their employee health department, local medical society, or licensing authority about how to proceed. The goal is to enroll the individual in a formal rehabilitation program. The possibility that one may lose one's medical license and be unable to return to practice provides powerful motivation. Some diversion programs report a success rate of approximately 70%; however, most rehabilitation programs report a recurrence rate of at least 25%. Long-term compliance often involves continued participation in support groups (eg, Narcotics Anonymous), random urine testing, and oral naltrexone therapy (a long-acting opioid antagonist). Effective prevention strategies are difficult to formulate; drug and alcohol addiction are immensely powerful behavioral drives, and "better" control of drug availability is unlikely to deter a determined individual. Despite the well-intentioned requirements of the Residency Review Committee, it is unlikely that education about the severe consequences of substance abuse will bring new and reliable behavior-altering information to the potential drug-abusing anesthesia provider. There remains controversy regarding the rate at which anesthesia staff will experience recidivism. Many experts argue for a "one strike and you're out" policy for anesthesiology residents who abuse injectable drugs. The decision as to whether a fully trained and certified physician who has been discovered to abuse injectable drugs should return to anesthetic practice after completing a rehabilitation program varies and depends on the rules and traditions of the practice group, the medical center, the relevant medical licensing board, and the perceived likelihood of recidivism. Physicians returning to practice following successful completion of a program must be carefully monitored over the long term as relapses can occur years after apparent successful rehabilitation. Alcohol abuse is a common problem among physicians and nurses, and anesthesia personnel are no exception. Interventions for alcohol abuse, as is true for injectable drug abuse, must be carefully orchestrated. Guidance from an addiction specialist, the employee health program, local medical society, or licensing authority is highly recommended.

4. Ionizing Radiation Exposure

The frequent use of imaging equipment (eg, fluoroscopy) during surgery and with procedural care outside of the operating room exposes the anesthesia provider to the risks of ionizing radiation. 12 The three most important methods of minimizing radiation doses are limiting total exposure time during procedures, using proper barriers, and maximizing one's distance from the source of radiation. Anesthesiologists who routinely perform fluoroscopic image-guided invasive procedures and anesthesia providers who routinely provide care for image-guided procedures involving ionizing radiation should consider wearing protective eyewear incorporating radiation shielding. Lead glass partitions or lead aprons with thyroid shields are mandatory for all personnel who are exposed to ionizing radiation. The inverse square law states that the dosage of radiation varies inversely with the square of the distance. Thus, the exposure at 4 m will be one-sixteenth that at 1 m. The maximum recommended occupational whole-body exposure to radiation is 5 rem/y. This should be monitored with an exposure badge. The health impact of exposure to electromagnetic radiation remains unclear. Vertigo and nausea have been reported in staff exposed to magnetic fields.

CASE DISCUSSION

Unexplained Intraoperative Tachycardia & Hypertension

A 73-year-old patient is scheduled for emergency relief of an intestinal obstruction from a sigmoid volvulus. The patient had a myocardial infarction 1 month earlier that was complicated by congestive heart failure. The blood pressure is 160/90 mm Hg, pulse is 110 beats/min, respiratory rate is 22 breaths/min, and temperature is 38.8°C.

Why is this case an emergency?

Strangulation of the bowel begins with venous obstruction but can quickly progress to arterial occlusion, ischemia, infarction, and perforation. Acute peritonitis could lead to severe dehydration, sepsis, shock, and multiorgan failure.

What special monitoring is appropriate for this patient?

Because of the history of recent myocardial infarction and congestive heart failure, an arterial line would be useful. Transesophageal echocardiography (TEE) and pulse contour analysis monitors of cardiac output could be used. Pulmonary arterial flotation catheters have often been used in the past, but they are associated with significant complications, and their use does not improve patient outcomes. Large fluid shifts should be anticipated. Furthermore, information regarding myocardial oxygen supply (diastolic blood pressure) and demand (systolic blood pressure, left ventricular wall stress, heart rate) should be continuously available.

What cardiovascular medications might be useful during general anesthesia?

Severe tachycardia or extremes in arterial blood pressure should be avoided. During the laparotomy, gradual increases in heart rate and blood pressure are noted. ST-segment elevations appear on the electrocardiogram. A nitroglycerin infusion is started. The heart rate is now 130 beats/min, and the blood pressure is 220/140 mm Hg. The concentration of volatile anesthetic is increased, and metoprolol is administered intravenously in 1-mg increments. This results in a decline in heart rate to 115 beats/min, with no change in blood pressure. Suddenly, the rhythm converts to ventricular tachycardia, with a profound drop in blood pressure. As amiodarone is being administered and the defibrillation unit prepared, the rhythm degenerates into ventricular fibrillation.

What can explain this series of events?

A differential diagnosis of pronounced tachycardia and hypertension might include pheochromocytoma, malignant hyperthermia, or thyroid storm. In this case, further inspection of the nitroglycerin infusion reveals a labeling error: although the tubing was labeled "nitroglycerin," the infusion bag was labeled "epinephrine."

How does this explain the paradoxical response to metoprolol?

Metoprolol is a β_1-adrenergic antagonist. It inhibits epinephrine's β_1-stimulation of heart rate, but it does not antagonize α-induced vasoconstriction. The net result is a decrease in heart rate and a sustained increase in blood pressure.

What is the cause of the ventricular tachycardia?

An overdose of epinephrine can cause life-threatening ventricular arrhythmias. In addition, if a central venous catheter were to be malpositioned with its tip in the right ventricle, the catheter tip could have stimulated ventricular arrhythmias.

What other factors may have contributed to this anesthetic mishap?

Multiple factors will often combine to create an anesthetic misadventure. Incorrect drug labels are but one example of errors that can result in patient injury. Inadequate preparation, technical failures, knowledge deficits, and practitioner fatigue or distraction can all contribute to adverse outcomes. Careful adherence to hospital policies, checklists, patient identification procedures, and surgical and regional block timeouts can all help prevent iatrogenic complications.

GUIDELINES

Institute for Healthcare Improvement. PDSA cycles. http://www.ihi.org/resources/pages/tools/plandostudyactworksheet.aspx. Accessed October 18, 2017.

Practice advisory for the prevention of perioperative peripheral neuropathies: a report by the American Society of Anesthesiologists Task Force on prevention of peripheral neuropathies. *Anesthesiology*. 2011;114:1.

Practice advisory for perioperative visual loss associated with spine surgery 2019: an updated report by the American Society of Anesthesiologists task force on perioperative visual loss, the North American Neuro-Ophthalmology Society, and the Society for Neuroscience in Anesthesiology and Critical Care. *Anesthesiology*. 2019;130:12.

SUGGESTED READINGS

Berge E, Seppala M, Lanier W. The anesthesiology community's approach to opioid and anesthetic abusing personnel: time to change course. *Anesthesiology*. 2008;109:762.

Bhananker S, Liau D, Kooner P, et al. Liability related to peripheral venous and arterial catheterization; a closed claims analysis. *Anesth Analg*. 2009;109:124.

Bhananker S, Posner K, Cheney F, et al. Injury and liability associated with monitored anesthesia care. *Anesthesiology*. 2006;104:228.

Bishop M, Souders J, Peterson C, et al. Factors associated with unanticipated day of surgery deaths in Department of Veterans Affairs hospitals. *Anesth Analg*. 2008;107:1924.

Bryson E, Silverstein J. Addiction and substance abuse in anesthesiology. *Anesthesiology*. 2008;109:905.

Caplan RA, Ward RJ, Posner K, Cheney FW. Unexpected cardiac arrest during spinal anesthesia: a closed claims analysis of predisposing factors. *Anesthesiology*. 1988;68:5.

Cheesman K, Brady J, Flood P, Li G. Epidemiology of anesthesia-related complications in labor and delivery, New York state, 2002–2005. *Anesth Analg*. 2009;109:1174.

Cheney F, Posner K, Lee L, et al. Trends in anesthesia-related death and brain damage. *Anesthesiology*. 2006;105:1071.

Chui J, Murkin JM, Posner KL, Domino KB. Perioperative peripheral nerve injury after general anesthesia: a qualitative systematic review. *Anesth Analg*. 2018;127:134.

Cima R, Brown M, Hebl J, et al. Use of Lean and Six Sigma methodology to improve operating room efficiency in a high volume tertiary care academic medical center. *J Am Coll Surg*. 2011;213:83.

Cook T, Bland L, Mihai R, Scott S. Litigation related to anaesthesia: an analysis of claims against the NHS in England 1995-2007. *Anaesthesia*. 2009;64:706.

Cook T, Scott S, Mihai R. Litigation related to airway and respiratory complications of anaesthesia: an analysis of claims against the NHS in England 1995–2007. *Anaesthesia*. 2010;65:556.

Cranshaw J, Gupta K, Cook T. Litigation related to drug errors in anaesthesia: an analysis of claims against the NHS in England 1995–2009. *Anaesthesia*. 2009;64:1317.

Crosby E. Medical malpractice and anesthesiology: literature review and role of the expert witness. *Can J Anesth*. 2007;54:227.

Davies J, Posner K, Lee L, et al. Liability associated with obstetric anesthesia. *Anesthesiology*. 2009;110:131.

Fitzgibbon DR, Posner KL, Domino KB, et al. Chronic pain management: American Society of Anesthesiologists Closed Claims Project. *Anesthesiology*. 2004;100:98.

Fitzsimons MG, Baker K, Malhotra R, Gottlieb A, Lowenstein E, Zapol WM. Reducing the incidence of substance use disorders in anesthesiology residents: 13 years of comprehensive urine drug screening. *Anesthesiology*. 2018;129:821.

Gayer S. Prone to blindness: answers to postoperative visual loss. *Anesth Analg*. 2011;112:11.

Grocott M, Mythen M. Perioperative medicine: the value proposition for anesthesia? *Anesthesiol Clin*. 2015;33:617.

Hawkins J, Chang J, Palmer S, et al. Anesthesia-related maternal mortality in the United States: 1979–2002. *Obstet Gynecol*. 2011;117:69.

Hewson DW, Bedforth NM, Hardman JG. Peripheral nerve injury arising in anaesthesia practice. *Anaesthesia*. 2018;73 Suppl 1:51.

Honardar M, Posner K, Domino K. Delayed detection of esophageal intubation in anesthesia malpractice claims; brief report of a case series. *Anesth Analg*. 2017;125:1948.

Hyman SA, Shotwell MS, Michaels DR, et al. A survey evaluating burnout, health status, depression, reported alcohol and substance use, and social support of anesthesiologists. *Anesth Analg*. 2017;125:2009.

Jimenez N, Posner K, Cheney F, et al. An update on pediatric anesthesia liability: a closed claims analysis. *Anesth Analg*. 2007;104:147.

Jones PM, Cherry RA, Allen BN, et al. Association between handover of anesthesia care and adverse postoperative outcomes among patients undergoing major surgery. *JAMA*. 2018;319:143.

Kannan J, Bernstein J. Perioperative anaphylaxis: diagnosis, evaluation and management. *Immunol Allergy Clin N Am*. 2015;35:321.

Kent CD, Posner KL, Mashour GA, et al. Patient perspectives on intraoperative awareness with explicit recall: report from a North American anaesthesia awareness registry. *Br J Anaesth*. 2015;115 Suppl 1:i114-i121.

Kla K, Lee L. Perioperative visual loss. *Best Pract Res Clin Anesthesiol*. 2016;30:69.

Kovacheva VP, Brovman EY, Greenberg P, Song E, Palanisamy A, Urman RD. A contemporary analysis of medicolegal issues in obstetric anesthesia between 2005 and 2015. *Anesth Analg*. 2019;128:1199.

Lee LA, Rothe S, Posner KL, et al. The American Society of Anesthesiologists Postoperative Visual Loss Registry: Analysis of 93 spine surgery cases with postoperative visual loss. *Anesthesiology*. 2006;105:652.

Li G, Warner M, Lang B, et al. Epidemiology of anesthesia-related mortality in the United States 1999–2005. *Anesthesiology*. 2009;110:759.

Liang B. "Standards" of anesthesia: Law and ASA guidelines. *J Clin Anesth*. 2008;20:393.

Lineberger C. Impairment in anesthesiology: awareness and education. *Int Anesth Clin*. 2008;46:151.

Mackey DC, Carpenter RL, Thompson GE, Brown DL, Bodily MN. Bradycardia and asystole during spinal anesthesia: a report of three cases without morbidity. *Anesthesiology*. 1989;70:866.

Malafa MM, Coleman JE, Bowman RW, Rohrich RJ. Perioperative corneal abrasion: updated guidelines for prevention and management. *Plast Reconstr Surg*. 2016;137:790e.

María LT, Alejandro GS, María Jesús PG. Central venous catheter insertion: review of recent evidence. *Best Pract Res Clin Anaesthesiol*. 2021;35:135.

Martin L, Mhyre J, Shanks A, et al. 3,423 emergency tracheal intubations at a university hospital: airway outcomes and complications. *Anesthesiology*. 2011;114:42.

McCombe K, Bogod DG. Learning from the law. A review of 21 years of litigation for nerve injury following central neuraxial blockade in obstetrics. *Anaesthesia*. 2020;75:541.

McCombe K, Bogod D. Regional anaesthesia: risk, consent, and complications. *Anaesthesia*. 2021;76 Suppl 1:18.

Mertes P, Demoly P, Malinovsky J. Hypersensitivity reactions in the anesthesia setting/allergic reactions to anesthetics. *Curr Open Allergy Clin Immunol*. 2012;12:361.

Mertes PM, Volcheck GW, Garvey LH, et al. Epidemiology of perioperative anaphylaxis. *Presse Med*. 2016;45:758.

Metzner J, Posner K, Domino K. The risk and safety of anesthesia at remote locations: the US closed claims analysis. *Curr Opin Anaesthesiol*. 2009;22:502.

Moellman J, Bernstein J, Lindsell C, et al. A consensus parameter for the evaluation and management of angioedema in the emergency department. *Acad Emerg Med*. 2014;21:469.

Monitto C, Hamilton R, Levey E, et al. Genetic predisposition to natural rubber latex allergy differs between health care workers and high-risk patients. *Anesth Analg*. 2010;110:1310.

Ramamoorthy C, Haberkern C, Bhananker S, et al. Anesthesia-related cardiac arrest in children with heart disease: data from the pediatric perioperative cardiac arrest (POCA) registry. *Anesth Analg*. 2010;110:1376.

Robinson S, Kirsch J. Lean strategies in the operating room. *Anesthesiol Clin*. 2015;33:713.

Rose G, Brown R. The impaired anesthesiologist: not just about drugs and alcohol anymore. *J Clin Anesthesiol*. 2010;22:379.

Savic L, Stannard N, Farooque S. Allergy and anaesthesia: managing the risk. *BJA Educ*. 2020;20:298.

Schulz CM, Burden A, Posner KL, et al. Frequency and type of situational awareness errors contributing to death and brain damage: a closed claims analysis. *Anesthesiology*. 2017;127:326.

Sprung J, Bourke DL, Contreras MG, et al. Perioperative hearing impairment. *Anesthesiology*. 2003;98:241.

Stojiljkovic L. Renin-angiotensin system inhibitors and angioedema: anesthetic implications. *Curr Opin Anesthesiol*. 2012;25:356.

Szokol JW, Chamberlin KJ. Value proposition and anesthesiology. *Anesthesiol Clin*. 2018;36:227.

Tanaka KA, Mondal S, Morita Y, Williams B, Strauss ER, Cicardi M. Perioperative management of patients with hereditary angioedema with special considerations for cardiopulmonary bypass. *Anesth Analg*. 2020;131:155.

van Cuilenborg VR, Hermanides J, Bos EME Drs, et al. Perioperative approach of allergic patients. *Best Pract Res Clin Anaesthesiol*. 2021;35:11.

Vorobeichik L, Weber EA, Tarshis J. Misconceptions surrounding penicillin allergy: implications for anesthesiologists. *Anesth Analg*. 2018;127:642.

Welch M, Brummett C, Welch T, et al. Perioperative nerve injuries: a retrospective study of 380,680 cases during a 10-year period at a single institution. *Anesthesiology*. 2009;111:490.

Wilson SR, Shinde S, Appleby I, et al. Guidelines for the safe provision of anaesthesia in magnetic resonance units 2019: Guidelines from the Association of Anaesthetists and the Neuro Anaesthesia and Critical Care Society of Great Britain and Ireland. *Anaesthesia*. 2019;74:638.

Winters M, Rosenbaum S, Vilke G, et al. Emergency department management of patients with ace inhibitor angioedema. *J Emergency Med*. 2013;45:775.

Woodward ZG, Urman RD, Domino KB. Safety of non-operating room anesthesia: a closed claims update. *Anesthesiol Clin*. 2017;35:569.

Cardiopulmonary Resuscitation

CHAPTER

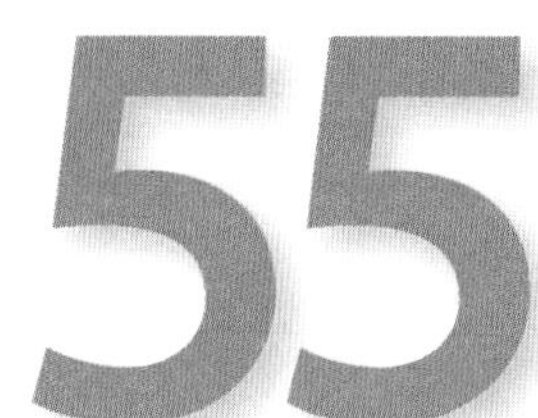

George W. Williams, MD, FASA, FCCM, FCCP

KEY CONCEPTS

1. Cardiopulmonary resuscitation (CPR) and emergency cardiovascular care (ECC) should be considered any time an individual cannot adequately oxygenate or perfuse vital organs—not only following cardiac or respiratory arrest.
2. Regardless of which transtracheal jet ventilation system is chosen, it must be readily available, use low-compliance tubing, and have secure connections.
3. Chest compressions should not be delayed; intubation may take place during CPR or during the pulse check.
4. Attempts at intubation should not interrupt ventilation for more than 10 s.
5. Chest compressions should begin before the delivery of breaths in the pulseless patient. Circulation takes precedence over airway interventions and breathing in the cardiac arrest patient.
6. Whether adult resuscitation is performed by a single rescuer or by two rescuers, two breaths are administered every 30 compressions (30:2), allowing 3 to 4 s for every two breaths. The cardiac compression rate should be 100 to 120/min regardless of the number of rescuers.
7. Health care personnel working in hospitals and ambulatory care facilities must be able to provide early defibrillation to patients with ventricular fibrillation as soon as possible. The time from collapse to defibrillation is the most important determinant of survival. The chances for survival decline 7% to 10% for every minute without defibrillation.
8. If intravenous cannulation is difficult, an intraosseous infusion can provide emergency vascular access in children and adults.
9. Lidocaine, epinephrine, atropine, naloxone, and vasopressin (but *not* sodium bicarbonate) can be delivered via a catheter whose tip extends past the endotracheal tube. Dosages 2 to 2½ times higher than recommended for intravenous use, diluted in 5 to 10 mL of normal saline or distilled water, are recommended for adult patients.
10. Because carbon dioxide, but not bicarbonate, readily crosses cell membranes and the blood–brain barrier, arterial hypercapnia causes intracellular tissue acidosis.
11. A wide QRS complex following a pacing spike signals electrical capture, but mechanical (ventricular) capture must be confirmed by an improving pulse or blood pressure.

TABLE 55–1 Emergency cardiac care (ECC).

1. Recognition of impending event
2. Activation of emergency response system
3. Basic life support
4. Defibrillation
5. Ventilation
6. Pharmacotherapy

1 **Cardiopulmonary resuscitation (CPR) and emergency cardiovascular care (ECC) should be considered any time an individual cannot adequately oxygenate or perfuse vital organs—not only following cardiac or respiratory arrest.**

This chapter presents an overview of the **2020 American Heart Association (AHA) Guidelines Update for Cardiopulmonary Resuscitation and Emergency Cardiovascular Care**, which provides revised recommendations for establishing and maintaining the *CABDs* of cardiopulmonary resuscitation: *Circulation, Airway, Breathing, and Defibrillation* (Table 55–1, Figures 55–1 and 55–2). The 2020 CPR-ECC guidelines have been updated with new evidence-based recommendations. Points of particular importance for the layperson are that the pulse should not be checked, and chest compression without ventilation may be as effective as compression with ventilation for the first several minutes. If a second lay rescuer is unavailable to perform mouth-to-mask ventilation, chest compressions alone are preferred to the primary rescuer attempting to do both. For the qualified health care provider, defibrillation using biphasic electrical current works best, and endotracheal tube (ETT) placement should be confirmed with a quantitative capnographic waveform analysis. More importantly, in the new guidelines, emphasis has been placed on the quality and adequacy of compressions, minimizing the interruption time of compressions and minimizing the *preshock pause* (the time taken from the last compression to the delivery of shock).

The sequence of steps in resuscitation has been changed since the 2010 guidelines from ABC (airway and breathing first, before compression) to CAB (compression first, with airway and breathing treated later). The previous guidelines opine that titrating resuscitative efforts to physiological parameters does not improve outcomes. Nonetheless, physiological monitoring methods to optimize CPR quality and *return of spontaneous circulation* (*ROSC*) are still useful. **The *rule of tens and multiples* can be applied: less than 10 s to check for a pulse; less than 10 s to place and secure the airway; target chest compression adequacy to maintain end-tidal pressure of carbon dioxide (P_{ETCO_2}) greater than 10 mm Hg; and target chest compression to maintain arterial diastolic blood pressure greater than 20 mm Hg and central venous oxygen saturation (S_{CVO_2}) greater than 30%.** The current guidelines suggest that a lack of a PET_{CO_2} greater than 10 mm Hg after 20 min in an intubated patient is associated with reduced likelihood of ROSC. An exception to this determination applies to nonintubated patients, in whom a specific P_{ETCO_2} cutoff should not be used to aid in the decision to end resuscitative efforts.

Changes in drug recommendations are a notable reaffirmation of epinephrine during cardiac arrest. Additionally, vasopressin, alone or in combination with epinephrine, offers no advantage over normal-dose epinephrine (1 mg every 3–5 min) in adult resuscitation following cardiac arrest. Amiodarone or lidocaine may be considered for ventricular fibrillation that is unresponsive to resuscitative efforts.

Although the use of extracorporeal membrane oxygenation (ECMO, also referred to as *extracorporeal cardiopulmonary resuscitation* [ECPR]) has been a topic of great interest and is increasingly available, the routine use of ECPR for cardiac arrest is not yet recommended. However, the guidelines suggest that when the etiology of the cardiac arrest is potentially reversible, the use of ECPR may be considered. The guidelines also allow for the use of point-of-care ultrasound but do not require it. Ultrasound techniques should only be performed by qualified personnel, and ultrasound interventions should not disrupt normal resuscitative practices and protocols. Of note, the use of ultrasonography has been found to increase interruptions in chest compressions.

This chapter is not intended as a substitute for a formal course in either life support without the use of special equipment (Basic Life Support [BLS]) or with the use of special equipment and drugs

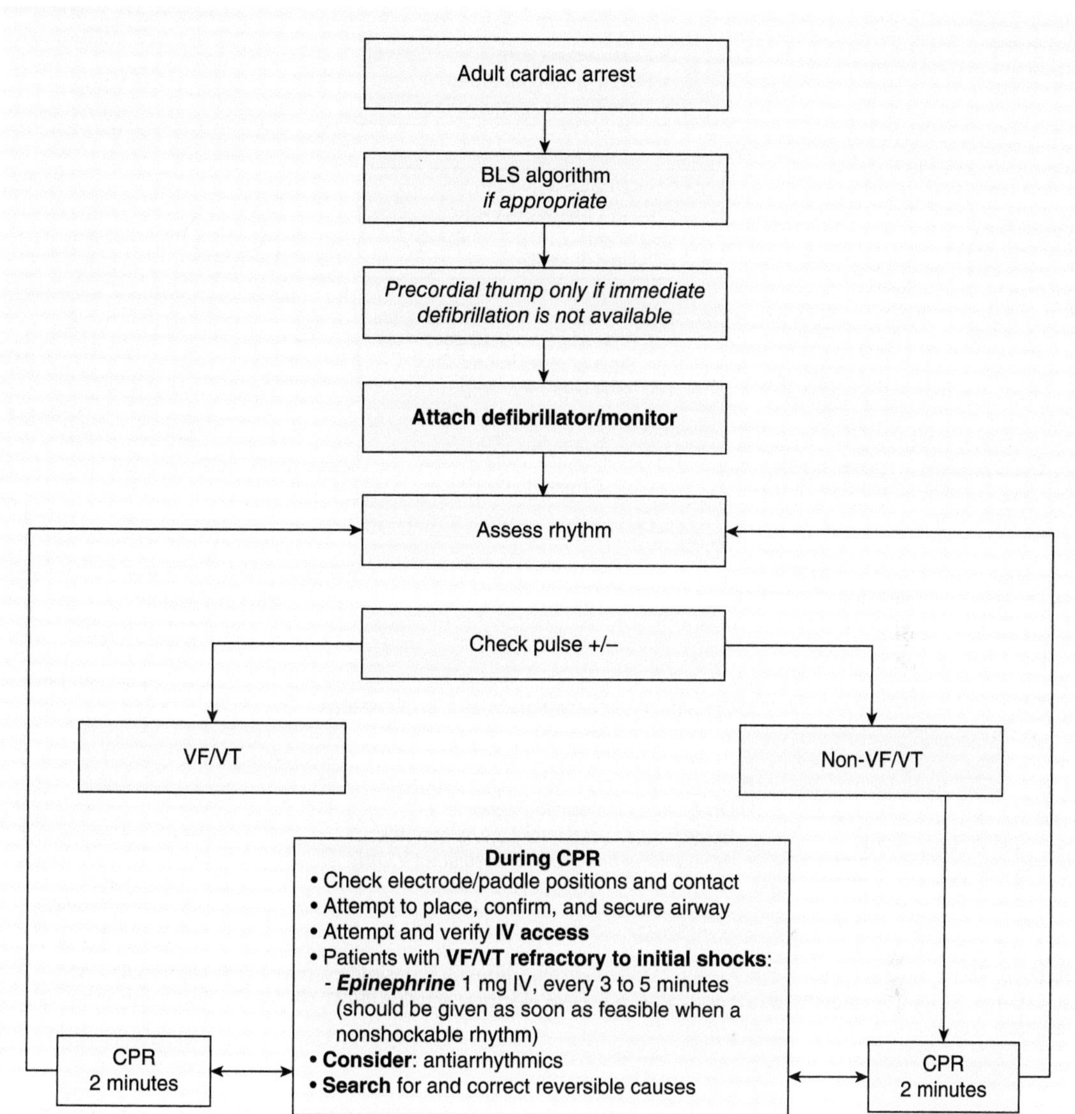

FIGURE 55–1 Universal algorithm for adult emergency cardiac care. ACS, acute coronary syndrome; BLS, basic life support; CPR, cardiopulmonary resuscitation; IV, intravenous; OD, overdose; VF/VT, ventricular fibrillation and pulseless ventricular tachycardia. (Data from Panchal AR, Bartos JA, Cabañas JG, et al: Part 3: Adult Basic and Advanced Life Support: 2020 American Heart Association Guidelines for Cardiopulmonary Resuscitation and Emergency Cardiovascular Care, *Circulation*. 2020 Oct 20;142(16_suppl_2): S366-S468.)

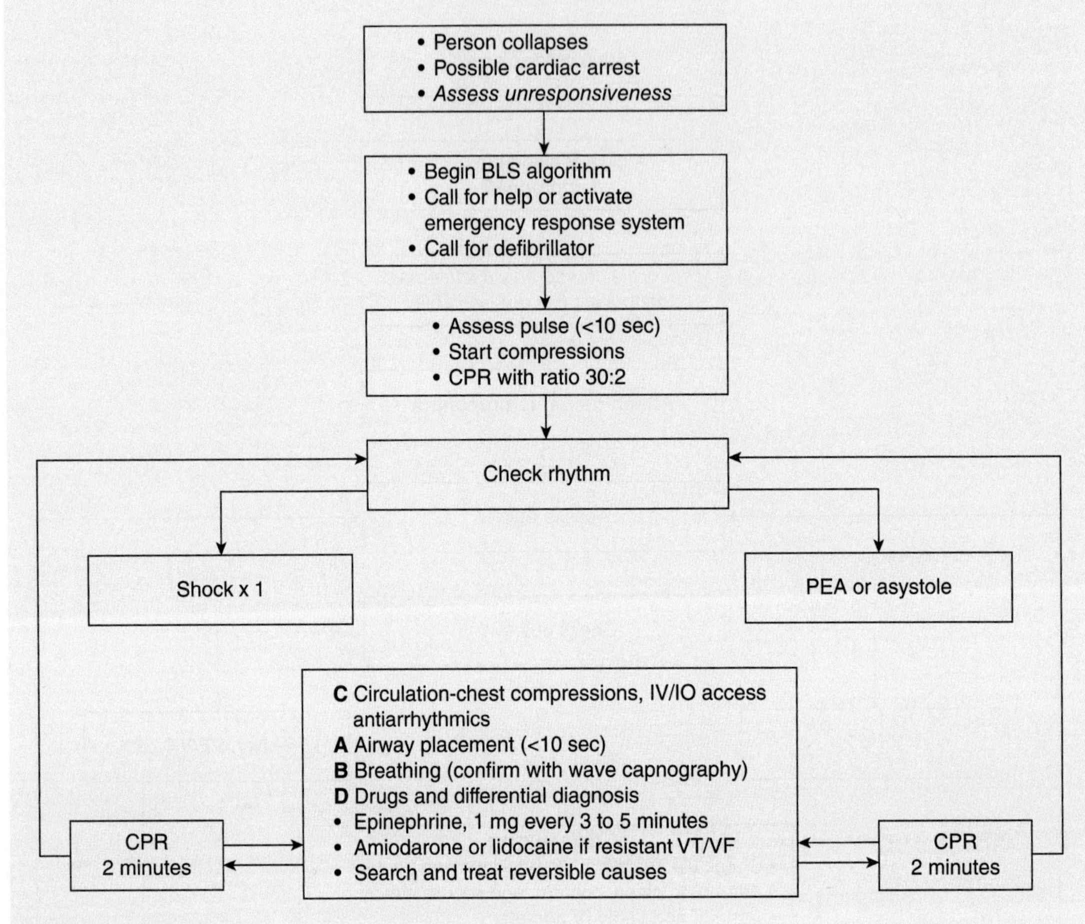

FIGURE 55–2 Comprehensive emergency cardiac care algorithm. BLS, basic life support; CPR, cardiopulmonary resuscitation; IO, intraosseous; IV, intravenous; PEA, pulseless electrical activity; VF/VT, ventricular fibrillation and pulseless ventricular tachycardia.

(Advanced Cardiac Life Support [ACLS]). Neonatal resuscitation is described in Chapter 41.

AIRWAY

Before CPR is initiated, the rescuer should determine that the victim is unresponsive and activate the emergency response system. *During low blood flow states such as cardiac arrest, oxygen delivery to the heart and brain is limited by blood flow rather than by arterial oxygen content; thus, current guidelines place greater emphasis on immediate initiation of chest compressions than on rescuer breaths.*

The patient is positioned supine on a firm surface. After initiation of chest compressions, the airway is evaluated. *The airway is most commonly obstructed by posterior displacement of the tongue or epiglottis.* If there is no evidence of cervical spine instability, a head-tilt chin-lift should be tried first (Figure 55–3). One hand (palm) is placed on the patient's forehead, applying pressure to tilt the head back while lifting the chin with the forefinger and index finger of the opposite hand. The jaw-thrust

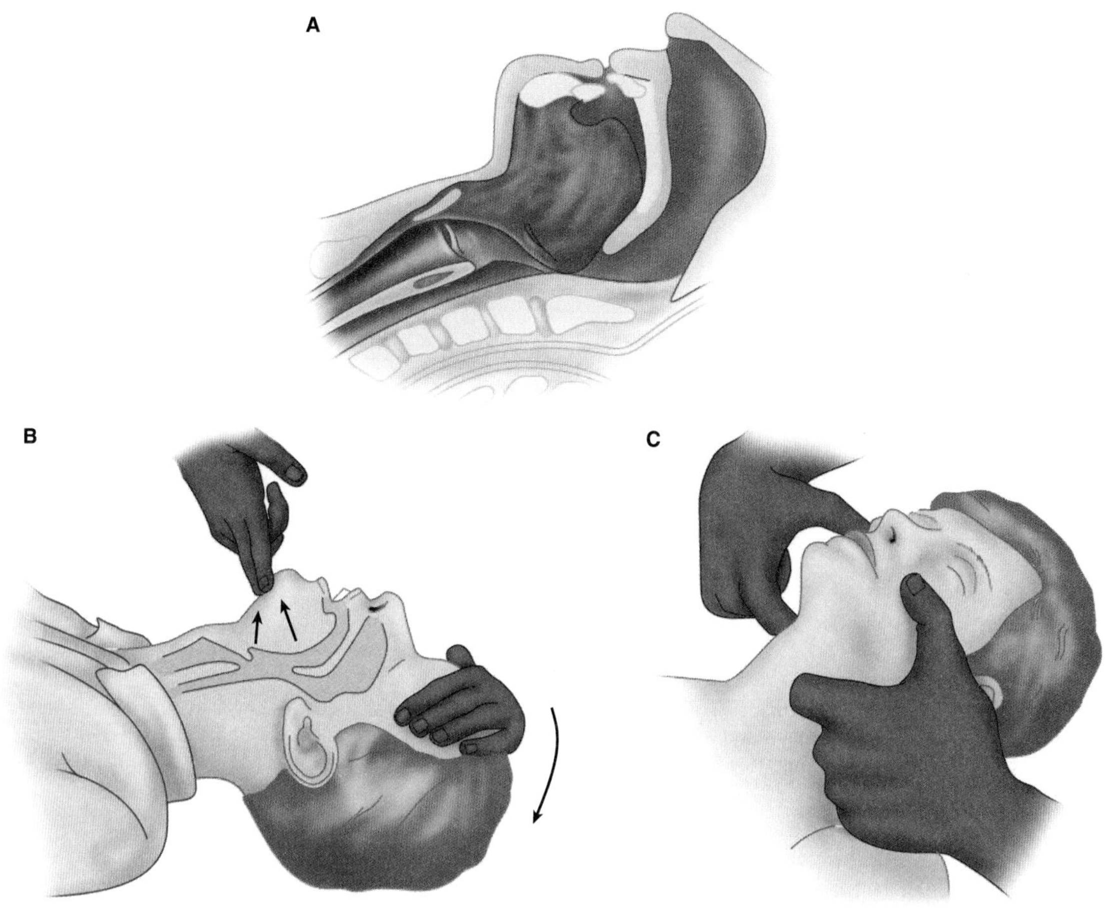

FIGURE 55–3 Loss of consciousness is often accompanied by loss of submandibular muscle tone (**A**). Occlusion of the airway by the tongue can be relieved by a head-tilt chin-lift (**B**) or a jaw-thrust (**C**). In patients with possible cervical spine injury, the angles of the jaw should be lifted anteriorly without hyperextending the neck.

may be more effective in opening the airway and is executed by placing both hands on either side of the patient's head, grasping the angles of the jaw, and lifting. Basic airway management is discussed in detail in Chapter 19, and additional airway management issues specifically related to trauma care are reviewed in Chapter 39.

Any vomitus or foreign body visible in the mouth of an unconscious patient must be removed. If the patient is conscious or if the foreign body cannot be removed by a finger sweep, the *Heimlich maneuver* is recommended. This subdiaphragmatic abdominal thrust elevates the diaphragm, expelling a blast of air from the lungs that displaces the foreign body (Figure 55–4). Complications of the Heimlich maneuver include rib fracture, trauma to internal viscera, and regurgitation with aspiration. A combination of back blows and chest thrusts is recommended to clear foreign body obstruction in infants (Table 55–2).

If after opening the airway breathing remains inadequate, the rescuer must initiate assisted ventilation by inflating the victim's lungs with each breath using a bag-mask device (see Chapter 19).

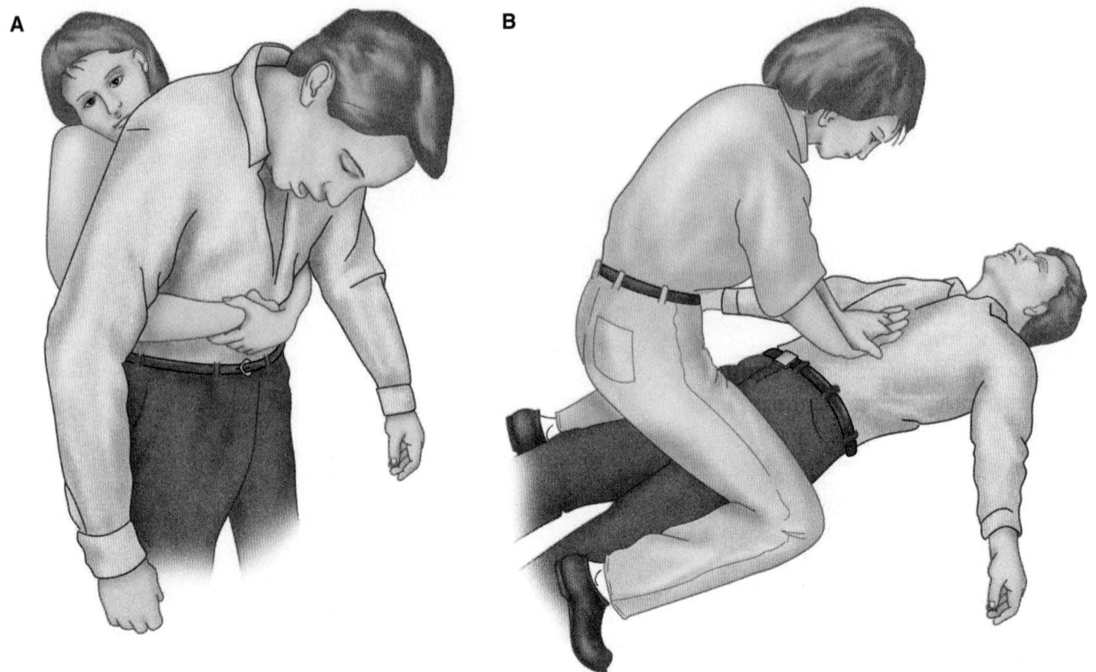

FIGURE 55–4 The Heimlich maneuver can be performed with the victim standing (**A**) or lying down (**B**). The hands are positioned slightly above the navel and well below the xiphoid process and then pressed into the abdomen with a quick upward thrust. The maneuver may need to be repeated.

Breaths are delivered slowly (inspiratory time of ½–1 s) at a rate of about 10 breaths/min, with smaller tidal volumes [VT] so as to minimize the adverse effect on cardiac preload. *Chest compressions (100–120/min) should not be suspended during two-person CPR to permit ventilation unless ventilation is not possible during compressions.*

Gastric inflation with subsequent regurgitation and aspiration is possible with positive-pressure mask ventilation, even with a small VT. Therefore, the airway should be secured with an ETT as soon as feasible, or, if that is not possible, an alternative airway should be inserted. There is inadequate evidence to support the optimal timing of the placement of an advanced airway (supraglottic device, ETT); however, chest compressions should not be interrupted for more than 10 s to place any advanced airway device. The benefit of an advanced airway must be considered in light of the risk of potential interruption in compressions. Advanced airways include the esophageal–tracheal Combitube (ETC), laryngeal mask airway (LMA), pharyngotracheal lumen airway, King laryngeal tube, and cuffed oropharyngeal airway. The ETC and LMA, along with oral and nasopharyngeal airways, face masks, laryngoscopes, and ETTs, are discussed in Chapter 19. Of these, the LMA is increasingly preferred for in-hospital arrests. The choice of bag-mask ventilation versus placement of an advanced airway is dependent upon the skills of the providers. Studies conflict as to the optimal use of advanced airway management techniques in comparison with bag-mask ventilation.

Independent of which airway adjunct is used, the guidelines state that rescuers must confirm ETT placement with a P_{ETCO_2} detector—an indicator, a capnograph, or a capnometric device. The preferred choice for confirmation of ETT placement is continuous capnographic waveform analysis. All confirmation devices are considered adjuncts to clinical confirmation techniques (eg, auscultation). *Once an artificial airway is successfully placed, it must be*

TABLE 55–2 Summary of recommended basic life support techniques.

	Infant (1–12 mo)	Child (>12 mo)	Adult
Breathing rate	20–30 breaths/min	20–30 breaths/min	6 breaths/min[1]
Pulse check	Brachial	Carotid	Carotid
Compression rate	>100/min	100/min	100–120/min
Compression method	Two or three fingers or thumb-encircling hands technique	Heel of one hand	Hands interlaced
Compression/ventilation ratio	30:2	30:2	30:2
Foreign body obstruction	Back blows followed by chest thrusts	Heimlich maneuver	Heimlich maneuver

[1]Decrease to 8–10 breaths/min if the airway is secured with a tracheal tube.

carefully secured with a tie or tape because up to 25% of airways are displaced during transportation.

Some causes of airway obstruction may not be relieved by conventional methods. Furthermore, endotracheal intubation may be technically impossible to perform in certain circumstances (eg, severe facial trauma), or repeated attempts may be unwise (eg, cervical spine trauma). Cricothyrotomy or tracheotomy may be necessary in situations such as these. *Cricothyrotomy* involves placing a large intravenous catheter or a commercially available cannula into the trachea through the midline of the cricothyroid membrane (Figure 55–5). Proper location is confirmed by aspiration of air. A 12- or 14-gauge catheter requires a driving pressure of 50 psi to generate sufficient gas flow for transtracheal jet ventilation. The catheter must be adequately secured to the skin because the jet ventilation pressure can otherwise easily propel the catheter out of the trachea and, if the tip remains beneath the skin, lead to massive subcutaneous emphysema.

Various systems are available that connect a high-pressure source of oxygen (eg, central wall oxygen, tank oxygen, or the anesthesia machine fresh gas outlet) to the catheter (Figure 55–6). A hand-operated jet injector or the oxygen flush valve of an anesthesia machine controls ventilation. The addition of a pressure regulator minimizes the risk of barotrauma.

2 **Regardless of which transtracheal jet ventilation system is chosen, it must be readily available, use low-compliance tubing, and have secure connections.** Direct connection of a 12- or 14-gauge intravenous catheter to the anesthesia circle system does not allow adequate ventilation because of the high compliance of the corrugated breathing tubing and breathing bag. Similarly, one cannot reliably deliver acceptable ventilation through a 12- or 14-gauge catheter with a self-inflating resuscitation bag. Approaches regarding front-of-neck airway access are reviewed in detail in Chapter 19.

Adequacy of ventilation—particularly expiration—is judged by observation of chest wall movement and auscultation of breath sounds. Acute complications include pneumothorax, subcutaneous emphysema, mediastinal emphysema, bleeding, esophageal puncture, aspiration, and respiratory acidosis. Long-term complications include tracheomalacia, subglottic stenosis, and vocal cord changes. Cricothyrotomy is not generally recommended in children younger than 10 years of age.

Tracheotomy can be performed in a more controlled fashion after oxygenation has been restored by cricothyrotomy (see Chapter 19).

BREATHING

3 Assessment of spontaneous breathing should immediately follow the opening or the establishment of the airway. **Chest compressions and ventilation should not be delayed for intubation if a patent airway is established by a jaw-thrust maneuver; intubation may take place during CPR or the pulse check.** Apnea is confirmed by lack of chest movement, absence of breath sounds, and lack of

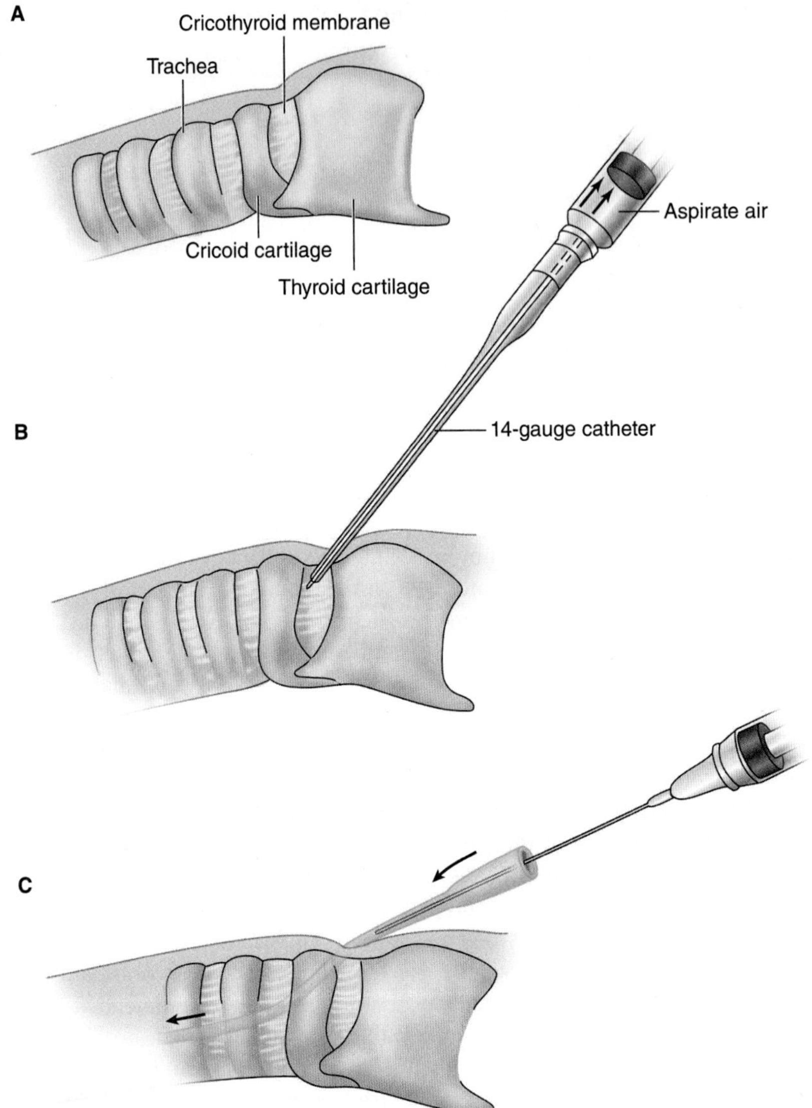

FIGURE 55–5 Percutaneous cricothyrotomy with a 14-gauge over-the-needle intravenous catheter. **A**: Locate the cricothyroid membrane. **B**: Puncture the membrane at the midline while stabilizing the trachea with the other hand. Proper location is confirmed by easy aspiration of air. **C**: Advance the catheter and withdraw the needle. Attach the syringe to the catheter, and aspirate again after the catheter is advanced to confirm that the catheter remains in the tracheal lumen.

airflow; it is important to note that agonal breathing is frequently seen in cardiac arrest and does not indicate true respiratory effort. Regardless of the airway and breathing methods employed, a specific regimen of ventilation has been proposed for the apneic patient and described earlier in this chapter. Initially, two breaths are slowly administered (2 s per breath in adults, 1–1½ s in infants and children). If these breaths cannot be delivered, either the airway is still obstructed and the head and neck need

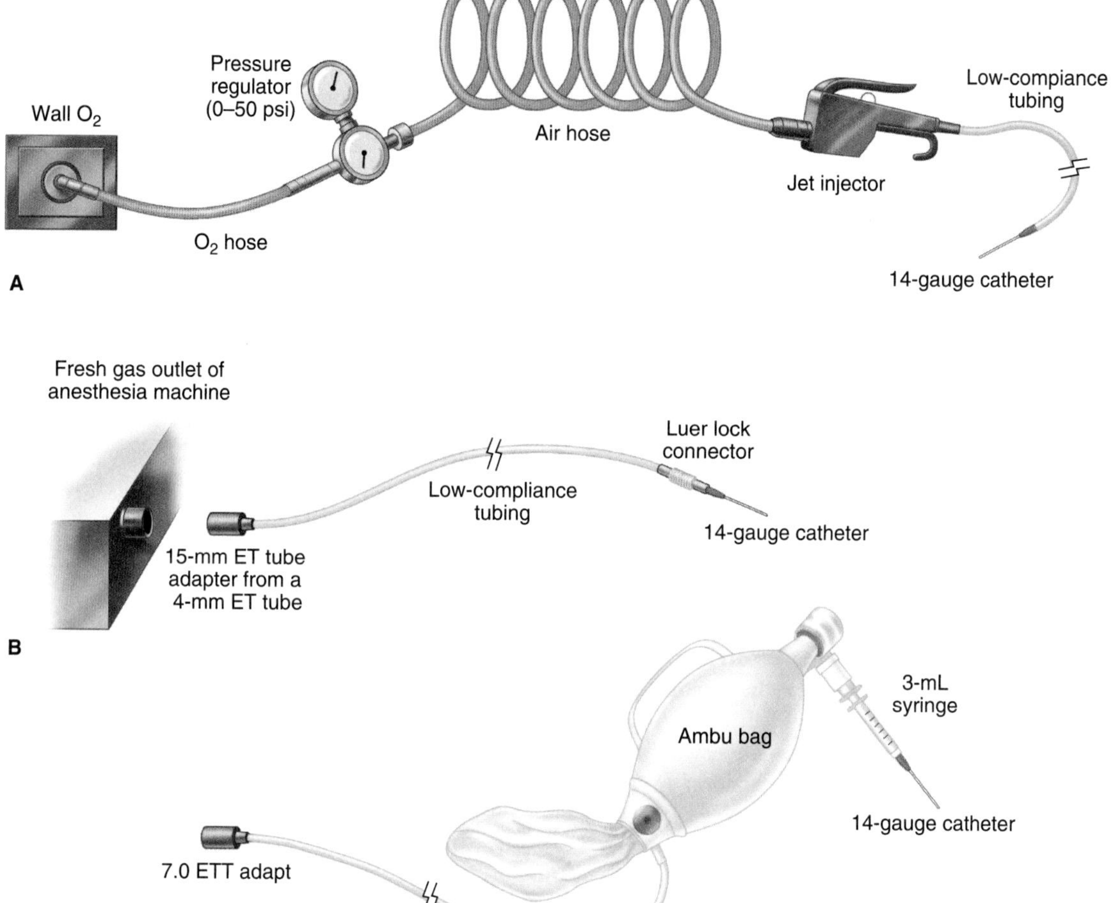

FIGURE 55–6 **A, B**: Two systems for transtracheal jet ventilation after cricothyrotomy (see **Figure 55–5**). A jet ventilator and pressure regulator (as shown in A) provide better control of the inspiratory cycle. Both systems use low-compliance tubing and a high-pressure source of oxygen. **C**: The hub from a 7.0 endotracheal tube (ETT) may be adapted to connect with a 14-gauge catheter and 3-mL syringe to provide jet ventilation with oxygen when outside the operating room or when jet ventilation is not available.

repositioning and possibly an oral airway placed, or a foreign body is present that must be removed.

Bag-mask rescue breathing should be instituted in the apneic patient when these devices are immediately available. Supplemental oxygen, preferably 100%, should always be used if available. Successful rescue breathing, *500 to 600 mL Vt, 6 times per minute in an adult with a secured airway and a ratio of 30 compressions to 2 ventilations if the airway is unsecured*, is confirmed by observing the chest rising and falling with each breath and hearing and feeling the escape of air during expiration

Devices that avoid use of the provider's mouth should be immediately available everywhere in the hospital. Ventilation with a mask may be performed in most patients by adjusting the airway or making the airtight seal more effective (see Chapter 19). Use of cricoid pressure to prevent regurgitation during cardiac arrest resuscitation may be considered; however, there are no data to support its efficacy in this (or any other) circumstance, and we do not recommend its routine use.

Endotracheal intubation by competent personnel should be attempted as soon as practical. 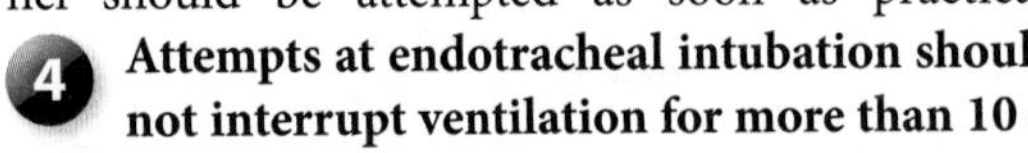 **Attempts at endotracheal intubation should not interrupt ventilation for more than 10 s.** After intubation, the patient can be ventilated with high oxygen concentrations. A rate of 6 breaths/min should be maintained because greater ventilatory rates may impede cardiac output during CPR in a cardiac arrest situation.

The ratio of physiological dead space to tidal volume (VD/VT) reflects the efficiency of CO_2 elimination. VD/VT increases during CPR as a result of low pulmonary blood flow and high alveolar pressures. Thus, minute ventilation may need to be increased by 50% to 100% once circulation is restored as CO_2 from the periphery is brought back to the lungs.

CIRCULATION

5 **Circulation takes precedence over airway interventions and breathing in the cardiac arrest patient. As previously noted, chest compressions should begin prior to the delivery of breaths.** Subsequent actions to assess circulation may then vary depending on whether the responder is a layperson or health care provider. *Although lay rescuers should assume that an unresponsive patient is in cardiac arrest and need not check the pulse, health care providers should assess for the presence or absence of a pulse.*

If the patient has an adequate pulse (carotid artery in an adult or child, brachial or femoral artery in an infant) or blood pressure, breathing is continued at 6 breaths/min for an adult or a child older than 8 years and 20 to 30 breaths/min for an infant or a child younger than 8 years of age (see **Table 55–2**). If the patient is pulseless or severely hypotensive, the circulatory system must be supported by a combination of external chest compressions, intravenous drug administration, and defibrillation when appropriate. Initiation of chest compressions is mandated by the inadequacy of peripheral perfusion, and drug choices and defibrillation energy levels often depend on an electrocardiographic diagnosis of arrhythmias.

External Chest Compression

Chest compressions force blood to flow either by increasing intrathoracic pressure (thoracic pump) or by directly compressing the heart (cardiac pump). During CPR of short duration, the blood flow is created more by the cardiac pump mechanism; as CPR continues, the heart becomes less compliant, and the thoracic pump mechanism becomes more important. As important as the rate and force of compression are for maintaining blood flow, effective perfusion of the heart and brain is best achieved when chest compression consumes 50% of the duty cycle, with the remaining 50% devoted to the relaxation phase (allowing blood return into the chest and heart). Real-time audiovisual feedback (ie, verbal or with a metronome) during CPR may improve performance and patient survival as there can be significant variability in chest compression rate, especially as compressors experience fatigue.

To perform chest compressions in the unresponsive or pulseless patient, the xiphoid process is located, and the heel of the rescuer's hand is placed over the lower half of the sternum. The other hand is placed over the hand on the sternum with the fingers either interlaced or extended, but off the chest. The rescuer's shoulders should be positioned directly over the hands with the elbows locked into position and arms extended so that the weight of the upper body is used for compressions. With a straight downward thrust, the sternum is depressed approximately 2 inches (5 cm) in adults and 1 to 1½ inches (2–4 cm) in children and then allowed to return to its normal position. For an infant, compressions ½ to 1 inches (1½–2½ cm) in depth are made with the middle and ring fingers on the sternum one fingerbreadth below the nipple line. Compression and release times should be equal.

6 **Whether adult resuscitation is performed by a single rescuer or by two rescuers, two breaths are administered every 30 compressions (30:2), allowing 3 to 4 s for the two breaths. The cardiac compression rate should be 100/min regardless of the number of rescuers. A slightly higher compression rate of more than 100/min is suggested for infants, with two breaths delivered every 30 compressions.**

Assessing the Adequacy of Chest Compressions

Adequacy of cardiac output can be estimated by monitoring P_{ETCO_2} (>10 mm Hg), S_{CVO_2} (>30%), and/or arterial pulsations (with arterial diastolic relaxation pressure >20 mm Hg). Arterial pulsations during chest compressions are not a good measure of adequate chest compression; however, spontaneous arterial pulsations are an indicator of ROSC. Physiological parameters, such as P_{ETCO_2}, S_{CVO_2}, and diastolic arterial pressure, may aid in assessing the adequacy of chest compressions but cannot be used exclusively to determine if CPR should be discontinued.

1. **P_{ETCO_2}**—In an intubated patient, a P_{ETCO_2} greater than 10 mm Hg indicates good-quality chest compressions; a P_{ETCO_2} less than 10 mm Hg has been shown to be a predictor of poor outcomes of CPR (decreased chance of ROSC) in CPR of more than 20 min duration. A transient increase in P_{ETCO_2} may be seen with the administration of sodium bicarbonate; however, an abrupt and sustained rise of P_{ETCO_2} is an indicator of ROSC.
2. **Coronary perfusion pressure (CPP)**—This is the difference between the aortic diastolic pressure and the right atrial diastolic pressure. Arterial diastolic pressure in the radial, brachial, or femoral artery is a good indicator of CPP. Arterial diastolic pressure greater than 20 mm Hg is an indicator of adequate chest compressions.
3. **S_{CVO_2}**—An S_{CVO_2} less than 30% in the jugular vein is associated with poor outcomes. If the S_{CVO_2} is less than 30%, attempts to improve the quality of CPR, either by improving the quality of compressions or through administration of medications, must be considered.

DEFIBRILLATION

Ventricular fibrillation is found most commonly in adults who experience nontraumatic cardiac arrest. The time from collapse to defibrillation is the most important determinant of survival. The chances for survival decline 7% to 10% for every minute without defibrillation (Figure 55–7). **Therefore, patients who** 7 **have cardiac arrest should be defibrillated at the earliest possible moment. Health care personnel working in hospitals and ambulatory care facilities must be able to provide early defibrillation to collapsed patients with ventricular fibrillation as soon as possible.** Shock should be delivered the moment the chest compressor removes their hands from the chest.

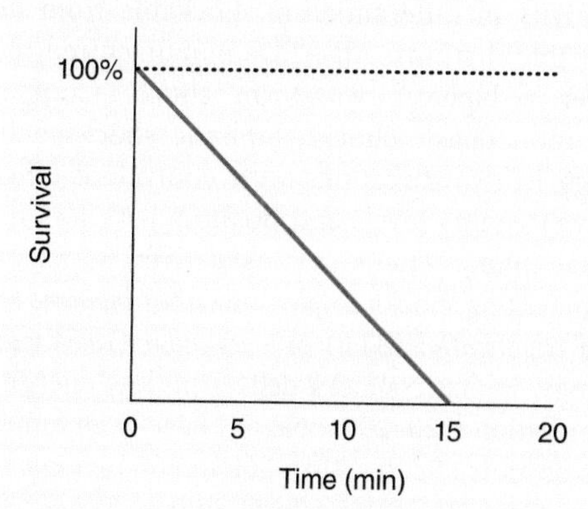

FIGURE 55–7 Success of defibrillation versus time. The chance of successful defibrillation of a patient in ventricular fibrillation decreases 7% to 10% per minute.

There is no definite relationship between the energy requirement for successful defibrillation and body size. A shock with too low an energy level will not successfully defibrillate; conversely, too high an energy level may result in myocardial injury. Defibrillators deliver energy in either monophasic or biphasic waveforms. Biphasic waveforms are recommended for cardioversion as they achieve the same degree of success but with less energy and theoretically less myocardial damage; newly manufactured defibrillators use biphasic waveforms.

Automated external defibrillators (AEDs) are available in many institutions. Such devices are increasingly being used throughout communities by police, firefighters, security personnel, sports marshals, ski patrol members, and airline flight attendants, among others. They are commonly placed in any public location where 20,000 or more people pass by every day. AEDs are microprocessor-controlled devices that are capable of electrocardiographic analysis with very high specificity and sensitivity in differentiating shockable from nonshockable rhythms. All AEDs manufactured today deliver a biphasic waveform shock. Compared with monophasic shocks, biphasic shocks deliver energy in two directions with equivalent efficacy at lower energy levels and possibly with less myocardial injury. These devices deliver impedance-compensating shocks employing either *biphasic truncated exponential* (BTE) or *rectilinear* (RBW) morphology. Biphasic shocks delivering low energy for defibrillation (120–200 joule [J]) have been found to be as or more effective than 200 to 360 J *monophasic damped sine* (MDS) waveform shocks. When using AEDs, one electrode pad is placed beside the upper right sternal border, just below the clavicle, and the other pad is placed just lateral to the left nipple, with the top of the pad a few inches below the axilla.

A decrease in time delay between the last compression and the delivery of a shock (the *preshock pause*) has received special emphasis in the 2020 guidelines. *Double sequential defibrillation* (delivering two or more shocks in immediate succession without intervening compressions) has not been shown to improve outcomes and increases the time to the next compression. Furthermore, it has been noted that the first shock is usually associated with a 90% efficacy. *Thus, the guidelines are for a single shock, followed by immediate resumption of chest compressions.*

For cardioversion of atrial fibrillation, 120 to 200 J can be used initially with escalation if needed. For atrial flutter or paroxysmal supraventricular tachycardia (PSVT), an initial energy level of 50 to 100 J is often adequate. All monophasic shocks should start with 200 J. Manufacturer instructions typically provide the recommended starting shock energy level specific to the device.

Ventricular tachycardia, particularly monomorphic ventricular tachycardia, responds well to shocks at initial energy levels of 100 J. For polymorphic ventricular tachycardia or for ventricular fibrillation, initial energy can be set at 120 to 200 J, depending upon the type of biphasic waveform being used. Stepwise increases in energy levels can be used if the first shock fails, though some AEDs operate with a fixed-energy protocol of 150 J with very high success in terminating ventricular fibrillation (see **Table 55–3**).

Cardioversion should be synchronized with the QRS complex and is recommended for hemodynamically stable, wide-complex tachycardia requiring cardioversion, PSVT, atrial fibrillation, and atrial flutter. Polymorphic ventricular tachycardia should be treated as ventricular fibrillation with unsynchronized shocks.

Invasive Cardiopulmonary Resuscitation

Thoracotomy and open-chest cardiac massage are not part of routine CPR because of the frequent incidence of complications. Nonetheless, these invasive techniques can be helpful in specific life-threatening circumstances that preclude effective closed-chest massage. Possible indications include cardiac arrest associated with penetrating or blunt chest trauma, penetrating abdominal trauma, severe chest deformity, pericardial tamponade, or pulmonary embolism. Extracorporeal membrane oxygenation is increasingly employed when the cause of arrest (eg, local anesthetic systemic toxicity) is reversible.

Intravenous Access

Establishing reliable intravenous access is a high priority, but it should not take precedence over initial chest compressions, airway management, or defibrillation. A preexisting internal jugular or subclavian catheter is ideal for venous access during resuscitation. If there is no central line access, an attempt should be made to establish peripheral intravenous access in either the antecubital or the external jugular vein. Peripheral intravenous sites are associated with a significant delay of 1 to 2 min between drug administration and delivery to the heart, as peripheral blood flow is drastically reduced during CPR. Administration of drugs given through a peripheral intravenous line should be followed by an intravenous flush (eg, a 20-mL fluid bolus in adults) or elevation of the extremity for 10 to 20 s, or both. Establishing central vein access can potentially cause interruption of CPR but should be considered if an inadequate response is seen to peripherally administered drugs.

If intravenous cannulation is difficult, an *intraosseous infusion* can provide emergency

vascular access in children and adults. A rigid 18-gauge spinal needle with a stylet or a small bone marrow trephine needle can be inserted into the distal femur or proximal tibia. If the tibia is chosen, a needle is inserted 2 to 3 cm below the tibial tuberosity at a 45° angle away from the epiphyseal plate (Figure 55–8). Once the needle is advanced through the cortex, it should stand upright without support. Correct placement is confirmed by the ability to aspirate marrow through the needle and deliver a smooth infusion of fluid. A network of venous sinusoids within the medullary cavity of long bones drains into the systemic circulation by way of nutrient or emissary veins. This route is very effective for the administration of drugs, crystalloids, colloids, and blood and can achieve flow rates exceeding 100 mL/h under gravity. Much higher flow rates are possible if the fluid is placed under pressure (eg, 300 mm Hg) with an infusion bag. The onset of drug action may be slightly delayed compared with intravenous or tracheal administration. The intraosseous route may require a higher dose of some drugs (eg, epinephrine) than recommended for intravenous administration. The use of intraosseous infusion for induction and maintenance of general anesthesia, antibiotic therapy, seizure control, and inotropic support has been described. (Note that most studies have evaluated the placement of intraosseous access in patients with intact hemodynamics or hypovolemic states, not in cardiac arrest situations.) Because of the risks of osteomyelitis and compartment syndrome, however, intraosseous infusions should be replaced by a conventional intravenous route as soon as possible. In addition, because of the theoretical risk of bone marrow or fat emboli, intraosseous infusions should be avoided if possible in patients with right-to-left shunts, pulmonary hypertension, or severe pulmonary insufficiency. Some resuscitation drugs are

9 fairly well absorbed following administration through an ETT. **Lidocaine, epinephrine, atropine, naloxone, and vasopressin (but *not* sodium bicarbonate) can be delivered via a catheter whose tip extends past the ETT. Notably, the American Heart Association recommends endotracheal dosing only when IV and intraosseous dosing cannot be accomplished. Dosages 2 to 2½ times higher than recommended for intravenous use, diluted in 5 to 10 mL of normal saline or distilled water, are recommended for adult patients.** It is important to note that some volume regurgitation can occur into the ETT, which may cause inaccurate $ETCO_2$ indications.

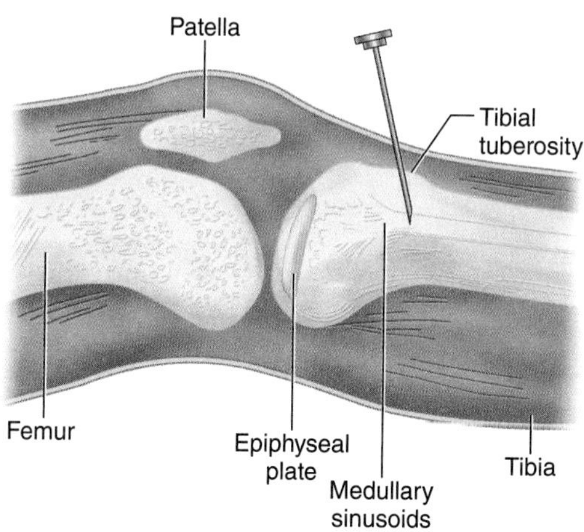

FIGURE 55–8 Intraosseous infusions provide emergency access to the venous circulation in pediatric patients by way of the large medullary venous channels. The needle is directed away from the epiphyseal plate to minimize the risk of injury.

Arrhythmia Recognition

Interpreting rhythm strips in the midst of a resuscitation situation is frequently complicated by artifacts and variations in monitoring techniques (eg, lead systems, equipment, motion). However, successful pharmacological and electrical treatment of cardiac arrest (Figure 55–9) depends on the definitive identification of the underlying arrhythmia.

Drug Administration

Many of the drugs administered during CPR have been described elsewhere in this text. Table 55–3 summarizes the cardiovascular actions, indications, and dosages of drugs commonly used during resuscitation.

Atropine is reasonable for treatment for symptomatic bradycardia. Infusions of chronotropic drugs (eg, dopamine, epinephrine, isoproterenol) can be

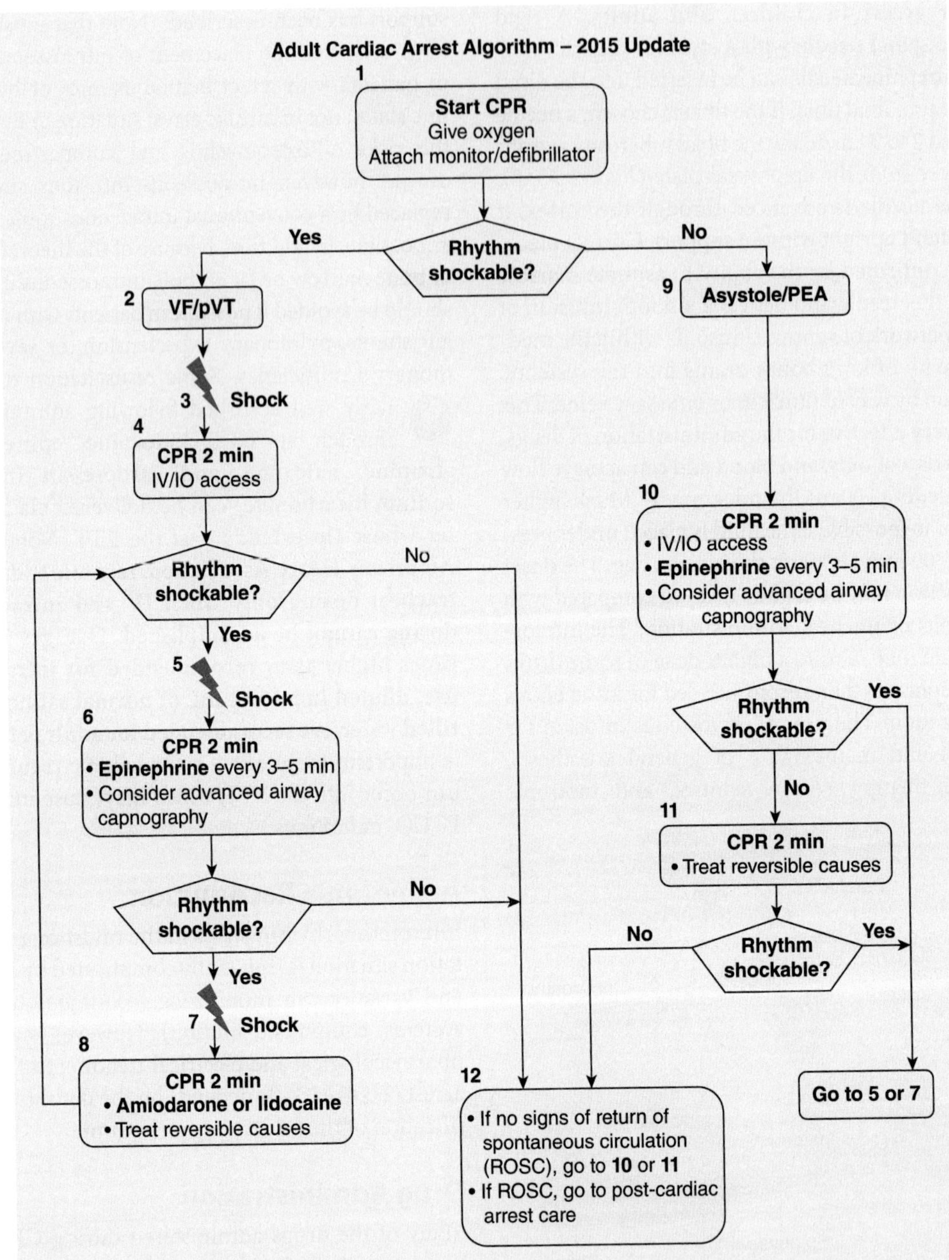

FIGURE 55–9 Adult cardiac arrest algorithm—2020 update. Algorithm for treating ventricular fibrillation and pulseless ventricular tachycardia (VF/VT). Pulseless ventricular tachycardia should be treated in the same way as ventricular fibrillation. Note: This figure and **Figures 55–1** and **55–2** emphasize the concept that rescuers and health care providers must assume that all unmonitored adult cardiac arrests are due to VF/VT. In each figure, the flow of the algorithm assumes that the arrhythmia is continuing. CPR, cardiopulmonary resuscitation; IV/IO, intravenous or intraosseous; PEA, pulseless electrical activity; VF/pVT, ventricular fibrillation and pulseless ventricular tachycardia. (Reproduced with permission from Panchal AR, Bartos JA, Cabañas JG, et al: Part 3: Adult Basic and Advanced Life Support: 2020 American Heart Association Guidelines for Cardiopulmonary Resuscitation and Emergency Cardiovascular Care. *Circulation*. 2020 Oct 20;142(16_suppl_2):S366-S468.)

CPR Quality

- Push hard (≥2 inches [5 cm]) and fast (≥100/min) and allow complete chest recoil
- Minimize interruptions in compressions
- Avoid excessive ventilation
- Rotate compressor every 2 minutes
- If no advanced airway, 30:2 compression-ventilation ratio
- Quantitative waveform capnography
- $PETCO_2$<10 mm Hg after 20 minutes suggests poor outcome and may be used in combination with other clinical factors (multimodal approach) to consider discontinuation of rescucitation

Intra-arterial Pressure

- If relaxation phase (diastolic) pressure <20 mm Hg, attempt to improve CPR quality Return of Spontaneous Circulation (ROSC)
- Pulse and blood pressure
- Abrupt sustained increase in $PETCO_2$ (typically ≥40 mm Hg)
- Spontaneous arterial pressure waves with intra-arterial monitoring

Shock Energy

- Biphasic: Manufacturer recommendation (eg, initial dose of 120–200 J); if unknown, use maximum available. Second and subsequent doses should be equivalent, and higher doses may be considered.
- Monophasic: 360 J

Drug Therapy

- Epinephrine IV/IO dose:
  1 mg every 3–5 minutes
- Amiodarone IV/IO dose:
  First dose: 300-mg bolus
  Second dose: 150-mg (hold extra dose of amiodarone if MI is suspected)
    - Lidocaine IV/IO dose:
    First dose: 1–1.5mg/kg
    Second dose: 0.5–0.75 mg/kg

Advanced Airway

- Supraglottic advanced airway or endotracheal intubation
- Waveform capnography to confirm and monitor ET tube placement
- 8–10 breaths per minute with continuous chest compressions

Reversible Causes

- Hypovolemia
- Hypoxia
- Hydrogen ion (acidosis)
- Hypo-/hyperkalemia
- Hypothermia
- Tension pneuomothorax
- Tamponade, cardiac
- Toxins
- Thrombosis, pulmonary
- Thrombosis, coronary

FIGURE 55–9 *(Continued)*

considered as an alternative to pacing if atropine is ineffective in the setting of symptomatic bradycardia. *Calcium chloride, sodium bicarbonate, and bretylium are conspicuously absent from this table.* Calcium (2–4 mg/kg of the chloride salt) is helpful in the treatment of documented hypocalcemia, hyperkalemia, hypermagnesemia, or a calcium channel blocker overdose. When used, 10% calcium chloride can be given

TABLE 55–3 Cardiovascular effects, indications, and dosages of resuscitation drugs.

			Initial Dose		
Drug	**Cardiovascular Effects**	**Indications**	**Adult**	**Pediatric**	**Comments**
Adenosine	Slows AV nodal conduction	Narrow complex tachycardias, stable supraventricular tachycardia, and wide-complex tachycardias if supraventricular in origin	6 mg over 1–3 s; 12 mg repeat dose	Initial dose 0.1–0.2 mg/kg; subsequent doses doubled to maximum single dose of 12 mg	Recommended as diagnostic or therapeutic maneuver for supraventricular tachycardias; give as rapid IV bolus. Vasodilates, BP may decrease. Theoretical risk of angina, bronchospasm, proarrhythmic action. Drug–drug interaction with theophylline, dipyridamole.
Atropine	Anticholinergic (parasympatholytic). Increases sinoatrial node rate and automaticity; increases AV node conduction	Symptomatic bradycardia, AV block	0.5–1.0 mg repeated every 3–5 min	0.02 mg/kg	Repeat atropine doses every 5 min to a total dose of 3 mg in adults or 0.5 mg in children, 1 mg in adolescents. The minimum pediatric dose is 0.1 mg. Do not use for infranodal (Mobitz II) block.
Epinephrine	α-Adrenergic effects increase myocardial and cerebral blood flow. β-Adrenergic effects may increase myocardial work and decrease subendocardial perfusion and cerebral blood flow	VF/VT, electromechanical dissociation, ventricular asystole, severe bradycardia unresponsive to atropine or pacing Severe hypotension	1 mg IV 0.03 mcg/kg/min in an infusion increased to effect	Initial dose 0.01 mg/kg IV; repeat same for subsequent doses 1 mcg/kg	Repeat doses every 3–5 min as necessary. An infusion of epinephrine (eg, 1 mg in 250 mL D_5W or NS, 4 mcg/mL) can be titrated to effect in adults (1–4 mcg/min) or children (0.1–1 mcg/kg/min). Administration down a tracheal tube requires higher doses (2–2.5 mg in adults, 0.1 mg/kg in children). High-dose epinephrine (0.1 mg/kg) in adults is recommended only after standard therapy has failed.
Lidocaine	Decreases rate of phase 4 depolarization (decreases automaticity); depresses conduction in reentry pathways. Elevates VF threshold. Reduces disparity in action potential duration between normal and ischemic tissue. Reduces action potential and effective refractory period duration	VT that has responded to defibrillation; premature ventricular contractions. Use only after ROSC; found to be less effective than amiodarone in VF or pulseless VT following OHCA	1–1.5 mg/kg	1 mg/kg	Doses of 0.5–1.5 mg/kg can be repeated every 5–10 min to a total dose of 3 mg/kg. After infarction or successful resuscitation, a continuous infusion (eg, 1 g in 500 mL D_5W, 2 mg/mL) should be run at a rate of 20–50 mcg/kg/min (2–4 mg/min in most adults). Therapeutic blood levels are usually 1.5–6 mcg/mL.

Vasopressin	Nonadrenergic peripheral vasoconstrictor; direct stimulation of V_1 receptors	Bleeding esophageal varices; adult shock-refractory VF; hemodynamic support in vasodilatory (septic) shock	40 units IV, single dose, 1 time only	Not recommended	Given alone or in combination with epinephrine may be considered; however there is no advantage as replacement for epinephrine in cardiac arrest; has a 10–20 min half-life.
Procainamide	Suppresses both atrial and ventricular arrhythmias	AF/flutter; preexcited atrial arrhythmias with rapid ventricular response; wide-complex tachycardia that cannot be distinguished as SVT or VT	20 mg/min until arrhythmia suppressed, hypotension develops, QRS complex increases by >50%, or total dose of 17 mg/kg has infused. In urgent situations, 50 mg/min may be used to a maximum of 17 mg/kg. Maintenance infusion, 1–4 mg/min	Loading dose: 15 mg/kg; infusion over 30–60 min; routine use in combination with drugs that prolong QT interval is not recommended	Contraindicated in overdose of tricyclic antidepressants or other antiarrhythmic drugs. Bolus doses can result in toxicity. Should not be used in preexisting QT prolongation or torsades de pointes. Blood levels should be monitored in patients with impaired kidney function and when constant infusion >3 mg/min for >24 h.
Amiodarone	Complex drug with effects on sodium, potassium, and calcium channels as well as α- and β-adrenergic blocking properties	SVT with accessory pathway conduction; unstable VT and VF; stable VT, polymorphic VT, wide-complex tachycardia of uncertain origin; AF/flutter with CHF; preexcited AF/flutter; adjunct to electrical cardioversion in refractory PSVTs, atrial tachycardia, and AF	150 mg over 10 min, followed by 1 mg/min for 6 h, then 0.5 mg/min, with supplementary infusion of 150 mg as necessary up to 2 g. For pulseless VT or VF, initial administration is 300 mg rapid infusion diluted in 20–30 mL of saline or dextrose in water	5 mg/kg for pulseless VT/VF; for perfusing tachycardia loading dose, 5 mg/kg IV/IO; maximum dose, 15 mg/kg/d	Antiarrhythmic of choice, particularly if cardiac function is impaired, EF <40%, or CHF. Routine use in combination with drugs prolonging QT interval is not recommended. Most frequent side effects are hypotension and bradycardia.

(*continued*)

TABLE 55–3 Cardiovascular effects, indications, and dosages of resuscitation drugs. (Continued)

			Initial Dose		
Drug	**Cardiovascular Effects**	**Indications**	**Adult**	**Pediatric**	**Comments**
Verapamil	Calcium channel blocking agent used to slow conduction and increase refractoriness in AV node, terminating reentrant arrhythmias that require AV nodal conduction for continuation	Controls ventricular response rate in AF/flutter and MAT; rate control in AF; terminating narrow-complex PSVT	2.5–5 mg IV over 2 min; without response, repeat dose with 5–10 mg every 15–30 min to a max of 20 mg		Use only in patients with narrow-complex PSVT or supraventricular arrhythmia. Do not use in presence of impaired ventricular function or CHF.
Diltiazem	Calcium channel blocking agent used to slow conduction and increase refractoriness in AV node, terminating reentrant arrhythmias that require AV nodal conduction for continuation	Slows conduction and increases refractoriness in AV node. May terminate reentrant arrhythmias. Controls ventricular response rate in AF/flutter and MAT	0.25 mg/kg, followed by second dose of 0.35 mg/kg if necessary; maintenance infusion of 5–15 mg/h in AF/flutter		May exacerbate CHF in severe LV dysfunction; may decrease myocardial contractility, but less so than verapamil.
Dobutamine	Synthetic catecholamine and potent inotropic agent with predominant β-adrenergic receptor-stimulating effects that increase cardiac contractility in a dose-dependent manner, accompanied by a decrease in LV filling pressures.	Severe systolic heart failure	5–20 mcg/kg/min		Hemodynamic end points rather than specific dose is goal. Older adults have significantly reduced response. May induce or exacerbate myocardial ischemia with increases in heart rate.
Flecainide	Potent sodium channel blocker with significant conduction-slowing effects	AF/flutter, ventricular arrhythmias and supraventricular arrhythmias without structural heart disease, ectopic atrial heart disease, AV nodal reentrant tachycardia, SVTs associated with an accessory pathway, including preexcited AF	2 mg/kg at 10 mg/min (IV use not approved in the United States)		Should not be used in patients with impaired LV function, or when coronary artery disease is suspected.

Ibutilide	Short-acting antiarrhythmic, prolongs the action potential duration and increases the refractory period	Acute conversion or adjunct to electrical cardioversion of AF/flutter of short duration	In patients >60 kg, 1 mg (10 mL) over 10 min; a second similar dose may be repeated in 10 min. In patients <60 kg, initial dose is 0.01 mg/kg		Patients should be monitored for arrhythmias for 4–6 h, and longer in those with hepatic dysfunction.
Magnesium	Hypomagnesemia associated with arrhythmias, cardiac insufficiency, and sudden death; can precipitate refractory VF; can hinder K^+ replacement	Torsades de pointes with prolonged QT, even with normal serum levels of magnesium	1–2 g in 50–100 mL D_5W over 15 min	500 mg/mL–IV/IO: 25–50 mg/kg; maximum dose: 2 g per dose	Rapid IV infusion for torsades de pointes or suspected hypomagnesemia not recommended in cardiac arrest except when arrhythmia suspected.
Propafenone	Significant conduction slowing and negative inotropic effects. Nonselective β-adrenergic–blocking properties	AF/flutter, ventricular arrhythmias and supraventricular arrhythmias without structural heart disease, ectopic atrial heart disease, AV nodal reentrant tachycardia, SVTs associated with an accessory pathway	2 mg/kg at 10 mg/min (IV use not approved in the United States)		Should be avoided with impaired LV function or when CAD suspected.
Sotalol	Prolongs action potential duration and increases cardiac tissue refractoriness. Nonselective β-adrenergic blocking properties	Preexcited AF/flutter, ventricular and supraventricular arrhythmias	1–1.5 mg/kg at a rate of 10 mg/min		Limited by need to be infused slowly. Avoid in patients with prolonged QT syndrome.

AF, atrial fibrillation; AV, atrioventricular; BP, blood pressure; CAD, coronary artery disease; CHF, congestive heart failure; EF, ejection fraction; IV/IO, intravenous/intraosseous; LV, left ventricular; MAT, multifocal atrial tachycardia; OHCA, out-of-hospital cardiac arrest; PEA, pulseless electrical activity; PSVT, paroxysmal supraventricular tachycardia; ROSC, return of spontaneous circulation; SVT, supraventricular tachycardia; VF, ventricular fibrillation; VT, ventricular tachycardia.

Data from Link MS, Berkow LC, Kudenchuk PJ, et al: Part 7: Adult Advanced Cardiovascular Life Support: 2015 American Heart Association Guidelines Update for Cardiopulmonary Resuscitation and Emergency Cardiovascular Care, *Circulation*. 2015 Nov 3;132(18 Suppl 2):S444-S464.

at 2 to 4 mg/kg every 10 min. *Sodium bicarbonate (0.5–1 mEq/kg) is not recommended in the guidelines and should be considered only in specific situations such as preexisting metabolic acidosis or hyperkalemia or in the treatment of tricyclic antidepressant or barbiturate overdose.* Sodium bicarbonate elevates plasma pH by combining with hydrogen ions to form carbonic acid,
10 which readily dissociates into CO_2 and water. **Because CO_2, but not bicarbonate, readily crosses cell membranes and the blood–brain barrier, arterial hypercapnia causes intracellular tissue acidosis.** Although successful defibrillation is not related to *arterial* pH, increased *intramyocardial* CO_2 may reduce the possibility of successful cardiac resuscitation. Furthermore, bicarbonate administration can lead to detrimental alterations in osmolality and the oxygen–hemoglobin dissociation curve. *Therefore, effective alveolar hyperventilation and adequate tissue perfusion are the treatments of choice for the respiratory and metabolic acidosis that accompany resuscitation.*

Intravenous fluid therapy with either colloid or balanced salt solutions is indicated in patients with intravascular volume depletion (eg, acute blood loss, diabetic ketoacidosis, thermal burns). Dextrose-containing solutions may worsen neurological outcomes and may lead to hyperosmotic diuresis. They should be avoided unless hypoglycemia is suspected. Likewise, administration of free water (eg, D_5W) may lead to cerebral edema.

Emergency Pacemaker Therapy

Transcutaneous cardiac pacing (**TCP**) is a noninvasive method of rapidly treating arrhythmias caused by conduction disorders or abnormal impulse. TCP is not routinely recommended in cardiac arrest. TCP use may be considered to treat asystole, bradycardia caused by heart block, or tachycardia from a reentrant mechanism. If there is concern about the use of atropine in high-grade block, TCP is always appropriate. If the patient is unstable with marked bradycardia, TCP should be implemented immediately while awaiting treatment response to drugs. A pacemaker unit has become a built-in feature of some defibrillator models. Disposable pacing electrodes are usually positioned on the patient in an anterior–posterior manner. The placement of the negative electrode corresponds to a V_2 electrocardiograph position, whereas the positive electrode is placed on the left posterior chest beneath the scapula and lateral to the spine. Note that this positioning does not interfere with paddle placement during defibrillation. Failure to capture may be due to electrode misplacement, poor electrode-to-skin contact, or increased transthoracic impedance (eg, barrel-shaped chest, pericardial effusion). Current output is slowly increased until the pacing stimuli obtain electrical and mechanical capture. A wide
11 QRS complex following a pacing spike signals *electrical* capture, but *mechanical* (ventricular) capture must be confirmed by an improving pulse or blood pressure. Conscious patients may require sedation to tolerate the discomfort of skeletal muscle contractions. Transcutaneous pacing can provide effective temporizing therapy until transvenous pacing or other definitive treatment can be initiated. TCP has many advantages over transvenous pacing because it can be used by almost all acute care providers, it can be initiated quickly at the bedside, and it does not involve the risk and placement time associated with central venous access.

Precordial Thump

The precordial thump is to be considered only in witnessed, monitored, pulseless ventricular tachycardia when a defibrillator is not immediately available. It provides only 5 to 10 J of mechanical energy to the heart. Recent studies suggest the precordial thump rarely results in ROSC and usually results in either no change in rhythm or deterioration into ventricular fibrillation or asystole. The latter situation may represent the phenomenon known as *commotio cordis*, where blunt impact to the chest without structural trauma results in ventricular arrhythmias or asystole.

Cardiac Arrest in Pregnancy

The priority in the pregnant patient is administering high-quality CPR and achieving resolution of aortocaval compression. Greater priority is given to airway management than in the general adult as pregnant patients are more prone to hypoxia (and oxygen consumption is 30% above normal in a pregnant patient). Fetal monitoring should not be attempted during CPR. At the start of the arrest, if the patient is beyond the second half of the pregnancy, local resources for a cesarean section should be immediately summoned. If ROSC is not achieved even after left uterine displacement or in the setting of nonsurvivable trauma, a *resuscitative hysterostomy* (perimortem cesarean delivery) should be attempted within 5 min of the arrest if appropriate personnel are available.

RECOMMENDED RESUSCITATION AND POST–CARDIAC ARREST CARE PROTOCOLS

During every resuscitation, there should be a team leader who integrates the assessment of the patient, including the historical information available and the electrocardiographic diagnosis, with the electrical and pharmacological therapy (Table 55–4). This person must have a firm grasp of the guidelines

TABLE 55–4 Steps for synchronized cardioversion.

Synchronized Cardioversion
Synchronized cardioversion is the treatment of choice when a patient has a symtomatic (unstable) reentry SVT or VT with pulses and is recommended to treat unstable atrial fibrillation and flutter.
Cardioversion is unlikely to be effective for treating junctional tachycardia or ectopic or multifocal atrial tachycardia because these rhythms have an automatic focus arising from cells that are spontaneously depolarizing at a rapid rate. Delivering a shock generally cannot stop these rhythms and may actually increase the rate of the tachyarrhythmia.
In synchronized cardioversion, shocks are administered through adhesive electrodes or handheld paddles with the defibrillator/monitor in synchronized (sync) mode. The sync mode delivers energy just after the R wave of the QRS complex.
Follow these steps to perform synchronized cardioversion, modifying the steps for your specific device.
1. Sedate all conscious patients unless unstable or deteriorating rapidly.
2. Turn on the defibrillator (monophasic or biphasic).
3. Attach monitor leads to the patient and ensure proper display of the patient's rhythm. Position adhesive electrode (conductor) pads on the patient.
4. Press the sync control button to engage the synchronization mode.
5. Look the markers of the R wave indicating sync mode.
6. Adjust monitor gain if necessary until sync markers occur with each R wave.
7. Select the appropriate energy level. Deliver synchronized shocks according to your device's recommended energy level to maximize the success of the first shock.
8. Announce to team members: "Charging defibrillator—stand clear!"
9. Press the charge button.
10. Clear the patient when the defibrillator is charged
11. Press the shock button(s).
12. Check the monitor. If tachycardia persists, increase the energy level (joules) according to the device manufacturer's recommendations.
13. Activate the sync mode after delivery of each synchronized shock. Most defibrillators default back to the unsynchronized mode after delivery of a synchronized shock. This default allows an immediate shock if cardioversion produces VF.

SVT, supraventricular tachycardia; VF, ventricular fibrillation; VT, ventricular tachycardia.

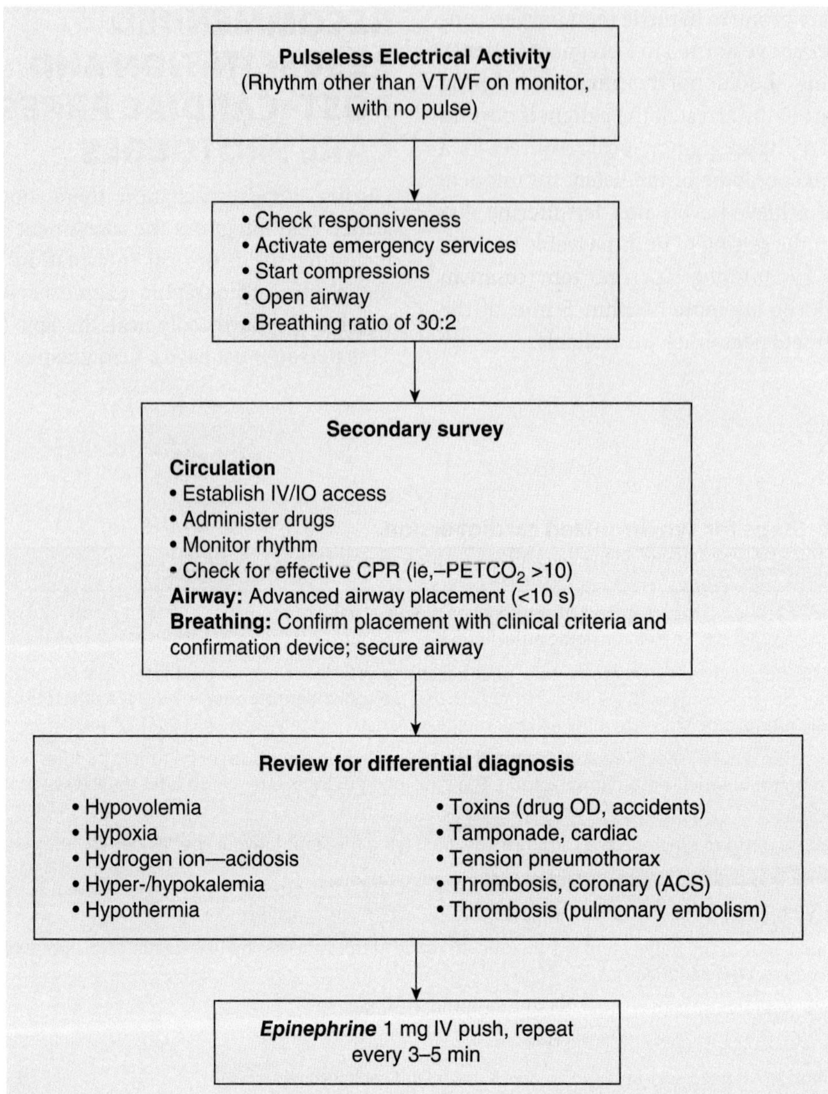

FIGURE 55–10 Pulseless electrical activity (PEA) algorithm. ACS, acute coronary care; CPR, cardiopulmonary resuscitation; IV/IO, intravenous or intraosseous; OD, overdose; P_{ETCO_2}, end-tidal carbon dioxide; VF/VT, ventricular fibrillation and pulseless ventricular tachycardia.

for cardiac arrest presented in the CPR-ECC algorithms (Figures 55–9 to 55–13). Of note, ACLS in the COVID-19 pandemic has triggered discussion about ethical boundaries of the discussion of DNR status and ensuring the safety of health care personnel; at this time, however, there are no accepted modifications in ACLS guidelines for patients infected with COVID-19. The 2020 guidelines place emphasis on post–cardiac arrest care and the resulting transition to critical care management. Rapid attention to cardiac intervention or neuroprotection should be promptly initiated, as shown in Figure 55–14. In addition, post event debriefing of rescue team members should take place to provide emotional and psychological relief and optimize future team function.

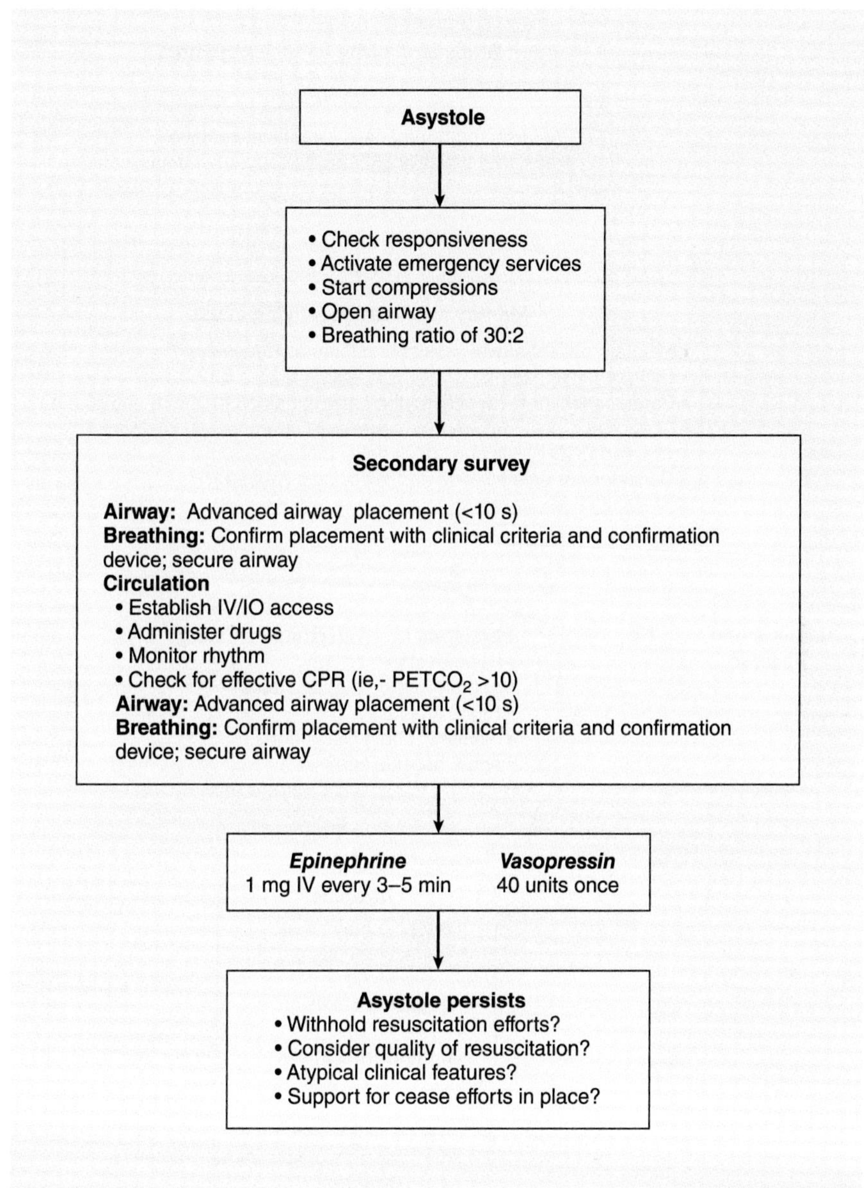

FIGURE 55–11 Asystole: The silent heart algorithm. DP, diastolic pressure; IV/IO, intravenous or intraosseous; P_{ETCO_2}, end-tidal carbon dioxide; S_{CVO_2}, central venous oxygen saturation; VF/VT, ventricular fibrillation and pulseless ventricular tachycardia.

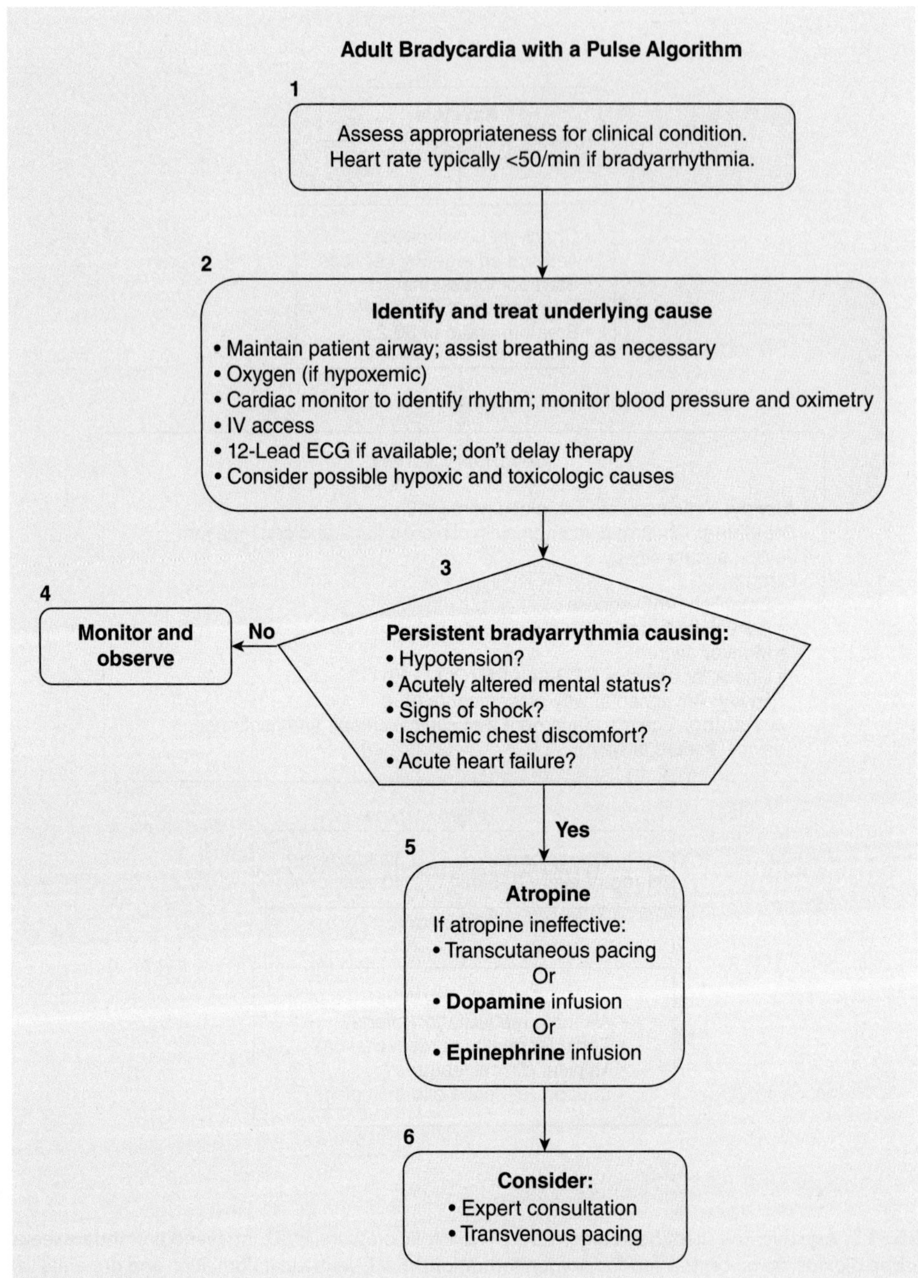

FIGURE 55–12 Adult bradycardia with a pulse algorithm. AV, atrioventricular; ECG, electrocardiogram; IV, intravenous. (Reprinted with permission *ACLS Advanced Cardiovascular Life Support Provider Manual* ©2020 American Heart Association, Inc.)

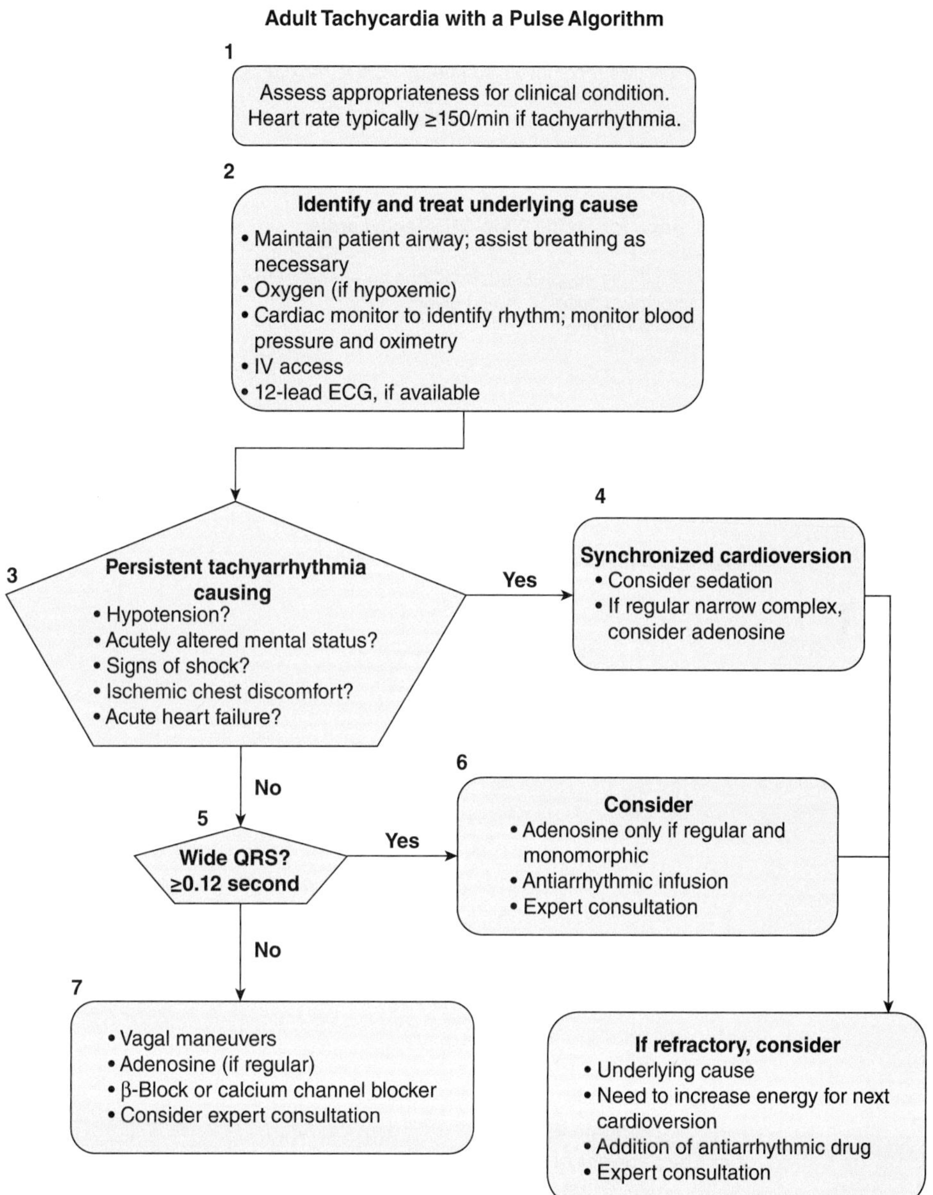

FIGURE 55–13 Adult tachycardia with a pulse algorithm. CHF, congestive heart failure; ECG, electrocardiogram; IV, intravenous; VT, ventricular tachycardia; WPW, Wolff-Parkinson-White syndrome. (Reprinted with permission *ACLS Advanced Cardiovascular Life Support Provider Manual* ©2020 American Heart Association, Inc.)

Doses/Details

Synchronized cardioversion:
Refer to your specific device's recommended energy level to maximize first shock success

Adenonsine IV dose:
First dose: 6 mg rapid IV push; follow with NS flush
Second dose: 12 mg if required

Antiarrhythmic Infusions for Stable Wide-QRS Tachycardia
Procainamide IV dose:
20–50 mg/min until arrhythmia suppressed, hypotension ensues, QRS duration increases >50%, or maximum dose 17 mg/kg given.
Maintenance infusion: 1–4 mg/min.
Avoid if prolonged QT or CHF.

Amiodarone IV dose:
First dose: 150 mg over 10 minutes.
Repeat as needed if VT recurs.
Follow by maintenance infusion of 1 mg/min for first 6 hours.

Sotalol IV dose:
100 mg (1.5 mg/kg) over 5 minutes.
Avoid if prolonged QT.

FIGURE 55–13 *(Continued)*

CASE DISCUSSION

Intraoperative Hypotension & Cardiac Arrest

A 16-year-old male is rushed to the operating room for an emergency laparotomy and thoracotomy after sustaining multiple abdominal and thoracic stab wounds. In the field, paramedics intubated the patient, started two large-bore intravenous lines, began fluid resuscitation, and inflated a pneumatic antishock garment. Upon arrival in the operating room, the patient's blood pressure is unobtainable, heart rate is 128 beats/min (sinus tachycardia), and respirations are being controlled by a bag-valve device.

What should be done immediately?

Cardiopulmonary resuscitation must be initiated immediately; external chest compressions should be started as soon as the arterial blood pressure is found to be inadequate for vital organ perfusion. Because the patient is already intubated, the location of the endotracheal tube must be confirmed with chest auscultation and quantitative waveform capnography (if available, to both confirm tube placement and assess the adequacy of CPR), and 100% oxygen should be delivered.

Which CPR sequence best fits this situation?

Pulselessness in the presence of sinus rhythm suggests severe hypovolemia, cardiac tamponade, ventricular rupture, dissecting aortic aneurysm, tension pneumothorax, profound hypoxemia and acidosis, or pulmonary embolism. Epinephrine, 1 mg, should be administered intravenously.

What is the most likely cause of this patient's profound hypotension?

The presence of multiple stab wounds strongly suggests hypovolemia. Point-of-care abdominal ultrasonography can rapidly identify a collapsed

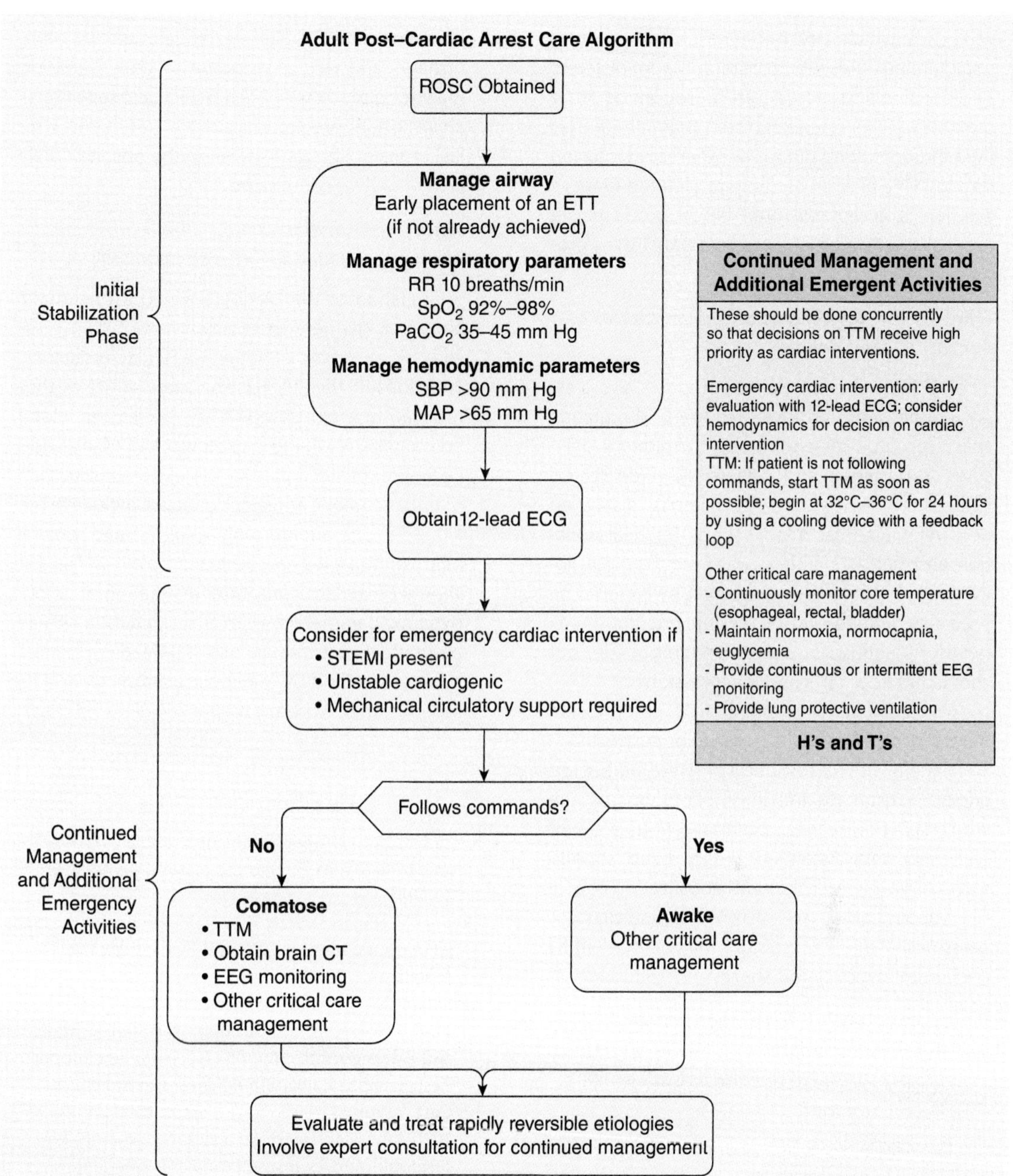
Adult Post–Cardiac Arrest Care Algorithm
Initial Stabilization Phase
ROSC Obtained
Manage airway
Early placement of an ETT
(if not already achieved)
Manage respiratory parameters
RR 10 breaths/min
SpO2 92%–98%
PaCO2 35–45 mm Hg
Manage hemodynamic parameters
SBP >90 mm Hg
MAP >65 mm Hg
Obtain12-lead ECG
Continued Management and Additional Emergency Activities
Consider for emergency cardiac intervention if
• STEMI present
• Unstable cardiogenic
• Mechanical circulatory support required
Follows commands?
No
Yes
Comatose
• TTM
• Obtain brain CT
• EEG monitoring
• Other critical care management
Awake
Other critical care management
Evaluate and treat rapidly reversible etiologies
Involve expert consultation for continued management
Continued Management and Additional Emergent Activities
These should be done concurrently so that decisions on TTM receive high priority as cardiac interventions.
Emergency cardiac intervention: early evaluation with 12-lead ECG; consider hemodynamics for decision on cardiac intervention
TTM: If patient is not following commands, start TTM as soon as possible; begin at 32°C–36°C for 24 hours by using a cooling device with a feedback loop
Other critical care management
- Continuously monitor core temperature (esophageal, rectal, bladder)
- Maintain normoxia, normocapnia, euglycemia
- Provide continuous or intermittent EEG monitoring
- Provide lung protective ventilation
H's and T's

FIGURE 55-14 Adult post–cardiac arrest care algorithm. CT, computed tomography; ECG, electrocardiogram; EEG, electroencephalogram; ETT, endotracheal tube; MAP, mean arterial pressure; ROSC, return of spontaneous circulation; RR, respiration rate; SBP, systolic blood pressure; STEMI, ST-elevation myocardial infarction; TTM, targeted temperature management.

vena cava, which is pathognomonic of hypovolemia. Warmed fluids should be rapidly administered. Additional venous access can be sought as other members of the operating room team administer fluid through blood pumps or other rapid infusion devices. Five percent albumin or lactated Ringer's solution is acceptable until blood products are available. Activation of a massive transfusion protocol is indicated.

What are the signs of tension pneumothorax and pericardial tamponade?

The signs of *tension pneumothorax*—the presence of air under positive pressure in the pleural space—include increasing peak inspiratory pressures, tachycardia and hypotension (decreased venous return), hypoxia (atelectasis), distended neck veins, unequal breath sounds, tracheal deviation, and mediastinal shift away from the pneumothorax. Point-of-care ultrasonography can also be used for identification of tension pneumothorax (and for diagnosis of pericardial tamponade) but should not interrupt chest compressions.

Pericardial tamponade—cardiac compression from pericardial contents—should be suspected in any patient with narrow pulse pressure, *pulsus paradoxus* (>10 mm Hg drop in systolic blood pressure with inspiration), elevated central venous pressure with neck vein distention, distant heart sounds, tachycardia, hypotension, and equalization of central venous, atrial, and ventricular end-diastolic pressures. Many of these signs may be masked by concurrent hypovolemic shock.

Fluid administration and properly performed external cardiac compressions do not result in satisfactory carotid or femoral pulsations. What else should be done?

Because external chest compressions are often ineffective in trauma patients, an emergency thoracotomy should be performed as soon as possible to clamp the thoracic aorta, relieve a tension pneumothorax or pericardial tamponade, identify possible intrathoracic hemorrhage, and perform open-chest cardiac compressions. Cross-clamping of the thoracic aorta increases brain and myocardial perfusion and decreases subdiaphragmatic hemorrhage, and lack of response to cross-clamping is a strong predictor of demise. Patient selection is an important predictor of survival as patients who lack signs of life upon arrival to the hospital rarely (~2%) survive to discharge.

What is the function of the pneumatic antishock garment, and how should it be removed?

Inflation of the bladders within a pneumatic antishock garment increases arterial blood pressure by elevating peripheral vascular resistance. Functionally, the suit has the same effect as thoracic aorta cross-clamping by decreasing blood flow and hemorrhage in the lower half of the body. Complications of inflating the abdominal section of the pneumatic antishock garment include acute kidney injury, altered lung volumes, and visceral injury during external chest compressions. The suit should be deflated only after restoration of hemodynamic parameters. Even then, deflation should be gradual as it may be accompanied by marked hypotension and by metabolic acidosis caused by reperfusion of ischemic tissues.

GUIDELINES

Kwon OY. The changes in cardiopulmonary resuscitation guidelines: from 2000 to the present. *J Exerc Rehabil.* 2019;15:738.

Lavonas E, Magid D, Aziz K et al. Highlights of the 2020 AHA Guidelines for CPR and ECC. American Heart Association; 2020.

Merchant RM, Topjian AA, Panchal AR, et al; Adult Basic and Advanced Life Support, Pediatric Basic and Advanced Life Support, Neonatal Life Support, Resuscitation Education Science, and Systems of Care Writing Groups. Part 1: Executive summary: 2020 American Heart Association guidelines for cardiopulmonary resuscitation and emergency cardiovascular care. *Circulation.* 2020;142(Suppl 2): S337.

Panchal AR, Bartos JA, Cabañas JG, et al; Adult Basic and Advanced Life Support Writing Group. Part 3: Adult Basic and Advanced Life Support: 2020 American Heart Association Guidelines for cardiopulmonary resuscitation and emergency cardiovascular care. *Circulation.* 2020;142(Suppl 2):S366.

Topjian AA, Raymond TT, Atkins D, et al; Pediatric Basic and Advanced Life Support Collaborators. Part 4: Pediatric basic and advanced life support: 2020 American Heart Association guidelines for cardiopulmonary resuscitation and emergency cardiovascular care. *Circulation*. 2020;142(Suppl 2): S469.

SUGGESTED READINGS

ATLS Subcommittee; American College of Surgeons Committee on Trauma; International ATLS Working Group. Advanced trauma life support (ATLS): the ninth edition. *J Trauma Acute Care Surg*. 2013;74:1363.

Bornstein K, Long B, Porta AD, et al. After a century, epinephrine's role in cardiac arrest resuscitation remains controversial. *Am J Emerg Med*. 2021;39:168.

Kramer DB, Lo B, Dickert NW. CPR in the Covid-19 era—an ethical framework. *N Engl J Med*. 2020;383:e6.

Kumar A, Avishay DM, Jones CR, et al. Sudden cardiac death: epidemiology, pathogenesis and management. *Rev Cardiovasc Med*. 2021;22:147.

Mody P, Brown SP, Kudenchuk PJ, et al. Intraosseous versus intravenous access in patients with out-of-hospital cardiac arrest: insights from the resuscitation outcomes consortium continuous chest compression trial. *Resuscitation*. 2019;134:69.

Polat O, Oguz AB, Eneyli MG, et al. Applied anatomy for tibial intraosseous access in adults: a radioanatomical study. *Clin Anat*. 2018;31:593.

Scrivens A, Reynolds PR, Emery FE, et al. Use of intraosseous needles in neonates: a systematic review. *Neonatology*. 2019;116:305.

Sinz E, Navarro K, Cheng A et al. *Advanced Cardiovascular Life Support Instructor Manual*. American Heart Association; 2020.

Sinz E, Navarro K, Cheng A et al. *Advanced Cardiovascular Life Support Provider Manual*. American Heart Association; 2020.

Tyler JA, Perkins Z, De'Ath HD. Intraosseous access in the resuscitation of trauma patients: a literature review. *Eur J Trauma Emerg Surg*. 2021;47:47.

Whitney R, Langhan M. Vascular Access in Pediatric Patients in the emergency department: types of access, indications, and complications. *Pediatr Emerg Med Pract*. 2017;14:1.

C H A P T E R

56

Postanesthesia Care

KEY CONCEPTS

1. Patients emerging from anesthesia should not leave the operating room until they have a patent airway, have adequate ventilation and oxygenation, and are hemodynamically stable. Qualified anesthesia personnel must attend the transfer to the postanesthesia care unit (PACU).

2. Before the recovering patient is fully awake, pain may be manifested as postoperative restlessness or agitation. Significant systemic disturbances (eg, hypoxemia, respiratory or metabolic acidosis, hypotension), bladder distention, or a surgical complication (eg, occult intraabdominal hemorrhage) must be considered in the differential diagnosis of postoperative restlessness or agitation.

3. Postoperative nausea and vomiting (PONV; see Chapter 17) is the most common immediate complication following general anesthesia, occurring in approximately 30% or more of all patients.

4. Intense shivering causes precipitous rises in oxygen consumption, carbon dioxide (CO2) production, and cardiac output, which may be poorly tolerated by patients with cardiac and/or pulmonary impairment.

5. Respiratory problems are the most frequently encountered serious complications in the PACU. The overwhelming majority are related to airway obstruction, hypoventilation, hypoxemia, or a combination of these problems.

6. Hypoventilation in the PACU is most commonly due to the residual depressant effects of anesthetic and analgesic agents on respiratory drive, often made worse by preexisting obstructive sleep apnea.

7. Hypoventilation with obtundation, circulatory depression, and severe acidosis (arterial blood pH <7.15) is an indication for immediate and decisive ventilatory and hemodynamic intervention, including airway and inotropic support as needed.

8. Following naloxone administration, patients should be observed closely for recurrence of opioid-induced respiratory depression ("renarcotization"), as naloxone has a shorter duration of action than many opioids.

9. Increased intrapulmonary shunting from a decreased functional residual capacity relative to closing capacity is the most common cause of hypoxemia following general anesthesia.

10. The possibility of a postoperative pneumothorax should always be considered following central line placement, supraclavicular or intercostal blocks, abdominal or chest trauma (including rib fractures), neck dissection, thyroidectomy (especially if thyroid dissection extends into the thorax), tracheostomy, nephrectomy, or other retroperitoneal or intraabdominal procedures (including laparoscopy),

—*Continued next page*

Continued—

especially if the diaphragm may have been penetrated or disrupted.

11 Hypovolemia is the most common cause of hypotension in the PACU and can result from hemorrhage, wound drainage, or inadequate fluid replacement.

12 Noxious stimulation from incisional pain, endotracheal intubation, bladder distention, or preoperative discontinuation of antihypertensive medication is usually responsible for postoperative hypertension.

Historically, the routine expectation of specialized postanesthesia nursing care was prompted by the recognition that many preventable deaths occurred immediately following anesthesia and surgery. The World War II experience of providing surgical care to battle casualties contributed to the postwar trend for centralized recovery rooms, where skilled nurses could closely and simultaneously attend several postoperative patients. Recently, some postoperative patients are more frequently cared for overnight in a postanesthesia care unit (PACU), or the equivalent, when there is a shortage of surgical intensive care beds.

Another recent change in postanesthesia care is related to the shift from inpatient to outpatient surgery. Now, more than 70% of surgical procedures in the United States are performed on an outpatient basis. Two phases of recovery may be recognized for outpatient surgery. *Phase 1* is the immediate care for patients during emergence and awakening from anesthesia that continues until standard PACU discharge criteria are met (see Discharge Criteria, later in the chapter). *Phase 2* is lower-level care that continues until the patient is ready to go home. "Fast-tracking" of select outpatients may allow them to safely bypass phase 1 recovery and go directly to the phase 2 level of care.

In many institutions, the PACU also functions as a more intensely monitored location for perioperative and chronic pain patients undergoing procedures such as single-shot nerve blocks and placement of epidural and peripheral nerve catheters, as well as for patients undergoing other invasive procedures such as central line placement, electroconvulsive therapy, thoracentesis, paracentesis, or cardioversion. The PACU must be appropriately staffed and equipped to manage such patients and their potential complications. For example, in areas where regional and epidural blocks are administered, Intralipid should be stocked in anticipation of potentially treating systemic local anesthetic toxicity.

This chapter reviews the essential components of a modern PACU, the general care of patients acutely recovering from anesthesia and surgery, and the respiratory and circulatory complications most commonly encountered in the PACU.

THE POSTANESTHESIA CARE UNIT

At the conclusion of any procedure requiring anesthesia, the emerging patient is taken to the PACU by one or more qualified anesthesia providers, often assisted by other personnel. During transport, supplemental oxygen is given by nasal cannula or mask, and the patient is monitored with pulse oximetry. Following general anesthesia, if an endotracheal tube or laryngeal mask airway (LMA) was utilized, the endotracheal tube or LMA will usually be removed prior to transport. Patients are also routinely observed in the PACU following regional anesthesia or monitored anesthesia care (local anesthesia with sedation). Most facilities have protocols that require patients to be admitted to the PACU following any type of anesthesia, except by specific order of the attending anesthesiologist. After a brief "hand-off" report to the PACU nurse, the patient will remain in the PACU until the major effects of the anesthesia have worn off and any anesthesia- or surgery-related complications of significance have been adequately addressed. This period requires heightened vigilance because it is characterized by an increased incidence of potentially life-threatening respiratory and circulatory complications.

Anesthesia is often delivered in areas remote from the main operating room suite, such as gastrointestinal and pulmonary endoscopy, interventional radiology, and magnetic resonance imaging suites. Patients recovering from anesthesia delivered in these areas must receive the same standard of care as surgical patients recovering from anesthesia. Some institutions have "satellite" PACUs to serve each of these remote areas individually, and others send patients from their various procedural areas to one centralized PACU; however, *the standard of postanesthesia care delivery must be the same for all PACUs within a given institution.*

Design

The PACU must be located near the operating rooms and procedure areas. A central location in the surgical suite is desirable as it ensures that the patient can be promptly transported back to surgery if needed and that members of the operating room team can quickly respond to urgent or emergent patient care issues in the PACU. Proximity to radiographic, laboratory, and other intensive care facilities is also important. Prolonged transfers to or from remote locations subject critically ill patients to increased jeopardy from urgent problems that may arise along the way.

An open-ward design facilitates observing multiple patients simultaneously. However, individually enclosed spaces are required for patients needing isolation for infection control. Many institutions constructing new PACUs choose to fully enclose all the PACU patient beds for infection control and privacy (important discussions between the patient, family, and care team often involve sensitive and confidential issues). A ratio of 1.5 PACU beds per operating room is customary, though this ratio will vary depending on the respective operating room suite's case type and volume, average case duration, and patient acuity. Each patient space should be well lit and large enough to allow easy access to patients for intravenous infusion pumps, ventilators, and imaging equipment. Construction guidelines typically specify a minimum of 7 ft between beds and 120 sq ft per patient. Multiple electrical outlets, including at least one with backup emergency power and at least one outlet each for oxygen and suction, should be present at each bed space.

Equipment

Inadequate monitoring in the PACU can lead to serious injury or death. Pulse oximetry (SpO_2), electrocardiogram (ECG), and automated noninvasive blood pressure (NIBP) monitors are mandatory for each patient. Although ECG, SpO_2, and NIBP must be utilized for every patient in the initial phase of recovery from anesthesia (phase 1), less intense monitoring may be adequate thereafter. Appropriate equipment must be available for those patients with intraarterial, central venous, pulmonary artery, or intracranial pressure monitoring. Capnography is increasingly used for both intubated and extubated patients. Patient body temperature must be assessed. A forced-air warming device, heating lamp, or warming/cooling blanket should be available.

The PACU must have its own supplies of basic and emergency equipment, separate from that of the operating room, including airway equipment and supplies, such as oxygen cannulas, a selection of masks, oral and nasal airways, laryngoscopes, endotracheal tubes, LMAs, a cricothyrotomy kit, and self-inflating bags for ventilation. Respiratory therapy equipment for aerosol bronchodilator treatments, continuous positive airway pressure (CPAP), and ventilators should be in close proximity to the recovery room. A difficult airway equipment and supplies cart with a bronchoscope and a video laryngoscope must be immediately available.

A readily available supply of catheters for venous, arterial, and central venous cannulation is mandatory in an inpatient setting. A cardiac defibrillator with transcutaneous pacing capabilities, and an emergency cart with drugs and supplies for advanced life support (see Chapter 55) and infusion pumps must be present and periodically inspected according to accreditation standards. Transvenous pacing catheters, pulse generators, and tracheostomy, chest tube, and vascular cut-down trays are typically present, depending on the surgical patient population. Point-of-care ultrasonography equipment should be available for central line and perineural catheter placement, assessment of hemodynamic status, endotracheal tube placement, gastric and bladder volume, and detection of pleural effusion, pneumothorax, and other pulmonary pathology.

Staffing

Inadequate staffing is often cited as contributing to PACU mishaps. The PACU should be staffed by nurses specifically trained and credentialed in the care of patients emerging from anesthesia. They should have expertise in airway management and advanced cardiac life support, as well as in problems commonly encountered in surgical patients relating to wound care, drainage catheters, and postoperative hemorrhage.

Patients in the PACU should be under the medical direction of a physician, usually an anesthesiologist, who must be immediately available to respond to urgent or emergent patient care problems. High-volume tertiary care surgical institutions may have an anesthesiologist assigned full time to the PACU. Appropriate management of a patient in the PACU may require a coordinated effort involving anesthesia providers, surgeons, nurses, respiratory therapists, and appropriate consultants. The anesthesia team emphasizes the management of analgesia, airway, cardiac, pulmonary, and metabolic problems, whereas the surgical team generally manages any problems directly related to the surgical procedure itself. A ratio of one nurse for two recovering patients is generally satisfactory; however, staffing should be tailored to the unique requirements of each patient and each facility. If the operating room schedule regularly includes pediatric patients or frequent short procedures, a ratio of one nurse to one patient is often needed. A charge nurse should be assigned to ensure optimal staffing resource management at all times, including the appropriate response to urgent or emergent patient care problems.

Care of the Patient

EMERGENCE FROM GENERAL ANESTHESIA

Emergence from general anesthesia is ideally characterized by smooth and gradual awakening in a controlled environment. However, problems such as airway obstruction, shivering, agitation, delirium, pain, nausea and vomiting, hypothermia, and autonomic lability are frequently encountered. Patients receiving spinal or epidural anesthesia may experience decreases in blood pressure during transport or recovery; the sympatholytic effects of major conduction blocks may prevent compensatory reflex vasoconstriction when patients are moved or when they sit up.

Following an inhalational anesthetic, the speed of emergence is directly proportional to alveolar ventilation but inversely proportional to the agent's blood solubility (see Chapter 8). Hypoventilation delays emergence from inhalational anesthesia. As the duration of anesthesia increases, emergence also becomes increasingly dependent on total tissue uptake, which is a function of agent solubility, the average concentration used, and the duration of exposure to the anesthetic. Recovery from most intravenous agents is dependent primarily on redistribution rather than metabolism and elimination. As the total administered dose increases, however, cumulative effects become clinically apparent in the form of prolonged emergence, and the termination of action becomes increasingly dependent on the metabolism or elimination. This is the basis for the concept of a *context-sensitive half-time* (see Chapter 7). Advanced age or kidney or liver disease can prolong emergence (see Chapter 9). Short- and ultrashort-acting anesthetic agents, such as propofol and remifentanil, significantly shorten emergence and time to discharge. The use of a bispectral index (BIS) monitor (see Chapter 6) may reduce total drug dosage and shorten recovery and time to discharge. The speed of emergence can also be influenced by preoperative medications. Premedication with agents that outlast the procedure (eg, lorazepam) may be expected to prolong emergence. The short duration of action of midazolam makes it a suitable premedication agent for short procedures.

Delayed Emergence

The most frequent cause of *delayed emergence* (when the patient fails to regain consciousness within an expected period of time after general anesthesia) is residual drug effect. Delayed emergence may occur as a result of an absolute or relative drug overdose. The effects of preoperative sleep deprivation or drug ingestion (alcohol, sedatives) can be additive to those of anesthetic agents in producing prolonged emergence. Intravenous naloxone (in 80-mcg increments in adults) and flumazenil (in 0.2-mg increments in adults) will readily reverse the effects of an opioid or benzodiazepine, respectively. Intravenous physostigmine (1–2 mg) may partially reverse the effect of other agents. A nerve stimulator can be used to exclude persisting neuromuscular blockade in poorly responsive patients on a mechanical ventilator who have inadequate spontaneous tidal volumes.

Less common causes of delayed emergence include hypothermia, marked metabolic disturbances, and perioperative stroke. A core temperature of less than 33°C has an anesthetic effect and greatly potentiates the actions of central nervous system depressants. Forced-air warming devices are most effective in raising body temperature. Hypoxemia and hypercarbia are readily excluded by pulse oximetry, capnography, and/or blood gas analysis. Hypercalcemia, hypermagnesemia, hyponatremia, hypoglycemia, and hyperglycemia are less common causes of delayed emergence that require laboratory measurements for diagnosis. Perioperative stroke is rare, except after neurological, cardiac, and cerebrovascular surgery (see Chapter 28); diagnosis is facilitated by neurological evaluation and radiological imaging.

TRANSPORT FROM THE OPERATING ROOM TO THE PACU

This seemingly short period may be complicated by the lack of adequate monitoring, medication access, or airway and resuscitative equipment. Patients
1 emerging from anesthesia should not leave the operating room until they have a patent airway, have adequate ventilation and oxygenation, and are hemodynamically stable; qualified anesthesia personnel must attend the transfer to the PACU. Transient hypoxemia (SpO_2 <90%) may develop in as many as 30% to 50% of otherwise "normal" patients during transport while breathing room air; we recommend supplemental oxygen for all transported patients, especially if the PACU is not in immediate proximity to the operating room. Unstable patients should remain intubated and should be transported with a portable monitor (ECG, SpO_2, and blood pressure) and a supply of emergency drugs. Since the transfer of intubated patients will always include the risk of unintended endotracheal tube dislodgement, appropriate airway equipment and supplies should be included in the transfer process, especially if the transfer travel distance is lengthy or includes an elevator ride.

All patients should be taken to the PACU on a bed or gurney that can be placed in either the head-down (Trendelenburg) or back-up position. The head-down position is useful for the management of hypovolemic patients, whereas the back-up position is useful for patients with underlying pulmonary dysfunction (see Chapters 20 and 23). Patients at increased risk of vomiting or upper airway bleeding (eg, following tonsillectomy) should be transported in the lateral position, which helps prevent airway obstruction and facilitates drainage of secretions.

ROUTINE RECOVERY

General Anesthesia

Airway patency, vital signs, oxygenation, and level of consciousness must be assessed immediately upon PACU arrival. Subsequent blood pressure, heart rate, and respiratory rate measurements are routinely made at least every 5 min for 15 min, or until stable, and every 15 min thereafter. Pulse oximetry and ECG are monitored continuously in all patients. In awake PACU patients, neuromuscular function should be assessed clinically (eg, head-lift and grip strength). At least one temperature measurement must also be obtained. Pain, the presence or absence of nausea or vomiting, and the adequacy of hydration and output (including urine flow, surgical drainage, and bleeding) should be assessed.

After initial vital signs have been recorded, the anesthesia provider should give a report to the PACU nurse that includes (1) relevant preoperative history (including mental status and any communication problems, such as language barriers, deafness, blindness, or mental disability); (2) pertinent intraoperative events (type of anesthesia, the surgical procedure, blood loss, fluid replacement, antibiotic and other relevant medication administration, and any complications); (3) any expected postoperative problems; (4) any anticipated need for PACU medication administration, such as antibiotics; and (5) postanesthesia orders. Postoperative orders should address analgesia and nausea/vomiting therapy; epidural or perineural catheter care, including the need for acute pain service involvement; administration of fluids or blood products; postoperative ventilation; and chest radiographs for follow-up of central venous catheterization.

All patients recovering from general anesthesia must receive supplemental oxygen and pulse oximetry monitoring during emergence because transient hypoxemia can develop even in healthy patients. A decision regarding the continuation of supplemental oxygen therapy at the time of PACU discharge can be made based on SpO_2 readings on room air. Arterial blood gas measurements may be obtained to confirm abnormal oximetry readings, but they are not usually necessary. Oxygen therapy should be carefully controlled in patients with a potential for CO_2 retention. Patients should generally be nursed in the back-up position to optimize oxygenation. However, elevating the head of the bed before the patient is responsive can lead to airway obstruction. In such cases, a preexisting oral or nasal airway should be left in place until the patient is awake and able to maintain the airway. Deep breathing and coughing should be encouraged periodically.

Regional Anesthesia

Patients who are heavily sedated or hemodynamically unstable following regional anesthesia should also receive supplemental oxygen in the PACU. Sensory and motor levels should be periodically recorded following regional anesthesia to document regression of the block. Precautions in the form of padding or repeated warning may be necessary to prevent self-injury from uncoordinated arm movements following brachial plexus blocks. Blood pressure should be closely monitored following spinal and epidural anesthesia. Bladder catheterization may be necessary for patients who have had spinal or epidural anesthesia.

Pain Control

Moderate to severe postoperative pain is commonly treated with oral or parenteral opioids. However, perioperative opioid administration is associated with side effects (nausea and vomiting, respiratory depression, pruritis, ileus, and urinary retention), which often have significant adverse effects on postoperative convalescence. In response to this problem, a variety of *opioid-sparing* strategies have been embraced over the past two decades to decrease opioid dosing and opioid-related side effects while maintaining satisfactory analgesia (see Chapter 47). Preoperative oral administration of nonsteroidal anti-inflammatory drugs (NSAIDs), acetaminophen (paracetamol), and gabapentin or pregabalin may significantly reduce postoperative opioid requirements, and these medications may be readministered postoperatively when the patient can resume oral medication. Additional analgesic modalities utilizing local anesthetics also reduce postoperative opioid analgesic requirements and thus reduce opioid-related side effects.

Mild to moderate postoperative pain can be treated orally with acetaminophen, an NSAID, hydrocodone, or oxycodone. Alternatively, ketorolac (15–30 mg in adults), an equivalent dose of diclofenac or ibuprofen, or acetaminophen (15 mg/kg, or 1 g if the patient is >50 kg) may be administered intravenously.

In situations where moderate to severe postoperative pain is present or oral analgesia is not possible, parenteral or intrathecal opioids, single-shot or continuous nerve blocks, wound infiltration, field blocks, intravenous lidocaine infusion, or continuous epidural analgesia are used, often in combination techniques (see Section IV). Parenteral opioids are most safely administered by careful titration of small doses. Considerable variability in opioid requirements should be expected, and adequate analgesia must be balanced against the risk of excessive sedation and respiratory depression. Intravenous opioids of intermediate to long duration, such as hydromorphone, 0.25 to 0.5 mg (0.015–0.02 mg/kg in children), or morphine, 2 to 4 mg (0.025–0.05 mg/kg in children), are most commonly used. Intravenous meperidine is used in small doses to treat postoperative shivering. We frequently encounter postoperative patients with a history of chronic opioid use, and opioid requirements are often markedly increased in these patients because of opioid tolerance and, especially, psychological dependence. Consultation with a pain specialist is often helpful in these situations. If liposomal bupivacaine (Exparel) wound infiltration is used, appropriate written and verbal communication must be employed to prevent the use of additional local anesthetics that could lead to systemic local anesthetic toxicity.

Analgesic effects of intravenous opioids usually peak within minutes of administration, though maximal respiratory depression, particularly with morphine and hydromorphone, may not occur until 20 to 30 min later. Patient-controlled analgesia can be instituted for inpatients when they are fully awake. Intramuscular administration of opioids is disadvantageous because of delayed and variable onset (10–20 min or longer) and delayed respiratory depression (up to 1 h).

When an epidural catheter is used, epidural bolus administration of fentanyl (50–100 mcg) or sufentanil (10–20 mcg) with 5 to 10 mL of 0.1% bupivacaine can provide excellent pain relief in adults. Epidural morphine (3–5 mg) may also be used, but delayed respiratory depression with epidural administration of this opioid mandates close monitoring for 24 h afterward (see Chapter 48).

Agitation

2 **Before the recovering patient is fully awake, pain may be manifested as postoperative restlessness or agitation. Significant systemic disturbances (eg, hypoxemia, respiratory or metabolic acidosis, hypotension), bladder distention, or a surgical complication (eg, occult intraabdominal hemorrhage) must also be considered in the differential diagnosis of postoperative restlessness or agitation.** Marked agitation may necessitate arm and leg restraints to avoid self-injury, particularly in children. When serious physiological disturbances have been excluded, cuddling and kind words from a sympathetic attendant or, preferably, a parent often calms the pediatric patient. Other contributory factors to agitation include marked preoperative anxiety and fear as well as adverse drug effects (large doses of central anticholinergic agents, phenothiazines, or ketamine). Physostigmine, 1 to 2 mg intravenously (0.05 mg/kg in children), is most effective in treating delirium due to atropine and scopolamine. If serious systemic disturbances and pain are excluded, persistent agitation may require sedation with intermittent intravenous doses of midazolam, 0.5 to 1 mg (0.05 mg/kg in children).

Nausea & Vomiting

3 **Postoperative nausea and vomiting (PONV; see Chapter 17) is the most common immediate complication following general anesthesia, occurring in approximately 30% or more of all patients.** Moreover, PONV occurs at home within 24 h of an uneventful discharge (*postdischarge nausea and vomiting*) in many ambulatory surgery patients. The etiology of PONV is usually multifactorial and associated with anesthetic and analgesic agents, the type of surgical procedure, and intrinsic patient factors, such as a history of motion sickness. It is also important to recognize that nausea is commonly reported at the onset of hypotension, particularly following spinal or epidural anesthesia.

Table 56–1 lists commonly recognized risk factors for PONV. A preoperative history of smoking lessens the likelihood of PONV, and propofol anesthesia decreases the incidence of PONV. The greatest incidence seems to be in young women. Opioid administration and intraperitoneal (especially laparoscopic), breast, or strabismus surgery increases the risk of PONV. Increased vagal tone manifested as sudden bradycardia commonly precedes, or coincides with, emesis. Selective 5-hydroxytryptamine (serotonin) receptor 3 (5-HT_3) antagonists, such as ondansetron, 4 mg (0.1 mg/kg in children), granisetron, 0.01–0.04 mg/kg, and dolasetron, 12.5 mg (0.035 mg/kg in children), are effective in preventing PONV, and, to a lesser extent, in treating established PONV. It should be noted that unlike ondansetron, which is usually effective immediately, dolasetron requires 15 min for onset of action. An orally disintegrating

TABLE 56–1 Risk factors for postoperative nausea and vomiting.

Patient factors
Young age
Female gender, particularly if menstruating on day of surgery or in first trimester of pregnancy
Large body habitus
History of prior postoperative emesis
History of motion sickness
Anesthetic techniques
General anesthesia
Drugs
Opioids
Volatile agents
Nitrous oxide
Surgical procedures
Strabismus surgery
Ear surgery
Laparoscopy
Orchiopexy
Ovum retrieval
Tonsillectomy
Breast surgery
Postoperative factors
Postoperative pain
Hypotension

tablet preparation of ondansetron (8 mg) may be useful for the treatment of, and prophylaxis against, postdischarge nausea and vomiting. Metoclopramide (0.15 mg/kg) is a less effective alternative to 5-HT_3 antagonists, which are not associated with the acute extrapyramidal (dystonic) manifestations and dysphoric reactions that may be encountered with metoclopramide or phenothiazine-type antiemetics. Transdermal scopolamine is effective, but it can be associated with side effects, including sedation, dysphoria, blurred vision, dry mouth, urinary retention, or exacerbation of glaucoma, particularly in older adult patients. Intravenous dexamethasone, 4 to 10 mg (0.10 mg/kg in children), when used as an antiemetic, has the additional advantages of providing a varying degree of analgesia and a sense of patient well-being or mild euphoria. Moreover, it seems to be effective for up to 24 h and thus may be useful for postdischarge nausea and vomiting. Oral aprepitant (Emend, 40 mg) may be administered within 3 h prior to anesthesia induction. Intravenous droperidol, 0.625 to 1.25 mg (0.05–0.075 mg/kg in children), when given intraoperatively, significantly decreases the likelihood of PONV. Unfortunately, droperidol carries a U.S. Food and Drug Administration "black box" warning, indicating that large (5–15 mg) doses can prolong the QT interval and lead to fatal cardiac arrhythmias. Nonpharmacological prophylaxis against PONV includes ensuring adequate hydration and stimulation of the P6 acupuncture point (volar aspect of wrist). The latter may include the application of pressure, electrical current, or injections.

Controversy exists regarding routine PONV prophylaxis for all patients. Because of the cost of treatment of established PONV, it appears cost-effective to provide prophylaxis to all patients in certain populations (eg, outpatients). Clearly, patients with multiple risk factors should receive prophylaxis. In addition, the use of two or three agents that act on differing receptors is more effective than single-agent prophylaxis.

Shivering & Hypothermia

Shivering can occur in the PACU as a result of intraoperative hypothermia or the effects of anesthetic agents, or both, and it is also common in the immediate postpartum period. The most important cause of hypothermia is a redistribution of heat from the body core to the peripheral compartments (see Chapter 52). A relatively cool ambient operating room temperature, prolonged exposure of a large wound, and use of large amounts of unwarmed intravenous fluids or high flows of unhumidified gases can also be contributory. Nearly all anesthetics, particularly volatile agents and spinal and epidural anesthesia, decrease the normal vasoconstrictive response to hypothermia by decreasing sympathetic tone. Although anesthetic agents also decrease the shivering threshold, shivering commonly observed during or after emergence from general anesthesia often represents the body's effort to increase heat production and raise body core temperature, and it may be associated with intense vasoconstriction. Emergence from even brief general anesthesia is sometimes also associated with shivering, and although the shivering can be one of several nonspecific neurological signs (eg, posturing, clonus, Babinski sign) that are sometimes observed during emergence, it is most often due to hypothermia. Regardless of the mechanism, shivering seems to be related to the duration of surgery and the use of a volatile agent. Shivering may occasionally be sufficiently intense to cause hyperthermia (38–39°C) and significant metabolic acidosis, both of which promptly resolve when the shivering stops. Other causes of shivering should be excluded, such as bacteremia and sepsis, drug allergy, or transfusion reaction.

Hypothermia should be treated with a forced-air warming device or (less satisfactorily) with warming lights or heating blankets to raise body temperature to normal. Intense shivering causes precipitous rises in oxygen consumption, CO_2 production, and cardiac output, which may be poorly tolerated by patients with cardiac or pulmonary impairment. Hypothermia has been associated with an increased incidence of myocardial ischemia, arrhythmias, coagulopathy with increased transfusion requirements, and prolonged muscle relaxant effects. Small intravenous doses of meperidine (10–25 mg) can reduce or even stop shivering. Intubated, mechanically ventilated, and sedated patients can be given a muscle relaxant (a small dose just sufficient to resolve the shivering) until normothermia is reestablished by active rewarming.

Discharge Criteria

A. PACU

Standards for discharging patients from the PACU are established by the department of anesthesiology and the hospital medical staff. They may allow PACU nurses to determine when patients may be transferred without the presence of a qualified anesthesia provider if all PACU discharge criteria have been met. Criteria can vary according to whether the patient is going to be discharged to an intensive care unit, a regular ward, phase 2 recovery, or directly to home.

Before PACU discharge, patients should have been observed for respiratory depression for at least 20 to 30 min after the last dose of parenteral opioid. Other minimum discharge criteria for patients recovering from general anesthesia usually include the following:

1. Easy arousability
2. Full orientation
3. The ability to maintain and protect the airway
4. Stable vital signs for at least 15 to 30 min
5. The ability to call for help, if necessary
6. No obvious surgical complications (such as active bleeding)

Postoperative pain, nausea, and vomiting must be controlled, and normothermia should be reestablished prior to PACU discharge. PACU patient scoring systems are widely used. Most assess SpO_2 (or color), consciousness, circulation, respiration, and motor activity (Table 56–2). Most patients meet discharge criteria within 60 min of PACU arrival, and efforts should be made to dismiss them promptly to save costs and increase PACU bed availability. Patients to be transferred to other intensive care areas need not meet all requirements.

In addition to the preceding criteria, patients receiving regional anesthesia should also be assessed for regression of both sensory and motor blockade. Complete resolution of the block prior to PACU dismissal avoids accidental injuries due to motor weakness or sensory deficits; however, many institutions have protocols that allow earlier discharge to appropriately monitored areas. Patients may be discharged with peripheral nerve blocks from single-shot or continuous perineural catheter infusions for the purpose of regional analgesia. Documenting regression of a block is important. Failure of a spinal or epidural block to resolve 6 h after the last dose of local anesthetic raises the possibility of spinal subdural or epidural hematoma, which should be excluded by prompt neurological evaluation and radiological imaging.

A major goal of most anesthetics should be rapid, comfortable emergence with minimal risk of PONV and postoperative pain to minimize the time needed in recovery and facilitate transfer to the next stage of recovery. Outpatients who meet the discharge criteria when they exit the operating room may be "fast-tracked," bypassing the PACU and proceeding directly to the phase 2 recovery area. Similarly, inpatients who meet the same criteria may be transferred directly from the operating room to their ward if appropriate staffing and monitoring are present.

TABLE 56–2 Postanesthetic Aldrete recovery score.[1]

Original Criteria	Modified Criteria	Point Value
Color	**Oxygenation**	
Pink	SpO_2 >92% on room air	2
Pale or dusky	SpO_2 >90% on oxygen	1
Cyanotic	SpO_2 <90% on oxygen	0
Respiration		
Can breathe deeply and cough	Breathes deeply and coughs freely	2
Shallow but adequate exchange	Dyspneic, shallow, or limited breathing	1
Apnea or obstruction	Apnea	0
Circulation		
Blood pressure within 20% of normal	Blood pressure ± 20 mm Hg of normal	2
Blood pressure within 20% to 50% of normal	Blood pressure ± 20–50 mm Hg of normal	1
Blood pressure deviating >50% from normal	Blood pressure more than ± 50 mm Hg of normal	0
Consciousness		
Awake, alert, and oriented	Fully awake	2
Arousable but readily drifts back to sleep	Arousable on calling	1
No response	Not responsive	0
Activity		
Moves all extremities	Same	2
Moves two extremities	Same	1
No movement	Same	0

[1]Ideally, the patient should be discharged when the total score is 10, but a minimum of 9 is required.

Data from Aldrete JA, Kronlik D. A postanesthetic recovery score. *Anesth Analg.* 1970;49:924; and Aldrete JA. The post-anesthesia recovery score revisited. *J Clin Anesth.* 1995 Feb;7(1):89.

B. Outpatients

In addition to emergence and awakening, recovery from anesthesia following outpatient procedures includes two additional stages: home readiness (phase 2 recovery) and complete psychomotor recovery. A scoring system has been developed to help assess home readiness discharge (Table 56–3). Recovery of proprioception, sympathetic tone, bladder function, and motor strength are additional criteria following regional anesthesia. For example, intact proprioception of the big toe, minimal orthostatic blood pressure or heart rate changes, and normal plantar flexion of the foot are important signals of recovery following spinal anesthesia. Urination and drinking or eating before discharge are usually no longer required; exceptions include patients with a history of urinary retention and those with diabetes.

Following general anesthesia, all outpatients must be discharged home in the company of a responsible adult who will stay with them overnight. Patients and their adult accompaniment must be provided with written postoperative instructions covering both routine follow-up care and urgent/emergency assistance. The assessment of home readiness is the responsibility of a qualified anesthesia provider, though authority to discharge a patient to home can be delegated to a nurse if approved discharge criteria are applied.

Home readiness does not imply that the patient has the ability to make important decisions, drive, or return to work. These activities require complete psychomotor recovery, which is often not achieved until 24 to 72 h postoperatively. All outpatient centers must use some system of postoperative

TABLE 56–3 Postanesthesia discharge scoring system (PADS).[1]

Criteria	Points
Vital signs	
Within 20% of preoperative baseline	2
Within 20% to 40% of preoperative baseline	1
>40% of preoperative baseline	0
Activity level	
Steady gait, no dizziness, at preoperative level	2
Requires assistance	1
Unable to ambulate	0
Nausea and vomiting	
Minimal, treated with oral medication	2
Moderate, treated with parenteral medication	1
Continues after repeated medication	0
Pain: minimal or none, acceptable to patient, controlled with oral medication	
Yes	2
No	1
Surgical bleeding	
Minimal: no dressing change required	2
Moderate: up to two dressing changes	1
Severe: three or more dressing changes	0

[1]Score ≥9 is required for discharge.

Modified with permission from Marshall SI, Chung F. Discharge criteria and complications after ambulatory surgery. *Anesth Analg.* 1999 Mar;88(3):508-517.

follow-up, preferably phone contact or, increasingly, a smartphone/web app the day after discharge.

Management of Complications

RESPIRATORY COMPLICATIONS

5 **Respiratory problems are the most frequently encountered serious complications in the PACU. The overwhelming majority are related to airway obstruction, hypoventilation, hypoxemia, or a combination of these problems.** Because hypoxemia is the final common pathway to serious injury or death, routine monitoring of pulse oximetry in the PACU leads to earlier recognition of these complications and fewer adverse outcomes and should be used with all PACU patients. Capnography is increasingly used on a routine basis following deep sedation or general anesthesia.

Airway Obstruction

Airway obstruction in unconscious patients is most commonly due to the tongue falling back against the posterior pharynx and is often seen in patients with obstructive sleep apnea (see Chapter 19). *Other causes of airway obstruction include laryngospasm, glottic edema, aspirated vomitus, a retained throat pack, secretions or blood in the airway, or external pressure on the trachea (eg, from a neck hematoma).* Partial airway obstruction usually presents as sonorous respiration. Near-total or total obstruction causes cessation of airflow and an absence of breath sounds and may be accompanied by *paradoxical* (rocking) movement of the chest. The abdomen and chest should normally rise together during inspiration; however, with airway obstruction, the chest descends as the abdomen rises during each inspiration (paradoxical chest movement). Patients with airway obstruction should receive supplemental oxygen while corrective measures are undertaken. A combined jaw-thrust and head-tilt maneuver pulls the tongue forward and opens the airway, and insertion of an oral or nasal airway often alleviates the problem. Nasal airways may be better tolerated than oral airways by patients emerging from anesthesia, especially when lidocaine-containing lubricant is used, and may decrease the likelihood of trauma to the teeth if the patient bites down. Nasal airways are easier to insert, with less risk of significant nasal bleeding, if a nasal spray vasoconstrictor such as phenylephrine or oxymetazoline (Afrin) is first administered. They should be inserted with caution, if at all, in patients with coagulopathy.

Laryngospasm should be considered if the aforementioned maneuvers fail to reestablish a patent airway. Laryngospasm is usually characterized by high-pitched crowing noises during ventilation but will be silent with complete glottic closure. Spasm of the vocal cords is more apt to occur following airway trauma, repeated instrumentation, or stimulation from secretions, blood, or other foreign material in the airway. The jaw-thrust maneuver, particularly when combined with gentle positive airway pressure via a tight-fitting face mask, usually breaks laryngospasm. Insertion of an oral or nasal airway is also helpful in ensuring a patent airway down to the level of the vocal cords. Secretions, blood, or other foreign material in the hypopharynx should be suctioned to prevent recurrence. Refractory laryngospasm should be treated with a small dose of intravenous succinylcholine (10–20 mg in adults) and positive-pressure ventilation with 100% oxygen. Endotracheal intubation may occasionally be necessary to reestablish adequate ventilation; emergency cricothyrotomy or transtracheal jet ventilation is indicated if intubation is unsuccessful in such instances.

Glottic edema following airway instrumentation is an important cause of airway obstruction in infants and young children because of the relatively small airway lumen. Significant pharyngeal and glottic edema and irritability, with friable, oozing oropharyngeal mucosa, is common in patients undergoing head and neck radiation therapy. Intravenous corticosteroids (dexamethasone, 0.5 mg/kg, 10-mg dose maximum) and/or aerosolized racemic epinephrine (0.5 mL of a 2.25% solution with 3 mL of normal saline) is often useful in such cases. Postoperative wound hematomas following thyroid, carotid artery, and other neck procedures can quickly compromise the airway, and opening the wound immediately relieves tracheal compression in most cases. Rarely, a gauze "throat pack" may be unintentionally left in the hypopharynx following oral surgery and can cause immediate or delayed complete airway obstruction.

Decannulation of a fresh tracheostomy is hazardous because recannulation may be difficult or impossible when the wound has not yet healed into a well-formed track. When a tracheostomy has been performed within the previous 4 weeks, intentional replacement of a tracheostomy cannula should only be performed with a surgeon at the bedside and with a tracheostomy instrument set, along with additional, appropriate difficult airway equipment, immediately available.

Hypoventilation

Hypoventilation, which is generally defined as a $PaCO_2$ greater than 45 mm Hg, is common following general anesthesia. In most instances, such hypoventilation is mild and not recognized. Significant hypoventilation commonly presents with clinical signs when the $PaCO_2$ is greater than 60 mm Hg or arterial blood pH is less than 7.25, including excessive somnolence, airway obstruction, slow respiratory rate, tachypnea with shallow breathing, or labored breathing. Mild to moderate respiratory acidosis may cause tachycardia, hypertension, and cardiac irritability via sympathetic stimulation, but more severe acidosis produces circulatory depression (see Chapter 50). If medically important hypoventilation is suspected, assessment and management are facilitated by capnography or arterial blood gas measurement, or both.

6 **Hypoventilation in the PACU is most commonly due to the residual depressant effects of anesthetic and analgesic agents on respiratory drive, often made worse by preexisting obstructive sleep apnea.** Opioid-induced respiratory depression characteristically produces a slow respiratory rate, often with large tidal volumes. The patient is somnolent but often responsive to verbal and physical stimuli and able to breathe on command. Delayed occurrence of respiratory depression has been reported with all opioids. Proposed mechanisms include variations in the intensity of stimulation during recovery and delayed release of the opioid from peripheral tissue compartments as the patient rewarms or begins to move.

Causes of residual muscle weakness in the PACU include inadequate muscle relaxant reversal, drug interactions that potentiate muscle relaxants, altered muscle relaxant pharmacokinetics (due to hypothermia, altered volumes of distribution, and kidney or liver dysfunction), and metabolic factors such as hypokalemia, hyper- or hypomagnesemia, or respiratory acidosis. Regardless of the cause, generalized weakness, uncoordinated movements ("fish out of water"), shallow tidal volumes, and tachypnea are usually apparent. The diagnosis of inadequate neuromuscular blockade reversal can be made with a nerve stimulator in unconscious patients; head lift and grip strength can be assessed in awake and cooperative patients. Splinting due to incisional pain, diaphragmatic dysfunction following upper abdominal or thoracic surgery, abdominal distention, and tight abdominal dressings are other factors that can contribute to hypoventilation. Increased CO_2 production from shivering, hyperthermia, or sepsis can also increase $PaCO_2$, even in normal patients recovering from general anesthesia. Marked hypoventilation and respiratory acidosis can result when these factors are superimposed on an impaired ventilatory reserve due to preexisting pulmonary, neuromuscular, or neurological disease.

Treatment of Hypoventilation

Treatment should generally be directed at the underlying cause, but marked hypoventilation always requires assisted or controlled ventilation until causal factors are identified and corrected. 7 **Hypoventilation with obtundation, circulatory depression, and severe acidosis (arterial blood pH <7.15) is an indication for immediate and decisive ventilatory and hemodynamic intervention, including airway and inotropic support as needed.** If intravenous naloxone is used to reverse opioid-induced respiratory depression, titration in small increments (80 mcg in adults) usually avoids complications and minimizes the likelihood that analgesia will be completely reversed. Antagonism of opioid-induced depression with large doses of naloxone often results in sudden pain and a marked increase in sympathetic tone. The latter can precipitate a hypertensive crisis, pulmonary edema, and myocardial ischemia or infarction. 8 Following naloxone administration, patients should be observed closely for recurrence of opioid-induced respiratory depression ("renarcotization"), as naloxone has a shorter duration of action than many opioids. If residual muscle paralysis is present, sugammadex (if rocuronium or vecuronium has been administered) or an additional cholinesterase inhibitor may be administered. Inadequate reversal despite a full dose of sugammadex or a cholinesterase inhibitor necessitates controlled ventilation under close observation until adequate recovery of muscle strength occurs. Hypoventilation due to pain and splinting following upper abdominal or thoracic procedures should be treated with multimodal analgesia, including intravenous or intraspinal opioid administration, intravenous acetaminophen, or NSAIDs, or with regional anesthesia techniques.

Hypoxemia

Mild hypoxemia is common in patients recovering from anesthesia without administration of supplemental oxygen. Mild to moderate hypoxemia (PaO_2 50–60 mm Hg) in young, healthy patients may be well tolerated initially, but with increasing duration or severity, the initial sympathetic stimulation often seen is replaced with progressive acidosis and circulatory depression. Cyanosis may not be detected if the hemoglobin concentration is reduced. Hypoxemia may also be suspected from restlessness, agitation, tachycardia, or atrial or ventricular dysrhythmias. Obtundation, bradycardia, hypotension, and cardiac arrest are late signs. Pulse oximetry facilitates the early detection of hypoxemia and must be routinely utilized in the PACU. Arterial blood gas measurements may be performed to confirm the diagnosis and guide therapy.

Hypoxemia in the PACU is usually caused by hypoventilation with or without obstruction, increased right-to-left intrapulmonary shunting, or both. A decrease in cardiac output or an increase in oxygen consumption (as with shivering) will accentuate hypoxemia. *Diffusion hypoxia* (see Chapter 8) is an uncommon cause of hypoxemia when recovering patients are given supplemental oxygen. Hypoxemia due exclusively to hypoventilation without obstruction is also unusual in patients receiving supplemental oxygen unless marked hypercapnia or a concomitant increase in intrapulmonary shunting is present. 9 **Increased intrapulmonary shunting from a decreased functional residual capacity (FRC) relative to closing capacity is the most common cause of hypoxemia following general anesthesia.** The greatest reductions in FRC occur following upper abdominal and thoracic surgery. The loss of lung volume is often attributed to microatelectasis, as atelectasis is often not identified on a chest radiograph. A semi-upright position helps maintain FRC.

Marked right-to-left intrapulmonary shunting $\dot{Q}_S/\dot{Q}_T$ is usually caused by atelectasis from prolonged intraoperative hypoventilation with low tidal volumes, unintentional endobronchial intubation, lobar

collapse from bronchial obstruction by secretions or blood, pulmonary aspiration, pulmonary edema, large pleural effusion, or pneumothorax. Postoperative pulmonary edema may present with wheezing or pink frothy fluid in the airway. Pulmonary edema may be due to left ventricular failure (cardiogenic), acute respiratory distress syndrome, or relief of prolonged airway obstruction (*negative-pressure pulmonary edema*). In contrast to wheezing associated with pulmonary edema, wheezing due to primary obstructive lung disease, which also often results in large increases in intrapulmonary shunting, is not associated with edema fluid in the airway or infiltrates on the chest
10 radiograph. **The possibility of a postoperative pneumothorax should always be considered following central line placement, supraclavicular or intercostal blocks, abdominal or chest trauma (including rib fractures), neck dissection, thyroidectomy (especially if the thyroid dissection extends into the thorax), tracheostomy, nephrectomy, or other retroperitoneal or intraabdominal procedures (including laparoscopy), especially if the diaphragm may have been penetrated or disrupted. Patients with subpleural blebs or large bullae can also develop pneumothorax during positive-pressure ventilation.**

Treatment of Hypoxemia

Oxygen therapy, with or without positive airway pressure, and relief of any existing airway obstruction with airway maneuvers, an oral or nasal airway, or oropharyngeal suctioning, provide the cornerstones of treatment for hypoxemia. Routine administration of 30% to 60% oxygen is usually enough to prevent hypoxemia with even moderate hypoventilation and hypercapnia. Importantly, clinical signs of hypoventilation and hypercapnia may be masked by routine oxygen administration. Patients with underlying pulmonary or cardiac disease may require higher concentrations of oxygen; oxygen therapy should be guided by SpO_2 or arterial blood gas measurements. Oxygen concentration must be closely controlled in patients with chronic CO_2 retention to avoid precipitating acute respiratory failure. Patients with severe or persistent hypoxemia should be given 100% oxygen via a nonrebreathing mask, LMA, or endotracheal tube until the cause is established and appropriate therapy is instituted; controlled or assisted mechanical ventilation may also be necessary. The chest radiograph (preferably with the patient positioned sitting upright) is valuable in assessing lung volume and heart size and in demonstrating pneumothorax, atelectasis, or pulmonary infiltrates. However, in cases of pulmonary aspiration, infiltrates are usually initially absent. If pneumothorax is suspected, a chest radiograph taken at end-expiration helps highlight the pneumothorax by providing the greatest contrast between lung tissue and adjacent air in the pleural space. In the intubated patient with hypoxemia, a chest radiograph should be used to verify proper endotracheal tube position. Point-of-care transthoracic ultrasonography is a valuable alternative tool for rapid, accurate assessment of endotracheal tube placement and for diagnosis of lobar consolidation, pleural effusion, and pneumothorax.

Additional treatment of hypoxemia should be directed at the underlying cause. A chest tube or Heimlich valve should be inserted for any symptomatic pneumothorax or one that is greater than 15% to 20%. An asymptomatic pneumothorax may be aspirated or followed by observation. Bronchospasm should be treated with aerosolized bronchodilator therapy, and potential or partial obstruction secondary to glottic or pharyngeal edema can be treated with racemic epinephrine or corticosteroids, or both. Diuretics should be given for fluid overload. Persistent hypoxemia in spite of 50% oxygen generally is an indication for positive end-expiratory pressure ventilation or continuous positive airway pressure. Therapeutic bronchoscopy is often useful in reexpanding lobar atelectasis caused by bronchial plugs or particulate aspiration. In the setting of an intubated patient, secretions or debris must be removed by suction and also by lavage, if necessary, and a malpositioned endotracheal tube must be appropriately repositioned.

CIRCULATORY COMPLICATIONS

The most common circulatory disturbances in the PACU are hypotension, hypertension, and arrhythmias. *The possibility that the circulatory abnormality is secondary to an underlying respiratory disturbance should always be considered before any other intervention, especially in children.*

Hypotension

Hypotension is usually due to hypovolemia, left
11 **ventricular dysfunction, or excessive arterial vasodilatation. Hypovolemia is the most common cause of hypotension in the PACU and can result from inadequate fluid replacement, wound drainage, or hemorrhage.** Vasoconstriction from hypothermia may mask hypovolemia until the patient's temperature begins to rise; subsequent peripheral vasodilation during rewarming unmasks the hypovolemia and results in hypotension. Spinal and epidural anesthesia produce hypotension from a combination of arterial vasodilation and venous pooling of blood. Much like nitroglycerine, neuraxial blocks produce venous pooling and reduce the effective circulating blood volume, despite an otherwise normal intravascular volume (see Chapter 45). Hypotension associated with sepsis and allergic reactions is usually the result of both hypovolemia and vasodilation. Hypotension from a tension pneumothorax or cardiac tamponade is the result of impaired venous return to the right atrium. Removal of more than 500 to 1000 mL of ascites fluid during surgical procedure or paracentesis may result in subsequent hypotension as additional fluid migrates from the intravascular space into the abdomen.

Left ventricular dysfunction in previously healthy persons is unusual unless associated with severe metabolic disturbances (hypoxemia, acidosis, sepsis). Hypotension due to ventricular dysfunction is primarily encountered in patients with underlying coronary artery or valvular heart disease or congestive heart failure and is usually precipitated by fluid overload, myocardial ischemia, acute increases in afterload, or arrhythmias.

Treatment of Hypotension

Mild hypotension during recovery from anesthesia is common and typically does not require intensive treatment. Significant hypotension is often defined as a 20% to 30% reduction in blood pressure below the patient's baseline level and usually requires correction. Treatment depends on the ability to assess intravascular volume. We advocate bedside ultrasound. An increase in blood pressure following a fluid bolus (250–500 mL crystalloid or 100–250 mL colloid) generally confirms hypovolemia. With severe hypotension, a vasopressor or inotrope (dopamine or epinephrine) may be necessary to increase arterial blood pressure until the intravascular volume deficit can be at least partially corrected. Signs of cardiac dysfunction should be sought in patients with known heart disease or cardiac risk factors. Failure of a patient with severe hypotension to promptly respond to initial treatment mandates echocardiographic examination or invasive hemodynamic monitoring (see Chapter 5). Manipulations of cardiac preload, contractility, and afterload are, at times, all required to restore the blood pressure to acceptable levels. The presence of a tension pneumothorax, as suggested by hypotension with unilaterally decreased breath sounds, hyperresonance, and tracheal deviation, is an indication for immediate pleural space aspiration, even before ultrasound or radiographic confirmation. Similarly, hypotension due to cardiac tamponade, usually following chest trauma or thoracic surgery, often necessitates immediate pericardiocentesis or surgical exploration.

Hypertension

Postoperative hypertension is common in the PACU and typically occurs within the first 30 min after
12 admission. Noxious stimulation from incisional pain, endotracheal intubation, bladder distention, or preoperative discontinuation of antihypertensive medication is usually responsible. Postoperative hypertension may also reflect the neuroendocrine stress response to surgery or increased sympathetic tone secondary to hypoxemia, hypercapnia, or metabolic acidosis. Patients with a history of hypertension are more likely to develop hypertension in the PACU. Fluid overload or intracranial hypertension may also occasionally present as postoperative hypertension.

Treatment of Hypertension

Mild hypertension generally does not require treatment, but a reversible cause should be sought. Marked hypertension can precipitate postoperative bleeding, myocardial ischemia, heart failure, or intracranial hemorrhage. Although decisions to treat postoperative hypertension should be individualized, in general, elevations in blood pressure greater than 20% to 30% of the patient's baseline, or those associated with adverse effects such as myocardial ischemia, heart failure, or bleeding, should be treated. After pain and potential bladder distention have been addressed, mild to moderate elevations can be treated with intravenous labetalol, an angiotensin-converting enzyme inhibitor such as enalapril, or a calcium channel blocker such as nicardipine. Hydralazine and sublingual nifedipine (when administered to patients not receiving β-blockers) may cause tachycardia and myocardial ischemia and infarction. Marked hypertension in patients with limited cardiac reserve requires direct intraarterial pressure monitoring and should be treated with an intravenous infusion of nitroprusside, nitroglycerin, nicardipine, clevidipine, or fenoldopam. The endpoint for treatment should be consistent with the patient's own normal blood pressure.

Arrhythmias

Respiratory disturbances, particularly hypoxemia, hypercarbia, and acidosis, will commonly provoke cardiac arrhythmias. Residual effects from anesthetic agents, increased sympathetic nervous system activity, other metabolic abnormalities, and preexisting cardiac or pulmonary disease also predispose patients to arrhythmias in the PACU.

Bradycardia often represents the residual effects of cholinesterase inhibitors, opioids, or β-adrenergic blockers. Tachycardia in the PACU is most commonly caused by pain, hypovolemia, or fever but may also be due to the effects of an anticholinergic agent, a β-agonist such as albuterol, or reflex tachycardia from hydralazine. Anesthetic-induced depression of baroreceptor function makes heart rate an unreliable monitor of intravascular volume in the PACU.

Premature atrial and ventricular beats may be the result of hypokalemia, hypomagnesemia, increased sympathetic tone, or, less commonly, myocardial ischemia. The latter can be diagnosed with a 12-lead ECG. Premature atrial or ventricular beats noted in the PACU without discernable cause will often also be found on the patient's preoperative ECG if one is available. Supraventricular tachyarrhythmias, including paroxysmal supraventricular tachycardia, atrial flutter, and atrial fibrillation, are typically encountered in patients with a history of these arrhythmias and are more commonly encountered following thoracic surgery. The management of arrhythmias is discussed in Chapters 21 and 55.

CASE DISCUSSION

Fever & Tachycardia in a Young Adult Man

A 19-year-old man sustained a closed fracture of the femur in a motor vehicle accident. He was placed in traction for 3 days prior to surgery. During that time, a persistent low-grade fever (37.5–38.7°C orally), mild hypertension (150–170/70–90 mm Hg), and tachycardia (100–126 beats/min) were noted. His hematocrit remained at 30%. Broad-spectrum antibiotic coverage was initiated.

He is scheduled for open reduction and internal fixation of the fracture. When the patient is brought into the operating room, vital signs are as follows: blood pressure 160/95 mm Hg, pulse 150 beats/min, respirations 20 breaths/min, and oral temperature 38.1°C. He is sweating and is anxious. On close examination, he is noted to have a slightly enlarged thyroid gland.

Should the surgical team proceed with the operation?

The proposed operation is elective; therefore, significant abnormalities should be diagnosed and properly treated preoperatively, if possible, to optimally prepare the patient for surgery. If the patient had an open fracture, the risk of infection would clearly mandate immediate operation. Even with a closed femoral fracture, cancellations or delays should be avoided because nonoperative treatment potentiates risks associated with bed rest, including atelectasis, pneumonia, deep venous thrombosis, and potentially lethal pulmonary thromboembolism. In deciding whether to proceed with the surgery, the anesthesia provider must ask the following questions:

1. What are the most likely causes of the abnormalities based on the clinical presentation?
2. What, if any, additional investigations or consultations might be helpful?
3. How would these or other commonly associated abnormalities affect anesthetic management?
4. Are the potential anesthetic interactions serious enough to delay surgery until a suspected cause is conclusively excluded? The tachycardia of 150 beats/min and the low-grade fever therefore require further evaluation prior to surgery.

What are the likely causes of the tachycardia and fever in this patient?

These two abnormalities may reflect one process or separate entities (Tables 56–4 and 56–5). Moreover, although multiple factors can often be simultaneously identified, their relative contribution is often not readily apparent. Fever commonly follows major trauma; contributory factors can include the inflammatory reaction to the tissue trauma, superimposed infection (most commonly wound, pulmonary, or urinary), antibiotic therapy (drug reaction), or thrombophlebitis. Infection must be seriously considered in this patient because of the risk of bacteria seeding and infecting the metal fixation device placed during surgery. Although tachycardia is commonly associated with a low-grade fever, it is usually not of this magnitude in a 19-year-old patient. Moderate to severe pain, anxiety, hypovolemia, or anemia may be other contributory factors. Pulmonary embolism should also be considered in any patient with long bone fracture, particularly when hypoxemia, tachypnea, or mental status changes are present. Lastly, the possibly enlarged thyroid gland, sweating, and anxious appearance, together with both fever and tachycardia, suggest thyrotoxicosis.

What (if any) additional measures may be helpful in evaluating the fever and tachycardia?

Arterial blood gas measurements, echocardiography, and a chest radiograph would be helpful in the identification of pulmonary embolism.

TABLE 56–4 Perioperative causes of tachycardia.

Anxiety
Pain
Fever (see Table 56–5)
Respiratory
Hypoxemia
Hypercapnia
Circulatory
Hypotension
Anemia
Hypovolemia
Congestive heart failure
Cardiac tamponade
Tension pneumothorax
Thromboembolism
Drug-induced
Antimuscarinic agents
β-Adrenergic agonists
Vasodilators
Allergy
Drug withdrawal
Metabolic disorders
Hypoglycemia
Thyrotoxicosis
Pheochromocytoma
Adrenal (addisonian) crisis
Carcinoid syndrome
Acute porphyria

TABLE 56–5 Perioperative causes of fever.

Infections
Immunologically mediated processes
Drug reactions
Blood reactions
Tissue destruction (rejection)
Connective tissue disorders
Granulomatous disorders
Tissue damage
Trauma
Infarction
Thrombosis
Neoplastic disorders
Metabolic disorders
Thyroid storm (thyroid crisis)
Adrenal (addisonian) crisis
Pheochromocytoma
Malignant hyperthermia
Neuroleptic malignant syndrome
Acute gout
Acute porphyria

A repeat hematocrit or hemoglobin concentration measurement would exclude worsening anemia; significant tachycardia may be expected when the hematocrit is below 25% to 27% (hemoglobin <8 g/dL) in most patients. The response to an intravenous fluid challenge with 250 to 500 mL of a colloid or crystalloid solution may be helpful; a decrease in heart rate after the fluid bolus would be strongly suggestive of hypovolemia. Similarly, response of the heart rate to sedation and additional opioid analgesia would be helpful in excluding anxiety and pain, respectively, as causes. Although a tentative diagnosis of hyperthyroidism can be made based on clinical grounds, confirmation requires the measurement of serum thyroid hormones. Signs of infection—such as increased inflammation or purulence in a wound, purulent sputum, an infiltrate on the chest film, pyuria, or leukocytosis with premature white cells on a blood smear ("shift to the left")—should prompt cultures and a delay of surgery until the results are obtained and correct antibiotic coverage is confirmed.

The patient is transferred to the PACU for further evaluation. A 12-lead ECG confirms sinus tachycardia of 150 beats/min. A chest film is normal. Arterial blood gas measurements on room air are normal (pH 7.44, $PaCO_2$ 41 mm Hg, PaO_2 87 mm Hg, and HCO_3^- 27 mEq/L). The hemoglobin concentration is found to be 11 g/dL. Blood for thyroid function tests is sent to the laboratory. The patient is sedated intravenously with midazolam (2 mg) and fentanyl (50 mcg) and is given 500 mL of 5% albumin. He seems to be relaxed and pain free, but the heart rate decreases only to 144 beats/min. The decision is made to proceed with surgery using continuous lumbar epidural anesthesia with 2% lidocaine. Esmolol is administered slowly until his pulse decreases to 120 beats/min, and a continuous esmolol infusion is administered at a rate of 300 mcg/kg/min.

The procedure is completed in 3 h. Although the patient did not report pain during the procedure and was given only minimal additional sedation (midazolam, 2 mg), he is delirious upon admission to the PACU. The esmolol infusion is continuing at a rate of 500 mcg/kg/min. Estimated blood loss was 500 mL, and fluid replacement consisted of 2 units of packed red blood cells, 500 mL of 5% albumin solution, and 2000 mL of lactated Ringer's injection. Vital signs are as follows: blood pressure 105/40 mm Hg, pulse 124 beats/min, respirations 30 breaths/min, and rectal temperature 38.8°C. Arterial blood gas measurements are reported as follows: pH 7.37, $PaCO_2$ 37 mm Hg, PaO_2 91 mm Hg, and HCO_3^- 22 mEq/L.

What is the most likely diagnosis?

The patient appears to be in a hypermetabolic state manifested by excessive adrenergic activity, fever, and a worsening mental status. The absence of major metabolic acidosis and lack of exposure to a known triggering agent exclude malignant hyperthermia (see Chapter 52). Other possibilities include a transfusion reaction, sepsis, or an undiagnosed pheochromocytoma. The sequence of events makes the first two unlikely, and the decreasing prominence of hypertension (now replaced with relative hypotension) and increasing fever also make the latter unlikely. The clinical presentation now suggests thyroid storm. He has also received a very large dose of esmolol for several hours, and this may be contributing to the relatively low blood pressure despite aggressive fluid administration.

Emergency consultation is obtained with an endocrinologist, who concurs with the diagnosis of thyroid storm and assists with its management. How is thyroid storm managed?

Thyroid storm (crisis) is a medical emergency that carries a 10% to 50% mortality rate. It is usually encountered in patients with poorly controlled or undiagnosed Graves disease. Precipitating factors include (1) the stress of surgery and anesthesia, (2) labor and delivery, (3) severe infection, and, rarely, (4) thyroiditis 1 to 2 weeks following administration of radioactive iodine. Manifestations usually include mental status changes (irritability, delirium, coma), fever, tachycardia, and hypotension. Both atrial and ventricular arrhythmias are common, particularly atrial fibrillation. Congestive heart failure develops in 25% of patients. Hypertension that often precedes hypotension, heat intolerance with profuse sweating, nausea and vomiting, and diarrhea may be prominent initially. Hypokalemia is present in up to 50% of patients. Levels of thyroid hormones are high in plasma but correlate poorly with the severity of the crisis. The sudden exacerbation of thyrotoxicosis may represent a rapid shift of the hormone from the protein-bound to the free state or increased responsiveness to thyroid hormones at the cellular level.

Treatment is directed toward reversing the crisis and its complications. Large doses of corticosteroids inhibit the synthesis, release, and peripheral conversion of thyroxine (T_4) to the more active triiodothyronine (T_3). Corticosteroids also prevent relative adrenal insufficiency secondary to the hypermetabolic state. Propylthiouracil is administered to inhibit the synthesis of thyroid hormone, and iodide is given to inhibit the release of thyroid hormones from the gland. Propranolol not only antagonizes the peripheral effects of the thyrotoxicosis but may also inhibit the peripheral conversion of T_4. Combined β_1- and β_2-blockade is preferable to selective β_1-antagonism (esmolol or metoprolol) because excessive β_2-receptor activity is responsible for the metabolic effects. β_2-Receptor blockade also reduces muscle blood flow and may decrease heat production. Supportive measures include surface cooling (cooling blanket), acetaminophen (aspirin is not recommended because it may displace thyroid hormone from plasma carrier proteins), and generous intravenous fluid replacement. Vasopressors are often necessary to support arterial blood pressure.

Ventricular rate control is indicated in patients with atrial fibrillation. Echocardiography and hemodynamic monitoring may facilitate the management of patients with signs of congestive heart failure or persistent hypotension. β-Adrenergic blockade is contraindicated in patients with congestive heart failure.

Propranolol, dexamethasone, propylthiouracil, and sodium iodide are given; the patient is admitted to the intensive care unit, where treatment is continued. Over the next 3 days, his mental status markedly improves. The T_3 and total T_4 levels on the day of surgery were both elevated to 250 ng/dL and 18.5 ng/dL, respectively. He was discharged home 6 days later to endocrinologist follow up on a regimen of propranolol and propylthiouracil, with a blood pressure of 124/80 mm Hg, a pulse of 92 beats/min, and an oral temperature of 37.3°C.

SUGGESTED READINGS

Apfelbaum J, Silverstein J, Chung F, et al. Practice guidelines for postanesthetic care: an updated report by the American Society of Anesthesiologists Task Force on Postanesthetic Care. *Anesthesiology*. 2013;118:291.

Chen Q, Chen E, Qian X. A narrative review on perioperative pain management strategies in enhanced recovery pathways—the past, present, and future. *J Clin Med*. 2021;10:2568.

Doleman B, Leonardi-Bee J, Heinink TP, et al. Pre-emptive and preventive NSAIDs for postoperative pain in adults undergoing all types of surgery. *Cochrane Database Syst Rev*. 2021;6:CD012978.

Dwyer-Hemmings L, Hampson A, Fairhead C, et al. A systematic review and meta-analysis of post-operative urinary retention with anaesthetic and analgesic modalities. *J Clin Anesth*. 2021;72:110280.

Elhassan MG, Chao PW, Curiel A. The conundrum of volume status assessment: revisiting current and future fools available for physicians at the bedside. *Cureus*. 2021;13:e15253.

Gali B, Gritzner SR, Henderson AJ, et al. Respiratory depression following ambulatory urogynecologic procedures: a retrospective analysis. *Mayo Clin Proc Innov Qual Outcomes*. 2019;3:169

Halterman RS, Gaber M, Janjua MST, et al. Use of a checklist for the postanesthesia care unit patient handoff. *J Perianesth Nurs*. 2019;34:834.

Ludbrook G, Lloyd C, Story D, et al. The effect of advanced recovery room care on postoperative outcomes in moderate-risk surgical patients: a multicentre feasibility study. *Anaesthesia*. 2021;76:480.

Luo J, Min S. Postoperative pain management in the postanesthesia care unit: an update. *J Pain Res*. 2017;10:2687.

Ramsingh D, Christian Fox J, Wilson WC. Perioperative point-of-care ultrasonography: an emerging technology to be embraced by anesthesiologists. *Anesth Analg*. 2015;120:990.

Schlesinger T, Weibel S, Meybohm P, et al. Drugs in anesthesia: preventing postoperative nausea and vomiting. *Curr Opin Anaesthesiol*. 2021;34:421.

Urits I, Peck J, Giacomazzi S, et al. Emergence delirium in perioperative pediatric care: a review of current evidence and new directions. *Adv Ther*. 2020;37:1897.

Wei B, Feng Y, Chen W, et al. Risk factors for emergence agitation in adults after general anesthesia: a systematic review and meta-analysis. *Acta Anaesthesiol Scand*. 2021;65:719.

CHAPTER 57

Common Clinical Concerns in Critical Care Medicine

Pranav Shah, MD

KEY CONCEPTS

1. Pulmonary edema usually results from either an increase in the net hydrostatic pressure across the capillaries (hemodynamic or cardiogenic pulmonary edema) or an increase in the permeability of the alveolar–capillary membrane (increased permeability edema or noncardiogenic pulmonary edema).
2. Reduced tidal volumes are associated with the greatest improvement in outcome after acute respiratory distress syndrome (ARDS) of any intervention subjected to a randomized clinical trial to date.
3. Early elective tracheal intubation is advisable when there are obvious signs of heat injury to the airway. Patients with hoarseness and stridor require immediate tracheal intubation or a surgical airway.
4. The criteria developed by the Acute Kidney Injury Network are now most often used to stage acute kidney injury (AKI). AKI is diagnosed by documenting an increase in serum creatinine of more than 50%, or an absolute increase of 0.3 mg/dL, and a reduction in urine output to less than 0.5 mL/kg/h for 6 h or longer, with all findings developing over 48 h or less.
5. *Septic shock* is defined as acute circulatory failure in a patient with sepsis or, more specifically, systolic blood pressure less than 90 mm Hg that is not responsive to volume resuscitation and requiring vasopressors for life support.
6. Critically ill patients frequently have abnormal host defenses from advanced age, malnutrition, drug therapy, loss of integrity of mucosal and skin barriers, and underlying diseases. Thus, age greater than 70 years, corticosteroid therapy, chemotherapy of malignancy, prolonged use of invasive devices, respiratory failure, kidney failure, head trauma, and burns are established risk factors for nosocomial infections.
7. Systemic pooling of blood and transudation of fluid into tissues result in relative hypovolemia in patients with sepsis.

Scope

The range of conditions that specialists in critical care medicine must address is extraordinarily broad. Many frequent concerns of the intensivist are covered in other chapters and will not be discussed here to avoid duplication. Therefore, for an overview of critical care medicine, the reader will need to refer to chapters where airway management (Chapter 19), inhalation therapy and ventilator management (Chapter 58), adrenergic agonists (Chapter 14), vasodilators (Chapter 15), fluids and electrolytes (Chapters 49–51), burn injury (Chapter 39), arrhythmias (Chapter 21), acute hypertension (Chapter 21), asthma and chronic obstructive pulmonary disease (Chapter 24), liver failure (Chapter 34), kidney disease (Chapter 31), resuscitation (Chapter 55), traumatic brain injury and intracranial pressure monitoring (Chapter 39), spinal cord injury (Chapter 39), diabetes (Chapter 35), nutrition (Chapter 53), and delirium (Chapters 28 and 54) are discussed.

Poisoning and drug overdosage are common reasons patients are admitted to the critical care unit, and this chapter contains such a case description. The initial treatment of such patients is most often initiated in the emergency department. The possible drugs (and drug combinations) are so great in number that we must refer interested readers to other sources. Specifics regarding overdosage with anesthetic drugs are discussed in Chapters 7 and 10. Hypothermia and malignant hyperthermia are discussed in Chapter 52. There is increasing interest in preventing post-traumatic stress disorder (PTSD) after critical illness. Studies have shown that this may occur in as many as 25% of patients surviving a stay in the intensive care unit (ICU). This edition was completed during the SARS-CoV-2 pandemic, during which standard intensive therapies changed frequently. Finally, there is increasing interest in preventing PTSD and "burnout" in the physicians, nurses, and therapists who care for patients with critical illness. The SARS-CoV-2 pandemic greatly exacerbated this latter concern. Thus, the scope of critical care is enormous, and not all of the important topics can be covered here.

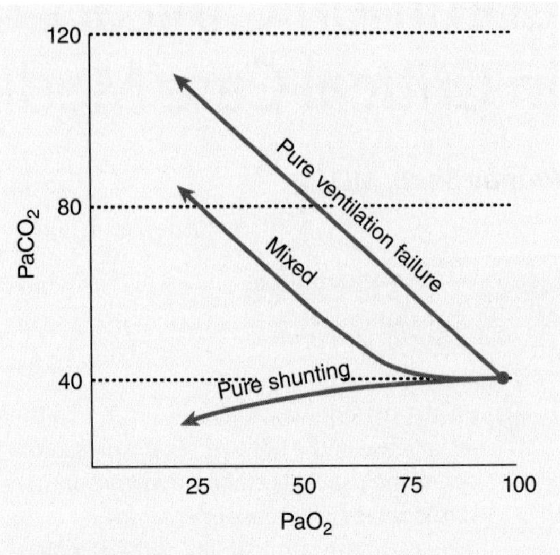

FIGURE 57–1 Arterial gas tension (room air) patterns during acute respiratory failure.

Respiratory Failure

Respiratory failure may be defined as a disorder of gas exchange severe enough to require acute therapeutic intervention. Definitions based on arterial blood gas measurements may not apply to patients with chronic pulmonary diseases. For example, dyspnea and progressive respiratory acidosis may be present in patients with chronic carbon dioxide (CO_2) retention. Arterial blood gases typically follow one of several patterns in patients with respiratory failure (Figure 57–1). At one extreme, the derangement primarily affects oxygen transfer from the alveoli into blood, giving rise to hypoxemia (hypoxic respiratory failure); in these patients, CO_2 elimination is typically normal or even enhanced unless severe ventilation/perfusion mismatching is present. At the other extreme, pure ventilatory failure primarily affects CO_2 elimination, resulting in hypercapnia; mismatching of ventilation to perfusion is typically absent or minimal. Hypoxemia, however, can occur with pure ventilatory failure when arterial CO_2 tension reaches 75 to 80 mm Hg in patients breathing room air (see the alveolar gas equation in Chapter 23). Few patients with respiratory failure display a pattern as "pure" as these extreme examples.

Treatment

Regardless of the disorder, the treatment of respiratory failure is primarily supportive while the reversible components of underlying disease(s) are treated. Hypoxemia is treated with oxygen therapy, positive airway pressure (if functional residual capacity is decreased), or perhaps "proning," whereas hypercarbia (ventilatory failure) is treated with mechanical ventilation when there is no effective pharmacological countermeasure (eg, naloxone for milder degrees of opioid overdosage). Other general measures may include using aerosolized bronchodilators, intravenous antibiotics, and diuretics for fluid overload, therapy to improve cardiac function, and nutritional support.

PULMONARY EDEMA

Pathophysiology

Pulmonary edema results from transudation of fluid, first from pulmonary capillaries into interstitial spaces and then from the interstitial spaces into alveoli. Fluid within the interstitial space and alveoli is collectively referred to as *extravascular lung water.* The movement of water across the pulmonary capillaries is similar to what occurs in other capillary beds and can be expressed by the Starling equation:

$$Q = K \times [(Pc' - Pi) - \sigma(\pi c' - \pi i)]$$

in which Q is net flow across the capillary; Pc′ and Pi are capillary and interstitial hydrostatic pressures, respectively; $\pi c'$ and πi are capillary and interstitial oncotic pressures, respectively; K is a filtration coefficient related to effective capillary surface area per mass of tissue; and σ is a reflection coefficient that expresses the permeability of the capillary endothelium to albumin. Albumin is particularly important in this context because more water will be lost to the interstitium when albumin is also lost to the interstitium. A σ with a value of 1 implies that the endothelium is completely impermeable to albumin, whereas a value of 0 indicates free passage of albumin and other particles/molecules. The pulmonary endothelium normally is partially permeable to albumin, such that interstitial albumin concentration is approximately one-half that of plasma; therefore, under normal conditions πi must be about 14 mm Hg (one-half that of plasma). Pulmonary capillary hydrostatic pressure is gravity dependent and thus depends on vertical height in the lung. It normally varies from 0 to 15 mm Hg (average, 7 mm Hg). Because Pi is thought to be normally about −4 to −8 mm Hg, the forces favoring transudation of fluid (Pc′, Pi, and πi) are usually almost balanced by the forces favoring reabsorption ($\pi c'$). The net amount of fluid that normally moves out of pulmonary capillaries is small (about 10–20 mL/h in adults) and is rapidly removed by pulmonary lymphatics, which return it into the central venous system.

The alveolar epithelial membrane is usually permeable to water and gases but is impermeable to albumin (and other proteins). A net movement of water from the interstitium into alveoli occurs only when the normally negative Pi becomes positive (relative to atmospheric pressure). Fortunately, because of the lung's unique ultrastructure and its capacity to increase lymph flow, the pulmonary interstitium usually accommodates large increases in capillary transudation before Pi becomes positive. When this reserve capacity is exceeded, pulmonary edema develops.

Causes of Pulmonary Edema

1 Pulmonary edema usually results from either an increase in the net hydrostatic pressure across the capillaries (hemodynamic or cardiogenic pulmonary edema) or an increase in the permeability of the alveolar–capillary membrane (increased permeability edema or noncardiogenic pulmonary edema). If a pulmonary artery catheter is present, the distinction can be based on the pulmonary artery occlusion pressure, which if greater than 18 mm Hg indicates that hydrostatic pressure is involved in forcing fluid across the capillaries into the interstitium and alveoli. However, the pulmonary artery catheter may provide incorrect guidance regarding etiology: In the case of "flash" pulmonary edema, the pulmonary artery occlusion pressure may now be normal, despite it having been elevated at the point in time when the pulmonary edema was induced. The protein content of the edema fluid can also help differentiate the two. Fluid due to hemodynamic edema has a low protein content, whereas that due to permeability edema has a high protein content.

Less common causes of edema include prolonged severe airway obstruction (negative pressure pulmonary edema), sudden reexpansion of a collapsed lung, high altitude, pulmonary lymphatic obstruction, and severe head injury, though the same mechanisms (ie, changes in hemodynamic parameters or capillary permeability) also account for these diagnoses. Pulmonary edema associated with airway obstruction may result from an increase in the transmural pressure across pulmonary capillaries associated with a markedly negative interstitial hydrostatic pressure. Neurogenic pulmonary edema appears to be related to a marked increase in sympathetic tone, which causes severe pulmonary hypertension and disruption of the alveolar–capillary membrane.

1. Increased Transmural Pressure Pulmonary Edema ("Cardiogenic" Pulmonary Edema)

Significantly increased Pc′ may increase extravascular lung water and result in pulmonary edema. As can be seen from the Starling equation, a decrease in $\pi c'$ may accentuate the effects of any increase in Pc′. Two major mechanisms increase Pc′: pulmonary venous hypertension and a markedly increased pulmonary blood flow. Any elevation of pulmonary venous pressure is transmitted passively backward to the pulmonary capillaries and secondarily increases Pc′. Pulmonary venous hypertension may result from left ventricular failure, mitral stenosis, or left atrial obstruction. Increases in pulmonary blood flow that exceed the capacity of the pulmonary vasculature will also raise Pc′. Marked increases in pulmonary blood flow can be the result of large left-to-right cardiac or peripheral shunts, hypervolemia (fluid overload), or extremes of anemia or exercise.

Treatment

Management of cardiogenic pulmonary edema involves decreasing the pressure in the pulmonary capillaries. Generally, this includes measures to improve left ventricular function, correct fluid overload with diuretics, or reduce pulmonary blood flow. Pharmacological treatment of acute cardiogenic pulmonary edema has included oxygen, morphine, diuretics (especially loop diuretics), vasodilators such as nitrates, and inotropes such as dobutamine or milrinone. By reducing left atrial pressure, pulmonary congestion is relieved; by reducing systemic vascular resistance, cardiac output may be improved. Positive airway pressure therapy is also a useful adjunct for improving oxygenation. When pulmonary edema is a consequence of left ventricular failure from acute coronary ischemia, intraaortic balloon counterpulsation or other cardiac assist devices may be needed in addition to thrombolysis and revascularization.

2. Increased Permeability Pulmonary Edema (Noncardiogenic Pulmonary Edema): Acute Lung Injury & Acute Respiratory Distress Syndrome

Extravascular lung water increases in patients with pulmonary edema from enhanced permeability or disruption of the capillary–alveolar membrane. The protective effect of plasma oncotic pressure is lost as increased amounts of albumin "leak" into the pulmonary interstitium; normal—or even low—capillary hydrostatic pressures are unopposed and result in transudation of fluid into the lungs. Permeability edema is seen with *acute lung injury* (PaO_2:FiO_2 ratio ≤300) and is often associated with sepsis, trauma, and pulmonary aspiration; when severe (PaO_2:FiO_2 ratio <200), it is referred to as *acute respiratory distress syndrome* (ARDS).

Pathophysiology

Acute lung injury and ARDS arise from severe injury of the capillary–alveolar membrane, commonly from systemic inflammatory response syndrome (SIRS). Regardless of the inciting cause of SIRS, the lung appears to respond similarly to the ensuing inflammatory response. The released secondary mediators increase pulmonary capillary permeability, induce pulmonary vasoconstriction, and inhibit hypoxic pulmonary vasoconstriction. Destruction of alveolar epithelial cells is prominent. Alveolar flooding with decreased surfactant production (due to loss of type II pneumocytes) leads to alveolar collapse. The exudative phase of ARDS will persist for a varying period and is often followed by a fibrotic phase (fibrosing alveolitis), which may lead to permanent scarring.

Clinical Manifestations

The diagnosis of acute lung injury or ARDS requires a PaO_2:FiO_2 ratio less than 300 (acute lung injury) or less than 200 (ARDS) and the presence of diffuse infiltrates on chest radiograph, while also excluding significant left ventricular dysfunction. The lung is often affected in a nonhomogeneous pattern, though dependent areas tend to be most affected.

Acute lung injury and ARDS are commonly seen in association with sepsis or trauma. Patients present with severe dyspnea and labored respirations. Hypoxemia due to intrapulmonary shunting is universal. Although dead space ventilation is increased, arterial CO_2 tension is typically decreased because of a marked increase in minute ventilation. Ventilatory failure may be seen in severe cases due to respiratory muscle fatigue or marked destruction of the capillary–alveolar membrane. Pulmonary hypertension and low or normal left ventricular filling pressures are characteristic hemodynamic findings.

Treatment

In addition to intensive respiratory care, treatment should be directed at reversible processes such as sepsis or hypotension. Hypoxemia is treated with oxygen therapy. Milder cases may be treated with noninvasive respiratory support, but most patients require intubation and mechanical ventilation. **Increased P_{plt} pressures (>30 cm H_2O) and high V_T (>6 mL/kg) should be avoided because overdistention of alveoli can induce iatrogenic lung injury, as (likely) can FiO_2 greater than 0.5.** Although injury from increased FiO_2 has not been conclusively demonstrated in humans, V_T of 12 mL/kg was associated with greater mortality than V_T of 6 mL/kg (and P_{plt} of less than
2 30 cm H_2O) in patients with ARDS. Thus, reduced tidal volumes are associated with the greatest improvement in outcome after ARDS of any intervention subjected to a randomized clinical trial to date.

If possible, the FiO_2 should be maintained at 0.5 or less, primarily by increasing positive end-expiratory pressure (PEEP). Other maneuvers to improve oxygenation may include the use of inhaled nitric oxide, inhaled prostacyclin or prostaglandin E_1 (PGE_1), and ventilation in the prone position. These three techniques improve oxygenation in many such patients but are not risk free. A meta-analysis concluded that moderate doses of corticosteroids likely improve morbidity and mortality outcomes in ARDS, but the underlying data remain controversial. Steroids have been shown to be beneficial in patients with COVID-19 lung disease. Patients with COVID-19 are at increased risk of pulmonary embolism, and anticoagulant therapy is likewise a part of the management regimen of critically ill patients. Prone positioning has also been shown to improve oxygenation in this patient population. Additional COVID-19 therapies are being developed at the time of this writing, and readers are advised that guidelines and recommendations for the ICU care of patients with COVID-19 are evolving.

Morbidity and mortality from ARDS usually arise from the precipitating cause or from complications rather than from the respiratory failure itself. Among the most common serious complications are sepsis, acute kidney failure, and gastrointestinal hemorrhage. Nosocomial pneumonia is often difficult to diagnose; antibiotics are generally indicated when there is a high index of suspicion (fever, purulent secretions, leukocytosis, change in chest radiograph). Brushings and bronchoalveolar lavage sampling via a flexible bronchoscope may be useful. Breach of mucocutaneous barriers by catheters, malnutrition, and altered host immunity contribute to a frequent incidence of infection. Acute kidney failure may result from various combinations of inadequate renal blood flow and perfusion pressure, sepsis, or nephrotoxins. Kidney failure increases the mortality rate for ARDS to more than 60%. Prophylaxis against gastrointestinal hemorrhage is recommended.

3. Negative Pressure Pulmonary Edema

Forceful inspiration against a closed glottis or an obstructed airway may lead to negative pressure pulmonary edema. In adults, this is often the consequence of laryngospasm during or after a general anesthetic, whereas in children, it is often a consequence of airway obstruction from infection (eg, epiglottitis) or tumor. Other potential causes include endotracheal tube obstruction or occlusion and virtually any other cause of airway obstruction. In adults, the incidence seems greater in healthier (American Society of Anesthesiologists class 1 or 2) than sicker patients and greater in males than females, which is probably a consequence of more forceful inspiratory efforts by healthy male patients. The onset is extremely rapid, and with appropriate treatment, the recovery may also be much more rapid than for other forms of pulmonary edema.

4. Neurogenic Pulmonary Edema

Head injury, intracranial bleeding, and abrupt reversal of opioid overdosage with naloxone can all precipitate pulmonary edema. Although the precise pathophysiology of this condition is not well understood, it has long been assumed that an abrupt, large increase in sympathetic tone is the precipitating event. Often, neurogenic pulmonary edema presents very rapidly after the inciting event and then dissipates over 24 h or so. In other cases, the presentation may be delayed by 12 to 18 h. Major neurological injuries may produce effects on the heart, so distinguishing between neurogenic and cardiogenic pulmonary edema is not always easy, and the two conditions may overlap.

DROWNING & NEAR-DROWNING

Drowning is asphyxia and death while submerged in water. Near-drowning is suffocation while submerged with (at least temporary) survival. Survival depends on the intensity and duration of the hypoxia and on the water temperature.

Pathophysiology

Both drowning and near-drowning can occur whether or not inhalation (aspiration) of water occurs. If water does not enter the airways, the patient primarily experiences asphyxia; however, if the patient inhales water, marked intrapulmonary shunting also takes place. Ninety percent of drowned patients aspirate fluid: fresh water, seawater, brackish water, or other fluids. Although the amount of liquid aspirated is generally small, marked ventilation/perfusion mismatching can result from fluids in the lung, reflex bronchospasm, and loss of pulmonary surfactant. Aspiration of gastric contents can also complicate drowning before or after loss of consciousness or during resuscitation.

The hypotonic water aspirated following freshwater drowning is rapidly absorbed by the pulmonary circulation; water cannot usually be recovered from the airways. If a significant amount is absorbed (>800 mL in a 70-kg adult), transient hemodilution, hyponatremia, and even hemolysis may occur. In contrast, aspiration of salt water (which is hypertonic) draws out water from the pulmonary circulation into the alveoli, flooding them and sometimes also causing hemoconcentration and hypernatremia. Hypermagnesemia and hypercalcemia have also been reported following near-drowning in salt water.

Patients who experience cold water near-drowning lose consciousness when core body temperature decreases below 32°C. Ventricular fibrillation occurs at about 28°C to 30°C, but relative to normothermic near-drowning, hypothermia has a protective effect on the brain and may improve outcomes provided that resuscitation is successful.

Clinical Manifestations

Nearly all patients with a true near-drowning episode will have hypoxemia and hypercarbia with metabolic and respiratory acidosis. Patients may also sustain other injuries, such as spine fractures following diving accidents. Brain damage is generally related to the duration of submersion and severity of asphyxia. Cerebral edema often complicates resuscitation after prolonged asphyxia. Acute lung injury and ARDS develop in many patients following successful resuscitation.

Treatment

Initial treatment of near-drowning is directed at restoring ventilation, perfusion, oxygenation, and acid–base balance as quickly as possible. Immediate measures include establishing a secure and unobstructed airway, administering oxygen, and initiating cardiopulmonary resuscitation. In-line stabilization of the cervical spine is necessary when intubating patients who experience near-drowning following a dive. Institution of cardiopulmonary resuscitation should not be delayed by attempts to drain salt water from the lungs. Resuscitation efforts should not be suspended for futility until the patient is rewarmed following cold water near-drowning. Complete recovery is possible in such instances, even after prolonged periods of asphyxia. After the initial resuscitation, further management will usually include positive-pressure ventilation and PEEP. Bronchospasm should be treated with bronchodilators, electrolyte abnormalities corrected, and acute lung injury and ARDS treated as previously discussed.

SMOKE INHALATION

Smoke inhalation is the leading cause of death from fires. Affected persons may or may not have sustained a burn. Burn victims who suffer from smoke inhalation have a mortality rate greater than other comparably burned patients without smoke inhalation. Any exposure to smoke in a fire requires a presumptive diagnosis of smoke inhalation until proved otherwise. A suggestive history might include loss of consciousness or disorientation in a patient exposed to a fire or with a burn acquired in a closed space.

Pathophysiology

The consequences of smoke inhalation are complex because they can involve three types of injuries: heat injury to the airways, exposure to toxic gases, and a chemical burn with deposition of carbonaceous particulates in the lower airways. The pulmonary response to smoke inhalation is equally complex and depends on the duration of the exposure, the composition of the material that burned, and the presence of any underlying lung disease. Combustion of synthetic materials may produce toxic gases such as carbon monoxide, hydrogen cyanide, hydrogen sulfide, hydrogen chloride, ammonia, chlorine, benzene, and aldehydes. When these gases react with water in the airways, they can produce hydrochloric, acetic, formic, and sulfuric acids. Carbon monoxide and cyanide poisoning are common.

After smoke inhalation, a direct mucosal injury may result in edema, inflammation, and sloughing. Loss of ciliary activity impairs the clearance of mucus and bacteria. Manifestations of acute lung injury and ARDS typically appear 2 to 3 days after the injury and seem related to the delayed development of SIRS rather than the acute smoke inhalation itself.

Clinical Manifestations

Patients may have minimal initial symptoms after smoke inhalation. Suggestive physical findings include facial or intraoral burns, singed nasal hairs, cough, carbonaceous sputum, and wheezing. The diagnosis is confirmed when bronchoscopy of the upper airway and the tracheobronchial tree reveals erythema, edema, mucosal ulcerations, and carbonaceous deposits. Arterial blood gases initially may be normal or reveal only mild hypoxemia and metabolic acidosis due to carbon monoxide. The chest radiograph is often normal on presentation.

Heat injury to the airways is usually confined to supraglottic structures unless there is prolonged exposure to steam. Progressive hoarseness and stridor suggest impending airway obstruction, which may develop over 12 to 18 h. Fluid resuscitation of burn injury will frequently exacerbate airway edema.

Carbon monoxide poisoning is usually defined as greater than 15% carboxyhemoglobin in the blood. The diagnosis is made by co-oximetry of arterial blood. Carbon monoxide has 210 times the affinity of oxygen for hemoglobin. When a CO molecule combines with hemoglobin to form carboxyhemoglobin, it decreases the affinity of the other binding sites for oxygen, shifting the hemoglobin dissociation curve to the right. The net result is a marked reduction in the oxygen-carrying capacity of blood. Carbon monoxide also has a 60-fold greater affinity than oxygen for myoglobin, which may lead to myocardial depression.

Carbon monoxide dissociates slowly from hemoglobin: The half-life of approximately 5 h when breathing room air decreases to 72 min when breathing 100% oxygen. Clinical manifestations result from tissue hypoxia from impaired oxygen delivery. Carboxyhemoglobin levels greater than 20% to 40% are associated with neurological impairment, nausea, fatigue, disorientation, and shock. Lower levels may also produce symptoms because carbon monoxide also binds cytochrome c and myoglobin. Compensatory mechanisms include increased cardiac output and peripheral vasodilation.

Cyanide toxicity may occur after fires that contain synthetic materials, particularly those containing polyurethane. After cyanide is inhaled or absorbed through mucosal surfaces and skin, it binds the cytochrome enzymes and inhibits cellular production of adenosine triphosphate (ATP). Patients present with neurological impairment and lactic acidosis, often accompanied by arrhythmias, increased cardiac output, and marked vasodilation.

A chemical burn of the respiratory mucosa follows the inhalation of large amounts of burned or burning debris, particularly when combined with toxic fumes. Inflammation of the airways results in bronchorrhea and wheezing. Bronchial edema and sloughing of the mucosa lead to obstruction of the lower airways and atelectasis. Progressive ventilation/perfusion mismatching can lead to marked hypoxemia over the course of 24 to 48 h, sometimes meeting the criteria for acute lung injury or ARDS.

Treatment

Bronchoscopy can diagnose an inhalation injury. In patients who are not intubated, we suggest performing it with a tracheal tube loaded over the bronchoscope so that intubation can quickly be performed if edema threatens the patency of the airway. Early 3 elective tracheal intubation is advisable when there are obvious signs of heat injury to the airway. Patients with hoarseness and stridor require immediate tracheal intubation or a surgical airway.

Carbon monoxide or cyanide poisoning accompanied by obtundation or coma also requires prompt tracheal intubation and ventilation with oxygen. The diagnosis of carbon monoxide poisoning requires co-oximetry: pulse oximeters cannot reliably differentiate between carboxyhemoglobin and oxyhemoglobin. The half-life of carboxyhemoglobin is markedly reduced with 100% oxygen, and hyperbaric oxygen therapy is useful when the patient does not respond to 100% oxygen. The diagnosis of cyanide poisoning is difficult because reliable measurements of cyanide are not readily available (normal levels are <0.1 mg/L). The enzyme rhodanese normally converts cyanide to thiocyanate, which is subsequently eliminated by the kidneys. Treatment for severe cyanide toxicity consists of administering sodium nitrite, 300 mg intravenously as a 3% solution over 3 to 5 min, followed by sodium thiosulfate, 12.5 g intravenously in the form of a 25% solution over 1 to 2 min. Sodium nitrite converts hemoglobin to methemoglobin, which has a higher affinity for cyanide than cytochrome oxidase; the cyanide, which is slowly released from cyanomethemoglobin, is converted by rhodanese to the less toxic thiocyanate.

Marked hypoxemia due to intrapulmonary shunting should be managed with tracheal intubation, oxygen therapy, bronchodilators, positive-pressure ventilation, and PEEP. Corticosteroids are ineffective and increase the rate of infections, so they should not be used.

Acute Myocardial Infarction

Acute myocardial infarction (AMI) is a dreaded complication of ischemic heart disease, with an overall mortality rate of 25%. More than one-half of these deaths occur shortly after onset, usually due to arrhythmias (ventricular fibrillation). With recent advances in interventional cardiology, the in-hospital mortality rate has been reduced to less than 10%.

Diagnosis of AMI can be made with combinations of increased troponin concentrations in blood, electrocardiogram findings, and clinical history. Perioperative diagnosis can be vexing and may depend primarily on troponin measurements. AMIs are divided into those associated with ST-segment elevation (STEMI) and those that are not associated with ST-segment elevation (NSTEMI). The latter are usually diagnosed by elevations of biomarkers, most commonly troponin. An increasingly popular classification scheme divides AMI into five types (type 1, from a spontaneous event such as plaque rupture; type 2, from increased demand or decreased oxygen supply; type 3, sudden cardiac death associated with symptoms or postmortem evidence of myocardial ischemia; type 4, AMI in association with percutaneous coronary interventions; type 5, AMI in association with coronary artery bypass surgery).

Pathophysiology

Most myocardial infarctions occur in patients with more than one severely narrowed (>75% narrowing of the cross-sectional area) coronary artery. STEMIs (most often type 1 AMIs) occur in an area distal to a complete occlusion. Patients who die within 24 h after AMI may have coronary atherosclerosis as the only cardiac abnormality identified upon necropsy. The occlusion is nearly always due to thrombosis at a stenotic atheromatous plaque. Coronary emboli or severe spasm is less commonly the cause. NSTEMIs (type 2 AMIs) more often occur in the setting of reduced myocardial perfusion due to hypotension or intimal hemorrhage, often in a situation of increased myocardial oxygen demand, and less commonly follow coronary plaque rupture and thrombosis. The size and location of the infarct depend on the distribution of the obstructed vessel and whether collateral vessels have formed. Anterior, apical, and septal infarcts of the left ventricle are usually due to thrombosis in the left anterior descending circulation; lateral and posterior left ventricular infarcts result from occlusions in the left circumflex system, whereas right ventricular and posterior–inferior left ventricular infarcts result from thrombosis in the right coronary artery.

Following brief episodes of severe ischemia, persisting myocardial dysfunction with only a slow and incomplete return of contractility can be observed. This phenomenon of "stunning" can contribute to ventricular dysfunction following AMI. Relief of the ischemia in these areas can restore contractile function, albeit not immediately. Stunning may be observed following aortic cross-clamping during cardiopulmonary bypass as a reduced cardiac output upon attempted separation from bypass (see Chapter 22). When severe hypokinesis or akinesis is observed in the setting of severe chronic ischemia, the myocardium in these noninfarcted but poorly contractile areas may be said to be "hibernating." This diagnosis can be confirmed by observing viable tissue with positron emission tomography or by showing that the hypocontractile myocardium responds to dobutamine.

Treatment

In the absence of contraindications (eg, a contradictory advanced directive) the immediate treatment of STEMI is thrombolysis and percutaneous coronary intervention in the cardiac catheterization laboratory. Oxygen was formerly routinely administered to all patients with AMI but now is reserved for those with reduced arterial saturation. Because the prognosis following AMI is generally inversely proportionate to the extent of necrosis, the focus in the management of an evolving STEMI remains on prompt reperfusion. Based on local resources, timing, and anatomic findings during angiography, stenting or coronary artery bypass surgery may be indicated. NSTEMI treatment varies, depending on the time of diagnosis and the perceived risk of progression. Guidelines for treatment of AMI change frequently and are regularly published by the American College of Cardiology/American Heart Association and by the European Society of Cardiology. We strongly recommend that current guidelines be consulted.

Current guidelines specify that following AMI all patients without contraindications should receive aspirin and β-blockers. Other medications and treatments such as angiotensin-converting enzyme (ACE) inhibitors, statins, and cessation of smoking are key to secondary prevention. Patients who have recurrent angina should be given nitrates. If angina persists or if there is a contraindication to β-blockers, calcium channel blockers should be administered. Persistent or recurrent angina signals the need for angiography.

Intraaortic balloon counterpulsation was in the past commonly used for hemodynamically compromised patients with refractory ischemia; however, there is limited evidence for improved outcomes with this therapy. Temporary pacing following AMI is indicated for Mobitz type II and complete heart block, a new bifascicular block, and bradycardia with hypotension. Emergency treatment of arrhythmias constantly evolves, and we recommend that the guidelines for Advanced Cardiac Life Support be followed. In general, ventricular tachycardia, if treated medically, is best managed with amiodarone (150 mg intravenous bolus over 10 min). Synchronized cardioversion may be used in patients with ventricular tachycardia and a pulse. Patients with stable narrow-complex supraventricular tachycardia should be treated with amiodarone. Patients with paroxysmal supraventricular tachycardia whose ejection fraction is preserved should be treated with a calcium channel blocker, a β-blocker, or direct current (DC) cardioversion. Unstable hypotensive patients should be cardioverted. Patients with ectopic or multifocal atrial tachycardia should not receive DC cardioversion; rather, they should be treated with calcium channel blockers, a β-blocker, or amiodarone.

Acute Kidney Injury & Failure

Acute kidney injury (AKI) is a rapid deterioration in kidney function that is not immediately reversible by normalizing blood pressure, intravascular volume, or cardiac output or by relieving urinary obstruction. The hallmark of AKI is azotemia, frequently accompanied by oliguria. Azotemia may be classified as prerenal, renal, or postrenal. The diagnosis of renal azotemia is one of exclusion: Prerenal and postrenal causes must always be excluded. However, not all patients with acute azotemia have kidney failure. Likewise, urine output of more than 500 mL/d does not imply that kidney function is normal. Basing the diagnosis of AKI on creatinine levels or an increase in blood urea nitrogen (BUN) is also problematic because creatinine clearance is not always a good measure of glomerular filtration rate. The criteria developed by the Acute Kidney Injury Network are now most often used to stage AKI (see Chapter 30). AKI is diagnosed by documenting an increase in serum creatinine of more than 50%, or an absolute increase of 0.3 mg/dL, and a reduction in urine output to less than 0.5 mL/kg/h for 6 h or longer, with all findings developing over 48 h or less.

4

TABLE 57–1 Potentially reversible causes of azotemia.

Prerenal
- Decreased renal perfusion
  - Hypovolemia
  - Reduced cardiac output
  - Hypotension
  - Abdominal compartment syndrome
- Increased renal vascular resistance
  - Neural
  - Humoral/pharmacological
  - Thromboembolic

Postrenal
- Urethral obstruction
- Bladder outlet obstruction
  - Neurogenic bladder
- Bilateral ureteral obstruction
  - Intrinsic
    - Calculi
    - Tumor
    - Blood clots
    - Papillary necrosis
  - Extrinsic
    - Abdominal or pelvic tumor
    - Retroperitoneal fibrosis
    - Postsurgical (ligation)

PRERENAL AZOTEMIA

Prerenal azotemia results from hypoperfusion of the kidneys; if untreated, it progresses to AKI. Renal hypoperfusion is typically the result of decreased arterial perfusion pressure, markedly increased venous pressure, or renal vasoconstriction (Table 57–1). Decreased perfusion pressure is usually associated with the release of norepinephrine, angiotensin II, and vasopressin. These hormones constrict cutaneous muscle and splanchnic vasculature and promote salt and water retention. The synthesis of vasodilating prostaglandins (prostacyclin and prostaglandin E_2 [PGE_2]) and nitric oxide in the kidneys and the intrarenal action of angiotensin II help maintain glomerular filtration. In the setting of marked prerenal azotemia, the use of cyclooxygenase inhibitors (eg, ketorolac for postoperative pain control) or ACE inhibitors can precipitate AKI. The diagnosis of prerenal azotemia is usually suspected from the clinical setting and confirmed by urinary laboratory indices (Table 57–2). Treatment of prerenal azotemia includes correcting intravascular volume deficits, improving cardiac function, restoring normal blood pressure, and reversing

TABLE 57–2 Urinary indices in azotemia.

Index	Prerenal	Renal	Postrenal
Specific gravity	>1.018	<0.012	Variable
Osmolality (mmol/kg)	>500	<350	Variable
Urine/plasma urea nitrogen ratio	>8	<3	Variable
Urine/plasma creatinine ratio	>40	<20	Variable
Urine/sodium (mEq/L)	<10	>40	Variable
Fractional excretion of sodium (%)	<1	>3	Variable
Renal failure index	<1	>1	Variable

increases in renal vascular resistance. *Hepatorenal syndrome* is discussed in Chapter 33.

POSTRENAL AZOTEMIA

Azotemia due to urinary tract obstruction is termed *postrenal azotemia*. Obstruction of urinary flow from both kidneys is usually necessary for azotemia and oliguria/anuria in these conditions. Complete obstruction eventually develops into AKI and kidney failure, whereas prolonged partial obstruction leads to chronic renal impairment. Rapid diagnosis and relief of acute obstruction usually restore normal renal function, often accompanied by a postobstructive diuresis. Obstruction may be diagnosed by a physical examination (the upper margin of the bladder can be percussed) or point-of-care ultrasound showing a distended bladder, or suggested by a radiograph of the abdomen (revealing bilateral renal calculi), but is definitively diagnosed by demonstrating dilation of the urinary tract proximal to the site of obstruction on imaging studies. Treatment depends on the site of obstruction. Obstruction at the bladder outlet can be relieved with catheterization of the bladder or suprapubic cystostomy, whereas ureteral obstruction requires nephrostomy or ureteral stents.

REVERSIBLE AZOTEMIA VERSUS AKI

In addition to physical diagnosis and imaging, diagnosis and treatment may be facilitated by analysis of urine (see **Table 57–2**); urinary composition in postrenal azotemia is variable and depends on the duration and severity of obstruction. In prerenal azotemia, tubular concentrating ability is preserved and reflected by a low urinary sodium concentration and high urine/serum creatinine ratio. Calculation of the *fractional excretion of filtered sodium* (FENa^+) may also be extremely useful in the setting of oliguria:

$$\mathrm{FENa}^+ = \frac{\text{Urine sodium/serum sodium}}{\text{Urine creatinine/serum creatinine}} \times 100\%$$

FENa^+ is less than 1% in oliguric patients with prerenal azotemia but typically exceeds 3% in patients with oliguric AKI. Values of 1% to 3% may be present in patients with nonoliguric AKI. The *renal failure index*, which is the urinary sodium concentration divided by the urine/plasma creatinine ratio, is a sensitive index for diagnosing kidney failure. The use of diuretics increases urinary sodium excretion and invalidates indices that rely on urinary sodium concentration as a measure of tubular function. Moreover, intrinsic kidney diseases that primarily affect renal vasculature or glomeruli may not affect tubular function and therefore are associated with indices that are similar to prerenal azotemia. Measurement of creatinine clearance can estimate the residual glomerular filtration rate but may underestimate the degree of renal impairment when the serum creatinine concentration is still rising.

Etiology of AKI

Causes of AKI are listed in Table 57–3. Up to 50% of cases follow major trauma or surgery; in most instances, ischemia and nephrotoxins are responsible.

TABLE 57–3 Causes of acute kidney injury.

Renal ischemia
Hypotension
Hypovolemia
Impaired cardiac output
Abdominal compartment syndrome
Nephrotoxins
Endogenous pigments
Hemoglobulin (hemolysis)
Myoglobin (rhabdomyolysis from crush injury and burns)
Radiographic contrast agents
Drugs
Antibiotics (aminoglycosides, amphotericin)
Nonsteroidal anti-inflammatory drugs
Chemotherapeutic agents (cisplatin, methotrexate)
Tubular crystals
Uric acid
Oxalate
Sulfonamides
Heavy metal poisoning
Organic solvents
Myeloma protein
Intrinsic kidney disease
Glomerular disease
Interstitial nephritis

AKI associated with ischemia has been termed *acute tubular necrosis*. Postischemic AKI follows certain surgical procedures more frequently than others: open abdominal aortic aneurysm resection, cardiac surgery with cardiopulmonary bypass, and operations to relieve obstructive jaundice. Aminoglycosides, amphotericin B, radiographic contrast dyes, cyclosporine, and cisplatin are the most commonly implicated exogenous nephrotoxins. Amphotericin B, contrast dyes, and cyclosporine also appear to produce direct intrarenal vasoconstriction. Hemoglobin and myoglobin are potent nephrotoxins when they are released during intravascular hemolysis and rhabdomyolysis, respectively. Nonsteroidal anti-inflammatory drugs may play an important role in some patients. Inhibition of prostaglandin synthesis by the latter group of agents decreases prostaglandin-mediated renal vasodilation, allowing unopposed renal vasoconstriction. Other factors predisposing to AKI include preexisting renal impairment, advanced age, atherosclerotic vascular disease, diabetes, and dehydration.

Pathogenesis of AKI

The sensitivity of the kidneys to injury may be explained by their very high metabolic rate and ability to concentrate potentially toxic substances. The pathogenesis of AKI is complex and probably has both a vascular endothelial and a renal epithelial (tubular) basis. Inadequate oxygen delivery to the kidney is the likely triggering event, leading to afferent arteriolar constriction, decreased glomerular permeability, increased vascular permeability, altered coagulation, inflammation, leukocyte activation, direct epithelial cell injury, and tubular obstruction. All can decrease glomerular filtration. A leak of filtered solutes through damaged portions of renal tubules may allow reabsorption of creatinine, urea, and other nitrogenous wastes.

Oliguric versus Nonoliguric AKI

AKI is often classified as nonoliguric (urinary volume >400 mL/d), oliguric (urinary volume <400 mL/d), or anuric (urinary volume <100 mL/d). Nonoliguric AKI accounts for up to 50% of cases. Urinary sodium concentrations in patients with nonoliguric AKI are typically lower than those in oliguric patients. For years it was speculated that one could convert oliguric AKI into nonoliguric AKI by administering mannitol, furosemide, "renal" doses of dopamine (1–2 mcg/kg/min), or fenoldopam. Theoretically, the resulting increase in urinary output might be therapeutic by preventing tubular obstruction. However, recent studies have found increased mortality in patients with AKI who received diuretics, and a meta-analysis showed no improvement in mortality or decrease in need for dialysis; therefore, diuretics should not be routinely administered to patients with AKI.

Treatment of AKI

AKI accounts for approximately 15% of ICU admissions. The mortality rate and cost of care for AKI remain high, and management is primarily supportive. Diuretics continue to be useful for conventional medical indications (eg, volume overload or rhabdomyolysis). AKI due to glomerulonephritis or vasculitis may respond to glucocorticoids. Standard treatment for oliguric and anuric patients includes restriction of fluid, sodium, potassium, and phosphorus. Daily weight measurements help guide fluid therapy. Hyponatremia can be treated with water restriction. Hyperkalemia may require the administration of an ion-exchange resin (sodium polystyrene), glucose and insulin, calcium gluconate, or sodium bicarbonate. Sodium bicarbonate therapy may also be necessary for metabolic acidosis when the serum bicarbonate level decreases to less than 15 mEq/L. Hyperphosphatemia requires dietary phosphate restriction and phosphate binders such as aluminum hydroxide, calcium carbonate, or calcium acetate. The dosages of drugs subject to renal excretion should be adjusted to the estimated glomerular filtration rate or measured creatinine clearance.

Renal replacement therapy may be employed to treat or prevent uremic complications (see Table 31–7). A double-lumen catheter placed in the internal jugular, subclavian, or femoral vein is usually used. The high morbidity and mortality rates associated with AKI would seem to argue for early dialysis, but dialysis does not appear to hasten recovery and may aggravate kidney injury if hypotension occurs or too much fluid is removed.

Because of concern that intermittent hemodialysis associated with hypotension may perpetuate kidney injury, continuous renal replacement therapy (CRRT; continuous venovenous hemofiltration or continuous venovenous hemodialysis, which removes fluid and solutes at a slow, controlled rate) has been used in critically ill patients with uremic AKI who do not tolerate the hemodynamic effects of intermittent "standard" hemodialysis. The main problem associated with CRRT is the expense, as the membrane is prone to clot formation and therefore must be periodically replaced. Despite this limitation, many experts believe CRRT is the best way to manage uremic ICU patients with AKI. The indications for CRRT are being expanded from oliguria and uremia to metabolic acidosis, fluid overload, and hyperkalemia. Nevertheless, we note that clinical trials have failed to show benefit of continuous technique over intermittent hemodialysis in these critically ill patients.

The nutritional management of AKI with uremia continues to evolve. There is now consensus among nephrologists, intensivists, and nutritionists that nutrition should be provided, and 1 to 1.5 g/kg/d of protein can be given, particularly for patients on CRRT.

Infections & Sepsis

The systemic inflammatory response to infection, termed *sepsis syndrome* (Figure 57–2), does not necessarily indicate the presence of bacteremia. Moreover, the inflammatory response is not unique to severe infections: Similar manifestations may be encountered with noninfectious illnesses. While the use of the term *systemic inflammatory response syndrome* (SIRS) was suggested by the Society of Critical Care Medicine (SCCM), European Society of Intensive Care Medicine (ESICM), American College of Chest Physicians (ACCP), American Thoracic Society (ATS), and Surgical Infection Society (SIS), these and other groups are now moving away from an emphasis on SIRS in the identification and treatment of patients with sepsis (see the ESICM's and SCCM's Third International Consensus Definitions for Sepsis and Septic Shock [Sepsis-3]) (Table 57–4).

Sepsis may be classified based on predisposition, insult, infection, response, and organ dysfunction.

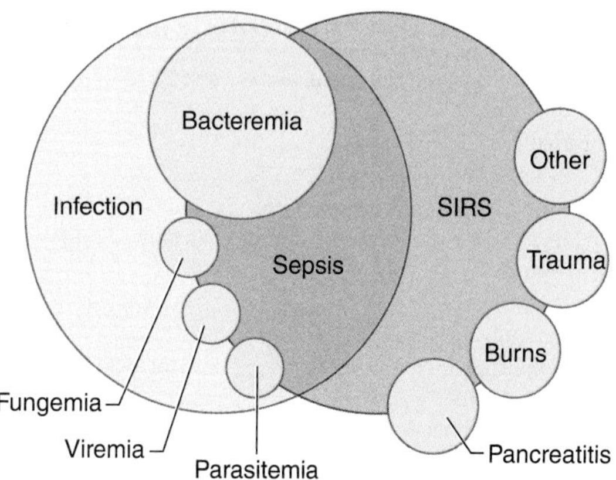

FIGURE 57–2 The relationship between infection, sepsis, and systemic inflammatory response syndrome (SIRS). (Modified with permission from American College of Chest Physicians/Society of Critical Care Medicine Consensus Conference: Definitions for sepsis and organ failure and guidelines for the use of innovative therapies in sepsis. *Crit Care Med.* 1992 Jun;20(6):864-874.)

Severe sepsis includes organ dysfunction. The term *multiple organ dysfunction syndrome* (MODS) has been suggested to describe the dysfunction of two or more
5 organs associated with sepsis. *Septic shock* is defined as acute circulatory failure in a patient with sepsis or, more specifically, systolic blood pressure less than 90 mm Hg that is not responsive to volume resuscitation and requiring vasopressors for life support.

Pathophysiology of SIRS

A mild systemic inflammatory response to an injury, infection, or another bodily insult may normally have salutatory effects. However, a marked or prolonged response, such as that associated with severe infections, can result in widespread organ dysfunction. Although gram-negative organisms account for most cases of infection-related SIRS, many other infectious agents are capable of inducing the same syndrome. These organisms either elaborate toxins or stimulate the release of substances that trigger this response. The most commonly recognized initiators are lipopolysaccharides released by gram-negative bacteria. Lipopolysaccharides are composed of an O polysaccharide, a core, and lipid A. Lipid A, an endotoxin, is responsible for the compounds' toxicity, which can affect nearly every organ.

TABLE 57–4 Diagnostic criteria for sepsis.[1,2]

Infection,[3] documented or suspected, and some of the following:
General variables
Fever (core temperature >38.3°C)
Hypothermia (core temperature <36°C)
Heart rate >90/min or >2 SD above the normal value for age
Tachypnea
Altered mental status
Significant edema or positive fluid balance (>20 mL/kg over 24 h)
Hyperglycemia (plasma glucose >120 mg/dL or 7.7 mmol/L) in the absence of diabetes
Inflammatory variables
Leukocytosis (WBC count >12,000/μL)
Leukopenia (WBC count <4000/μL)
Normal WBC count with >10% immature forms
Plasma C-reactive protein >2 SD above the normal value
Plasma procalcitonin >2 SD above the normal value
Hemodynamic variables
Arterial hypotension[4] (SBP <90 mm Hg, MAP <70, or an SBP decrease >40 mm Hg in adults or <2 SD below normal value for age)
$S\bar{v}o_2$ >70%[4]
Cardiac index[4] >3.5 L/min per m^2
Organ dysfunction variables
Arterial hypoxemia (PaO_2/FiO_2 < 300)
Acute oliguria (urine output <0.5 mL/kg/h or 45 mmol/L for at least 2 h)
Creatinine increase >0.5 mg/dL
Coagulation abnormalities (INR >1.5 or aPTT >60 s)
Ileus (absent bowel sounds)
Thrombocytopenia (platelet count <100,000/μL)
Hyperbilirubinemia (plasma total bilirubin >4 mg/dL or 70 mmol/L)
Tissue perfusion variables
Hyperlactatemia (>1 mmol/L)
Decreased capillary refill or mottling

[1]aPTT, activated partial thromboplastin time; INR, international normalized ratio; MAP, mean arterial blood pressure; SBP, systolic blood pressure; SD, standard deviation; $S\bar{v}o_2$, mixed venous oxygen saturation; WBC, white blood cell.

[2]Diagnostic criteria for sepsis in the pediatric population are signs and symptoms of inflammation plus infection with hyper- or hypothermia (rectal temperature >38.4°C or <35°C), tachycardia (may be absent in hypothermia patients), and at least one of the following indications of altered organ function: altered mental status, hypoxemia, increased serum lactate level, or bounding pulses.

[3]Infection defined as a pathological process induced by a microorganism.

[4]$S\bar{v}o_2$>70% (normally, 75–80%) and cardiac index 3.5–5.5 are normal in children; therefore, neither should be used as a sign of sepsis in newborns or children.

Reproduced with permission from Levy MM, Fink MP, Marshall JC, et al. 2001 SCCM/ESICM/ACCP/ATS/SIS International Sepsis Definitions Conference. *Crit Care Med.* 2003 Apr;31(4):1250-1256.

The central mechanism in initiating SIRS appears to be the abnormal secretion of cytokines. These low-molecular-weight peptides and glycoproteins function as intercellular mediators regulating such biological processes as local and systemic immune responses, inflammation, wound healing, and hematopoiesis. The resulting inflammatory response includes the release of potentially harmful phospholipids, the attraction of neutrophils, and activation of the complement, kinin, and coagulation cascades.

INFECTIONS IN THE ICU

Infections are a leading cause of death in patients with critical illness. Serious infections may be "community acquired" or subsequent to hospital admission for an unrelated illness. The term *nosocomial infection* describes hospital-acquired infections that develop at least 48 h following admission. Most nosocomial infections arise from the patient's endogenous bacterial flora. Furthermore, many critically ill patients may become colonized by resistant bacterial strains. Urinary infections, usually due to gram-negative organisms and typically associated with indwelling catheters or urinary obstruction, account for many nosocomial infections. The incidence of bloodstream and catheter-associated urinary tract infections has declined markedly with scrupulous attention to handwashing, aseptic placement of central venous catheters, and earlier removal of bladder catheters. Routine elevation of the head of the bed has led to a marked reduction in ventilator-associated pneumonia. Surgical site and other wound infections and community-acquired pneumonia continue to be vexing. Enteral nutrition reduces bacterial translocation across the gut and reduces the likelihood of sepsis (see Chapter 53) relative to either starvation or parenteral nutrition.

Strains of bacteria resistant to commonly used antibiotics are often responsible for infections in patients with critical illness. Host immunity plays an important role in determining not only the course of an infection but also the types of organisms that can cause infection. Thus, organisms that normally do not cause serious infections in immunocompetent patients can produce life-threatening infections in those who are immunocompromised (Table 57–5).

TABLE 57–5 Pathogens commonly associated with serious infections in patients in the intensive care unit.

Infection or Site	Pathogens
Pneumonia	
Community-acquired (nonimmunocompromised host)	*Streptococcus pneumoniae* *Haemophilus influenzae* *Moraxella catarrhalis* *Mycoplasma pneumoniae* *Legionella pneumophila* *Chlamydia pneumoniae* Methicillin-resistant *Staphylococcus aureus* (MRSA) Influenza virus
Health care–associated	MRSA *Pseudomonas aeruginosa* *Klebsiella pneumoniae* *Acinetobacter* species *Stenotrophomonas* species *L. pneumophila*
Immunocompromised host	
Neutropenia	Any pathogen listed above *Aspergillus* species *Candida* species
Human immunodeficiency virus	Any pathogen listed above *Pneumocystis jirovecii* (formerly *P. carinii*) *Mycobacterium tuberculosis* *Histoplasma capsulatum* Other fungi Cytomegalovirus
Solid organ transplant or bone marrow transplant	Any pathogen listed above (Can vary depending on timing of infection to transplant)
Cystic fibrosis	*H. influenzae (early)* *S. aureus* *P. aeruginosa* *Burkholderia cepacia*
Lung abscess	*Bacteroides* species *Peptostreptococcus* species *Fusobacterium* species *Nocardia* (immunocompromised patients) Amebic (when suggestive by exposure)
Empyema	
Usually acute	*S. aureus* *S. pneumoniae* Group A streptococci *H. influenzae*
Usually subacute or chronic	Anaerobic bacteria *Enterobacteriaceae* *M. tuberculosis*

(*continued*)

TABLE 57–5 Pathogens commonly associated with serious infections in patients in the intensive care unit. (Continued)

Infection or Site	Pathogens
Meningitis	
	S. pneumoniae *Neisseria meningitidis* *Listeria monocytogenes* *H. influenzae*
Neonates	*Escherichia coli* Group B streptococci
Postsurgical or post-trauma	*S. aureus* *Enterobacteriaceae* *P. aeruginosa*
Brain abscess	
	Streptococci *Bacteroides* species
Postsurgical or post-trauma	*Enterobacteriaceae* *S. aureus*
Immunocompromised or human immunodeficiency virus (HIV) infected	*Nocardia* *Toxoplasma gondii*
Encephalitis	
	West Nile virus Herpes simplex virus Arbovirus Rabies virus *Bartonella henselae*
Endocarditis	
	Streptococcus viridans *Enterococcus* species *S. aureus* *Streptococcus bovis*
Intravenous drug user, prosthetic valves	MRSA
Prosthetic valve	*Candida* species
Catheter-associated bacteremia	
	Candida species *S. aureus* *Enterococcus* species *Enterobacteriaceae* *P. aeruginosa*
Pyelonephritis	
	Enterobacteriaceae *E. coli* *Enterococcus* species
(This group catheter-associated, postsurgical)	*P. aeruginosa* *Acinetobacter* species

(*continued*)

TABLE 57–5 Pathogens commonly associated with serious infections in patients in the intensive care unit. (Continued)

Infection or Site	Pathogens
Peritonitis	
Primary or spontaneous	*Enterobacteriaceae* *S. pneumoniae* *Enterococcus* species Anaerobic bacteria (rare)
Secondary (bowel perforation)	*Enterobacteriaceae* *Bacteroides* species *Enterococcus* species *P. aeruginosa* (uncommon)
Tertiary (bowel surgery, hospitalized on antibiotics)	*P. aeruginosa* MRSA *Acinetobacter* species *Candida* species
Skin structure infections	
Cellulitis	Group A streptococci *S. aureus* *Enterobacteriaceae* (diabetic patients)
Decubitus ulcer	Polymicrobial *Streptococcus pyogenes* *Enterococcus* species *Enterobacteriaceae* Anaerobic streptococci *P. aeruginosa* *S. aureus* *Bacteroides* species
Necrotizing fasciitis	*Streptococcus* species *Clostridia* species Mixed aerobic/anaerobic bacteria
Muscle infection	
Myonecrosis (gas gangrene)	*Clostridium perfringens* Other *Clostridia* species
Pyomyositis	*S. aureus* Group A streptococci Anaerobic bacteria Gram-negative bacteria (rare)
Septic shock	
Community-acquired	*S. pneumoniae* *N. meningitidis* *H. influenzae* *E. coli* *Capnocytophaga* (with splenectomy)

(*continued*)

TABLE 57–5 Pathogens commonly associated with serious infections in patients in the intensive care unit. (Continued)

Infection or Site	Pathogens
Health care–associated	MRSA *P. aeruginosa* *Acinetobacter* species *Candida* species
Toxic shock syndrome	*S. aureus* *Streptococcus* species
Regional illness or special circumstances	Rickettsial species *Ehrlichia* species *Babesia* species *B. henselae* (immunocompromised hosts) *Yersinia pestis* *Francisella tularensis* *Leptospira* *Salmonella enteritidis* *Salmonella typhi*

Reproduced with permission from Gabrielli A, Layon AJ, Yu M. *Civetta, Taylor & Kirby's Critical Care.* 4th ed. Philadelphia, PA: Lippincott Williams & Wilkins; 2009.

6 Critically ill patients frequently have abnormal host defenses from advanced age, malnutrition, drug therapy, loss of integrity of mucosal and skin barriers, and underlying diseases. Thus, age greater than 70 years, corticosteroid therapy, cancer chemotherapy, prolonged use of invasive devices, respiratory failure, kidney failure, head trauma, and burns are established risk factors for nosocomial infections. Patients with burns involving more than 40% of body surface area have a significantly increased risk of mortality from infections. After burn injury, early removal of the necrotic eschar followed by skin grafting and wound closure appears to reverse immunological defects and reduce infection risk.

Nosocomial cases of pneumonia are usually caused by gram-negative organisms. Preservation of gastric acidity inhibits the overgrowth of gram-negative organisms in the stomach and their subsequent migration into the oropharynx. Tracheal intubation does not provide complete protection because patients may still aspirate gastric fluid despite a properly functioning endotracheal tube cuff. Nebulizers and humidifiers can also be sources of infection. Selective decontamination of the gut with nonabsorbable antibiotics may reduce the incidence of infection but does not change the outcome. As noted earlier, elevating the head of the bed 30° or more will reduce the likelihood of ventilator-associated pneumonia by reducing gastroesophageal reflux.

Wounds are common sources of sepsis in postoperative and trauma patients; restricting antibiotic prophylaxis to the immediate perioperative time appears to decrease the incidence of postoperative infections. Intraabdominal infections due to perforated ulcer, diverticulitis, appendicitis, and acalculous cholecystitis can develop in critically ill patients whether or not they are recovering from a surgical procedure. Intravascular catheter-related infections are most commonly caused by *Staphylococcus epidermidis, Staphylococcus aureus,* streptococci, *Candida* species, and gram-negative rods. Bacterial sinusitis may be an unrecognized source of sepsis in patients ventilated through nasotracheal tubes. The widespread administration of antibiotics has led to the development of microorganisms that are resistant to most standard antimicrobials. Organisms that were formerly rare such as *Clostridium difficile* ("c. diff.")

and multidrug-resistant organisms are now vexing problems for those who care for sick patients in tertiary hospitals.

SEPTIC SHOCK

The SCCM/ESICM/ACCP/ATS/SIS Consensus Conference defined *septic shock* as sepsis associated with hypotension (systolic blood pressure <90 mm Hg, mean arterial pressure <60 mm Hg, or systemic blood pressure <40 mm Hg from baseline) despite adequate fluid resuscitation.

Septic shock is usually characterized by inadequate tissue perfusion and widespread cellular dysfunction. In contrast to other forms of shock (hypovolemic, cardiogenic, neurogenic, or anaphylactic), cellular dysfunction in septic shock is not necessarily related to hypoperfusion. Instead, metabolic blocks at the cellular and microcirculation levels may contribute to impaired cellular oxidation. A different definition, chosen by the Third International Consensus Definitions for Sepsis and Septic Shock in 2016, deemphasized the role of systemic inflammation in making the diagnosis of sepsis while emphasizing the role of organ dysfunction, per se. At the present time, it is unclear who will win the debate regarding SIRS! Meanwhile, the qSOFA (quick Sepsis-related Organ Failure Assessment) score using only altered mental status (a Glasgow Coma Scale score of <15), tachypnea (respiratory rate of ≥20/min), and hypotension (systolic blood pressure of ≤100 mm Hg) for a maximum score of 3 and a minimum score of 0 is increasingly used to identify those patients with suspected infection who are at greater risk for a poor outcome.

Pathophysiology

An infectious process that induces severe or protracted systemic inflammation can result in septic shock. In hospitalized patients, septic shock most commonly follows gram-negative infections in either the genitourinary tract or the lungs. In up to 50% of cases of severe sepsis, no organisms can be cultured from blood. Hypotension is due to a decreased circulating intravascular volume resulting from a diffuse capillary leak. Patients may also have sepsis-induced myocardial depression. Activation of platelets and coagulation can lead to fibrin-platelet aggregates, further compromising tissue blood flow. Hypoxemia from ARDS accentuates tissue hypoxia. The release of vasoactive substances and the formation of microthrombi in the pulmonary circulation increase pulmonary vascular resistance.

Hemodynamic Subsets

The circulation in patients with septic shock is often described as either hyperdynamic or hypodynamic. In reality, both represent the same process, but their expression depends on preexisting cardiac function, intravascular volume, and the patient's response. 7 Systemic pooling of blood and transudation of fluid into tissues result in relative hypovolemia in patients with sepsis. Hyperdynamic septic shock is characterized by normal or elevated cardiac output and profoundly reduced systemic vascular resistance. Decreased myocardial contractility is often demonstrable by echocardiography, even in patients with markedly increased cardiac output. Mixed venous oxygen saturation is characteristically increased in the absence of hypoxemia and likely reflects the increased cardiac output and the cellular metabolic defect in oxygen utilization. Patients with septic shock usually require vasopressor support to maintain a mean arterial pressure of 65 mm Hg or greater despite adequate circulating blood volume, and they have serum lactate levels greater than 2 mmol/L.

It used to be accepted wisdom that decreased cardiac output with low or normal systemic vascular resistance was usually seen later in the course of shock. This view is false. It is more likely to be seen in severely hypovolemic patients and in those with underlying cardiac disease. Myocardial depression is prominent. Mixed venous oxygen saturation is reduced in these patients. Pulmonary hypertension is often prominent and may contribute to right ventricular dysfunction.

Clinical Manifestations

Clinical manifestations of septic shock appear to be primarily related to host response rather than the infective agent. Septic shock classically presents following an abrupt onset of chills, fever, nausea (and often vomiting), with decreased mental status, tachypnea, hypotension, and tachycardia. The patient may appear flushed and feel warm (hyperdynamic) or pale with cool and often cyanotic extremities (hypodynamic). In old, debilitated patients and in infants, the diagnosis often is less obvious, and hypothermia may be seen.

Leukocytosis with a leftward shift to premature cell forms is typical, but leukopenia, an ominous sign, can be seen with overwhelming sepsis. Progressive metabolic (usually lactic) acidosis may be partially compensated by a concomitant respiratory alkalosis. Elevated lactate levels reflect both increased production resulting from poor tissue perfusion and decreased uptake by the liver and kidneys. Hypoxemia may herald the onset of ARDS. Hypovolemia and hypotension may lead to oliguria that will often progress to AKI. Elevations in serum aminotransferases and bilirubin are due to hepatic dysfunction. Insulin resistance is uniformly present and produces hyperglycemia. Thrombocytopenia is common and is often an early sign of sepsis. Laboratory evidence of disseminated intravascular coagulation (DIC) is often present but is rarely associated with bleeding. Stress ulceration of gastric mucosa is common. Respiratory and kidney failure are the leading causes of death in septic patients.

Neutropenic patients (absolute neutrophil count 500/μL) may develop skin lesions that can ulcerate and become gangrenous (ecthyma gangrenosum). These lesions are commonly associated with *Pseudomonas* septicemia but can be caused by other organisms. Perirectal abscesses can develop very quickly in neutropenic patients with few external signs; conscious patients may report only perirectal pain.

Treatment

Septic shock is a medical emergency that requires immediate intervention. Treatment is threefold: (1) control and eradication of the infection by appropriate and timely intravenous antibiotics, drainage of abscesses, debridement of necrotic tissues, and removal of infected foreign bodies; (2) maintenance of adequate perfusion with intravenous fluids and inotropic and vasopressor agents; and (3) supportive treatment of complications such as ARDS, kidney failure, gastrointestinal bleeding, and DIC.

Antibiotic treatment usually is initiated before pathogens are identified but only after adequate cultures are obtained (commonly, blood, urine, wounds, and sputum). Pending the results of cultures and tests of antibiotic sensitivity, combination therapy with two or more antibiotics is generally indicated. The choice depends on which organisms are seen with the greatest frequency in one's medical center. Additional diagnostic studies may be indicated (eg, thoracentesis, paracentesis, lumbar puncture, or imaging), depending on the history and physical examination.

Empiric antibiotic therapy in immunocompromised patients should be based on pathogens that are generally associated with the immune defect (see **Table 57–5**). Vancomycin is added if an intravascular catheter-related infection is suspected. Clindamycin or metronidazole may be given to neutropenic patients if a rectal abscess is suspected. Many clinicians initiate therapy for a presumed fungal infection when an immunocompromised patient continues to experience fever despite antibiotic therapy. Granulocyte colony-stimulating factor or granulocyte–macrophage colony-stimulating factor may be used to shorten the period of neutropenia; granulocyte transfusion may occasionally be used in refractory gram-negative bacteremia. Diffuse interstitial infiltrates on a chest radiograph may suggest unusual bacterial, parasitic, or viral pathogens; many clinicians initiate empiric therapy with trimethoprim-sulfamethoxazole and erythromycin in such instances. Nodular infiltrates on a radiograph suggest fungal pneumonia and may warrant antifungal therapy. Antiviral therapy should be considered in septic patients who are more than 1 month post–bone marrow or solid organ transplantation. Consultation with an infectious disease specialist will be helpful.

In general, therapy should follow the most recent guidelines. The presence of inadequate perfusion is determined by measurement of blood lactate. Goal-directed fluid therapy was also recommended by many groups in the past, but multiple randomized clinical trials have failed to show benefit in septic shock. Now, most authors recommend a more restricted approach to fluid resuscitation and invasive monitoring. Packed red blood cell transfusions are given to keep hemoglobin levels at least 8 g/dL, especially when cardiac output and central venous oxygen saturation are below targets. Marked "third-spacing" has long been regarded as characteristic of septic shock, but currently there is debate regarding the actual existence of the third space and regarding whether administration of large volumes of intravenous fluid is cause or treatment. Colloid solutions more rapidly restore intravascular volume compared with crystalloid solutions but otherwise offer no proven additional benefit. **Vasopressor therapy is generally initiated if hypotension (mean arterial pressure <65 mm Hg) or elevated blood lactate levels persist following administration of intravenous fluids.** Norepinephrine is preferred; positive inotropic drugs (eg, epinephrine) are indicated when norepinephrine "fails" despite adequate volume resuscitation. Blood glucose should be controlled with a target value of less than 180 mg/dL. In patients with hypotension that is refractory to norepinephrine plus epinephrine, vasopressin may be administered to improve blood pressure. Severe acidosis may decrease the efficacy of inotropes and should therefore be corrected (pH >7.20) with bicarbonate or THAM infusion in patients with refractory hypotension. "Renal" doses of dopamine or fenoldopam may increase urinary output and reassure clinicians, but they do not improve or protect kidney function or patient outcomes. Clinical trials of naloxone, fibronectin, inhibitors of the coagulation cascade, and monoclonal antibodies directed against lipopolysaccharide have been uniformly disappointing in septic shock.

Gastrointestinal Hemorrhage

Acute gastrointestinal hemorrhage is a common reason for admission to the ICU. Older age (>60 years), comorbid illnesses, hypotension, marked blood loss (>5 units), and recurrent hemorrhage are associated with increased mortality. Management begins with resuscitation and rapid identification of the site of bleeding. The clinician should differentiate between upper and lower gastrointestinal bleeding. A history of hematemesis indicates bleeding proximal to the ligament of Treitz. Melena often indicates bleeding proximal to the cecum. Hematochezia (bright red blood from the rectum) indicates either very brisk upper gastrointestinal bleeding (likely to be associated with hypotension) or, more commonly, lower gastrointestinal bleeding. The presence of maroon stools usually localizes the bleeding to the area between the distal small bowel and the right colon.

At least one large-bore intravenous cannula should be placed, and blood should be sent for laboratory analysis and crossmatch. Fluid resuscitation guidelines are discussed in Chapter 51. Serial hemoglobin or hematocrit measurements may not accurately reflect acute blood loss during ongoing hemorrhage. Placement of a nasogastric tube may help identify an upper gastrointestinal source if bright red blood or "coffee grounds"–appearing material can be aspirated; inability to aspirate blood, however, does not rule out an upper gastrointestinal source.

Upper Gastrointestinal Bleeding

Lavage through a nasogastric tube can help assess the rate of bleeding and facilitate esophagogastroduodenoscopy (EGD). EGD should be performed when possible to diagnose the cause of bleeding. Arteriography should be performed if the site of bleeding cannot be visualized with endoscopy. In unselected patients, the more common causes of upper gastrointestinal bleeding, in decreasing order of likelihood, are duodenal ulcer, gastric ulcer, erosive gastritis, and esophageal varices. Erosive gastritis may be due to stress, alcohol, aspirin, nonsteroidal anti-inflammatory drugs, and corticosteroids. Less common causes of upper gastrointestinal bleeding include angiodysplasia, erosive esophagitis, Mallory–Weiss tear, gastric tumor, and aortoenteric fistula.

Both interventional endoscopy and interventional arteriography can be used therapeutically to find and stop bleeding from peptic ulcers (gastric or duodenal). Surgery (or, increasingly, interventional radiology) is generally indicated for severe hemorrhage (>5 units) and recurrent bleeding. H_2-receptor blockers and proton pump inhibitors are ineffective in stopping hemorrhage but may reduce the likelihood of rebleeding. Erosive gastritis is better prevented than treated. Proton pump inhibitors,

H_2-receptor blockers, antacids, and sucralfate are all effective for prophylaxis. However, overuse of proton pump inhibitors is associated with an increased incidence of hospital-acquired pneumonia. Data show that patients who require mechanical ventilation for more than 48 h or who are coagulopathic derive the greatest benefit from prophylaxis. Other groups of patients showing relative benefit from prophylaxis include those with AKI, sepsis, liver failure, hypotension, traumatic brain injury, a history of prior gastrointestinal hemorrhage, recent major surgery, or those receiving large-dose corticosteroid therapy.

Once bleeding has begun, there is generally no specific therapy other than embolization or coagulation. Interventional endoscopy or interventional angiography reduces blood transfusions, rebleeding, hospital stay, and the need for urgent surgery. Balloon tamponade (Sengstaken–Blakemore, Minnesota, or Linton tubes) may be used as adjunctive therapy for variceal bleeding but usually requires concurrent endotracheal intubation to protect the airway against aspiration.

Lower Gastrointestinal Bleeding

Common causes of lower gastrointestinal bleeding include diverticular disease, angiodysplasia, neoplasms, inflammatory bowel disease, ischemic colitis, infectious colitis, and anorectal disease (hemorrhoids, fissure, fistula). Inspection and sigmoidoscopy can usually diagnose the more distal lesions. Colonoscopy usually allows definitive diagnosis (particularly for more proximal bleeding sites) and is often useful therapeutically. Interventional endoscopy or interventional angiography are the usual first choices for persistent bleeding. Surgical treatment is reserved for severe or recurrent hemorrhage.

Delirium

In the past, patients with critical illness and delirium were typically mechanically restrained and given sedative or paralytic drugs, or both. All of these approaches have been associated with adverse consequences. Restraints are inhumane unless used only as a last resort for patient protection. Prolonged use of propofol has led to "propofol infusion syndrome," particularly in children. Prolonged use of neuromuscular blockers has been associated with critical illness myopathy. Fortunately, improved drugs for sedation (eg, dexmedetomidine) are more effective and have fewer adverse consequences.

Post-Traumatic Stress Disorder

Both surviving patients and caregivers find being in the critical care unit stressful. Increasing clinical and research attention is being paid to these concerns. PTSD has been a particular problem for caregivers during the COVID-19 pandemic.

End-of-Life Care

In the United States, death is a taboo subject for many people. Many attend to last wills and testaments, estate planning, and taxes, but fewer than 15% of the adult population has made advance decisions about restrictions on life-supporting measures. Yet surveys consistently show a widespread preference for a dignified, comfortable, and peaceful death at home and a widely shared wish to avoid dying in a hospital, particularly in an ICU.

The quandary about what to do is particularly vexing when it concerns a surgical patient who sought relief from symptoms, with improved functionality and a better quality of life, but who after suffering complications now requires ongoing life-supporting measures with little prospect of achieving the goals of the operation. Some physicians find it difficult to discuss such situations in a humane, nonadversarial manner and find it difficult to address the accusations, anger, and despair of family members and friends whose expectations have not been met. Good communication skills are the essential foundation. Communications with the family, friends, and all caregivers must be timely, consistent (having only one physician serve as the spokesman has great advantages), accurate, clear to laypersons, advisory without being dictatorial, focused on what is best for the patient, and aligned with the patient's wishes. A gradual stepwise approach over time allows family members and friends time to digest the information, get beyond their initial reactions to the bad news, and make the difficult decision to withdraw intensive support.

Finally, it is important to recognize two ethical principles that are relevant here. The first is the principle of double effect. All medical interventions have potential benefits as well as burdens and risks. If the doses of morphine or sedative drug required to relieve pain and agitation result in unintended side effects, we accept them, even if the result is death. *This is not euthanasia.* The second principle is that withdrawal of medical therapies and interventions is no different from withholding them: Both may be done to respect the patient's autonomy. There is a broad religious consensus that heroic measures are not mandated to support a heartbeat at the end of life.

CASE DISCUSSION

An Obtunded Young Woman

A 23-year-old woman is admitted to the hospital obtunded with slow respirations (7 breaths/min). Blood pressure is 90/60 mm Hg, and the pulse is 90 beats/min. She was found at home in bed with empty bottles of diazepam, acetaminophen with hydrocodone, and fluoxetine lying next to her.

How is the diagnosis of a drug overdose made?

The presumptive diagnosis of a drug overdose usually must be made from the history, circumstantial evidence, and any witnesses. Signs and symptoms may not be helpful. Confirmation of a suspected drug overdose or poison ingestion usually requires delayed laboratory testing for the suspected agent in body fluids. Intentional overdoses (self-poisoning) are the most common mechanism and typically occur in young adults who are depressed. Ingestion of multiple drugs is common. Benzodiazepines, antidepressants, aspirin, acetaminophen, and alcohol are the most commonly ingested agents.

Accidental overdoses frequently occur in intravenous drug abusers and children. Commonly abused substances include opioids, stimulants (cocaine and methamphetamine), and hallucinogens (ketamine and phencyclidine [PCP]). Younger children occasionally accidentally ingest caustic household alkali (eg, drain cleaner), acids, and hydrocarbons (eg, petroleum products), in addition to unsecured medications of all types. Organophosphate poisoning (parathion and malathion) usually occurs in adults following agricultural exposure. Overdoses and poisoning less commonly occur as an attempted homicide.

What are appropriate steps in managing this patient?

Regardless of the type of drug or poison ingested, the principles of initial supportive care are the same. Airway patency with adequate ventilation and oxygenation must be obtained. Unless otherwise contraindicated, oxygen therapy should be used to maintain normal arterial saturation. Hypoventilation and obtunded airway reflexes require tracheal intubation and mechanical ventilation. Many clinicians routinely administer naloxone (up to 2 mg), dextrose 50% (50 mL), and thiamine (100 mg) intravenously to all obtunded or comatose patients until a diagnosis is established; this may help exclude or treat opioid overdose, hypoglycemia, and Wernicke–Korsakoff syndrome, respectively. The dextrose can be omitted when a glucose measurement indicates it is not necessary. In this patient, intubation should be performed prior to naloxone because the respiratory depression is likely due to both the hydrocodone and the diazepam.

Blood, urine, and gastric fluid specimens should be obtained and sent for toxicology screening. Blood is also sent for routine hematological and chemistry studies (including liver function). Urine is usually obtained after bladder catheterization, and gastric fluid can be aspirated from a nasogastric tube; the latter should be placed after intubation to avoid pulmonary aspiration. Alternatively, emesis material may be tested for drugs in conscious persons.

Hypotension should generally be treated with intravenous fluids unless the patient is obviously in pulmonary edema; an inotrope or vasopressor may be necessary in some instances. Seizure activity may be the result of hypoxia or a pharmacological action of a drug (tricyclic antidepressants) or poison. Seizure activity is unlikely in this patient because she ingested diazepam, a potent anticonvulsant.

Should flumazenil be administered?

Flumazenil should generally not be administered to patients who overdose on both a benzodiazepine and an antidepressant and those who have a history of seizures. Reversal of the benzodiazepine's anticonvulsant action can precipitate seizure activity in such instances. Moreover, as is the case with naloxone and opioids, the half-life of flumazenil is shorter than that of benzodiazepines. Thus, it is often preferable to ventilate the patient until the benzodiazepine effect dissipates, the patient regains consciousness, and the respiratory depression resolves.

Should any other antidotes be given?

Because the patient also ingested an unknown quantity of acetaminophen (paracetamol), administration of N-acetylcysteine (NAC; Mucomyst) should be considered. Acetaminophen toxicity is due to the depletion of hepatic glutathione, resulting in the accumulation of toxic metabolic intermediates. Hepatic toxicity is usually associated with ingestion of more than 140 mg/kg of acetaminophen. NAC prevents hepatic damage by acting as a sulfhydryl donor and restoring hepatic glutathione levels. If the patient is suspected of having ingested a toxic dose of acetaminophen, an initial dosage of NAC (140 mg/kg orally or by nasogastric tube) should be administered even before plasma acetaminophen levels are obtained; additional doses are given according to the measured plasma level. If the patient cannot tolerate oral or gastric administration of NAC, if the patient is pregnant, or if the risk of hepatotoxicity is high, NAC should be given intravenously.

What measures might limit drug toxicity?

Toxicity might be reduced by decreasing drug absorption or enhancing elimination. Gastrointestinal absorption of an ingested substance can be reduced by emptying stomach contents and administering activated charcoal. Both methods can be effective up to 12 h following ingestion. If the patient is intubated, the stomach is lavaged carefully to avoid pulmonary aspiration. Emesis may be induced in conscious patients with syrup of ipecac 30 mL (15 mL in a child). Gastric lavage and induced emesis are generally contraindicated for patients who ingest caustic substances or hydrocarbons because of a high risk of aspiration and worsening mucosal injury.

Activated charcoal, 1 to 2 g/kg, is administered orally or by nasogastric tube with a diluent. The charcoal irreversibly binds most drugs and poisons in the gut, allowing them to be eliminated in stools. In fact, charcoal can create a negative diffusion gradient between the gut and the circulation, allowing the drug or poison to be effectively removed from the body.

Alkalinization of the serum with sodium bicarbonate for tricyclic antidepressant overdose is beneficial because, by increasing pH, protein binding is enhanced; if seizures occur, the alkalinization prevents acidosis-induced cardiotoxicity.

What other methods can enhance drug elimination?

The easiest method of increasing drug elimination is forced diuresis. Unfortunately, this method is of limited use for drugs that are highly protein bound or have large volumes of distribution. Mannitol or furosemide with saline may be used. Concomitant administration of alkali (sodium bicarbonate) enhances the elimination of weakly acidic drugs such as salicylates and barbiturates; alkalization of the urine traps the ionized form of these drugs in the renal tubules and enhances urinary elimination. Hemodialysis is usually reserved for patients with severe toxicity who continue to deteriorate despite aggressive supportive therapy.

WEBSITES

Acute Kidney Injury Network. http://www.akinet.org/

American Association of Poison Control Centers. http://www.aapcc.org/

American Heart Association. http://cpr.heart.org/AHAECC/CPRAndECC/ResuscitationScience/Guidelines/UCM_473201_Guidelines.jsp

Quick Sepsis-Related Organ Function Assessment. http://www.qsofa.org/

SOFA calculator. http://clincalc.com/IcuMortality/SOFA.aspx

Surviving Sepsis campaign. http://www.survivingsepsis.org/

SUGGESTED READINGS

Andrews LJ, Benken ST. COVID-19: ICU delirium management during SARS-CoV-2 pandemic-pharmacological considerations. *Crit Care.* 2020;24:375.

Aslakson RA, Curtis JR, Nelson JE. The changing role of palliative care in the ICU. *Crit Care Med.* 2014;42:2418.

Botti C, Lusetti F, Peroni S, et al. The role of tracheotomy and timing of weaning and decannulation in patients affected by severe COVID-19. *Ear Nose Throat J.* 2021;100(2_suppl):116S.

Dellinger RP, Levy MM, Rhodes A, et al; Surviving Sepsis Campaign Guidelines Committee including the Pediatric Subgroup. Surviving sepsis campaign: international guidelines for management of severe sepsis and septic shock: 2012. *Crit Care Med.* 2013;41:580.

Finsterer J. Neurological perspectives of neurogenic pulmonary edema. *Eur Neurol.* 2019;81:94.

Grigonis AM, Mathews KS, Benka-Coker WO, et al. Long-term acute care hospitals extend ICU capacity for COVID-19 response and recovery. *Chest.* 2021;159:1894.

Hasan Z. A review of acute respiratory distress syndrome management and treatment. *Am J Ther.* 2021;28:e189.

Kim L, Garg S, O'Halloran A, Whitaker M, et al. Risk factors for intensive care unit admission and in-hospital mortality among hospitalized adults identified through the US Coronavirus disease 2019 (COVID-19)-associated hospitalization surveillance network (COVID-NET). *Clin Infect Dis.* 2021;72:e206.

Leisman DE, Deutschman CS, Legrand M. Facing COVID-19 in the ICU: vascular dysfunction, thrombosis, and dysregulated inflammation. *Intensive Care Med.* 2020;46:1105.

Levey AS, James MT. Acute kidney injury. *Ann Intern Med.* 2017;167:ITC66.

Liu R, Wang J, Zhao G, Su Z. Negative pressure pulmonary edema after general anesthesia. *Medicine* (Baltimore). 2019;98:e15389.

Menk M, Estenssoro E, Sahetyat SK, et al. Current and evolving standards of care for patients with ARDS. *Intensive Care Med.* 2020;46:2157.

Michalsen A, Sadovnikoff N. *Compelling Ethical Challenges in Critical Care and Emergency Medicine.* Springer; 2020.

Musick S, Alberico A. Neurologic assessment of the neurocritical care patient. *Front Neurol.* 2021;12:588989.

Oropello JM, Pastores SM, Kvetan V. *Critical Care.* McGraw-Hill/Lange; 2017.

Seymour CW, Liu VX, Iwashyna TJ, et al. Assessment of clinical criteria for sepsis: for the Third International Consensus Definitions for Sepsis and Septic Shock (Sepsis-3). *JAMA.* 2016;315:762. Erratum in: *JAMA.* 2016;315:2237.

Sharif S, Owen JJ, Upadhye S. The end of early goal-directed therapy? *Am J Emerg Med.* 2016;34:292.

Singer M, Deutschman CS, Seymour CW, et al. The Third International Consensus definitions for sepsis and septic shock (Sepsis-3). *JAMA.* 2016;315:801.

Vijayan A. Tackling AKI: prevention, timing of dialysis and follow-up. *Nat Rev Nephrol.* 2021;17:87.

Vincent J-L, Abraham E, Kochanek P, et al, eds. *Textbook of Critical Care.* 7th ed. Elsevier Saunders; 2017.

CHAPTER 58

Inhalation Therapy & Mechanical Ventilation in the PACU & ICU

KEY CONCEPTS

1. Hyperoxia *and* hypoxia are risk factors for but not the primary causes of retinopathy of prematurity (ROP). Neonates' risk of ROP increases with low birth weight and complexity of comorbidities (eg, sepsis).
2. The disadvantage of conventional pressure control ventilation (PCV) is that tidal volume (V_T) is not guaranteed (though there are modes in which the consistent delivered pressure of PCV can be combined with a predefined volume delivery).
3. PCV is similar to pressure support ventilation in that peak airway pressure is controlled, but it is different in that a mandatory rate and inspiratory time are selected. As with pressure support, gas flow ceases when the pressure level is reached; however, the ventilator does not cycle to expiration until the preset inspiration time has elapsed.
4. Both nasotracheal and orotracheal intubation appear to be relatively safe for at least 2 to 3 weeks.
5. When left in place for more than 2 to 3 weeks, both orotracheal and nasotracheal tubes predispose patients to subglottic stenosis. If longer periods of mechanical ventilation are necessary, the endotracheal tube should generally be replaced by a cuffed tracheostomy tube.
6. The major effect of positive end-expiratory pressure (PEEP) on the lungs is to increase functional residual capacity (FRC). In patients with decreased lung volume, appropriate levels of either PEEP or continuous positive airway pressure (CPAP) will increase FRC and tidal ventilation above closing capacity. This will improve lung compliance and will correct ventilation/perfusion abnormalities.
7. Compared with a V_T of 12 mL/kg, a VT of 6 mL/kg and plateau pressure (P_{plt}) less than 30 cm H_2O have been associated with reduced mortality in patients with acute respiratory distress syndrome.
8. A higher incidence of pulmonary barotrauma is observed with excessive PEEP or CPAP at levels greater than 20 cm H_2O.
9. Maneuvers that produce sustained maximum lung inflation, such as the use of an incentive spirometer, can be helpful in inducing cough as well as preventing atelectasis and preserving normal lung volume.

Respiratory care includes both the delivery of pulmonary therapy and the performance of diagnostic tests. Respiratory therapists' scope of practice encompasses medical gas therapy, delivery of aerosolized medications, airway management, mechanical ventilation, positive airway pressure therapy, critical care monitoring, cardiopulmonary rehabilitation, and the application of various techniques collectively termed *chest physiotherapy*. The latter includes administering aerosols, clearing pulmonary secretions, reexpanding atelectatic lung, and preserving normal lung function postoperatively or during illness. Diagnostic services may include pulmonary function testing, arterial blood gas analysis, and evaluation of sleep-disordered breathing. These procedures and services are well described in clinical practice guidelines developed by the American Association for Respiratory Care.

MEDICAL GAS THERAPY

Therapeutic medical gases include oxygen at ambient or hyperbaric pressure, helium–oxygen mixtures (heliox), and nitric oxide. Oxygen is made available in high-pressure cylinders, via pipeline systems, from oxygen concentrators, as well as in liquid form. Heliox, because of its relatively low density, is occasionally used to reduce the increased work of breathing caused by partial upper airway obstruction. Nitric oxide is administered as a direct, selective pulmonary vasodilator.

The primary goal of oxygen therapy is to prevent or correct hypoxemia or tissue hypoxia. Table 58–1 identifies classic categories of hypoxia. Having a patient inhale an increased concentration of oxygen alone may not correct either hypoxemia or hypoxia. Continuous positive airway pressure (CPAP) or positive end-expiratory pressure (PEEP) may be required to recruit collapsed alveoli. Patients with profound hypercapnia may require ventilatory assistance. Increased concentrations of oxygen (possibly at hyperbaric pressures) may be indicated for conditions requiring removal of entrapped gas (eg, nitrogen) from body cavities or vessels. The short-term inhalation of increased concentrations of oxygen is relatively free of complications.

Supplemental oxygen is indicated for adults, children, and infants (older than 1 month) when PaO_2 is less than 60 mm Hg (8 kPa) or SaO_2 or SpO_2 is less than 90% while breathing room air. In neonates, therapy is recommended if PaO_2 is less than 50 mm Hg (6.7 kPa) or SaO_2 is less than 88% (or capillary PO_2 is less than 40 mm Hg [5.3 kPa]). Therapy may be indicated for patients when hypoxemia or hypoxia is suspected based on a medical history and physical examination. Supplemental oxygen is given during the perioperative period because general anesthesia commonly causes a decrease in PaO_2 secondary to increased pulmonary ventilation/perfusion mismatching and decreased functional residual capacity (FRC). Supplemental oxygen should be provided before procedures such as tracheal suctioning or bronchoscopy, which commonly cause arterial desaturation. There is evidence that

TABLE 58–1 Classification of hypoxia.[1]

Hypoxia	Pathophysiological Category	Clinical Example
Hypoxic hypoxia	$\downarrow P_{Barom}$ or $\downarrow FiO_2$ (<0.21)	Altitude, O_2 equipment error
	Alveolar hypoventilation	Drug overdose, COPD exacerbation
	Pulmonary diffusion defect	Emphysema, pulmonary fibrosis
	Pulmonary $\dot{V}/\dot{Q}$ mismatch	Asthma, pulmonary emboli
	R → L shunt	Atelectasis, cyanotic congenital heart disease
Circulatory hypoxia	Reduced cardiac output	Severe heart failure, dehydration
	Microvascular dysfunction	Sepsis, SIRS
Hemic hypoxia	Reduced hemoglobin content	Anemias
	Reduced hemoglobin function	Carboxyhemoglobinemia, methemoglobinemia
Demand hypoxia	$\uparrow O_2$ consumption	Fever, seizures
Histotoxic hypoxia	Inability of cells to utilize O_2	Cyanide toxicity, ↑TNF, late sepsis

[1]COPD, chronic obstructive pulmonary disease; FiO_2, fraction of inspired oxygen; O_2, oxygen; P_{Barom}, barometric pressure; R → L, right to left; SIRS, systemic inflammatory response syndrome; TNF, tumor necrosis factor; $\dot{V}/\dot{Q}$, ventilation/perfusion.

supplemental oxygen is effective in prolonging the survival of patients with chronic obstructive pulmonary disease (COPD) when their resting PaO_2 is less than 60 mm Hg at sea level. Supplemental oxygen therapy also appears to have a mild beneficial effect on the mean pulmonary arterial pressure and subjective indices of patients' dyspnea.

AMBIENT OXYGEN THERAPY EQUIPMENT

Classifying Oxygen Therapy Equipment

Oxygen given alone or in a gas can be mixed with air as a partial supplement to patients' tidal volume or serve as the entire source of the inspired volume. The devices or systems used for this are classified based on their maximal flow rates and a range of fractions of inspired oxygen (FiO_2). Other considerations in selecting an oxygen delivery technique include patient compliance, the presence and type of artificial airway, and the need for humidification or an aerosol delivery system.

A. Low-Flow or Variable-Performance Equipment

Oxygen (usually 100%) is supplied at a fixed flow that is only a portion of inspired gas. Such devices (eg, nasal "prongs") are usually intended for patients with stable breathing patterns. As ventilatory demands change, variable amounts of room air will dilute the oxygen flow. Low-flow systems are adequate for patients with:

- Minute ventilation less than or equal to 8 to 10 L/min
- Breathing frequencies greater than or equal to 20 breaths/min
- Tidal volumes (VT) less than or equal to 0.8 L
- Normal inspiratory flow (10–30 L/min)

B. High-Flow or Fixed-Performance Equipment

Inspired gas at a preset FiO_2 is supplied continuously at high flow or by providing a sufficiently large reservoir of premixed gas. Ideally, the delivered FiO_2 is not affected by variations in ventilatory level or breathing pattern. High-flow systems are indicated for patients who require:

- Consistent FiO_2
- Larger inspiratory flows of gas (>40 L/min)

1. Variable-Performance Equipment

Nasal Cannulas

The nasal cannula is available as either a single-ended soft plastic tube with an over-the-ear head-elastic or dual-flow (to both nares) with under-the-chin lariat adjustment. Sizes appropriate for adults, children, and infants are available. Cannulas are connected to flowmeters with small-bore tubing. The tubing should be adjusted to avoid pressure sores on the ears, cheeks, and nose. Patients receiving long-term oxygen therapy most commonly use a nasal cannula. The appliance is usually well tolerated, allowing unencumbered speech, eating, and drinking. Cannulas can be combined with spectacle frames for convenience or to improve cosmesis. Since oxygen flows continuously, approximately 80% of the gas is wasted during expiration.

The actual FiO_2 delivered to adults with nasal cannulas is determined by oxygen flow, nasopharyngeal volume, and the patient's inspiratory flow (the latter depends both on VT and inspiratory time) (Table 58–2). Oxygen from the cannula can fill the nasopharynx after exhalation, yet with inspiration, oxygen and entrained air are drawn into the trachea. The inspired percent oxygen in inspired air increases by approximately 2% (above 21%) per liter of oxygen flow with quiet breathing in adults; thus, cannulas can be expected to provide inspired oxygen concentrations up to 30% with normal breathing and oxygen flows of 4 L/min. Levels of 40% or greater can be attained with oxygen flows of 10 L/min or greater; however, flows greater than 5 L/min are poorly tolerated because of the discomfort of gas jetting into the nasal cavity and because of drying and crusting of the nasal mucosa.

Data from "normal-breathing subjects" may not be accurate for acutely ill tachypneic patients. Increasing VT and reducing inspiratory time will dilute the small flow of oxygen. Different proportions

TABLE 58–2 Oxygen delivery devices and systems.

Device/System	Oxygen Flow Rate (L/min)	FiO_2 Range[1]
Nasal cannula	1	0.21–0.24
	2	0.23–0.28
	3	0.27–0.34
	4	0.31–0.38
	5–6	0.32–0.44
Simple mask	5–6	0.30–0.45
	7–8	0.40–0.60
Mask with reservoir	5	0.35–0.50
Partial rebreathing mask-bag	7	0.35–0.75
	15	0.65–1.00
Nonrebreathing mask-bag	7–15	0.40–1.00
Venturi mask and jet nebulizer	4–6 (total flow = 15)	0.24
	4–6 (total flow = 45)	0.28
	8–10 (total flow = 45)	0.35
	8–10 (total flow = 33)	0.40
	8–12 (total flow = 33)	0.50

[1]FiO_2, fraction of inspired oxygen.

of mouth-only versus nose-only breathing and varied inspiratory flow can alter FiO_2 by up to 40%. In clinical practice, flow should be titrated according to vital signs and pulse oximetry or arterial blood gas measurements. Some patients with COPD tend to hypoventilate with even modest oxygen flows yet are hypoxemic on room air. They may do well with cannula flows of less than 2 L/min.

Special cannulas allow infants to nurse without interrupting supplemental oxygen, and these cannulas are less likely to traumatize the face and nose than oxygen masks. Because of the reduced minute ventilation of infants, flow through the cannula must be proportionately reduced. This generally requires a pressure-compensated flowmeter accurate at delivering oxygen flows in the less than 3 L/min range. Hypopharyngeal oxygen sampling from infants breathing with cannulas has demonstrated mean FiO_2 of 0.35, 0.45, 0.6, and 0.68 with flows of 0.25, 0.5, 0.75, and 1.0 L/min, respectively.

Nasal Mask

The nasal mask is a hybrid of the nasal cannula and a face mask. The lower edge of the mask's flanges rests on the upper lip, surrounding the external nose. Nasal masks provide supplemental oxygen equivalent to the nasal cannula under low-flow conditions in adult patients. Many patients find the nasal mask more comfortable than a nasal cannula. The nasal mask does not produce sores around the external nares, and dry oxygen is not "jetted" into the nasal cavity. The nasal mask should be considered if it improves patient comfort and compliance.

"Simple" Oxygen Mask

The "simple" oxygen mask is a disposable lightweight plastic device that covers both the nose and the mouth. It has no reservoir bag. Masks are secured to the patient's face by the adjustment of an elastic headband. The seal is rarely complete: usually there is "inboard" leaking. Thus, patients receive a mixture of oxygen and secondarily entrained room air, depending on the size of the leak, oxygen flow, and breathing pattern.

The body of the mask functions as a reservoir for both oxygen and expired carbon dioxide (CO_2). A minimum oxygen flow of approximately 5 L/min is applied to the mask to limit rebreathing and the resulting increased respiratory work. Wearing any mask appliance for long periods of time is uncomfortable. Speech is muffled, and drinking and eating are difficult.

It is difficult to predict delivered FiO_2 at specific oxygen flow rates. During normal breathing, it is reasonable to expect an FiO_2 of 0.3 to 0.6 with flows of 5 to 10 L/min, respectively. Oxygen levels can be increased with smaller V_T or slower breathing rates. With higher flows and ideal conditions, FiO_2 may approach 0.7 or 0.8.

Masks lacking oxygen reservoirs may be best suited for patients who require concentrations of oxygen not easily attainable using cannulas but who require oxygen therapy for short periods of time. Examples would include medical transport or therapy in the postanesthesia care unit or emergency department. It is not the device of choice for patients who are profoundly hypoxemic, tachypneic, or unable to protect their airway from aspiration.

Masks with Gas Reservoirs

Incorporating a gas reservoir expands the applicability of the simple mask. Two types of reservoir masks are commonly used: the partial rebreathing mask and the nonrebreathing mask. Both are disposable, lightweight, transparent plastic under-the-chin reservoirs. The difference between the two relates to the use of valves on the mask and between the mask and the bag reservoir. Mask reservoirs commonly hold less than 600 mL of gas volume. The phrase "partial rebreather" is used because "part" of the patient's expired VT refills the bag. Because expired gas is largely from "dead space ventilation," significant rebreathing of CO_2 usually does not occur.

The nonrebreather uses the same basic system as the partial rebreather but incorporates flap-type valves between the bag and mask and on at least one of the mask's exhalation ports. Inboard leaking is common, and room air will enter during brisk inspiratory flows, even when the bag contains gas. The lack of a complete facial seal and a relatively small reservoir limit the delivered oxygen concentration. The key factor in the successful application of the mask is to use a sufficiently high flow of oxygen so that the reservoir bag is at least partially full during inspiration. Typical minimum flows of oxygen are 10 to 15 L/min. Well-fitting partial rebreathing masks provide a range of FiO_2 from 0.35 to 0.60 with oxygen flows up to 10 L/min. With inlet flows of 15 L/min or more and ideal breathing conditions, FiO_2 may approach 1.0. Either style of mask is indicated for patients with significant hypoxemia but relatively normal spontaneous minute ventilation.

2. Fixed-Performance (High-Flow) Equipment

Profoundly dyspneic patients with gasping respiration may be served by a fixed-performance, high-flow oxygen system.

Anesthesia Bag or Bag-Mask-Valve Systems

Self-inflating bags consist of a roughly 1.5-L bladder, usually with an oxygen inlet reservoir. Anesthesia bags are 1-, 2-, or 3-L non–self-inflating reservoirs with a tailpiece gas inlet. Masks are designed to provide a comfortable leak-free seal for manual ventilation. The inspiratory/expiratory valve systems may vary. The flow to the reservoir should be kept high so the bags do not deflate substantially. When using an anesthesia bag, operators may frequently have to adjust the oxygen flow and exhaust valve to respond to changing breathing patterns or demands, particularly when maintaining a complete seal between the mask and face is difficult.

The most common systems for disposable and permanent self-inflating resuscitation bags use a unidirectional gas flow. Although these devices offer the potential for a constant FiO_2 greater than 0.9, tailpiece inlet valves will not open for a spontaneously breathing patient. Opening the valves requires negative-pressure bag recoil after compression. If this situation is not recognized, clinicians might be misled into thinking the patient is receiving a greater concentration of oxygen than is the case.

There are limits to the ability of each system to maintain its fixed-performance characteristics. Delivered FiO_2 can approach 1.0 with either anesthesia or self-inflating bags. Spontaneously breathing patients are allowed to breathe only the contents of the system if the mask seal is tight and the reservoir is adequately maintained.

Failure to maintain an adequate oxygen supply in the reservoir and inlet flow is a concern. The spring-loaded valve of anesthesia bags must be adjusted to prevent overdistention of the bag. Self-inflating bags look the same whether or not oxygen flow to the unit is adequate, and they will entrain room air into the bag, thus lowering the delivered FiO_2.

Air-Entraining Venturi Masks

Gas delivery with air-entraining masks is different than with an oxygen reservoir. The goal is to create an open system with high flow about the nose and mouth, with a fixed FiO_2. Oxygen is directed by small-bore tubing to a mixing jet; the final oxygen concentration depends on the ratio of air drawn in through entrainment ports. Manufacturers have developed both fixed and adjustable entrainment selections over an FiO_2 range. Most provide instructions for the operator to set a minimum flow of oxygen. Table 58–3 identifies total flow at various inlet flows and FiO_2.

TABLE 58–3 Air-entrainment mask input flow versus total flow at varying FiO_2.[1]

FiO_2	Inlet Oxygen Flow (Minimum)	Total Flow (L/min)
0.24	4	97
0.28	6	68
0.3	6	54
0.35	8	45
0.4	12	50
0.5	12	33
0.7	12	19
0.8	12	16
1.0	12	12

[1]FiO_2, fraction of inspired oxygen.

Despite the high-flow concept, actual FiO_2 can vary by up to 6% from the anticipated setting. Air-entraining masks are a logical choice for patients who require FiO_2 greater than can be provided by devices such as nasal cannulas. Patients with COPD who tend to hypoventilate with a moderate FiO_2 are candidates for the Venturi mask. Clinicians providing oxygen therapy with Venturi masks should be aware of the previously mentioned problems. FiO_2 can increase if the air entrainment ports are obstructed by the patient's hands, bedsheets, or water condensate. Clinicians should encourage the patient and caregivers to keep the mask on the face continuously: interruption of oxygen delivery may be life threatening in unstable patients with hypoxemia. Accurate analysis of the delivered FiO_2 during air-entrainment mask breathing is difficult. Pulse oximetry (or arterial blood gas analysis) and the patient's respiratory rate should guide clinicians as to whether the patient's demands are being met by the mask's flow.

Air-Entraining Nebulizers

Large-volume, high-output or "all-purpose" nebulizers have been used in respiratory care for many years to provide mist therapy with some control of the FiO_2. These units are commonly placed on patients following extubation for their aerosol-producing properties. Like the air-entraining masks, nebulizers use a pneumatic jet and an adjustable orifice to vary entrained air for varying FiO_2 levels. Many of these devices maximally allow 15 L/min when the source pressure is 50 psi. This means that on the 100% setting (no air entrainment) output flow is only 15 L/min. Only patients breathing slowly with small V_T will receive 100% oxygen. This problem has been addressed by high-flow, high-FiO_2 nebulizers. For more common applications that use an FiO_2 of 0.3 to 0.5, room air is entrained, reducing the FiO_2 and increasing the total flow output to 40 to 50 L/min.

Knowledge of the air/oxygen ratio and the input flow rate of oxygen allows the total outflow to be calculated. Nebulizer systems can be applied to the patient with many different devices, including tracheostomy dome/collar, face tent, and T-piece adapter. These appliances can all be attached via large-bore tubing to the nebulizer. This open system freely vents inspiratory and expiratory gases around the patient's face or out a distal port of a T-piece adapter. Unfortunately, the lack of any valves allows patients to secondarily entrain room air. It is common practice to use either a reservoir bag before the T-piece or a reservoir tube on the distal side of the T-piece to provide a larger volume of gas than that coming from the nebulizer. A typical concern of those applying air-entrainment aerosol therapy with controlled oxygen concentration is whether the system will provide adequate flow. Clinicians should observe the mist like a tracer to determine the adequacy of flow. When a T-piece is used and the visible mist (exiting the distal port) disappears during inspiration, the flow is inadequate.

A common clinical problem occurs when excess water collects in the tubing, completely obstructing gas flow or increasing resistance to flow. Other complications include bronchospasm or laryngospasm as a consequence of airway irritation from sterile water droplets (condensate of the aerosol). In such circumstances, a heated (nonaerosol) humidification system should be substituted.

High-Flow Air–Oxygen Systems

Dual air–oxygen flowmeters and air–oxygen blenders are commonly used for oxygen administration as well as freestanding CPAP and "add-on" ventilator systems. These systems differ from the air-entraining nebulizers because their total output flows do not diminish at FiO_2 greater than 0.4. With these high-flow systems, the total flow to the patient and FiO_2 can be set independently to meet patient needs. This can be done using a large reservoir bag or constant flows in the range of 50 to more than 100 L/min. Clinicians can use a variety of appliances with these systems, including aerosol masks, face tents, or well-fitted nonrebreathing system masks with air–oxygen blenders. Face-sealing mask systems can also be constructed with a reservoir bag and a safety valve to allow breathing if the blender fails. The high flows of gas require the use of heated humidifiers of the type commonly used on mechanical ventilators. Humidification offers an advantage for patients with reactive airways. Because of the high flows, such systems are used to apply CPAP or bilevel positive airway pressure (BiPAP) for spontaneously breathing patients.

Oxygen Hoods

Many infants and neonates will not tolerate facial appliances. Oxygen hoods cover only the head, allowing access to the child's lower body while still permitting the use of a standard incubator or radiant warmer. The hood is ideal for relatively short-term oxygen therapy for newborns and inactive infants. However, for mobile infants requiring longer-term therapy, the nasal cannula, face mask, or full-bed enclosure allow for greater mobility.

Normally, oxygen and air are premixed by an air–oxygen blender and passed through a heated humidifier. Nebulizers should be avoided. Most pneumatic jet-type nebulizers create noise levels (>65 dB) that may cause newborn hearing loss. Hoods come in different sizes. Some are simple Plexiglas boxes; others have elaborate systems for sealing the neck opening. There is no attempt to completely seal the system because a constant flow of gas is needed to remove CO_2 (minimum flow >7 L/min). Hood inlet flows of 10 to 15 L/min are adequate for most patients.

Helium–Oxygen Therapy

Helium–oxygen (heliox) mixtures are provided in several standard blends. The most popular mixture is 79%/21% helium–oxygen, which has a density that is 40% that of pure oxygen. Helium–oxygen mixtures are available in large-sized compressed gas cylinders.

In anesthetic practice, pressures needed to ventilate patients with small-diameter endotracheal tubes can be substantially reduced when the 79%/21% mixture is used. Heliox can provide patients with upper airway–obstructing lesions (eg, subglottic edema, foreign bodies, tracheal tumors) with relief from acute distress pending more definitive care. The benefit is less convincing in treating lower airway obstruction from COPD or acute asthma. Helium mixtures may also be used as the driving gas for small-volume nebulizers in bronchodilator therapy for asthma. However, with heliox, the nebulizer flow needs to be increased to 11 L/min versus the usual 6 to 8 L/min with oxygen. Patients' work of breathing can be reduced with heliox as compared with a conventional oxygen/nitrogen gas mixture.

Hyperbaric Oxygen

Hyperbaric oxygen therapy uses a pressurized chamber to expose the patient to oxygen tensions exceeding ambient barometric pressure (at sea level, the ambient pressure is 760 mm Hg). With a one-person hyperbaric chamber, 100% oxygen is usually used to pressurize the chamber. Larger chambers allow for the simultaneous treatment of multiple patients and for the presence of medical personnel in the chamber with patients. Multiplace chambers use air to pressurize the chamber, whereas patients receive 100% oxygen by mask, hood, or endotracheal tube. Common indications for hyperbaric oxygen where outcome benefits have been shown include decompression sickness (the "bends"), certain forms of gas embolism, gas gangrene, anaerobic bacterial infections, carbon monoxide poisoning, and treatment of certain chronic wounds.

3. Hazards of Oxygen Therapy

Oxygen (O_2) therapy can result in both respiratory and nonrespiratory toxicity. Important factors include patient susceptibility, the FiO_2, and the duration of therapy.

Hypoventilation

This complication is often seen in patients with COPD who have chronic CO_2 retention or in patients receiving opioids. Patients who retain CO_2 persistently have a respiratory drive that becomes at least partly dependent on the maintenance of relative hypoxemia. Elevation of arterial O_2 tension to "normal" can therefore trigger severe hypoventilation in these patients. O_2 therapy can be indirectly hazardous for patients being monitored with pulse oximetry while receiving opioids for pain. Opioid-induced hypoventilation may not cause arterial O_2 desaturation, despite markedly reduced respiratory rates. Thus, supplemental O_2 renders pulse oximetry a poor monitor for opioid-induced respiratory depression.

Absorption Atelectasis

High concentrations of O_2 can cause pulmonary atelectasis in areas of low $\dot{V}/\dot{Q}$ ratios. As nitrogen is "washed out" of the lungs, the lowered gas tension in pulmonary capillary blood results in increased uptake of alveolar gas and absorption atelectasis. If the area remains perfused but nonventilated, the resulting intrapulmonary shunt with increasing "venous admixture" can lead to progressive widening of the alveolar-to-arterial (A–a) gradient.

Pulmonary Toxicity

Prolonged exposure to high concentrations of O_2 may damage the lungs. Toxicity is dependent both on the partial pressure of O_2 in the inspired gas and the duration of exposure. Alveolar rather than arterial O_2 tension is most important in the development of O_2 toxicity. Although 100% O_2 for up to 10 to 20 h is generally considered safe, concentrations greater than 50% to 60% are undesirable for longer periods as they may lead to pulmonary toxicity.

O_2 toxicity is attributed to the intracellular generation of highly reactive O_2 metabolites (free radicals) such as superoxide and activated hydroxyl ions, singlet O_2, and hydrogen peroxide. A high concentration of O_2 increases the likelihood of generating toxic species. These metabolites are cytotoxic because they readily react with DNA, proteins, and lipids. Two cellular enzymes, superoxide dismutase and catalase, protect against toxicity by sequentially converting superoxide first to hydrogen peroxide and then to water. Additional protection may be provided by antioxidants and free radical scavengers; however, there is no good clinical evidence that these agents prevent pulmonary toxicity. O_2 toxicity may present as tracheobronchitis initially in some patients. Pulmonary O_2 toxicity in newborn infants is manifested as bronchopulmonary dysplasia. In experimental animals, O_2-mediated lung injury produces a condition indistinguishable from acute respiratory distress syndrome (ARDS).

Retinopathy of Prematurity

Retinopathy of prematurity (ROP), formerly termed *retrolental fibroplasia*, is a neovascular retinal disorder that develops in the great majority of premature survivors born at less than 28 weeks' gestation. ROP may include disorganized vascular proliferation and fibrosis and may lead to retinal detachment and blindness. ROP resolves in approximately 80% of these cases without visual loss from retinal detachments or scars. ROP was very common in the 1940s and 1950s when unmonitored high (>0.5 FiO_2) O_2 was often administered to premature infants.
1 However, it is now known that hyperoxia *and* hypoxia are risk factors for, but not the primary causes of, ROP. Neonates' risk of ROP increases with low birth weight and complexity of comorbidities (eg, sepsis). In contrast to pulmonary toxicity, ROP correlates better with arterial than with alveolar O_2 tension. The recommended arterial concentrations for premature infants receiving O_2 are 50 to 80 mm Hg (6.6–10.6 kPa). If an infant requires arterial O_2 saturations of 96% to 99% for cardiopulmonary reasons, fear about causing or worsening ROP is not a reason to withhold the O_2.

Hyperbaric O_2 Toxicity

The increased inspired O_2 tensions associated with hyperbaric O_2 therapy greatly accelerate O_2 toxicity. The risk and expected degree of toxicity are directly related to the pressures used as well as the duration of exposure. Prolonged exposure to O_2 partial pressures in excess of 0.5 atmosphere can cause pulmonary O_2 toxicity. This may present initially with retrosternal burning, cough, and chest tightness. There will be progressive impairment of pulmonary function with continued exposure. Patients exposed to O_2 at 2 atmospheres or greater are also at risk for central nervous system toxicity that may be expressed as behavior changes, nausea, vertigo, muscular twitching, or convulsions.

Fire Hazard

O_2 vigorously supports combustion. The potential for uncontained O_2 enriched gas mixtures to promote fires and explosions is discussed in Chapter 2.

MECHANICAL VENTILATION

Patients with critical illness often require mechanical ventilation to replace or supplement normal spontaneous ventilation. In some instances, the problem is primarily that of impaired CO_2 elimination (ventilatory failure). In other instances, mechanical ventilation may be used as an adjunct (usually to positive-pressure therapy, as discussed next) in the treatment of hypoxemia. The decision to initiate mechanical ventilation is made on clinical grounds, but certain parameters have been suggested as guidelines (Table 58–4).

TABLE 58–4 Indicators of the need for mechanical ventilation.

Criterion	Measurement
Direct measurement	
Arterial oxygen tension	<50 mm Hg on room air
Arterial CO_2 tension	>50 mm Hg in the absence of metabolic alkalosis
Derived indices	
PaO_2/FiO_2 ratio	<300 mm Hg
$PA–aO_2$ gradient	>350 mm Hg
VD/VT	>0.6
Clinical indices	
Respiratory rate	>35 breaths/min
Mechanical indices	
Tidal volume	<5 mL/kg
Vital capacity	<15 mL/kg
Maximum inspiratory force	>–25 cm H_2O (eg, –15 cm H_2O)

CO_2, carbon dioxide; FiO_2, fraction of inspired oxygen; PaO_2, partial pressure of oxygen in arterial blood; VD/VT, dead space to tidal volume ratio.

Of the two available techniques, positive-pressure ventilation and negative-pressure ventilation (*iron lung*), the former has much wider applications and is almost universally used. Although negative-pressure ventilation does not require tracheal intubation, it cannot overcome substantial increases in airway resistance or decreases in pulmonary compliance, and it also limits access to the patient.

During positive-pressure ventilation, lung inflation is achieved by periodically applying positive pressure to the upper airway through a tight-fitting mask (noninvasive mechanical ventilation) or through a tracheal or tracheostomy tube. Increased airway resistance and decreased lung compliance can be overcome by manipulating inspiratory gas flow and pressure. The major disadvantages of positive-pressure ventilation are altered ventilation-to-perfusion relationships, potentially adverse circulatory effects, and risk of pulmonary barotrauma and volutrauma. Positive-pressure ventilation increases physiological dead space because gas flow is preferentially directed to the more compliant, nondependent areas of the lungs, whereas blood flow (influenced by gravity) favors dependent areas. Reductions in cardiac output are primarily due to impaired blood return to the heart from increased intrathoracic pressure. Barotrauma is closely related to repetitive high peak inflation pressures and underlying lung disease, whereas volutrauma is related to the repetitive collapse and reexpansion of alveoli.

1. Positive-Pressure Ventilators

Positive-pressure ventilators periodically create a pressure gradient between the machine circuit and the alveoli resulting in inspiratory gas flow. Exhalation occurs passively. Ventilators and their control mechanisms can be powered pneumatically (by a pressurized gas source), electrically, or by both mechanisms. Gas flow is either derived directly from the pressurized gas source or produced by the action of a rotary or linear piston. This gas flow then either goes directly to the patient (single-circuit system) or, as commonly occurs with operating room ventilators, compresses a reservoir bag or bellows that is part of the patient circuit (double-circuit system).

All ventilators have four phases: inspiration, the changeover from inspiration to expiration (cycling), expiration, and the changeover from expiration to inspiration (trigger) (see Chapter 4). These phases are defined by VT, ventilatory rate, inspiratory time, inspiratory gas flow, and expiratory time.

Classification of Ventilators

Modern ventilators are complicated and defy simple classification. The incorporation of microprocessors into ventilators has further complicated this task. The complexity of ventilator nomenclature combined with a proprietary naming schema for similar ventilator functionality has led to calls for uniform taxonomy for ventilator modes. Chatburn provides one such nomenclature, and the salient points of his scheme are used to frame the following discussion on ventilator modes.

Phase Variables

The breathing period can be divided into four phases: (1) change from expiration to inspiration (trigger), (2) inspiration (target), (3) change from inspiration to expiration (cycle), and (4) expiration. The trigger variable starts inspiration when it (pressure, volume, flow, or time) reaches a preset value. When time is the trigger, breaths are initiated on a defined frequency regardless of patient effort (Figure 58–1). Alternatively, pressure, flow, or volume triggers initiate a breath when the ventilator detects a change in pressure, flow, or volume, respectively caused by patient effort.

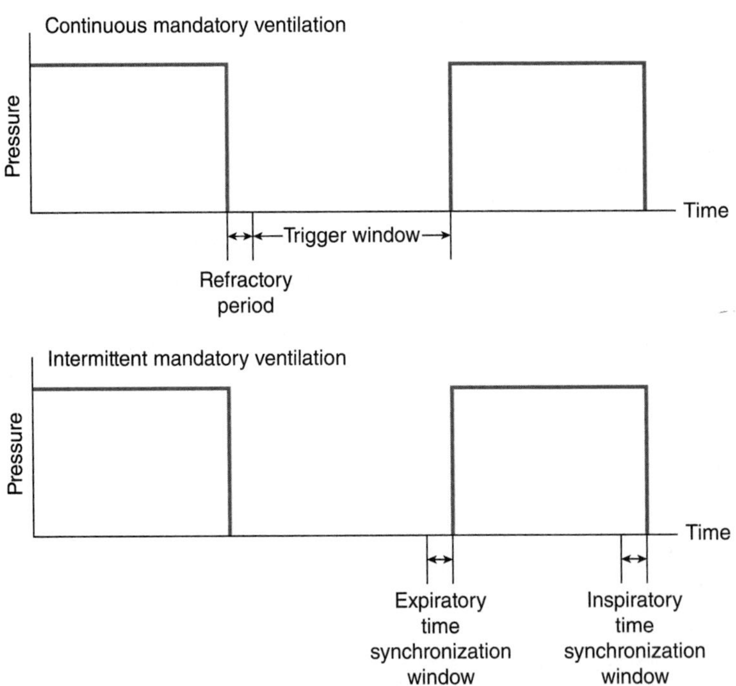

FIGURE 58–1 Trigger and synchronization windows. If a patient signal occurs within the trigger window, inspiration is patient triggered. If a patient signal occurs within a synchronization window, inspiration is ventilator triggered (or cycled if at the end of inspiration) and patient synchronized. Note that, in general, a trigger window is used with continuous mandatory ventilation, and a synchronization window is used with intermittent mandatory ventilation. (Reproduced with permission from Chatburn RL, Khatib M, Mireles-Cabodevila E. A taxonomy for mechanical ventilation: 10 fundamental maxims. *Resp Care.* 2014 Nov;59(11):1747-1763.)

The target variable (pressure, volume, or flow) must reach a specified level before inspiration ends. This used to be called "limit," but nomenclatures have changed. The target variable does not define the end of inspiration but only the upper boundary for each breath. When the cycle variable is reached, inspiration ends. Options include pressure, volume, flow, or time.

Pressure-cycled ventilators cycle into the expiratory phase when airway pressure reaches a predetermined limit. V_T and inspiratory time vary, being related to airway resistance and pulmonary and circuit compliance. A significant leak in the patient circuit can prevent the necessary rise in circuit pressure and machine cycling. Conversely, an acute increase in airway resistance or a decrease in pulmonary compliance or circuit compliance (eg, a kinked tube) causes premature cycling and decreases delivered V_T. Pressure-cycled ventilators have been most often used for short-term indications (eg, transport).

Volume-cycled ventilators terminate inspiration when a preselected volume is delivered. Many adult ventilators are volume cycled but also have secondary limits on inspiratory pressure to guard against pulmonary barotrauma. If inspiratory pressure exceeds the pressure limit, the machine cycles into expiration even if the selected V_T has not been delivered.

Properly functioning volume-cycled ventilators do not deliver the set V_T to the patient. A percentage of the set V_T is always lost due to expansion of the breathing circuit during inspiration. Circuit compliance is usually about 3 to 5 mL/cm H_2O; thus, if a pressure of 30 cm H_2O is generated during inspiration, 90 to 150 mL of the set V_T is lost to the circuit. Loss of V_T from expansion of the breathing circuit is therefore inversely related to lung compliance. For accurate measurement of the exhaled V_T, the spirometer must be placed at the tracheal tube rather than the exhalation valve of the ventilator.

Flow-cycled ventilators have pressure and flow sensors that allow the ventilator to monitor inspiratory flow at a preselected fixed inspiratory pressure; when this flow reaches a predetermined level (usually 25% of the initial peak mechanical inspiratory flow rate), the ventilator cycles from inspiration into expiration (see the later sections on pressure support and pressure-controlled ventilation).

Time-cycled ventilators cycle to the expiratory phase once a predetermined interval elapses from the start of inspiration. V_T is the product of the set inspiratory time and inspiratory flow rate. Time-cycled ventilators are commonly used for neonates and in the operating room.

Ventilator Modes

A ventilator mode is a combination of control variable, breath sequence, and target scheme. Additionally, to understand ventilator mechanics, one must consider the phase variables mentioned earlier.

Control Variables

The control variable is the independent variable in the ventilator mode (Figure 58–2). The choices are pressure, volume, and flow. In pressure-controlled ventilation (PCV), pressure is an independent variable, and pressure waveform is specified (eg, rectangular waveform). In volume-controlled ventilation (VCV), a volume waveform is defined. In common terminology, flow-controlled ventilation is not commonly used because flow is derivative of volume. When one directly controls volume, one indirectly controls flow.

Targeting Scheme

Targeting scheme is a feedback control design to deliver a specific pattern. A type of targeting scheme called *set point targeting* is the most basic. One sets a value, and the ventilator seeks to deliver it. For VCV, set points would be V_T and flow. For PCV, commonly it would be inspiratory pressure and inspiratory time.

Breath Sequence

Breath sequence is the pattern of mandatory or spontaneous breaths in a ventilator mode, or both (Figure 58–3). In a spontaneous breath, the patient determines both the timing and the size of the breath. Thus, it is patient-triggered and patient-cycled. A *mandatory breath* is any breath that is not spontaneous. An a*ssisted breath* is a breath in which the ventilator does some of the work for a patient-initiated breath.

There are three possible breath sequences. *Continuous spontaneous ventilation* (CSV) is a sequence

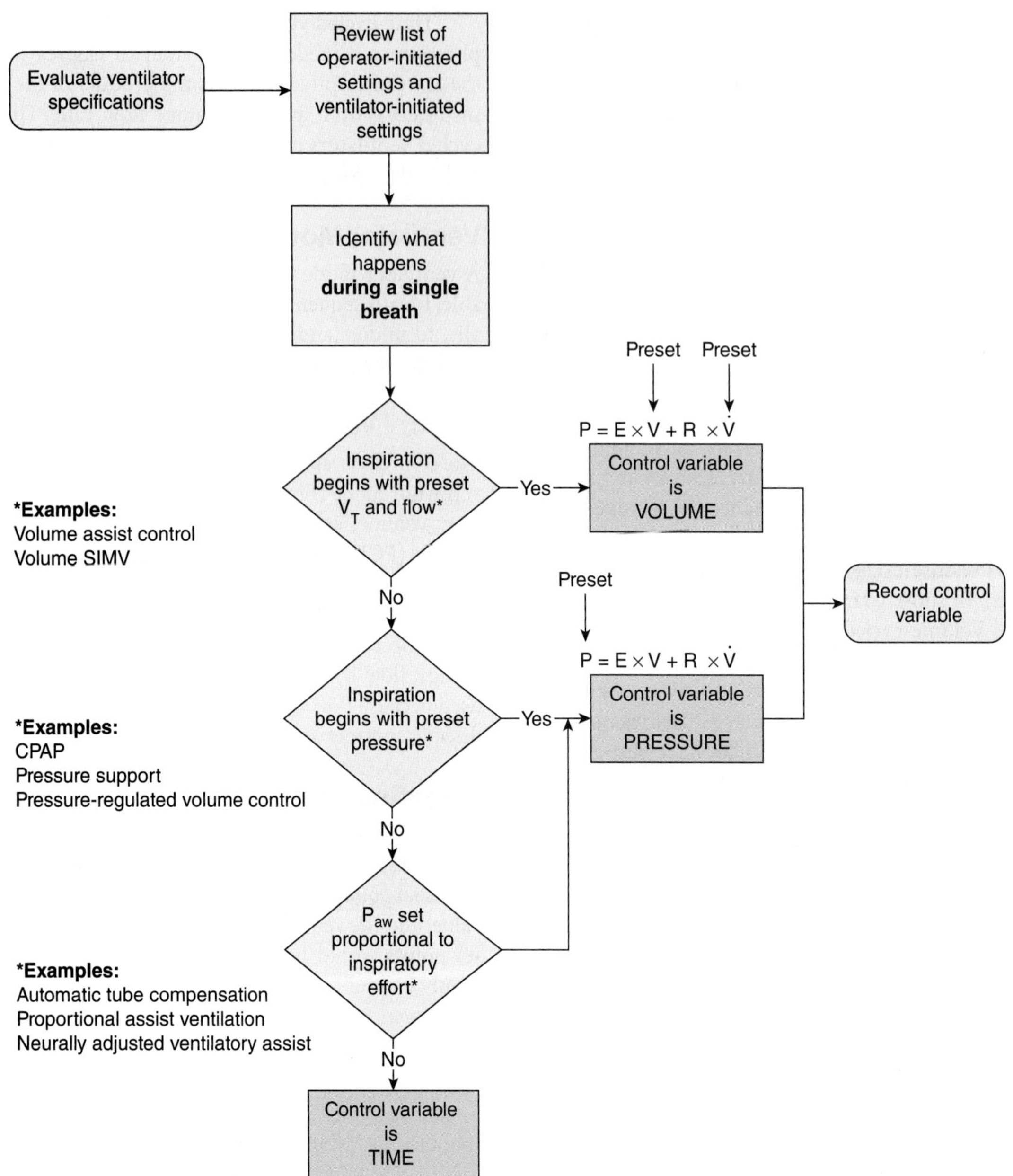

FIGURE 58–2 Rubric for determining the control variable of a mode. CPAP, continuous positive airway pressure; E, elastance; P, pressure; P_{aw}, airway pressure; R, resistance; SIMV, synchronized intermittent mandatory ventilation; V, volume; $\dot{V}$, inspiratory flow; V_T, tidal volume. (Reproduced with permission from Mandu Press. Cleveland, Ohio.)

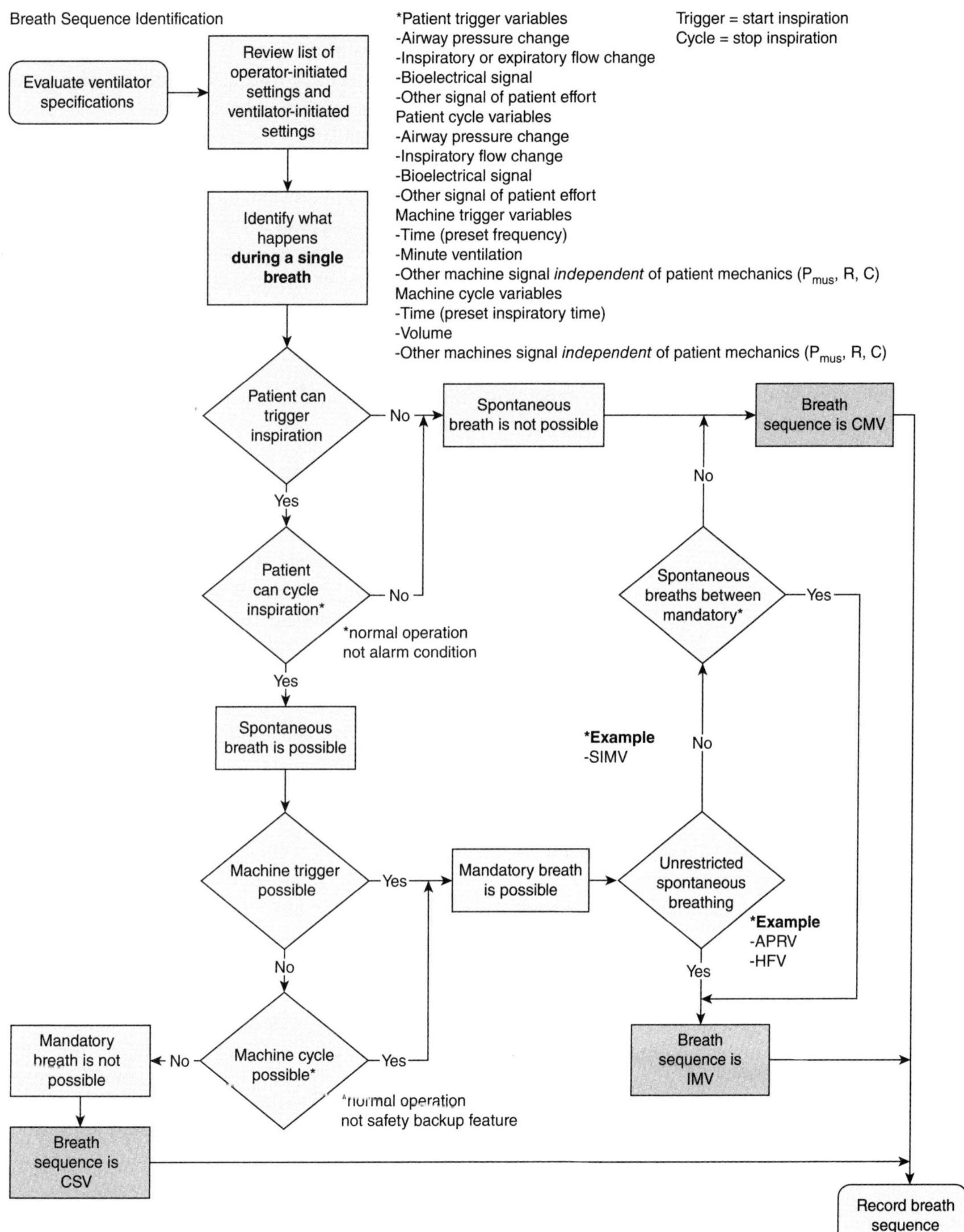

FIGURE 58–3 Rubric for determining the breath sequence of a mode. APRV, airway pressure release ventilation; C, compliance; CMV, continuous mandatory ventilation; CSV, continuous spontaneous ventilation; HFV, high-frequency ventilation; IMV, intermittent mandatory ventilation; P_{mus}, ventilatory muscle pressure; R, resistance. (Reproduced with permission from Mandu Press. Cleveland, Ohio.)

in which all breaths are spontaneous. *Intermittently mandatory ventilation* (IMV) is a sequence in which spontaneous breaths are permitted in between mandatory breaths. If a mandatory breath is triggered by the patient, it is a "synchronized" mandatory breath. In *continuous mandatory ventilation* (CMV), all breaths (including those by patient effort) are mandatory.

Combining the two types of control variables (pressure control [PC] and volume control [VC]) with three breath sequences gives us five breathing patterns: VC-CMV, VC-IMV, PC-CMV, PC-IMV, and PC-CSV. The sixth, VC-CSV, would mean that patient would specify the time and size of breath; however, in VC mode, a patient could not specify the size of breath.

A. IMV Breath Sequences

IMV permits spontaneous ventilation. A selected number of mechanical breaths (with fixed V_T) are given to supplement spontaneous breathing. At increased mandatory rates (10–12 breaths/min), IMV essentially provides all of the patient's ventilation; at reduced rates (1–2 breaths/min), it provides minimal mechanical ventilation and allows the patient to breathe almost independently. The frequency and V_T of spontaneous breaths are determined by the patient's ventilatory drive and muscle strength. The IMV rate can be adjusted to maintain the desired minute ventilation. IMV has found the greatest use as a weaning technique.

Synchronized intermittent mandatory ventilation (SIMV) times the mechanical breath, whenever possible, to coincide with the beginning of a spontaneous effort. Proper synchronization prevents superimposing (stacking) a mechanical breath in the middle of a spontaneous breath, which might otherwise result in a very large V_T. As with CMV and *assist-control (AC) ventilation* (discussed next), settings limiting inspiratory pressure guard against pulmonary barotrauma. The great advantage of SIMV over IMV is that it provides for increased patient comfort. When IMV or SIMV are used for weaning, machine breaths provide a backup if the patient becomes fatigued. However, if the rate is set too low (4 breaths/min), the backup may be insufficient, particularly for weak patients who cannot overcome the added work of breathing during spontaneous breaths.

IMV circuits provide a continuous flow of gas for spontaneous ventilation between mechanical breaths. Modern ventilators incorporate SIMV into their design, but older models required modification with a parallel circuit, a continuous flow system, or a demand flow valve. Regardless of the system, proper functioning of one-way valves and sufficient gas flow are necessary to prevent an increase in the patient's work of breathing, particularly when PEEP is also used.

Thus far, the discussion of IMV has assumed this to be a volume-limited format; however, IMV can also be provided in a pressure-limited format if desired (as described next).

B. Pressure-Controlled Breath Sequences (PC-CMV, PC-IMV, and PC-CSV)

PC breath sequences may be used in both the AC and IMV modes. In AC mode, all breaths (either machine initiated or patient initiated) are time cycled and pressure limited. In IMV, machine-initiated breaths are time cycled and pressure limited. The patient may breathe spontaneously between the set rate, and the V_T of the spontaneous breaths is determined by the patient. The advantage of PCV is that by limiting inspiratory pressure, the risks of barotrauma and volutrauma may be decreased. Also, by extending inspiratory time, better mixing and recruitment of collapsed or flooded alveoli may be achieved when used with adequate PEEP levels. 2 The disadvantage of conventional PCV is that V_T is not guaranteed (though there are modes in which the consistent delivered pressure of PCV can be combined with a predefined volume delivery). Changes in compliance or resistance will affect delivered V_T. This is a major concern in patients with acute lung injury because if the compliance decreases and the pressure limit is not increased, adequate V_T may not be attained. PCV has been used for patients with acute lung injury or ARDS, often with a prolonged inspiratory time or *inverse inspiratory/expiratory (I:E) ratio ventilation* (IRV) (see later discussion) in an effort to recruit collapsed and flooded alveoli. The disadvantage of using IRV with PCV is that patients will require deep sedation, perhaps with paralysis, to tolerate this ventilatory mode.

With PCV, pressure and inspiratory time are preset, whereas flow and volume are variable and dependent on the patient's resistance and compliance. With volume ventilation, on the other hand, inspiratory time is also preset, but flow and VT are also preset, and with increased resistance or reduced compliance, the inspiratory pressure can be greatly increased.

3 PCV is similar to pressure support ventilation (PSV) in that peak airway pressure is controlled but is different in that a mandatory rate and inspiratory time are selected. As with pressure support, gas flow ceases when the pressure level is reached; however, the ventilator does not cycle to expiration until the preset inspiration time has elapsed.

Mode Examples

A. Continuous Mandatory Ventilation (Example of VC-CMV Breathing Pattern)

In this mode, the ventilator cycles from expiration to inspiration after a fixed time interval. The interval determines the ventilatory rate. Typical settings on this mode provide a fixed VT and fixed rate (and, therefore, minute ventilation) regardless of patient effort because *the patient cannot breathe spontaneously*. Settings to limit inspiratory pressure guard against pulmonary barotrauma, and indeed CMV can be provided in a pressure-limited (rather than volume-limited) way. Controlled ventilation is best reserved for patients capable of little or no ventilatory effort. Awake patients with active ventilatory effort require sedation, possibly with muscle paralysis, to safely receive CMV.

B. Assist-Control Ventilation (Example of VC-CMV Breathing Pattern, or Can Be Set as PC-CMV)

Incorporation of a pressure sensor in the breathing circuit of AC ventilators permits the patient's inspiratory effort to be used to trigger inspiration. A sensitivity control allows the selection of the inspiratory effort required. *The ventilator can be set for a fixed ventilatory rate, but each patient effort of sufficient magnitude will trigger the set* VT. If spontaneous inspiratory efforts are not detected, the machine functions as if in the control mode. Most often, AC ventilation is used in a volume-limited format, but it can also be provided in a pressure-limited way (as discussed later).

C. Pressure Support Ventilation (Example of PC-CSV Breathing Pattern)

PSV was designed to augment the VT of spontaneously breathing patients and overcome any increased inspiratory resistance from the tracheal tube, breathing circuit (tubing, connectors, and humidifier), and ventilator (pneumatic circuitry and valves). Microprocessor-controlled machines have this mode, which delivers sufficient gas flow with every inspiratory effort to maintain a predetermined positive pressure throughout inspiration. When inspiratory flow decreases to a predetermined level, the ventilator's feedback (servo) loop cycles the machine into the expiratory phase, and airway pressure returns to baseline (Figure 58–4). The only setting in this mode is inspiratory pressure. The patient determines the respiratory rate, and VT varies according to inspiratory gas flow, lung mechanics, and the patient's own inspiratory effort. Low levels of PSV (5–10 cm H_2O) are usually sufficient to overcome any added resistance imposed by the breathing apparatus. Higher levels (10–40 cm H_2O) can function as a standalone ventilatory mode if the patient has sufficient spontaneous ventilatory drive and stable lung mechanics. The principal advantages of PSV are its ability to augment spontaneous VT, decrease the work of breathing, and increase patient comfort. However, if the

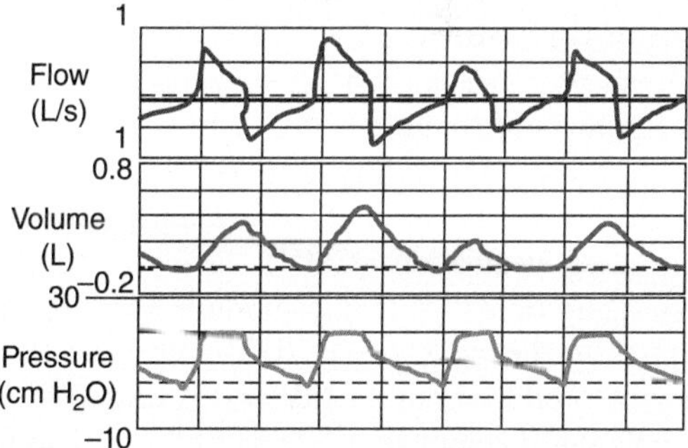

FIGURE 58–4 Pressure support ventilation. The patient initiates a breath; the machine is set to deliver 15 cm H_2O pressure (above 5 cm H_2O of continuous positive airway pressure [CPAP]). When flow ceases, the machine cycles into the expiratory mode.

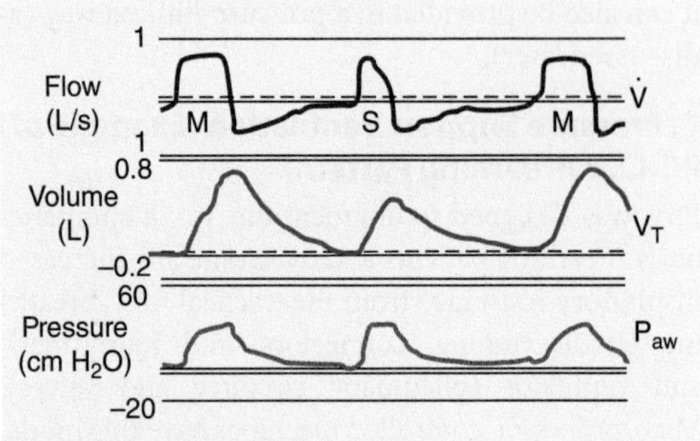

FIGURE 58–5 Intermittent mechanical ventilation with pressure support. M = machine breath → set tidal volume (VT) delivered. S = spontaneous breath, 15 cm of pressure support over 5 cm of positive end-expiratory pressure. VT depends on patient effort and lungh mechanics. V, flow; P_{aw}, partial airway pressure.

patient fatigues or lung mechanics change, VT may be inadequate, and there is no backup rate if the patient's intrinsic respiratory rate decreases (eg, after opioid dosing). Note that one can add "pressure support" to IMV breathing breath sequences (Figure 58–5). The IMV machine mandatory breaths provide backup, and a low level of pressure support is used to offset the increased work of breathing resulting from the endotracheal tube, breathing circuit, and machine during the spontaneous breaths.

D. Inverse I:E Ratio Ventilation Modes, Including Airway Pressure Release Ventilation (Usually Examples of PC-IMV Breathing Pattern)

IRV reverses the normal I:E time ratio of 1:3 or greater to a ratio of greater than 1:1 (eg, 1.5:1). This may be achieved by adding an end-inspiratory pause, by decreasing peak inspiratory flow during volume-controlled ventilation (CMV), or by setting an inspiratory time such that inspiration is longer than expiration during PCV (PC-IRV). Intrinsic PEEP may be produced during IRV and is caused by air trapping or incomplete emptying of the lung to the baseline pressure prior to the initiation of the next breath. This air trapping increases FRC until a new equilibrium is reached. This mode does not allow spontaneous breathing and requires heavy sedation or neuromuscular blockade. IRV with PEEP is effective for improving oxygenation in patients with decreased FRC.

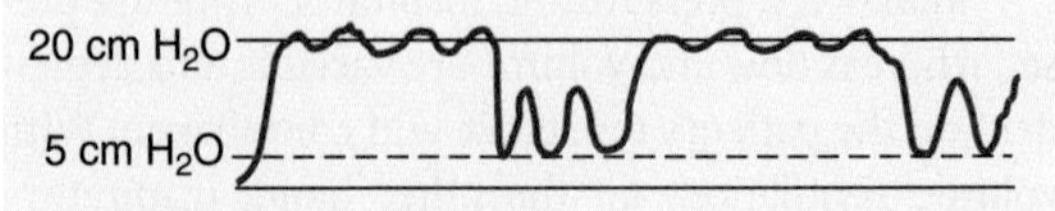

FIGURE 58–6 Airway pressure release ventilation.

E. Airway Pressure Release Ventilation

Airway pressure release ventilation (APRV), or bilevel ventilation, is a mode in which a relatively high PEEP is used, despite the patient being allowed to breathe spontaneously. Intermittently, the PEEP level decreases to help augment the elimination of CO_2 (Figure 58–6). The inspiratory and expiratory times, high and low PEEP levels, and spontaneous respiratory activity determine minute ventilation. Initial settings include a minimum PEEP of 10 to 12 cm H_2O and a release level of 5 to 10 cm H_2O. Commonly, 10 to 12 releases are chosen as a starting point, along with a time at low PEEP to allow only 50% to 70% of expiratory flow (to provide "auto PEEP"). Advantages of APRV appear to be less circulatory depression and pulmonary barotrauma as well as less need for sedation. This technique appears to be an attractive alternative to PC-IRV for overcoming problems with high peak inspiratory pressures in patients with reduced lung compliance.

Basic Mechanics of Ventilators

Most modern ventilators behave like flow generators. Constant flow generators deliver a constant inspiratory gas flow regardless of airway circuit pressure. Constant flow is produced by the use of either a solenoid (on–off) valve with a high-pressure gas source (5–50 psi) or via a gas injector (Venturi) with a lower-pressure source. Machines with high-pressure gas sources allow inspiratory gas flow to remain constant despite large changes in airway resistance or pulmonary compliance. Ventilator performance varies with airway pressure for gas injectors. Nonconstant flow generators consistently vary inspiratory flow with each inspiratory cycle (such as by a rotary piston); a sine wave pattern of flow is typical.

Constant-pressure generators maintain airway pressure constant throughout inspiration and irrespective of inspiratory gas flow. Gas flow ceases when airway pressure equals the set inspiratory pressure. Pressure generators typically operate at low gas pressures (just above peak inspiratory pressure).

Cycling (Changeover from Inspiration to Expiration)

Time-cycled ventilators cycle to the expiratory phase once a predetermined interval elapses from the start of inspiration. VT is the product of the set inspiratory time and inspiratory flow rate. Time-cycled ventilators are commonly used for neonates and in the operating room.

Volume-cycled ventilators terminate inspiration when a preselected volume is delivered. Many adult ventilators are volume cycled but also have secondary limits on inspiratory pressure to guard against pulmonary barotrauma. If inspiratory pressure exceeds the pressure limit, the machine cycles into expiration even if the selected volume has not been delivered.

Pressure-cycled ventilators cycle into the expiratory phase when airway pressure reaches a predetermined level. VT and inspiratory time vary, being related to airway resistance and pulmonary and circuit compliance. A significant leak in the patient circuit can prevent the necessary rise in circuit pressure and machine cycling. Conversely, an acute increase in airway resistance, or decrease in pulmonary compliance, or circuit compliance (kink) causes premature cycling and decreases the delivered VT.

Flow-cycled ventilators have pressure and flow sensors that allow the ventilator to monitor inspiratory flow at a preselected fixed inspiratory pressure; when this flow reaches a predetermined level (usually 25% of the initial peak mechanical inspiratory flow rate), the ventilator cycles from inspiration into expiration (see the earlier sections on pressure support and pressure-controlled ventilation).

Microprocessor-Controlled Ventilators

These versatile machines can be set to function in any one of a variety of inspiratory flow and cycling patterns. Microprocessor-controlled ventilators are the current norm in critical care units and on newer anesthesia machines.

High-Frequency Ventilation

High-frequency ventilation is sufficiently different from conventional modes of mechanical ventilation that its mechanics require separate mention. Three forms of high-frequency ventilation (HFV) are available. High-frequency positive-pressure ventilation involves delivering a small "conventional" VT at a rate of 60 to 120 breaths/min. High-frequency jet ventilation (HFJV) utilizes a small cannula at or in the airway through which a pulsed jet of high-pressure gas is delivered at a set frequency of 120 to 600 times/min (2–10 Hz). The jet of gas may entrain air (Bernoulli effect), which may augment VT. High-frequency oscillation employs a driver (usually a piston) that creates to-and-fro gas movement in the airway at rates of 180 to 3000 times/min (3–50 Hz).

These forms of ventilation all produce VT at or below anatomic dead space. The exact mechanism of gas exchange is unclear but is probably a combination of effects. Jet ventilation has found the widest use in the operating room for laryngeal, tracheal, and bronchial procedures. In the intensive care unit (ICU), HFJV may be useful in managing some patients with bronchopleural and tracheoesophageal fistulas when conventional ventilation has failed. Occasionally, HFJV or high-frequency oscillation is used in patients with ARDS to try to improve oxygenation. Inadequate heating and humidification of inspired gases during prolonged HFV, however, can be a problem. Initial settings for HFJV are typically a rate of 120 to 240 breaths/min, an inspiratory time of 33%, and a drive pressure of 15 to 30 psi. Mean airway pressure should be measured in the trachea at least 5 cm below the injector to avoid an artifactual error from gas entrainment. CO_2 elimination is generally increased by increasing the drive pressure, whereas adequacy of oxygenation relates to the mean airway pressure. An intrinsic PEEP effect is seen during HFJV at high drive pressures and inspiratory times greater than 40%.

Differential Lung Ventilation

This technique, also referred to as *independent lung ventilation*, may be used in patients with severe unilateral lung disease or those with bronchopleural fistulae.

The use of conventional positive-pressure ventilation and PEEP in such instances can aggravate ventilation/perfusion mismatching or, in patients with fistula, result in inadequate ventilation of the unaffected lung. In patients with restrictive disease of one lung, overdistention of the normal lung can lead to worsening hypoxemia or barotrauma. With the correct placement of a double-lumen endotracheal tube, positive-pressure ventilation can be applied to each lung independently using two ventilators. When two ventilators are used, the timing of mechanical breaths is often synchronized, with one ventilator, the "master," setting the rate for the "slave" ventilator.

2. Care of Patients Requiring Mechanical Ventilation

Tracheal Intubation

Tracheal intubation is most commonly undertaken in critically ill patients to manage pulmonary failure with mechanical ventilation. **4** Both nasotracheal and orotracheal intubation appear to be relatively safe for at least 2 to 3 weeks. When compared with orotracheal intubation, nasotracheal intubation may be more comfortable and more secure for the patient (fewer instances of accidental extubation). Nasal intubation, however, has its own set of associated adverse events, including nasal bleeding, transient bacteremia, submucosal dissection of the nasopharynx or oropharynx, and sinusitis or otitis media (from obstruction of sinus outflow or of the auditory tubes). Nasal intubations will also generally incorporate a smaller diameter tube than orotracheal intubations, and this can make it more difficult to clear secretions and can limit the clinician to smaller fiberoptic bronchoscopes.

Intubation often can be carried out without the use of sedation or muscle paralysis in agonal or unconscious patients. However, topical anesthesia of the airway and sedation are helpful in patients who still have active airway reflexes. More vigorous and uncooperative patients require varying degrees of sedation. Small doses of relatively short-acting agents are generally used; popular agents include midazolam, etomidate, dexmedetomidine, and propofol. If necessary, a neuromuscular blocker can be used for paralysis after a hypnotic is given.

The time of endotracheal intubation and initiation of mechanical ventilation can be periods of great hemodynamic instability. Hypertension, hypotension, bradycardia, or tachycardia may be encountered as a consequence of airway stimulation, drug effects, straining by the patient, and reduced venous return due to airway positive pressure. Careful monitoring is required during and immediately following intubation of patients with critical illness.

5 When left in place for more than 2 to 3 weeks, both orotracheal and nasotracheal tubes predispose patients to subglottic stenosis. If longer periods of mechanical ventilation are necessary, the endotracheal tube should be replaced by a cuffed tracheostomy tube. If it is clear that an endotracheal tube will be required for more than 2 weeks, a tracheostomy may be performed soon after intubation. While earlier tracheostomy does not reduce mortality, it may reduce the incidence of pneumonia, the duration of mechanical ventilation, and the length of stay.

Initial Ventilator Settings

Depending on the type of pulmonary failure, mechanical ventilation is used to provide either partial or full ventilatory support. For full ventilatory support, CMV, AC, or PCV is generally employed with a respiratory rate of 10 to 14 breaths/min, a VT of 6 mL/kg, and PEEP of 5 to 10 cm H_2O. These settings reduce the likelihood of high peak inflation pressures (greater than 35 to 40 cm H_2O), barotrauma, and volutrauma. Excessive airway pressures that overdistend alveoli (transalveolar pressure >35 cm H_2O) promote lung injury in experimental settings. **6** Likewise, compared with a VT of 12 mL/kg, a VT of 6 mL/kg and plateau pressure (P_{plt}) less than 30 cm H_2O reduces the likelihood of mortality in patients with ARDS. Partial ventilatory support is usually provided by lower SIMV settings (<8 breaths/min), either with or without pressure support. Lower P_{plt} (<20–30 cm H_2O) is recommended to better preserve cardiac output and lessen adverse effects on ventilation/perfusion relationships.

Patients breathing spontaneously on SIMV must overcome the additional resistances of the endotracheal tube, demand valves, and breathing circuit of the ventilator. These imposed resistances increase the work of breathing. Smaller tubes (<7.0 mm internal diameter in adults) increase resistance and should be avoided if possible. The simultaneous use of pressure support of 5 to 15 cm H_2O during SIMV can compensate for tube and circuit resistance.

The addition of 5 to 8 cm H_2O of PEEP during positive-pressure ventilation preserves FRC and gas exchange. This "physiological" PEEP is purported to compensate for the loss of a similar amount of intrinsic PEEP (and decrease in FRC) in patients following tracheal intubation. Periodic sigh breaths (large VT) are not necessary when a PEEP of 5 to 8 cm H_2O accompanies VT of appropriate volumes.

Sedation & Paralysis

Sedation and paralysis may be necessary for patients who become agitated and "fight" the ventilator. Repetitive coughing ("bucking") and straining can have adverse hemodynamic effects, can interfere with gas exchange, and may predispose to pulmonary barotrauma and self-inflicted injury. Sedation with or without paralysis may also be desirable when patients continue to be tachypneic despite high mechanical respiratory rates (>16–18 breaths/min).

Commonly used sedatives include opioids (morphine or fentanyl), benzodiazepines (usually midazolam), propofol, and dexmedetomidine. These agents may be used alone or in combination and are often administered by continuous infusion. Propofol is avoided for prolonged sedation due to concerns about *propofol infusion syndrome* (see Chapter 9). Nondepolarizing paralytic agents are used in combination with sedation when ventilation cannot otherwise be accomplished.

Monitoring

Critically ill patients receiving mechanical ventilation should be cared for in a head-up position to reduce the risk of ventilator-associated pneumonia unless prone positioning is required to optimize oxygenation (eg, patients with COVID-19). Mechanically ventilated patients require continuous monitoring for adverse hemodynamic and pulmonary effects arising from positive pressure in the airways. Continuous electrocardiography, pulse oximetry, and capnometry are nearly universal. Direct intraarterial pressure monitoring is often employed for sampling of arterial blood for respiratory gas analysis. Accurate recording of fluid intake and output is necessary to assess fluid balance. An indwelling urinary catheter will lead to an increased risk of urinary tract infections and should be avoided when possible, but it is helpful for monitoring urinary output. Chest radiographs are commonly obtained to confirm endotracheal tube and central venous catheter positions, evaluate for evidence of pulmonary barotrauma or pulmonary disease, and identify signs of pulmonary edema.

Airway pressures (baseline, peak, plateau, and mean), inhaled and exhaled VT (mechanical and spontaneous), and fractional concentration of O_2 should be closely monitored. Monitoring these parameters not only allows optimal adjustment of ventilator settings but also helps detect problems with the endotracheal tube, breathing circuit, or ventilator. For example, an increasing P_{plt} for a set VT can indicate worsening compliance. A declining blood pressure and increasing P_{plt} from dynamic hyperinflation (autoPEEP) can be quickly diagnosed and treated by disconnecting the patient from the ventilator. Inadequate suctioning of airway secretions and the presence of large mucus plugs are often manifested as increasing peak inflation pressures (a sign of increased resistance to gas flow) and decreasing exhaled VT. An abrupt increase in peak inflation pressure together with sudden hypotension strongly suggests a pneumothorax.

3. Discontinuing Mechanical Ventilation

There are two phases to discontinuing mechanical ventilation. In the first, "readiness testing," so-called weaning parameters and other assessments are used to determine whether the patient can tolerate progressive withdrawal of mechanical ventilator support. The second phase, "weaning" or "liberation," describes the way in which mechanical support is removed.

Readiness testing should include determining whether the process that necessitated mechanical ventilation has been reversed or controlled. Complicating factors including bronchospasm, heart failure, infection, malnutrition, increased CO_2

production due to increased carbohydrate loads, acid–base derangements, anemia, altered mental status, and sleep deprivation should be adequately treated. In addition to the listed conditions, chronic lung disease and respiratory muscle wasting from prolonged disuse (frailty) may lead to failed or prolonged weaning.

Weaning from mechanical ventilation should be considered when patients no longer meet the criteria for mechanical ventilation (see **Table 58–4**). In general, this occurs when patients have a pH greater than 7.25, show adequate arterial O_2 saturation while receiving FiO_2 less than 0.5, are able to spontaneously breathe, are hemodynamically stable, and have no current signs of myocardial ischemia. Additional mechanical indices have also been suggested (Table 58–5). Useful weaning parameters include arterial blood gas tensions, respiratory rate, and rapid shallow breathing index (RSBI). For successful weaning and extubation, intact airway reflexes are mandatory, and a cooperative patient is helpful, unless the patient will retain a cuffed tracheostomy tube. Similarly, adequate oxygenation (arterial O_2 saturation >90% on 40–50% O_2 with <5 cm H_2O of PEEP) is mandatory prior to extubation. When the patient is weaned from mechanical ventilation and extubation is planned, the RSBI is frequently used to help predict who can be successfully weaned from mechanical ventilation and extubated. With the patient breathing spontaneously on a T-piece, the V_T (in liters) and respiratory rate (*f*) are measured:

$$\text{RSBI} = \frac{f\,(\text{breaths/min})}{V_T(\text{L})}$$

TABLE 58–5 Mechanical criteria for weaning/extubation.

Criterion	Measurement
Inspiratory pressure	<–25 cm H_2O
Tidal volume	>5 mL/kg
Vital capacity	>10 mL/kg
Minute ventilation	<10 mL
Rapid shallow breathing index	<100

Most patients with an RSBI less than 105 breaths/min/L can be successfully extubated. Those with an RSBI greater than 120 should retain some degree of mechanical ventilator support.

The common techniques to wean a patient from the ventilator include SIMV, pressure support, or periods of spontaneous breathing alone on a T-piece or on low levels of CPAP. Many institutions use "automated tube compensation" to provide just enough pressure support to compensate for the resistance of breathing through an endotracheal tube. Newer mechanical ventilators have a setting that will automatically adjust gas flows to make this adjustment. In practice in adults breathing through conventionally sized tubes (7.5–8.5), the adjustment will typically amount to pressure support of 5 cm H_2O and PEEP of 5 cm H_2O.

Weaning with SIMV

With SIMV the number of mechanical breaths is progressively decreased (by 1–2 breaths/min) as long as the arterial CO_2 tension and respiratory rate remain acceptable (generally <45–50 mm Hg and <30 breaths/min, respectively). If pressure support is concomitantly used, it should generally be reduced to 5 to 8 cm H_2O. In patients with acid–base disturbances or chronic CO_2 retention, arterial blood pH (>7.35) is more useful than CO_2 tension. Blood gas measurements can be checked after a minimum of 15 to 30 min at each setting. When an IMV of 2 to 4 breaths is reached, mechanical ventilation is discontinued if arterial oxygenation remains acceptable.

Weaning with PSV

Weaning with PSV alone is accomplished by gradually decreasing the pressure support level by 2 to 3 cm H_2O while V_T, arterial blood gas tensions, and respiratory rate are monitored (using the same criteria as for IMV). The goal is to try to ensure a V_T of 4 to 6 mL/kg and an *f* of less than 30 with acceptable PaO_2 and $PaCO_2$. When a pressure support level of 5 to 8 cm H_2O is reached, the patient is considered weaned.

Weaning with a T-Piece or CPAP

T-piece trials allow observation while the patient breathes spontaneously without any mechanical breaths. The T-piece attaches directly to the endotracheal tube or tracheostomy tube and has corrugated tubing on the other two limbs. A humidified oxygen–air mixture flows into the proximal limb and exits from the distal limb. Sufficient gas flow must be given in the proximal limb to prevent the mist from being completely drawn back at the distal limb during inspiration; this ensures that the patient is receiving the desired oxygen concentration. The patient is observed closely during this period; obvious new signs of fatigue, chest retractions, tachypnea, tachycardia, arrhythmias, or hypertension or hypotension should terminate the trial. If the patient appears to tolerate the trial period and the RSBI is less than 105, mechanical ventilation can be discontinued permanently. If the patient can also protect and clear the airway, the endotracheal tube can be removed.

If the patient has been intubated for a prolonged period or has severe underlying lung disease, sequential T-piece trials may be necessary. Periodic trials of 10 to 30 min are initiated and progressively increased, typically by 5 to 10 min per trial as long as the patient appears comfortable, maintains acceptable arterial saturation, and does not become hypercarbic.

Many patients develop progressive atelectasis during prolonged T-piece trials. This may reflect the absence of a normal "physiological" PEEP when the larynx is bypassed by an endotracheal tube. If this is a concern, spontaneous breathing trials on low levels (5 cm H_2O) of CPAP can help maintain FRC and prevent atelectasis.

POSITIVE AIRWAY PRESSURE THERAPY

Positive airway pressure therapy can be used in patients who are breathing spontaneously as well as those who are mechanically ventilated. The principal indication for positive airway pressure therapy is a decrease in FRC resulting in absolute or relative hypoxemia. By increasing transpulmonary distending pressure, positive airway pressure therapy can increase FRC, improve (increase) lung compliance, and reverse ventilation/perfusion mismatching. Improvement in the latter parameter will show as a decrease in venous admixture and an improvement in arterial O_2 tension.

Positive End-Expiratory Pressure (PEEP)

Application of positive pressure during expiration as an adjunct to a mechanically delivered breath is referred to as *positive end-expiratory pressure* or *PEEP*. The ventilator's PEEP valve provides a pressure threshold that allows expiratory flow to occur only when airway pressure exceeds the selected PEEP level.

Continuous Positive Airway Pressure (CPAP)

Application of a positive-pressure threshold during both inspiration and expiration with spontaneous breathing is referred to as *CPAP*. Constant levels of pressure can be attained only if a high-flow (inspiratory) gas source is provided. When the patient does not have an artificial airway, tightly fitting masks can be used. Because of the risks of gastric distention and regurgitation, CPAP masks should be used only on patients with intact airway reflexes and with CPAP levels less than 15 cm H_2O (less than lower esophageal sphincter pressure in normal persons). Expiratory pressures greater than 15 cm H_2O should only be administered by tracheal or tracheostomy tube.

CPAP versus PEEP

The distinction between PEEP and CPAP is often blurred in the clinical setting because patients may breathe with a combination of mechanical and spontaneous breaths. Therefore, the two terms are often used interchangeably. In the strictest sense, "pure" PEEP is provided as a ventilator-cycled breath. In contrast, a "pure" CPAP system provides only sufficient continuous or "on-demand" gas flows (60–90 L/min) to prevent inspiratory airway pressure from falling perceptibly below the expiratory level during spontaneous breaths (Figure 58–7). Some ventilators with demand valve–based CPAP systems may not be adequately responsive and result in increased inspiratory work of breathing. This situation can be corrected by adding low levels of (inspiratory)

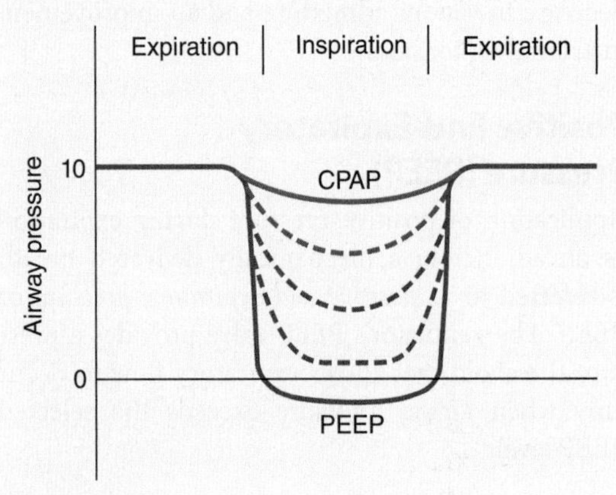

FIGURE 58–7 Airway pressure during positive end-expiratory pressure (PEEP) and continuous positive airway pressure (CPAP). Note that by increasing inspiratory gas flows, PEEP progressively becomes CPAP.

PSV if in a volume-targeted mode or changing to a pressure-targeted mode. In clinical practice, controlled ventilation, PSV, and CPAP/PEEP support can be delivered by most modern ICU ventilators. Manufacturers have also developed specific devices to deliver bilevel inspiratory positive airway pressure (IPAP) with expiratory positive airway pressure (EPAP) in either a spontaneous or time-cycled fashion. The term *bilevel positive airway pressure* (BiPAP) has become a commonly used phrase, adding to the confusion of airway pressure terminology.

Pulmonary Effects of PEEP & CPAP

7 The major effect of PEEP and CPAP on the lungs is to increase FRC. In patients with decreased lung volume, appropriate levels of either PEEP or CPAP will increase FRC and tidal ventilation above closing capacity, improve lung compliance, and correct ventilation/perfusion abnormalities. The resulting decrease in intrapulmonary shunting improves arterial oxygenation. The principal mechanism of action for both PEEP and CPAP appears to be the expansion of partially collapsed alveoli. Recruitment (reexpansion) of collapsed alveoli occurs at PEEP or CPAP levels above the inflection point, defined as the pressure level on a pressure–volume curve at which collapsed alveoli are recruited (open); with small changes in pressure, there are large changes in volume (Figure 58–8). Although neither PEEP nor CPAP decreases total extravascular lung water, studies suggest that they do redistribute extravascular lung water from the interstitial space between alveoli and endothelial cells toward peribronchial and perihilar areas. Both effects can potentially improve arterial oxygenation.

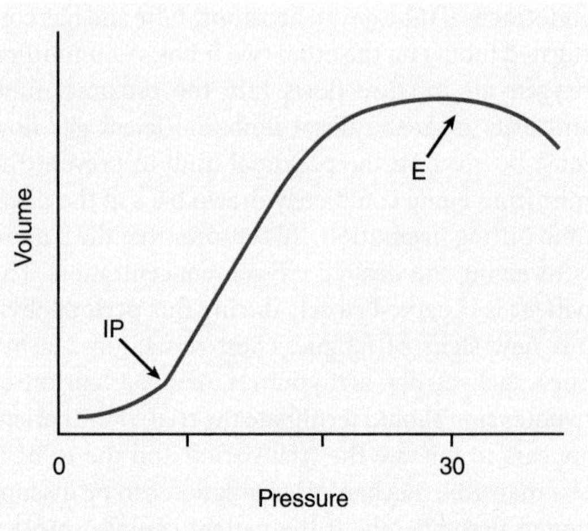

FIGURE 58–8 Pressure–volume curve for pulmonary system (eg, lung, thoracic). Inflection point (IP) above which the majority of alveoli are recruited. E, result of excessive pressure when alveoli are overdistended and pulmonary compliance decreases.

Excessive PEEP or CPAP, however, can overdistend alveoli (and bronchi), increasing dead space ventilation and reducing lung compliance; both effects can significantly increase the work of breathing. By compressing alveolar capillaries, overdistention of normal alveoli can also increase pulmonary vascular resistance and right ventricular afterload.

8 A higher incidence of pulmonary barotrauma is observed with PEEP or CPAP at levels greater than 20 cm H_2O. Disruption of alveoli allows air to track interstitially along bronchi into the mediastinum (pneumomediastinum). From the mediastinum, air can then rupture into the pleural space (pneumothorax) or the pericardium (pneumopericardium) or can dissect along tissue planes subcutaneously (subcutaneous emphysema) or into the abdomen (pneumoperitoneum or pneumoretroperitoneum). A bronchopleural fistula results when an air leak fails to seal (close). Although barotrauma

must be considered in any discussion of CPAP and PEEP, in fact, it may be more clearly associated with higher peak inspiratory pressures that result in increasing the level of PEEP or CPAP. Other factors that may increase the risk of barotrauma include underlying lung disease (asthma, interstitial lung disease, COPD), dynamic hyperinflation (too frequent breaths or too short expiratory times leading to intrinsic [or auto] PEEP), and excessive VT (>10–15 mL/kg).

Adverse Nonpulmonary Effects of PEEP & CPAP

Nonpulmonary adverse effects are primarily circulatory and the result of transmission of the elevated airway pressure to the contents of the chest. Transmission is directly related to lung compliance; thus, patients with decreased lung compliance (most patients requiring PEEP) are the least affected.

Progressive reductions in cardiac output may be seen as mean airway pressure and mean intrathoracic pressure rise. The principal mechanism appears to be inhibition of the return of venous blood to the heart from increased intrathoracic pressure. Other mechanisms may include reduced left ventricular filling from leftward displacement of the interventricular septum (when overdistention of alveoli and increased pulmonary vascular resistance lead to increased right ventricular volume). When this occurs, left ventricular compliance may be reduced, necessitating a higher filling pressure to achieve the same cardiac output. An increase in intravascular volume will usually at least partially offset the effects of CPAP and PEEP on cardiac output. Circulatory depression is most often associated with end-expiratory pressures greater than 15 cm H_2O.

PEEP-induced elevations in intrathoracic pressure and reductions in cardiac output decrease both kidney and liver blood flow. Urinary output, glomerular filtration, and free water clearance decrease.

Increased end-expiratory pressures impede blood return from the brain to the heart and may increase intracranial pressure in patients whose intracranial compliance is decreased. Therefore, with evidence of increased intracranial pressure, the level of PEEP must be carefully chosen to balance oxygenation requirements against potential adverse effects on intracranial pressure.

Optimum Use of PEEP & CPAP

The goal of positive-pressure therapy is to increase oxygen delivery to tissues while avoiding the adverse sequelae of excessively increased (>0.5) FiO_2. The need for excessive FiO_2 is most easily avoided with an adequate cardiac output and hemoglobin concentration. Ideally, mixed venous oxygen tensions should be followed. As we have repeatedly emphasized, the salutary effect of PEEP (or CPAP) on arterial oxygen tension must be balanced against any detrimental effect on cardiac output. Volume infusion or inotropic support may be necessary.

At optimal PEEP, the benefits of PEEP exceed any risks. Practically, PEEP is usually added in increments of 2 to 5 cm H_2O until the desired therapeutic endpoint is reached. The most commonly suggested endpoint is an arterial oxygen saturation of hemoglobin of greater than 88% to 90% on a nontoxic inspired oxygen concentration (≤50%). Many clinicians favor reducing the inspired oxygen concentration to 50% or less because of the potentially adverse effect of greater oxygen concentrations on the lung. Alternatively, PEEP may be titrated to the mixed venous oxygen saturation (>50–60%).

OTHER RESPIRATORY CARE TECHNIQUES

Other respiratory care techniques, including administration of aerosolized water or bronchodilators and clearing of pulmonary secretions, preserve or improve pulmonary function.

An aerosol mist is a gas or gas mixture containing a suspension of liquid particles. Aerosolized water may be administered to loosen inspissated secretions and facilitate their removal from the tracheobronchial tree. Aerosol mists are also used to administer bronchodilators, mucolytic agents, or vasoconstrictors (metered-dose inhalers are preferred for administration of bronchodilators). A normal cough requires an adequate inspiratory capacity, an intact glottis, and adequate muscle strength (abdominal muscles and diaphragm). Aerosol mists with or without bronchodilators may induce cough as well as loosen secretions. Instillation of hypertonic saline has been used as a mucolytic and to induce cough. Additional effective measures include chest percussion or vibration therapy and postural drainage of the various lung lobes.

9 Maneuvers that produce sustained maximum lung inflation, such as the use of an incentive spirometer, can be helpful in inducing cough as well as preventing atelectasis and preserving normal lung volume. Patients should be instructed to inhale maximally and hold their breath for 2 to 3 s before exhalation.

When thick, copious secretions are associated with atelectasis and hypoxemia, more aggressive measures may be indicated. These include suctioning the patient with a catheter or fiberoptic bronchoscope. When there is atelectasis without retention of secretions, a brief period of CPAP by mask or positive-pressure ventilation through a tracheal tube is often effective.

SUGGESTED READINGS

Chatburn RL, Khatib M Mireles-Cabodevila E. A taxonomy for mechanical ventilation: 10 fundamental maxims. *Resp Care*. 2014;59:1747.

Liu R, Wang J, Zhao G, Su Z. Negative pressure pulmonary edema after general anesthesia. *Medicine* (Baltimore). 2019;98:e15389.

Menk M, Estenssoro E, Sahetyat SK, et al. Current and evolving standards of care for patients with ARDS. *Intensive Care Med*. 2020;46:2157.

Vincent J-L, Abraham E, Kochanek P, et al, eds. *Textbook of Critical Care*. 7th ed. Elsevier Saunders; 2017.

C H A P T E R 59

Safety, Quality, & Performance Improvement

KEY CONCEPTS

1. In the 1980s, anesthesiology was recognized as the first medical specialty to adopt mandatory safety-related clinical practice guidelines. Adoption of these guidelines, which described standards for basic monitoring during general anesthesia, was associated with a reduction in the number of patients experiencing brain damage or death secondary to ventilation mishaps during general anesthesia.
2. In 1999 the Institute of Medicine of the (U.S.) National Academy of Sciences summarized available safety information in its report, *To Err Is Human: Building a Safer Healthcare System*, which highlighted many opportunities for improved quality and safety.
3. It has long been recognized that quality and safety are closely related to consistency and reduced practice variation.
4. In manufacturing and in medicine, there is a natural tendency to assume that errors can be prevented by better education or better management of individual workers (ie, to look at errors as individual failures made by individual workers) rather than as failures of a system or a process. To reduce errors, one changes the system or process to reduce unwanted variation so that random errors are less likely.

PATIENT SAFETY ISSUES

As a profession, anesthesiology has spearheaded efforts to improve patient safety. Some of the first studies to evaluate the safety of care focused on the provision and sequelae of anesthesia. When spinal anesthesia was virtually abandoned in the United Kingdom (as a response to two patients developing subsequent paraplegia), Drs Robert Dripps and Leroy Vandam helped prevent spinal anesthesia from being abandoned in North America by carefully reporting outcomes of 10,098 patients who received this technique. They determined that only one patient (who proved to have a previously undiagnosed spinal meningioma) developed severe, long-term neurological sequelae.

After halothane was introduced into clinical practice in 1954, concerns arose about whether it might be associated with an increased risk of hepatic injury. The National Halothane Study, performed long before the term *outcomes research* gained widespread use, demonstrated the remarkable safety of the then relatively new agent compared with the alternatives. This study failed, however, to settle the question of whether "halothane hepatitis" actually existed.

1 In the 1980s, anesthesiology was recognized as the first medical specialty to adopt *mandatory* safety-related clinical practice guidelines. Adoption of these guidelines was not without controversy, given that for the first time the American Society of Anesthesiologists (ASA) was "dictating" how

physicians should practice. Adoption of standards for basic monitoring during general anesthesia (that included detection of carbon dioxide in exhaled gas) was associated with a reduction in the number of patients experiencing brain damage or death secondary to ventilation mishaps. A fortunate associated result was that the cost of medical liability insurance coverage for American anesthesiologists also declined.

In 1984, Dr Ellison Pierce, then the president of the ASA, created the Patient Safety and Risk Management Committee. The Anesthesia Patient Safety Foundation (APSF), which celebrated its 35th anniversary in 2021, was also Dr Pierce's creation. The APSF continues to spearhead efforts to make anesthesia and perioperative care safer for patients and practitioners. Similarly, through its guidelines, statements, advisories, and practice parameters, the ASA continues to promote safety and provide guidance to clinicians. As Dr Pierce noted, "Patient safety is not a fad. It is not a preoccupation of the past. It is not an objective that has been fulfilled or a reflection of a problem that has been solved. Patient safety is an ongoing necessity. It must be sustained by research, training, and daily application in the workplace."

Meanwhile, other specialties of medicine began to place greater emphasis on quality and safety. **2** In 1999 the Institute of Medicine (IOM) of the (U.S.) National Academy of Sciences summarized available safety information in a report entitled *To Err Is Human: Building a Safer Healthcare System.* That document highlighted many opportunities for improved quality and safety in the U.S. health care system. A subsequent IOM report, *Crossing the Quality Chasm: A New Health System for the 21st Century,* explored the ways that unnecessary variation in medical practice reduced quality and safety. More recently, the Institute for Healthcare Improvement has been "motivating and building the will for change; identifying and testing new models of care in partnership with both patients and health care professionals; and ensuring the broadest possible adoption of best practices and effective innovations," as described on its website. Meanwhile, the ASA has continued its involvement in quality improvement by funding and sponsoring the Anesthesia Quality Institute, which allows individual practices and individual physicians to compare their performance with those in a national database of tens of millions of anesthetics.

QUALITY OF CARE & PERFORMANCE IMPROVEMENT ISSUES

3 It has long been recognized that quality and safety are closely related to consistency and reduced process variation. The quality and safety movement(s) in medicine have their origins in the work of Walter Shewhart and his associate W. Edwards Deming, who popularized the use of statistics and control charts in improving the reliability of industrial processes. In manufacturing (where these ideas were initially applied), reducing an error rate reduces the frequency of defective products, reduces the need for product inspections, and increases the customer's satisfaction with the product and the manufacturer. In medicine, reducing the error rate for everything from accurate timing and delivery of prophylactic antibiotics to ensuring "correct side and site" surgery or regional anesthetic blocks reduces preventable harm to patients, eliminates the additional costs resulting from those errors, and improves quality.

Strategies to Reduce Performance Errors

4 In manufacturing and in medicine, there is a natural tendency to assume that errors can be prevented by better education, better performance, or better management of *individual workers.* In other words, there is a tendency to look at errors as individual failures made by individual workers rather than as failures of a system or a process. This is exemplified by the so-called root cause analysis. Typically, there are multiple factors, not a single root cause, that lead to a system failure. As was first stated by Arthur Jones and then popularized by Paul Batalden, "All organizations are perfectly designed to get the results they get!" "Accidents" are included among the results about which he speaks! Therefore, in taking an organizational or systems point of view (as advocated by Deming) to reduce preventable errors, one changes the system or process to make these preventable errors less likely. An outstanding example of this is the "universal protocol" prior to invasive procedures. Adherence to the universal protocol ensures that the correct procedure is performed on the correct part of the correct patient by the correct physician, that the patient has given informed consent, that all needed equipment and images are available, and that (if needed) the correct prophylactic antibiotic was given at the correct time.

A related example of a simple approach to improve the safety and quality of a procedure is the use of a cognitive aid, such as a standardized checklist, as described in the popular press by Dr Atul Gawande. The importance of checklists is addressed elsewhere in this text, for example, in Chapter 2 in the context of developing a culture of safety in the operating room. Such checklists provide the "script" for the preprocedure universal protocol (Figure 59–1). Studies have shown that the incidence of catheter-related bloodstream infections can be reduced when central venous catheters are inserted after adequate cleansing and disinfection of the operator's hands by an operator wearing a surgical hat and mask, sterile gown, and gloves; using chlorhexidine (rather than povidone iodide) skin preparation of the insertion site; and with sterile drapes of adequate size to maintain a sterile field. Individual elements in this central line "bundle" are much less likely to be omitted when a checklist is required before every central line insertion; a sample checklist is shown in Figure 59–2.

Benefits of Good Communication

Checklists emphasize two important principles about improving quality and safety in the surgical environment. First, the proper use of a checklist requires that a physician *communicate* with other members of the team. Good communication among team members prevents errors, improves quality, and increases satisfaction with the work environment. It is easy to find examples of good communication strategies. By clearly and forcefully announcing that protamine infusion has been started (after extracorporeal perfusion has been discontinued during a cardiac operation), the anesthesiologist helps prevent the surgeon and perfusionist from making a critical error, such as using the "pump sucker" to aspirate blood from the surgical field or resuming extracorporeal perfusion without additional heparin. Accurate and complete "posting" of an intended surgical procedure provides another opportunity for good communication. In this way, the surgeon helps the operating room nurses prepare the necessary instrumentation for the procedure. Accurate and complete posting helps ensure that the appropriate regional anesthetic will be performed. We have selected these examples of good communication because we know of patients who were injured as a consequence of failure to transfer these specific points of information.

Participation in a checklist reminds every member of the surgical team that everyone has a stake in patient safety and good surgical outcomes. The team member who records the checklist "results" is usually not a physician but has the implicit authority to enforce adherence to the checklist. One may find excessive deference to authority figures on poorly functioning teams. Team members may feel that their opinions are not wanted or valued and may fear retaliation if they bring up safety concerns. On well-functioning teams, there is a "flattening" of the hierarchy such that every team member has the authority and every team member feels an obligation to halt the proceedings to prevent potential patient harm. The Toyota Corporation is famous for allowing any team member to shut down the automotive production line when a problem is suspected.

Quality Improvement & Quality Assurance Measures

In surgery, there are well-recognized indicators of good quality, such as a very low incidence of surgical site infections or of perioperative mortality. However, at present there is no consensus as to the important measurements that can be used to assess the quality of anesthesia care. Nevertheless, surrogate anesthesia indicators have been monitored by a variety of well-meaning agencies. Examples include the selection and timing of preoperative antibiotics and the temperature of patients in the postanesthesia care unit after colorectal surgery.

Name **MRN** **Patient Identification**	**Pre-Procedure and Time Out** Documentation

Procedure 1: ______________________________

Pre-Procedure Verification	**Circle**	**One**	
➢ Patient's identity confirmed using two identifiers	Yes	No	
➢ Procedure confirmed and consistent with documents, e.g. H&P, progress notes	Yes	No	
➢ Procedure site & side verified	Yes	No	NA
➢ Relevant images reviewed/available	Yes	No	NA
➢ Procedure site marked (required for procedures involving laterality, lesions, levels, digits)	Yes	No	NA
➢ Risk/benefits discussed and/or consent form completed	Yes	No	NA

Time Out Verification (Performed immediately prior to the procedure)		**Circle**	**One**
➢ Patient's identity confirmed using two identifiers	Yes	No	
➢ Procedure site and side verified	Yes	No	NA
➢ Correct procedure confirmed	Yes	No	
➢ Correct patient position confirmed	Yes	No	NA
➢ Availablility of Implants/special equipment confirmed	Yes	No	NA

______________________________ __________ __________
Signature & Printed Name or ID of Provider **Performing Procedure** Date Time

______________________________ __________ __________
Signature, Title & Printed Name of Person **Completing Form** Date Time

Procedure 2: ______________________________
(to be used for second block or any time patient position is changed (i.e., supine to prone)

Pre-Procedure Verification	**Circle**	**One**	
➢ Patient's identity confirmed using two identifiers	Yes	No	
➢ Procedure confirmed and consistent with documents, e.g. H&P, progress notes	Yes	No	
➢ Procedure site & side verified	Yes	No	NA
➢ Relevant images reviewed/available	Yes	No	NA
➢ Procedure site marked (required for procedures involving laterality, lesions, levels, digits)	Yes	No	NA
➢ Risk/benefits discussed and/or consent form completed	Yes	No	NA

Time Out Verification (Performed immediately prior to the procedure)		**Circle**	**One**
➢ Patient's identity confirmed using two identifiers	Yes	No	
➢ Procedure site and side verified	Yes	No	NA
➢ Correct procedure confirmed	Yes	No	
➢ Correct patient position confirmed	Yes	No	NA
➢ Availability of Implants/special equipment confirmed	Yes	No	NA

______________________________ __________ __________
Signature & Printed Name or ID of Provider **Performing Procedure** Date Time

______________________________ __________ __________
Signature, Title & Printed Name of Person **Completing Form** Date Time

Comments: ______________________________

____

FIGURE 59–1 The "time out" checklist used at the Virginia Commonwealth University Health System before all regional anesthesia procedures. There is space for two separate time outs. An additional time out is performed whenever a patient's position is changed for a second regional block (most commonly for lower extremity surgery). For convenience, the regional anesthesia time out checklist is printed on the reverse of the Consent for Anesthesia acknowledgment form. (Reproduced with permission from Virginia Commonwealth University Health System.)

PATIENT NAME

MRN
(or PATIENT LABEL)

QUALITY DOCUMENT. NOT PART OF THE PERMANENT MEDICAL RECORD.
Return to designated area on your unit.

Intravascular Access Catheter Insertion Checklist

Purpose: To work as a team to decrease patient harm from catheter-related blood stream infections
When: During all central venous catheter insertion or re-wirings
Who: Assistant to complete this form during catheter insertion

1. Date: ______________________ Time: ________________ a.m. p.m.

2. Procedure Site: _________________________________ ☐ New ☐ Re-wiring

3. Procedure is: ☐ Elective ☐ Emergent

4. Before procedure, did person(s) performing procedure:

➢ Wash hands immediately prior?	☐ Yes	☐ No
➢ Sterilize procedure site (chlorhexidine)?	☐ Yes	☐ No
➢ Drape entire patient in sterile fashion?	☐ Yes	☐ No

5. During procedure, did personnel performing procedure:

➢ Wear sterile gloves?	☐ Yes	☐ No
➢ Wear hat and mask?	☐ Yes	☐ No
➢ Wear sterile gown?	☐ Yes	☐ No
➢ Maintain a sterile field?	☐ Yes	☐ No

6. Did **all** personnel assisting with procedure follow the policy? ☐ Yes ☐ No

7. Procedure stopped at any time due to break in sterile field? ☐ Yes ☐ No

If yes, Corrective Actions Taken:
☐ Person performing procedure applied appropriate barrier, re-prepped and draped the pateint ☐ New checklist initiated
☐ Complete new set up: staff barriers, prep, drape new line ☐ New checklist initiated

☐ Attending/designee paged; problem corrected
☐ Attending/designee paged; problem not corrected

8. After procedure, were:

➢ Sterile dressings applied to the site?	☐ Yes	☐ No
➢ New IV bag & tubing set up?	☐ Yes	☐ No
➢ New stopcocks and access devices used?	☐ Yes	☐ No
➢ All ports closed with sterile dead enders?	☐ Yes	☐ No

9. Comments– Please note any additional corrective actions taken: ____________________________

STOP The assistant should **STOP** any procedure that does not meet this standard of care. The procedure should not continue until everyone is in compliance. The assistant will contact unit or division leadership immediately for anyone refusing to comply with this policy.

Name of Person Performing Procedure (& ID #)
PRINT NAME

Assistant Completing Checklist
PRINT NAME

FIGURE 59–2 Mandatory checklist for the insertion of central venous catheters in patients who are not currently undergoing anesthesia and surgery at the Virginia Commonwealth University Health System. A similar electronic document is contained within the Anesthesia Information Management electronic record for central venous lines. (Reproduced with permission from Virginia Commonwealth University Health System.)

The Physician Quality Reporting System (PQRS) encourages eligible professionals and practice groups to submit information on their quality of care to the U.S. Medicare program. PQRS was initiated by the Centers for Medicare and Medicaid Services in 2006 as a "pay for performance" program that paid bonuses to those who reported quality measures. Since 2015, PQRS no longer pays out bonuses for reporting, but it issues a 0.5% penalty for those who do not report these measures. Since 2013, all anesthesiologists, pain physicians, and certified registered nurse anesthetists must report Medicare PQRS quality measures.

Mindful of the importance of having accurate and relevant outcome measures, ASA charged the Anesthesia Quality Institute (in 2009) with developing and collecting valid quality indicators for anesthetic care that can be used for quality improvement programs. Aggregation of the large amount of data required for statistical validity is dependent on the widespread adoption of electronic medical records (EMRs) and anesthesia information management systems (AIMS) (discussed in Chapter 18). It is our hope that the data and indicators that are collected and aggregated will provide greater insight into how the quality of anesthesia care may influence clinical outcomes that are important to patients.

In any individual department or medical center there should be myriad opportunities to improve the quality of care; members of the anesthesiology department need to be involved with many of them. The Accreditation Council for Graduate Medical Education now specifies that house officers participate in quality improvement exercises. This is a very welcome development, but only a limited number of anesthesiologists are familiar with the methodology. The Institute for Health Care Improvement (IHI) offers a variety of teaching tools to facilitate performance improvement in health care.

We strongly recommend that every medical center use a standard format for planning and conducting such projects. Some medical centers favor the so-called 6 sigma program. This is a reasonable approach, but it does mandate more specialized training. We favor Dr Shewhart's (as adapted by Dr Deming and also by the IHI) plan-do-study-act (PDSA) cycles because they are simple, straightforward, and readily accomplished without the need for specialized training. Regardless of the rubric, success requires proper planning. Specifically, one cannot improve quality if one does not define a goal and define how success toward achieving that goal will be measured. On the other hand, a group cannot allow itself to be frozen in a perpetual state of planning. After "doing" the change and studying the results, the group can act on them in deciding how best to evolve the current process improvement plan. In a true "continuous quality improvement" program, unless the PDSA cycles continue indefinitely there will be an inevitable "drift" toward poorer performance.

SUGGESTED READINGS

Berwick DM. Controlling variation in health care: a consultation from Walter Shewhart. *Medical Care.* 1991;29:1212.

Dekker S. *Drift into Failure: From Hunting Broken Components to Understanding Complex Systems.* CRC Press; 2011.

Deming WE. *Out of the Crisis.* MIT Press; 1986.

Dripps RD, Vandam LD. Long-term follow-up of patients who received 10,098 spinal anesthetics: failure to discover major neurological sequelae. *JAMA.* 1954;156:1486.

Gawande A. *The Checklist Manifesto: How to Get Things Right.* Metropolitan Books/Henry Holt; 2009.

Institute of Medicine. *Crossing the Quality Chasm: A New Health System for the 21st Century.* National Academy Press; 2001. Available at http://www.nap.edu/

Institute of Medicine. *To Err Is Human: Building a Safer Healthcare System.* National Academy Press; 2000. Available at http://www.nap.edu/

Maltby JR, Hutter CDD, Clayton KC. The Woolley and Roe case. *Br J Anaesth.* 2000;84:121.

Methangkool E, Cole DJ, Cannesson M. Progress in patient safety in anesthesia. *JAMA.* 2020;324:2485.

Perrow C. *Normal Accidents: Living With High-risk Technologies.* Princeton University Press; 1999.

Pierce EC Jr. The 34th Rovenstine Lecture. 40 years behind the mask: safety revisited. *Anesthesiology.* 1996;84:965.

Summary of the National Halothane Study. Possible association between halothane anesthesia and postoperative hepatic necrosis. *JAMA.* 1966;197:775.

WEBSITES

American Society of Anesthesiologists standards, guidelines, statements, and other documents. https://www.asahq.org/quality-and-practice-management/standards-and-guidelines

Center for Medicare and Medicaid Services, "About PQRS." http://www.cms.gov

Institute for Healthcare Improvement. http://www.ihi.org.

The W. Edwards Deming Institute. https://www.deming.org/

Index

Note: Page numbers followed by *f* and *t* indicate figures and tables, respectively.

I

J

K

O

P

S

PERIPHERAL NERVE INNERVATION, ANTERIOR VIEW

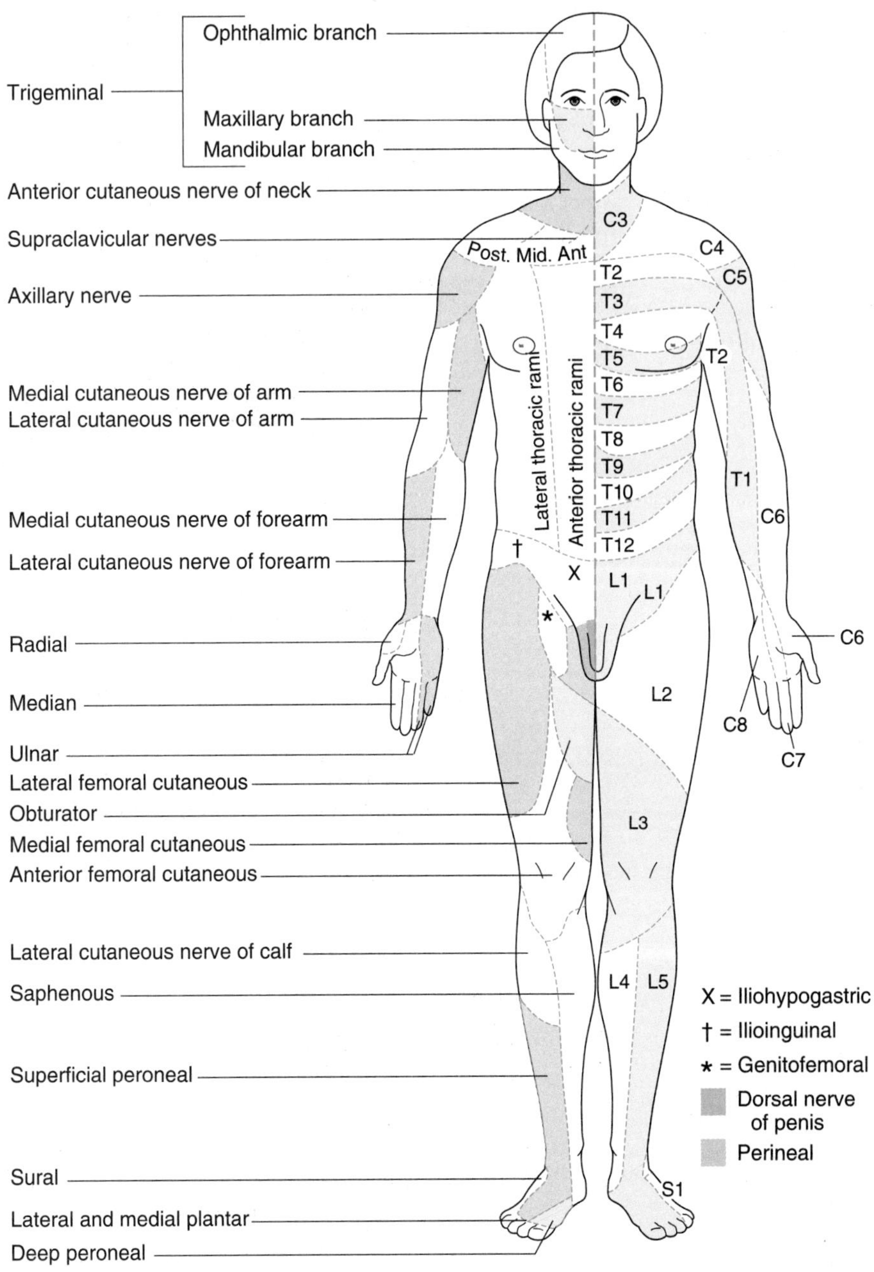

Peripheral nerve
Nerve root
Trigeminal
Ophthalmic branch
Maxillary branch
Mandibular branch
Anterior cutaneous nerve of neck
Supraclavicular nerves
Post. Mid. Ant
Axillary nerve
Medial cutaneous nerve of arm
Lateral cutaneous nerve of arm
Medial cutaneous nerve of forearm
Lateral cutaneous nerve of forearm
Radial
Median
Ulnar
Lateral femoral cutaneous
Obturator
Medial femoral cutaneous
Anterior femoral cutaneous
Lateral cutaneous nerve of calf
Saphenous
Superficial peroneal
Sural
Lateral and medial plantar
Deep peroneal
Lateral thoracic rami
Anterior thoracic rami
C3
C4
C5
T2
T3
T4
T5
T6
T7
T8
T9
T10
T11
T12
T1
C6
L1
L2
L3
L4
L5
S1
C8
C7
X = Iliohypogastric
† = Ilioinguinal
* = Genitofemoral
Dorsal nerve of penis
Perineal